Imaging
of
Orthopedic
Trauma

Second Edition

Imaging of Orthopedic Trauma

Second Edition

Editor

Thomas H. Berquist, M.D., F.A.C.R.

Professor of Radiology
Mayo Medical School
Chairman
Diagnostic Radiology
Mayo Clinic Jacksonville
Jacksonville, Florida

Raven Press ⚞ New York

Raven Press, Ltd., 1185 Avenue of the Americas, New York, New York 10036

Made in the United States of America

Library of Congress Cataloging in Publication Data

Imaging of orthopedic trauma/editor, Thomas H. Berquist.—2nd ed.
    p. cm.
  Rev. ed. of: Imaging of orthopedic trauma and surgery.
  Includes bibliographical references and index.
  ISBN 0-88167-805-8
  1. Radiography in orthopedics. 2. Musculoskeletal system—Wounds and injuries—Imaging. I. Berquist, Thomas H. (Thomas Henry), 1945–
II. Imaging of orthopedic trauma and surgery.
  [DNLM: 1. Bone and Bones—injuries. 2. Bone and Bones—
radiography. 3. Fractures—radiography. WE 200 I31]
RD734.5.R33I43 1991
617.1'5—dc20
DNLM/DLC
for Library of Congress   91-21827
                                                CIP

9 8 7 6 5 4 3 2 1

To my wife, Kay,
and sons, Aric, Matthew, and Andrew

Contents

Contributors ix

Preface xi

Acknowledgments xii

1. Diagnostic Techniques 1
Claire E. Bender, Thomas H. Berquist, John G. Stears,
Norlin T. Winkler, E. Meredith James, Manuel L. Brown,
Timothy J. Welch, Gerald R. May, and Glenn S. Forbes

2. Fracture Healing 39
James A. Rand and Thomas H. Berquist

3. Soft Tissue Injuries 83
Thomas H. Berquist and James K. DeOrio

4. The Spine 93
Thomas H. Berquist and Miguel E. Cabanela

5. The Pelvis and Hips 207
Thomas H. Berquist and Mark B. Coventry

6. The Femur and Thigh 311
Claire E. Bender, Donald C. Campbell II, and Thomas H. Berquist

7. The Knee 333
James A. Rand and Thomas H. Berquist

8. The Tibia, Fibula, and Calf 433
Claire E. Bender, Donald C. Campbell II, and Thomas H. Berquist

9. The Foot and Ankle 453
Thomas H. Berquist, Bernard F. Morrey, Joseph R. Cass,
and Kenneth A. Johnson

10. The Shoulder 579
Robert H. Cofield and Thomas H. Berquist

11. The Humerus and Arm 659
Claire E. Bender, Donald C. Campbell II, and Thomas H. Berquist

12. The Elbow 675
Bernard F. Morrey and Thomas H. Berquist

13. The Radius, Ulna, and Forearm 731
Claire E. Bender, Donald C. Campbell II, and Thomas H. Berquist

14. The Hand and Wrist 749
Michael B. Wood and Thomas H. Berquist

15. Imaging of Post-traumatic Infection 871
Thomas H. Berquist and Manuel L. Brown

16. Stress Fractures 881
Thomas H. Berquist, Kay L. Cooper, and Douglas J. Pritchard

Subject Index 895

Contributors

Claire E. Bender, M.D., *Department of Diagnostic Radiology, Mayo Medical School, Mayo Clinic, 200 First St. S.W., Rochester, Minnesota 55905*

Thomas H. Berquist, M.D., F.A.C.R., *Department of Diagnostic Radiology, Mayo Medical School, Mayo Clinic Jacksonville, 4500 San Pablo Rd., Jacksonville, Florida 32224*

Manuel L. Brown, M.D., *Department of Diagnostic Radiology and Laboratory Medicine, Mayo Medical School, Mayo Clinic, 200 First St. S.W., Rochester, Minnesota 55905*

Miguel E. Cabanela, M.D., *Department of Orthopedic Surgery, Mayo Medical School, Mayo Clinic, 200 First St. S.W., Rochester, Minnesota 55905*

Donald C. Campbell II, M.D., *Department of Orthopedic Surgery, Mayo Medical School, Mayo Clinic, 200 First St. S.W., Rochester, Minnesota 55905*

Joseph R. Cass, M.D., *Orthopedic Center, 1301 South Ninth Ave., Sioux Falls, South Dakota 57105*

Robert H. Cofield, M.D., *Department of Orthopedic Surgery, Mayo Medical School, Mayo Clinic, 200 First St. S.W., Rochester, Minnesota 55905*

Kay L. Cooper, M.D., *Department of Diagnostic Radiology, Mayo Medical School, Mayo Clinic, 200 First St. S.W., Rochester, Minnesota 55905*

Mark B. Coventry, M.D., *Department of Orthopedic Surgery, Mayo Medical School, Mayo Clinic, 200 First St., S.W., Rochester, Minnesota 55905*

James K. DeOrio, M.D., *Department of Orthopedic Surgery, Mayo Medical School, Mayo Clinic Jacksonville, 4500 San Pablo Rd., Jacksonville, Florida 32224*

Glenn S. Forbes, M.D., *Department of Diagnostic Radiology, Mayo Medical School, Mayo Clinic, 200 First St. S.W., Rochester, Minnesota 55905*

E. Meredith James, M.D., *Department of Diagnostic Radiology, Mayo Medical School, Mayo Clinic, 200 First St. S.W., Rochester, Minnesota 55905*

Kenneth A. Johnson, M.D., *Department of Orthopedic Surgery, Mayo Medical School, Mayo Clinic, 13400 E. Shea Blvd., Scottsdale, Arizona 85259*

Gerald R. May, M.D., *Department of Radiology, Providence Hospital, 500 17th Ave., Seattle, Washington 98124*

Bernard F. Morrey, M.D., *Department of Orthopedic Surgery, Mayo Medical School, Mayo Clinic, 200 First St. S.W., Rochester, Minnesota 55905*

Douglas J. Pritchard, M.D., *Department of Orthopedic Surgery, Mayo Medical School, Mayo Clinic, 200 First St. S.W., Rochester, Minnesota 55905*

James A. Rand, M.D., *Department of Orthopedic Surgery, Mayo Medical School, Mayo Clinic, 200 First St. S.W., Rochester, Minnesota 55905*

John G. Stears, R.T.(R), *Mayo School of Health Related Sciences, Radiology Program, Mayo Clinic, 200 First St. S.W., Rochester, Minnesota 55905*

Timothy J. Welch, M.D.,   *Department of Diagnostic Radiology, Mayo Medical School, Mayo Clinic, 200 First St. S.W., Rochester, Minnesota 55905*

Norlin T. Winkler, R.T.(R),   *Mayo School of Health Related Sciences, Mayo Medical School, Mayo Clinic, 200 First St. S.W., Rochester, Minnesota 55905*

Michael B. Wood, M.D.,   *Department of Orthopedic Surgery, Mayo Medical School, Mayo Clinic, 200 First St. S.W., Rochester, Minnesota 55905*

Preface

Since the first edition of this text, there have been many new developments in orthopedic radiology. New imaging techniques have progressed significantly, specifically magnetic resonance imaging. Other diagnostic and interventional techniques also have expanded over the last few years. The goal of this edition does not differ significantly from that of the first. Once again, communication between the imagers or radiologists and orthopedic surgeons is emphasized.

As in the first edition, the initial three chapters of this text discuss basic concepts in diagnostic imaging techniques, fracture healing, and soft tissue injury. The diagnostic technique section has been refined to concentrate more fully on those techniques used specifically for evaluation and follow-up of traumatic injuries. The chapter on diagnostic imaging, Chapter 1, is again intended to combine basic principles with sufficient detail to afford an understanding of the mechanics of these techniques so that repetition in later chapters is not necessary. A chapter on soft tissue injuries, Chapter 3, has been added largely because of the significant impact of MRI in evaluating these types of injuries. It is now important for the radiologist to understand the mechanisms of soft tissue injury and healing as well as certain classifications commonly used by orthopedic surgeons.

The main body of the text (Chapters 4–14) addresses imaging in adult trauma, including evaluation of post-reduction treatment techniques. The chapters are anatomically oriented with a review of essential musculoskeletal anatomy in the introductory section of each chapter, followed by a discussion of routine radiographic techniques and special techniques as they relate to the specific anatomic region. The clinical aspects of specific bone and soft tissue injuries are included in each section. The illustrations have been carefully selected to demonstrate how certain techniques are more pertinent for a specific clinical problem. Orthopedic classifications and treatment techniques are discussed as they apply to each anatomic area.

The final chapters, Chapters 15 and 16, discuss stress fractures and infection related to post-traumatic injury. Again, the emphasis is placed on imaging of these specific problems.

This text provides a comprehensive, well-referenced resource for radiologists, orthopedic surgeons and other clinicians, or residents in training who deal with trauma. The contributions of the radiologists and orthopedic surgeons in preparing each section of this text demonstrates the importance of communication and dialogue in daily clinical practice. The end result of this improved communication will be optimal use of the many imaging techniques in providing improved patient care.

Acknowledgments

Preparation of a comprehensive reference text requires the support of numerous individuals. Many colleagues provided daily assistance in obtaining representative material. I especially want to thank the residents in diagnostic radiology and orthopedic surgery who assisted in collecting these cases. William Mundstock, Ken McEwen, Tim Kodet, and their technology staff provided invaluable assistance in obtaining radiographs of special views frequently used in orthopedic practice. Both Sue Ramthun and Tim Kodet deserve special mention for their assistance in posing for demonstrations of radiographic positioning techniques.

The department of photographics provided quality radiographic prints for publication. James Martin and Tom Flood were especially helpful in this regard. The expertise of Elman Hanken was valuable in filming patient positioning techniques.

The medial graphics department headed by Bob Benassi, with direct assistance from Tammy Bell, John Hagen, John Hutchison, and Jack Nelson, provided excellent illustrations demonstrating classifications and specific injuries.

The manuscript was prepared by secretaries in diagnostic radiology and orthopedic surgery. Special thanks are due to my secretaries, Cindy Franke and Rebecca Richmond, for their diligence and patience in preparing the manuscript, tables, and lengthy bibliography.

Finally, I wish to thank Mary Rogers, my editor and the president of Raven Press, and the production staff, especially Nicholas Radhuber.

*Imaging of Orthopedic Trauma,
Second Edition*, edited by T.H. Berquist,
Mayo Clinic © 1992. Published
by Raven Press, Ltd., New York.

CHAPTER 1

Diagnostic Techniques

Claire E. Bender, Thomas H. Berquist, John G. Stears, Norlin T. Winkler,
E. Meredith James, Manuel L. Brown, Timothy J. Welch, Gerald R. May,
and Glenn S. Forbes

Routine Radiography, 1
  Equipment, 2
  Screen-Film Combinations, 3
  Radiation Protection, 7
  Film Labeling, 7
Tomography, 7
  Blurring and Section Thickness, 7
  Tube Motion in Orthopedic Tomography, 8
  Summary, 9
Magnification Radiography, 11
  Equipment and Principles of Magnification, 11
  Advantages and Limitations, 12
Ultrasound, 12
  Real-time Scanners, 12
  Doppler, 13
  Orthopedic Applications, 13
Skeletal Scintigraphy, 16
  Radiopharmaceuticals Used in Bone Scanning, 16
  Instrumentation, 17
  Clinical Applications, 17
  Trauma, 17
  Vascularity of Bone, 18
  Infection, 19
  Further Clinical Applications, 19

Computed Tomography, 19
  Equipment, 19
  Techniques, 20
  Indications, 22
Magnetic Resonance Imaging, 22
  Clinical Techniques, 23
  Patient Selection, 23
  Patient Positioning and Coil Selection, 24
  Pulse Sequences and Imaging Parameters, 25
  Clinical Applications, 25
Angiography, 26
  Equipment, 26
  Technique, 28
  Indications, 28
Myelography, 28
  Technique, 29
  Normal Myelographic Anatomy, 29
  Indications, 30
Introduction to Arthrography, 30
  Equipment, 31
  Contrast Material, 33
  Complications, 33
References, 33

There are multiple imaging techniques that are of diagnostic importance in evaluating orthopedic problems. Table 1-1 provides a list of the major techniques used in musculoskeletal evaluation. Proper application of these techniques is essential in obtaining optimal diagnostic information. In this chapter we will provide the background information and indications for each of the modalities listed in Table 1-1. This information will be applied in subsequent chapters in discussing the radiographic evaluation of orthopedic problems.

ROUTINE RADIOGRAPHY

Routine radiography remains the mainstay for diagnostic evaluation of orthopedic problems. This section will discuss equipment, radiation protection, film identi-

C. E. Bender, J. G. Stears, N. T. Winkler, E. M. James, T. J. Welch, G. S. Forbes: Department of Diagnostic Radiology, Mayo Medical School, Mayo Clinic, Rochester, Minnesota 55905.
  T. H. Berquist: Department of Diagnostic Radiology, Mayo Medical School, Mayo Clinic Jacksonville, Jacksonville, Florida 32224.
  G. R. May: Department of Radiology, Providence Hospital, Seattle, Washington 98124.

TABLE 1-1. *Diagnostic techniques in orthopedic trauma*

Routine radiography
Conventional tomography
  Linear motion
  Complex motion
Magnification radiography
Ultrasonography
Skeletal scintigraphy
Computed tomography
Magnetic resonance
  imaging
Angiography
Myelography
Arthrography
Tenography

fication, and other background material necessary for radiography of consistently high quality. Specific positioning techniques will be discussed in future chapters as appropriate.

Thorough radiographic evaluation of any condition requires high quality films. These cannot be obtained without properly functioning equipment, proper screen-film combinations, and technical consistency. Communication between the examining physician, the radiologist, and the technologist performing the examination is essential. The proper views will be obtained only if the information concerning the patient's situation is properly distributed.

Equipment

The following equipment is used in our department for routine orthopedic radiography: (1) a 3-phase, 12-pulse x-ray generator, (2) Eimac AZ92 x-ray tubes with a 0.6-mm focal spot, and (3) 4-way floating tables. Radiography of the axial skeleton is performed at a 48-inch source-to-film distance (Bucky grid technique, 16:1 ratio), with Kodak X-omatic cassettes, Lanex medium screens, and Kodak TML film. Extremity radiographs are obtained with Kodak Lanex fine screens, and Kodak TML film.

For the acutely traumatized patient we use a dedicated radiographic room adjacent to the emergency room. The equipment includes a Kermath Versitome table with a U-arm system capable of performing all routine radiographs as well as tomography in the lateral, oblique, anteroposterior (AP), and transaxial directions (Fig. 1-1). The room is also equipped with a modern life-support system. With such a dedicated emergency unit we can obtain radiographs in all directions without moving the patient. The same film and screens are used in the trauma room.

Selection of the proper recording medium (films and screens) is essential in obtaining radiographs of consistently high quality. The choice of screen-film combinations is complicated by the number of combinations available. There are approximately 40 different screens and 80 different films on the market. Various screen-film combinations can produce radiographs with a broad spectrum of sensitivity, contrast, and resolution characteristics. Generally, the optimum combination will be a compromise between the image quality desired, available equipment, and patient-exposure factors. The ideal combination would insure high speed, high detail, high contrast, and wide latitude. However, these factors tend to oppose one another. High-speed systems tend to

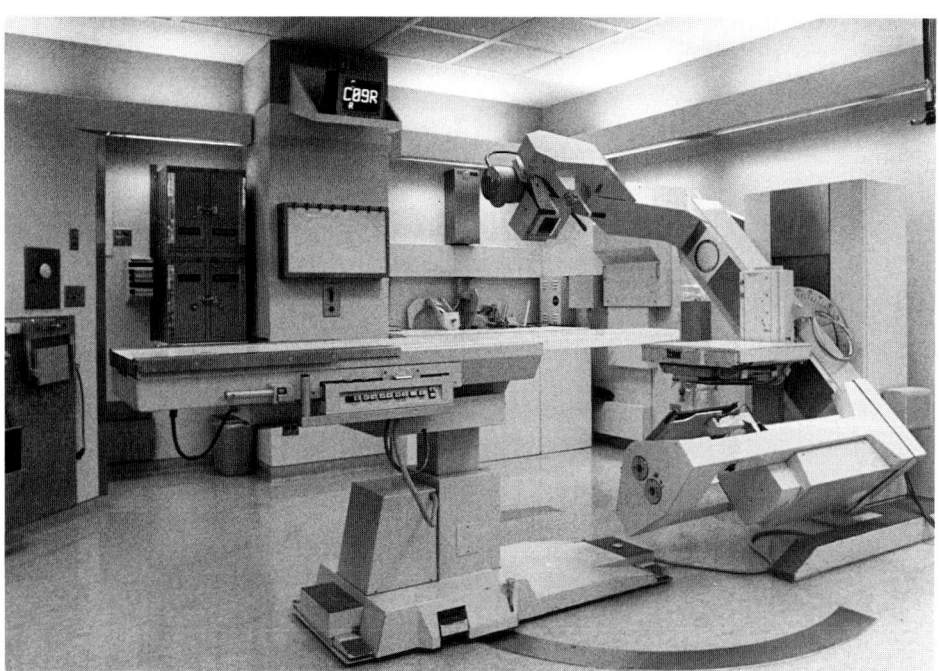

FIG. 1-1. Radiographic trauma unit. Versigraph with multiple angle tomographic capability, life-support equipment, and ample space for managing critically injured patients.

have lower resolution characteristics, and high-contrast systems are low in latitude. Institutions with small generators may have to sacrifice resolution for a higher-speed system because of equipment limitations (2).

Screen-Film Combinations

It is common to describe screen-film sensitivity or speed using a relative speed index (Fig. 1-2). The index is built around a par-speed calcium tungstate intensifying screen and par-speed film equaling 100, assuming optimal processing conditions. For comparison, a system is assigned a number that expresses its speed relative to the standard. Therefore, systems that are twice as fast as the standard (requiring half the exposure time) are 200 speed. Systems with one-half the speed (requiring twice the exposure time) are assigned a speed index of 50. Of the two components of the screen-film combination, the intensifying screen exerts the most influence on speed and resolution characteristics.

Many manufacturing processes are used in tailoring an intensifying screen for the desired characteristics. However, the phosphor material used in the screen is the major variable influencing the speed of the system. The currently used phosphors vary in their ability to convert photons to usable light and can be ranged in a scale of one to nine. In general, the calcium tungstate phosphors are least efficient and the rare earth phosphors most efficient, with other materials falling in between (6). Figure 1-2 lists some of the commonly used phosphor materials and the anticipated relative speed of the system.

The color of light emitted by the phosphor is an important consideration. Most of the phosphors, with the exception of the rare-earth family, emit light in the blue or ultraviolet range. Rare-earth phosphors emit light in the green region of the spectrum. However, activators used in the phosphors can be altered, resulting in a shift of the color into the blue portion of the spectrum. Care must be taken in selection of film to be certain that the film is sensitive to the color emitted by the screen.

In addition to the effects of spectral sensitivity, the film selected can also alter the speed of the system and the contrast of the radiographs. Excluding single-emulsion films, most manufacturers provide film that ranges in speed by a factor of two within the spectral-sensitivity groups. This variation in the speed of the film offers control over the contrast of the images, which can be adjusted through use of different types of film. These films are designated as latitude, medium-contrast, or high-contrast. Latitude films are designed to image a broad range of radiographic densities, such as soft tissue and bone. High-contrast films are designed to enhance subtle changes in contrast, and medium-contrast films range somewhere between latitude and high-contrast films.

In selecting a screen-film combination, the intensifying screen or screens should be chosen according to the required speed and resolution. Detail or extremity systems often use one intensifying screen. Desired image contrast and control of speed are options to be considered in the selection of radiographic films.

What is considered to be an optimal system should be determined within each institution. In theory, multiple screen-film combinations would be needed to obtain optimal results for each specific radiographic examination; however, this approach increases the potential for human error and inconsistency. Many departments select one screen-film system for all examinations or purchase different types of cassettes to assist in identification of the combinations within the department. In general, we use a 300-speed system for the axial skeleton and proximal extremities and an 80-speed system for the distal extremities. Proper choice of screen-film combinations will help maintain consistent radiographic quality. However, consistency in selecting proper exposure factors may be an even larger problem.

Patient size and the body part being examined specifi-

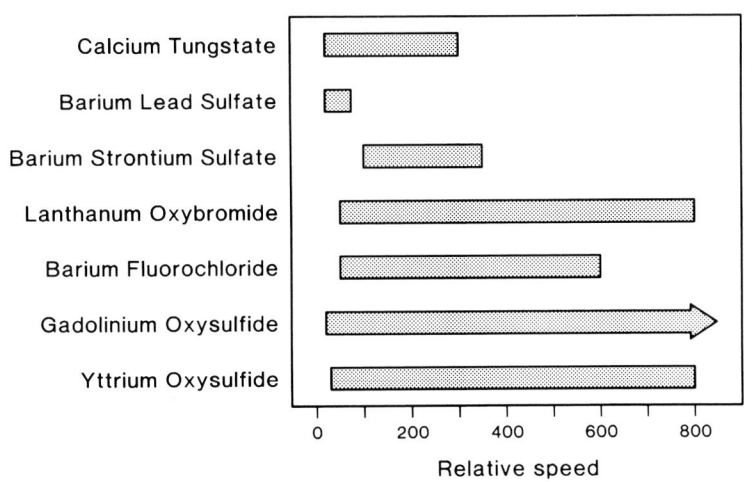

FIG. 1–2. Expected system speed by phosphor material for single or pairs of intensifying screens and single or double emulsion films. Exposure conditions, film processing, and match of spectral sensitivity are assured. The standard is the calcium tungstate screen (par speed) and par-speed film equalling 100.

KILOVOLTAGE vs MEASURED CENTIMETER THICKNESS

	SCALE 2	SCALE 1	CM	1/2 SCALE	1/4 SCALE	1/8 SCALE
		47	52	6	58	63	72
		48	53	7	59	64	73
		49	54	8	60	66	74
		50	55	9	61	68	76
SCALE 4	51	56	10	62	70	78
47	52	58	11	63	72	80
48	53	59	12	64	73	82
49	54	60	13	66	74	84
50	55	61	14	68	76	87
SCALE 8	51	56	62	15	70	78	91
47	52	58	63	16	72	80	95
48	53	59	64	17	73	82	98
49	54	60	66	18	74	84	101
50	55	61	68	19	76	87	105
51	56	62	70	20	78	91	110
52	58	63	72	21	80	95	115
53	59	64	73	22	82	98	120
54	60	66	74	23	84	101	125
55	61	68	76	24	87	105	130
56	62	70	78	25	91	110	135
58	63	72	80	26	95	115	140
59	64	73	82	27	98	120	
60	66	74	84	28	101	125	
61	68	76	87	29	105		
62	70	78	91	30	110		
63	72	80	95	31	115		
64	73	82	98	32	120		
66	74	84	101	33	125		
68	76	87	105	34	130		
70	78	91	110	35	135		
72	80	95	115	36	140		
73	82	98	120	37			
74	84	101	125	38			
76	87	105	130	39			
78	91	110	135	40			
80	95	115	140	41			

EXTREMITY CASSETTE

CM	kVp
1	45
2	47
3	49
4	52
5	55
6	58
7	61
8	64
9	67
10	70

EXTREMITY — Non-Bucky	TIME	mA	kVp	TFD	CASSETTE
REGULAR CASSETTE					
Ankle/Elbow				48″	24 x 30 cm
Tibia-Fibula				48″	14 x 17 in
Calcaneous				48″	8 x 10 in
Wrist-Carpal Tunnel				48″	8 x 10 in
Cast - Plaster				48″	
Cast - Fiberglass				48″	
EXTREMITY CASSETTE			SM MED LG		
Hand/Wrist PA/OBL				48″	24 x 30 cm
Hand/Wrist LAT				48″	8 x 10 in
Forearm				48″	7 x 17 in
Toes				48″	24 x 30 cm
Foot				48″	24 x 30 cm

A

FIG. 1–3. Kilovoltage versus centimeter thickness of the body part being examined. Charts are available in each filming station. **A** kVp chart and extremity techniques. **B** Skull, spine, and abdomen chart. **C** Pelvis, shoulder, femur, knee, chest, and ribs.

ROUTINE RADIOGRAPHIC TECHNIQUE

EXAMINATION	TIME	mA	kVp	mAs	TFD	CASSETTE
SKULL						
SKULL, AP, LAT Adult					48"	24 x 30 cm
CERVICAL SPINE						
Cervical AP 10°↑					48"	8 x 10 in
Lateral (Cross Table)					48"	24 x 30 cm
OBL (Table Top)					48"	24 x 30 cm
Swimmer's					48"	24 x 30 cm
Odontoid					30"	8 x 10 in
Piller 30°↓					48"	24 x 30 cm
THORACIC SPINE						
Thoracic AP (Filter)					48"	35 x 43 cm
Thoracic LAT (Filter)		↓			48"	35 x 43 cm
THIN ____mA AVERAGE ____mA PORTLY ____mA						
Thoracic Lower LAT (No Filter)					48"	24 x 30 cm
LUMBAR SPINE/ABDOMEN						
Lumbar AP 5°↑ and Abdomen						
– 18 cm					48"	35 x 43 cm
19 - 23 cm					48"	35 x 43 cm
24 cm -					48"	35 x 43 cm
Lumbar OBL 42° 5°↑						
– 18 cm					48"	24 x 30 cm
19 - 23 cm					48"	24 x 30 cm
24 cm -					48"	24 x 30 cm
Lumbar LAT Meas L-2					48"	30 x 35 cm
Lumbar Loc LAT Meas L-5					48"	8 x 10 in
Lumbar Graft LAT					48"	24 x 30 cm
Lumbar Flexion & Extension					48"	30 x 35 cm

B

FIG. 1–3. (*Continued.*)

cally affect exposure factors (kVp and mA-s) required for optimal radiographs. We prefer to use a system that can be applied throughout the department and provide uniform quality. Measuring the body part to be examined and referring to standardized charts (Fig. 1-3) available in each examining station results in more uniform quality. The charts remove the guesswork in deciding which exposure factors should be used.

In addition to using the proper exposure factors, certain basic principles of physics must be applied. The focal spot should be as small as practical in order to reduce geometric unsharpness, or blurring. The central portion of the beam should be as perpendicular to the cassette as possible in order to minimize distortion of the object being radiographed. This also assures that adjacent structures will be recorded in their true spatial relationships (Fig. 1-4). The body part to be examined should be placed parallel to the film to minimize magnification, blurring, and distortion. The body part should be placed as close as possible to the cassette.

Motion of either the equipment or the body part during the examination results in blurring of the image.

Date:

EXAMINATION	TIME	mA	kVp	mAs	TFD	CASSETTE
PELVIC REGION						
Pelvis & Hips AP / OBL 5°↓					48″	35 x 43 cm
Hips LAT					48″	24 x 30 cm
Sacrum AP 5°↑					48″	24 x 30 cm
Coccyx AP 10°↓					48″	24 x 30 cm
Sacrum, Coccyx LAT					48″	24 x 30 cm
S-I Joints (R & LPO 20°)					48″	24 x 30 cm
SHOULDER						
Shoulder AP					48″	24 x 30 cm
Neer View					48″	24 x 30 cm
Transthoracic Lateral					48″	35 x 43 cm
Axillary (Grid)					48″	24 x 30 cm
Scapula AP & LAT OBL					48″	24 x 30 cm
Clavical					48″	24 x 30 cm
Humerus					48″	35 x 43 cm
FEMUR, KNEE						
Femur					48″	35 x 43 cm
LAT & OBL for Vessels					48″	35 x 43 cm
Knee					48″	24 x 30 cm
Intercondylar Notch					48″	Non-Bucky
Patella (Merchants)					48″	Non-Bucky
CHEST						
AP Supine, All					48″	Non-Bucky
Bucky Chest						
Lateral Supine (Bucky)					48″	35 x 43 cm
Lateral Decubitus (Grid)					48″	35 x 43 cm
Lateral Sternum					48″	30 x 35 cm
RIBS						
Ribs Above Diaphragm		↓			48″	24 x 30 cm
	THIN _____mA	AVERAGE _____mA	PORTLY _____mA			
Ribs Below Diaphragm						
– 18 cm					48″	24 x 30 cm
19 - 23 cm					48″	24 x 30 cm
24 cm -					48″	24 x 30 cm

C

FIG. 1–3. (Continued.)

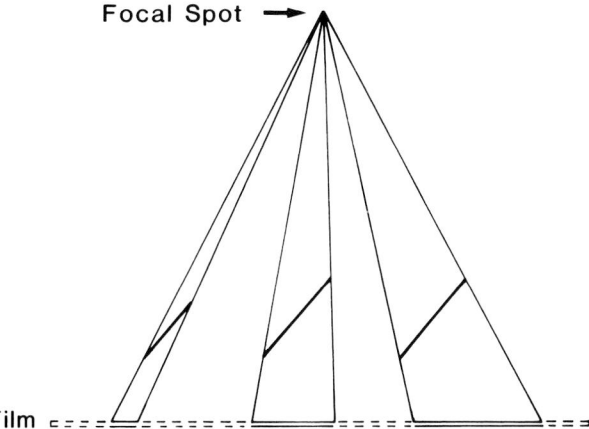

Focal Spot →

Film

FIG. 1–4. The size and shape of an object are dependent upon its location within the x-ray beam (10).

Thus short exposure times are necessary, especially in severely injured or uncooperative patients. This will assist in reducing the lack of clarity in the image due to motion. Proper positioning as well as reduced motion can also be aided by using positioning wedges and props. This not only assists the patient in maintaining the proper position but also assures consistency in positioning. Consistency in positioning is especially desirable in orthopedic radiology, as multiple follow-up studies are often performed. Slight changes in position may make observation of fracture healing and other orthopedic problems more difficult.

Radiation Protection

Proper radiation protection must be given to the patient, the radiology department staff, and any assistants who may be required to aid in patient positioning. When it is necessary to hold or position patients (as in acute trauma or when children are involved), it is often best to enlist the aid of persons not normally engaged in radiographic work. For instance, parents may be best able to calm and reassure children. Assistants should wear lead gloves and aprons during the procedure (1,2).

Multiple factors must be considered in discussing patient exposure. Proper positioning and exposure factors will prevent unnecessary retakes. Proper collimation not only decreases patient exposure but also increases image quality. Gonadal shielding should be undertaken when it will not obscure needed information. The Bureau of Radiological Health recommends shielding when the gonads lie within 5 cm of the primary beam in patients of reproductive age, assuming the objective of the examination will not be compromised (4).

Filtration with a minimum of 2.5 mm of aluminum equivalent is required with fluoroscopic and radiographic units capable of generating over 70 kVp. This

reduces the soft radiation that increases patient exposure but is of no diagnostic usefulness (4). Proper choice of screen-film combination may reduce patient exposure by as much as 400%. Technical factors such as high kVp also reduce patient exposure. Therefore, the highest practical kVp (the kVp that produces the needed subject contrast) should be used.

Film Labeling

Radiographic films must be properly labeled with the patient's name, registration number, and the date. If multiple films are to be taken on the same date they should be properly numbered chronologically or have the time imprinted on them. In larger departments it is also helpful to include the technologist's initials on the film. The films should be labeled as to right or left, and if specific positions were used they should be indicated (1,4).

TOMOGRAPHY

Tomography, or body-section radiography, provides a method of blurring out unwanted information in order to better visualize the desired structures. *Laminography, planography,* and *stratigraphy* are terms that have been applied to this technique. The technique was developed by two Dutch investigators Ziedes des Plantes and Bartelink, in 1931 (8). During the exposure the x-ray tube and film move in two parallel planes but in opposite directions. Speeds are maintained at a constant relationship.

Most skeletal structures can be readily evaluated with routine radiographs or films obtained with fluoroscopic monitoring (15). Tomography is a useful addition to conventional films when more detailed information is required (7,9,13,14). Conventional tomography provides an image of any selected plane in the body while blurring structures above and below that plane (11,12). Basic equipment includes (1) x-ray tube, (2) a connecting rod that moves about a fixed fulcrum, and (3) a cassette and film (Fig. 1-5). As the film moves in one direction, the tube moves in the opposite direction. The plane of interest within the patient (*shaded area* in Fig. 1-5) is most commonly selected by adjusting the fulcrum level. Less commonly, the apparatus includes an elevating table top to position the plane of interest at a fixed level. Only the plane of interest remains in sharp focus on the tomogram. Planes above and below (Fig. 1-5) will be blurred. Commonly used tomographic motions include simple (linear) and complex (circular, hypocycloidal, elliptical, and trispiral) (Fig. 1-6).

Blurring and Section Thickness

A better understanding of tomography requires a basic understanding of blurring and section thickness. Blur-

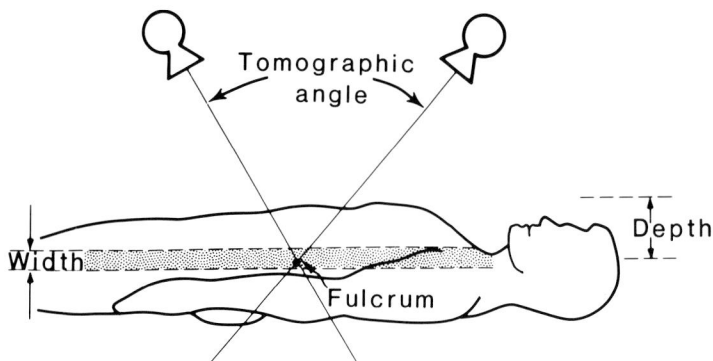

FIG. 1–5. Linear tomography. The fulcrum (focal plane), tomographic angle, and motion of the tube and film are demonstrated (12).

ring refers to the effect of the tomographic system on objects outside the focal plane (10). It depends upon (1) the amplitude of tube travel, (2) its orientation (Fig. 1-7), and (3) the distance of the tube from the focal plane. Section thickness refers to the plane that is in sharp focus on the film (10). It is inversely dependent (but not proportional) to the amplitude of tube travel. Therefore, the greater the tomographic angle, the thinner the section (10).

For evaluating skeletal structures (which have high inherent contrast), wide-angle tomography using an arc of 30°–50° is usually preferred. With the wide angle, maximum blurring of objects outside the focal plane occurs, and therefore phantom images (unwanted images) are less likely to be produced. For standard skeletal tomography we use a CGR Stratomatic, which is capable of performing linear (longitudinal, transverse, and diagonal), circular, and trispiral motions. Linear and circular tube travel may be 20°, 30°, or 45°. In trispiral studies the angle is always 45°. 3M XUD film with Lanex regular screens (200 speed system) in special carbon-fiber front cassettes are used at a 48-inch source-to-film distance. A Bucky grid with a 12:1 ratio is used. Exposure factors will vary with the body part being studied.

Tube Motion in Orthopedic Tomography

In orthopedic practice tomography is frequently used to evaluate subtle fractures (Fig. 1-8) (7,14). Fracture healing and other clinical problems are also effectively studied with tomography (Table 1-2). In most orthopedic tomography the detail is improved with trispiral or other complex motion. Occasionally, especially in patients with metal internal or external fixation devices, linear motion may be more useful (Fig. 1-9). Trispiral motion (Fig. 1-9A) can cause significant loss of bone detail adjacent to the metal. Linear motion parallel to the metal (Fig. 1-9C) and linear motion perpendicular to the metal (Fig. 1-9B) demonstrate that the metal artifact is reduced when the motion of the tube is parallel to the metal. Note that the adjacent bone and bone graft (Fig. 1-9C) are better defined with linear motion parallel to the metal. In certain cases the configuration of the fixation device is such that examination choices are more difficult. Tomography is still useful in providing increased detail in these situations.

In the immobilized patient with acute trauma we use the Kermath Versitome system (Fig. 1-1). It provides multiple-projection radiography (AP, lateral, oblique) in the supine patient; and, in addition, through the use of an angulated cassette holder, it allows tomograms to be obtained in the exact plane of interest. Linear (longitudinal AP, transverse AP, transverse oblique, and transverse lateral) and transverse axial tomography are available (Fig. 1-10). This versatility is useful in the acutely

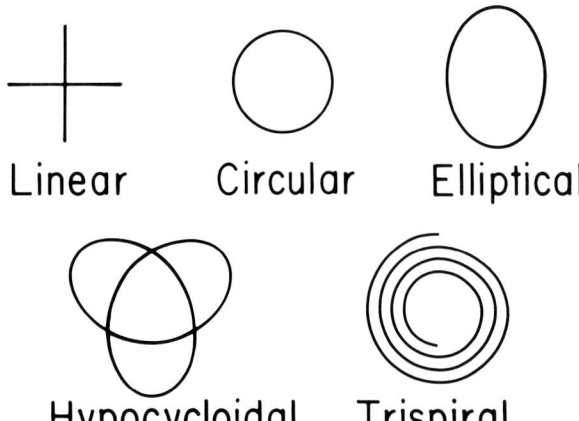

FIG. 1–6. Illustration of commonly used tomographic motions (12).

TABLE 1–2. *Tomography: orthopedic indications*

Trispiral or complex motion
Subtle fractures
Stress fractures
Fracture healing
Metabolic bone disease
Neoplasms
Arthritis
Linear motion
Acute trauma (Versitome)
Metal fixation devices

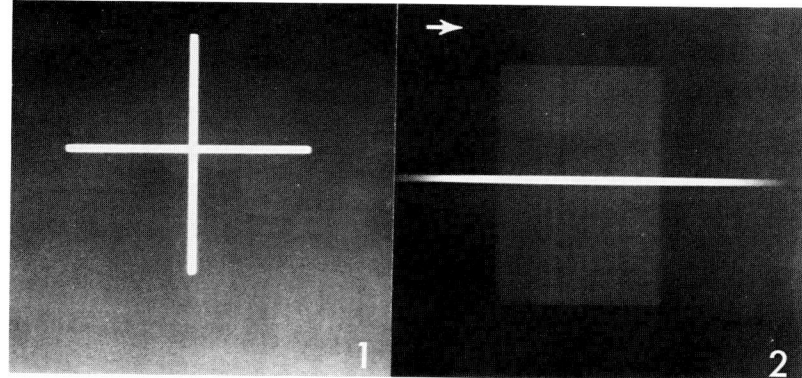

FIG. 1–7. Tomographic blur in linear tomography. The tube motion is transverse (*white arrow* in number 2). Both wires of the cross pattern are in focus in plane number 1 (*left*). When the fulcrum is above the wire pattern, the blurring is less evident in the wire pattern parallel to the tube motion (number 2, *right*) (12).

injured patient, for it is often necessary to define the extent of the injury with tomography so that proper treatment can be instituted prior to moving the patient. The Versitome also provides a linear-sweep range of 8°–50°. We commonly use the 50° angle for skeletal tomography. Narrower angles (10° amplitude) may be used in uncooperative patients, as the exposure time is reduced with narrow-angle tomography. With transverse axial tomography, the tube travels 180°. Kodak OG film with Lanex regular screens (400 speed system) and 52-inch source-film distance are used.

Summary

The type of tomographic motion used may greatly influence the radiographic findings. There are advantages to simple and complex motion studies. Increased blurring of objects occurs outside the plane in focus because of the greater distance the tube-film moves during the complex motion exposure. This results in elimination of streaking (incomplete blur) in images of structures when their long axis is aligned with the tube-film motion, as seen in linear tomography (10). Complex motion has a

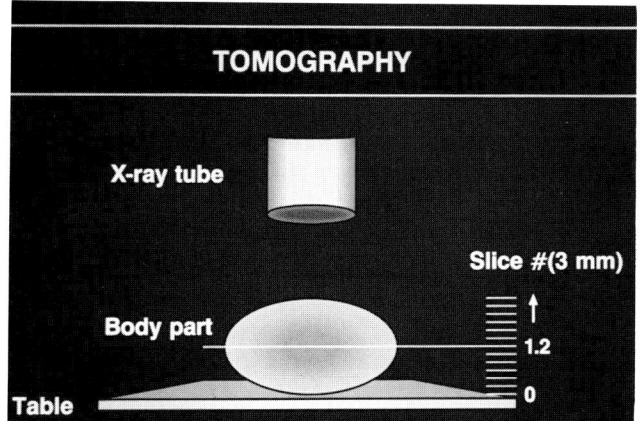

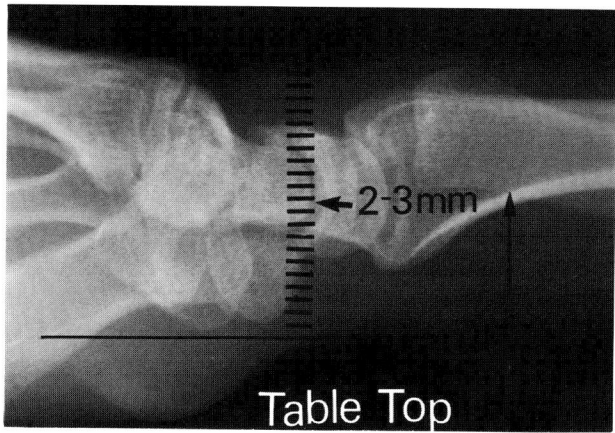

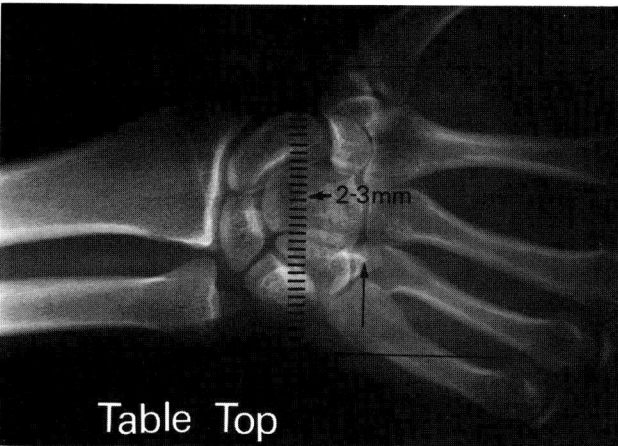

FIG. 1–8. A: Illustration of body part and distance from table top for selecting tomographic sections. Wrist positioned for 2–3 mm thick PA (**B**) and lateral (**C**) tomograms. It is important to obtain two projections and carefully monitor films to be certain that all structures are completely included on the tomographic sections.

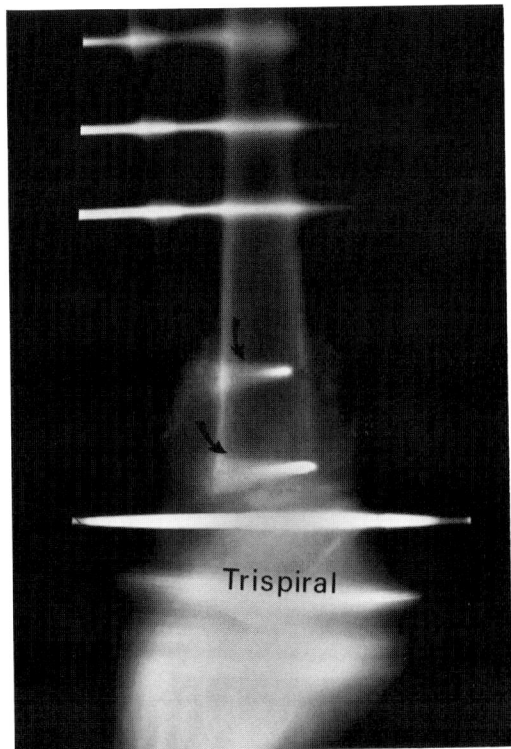

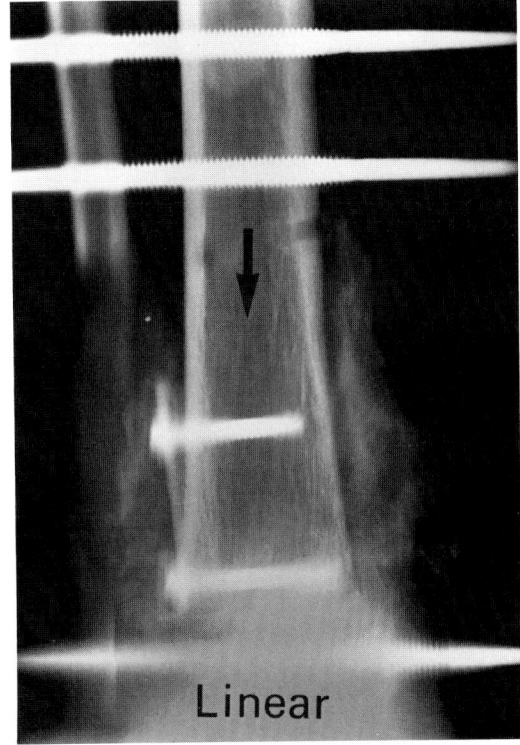

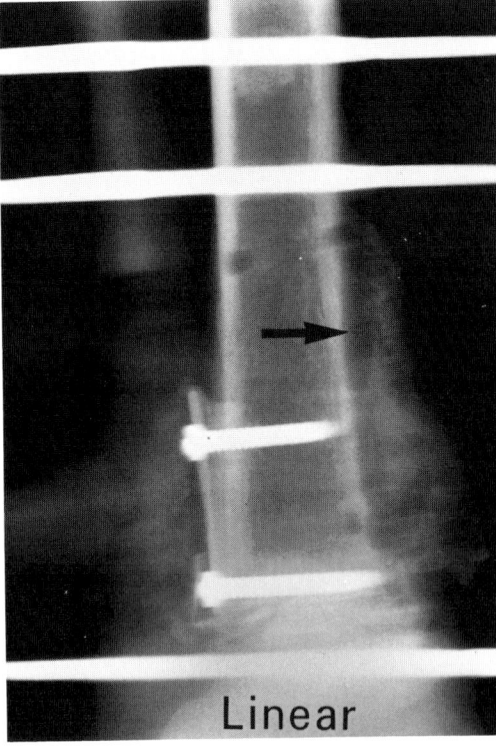

FIG. 1–9. Tomography of the distal tibia and fibula with bone grafts, internal fixation screws, and external fixation pins in place. **A:** Trispiral tomography causes blurring of the pins, which obscures adjacent bone detail. With linear motion perpendicular to the pins and screws (**B**) the problem is reduced. The most optimal detail is obtained with motion parallel to the fixation devices (*arrow*, **C**).

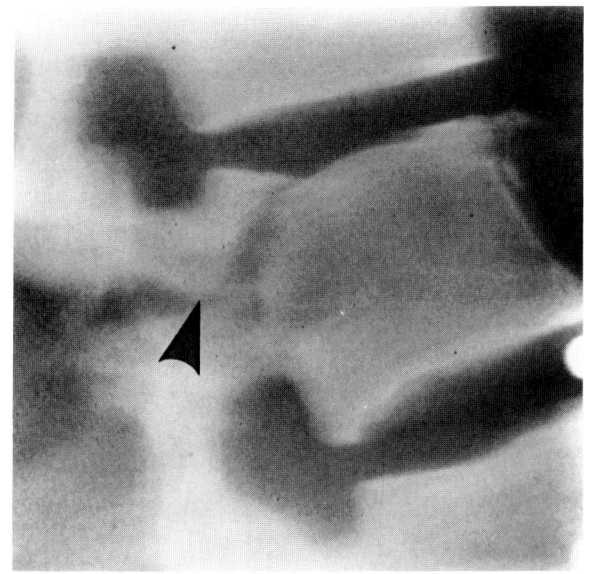

FIG. 1-10. Linear lateral tomogram of the upper lumbar spine (patient supine on versitome) demonstrating a Chance fracture with separation of the pedicles (*arrowhead*).

damage under heavy exposure conditions. A three-phase generator is also preferred.

For magnification hand films we use (1) 44-inch source-film distance, (2) Kodak NMB single emulsion film, (3) Kodak single Min-r intensifying screens (used as a rear screen), and (4) exposure factors of 60 kVp, 30 mA-s, and 1.25 sec. The patient's hand is supported on a Lucite stand 24 inches above the film. This results in a 2.2:1 magnification factor (Fig. 1-11).

Magnification radiography is based on two geometric principles. First, the size of the image is proportional to the distance between the object and the film; and second, the smaller the focal spot of the x-ray tube, the sharper the image (16,23,24). A focal spot size of 0.30 mm or less is required for magnification radiography. Increased image size occurs as the distance between the object and film increases and as the distance between the focal spot and the object decreases, other factors remaining constant (16,23). Geometric magnification is defined as the ratio of the source-film distance to the source-object distance for a point-source focal spot (Fig. 1-12).

decreased tendency to produce phantom images (unreal or unwanted images). The more complex the motion, the less the likelihood of phantom images. Linear tomography has the advantage of shorter exposure time, which may be useful in uncooperative patients. Linear motion may also be more useful when metal fixation devices are in place.

MAGNIFICATION RADIOGRAPHY

Magnification radiography was first introduced in 1940 but did not gain popularity until the last few decades (16). The primary indication for this technique is small vessel angiography, but it is also useful in skeletal radiography. The technique provides accurate and detailed assessment of subtle skeletal abnormalities in articular, metabolic, infectious, neoplastic, and traumatic disorders (17-22,25).

Equipment and Principles of Magnification

A thorough understanding of the equipment and principles of magnification is necessary in order to obtain high-quality magnification radiographs. Proper selection of the x-ray tube is the key to success. We use a Machlett DX78E tube with a 0.20-mm focal spot (as specified by the manufacturer). The actual focal spot size (grid-biased) measured 0.10 mm using a star text pattern in accordance with the specifications of the National Electrical Manufacturers Association (16,24). High-speed rotation of the anode is necessary to prevent x-ray tube

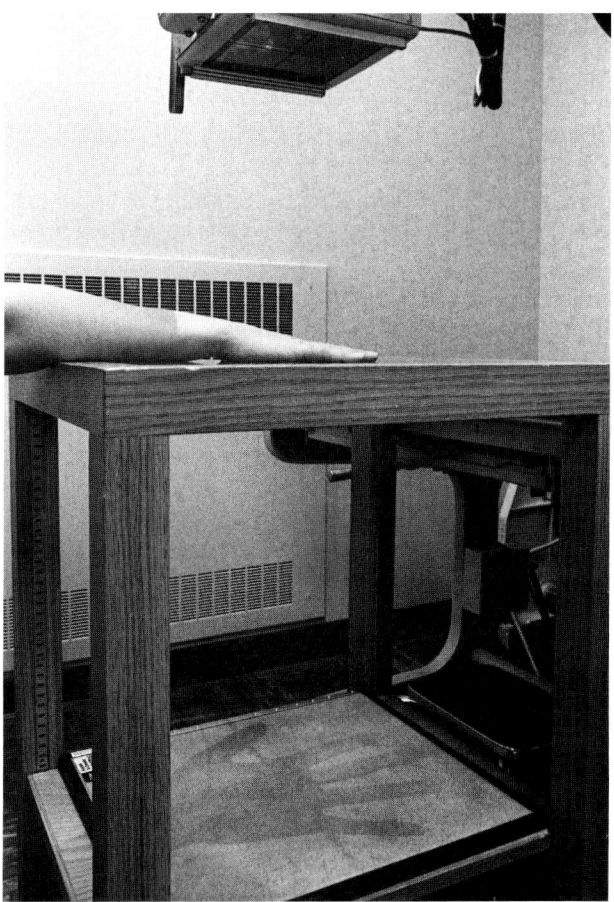

FIG. 1-11. Radiographic magnification unit. X-ray tube with a lucite plate for positioning the body part and a 14 × 17 in. cassette in the lower portion of the support frame. The hand is positioned for filming. Note the size of the shadow cast on the cassette.

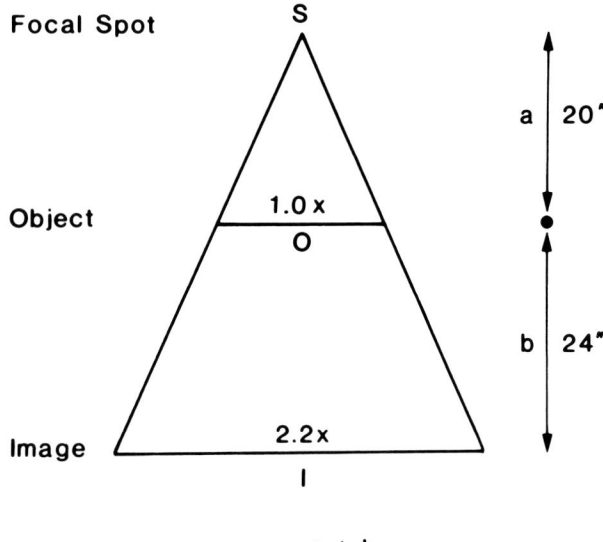

Focal Spot

S

a | 20″

Object

1.0 x

O

b | 24″

Image

2.2 x

I

$$\text{Magnification} = \frac{a + b}{a} = 2.2$$

FIG. 1-12. Principles of magnification. Note the source (S) to image (I) distance (a + b) divided by the source (S) to object (O) distance (a) equals a magnification factor of 2.2.

Advantages and Limitations

Radiation exposure to the skin is increased in magnification radiography because of the short source-to-skin distance. However, the size of the entrance field (in skull and abdominal magnification) is significantly reduced, thereby lowering total body exposure to nearly the equivalent dose obtained with conventional techniques. Entrance exposure to the skin for the magnified hand using our technique measures 246 mR.* This exposure is higher than the routine hand films (26 mR) but is accepted, as the magnification technique is used only in selected cases (19,24). Also, the hand is among the least radiosensitive body parts. The overall high-quality image is the advantage of this technique (Fig. 1-13). Increased effective sharpness, reduced effective noise, increased subject contrast (the air gap reduces the scattered radiation reaching the film), and improved visual effect of the enlargement contribute to high-quality radiographs. When the technique is properly performed, anatomic structures are better defined than those visualized in conventional radiographs observed with a magnifying lens. Use of a magnifying lens results in magnification of the inherent unsharpness of the screen-film combination and graininess along with magnification of the anatomic detail (16,22).

Limitations of magnification are (1) imaging is limited to small areas, (2) proper positioning of the area of interest may be difficult, (3) high relative skin exposure and

---

* Webbels W: Exposure data, St. Mary's Hospital, 1988

long exposure times may result in limited tube-loading capabilities (22).

ULTRASOUND

The term *ultrasound* refers to mechanical vibrations whose frequencies are above the limit of human audible perception (about 20,000 Hz or cycles per second). Medical ultrasound imaging utilizes frequencies in the range of 2–10 MHz (35,42). A central component of any ultrasound instrument is the transducer, which contains a small piezoelectric crystal. It serves as both the transmitter of sound waves into the body and the receiver of the returning echoes. When a brief alternating current is applied to the crystal, it vibrates at a characteristic frequency. By applying this vibrating transducer to the skin surface (through an acoustic coupling medium such as mineral oil or gel), the mechanical energy is transmitted into the body as a brief pulse of high-frequency sound waves. The advancing wave front interacts with tissues in various poorly understood ways and generates small reflected waves that return to the transducer. These cause the crystal to vibrate again, thereby generating an electrical signal that is conducted back to the machine where it is processed and displayed. With B-mode ultrasound imaging, the returning echoes are displayed as dots of light on a television screen, with the position of the dot on the screen corresponding to the position in the body where the echo was generated. In this way, the ultrasound image represents a cross-sectional display of the underlying anatomy. Unlike computed tomography, in which the geometric constraints of the scanner itself limit the possible scanning planes obtainable, any conceivable plane or section can be obtained with modern ultrasound instruments. Such scanning flexibility can be of great value in demonstrating the continuity or discontinuity of adjacent structures (42,45).

Real-time Scanners

Real-time ultrasound scanners generate rapid, sequential B-scan images that permit high-speed continuous viewing (26,29,33,42,43,45). These instruments can display dynamic events, such as a pulsating vessel, or can be moved across the body to provide continuous viewing of the underlying anatomy. Grey-scale image processing is utilized, whereby the returning echoes (depending on their amplitude) are assigned one of up to 64 shades of grey for final display. The resulting images, therefore, demonstrate not only the major boundaries between soft tissue structures but also their internal parenchymatous texture. This permits characterization of diffuse pathologic processes as well as detection of space-occupying lesions.

High-resolution images of superficial soft tissue struc-

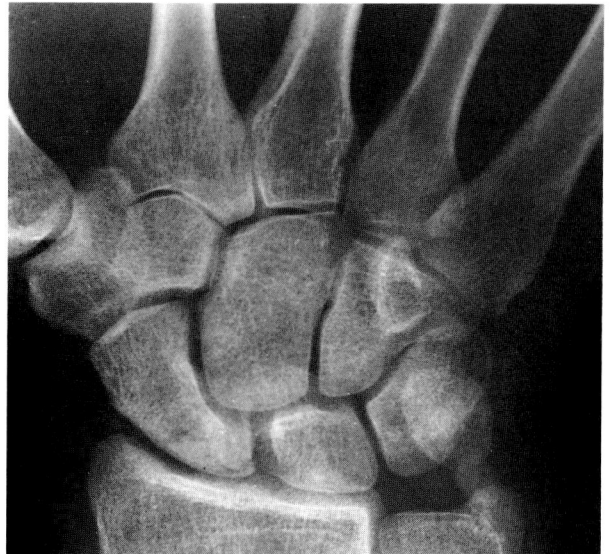 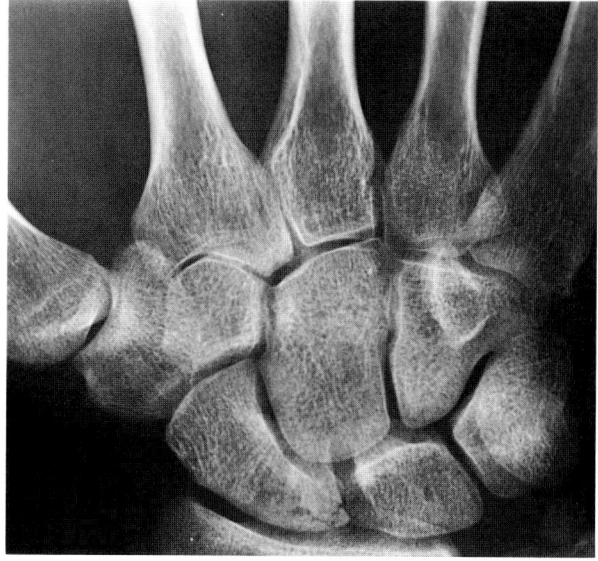

FIG. 1–13. PA views of the wrist in a patient with fragmentation and avascular necrosis of the proximal scaphoid. **A:** Routine technique. **B:** Magnification technique.

tures can be obtained by using high-frequency sound waves (up to about 10 MHz) (40). It is a fundamental principle of ultrasound that the higher the frequency of the sound, the better the resolution of the images. However, it is also fundamentally true that high-frequency sound waves are attenuated more rapidly in the soft tissues and therefore cannot penetrate very deeply. The result of these counterbalancing effects is that one can obtain submillimeter resolution, but only for structures located within about 5 cm of the skin surface.

Transmission ultrasonography is an additional static imaging technique that is not commonly used clinically. The basic difference between these techniques is that conventional ultrasound depicts reflected echoes from tissue while transmission ultrasonography utilizes transmitting and receiving transducers to measure attenuation of ultrasonic waves (35). These images are similar to radiographs and provide more detail than conventional ultrasonographic images (Fig. 1-14).

Doppler

Doppler ultrasound techniques reflect changes in frequency of moving structures. This technique is commonly used to evaluate blood flow. The Doppler effect is based on change in observed frequency owing to either object or observer motion. Changes in frequency indicate that motion or flow is present. When flow is moving toward the ultrasound source, Doppler frequency is increased. If flow or motion is in the opposite direction of the emitted wave (away from the source) the frequence decreases (Fig. 1-15). Most new vascular ultrasound imagers offer both Doppler and color-flow techniques.

This provides more accurate assessment of vascular disease and flow abnormalities.

Orthopedic Applications

Perhaps the most severe limitation of diagnostic ultrasound imaging is due to the inability of sound waves to penetrate gas and bone. The strength of an echo generated at the boundary between any two tissues is related to differences in the acoustic impedance of the tissues (a physical property generally dependent on density). Because the acoustic impedances of bone and air are so different from those of human soft tissues, almost all sound energy is reflected off a soft tissue-bone or soft tissue-gas interface, leaving essentially no sound energy left to penetrate, and thus image, deeper structures. The strong echo reflected off such an interface "overwhelms" the transducer and is displayed as useless noise or artifact in the image.

Because this fundamental physical principle prevents ultrasound from passing from soft tissue into bone, the applications of this modality to orthopedics are generally limited to the soft tissues (35,42).

The most frequent, early musculoskeletal application of ultrasound was to distinguish fluid from solid tissue, which is particularly useful in the characterization of the internal consistency of masses (Fig. 1-16) (27). A simple fluid collection, such as an uncomplicated cyst, will be represented sonographically as an echo-free area, while solid tissue, or the cells and debris within some fluid masses (such as abscesses), will provide interfaces for sound reflection and will therefore be echogenic. Some masses, of course, will demonstrate a complex pattern

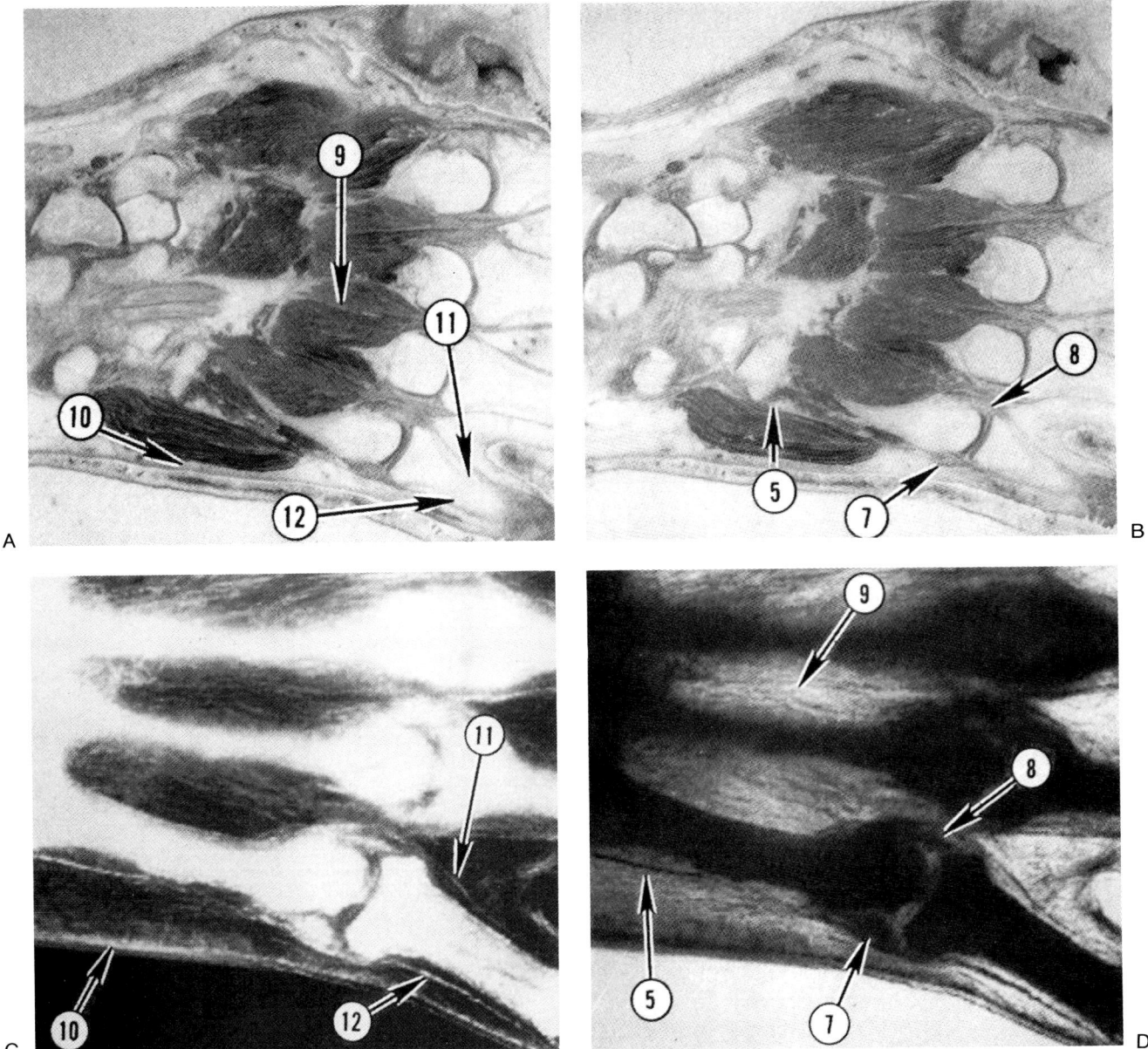

FIG. 1–14. Anatomic sections (**A**) and (**B**) and corresponding ultrasonographic images (**C**) and (**D**) of the hand. Abductor digiti minimi fascia (5), ulnar collateral ligament (7), radial collateral ligament (8), interosseous fascia (9), junction of abductor digiti minimi and subcutaneous fat (10), extensor muscles (11 and 12) (35).

with both solid and cystic elements. In addition to characterizing a mass by the number of echoes generated within it, it is also important to assess the manner in which sound is transmitted through the mass. Fluid-containing structures cause little attenuation of the sound beam and thereby demonstrate a characteristic ultrasound finding: so-called "enhanced through-transmission." This finding takes the form of stronger or brighter echoes deep to the fluid structure. Solid lesions cause greater attenuation of sound and therefore lack the finding of acoustic enhancement. By evaluating both the internal echogenicity of a mass and the ease of sound

propagation through it, one can, in virtually all instances, characterize the basic contents of the mass as fluid, solid, or mixed. While such a broad categorization is by no means histologically specific, such information, combined with appropriate clinical data, can often be very helpful in patient management.

A common anatomic region where ultrasound has come to play a key role in diagnostic soft tissue evaluation is the popliteal fossa (28,32,36,39). Masses or swelling in this area, whether pulsatile or not, can be difficult diagnostic problems for the clinician. Ultrasound has been successful in imaging popliteal artery aneurysms,

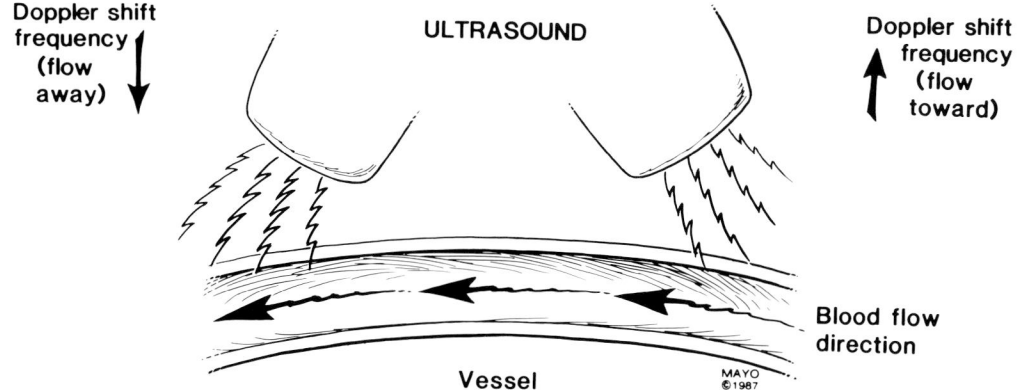

FIG. 1-15. Illustration of Doppler ultrasound showing relationship of flow direction to transducer. [From Berquist, T. H. (1989): *Radiology of the Foot and Ankle,* New York, Raven Press.]

popliteal cysts, abscesses, hematomas, and malignant tumors. In addition, patients with acute calf pain can be evaluated by ultrasound to differentiate pseudothrombophlebitis (due to ruptured popliteal cyst) from true thrombophlebitis (41,44).

The patient is positioned prone on the examining table, and both transverse and longitudinal scans are obtained on the posterior surface of the lower extremity from the lower thigh to the mid-calf. Because the popliteal artery can virtually always be visualized, an aneurysm involving this vessel is readily appreciated by not-

ing continuity of the "mass" with the vessel above and below. Doppler evaluation can confirm arterial flow. A popliteal cyst usually appears sonographically as an echo-free mass exhibiting acoustic "enhancement" behind it, which is located separate from the popliteal artery (Fig. 1-17) (28,32,36,39). If large, it can dissect for a considerable length into the calf. Occasionally, the cyst may contain scattered internal echoes, representing fibrin strands or other debris. Such an appearance can be indistinguishable from an abscess, but the clinical presentation usually permits differentiation.

Numerous studies have confirmed the accuracy of ultrasound in detecting popliteal cysts when compared with the results of arthrography. In patients with rheumatoid arthritis, ultrasound has also been reported to be useful in distinguishing proliferative synovial tissue from simple effusion in the suprapatellar recess of the joint space (29,38).

In recent years, the musculoskeletal applications for ultrasonography have expanded significantly (Table 1–3) (30,31,34,35,37). Musculoskeletal injuries, such as rotator cuff tears, and other muscle, tendon, and ligament injuries are more frequently investigated with ultrasound. Complications of trauma, particularly venous

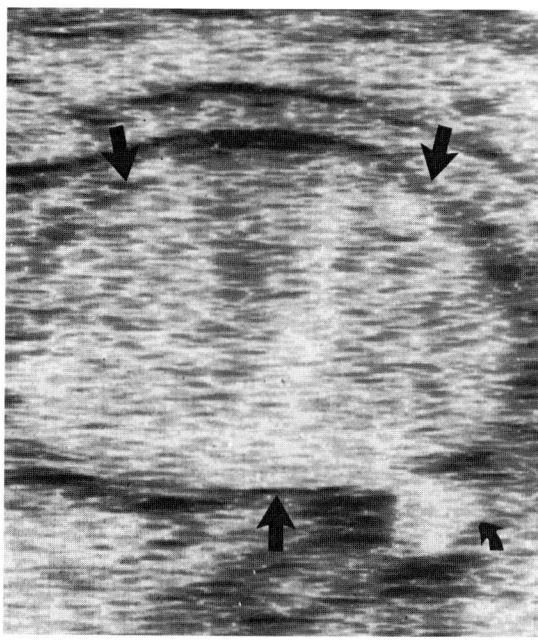

FIG. 1-16. Transverse image of the upper arm using a small-parts scanner demonstrates an oval shaped, well-circumscribed solid mass (*straight arrows*). Small hash marks at the bottom of the image represent a 1 mm scale. *Curved arrow* points to the brachial artery, deep to the mass. Diagnosis: neurofibroma.

TABLE 1-3. *Ultrasonography**

Musculoskeletal applications
Soft tissue masses (cystic vs. solid)
Trauma
Muscle tears
Hematomas
Foreign bodies
Wood, glass, metal
Vascular disease
Joint effusions
Arthropathies

* From refs 34,35,42.

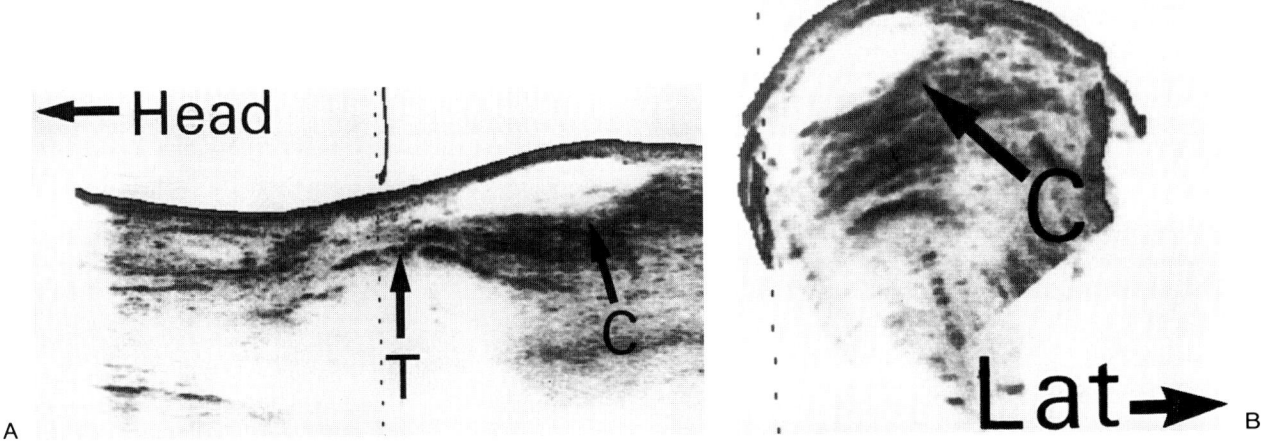

FIG. 1–17. Popliteal cyst. Longitudinal (**A**) and transverse (**B**) ultrasound images of the popliteal fossa with the patient laying prone show an elongated echo-free cystic mass (C) posteromedially. The posterior surface of the tibia (T) produces a strong acoustic interface that prevents further penetration of sound.

thrombosis, can also be assessed with ultrasonography (30,34). These applications will be discussed more completely in specific anatomic chapters.

SKELETAL SCINTIGRAPHY

Bone scintigraphy developed by way of a progression that began with P-32 orthophosphate tissue distribution studies in the 1930s. Early nuclides of calcium were first used in the 1940s to study bone mineral metabolism. The earliest attempts at external detection included surface counting of the distribution of P-32 orthophosphate and manual scanning with a Geiger-Müller tube of the distribution of gallium-72, and later strontium-85. Strontium-85, strontium-87m, and fluorine-18 all played major roles in the development of clinical bone scanning in the 1960s and early 1970s. Current bone imaging is a spin-off of the early work with phosphate compounds and has its origins with Subramanian's introduction of tripolyphosphate (74,75).

Radiopharmaceuticals Used in Bone Scanning

Radiopharmaceuticals currently used in bone scanning include compounds with P—O—P bonds (phosphates) and P—C—P bonds (phosphonates). The phosphonates are the current agents of choice because of their better stability and soft tissue clearance rates. The phosphate and phosphonate reagents come in sterile pyrogenfree lyophilized form with stannous ion as a reducing agent. Tc-99m is reduced from the +7 to the +4 state and forms a chelate with the diphosphonate. After compounding, the material is checked for acceptability by quality control procedures commonly using thin-layer

or paper chromatography. The material is injected intravenously. Its localization in bone is dependent on blood flow and osteoblastic activity. The most widely accepted mechanism of localization is felt to be chemiadsorption to the hydroxyapatite crystals of the bone mineral matrix. Approximately 50% of the mineral is cleared by the kidneys and excreted in the urine. Good hydration and an appropriate interval between administration and scanning of approximately 3 hours allow for soft tissue clearance and improved target-to-background ratios.

Another important radiopharmaceutical in the case of orthopedic patients with suspected infection is gallium-67 citrate. In the 1950s gallium isotopes were originally studied as potential bone-scanning agents. Although they do localize in bone, the available isotopes at that time were not satisfactory for imaging. Later, gallium-67 was shown to localize in tumors and sites of infection, its major role today. The mechanism of localization of gallium in infection sites is not well understood, but it appears to be related to the binding of gallium to transferrin and lactoferrin, leukocyte labeling, and/or direct bacterial uptake (60). The optimal time from injection to scan is 24–48 hours. Since we know that gallium is deposited in bone, care must be taken in the interpretation of gallium-uptake when looking for bone or joint infections. A sequence of Tc-99m and gallium scans may be necessary to differentiate reactive bone from inflammatory lesions.

A new agent that has proved useful in bone and joint infections is indium-111-labeled autologous white blood cells (62,65–67,70). The method of cell labeling is beyond the scope of this chapter, but the primary method is based on the work of Thakur (78,79). White blood cells migrate to sites of infection, and localization in the area of bone implies an infectious process. Images may be taken at 4 and 24 hours after the administration of the labeled white cells. Another new agent that may prove useful in bone and joint infections is In-111 polyclonal human IgG (66,70).

Instrumentation

The Anger-gamma camera is the imaging instrument used for all bone imaging. The camera allows total-body surveys with a moving table or moving detector. Selected views can also be obtained with this instrument. Radioactivity from the patient passes through a lead collimator and enters a sodium iodide crystal. The photon deposits its energy in the crystal. It in turn gives off photons of light, which are converted to electrons by the photocathode of the photomultiplier tubes. These electrons are amplified by the photomultiplier tubes and processed, with the resulting data being placed on film or entered into a computer for further analysis.

Collimators are designated according to the resolution and energy levels at which they can be used (i.e., low energy for Tc-99m agents, medium energy for indium-111 labeled white cells or gallium-67 studies, and high energy for iodine-131 agents). Collimator holes can be parallel or nonparallel; converging collimators magnify slightly. The pinhole collimator is a single hole that allows for magnification of an area of interest with some geometric distortion.

Clinical Applications

Although there are many indications for the use of bone scanning in clinical practice, the most common use is in oncology for detection and follow-up of metastatic bone disease primarily from prostatic, breast, and lung cancer or primary bone tumors (51). The orthopedic uses of bone scanning primarily include diagnosis of trauma and infection, determination of vascularity, compartmental evaluation of degenerative arthritis of joints, and evaluation of patients with painful prosthesis (46–48,52–55,71,77,80). Secondary uses include evaluation of elevated alkaline phosphatase and diagnosis of patients who present with bone pain of undetermined etiology (49,50).

Trauma

Bone scanning can provide important information in patients with known or suspected trauma (48,56). Routine radiographs will easily demonstrate the site of fracture in most patients with a clinical history of trauma. In these uncomplicated cases, bone scintigraphy will not add significant additional information. However, when the initial x-rays are normal, as may occur with subtle fractures of the pelvis (Fig. 1-18), proximal femurs, or

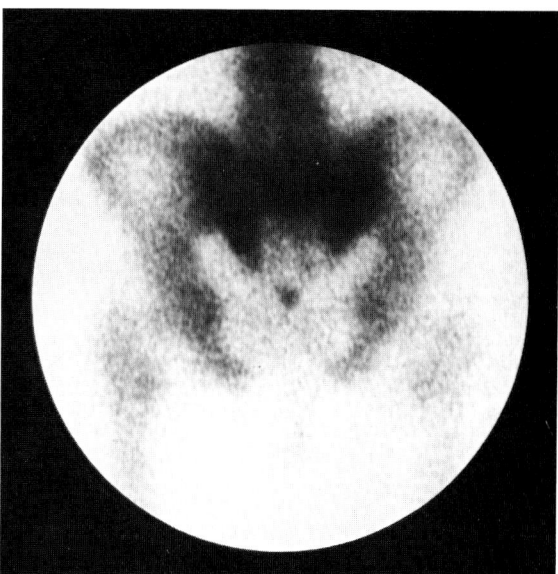

FIG. 1–18. Pelvic x-ray and tomograms of the right hip were normal in this elderly female with hip pain following a fall. Tc-99m MDP scan shows increased uptake in the mid sacrum and both sacroiliac joints due to fractures.

carpal bones (Fig. 1-19) (54), the bone scan may play a role in directing the course of management. Fractures will show focal areas of increased uptake early, with 80 percent visible in 24 hours and 95 percent in 72 hours (59,63), although in elderly patients more time is often required for the onset of activity to occur at the fracture

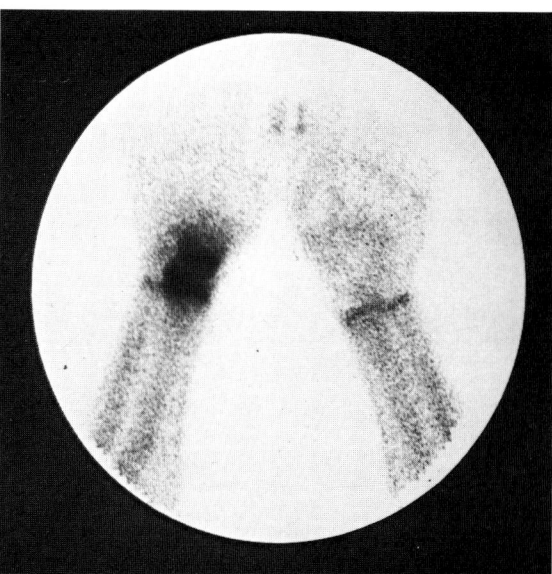

FIG. 1–19. X-ray and tomograms were normal in a 16-year-old male with left wrist pain following a fall. The Tc-99m DDP bone scan shows marked focal areas of increased uptake in the distal radius and scaphoid. Repeat tomograms showed a fracture of the distal radius and scaphoid.

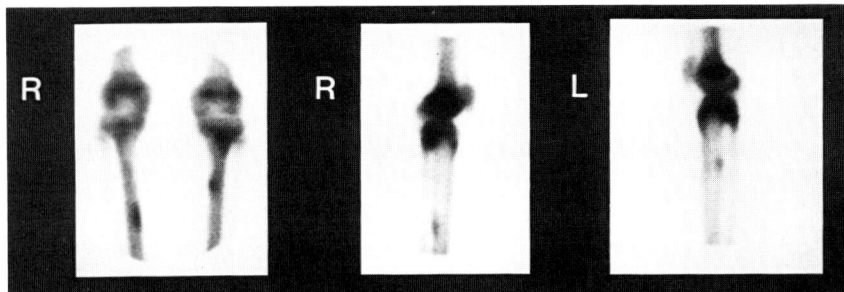

FIG. 1-20. Tc-99m MDP scan in a 22-year-old jogger with left lower leg pain reveals increased uptake in the posterior aspect of both tibias due to stress fractures.

site. Bone scanning is also very helpful in patients suspected of having stress fractures. The scan will detect stress fractures earlier than radiography, and if cessation of the stress is instituted, the radiograph may never become positive (Fig. 1-20) (56,73,81). A negative scan implies that the symptoms are not due to a stress fracture. Finally, in the battered-child syndrome, the bone scan may show the extent of the bone trauma, allowing for directed radiographic confirmation. The scan may also demonstrate bone contusion not seen radiographically.

Other uses for bone scanning are currently being explored. Animal models show that sequential studies can use radionuclide imaging to evaluate fracture healing (59), although this has not been convincingly demonstrated in humans. The question of bone viability following trauma, such as in the formal neck fracture, can also be evaluated with bone scanning (Fig. 1-21) (57,58). Finally, focal areas of intense increased uptake in the spine may indicate pseudarthrosis in patients with ankylosing spondylitis or following fusion. This finding on an otherwise normal patient may indicate spondylosis (64).

Vascularity of Bone

The vascularity of bone can be assessed with the use of radiotracers. As mentioned above, bone scanning has a potential clinical role in evaluating femoral head vascularity following fracture. In a patient suspected of having Legg-Calve-Perthes disease, the bone scan will demonstrate a lack of tracer earlier than the appearance of the radiographic findings (Fig. 1-22) (52,55,76). The results of one large series showed a sensitivity of 98 percent, a specificity of 95 percent, and an accuracy of 96 percent (76). After revascularization, the bone scan may reveal increased activity in the femoral head. Elderly patients with painful knees may show intense activity in the metaphysis of the tibia or femur due to osteonecrosis (61). Bone scintigraphy may also play a role in the early evaluation of bone grafts, detecting vascularity in the first postoperative week (47). Studies performed later may not be accurate since uptake may occur in a thin area of new cortical bone and may not demonstrate true graft viability.

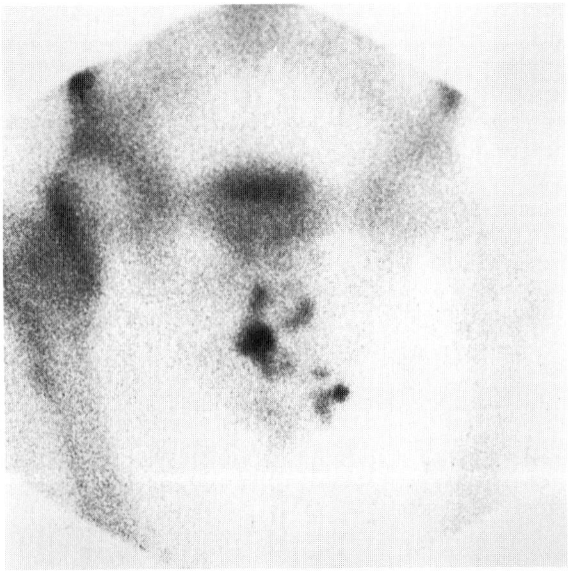

FIG. 1-21. Tc-99m MDP scan in a 44-year-old female with a fractured right femur from a skating accident. There is also decreased uptake in the femoral head due to loss of vasculature. Several months later the typical radiographic features of avascular necrosis appeared.

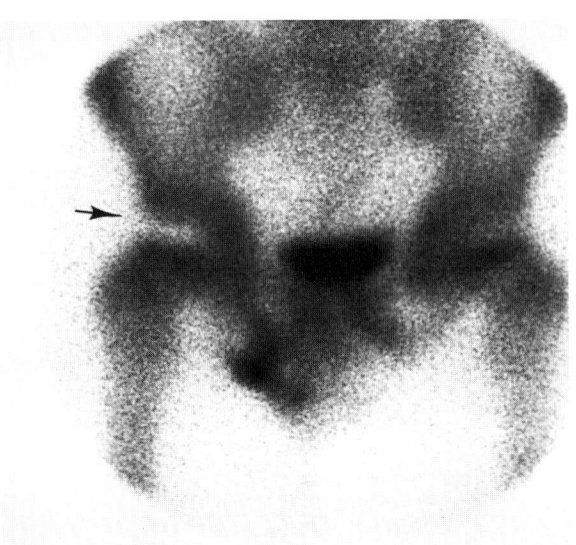

FIG. 1-22. Tc-99m MDP scan in a 7-year-old male with a limp and hip pain shows a well-defined photon deficient area in the right femoral head (*arrow*). Radiographic findings were consistent with Legg-Calvé-Perthes disease.

Infection

Bone scanning is helpful in the evaluation of patients with suspected osteomyelitis (69,72). However, there are pitfalls in its use, especially in neonatal osteomyelitis, in patients with orthopedic appliances, and in patients with recent trauma or surgery. Gallium and indium-labeled white cells can be helpful in these instances. This topic will be covered in detail in the chapter on osteomyelitis (Chapter 14).

Further Clinical Applications

The bone scanning agents accumulate in the arthritides. Although the pattern of localization may help differentiate between rheumatoid arthritis and the rheumatoid variants, the scan is less specific than radiographic findings, and its ability to aid in the diagnosis and follow up of patients with arthritis is uncertain. When it is important to assess accurately the compartmental involvement of osteoarthritis of the knee, the bone scan is more sensitive than radiographs or arthrography (80).

Following joint replacement, the bone scan may show increased activity for 6–12 months as the bone readjusts to the new stresses of the arthroplasty. Following the appropriate interval, increased uptake in the components implies loosening or infection (62,65,68). The injection of a trace into the joint at the time of arthrography can aid in detecting component loosening.

COMPUTED TOMOGRAPHY

The introduction of computed tomography (CT) has played a major role in improving imaging of most structures in the body and has resulted in a decrease in the use of more invasive imaging modalities, such as angiography. It has a secondary role in skeletal imaging, as in most areas it has not supplanted the routine radiograph. CT of the skeletal system, however, can add additional information to the plain film examination in a number of skeletal abnormalities (82,93,94,96,101). Initial experience in CT scanning of the musculoskeletal system was directed mainly toward the evaluation of neoplasms. This function has been largely supplanted by magnetic resonance imaging (89,91). Experience with CT has demonstrated its usefulness in trauma and certain other orthopedic problems (82,87,90,95,103).

Equipment

CT scanners use highly collimated x-ray beams, highly efficient detectors, and computer-image reconstruction and display to produce images that have superior contrast resolution but slightly less spatial resolution

than routine radiographs. CT thus provides better display of soft tissues than any plain film technique. In addition, the transverse axial orientation of the images is a useful supplement to the plain film examination of skeletal structures.

All CT scanners have three components: (1) the scanning gantry, (2) the computer, (3) the display console. The scanning gantry contains the x-ray source, detectory system, and couch and positioning system for the patient. The patient lies on the horizontal couch and moves through a circular opening in the vertically oriented scanning gantry, passing through the x-ray source and detectors. Although many gantry systems can be tilted a few degrees from the vertical, the orientation of the system permits only transverse axial images to be obtained in most cases. Therefore, sagittal and coronal images are usually obtained by computer reformatting of the transverse axial image data rather than by direct scanning. Certain regions such as the facial bones and peripheral extremities can be positioned to obtain direct coronal or sagittal data. In a typical CT scanner the x-ray tube moves through 360° at small increments (as many as 1200 or more) during a single CT scan slice (Fig. 1-23). The x-ray detectors (which can be fixed or rotate opposite the x-ray tube) take several hundred measurements of x-ray transmission at each increment. Once slice requires one or more seconds depending upon the scanner used. In critically injured patients or patients with respiratory difficulty, fast scanners are required. The advent of electron beam CT scanning, in which there are no moving parts, allows for scan times as short as 50 milliseconds. The use of subsecond scan times greatly enhanced CT images in this patient population (85). Dynamic images of the extremities can also be obtained in this manner.

The data from the x-ray detectors is processed by a

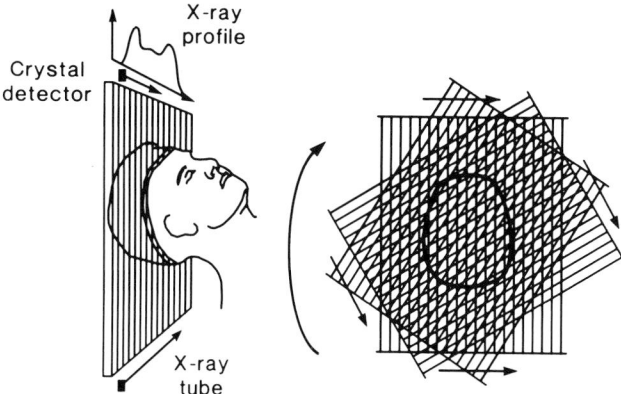

FIG. 1–23. Basic data collection method used in computed tomography consists of collecting a series of contiguous transmission measurements (called a *profile*) repeated at various angles about the subject (*right*). (Courtesy of E. C. McCullough, Mayo Clinic, Rochester, Minnesota).

computer that uses an algorithm (a series of mathematical formulas) to manipulate the data and reconstruct an image of the scanned object. Reconstruction time for a single image varies from 1–60 seconds. The computer divides the scanned area into a matrix (e.g., 256 × 256 or 512 × 512) of small squares (picture elements or pixels). An x-ray attenuation coefficient is determined for each square by applying the reconstruction algorithm to the data obtained by the detectors. Each square is then assigned a CT number related to the attenuation coefficient (with the CT number of water being 0). The numbers are displayed on the final image as various shades of grey with the highest numbers (e.g., air) being black.

Since the x-ray beam in the scanner has a finite thickness (from 3–13 mm for most scanners), the x-ray attenuation coefficient calculated by the computer for each pixel actually represents the average coefficient of a volume of tissue rather than a plane. The pixel thus actually represents a volume element or voxel. This can introduce a significant artifact, called a *partial volume effect,* into the final image (Fig. 1-24). This occurs when two objects that have different x-ray attenuation coefficients (e.g., bone and fat) are both included in the volume scanned. Since the pixels displayed on the monitor screen are represented as the average attenuation coefficient of the contents of the voxel, the number for the voxel containing both bone and fat will be somewhere between the actual attenuation coefficients of fat and bone. This partial volume artifact can result in significant errors. For example, a fracture line in the transverse plane of the scan can be missed because it is averaged in with the bone in the rest of the voxel.

The reconstructed image is displayed on a console that allows the operator to manipulate the window width (range of CT numbers in the grey scale) and the window

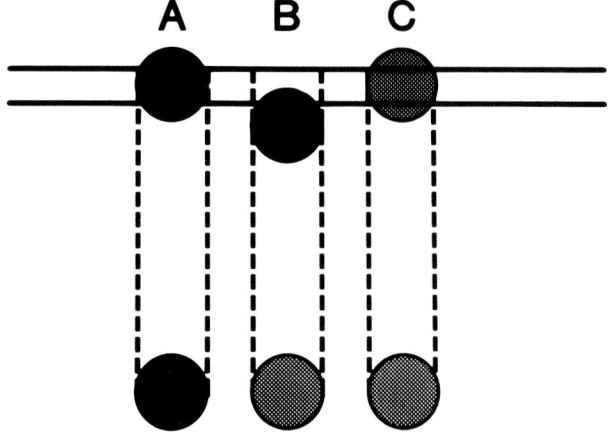

FIG. 1–24. Concept of partial volume effect in which a highly attenuating structure partially occupying the scan slice width (**B**) appears to be the same density as the lower attenuating structure (**C**) fully occupying the scan slice width. (Courtesy of E. C. McCullough, Mayo Clinic, Rochester, Minnesota).

level (center of the grey scale) optimally to display either bone detail or soft tissues. In addition, the operator can obtain sagittal or coronal reconstructions of the scanned object using computer reconstruction of the transverse image data.

Many CT scanners can also produce digital radiographs of any area of the body by moving the patient through the x-ray beam with sampling at intervals from the x-ray detectors. These digital images (Fig. 1-25) are of lesser quality than routine radiographs but can be quite useful for localization purposes.

The x-ray dose delivered by a CT scan varies with a number of factors, some related to the CT unit (e.g., transverse spatial resolution, slice thickness, scan noise) and some related to the individual examination, such as the number of slices obtained and the degree of overlap of the slices. In general, the dose is greater than that for a single radiograph but less than that for conventional tomograms of the same body part. CT doses may vary from less than 1 rad to greater than 10 rads (83,100).

Techniques

The radiologist should review the patient's history and the indication for the examination in order to tailor the procedure to the patient's problem. In most cases, contiguous slices 1 cm thick are adequate, although in evaluation of small lesions or anatomically complex areas such as the spine, thinner slices at overlapping intervals are required. The latter is especially important if three-dimensional reconstruction is contemplated (90,92, 103,106). Anatomic symmetry is very useful in evaluating CT images of the skeletal system and therefore care should be taken to position the patient symmetrically within the scanner. The contralateral side should be included whenever possible. The gastrointestinal tract can be opacified with oral or rectal contrast if a lesion in the abdomen or pelvis is suspected. Intravenous contrast by rapid infusion or bolus technique with rapid acquisition of multiple slices may be useful in detecting subtle soft tissue lesions or in detecting the relationship of pathology to major vessels. Non-ionic contrast material has supplanted ionic contrast material in patients with contrast allergy, significant cardiovascular disease or certain other specific indications. In these patient groups it provides an increased margin of safety. The radiologist should monitor the procedure and manipulate the display controls (window level and window width) to insure optimal display of both bones and soft tissues. Images of bones should be viewed at wide window width settings and high window levels, while soft tissues are best displayed at narrower window widths and lower levels.

The quality of the CT image is affected by a number of variables beyond the control of the examiner. In general, individual muscles, vessels, and nerves are optimally

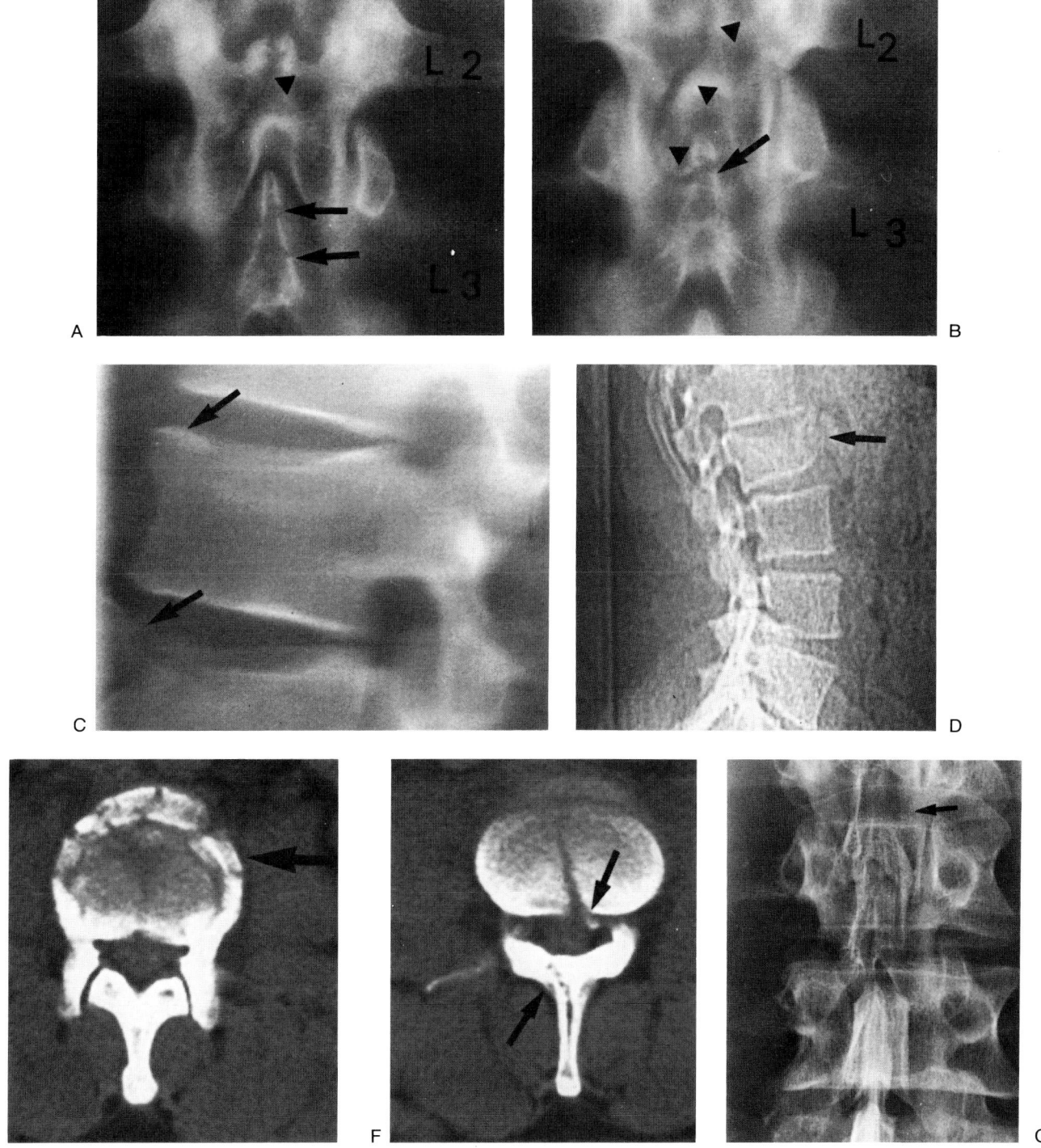

FIG. 1–25. Complex lumbar spine fracture. AP (**A, B**) and lateral (**C**) tomograms demonstrate compression of several lumbar vertebrae (*arrows,* **C**) and posterior element fractures (*arrows,* **A, B**). CT scout (**D**) and axial images (**E, F**). The CT images (**E, F**) demonstrate the position of the fragments and spinal canal involvement to better advantage (*arrows*). Myelogram preoperatively (**G**) demonstrates a block (*arrow*) at the L2-L3 level.

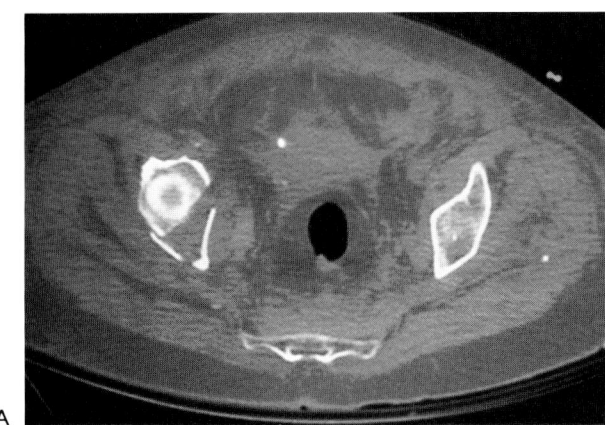 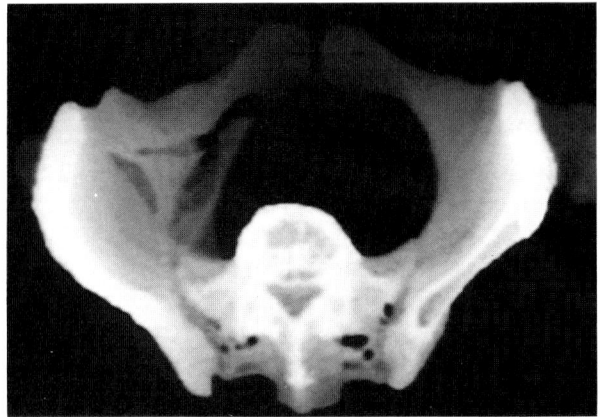

A   B

FIG. 1-26. Complex acetabular fracture. Axial CT image (**A**) and three-dimensional reconstruction (**B**). The relationship of the fragments is more easily appreciated after reconstruction.

imaged when surrounded by fat. Thus, the scan is less helpful in examining thin patients, infants, or the distal extremities (83,91). Patient motion produces significant degradation of image quality. This can be especially troublesome in attempting to evaluate a severely injured or uncooperative patient. Metallic objects such as joint prostheses, internal-fixation devices, and surgical clips produce artifacts that may obscure detail in the region of interest (92).

Indications

CT is particularly useful in examination of the bones in areas of complex anatomy such as the pelvis, hips, sacrum, spine, shoulders, and face (84,90,96,98,99,101, 106). In addition, some areas that cannot be easily displayed on routine radiographs, such as the sternoclavicular joints, are optimally seen on the cross-sectional images obtained by CT (88). Occult fractures not visible on plain film or tomography may be detected, especially in the spine (82,86,87,96,97,102). Some authors have found CT more useful than plain film tomography in the evaluation of the vertebral column following trauma (82). Most have found that CT adds valuable information to routine radiographs in the majority of cases, although most cases studied by CT were selected instances rather than consecutive cases of trauma. In addition to the presence of a fracture, CT can demonstrate bone, disk, blood, or foreign bodies in the spinal canal (90,97). Non-ionic contrast may be introduced for better delineation of the spinal canal (103). Plain films are still essential, as CT may miss horizontal fractures (fractures parallel to the plane of the scan slice), such as odontoid fractures, owing to the partial volume effect or improper slice selection. In addition, it is difficult to detect vertebral body compression fractures, subluxations, and increased intervertebral distance on CT scans alone (97).

CT scans of the shoulder, hip, or pelvis after trauma aid in the display of the spatial relationships of the fracture fragments before and after reduction. CT may detect intraarticular fragments that prevent reduction and require operative intervention (123,129,132,133,138). Three-dimensional reconstruction is most often used to assist with surgical planning of these complex fractures (Fig. 1-26) (90,104,106).

CT can accurately detect soft tissue injuries and is especially important in evaluating the abdomen after trauma (105). CT has replaced other imaging modalities as the procedure of choice in trauma patients. CT may also be useful in detecting some vascular injuries (such as thoracic aortic pseudoaneurysm). CT also played an increasing role in managing patients because of the widespread application of biopsy and aspiration techniques using CT guidance. CT biopsy and aspiration gives accurate results with few complications in suspected tumors, metastasis, or fluid collections (107).

MAGNETIC RESONANCE IMAGING

Resonance properties of nuclei were first reported by Block and Purcell. Clinical interest in magnetic resonance as an imaging modality has increased rapidly. Early work in the field was initiated by Damadian and Lauterbur. Technological advancements have progressed significantly resulting in improved image quality, patient throughput and in some cases improved specificity since the first edition of this text (108–117, 122,125,126).

The principles of magnetic resonance imaging (MRI) are beyond the scope of this small chapter. The reader is referred to more detailed discussions for a more thorough evaluation of the principles of magnetic resonance imaging (111,127,130).

Clinical Techniques

Magnetic resonance imaging has rapidly become an accepted technique in evaluation of the musculoskeletal system, specifically soft tissue trauma, but also articular and skeletal injuries (110,111,119,123). Respiratory motion is not a significant problem in the extremities as it is in the chest and upper abdomen and, therefore, examination of the extremities is easily accomplished with MRI. Images can be obtained in the coronal, sagittal, oblique, and transaxial planes. In addition, soft tissue contrast is superior to computed tomography and other imaging techniques.

Using conventional pulse sequences, normal anatomic tissues have fairly characteristic signal intensities using magnetic resonance imaging. Fat and medullary bone have the highest signal intensity and appear nearly white on magnetic resonance images. Signal intensity of articular cartilage is between muscle and medullary bone. It has been suggested that the different image appearance of articular meniscal cartilage is probably due to variations in the type of collagen and water content of these structures (120). Water content of articular cartilage is higher (75–80%) than menisci. Menisci, ligaments, and tendons appear black on MRI images. These structures are composed of predominantly type I collagen (articular cartilage is type II) and contain less water (120). Therefore, articular cartilage typically has a gray appearance on MR images while the latter tend to appear dark or black. Blood vessels also appear black if flow is normal. However, signal intensity in vascular structures may vary depending upon the velocity of flow and other pulse sequence variables. Cortical bone is white on CT images and often causes a significant beam hardening artifact decreasing the ability to evaluate juxta cortical soft tissues. Cortical bone is black on MR images and there is no artifact. This allows adjacent soft tissues to be more easily evaluated.

MR examinations must be conducted differently than conventional radiographic or CT examinations. Patient selection, patient positioning, coil selection, and pulse sequences must be carefully considered to optimize image information and patient throughput (109,111).

Patient Selection

The MR imaging gantry is more confining than a conventional fluoroscopic unit or CT scanner. Patients are typically positioned in the center of the cylindrical magnet during the examination. Despite this apparent drawback, we note problems with claustrophobia in only about 2–5% of patients (111). Patients with claustrophobic tendencies seem to tolerate MR examinations more easily when they are in the prone position. The prone position makes positioning of the foot and ankle more difficult and this should be considered when evaluating patients with disorders in this region. When necessary, mild sedation with oral Valium may be helpful in patients with some degree of claustrophobia.

The patient's clinical status must also be considered. When significant discomfort or inability to maintain necessary positions is a problem, the examination may be difficult to complete. Premedication with Valium or Demerol may be useful in these cases. Initially there was concern that severely ill patients requiring cardiac and respiratory monitoring may be difficult if not impossible to examine. Remember, ferramagnetic anesthesia equipment cannot be moved into the magnet room or near the gantry without affecting the images. Our experience shows that patients can be successfully monitored with proper equipment. Typical equipment includes blood pressure cuff with plastic connectors, chest bellows for respiratory evaluation, and an ECG telemetry system. Respiratory rate and ECG are monitored on a saturn monitor. Generally satisfactory monitoring can be achieved in patients without affecting image quality (111).

Magnetic fields may affect certain metallic implants and electrical devices. In most situations, the exact chemical structure of surgically implanted materials cannot be determined (121). Fortunately, early efforts to determine which implants are potentially dangerous to the patient or may affect image quality have been successful (109,111,117,123–125). Synchronous pacemakers convert to the asynchronous mode when placed in a magnetic field. Pacemaker power pack may also torque in the magnetic field. In addition, significant degradation may occur if the power pack is in the region being examined (125). Numerous heart valves and other metallic materials have been studied and artifacts created are negligible without significant risk to the patient (111,124).

The majority of surgical clips at our institution are not ferromagnetic (Fig. 1–27). However, a significant number of aneurysm clips (approximately 75%) are ferromagnetic and torquing can be demonstrated in a magnetic environment (124). Therefore, patients with aneurysm clips or pacemakers are currently not examined.

Manufacturers of most orthopedic appliances (plate and screws, joint prostheses, etc.) generally use high-grade stainless steel, cobalt/acromion, titanium, or multiphase alloys. These materials are usually not ferromagnetic but may contain small quantities of iron impurities. All of the orthopedic appliances at our institution have been tested for magnetic properties including heating. No heating or magnetic response could be detected (111).

Metal materials with ferromagnetic impurities can cause significant artifact on both CT and MR images (111,117). Nonferromagnetic materials cause areas of no

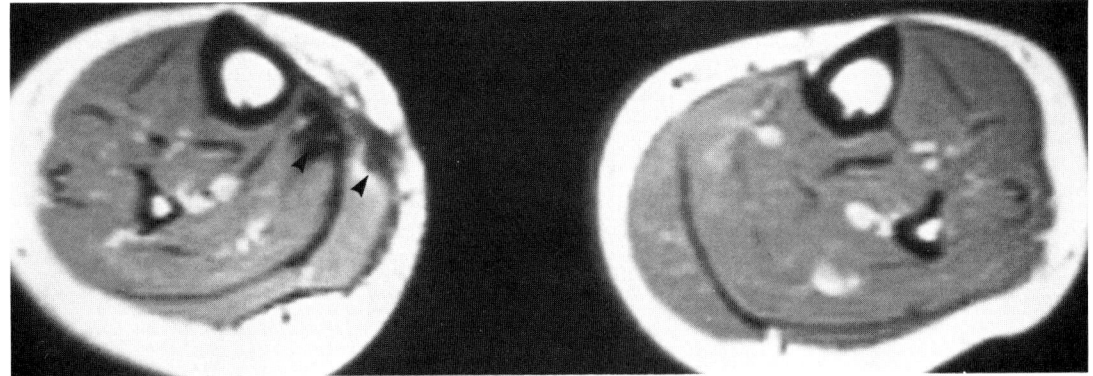

A

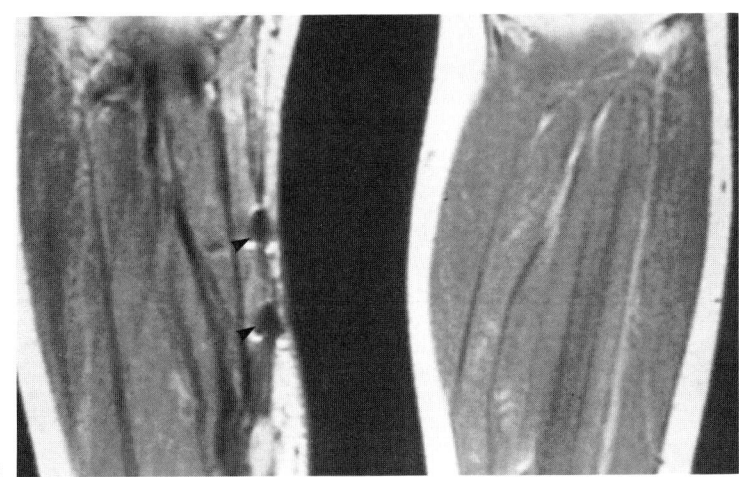

B

FIG. 1-27. Axial (**A**) and coronal (**B**) SE 500/20 images of the calves in a patient with surgical clips in the right calf medially. Note the minimal artifact (*arrows*) (111).

signal but less artifact. The degree of artifact is dependent on the size and configuration of the metal (Fig. 1–28). When imaging a hip prosthesis, more artifact is created by the large irregular neck and head region than the more regular and small femoral portion. There are also significant artifacts created by orthopedic screws, probably related to configuration of the screw, increased ferromagnetic impurities and fragments from metal bits used for drilling. Even these small amounts of ferromagnetic material can cause significant artifact (111,124). Early experience with metal implants at low and high field strength (0.15–1.5T) shows that artifacts are more significant at higher field strengths (111). Evaluation of patients with casts and bulky dressings is also possible with MRI without causing significant problems with image quality.

External fixation devices, although bulky, may not be ferromagnetic and can be easily checked with a hand-held magnet prior to imaging.

Patient Positioning and Coil Selection

Patient positioning considerations include body part, size, and expected examination time. Typically the patient is examined with the most closely coupled coil possi-

ble to achieve the maximum signal-to-noise ratio and best basal resolution (109,111,118). Signal-noise ratios may increase four to six times with a limb coil compared to the head or body coils (118). The knees, legs, foot, and ankle can be examined in the circumferential extremity coil or with flat coils (Fig. 1-29). Both are available with high field magnets and should be used when they fit the clinical setting. With noncircumferential surface coils (flat or incomplete circle), the depth of view is limited. This can result in loss of uniform signal in structures farther from the coil. As a rule, the depth of view of the flat coils is approximately one-half the diameter or width of the coil (118). A larger head coil may be used when comparison with the opposite extremity is required. More recently, dual coils have become available for evaluation of both extremities simultaneously.

Position and course of the anatomic structures being studied must also be considered. The coronal and sagittal images do not necessarily mean that partial volume effects are less significant than previously demonstrated with axial CT images. This must be kept in mind when evaluating the extent of disease processes in the coronal and sagittal planes. When possible, image planes should be chosen to fit the structure being studied. This may require off-axis oblique planes to best evaluate these anatomic regions.

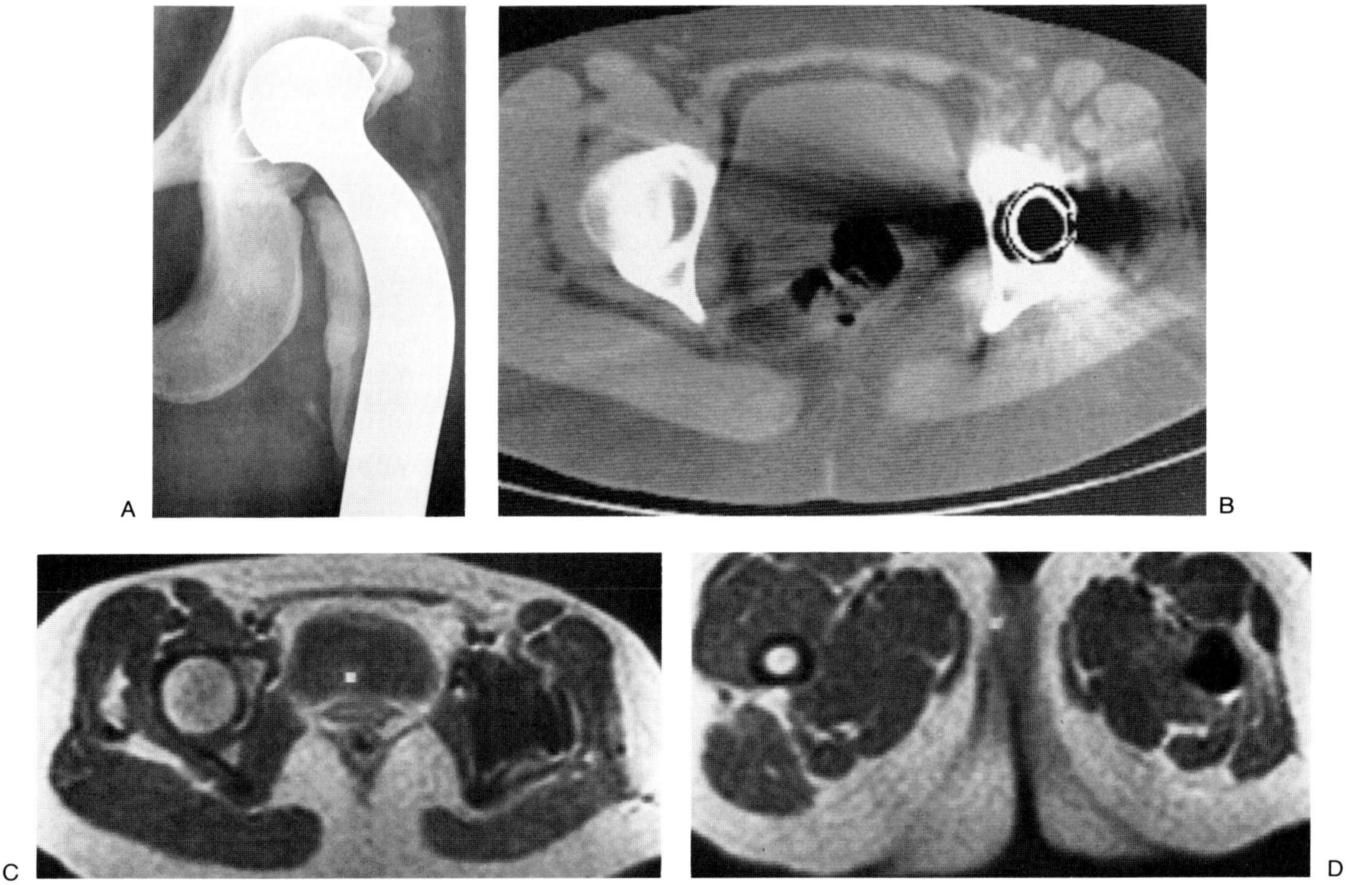

FIG. 1–28. Custom total hip arthroplasty. AP radiograph (**A**) demonstrates the amount of metal present. **B:** Axial CT image with considerable artifact due to the metal component. Low field (0.15T) MR images through the femoral head (**C**) and stem of the component (**D**) show only minimal local signal loss (111).

Pulse Sequences and Imaging Parameters

Use of different pulse sequences (inversion recovery, spin echo, partial saturation, chemical shift, and gradient echo techniques) and many available TE and TR selections at first seem cumbersome. However, current experience indicates that most musculoskeletal pathology can be evaluated with simple T1- and T2-weighted spin-echo sequences (111). Short TE, TR spin-echo sequences are T1-weighted and can be performed quickly providing excellent anatomic detail. Long TE, TR sequences are T2-weighted and are particularly useful for evaluating hemorrhage and other traumatic changes in the muscles, tendons, ligaments, and other soft tissues. More specific information regarding pulse sequences will be presented in the anatomic chapters when discussing imaging evaluation of specific traumatic conditions.

Clinical Applications

Superior soft tissue contrast, multiple image planes, and excellent spatial resolution give MR many advantages over other techniques in evaluating soft tissue (Fig. 130), articular (Fig. 1–31) and even subtle osseous (Fig.

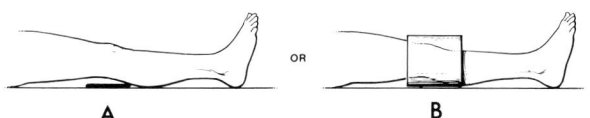

FIG. 1–29. Illustration of flat (**A**) and circumferential (**B**) coils for examination of the knee (111).

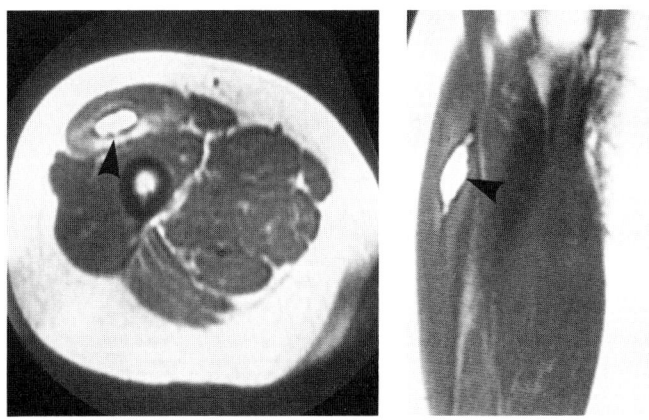

FIG. 1–30. Axial (**A**) and sagittal (**B**) SE 2000/30 images of the thigh demonstrating a post-traumatic hematoma (*arrows*).

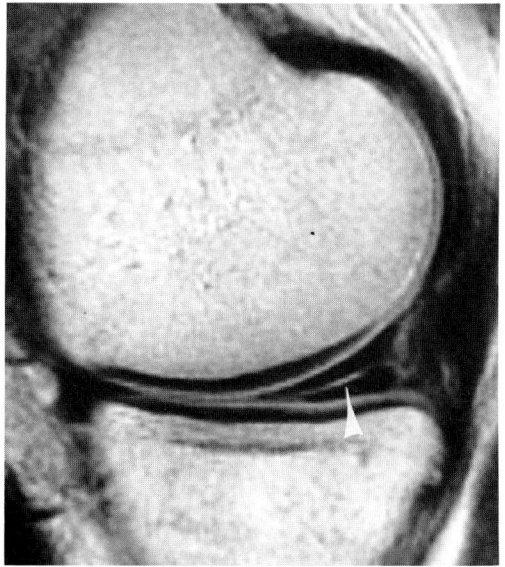

FIG. 1–31. Sagittal SE 2000/20 image of the knee demonstrating a longitudinal meniscus tear (*arrow*).

1-32) trauma. All structures can be examined compared to ultrasound, which is less versatile. MRI is also of value in evaluating conditions that may be associated with trauma such as osteonecrosis and infection. Specific changes seen with these conditions will be described later in specific anatomic chapters.

ANGIOGRAPHY

Angiography is useful in the diagnosis and treatment of vascular injuries following blunt, penetrating, or operative trauma (139,140,145). Vascular injuries include intimal injury, arterial transection or thrombosis, pseu-

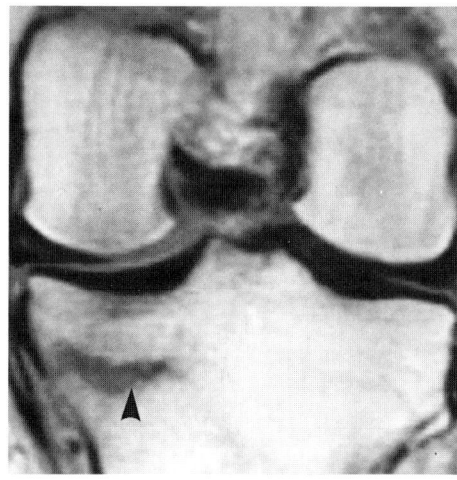

FIG. 1–32. Coronal SE 500/20 image of the knee demonstrating a medial tibial stress fracture (*arrow*).

doaneurysm, arteriovenous fistula, and venous thrombosis or transection (149). Vascular trauma may be asymptomatic or may result in hemorrhage, pulse defects, expanding masses, bruits, or signs of distal ischemia (143). In addition, repetitive minor trauma, usually occupationally related, may result in vascular injury as serious as that produced by major trauma (131). Ultrasound and computed tomography have reduced the necessity for diagnostic angiography in many of the above conditions.

In addition to diagnosis, angiography can be used to treat some of the arterial lesions by transcatheter introduction of embolic materials to produce temporary or permanent vessel occlusion (132,133–138,141,142,146–148,150,152). These techniques are most helpful in the patient with post-traumatic pelvic hemorrhage, the majority of which is due to arterial sources. The bleeding arteries can be accurately localized and then occluded through the catheter, resulting in a high rate of successful cessation of the hemorrhage (Fig. 1-33). In addition, some cases of pseudoaneurysm and arteriovenous fistula can be treated by transcatheter embolization.

Equipment

The angiogram should be performed on dedicated angiographic equipment if possible, since this results in the highest quality films and the most flexibility in obtaining multiple views and a variety of film series. A variety of contrast media and catheter shapes are available, depending upon the type of study performed and the preference of the angiographer.

Transcatheter occlusion of blood vessels requires a variety of agents whose use depends upon the specific clinical situation and the experience and preference of the angiographer. The occluding agents include particles of Gelfoam, Ivalon, or blood clot, and mechanical devices, such as the mechanical coils or detachable balloons (142,144,151). Selection and preparation of the embolic material depends upon the size of the blood vessel occluded, and the duration of occlusion varies from a few days for blood clot to a few weeks for Gelfoam. Permanent occlusion can be accomplished with coils, balloons, and Ivalon. In most cases of hemorrhage a temporary agent such as blood clot or Gelfoam is adequate. For arteriovenous fistula or pseudoaneurysm, a permanent agent should be used. The development of smaller catheter systems has extended the use of embolization in many patients that were technically not possible previously (142,150,151).

Digital subtraction angiography (DSA) can image vessels using less contrast than traditional film scans (134). This technique links a computer of an X-ray fluoroscope and allows high-quality images of arteries to be made after intra-arterial injection of contrast medium. The in-

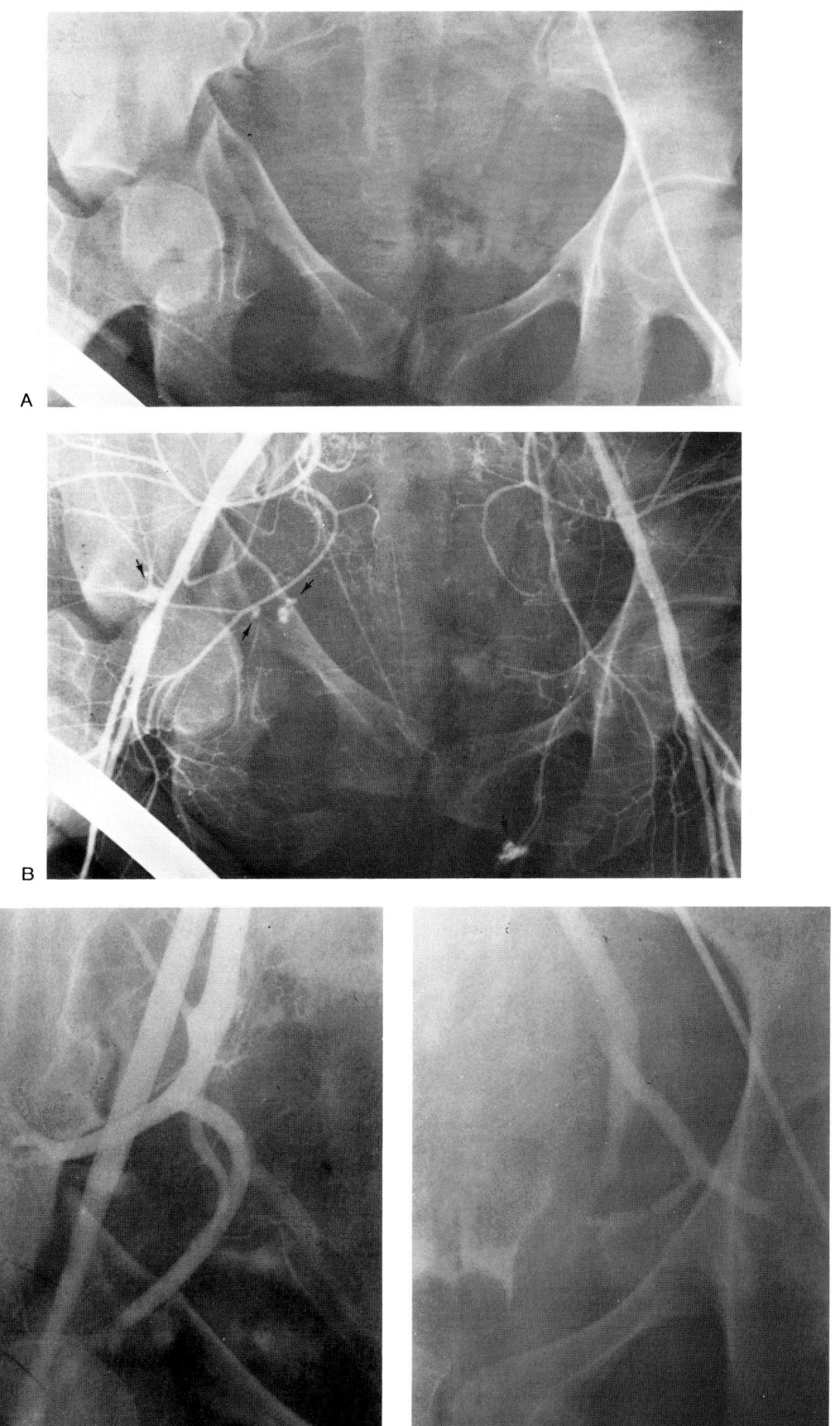

FIG. 1–33. Class III pelvic fracture: **A:** AP radiograph with angiographic catheter in place on the left. There is a complex right acetabular and anterior pelvic fracture. **B:** Angiogram demonstrates multiple bleeding sites (*arrows*). Following embolization with gelfoam the bleeding vessels have been occluded on the right (**C**) and left (**D**).

27

formation from the fluoroscopic images is digitized, and the computer then subtracts an image made before injection of contrast material from images made after injection. The only difference between the two images, the contrast in the blood vessels, is then enhanced by the computer, allowing excellent vascular images to be obtained. Initially, this technique was used with intravenous injections, but due to poor image quality this has been largely abandoned. Currently DSA studies use intra-arterial injections of contrast. The images obtained are perfectly adequate for the diagnosis of arterial occlusion in most areas of the body and in many cases will also allow detection of fine detail, such as intimal injuries. The main role of DSA in trauma patients is to decrease the amount of contrast used since these patients have multiple injections of contrast for various diagnostic tests (134).

Technique

The angiographic examination and all other imaging examinations should be tailored to the clinical problems of the patient. The imaging evaluation should be designed in such a way that no tests that might interfere with a subsequent angiogram are performed. For example, oral or rectal contrast media should not be administered prior to the angiogram. In addition, care should be exercised in the amount of intravenous contrast material given both before and during the angiogram, as large volumes of intravenous contrast material can have serious effects on renal function. One should be certain that the patient's other injuries can be stabilized long enough to allow angiography to be performed before surgical intervention is required. If not, the angiogram can be delayed. The angiographer should direct attention initially to the area of greatest clinical suspicion; survey examinations of the rest of the body should be performed afterward if the patient's condition and the amount of contrast medium used permits.

In most cases, a transfemoral route using the Seldinger technique with selective catheterization of the affected vessel is the preferred approach for performance of the angiographic exam. In a few cases this route is not available owing to the extent of pelvic trauma or to coexisting vascular disease. In these cases an axillary approach can be used. Complications of these techniques can occur at the puncture site (hemorrhage, arterial obstruction, pseudoaneurysm, arteriovenous fistula), or result from the guide wire or catheter (vessel perforation or intimal damage, distal embolization), or may be systemic (contrast medium reactions, cardiac and neurologic abnormalities). The incidence of complications is higher with the axillary than the transfemoral approach mainly because of an increase in the number of puncture sites and neurologic complications (135).

Great care and attention to technical detail are required when attempting transcatheter embolization. In general, only the affected artery should be occluded and the agent used should provide a duration of occlusion that is sufficient to resolve the clinical problem. (Fig. 1-33) In pelvic bleeding, which is the most common indication for embolization after trauma, only those branches of the internal iliac artery from which the hemorrhage is occurring should be occluded, although selective catheterization is not possible in all cases. In some cases, occlusion of the entire internal iliac is all that is possible. Agents that produce occlusions of short duration (blood clots and Gelfoam) should be used. If both internal iliac arteries must be occluded, the risk of such complications as impotence or ischemic necrosis of the bladder increases; but in these instances the procedure may be necessary to save the patient's life.

Indications

Angiography can accurately identify the vast majority of trauma-induced arterial lesions. Unfortunately, despite years of experience with its use, the indications for angiography after trauma are still not well defined. In extremity trauma, some physicians advocate performing angiography in every case of blunt or penetrating trauma that occurs near a major vessel, whereas others favor angiography only when physical findings such as pulse deficit or bruit are present (143,145). The indications for angiography in thoracic trauma are equally varied depending on the series quoted (133). Pelvic angiography, for the diagnosis and treatment of bleeding after pelvic trauma, is very useful. Embolization is required in 1% of pelvic fracture patients. It is reserved for those patients with life-threatening bleeding. The majority of patients can be managed with conservative therapy or external fixation (144). Venography may be useful in a few cases to define venous injuries, especially in the case of expanding pelvic hematomas with negative angiograms (147).

The performance of these examinations will probably continue to depend upon local experience and the availability of angiographic and surgical expertise.

MYELOGRAPHY

Positive contrast myelography has been accomplished for many years and provides useful information regarding the bony spinal canal, spinal cord, and nerve roots (see Fig. 1-25). Until recently positive contrast examination of the spinal canal was performed with film or fluoroscopic studies. The advent of computed tomography of the spine has added a new imaging technique. The combination of CT and intrathecal contrast medium has provided an additional technique for evaluation of the posterior spinal structures that is complementary to conventional myelography and occasionally more definitive (156,158).

Two contrast agents were primarily used for myelography in the United States. Iophendylate (Pantopaque) is an oil-based medium and has a long history of established use in myelography. Metrizamide (Amipaque), a water-soluble agent, followed and was widely accepted. The water-soluble agent generally has more irritating side effects on the central nervous system; however, it is less viscous, thus providing better visualization of nerve roots. Also, because of its water solubility, metrizamide does not have to be removed from the spinal canal, as does its counterpart iophendylate. Both materials have advantages in different situations. Either of the contrast agents is adequate, and selections should be based on the practice and the patient's clinical situation (157). Now, new low osmolality contrast agents have replaced both of the above agents in most situations (159).

Technique

Routine myelography is accomplished with the patient in the prone position on a radiographic table equipped for 90° tilt in either direction. Plain films should be thoroughly examined prior to the examination, as subtle changes on these films may dictate changes in filming sequence and the appropriate needle placement for the myelogram. Routinely a 20–22-gauge needle is introduced into the L2-L3 interspace. Because of the level of the conus, puncture at a higher site is undesirable. If the needle is placed in a lower position, it may create artifacts, making it difficult to identify L4 and L5 pathology. This is, of course, a common location for lumbar disk disease. Spinal puncture should be made with fluoroscopic guidance to insure an ideal midline position for the needle. This allows better position of the needle for injection in the subarachnoid space. Following a single-wall midline puncture, cerebral spinal fluid should be collected for laboratory studies. The contrast material is then injected under fluoroscopic observation to confirm its presence in the subarachnoid space. In most cases, 12–14 ml of contrast agent is all that is required. Fourteen to 20 ml of low osmolality contrast medium (Isovue 200) may be needed if the entire spine is being studied.

Filming for myelograms consists of a series of AP, cross-table lateral, and oblique exposures through the region of potential disease. Tilting the table under fluoroscopic control produces gravity-directed flow of the contrast material, allowing one to evaluate the site of interest.

With low osmolality (non-ionic) water soluble myelography, several changes from the older pantopaque technique are employed (153,155,157,159). The patient should be well hydrated, and the patient's anti-convulsant therapy should be continued.

A smaller needle is used (20–22 gauge), since the contrast agent is less viscous. A major advantage of the new non-ionic and water soluble contrast agents (metrizamide) is that they need not be removed from the spinal canal following the procedure. Contrast agent is totally absorbed from the cerebral spinal fluid space and excreted through the kidneys in 24–48 hours. Although these agents are more directly irritating to the central nervous system than iophendylate, it is considered to have less potential for the feared late complication of arachnoiditis. Arachnoiditis has been attributed to iophendylate in certain cases. The lesser risk of arachnoiditis with use of metrizamide is primarily due to the total disappearance of metrizamide through its early resorption (160).

Following myelography with water soluble agents, the patient should be kept well hydrated and the head should be elevated at approximately 45° for several hours. This prevents the immediate ascent of a bolus of contrast medium into the intracranial region. If this should occur, the incidence of complications such as seizure is significantly higher. With iophendylate, the patient should be kept supine, well hydrated, and still with as little head movement as possible for at least 6–8 hours. If headaches occur following the myelogram, they should be treated supportively.

Although myelography is rarely indicated immediately following acute spinal trauma, in such cases the procedure is conducted quite differently. The needle must be positioned away from the lesion, often resulting in a lower puncture site or a C1 puncture (158). Only a small amount of cerebral spinal fluid should be removed in cases of potential obstruction. The fluid should be examined carefully, and if blood is present the significant risk of arachnoiditis must be recognized. In these situations, the water soluble agents are contrast materials of choice (162).

Patient positioning may be a significant problem following acute injury. This may require additional equipment to stabilize the spine and assist in controlled patient motion in directing dye flow.

Normal Myelographic Anatomy

The cord and proximal nerve roots entering the neural canals are demonstrated myelographically as negative filling defects (Fig. 1-34). The spinal cord is widest at the C5-C6 level, occupying up to 75% of the transverse diameter of the sac on the AP view (Fig. 1-34). The spinal canal is smaller in the thoracic region and the conus is best demonstrated with the supine AP views at the T12 level (Fig. 1-35). The opacified subarachnoid space is separated from the bony walls of the canal by fat, liga-

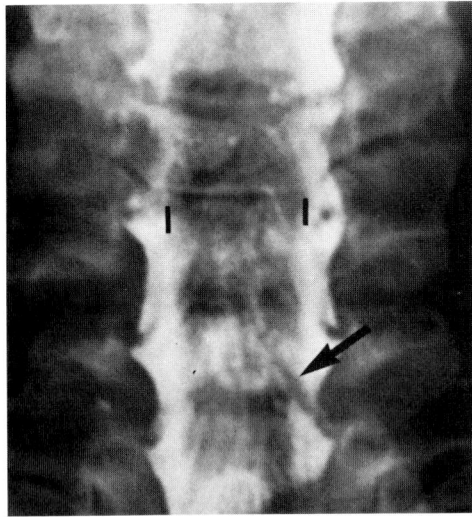

FIG. 1–34. Normal AP cervical myelogram. Note the nerve roots (*arrow*) and width of the spinal canal (*vertical lines*).

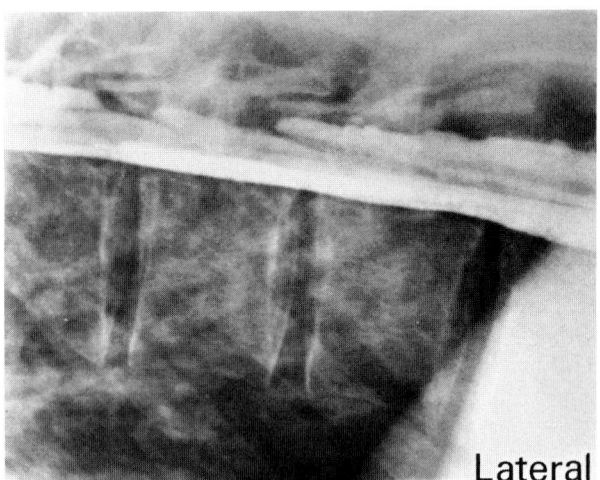

FIG. 1–36. Normal lateral thoracic myelogram.

ments, and the veins of the epidural space. On the lateral view, smooth indentations may be seen at the interspaces owing to the posterior longitudinal ligament (Fig. 1-36). Draining veins may be seen on occasion near the conus in the thoracic region.

Indications

In practice, myelography is most commonly used for definitive diagnosis or exclusion of herniated disks. This has changed significantly in recent years owing to the increased application of computed tomography, with or without metrizamide, in evaluation of the spinal canal

(156,158). Other indications for conventional myelography include spondylosis or spinal stenosis, spinal tumors, congenital malformations, and arteriovenous malformations (Table 1-4). Myelography is rarely indicated following acute spinal trauma. Computed tomography and conventional tomography will usually provide the necessary information. In selected patients, myelography may be useful in defining the level of epidural obstruction (see Fig. 1-25) following trauma or surgery (Fig. 1-37) and in localizing cervical nerve root avulsions (158,161).

INTRODUCTION TO ARTHROGRAPHY

This section provides the necessary background information for arthrography regardless of the joint being

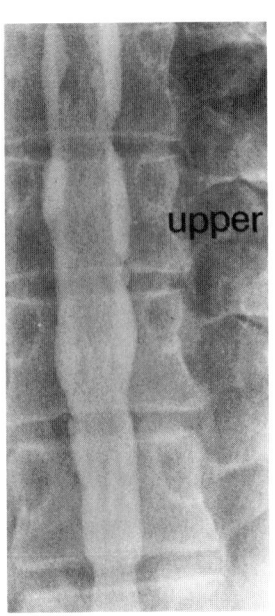

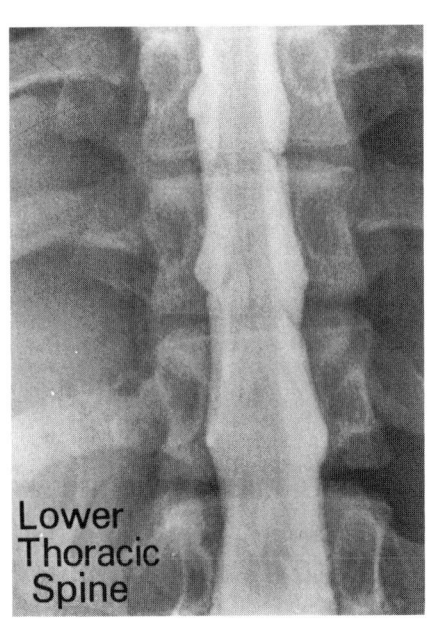

FIG. 1–35. Normal AP thoracic myelogram with views of the upper (**A**) and lower (**B**) thoracic spine.

TABLE 1-4. *Myelography: common indications*

Disk disease
Spondylosis and spinal stenosis
Spinal neoplasms
Primary
Metastatic
Congenital malformations
Arachnoid cysts
Arteriovenous malformations
Arachnoiditis
Trauma
Epidural obstruction
Nerve root avulsion

TABLE 1-5. *Arthrography: commonly studied joints*

Knee*
Shoulder*
Hip
Wrist
Ankle
Hand
Elbow
Foot
Tarsal
Metatarsophalangeal
Lumbar facet
Temporomandibular*
Sacroiliac
Pubic symphysis

* In order of decreasing frequency prior to MRI.

studied. Details involving procedural techniques will be reserved for specific anatomic chapters.

Arthrography is an extremely useful, benign procedure. Prior to MRI, this technique was most frequently employed in the knee, shoulder, and hip; however, almost any accessible articulation may be evaluated. In recent years MRI has replaced knee arthrography and MRI is also becoming an accepted technique for the shoulder. Table 1-5 lists the joints most frequently studied at the Mayo Clinic in order of decreasing frequency.

In order to obtain the maximum information, arthrography or tenography should be performed by an experienced arthrographer with a thorough understanding of the patient's clinical situation. Review of routine radiographs is essential. These films may provide clues that dictate subtle changes in film technique, views that may be required, and the contrast medium that may be best suited for the procedure. Simply stated, these techniques should be tailored to the individual patient and not performed as a set procedure.

Equipment

Radiographic equipment should provide excellent detail and allow adequate work space to simplify patient positioning and needle placement. We prefer an overhead fluoroscopic tube with a small focal spot (no larger than 0.6 mm) and a 48-inch source-to-target distance (Fig. 1-38). This provides better geometric positioning and resulting film quality than a conventional fluoroscopic suite with the x-ray tube under the table. The overhead tube allows better access to the patient, making the procedure less difficult to perform. This table, which is movable, can be used for all types of arthrography and interventional orthopedic procedures.

The arthrogram set (Fig. 1-39) is devised so that all arthrograms, injections, and biopsies can be performed with the same tray. The tray includes the following

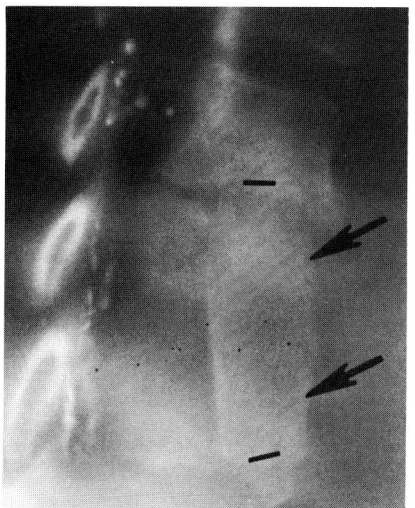
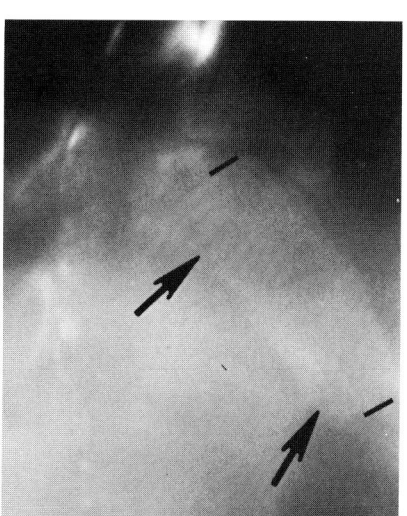
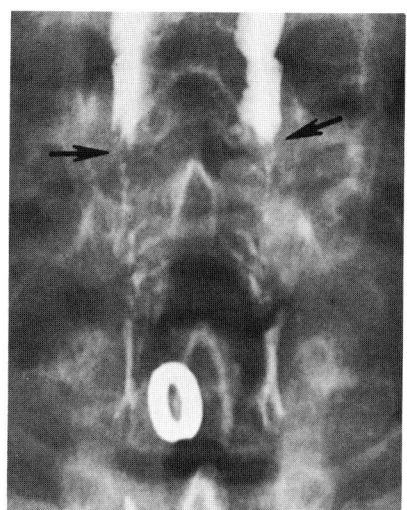

A   B   C

FIG. 1-37. A: Postoperative anterior bone graft cervical fusion (*arrows*) demonstrated on lateral tomogram. Several weeks later tomograms (**B**) demonstrate displacement of the graft (*arrows*) and a myelogram (**C**) demonstrates obstruction (*arrows*) at the operative site.

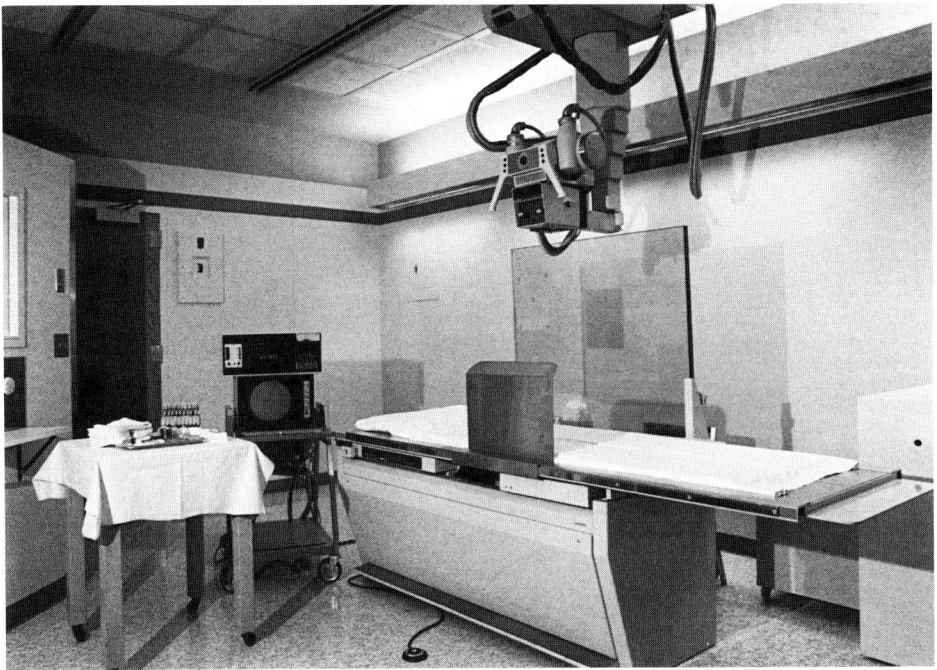

FIG. 1–38. Arthrographic and interventional fluoroscopic suite with overhead fluoroscopic tube to allow greater patient access.

items: four sterile drapes, one sterile drape with a 4-inch center hole, six absorbent 6 × 6 gauze sponges, one 5 ml syringe, two 10 ml syringes, one 30 ml syringe, one cup for contrast material, and extension tubing. A needle box is kept in the room. This contains 22- and 18-gauge spinal needles, $1\frac{1}{2}$-inch 18- and 22-gauge needles, and $\frac{5}{8}$-inch 25-gauge needles. Needle selection will vary depending on the joint to be studied and the size of the patient.

Additional items include vials of nonbacteriostatic sa-line solution for joint aspiration and irrigation, culture vials for aerobic and anaerobic bacterial and fungal studies, specimen tubes for synovial fluid analysis, and 1% lidocaine (Xylocaine). Betamethasone (Celestone) and 0.25% bupivacaine (Marcaine) are also stocked for diagnostic and therapeutic injections. Sterile conventional and leaded surgical gloves are also available in the arthrographic suite. An additional necessity is an emergency tray or cart in case of contrast medium reactions or other unforeseen emergencies.

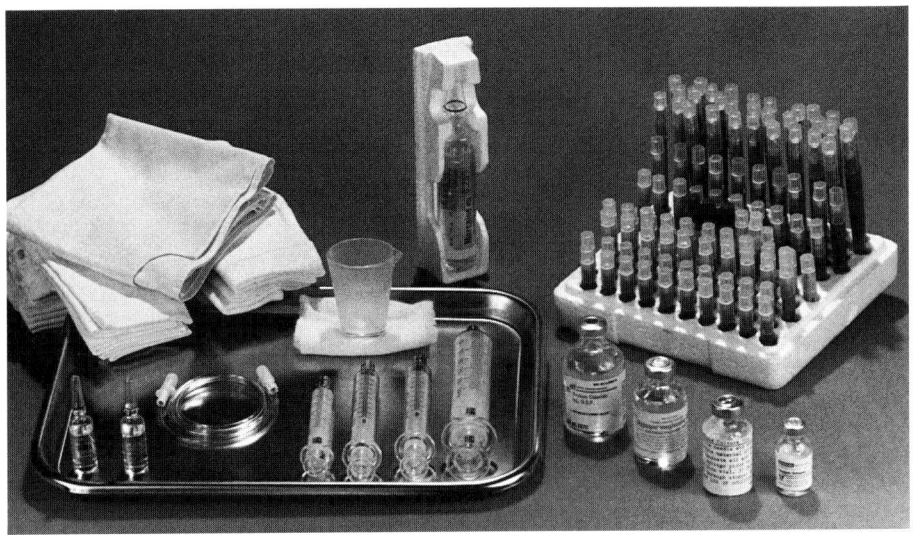

FIG. 1–39. Arthrogram set with syringes, needles, anesthetic vials, culture bottles, Celestone, and other items needed for arthrography and tenography.

Contrast Material

Arthrography may be performed with positive-contrast material, air, or double-contrast techniques that use both a positive contrast medium and air or CO_2. Several contrast media are available. We most commonly use Hypaque-M-60 (Winthrop). Renografin-60 and Reno M-60 (Squibb) may also be used. Iodine content, approximately 47% with Hypaque-M-60, does not differ significantly from that in other arthrographic contrast media. However, sodium content with these contrast agents is less than with other diatrizoates, resulting in less irritation. Extracapsular injection is particularly painful if the sodium content of the contrast medium is too high. New non-ionic low osmolality agents are not frequently used in our practice.

Because of increased osmolality and rapid absorption, contrast medium becomes rapidly diluted in joints and tendon sheaths, resulting in loss of detail on the radiographs. This may occur in 5–10 minutes following the injection. If an effusion is present in the joint, the detail may deteriorate even more rapidly. This can be prevented to some degree by combining 0.3 ml of 1:1000 epinephrine with the contrast material (165). However, epinephrine may cause systemic side effects and should not be used in patients with cardiac disease. We generally reserve the use of epinephrine for cases that require tomography or CT in addition to the conventional views. Tomography requires significantly more time, and if epinephrine is not used the image quality may be decreased.

Improved contrast agents are being investigated but are not commonly used at this time. PhDZ 59B was studied in Sweden, and it demonstrated prolonged duration in the joints (163). Metrizamide, used in myelography, is a water-soluble contrast medium that has also been investigated for arthrographic purposes. Metrizamide also remains in the joint longer and has a lower incidence of postarthrographic effusion compared to Urografin-60 and Conray-282 (170,171).

In the shoulder, knee, and elbow, double-contrast technique provides increased articular detail. We routinely use room air rather than CO_2. Room air is less expensive and readily available, and we have not experienced any complications. Mink reported a lower incidence of postarthrographic pain with room air compared to CO_2 (173). Rarely, room air alone is used in patients with a significant history of allergy to contrast media.

Complications

Articular and tendon sheath injections are benign procedures with little risk of significant complications. Freiberger reported an incidence of infection of 1:25,000 cases (165). Newberg et al. (175), reported three infections and 61 cases of hives in 126,000 patients. Effusions may occur following arthrography, whether contrast medium or air alone is used. The effusion usually appears within 12 hours of the arthrogram and results in pain and stiffness of the involved joint (165,174). Murray reported transient eosinophilia in the knee following pneumoarthrography, which is often combined with a turbid fluid owing to the high eosinophil count (normally 2%, 75% following pneumoarthrography). No infection could be detected (174,176). Eosinophilic infiltration of the synovium has also been demonstrated (169,176) and may explain the postarthrographic pain and swelling. Mink postulates that pH decreases in the synovial fluid following arthrography may be responsible for the discomfort experienced by some patients (173). Regardless of the etiology of the effusion and discomfort, this is not usually a significant problem, especially when compared with the diagnostic usefulness of the procedure (168,173). This difficulty seems to be less of a problem following double-contrast studies, perhaps because of the smaller volumes of contrast medium used with this technique (167). Also, air may remain in the joint for up to 10 days (174), which will result in increased crepitation in the joint.

Patients should be questioned concerning allergies to iodinated contrast media prior to having the arthrogram performed. Allergy to contrast agents must be considered but is extremely rare, numbering fewer than 1 per 1000 studies in Freiberger's series (165). Urticaria is the usual reaction experienced and often no treatment is required. Antihistamines may be used in more severe cases of urticaria. Most reactions to contrast medium develop within 15–30 minutes following the injection. When necessary, premedication with steroids can be useful (172). However, MRI makes these steps unnecessary in most situations.

REFERENCES

Routine Radiography

1. Ballinger PW. *Merrill's atlas of roentgenographic positions and standard radiologic procedures.* St. Louis: C.V. Mosby, 1982.
2. Bernau A, Berqusit TH. *Orthopedic positioning in diagnostic radiology.* Baltimore: Urban & Schwarzenberg, 1983.
3. Eastman Kodak Co.: *The fundamentals of radiology.* 12th Ed. Rochester, NY, 1980.
4. Gonadal shielding in diagnostic radiology. Publication No. (FDA) 75-8024, Rockville, Bureau of Radiological Health, 1975.
5. Orhan HS, Showalter CK, Koustenis GH, et al. A sensitometric evaluation of film-screen-chemistry-processor systems in the state of New Jersey. Bureau of Radiological Health, Rockville, 1982.
6. Picus D, McAlister WH, Smith E, Rodewald S, Jost GR, Evens RG. Plain radiography with a rare-earth screen: Comparison with calcium tungstate screen. *AJR* 1984;143:1335–1338.

Tomography

7. Apple JS, Martinez S, Allen NB, Caldwell DS, Rice JR. Occult fractures of the knee: Tomographic evaluation. *Radiology* 1983;148:383–387.

8. Berrett A, Brunner S, Valvassori GE. *Modern thin section tomography.* Springfield, IL: Charles C. Thomas, 1973.
9. Bokstrom I. Principles of vertebral tomography. *Acta Radiol Suppl* 1953;103:5–109.
10. Curry TS, Dowdey JE, Murry JR. *An introduction to the physics of diagnostic radiology.* 3rd ed. Philadelphia: Lea & Febiger, 1990.
11. Eastman Kodak Co. *Fundamentals of radiology.* 12th Ed. Rochester, New York, 1980.
12. McCullough EC, Coulam CM. Physical and dosimetric aspects of diagnostic geometrical and computer-assisted tomographic procedures. *Radiol Clin North Am* 1976;14:3–24.
13. Norman A. The value of tomography in the diagnosis of skeletal disorders. *Radiol Clin North Am* 1970;8:251–258.
14. Pavloy H, Torg JS, Freiberger RH. Tarsal navicular stress fractures: Radiographic evaluation. *Radiology* 1983;148:641–645.
15. Resnick D, Niwayama G. *Diagnosis of bone and joint disorders.* Philadelphia: W.B. Saunders Co., 1988.

Magnification Radiography

16. Curry TS, Dowdey JE, Murry JR. *An introduction to the physics of diagnostic radiology.* 3rd Ed. Philadelphia: Lea & Febiger, 1984.
17. Fletcher DE, Rowley KA. Radiographic enlargements in diagnostic radiology. *Br J Radiol* 1951;24:598–604.
18. Genant HK, Kunio D, Mall JC, Sickles EA. Direct magnification for skeletal radiography. *Radiology* 1977;123:47–55.
19. Gordon SL, Greer RB, Wiedner WA. Magnification roentgenographic technique in orthopedics. *Clin Orthop* 1973;91:169–173.
20. Milne E. Magnification radiology, editorial. *Applied Radiol* 1976; Jan-Feb:12,
21. Nemet A, Cox WF. The improvement of definition of x-ray image magnification. *Br J Radiol* 1956;29:335–337.
22. Resnick D, Niwayama G. *Diagnosis of bone and joint disorders.* Philadelphia: W.B. Saunders Co., 1988.
23. Eastman Kodak Co. *The fundamentals of radiology.* 12th Ed. Rochester, New York, 1980.
24. Wagner LK, Cohen G, Wong W, Amtey SR. Dose efficiency and the effects of resolution and noise detail perceptibility in radiographic magnification. *Med Phys* 1981;8:24–32.
25. Weiss A. A technique for demonstrating fine detail in the bones of the hand. *Clin Radiol* 1972;23:185–187.

Ultrasound

26. Bluth EI, Merritt CRB, Sullivan MA. Gray scale ultrasound evaluation of the lower extremities. *JAMA* 1982;247:3127–3129.
27. Braunstein EM, Silver TM, Martel W, Jaffe M. Ultrasonographic diagnosis of extremity masses. *Skeletal Radiol* 1981;6:157–163.
28. Carpenter JR, Hattery RR, Hunder GG, Bryan RS, McLeod RA. Ultrasound evaluation of the popliteal space. Comparison of arthrography and physical examination. *Mayo Clin Proc* 1976;51:498–503.
29. Cooperberg PL, Tsang L, Truelove L, Knickerbocker WJ. Grey scale ultrasound in the evaluation of rheumatoid arthritis of the knee. *Radiology* 1978;126:759–763.
30. Dorfman GS, Froelich JA, Cronan JJ, Urbanek PJ, Herndon JH. Lower extremity venous thrombosis in patients with acute hip fractures: Determination of anatomic location and time onset with compression sonography. *AJR* 1990;154:851–855.
31. Fornage BD, Scheruberg FL, Rifkin MD. Ultrasound examination of the hand. *Radiology* 1985;155:785–788.
32. Gordon GV, Edell S. Ultrasonic evaluation of popliteal cysts. *Arch Intern Med* 1980;140:1453–1455.
33. Gompels BM, Darlington LG. Grey scale ultrasonography and arthrography in evaluation of popliteal cysts. *Clin Radiol* 1979;30:539–545.
34. Harcke HT, Grissom LE, Furkelstein MS. Evaluation of the musculoskeletal system with sonography. *AJR* 1988;150:1253–1261.
35. Hentz VR, Green PS, Arditi M. Imaging studies of the cadaver hand using transmission ultrasound. *Skel Radiol* 1987;16:474–480.
36. Hermann G, Yeh HC, Lehr-James C, et al. Diagnosis of popliteal cysts: Double contrast arthrography and sonography. *AJR* 1981;137:369–372.
37. Holder J, Fretz CJ, Terrier F, Gerber C. Rotator cuff tears: Correlation of sonographic and surgical findings. *Radiology* 1988;169:791–794.
38. Kaufman RA, Tarskins RB, Babcock DS, Crawford AH. Arthrosonography in the diagnosis of pigmented villonodular synovitis. *AJR* 1982;139:396–398.
39. Lawson TL, Mittler S. Ultrasonic evaluation of extremity soft tissue lesions with arthrographic correlation. *J Can Assoc Radiol* 1978;29:58–61.
40. Leopold GR. Ultrasonography of superficially located structures. *Radiol Clin North Am* 1980;18:161–173.
41. McDonald DG, Leopold GR. Ultrasound B-scanning in the differentiation of Baker's cyst and thrombophlebitis. *Br J Radiol* 1972;45:729–732.
42. Sarti DA, Sample WF. *Diagnostic ultrasound, text and cases.* Boston: G.K. Hall and Co., 1980.
43. Silber TM, Washburn RL, Stanley JC, et al. Grey scale ultrasound evaluation of popliteal artery aneurysms. *AJR* 1977;129:1003–XXX.
44. Swett HA, Jaffe RB, McIff EB. Popliteal cysts: Presentation as thrombophlebitis. *Radiology* 1975;115:613–615.
45. Winsberg F, Cooperberg PL. *Real time ultrasonography.* New York: Churchill Livingstone, 1982.

Skeletal Scintigraphy

46. Ash JM, Gilday DL, Reilly BJ. Pinhole imaging of hip disorders in children. *J Nucl Med* 1975;16:512.
47. Berggren A, Weiland AJ, Ostrup LT. Bone scintigraphy in evaluating the viability of composite bone grafts revascularized by microvascular anastomosis, conventional autologous bone grafts, and free nonrevascularized periosteal grafts. *J Bone Joint Surg* 1982;64A:799–809.
48. Campbell G, Warnekros W. Tarsal stress fracture in a long distance runner. *J Am Pediatry Assoc* 1983;73:532–536.
49. Collier BD, Kir MK, Mills BJ, et al. Bone scan: A useful test for evaluating patients with low back pain. *Skel Radiol* 1990;19:267–270.
50. Collier BD, Johnson RP, Carrera GF, et al. Chronic knee pain assessed by SPECT: Comparison with other modalities. *Radiology* 1985;157:795–802.
51. Collins JD, Bassett L, Main GD, Kagan C. Percutaneous biopsy following positive bone scans. *Radiology* 1979;132:439–442.
52. Danigelis JA. Pinhole imaging in Legg-Perthes disease: Further observations. *Semin Nucl Med* 1976;6:69–82.
53. Desai A, Alavi A, Dalinka M, Brighton C, Esterhai J. Role of bone scintigraphy in the evaluation and treatment of nonunited fractures: Concise communication. *J Nucl Med* 1980;21:931–934.
54. Ganel A, Engel J, Oster Z, Farine I. Bone scanning and assessment of fractures of the scaphoid. *J Hand Surg* 1979;4:540–543.
55. Gelman MI, Coleman RE, Stevens PM, Davey BW. Radiography, radionuclide imaging and arthrography in evaluation of total hip and knee replacement. *Radiology* 1978;128:677–682.
56. Geslien JE, Thrall JH, Espinosa JL, Older RA. Early detection of stress fractures using Tc-99m polyphosphate. *Radiology* 1976;121:683–687.
57. Greiff J. Determination of the vitality of the femoral head with Tc-99m-SN-pyrophosphate scintigraphy. *Acta Orthop Scand* 1980;51:109–117.
58. Greiff J, Lanng S, Hoilund-Carlsen PF. Early detection by Tc-99m-Sn-pyrophosphate scintigraphy of femoral head necrosis following medial femoral neck fractures. *Acta Orthop Scand* 1980;51:119.
59. Gumerman LW, Fogel SR, Goodman MA, et al. Experimental fracture healing: Evaluation of radionuclide bone imaging: Concise communication. *J Nucl Med* 1978;19:1320–1323.

60. Hoffer P. Gallium: Mechanisms. *J Nucl Med* 1980;21:282–285.
61. Lotke PA, Ecker ML, Alavi A. Painful knees in older patients: Radionuclide diagnosis of possible osteonecrosis with spontaneous resolution. *J Bone Joint Surg* 1977;59A:617–621.
62. Magnuson JE, Brown ML, Hauser MF, Berquist TH, Fitzgerald RH, Klee GG. In-111 labeled leukocyte scintigraphy in suspected orthopedic prosthesis infection: Comparison with other imaging modalities. *Radiology* 1988;168:235–239.
63. Matin P. The appearance of bone scans following fractures, including immediate and long-term studies. *J Nucl Med* 1979;20:1227–1231.
64. McMaster MJ, Merrick MV. A scintigraphic assessment of the scoliotic spine after fusion. *J Bone Joint Surg* 1980;62B:65–72.
65. Merkel KD, Brown ML, Dewanjee MK, Fitzgerald RH. Comparison of indium-labeled leukocyte imaging with sequential technetium-gallium scanning in the diagnosis of low-grade musculoskeletal sepsis. *J Bone Joint Surg* 1985;67A:465–476.
66. Oyen WJG, Claessens RAMJ, vanHorn JR, van der Meer, JWM. Scintigraphic detection of bone and joint infections with Indium-111 labeled nonspecific polyclonal human immunoglobulin. *J Nucl Med* 1990;31:403–412.
67. Pring DJ, et al. Indium-granulocyte scanning in the painful prosthetic joint. *AJR* 1986;146:167–172.
68. Rosenthall L, Lisbona R, Hernandez M, Hadjipavlou A. Tc-99m-pp and Ga-67 imaging following insertion of orthopedic devices. *Radiology* 1979;133:717–721.
69. Rosenthal L, Kloiber R, Damten B, Al-Majed H. Sequential use of radiophosphate and radiogallium imaging in the differential diagnosis of bone, joint, and soft tissue infection: Quantitative analysis. *Diagn Imaging* 1982;51:249–258.
70. Rubin RH, Fischman AJ, Callahan RJ., et al. ^{111}In-labeled nonspecific immunoglobulin scanning in detection of focal infection. *N Engl J Med* 1989;321:935–940.
71. Schaffer DL, Pendergrass HP. Comparison of enzyme clinical, radiographic, and radionuclide methods of detecting bone metastasis from carcinoma of the prostate. *Radiology* 1976;121:431–434.
72. Seabold JE, et al. Detection of osteomyelitis at fracture nonunion sites: Comparison of two scintigraphic methods. *AJR* 1989;152:1021–1027.
73. Spencer RB, Levinson ED, Baldwin RD, Sziklas JJ, Witek JT, Rosenberg R. Diverse bone scan abnormalities in "shin splints". *J Nucl Med* 1979;20:1271–1272.
74. Subramanian G, McAfee JG. A new complex for skeletal imaging. *Radiology* 1971;99:192–196.
75. Subramanian G, McAfee JG, Bell EG, Blair RJ, Omara RE, Ralston PH. Tc-99m-labeled polyphosphate as a skeletal imaging agent. *Radiology* 1972;102:701–704.
76. Sutherland AD, Savage JP, Paterson DC, Foster BK. The nuclide bone scan in the diagnosis and management of Perthes disease. *J Bone Joint Surg* 1980;62B:300–306.
77. Swee RG, McLeod RA, Beabout JW. Osteoid osteoma. Detection, diagnosis and localization. *Radiology* 1979;130:117–123.
78. Thakur ML, Coleman RE, Mayhall CG, Welch MJ. Preparation and evaluation of 111In-labeled leukocytes as an abscess imaging agent in dogs. *Radiology* 1976;119:731–732.
79. Thakur ML, Coleman RE, Welch MJ. Indium-111-labeled leukocytes for the localization of abscesses: Preparation, analysis, tissue distribution in comparison with gallium-67 citrate in dogs. *J Lab Clin Med* 1977;89:217–228.
80. Thomas RH, Resnick D, Naomi PA, Alazraki NP, Daniel D, Greenfield R. Compartmental evaluation of osteoarthritis of the knee. A comparitive study of available diagnostic modalities. *Radiology* 1975;116:585–594.
81. Wilcox JR, Moniot AL, Green JP. Bone scanning and the evaluation of exercise-related injuries. *Radiology* 1977;123:699–703.

Computed Tomography

82. Brant-Zawadski M, Miller EM, Federle MP. CT in the evaluation of spine trauma. *AJR* 1981;136:369–375.
83. Brasch RC, Boyd DP, Gooding CA. Computed tomographic scanning in children: Comparison of radiation dose and resolving power of commercial CT scanners. *AJR* 1978;131:95–101.
84. Canale ST, Manugian AH. Irreducible traumatic dislocations of the hip. *J Bone Joint Surg* 1979;61A:7–14.
85. Chang W. Slice characteristics of the Imatron cine-CT scanner. *JCAT* 1987;11:554.
86. Coin CG, Pennink M, Ahmad WD, Keranen VJ. Diving type injury to the cervical spine: Contribution of computed tomography to management. *J Comp Assist Tomogr* 1979;3:362–372.
87. Colley DP, Dunsker SB. Traumatic narrowing of the dorsolumbar spinal canal demonstrated by computed tomography. *Radiology* 1978;129:95–98.
88. Destouet JM, Gilula LA, Murphy WA, Sagel SS. Computed tomography of the sterno-clavicular joint and sternum. *Radiology* 1981;138:123–128.
89. Dooms GC, Fisher MR, Hricak H, Higgins CB. MR imaging of intramuscular hemorrhage. *J Comp Assist Tomogr* 1985;9:908–913.
90. Drebin RA, Magid D, Robertson DD, Fishman EK. Fidelity of three dimensional CT imaging for detecting fracture gaps. *JCAT* 1989;13:487–489.
91. Ehman RL, Berquist TH. Magnetic resonance imaging of musculoskeletal trauma. *Radiol Clin North Am* 1986;24:291–319.
92. Fishman EK, Magid D, Robertson DD, et al. Metallic implants: CT with multiplanar reconstruction. *Radiology* 1986;160:675–681.
93. Genant HK. Computed tomography. In: Resnick D. and Niwayama, G.: *Diagnosis of bone and joint disorders*. Philadelphia: W.B. Saunders Co., 1981.
94. Genant HK, Cann CE, Chafetz NI, Helms CA. Advances in computed tomography of the musculoskeletal system. *Radiol Clin North Am* 1981;19:645–674.
95. Gilula LA, Murphy WA, Chandrakant CT, Patel RB. Computed tomography of the osseous pelvis. *Radiology* 1979;132:107–114.
96. Griffiths HJ, Hamlin DJ, Kiss S, Lovelock J. Efficacy of CT scanning in a group of 174 patients with orthopedic and musculoskeletal problems. *Skeletal Radiol* 1981;7:87–98.
97. Handel SF, Lee YY. Computed tomography of spinal fractures. *Radiol Clin North Am* 1981;19:69–89.
98. Lange TA, Alter AJ. Evaluation of complex acetabular fractures by computed tomography. *J Comp Assist Tomogr* 1980;4:849–852.
99. Lasda NA, Levinsohn EM, Yuan HA, Bunnell WP. Computerized tomography in disorders of the hip. *J Bone Joint Surg* 1978;60A:1099–1102.
100. McCullough EC, Payne JT. Patient dosage in computed tomography. *Radiology* 1978;129:457–463.
101. McLeod RA, Stephens DH, Beabout JW, Sheedy PF III, Hattery RR. Computed tomography in the skeletal system. *Semin Roentgenol* 1978;13:235–247.
102. O'Callaghan JP, Ulrich CG, Yuan HA. CT of facet distraction if flexion injuries of the thoracolumbar spine: The naked facet. *AJR* 1980;134:563–572.
103. O'Connor JF, Cohen J. Computerized tomography in orthopedic surgery. *J Bone Joint Surg* 1978;60A:1096–1098.
104. Pate D, Resnick D, Andre M, et al. Perspective: Three dimensional imaging of the musculoskeletal system. *AJR* 1986;147:545–551.
105. Toombs BD, Lester RG, Ben-Menachem Y, Sandler CM. Computed tomography in blunt trauma. *Radiol Clin North Am* 1981;19:17–35.
106. Totty WG, Vannier MW. Complex musculoskeletal anatomy: Analysis using three dimensional surface reconstruction. *Radiology* 1984;150:173–177.
107. Welch TJ, Sheedy PF II, Johnson CD, et al. CT guided biopsy: Prospective analysis of 1,000 procedures. *Radiology* 1989;171:493–496.

Magnetic Resonance Imaging

108. Alfidi RJ, Haaga JR, El Yousef SJ, et al. Preliminary experimental results in humans and animals with superconducting, whole-

body nuclear magnetic resonance scanner. *Radiology* 1982; 143:175–181.

109. Beltran J, Nato AM, Mosure JC, Shaman OM, Weiss KL, Suegler WA. Surface coil imaging at 1.5T. *Radiology* 1986;161:203–209.

110. Berquist TH. Magnetic resonance imaging: Preliminary experience in orthopedic radiology. *Mag Res Imag* 1984;2:41–52.

111. Berquist TH. Magnetic resonance of the musculoskeletal system. New York: Raven Press, 1990.

112. Block F. Nuclear induction. *Physical Review* 1948;70 (7 and 8).

113. Bydder GM, Steiner RE, Young IR. Clinical NMR images of the brain: 140 cases. *AJR* 1982;139:215–236.

114. Crooks LE, Arakawa M, Hoenninger J, et al. Nuclear magnetic resonance whole-body images operating at 3.5 Kgauss. *Radiology* 1982;143:169–174.

115. Crooke LE, Ortendahl DA, Kaufman L, et al. Clinical efficacy of nuclear magnetic resonance imaging. *Radiology* 1983;146:123–128.

116. Damadian R. Tumor detection by nuclear magnetic resonance. *Science* 1971;171:1151–1153.

117. Davis PL, Crooks L, Arakawa M, McKee R, Kaufman L, Margulis A. Potential hazards of magnetic resonance imaging. *AJR* 1981;137:857–860.

118. Fisher MR, Barker B, Amparo E, et al. MR imaging using specialized coils. *Radiology* 1985;157:443–447.

119. Fletcher BD, Scoles PV, Nelson DA. Osteomyelitis in children: Detection by magnetic resonance imaging. *Radiology* 1984; 150:57–60.

120. King CL, Henkelman RM, Poon PY, Rubenstein J. MR imaging of the normal knee. *J Comput Assist Tomogr* 1984;8:1147–1154.

121. Lackman RW, Kaufman B, Hans JS, et al. MR imaging in patients with metallic implants. *Radiology* 1985;157:711–714.

122. Lauterbur P. Magnetic resonance zeugmatography. *Pure and Applied Chem* 1975;40(2):40.

123. Moon KL, Genant HK, Helms CA, Chafetz NI, Crooks LE, Kaufman L. Musculoskeletal applications of magnetic resonance imaging. *Radiology* 1983;147:161–171.

124. New PFJ, Rosen BR, Brady TJ, et al. Potential hazards and artifacts of ferromagnetic and nonferromagnetic surgical and dental materials and devices in magnetic resonance imaging. *Radiology* 1983;147:139–148.

125. Pavlicek W, Geisinger M, Castle L, et al. The effects of magnetic resonance imaging on patients with cardiac pacemakers. *Radiology* 1983;147:149–153.

126. Purcell EM, Torrey HC, Pound RV. Resonance absorption by nuclear magnetic moments in a solid. *Phys Rev* 1946;69:37–38.

127. Pykett I, Newhouse JH, Buonanno FS, et al. Principles of nuclear magnetic resonance imaging. *Radiology* 1982;143:157–168.

128. Ranade SS, Shah S, Advani SH, Kasturi SR. Pulsed nuclear magnetic resonance studies of human bone marrow. *Physiol Chem Phys* 1977;9:297–299.

129. Saunders RD. Biological effects of NMR clinical imaging. *Applied Radiol* 1982;11:43–46: Sept/Oct.

130. Schwartz JL, Crooks LE. NMR imaging produces no observable mutation or cytotoxicity on mammalian cells. *AJR* 1982; 139:583–585.

Angiography

131. Conn J, Bergan JJ, Bell JL. Hypothenar hammar syndrome: Post-traumatic digital ischemia. *Surgery* 1970;68:1122–1128.

132. Crossland SG, Slovin AJ. The role of arteriography in diagnosing unsuspected vascular injuries. *Am Surg* 1978;44:98–103.

133. Fisher RG, Hadlock F, Ben-Menachem Y. Laceration of the thoracic aorta and brachiocephalic arteries by blunt trauma. *Radiol Clin North Am* 1981;19:91–110.

134. Foley WD, Milde MW. Intra-arterial digital subtraction angiography. *Radiol Clin North Am* 1985;23:293–319.

135. Hessel SJ. Complications of angiography and other catheter procedures. In Abrams HL, *Angiography.* Boston: Little, Brown and Co., 1983.

136. Kam J, Jackson H, Ben-Menachem Y. Vascular injuries in blunt pelvic trauma. *Radiol Clin North Am* 1981;19:171–186.

137. Long EK. Pelvic angiography. In: Abrams, HL, *Angiography.* Boston: Little, Brown and Co., 1983.

138. Lang EK. Transcatheter embolization of pelvic vessels for control of intractable hemorrhage. *Radiology* 1981;140:331–339.

139. Lang EK. The role of arteriography in trauma. *Radiol Clin North Am* 1976;14:353–370.

140. Love L. Arterial trauma. *Semin Roentgenol* 1970;5:267–283.

141. Margolies MN, Ring EJ, Waltman AC, Kerr WS, Baum S. Arteriography in the management of hemorrhage from pelvic fractures. *N Engl J Med* 1972;287:317–321.

142. Mazer M, Smith CW, Martin VN. Distal splenic artery embolization with flow directed balloon catheter. *Radiology* 1985; 154:245.

143. McDonald EJ, Goodman PC, Winestock DP. The clinical indications for arteriography in trauma to the extremity. *Radiology* 1975;116:45–47.

144. Mucha P, Welch TJ. Hemorrhage in major pelvic fractures. *Surg Clin North Am* 1988;68:757–773.

145. Reid JDS, Redman HC, Wergelt JA, Thal ER, Frances H III. Value of angiography in detection of arterial injury. *AJR* 1988;151:1035–1039.

146. Ring EJ, Athanasoulis C, Waltman AC, Margolies MN, Baum S. Arteriographic management of hemorrhage following pelvic fractures. *Radiology* 1973;109:65–70.

147. Ring EJ, Waltman AC, Athanasoulis C, Smith JC, Baum S. Angiography in pelvic trauma. *Surg Gynecol Obstet* 1974;139:375–380.

148. Rubin BE, Fortune WP, May MM. Therapeutic embolization of post-operative hemorrhage about the hip of a patient with pseudomonas infection. *J Bone Joint Surg* 1978;60A:988–991.

149. Slaney G, Ashton F. Arterial injuries and their management. *Postgrad Med* 1971;47:257–269.

150. Taki W, Handa H, Moyake H, et al. New detachable balloon technique for traumatic carotid-cavernous sinus fistula. *AJNR* 1985;6:961–964.

151. Uflacker R. Transcatheter embolization of arterial aneurysms. *Br J Radiol* 1986;59:317–324.

152. van Urk H, Perlberger RR, Muller H. Selective arterial embolization for control of traumatic pelvic hemorrhage. *Surgery* 1978;83:133–137.

Myelography

153. Ahn HS, Rosenbaum AE. Lumbar myelography with metrizamide supplemental techniques. *Am J Neuroradiol* 1981;136:547–551.

154. DiChiro G, Fisher RL. Contrast radiography of the spinal cord. *Arch Neurol* 1964;11:125–143.

155. Fox AJ, Venulia F, Debrun G. Complete myelography with metrizamide. *Am J Neuroradiol* 1981;2:79–84.

156. Genant HK, Chefetz N, Helms CA. *Computed tomography of the lumbar spine. Diagnosis and therapeutic implications for the radiologist, orthopedist, and neurosurgeon.* San Francisco: University of California Press, 1982.

157. Kieffer SA, Binet EF, Esquerra JV, Hantman RP, Gross CE. Contrast agents for myelography: Clinical and radiographic evaluation of Ampipaque and Pantopaque. *Radiology* 1978;129:695–705.

158. Leo JS, Bergeron RT, Kricheff II, Benjamin MV. Metrizamide myelography for cervical spinal cord injury. *Radiology* 1978;129:707–711.

159. McClennan BL. Low osmolality contrast media: Premises and promises. *Radiology* 1987;162:1–8.

160. Paling MR, Quindlin EA, DiChiro G. Spinal seizures after metrizamide myelography in a patient with spinal block. *Am J Neuroradiol* 1980;1:473.

161. Pay NT, George AE, Benjamin MV, Bergeron T, Lin JP, Kricheff II. Positive and negative contrast myelography in spinal trauma. *Radiology* 1977;123:103–111.

162. Skalpe IO. Adhesive arachnoiditis following lumbar radiculography with water soluble contrast agents. A clinical report with special reference to metrizamide. *Radiology* 1976;121:647–651.

Introduction to Arthrography and Tenography

163. Bjork L, Erikson U, Ingelman B. A new type of contrast medium in arthrography. *AJR* 1970;109:606–610.
164. Evans GA, Frenyo SD. The stress tenogram in diagnosis of ruptures of the lateral ligament of the ankle. *J Bone Joint Surg* 1979;61B:347–351.
165. Freiberger RH, Kaye J. *Arthrography.* New York: Appleton-Century-Crofts, 1979.
166. Gilula LA, Oloff L, Caputi R, Destouet JM, Jacobs A, Solomon MA. Ankle tenography: A key to unexplained symptomatology. *Radiology* 1984;151:581–587.
167. Hall FM. Morbidity from shoulder arthrography. *AJR* 1981; 136:59.
168. Hall FM, Goldberg RP, Wyshak G, Kilcogne RF. Shoulder arthrography: Comparison of morbidity after use of various contrast media. *Radiology* 1985;154:339–341.
169. Hasselbacher P, Schumacher HR. Synovial fluid eosinophilia following arthrography. *J Rheumatol* 1978;5:173–176.
170. Johansen JC. Arthrography with Amipaque and other contrast media. *Invest Radiol* 1976;11:534–540.
171. Katzberg RW. Evaluation of various contrast agents for improved arthrography. *Invest Radiol* 1976;11:528–533.
172. Lasser EC. Pretreatment with corticosteroids to prevent reactions to IV contrast material: Overview and implications. *AJR* 1988;150:257–259.
173. Mink JH. Air vs CO_2 for knee arthrography. *AJR* 1980;134:991–993.
174. Murray RC, Forral E. Transitory eosinophilia localized to the knee joint. *J Bone Joint Surg* 1950;32B:74–83.
175. Newberg AH, Munn CS, Robbins AH. Complications of arthrography. *Radiology* 1985;155:605–606.
176. Pastershank SP, Resnick D, Niwayama G, Danzig L, Haghighi P. The effect of water soluble contrast media on the synovial membrane. *Radiology* 1982;143:331–334.

Imaging of Orthopedic Trauma,
Second Edition, edited by T.H. Berquist,
Mayo Clinic © 1992. Published
by Raven Press, Ltd., New York.

CHAPTER 2

Fracture Healing

James A. Rand and Thomas H. Berquist

Types of Fractures, 39
Radiographic Description of Fractures and Fracture-
  Dislocation, 43
Phases of Fracture Healing, 46
Vascular Supply to Bone, 47
Blood Flow in Bone, 48
Physiology of Fracture Healing, 49
  The Vascular Response to Fracture, 49
  Cellular Response to Fracture, 51
Biomechanics of Fracture Healing, 52
  Biomechanics of Normal Bone, 52
  Fracture Healing, 53
  Biologic Signs for Fracture Healing, 55
  Electrical Signals, 55
  Bone-Inductive Signal, 56
Fracture Fixation, 57
  Compression-Plate Fixation of Fractures, 57
  Mechanism of Action of Compression-Fixation, 58
  Morphologic Findings of Primary Bone Healing with
    Compression-Plate Fixation, 59
  Effect of a Plate on Bone-Blood Flow, 59

Biomechanics of Plate Fixation, 59
Adverse Effects of a Compression Plate, 60
Intramedullary Nail Fixation of Fractures, 62
Effect of an Intramedullary Nail on Bone-Blood
  Flow, 62
Morphologic Findings in Union through
  Intramedullary Nail Fixation, 63
Biomechanics of Intramedullary Nail Fixation, 64
Complications of Intramedullary Nailing, 64
Comparisons of Intramedullary Nail and Plate
  Fixation of Fractures, 65
External Fixation, 67
Imaging of Orthopedic Fixation Devices, 69
Fracture Union and Non-union, 71
  Definition of Union and Non-union, 71
  Etiologic Factors in the Pathogenesis of Non-union,
    71
  Diagnosis and Classification of Non-union, 73
  Treatment Modalities, 74
References, 77

Trauma is a frequent occurrence in our highly mechanized society. Injuries to the axial skeleton and limbs are common problems for the orthopedic surgeon and radiologist. Fracture recognition, assessment of the etiologic mechanism, and determination of the extent of healing are essential in patient management. Accurate description of the fractures and changes noted on the postreduction radiographs is an essential part of communication between the radiologist and the orthopedic surgeon. Recognition of the failure or orderly progress of fracture union will aid in deciding upon an appropriate course of management. This requires a thorough understanding of clinical findings and method used for reduction (i.e., internal fixation, type of appliance, etc.) so that the proper imaging techniques can be chosen.

Types of Fractures

There are many common labels that describe the various types of fractures and fracture-dislocations. Terms such as *clay shoveler's fracture, Monteggia fracture,* and *greenstick fracture* may be well understood (10,48,145,162,200). However, these labels are often misused, and a proper description of the bony and ligamentous injury is preferred. The detection of fractures may be somewhat difficult, although in most situations the abnormality is readily identified. All too often, however, the interpreter of the film gives a less than complete description of the injury.

J. A. Rand: Department of Orthopedic Surgery, Mayo Medical School, Mayo Clinic, Rochester, Minnesota 55905.

T. H. Berquist: Department of Diagnostic Radiology, Mayo Medical School, Mayo Clinic Jacksonville, Jacksonville, Florida 32224.

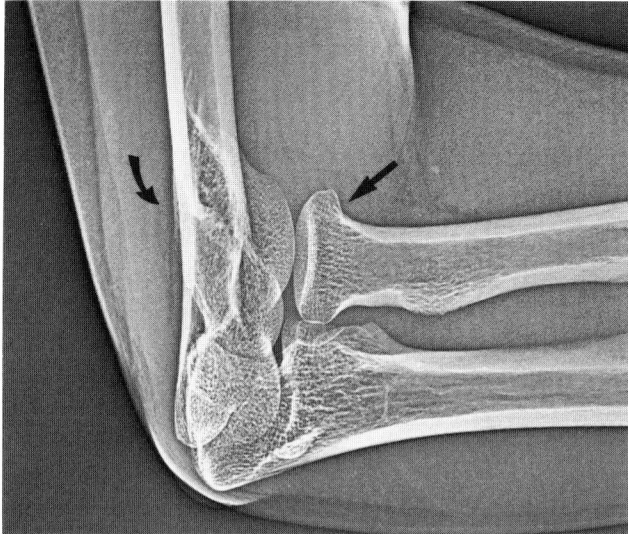

FIG. 2-1. Radial head view of the elbow demonstrating displaced anterior (*straight arrow*) and posterior fat pads (*curved arrow*). Note the subtle radial head fracture.

Evaluation of skeletal trauma should begin with a thorough evaluation of the soft tissues, tissue planes, and fat pads. The skin and soft tissues are intact in closed fractures. Disruption of the soft tissues results in an open or compound fracture (202). Displacement of the fat pads of the elbow (Fig. 2-1), the pronator fat stripe of the distal radius (Fig. 2-2), and the navicular fat stripe may be the only clues to the presence of subtle fractures. Another helpful finding is the presence of a lipohemarthrosis (fat blood level) in the joint, which indicates an intracapsular fracture (Fig. 2-3).

Fractures may be complete (both cortices interrupted) or incomplete (one cortex fractured). Incomplete fractures generally occur in children. The following is a list of the commonly encountered incomplete fractures:

1. Torus fracture. An incomplete fracture resulting in buckling of the cortex (Fig. 2-4 and 2-5).
2. Greenstick fracture. Interruption of one cortex with angulation resembling a broken branch (Fig. 2-6).

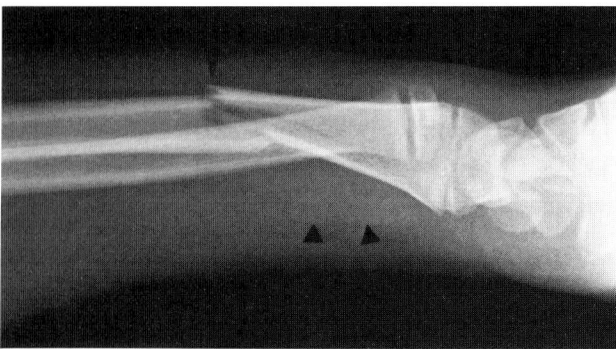

FIG. 2-2. Fracture of the distal radial shaft (*arrow*). The pronator fat stripe is displaced (*double arrows*). In certain cases the displaced fat stripe may be the only indication of injury.

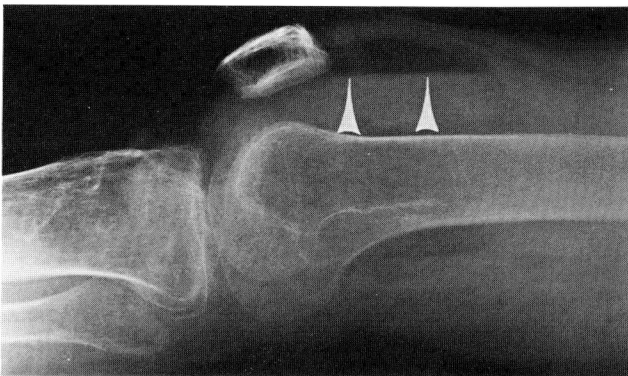

FIG. 2-3. Cross table lateral view of the knee in a patient with a subtle intra-articular fracture. Note the obvious (*arrowheads*) lipohemarthrosis.

3. Microfracture or bowing fracture. A bending fracture that commonly involves the radius and ulna (Fig. 2-7). Often there is no obvious fracture line (28,29).
4. Growth plate or physeal fracture. A subtle fracture of the growth plate and associated metaphysis or epiphysis that can be easily overlooked. This group of fractures has been classified by Salter and Harris (Fig. 2-8) (198). In Type I, the fracture involves the growth plate but spares the epiphysis and metaphysis. In Type II, the fracture involves the growth plate and exits through the metaphysis (Fig. 2-9). In Type III, the fracture involves the growth plate and exits through the epiphysis. In Type IV, the fracture line extends through the epiphysis, growth plate, and metaphysis (Fig. 2-10). Finally, in Type V, the growth plate is impacted or crushed.

Recently, a new, subtle injury has been described. The radiograph is normal in these patients. However, magnetic resonance images (MRI) demonstrate medullary signal intensity changes. This symptomatic fracture has been called *bone bruise* (Fig. 2-11). It probably represents trabecular compression due to local axial loading.

Complete fractures involve both cortices with a lucent

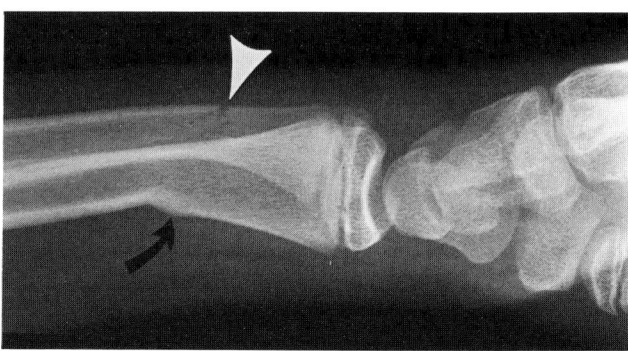

FIG. 2-4. Lateral view of the wrist. There is a torus fracture of the distal radius (*curved black arrow*) and a greenstick fracture of the dorsal ulna (*large white arrowhead*). Note the displaced pronator fat stripe.

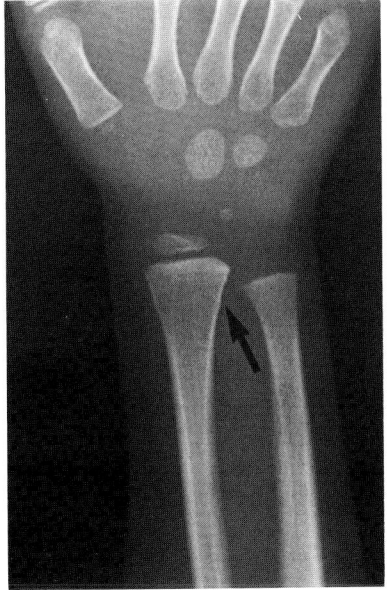 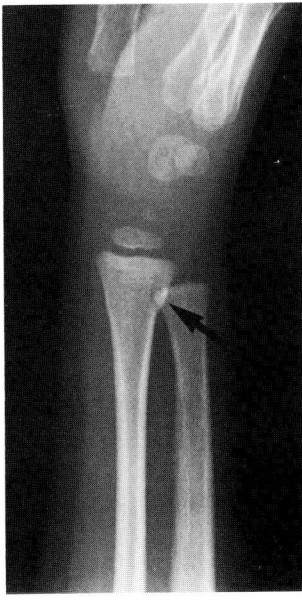

A   B

FIG. 2–5. PA (**A**) and lateral (**B**) views of the wrist demonstrating a subtle torus fracture (*arrow*) in the distal radius.

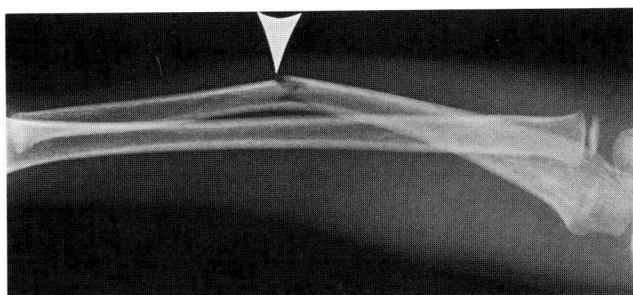

FIG. 2–6. Forearm. There is a greenstick fracture (*white arrowhead*) of the ulnar midshaft.

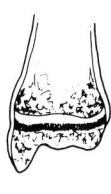 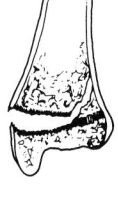 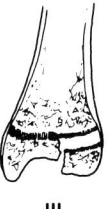

I   II   III

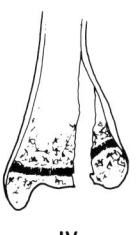 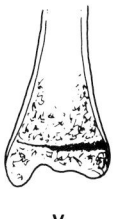

IV   V

FIG. 2–8. Illustration of the Salter-Harris type of growth-plate fracture.

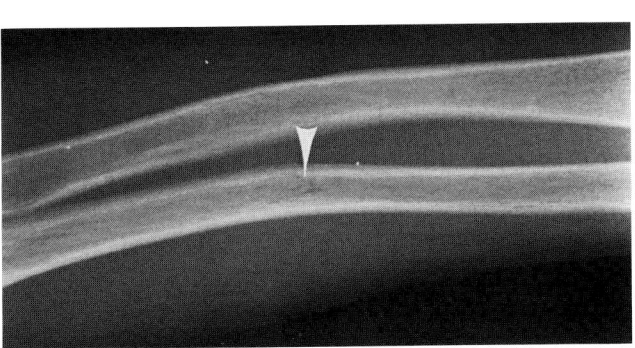

FIG. 2–7. Forearm. Bowing fractures of the radius and ulna are present. A small lucent fracture line (*white arrowhead*) is evident in the mid ulna.

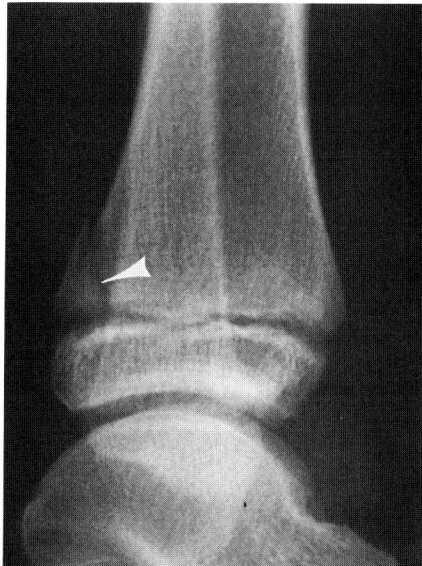

FIG. 2–9. Lateral view of the ankle demonstrating atypical Salter-Harris II fracture involving the metaphysis (*arrowhead*) of the distal tibia.

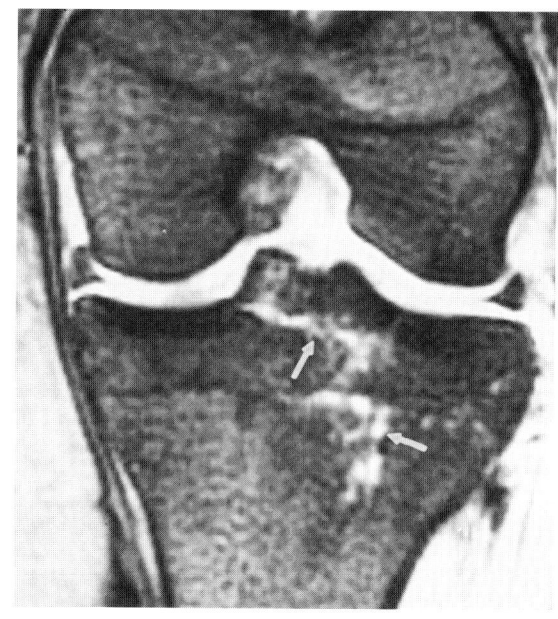

FIG. 2–11. Gradient echo (MPGR) coronal image of the knee in a patient with normal radiographs and suspected meniscal injury. There is a stelate mid tibial marrow fracture (*arrows*).

line through the medullary portion of the bone. These fractures may be transverse, oblique, spiral, or comminuted. Depression fractures, such as those seen with cancellous bone in the region of the tibial plateau, also occur (Fig. 2-12). Compression fractures occur in the vertebral body and may involve the anterior or lateral cortex (Fig. 2-13). Avulsion fractures occur at the insertion of ligaments or tendons (Fig. 2-14). The fracture results from an abrupt tensile force from the muscle tendon unit. Avulsion fractures will be discussed more thoroughly in

anatomic chapters (215). Pathologic fractures involve bone with some underlying abnormality such as metabolic disease or neoplasm (Fig. 2-15). Stress fractures are incomplete fractures due to chronic overuse of normal bone and are most often seen in the metatarsals of military recruits and in the femoral necks, pubic rami, and tibias of long-distance runners (Fig. 2-16) (66,150,202). (See Chapter 16, Stress Fractures.) The insufficiency fracture is a special example of the stress fracture (172). Abnormal bone gives way under stresses that would not

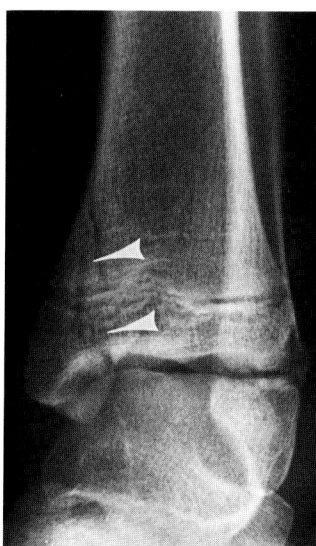

FIG. 2–10. Oblique of the ankle demonstrating a Salter-Harris IV fracture involving the epiphysis and metaphysis (*arrowheads*).

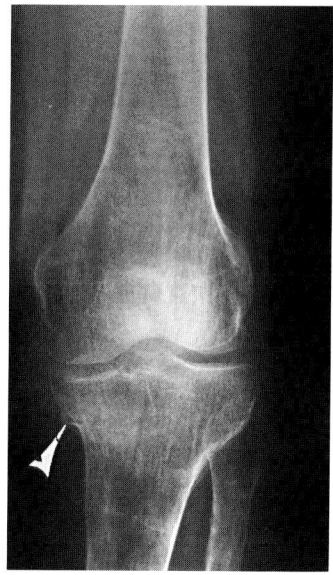

FIG. 2–12. AP view of the knee. There is a depressed cortical fracture of the upper tibia medially (*arrowhead*).

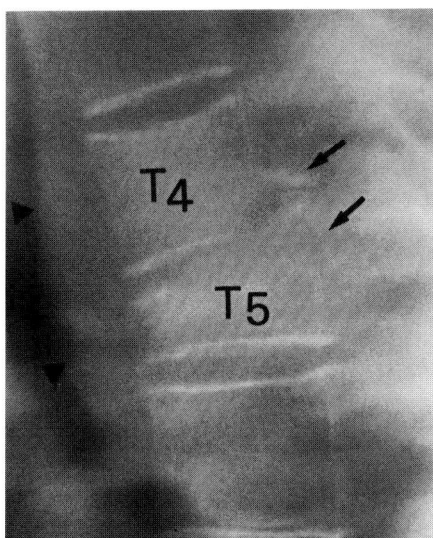

FIG. 2–13. Lateral tomogram of the upper thoracic spine demonstrating a T5 compression fracture. Note the posterior fragments (*arrows*) and anterior soft tissue swelling (*arrowheads*).

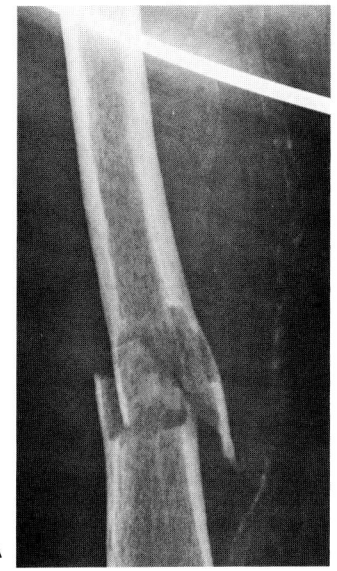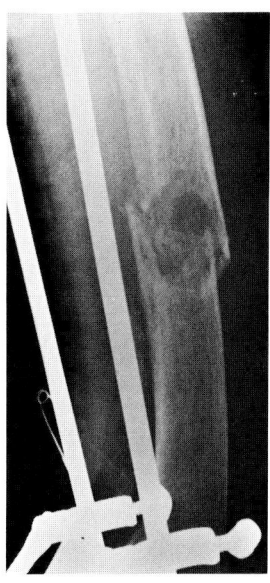

FIG. 2–15. AP (**A**) and lateral (**B**) views of the mid femur taken in traction. There is a large lytic lesion with a complete pathologic fracture through the metastatic neoplasm.

be excessive under normal circumstances. An example is a stress fracture affecting the tibia or femoral neck in a patient with rheumatoid arthritis who becomes too active too soon after total joint arthroplasty.

Radiographic Description of Fractures and Fracture-Dislocations

Table 2-1 offers an outline approach to the description of fractures or fracture-dislocations (180). A general de-

scription of the fracture should be provided first. This should include the date, time of day, and projections obtained. Is the fracture transverse or oblique? Is there significant soft tissue involvement? The locations should be specified (epiphysis, metaphysis, or shaft). Fractures of the shaft can be conveniently divided into mid, proximal or distal thirds (Fig. 2-17A). The anatomic description of the position of the fracture fragments should be given. This includes the apposition of the fragments and whether there has been any change in the anatomic length of the part (Fig. 2-18). Fractures may be impacted, which imparts some degree of stability (Fig. 2-19). Distraction or separation of the fracture fragments may be the result of traction devices or soft tis-

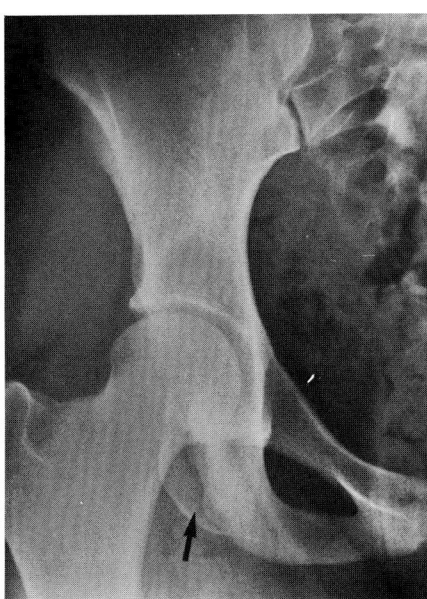

FIG. 2–14. Avulsion fracture of the ischium (*arrow*) at the origin of the hamstring muscles.

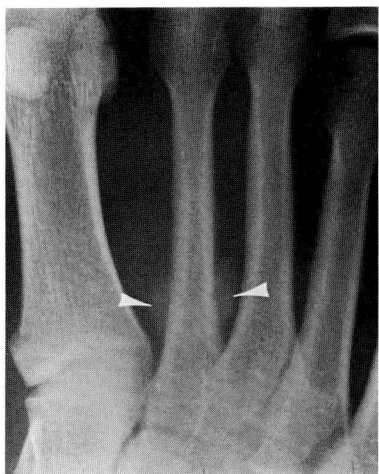

FIG. 2–16. Healing stress fracture of the proximal second metatarsal with callus formation (*arrows*).

TABLE 2-1. *Skeletal injury: Radiographic description of fractures and fracture dislocations*

I. Fractures
A. General description
1. Date and time
2. Projections obtained
3. Type of fracture
4. Soft tissue evaluation
B. Location
C. Anatomic position of fragments
1. Length and apposition
2. Angulation
3. Displacement
4. Rotation
D. Further imaging techniques
II. Subluxation/dislocation
A. Degree of displacement
B. Joint space
C. Associated fractures
1. Location
2. Articular involvement

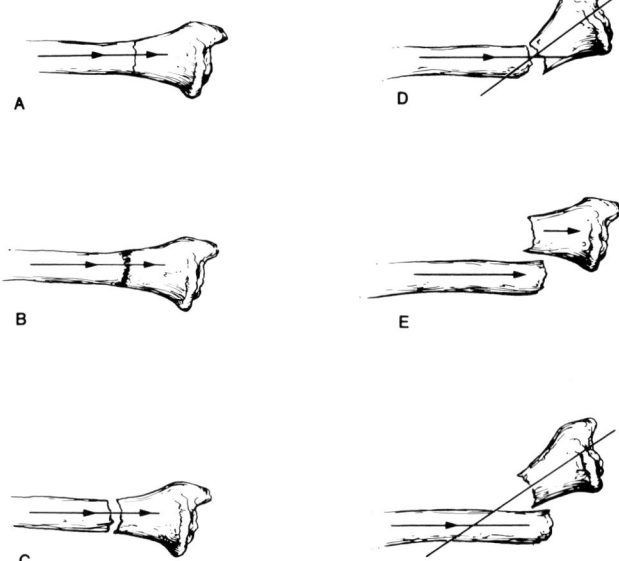

FIG. 2-18. Illustration of fractures. **A:** An undisplaced complete fracture with normal alignment and no displacement. **B:** An impacted fracture with slight shortening (*dark zone*) and normal alignment. There is no angulation. **C:** A distracted fracture with normal alignment and no angulation. **D:** Distal shaft fracture with angulation. **E:** Transverse fracture with no apposition of the fracture fragments. No angulation or rotation. Shortening or overriding is present. **F:** Distal shaft fracture with shortening, angulation, and displacement.

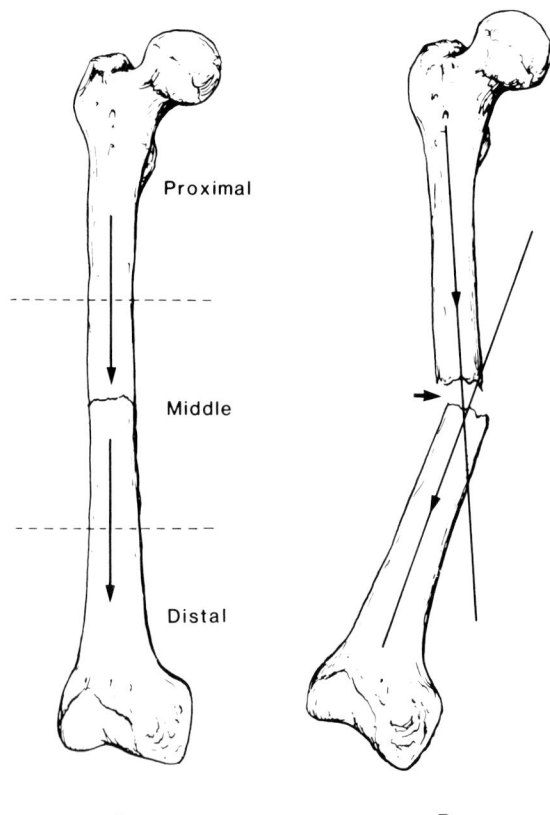

FIG. 2-17. A: The femoral shaft and other long bones can be divided into thirds for purposes of fracture description. When discussing alignment the longitudinal axis is described (*arrow*). **B:** A transverse fracture of the femoral midshaft is demonstrated. Angulation may be described by the direction of the apex, in which case there is medial angulation (*arrow*) and distraction of the fracture fragments. Angulation may also be described by the position of the distal fragment. In this illustration the distal fragment is laterally angulated.

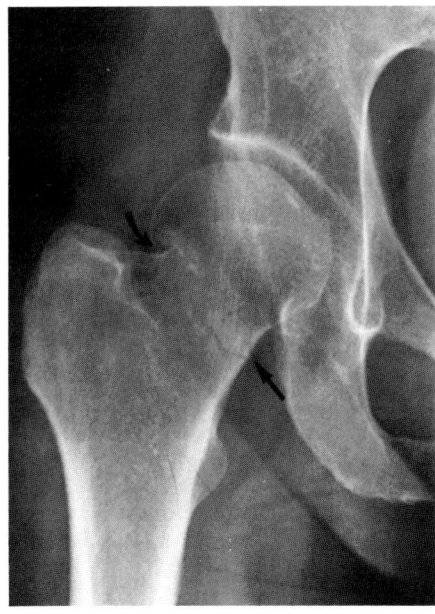

FIG. 2-19. AP view of the right hip. The subcapital fracture (*arrow*) is complete with impaction of the lateral cortex (*curved arrow*).

sue interposition. These factors should be carefully reported (84).

Any angulation of the fracture fragments should also be discussed in the radiographic report (Figs. 2-17B, 2-18, and 2-20). There are two commonly used methods for describing fracture angulation (180). We prefer to describe angulation according to the direction of the apex of the fracture fragments (Fig. 2-20). One may also report angulation according to the direction of the distal fragment. For example, fragments can be said to be angulated medially (varus) (Fig. 2-20), or alternatively, the distal fragment can be said to be angulated laterally (valgus). Displacement describes any change in the anatomic axis of the components of the fracture. Overriding or displacement of comminuted fragments should be noted. Rotation of the fragments, particularly common with spiral fractures of the metacarpals and tibia, may pose significant treatment problems. The fracture of the femur in Fig. 2-20 is rotated. Note that the proximal fragment is visualized in the anteroposterior (AP) projection, and the distal fragment is seen laterally. The thickness of the cortex at the fracture site is also an important indicator of rotation (84).

Descriptions of subluxations and dislocations should include the degree of displacement of the articular surfaces. If the subluxation involves the spine (Fig. 2-21), the upper vertebral body should be described in relation to the body below. In the peripheral skeleton the distal

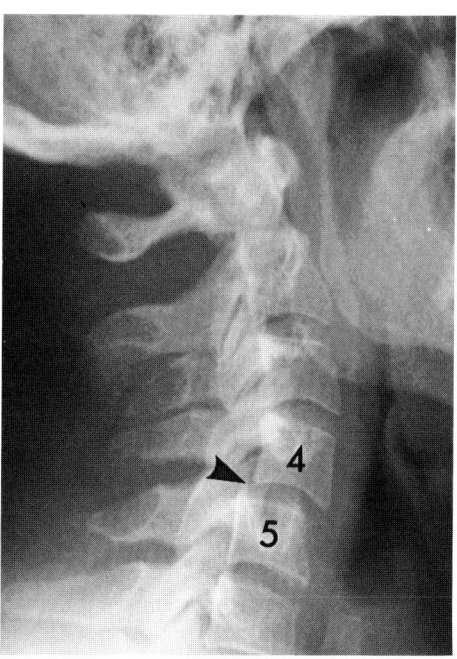

FIG. 2–21. Lateral view of the cervical spine demonstrating anterior subluxation of C4 on C5.

fragment is described in relation to the proximal fragment. Figure 2-22 demonstrates dorsal dislocation of the middle phalanx in relation to the proximal phalanx. Evaluation of the joint space should also be discussed, as ligament interposition or osteochondral fragments may result in joint-space widening. This is especially important following reduction. The location and the degree of articular involvement of any associated fractures should also be described.

Careful reporting of post-reduction views is also important (Table 2-2). Any interval changes in position of the fracture fragments should be noted. Has there been a change in bony apposition or angulation? Fractures treated with traction may demonstrate these changes as well as increased distraction (as a result of soft tissue interposition or excessive traction). Evidence of callus formation should be mentioned, although the diagnosis

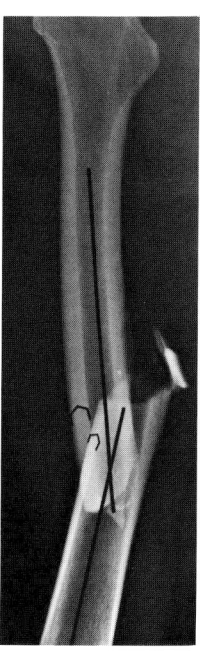

FIG. 2–20. AP view of the right femur. There is a comminuted overriding fracture of the femur at the junction of the mid and distal thirds. The fracture is angulated medially with considerable rotation of the distal fragment. (Note upper shaft in AP and lower shaft in lateral position.) Cortical thickness (*brackets*) at the fracture site is not uniform, which is another indication of rotation.

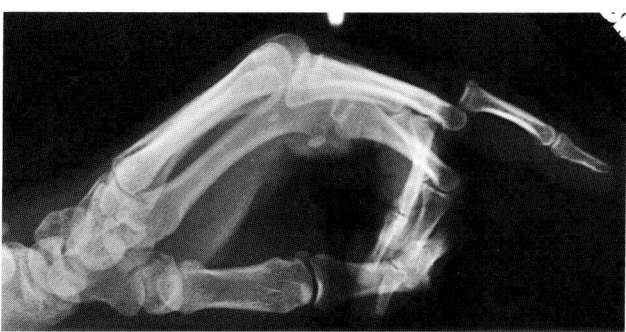

FIG. 2–22. Lateral view of the middle finger. There is dorsal dislocation of the middle phalanx on the proximal phalanx. The articular surfaces are completely disrupted.

TABLE 2-2. *Skeletal injury: A structured approach to interpretation of post-reduction radiographs*

I. Interval change
  A. Change in apposition
  B. Change in angulation
  C. Distraction or impaction
II. Healing process
  A. Callus formation
  B. Evidence of delayed, or non-union
III. Assessment of fixation devices (position of rods, screws, pins, etc.)
IV. Additional imaging techniques

of fracture healing is made clinically. If an internal or external fixation device is in place, the position of the device should be compared with that of previous films. Evidence of loosening, metal fracture, or improper positioning should be noted (Figs. 2-23 and 2-24). Irregularity and sclerosis of the opposing fracture fragments may indicate delayed union or non-union. Serial films are most helpful in this determination. As with prereduction radiographs, additional images may be helpful in evaluating the healing process. Tomography, computerized tomography (CT), isotope, or MRI studies may be indicated if evidence of delayed union or non-union, or infection, is present. Comments regarding direct care of the patient, such as acceptability of the position of the fragments, should be avoided (180). Radiographs do not present the entire clinical picture. In detection and follow-up, patient care is enhanced when close communica-

tion occurs between clinicians (orthopedic surgeons) and radiologists (21,22,46).

Phases of Fracture Healing

Fracture healing may be divided into three phases: (1) inflammatory, (2) reparative, and (3) remodeling (Fig. 2-24) (54).

The inflammatory phase comprises 10%, the reparative phase 40%, and the remodeling phase 70% of the time to fracture union (54). These phases are not distinct, there being a significant overlap between them. The inflammatory phase consists of hematoma formation, osteocyte death, vasodilatation, and migration of acute inflammatory cells into the wound (54). There is a prominent hematoma present as well as necrotic fracture ends. The reparative phase consists of vascular dilatation, which involves the entire vascular bed of the affected limb, new vessel proliferation, mesenchymal cell proliferation, change from an acid to alkaline pH, and collagen production in the wound (54). There is prominent granulation tissue present as well as early cartilage and bone formation. The remodeling phase consists of osteoblastic resorption and new bone formation (54). During this late phase in fracture healing, there is prominent endosteal and periosteal callus formation. Revascularization of the bone occurs.

Fracture repair may be conceptually divided into those events associated with the soft tissue proliferation and those related to mineralization of the callus. The

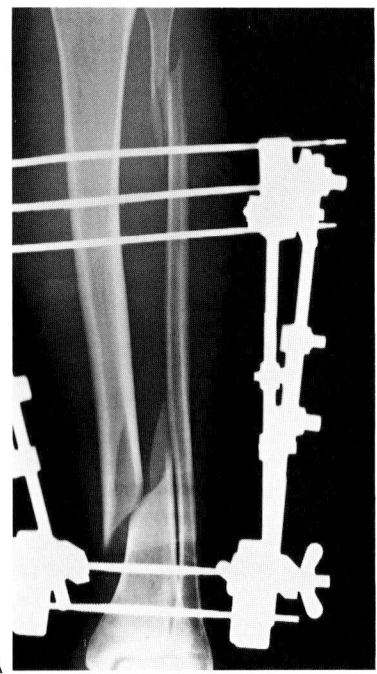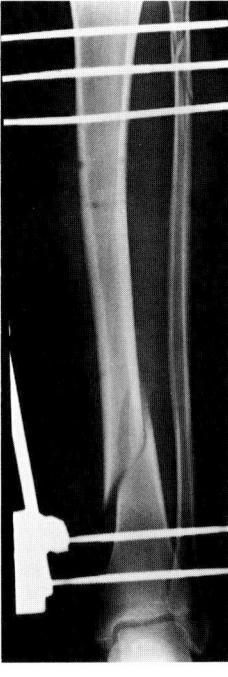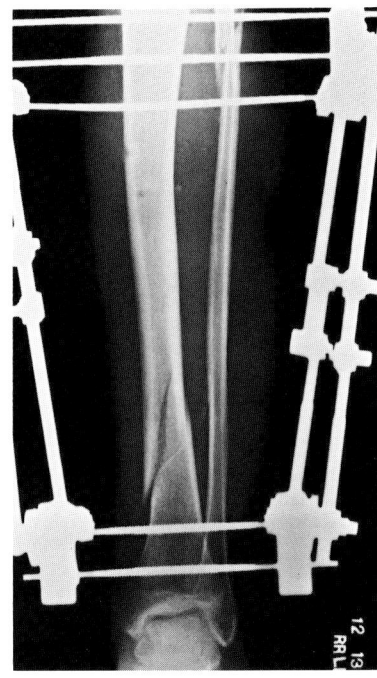

FIG. 2-23. Spiral fractures of the distal tibia and upper fibula with Hoffman external fixation. Sequential radiographs demonstrate change in position of the fragments (**A-C**). With proper adjustment of the fixateur, the position and alignment are clearly improved in **C**.

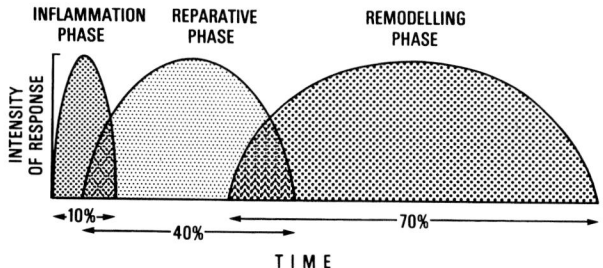

FIG. 2–24. Phases of fracture healing (54).

initial fibroblastic proliferation is associated with an increase in proteoglycans. As chondroblasts and osteoblasts proliferate, collagen production increases and is associated with a decrease in proteoglycans. Mineralization of the matrix occurs later. Finally, bone remodeling results in a return to normal.

The healing process clinically and radiographically can differ significantly. The fracture margins are generally well defined acutely. Over a period of 10–20 days the fracture line becomes wider and more irregular due to hyperemia and resorption of necrotic bone at the fracture margin. The fracture is healed radiographically when the callus is solid and trabecular bone bridges the fracture site. The patient is generally allowed to bear weight and/or the fracture is clinically healed well before these radiographic changes occur (9,84). MRI allows soft tissue changes and the healing process to be more effectively observed and may play a significant role in fracture assessment in the future.

Vascular Supply to Bone

A knowledge of the normal blood supply of a long bone is the key to understanding fracture repair. The normal afferent blood supply to a mature, mammalian tubular bone consists of three parts: (1) the nutrient artery, (2) the metaphyseal arteries, and (3) the periosteal arteries (Fig. 2-25) (39,115,156,187,201). Upon entering the medullary cavity, the nutrient artery divides into two major branches that ascend and descend within the shaft. Arterial sub-branches form two parallel arterial supplies, one to the cortex and another to the marrow (136,211). The cortical branches give rise to branches oriented parallel to the shaft as well as to radially directed vessels (140,221). Conduit vessels connect the arteriolar system with the periosteal vessels (Fig. 2-26) (140). The smaller arterioles supply capillaries to the haversian canals (115,140). The haversian canals are connected to osteocytes via canaliculi (94). Some authors have suggested that the inner two-thirds to three-quarters of the cortex is supplied by the nutrient system (39,110, 187,192,224), while the outer one-third is supplied by the periosteal vessels (186,224). More recent authors state that the endosteal system supplies the majority of blood to the cortex (140,221). The metaphyseal arteries supply blood to the metaphysis and anastomose with the medullary arteries (187,224).

The efferent or venous drainage of a long bone consists of three parts: (1) the emissary veins and the vena comitans of the nutrient artery, (2) the cortical venous channels, and (3) the periosteal capillaries (187). The emissary veins and vena comitans of the nutrient artery are derived from the central venous sinus in the medullary canal and are involved primarily in drainage of the marrow (140,187). The majority of the cortical bone venous drainage takes place through the periosteal capillaries (140). In contrast, Trias and colleagues feel that the majority of the cortical venous drainage is centripetal into the sinusoidal system in the marrow (221).

The normal circulatory pattern of diaphyseal cortex is

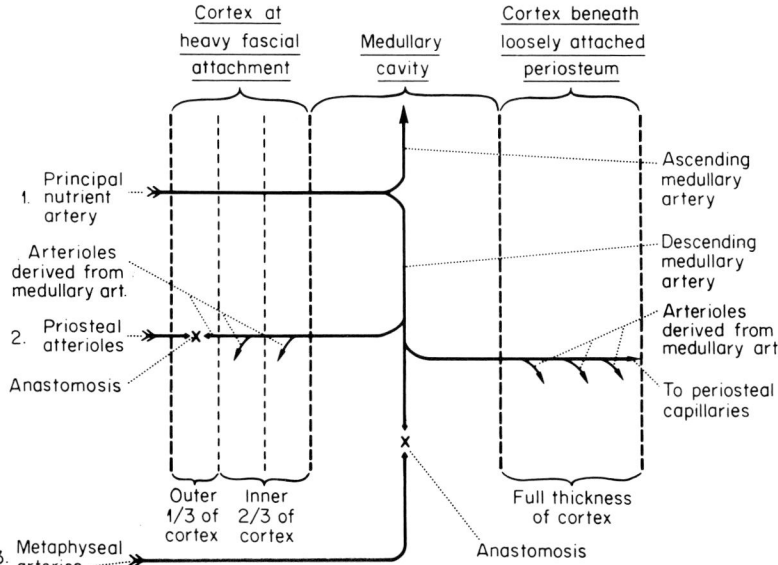

FIG. 2-25. Afferent blood supply of bone and sites of anastomosis. The afferent vascular system brings blood to every portion of a long bone and includes three primary components that together form the total nutrient supply. The components include: 1) the principle nutrient artery, 2) the metaphyseal arteries, and 3) the periosteal arterioles (187).

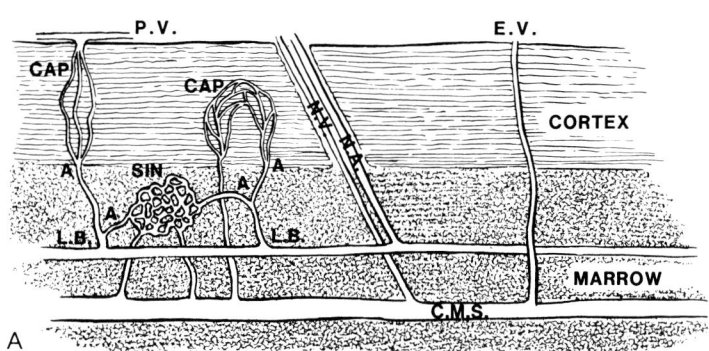
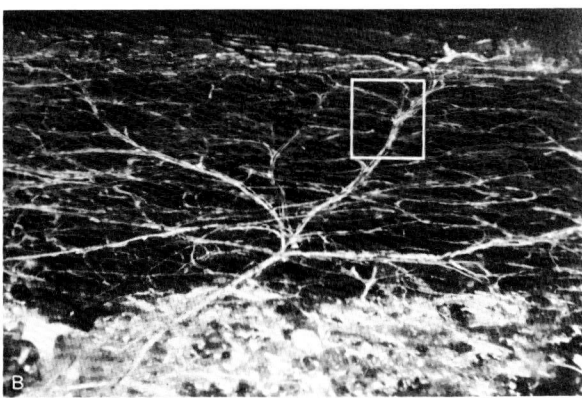

FIG. 2–26. A: Circulation of the tibial diaphysis. NA, nutrient artery; NV, nutrient vein; CMS, central medullary sinus; LB, lateral branches of nutrient artery; CAP, haversian capillaries; PV, periosteal vein; EV, emissary vein. **B:** Branches of nutrient artery in diaphyseal cortex (140).

one of centrifugal flow from the endosteum to the periosteum (Fig. 2-27) (39,187,188). This pattern of flow may be reversed in pathologic conditions, such as after fracture (39).

Key sites of anastomosis between the three components of the afferent vascular system exist (156,187,224). An anastomosis exists between the nutrient medullary vessels and the metaphyseal vessels at the end of the medullary cavity. An anastomosis also exists between the nutrient-medullary system and the periosteal vessels in the outer cortex. These anastomoses are of key importance when one of these vascular systems is disrupted, as in the period following fracture.

The relative importance of the three afferent components for maintenance of viability of the diaphyseal cortex has been investigated. In the adult mammal, the primary source of blood supply to the diaphyseal cortex is the nutrient system (110,167). Shim and colleagues have shown that the nutrient artery supplies at least 46% of the total blood supply of the femur (206). The nutrient artery supplies at least 71% of the total blood supply of the shaft and 35% of the total blood supply of the metaphyseal-epiphyseal area. After nutrient-artery ligation, 63% of the normal flow through the upper epiphysis, 30% of the flow through the shaft, and 67% of the flow

through the lower epiphysis and metaphysis are still intact (206). The nutrient artery is responsible for 70% and the epiphyseal-metaphyseal system for 30%, of the blood flow to a long bone (206). The metaphyseal vessels are second in importance after the nutrient system, and the periosteal vessels are least important (110). Although the periosteal vessels are of minor importance in supplying blood to the normal cortex, they do supply the vessels for the development of new haversian systems on the external surface of the cortex (156).

Blood Flow in Bone

The circulation of blood through bone is necessary for osteogenesis, the maintenance of bone vitality, bone growth, and repair of fractures (205). Blood flow in the entire skeleton of animals has been estimated to be between 4% and 10% of the resting cardiac output (205) and 5.2–6.9% in the dog (235). In the conscious dog, bone blood flow is 9.6% (mature) and 10.3% (immature) of the cardiac output (151). In humans, skeletal blood flow has been estimated as 5% of the resting cardiac output (208).

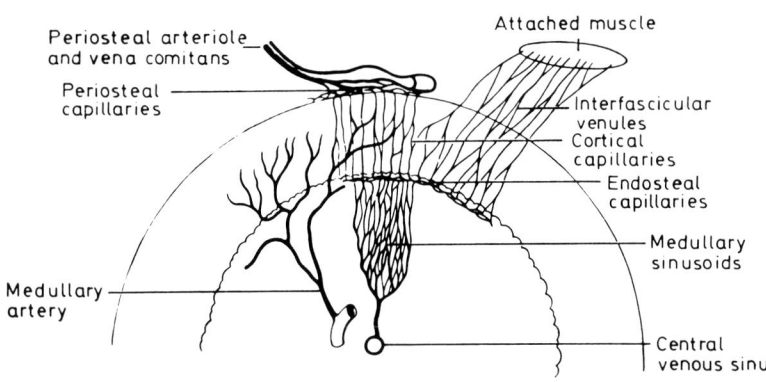

FIG. 2–27. Centrifugal flow of blood from endosteum to periosteum. (From Brookes M. *The blood supply of bone.* London: Butterworth, 1971, p. 119.)

Blood flow through various regions of bone varies, as does blood flow between different bones within an animal and blood flow in immature as opposed to mature animals. Weinman and colleagues noted blood flows of 7.7 ml per min per 100 gm in the tibias of immature dogs compared with 5.6 ml per min per 100 gm in mature dogs (235). Morris and Kelly, using microspheres in mature dogs, found blood-flow values of 2.46 ml per min per 100 gm in cortical bone and 38.3 ml per min per 100 gm in cancellous bone (151). Higher perfusion values have been noted for immature as opposed to mature dogs (237). Kane and Grim, using potassium-42 and rubidium-86 clearance in dogs, noted considerable variation in blood-flow rates in ml per min per 100 gm between the humerus, tibia, and femur (113). They also noted variation in blood flow in various regions of bone, with the epiphysis having a higher rate of blood flow than the shaft, and the marrow having a higher rate of flow than the cortex (113). Whiteside and colleagues noted a higher flow in the metaphysis than in the epiphysis and least flow in the diaphysis (237). Brookes, using chromium-51-labeled red cells in the femur of rats, noted greatest to least blood flow in the following order: inferior metaphysis, marrow, superior metaphysis, inferior epiphysis, and finally cortex (38). Since there was a variation in blood-flow rate in compact and cancellous bone, Brookes felt that vascular factors might have a major function in the local control of normal bone formation and bone repair (38). Whiteside and colleagues, using hydrogen washout in rabbits, noted a positive correlation between blood-flow rate and the histologic level of osteoblastic activity in the skeleton (237). Another possible function of the heterogeneity of bone blood flow might be to regulate the mineral reservoir in order to stabilize ion levels in bone (31).

Various factors may contribute to the regulation of blood flow. Shim and Patterson have noted that the osseous circulation is affected by changes in the systemic cardiovascular condition, such as local femoral arterial occlusion and systemic hypoxia and hypercapnia (Table 2-3) (209). They felt that neutral, hormonal, and metabolic factors, both local and systemic, control blood flow. Shim and colleagues have also noted that sympathetic nerve stimulation and skeletal muscle contraction affect blood flow (207).

Many different methods of studying the rate of normal blood flow have been used, and estimates of blood flow in normal bone vary widely. Direct and indirect methods

of measuring blood flow in bone have been used (44). Excellent summaries of the various techniques and their limitations have been published by Kelly (115) and Shim (205).

PHYSIOLOGY OF FRACTURE HEALING

The Vascular Response to Fracture

The vasculature serves a key function in fracture healing. Albrecht von Haller, in 1763, stated that "the origin of bone is the artery carrying the blood and in it the mineral elements" (92). The most important histologic elements for bony callus formation are osteoblasts and the vascular proliferation that occurs after fracture (216). Blaisdell and Cowan felt that the manner and branching of the new blood vessels determined the orientation and position of the early bony trabeculae (24). Osteogenesis is carried on by cells carried into the fibrocartilaginous callus by the proliferating vasculature (229). Trueta believed that the endothelial cells of the new blood vessels divide at both ends and along large sections of the vessel walls, laying down a progeny of osteoblasts (222). These cells remain attached by cytoplasmic processes that are retained in bone as bone matrix is laid down around the cells (217). The new vessels invade and resorb dead bone, with new bone formation occurring adjacent to them (178). The new vasculature appears at the fracture ends and the pericallus soft tissue (216). As maturation of the cells occurs, the vessels are oriented parallel to the bone axis, anastomoses develop, and normal vascularization is restored (217).

Along with vascular proliferation following fracture, blood flow also undergoes a local change. Wray and Lynch noted an increase in the vascular volume of the affected limb by the third day after fracture, with a peak at 9 days, followed by a gradual return to normal levels (245). Laurnen and Kelly noted an increase in blood flow to bone in canine tibial fractures by the first day after fracture, with a peak of six times normal at 2 weeks, followed by a gradual return to normal (Fig. 2-28) (132). They did not find any significant changes in oxygen, carbon dioxide, or pH levels. They concluded that an increase in blood flow in bone was the primary homeostatic mechanism responsible for supplying the increased metabolic requirements of the healing fracture. Paradis and Kelly found a significant correlation between blood flow in bone and mineral deposition in canine tibial fractures (169). They also noted an increase in blood flow in bone with a peak 10 days after fracture. Hughes and colleagues found that the increase in blood flow following a fracture represents recruitment of capillaries (103). Thus, following a fracture, vessels increase in size and number, and blood flow also increases.

The importance of the three afferent sources of blood supply to a long bone in contributing to fracture healing

TABLE 2–3. *Factors involved in blood flow regulation*

Systemic	Local
Cardiovascular condition	Arterial occlusion
Hypoxia	Muscle contracture
Hypercapnia	Sympathetic nerve
Hormonal	stimulation

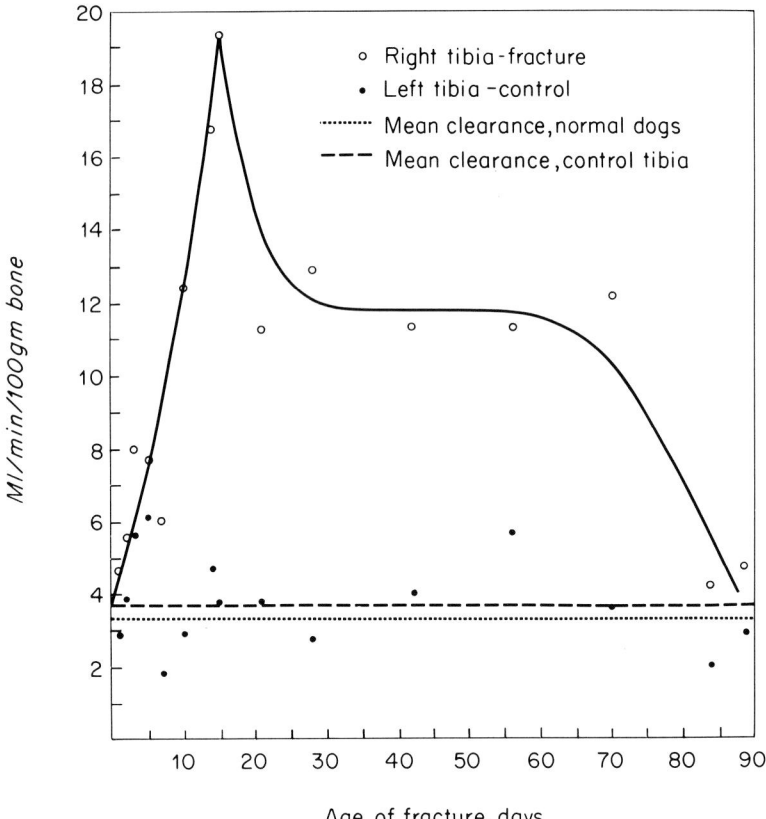

FIG. 2–28. Vascular response following fracture (132).

has been debated. Cavadias and Trueta performed vascular suppression of two of the three afferent sources of blood supply to healing osteotomies of the radius in rabbits (44). When the nutrient vessels were the only source of blood supply to the fracture, no periosteal callus was noted, union occurred by endosteal callus and was delayed compared with that in controls, and there was decreased breaking strength of the callus. When the metaphyseal-epiphyseal vessels were the only source of blood supply, extensive necrosis of the cortex occurred despite patent medullary vessels on arteriograms, and union was delayed. When the periosteal vessels were the only source of blood supply, the periosteal callus appeared normally, necrosis of the inner one-half of the cortex occurred, no endosteal callus was present, union occurred by periosteal callus, and a late revascularization of the inner cortex by the periosteal vessels occurred. Johnson studied the repair of canine tibial defects after suppression of blood supply to bone (110). He found that the nutrient vessels alone would maintain viability of the inner one-half of the cortex and allow active repair of the defect. The metaphyseal vessels would maintain viability of the medulla but would not support active repair of the defect. The periosteal vessels alone were not able to support any active repair or serve as a collateral source of blood supply during the four weeks of the experiment. Johnson concluded that the nutrient vessels were the most important, the metaphyseal vessels of in-

termediary importance, and the periosteal vessels of least importance in the repair of a bone defect (110).

The relative importance of the periosteal compared with the endosteal blood supply in contributing to fracture union has been contested. Kolodny felt that the periosteal blood supply was essential for normal union of osteotomies of the radius in dogs and that the periosteal callus was more important than the endosteal callus for fracture union (121). Destruction of the nutrient artery affected fracture healing only in cases in which the periosteal vessels had been destroyed (121). Wray, in studying rabbit tibial fractures, felt that the periosteal vascular system as augmented by vessels from the surrounding soft tissues was the major source for vascularization of the forming callus (244). He felt that the interosseous circulation was not important in fracture healing. Holden emphasized the importance of the vessels derived from the surrounding soft tissues (102). In rabbits with segmental-displaced fractures of the radius, he noted the revascularization of the entire thickness of the cortex occurred by periosteal vessels prior to re-establishment of continuity of the medullary vessels. If the surrounding muscles were made ischemic, revascularization of the bone was delayed until after revascularization of the muscle had occurred.

In contrast, other authors have thought that the medullary vascular system is more important for fracture healing than the periosteal system. Ladanyi and Hidvegi, in studying osteotomies of the ulna in dogs, found that response from the medullary vascular system appeared earlier in the fracture area and was consistently richer than the periosteal response (127). Rhinelander believes that the medullary arterial system derived from the nutrient and metaphyseal vessels remains dominant throughout fracture healing (189). He claims that the periosteal vessels play a significant role only in the vicinity of fascial attachments and that this new external blood supply is distinct from the normal one. Rhinelander stated that the new periosteal blood supply is derived entirely from extraosseous arterial systems and is only facultative in regard to its bone function. This extraosseous blood supply is derived from ruptured capillaries and arterioles in torn muscle that combine with torn periosteal arterioles. The extraosseous blood supply is transitory and persists only until the medullary vessels have regenerated and restored the normal centrifugal flow of blood through the cortex.

A partial explanation for the discrepancy of opinion concerning the relative importance of the periosteal and medullary systems for fracture union may be found if differences in displaced and undisplaced fractures are taken into account. The vascular changes in the healing of displaced and undisplaced diaphyseal fractures differ. In undisplaced fractures, not all vascular connections adjacent to the fracture are served (190). The majority of the blood supply for revascularization is derived from the medullary circulation, which furnishes the major portion of the blood supply to the uniting callus and revascularizes the necrotic cortex at the fracture (190). The majority of the blood supply for revascularization is derived from the medullary circulation, which furnishes the major portion of the blood supply to the uniting callus and revascularizes the necrotic cortex at the fracture (190). The medullary vascular system remains dominant throughout all stages of healing, and the periosteal vessels have only a limited role (180). In contrast, in displaced fractures the proliferation of the disrupted endosteal vessels is initially blocked by the hematoma (192). The periosteal circulation, augmented by vessels from the surrounding soft tissues, is the initial source of blood supply to the fracture and supplies the external callus. If stable reduction is maintained, early regeneration of the medullary vessels may occur; but if reduction is unstable, regeneration of medullary vessels is delayed by the interposition of fibrocartilage in the fracture site. As the medullary vessels regenerate, they become dominant and supply the area of earliest osseous union. Therefore, in both undisplaced and displaced fractures, the medullary circulation remains dominant and supplies the area of earliest osseous union (192).

The function of the vascular dilatation after fracture is to supply nutrients to the healing fracture. Oxygen is a prime nutrient, yet controversy exists concerning the optimum oxygen concentrations for fracture union. Sim

and Kelly, in comparing bone remodeling, oxygen consumption, and blood flow in canine tibias, found the arteriovenous oxygen difference (i.e., oxygen extraction) unchanged in high, normal, or low remodeling states (210). However, they did note a close correlation between the rate of bone remodeling, oxygen consumption, and the rate of blood flow in bone. In high remodeling states there was an increase in oxygen consumption, which correlated with an increased rate of blood flow. They concluded that alterations in blood flow were important in meeting the nutritional demands of active tissue.

Brighton and Krebs studied oxygen tension in healing fibular fractures in the rabbit (36). They noted the lowest oxygen tension in newly formed cartilage and fiber bone, and the highest values in fibrous tissue in the callus. Biomechanical evaluation of fracture stiffness in a three-point bending test revealed a return to control levels of stiffness prior to an increase in oxygen tension at the fracture site. Oxygen tension at the fracture site did not rise to normal diaphyseal levels until the medullary canal was reconstituted. They concluded that the low oxygen tension at the fracture site might be a stimulus to osteoblast proliferation and calcium release.

In contrast, Ham felt that osteogenic cells in the presence of an adequate blood supply and calcium would form bone but in the absence of an adequate blood supply and calcium would form cartilage (93). Bassett, in studying chick mesenchymal cells in tissue culture, noted cellular differentiation into bone in the presence of a high-oxygen environment, whereas cartilage was formed in a low-oxygen environment (15). Heppenstall and colleagues studied the effect of chronic hypoxia on the healing of fibular fractures in the dog (98). They noted decreased new bone formation and decreased biomechanical strength of the fracture in the hypoxic dogs as compared with controls. They felt that the poor fracture healing in these dogs might be attributable to a loss of the normal oxygen gradient across the fracture.

Biochemical studies have shown the importance of oxidative metabolism for fracture healing. Kuhlman and Bakowski, in studying the enzyme content of fracture callus, noted that the process of bone repair relied upon oxidative carbohydrate metabolism, which indicated the importance of an adequate blood supply for fracture healing (122). Ketenjian and Arsenis noted that a shift to oxidative glycolysis occurred with cartilage maturation in the callus (116). They felt that this finding supported the concept of oxybiotic metabolism in the fracture during the early stages of vascular invasion.

Cellular Response to Fracture

The basic requirements for bone formation are the presence of free circulatory elements, adequate surfaces on which bone formation may take place, and cells with osteogenic potency (219). The origin of the cells involved in fracture repair and the relative contributions of the periosteum and the endosteum have been the subject of controversy. As early as 1740, Duhamel considered the periosteum as osteogenic, while Haller considered the endosteum and haversian canals as most significant for fracture union (67,92). Todd and Iler felt that both the periosteal and endosteal cells were of major importance, while the cells of compact bone were of minor importance (217). Enneking found that periosteal activity following a fracture preceded endosteal cellular activity (72). The endosteal reaction followed the periosteal reaction by 48 hours but was of equal intensity and duration (72). Slätis and Rokkanen stated that the intense proliferation of the periosteal osteogenic cells was responsible for the majority of the initial callus (212).

The cells involved in the repair of a fracture include osteogenic cells derived from the cambium layer of the periosteum, from Volkmann's and haversian canals, and from the endosteum (20,72,229). Undifferentiated surrounding mesenchymal cells as well as cells derived from the new vasculature may play a role (Table 2-4) (222,229). Bassett and Ruedi have shown that bone formation may occur in a bone defect isolated from the periosteum and endosteum, indicating the osteogenic potential of cells lining Volkmann's and haversian canals (18).

Controversy has also surrounded the relative importance of the endosteal and periosteal callus in securing fracture union. Lexer felt that the periosteal callus was most important in fracture union (136), while Bier felt that the endosteal callus was most important (121). The periosteum has been noted to form the earliest callus following a fracture, while the endosteum forms callus only after the intraosseous circulation has recovered (121). Phemister thought that the periosteum was very important for fracture healing and noted that excision of the periosteum delayed callus formation and ossification and predisposed to delay union (178). Subperiosteal osteoblasts play a very active role in periosteal callus formation (203). Therefore, excessive periosteal stripping at operation should be avoided to prevent damage to the blood supply of the bone (83). Periosteal stripping may devitalize the underlying bone and damage the cambium layer of the periosteum (217). In healing of bone defects, the presence of periosteum allows union; in the absence of periosteum, non-union occurs (155). It has been

TABLE 2-4. Cells involved in fracture repair

Undifferentiated menenchymal
Cambium layer of periosteum
Volkmann's canals
Haversian canals
Endosteum
Vascular

stated that mineralized periosteal callus is the first callus to span the fracture gap (158). In contrast, other authors have found that the endosteal callus unites the fracture prior to the bridging of the fracture gap by the periosteal callus (71,189). Rhinelander stated that the medullary callus was always the first to accomplish osseous union, with the periosteal callus functioning as an ancillary external support (189).

Thus, both periosteal and endosteal callus are important in fracture union, with their relative contributions depending upon the initial displacement of the fracture, the degree of initial trauma, and the stability of immobilization during treatment.

BIOMECHANICS OF FRACTURE HEALING

Biomechanics of Normal Bone

A knowledge of the effect of various stresses upon normal bone and its general mechanical properties is important for understanding the response of bone to fracture and internal fixation. As Wolff pointed out in 1892, "Every change in the form and function of a bone, or of its function alone, is followed by certain definite changes in its internal architecture and equally definite secondary alterations in the external conformation in accordance with mathematical laws" (242). The ability of bone to adapt to stress becomes progressively more apparent when the morphology of the trabecular pattern of the femoral neck and head is viewed on a phylogenetic basis (220). A similar phenomenon may be seen during normal growth and development. A change in the posture of the human infant is reflected in changes in the trabecular pattern of the femoral head (220).

Various theories have been advanced to explain the mechanical basis for these morphological findings. According to Scott, there are five theories concerning the mechanical structure of bone (203). Bone may be formed along lines of tension or pressure stress. Pressure from either weight-bearing or muscle action may determine bone structure. The internal architecture of bone may follow its external conformation, with functional demands playing only a secondary role in its modification. The vascular pattern may determine bony architecture. Or, finally, the elastic recoil of bone following loading may affect bone structure. The actual mechanical structure of bone is probably affected by all of the factors mentioned in these various theories. Most important, bone is able to respond to applied stress. Glucksmann has shown experimentally that bone growth may be affected by applied forces (85). *In vitro* endosteal chick cultures, when subjected to tension, form bone oriented perpendicularly to the tension force; when subjected to compression, the endosteal cultures form bone oriented parallel to the compression force (85). If the longitudinal growth of chick rudiments is inhibited *in vitro,* ossification will always be greater on the convex side (86). Thus bone formation responds to applied stresses. Additionally, Bassett has shown that *in vitro* mesenchymal cell differentiation is affected by the mechanical environment (Table 2-5) (15). In the presence of compression plus adequate oxygen, bone is formed. In contrast, in the presence of tension plus adequate oxygen, fibrous tissue is formed.

The material properties of bone are unique and must be considered when analyzing the mechanical structure of bone. Bone is nonisotropic and viscoelastic (42,65). As a nonisotropic material, it has different properties in different directions. As a viscoelastic material, it is a material whose characteristic constants are affected by the rate of deformation. Any material, including bone, may be characterized by three such constants (184). First, Young's modulus or stiffness is the slope of the stress-strain curve obtained from a uniaxial tension test. Second, Poisson's ratio is the negative of the ratio of transverse strain to longitudinal strain in the direction of uniaxial loading and is a measure of the ability of a material to conserve volume when loaded in one direction. Finally, the shear modulus is the ratio of the induced shear to the resulting shear strain and is determined from torsional testing. Values for human bone of Young's modulus (14.1×10^9 N/m^2), Poisson's ratio (0.08 to 0.45), and the shear modulus (0.31×10^9 N/m^2) have been reported (184). Additionally, maximum shear stress may be obtained by torsional testing.

The nonisotropic nature of bone is reflected in variations in mechanical properties from one region to another in a given bone, differences in the same region between different individuals, and differences from one bone to another within an individual (65,74). Therefore, both the type of testing and the site of bone sampling influence results. Careful selection of samples, preferably mirror segments within an animal, is thus necessary for comparison testing. The physical factors that affect such variations in bone strength include the number of collagen fibrils, the axial direction of these fibrils, the number of osteones, and the mineral content of the bone (75). Thus, bending strength increases as the ash (mineral) content of the bone increases (55). Totally haversian bone is 30% weaker than lamellar bone in tensile strength (55). Tensile strength in the longitudinal direction (i.e., oriented parallel to the haversian canals) differs from that in the transverse direction (186). Compression

strength also differs, depending upon the direction of loading, with bone being 50% stronger when loaded parallel to the osteones as opposed to transverse loading (62). Age has an effect, with the tensile strength of human femoral bone decreasing approximately 4% per decade (146).

Similarly, the mechanical principles involved in the initiation of a fracture vary according to the type of stress applied and its rate of application. In tension, plastic deformation is exhibited by the bone and failure occurs by a transverse fracture (42). In pure compression, an oblique fracture occurs, with a shear initiation as the mode of failure (42). Burstein and colleagues have noted microfractures at an angle of 45° to the direction of compressive loading along the lines of principal shear stress (42). These cracks are more numerous if the stress-field is nonuniform (42). Failure in both tension and compression is consistent with such a multiphasic material as bone, which exhibits yield by means of a pullout that creates voids and crazes (42). Torsional loading results in pure shear stress, giving rise to a spiral fracture along the plane of maximum shear stress (42). Pugh felt that torsional loading resulted in a failure at 45° because this angle marked a tension plane (181). Burstein noted that in torsional failure the vascular network between lamellae acted as a surface of fracture initiation (42,184).

In fact, bone has a high resistance to bending and torsion, largely because the bony material is located at the periphery, where the stresses are highest (181). The rigidity-efficiency of the tissue increases with the fourth power of the distance from the center of rotation or bending (173). Therefore, endosteal callus is less efficient than interfragmentary bone, which in turn is less efficient than periosteal callus, provided that the repair tissue is of equal quality (173). Fractures tend to occur along planes of tension or shear because bone is weakest in tension and shear and strongest in compression (181). If a bone is loaded purely in bending, the initiation of fracture always begins on the tensile side because its tensile strength is less than its compressive strength (62).

Other factors besides the plane of the fracture provide information concerning the initiating forces. Flat smooth surfaces result from a quickly traveling crack or a brittle fracture process with low energy absorption (184). Rough surfaces with pull-out of constituents indicate a slower fracture process and more energy absorption. Since bone is a viscoelastic material, it is stiffer at higher rates of loading and its fracture strength is higher (181). Therefore, in high-loading rate injuries more energy is absorbed, resulting in a comminuted fracture (181).

TABLE 2–5. *Mechanical and biologic factors affecting osteogenic cell differentiation*

Environment	Tissue formed
Compression + high O$_2$	Bone
Compression + low O$_2$	Cartilage
Tension + high O$_2$	Fibrous tissue

Fracture Healing

When is the fracture healed? This is the key question that confronts the surgeon when treating a patient with a fracture. Clinical criteria are useful in framing an answer but are difficult to quantitate. A knowledge of the changes in the biomechanical characteristics of a healing fracture is useful both for clinical treatment and for experimental studies in which quantitative comparisons between treatment methods can be performed.

In healing fibular fractures in rabbits, Brighton and Krebs found a progressive increase in bending strength and rigidity as healing progressed (36). Lindsay studied healing fibular fractures in rats by subjecting the healing fractures to a simple bending test (Fig. 2-29) (139). He noted a progressive increase in strength until the twenty-first day following fracture, which correlated with increasing mineralization of the fracture and increasing callus area. After the twenty-first day, there was a small decrease in strength in conjunction with a decrease in callus area. This was followed by a gradual increase in strength to control levels despite a further decrease in callus area (139). Lindsay felt that the decrease followed by an increase in bone strength correlated with the phases of fracture remodeling (138). In further studies, Lindsay found a direct correlation between the breaking strength of the healing fracture and the size and weight of the bone (138). He noted that the breaking strength varied according to three phases of fracture healing: fibrosis, calcification, and structural reorganization (138).

In healing osteotomies of the radius in rabbits, Falkenberg noted a peak in callus area and ash weight of the fracture between 20 and 30 days following fracture (75). From 20 to 60 days following fracture, the callus area decreased 50% and the ash weight decreased 25%, but the absolute tensile strength of the callus increased 100% (75). An increase in mineral content paralleled the increase in bone strength in the later stages of fracture healing (75). Also, hydroxyapatite crystals were reorganized during fracture remodeling from an initially random ori-

entation of the C-axis of the crystals to an orientation parallel to the longitudinal axis of the bone (158). Falkenberg concluded that an initial rapid increase in the absolute tensile strength of the callus occurs with increasing callus area, but the actual quality of the callus improves more slowly in conjunction with fracture remodeling (75). A combination of increasing mineral content, reorientation of the hydroxyapatite crystals, and secondary osteone formation contributes to the increase in strength of the healing fracture.

White and colleagues have classified fracture healing into four biomechanical stages based upon torsional testing of the healing fracture (Fig. 2-30) (236). Stage I displays failure through the original fracture site with low stiffness. Stage II displays failure through the original fracture site with high stiffness. Stage III displays failure partially through the original fracture site with high stiffness. Stage IV displays failure entirely through intact bone with high stiffness. A progressive increase in the maturity of fracture healing is present from Stages I to IV.

Different mechanical forces also have different effects upon fracture healing. Yamagishi and Yoshimura found that a neutral force resulted in healing by direct transformation of mesenchymal cells into osteoblasts, but healing was slow (247). A compression force resulted in rapid healing by endochondral ossification unless the force was excessive, in which case healing was delayed (247). If a distraction force was applied, fibrous tissue formed and healing was also delayed (247). The worst loading configuration was shear combined with intermittent compression, which resulted in pseudarthrosis (247). Friedenberg and French attempted to quantitate the effects of compression forces on fracture healing (80). They found that an optimum range of compression existed, in which fracture union occurred in two-thirds of their experimental

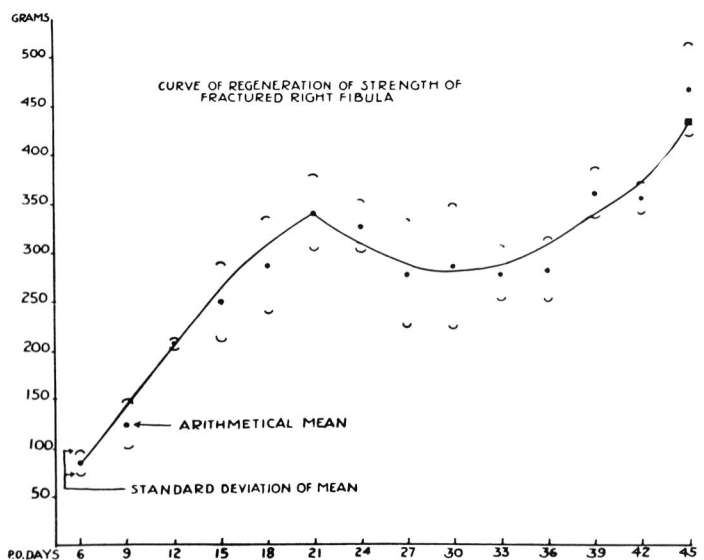

FIG. 2-29. Healing strength of a fracture (139).

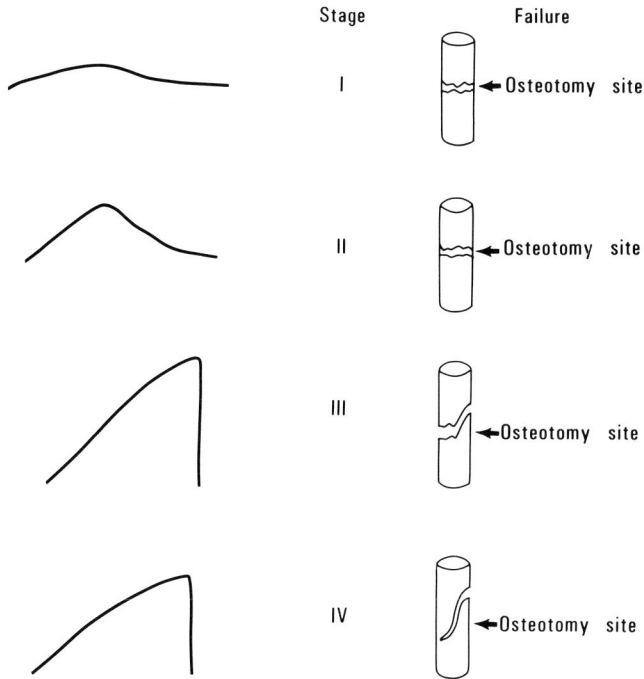

Stage   Failure

I   ←Osteotomy site

II   ←Osteotomy site

III   ←Osteotomy site

IV   ←Osteotomy site

FIG. 2–30. Biomechanical stages of fracture healing (Modified from 236).

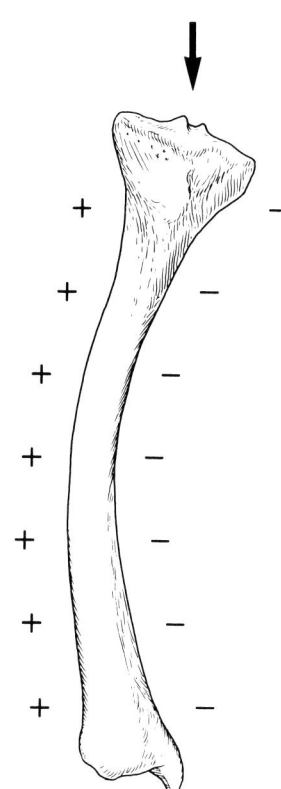

FIG. 2–31. Stress-generated potential in bone.

animals (80). Higher or lower compression resulted in a lower rate of union (80).

Therefore, mechanical forces affected the rate of fracture union. Fracture healing progresses through several stages with a gradual increase in strength. The increase in strength correlates with callus area initially but in later stages relates to fracture remodeling.

Biologic Signs for Fracture Healing

The nature of the signal that induces fracture healing is poorly understood. Two concepts have been advanced as a potential initiating signal for fracture healing. The first is a series of electrical signals, and the second involves a bone-inductive substance. It is beyond the scope of this review to give a detailed discussion of these concepts, but they will be briefly summarized.

Electrical Signals

Two types of electrical signals or potentials are found in bone: (1) stress-generated or strain-generated potentials, and (2) bioelectric or standing potentials. Stress-generated potentials arise when bone is stressed, and they are not dependent upon cell viability. Areas of compression are electronegative, while areas of tension are electropositive (Fig. 2-31) (79). These electrical signals arise from the organic component of the bone and are not derived from the mineral component. In normal in-

tact bone, Friedenberg and colleagues have shown that electrical polarity exists with the ends of the bone being electronegative in comparison to the midshaft (79). Following fracture or osteotomy the electrical polarity will change. The entire surface of the bone becomes electronegative with a peak of electronegativity occurring over the fracture site (Fig. 2-32) (79). This change in electrical potentials will remain until the fracture heals. A second peak of electronegativity will also occur over the opposite physis (79). The bioelectrical potentials are dependent upon cell viability. If the cells are killed or damaged there will be a significant drop in the electrical potentials in the area.

Friedenberg has shown with implantable electrodes that bone will form immediately around the negative electrode or cathode (79). However, there is an optimal amperage below which no bone will form and above which bone formation will give way to cell necrosis. Surrounding the positive electrode or anode only bone necrosis will occur. In the rabbit fibula, electrical stimulation will result in a significant increase in fracture healing, as evidenced by an increased maximum resistance to bending (81). Using this semi-invasive technique, the amount of new bone formed is related to the true current density and change (35). The amount of bone formed is linearly related to charge. In fact, a variety of forms of electricity will produce osteogenesis. In addition to di-

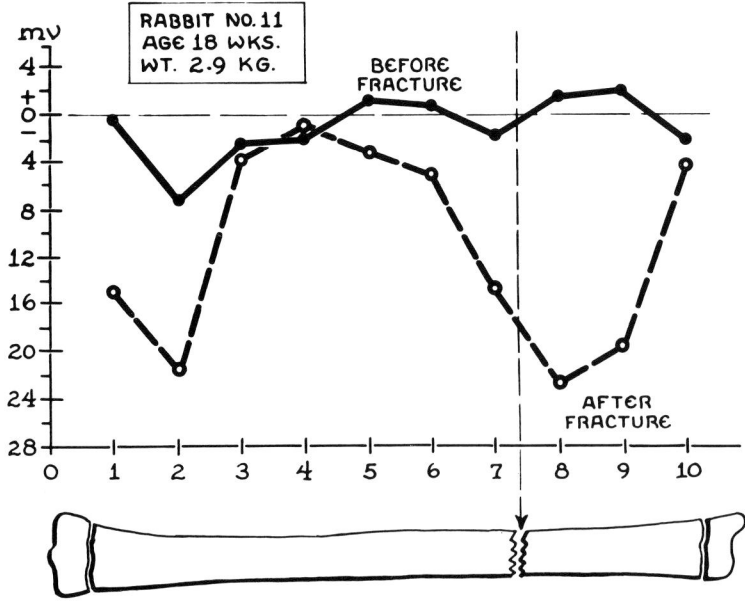

FIG. 2-32. Negative potential at the fracture site (79).

rect current of varying amplitude, pulse width, and frequency, noninvasive techniques using electromagnetic fields, as advocated by Bassett, have proved successful both experimentally and clinically (16). The mechanism of action of the electrical stimulation of bone cells is poorly understood, but two potential mechanisms are (1) direct cellular changes induced by the electrical current possibly acting through cyclic AMP, or (2) indirect changes produced in the microenvironment (82). Friedenberg and colleagues feel that a change in the oxygen concentration in the microenvironment is a probable mechanism of action (82).

Jacobs and colleagues studied the mechanism of healing of non-unions treated by the semi-invasive technique of implanted electrodes in non-union of canine ulnae (107). In hypertrophic non-unions, bone formation was twice as great in the electrically stimulated non-unions as compared with controls. In oligotrophic non-unions, bone formation was increased 22% as compared with controls. Bone did not form in fibrous tissue alone but always arose by appositional growth from existing bone. Jacobs and colleagues concluded that electrical stimulation functioned through a cell-mediated rather than physiochemical mechanism (107).

Bassett and colleagues studied the effects of pulsating electromagnetic fields upon acute fracture repair (19). They found that the biologic response was dependent upon a specific type of wave form. Osteogenesis was not directly stimulated. The major effect of electrical stimulation was an increased rate of mineralization of existing fibrocartilage. A similar mechanism of action has been suggested for pulsating electromagnetic fields used in treating non-unions (17).

Bone-Inductive Signal

As mentioned earlier, bone-inducing material has been advocated as an alternative signal for fracture healing. Induction refers to the capacity of one living cell to influence the differentiation of another living cell. Three conditions must be met for bone induction to occur (45). First, an inducing agent must be present. Second, viable osteogenic precursor cells must be available. Third, the environment must be permissive for osteogenesis. Extraskeletal implantation of decalcified bone matrix will induce surrounding pleuripotent host cells to differentiate into osteoblasts and form bone (227). The inducer cells and the induced cells are felt to be derived from the host bed rather than from the bone graft (227). The osteogenic cells arise from a competent mesenchymal cell population residing in the host tissue rather than from blood-borne or vascular cells (18,228).

A variety of substances have been sought that might act to induce bone. The concept of a bone-induction substance has been experimentally studied by a variety of authors. Urist has identified a substance that he terms *bone morphogenic protein* (BMP) (228). The bone morphogenic principle will induce the formation of new bone as old bone is resorbed. Even in the absence of living cells, the organic matrix of bone contains this protein, which can induce formation of new bone adjacent to living bone. BMP has a molecular weight of approximately 10,000 and can diffuse across a Millipore filter. It appears to play a role in osteoinduction, which depends upon a substrate-cell interaction that induces competent mesenchymal cells to differentiate into osteoblasts. More generally, a variety of factors have been noted to influence bone induction. Induction is accelerated by the demineralization, freezing, and heat denaturation of bone; and it is inhibited by irradiation, proteolytic enzyme degradation, or the presence of minerals (228). Heterotopic ossification is an example of bone induction in muscle.

The most frequent use of the bone-induction principle in orthopedics involves bone grafting. Three factors act in bone grafting: cellular proliferation, prevention of fibrous ingrowth, and induction (97). Both the host and graft contribute cells that form new bone about the transplant (97). Some of the potential sources of osteogenic cells include surface osteoblasts in the graft and recipient bone, marrow cells, soft tissues in the recipient bed, and free circulatory elements in the blood (40). The contribution of each osteogenic cell population in the cancellous bone graft has been studied by Gray and Elves (89). Endosteal lining cells and marrow stroma contribute 60% to osteogenesis and periosteal cells 30% (89). The least osteogenic tissues are marrow cells and osteocytes (89). The rate of osteogenesis is 2.2 times higher in cancellous than in cortical bone grafts (89).

The type of bone graft used has an effect upon the results. Autogenous bone graft is the most osteogenic, followed by freeze-dried homogeneous bone (96). Autogenous cancellous or corticocancellous grafts contribute to bone formation, are free from immunologic response and allow bone induction in the recipient bed (40).

FRACTURE FIXATION

Compression-Plate Fixation of Fractures

Plate fixation of fractures is designed to immobilize the fracture while allowing mobility of the soft tissues of the injured limb. The first use of a bone plate has been attributed to Hansmann in 1886 (95). A variety of bone plates subsequently became available in the early part of the twentieth century, such as the Lane and Sherman plates. Many modifications of bone plates have been devised in an attempt to improve the quality of fixation (Figs. 2-33 and 2-34).

The significance of compression in promoting bone union was first advocated by Key in 1932 in arthrodesis of the knee (117). Key felt that the factors acting in compression arthrodesis were apposition of the bone surfaces, fixation of the fragments, and compression itself. In 1946, Eggers made the first attempt to use compression to aid healing of fractures immobilized by plates (68). He devised a plate termed the *contact split* that allowed sliding contact of the fracture fragments and physiologic compression of the fragments from muscular action (69). According to Eggers, excessive compression would cause necrosis of bone, while lack of compression would fail to stimulate osteogenesis; physiologic compression from muscular action, however, would be optimal for stimulating bone union (70,71). Key and Reynolds found slightly more rapid union with an Eggers plate than with a standard bone plate (118). Close approximation and continuous immobilization of the fracture ends were felt to be advantages of the Eggers plate. In fact, primary bone union without an intermediary cartilaginous state was noted in some fractures treated with the Eggers plate (118). The major difficulty with the Eggers contact splint, however, was its inability to control the quantity of compression and degree of immobilization of the fracture site.

Danis, in 1947, stated that the key principles of internal fixation were rigid immobilization, axial pressure, and coaptation of the bone fragments (59). In 1949, Danis described the first true compression plate and reported satisfactory results in its use in treating forearm

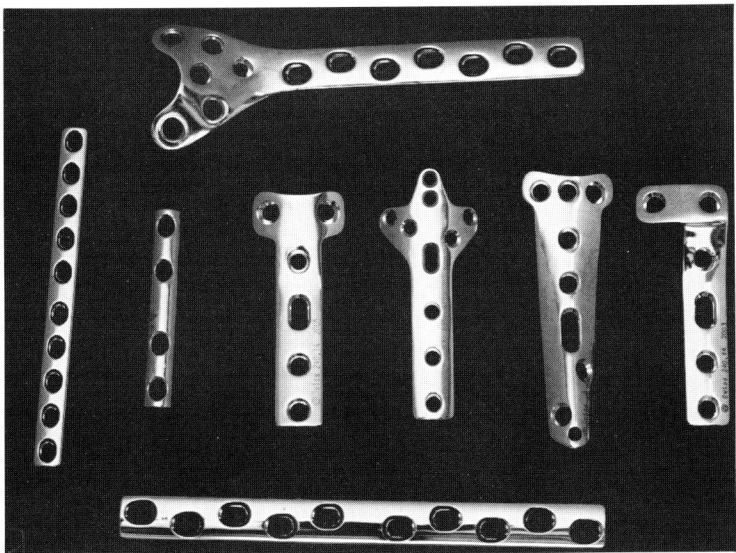

FIG. 2–33. Types of bone plates. *Upper:* condylar buttress; *middle* (*left to right*) 3.5 mm DCP (dynamic compression plate), semitubular, T-plate, cloverleaf, spoon, L-plate; *lower:* 4.5 mm DCP.

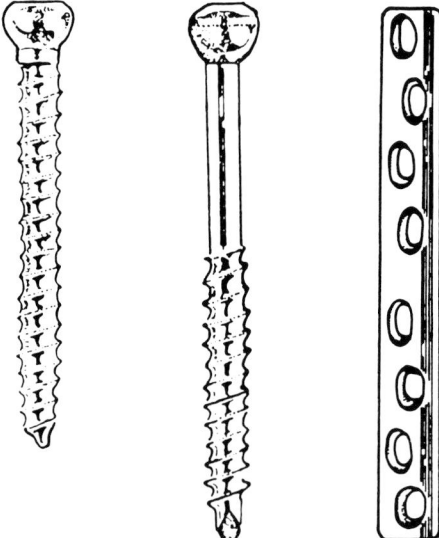

FIG. 2–34. Illustration of cortical (*left*) and cancellous (*middle*) screws, and the oval holes in a dynamic compression plate (DCP) (193).

fractures (60). Venable believed that impacted coaptation of the fracture fragments was essential for early healing and that excessive callus was evidence of insufficient stability or insufficient blood supply to the fracture (231). Venable also devised a compression plate to achieve rigid stabilization of the fracture. Bagby devised a plate that was self-compressing upon application owing to impaction of the screws against the screw holes in the plate (11). He found that union occurred earlier in experimental fractures treated with a compression plate than in those treated with a standard bone plate. Bagby felt that the effect of compression on fracture healing might be either a direct effect of the compression or more likely an indirect effect. Compression would result in close approximation of the fracture fragments, which would decrease the fracture gap and might stimulate osteogenesis and would also provide rigid immobilization (11,12,13).

Müller, in 1962, reported on primary bone healing using the AO compression plate (152). There was no resorption of the fracture site, no radiologically evident callus, and primary bone healing occurred in 79% of 188 tibial fractures. He believed that compression improved stability, but he was unable to prove that compression actually stimulates bone union. Allgower and Perren reported on the dynamic compression plate (DCP) in 1969, which was similar in principle to the plate previously designed by Bagby (6,175,177). The major advantages of the DCP when compared with the standard AO compression plate include improved engineering (which allows greater versatility in the angle of screw placement and compression between any two screw holes in the plate) compression with limited surgical exposure, and absence of unpredictable change in com-

pression—a problem in the removal of the standard compression device (174). The advocates of the DCP and standard AO compression plates stress the advantages of maintaining rigid fixation of the fractures with these implants.

Mechanism of Action of Compression-Fixation

The mechanism of action and the optimum quantity of compression for fracture healing have been investigated. In experimental fractures, it has been suggested that there is an optimal range of compression in which union is stimulated. Higher pressures cause bone necrosis and lower pressures fail to stimulate bone union (70,80,128,149). Friedenberg and French found an increased rate of union from compression-fixation, which was attributed to enhanced mobility of the fracture fragments, enhanced immobility of the fracture combined with close contact of fragments, and a possible stimulation of osteogenesis at the fracture site from the pressure (80). In contrast, Laurin was unable to demonstrate more rapid union in experimental fractures subjected to compression. Lettin found a similar rate of union in fractures fixed with a bone plate, whether compression was applied or not (134). Ford and Key were unable to demonstrate more rapid union with compression across experimental canine fractures of the ilium and did not observe bone necrosis from high pressure (77). Anderson, in comparing compression- and noncompression-plate fixation of canine femoral osteotomies, found more rapid union and less periosteal callus in those fractures treated with compression (8). Prominent endosteal callus was responsible for the area of earliest osseous union with both types of plate fixation. However, there was no significant difference in tensile strength between those fractures treated with compression and those without (8). Allgower and Perren, in studying compression-plate fixation of experimental fractures, noted that, despite the high loads applied to the bone by the compression plate and at the screw-bone interface, no bone necrosis occurred (5).

The biomechanical properties of bone help explain the variable effects of compression. The pressure beneath a compression plate decreases approximately 20% initially owing to the viscoelastic behavior of bone and then gradually decreased by 50% over the next 8 weeks in conjunction with haversian remodeling (175). Coletti found that bone loaded with compression of greater than 318 psi responded with formation of bone beneath the pressure site (47). The area of bone formation correlated with areas of tensile stress, and there was no evidence of bone necrosis. Given this relation between pressure and bone formation, a unique mechanical explanation for the mechanism of action of compression has been suggested by Pinter (179). X-ray diffraction studies of bovine bone *in vitro* revealed an association between an increase in the total quantity and crystalline material in bone and a decrease in the quantity of amorphous material present when the bone was subjected to compressive loading (179). Pinter believed that the beneficial action of compression might be a purely physical process of oriented crystal growth superimposed upon cellular activity (179).

Morphologic Findings of Primary Bone Healing with Compression-Plate Fixation

The morphologic findings and characteristics of fracture union after compression-plate fixation have been termed *soudre autogéne,* or *primary fracture healing* (200). Some authors consider primary fracture healing the ideal mode of healing. Under rigid internal fixation, primary angiogenic ossification may occur, in which the ingrowing capillary network is protected from motion and thus disruption. This allows osteoblastic proliferation and direct bone union of the fracture gap (200). Histologically, secondary osteones directly cross the fracture site without the presence of intervening cartilage. New osteone formation is estimated to occur within 5 to 6 weeks in the dog and within 3 months in humans (143,200). The osteoblastic "cutter head" forming the secondary osteone progresses at a rate of 50 to 80 microns in 24 hours (200). The advantage of primary fracture healing is that the restoration of the original bone structure of the cortex begins earlier than in fracture healing without rigid fixation. Therefore, the main features of primary bone healing include primary bone union in interfragmental gaps, minimal resorption of the bone ends without widening of the fracture gap, longitudinally directed secondary osteones crossing the fracture, and minimal external callus (178). Minimal external callus is seen on radiographs associated with a gradual obliteration of the fracture line.

Primary bone healing has been observed by several authors using other modes of fixation than the compression plate, including external fixation with pins and a compression spring (80,247). Blockey, as well as Burwell, reported primary fracture healing using a noncompression Burns plate that provided rigid internal fixation (25,43). Primary bone healing similar to that observed with the standard AO compression plate has been reported using the DCP plate (6,175).

Bone healing beneath a compression plate occurs in two distinct forms. Immediately beneath the plate, primary bone healing occurs where the cortical fragments are in direct contact. This involves the direct bridging of the fracture by secondary osteones with minimal periosteal callus but significant bridging medullary callus. This is contact healing (176,189). Union of the cortex opposite the plate involves a different mechanism. A slight gap exists between the fracture fragments and union here is termed *gap healing* (176,182,189). In gap healing, direct bone formation occurs oriented perpendicularly to the long axis of the bone and must later be remodeled into longitudinal osteones. The vascular supply for gap healing receives an important contribution from the periosteal circulation, whereas in contact healing the endosteal circulation is most important (182). In both cases primary bone healing occurs only in the presence of an adequate blood supply and rigid stabilization of the fracture (189). Enhancement of stabilization that protects the regenerating blood vessels is the major contribution of compression-fixation (187).

Effect of a Plate on Bone-Blood Flow

The effect of internal fixation of the blood supply of a long bone has been the subject of extensive investigation. Rhinelander believes that, of the methods of secure internal fixation, plating disturbs the blood supply least (189). He has noted reconstitution of medullary vessels across an osteotomy within 1 week of internal fixation with a plate (189). However, because it blocks the venous drainage from the bone, the plate does reduce vascularization of the entire thickness of the cortex immediately beneath the plate (187,189,194). Screws do not significantly disturb the circulation (189). Olerud found avascular regions extending over one-half the thickness of the cortex beneath a compression plate (160,161). He noted revascularization occurring from periosteal, endosteal, and haversian vessels. Endosteal vessels are responsible for 80% of the revascularization of a fracture fixed with a compression plate (141,142).

Biomechanics of Plate Fixation

Biomechanical analysis of the fixation achieved with various plates has been performed. Lindahl found that the AO plate ranked among the top three plates tested for resistance to bending and torsion (137). He felt that the anchorage of a plate should satisfy the following requirements: the rigidity and shape of the plate should be such that the strength of immobilization is roughly equal to bone; enough screws must be used and the shear area should be large; and the material should be as nonirritating as possible (137). According to Lindahl, the AO plate best fulfilled these requirements. The cross-sectional area of the plate is important. The broader the plate, the greater the rigidity of fixation without regard to the other aspects of fixation (159). More rapid healing of experimental fractures has been observed with the use of a broad, as opposed to narrow, compression plate (159).

The mechanical effect of a compression plate is to create compression of the cortex beneath the plate and a bending moment in which tensile forces lead to distraction of the cortex opposite the plate (239,240). Therefore, only 17.4–21.6% of the total cross-sectional area of the bone is in actual contact (239,240). Rybicki and colleagues, using a finite-element analysis, predicted a 9% contact of the fracture surfaces for an oblique fracture treated with a compression plate (197). Stabilization with a compression plate is based upon local pressure and transmission of force between the implant and bone (176). In addition to friction between the implant and bone, friction between the fracture surfaces is also important. If a plate is placed on the tension side of the bone as a "tension band" and is applied with a "prebend", compression will tend to be applied to the cortex opposite the plate as well as to the cortex beneath the plate, resulting in greater bony contact and stability (176). If prebending and compression are used, a gap may occur on the cortex beneath the plate, but the potential gap on the cortex opposite the plate is closed (159). Prebending of the plate generates interfragmental friction in the opposite cortex, which results in increased torsional load stability. An increased rate of histologic union has been observed using prebending of the plate combined with compression as opposed to use of compression alone (159). Compression of any two surfaces produces friction that preloads the surfaces, keeping them in motionless coaptation. The friction generated by compression protects against the shearing forces generated by torsional stresses (173). In a transverse fracture, Rybicki noted that in the ideal compression-loading configuration 80% of the applied load was supported by the bone (196). He found that the cortex beneath the plate was protected from 75% of the applied stress, while the cortex opposite the plate was subjected to 1.5 times the applied stress value.

Adverse Effects of a Compression Plate

Adverse effects of the underlying bone have been observed in fractures treated with rigid compression plates. A major clinical concern is a diminution of bone strength according to Wolff's law due to stress protection of the bone by the plate. Spongious transformation of the cortex may occur beneath a compression plate because the rate of bone resorption exceeds the rate of bone formation. In experimental canine femoral fractures treated with rigid compression plates, Uhthoff and colleagues noted that there was osteopenia of the cortex beneath the plate, a reduction in shaft caliber, and persistent woven bone at the fracture site (Fig. 2-35) (226). Eighteen months after compression-plate fixation of forearm fractures, Mathews found satisfactory mineralization of the bone but also atrophy of cortical bone (143). In contrast, Stromberg felt that a decrease in bone mineral occurred beneath the plate with an increase in bone mineral proximal to the plate (213,214). A 50% decrease in thickness of the cortex from intracortical resorption and a 15% decrease in calcium content beneath the plate were observed in intact rabbit femora 17 weeks following application of an ASIF compression plate (165). A decrease in cortical thickness by 11.2% due to endosteal resorption and a 15.9% decrease in ash weight (mineral content) has been reported in unfractured canine femora following application of a compression plate for 7 months (165,166).

These changes in underlying bone have biomechanical consequences. Tonino and colleagues found a 17% decrease in bone mineral and a 30% decrease in mechanical strength in bending tests in intact canine femora treated with a steel AO compression plate as opposed to a plastic plate (218). A reduction in torque moment of 53% and angular deformation of 26.3% was observed after application of a rigid DCP plate to intact rabbit tibias with or without compression (167). Stromberg found a reduction in maximum torque capacity of 18% and maximum angle of torsion of 22% in plated bones compared with those in controls (213,214). Akeson and colleagues found that a bone treated with a compression plate showed no change in its mechanical properties, such as the ultimate bending strength or modulus of elasticity; but significant alterations were visible in the structural properties of the bone, such as the maximum bending load and energy absorption (2). They did not find

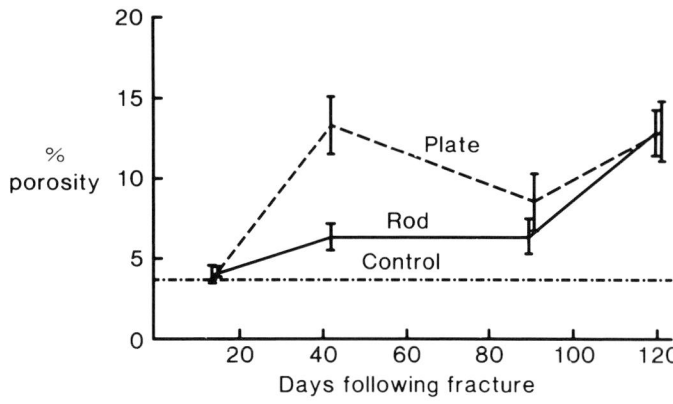

FIG. 2–35. Bone porosity following internal fixation of canine tibial fractures (183).

any change in the porosity of the bone but did find a thinning of the cortical wall.

In comparing plates with different degrees of stiffness and therefore rigidity of fixation, less adverse structural changes were noted with a less stiff plate (1,2). A 70% reduction of bone stress occurs near a steel plate and a 60% reduction of stress near a less stiff titanium plate (176). Double plating results in a marked reduction in bone strength (120). Woo and Akeson reported that a special composite plate with a low modulus of elasticity (i.e., stiffness) resulted in healed fractures that did not display any significant differences from controls upon biomechanical testing (243). However, Hutzschenreuter found that a thick (i.e., stiff) plate allowed bone union without resorption of the fragment ends and minimal callus, whereas a thin (i.e., less stiff) plate resulted in marked bone resorption and marked callus formation (104).

The effect of rigid plates on intact bone has also been investigated. Woo and colleagues noted a decrease in the structural properties of the bone due to thinning of the cortex, whereas mechanical properties remained unchanged from controls (243,247). Slatis and colleagues performed a study of the effect of the DCP plate on intact rabbit tibias. They found an increase in bone porosity within 3 weeks, and by 36 weeks resorption cavities occupied 40.6% of the cortex (211). A thinning of the cortical wall occurred along with an increase in the diameter of the bone. These changes in the bone were more marked in the cortex beneath the plate than in the opposite cortex. Similar morphologic changes occurred in the presence of a standard rigid plate or a compression plate. Slätis and colleagues concluded that the morphologic bone changes were a product of the rigid plate and were not influenced by compression (211). Application of a plate to intact bone also results in an acceleration of bone turnover rates (53). The addition of compression or distraction does not significantly change this effect of the plate. Bone porosity increases above control values regardless of the mode of plate application (53). The hydroxyproline content increases with a decrease in the calcium-hydroxyproline ratio, indicating active remodeling of bone tissue (164). Two explanations for the increase in porosity observed beneath a plate have been suggested: the porosity may reflect mechanical unloading or the remodeling process (173).

Since adverse structural changes occur in bone subjected to rigid internal fixation, the danger of bone refracture exists. Therefore, the timing of removal of the internal fixation device must be considered. Bone refracture may occur following plate fixation by two mechanisms (78). First, bone may fail at its weakest section. Second, local stress risers may be present near the fracture site. Stress risers include screw holes, which induce local stresses two to three times greater than those present in adjacent bone areas, and compact dense callus

with a different modulus of elasticity (Fig. 2-36) (78). Hutzschenreuter and colleagues reported early refracture of the bone at the end of the plate in an animal fixed with a rigid plate (104). They attributed the fracture to increased stress at the junction of the rigidly plated bone segment with the normal elastic bone. Stromberg cautioned concerning refracture after plate removal because the load distribution on the bone underlying the plate will suddenly alter (213). Since the bone will be unprepared to deal with the normal load, the possibility of refracture exists.

Convent believed that any implant material should be removed in younger persons and that removal should be carefully timed (50). An overly late removal might lead to refracture because of spongious transformation of the bone. However, he believed that a period of 1–2 years should elapse prior to plate removal, and a period of protected usage for 6–8 weeks should follow removal of the plate. Convent stated that the majority of refractures were due to screw holes acting as stress risers in the bone (50). Huys and colleagues stated that plates should be routinely removed only in athletes or children, or in cases in which they are symptomatic (105). If an implant is removed, the limb should be protected for a period of time to prevent refracture. In the lower extremity, the AO group recommends routine removal of the implant after 1–2 years because of stress protection of the bone by the implant (154).

In summary, the advantages of compression-plate fixation include rigid immobilization of the fracture and a decrease in the fracture gap. The regenerating blood sup-

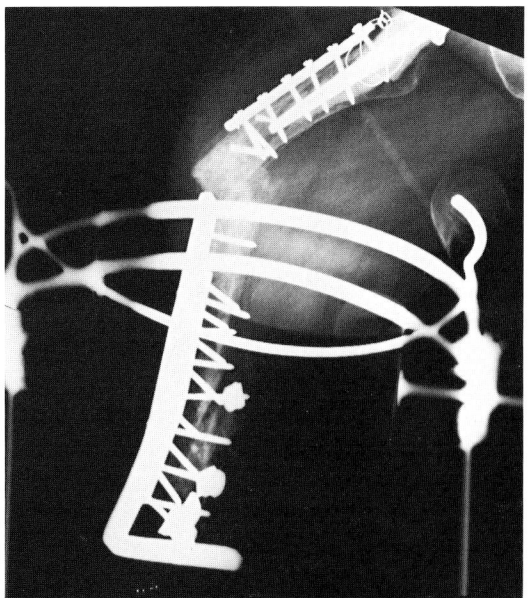

FIG. 2-36. Stress riser between two rigid plated segments of the femur. (From Rand JA, Ank N, Chao EYS, Kelly PJ. Biomechanical factors in fracture healing. *Minn Med* 1982;65:558.)

ply is protected, allowing primary bone healing across the fracture at an early time following injury. The disadvantages are local interference with the venous drainage of the bone, stress protection of the bone by the rigid implant, and the need for exposure of the bone with resultant disturbance of its blood supply and risk of infection.

Intramedullary Nail Fixation of Fractures

The technique of intramedullary nail fixation of fractures was used as early as 1897 by Nicolayson, in 1906 by Delbet, and in 1913 by Lambotte (232). The use of massive nails in the medullary cavity was introduced by Hey Groves in 1916 (232). A variety of materials were used for the early intramedullary nails, including ivory, bone, and metal, but they caused tissue reaction to the implant. Rush and Rush used a round Steinmann pin for intramedullary fixation in 1939 (174,195). However, intramedullary nail fixation was not popularized until the reports of Küntscher in the early 1940s. Since that time, many different designs of intramedullary nails have been devised and this method of fracture treatment is widely used (Fig. 2-37). The reports of Lauritzen and Watson-Jones give excellent historical reviews (131,232).

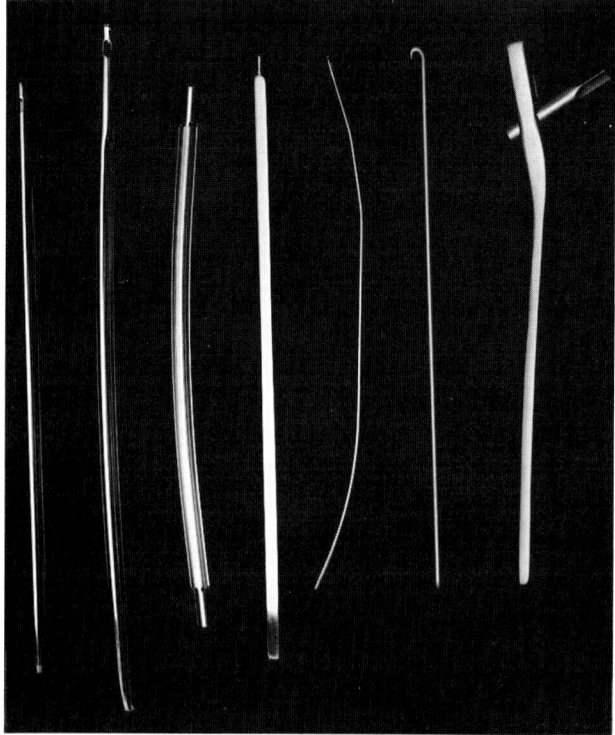

FIG. 2–37. Types of intramedullary nails. *Left to right:* Klintscher, ASIF, Sampson, Hansen-Street, Enders, Rush, Zickel.

Effect of an Intramedullary Nail on Bone-Blood Flow

The effect of an intramedullary nail on the blood supply of a healing fracture has been a source of concern and investigation. Trueta and Cavadais compared intramedullary nail-fixed and unfixed osteotomies of the radius in rabbits, in which the metaphyseal blood supply in each had been suppressed (223). The nutrient artery was never reconstructed in the nailed fractures, and necrosis of the marrow and inner one-third to two-thirds of the cortex occurred. Large portions of necrotic cortex persisted for up to 8 months following nailing. However, the number of small vessels at the fracture site appeared similar in both the nailed and unfixed fractures. The new vessels on the nailed side were derived from the periosteal circulation. Large quantities of periosteal callus but no endosteal callus formed on the nailed side. In contrast, large quantities of endosteal callus formed on the unfixed side. In spite of differences in vascularity and callus formation, delayed union did not occur in any of the nailed fractures.

Gothman studied intramedullary nailing of the tibia in rabbits (88). In unfractured tibias subjected to intramedullary nailing, active medullary vessels were noted to persist after introduction of the nail. One week following fracture and intramedullary nailing, the cortex showed evidence of a vascular reaction derived largely from the periosteal circulation and to a small extent from the persisting medullary arteries. The arterial reaction displayed a peak response between 2 and 4 weeks following nailing, with the majority of vessels being derived from the surrounding soft tissues. Minimal vascular reaction was noted from the medullary vessels. In tibial fractures in monkeys treated with intramedullary nail fixation, the vascular response was similar to the case of the rabbit, with vessels derived from the surrounding soft tissues being of major importance (87,88). Although segments of the medullary vessels remained patent via anastomoses with metaphyseal vessels, they frequently did not reach the fracture site. Callus formation largely followed the new vessels derived from the soft tissues.

Rhinelander studied the effect of loose- and tight-fitting intramedullary nails on fracture-site revascularization (187–190,192). In the presence of a loose-fitting intramedullary nail, the inner two-thirds to three-fourths of the cortex in contact with the nail became avascular. The outer one-third of the cortex remained vascularized by vessels derived from the periosteal circulation. Medullary vessels were regenerated in spaces surrounding the nail to revascularize the cortex. If medullary reaming was performed and a tight-fitting nail inserted, the cortex became devascularized except for areas of fascial attachments and a small external layer of the cortex. Revascularization occurred through a regenerative endosteal membrane formed around the nail, through the external callus at its junction with the cortex via the periosteal circulation, and through the substance of the cortex via regenerating nutrient vessels. Six weeks following intramedullary reaming and tight nailing, the significant component of the regenerative blood supply was derived from the medullary circulation. Since a tight nail results in almost total medullary blockage, regeneration of the nutrient vascular supply occurs through intracortical arteries.

Rhinelander also noted that intramedullary nailing delays fracture healing because nailing results in almost total devascularization of the fracture ends, damaging the medullary vessels, and also strips away the fascial attachments that carry the periosteal arterioles. In addition, an intramedullary nail inhibits the endosteal callus formation that is responsible for the area of earliest osseous union (189). Delayed union was observed frequently with a Küntscher nail, whereas union occurred earlier with a four-fluted Schneider nail. The nutrient artery was able to regenerate between the flutes, providing a more favorable situation for revascularization than the cloverleaf nail. Danckwardt-Lilliestrom and colleagues found that osteotomy plus intramedullary reaming resulted in total avascularity of the fracture ends (57). Initially, the normal centrifugal flow of blood through the cortex was replaced by a centripetal flow derived from the periosteal circulation. If stable fixation was maintained, revascularization occurred by way of longitudinally directed vessels penetrating through the cortex (the so-called *cutter head* formation), by connections with pre-existing intracortical vessels, by vessels surrounding the nail, and by vessels penetrating through the fracture gap. Immediate bone formation occurred in the fracture gap followed by remodeling of the fracture area by longitudinal secondary osteones.

The effects of intramedullary reaming have been studied (56,57,189). Intramedullary reaming, in the absence of fracture or nailing, almost completely destroys the medullary blood vessels of the diaphysis. Three days following reaming of the medullary cavity, from 10–60% of the cross-sectional area of the cortex is avascular (57). High intramedullary pressures of up to 300 mg of Hg are generated during reaming, resulting in fat embolization into the cortex that obstructs the intracortical vessels. Some marrow is forced subperiosteally, resulting in increased periosteal new bone formation (56). However, if low intramedullary pressures are maintained during reaming by applying a negative pressure to the medullary cavity, intracortical fat embolism may be minimized, allowing more rapid bone revascularization (58).

Morphologic Findings in Union through Intramedullary Nail Fixation

Morphologic studies of fracture union have revealed several differences between nailed and unfixed fractures.

In nailed fractures, Fitts and colleagues found extensive periosteal callus at a distance from the fracture site (76). Maximum callus at the fracture site was greater in the unfixed than in the nailed fractures. However, callus appeared earlier and union occurred more rapidly in the nailed fractures. They concluded that the immobilization provided by the nail was the factor determining more rapid union in the nailed group. Sharma and Kumar noted greater periosteal callus formation in unfixed than in nailed fractures (204). Nailed fractures united by periosteal callus because the nail blocked endosteal callus formation. Union generally occurred by endochondral ossification, but one fracture, in which rigid fixation was maintained, displayed union by direct bone formation. In fractures treated with an intramedullary nail, Rhinelander found that greater periosteal callus formed when rotation was not controlled compared with fractures with rotational stability (191). Anderson and colleagues noted excessive periosteal new bone formation with sequestration of the cortical fracture ends and delayed union in the presence of a loose intramedullary nail. Union occurred by endochondral ossification (9). In the presence of a tight intramedullary nail, there was less periosteal new bone formation, minimal cortical bone resorption, and rapid fracture union. Union occurred by direct bone formation. Anderson concluded that the insertion of an intramedullary nail is basically unsound physiologically because it destroys the medullary blood supply and prevents endosteal callus formation (8). Varma and Mehta found that union was delayed in nailed fractures when compared with unfixed fractures (230). However, union occurred more rapidly in nailed fractures with secure fixation than in fractures without adequate fixation. In the presence of stable fixation, union occurred by direct bone formation. In the presence of unstable fixation, union occurred by endochondral ossification. They stressed the importance of stable intramedullary fixation.

In clinical studies, Küntscher recognized that endosteal callus was inhibited by the intramedullary nail and that union occurred by more extensively formed periosteal callus (124). Küntscher believed that periosteal callus was most important for fracture repair (126). He believed that even complete destruction of the endosteum during intramedullary nailing did not prevent fracture union. In experimental studies in dogs, he noted that endosteal callus completely encircled the intramedullary nail (126). The technique of closed intramedullary nailing was developed to avoid damaging the periosteum, which might interfere with periosteal callus formation. In an extensive review of clinical material, Lauritzen was unable to find evidence of more rapid or delayed callus formation due to intramedullary nailing (131). Rhinelander stated that an intramedullary nail always results in a delay in fracture healing because it limits the formation of the medullary bridging callus that is responsible for the earliest osseous union (189). Union is effected by periosteal bridging callus that requires an abundance of extraosseous blood supply. Since stripping of the periosteum and fascial attachments from the fracture ends may occur at the time of injury or surgery, revascularization of the fracture site may be delayed.

Danckwardt-Lilliestrom studied the effect of intramedullary reaming on the healing of a cortical defect (56). When the medullary cavity was intact, the defect was rapidly bridged and filled by woven bone. However, if the medullary cavity had been destroyed by intramedullary reaming, the defect was bridged by periosteal callus, which occurred at a later time than if the medullary cavity were intact.

Biomechanics of Intramedullary Nail Fixation

Biomechanical evaluation of intramedullary nails and the mechanical aspects of nail fixation have been performed. Küntscher believed that the basic principle of stable intramedullary fixation was flexible impingement of the nail in the bone (124). Reaming of the canal might be necessary to achieve stable fixation. Küntscher stated that a nail must be strong enough to resist the stresses caused by muscle contraction, joint movement, and weight bearing. It must have sufficient elasticity to be compressed during insertion and to re-expand once in place, both to prevent rotation of the fracture and to fill the medullary cavity if bone resorption occurs around the nail (125). Küntscher believed that a V-profile or cloverleaf pattern best fit these criteria. The intramedullary nail has been suggested as a favorable method of fixation because the nail absorbs shearing and bending stress but allows compressive stress across the fracture line (126). Lauritzen believed that a good nail should have flexibility to allow oblique insertion in curved bones, strength to provide fracture stability, and resistance against corrosion (131). The thickness of the nail should not be so large that the nail becomes inflexible, which would increase the risk of impaction.

One of the difficulties with intramedullary nails has been the bending and breaking of the implant. Intramedullary reaming was introduced to allow the use of larger, stronger nails, as well as to improve contract between the nail and the bone. An 11-mm Küntscher nail has twice the resistance to bending as a 9-mm nail (238). The strength of a nail depends not only on its design but also on its orientation in the bone and the mode of testing (4). A diamond-shaped or Schneider nail is more rigid in torsion than a Küntscher nail, although a Küntscher nail is stronger in bending. Placing the slot of the Küntscher nail on the tension side of the bone results in greater strength than placing the slot on the compression side. The "working length" of the nail (that portion of the nail crossing the fracture between the two areas of contact in the proximal and distal fracture fragments) affects the rigidity of fixation (4). The stiffness in bending and torsional rigidity are inversely proportional to the working length. Doubling the working length will halve the rigidity in torsion.

The most recently developed intramedullary nail is a fluted nail that is extremely rigid and provides rotational control. Allen and colleagues stated that the fluted nail was designed to overcome the following difficulties of conventional nails: too much flexibility for optimum healing; poor torsional load transmission; poor fixation of the nail in the intramedullary canal; and an appreciable incidence of non-union, malunion, and implant failure if the canal is not reamed to the larger sizes (3). This nail has greater bending rigidity and bending strength than conventional nails and provides significant torsional rigidity, which no other nail provides. However, the bending stiffness of this nail remains 25% less than that of the femur. The stiffness of the nail allows three-point fixation with a secure fit even if the canal is reamed to a larger diameter than the nail. The rigidity of fixation with the fluted nail is approached only by dual-compression plating.

Comparative biomechanical evaluation of the quality of fracture union in either unfixed fractures or fractures fixed with an intramedullary nail was performed by Falkenberg (75). A linear increase in the tensile strength of both the nailed and unfixed fractures occurred beginning on the tenth day following fracture. In the initial phases of healing, the nailed fractures were stronger than the unfixed fractures. This was attributed to the improved stability of the nailed fractures. After the fortieth day following fracture, the absolute tensile strength of the unnailed fracture was greater than the nailed fracture, and, by the sixtieth day, the difference was highly significant ($p < 0.001$). Callus formation was 25% less in the nailed than in the unfixed fractures 30 days following fracture, and a marked retardation of endosteal callus was noted in the nailed fractures. When adjustments for cross-sectional area were made, the strength of the nailed fractures remained less than that of the unfixed fractures.

Complications of Intramedullary Nailing

Many complications of intramedullary nailing have been reported. Reported complications include infection, impaction of the nail, impaction of the guide wire, vascular injury, neural injury, distraction of the fracture, splintering of bone, migration of the nail, penetration of the joint by the nail, bending of the nail, failure to engage the distal fragment, radiation burns, delayed union, nonunion, bursitis around the protruding portion of the nail, and fat embolism. Böhler believed that most complications were related to use of too thick, thin, short, or long a nail (26). Dencker reported the complications encountered in open intramedullary nailing in 432 fractures of the femur (63). Technical errors were encountered in 14% of the cases, with too short a nail as the most frequent error. Complications included inadequate fixation in 5.7%, nail impaction in 5.5%, splintering of the femur in 1.4%, penetration of the joint by the nail in 0.7%, and failure to engage the distal fragment in 0.5% of the cases. The incidence of infection following intramedullary nailing has been estimated at 5% (232). Refracture following intramedullary nailing may occur. Convent stated that the risk of refracture over a 10-year period was 1% in nail-fixed fractures compared with 5% with plate-fixed fractures (50). Böhler believed that an intramedullary nail inhibited callus formation and therefore that nail removal should be delayed for at least 1 year to minimize the risk of refracture (26). Huys and colleagues noted that osteoporosis due to stress protection of the bone occurs with intramedullary nail fixation as well as with plate fixation (108).

In summary, intramedullary nail fixation has proved useful in the clinical treatment of fractures. However, intramedullary nailing and reaming damage the nutrient vessels and medullary circulation as well as inhibit endosteal callus formation. Rotational stability is a problem with nails other than the new fluted nail. In the presence of secure fixation with an intramedullary nail, union with primary bone healing may occur.

Comparisons of Intramedullary Nail and Plate Fixation of Fractures

Few comparisons between intramedullary nail and plate fixation of experimental fractures have been reported. Barron and colleagues studied blood flow and fracture healing in osteotomies of the ulna in dogs treated with either a standard plate or an intramedullary Steinmann pin (14). At 14 days following fracture, they found that fracture-site blood flow was greater on the plate side, whereas whole-bone blood flow was greater on the nail side. At 14 days, new bone formation was greater on the plate than the nail side. However, at 90 days following fracture, there was no difference in blood flow, new bone formation, or fracture union between the two sides. Barron and colleagues concluded that an intramedullary nail decreases blood flow to a fracture site and that plate fixation results in increased quantities of endosteal and periosteal new bone. Therefore, they believed that a plate was a more physiologically sound method of fixation than an intramedullary nail (14).

Mihula compared the intramedullary nail to plate fixation in osteotomies of the canine radius (148). Revascularization of plate-fixed fractures occurred by medullary vessels, while nail-fixed fractures were revascularized both by medullary vessels and by vessels derived from the periosteal system and soft tissues. The most rapid

union occurred in the fractures treated with a plate. He concluded that plate fixation was the more physiologically sound mode of internal fixation. Rhinelander, on the other hand, noted that both plates and intramedullary nails have an adverse effects on fracture-site revascularization (192). He stated that the cortex beneath a tightly applied plate becomes avascular and the endosteum in contact with a tight-fitting intramedullary nail becomes avascular.

Reynolds and Key compared healing of canine femoral osteotomies treated with standard plates, slotted Eggers plates, and intramedullary nails (185). They noted an inhibition of endosteal callus formation by the intramedullary nail. If the nail fixation was secure, only a small quantity of periosteal callus formed; but if the nail was loose, large quantities of periosteal callus formed. Union occurred most rapidly in the fractures treated with the Eggers plate. However, they concluded that if approximation and continued immobilization of the bone ends was achieved, union would occur in approximately the same time regardless of the type of internal fixation employed (64).

Gustilo and colleagues compared intramedullary nail and plate fixation in femoral osteotomies in the dog (91). On the nail side, avascularity of almost the entire diaphyseal cortex occurred, with cortical necrosis persisting for 6 to 12 weeks following fracture. The nailed fracture displayed marked periosteal proliferation and an inhibition of endosteal callus formation. Union occurred within 3 months on the plate side compared with 6 months on the nail side.

Braden and Brinker studied healing of canine femoral osteotomies fixed with an intramedullary pin alone, an intramedullary pin plus a one-half Kirschner wire (to control rotation), and a compression plate (31). Fractures treated with a plate displayed less callus, earlier revascularization, and earlier union than fractures treated with the other methods of fixation. The overall success rate was 91% with the plate (one plate loosened owing to screw failure), 100% with the intramedullary pins plus a one-half Kirschner wire, and 64% with the intramedullary pin alone. They concluded that plate fixation was the best mode of treatment. A comparative study of fractures of the radius in rabbits treated with either an intramedullary nail or a subperiosteal plate or left unfixed did not reveal any significant differences in return of mechanical strength as evidenced by a four-point bending test (198). Fracture stiffness returned more rapidly than strength.

Anderson compared various methods of fracture treatment in canine femoral osteotomies (7). The femora treated without fixation displayed a large quantity of callus. Delayed union and non-union occurred frequently. In the presence of a loose-fitting intramedullary nail that did not control rotation, necrosis of the fracture ends occurred, a large quantity of periosteal callus formed, and endosteal callus was severely inhibited. Healing occurred by endochondral ossification, with delayed union and non-union occurring frequently. In the presence of a tight-fitting intramedullary nail, little periosteal or endosteal callus formed. Union occurred by direct primary bone formation at the fracture site. Fractures treated with a standard noncompression plate displayed moderate periosteal callus and a large quantity of endosteal callus. Union occurred by cartilaginous endosteal callus. The fractures treated with compression plates united with minimal periosteal callus, a large quantity of endosteal callus, and direct primary bone formation. Therefore, union occurred by direct bone formation in the tight-fitting intramedullary nail group and the compression-plate group. In both groups, rigid immobilization of the fracture was present.

Comparative biomechanical evaluation of the quality of fixation provided by intramedullary nails and plates was performed by Laurence and colleagues (129). Küntscher intramedullary nails provided greater bending stiffness than any onlay plate but were unable to provide rotational stiffness. Addition of a keel to the nail did not significantly improve torsional resistance. Biomechanical evaluation of the quality of bone union after either intramedullary nail or plate fixation was performed by Braden and colleagues (32). Upon torsional testing 10 weeks following fracture, the fractures fixed with an intramedullary pin plus a one-half Kirschner wire to control rotation has regained 80.2% of the control value for ultimate strength. The group fixed with only an intramedullary pin regained 61.9%, and the plate group regained 36% of the control value for ultimate strength. A significant difference ($p < 0.01$) was noted between the intramedullary pin combined with a one-half Kirschner wire group and the plate group. Bra-

den and colleagues attributed the lower strength of the plate group to stress protection of the bone by the plate.

Rand and colleagues compared open intramedullary nailing after reaming and compression-plate fixation with regard to fracture-site blood flow, rate of fracture union, and biomechanical quality of fracture union (183). The rod-fixed side displayed significantly higher whole-bone and fracture-site blood flow (Fig. 2-38). Significantly more endosteal new bone was present on the plate side than on the rod side, while more periosteal new bone was seen on the rod side rather than the plate side (Fig. 2-39). There was a general tendency for the rod side to display a less mature biomechanical stage of union than the plate side at all three time interval studies (Fig. 2-40). The conclusion from this study was that fractures fixed with an intramedullary rod displayed higher values for a longer time for bone blood flow than do those fractures fixed by a rigid plate. The high, prolonged blood flow on the rod side may reflect a compensatory mechanism to increase blood flow to bone because the medullary circulation is blocked by the intramedullary rod (183). The delay in biomechanical maturation of a rod-fixed fracture may reflect an inhibition of endosteal callus formation rather than an effect upon bone blood flow (183).

The appropriate management of the fracture with failed internal fixation depends upon identifying the reasons for failure, whether mechanical or biologic. Secondary surgical intervention must obtain adequate mechanical stability while minimizing adverse biologic consequences. Karlstrom and Olerud have studied the biologic effects of secondary internal fixation (112). They studied the effects of primary plate fixation followed by intramedullary nailing after reaming in osteotomies of the rabbit tibia. They then compared these re-

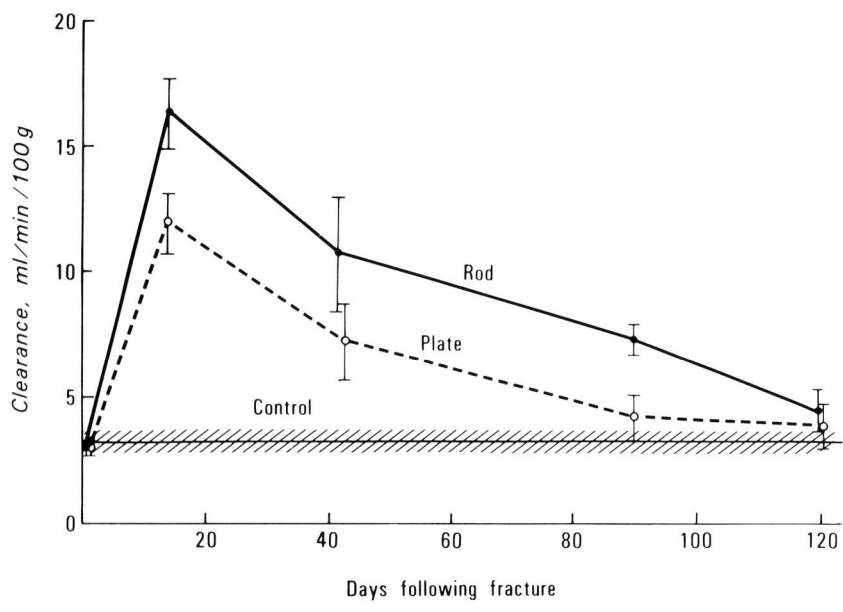

FIG. 2-38. Increased blood flow on the rod-fixed side of a canine tibial fracture as opposed to the plate-fixed side (183).

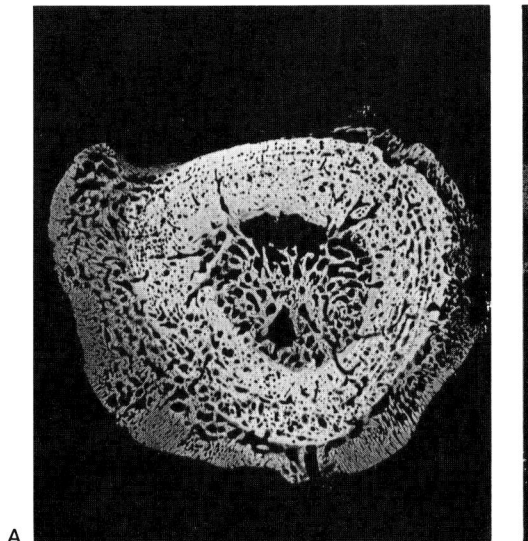 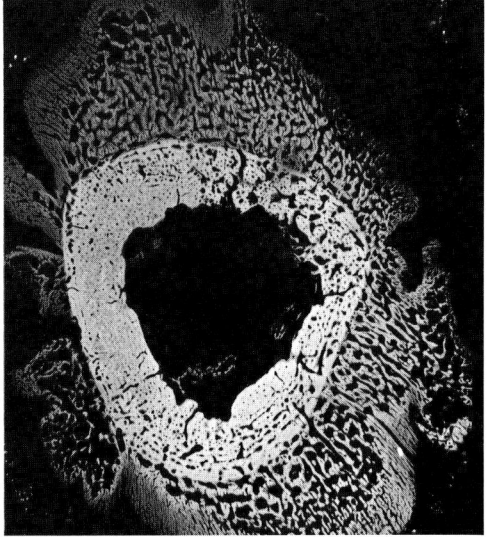

FIG. 2–39. A: Moderate periosteal and extensive endosteal callus seen in a transverse section of a 90-day plate-fixed canine tibial fracture. **B:** Extensive periosteal callus and minimal endosteal callus seen in a transverse section of a 90-day rod-fixed canine tibial fracture (183).

sults with primary intramedullary nailing after reaming followed by secondary plate fixation. The vascular damage of each procedure was not additive. The reparative process of revascularization following the first operation limited the area of cortical avascularity after the second operation. They concluded that in clinical practice secondary internal fixation by an intramedullary nail was preferable to a plate because it protected against refracture of the bone owing to cancellous transformation of the bone.

The clinical correlation of these studies is evident. The requirements for fracture healing include accurate reduction and close contact of the fracture fragments, an adequate blood supply, the presence of osteogenic cells, and stability of the fracture site. If internal fixation of a fracture is performed, accurate reduction, close contact, and stability may be obtained. However, the internal fixation will significantly alter bone blood flow with possible adverse consequences on fracture healing. One should avoid excessive internal fixation with damage to periosteal and endosteal vascular supplies, as non-union may result.

External Fixation

External fixation is in frequent use for stabilizing fractures (Fig. 2-41). Indications for external fixation include open fractures, severely unstable comminuted fractures, infected non-unions, arthrodesis, and leg

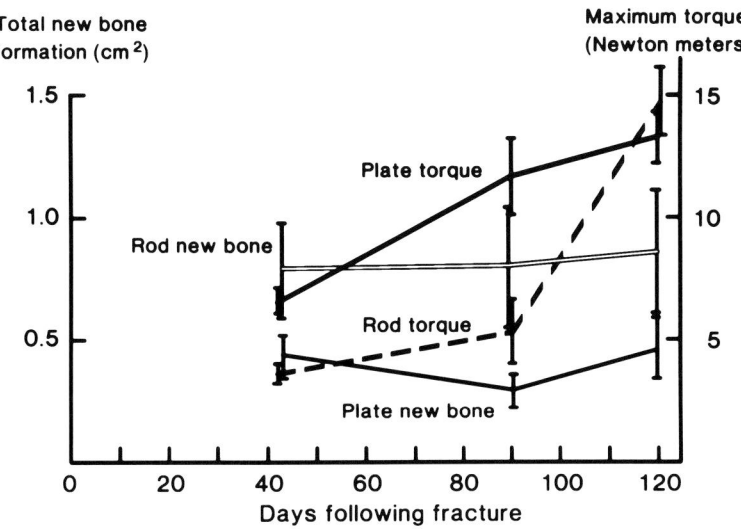

FIG. 2–40. Increased strength of a plate-fixed compared to a rod-fixed canine tibial fracture at 42 and 90 days despite greater new bone formation on the rod side (183).

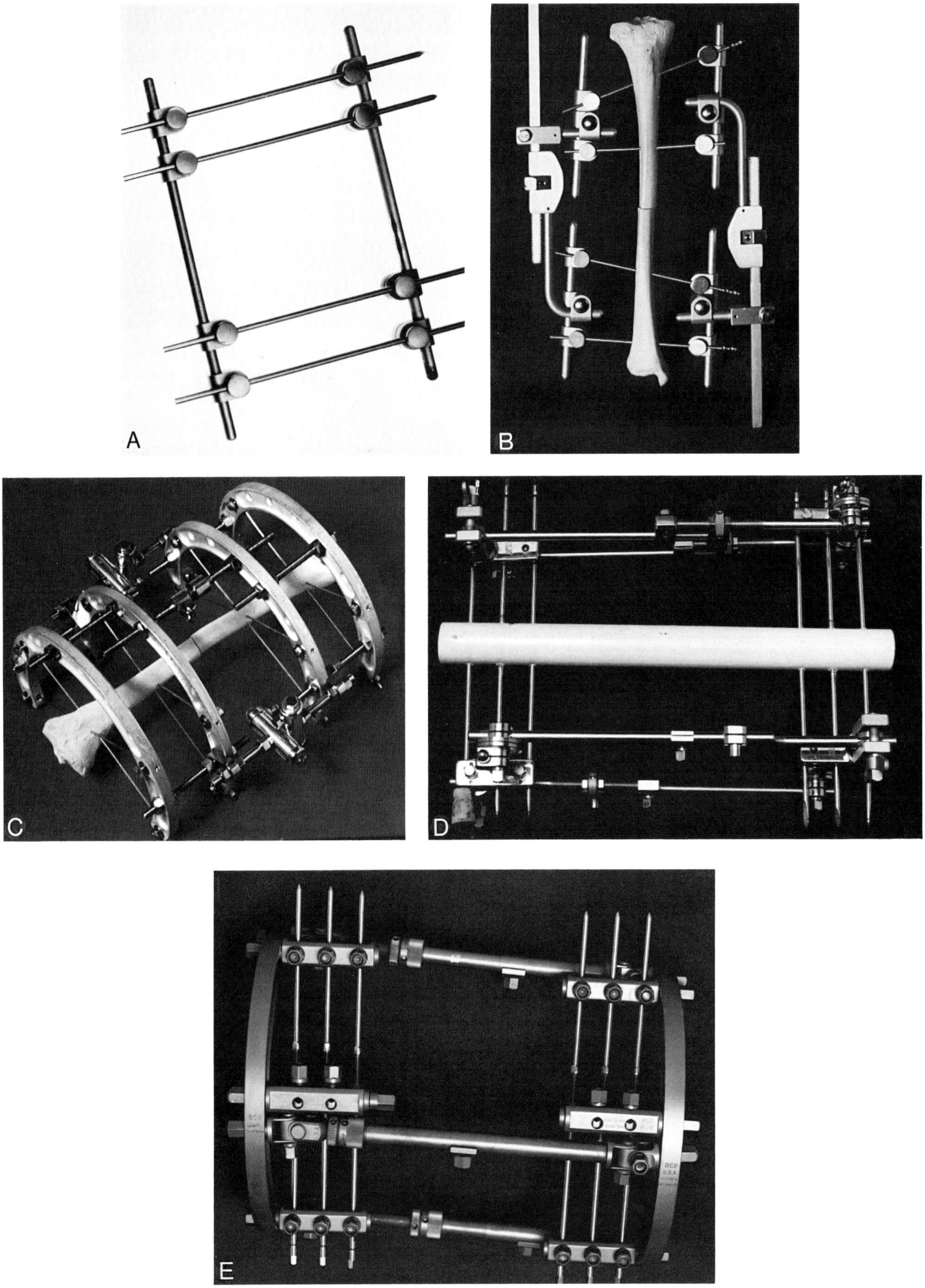

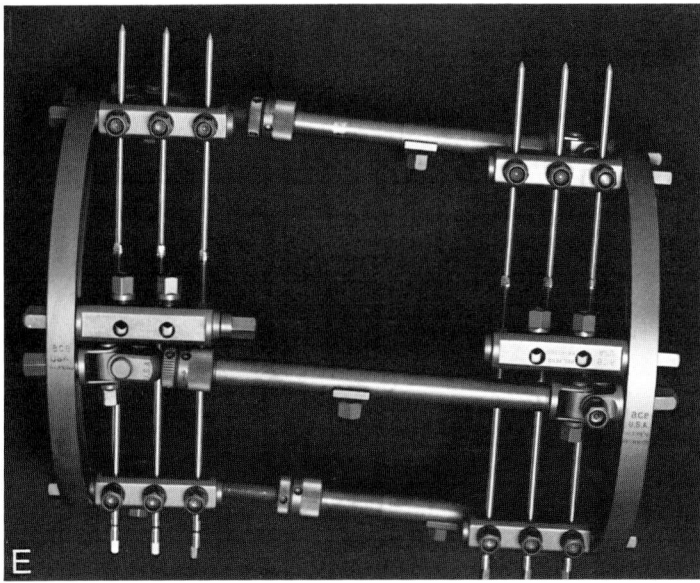

FIG. 2–41. External fixation devices. **A:** Original Roger-Anderson; **B:** new Roger-Anderson allowing compression of fracture surfaces; **C:** Volkov-Oganision device; **D:** Hoffman quadralateral frame; **E:** Fischer apparatus.

lengthening. External fixation is advantageous in that it requires minimal operative trauma for application, is remote from the fracture, requires a minimum of foreign material, and is adjustable after application. External fixation also allows wound care, preserves joint motion, and provides mobilization of the patient. However, complications of pin loosening, pin infection, and neurovascular injury may occur (90). The majority of reports concerning external fixation of fractures are clinical with little scientific basis.

Yamagishi and Yoshimura studied rabbit tibial fractures treated with external fixation using varying mechanical conditions (247). For optimal healing, moderate intermittent compression was the preferred mechanical environment. Laurin and colleagues studied a similar model, using pins and plaster supplemented by an intramedullary pin (130). They found three phases in fracture healing: (1) hematoma with instability; (2) periosteal callus formation with increasing strength; and (3) endosteal callus that provided little additional stability. They concluded that compression did not hasten callus formation (130). A comparison between cast immobilization and unilateral single-sidebar external fixation in rabbit tibial osteotomies revealed increased blood flow at 7 weeks on the cast-immobilized side (52). The relative rigidity of the fixation was felt to decrease the tendency to form callus and thus to lessen the need for blood supply (52).

A comparison of unilateral external fixation and compression-plate fixation in canine tibial osteotomies revealed less rigid fixation with the external fixation device (135). The less rigid external fixation correlated with a persistently elevated blood flow and less mature biomechanical strength (135). In another study, the effect of varying rigidity of external fixation devices was analyzed using a canine tibial-fracture model (246). The less rigid external fixation resulted in an increased periosteal callus and increased bone porosity but no difference in bone blood flow or mechanical strength (246). Finally, cyclic loading has been compared with constant compression using external fixation in rabbit tibial osteotomies (168,241). The cyclic compression-treated bones exhibited improved mechanical strength and a 27% saving in healing time compared with the constant-compression group (168,241).

Mechanical monitoring of fracture healing has also been performed in fractures treated with external fixation devices. In sheep tibial osteotomies, there was an initial slow decrease followed by a rapid decrease in the ability to displace the fracture upon stress (109). The changes in mechanical properties were attributed to progressive mineralization of the fracture callus (109). Jorgenson has used a similar technique to study healing human tibial fractures treated with external fixation (111). Five different shapes of healing curves were found and could be related to the type of fracture, extent of weight

bearing by the patient, and quality of treatment. He felt that this technique was applicable to determine the appropriate time for weight bearing and removal of the external device (111). Burny identified eight types of deformation curves in healing human tibial fractures (41). He recognized three segments in the healing of a fracture treated with external fixation. There was an initial increase in mobility during the first 3 weeks related to resorption of the bone ends. Next, there was a decrease in mobility related to interfragmentary union. Finally, a plateau level was reached, in which the mechanical properties of the callus were approximately 50% that of normal bone (41).

In summary, although external fixation is in frequent use, additional information is required in order to determine the optimal external-fixation configuration, mode of application, and duration of use. Mechanical monitoring of the fracture site may prove to be a useful technique for assessing the appropriate timing for weight bearing and removal of the external device. Monitoring can also be used for demonstrating problems in fracture union at a time that will allow early intervention by the treating physician.

Imaging of Orthopedic Fixation Devices

Physicians who are not familiar with the indications for their use and appearance of orthopedic fixation devices (see Figs. 2-34, 2-37, and 2-41) may find evaluation of radiographs and other imaging modalities difficult to interpret. Tables 2-6 and 2-7 list the commonly used orthopedic devices and indications for operative therapy (193).

Routine radiographs provide the basis for following the healing process and for noting any problems with fixation devices in most areas. On occasion computed tomography, conventional tomography, or radionuclide studies are required to evaluate subtle changes, specifically retarded healing and/or infection (65,123). MRI has limited utility, especially with high-field imagers (≥1.0 Tesla) due to the significant artifact created by certain fixation devices (see "Magnetic Resonance Imaging", Chapter 1) (23).

TABLE 2-6. *Indications for operative fixation**

Operative fixation is employed
1. When closed methods have failed.
2. When experience dictates that closed methods will fail.
3. When articular surfaces are fractured and displaced.
4. When a fracture is due to tumor metastasis or such a fracture appears imminent.
5. When there is associated neurovascular injury.
6. When multiple injuries are present.
7. When continued confinement to bed is undesirable.
8. When the cost of treatment may be substantially reduced.

* From 193, with permission.

TABLE 2–7. *Classification of fixation devices**

Internal		External
Wire	Intramedullary fixation	Tibia
Cerclage wiring	Reamed nails	Radius
Tension band wiring	Standard (Kuntscher)	Pelvis
Parham bands	Interlocking	
Screws and plates	Unreamed nails	
Screws	Rush	
Cortical	Ender's	
Cancellous	Huckenthal	
Plates	Lottes	
Dynamic compression plate	Pins and wires	
Blade plate	Knowles pins	
Buttress plates multiple (by	Hagey pins	
anatomic location)	Steinman pins	
	Kirschner wires	
Dynamic hip screw	Spinal fixation	
	Harrington rods	
	Luque rods	
	Dwyer device	
	Zielke device	

* From 193, with permission.

Certain basic concepts can be applied to evaluating fixation devices on routine radiographs. Obviously, serial radiographs are essential to evaluate changes in fracture fragments (see Fig. 2-23) and change in the position of the fixation devices (Fig. 2-42). At least two views, typically AP and lateral, are required. The entire fixation device and preferrably the entire long bone with articulations should be included on the film (193). Consistent exposure factors and positioning are equally important on each follow-up study (193,198).

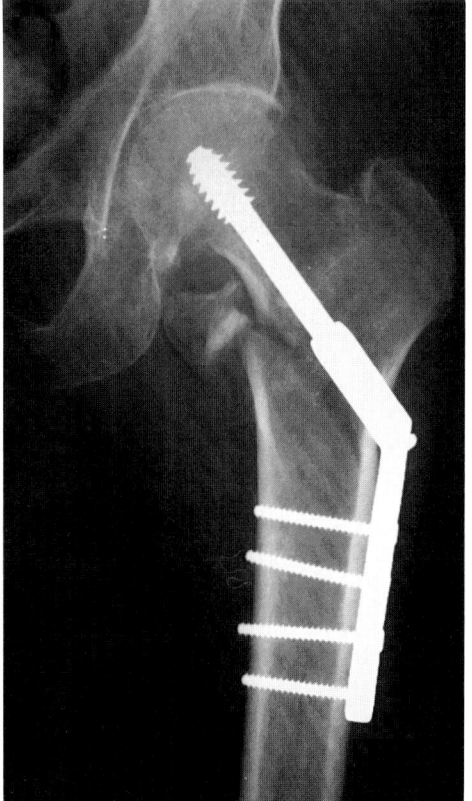
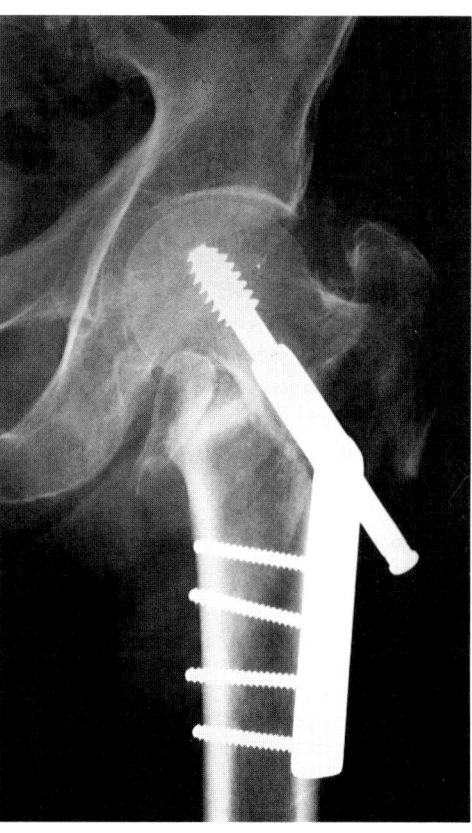

A   B

FIG. 2–42. A: Comminuted subtrochanteric fracture reduced with a dynamic sliding screw and side plate. **B:** Several weeks later the reduction has failed with lateral displacement of the upper fragments and marked shortening of the screw. Note the cortical screws in the side plate are well positioned through both cortices.

When compression plates and screws are used, it is important to note the initial position of the device, especially the screws. Most screws in a given plate should pass through both cortices to achieve adequate fixation. Screws or pins (Knowles pins) used near articular surfaces should not penetrate the articular surface. Multiple oblique views or fluoroscopic positioning may be necessary to detect subtle articular penetration (199).

Medullary nails are commonly used for fixation (191,198) of long bone shaft fractures. These devices may be fixed with interlocking screws to prevent rotation of fragments and assist in maintaining reduction.

External fixation devices are generally used for reduction of comminuted or open fractures. These devices (see Fig. 2-23) are not difficult to evaluate on images. However, positioning for radiographs can be hindered by these bulky fixateurs. Radiographs should be evaluated to be certain that the threaded portion of the pins are intracortical. Fracture of the pins or fracture fragment motion needs to be evaluated. Pin tract infections and thermal necrosis of adjacent bone have also been reported. Infection is difficult to evaluate when the pin is in place. Ring sequestra have been described in pin tracts after pin removal. Thermal necrosis causes sclerosis adjacent to the pin tract (84,144,157,193).

FRACTURE UNION AND NON-UNION

Definition of Union and Non-union

One of the most difficult decisions facing the clinician is the determination of fracture union. Union may be defined in many ways. Clinically, union may occur when there is no local tenderness and the fractured bone ends can no longer be moved by the examining physician. Union may also be defined as the time when the individual is able to bear full weight with or without aids. The problem with both of these definitions of clinical union is that a firm fibrocartilaginous union can prevent motion between the fractured bone ends and allow weight bearing even when true bony union has not occurred. While a fracture does not obtain adequate strength without bone bridging and fracture remodeling, clinical weight bearing can occur when the fracture has regained only approximately 50% of the strength of normal bone. Thus clinical union frequently precedes radiographic union and may be present as early as 6–8 weeks after injury (233). Therefore, although clinical union is useful in deciding treatment options such as time of weight bearing, it is inadequate as an end point for following the patient's fracture.

Union may also be defined radiographically. Is bridging callus across a fracture an adequate end point for deciding union? How much callus should be present? Does the presence of a fracture line affect the decision regarding union? Even with radiographic information, many questions can be raised regarding the end point for union. Unfortunately, fixed criteria that are applicable to all situations are difficult to define. Complete obliteration of the fracture line with evidence of fracture remodeling is a strict criterion for union. For practical purposes, a fracture with bridging callus surrounding 50% of the fracture site with no pain or motion on clinical testing may be considered united. However, such fracture strength, although adequate for function without external splintage, may be inadequate for vigorous sports activities without a risk of refracture. Fracture remodeling with obliteration of the fracture line is essential for optimal mechanical strength. Thus, stating a standard time for fracture union for even a specific bone with a single fracture type is difficult (233). Only the minimal period can be defined and fixed. The rate of union is never constant. It is affected by a variety of biologic variables.

Non-union may be easier to define. One must consider the definition of delayed union, non-union, and pseudarthrosis. A delayed union occurs when a fracture has not united at the average time for the location and type of fracture (33). It is important to specify the type of fracture in deciding upon the definition of a delayed union (Fig. 2-43). A nondisplaced transverse fracture without comminution may be expected to heal more rapidly than a severely displaced comminuted fracture in the same location. A non-union exists when the repair process has completely stopped and union will not occur without surgical intervention (33). The term *pseudarthrosis* is often used synonymously with the term *non-union*. A more limited and perhaps more accurate usage would limit use of the term *pseudarthrosis* to a true synovial-lined cavity, the synovial pseudarthrosis. The distinction between fibrous tissue interposition and a true synovial pseudarthrosis is important. Electrical stimulation as a treatment method has a high failure rate in the presence of a synovial pseudarthrosis (34,73). The AO group has divided non-unions into two types: hypertrophic and avascular (154). The distinction is based upon radiographic appearance and the need for bone grafting to obtain union.

Etiologic Factors in the Pathogenesis of Non-union

The etiologic factors contributing to failure of fracture union may be considered as either systemic or local (Table 2-8). Systemic factors of importance include nutritional level, age, endocrine status, and medications. While nutrition is not really a significant problem in the United States, severe vitamin deficiencies, especially of A, C, and D, can alter fracture healing (97). Fractures tend to heal more slowly in the elderly than in the young. Endocrine abnormalities such as hypothyroidism can lead to a delay in fracture union (119). Systemic treat-

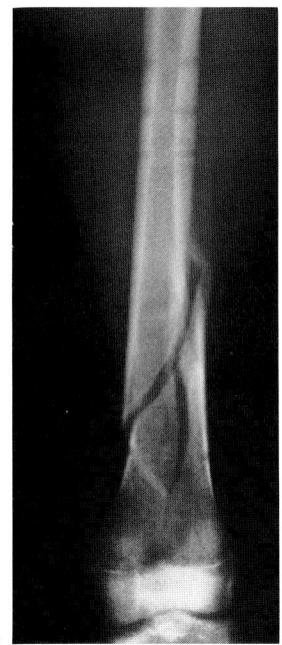
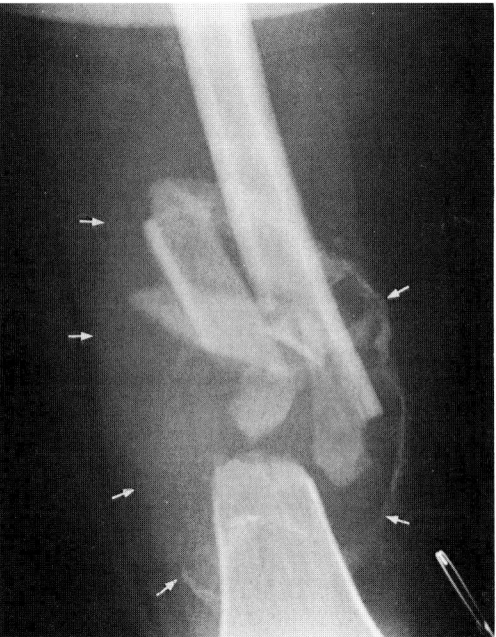
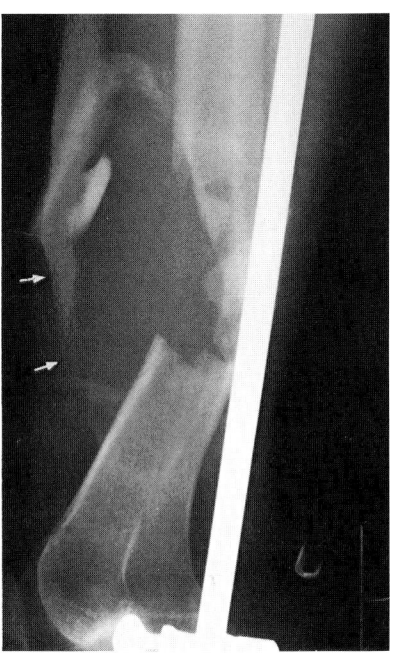

FIG. 2-43. A: Early union of a non-displaced spiral fracture of the femur. AP **(B)** and lateral **(C)** radiographs of a comminuted femoral fracture with callus forming in the large hematoma (*arrows*).

ment with diphosphonate for Paget's disease may lead to delayed mineralization and thus to a delay of union of normal bone that has sustained a fracture. Systemic metabolic bone disease may result in poor fracture healing due to inadequate mechanical strength but usually does not lead to a delayed rate of union.

Local factors are of much greater importance than systemic factors in the pathogenesis of non-union. Local factors of importance are displacement of bone ends, open fractures, infection, comminution with loss of bone substance, inadequate fixation, insufficient time, inappropriate surgical intervention, persistent angulation, inadequate blood supply, segmental fracture, soft tissue interposition, and distraction (33,97,233).

Distraction of the fracture ends allows fibrous tissue ingrowth and interposition of soft tissues, which mechanically interfere with bridging callus (93). Distraction may also lead to tension at the fracture site that impedes

bone formation (18). By preventing bone contact, distraction leads to inadequate immobilization. The converse of distraction, compression, leads to close bony contact and improved immobilization (59,60).

The importance of an adequate blood supply for fracture healing has been well emphasized (205). In the segmental or displaced fracture, the endosteal blood supply to the fracture site has been disrupted (192). This leads to a delayed rate of revascularization and subsequent union. Motion at the fracture site from inadequate immobilization may disrupt the initial endosteal vessels attempting to bridge the fracture site (97). Ill-performed open reduction and internal fixation may further disrupt the blood supply and provide insufficient stability to allow healing.

The advantages of open reduction in obtaining close contact and anatomic alignment must be weighed against the increased soft tissue damage incurred and the risk of infection. If internal fixation is chosen, an excellent reduction and stable internal fixation must be achieved. Displacement and comminution of the fracture as well as the soft tissue damage associated with an open fracture probably contribute to non-union by interfering with the local blood supply to the fracture (97). Jackson and MacNab correlated the time to union with the extent of displacement in tibial fractures (106). They found that fractures with minimal displacement healed in 4 months, whereas those with marked displacement frequently were not united before 6 months. Eighty-six percent of the closed tibial fractures united within 6 months, as compared with 66% of the open fractures (106). The type of fracture correlates with the time to

TABLE 2-8. *Factors affecting fracture healing*

Systemic	Local
Nutrition	Displacement
Age	Open or closed fracture
Endocrine status	Infection
Medication	Comminution
	Quality of fixation
	Surgical intervention
	Angulation
	Blood supply
	Soft tissue interposition
	Distraction
	Time

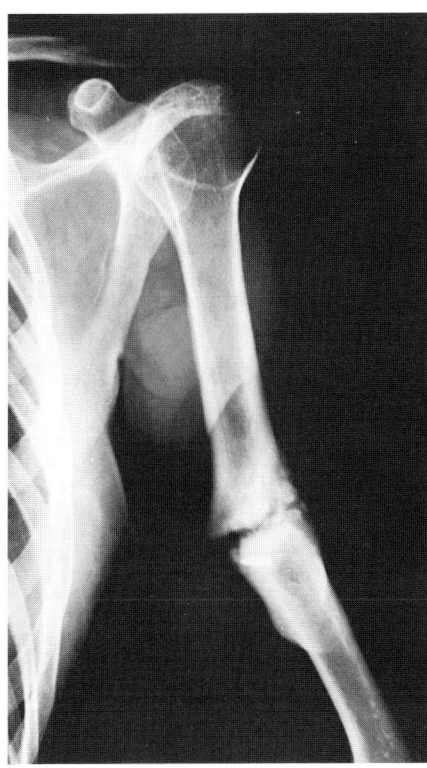

FIG. 2–44. Non-union of a transverse fracture of the humerus with sclerosis of the bone ends and visible fracture line.

union, requiring 13 weeks in transverse, 17 weeks in oblique, and 20 weeks in spiral and comminuted fractures of the tibia (106). Infection of the fracture site leads to a delayed rate of union. Infection may damage the local blood supply as well as interfere with callus formation (97).

Diagnosis and Classification of Non-union

The diagnosis of non-union can frequently be made by routine radiographs obtained in two planes. The

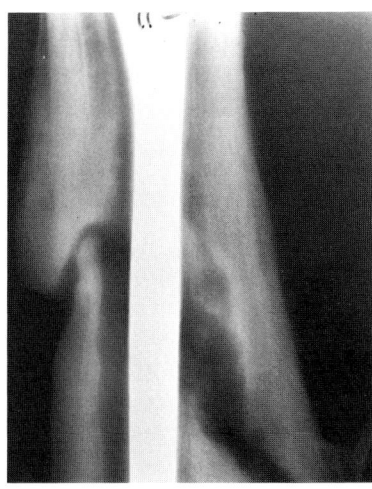

FIG. 2–45. AP tomogram of a hypertrophic non-union of the femur with a poorly fitting Zickel nail.

roentgenographic findings in non-union are sclerosis of the bone ends, sealing off of the medullary cavity, and sclerotic marginal proliferation of bone that does not bridge the fracture site (Fig. 2-44) (33). A lucency or gap may be present between the bone ends. Serial roentgenograms over a period of several months that fail to show progression of union are most helpful in the diagnosis (33). Additional stress roentgenograms and conventional or computed tomography are also helpful (Fig. 2-45) (33,123). Bone scintigraphy has been advocated as a useful technique for diagnosis of non-union (Fig. 2-46) (65,73). Three specific bone-scan patterns have been identified: (1) an intense activity at the fracture site, (2) a cold cleft between two intense areas of uptake, and (3) an indeterminate pattern in which a cold cleft cannot be identified with certainty (65,73). The pattern displaying a cold cleft between the bone ends is indicative of a synovial pseudarthrosis with a false positive rate of 10.8% (65,73). In the series of Esterhai and colleagues, an intense uniform uptake was present in 69.5%, the cold cleft

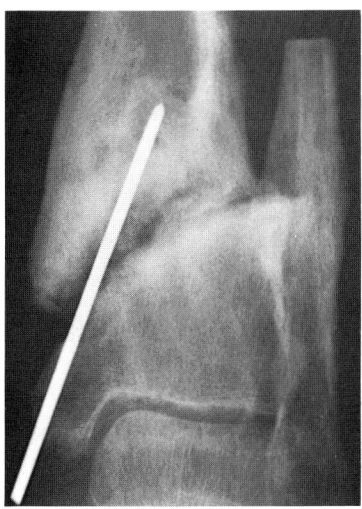 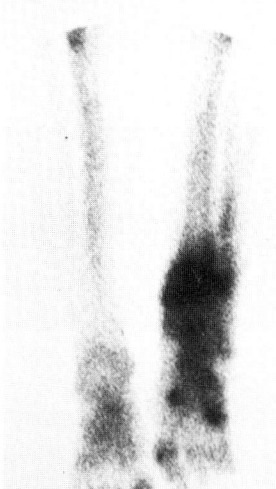

A B

FIG. 2–46. Radiograph of the ankle (A) and bone scan (B) of a distal tibial hypertrophic non-union.

type in 23.4%, and an indeterminate pattern in 7.1% of 157 scans (73). A synovial pseudarthrosis was most frequently present in non-unions of the humerus (57.1%) (73).

Non-unions may be divided into several types. Non-union may be considered with respect to the presence or absence of complicating infection, i.e., noninfected, previously infected, or infected (154). Non-unions may also be classified according to location, whether they are diaphyseal and metaphyseal (154). The diaphyseal pseudarthrosis may be subclassified into hypervascular and avascular types (154,234). The hypervascular non-union is vascular and capable of biologic reaction (Fig. 2-47) (234). The hypervascular non-union may be further subdivided into elephant foot, horse hoof, and oligotrophic types based upon the radiographic appearance (234). The elephant-foot type has hypertrophy of the bone ends and exuberant callus formation. It represents 85–90% of non-unions following nonoperative treatment (154). The horse hoof type has only mild callus formation and sclerosis is frequently present. This type is commonly associated with unstable internal fixation. The oligotrophic non-union has minimal callus formation. This type

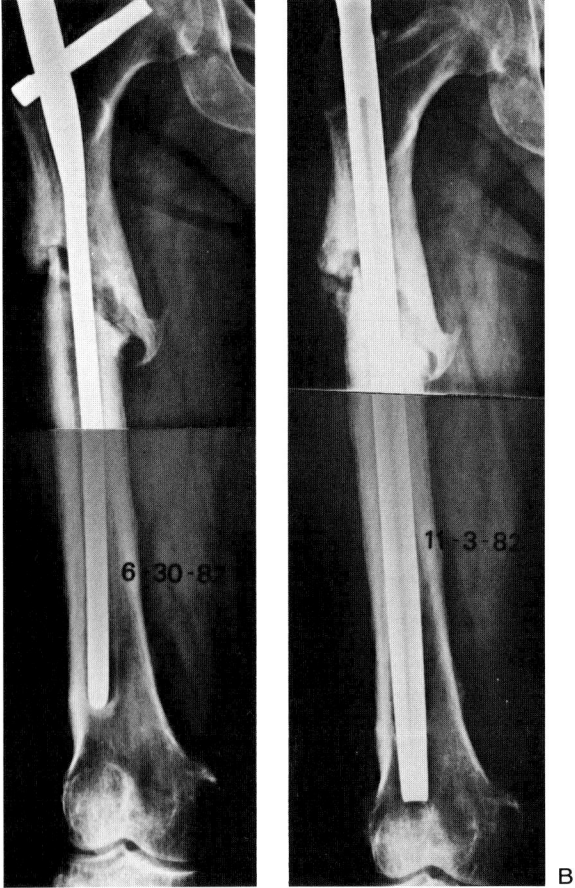

FIG. 2–47. A: Hypertrophic non-union with a poorly fitting Zickel nail. **B:** Repeat radiograph after revision with a large ASIF intramedullary nail.

occurs following major displacement of a fracture, distraction of the fragments, or internal fixation.

The avascular non-union has poor vascularity and is incapable of biologic reaction (Fig. 2-48). It may be subdivided into torsion wedge, comminuted, defect, and atrophic types (234). The torsion-wedge non-union has an avascular intermediate fragment that is healed to one main fragment but not to the other. The comminuted non-union is characterized by one or more necrotic intermediate fragments with absence of callus. A defect non-union is present when fibrosis seals the fracture ends, which remain osteoporotic and atrophic (234).

Treatment Modalities

A detailed discussion of the treatment of non-united fractures is beyond the scope of the present chapter. However, the available treatment modalities and their indications related to the type of non-union will be briefly reviewed. The principles of treatment of non-union are firm fixation, apposition of the fragments, and osteogenesis (27,31). The commonly used methods of treatment of the non-united fracture include bone grafting, rigid fixation (either internal or external), and electrical stimulation (30,37,49). A combination of these modalities may be used (Figs. 2-37, 2-49) (100,102,133,171). The hypervascular non-union is capable of biologic reaction and does not require bone grafting. The well-aligned hypervascular pseudarthrosis may be adequately treated with rigid internal fixation alone (Fig. 2-47). There is no need for removal of the intervening fibrous tissue and no need for external cast immobilization. In contrast, the avascular non-union requires rigid fixation plus extensive decortication and an autogenous cancellous bone graft (Fig. 2-48) (154). Using these techniques, Rosen reported an average healing time of 7.0 months in 59 hypervascular non-unions with 1 failure and 8.2 months in 67 avascular non-unions with 10 failures (194). The main reasons for bone grafting of a non-union are to bridge a gap or defect, to maintain or regain length, and to stimulate osteogenesis (194).

In the metaphyseal non-union, the joint must be mobilized, the articular surface reconstituted, and the fragment fixed to the shaft (154,194). Internal fixation with special plates or dual-onlay cortical cancellous bone grafts aids in achieving union.

The objectives in treatment of the infected non-union are eradication of the infection and healing through fracture union (147,154). The principles of treatment are to eliminate the infection, obtain bone stability, and employ a cancellous bone graft when necessary (147). Bone union can occur in the presence of infection, but the activity of infection must be decreased before attempts at achieving bone stability are made. Following this principle, Meyer and colleagues achieved union in 60 of 64

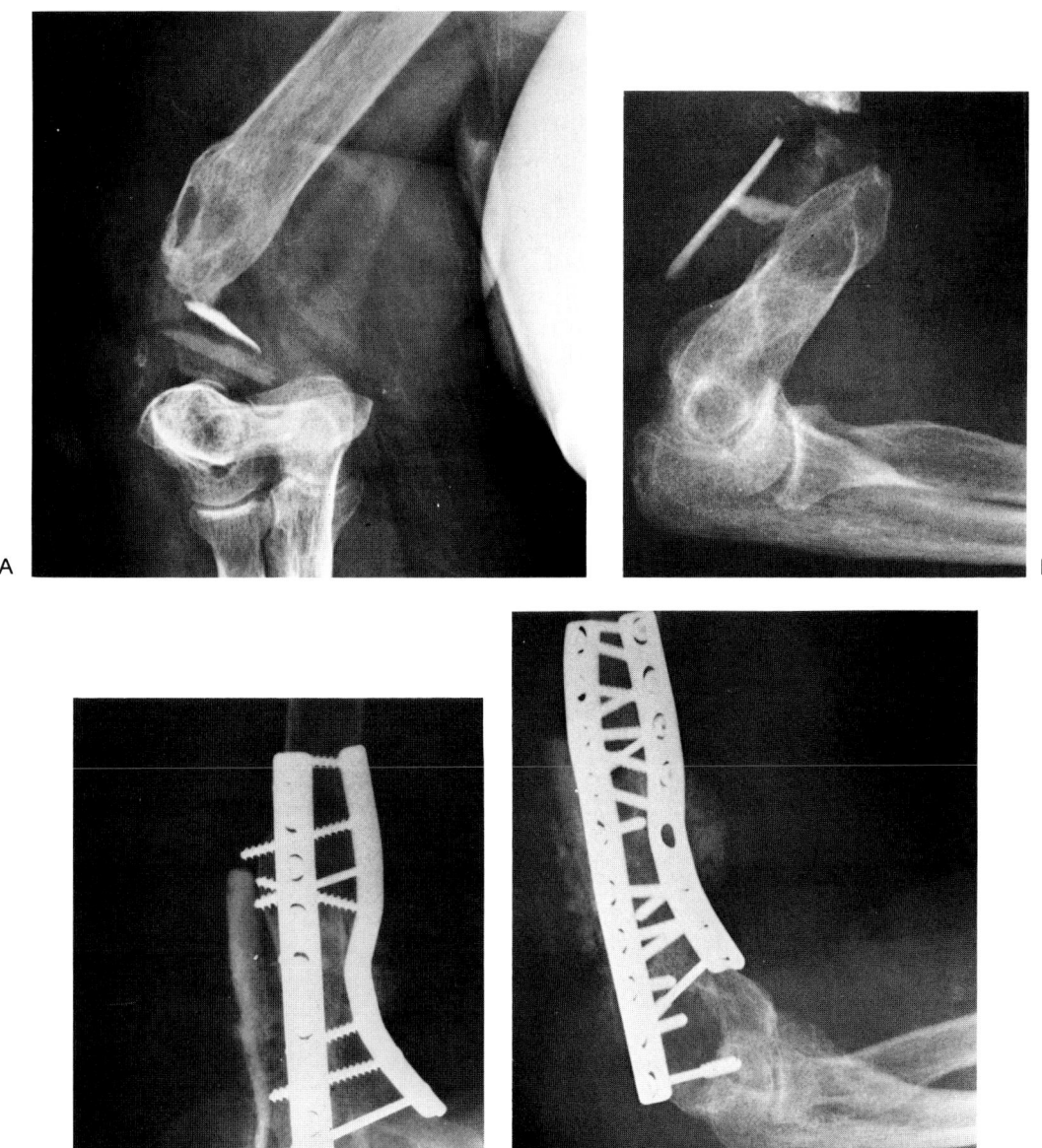

FIG. 2-48. AP (**A**) and lateral (**B**) radiograph of an atrophic non-union of the distal humerus. AP (**C**) and lateral (**D**) radiographs following dual compression plate fixation and bone grafting.

fractures (147). D'Aubigne has emphasized the importance of recognition of the history of previous or active infection in the prognosis of treatment of the non-united fracture (61). In his treatment of 814 non-unions, the failure rate was 2.5% in the uninfected fracture, 6.4% in cases with a history of previous infection, and 25.3% if there had been a history of previous sepsis combined with a septic flair postoperatively.

Electrical stimulation in the treatment of the non-united fracture has been used with increasing frequency (27,99,100,101). Three types of electrical stimulation devices are currently in use: noninvasive, semi-invasive, and invasive. The noninvasive technique utilizes externally placed electromagnetic coils that create pulsating electromagnetic fields (Figs. 2-50 and 2-51). The overall success rate of this technique has been reported as 75% in 332 patients (17). The advantage of this technique is that it does not require a surgical procedure for implantation. The semi-invasive technique consists of a percutaneous insertion of electrodes into the non-union site (Fig. 2-52) (37). A success rate of 83.7% in 178 non-unions has been reported using this technique (34). Infection and the presence of a synovial pseudarthrosis decrease the rate of success. The invasive technique consists of implantation of the entire electrical stimulation unit. The success of this technique has been reported as approximately 86% (170). The disadvantage of this technique is that it requires another surgical procedure for removal.

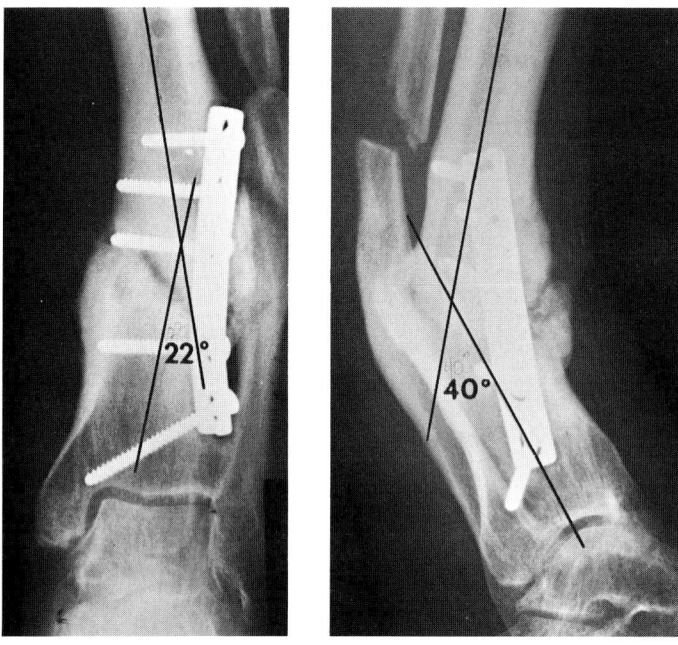
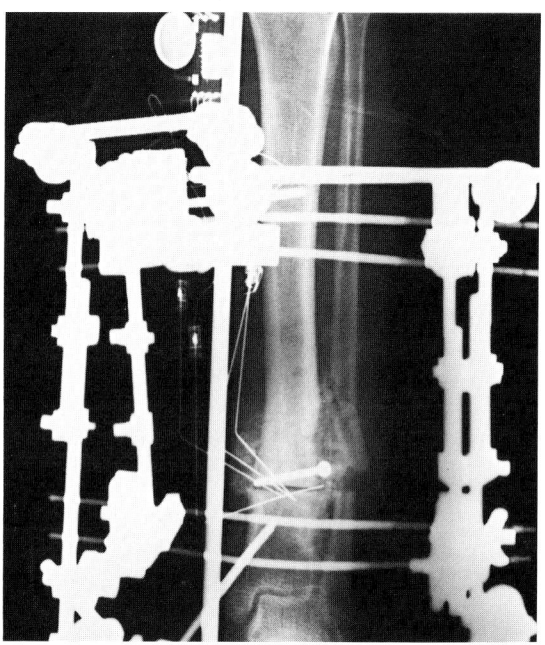

A   B   C

FIG. 2–49. AP (**A**) and lateral (**B**) radiographs of a hypertrophic tibial non-union with varus alignment and posterior angulation following plate fixation. **C:** Radiograph following correction of alignment with a Hoffman apparatus, bone grafting, and insertion of percutaneous electrodes for electrical stimulation.

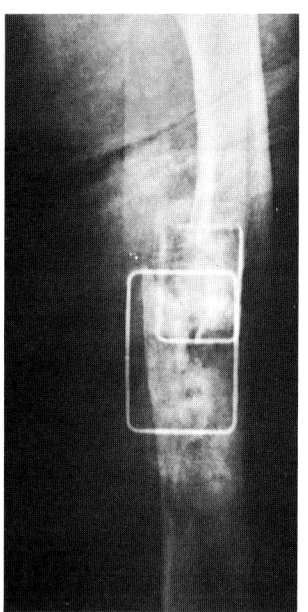
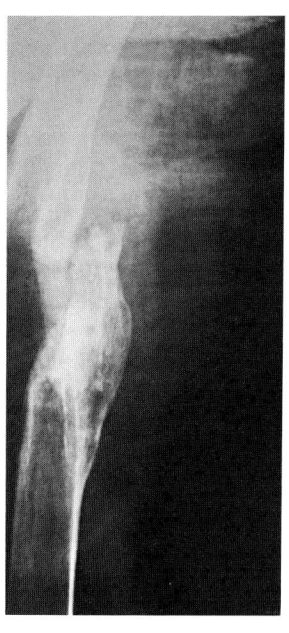

A   B

FIG. 2–50. A: External coil electrical stimulation of femoral non-union at the site of a pathologic fracture through an area of osteomyelitis. **B:** Bone bridging of the fracture gap six months following electrical stimulation.

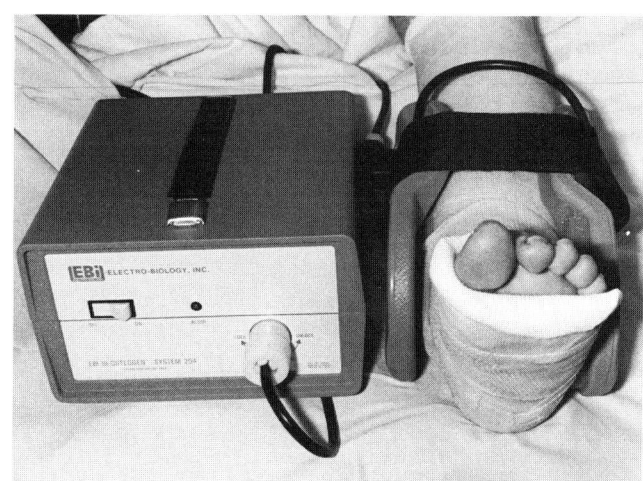

FIG. 2–51. External coil electrical stimulation device on a tibial non-union.

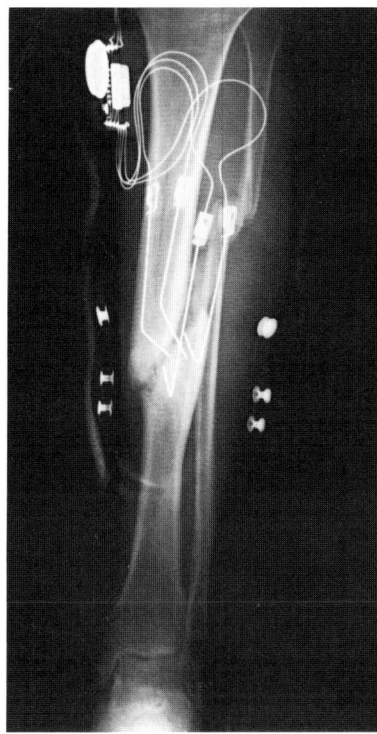

FIG. 2–52. Percutaneous electrical stimulation of a well aligned hypertrophic tibial non-union.

In summary, the factors involved in the pathogenesis of non-union should be recognized. Initial fracture treatment should strive to minimize those adverse factors beyond control of the surgeon and should not add iatrogenic factors that contribute to non-union. Once non-union has occurred, the type of non-union should be determined, the presence or absence of infection assessed, and a treatment plan devised.

REFERENCES

 1. Akeson WH, Woo S, Coutts RD, et al. Quantitative histological evaluation of early fracture healing of cortical bones immobilized by stainless steel and composite plates. *Calcif Tissue Res* 1975;19:27–37.
 2. Akeson WH, Woo S, Rutherford L, Coutts RD, Gonsalves M, Amiel D. The effects of rigidity of internal fixation plates on long bone remodeling. *Acta Orthop Scand* 1976;47:241–249.
 3. Allen WC, Heiple KC, Burstein AH. A fluted femoral intramedullary rod. *J Bone Joint Surg* 1978;60A:506–515.
 4. Allen WC, Piotrowski G, Burstein AH, Frankel VH. Biomechanical principles of intramedullary fixation. *Clin Orthop* 1968;60:13–20.
 5. Allgower M, Ehrsam R, Ganz R, Matter P, Perren SM. Clinical experience with a new compression plate "DCP". *Acta Orthop Scand* 1969;125:45–61.
 6. Allgower M, Perren S, Matter P. A new plate for internal fixation—the dynamic compression plate (DCP). *Injury* 1970;2:40–47.
 7. Anderson LD. Compression plate fixation and the effect of different types of internal fixation on fracture healing. *J Bone Joint Surg* 1965;47A:191–208.
 8. Anderson LD. Compression plate fixation and the effects of different types of internal fixation on fracture healing. *Instruct Course Lect* 1969;18:224–241.
 9. Anderson LD, Gilmer WS, Tooms RE. Experimental fractures treated with loose and tight fitting medullary nails. *Surg Forum* 1962;13:455–457.
10. Bado JL. *The Monteggia lesion.* Springfield, IL: Charles C. Thomas, 1962.
11. Bagby GW. Compression bone plating: Historical considerations. *J Bone Joint Surg* 1977;59A:625–631.
12. Bagby GW, Janes JM. An impacting bone plate. *Proc Staff Meetings, Mayo Clin* 1957;32:55–57.
13. Bagby GW, Hanes JM. The effect of compression of the rate of fracture healing using a special plate. *Am J Surg* 1958;95:761–771.
14. Barron SE, Robb RA, Taylor WF, Kelly PJ. The effect of fixation with intramedullary rods and plates on fracture-site blood flow and bone remodeling in dogs. *J Bone Joint Surg* 1977;59A:376–385.
15. Bassett CAL. Current concepts of bone formation. *J Bone Joint Surg* 1962;44A:1217–1244.
16. Bassett CAL. Augmentation of bone repair by inductively coupled electromagnetic fields. *Science* 1974;184:575–577.
17. Bassett CAL, Mitchell SN, Gaston SR. Pulsing electromagnetic field treatment in ununited fractures and failed arthrodesis. *JAMA* 1982;247:623–628.
18. Bassett CAL, Ruedi TP. Transformation of fibrous tissues to bone in vivo. *Nature* 1966;209:988.
19. Bassett CAL, Valdes MG, Hernandez E. Modification of fracture repair with selected pulsing electromagnetic fields. *J Bone Joint Surg* 1982;64A:888–895.
20. Bast TH, Sullivan WE, Geist FD. The repair of bone. *Anat Rec* 1925;31:255–280.
21. Berbaum KS, Franken EA, El-Khoury GY. Impact of history on radiographic detection of fractures: A comparison of radiologists and orthopedists. *AJR* 1989;153:1221–1224.
22. Berbaum KS, El-Khoury GY, Franken EA, Kathol M, Montgomery WJ, Hesson W. Impact of clinical history on fracture detection with radiography. *Radiology* 1988;168:507–511.
23. Berquist TH. *Magnetic resonance of the musculoskeletal system.* New York: Raven Press, 1990.
24. Blaisdell FE, Cowan JF. Healing of simple fractures. *Arch Surg* 1926;12:619–654.
25. Blockey NJ. The value of rigid fixation in the treatment of fractures of the adult tibial shaft. *J Bone Joint Surg* 1956;38B:518–527.
26. Böhler J. Results in medullary nailing of ninety-five fresh fractures of the femur. *J Bone Joint Surg* 1951;33A:670–678.
27. Böhler J. An approach to non-union of fractures. *Surg Ann* 1982;14:299–315.
28. Borden S IV. Traumatic bowing of the forearm in children. *J Bone Joint Surg* 1974;56A:611–616.
29. Borden S IV. Roentgen recognition of acute plastic bowing of the forearm in children. *AJR* 1975;125:524–530.
30. Boyd HB, Anderson LD, Johnston DS. Changing concepts in the treatment of non-unions. *Clin Orthop* 1965;43:37–54.
31. Braden TD, Brinker WO. Radiologic and gross anatomic evaluation of bone healing in the dog. *J Am Vet Med Assoc* 1976;169:1318–1323.
32. Braden TD, Brinker WO, Little RW, et al. Comparative biomechanical evaluation of bone healing in the dog. *J Am Vet Med Assoc* 1973;163:65–69.
33. Brasher HR. Diagnosis and prevention of non-union. *J Bone Joint Surg* 1965;47A:174–178.
34. Brighton CT, Black J, Friedenburg ZB. A multicenter study of the treatment of non-unions with constant direct current. *J Bone Joint Surg* 1981;63A:2–13.
35. Brighton CT, Friedenberg ZB, Black J, Esterhai JL, Mitchall JEJ, Mortigue F. Electrically induced osteogenesis. Relationship between charge, current density, and the amount of bone formed. *Clin Orthop* 1981;161:122–132.
36. Brighton CT, Krebs AG. Oxygen tension of healing fractures in the rabbit. *J Bone Joint Surg* 1972;54A:323–332.
37. Brighton CT. The semi-invasive method of treating nonunion with direct current. *Orthop Clin North Am* 1984;15:33–45.
38. Brookes M. Blood flow rates in compact and cancellous bone and bone marrow. *J Anat* 1967;101:533–541.

39. Brookes M, Elkin AC, Harrison RG, Heald CB. A new concept of capillary circulation in bone cortex. Some clinical applications. *Lancet* 1961;1:1078–1081.

40. Brown KLB, Cruess RL. Bone and cartilage transplantation in orthopedic surgery. *J Bone Joint Surg* 1982;64A:270–279.

41. Burny FL. Strain gauge measurement of fracture healing. In Brocker AF, Edwards CC. *External fixation: The current state of the art.* Baltimore: Williams and Wilkins, 1979.

42. Burstein AH, Reilly DT, Frankel VH. Failure characteristics of bone and bone tissue. In Kenedi RM. *Perspectives in biomedical engineering.* Baltimore: University Park Press, 1973.

43. Burwell HN. Plate fixation of tibial shaft fractures. *J Bone Joint Surg* 1971;53B:258–271.

44. Cavadias AX, Trueta J. An experimental study of the vascular contribution to the callus of fracture. *Surg Gynecol Obstet* 1965;120:731–747.

45. Chalmers J, Gray DH, Rush J. Observations on the induction of bone in soft tissues. *J Bone Joint Surg* 1975;57B:36–45.

46. Clinger NJ, Hunter TB, Hillman BJ. Radiology reporting: Attitudes of referring physicians. *Radiology* 1988;169:825–826.

47. Coletti JM Jr. Effects of sustained compression loading of cortical bone in vivo. *Surg Forum* 1969;20:471–473.

48. Coltart WD. "Aviator's Astragalus." *J Bone Joint Surg* 1952;34B:545–566.

49. Connolly JF. Selection, evaluation, and indications for electrical stimulation of ununited fractures. *Clin Orthop* 1981;161:39–53.

50. Convent L. On secondary fracture after removal of internal fixation material. *Acta Orthop Belg* 1977;43:89–93.

51. Copp DH, Shim SS. Extraction ratio and bone clearance of Sr[85] as a measure of effective bone blood flow. *Circ Res* 1965;16:461–467.

52. Court-Brown CM. An analysis of the Sukhtian-Hughes external fixation device and its effect on bone blood flow and healing. Unpublished data.

53. Coutts RD, Harris WH, Weinberg EH. Compression plating: Experimental study of the effect on bone formation rates. *Acta Orthop Scand* 1973;44:256–262.

54. Cruess RL, Dumont J. Fracture healing. *Can J Surg* 1975;18:403–413.

55. Currey JD. The mechanical properties of bone. *Clin Orthop* 1970;73:21.

56. Danckwardt-Lilliestrom G. Reaming of the medullary cavity and its effect on diaphyseal bone. *Acta Orthop Scand Suppl* 1969;128:1–153.

57. Danckwardt-Lilliestrom G, Lorenzi GL, Olerud S. Intramedullary nailing after reaming. *Acta Orthop Scand Suppl* 1970;134:1–78.

58. Danckwardt-Lilliestrom G, Lorenzi GL, Olerud S. Intracortical circulation after intramedullary reaming with reduction of pressure in the medullary cavity: A microangiographic study on the rabbit tibia. *J Bone Joint Surg* 1970;52A:1390–1394.

59. Danis R. The operative treatment of bone fractures. *J Chir* 1947;7:318–320.

60. Danis R. *Théorie et pratique de l'ostéosynthèse.* Paris: Masson & Cie, 1949.

61. D' Aubigne RM. Infection in the treatment of un-united fractures. *Clin Orthop* 1965;143:77–82.

62. Dempster WT, Liddecoat RT. Compact bone as a non-isotropic material. *Am J Anat* 1952;91:331–362.

63. Dencker H. Shaft fractures of the femur. *Acta Chir Scand* 1965;130:173–184.

64. Dencker H. Technical problems of medullary nailing. *Acta Chir Scand* 1965;130:185.

65. Desai A, Alavi A, Dalinka M, Brighton C, Esterhai J. Role of bone scintigraphy in the evaluation and treatment of non-united fractures. *J Nucl Med* 1980;21:931–934.

66. Devas M. Stress fractures. Edinburgh: Churchill Livingstone, 1975.

67. Duhamel HL. Cited by Keith A. in *Br J Surg* 1917;5:685–693.

68. Eggers GWN. The contact splint. *Trans South Surg Assoc* 1946;58:418–424.

69. Eggers GWN. Internal contact splint. *J Bone Joint Surg* 1948;30A:40–52.

70. Eggers GWN, Ainsworth WH, Shindler TO, Pomerat CM. Clini-cal significance of the contact-compression factor in bone surgery. *Arch Surg* 1951;62:467–474.

71. Eggers GWN, Shindler TO, Pomerat CM. The influence of the contact-compression factor on osteogenesis in surgical fractures. *J Bone Joint Surg* 1949;31A:693.

72. Enneking WF. The repair of complete fractures of rat tibiae. *Anat Rec* 1948;101:515–532.

73. Esterhai JL, Brighton CT, Heppenstall RB, Alvavi A, Desai AG. Detection of synovial pseudarthrosis by Tc[99] scintigraphy. *Clin Orthop* 1981;161:15–23.

74. Evans FG, LeBow M. Strength of human compact bone under repetitive loading. *J Appl Physiol* 1957;10:127–130.

75. Falkenberg J. An experimental study of the rate of fracture healing. *Acta Orthop Scand Suppl* 1961;50:1–98.

76. Fitts WT, Roberts B, Spoont SI, et al. The effect of intramedullary nailing on the healing of fractures. *Surg Gynecol Obstet* 1949;89:609–615.

77. Ford LT, Key JA. Experimental study of the effect of pressure on healing bone. *Arch Surg* 1954;69:627–634.

78. Frankel VH, Burstein AH. The biomechanics of refracture of bone. *Clin Orthop* 1968;60:221–225.

79. Friedenberg ZB, Brighton CT. Bioelectrical potentials in bone. *J Bone Joint Surg* 1966;48A:915–923.

80. Friedenberg ZB, French G. The effects of known compression forces on fracture healing. *Surg Gynecol Obstet* 1952;94:743–748.

81. Friedenberg ZB, Roberts PG, Didizian NH, Brighton CT. Stimulation of fracture healing by direct current in the rabbit fibula. *J Bone Joint Surg* 1971;53A:1400–1408.

82. Friedenberg ZB, Zemsky LM, Pollis RP, Brighton CT. The response of non-traumatized bone to direct current. *J Bone Joint Surg* 1974;56A:1023–1030.

83. Gallie WE, Robertson DE. The repair of bone. *Br J Surg* 1919;7:211–216.

84. Gelman MI. *Radiology of orthopedic procedures, problems, and complications.* Philadelphia: W.B. Saunders, 1984.

85. Glucksmann A. Studies of bone mechanics in vitro. *Anat Rec* 1938;72:97–114.

86. Glucksmann A. The role of mechanical stresses in bone formation in vitro. *J Anat* 1941;76:231–239.

87. Gothman L. Arterial changes in experimental fractures of the monkey's tibia treated with intramedullary nailing. *Acta Chir Scand* 1961;121:56–66.

88. Gothman L. Vascular reactions in experimental fractures. *Acta Chir Scand Suppl* 1961;284:1.

89. Gray JC, Elves MW. Donor cell's contribution to osteogenesis in experimental cancellous bone grafts. *Clin Orthop* 1982;163:261–271.

90. Green SA. Complications of external skeletal fixation. *Clin Orthop* 1984;180:109–116.

91. Gustilo RB, Nelson GE, Hamel A, Moe JH. The effect of intramedullary nailing of the blood supply of the diaphysis of long bones in mature dogs. *J Bone Joint Surg* 1964;46A:1362–1363.

92. Haller A. Cited by Keith A. in *Br J Surg* 1917;5:685–693.

93. Ham AW. A histological study of the early phases of bone repair. *J Bone Joint Surg* 1930;12:827–844.

94. Ham AW. *Histology.* 8th ed. Philadelphia: J. B. Lippincott Co., 1979.

95. Hansmann H. Cited by Bagby GW (13).

96. Heiple KG, Chase SW, Herndon CH. A comparative study of the healing process following different types of bone transplantation. *J Bone Joint Surg* 1963;45A:1593–1612.

97. Heiple KG, Herndon CH. The pathologic physiology of nonunion. *Clin Orthop* 1965;43:11–21.

98. Heppenstall RB, Goodwin CW, Brighton CT. Fracture healing in the presence of chronic hypoxia. *J Bone Joint Surg* 1976;58A:1153–1156.

99. Heppenstall RB: Constant direct current treatment for established non-union of the tibia. *Clin Orthop* 178:179–184, 1983.

100. Heppenstall RB, Brighton CT, Esterhai JL, Muller G. Prognostic factors in nonunion of the tibia: An evaluation of 185 cases treated with constant direct current. *J Trauma* 1984;24:790–795.

101. Heppenstall RB. The present role of bone graft surgery in treating nonunion. *Orthop Clin North Am* 1984;15:113–123.
102. Holden CEA. The role of blood supply to soft tissue in the healing of diaphyseal fractures. *J Bone Joint Surg* 1972;54A:993–1000.
103. Hughes SPF, Lemon GJ, Davis DR, Bassingthwaythe JB, Kelly PJ. Extraction of minerals after experimental fractures of the tibia in dogs. *J Bone Joint Surg* 1979;61A:857–866.
104. Hutzschenreuter P, Perren SM, Steinemann S. Some effects of rigidity of internal fixation on the healing pattern of osteotomies. *Injury* 1969;1:77–81.
105. Huys F, Martens M, Mulier JC. Should surgical implants be removed? *Acta Orthop Belg* 1977;43:Fascicle 1.
106. Jackson RW, MacNab I. Fractures of the shaft of the tibia. *Am J Surg* 1959;97:543–557.
107. Jacobs RR, Leuth U, Dueland RT. Electrical stimulation of experimental non-unions. *Clin Orthop* 1981;161:146–153.
108. Jensen JS, Johansen J, March A. Middle third femoral fractures treated with medullary nailing or AO compression plates. *Injury* 1977;8:174–181.
109. Jofe MH, Hayes WC, Beaupre GS, et al. Biomechanical monitoring of healing with external skeletal fixation. *Transactions* (28th annual meeting), *Orthop Res Soc* 1982.
110. Johnson RW. A physiological study of the blood supply of the diaphysis. *J Bone Joint Surg* 1927;9:153–184.
111. Jorgenson TE. A simple mechanical method of assessing fracture healing. In Brooker AF, Edwards CC. *External fixation: The current state of the art.* Baltimore: Williams and Wilkins, 1979.
112. Karlstrom G, Olerud S. Secondary internal fixation: Experimental studies on revascularization and healing in osteotomized rabbit tibias. *Acta Orthop Scand Suppl* 1979;175:3–39.
113. Kane WJ, Grim E. Blood flow to canine hind-limb bone, muscle and skin. *J Bone Joint Surg* 1969;51A:309–322.
114. Keith A. Bone growth and bone repair. *Br J Surg* 1917;5:685–693.
115. Kelly PJ. Anatomy, physiology and pathology of the blood supply of bones. *J Bone Joint Surg* 1968;50A:766–783.
116. Ketenjian AY, Arsenis C. Morphological and biomechanical studies during differentiation and calcification of fracture callus cartilage. *Clin Orthop* 1975;107:266–273.
117. Key JA. Positive pressure in arthrodesis for tuberculosis of the knee joint. *South Med* 1932;25:909–915.
118. Key JA, Reynolds FC. Contact splints vs. standard bone plates in the fixation of experimental fractures. *Ann Surg* 1953;137:911–919.
119. Khomullo GV. Regeneration of bone tissue in animals depending on the basal metabolic rate. *Bull Eksp Biol Med* 1962;53:97.
120. Kinzl L. Cited by Perren SM, Matter P, Ruedi R, et al. Biomechanics of fracture healing after internal fixation. *Surg Ann* 1975;7:361.
121. Kolodny A. The periosteal blood supply and healing of fractures. *J Bone Joint Surg* 1923;5:698–711.
122. Kuhlman RE, Bakowski MJ. The biomechanical activity of fracture callus in relation to bone production. *Clin Orthop* 1975;107:258–265.
123. Kuhlman JE, Fishman EK, Magid D, Scott WW, Brooker AF, Siegelman SS. Fracture nonunion: CT assessment with multiplanar reconstruction. *Radiology* 1988;167:483–488.
124. Küntscher GBG. The Kuntscher method of intramedullary fixation. *J Bone Joint Surg* 1958;40A:17–26.
125. Küntscher GBG. Intramedullary surgical technique and its place in orthopaedic surgery: My present concept. *J Bone Joint Surg* 1965;47A:809–818.
126. Küntscher GBG. The intramedullary nailing of fractures. *Clin Orthop* 1968;60:5–12.
127. Ladanyi J, Hidvegi F. Blood supply of experimental callus formation. *Acta Morphol* 1954;4:35–44.
128. Laros GS. Fracture healing: Compression vs fixation. *Arch Surg* 1974;108:698–702.
129. Laurence M, Freeman MAR, Swanson SAV. Engineering considerations in the internal fixation of fractures of the tibial shaft. *J Bone Joint Surg* 1969;51B:754–765.
130. Laurin CA, Sison V, Roque N. Mechanical investigation of experimental fractures. *Can J Surg* 1963;6:218–228.
131. Lauritzen F. Medullary nailing. *Acta Chir Scand* Suppl 1949;147:1–224.
132. Laurnen EL, Kelly PJ. Blood flow, oxygen consumption, carbon-dioxide production and blood-calcium and pH changes in tibial fractures in dogs. *J Bone Joint Surg* 1969;51A:298–308.
133. Lavine LS, Grodzinsky AJ. Electrical stimulation of repair of bone. *J Bone Joint Surg* 1987;69A:626–630.
134. Lettin AWF. The effects of axial compression on the healing of experimental fractures of the rabbit tibia. *Proc Roy Soc Med* 1954;58:30.
135. Lewallen DG, Chao EYS, Kasman RA, et al. Comparison of compression plates and external fixation on early bone healing. *J Bone Joint Surg* 1984;66A:1084–1091.
136. Lexer. Cited by Kolodny A. The periosteal blood supply and healing of fractures. *J Bone Joint Surg* 1923;5:698.
137. Lindahl O. The rigidity of fracture immobilization with plates. *Acta Orthop Scand* 1967;38:101–114.
138. Lindsay MK. Observations on fracture healing in rats. *J Bone Joint Surg* 1934;16:162–167.
139. Lindsay MK, Howes EL. The breaking strength of healing fractures. *J Bone Joint Surg* 1931;13:491–501.
140. Lopez-Curto JA, Bassingthwaighte JB, Kelly PJ. Anatomy of the microvasculature of the tibial diaphysis of the adult dog. *J Bone Joint Surg* 1980;62A:1362–1369.
141. Lottes JO. Medullary nailing of the tibia with the triflange nail. *Clin Orthop* 1974;105:253–266.
142. MacEwen W. Cited by Keith A in *Br J Surg* 1917;5:685–693.
143. Mathews RS, Cooper EM. Cortical bone atrophy secondary to compression plate fixation: A clinical and pathophysiologic study. *Surg Forum* 1976;27:523–525.
144. Matthews LS, Green CA, Goldstein SA. The thermal effects of skeletal fixation pre insertion in bone. *J Bone Joint Surg* 1984;66A:1077–1083.
145. McKellar-Hall RD. Clay shovelers fracture. *J Bone Joint Surg* 1940;22:63–75.
146. Melick RA, Miller DR. Variations of tensile strength of human cortical bone with age. *Clin Sci* 1966;30:243–248.
147. Meyer S, Weland AJ, Willenegger H. The treatment of infected non-unions of fractures of long bones. *J Bone Joint Surg* 1975;57A:836–842.
148. Mihula A. The sources of healing of a fracture of tubular bone in different types of osteosyntheses from the standpoint of vessel supply. *Rozhl Chir* 1973;52:35–41.
149. Milner JC, Rhinelander FW. Compression fixation and primary bone healing. *Surg Forum* 1968;19:453–456.
150. Morris JM, Blickenstaft LD. *Fatique fractures.* Springfield, IL: Charles C. Thomas, 1967.
151. Morris MA, Kelly PJ. Use of tracer microspheres to measure bone blood flow in conscious dogs. *Calcif Tiss Int* 1980;32:69–76.
152. Müller ME. Internal fixation for fresh fractures and for non-union. *Proc R Soc Med* 1963;56:455–459.
153. Müller ME. Treatment of non-unions by compression. *Clin Orthop* 1965;43:83–92.
154. Müller ME, Allgower M, Willenegger H. *Manual of internal fixation.* New York: Springer-Verlag, 1970.
155. Narang R, Laskin DM. Experimental osteogenesis at fracture sites and gaps. *J Oral Surg* 1976;34:225–231.
156. Nelson GE, Kelly PJ, Peterson LFA, James JM. Blood supply of the human tibia. *J Bone Joint Surg* 1960;42A:625–636.
157. Nguyen VD, London J, Cone RO III. Ring sequestrum: Radiologic characteristics of skeletal pin-tract osteomyelitis. *Radiology* 1986;158:129–131.
158. Nilsonne U. Biophysical investigations of the mineral phase in healing fractures. *Acta Orthop Scand Suppl* 1959;37:1–81.
159. Nunamaker DM, Perren SM. A radiological and histological analysis of fracture healing using prebending of compression plates. *Clin Orthop* 1979;138:167–174.
160. Olerud S, Danckwardt-Lilliestrom G. Fracture healing in compression osteosynthesis in the dog. *J Bone Joint Surg* 1968;50B:844–851.
161. Olerud S, Danckwardt-Lilliestrom G. Fracture healing in compression osteosyntheses. *Acta Orthop Scand Suppl* 1971;137:1–44.

162. Ollier L. Cited by Keith A, in *Br J Surg* 1917;5:685–693.
163. O'Sullivan ME, Chao EYS, Kelly PJ. The effects of fixation on fracture healing. *J Bone Joint Surg* 1989;71A:306–310.
164. Ozonoff MB. *Pediatric orthopedic radiology.* Philadelphia: W. B. Saunders Co., 1979.
165. Paavolainen P, Karaharju E, Slatis P, Ahonen J, Holmström T. Effect of rigid plate fixation on stricture and mineral content of cortical bone. *Clin Orthop* 1978;136:287–293.
166. Paavolainen P, Slatis P, Ahonen J, Karaharju E. Changes in calcium and hydroxyproline content of cortical bone after compression and neutral plate fixation. *Acta Orthop Scand* 1978;49:492–496.
167. Paavolainen P, Slatis P, Karaharju E, Holstrom T. Studies on mechanical strength of bone. *Acta Orthop Scand* 1978;49:506–511.
168. Panjabi MM, White AA, Wolf JW. A biomechanical comparison of the effects of constant and cyclic compression on fracture healing in rabbit long bones. *Acta Orthop Scand* 1979;50:653–661.
169. Paradis GR, Kelly PJ. Blood flow and mineral deposition in canine tibial fractures. *J Bone Joint Surg* 1975;57A:220–226.
170. Paterson DC, Lewis GN, Cass CA. Treatment of delayed union and non-union with an implanted direct current stimulator. *Clin Orthop* 1980;148:117–128.
171. Paterson DC. Treatment of nonunion with a constant direct current. A totally implantable system. *Orthop Clin North Am* 1984;15:47–59.
172. Pentecost RL, Murray RA, Brindley HH. Fatigue, insufficiency and pathological fractures. *JAMA* 1964;187:1001–1004.
173. Perren SM. Physical and biological aspects of fracture healing with special reference to internal fixation. *Clin Orthop* 1979;138:175–179.
174. Perren SM, Allgower M, Cordey J, et al. Developments of compression plate techniques for internal fixation of fractures. *Prog Surg* 1973;12:152–179.
175. Perren SM, Huggler A, Russenberger M, et al. The reaction of cortical bone to compression. *Acta Orthop Scand Suppl* 1969;125:19–28.
176. Perren SM, Matter P, Ruedi R, et al. Biomechanics of fracture healing after internal fixation. *Surg Annu* 1975;7:361–390.
177. Perren SM, Russenberger M, Steinemann S, Müller ME, Allgöwer M. A dynamic compression plate. *Acta Orthop Scand Suppl* 1969;125:31–41.
178. Phemister DB. Bone growth and repair. *Ann Surg* 1935;102:261–285.
179. Pinter J, Rischak G, Lenart G. The effect of compression on bone mineral. *Clin Orthop* 1972;83:286–291.
180. Pitt MJ, Speer DP. Radiologic reporting of orthopedic trauma. *Med Radiogr Photogr* 1982;58:14–18.
181. Pugh J. An introduction to the biomechanics and biomaterials of bone, joints, and implants. *Bull Hosp Joint Dis* 1976;37:124–148.
182. Rahn BA, Gallinaro P, Baltensperger A, Perren SM. Primary bone healing. *J Bone Joint Surg* 1971;53A:783–786.
183. Rand JA, An KN, Chao EYS, Kelly PJ. A comparison of the effects of open intramedullary nailing and comparison-plate fixation on fracture-site blood flow and fracture union. *J Bone Joint Surg* 1981;63A:427–442.
184. Reilly DT, Burstein AH. The mechanical properties of cortical bone. *J Bone Joint Surg* 1974;56A:1001–1021.
185. Reynolds FC, Key JA. Fracture healing after fixation with standard plates, contact splints and medullary nails. *J Bone Joint Surg* 1954;36A:577–587.
186. Rhinelander FW. The normal microcirculation of diaphyseal cortex and its response to fracture. *J Bone Joint Surg* 1968;50A:784–800.
187. Rhinelander FW. Circulation in bone. In Bourne GH. *The biochemistry and physiology of bone,* Vol. II, Chapter 1. New York: Academic Press, 1971, pp. 1–77.
188. Rhinelander FW. Effects of medullary nailing on the normal blood supply of diaphyseal cortex. *Instruct Course Lect* 1973;22:161–187.
189. Rhinelander FW. Tibial blood supply in relation to fracture healing. *Clin Orthop* 1974;105:34–81.
190. Rhinelander FW, Baraby RA. Microangiography in bone healing. I. Undisplaced closed fractures. *J Bone Joint Surg* 1962;44A:1273–1298.
191. Rhinelander FW, Gracilla RV, Phillips RS. Microangiography in bone healing. III. Osteotomies with internal fixation. *J Bone Joint Surg* 1967;49A:1006.
192. Rhinelander FW, Phillips RS, Steel WM, Beer JC. Microangiography in bone healing. II. Displaced closed fractures. *J Bone Joint Surg* 1968;50A:643–662.
193. Richardson ML, Kilcoyne RF, Mayo KA, Lamont JG, Hastrup W. Radiographic evaluation of modern fixation devices. *Radiographics* 1987;7:685–701.
194. Rosen H. Compression treatment of long bone pseudarthrosis. *Clin Orthop* 1979;138:154–166.
195. Rush LV, Rush HL. A technique for longitudinal pin fixation of certain fractures of the ulna and of the femur. *J Bone Joint Surg* 1939;21:619–626.
196. Rybicki EF, Mills EJ, Hassler CR, et al. Mathematical and experimental studies on the mechanics of plated transverse fractures. *J Biomech* 1974;7:377–384.
197. Rybicki EF, Simonen FA. Mechanics of oblique fracture fixation using a finite-element model. *J Biomech* 1977;10:141–148.
198. Salter RB, Harris R. Injuries involving the epiphyseal plate. *J Bone Joint Surg* 1963;45A:587–622.
199. Sartoris DJ, Kerr R, Goergen T, Resnick D. Sliding screw fixation of proximal femoral fractures: Radiographic assessment. *Skel Radiol* 1985;14:104–110.
200. Schenk R, Willenegger H. Morphological findings in primary bone healing. *Symp Biol Hung* 1967;7:75–86.
201. Schneider M, Hansen ST, Winquist RA. Closed intramedullary nailing of fractures of the femoral shaft. *Instruct Course Lect* 1978;27:88–108.
202. Schultz RJ. *The language of fractures.* Baltimore: Williams and Wilkins, 1972.
203. Scott JH. The mechanical basis of bone formation. *J Bone Joint Surg* 1957;39B:134–144.
204. Sharma OP, Kumar R. An experimental study of fracture healing after intramedullary nailing. *Ind J Surg* 1975;37:260–263.
205. Shim SS. Physiology of blood circulation of bone. *J Bone Joint Surg* 1968;50A:812–824.
206. Shim SS, Copp DH, Patterson FP. Measurement of the rate and distribution of the nutrient and other arterial blood supply in long bones of the rabbit. *J Bone Joint Surg* 1968;50B:178–183.
207. Shim SS, Hawk HE, Yu WY. The relationship between blood flow and marrow cavity pressure of bone. *Surg Gynecol Obstet* 1972;135:353–360.
208. Shim SS, McPherson GD, Schwigel JF. The rates of blood flow of bones and skeleton in man with emphasis on a radioisotopic method of measurement. *Ann R Coll Phys Surg Can* 1970;3:74–75.
209. Shim SS, Patterson FP. A direct method of qualitative study of bone blood circulation. *Surg Gynecol Obstet* 1967;125:261–268.
210. Sim FH, Kelly PJ. Relationship of bone remodeling, oxygen consumption, and blood flow in bone. *J Bone Joint Surg* 1970;52A:1377–1390.
211. Slätis P, Karaharju E, Holstrom T, et al. Structural changes in intact tubular bone after application of rigid plates with and without compression. *J Bone Joint Surg* 1978;60A:516–522.
212. Slätis P, Rokkanen P. The normal repair of experimental fractures. *Acta Orthop Scand* 1965;36:221–229.
213. Stromberg NEL. Diaphyseal bone in rigid internal plate fixation: Experimental study of the weakening of canine long bone. *Acta Chir Scand Suppl* 1976;456:1–34.
214. Stromberg NEL, Dalen N. Influence of a rigid plate for internal fixation on the maximum torque capacity of long bones. *Acta Chir Scand* 1976;142:115–122.
215. Tehranzadeh J. The spectrum of avulsion and avulsion-like injuries of the musculoskeletal system. *Radiographics* 1987;7:945–974.
216. Teneff S. Experimental studies on vascularization of bony calluses. *J Intern Coll Surg* 1950;13:186–190.
217. Todd TW, Iler DH. The phenomena of early stages in bone repair. *Ann Surg* 1927;86:715–736.

218. Tonino AJ, Davidson CL, Klopper PJ, et al. Protection from stress on bone and its effects. *J Bone Joint Surg* 1976;58B:107–113.

219. Tonna EA, Cronkite EP. Cellular response to fracture studied with tritiated thymidine. *J Bone Joint Surg* 1961;43A:352–361.

220. Townsley W. The influence of mechanical factors on the development and structure of bone. *Am J Phys Anthropol* 1948;6:25–45.

221. Trias A, Fery A. Cortical circulation of long bones. *J Bone Joint Surg* 1979;61A:1052–1059.

222. Trueta J. The role of the vessels in osteogenesis. *J Bone Joint Surg* 1963;45B:402–418.

223. Trueta J, Cavadias AX. Vascular changes caused by the Kuntscher type of nailing. An experimental study in the rabbit. *J Bone Joint Surg* 1955;37B:492–505.

224. Trueta J, Cavadias AX. A study of the blood supply of the long bones. *Surg Gynecol Obstet* 1964;118:485–498.

225. Udupa KN, Prasad GC. Chemical and histochemical studies on the organic constituents in fracture repair in rats. *J Bone Joint Surg* 1963;45B:770–779.

226. Uhthoff HK, Dubuc FL. Bone structure changes in the dog under rigid internal fixation. *Clin Orthop* 1971;81:165–170.

227. Urist MR. Bone formation by auto-induction. *Science* 1965;150:893–899.

228. Urist MR, Hay PH, Dubuc F, Buring K. Osteogenic competence. *Clin Orthop* 1969;64:194–220.

229. Urist MR, McLean FC. Calcification and ossification. I. Calcification in the callus in healing fractures in normal rats. *J Bone Joint Surg* 1941;23:1–16.

230. Varma BP, Mehta SH. Fracture healing with intramedullary nail fixation of the long bones: An experimental study. *Acta Orthop Scand* 1967;38:419–433.

231. Venable CS. An impacting bone plate to attain closed coaptation. *Ann Surg* 1951;133:808–813.

232. Watson-Jones R, Bonnin JG, King T, et al. Medullary nailing of fractures after 50 years. *J Bone Joint Surg* 1950;32B:694–729.

233. Watson-Jones R, Coltart WD. Slow union of fractures with a study of 804 fractures of the shafts of the tibia and femur. *Clin Orthop* 1982;168:2–16.

234. Weber BC, Chech O. *Pseudarthrosis.* Bern: Hans, Huber, 1976.

235. Weinman DT, Kelly PJ, Owen CA, Orvis AL. Skeletal clearance of Ca^{47} and Sr^{85} and skeletal blood flow in dogs. *Proc Staff Meet Mayo Clin.* 1963;38:559–570.

236. White AA, Panjabi MM, Southwick WO. The four biomechanical stages of fracture repair. *J Bone Joint Surg* 1977;59A:188–192.

237. Whiteside LA, Simmons DJ, Lesker PA. Comparison of regional bone blood flow in areas with differing osteoblastic activity in the rabbit tibia. *Clin Orthop* 1977;124:267–270.

238. Wickstrom J, Corban MS. Intramedullary fixation for fractures of the femoral shaft. *J Trauma* 1967;7:551–583.

239. Wirth CR, Campbell CJ, Askew MJ, et al. Biomechanics of compression plating. *Surg Forum* 1973;24:470–471.

240. Wirth CR, Campbell CJ, Askew MJ, et al. The biomechanical effects of compression plates applied to fractures. *J Trauma* 1974;14:563.

241. Wolff JW, White AA, Panjabi MM, Southwick WO. Comparison of cyclic loading versus constant compression in the treatment of long bone fractures in rabbits. *J Bone Joint Surg* 1981;63A:805–810.

242. Wolff J. *Das Gesetz der Transformation der knochen.* Berlin: Hirschwold, 1892.

243. Woo S, Akeson WH, Leventz B, et al. Potential application of graphite fiber and methyl methacrylate resin composites as internal fixation plates. *J Bomed Mater Res* 1974;8:321–338.

244. Wray JB. Vascular regeneration in the healing fracture. *Angiology* 1963;14:134–138.

245. Wray JB, Lynch CJ. The vascular response to fracture of the tibia in the rate. *J Bone Joint Surg* 1959;41A:1143–1148.

246. Wu JJ, Shry HS, Chao EYS, et al. Comparison of osteotomy healing under external fixation devices with varying stiffness. *J Bone Joint Surg* 1984;66A:1258–1264.

247. Yamagishi M, Yoshimura Y. The biomechanics of fracture healing. *J Bone Joint Surg* 1955;37A:1035–1068.

*Imaging of Orthopedic Trauma,
Second Edition*, edited by T.H. Berquist,
Mayo Clinic © 1992. Published
by Raven Press, Ltd., New York.

CHAPTER 3

Soft Tissue Injuries

Thomas H. Berquist and James K. DeOrio

Categories of Soft Tissue Injury, 83
    Contusion, 83
    Hemorrhage, 83
    Hematoma, 84
    Strain, 84
    Sprain, 84
    Tenosynovitis, 84
    Bursitis, 84
    Nerve Injury, 84
    Myositis Ossificans, 84
    Rhabdomyolisis, 84
    Compartment Syndrome, 84

Classification of Soft Tissue Injuries, 84
Healing of Soft Tissue Injuries, 85
Imaging of Soft Tissue Injuries, 86
    Hemorrhage-Hematoma, 86
    Muscle, Tendon, Ligament Injuries, 87
    Myositis Ossificans, 87
    Rhabdomyolysis, 87
    Miscellaneous Conditions, 90
References, 90

With the increasing interest in physical fitness by the general population and increased and earlier training regimens for organized athletics, the incidence of soft tissue injuries has steadily increased. This has resulted in an expanding effort to better define the nature of these injuries, both from the standpoint of prevention and treatment (3,13,21,22,29).

In recent years, diagnosis of these injuries has also been improved by the new imaging capabilities provided by ultrasound, computed tomography (CT), and especially magnetic resonance imaging (MRI). Although clinical evaluation is often an accurate method of determining the extent of injury, new imaging modalities have provided more definitive information regarding the diagnosis and degree of the injury. The healing process can also be more closely monitored, which is particularly important in determining when the injury is healed or when the athlete can return to normal activities. With this in mind, it is increasingly important that communication between the clinician (orthopedic surgeon, emergency room physician, physical medicine physician, or sports medicine physician) and the radiologist be as complete as possible. This requires an understanding of the terms and classifications used in describing soft tissue injuries. The imaging appearance of soft tissue injuries will also be discussed.

CATEGORIES OF SOFT TISSUE INJURY

Contusion

A contusion typically occurs as a result of a direct blow against the extremity resulting in bruising of the skin and the underlying soft tissues. This results in rupture of capillaries and an infiltrative type of bleeding that is followed by edema and inflammatory reaction. Resulting swelling may be either superficial or deep (4,16,23).

Hemorrhage

We prefer to separate hemorrhage and hematoma as their image appearance and prognosis appear to differ. Hemorrhage should be defined as tracking of blood through the tissues without localized or walled-off collections of blood. This typically occurs with a direct blow or stretching injury to a muscle, tendon, or ligament (4,9,27).

T. H. Berquist and J. K. DeOrio: Departments of Diagnostic Radiology and Orthopedic Surgery, Mayo Medical School, Mayo Clinic Jacksonville, Jacksonville, Florida 32224.

Hematoma

Hematoma is a well defined and restricted collection of blood. This should be differentiated from a hemarthrosis, which is a pooling of blood in the joint. Muckle categorized hematomas depending upon their location (21). He grouped hematomas into intermuscular, intramuscular, and mixed. The value of this on a clinical basis is questionable.

Strain

Strain is defined as damage to a part of a muscle or tendon unit (23). This may result from acute injury, episodic overuse, or chronic strain. It has been demonstrated that strains are almost always continued to the musculotendinous junction. Even injuries within the muscle belly are felt to be myotendinous junction injuries occurring in mid-muscle myotendinous attachments (12). Classification of this injury and the grading system will be described below (7,20,23).

Sprain

Sprains are injuries to a ligament resulting in variable degrees of ligament disruption (4,7,20,23).

Tenosynovitis

Tenosynovitis is defined as inflammation of the synovium surrounding the tendon. This may be due to acute or chronic overuse or to direct trauma (23).

Bursitis

Bursitis is defined as an inflammatory reaction in a bursa. These are typically the result of overuse syndromes and occur most frequently in the subacromial region, greater trochanter, and over the olecranon (4,23).

Nerve Injury

Nerve injuries may result from direct contusion of the nerve, compression of the nerve within a fixed compartment, or from stretching injury. The latter is generally associated with overstretching of the nerve such as the axillary nerve following shoulder dislocations, or sciatic nerve after posterior hip dislocation (16,23).

Myositis Ossificans

This term is often used to describe several conditions that differ considerably. As described, it implies inflammation of the muscle followed by ossification. More commonly, ossification of infiltrated blood or hematoma at the origin or insertion of a muscle to bone more likely occurs. A second form of myositis ossificans occurs when there is actually layering of new bone formation within a muscle that is separated from the bone by a layer of muscle or soft tissue. This may be related to invasion of periosteal cells into the hematoma at the time of injury. A third form of myositis ossificans occurs following trauma to a joint or fracture site. Hematoma in these locations may ossify as a result of repeated trauma to the healing tissue (1,16,23).

Rhabdomyolisis

Rhabdomyolisis is defined as skeletal muscle injury, reversible or irreversible, that alters the integrity of cell membranes sufficiently to allow the escape of cell contents into the extracellular fluid. The most frequent etiologies of this condition are crush injuries, extreme exercise, burn or electrical injuries, seizures, and drug abuse. If unrecognized clinically this condition may lead to renal failure, hyperkalemia, or hypocalcemia.

Compartment Syndrome

Compartment syndrome is defined as soft tissue injury with increased pressure within a fascial compartment. This is usually the result of trauma with hemorrhage and/or edema that elevates the compartment pressure and can lead to significant ischemia due to circulatory compromise. Exertional compartment syndromes have also been described in athletes (11). The calf and thigh are most commonly involved (3,20,22,23,27,28,34).

CLASSIFICATION OF SOFT TISSUE INJURIES

There are numerous methods for classification of soft tissue injuries. Some use anatomic change while others use etiology or clinical symptomatology. Clinically injuries may be graded from 1 to 4 based upon their symptomatology. Patients with grade 1 injuries typically have transient pain or discomfort that occurs shortly after the injury. The patient may experience local tenderness on physical examination either with palpation or stretching of the injured tissue. Grade 2 injuries are more intense with pain symptoms lasting several weeks after the initial episode. If exercise patterns continue, the pain typically presents late in the exercise program or immediately following the program. Physical examination reveals more localized pain. Grade 3 injuries tend to last several weeks after the initial incident. Pain is usually present in the middle of activity but becomes progressively more obvious with initiation of the activity associated with the injury. Grade 4 injuries are those in which pain is present for more than four weeks. Pain typically occurs before or early in each exercise program. At this stage, physical findings include reduced range of motion and, in some cases, atrophy of muscle groups. McKeag further defined these pathophysiological events in an attempt to demonstrate the appropriateness in imaging procedures (19). Typically with grade 1 and 2 injuries, there is muscle inflammation and some breakdown with release of lactic acid. With grade 3 injuries, periostitis may be evident. Bone involvement with potential stress fracture occurs with grade 3 and grade 4 injuries. Therefore, it is at this point where imaging may be more appropriate (16,19).

Injuries vary with etiology. The etiology of direct soft tissue injury may be direct trauma. This can lead to contusion of the underlying tissues. Indirect injuries may be acute or chronic. Acute injuries occur with sudden overloading of muscles, tendons, or ligaments. "Overuse" injuries are due to repeated overload or frictional resistance. Tendonitis and bursitis are usually examples of overuse, but they can occur with acute trauma (16,19, 23,24).

Injuries to muscle tendon units and ligaments are classified in a similar fashion (Fig. 3-1). Terms that are used to describe the two different anatomic sites differ although the grading system is similar. Injuries to muscle

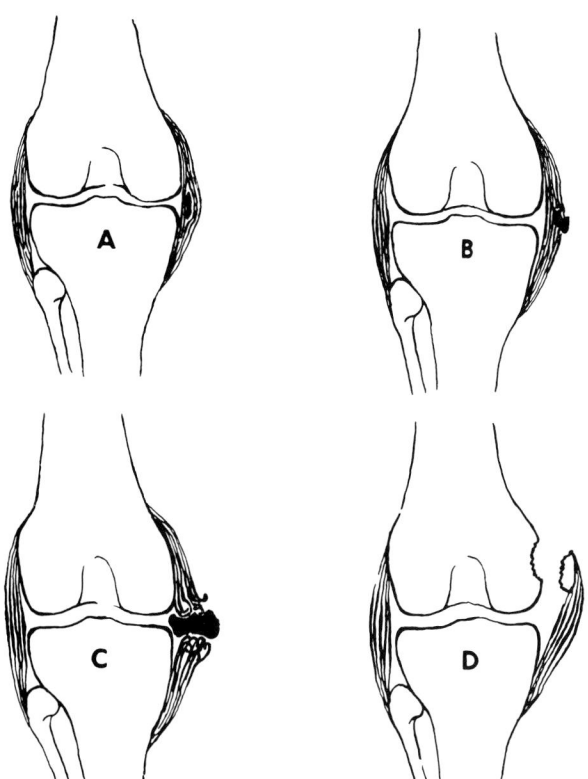

FIG. 3-1. Illustration of the classification used for ligament sprains. A: Grade 1: minimal disruption of fibers; B: Grade 2: ≤50% of fibers involved; C: Grade 3: complete disruption; D: fracture-sprain-avulsed fragment of bone with ligament separation (23).

tendon units are classified as strains and can be grouped into three general categories. A grade 1 strain indicates a minor injury to a muscle or tendon unit with only minimal fiber disruption. A grade 2 strain indicates a more significant injury with up to 50% of the muscle or tendon fibers involved. Grade 3 strains are complete disruptions of the muscle tendon unit. Ligament injuries are referred to as *sprains* and classified using the same system. A fourth category available for ligaments is the avulsion sprain. This category indicates an avulsion fracture with ligament attached (4,17,23).

HEALING OF SOFT TISSUE INJURIES

An understanding of the time required and the number of pathophysiologic changes that occur for healing of soft tissue injuries is important. This is especially useful when evaluating imaging techniques in patients with soft tissue injuries. For instance, phases of ligament healing similar to those described for fracture healing are generally divided into three stages. First is the acute *inflammatory* phase, followed by the *reparative* phase, and finally the *remodeling* phase. The acute inflammatory phase generally occurs within the first 72 hours but may last longer depending upon the severity of the injury. During this phase, cellular and four major humoral components are responsible for the changes in the injured area. First, intrinsic coagulation factors are stimulated by damaged surfaces of exposed collagen in the wall of the damaged blood vessels. The fibrinolinic system and kinin system also play a part. The latter has a strong vasodilatory effect on blood vessels in the region of the trauma, which results in the edema secondary to the increased vascular permeability. The complement system initiates an antigen antibody complex that stimulates the process of phagocytosis for removal of damaged tissue (16,23,32).

The reparative phase, or phase 2, varies with the extent of injury. This phase begins 48–72 hours after injury and may last up to six weeks. This phase is characterized by generation and deposition of collagen in the injured area. The remodeling phase may last up to a year or more. With healing, the ligament contracts providing increased tensil strength. At 12 months, however, only 50–75% of the original strength is retained (35). The effect of activity on collagen formation in the remodeling phase is critical. An exercise program designed to stress the ligament will be likely to stimulate the healing and, thus, increase strength of the injured area (2,16,23,32,35).

Normal ligaments differ from repaired ligaments in the type of collagen that is present. Normal ligaments are composed primarily of Type I collagen, whereas damaged or healing ligaments contain a large portion of immature, or Type III collagen. The concentration of Type I collagen becomes predominant upon complete healing (35). Studies of collagen repair have found that healing collagen is deficient in both content and quantity for at least 40 weeks following injuries (16).

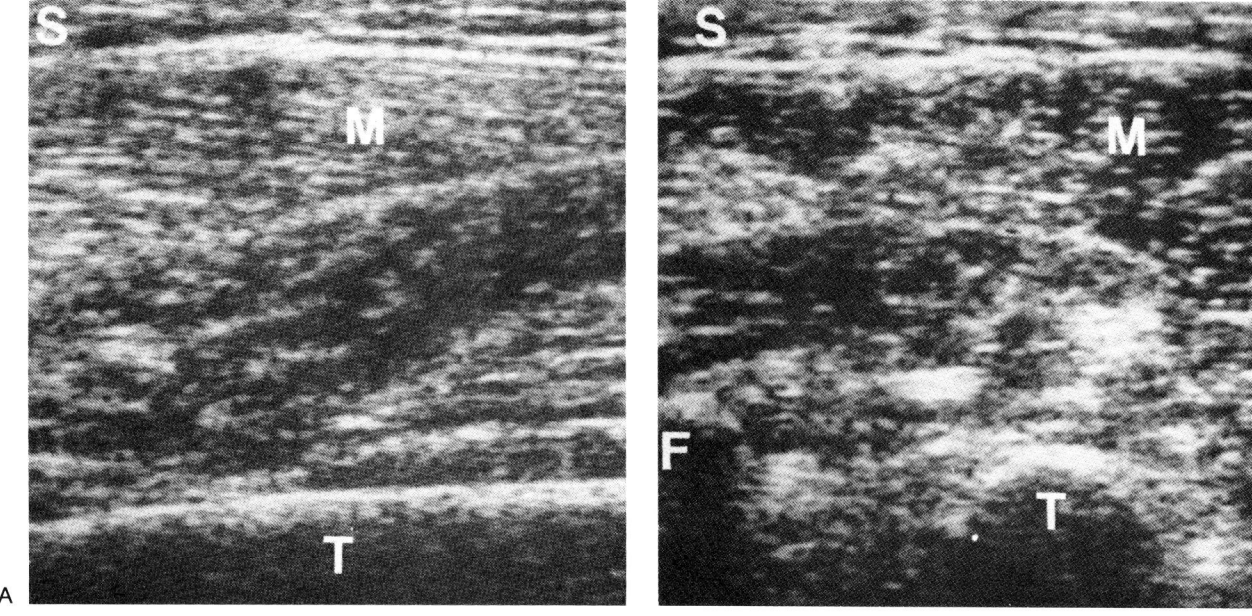

FIG. 3-2. Ultrasonography of normal muscle and tendon. **A:** Longitudinal and **(B)** transverse sonogram of the normal leg. (S, subcutaneous tissue; M, muscle; T, tibia) (From 13, used with permission.)

IMAGING OF SOFT TISSUE INJURIES

New imaging techniques, specifically MRI, have increased our ability to detect and follow post-traumatic extra-articular soft tissue conditions (4,8–10). Specific anatomic features will be discussed more fully in later chapters. However, general image features are most appropriately discussed in this section.

Hemorrhage-Hematoma

Imaging of contusions and minor hemorrhages into muscle or other soft tissues is generally not required. However, evaluating the extent of injury and separation of minor injury from hematoma may be important (8–10,22,23). These injuries may be identified by distortion of soft tissue plains on routine radiographs. However, more commonly, ultrasonography, CT, or MRI is used to evaluate soft tissue injuries (4,10,13,15).

Ultrasonography is useful for differentiating solid and cystic lesions. More recently superficial tendon, ligament, and muscle injuries have also been evaluated with ultrasound, i.e., the Achilles tendon and rotator cuff (13,15). Subcutaneous fat is more echogenic than the underlying muscle. Normal muscle typically contains fine parallel echoes (15). The overlying fascia forms a fine echogenic layer over the muscle (Fig. 3-2). Echogenicity varies with muscle contraction so that, when contracted, the volume increases but echogenicity frequently decreases (13,15). Tendons and ligaments have a fibrillar echo pattern (Fig. 3-3) (13,15). The ultrasound appearance of hemorrhage and hematoma vary with the

degree of injury and clot present. Organized clot is more echogenic than lysed clot or fluid, which tends to appear echoic (15). Organized hematomas have well-defined margins (Fig. 3-4), whereas hemorrhage is more irregular with enlargement of the muscle bundle (13,15).

MRI has replaced CT for evaluation of many soft tissue lesions, including post-traumatic hemorrhage and hematoma (4,10). Acute hemorrhage into a muscle is usually hyperdense on CT with increased volume of the involved muscle compared to the opposite extremity. Changes may be subtle. The MR features of soft tissue injury have been well documented (4,8,10). Normal

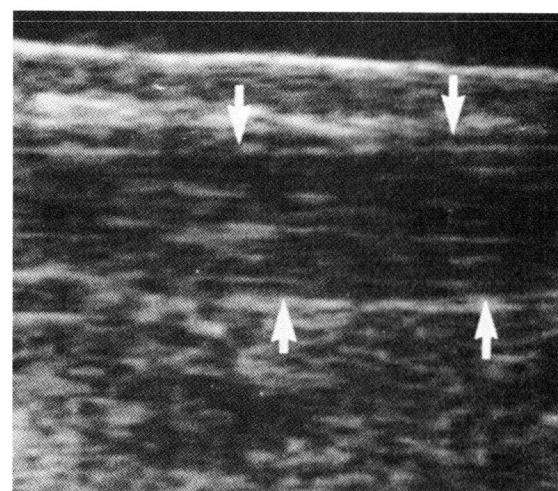

FIG. 3-3. Longitudinal sonogram of a normal Achilles tendon demonstrating the normal parallel linear echoes (From 15, used with permission).

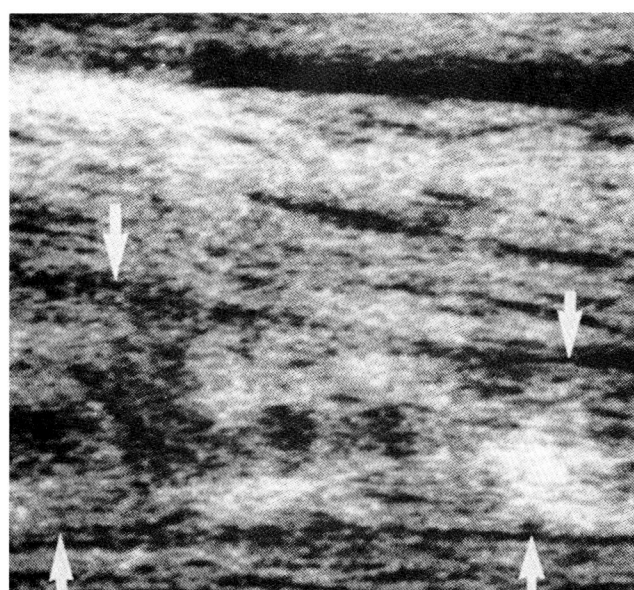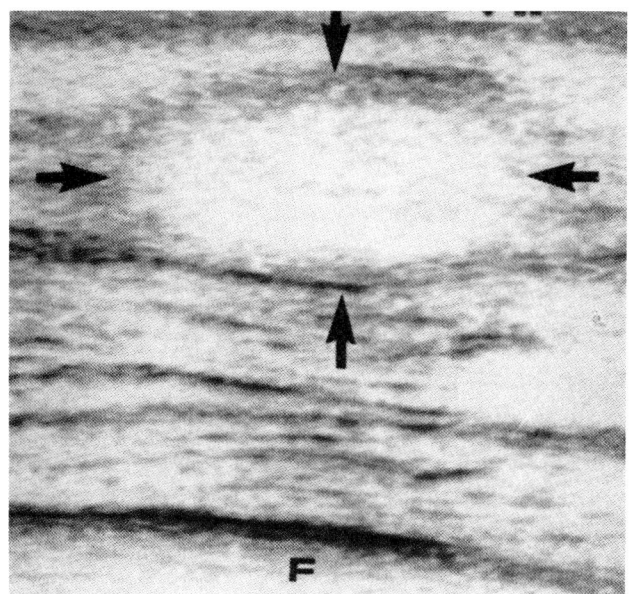

A   B

FIG. 3–4. Sonogram of a biceps hematoma (**A**) with loss of normal muscle echo texture and areas of mixed echogenicity (*arrows*). **B:** Longitudinal sonogram of an oval hypoechoic hematoma (*arrows*) (F, femur). (From 15 used with permission.)

muscle has intermediate signal intensity on MR images. Fat and marrow are high intensity, and ligaments, tendons, and bone have no signal and appear black on MR images (4). Hemorrhage has a feathery high signal intensity appearance on T2-weighted images (Fig. 3-5) and may be lower intensity or isointense with muscle on T1-weighted sequences. With time, the signal intensity returns to normal if no further injury occurs (4,33).

Hematomas are well-defined collections of variable signal intensity. Signal intensity varies with the field strength of the magnet and the age of the hematoma (4,6,8,30,33). The signal intensity is effected by the presence of paramagnetic substances. The relaxation times of oxygenated blood are long (low intensity on T1- and high intensity on T2-weighted images) compared to normal solid tissues (8). At high fields (≥ 1.0T), deoxygenated hemoglobin contains iron in the high-spin ferrous state. When red cell membranes are intact, the diffusing water molecules experience shifts in resonant frequency due to the presence of a field gradient that causes T2 relaxation shortening. This results in areas of low intensity in hematomas on high field imagers (Fig. 3-6). With time, methemoglobin formation occurs, which contains iron in the ferric (strongly paramagnetic) form. This tends to reduce T1 relaxation time greater than T2 relaxation time (6,8,9). Therefore, methemoglobin can cause areas of high intensity or T1-weighted images and low intensity on T2-weighted images (Fig. 3-7). In some cases, hematomas resolve more slowly than hemorrhage and may remain symptomatic for months to years if improperly treated (4).

Muscle, Tendon, Ligament Injuries

Ultrasound, CT, and MRI are effective for evaluating sprains and strains (4,5,8,29). Tendon and ligament tears are seen as localized areas of increased echo texture (13,15). MRI and CT may also demonstrate these defects. However, because of the superior soft tissue contrast, MRI is superior to CT in classifying the grade of injury. T2-weighted images clearly demonstrate the width of the normal low intensity tendon or ligament. Ruptures are demonstrated as areas of high intensity (Fig. 3-8). By using both axial and either coronal or sagittal images, the grade (1, 2, or 3) of tear can be defined. T1-weighted images are usually not necessary (4).

Myositis Ossificans

Computed tomography is the technique of choice for evaluating myositis ossificans. The features are not as well described with MRI. Early peripheral ossification or calcification is more easily detected with CT when radiographic features are not typical and do not need clarification (1).

Rhabdomyolysis

Imaging of rhabdomyolysis can be accomplished with radionuclide scans. Delayed Tc-99 mHDP bone scans demonstrate areas of increased soft tissue uptake. Increased uptake of isotopes in muscle may be related to

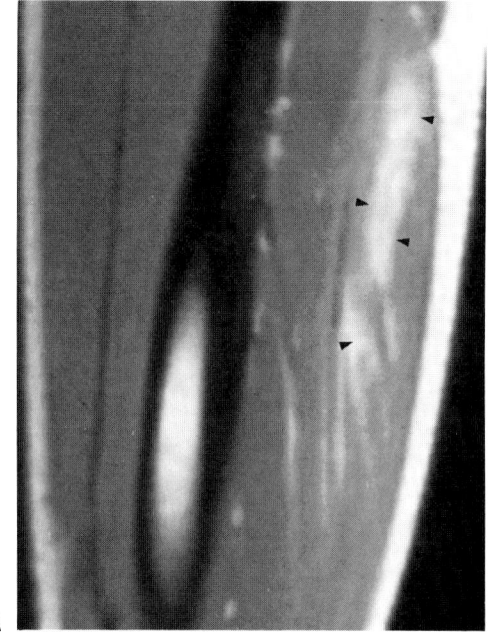

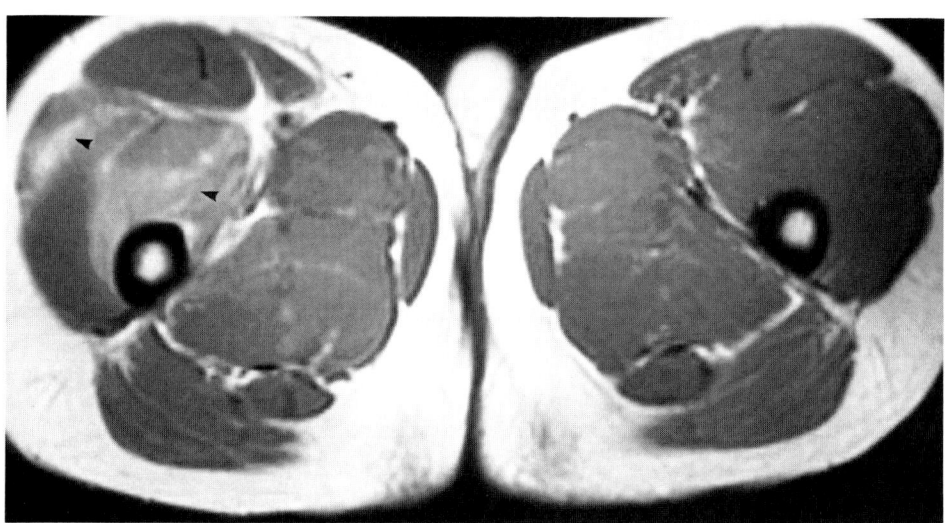

FIG. 3–5. A: T2-weighted (SE 2000/60) sagittal image of the thigh demonstrating an irregular area of increased signal intensity (*arrowheads*) due to hemorrhage into the hamstring muscles. **B:** Axial spin density (SE 2000/30) image of the thighs showing the normal left thigh and irregular increased intensity on the right (*arrowheads*) due to hemorrhage.

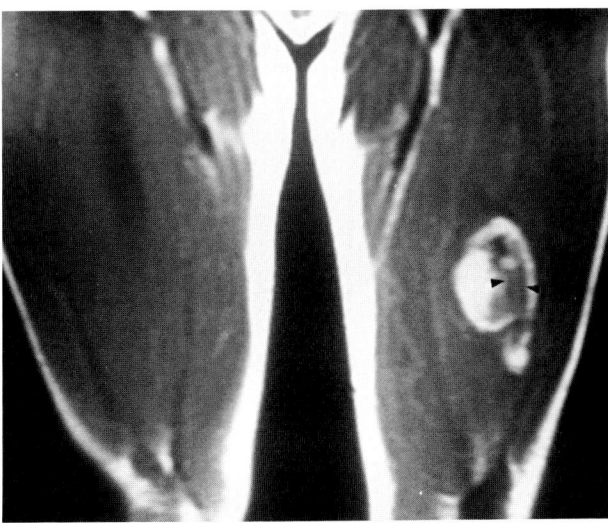

FIG. 3-6. Coronal T2-weighted image of a thigh hematoma with low intensity in the center (*arrowheads*) due to paramagnetic effects.

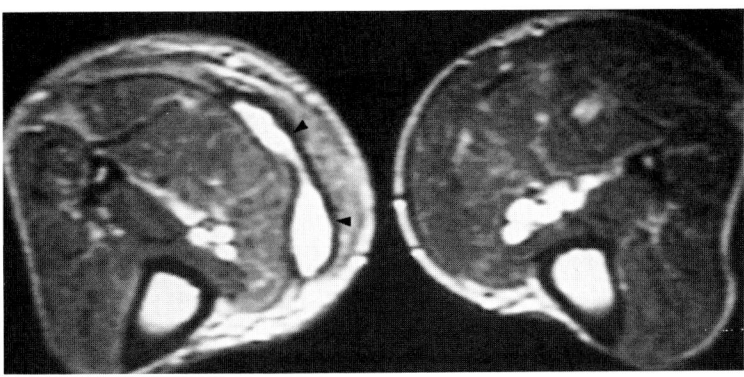

FIG. 3-7. Chronic hematoma (SE 2000/60) in the calf between the soleus and gastrocnemius due to a plantaris muscle tear. The margin (*arrowheads*) is low intensity that can be seen with macrophage ladened with methemoglobin or a fibrous capsule.

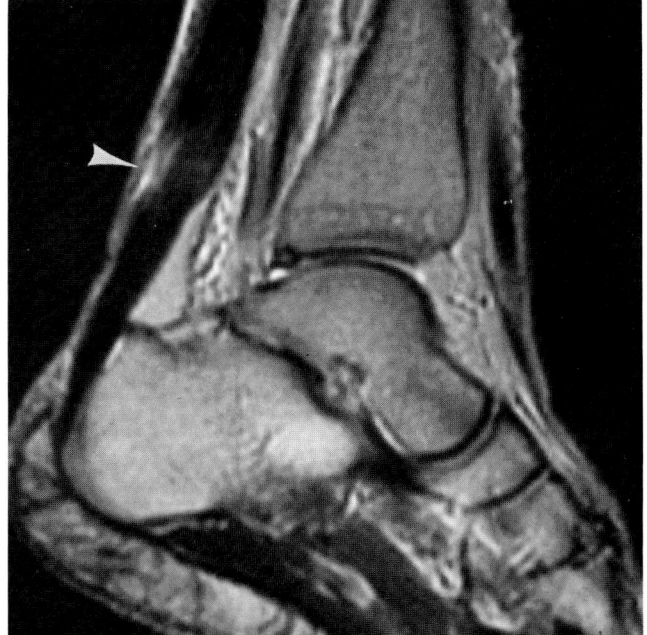
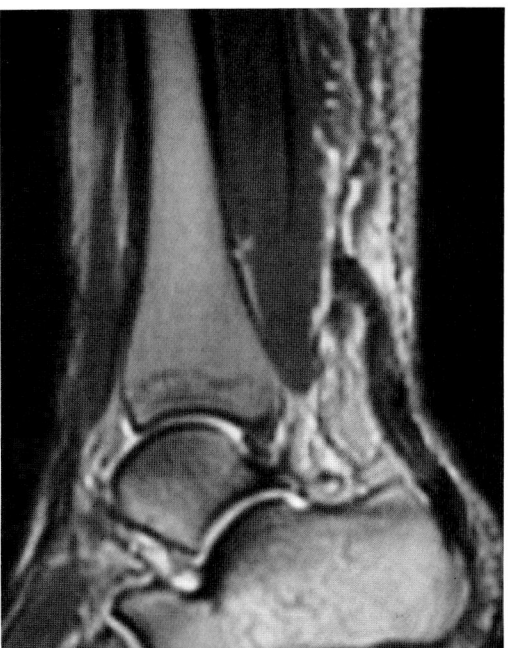

FIG. 3-8. Sagittal SE 2000/60 images of Achilles tendon tears. **A:** Grade 1 tear (*arrow*) with thickening of the tendon. **B:** Complete tear with loss of integrity and laxity of the distal segment.

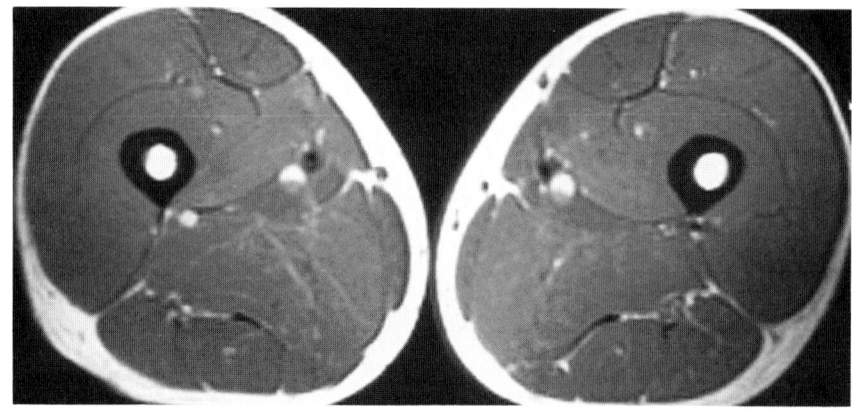

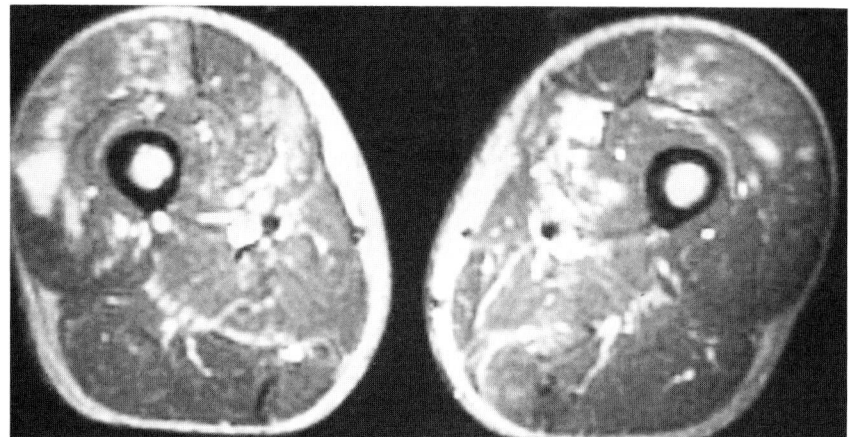

FIG. 3–9. Rhabdomyolysis due to overuse. **A:** T1-weighted (SE 500/20) image of the thighs is normal. **B:** T2-weighted (SE 2000/60) image shows multiple interstitial and focal areas of increased signal intensity. Changes are most extensive in the quadriceps group.

hyperemia, altered capillary permiability, or binding to hormone or enzyme receptors (14,18).

CT and MRI provide superior spatial resolution, and the contrast advantages of MRI make this technique ideal for determining the muscle groups that are involved. It is important to obtain T2-weighted (SE ≥ 2000, ≥60) in order to clearly define the soft tissue involvement. Rhabdomyolysis may be easily overlooked on T1-weighted images (Fig. 3-9).

Miscellaneous Conditions

Other overuse syndromes such as tenosynovitis, bursitis, etc. may not require imaging studies. However, MRI is capable of defining many bone, joint, and soft tissue disorders. Therefore, it is an excellent screening technique for evaluating musculoskeletal injuries (4,8,10).

REFERENCES

1. Amendola MA, Glazer GM, Agha FP, Frances IR, Weatherbee L, Wartel W. Myositis ossificans circum script: Computed tomographic diagnosis. *Radiology* 1983;149:775–779.
2. American Academy of Orthopedic Surgeons, Orthopedic Knowledge Update 3: Home Study Syllabus. Park Ridge, American Academy of Orthopedic Surgeons, January, 1990.
3. Baker BE. Current concepts in diagnosis and treatment of musculotendinous injuries. *Med Sci Sports Exerc* 1984;16:323–327.
4. Berquist TH. *Magnetic resonance of the musculoskeletal system.* New York: Raven Press, 1990.
5. Daffner RH, Reimer BL, Lupetin AR, Dash N. Magnetic resonance imaging of acute tendon ruptures. *Skel Radiol* 1986;15:619–621.
6. Dooms GC, Fisher MR, Hricak H, Higgins CB. MR imaging of intramuscular hemorrhage. *J Comput Assist Tomogr* 1985;9:908–913.
7. Dyment PG. Athletic injuries. *Sports Med* 1989;10:291–299.
8. Ehman RL. Interpretation of MR images. In Berquist TH. *Magnetic resonance of the musculoskeletal system.* New York: Raven Press, 1990.
9. Ehman RL, Berquist TH. Magnetic resonance imaging of musculoskeletal trauma. *Radiol Clin North Am* 1986;24:291–320.
10. Fleckstein JL, Weatherall PT, Partey RW, Payne JA, Pesbock RM. Sports related muscle injuries: Evaluation with MR imaging. *Radiology* 1989;172:793–798.
11. Fronek J, Marabak SJ, Hargens AR, Lee YF, Gersheeni PH, Garfen MA, Akeson WH. Management of chronic exertional anterior compartment syndrome of the lower extremity. *Clin Orthop* 1987;220:217–227.
12. Garrett WE, Nicholau PK, Ribbeck BM, Glisson RR, Seaber AV. The effect of muscle architecture on the biomechanical failure properties of skeletal muscle under passive extension. *Am J Sports Med* 1988;16:7–12.
13. Harcke HT, Grissom LE, Furkelstein MS. Evaluation of the musculoskeletal system with sonography. *AJR* 1988;150:1253–1261.
14. Herfhens RJ, Sievers R, Kaufman L. Nuclear magnetic resonance imaging of the infarcted muscle: A rat model. *Radiology* 1983;147:761–764.
15. Kaplan PA, Matamoros A, Anderson JC. Sonography of the musculoskeletal system. *AJR* 1990;155:237–245.

16. Kelle HJ. Acute soft tissue injuries—a review of the literature. *Med Sci Sports Exerc* 1985;86:489–500.
17. Marcinik EJ, Hodgdon JA, O'Brien JJ. A comparison of sprain and strain injury rates during aerobic/calisthenic and aerobic/circuit weight training programs. *Mil Med* 1987;152:252–254.
18. Martin P, Lang G, Caretta R, Simon G. Scintigraphic evaluation of muscle damage following extreme exercise. *J Nucl Med* 1983;24:308–311.
19. McKeag DB. The concept of overuse: Primary care aspects of overuse syndromes in sports. *Primary Care* 1984;11:43–59.
20. McMaster PE. Tendon and muscle ruptures. *J Bone Joint Surg* 1933;15:705–722.
21. Muckle DS. Injuries in sport. *Royal S Health* 1982;102:93–94.
22. Oakes BW. Hamstring muscle injuries. *Aust Fam Physician* 1984;13:587–591.
23. O'Donoghue DH. *Treatment of injuries to athletes.* 4th Ed., Philadelphia: W.B. Saunders, 1984.
24. Puffer JC, Zachazewski JE. Management of overuse injuries. *Prac Ther* 1988;38:225–232.
25. Radirs EL. Role of muscles in protecting athletes from injury. *Acta Med Scand Suppl* 1986;711:143–147.
26. Raether PM, Luther LD. Recurrent compartment syndrome in the posterior thigh. *Am J Sports Med* 1982;10:40–43.
27. Renstrom P. Swedish research in sports traumatology. *Clin Orthop* 1984;191:144–158.
28. Rooser B. Quadriceps contusion with compartment syndrome. *Acta Orthop Scand* 1987;58:170–172.
29. Rosenberg ZS, Feldman F, Singson RD. Peroneal tendon injuries: CT analysis. *Radiology* 1986;161:743–748.
30. Rubin JI, Gomori JM, Grossman RI, Gefter WB, Kressel HY. High-field MR imaging of extracranial hematomas. *AJR* 1987;148:813–817.
31. Ryan AJ. Medical aspects of sports. *JAMA* 1965;194:643–645.
32. Smith GH. The treatment and management of soft tissue injuries. *Practitioner* 1987;58:170–172.
33. Swensen SJ, Keller PJ, Berquist TH, McLeod RA, Stephens DH. Magnetic resonance of hemorrhage. *AJR* 1985;145:921–927.
34. Whitesides TE, Haney TC, Moremoto K. Tissue pressure measurements as a determinator for need for fasciotomy. *Clin Orthop* 1975;113:43–51.
35. Woos LY, Orlando CA, Gomez MA, Frank CB, Akeson WA. Tensile properties in the medial collateral ligament in a function of age. *J Orthop Res* 1986;4:133–141.

Imaging of Orthopedic Trauma,
Second Edition, edited by T.H. Berquist,
Mayo Clinic © 1992. Published
by Raven Press, Ltd., New York.

CHAPTER 4

The Spine

Thomas H. Berquist and Miguel E. Cabanela

Anatomy, 93
  Osteology, 93
  Cervical Vertebrae, 96
  Thoracic Vertebrae, 96
  Lumbar Vertebrae, 96
  Sacrum, 99
  Ligamentous Anatomy, 100
  Neurovascular Anatomy, 101
Radiographic Evaluation of Spinal Trauma, 104
  Routine Radiography of the Cervical Spine, 104
  Routine Radiography of the Thoracic and Lumbar
    Spine, 115
  Conventional and Computed Tomography (CT), 119
  Magnetic Resonance Imaging (MRI), 121
  Radionuclide Scanning, 123
Cervical Spine Trauma, 123
  Mechanism of Injury, 123
  Cervical Spine Fractures and Fracture-Dislocations,
    129

Upper Cervical Spine, 129
Lower Cervical Spine (C3-C7), 151
Cervical Spine Trauma—Associated Injuries, 161
Cervical Spine Injuries—Essentials of Management,
  163
Thoracic and Lumbar Spine Trauma, 169
  Mechanism of Injury, 170
  Thoracic and Lumbar Injuries—Essentials of
    Management, 185
  Management of Specific Injuries, 186
  Radiographic Evaluation of Fusion Complications,
    190
Spondylolysis and Spondylolisthesis, 194
  Treatment of Spondylolysis and Spondylolisthesis,
    198
Ankylosing Spondylitis, 199
References, 201

ANATOMY

Review of the anatomic features of the spine is critical for proper interpretation and utilization of imaging techniques. Although a complete review of spinal anatomy is beyond the scope of this chapter, we will discuss essential anatomy required for radiographic interpretation.

Osteology

The vertebral column is composed of 7 cervical, 12 thoracic, 5 lumbar, 5 sacral, and 4 coccygeal segments (Fig. 4-1). The lateral masses of C1 (atlas) articulate with the occipital condyles at the base of the skull. The sacrum articulates with the innominate bones of the pelvis.

T. H. Berquist: Department of Diagnostic Radiology, Mayo Medical School, Mayo Clinic Jacksonville, Jacksonville, Florida 32224.
M. E. Cabanela: Department of Orthopedic Surgery, Mayo Medical School, Mayo Clinic, Rochester, Minnesota 55905.

The vertebral column supports the weight of the trunk and provides a bony protective covering for the spinal cord (3,4,9,10). Two major structures, the anterior body and posterior neural arch, make up the typical vertebra. The anterior body develops from one ossification center and the neural arch from two symmetric ossification centers (Fig. 4-2) (4). The neural arch normally fuses dorsally at 1 year of age. Fusion of the two posterior components with the anterior body usually occurs by 3 years of age. During puberty, secondary ossification centers appear on the spinous process, on the transverse processes, and at the margins of the superior and inferior articular facets. Ring epiphyses develop on the superior and inferior margins of the vertebral body. These centers usually fuse by age 25 (3–5). Failure of ossification centers to fuse can be difficult to differentiate from fracture (Fig. 4-3).

The typical vertebral body (Fig. 4-4) consists of the anterior body with the vertebral arch, which is composed of two pedicles and two paired laminae. The laminae

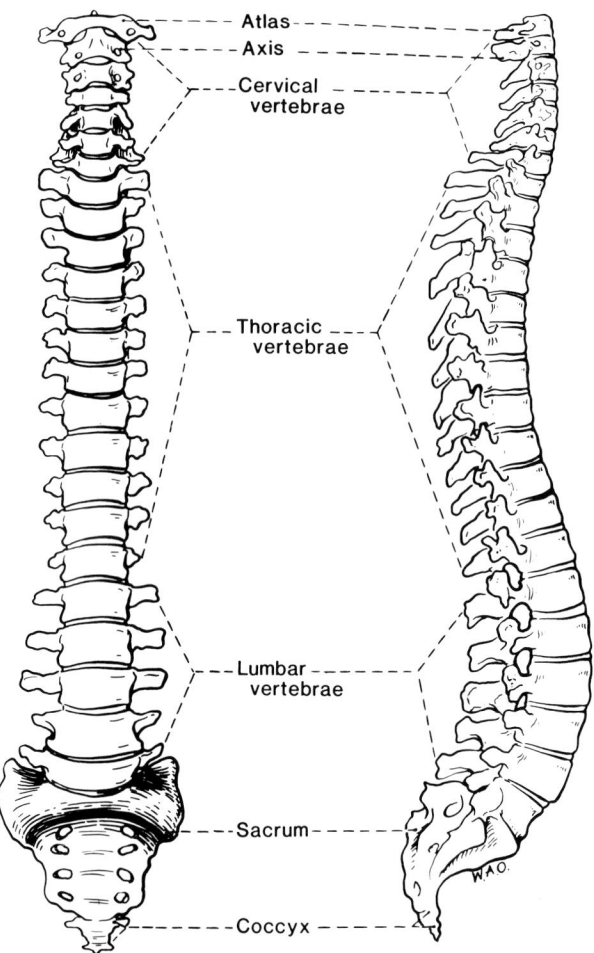

FIG. 4–1. Illustration of the AP and lateral views of the spinal column. The normal cervical and lumbar lordotic curves are demonstrated (5).

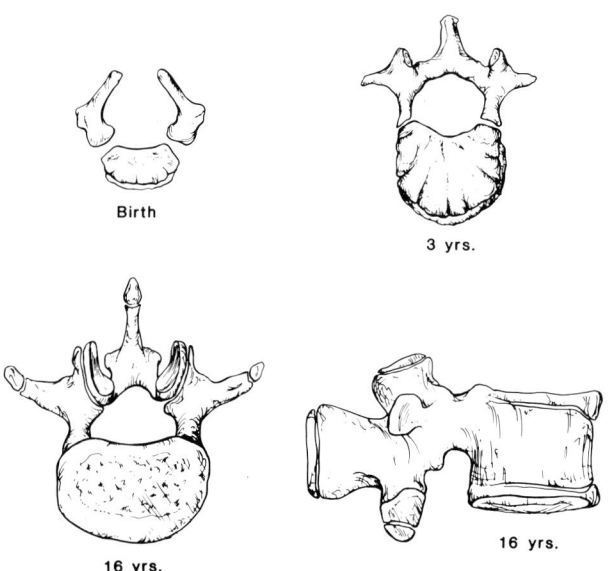

FIG. 4–2. Ossification centers of the vertebra.

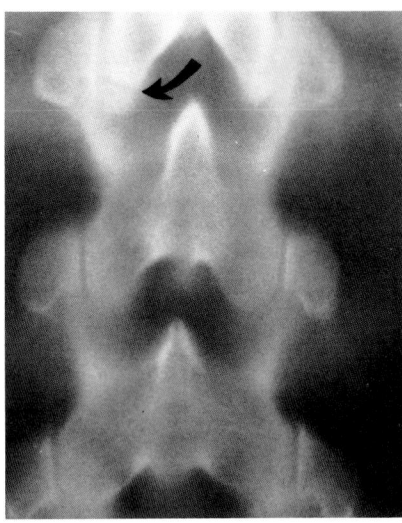

FIG. 4–3. Tomogram of the lumbar spine. There is an unfused ossification center (*arrow*). This should not be confused with a fracture.

join posteriorly to form the spinous process. In addition, there are transverse processes bilaterally. Four extensions from the lamina-pedicle junction form the apophyseal or facet joints. The facets articulate with the vertebrae above and below. These apophyseal joints play an important role in determining the range and direction of motion of the vertebral column (3). Most of the weight-bearing function is provided by the vertebral bodies and interposed elastic vertebral disks. However, the apophyseal joints are also involved in weight bearing, especially when one changes from the sitting to the standing position.

There are several anatomic features that distinguish the regions of the spine. The bodies of the cervical and lumbar vertebrae are wider in transverse than in AP diameter (Fig. 4-5). The thoracic vertebral body is more uniform in AP and lateral diameter. In the upper thoracic region the vertebral bodies are somewhat heart shaped. The spinal canal in the cervical and lumbar region is triangular compared with the smaller circular configuration in the thoracic region (4,5,8). The transverse processes in the cervical region contain anterior and posterior tubercles as well as a distinguishing feature, the foramen transversarium. The vertebral artery traverses this foramen from C7 to C1. The transverse processes in the thoracic region are directed dorsally, and T1 through T10 contain facets for rib articulation (Fig. 4-5B). Transverse processes in the lumbar region project almost straight laterally and increase in size from L1 to L3. The L4 transverse process is shorter and directed more cephalad. The transverse process of L5 is broader, more sturdy, and also directed dorsally (Fig. 4-6).

Spinous processes are short and often bifid in the cervical spine. The spinous process of C7 is the longest and most prominent, whereas the spinous process of C2 is

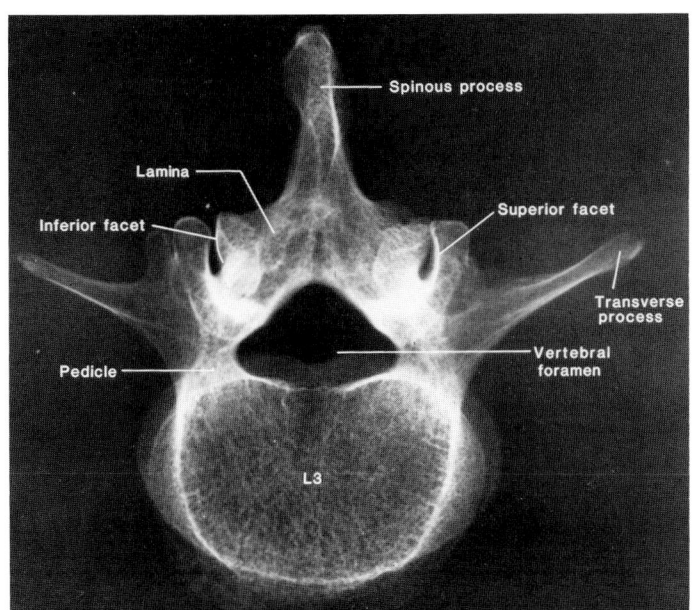

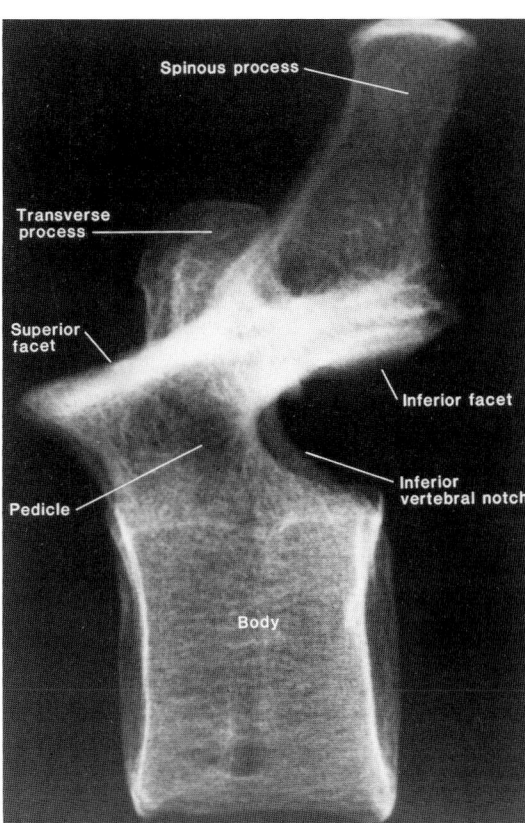

FIG. 4-4. Radiographs of dried skeletal specimens. **A**: Axial view of L3. **B**: Lateral view of L1.

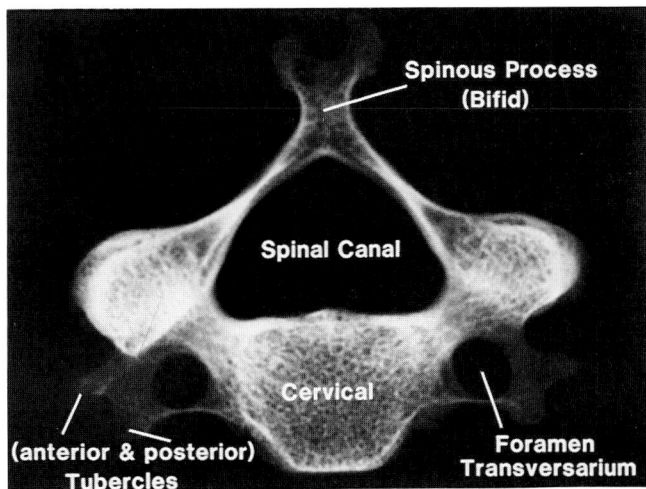

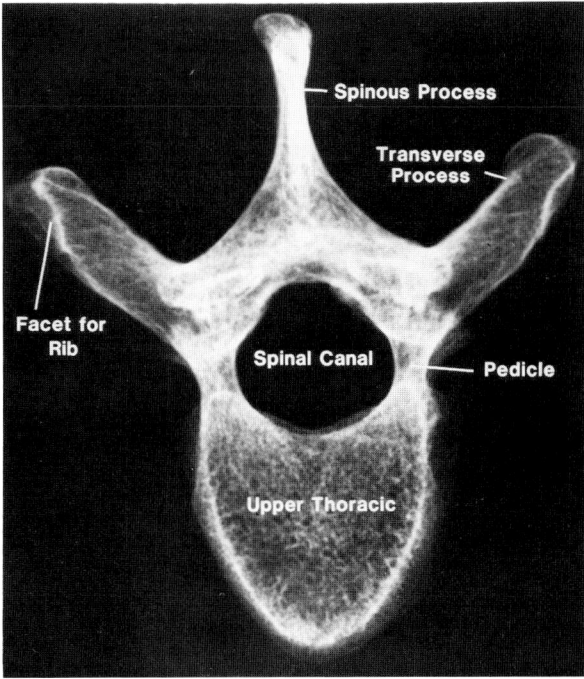

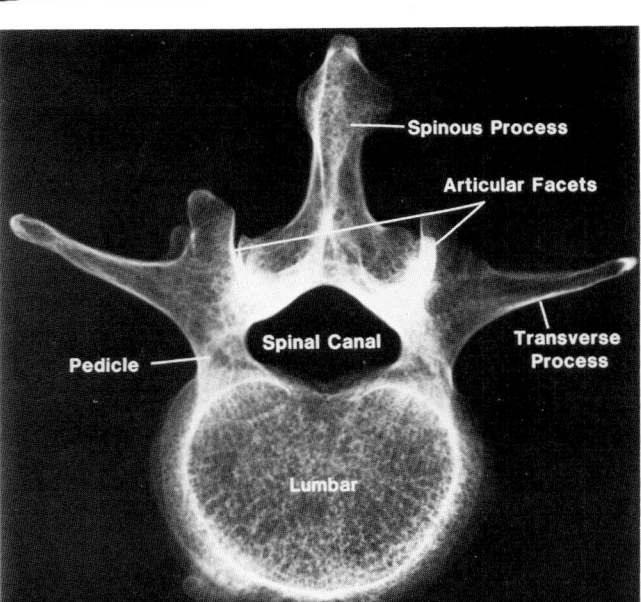

FIG. 4-5. Axial radiographs demonstrating features of the cervical (**A**), thoracic (**B**), and lumbar (**C**) vertebrae.

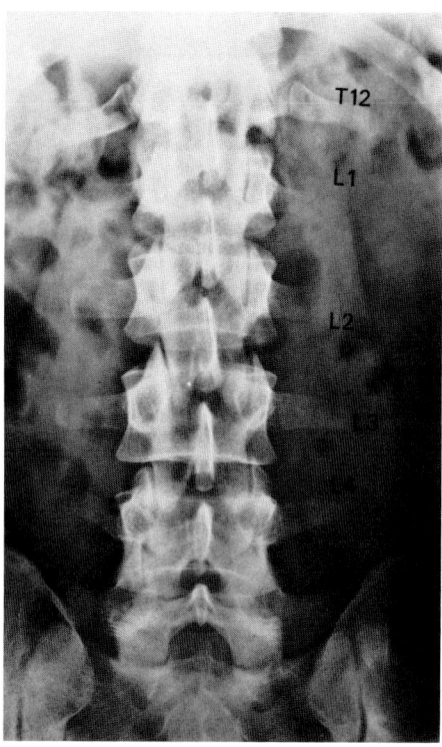

FIG. 4–6. AP radiograph of the lumbar spine demonstrating the typical appearance of the transverse process.

short and bulbous (see Figs. 4-5 and 4-9). Spinous processes in the thoracic region are directed sharply caudad; they are long and narrow compared with the broad-based short spinous processes in the lumbar region.

The articular facets differ significantly in the cervical, thoracic, and lumbar region. In the cervical spine, the articular facets angle approximately 20° in a caudad direction with the facet directed posteriorly. A similar but steeper angle is present in the thoracic region, and the facets are angled slightly dorsolaterally. The facet joints in the lumbar region change abruptly, with the superior facets directed dorsally and medially and the inferior facets directed ventrally and laterally (see Fig. 4-4A). This results in restricted rotation in the lumbar region (3–5,9).

Cervical Vertebrae

The distinguishing feature of the cervical vertebrae is the foramen transversarium. In addition, there are several significant anatomic differences between C1, C2, C7, and the remaining cervical vertebrae (C3 to C6). The atlas (Fig. 4-7) has no vertebral body and lacks a true spinous process (1,3,4,5). C1 (atlas) is a ringlike structure with a large vertebral foramen bounded by the anterior and posterior arches. There are two large lateral masses that contain a superior articular facet. This facet articulates superiorly and medially with the occipital condyle. The inferior facet is directed medially and articulates with the superior facet of C2. Medial to the lateral masses are tubercles for the attachment of the strong transverse

ligament. The transverse processes of C1 are also much larger when compared with the remaining cervical vertebrae (Fig. 4-7A).

C2 has several distinguishing features. These include a prominent but short spinous process that is helpful in differentiating the level of the upper cervical spine when the entire spine is not included on a radiographic film (Fig. 4-8). The odontoid or dens projects superiorly from the body of C2 and articulates with the anterior ring of C1. The spinal canal at C2 is significantly smaller and rounder than C1. The articular facets of C2 are also atypical when compared with the remaining cervical spine. The superior facets are directed in a superior lateral direction with an angle of approximately 20° in a lateral and caudad direction (Fig. 4-8) (1,3).

The C3 through C6 vertebrae are typical cervical vertebrae (Fig. 4-9) with triangular vertebral foramina and typically the facet joints are directed inferiorly approximately 20°. C7 can be distinguished by its prominent spinous process (Fig. 4-9). In 2% of cases there is a tubercle on the transverse process of C7 for a cervical rib (4,5).

Thoracic Vertebrae

The upper and lower thoracic vertebrae have some features similar to the cervical or lumbar vertebrae. Thus, the middle four thoracic vertebral bodies are most typical. In the upper thoracic spine the vertebral bodies are more triangular or heart shaped, with the apex of the triangle directed ventrally (see Fig. 4-5). The vertebral bodies in the thoracic spine are typically larger in AP than in transverse diameter. The height of the thoracic vertebral body is 1.5–2 mm less ventrally than dorsally (Fig. 4-10). This normal feature should not be confused with a compression fracture (1,3,4,5). Costal facets for rib articulations are a distinguishing feature of thoracic vertebrae. These are located on the inferior or ventral surface of the transverse process from T1 to T10 and at the junction of the body and pedicle from T1 to T12. The last two ribs do not typically articulate with the transverse processes. The pedicles in the thoracic spine are short and thin, and the vertebral foramina are smaller and more circular than those in either the cervical or lumbar region. The transverse processes typically decrease in length as one progresses from T1 to T12. Orientation of the facets in the thoracic region is almost vertical. They are directed posteriorly and slightly laterally throughout the thoracic spine except at the T12 level. Here the inferior facets face laterally to articulate with the superior facets of L1.

Lumbar Vertebrae

The lumbar vertebral bodies are larger than the thoracic vertebrae and are typically kidney shaped, with the transverse diameter greater than the AP diameter (see Figs. 4-4 and 4-5). The vertical dimension of L5 is

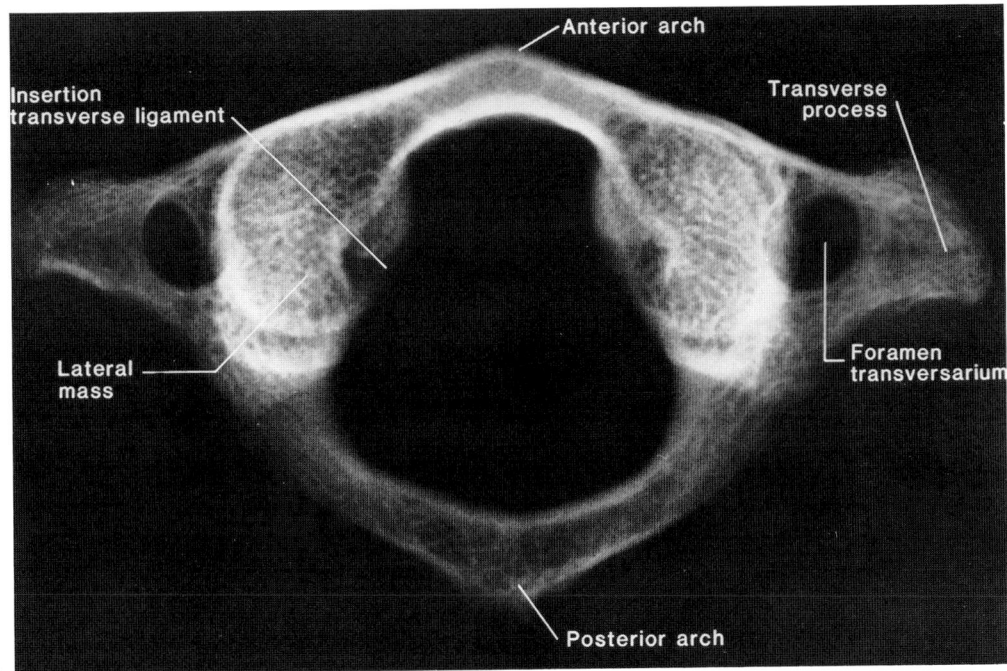

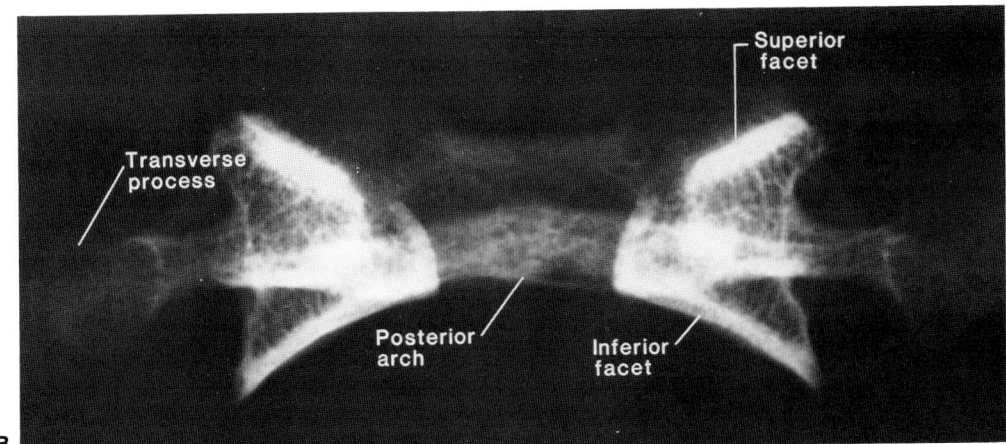

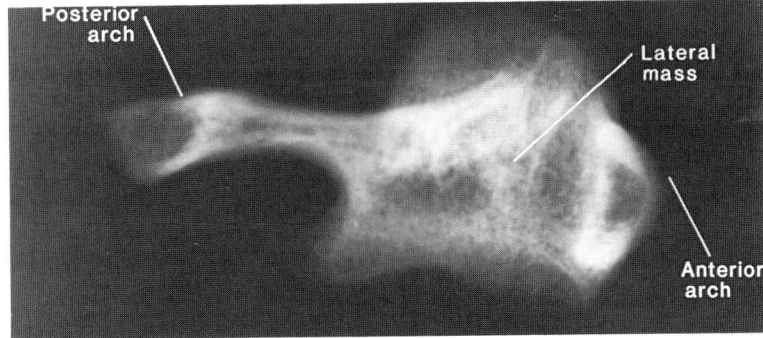

FIG. 4–7. Radiographs of the atlas (C1). **A**: Axial view; **B**: AP view; **C**: lateral view.

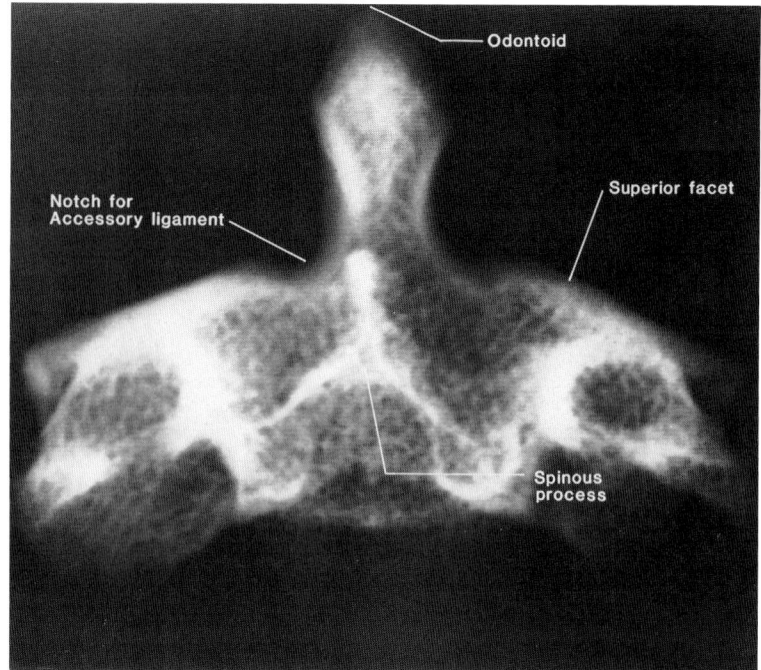

A

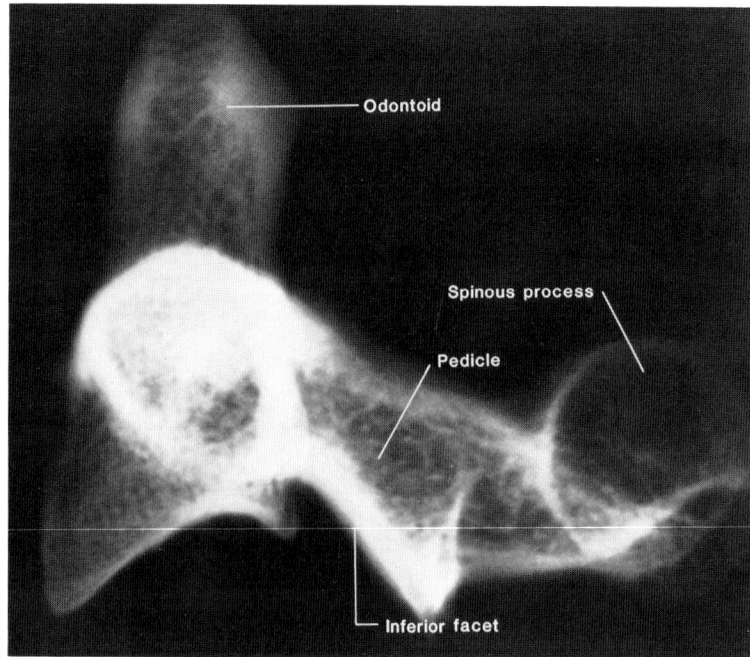

B

FIG. 4-8. Radiographs of C2 in the AP (**A**) and lateral (**B**) projections.

THE SPINE / 99

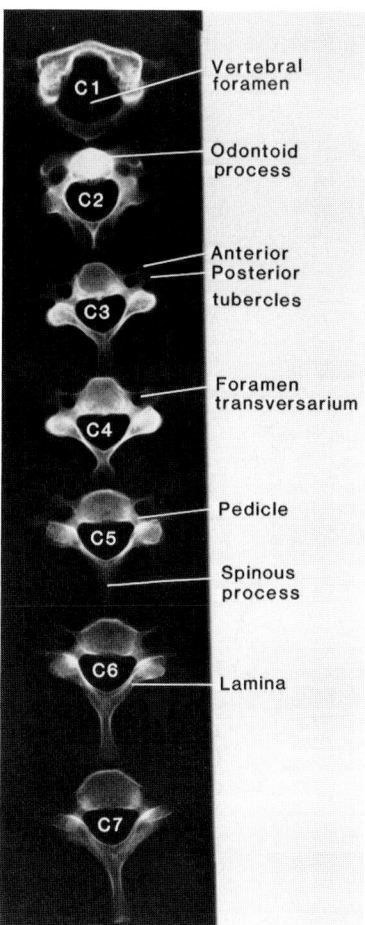

FIG. 4-9. Axial radiographs of the cervical vertebrae.

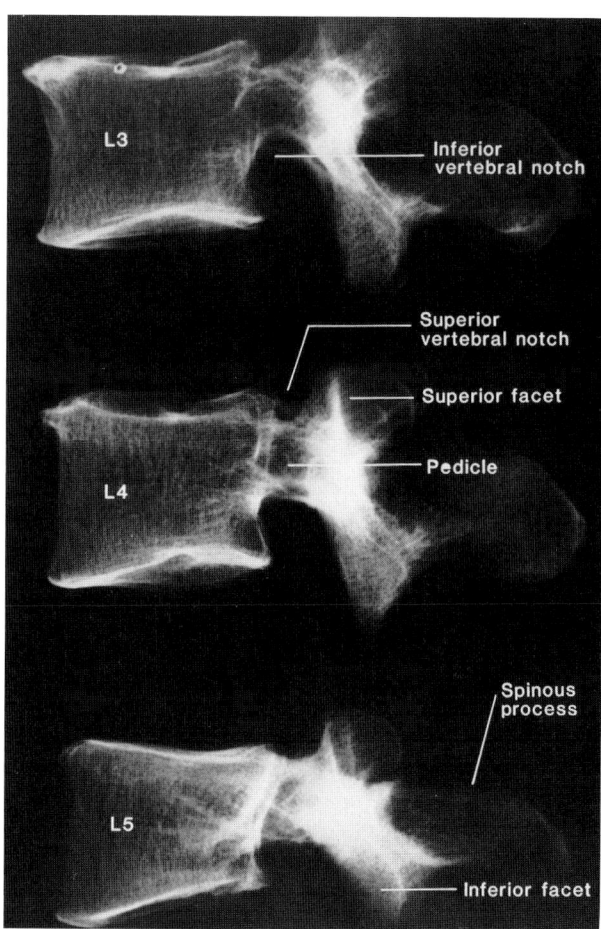

FIG. 4-11. Lateral radiographs of L3-L5.

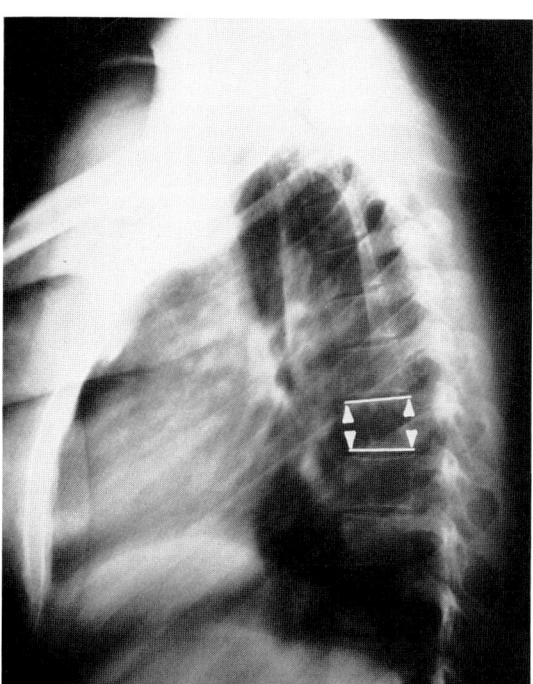

FIG. 4-10. Lateral view of the thoracic spine demonstrating the reduced height of the anterior vertebral body (*arrows* at anterior and posterior margins).

greater anteriorly than posteriorly (Fig. 4-11). As in the case of the cervical spine, the spinal canal or the vertebral foramen is triangular in the lumbar region. The laminae in the lumbar region are strong and often asymmetric. The pedicles are short and thick. The apophyseal joints arise from the lamina-pedicle junction. The superior facets are directed posteriorly and medially and the inferior facets, posteriorly and laterally. The lumbar vertebrae have no costal facets and no foramen transversarium. The transverse processes of the first three lumbar vertebrae are straight and project almost directly laterally, increasing in length from L1 through L3. At L4 and L5 the transverse processes are shorter, with the transverse process of L4 being directed somewhat dorsally and superiorly compared with the short, stout transverse process of L5 (Fig. 4-6) (3,4,5,9).

Sacrum

In adults, the sacrum is composed of 5 nonmovable segments (Fig. 4-12). The disks are ossified and fused. The first sacral segment and C1 are the only vertebrae with true lateral masses (3,4). The sacrum articulates with the ilia, forming paired synovial sacroiliac joints. Superiorly, two facets articulate with the inferior facets

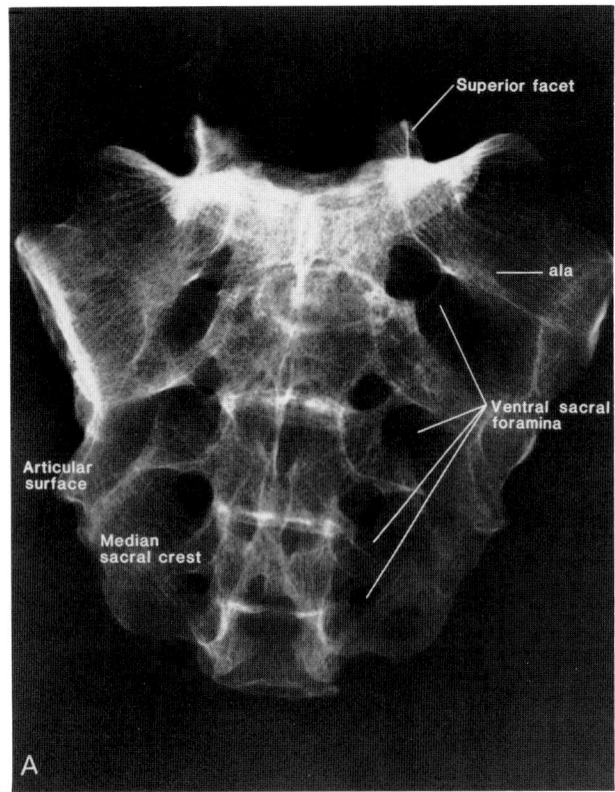 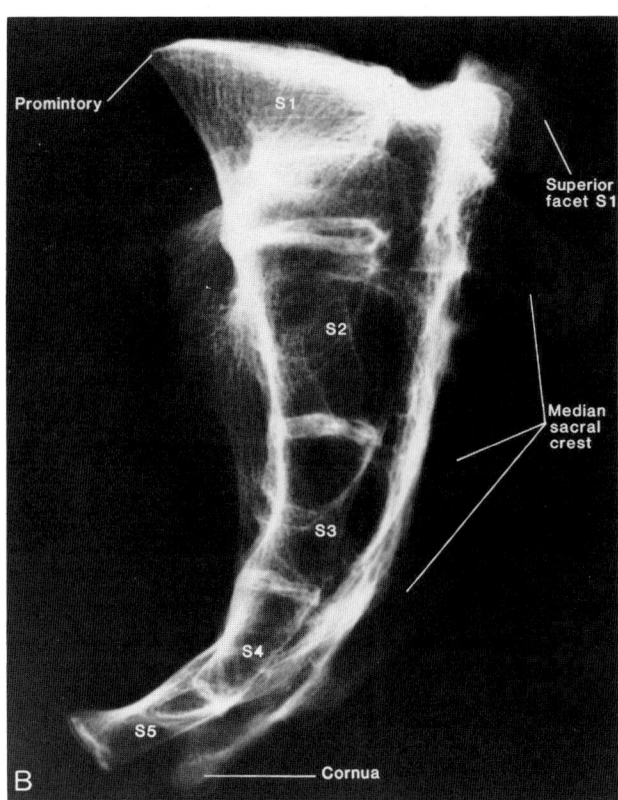

FIG. 4-12. Radiographs of the sacrum. AP (**A**) and lateral views (**B**) of dried skeletal specimens.

of L5. Of the five sacral segments, the first is the largest. The size of the segments diminishes as one progresses inferiorly. The costal elements and transverse processes are fused. On the AP or frontal view the ventral sacral foramina (four pairs) can be clearly visualized (1,5).

Ligamentous Anatomy

The fibrocartilaginous intervertebral disks are the main connecting segments between the vertebral bodies from C2 through the sacrum. There may be rudimentary disks at the sacral levels; however, the sacral segments are usually completely fused.

The nucleus pulposus and annulus fibrosus are derived from the notochord embryologically. The disks, composed of the nucleus pulposus and annulus, contribute approximately one-fourth to one-third of the height of the vertebral column (4). The configuration of the disk varies somewhat, depending upon the region of the vertebral column in which it is located. In the cervical region, the disks are taller ventrally than dorsally. A similar situation is present in the lumbar region (see Figs. 4-19, 4-31, and 4-32). In the thoracic region the disks are approximately equal in height anteriorly and posteriorly (Fig. 4-10). The thickness of the disk in the lumbar region increases slightly as one progresses from L1 to L4 with the disk at the L4 level being the largest (see Fig. 4-31B). The L5-S1 disk is triangular and much thicker ventrally. The fibers of the annulus fibrosus develop in

concentric rings running obliquely, with the superficial fibers blending into the anterior and posterior longitudinal ligaments (1,3,4,5,9).

The anterior longitudinal ligament is stronger and wider than the posterior longitudinal ligament (Fig. 4-13). It is narrowest at its origin at the base of the skull and gradually widens to the level of its insertion of the pelvic surface of the sacrum.

The posterior longitudinal ligament lies within the vertebral foramen along the posterior surface of the vertebral body (Fig. 4-13). This ligament is contiguous with the tectorial membrane superiorly and extends caudally into the sacral canal. The posterior longitudinal ligament blends with the fibers of the annulus fibrosus but is separated from the vertebral body by a venous plexus (5). The narrow width and central location of the posterior longitudinal ligaments may explain the increased incidence of posterolateral disk protrusions as opposed to central disk protrusions.

The ligamentum flavum is an elastic, thick, paired ligament that extends between the lamina of the adjacent vertebra. The ligaments blend with the articular capsules of the apophyseal joints (Fig. 4-13). Posterior to the ligamentum flavum is the thinner intraspinous ligament, which joins the spinous processes and blends superficially with the supraspinous ligament (Fig. 4-13). The supraspinous ligament in the cervical region is stronger and is called the ligamentum nuchae (Fig. 4-14). The latter structure extends from the external occipital pro-

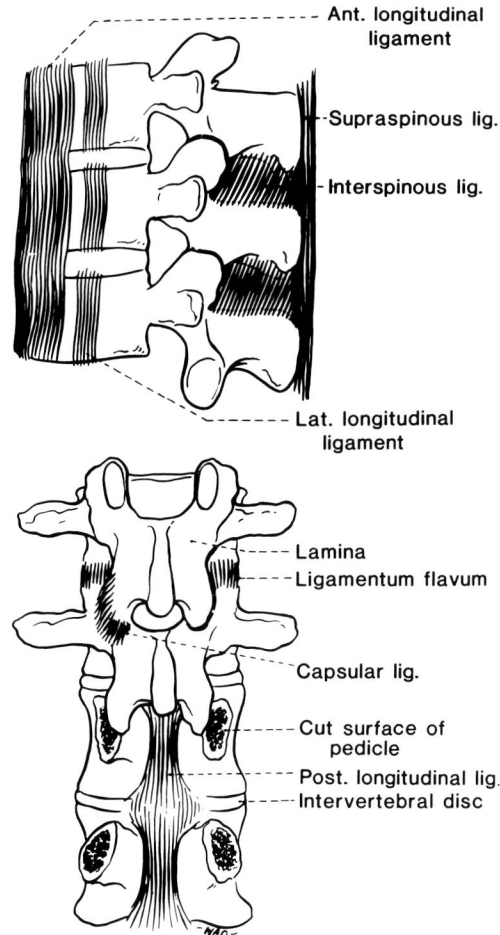

FIG. 4–13. Illustration of the ligament anatomy (5).

Labels for top illustration:
Ant. longitudinal ligament
Supraspinous lig.
Interspinous lig.
Lat. longitudinal ligament

Labels for bottom illustration:
Lamina
Ligamentum flavum
Capsular lig.
Cut surface of pedicle
Post. longitudinal lig.
Intervertebral disc

tuberance to the spinous process of C7. Extending between the transverse processes are the intertransverse ligaments, which are best developed in the thoracic and lumbar region and essentially nonexistent in the cervical region. Also, in the cervical region the interspinous ligament may be sparse and disappear with age, resulting in

a questionable significance if this ligament were torn secondary to trauma (3,4,5,7).

The apophyseal or facet joints are synovial joints with a fibrous capsule. Internally there are meniscuslike tabs composed primarily of synovium and fatty tissue that project from the capsule into the joints. The articular capsules are more lax in the cervical spine, allowing more motion than in the remainder of the spine.

The ligamentous anatomy in the atlantoaxial region is more complex, requiring more emphasis (Fig. 4-15). The posterior longitudinal ligament is continuous with the tectorial membrane that extends cephalad to the inner aspect of the foramen magnum. The transverse ligament lies ventral to the tectorial membrane. It is a strong fibrous band that connects the tubercles of the lateral masses of C1 posteriorly and maintains the relationship of the odontoid to the anterior ring of C1. There are synovial joints between the odontoid and anterior ring at C1 and between the odontoid and transverse ligament. In addition, there are three ligaments extending vertically from the tip of the odontoid (Fig. 4-15). The apical ligament extends superiorly and attaches to the occipital bone. The two alar or check ligaments extend from the apex of the odontoid in a dorsilateral direction. The accessory ligament is a significant structure attaching at the base of the odontoid on either side. It is through this ligament that the odontoid receives part of its blood supply (3–5,7,9).

Neurovascular Anatomy

The blood supply of the spinal cord is derived from the anterior and posterior spinal arteries (2,6). In the cervical region, these branches are supplied by the vertebral arteries. In the thoracic and lumbar region the arterial supply is derived from the paired intercostal and lumbar vessels. The artery of Adamkiewicz is generally the largest anterior spinal artery. This vessel arises from a lower inter-

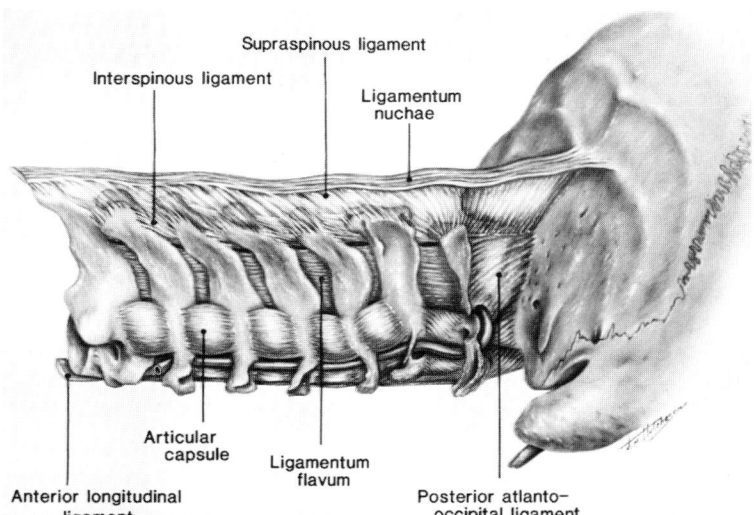

Labels:
Interspinous ligament
Supraspinous ligament
Ligamentum nuchae
Articular capsule
Ligamentum flavum
Anterior longitudinal ligament
Posterior atlanto-occipital ligament

FIG. 4–14. Ligaments of the cervical spine (7).

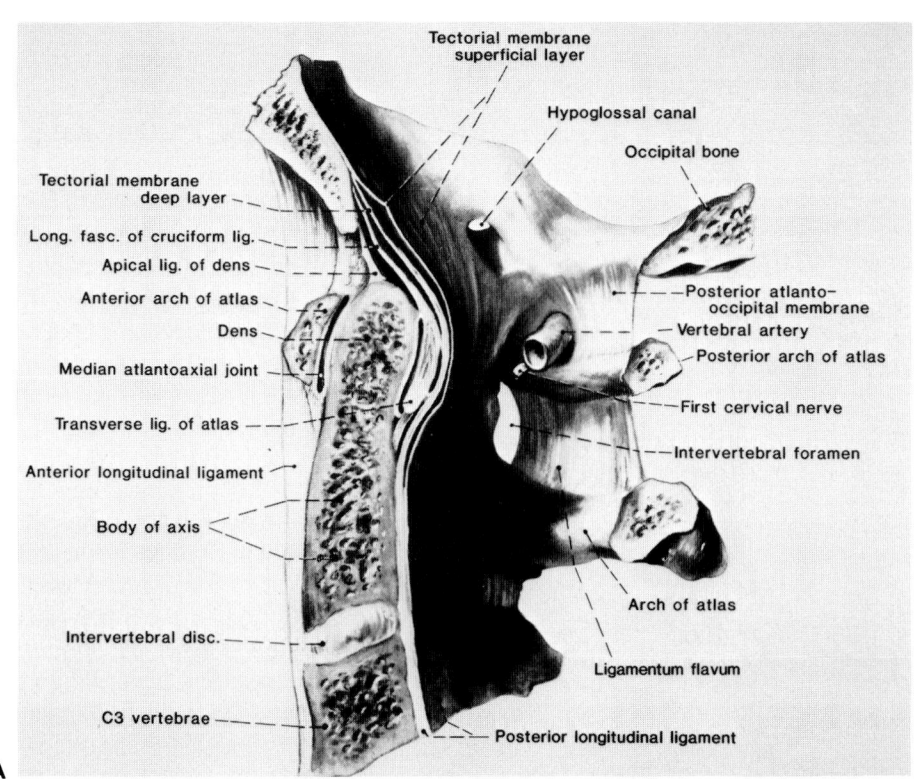

Tectorial membrane
superficial layer

Hypoglossal canal

Occipital bone

Tectorial membrane
deep layer

Long. fasc. of cruciform lig.

Apical lig. of dens

Anterior arch of atlas

Dens

Median atlantoaxial joint

Transverse lig. of atlas

Anterior longitudinal ligament

Body of axis

Intervertebral disc.

C3 vertebrae

Posterior atlanto-
occipital membrane

Vertebral artery

Posterior arch of atlas

First cervical nerve

Intervertebral foramen

Arch of atlas

Ligamentum flavum

Posterior longitudinal ligament

A

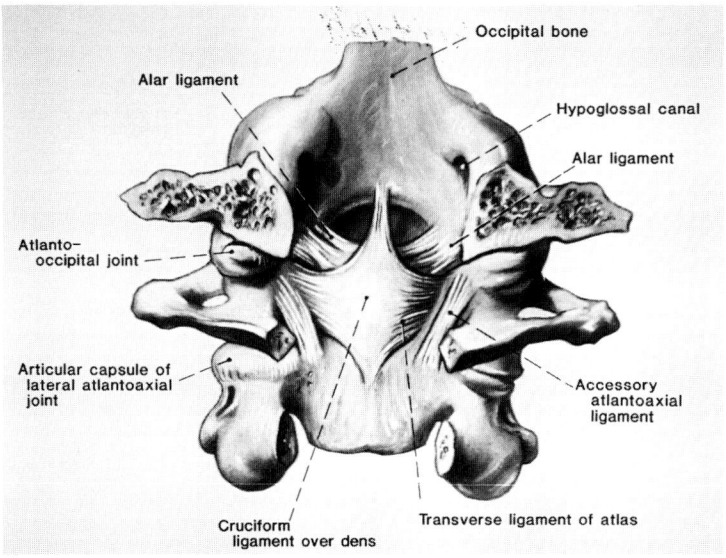

Occipital bone

Alar ligament

Hypoglossal canal

Alar ligament

Atlanto-
occipital joint

Articular capsule of
lateral atlantoaxial
joint

Accessory
atlantoaxial
ligament

Cruciform
ligament over dens

Transverse ligament of atlas

B

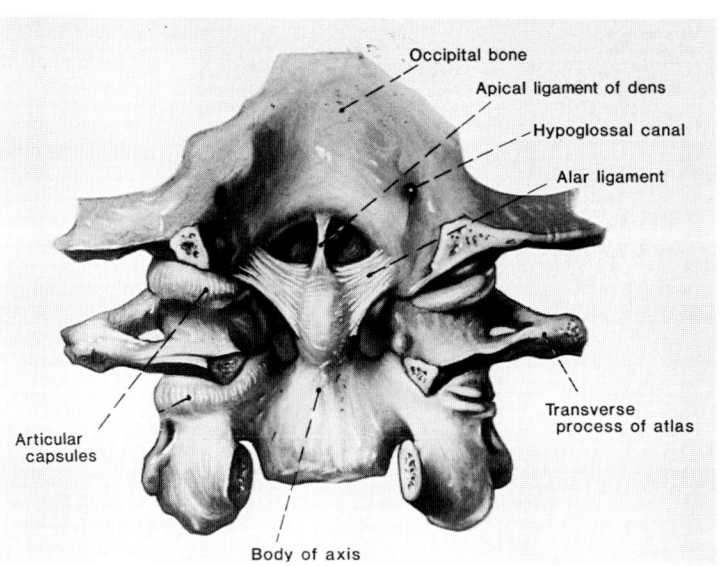

Occipital bone

Apical ligament of dens

Hypoglossal canal

Alar ligament

Transverse
process of atlas

Articular
capsules

Body of axis

C

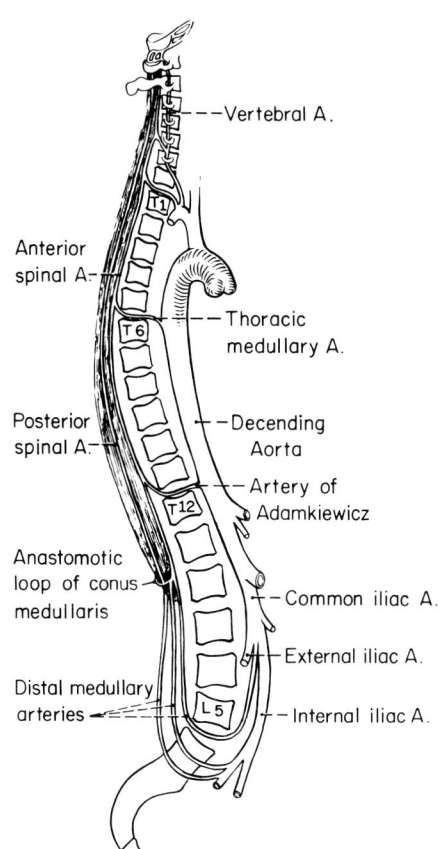

FIG. 4–16. Illustration of the vascular supply of the spinal cord (6).

TABLE 4-1. *Radiographic evaluation of spinal trauma*[a]

Routine Radiography
  Cervical Spine
    AP, lateral, oblique, open-mouth odontoid view[b]
    Swimmers view
    Angled AP views
    Pillar views
    Upright lateral[b]
    Fluoroscopic flexion and extension
  Thoracic
    AP, lateral[b]
    Oblique
  Lumbar
    AP, lateral[b]
    Oblique
Tomography (conventional)
  AP, lateral, oblique
Computed tomography
Myelography
Magnetic resonance imaging
Radionuclide scans

[a] (19,26); [b] routine procedure for acute trauma.

costal or upper lumbar artery (Fig. 4-16) (4,6). The blood supply in the sacral region is supplied by paired sacral vessels (Fig. 4-16). Multiple perforating arteries arise from these major vessels and supply the anterior portion of the vertebral body. Lateral to the vertebral body there is a dorsal segmental branch that supplies the posterior musculature (Fig. 4-17).

A portion of the venous drainage of the vertebral body occurs through the middle posterior surface in the same region as the chief entrance of the arterial supply (Fig. 4-17). The venous plexus is a valveless plexus lying between the spinal cord and body neural arch. The previously described plexus lying between the posterior longitudinal ligament and posterior aspect of the vertebral body drains the central tributaries from the vertebral body. There is also an internal plexus anteriorly and posteriorly that is connected to a series of circular venous channels. The internal plexus is continuous with the external plexus via the intervertebral foramina.

The spinal cord with its meningeal envelope lies within the vertebral foramen and extends in the adult from the foramen magnum to the upper border of L2 (2,3). The vertebral foramen is bordered by the body anteriorly, the pedicles laterally, and the lamina posteriorly. The size of the vertebral foramen is largest in the lumbar and cervical regions, which coincides with the nerve distribution to the upper and lower extremities. The spinal cord occupies approximately 50% of the vertebral foramen. The remainder of the space is occupied by the epidural venous plexus, which is intermixed with fat, connective tissue, and the protective meningeal portions of the spinal cord. The dura is a dense fibrous tube contiguous with the foramen magnum and extends to the level of the third sacral segment. The dural sleeves surround each set of spinal nerve roots as they exit the dural sac. The pia mater is the thin innermost layer of the meninges that is applied to the spinal cord and nerve roots as they cross the subarachnoid space. More peripheral to the pia mater is the arachnoid, which encloses the subarachnoid space. The arachnoid, pia, and dura are united by the dentate ligaments that pass from the spinal cord to the dura. In the adult the spinal cord proper terminates at the conus medullaris. The filum terminale continues caudally until it blends with the posterior ligament and sacral canal. Both structures are enveloped in the dural sac to the S2 level.

There are 31 pairs of spinal nerves: 8 cervical, 12 thoracic, 5 lumbar, 5 sacral, and 1 coccygeal. Cervical nerve roots exit above the level of the adjacent vertebral body (C8 exits between C7 and T1). In the remainder of the spine, the nerve roots exit below the adjacent bodies (T1 exits at the intervertebral foramen between T1 and T2).

FIG. 4–15. Ligament anatomy of the upper cervical spine. **A:** Sagittal illustration with anatomy labelled. **B, C:** Posterior coronal illustrations (5).

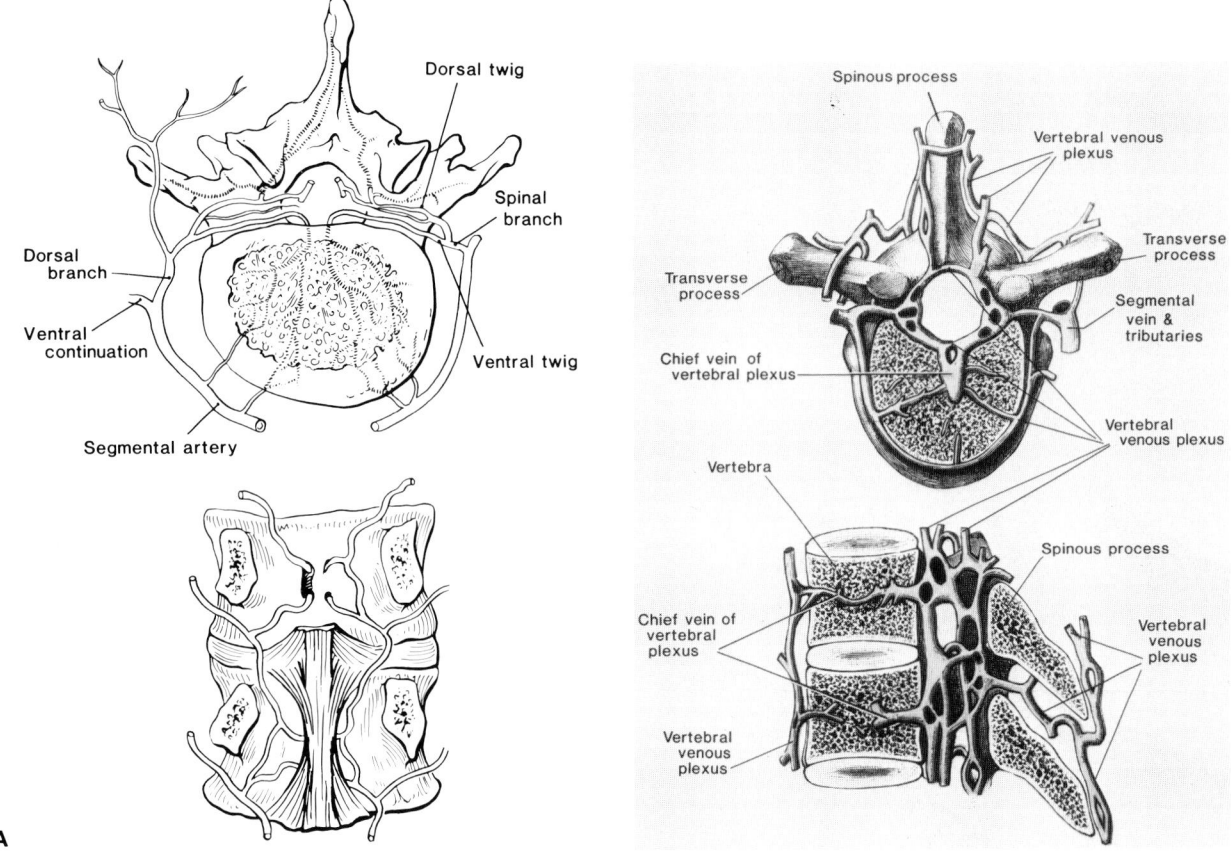

FIG. 4-17. Illustration of arterial (**A**) and venous (**B**) anatomy of the vertebra (5).

RADIOGRAPHIC EVALUATION OF SPINAL TRAUMA

Acutely injured patients with suspected spinal trauma must be properly immobilized until the radiographic examination is complete and treatment instituted. Radiographic evaluation can be accomplished only when close communication between the radiologist and clinicians (orthopedic surgeons and neurosurgeons) is maintained (19,59,72). A well-organized approach will ensure optimal use of routine films, tomography, computed tomography (CT), magnetic resonance imaging (MRI), and other techniques in determining the extent of injury and stability of the lesion (Table 4-1).

A simple radiographic table with an overhead tube capable of being positioned at different angles is sufficient for evaluation of the spine. The necessary views for evaluation of the cervical, thoracic, and lumbar spine can be easily obtained. We utilize a C-arm Versigraph, which allows AP, lateral, and oblique views without moving the patient. In addition, tomograms can be obtained in the AP, lateral, oblique, and transaxial projections. Conventional radiographic equipment would require the patient to be placed in the oblique or lateral position in order to obtain tomograms in these projections.

Routine Radiography of the Cervical Spine

Routine radiographs remain the most effective screening technique for evaluating spinal trauma (19,26). Radiographic evaluation of the cervical spine should be thoroughly and completely monitored by the radiologist

TABLE 4-2. *Lateral radiograph in cervical spine trauma[a]*

Injuries that can be identified	Injuries that are typically not identified
Upper cervical spine	Upper cervical spine
Atlanto-occipital dislocation	CI fractures
C1-C2 dislocation	Jefferson's fracture
C1 Fractures	Lateral mass
Anterior arch	Transverse process
Posterior arch	Lower cervical spine
C2 Fractures	Uncinate process
Odontoid	fracture
Vertebral body	Laminar fracture
Hangman's fracture	Pedicle fracture
Lower cervical spine	Pillar fracture
Compression fracture	Transverse
Burst fracture	process fracture
Spinous process fracture	
Locked facets	
Soft tissue injuries	
Flexion compression	
Flexion distraction	
Hyperextension	

[a] (19,29,40).

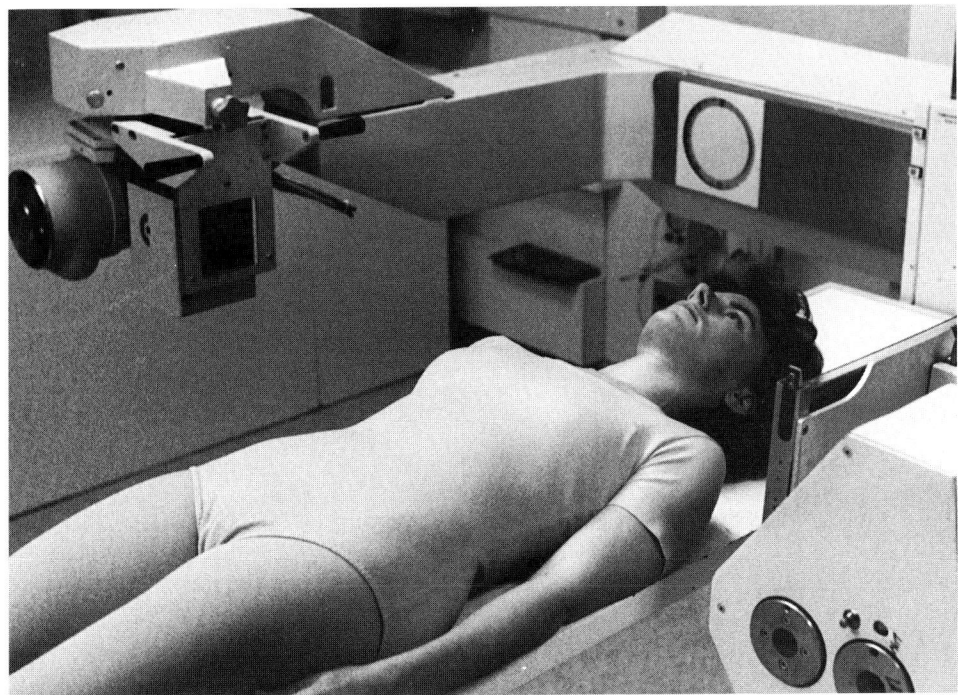
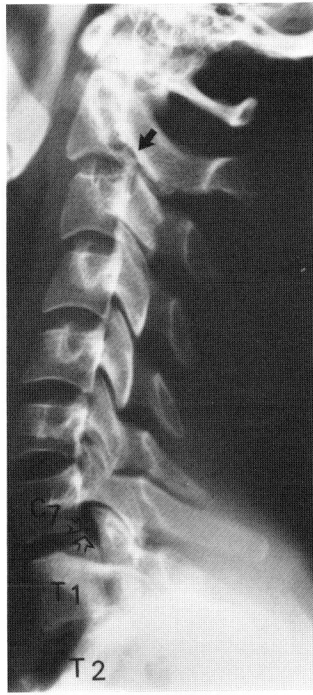

A

B

FIG. 4–18. Lateral view of the cervical spine. A: Patient positioned on the Versigraph with the C-arm horizontally oriented for the lateral view. B: Lateral view of the cervical spine demonstrating the difference in size of C7 and T1. Note also the normal subluxation of C2 on C3 in this teenage patient (*upper arrow*).

until the degree of injury has been established. Such an evaluation demands that the examination be tailored to the patient's clinical symptoms. The initial evaluation should include lateral, oblique, AP, and odontoid views (Table 4-1). Pillar views may also be indicated. However, the head must be turned for pillar views. Therefore, the other views should be studied first to determine whether it is safe or necessary to move the head for pillar views.

Lateral View

The initial lateral view is obtained with the patient supine using a cross-table lateral technique (Fig. 4-18). This view is the most important radiographic view, as most significant pathology can be detected on it (19,26,40,44). In our review of 420 cervical spine fractures, the lateral view was positive in approximately 90% (Table 4-2). Others report that at least 67% of injuries can be detected on the lateral view (26,40).

There are many features that should be carefully examined on the lateral view. It is essential that all seven cervical vertebrae be well demonstrated. Ideally, T1 should also be visible on the lateral view. The lateral view allows assessment of the following structures: the anterior and posterior arches of C1, the odontoid, vertebral bodies, disk spaces, facet joints, and spinous processes. The lateral radiograph shows that the body of T1 is larger than C7, which can give the false impression of subluxation (Fig. 4-18). This fact must be kept in mind in evaluating patients with flexion injuries.

The features demonstrated on the lateral view must be studied systematically as shown in Table 4-3. In the upper cervical region there are several relationships and measurements that must be checked routinely. These are better demonstrated on the lateral view of the head owing to better centering of the radiographic beam. A line drawn along the clivus to the tip of the odontoid should point to the tip of the odontoid at the junction of the anterior and middle thirds (Fig. 4-19). A line drawn tangentially to the lamina of C1 should intersect the posterior foramen magnum (19,25). The space between the odontoid and anterior ring of C1 measured at its most inferior margin should not exceed 2 mm in adults (19,25,40,44). This measurement may be as much as 4.5 mm in children (24,44).

Careful attention should also be paid to the soft tissues in the prevertebral space (19). In the adult, the measurement of the soft tissue from the anterior inferior margin of C2 to the retropharyngeal wall should not exceed 7 mm (19,40,44). The distance from the posterior wall of the trachea to the anterior inferior margin of C6 should not exceed 14 mm in children or 22 mm in adults (40). Care must be taken in measuring this distance in young people and children, because change in inspiration can simulate swelling. Nasogastric and endotracheal tubes invalidate measurements of the retropharyngeal space (Fig. 4-20) (40). The posterior portions of the maxillary antra and mandible may also provide a clue to the mechanism of injury. These structures can be partially studied on most lateral views of the cervical spine. Mandibular

TABLE 4-3. *Cervical spine trauma: Lateral radiographic evaluation*[a]

Upper cervical spine (occipital condyles to C2)	Lower cervical spine (C3-C7)

Clivo-odontoid relationship
C1-odontoid measurement
   2–2.5 mm in adults
   4–4.5 mm in children
Retropharyngeal space
Posterior pharyngeal wall to anterior inferior body
   of C2 = 7 mm adults, 7 mm children
	Anterior inferior margin C3 to pharyngeal
	   airway = 4–5 mm
	Prevertebral fat stripe
	Retrotracheal spaces (posterior tracheal wall
	   to anterior inferior body C6)
	   Normal in adults ≤ 22 mm
	   Normal in children ≤ 14 mm
	Anterior spinal line
	Posterior spinal line
	Spinolaminar line
	Disk spaces
	Facet joints
	Spinous processes and interspinous distance

[a] (19,40,44,71).

fractures are often associated with hyperextension injuries (46).

Perhaps a more useful and readily accessible tool than these varied measurements is the prevertebral fat stripe. This can be identified in most adults as it courses along the anterior margin of the anterior longitudinal ligament. At the C6 level it deviates anteriorly over the scalene muscles (Fig. 4-21) (40,76). Hemorrhage from hyperextension injuries will displace the fat stripe anteriorly (37,76). This may be the only indication of injury. The fat stripe is less frequently seen in children (19).

Although it is important to evaluate the prevertebral soft tissues, there is obviously overlap between normal and abnormal (see Fig. 4-20) (19,53,71). Templeton et al. (71) demonstrated considerable variation in normal

measurements. However, as a rule, if the soft tissues are abnormal one should proceed with further studies, including CT and MRI to be certain that an injury is not overlooked (53,71). When the prevertebral soft tissue measurements at the anterior inferior margins of C2, C3, C4 are 7–10 mm, further studies should be considered. If the measurement exceeds 10 mm, further imaging evaluation is definitely indicated (71).

The normal lordotic curve of the cervical spine can be followed along the anterior margins of the vertebral bodies (anterior spinal line), the posterior margins of the bodies (posterior spinal line), and the laminal spinolaminar line (Fig. 4-21) (41). Disruption in these lines can indicate instability or ligament injury with resulting subluxation (Fig. 4-22). One must be careful, however, not to confuse normal positional changes with pathology. In

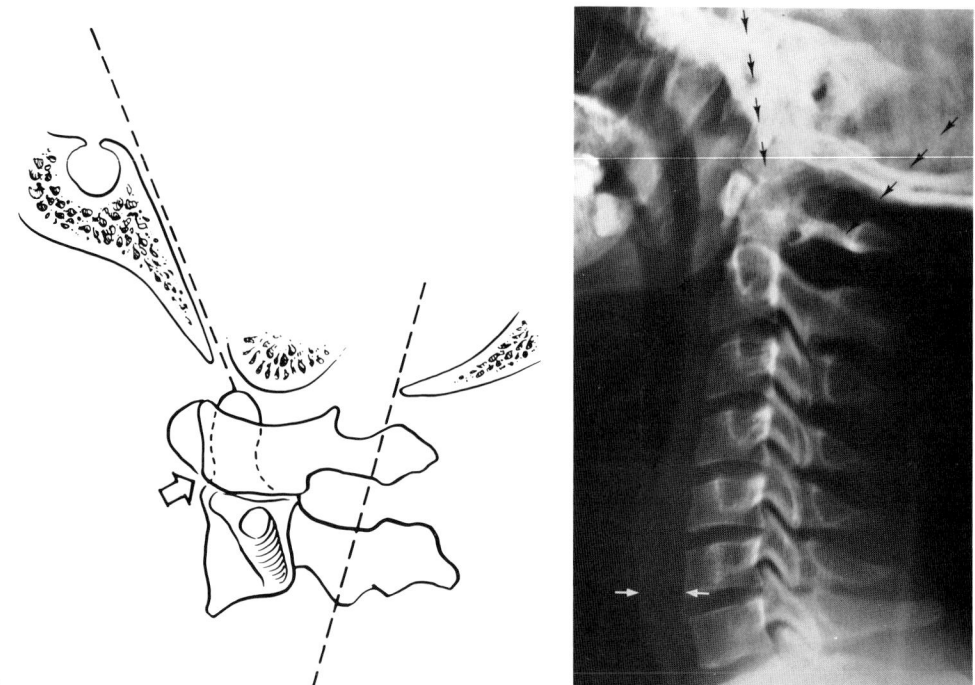

FIG. 4-19. A: Illustration of normal anatomic relationship in the upper cervical spine. **B**: Normal lateral cervical spine showing the lines of the lamina and clivus (*arrows*) and normal retrotracheal soft tissues.

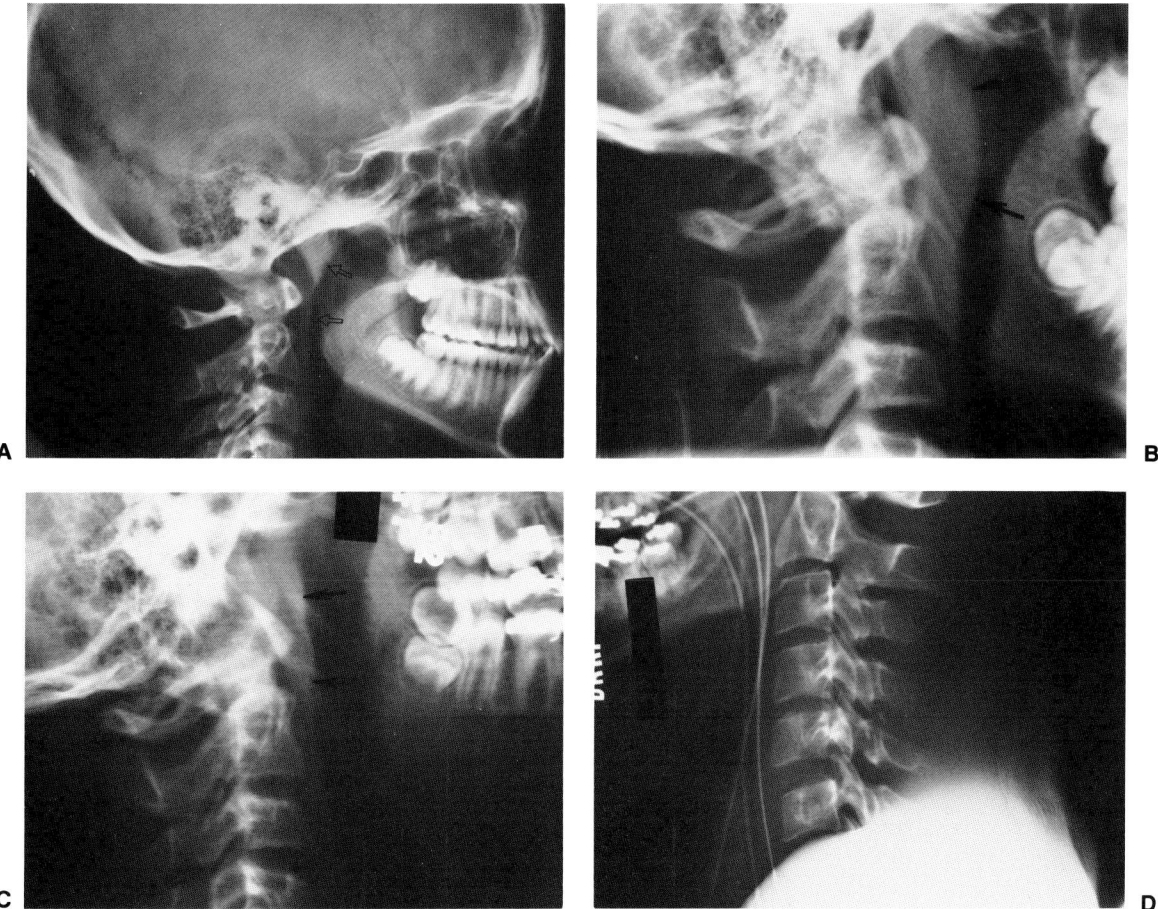

FIG. 4–20. A: Lateral view of the skull demonstrating normal retropharyngeal soft tissues. With slight flexion (**B**) the soft tissue appears prominent. In extension (**C**) the tissue is normal. If nasogastric or endotracheal tubes (**D**) are in place, accurate measurement is not possible.

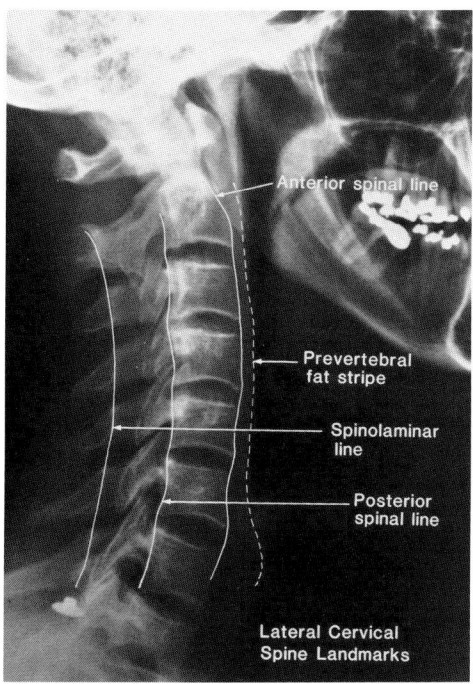

FIG. 4–21. Lateral view of the cervical spine demonstrating the normal cervical lines and prevertebral fat stripe.

the supine position, patients have a tendency to lose the normal cervical lordotic curve, which can be misinterpreted as evidence of a ligament injury (Fig. 4-22A). Muscle spasm may result in straightening of the normal cervical lordotic curve. In addition, there is normally slight ligament laxity at C2-C3 and C3-C4 in children and teenagers (see Fig. 4-18B). This can result in slight anterior subluxation of C2 on C3 or C3 on C4 until at least age 18.

Evaluation of the disk spaces, facet joints, and spinous processes is an important factor in determining treatment and prognosis of spinal injury (40,41). These areas can be fairly accurately assessed on the lateral view (Figs. 4-22B and 4-23). Lateral radiographs reveal instability, which can be defined as abnormal motion between vertebrae whether clinical symptoms are present or not (40,77). Findings indicating instability include narrowing of the disk space, compression of the vertebral body exceeding 25%, subluxation of greater than 3 mm, and increase in the rotational angle of adjacent vertebrae beyond 11° (46,69,77). An additional feature is widening of the interspinous distance, which normally decreases as one progresses caudally from C1 to C7 (Fig. 4-23). More recently, Young et al. (81) demonstrated

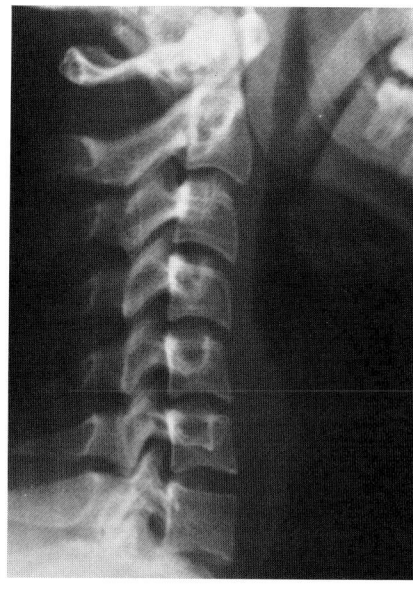 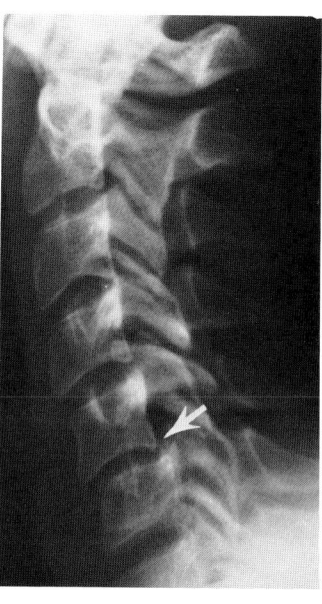

FIG. 4–22. **A**: Loss of the normal cervical lordotic curve in the supine position. Note the neck is slightly flexed. No lesions were present. **B**: Subtle subluxation of C5 on C6. There is interruption of the posterior spinal line (*arrow*) and narrowing of the disc space. The pillar of C5 is rotated off axis.

that variation in the distance between the spinolaminar line and articular pillars (Fig. 4-24) was useful for identification of rotational soft tissue injuries.

How many of these signs need to be identified before the diagnosis of instability should be considered? This is a valid question and has resulted in confusion over the years. Denis popularized the three column approach that assists in simplifying this problem (19,27). The spine can be divided into three columns. The anterior column includes the anterior longitudinal ligament, anterior half of the vertebral body, and the anterior disk. The middle column includes the posterior vertebral body, disk, and posterior longitudinal ligament. The posterior column is made up of the facet joints, posterior osseous structures and ligaments (Fig. 4-25). Disruption of two adjacent columns indicates instability. Identification of widening of the interspinous distance, subluxation (>3 mm), or

widened facet joints as single injuries is also indicative of instability as two columns are generally involved for these changes to occur (19,27).

Sometimes it is difficult to obtain a radiograph that includes the entire cervical spine. Penetration of the shoulders may be difficult owing to muscle spasm in the neck or shoulder injuries. However, the arms can be pulled distally in some patients, which may allow better visualization of the lower cervical spine (Fig. 4-26). This requires more attendants in the room and exposes the "puller" to radiation. Kaufman has stated that this technique should not be used unless there is a low suspicion of injury (48). Distraction of the arms can cause hyperextension of the cervical spine, thereby exacerbating an existing injury.

We routinely obtain swimmer's views on all patients if C7 and T1 are not visible on the lateral view (Fig. 4-27).

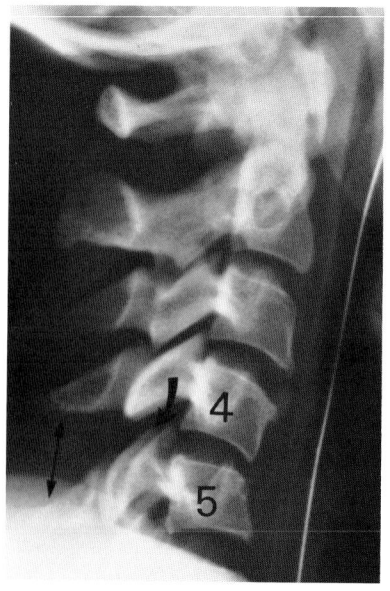 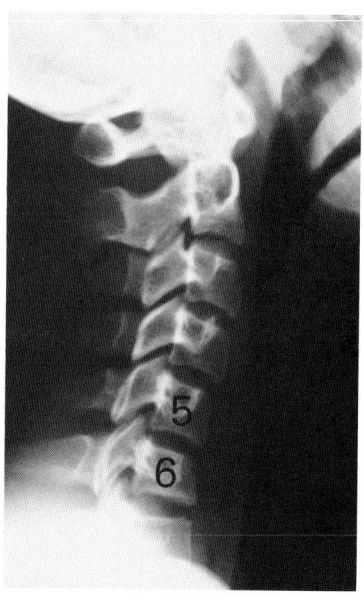

FIG. 4–23. **A**: Disruptive hyperflexion injury with widening of the interspinous distance (*straight arrow*), facet joints (*curved arrow*) and narrowing of the disk space at C4-C5. **B**: Subtle subluxation of C5 on C6 (widened interspinous distance, facet joints, and slight disk space narrowing due to a posterior ligament tear).

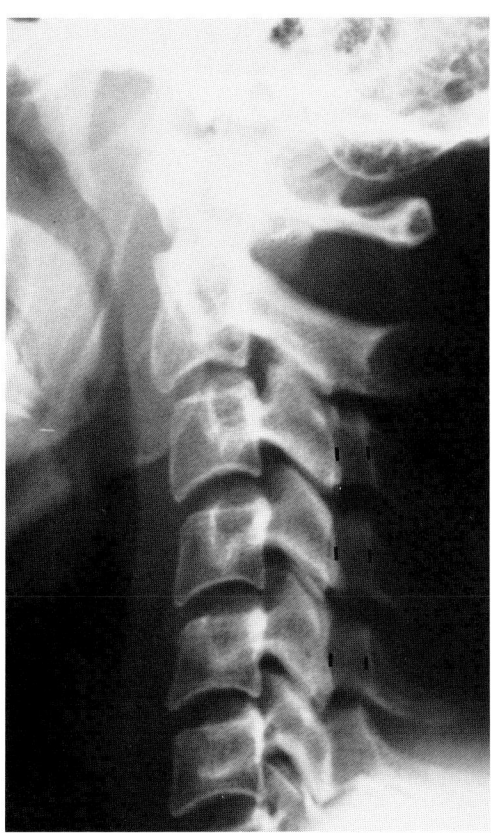

FIG. 4–24. Lateral view of the cervical spine demonstrating normal laminar spaces (spinolaminal line to articular pillars). Abrupt change in distance indicates a rotational injury.

This view is taken with the patient supine and the arm closest to the film elevated above the head (Fig. 4-27A). Occasionally even this technique is inadequate. In such cases lateral tomography can be performed with the Versigraph without moving the patient.

AP View

The AP view is obtained by angling the tube 5°–20° to the head. The beam is centered just below the thyroid cartilage (12,13). The cassette (8 × 10 cm) is placed under the cervical spine, either in a Bucky tray or in the lower C-arm of the Versigraph. This view allows visualization of the vertebral bodies, uncinate processes, articular pillars, and spinous processes from C7 to C3 (Fig. 4-28). The upper cervical spine is rarely visualized on this view. In the normal cervical spine, the articular pillars should form a smooth undulating margin bilaterally, and the spinous processes should be centered and equally spaced (Fig. 4-28B). Deviation of the spinous process from the midline (Fig. 4-28C) may indicate a unilateral locked facet secondary to a flexion-rotation injury. These injuries can be subtle and are frequently missed (66). Widening of the interspinous distance may indicate subluxation or dislocation (Fig. 4-28D). Naidich and colleagues have stated that an interspinous dis-

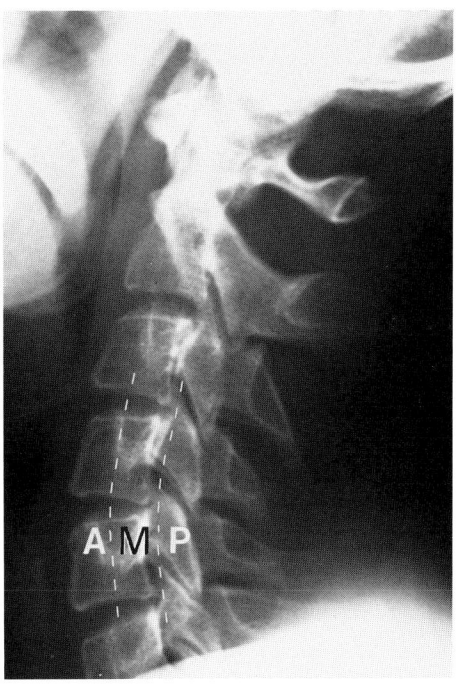

FIG. 4–25. Lateral view of the cervical spine demonstrating the three columns used in evaluating instability. A (anterior column): anterior longitudinal ligament, anterior body, anterior disk; M (mid column): posterior body, disk, and posterior longitudinal ligament; P (posterior column): posterior ligaments and bony structures.

tance 1.5 times that of the interspinous distance above and below indicates dislocation (61). A double spinous process may be seen on the AP view in spinous process fractures (Fig. 4-28E and F) (23). Careful attention to detail on the AP view of the lower cervical spine may be most helpful. Changes detected may be the only clue to more serious, unstable injuries that may be partially obscured on the lateral view.

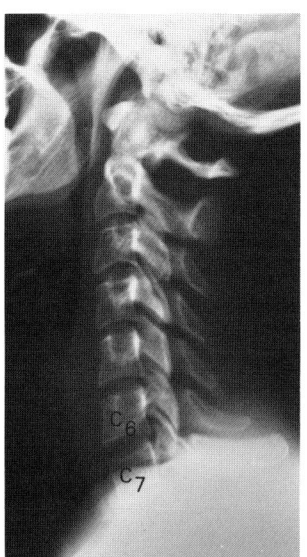
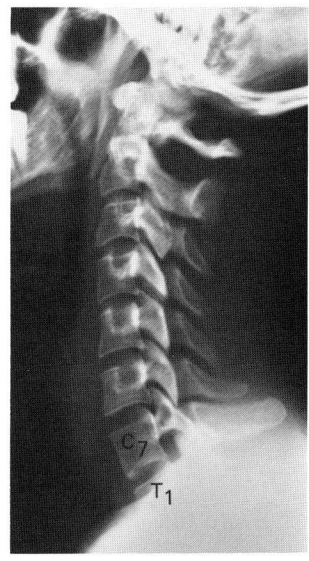

A   B

FIG. 4–26. Lateral view of the cervical spine (A) and after pulling down on the arms (B).

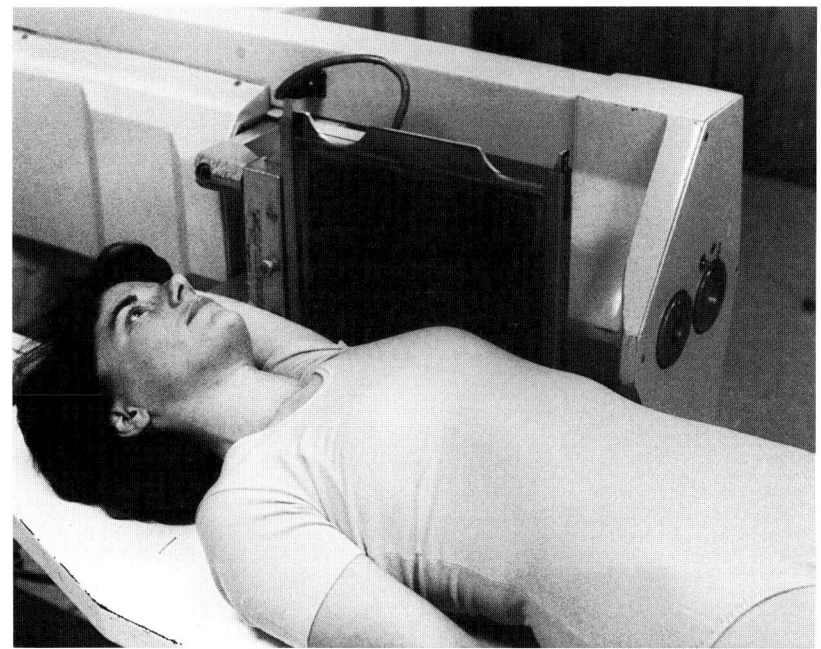

A

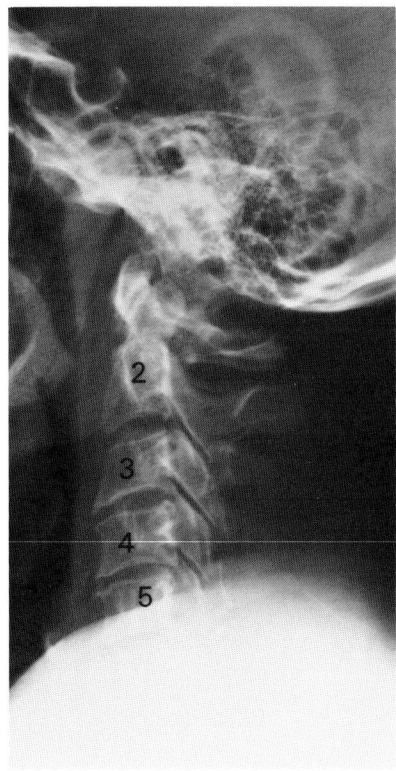

B

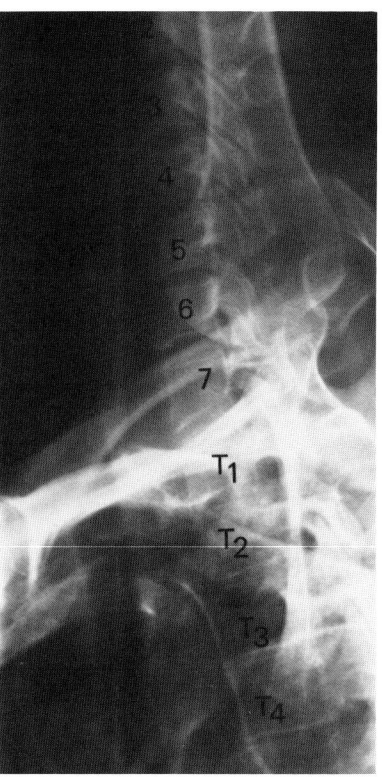

C

FIG. 4–27. A: Patient positioned for the swimmer's view. The C-arm is horizontal and centered on the lower cervical spine. The arm closest to the film is elevated. B: Lateral view demonstrating only five cervical vertebrae. C: The swimmers view demonstrates the entire cervical spine and upper thoracic spine.

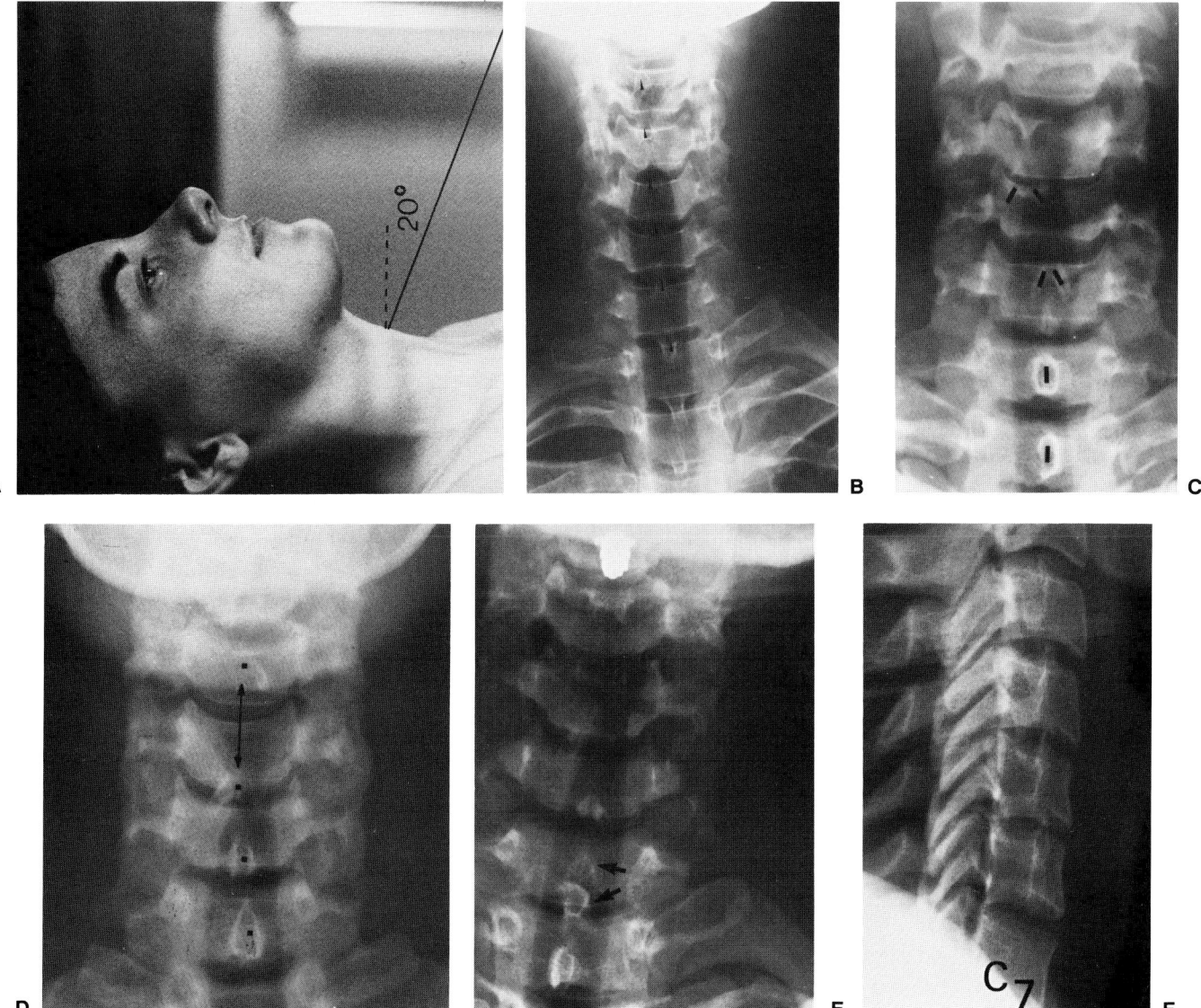

FIG. 4–28. A: Patient positioned for the AP view. Beam is angled 20° toward the head. **B**: Normal AP view of the spine. The spinous processes (·) are equidistant. **C**: Normal positioning of the spinous process from T1 to C6. The C5 spinous process is rotated to the right due to a unilateral locked facet. **D**: Increased interspinous distance between C4 and C5 due to anterior subluxation. **E**: Double spinous process due to fracture of C7. This is not well seen on the lateral view (**F**).

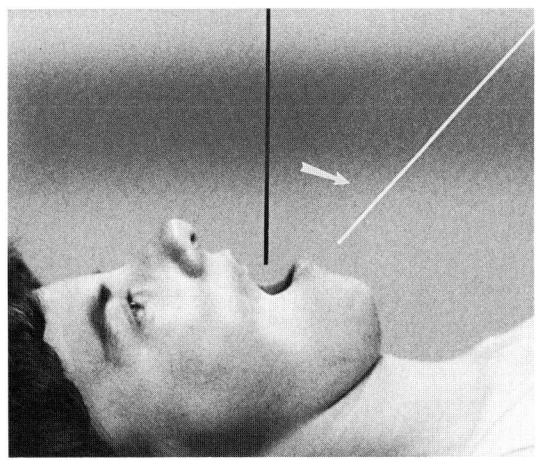
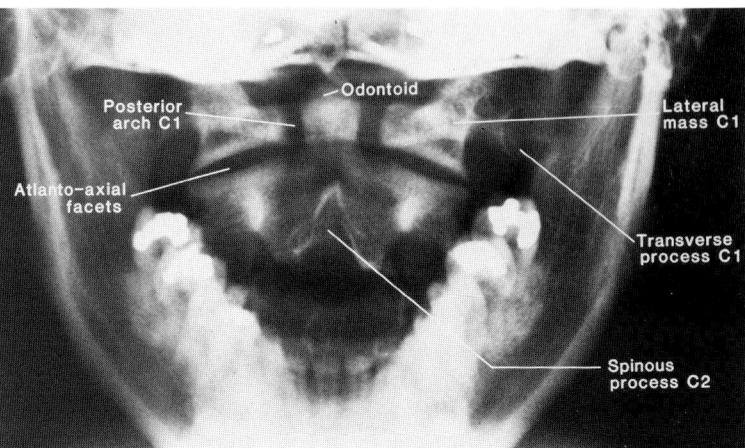

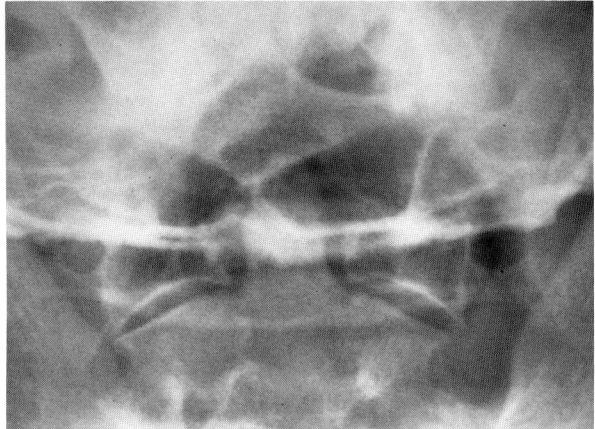
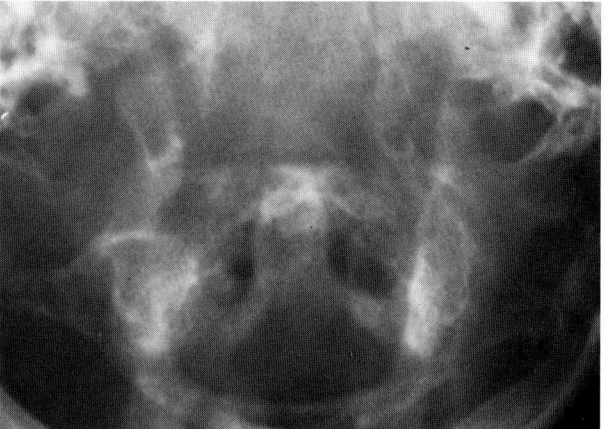

FIG. 4–29. Open mouth AP view of the odontoid. **A**: Patient positioned for the odontoid view. **B**: Normal radiograph. Increasing the angle (*white line, 4-29A*) may be useful when overlap of osseous structures obscures the odontoid (**C**). When the angle is increased the odontoid and C1 are seen to better advantage (**D**).

Odontoid View

The odontoid view is obtained with the patient's mouth open as wide as possible. The beam is centered over the open mouth and aligned perpendicularly to the cassette (Fig. 4-29A) (16,18,65).

The neck should not be extended or the posterior occiput may obscure the odontoid (25). This view (Fig. 4-29B) allows one to study the odontoid, lateral masses, and transverse processes of C1. If the patient and tube are properly aligned, the spinous process of C2 will be midline. Spaces between the teeth and the inferior margin of the posterior arch of C1 may overlap the odontoid and should not be confused with fractures (25). If the odontoid is not well demonstrated (Fig. 4-29C), the tube can be angled (Fig. 4-29A—*white line*) to reduce bony overlap (25,32).

Oblique Views

The oblique views, following acute trauma, are obtained by angling the C-arm 45° from the horizontal (Fig. 4-28A). In the upright position the patient is rotated (Fig. 4-28B), so that the side away from the film is demonstrated (16,18). Detail is improved on the Versigraph. Also, magnification caused by the distance between the patient and the film may assist in detecting subtle fractures. Using a conventional table, oblique views are obtained by angling the tube 35°–40° to the horizontal with a 15° cranial angle (11,16,27). The oblique views provide excellent detail of the uncinate processes, pedicles, lamina, and alignment of facet joints (Fig. 4-28C). These views are particularly important in detecting facet subluxations and dislocations (18,25,40,41).

Pillar Views

A significant number of cervical spine fractures (50% in Gehweiler's series) involve the posterior arch (40). Pillar views are useful in evaluation of the articular pillars and lamina. This view is obtained by angling the tube 25°–30° toward the feet and can be performed with the patient's neck extended or rotated 45° (Fig. 4-31A). The central beam is centered on C7 and enters near the thy-

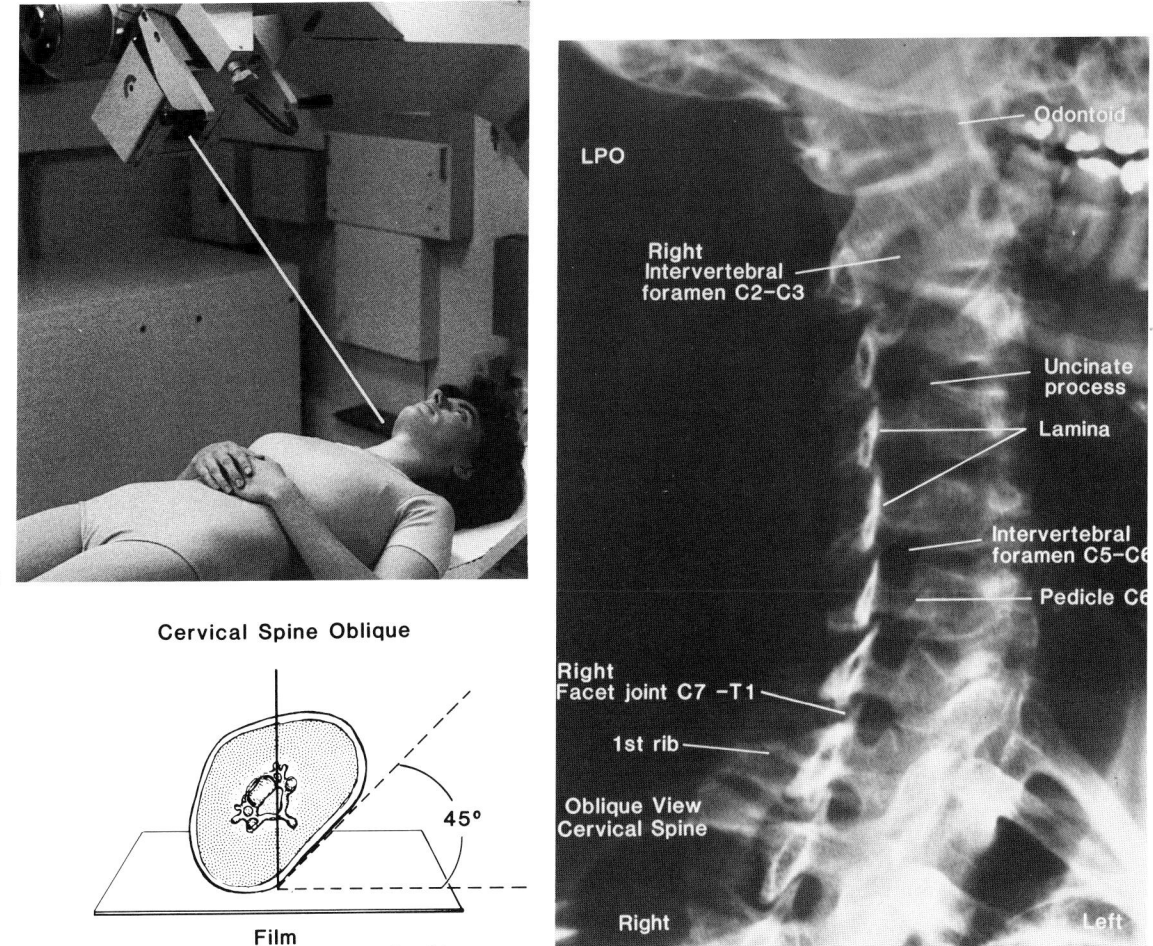

FIG. 4–30. A: Patient positioned for oblique view with the C-arm angled 45°. The posterior elements closest to the film will be noted on the film. **B**: Routine oblique view demonstrates the posterior elements farthest from the film. **C**: Oblique view of the cervical spine taken on the Versigraph.

roid cartilage. The AP, lateral, and oblique views must be reviewed first to be certain there is no unstable or significant injury. Rotation of the head or extension of the neck should be avoided if a significant injury is evident on initial views (Fig. 4-30). Pillar fractures, if present, are almost always stable but can result in significant pain and radiculopathy (12,57,69,74). The articular pillars should be symmetric in height. A difference in height of 2 mm in the same vertebral unit may indicate a fracture (74). Changes in height and wedging can be seen frequently in elderly patients with chronic degenerative changes, and it is best not to diagnose a fracture unless an actual fracture line can be seen (Fig. 4-31). The measurements given here may be helpful as a secondary sign.

It is obvious from Fig. 4-31 that obtaining high-quality pillar views can be difficult. Wales and colleagues found tomography more useful (75). They reported that pillar views missed 65% of posterior-element fractures demonstrated by tomography.

Flexion and Extension Views

Flexion and extension views of the cervical spine are performed to evaluate stability. The examination is most often indicated to exclude ligament instability following trauma or to determine whether fractures are healed or stable. This examination should be performed fluoroscopically, so that a true lateral position can be properly attained and the degree of motion monitored. Some authors perform upright lateral views prior to clearing patients with otherwise normal cervical spine series (27).

The patient should sit or stand. Physiologic extension and flexion in the lateral position are monitored fluoroscopically. The extension maneuver is performed initially, and alignment of the vertebrae and anterior ligament structures are studied. The patient is then asked to flex the cervical spine slowly so that alignment, subluxation, facet joint widening, and spinous process motion can be carefully observed. The criteria discussed in rou-

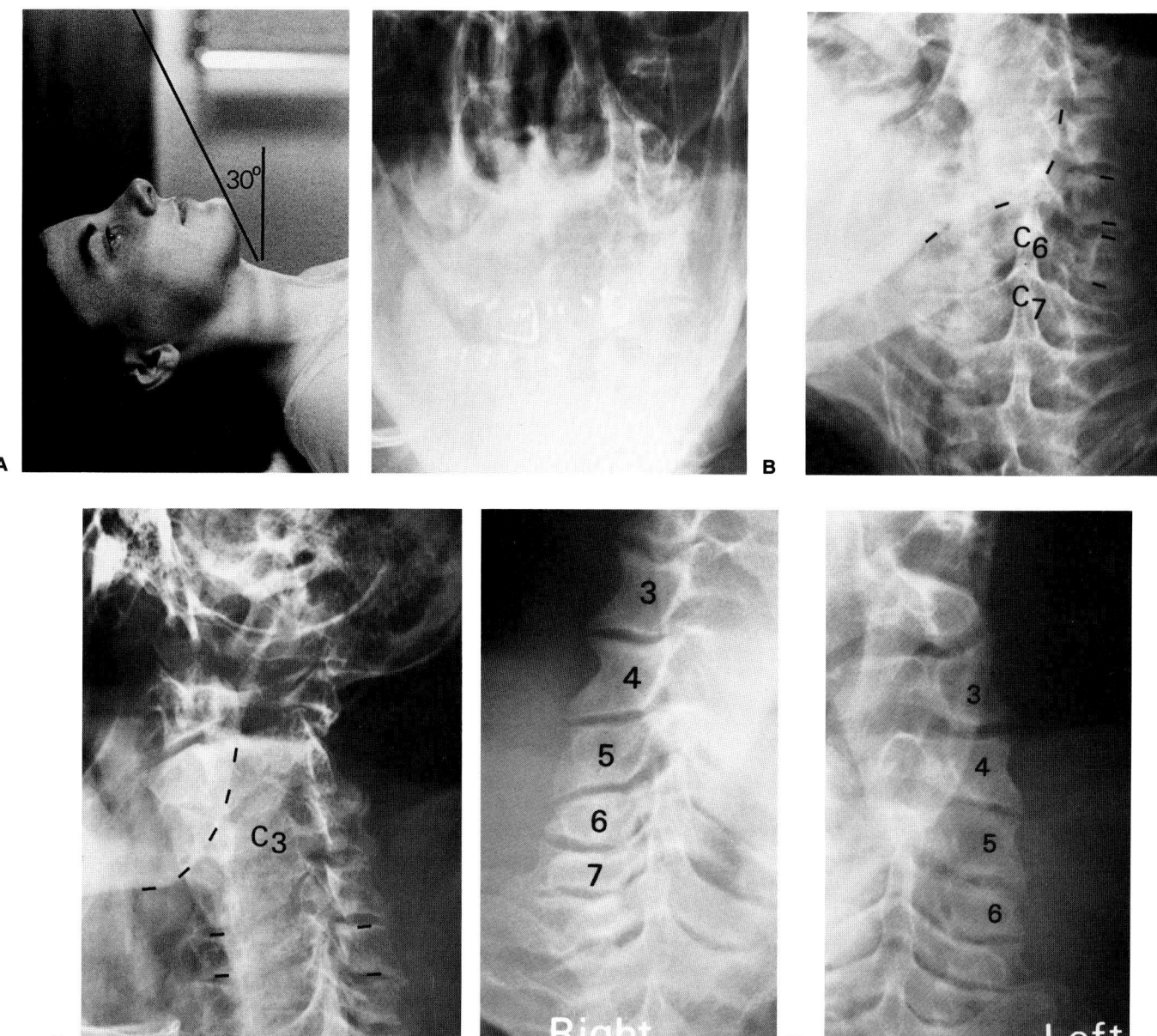

FIG. 4–31. A: Patient positioned for pillar view with head in neutral position and with beam angled 30° toward the feet. **B**: Radiograph with the head in anatomic position. The mandible obscures the cervical spine. **C**: Head rotated 45° to the right. The lower articular pillars on the left are demonstrated, but the pillars on the right are obscured (mandible, *broken line*). **D**: Elevating the chin alleviates this problem to some degree. Normally views should be taken with the head rotated both right (**E**) and left (**F**).

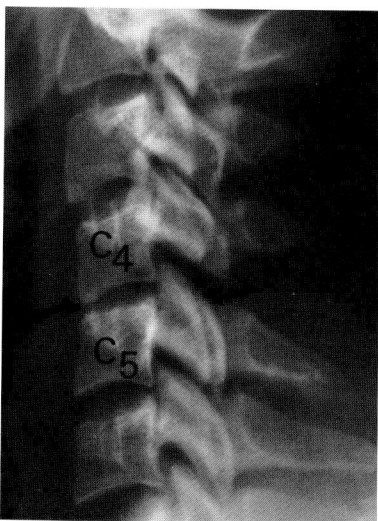

FIG. 4-32. Flexion view of the cervical spine with instability. There is widening of the facet joint and disk space narrowing at C4-C5.

tine evaluation of the lateral cervical spine (see Table 4-3) can be applied (Fig. 4-32). However, subtle changes may be important, and care must be taken not to overlook posterior ligament damage. Vertebral body subluxation in flexion should not exceed 1 mm (34,40,41).

Flexion and extension views are often inaccurate immediately following injury. Muscle spasm can result in reduced motion and a false negative examination. There-fore, this examination should not be performed until the spasm has subsided. This may require use of a cervical collar for several days.

Routine Radiography of the Thoracic and Lumbar Spine

In the acutely injured patient, AP and lateral views of the thoracic and lumbar spine are routinely obtained. Occasionally, oblique views and tomography are required. The AP thoracic view is obtained with the tube centered over the midthoracic spine. The greater thickness of structures in the lower spine often produces underexposure; over-exposure is more common in the upper thoracic spine. Fuchs places the anode at the superior portion of the spine, utilizing the "heal effect" to obtain a more uniform radiograph (38).

In examining the AP view of the thoracic spine (Fig. 4-33A), one should pay careful attention to the alignment and configuration of the vertebral bodies. Traumatic compression may be asymmetrical (Fig. 4-34). Occasionally, lateral wedging can occur, which may be subtle and best seen on the AP view. Also, changes in the interpedicular distance should be observed (Fig. 4-35), as this may indicate fracture of the posterior elements. The spinous processes can also be seen in the midline posteriorly. The transverse processes in the thoracic spine are best seen on the AP view and normally decrease in length as one progresses caudally. Careful evaluation of the intracostal distances may be helpful, especially in the up-

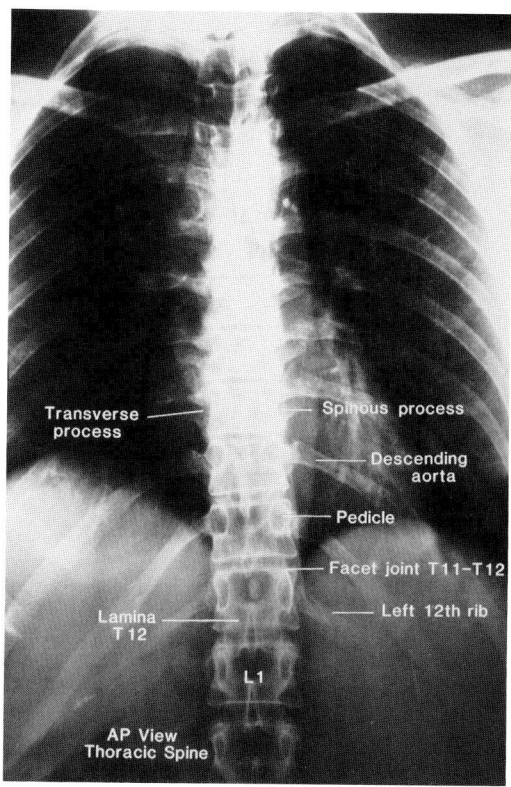

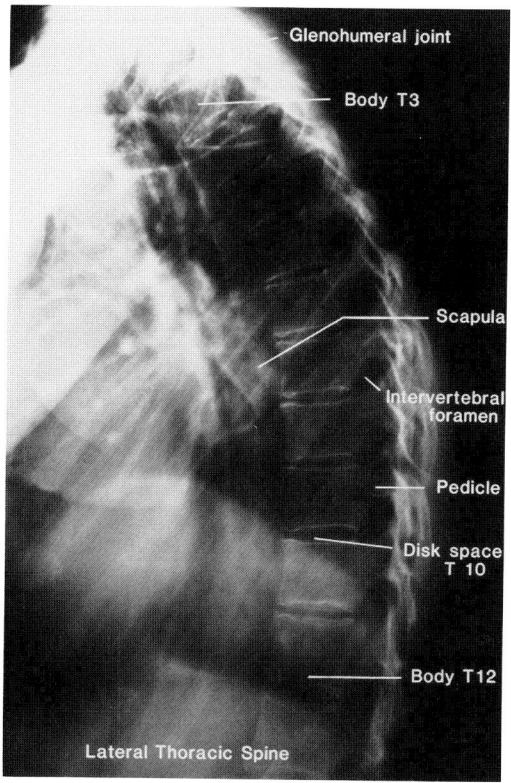

FIG. 4-33. AP (A) and lateral (B) view of the thoracic spine.

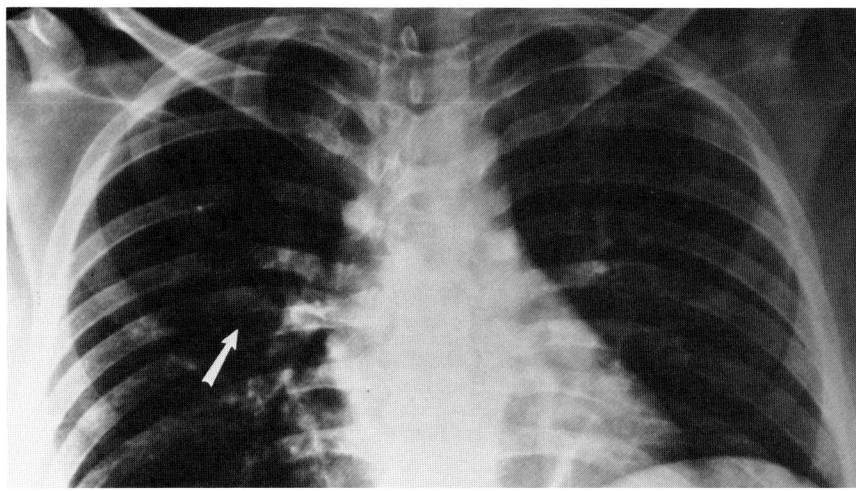

FIG. 4–34. AP view of the spine demonstrates asymmetry in the intercostal distance on the right (*arrow*) due to anterior subluxation of T5 on T6.

per thoracic spine (Fig. 4-34). This may provide the only clue to subluxation in a patient in whom lateral views may be difficult to obtain. Finally, on the AP view the height of each disk space in the thoracic region is usually the same.

Evaluation of the paraspinal soft tissues is very important (Fig. 4-36). Soft tissue swelling may be the only clue to vertebral fracture. Also, aortic rupture should be considered in this setting (19,30).

The lateral view of the thoracic spine can be obtained using cross-table technique if rotating the patient is not possible. On the lateral view (Fig. 4-33B), one can evaluate the alignment of the vertebral bodies, pedicles, lamina, and spinous processes. The posterior vertebral margin should be straight or concave (28). The height of the posterior edge of the vertebral body is 1–1.5 mm greater

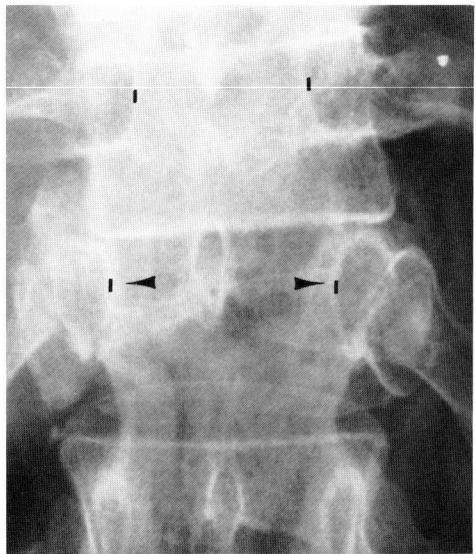

FIG. 4–35. AP view of the lower thoracic spine demonstrating increased interpedicular distance (*vertical lines*) due to a burst fracture of T12.

than that of the anterior edge (25,52). This should not be misinterpreted as acute traumatic compression.

The AP view of the lumbar spine is obtained with the tube centered over the umbilicus (Fig. 4-37A). To avoid distortion from the lordotic curve, the knees can be flexed 45° or more (18,25). Often, this may not be possible in a severely injuried patient. In the lumbar spine, the interpedicular distance normally widens slightly as one progresses from L1 to L5. Careful attention must also be given to the spinous processes and "butterfly" configuration of the lamina and apophyseal facets. Interruption of these strictures may be the only clue to a posterior fracture-dislocation (Fig. 4-38). The transverse processes are clearly seen and usually increase in length from L1 to L3. The transverse processes of L4 are directed slightly cephalad, and those of L5 are much shorter and also directed slightly cephalad (Fig. 4-38; see also Fig. 4-6). The lateral view of the lumbar spine can be obtained with a cross-table technique, turning the patient (if possible) to the lateral position or utilizing the C-arm Versigraph. The cross-table technique is preferred following trauma.

On the lateral view of the lumbar spine the bodies, pedicles, facet joints, and spinous processes can be clearly demonstrated. It should be noted that the body of L1 is often slightly wedged anteriorly. On occasion this may be difficult to differentiate from an acute injury (Fig. 4-37). As in the remainder of the spine, alignment of the vertebral bodies is also well demonstrated on the lateral view. A coned-lateral view of L5-S1 is also helpful, as better detail can be obtained. There is less scatter and geometric resolution is improved with this technique.

Oblique views are commonly obtained in the lumbar region and are extremely helpful in evaluating the facet joints, lamina, and pars interarticularis. Oblique views are obtained by angling the tube on the Versigraph or rotating the patient 45° into both the left posterior and right posterior oblique positions. The left oblique view

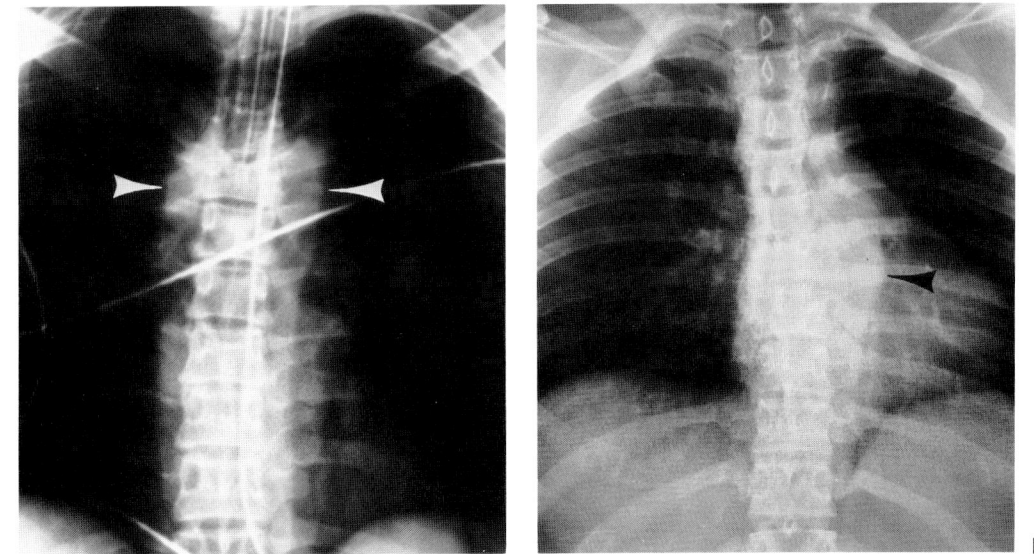

FIG. 4-36. Paraspinal hematomas (*arrows*) due to upper (**A**) and mid (**B**) thoracic fractures.

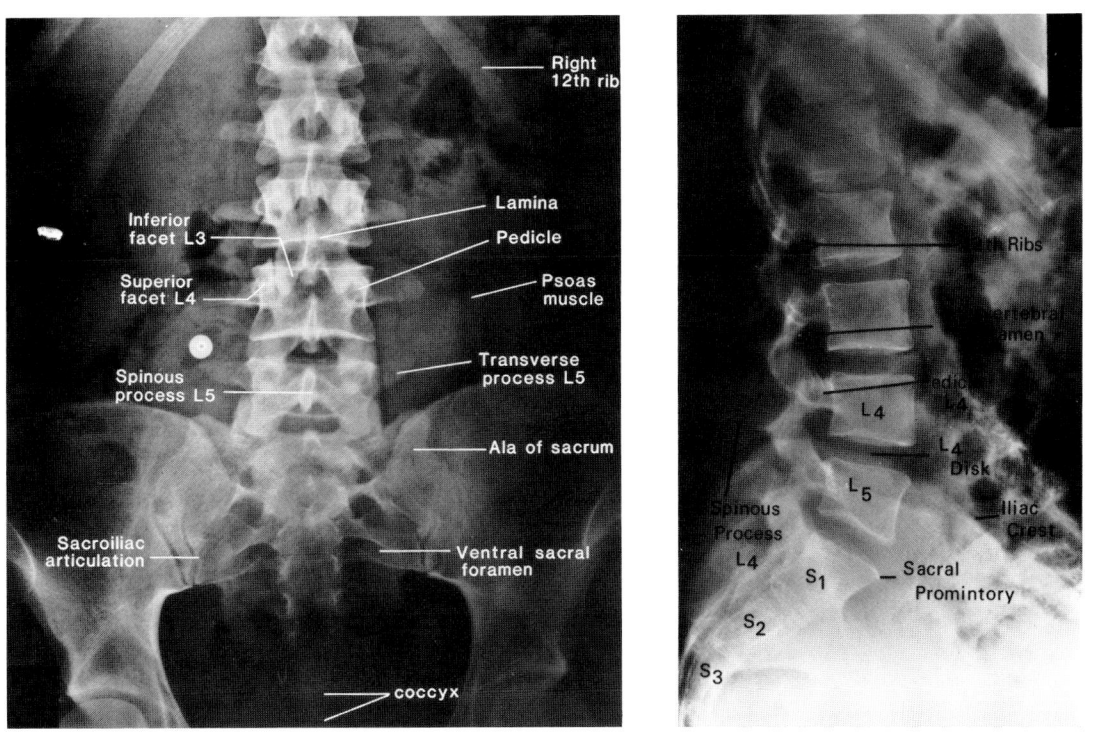

FIG. 4-37. Normal AP (**A**) and lateral (**B**) views of the lumbar spine.

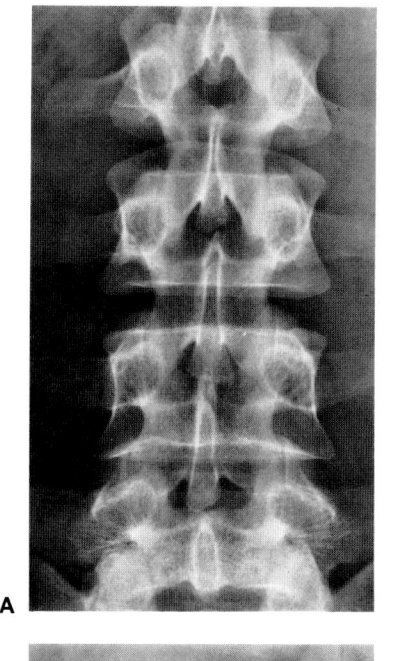

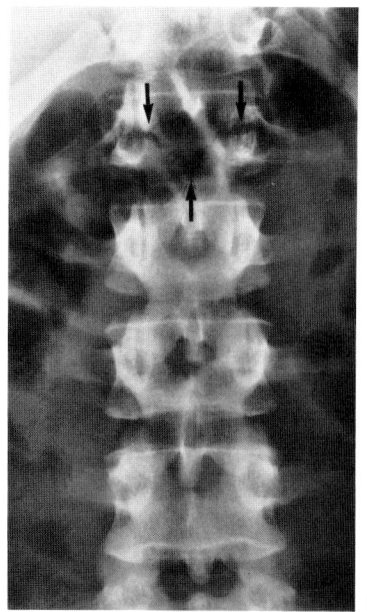

A

B

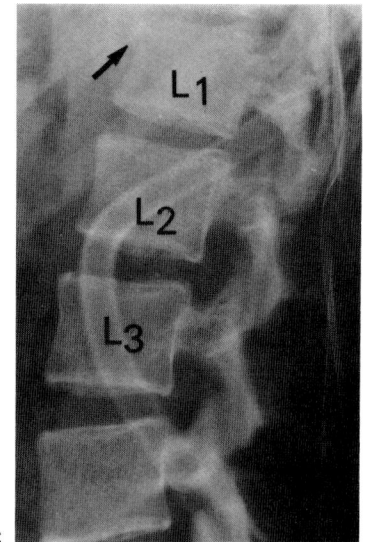

L1

L2

L3

C

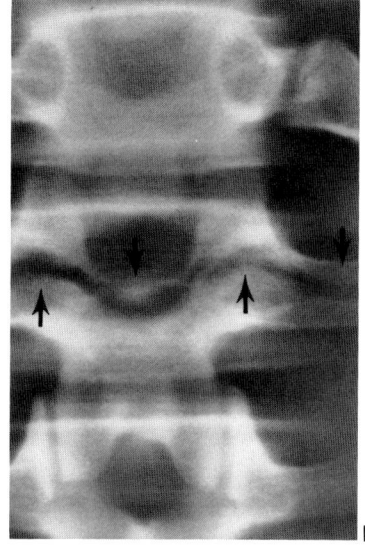

D

FIG. 4–38. A: Normal AP view of the lumbar spine. Note the normal interpendicular distance and "butterfly" configuration of the lamina and articular processes. The spinous process is the "body of the butterfly." **B**: AP view of the lumbar spine demonstrating a transverse fracture through the neural arch at L1 (*arrows*). **C**: Lateral view demonstrates mild compression of L1 with cortical collapse anteriorly. **D**: A tomogram clearly demonstrates the transverse fracture extending through the pedicles and transverse processes bilaterally (*arrows*).

demonstrates the left side of the posterior arch and the right oblique, the right side (Fig. 4-39).

This view demonstrates the "Scotty dog" (25). The nose is the transverse process, the eye is the pedicle, the ear is the superior facet, and the neck is the pars interarticularis. The lamina is the body, and the inferior facet is the front leg. The opposite superior facet (side farthest from the film) is the tail, and the opposite inferior facet is the hind leg (25).

AP and lateral views of the sacrum can be obtained by centering the tube over the sacrum with the central beam perpendicular to the cassette (Fig. 4-40). On the AP view,

the arcuate lines and ventral sacral foramina should be carefully studied. Interruption in the arcuate lines may be the only sign of fracture (see Chapter 5). The lateral view is useful in demonstrating displacement of sacral fractures and in detecting fractures or dislocations of the coccyx.

Conventional and Computed Tomography (CT)

Tomographic techniques and CT are often helpful in determining the full extent of injury (21,22,35,49, 64,68,70,78,80). Computed tomography is most frequently selected, but conventional tomography is pre-

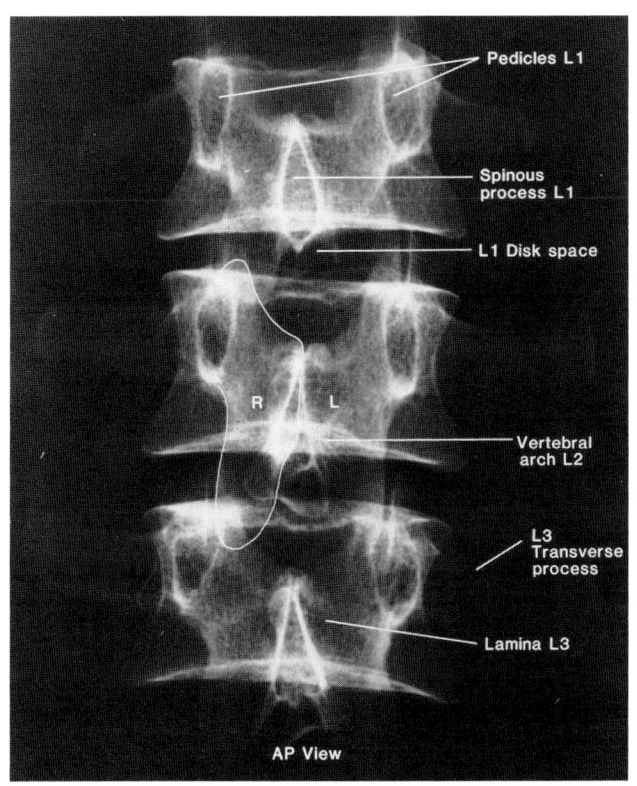

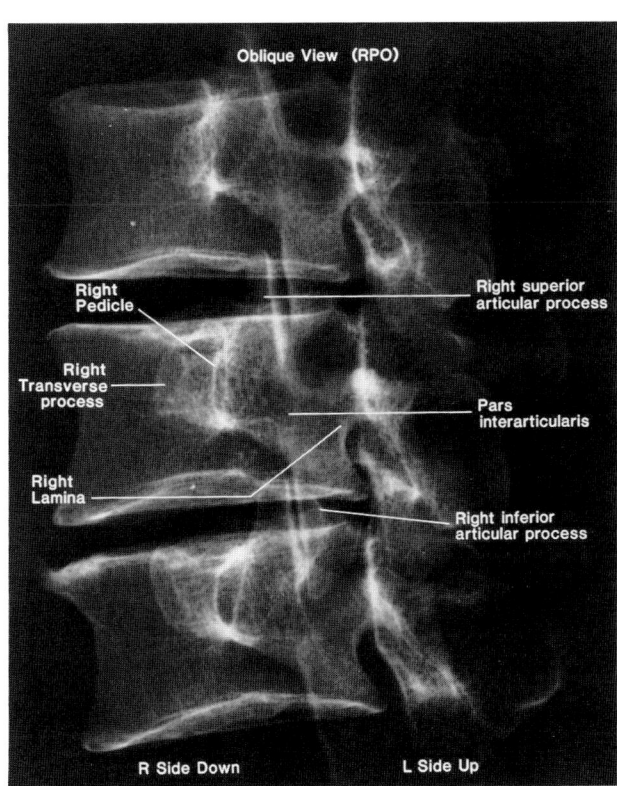

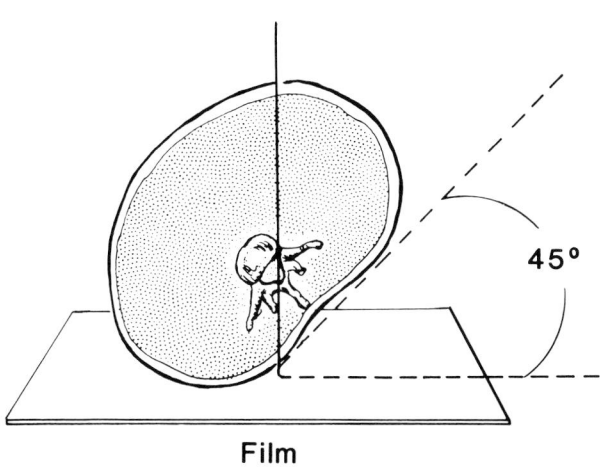

Lumbar Spine Oblique

FIG. 4-39. **A**: AP view of skeletal specimens L1 to L3. The right side of the posterior arch is marked (*white line*) at L2. **B**: Illustration of position for oblique view. **C**: Oblique view with right side closest to the film. The right side of the posterior arch forms the head, neck, front leg of the "Scotty dog."

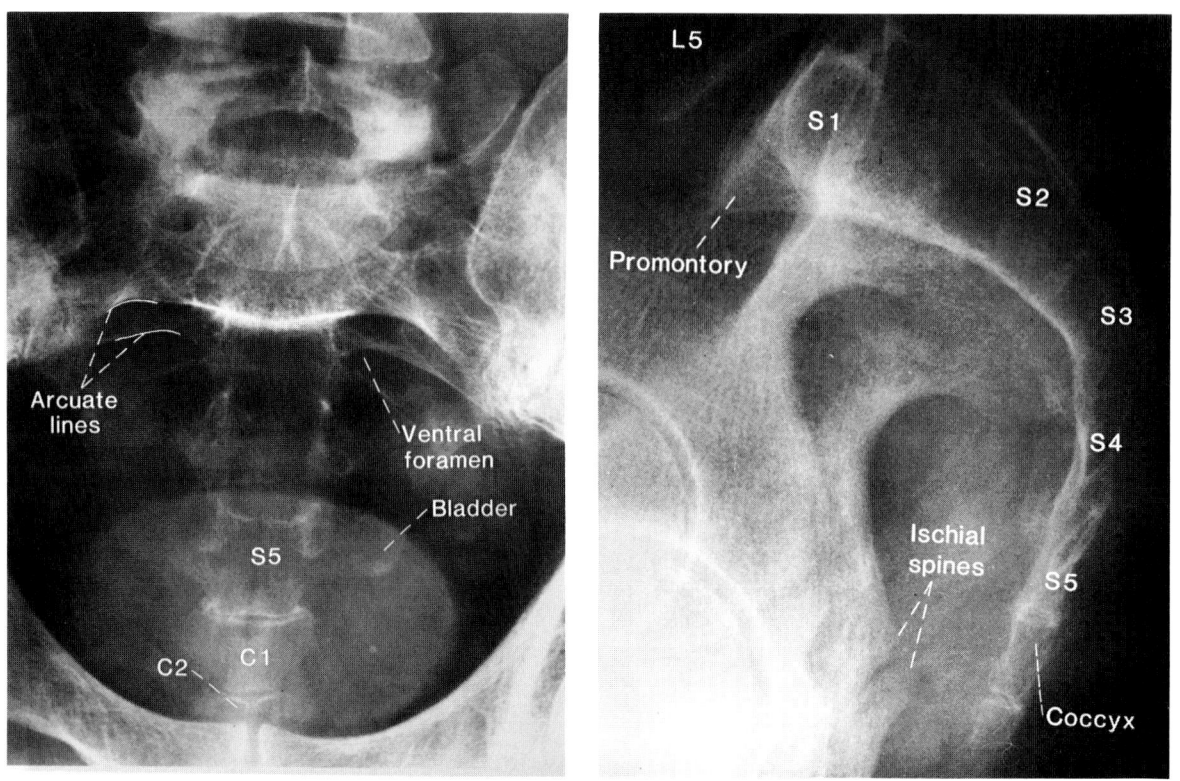

FIG. 4–40. AP (**A**) and lateral (**B**) views of the sacrum.

ferred in patients with suspected odontoid fractures or when the fracture line may be parallel to the CT image plane. In this setting, fractures may be overlooked due to partial volume effects (Fig. 4-41) (19).

The choice of examination is based on several factors

including patient status, type of injury suspected, and equipment availability (Table 4-4). Most skeletal tomography is performed using complex motion techniques as opposed to linear tomography. This would require moving the patient. The C-arm unit permits linear tomogra-

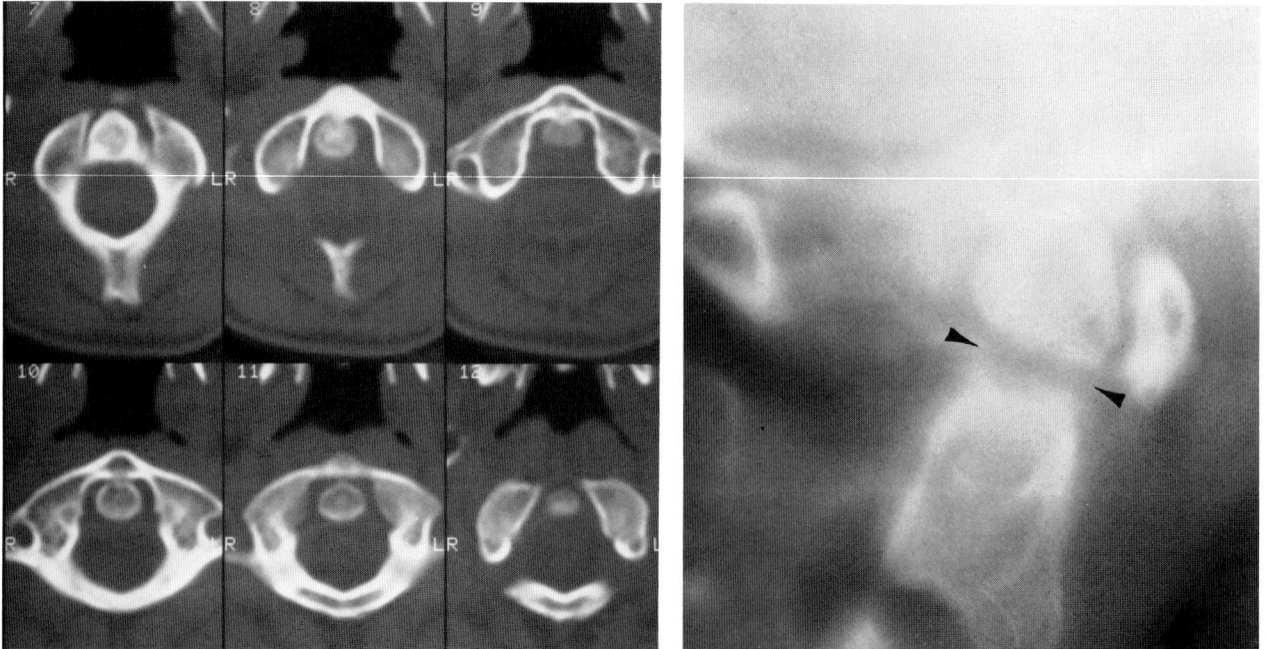

FIG. 4–41. Type II odontoid fracture. CT images (**A**) are normal. Lateral tomogram (**B**) clearly demonstrates the fracture (*arrows*).

TABLE 4-4. *Conventional vs. computed tomography*

Patient status
  Pain
  Neurological deficit
Mechanism of injury
Location of injury
  Upper cervical spine
  Lower cervical spine
  Anterior vs. posterior structures
Availability of equipment
  Type of CT scanner
  C-arm vs. conventional tomography (patient can be studied in AP, lateral, and oblique planes with C-arm)

TABLE 4-5. *Conventional vs. computed tomography applications*[a]

Conventional tomography	Computed tomography
Confirm suspected fractures	Spinal canal assessment
Odontoid	Bone fragments
Posterior elements	Hematoma
Facet fractures	Dural tears (with contrast)
Perched or locked facets	Operative planning
Classification of injuries (contiguous segments useful in determining mechanism of injury)	Three-dimensional reconstruction

[a] (19).

phy in the AP, lateral, oblique, and axial planes without moving the patient. Routinely, we obtain AP and lateral tomograms. Tomography (Table 4-5) is most useful for evaluating odontoid fractures, fractures in the plane of CT imaging (Fig. 4-42), the facet joints (Fig. 4-43), and for demonstrating contiguous segments (19,20,80).

Computed tomography (Table 4-5) is most useful for evaluating patients with neurologic deficits, bone fragments in the spinal canal (Fig. 4-44), or neural foramina, and for preoperative planning of complex injuries (13,14,31,55,63,73). On occasion intrathecal contrast plus CT are used to evaluate dural tears and nerve root injuries (39,47,60). Non-ionic water soluble contrast can be injected via the lumbar route or by C1-C2 puncture in the immoblized patient. In most patients, 5-mm-thick contiguous slices are adequate for evaluating spinal fractures. If reconstruction in the coronal and sagittal planes or three-dimensional processing are required, much thinner slices should be obtained. Three millimeter slices at 2-mm intervals or 1.5-mm contiguous slices provide superior reconstructed images (19,79).

Magnetic Resonance Imaging (MRI)

MRI is an established technique for evaluating the musculoskeletal system (17,19,26,36,45). Soft tissue contrast is superior to CT and images can be obtained in the axial, coronal, oblique, and sagittal planes. Fine bone detail (i.e., the thin cortical bone of vertebral bodies) is not as well demonstrated with MRI compared to CT (58). Also, the confining nature of the MR gantry reduces patient access, especially on high field (>1.0 Tesla) imagers. Therefore, MRI is not as frequently utilized in the acutely injured patient with multiple trauma.

MR imaging techniques have improved significantly over the past several years. Although there are numerous sequences to choose from, most utilize both T1- and T2-weighted images to completely evaluate the osseous and soft tissue anatomy (15,19,33). Sagittal T1-weighted images (SE 500/20) provide a good screening technique for changes in the vertebral body (Fig. 4-45). T2-weighted images are more useful for evaluation of the spinal cord and disks (Fig. 4-46). Muscle tears and liga-

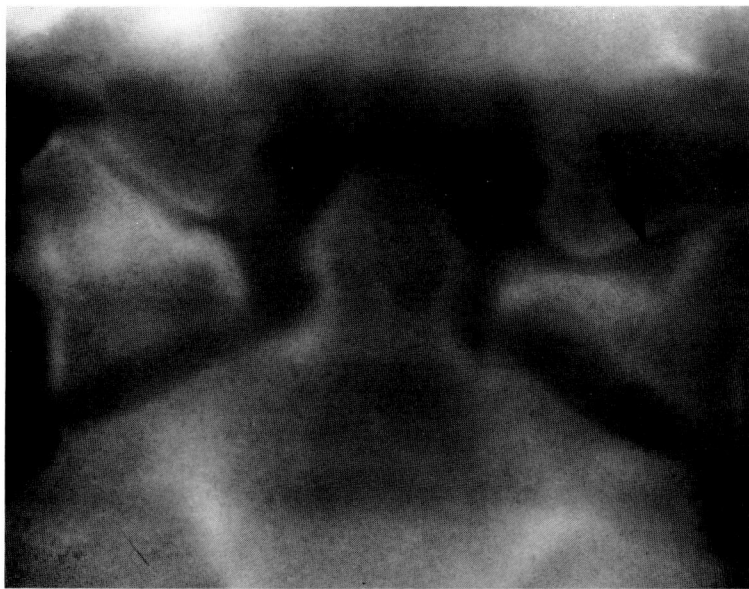

FIG. 4-42. AP tomogram demonstrating an impaction fracture of the left lateral mass of C1 (*arrow*). This was overlooked on CT.

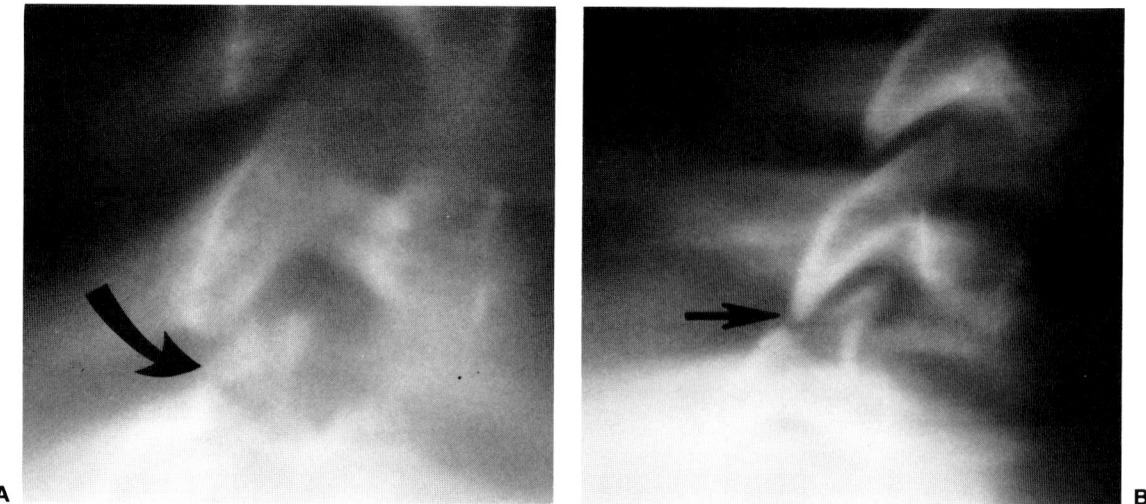

FIG. 4–43. Lateral tomograms of the facet joints demonstrating bilateral fracture subluxations (**A, B**).

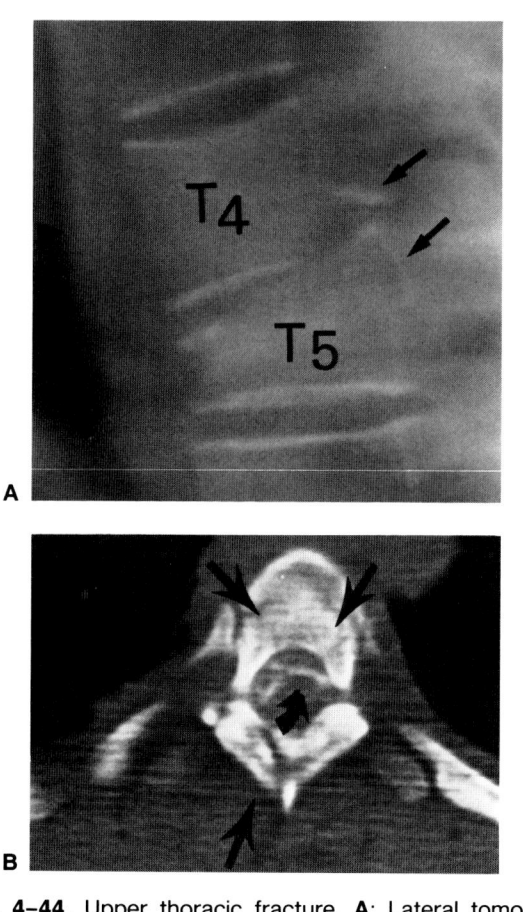

FIG. 4–44. Upper thoracic fracture. **A**: Lateral tomogram demonstrates a T4-T5 fracture subluxation with posterior fragments (*arrows*) and prevertebral swelling (*arrowheads*). **B**: CT image shows the fractures (*arrows*) and fragments in the spinal canal (*curved arrow*) more clearly.

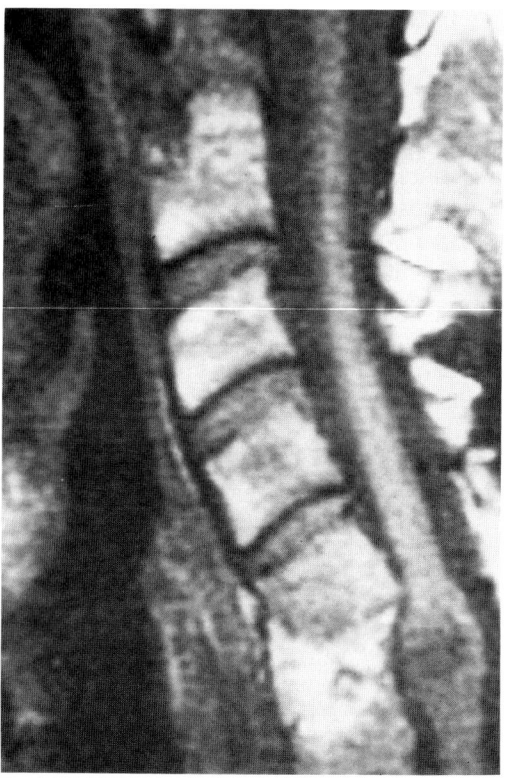

FIG. 4–45. Sagittal T1 (SE 500/20) image of the cervical spine demonstrating a C5-C6 flexion compression injury with a post traumatic syrinx in the spinal cord.

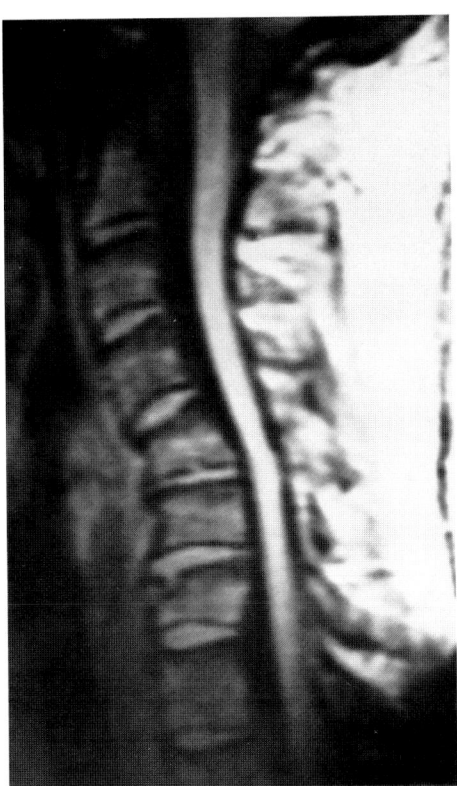

FIG. 4-46. Sagittal MPGR (multiplanar grass) image with C5 and C7 compression fractures. The spinal cord is normal.

ment injuries should also be more easily appreciated on T2-weighted images (50,51). Spin-echo T2-weighted images (SE ≥ 2000, ≥60) require 9–16 minutes of image time. New gradient echo techniques with reduced flip angles can provide images with T2* weighting in about 4 minutes, which is advantageous in patients with spinal cord injury (Fig. 4-46) (15,33). Gadolinium diethylenetriamine penta-acetic acid (DTPA) with T1-weighted images is also useful for more complete evaluation of the spinal cord.

To date, MRI has been most useful for evaluation of the spinal cord and disks (42,43). Kulkarni et al. (50,51) described patterns of cord abnormality (edema and hemorrhage) that were useful in predicting neurological recovery. The potential for evaluating posterior muscle and ligament injury also exists. However, results are preliminary at this time. Currently, MRI is most often used in patients with stable injuries, or normal radiographs with evidence of spinal cord involvement (42,43).

Radionuclide Scanning

Technetium bone scans are rarely indicated in acute spinal trauma. Bone and soft tissue injuries are more effectively evaluated with radiographic techniques described above. However, technetium-99m diphosphonate studies can be useful for detection of subtle poste-rior element fractures, especially in the presence of normal radiographs (62).

CERVICAL SPINE TRAUMA

Approximately 65% of spinal injuries involve the cervical region (91). A team approach is essential in proper management of patients with acute cervical spine fracture or fracture-dislocation. This dictates that radiologists and clinicians must thoroughly discuss the patient's clinical condition. Delay in diagnosis of the severity of the lesion may result in instability and neurologic complications. Subtle posterior ligament injuries are particularly difficult and, if initially missed, these may result in significant deformity and neurological sequelae (89).

Mechanism of Injury

A thorough understanding of the mechanism of injury is essential in proper management of cervical spine trauma. Unfortunately, the classifications available in the literature are numerous and often confusing (83–88,91,92,97,98,101,102,107,111). In-depth discussions of this topic have been presented by Gehweiler (97), Brackman and Penning (87), and Holdsworth (101). The details described in these studies are extremely valuable in understanding fractures and fracture-dislocations of the cervical spine. However, at times the classifications proposed are cumbersome. The mechanism of injury is rarely pure (e.g., flexion or extension alone without compression or rotation). One must guard against oversimplification, but categories of injury can become so complex that they become impractical. Classifications should be easily understood and yet remain accurate. The ultimate goal should be a standard classification that is accurate for determining the proper treatment and prognosis of the injury.

In our series of 420 cervical spine fractures and fracture-dislocations, most injuries could be classified into four groups (Table 4-6). Hyperextension occurred in 38% of patients. Hyperflexion injuries were somewhat more common (46%). Most were flexion-compression or disruptive hyperflexion injuries. This group included 12% of the total series who had unilateral facet locking or perching. Vertical compression injuries occurred in 4% of the 420 patients. Radiographic classification could not be accomplished in 10%–12% of cases. These patients presented with radiographic findings that did not allow exact determination of the mechanism of injury. Injuries included nondisplaced odontoid fractures, in which the radiographic features were insufficient to determine the mechanism of injury even when combined with clinical data. Spinous process fractures may result from flexion, extension, or direct trauma. If there are no

TABLE 4-6. *Classification and radiographic features of cervical spine injuries*[a]

Type of injury	Incidence (%)[b] in 420 patients
Hyperflexion	46%
A. Disruptive hyperflexion	
Hyperflexion sprain	
(transient dislocation)	
Hyperflexion dislocation	
Locked facets (12% unilateral)[c]	
Spinous process fracture	
B. Compressive hyperflexion	
Vertebral wedge fracture	
Teardrop fracture	
Fracture dislocation	
C. Shearing injuries	
Anteriorly displaced odontoid fracture	
Hyperextension	38%
A. Disruptive hyperflexion	
Hangman's fracture	
Hyperextension sprain	
Anterior inferior vertebral body fracture	
B. Compressive hyperflexion	
Posterior arch fractures	
Hyperextension fracture dislocation	
C. Shearing injuries	
Posteriorly displaced odontoid fracture	
Axial Compression	4%
Jefferson's fracture	
Burst fractures	
Hyper-rotation Injuries	
Rotary fixation C1 on C2	
Anterior and posterior ligament disruptions	
Lateral Flexion Injuries	
Uncinate process fracture	
Transverse process fracture	
Lateral wedge fracture	
Brachial plexus avulsion	
Indeterminate	10–12%

[a] (88,91,97,100).
[b] 10–12% indeterminate based on radiograph alone (spinous process fractures, undisplaced odontoid fractures, etc.).
[c] 12% of hyperflexion injuries were due to flexion-rotation with unilateral facet locking.

associated fractures, classification is difficult in this case as well.

Daffner describes similar findings in 646 cervical spine injuries. Radiographic features allowed identification of four basic mechanisms of injury (flexion, extension, shearing, and rotation) in the majority of patients (91,92).

Hyperflexion Injuries

There are many descriptive terms in the literature that attempt to define the motion of the cervical spine and the direction of the force that results in injury. Certain of these terms are extremely helpful and others are confusing. Flexion injuries have been classified as (1) disruptive, (2) compressive, and (3) shearing in nature (Table 4-6) (82,87,97). Disruptive hyperflexion indicates that the blow was directed upward toward the occipital re-

gion, resulting in forward flexion of the head. The major force is applied to the posterior ligaments and spinous processes, resulting in distraction of the spinous processes (Fig. 4-47). If the force is sufficient and the motion of the head continues, the posterior ligaments are interrupted, resulting in an unstable injury. The cervical spine may then return to its near normal position, depending upon the extent of force applied. In this case, the lateral radiograph may demonstrate kyphosis, with widening of the interspinous distance and facet joints (Fig. 4-47B). If the disruptive force continues, however, unilateral or bilateral locking of the facets occurs, depending on the degree of associated rotation (Fig. 4-48). We prefer to consider unilateral locking as a flexion-rotation injury (Fig. 4-48). As mentioned earlier, this type of injury occurred in 12% of 420 patients in our series. Flexion-rotation injuries may be subtle, with only minimal anterior subluxation (105). On the lateral view, the facet

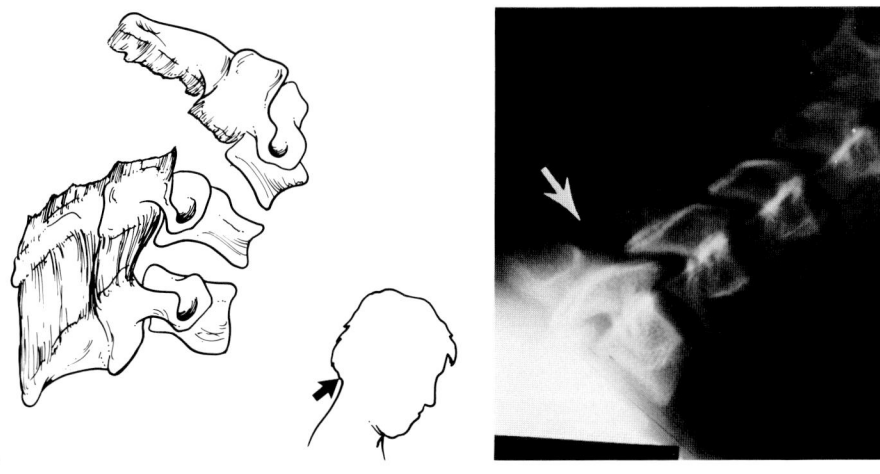

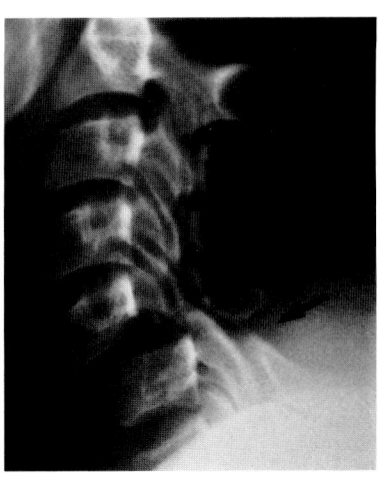

FIG. 4–47. A: Illustration of disruptive hyperflexion injury. The majority of the force is transmitted to the posterior ligaments. **B**: Posterior ligament injury with subtle kyphotic angulation to C5-C6. Note the widened interspinous distance (*arrow*). **C**: Bilateral locked facets are due to disruptive hyperflexion. The subluxation (C5 on C6) is typically at least one-half the AP diameter of the vertebral body.

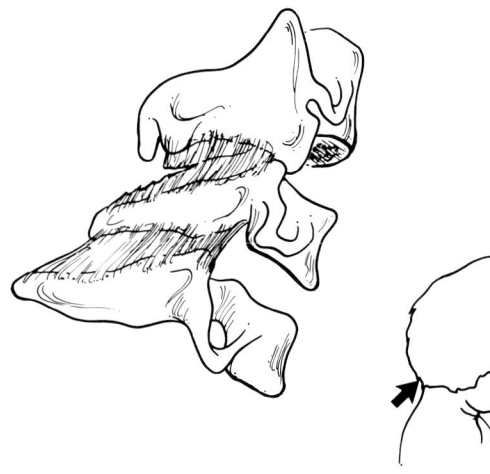

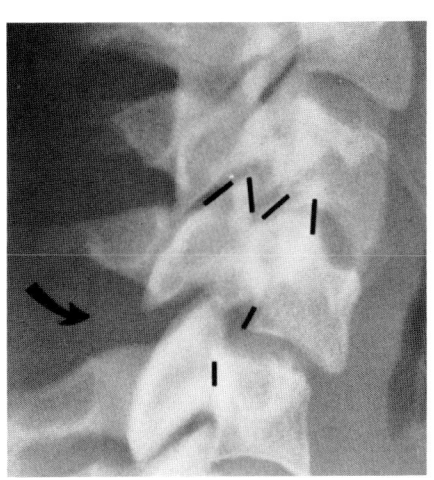

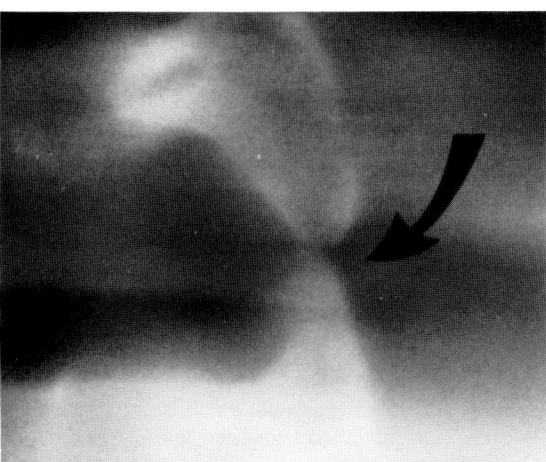

FIG. 4–48. A: Illustration of flexion rotation injury. **B**: Lateral radiograph of unilateral locked facet at C4-C5. The facets of C4 are rotated with a "bow tie" configuration. There is widening of the interspinous distance (*curved arrow*) and subluxation due to ligament disruption. **C**: Tomogram of the cervical spine following a flexion rotation injury. The facets are perched (*arrow*) but not locked.

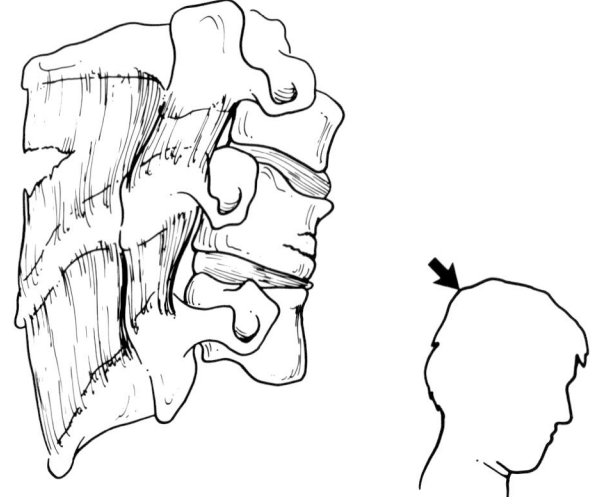

FIG. 4–49. Illustration of flexion compression injury. More force is transmitted to the anterior vertebral body.

joints at the level of the injury rotate, giving a "bow tie" appearance (Fig. 4-48B) (99). Oblique views will usually demonstrate the injury more clearly. Conventional or computed tomography is frequently needed for complete evaluation of these injuries (Fig. 4-48C).

Compressive hyperflexion injuries occur when a force is applied to the top of the head, resulting in forward arching of the head (Fig. 4-49). The main force is distributed along the vertebral bodies. As described earlier, the force is mainly compressive and thus the posterior liga-

ments may remain intact. Wedge fractures of the bodies, teardrop fractures, and fracture-dislocations may result. Harris states that the flexion teardrop injury is the most unstable lesion of all (100). In this situation the vertebrae above the injury move anteriorly, and the vertebrae below posteriorly, in a circular direction (Fig. 4-50).

Compressive shearing forces result from a force directed to the back of the head with the head moving forward. The result may be an anteriorly displaced fracture of the odontoid. Atlantoaxial and atlanto-occipital dislocations are rare but may also occur in this type of injury.

Gehweiler (98) classified hyperflexion injuries as follows: Type I, anterior fracture-dislocation of the odontoid; Type II, hyperflexion sprain; Type III, locked facets, Type IV, teardrop fracture-dislocation. These injuries are all basically due to hyperflexion. The important feature is the potential instability and frequency of neurologic complications, especially in the low cervical injuries. It has been reiterated many times in the literature that flexion alone will not result in disruption of the posterior ligaments (98,99,111). The mechanism of injury is rarely pure. In our experience (420 cases) most hyperflexion injuries were of the flexion-compression variety. Regardless of the exact mechanism, one must be aware of the potential significance of hyperflexion injuries. They are frequently unstable and require aggressive treatment. This usually indicates halo immobilization frequently followed by posterior fusion. In our series the incidence of significant neurologic complications follow-

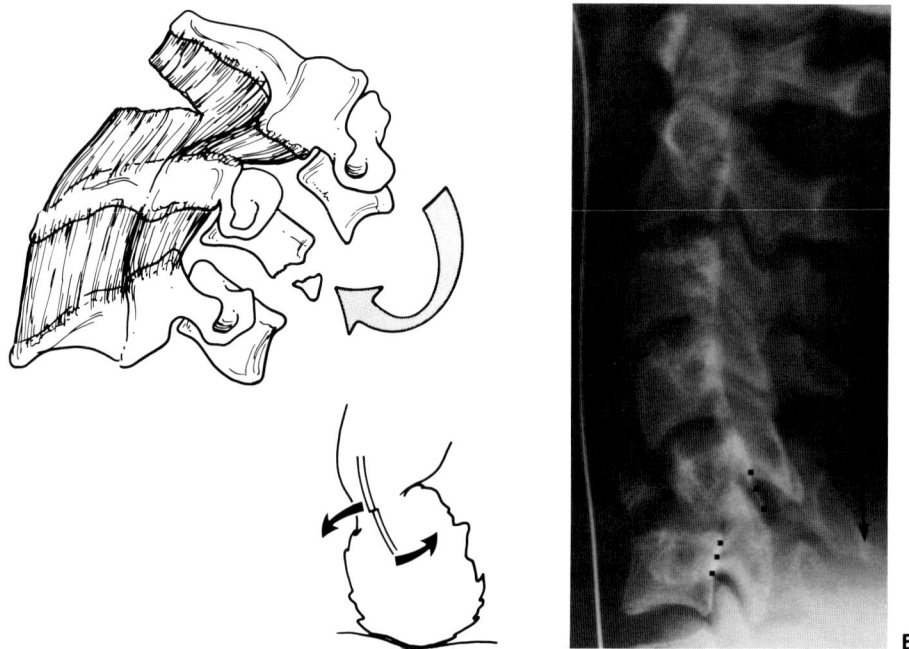

FIG. 4–50. A: Illustration of forces in hyperflexion "teardrop" injury. **B:** Lateral radiograph following hyperflexion compression injury with teardrop fracture of C5. Note the subluxation of C5 on C6 and marked widening of the interspinous distance due to tearing of the posterior ligaments. This degree of widening would not be seen with a hyperextension injury.

TABLE 4-7. *Cervical spine trauma: Indicators of instability on the lateral radiograph[a]*

Vertebral subluxation > 3 mm[b]
Angular deformity > 11°
Increased interspinous distance[b]
Narrowed disk space
Facet joint widening[b]
Vertebral compression > 25%

[a] (91,92,98,100,110).
[b] Indicate instability more reliably.

ing flexion-compression injuries was 72%. Other series have also reported a high incidence of neurologic complications with flexion injuries (99). Delayed instability is also a feared complication of subtle posterior ligament injuries (85,89,106,108).

Radiographic findings on the lateral view are useful in evaluating instability (Table 4-7). These findings include anterior subluxation greater than 3.5 mm, angular deformity greater than 11°, widening of the interspinous distance, compression of the vertebral body greater than 25%, and disk space narrowing. Harris has classified bilateral locked facets and hyperflexion-teardrop injuries as unstable (100). Both injuries fulfill the above criteria, and the latter injury is fraught with frequent neurologic complications. Indentification of widened interspinous distance, widened facet joints, or subluxation (>3 mm) alone are sufficient to make the diagnosis of instability. Widening of the interpedicular distance on the AP view (burst fracture) also indicates instability (92). These changes essentially indicate two column involvement as describes by Denis (see Fig. 4-25) (93).

Hyperextension Injuries

Hyperextension injuries were once thought to be uncommon; however, in our experience and according to other authors as well, hyperextension injuries are nearly as common as hyperflexion (83,96–98,111). In our series 38% of the patients sustained hyperextension injuries (see Table 4-6).

If a force is applied to the mandible in an upward direction, disruption of the anterior longitudinal ligament and disk may result (Fig. 4-51). The lateral radiograph may be normal or reveal soft tissue swelling with displacement of the prevertebral fat stripe (97,109). Widening of the anterior disk space may also be evident (Fig. 4-51B) (90). A small chip fracture, usually from the anterior inferior aspect of the vertebral body, may be noted (Fig. 4-52). Unfortunately, the radiographic changes may be very subtle, with further confusion added by the presence of significant neurologic deficits. Neurologic damage often is the result of anteroposterior compression of the cord, leading to a decrease in the AP diameter of the spinal canal and vascular compromise to the cord (central cord syndrome). This could occur in spondylotic or normal spines (see Fig. 4-51) (86,97,111). Marar suggested that infolding of the ligamentum flavum may also play a part in the cord impingement (104). The incidence of cord compromise with hyperextension injury from C3 to C7 was 22% in our series. In the upper cervical spine, the most common hyperextension injury is the "hangman's" fracture, in which neurologic findings are uncommon. No permanent neurologic deficits were evi-

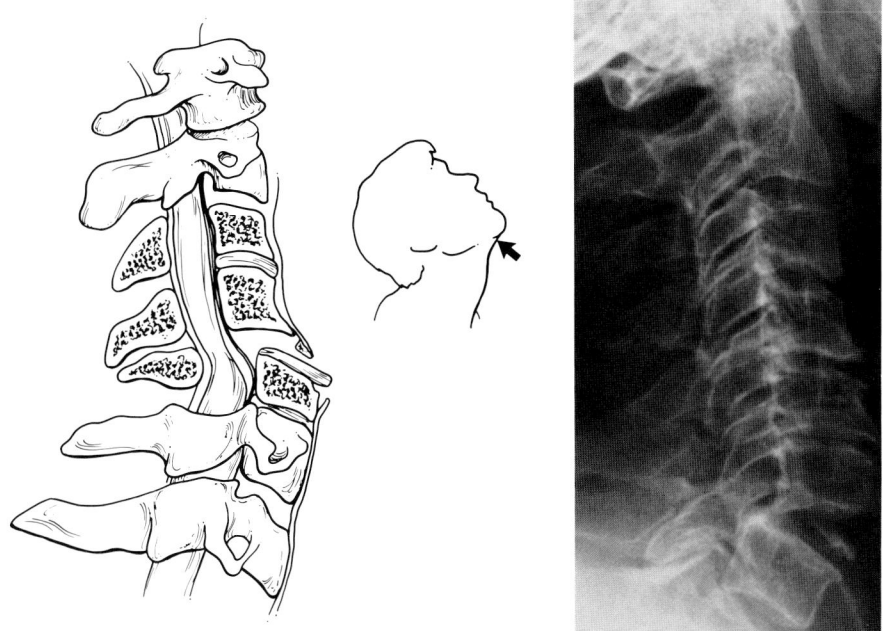

A   **B**

FIG. 4–51. A: Illustration of disruptive hyperextension injury. The cord may be compressed with this injury. **B:** Lateral radiograph demonstrating anterior widening of the interspace with a chip fracture due to disruptive hyperextension.

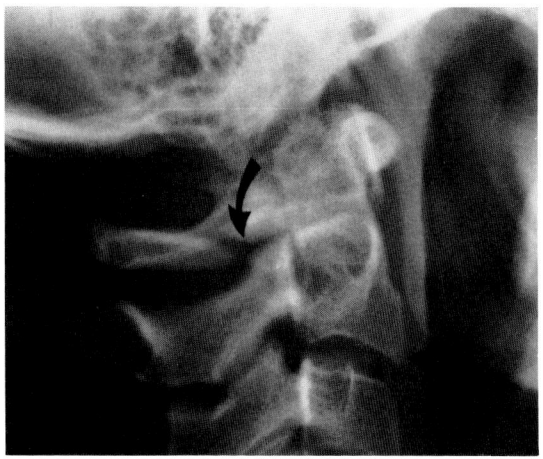

FIG. 4–52. Lateral radiograph demonstrating a subtle anterior inferior fracture of the body of C2 (*straight arrow*). There is a congenital defect in the posterior ring of C1 (*curved arrow*).

Hyperextension may also result from blows directed to the vertex of the skull, when most of the force is absorbed by the posterior arch. Fractures of the spinous process, lamina, pedicles, and articular pillars may result (Fig. 4-53). Anterior subluxation may occur, which on the lateral radiograph could be mistaken for a flexion injury. Oblique and pillar views will demonstrate the posterior arch fractures and aid in differentiating the mechanism of injury (97,111). In these cases, conventional tomography or computed tomography is often needed to evaluate the neural arch (Fig. 4-53). Facial injuries are also common in patients with hyperextension injuries (96,111). Finally, anterior shearing forces result in posterior fracture-dislocations in the upper cervical spine.

Most hyperextension injuries are stable. Unstable injuries include some of the hangman's fractures, hyperextension fracture-dislocations, and hyperextension sprain. The last is stable in flexion but unstable during extension (100).

dent in upper (C1-C2) cervical injuries, although 10% did develop transient neurologic symptoms. As noted previously, MRI is an extremely valuable technique for evaluating cord injury, especially in patients with stable injuries.

Vertical-Compression Injuries

Pure vertical compression may result in a typical Jefferson's fracture (see Fig. 4-54) or a burst fracture in the

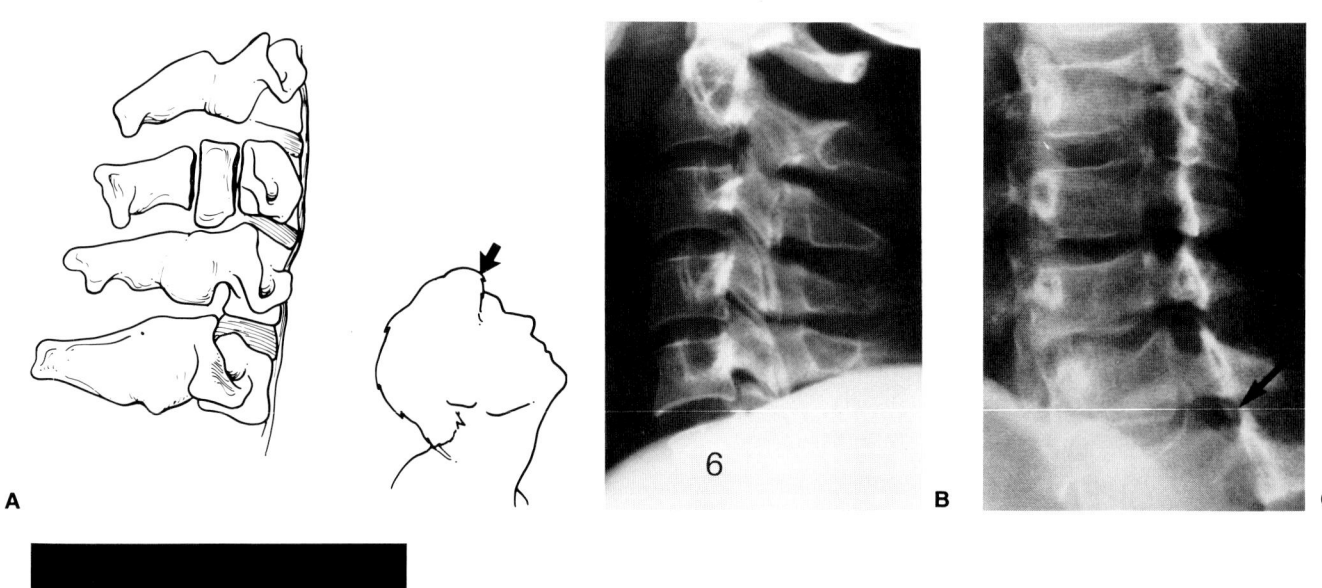

A

B

C

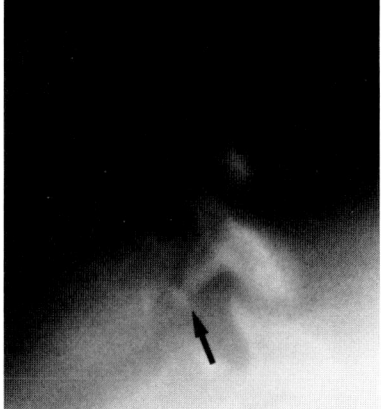

D

FIG. 4–53. A: Illustration of compressive hyperextension with neural arch fracture. **B**: Lateral view demonstrates only the upper six cervical vertebrae with widening of the C5 interspace. **C**: Oblique view demonstrates a fracture of the superior facet of C5. **D**: Tomograms demonstrate a pedicle fracture (*arrow*) assisting in diagnosing an extension injury.

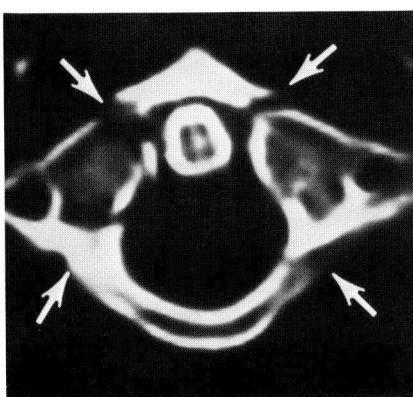

FIG. 4-54. Axial CT image demonstrating a typical Jeffersons fracture with multiple breaks (*arrows*) in the ring of C1.

lower cervical spine. The spine must be in near neutral positions at the time the vertical force is applied. These injuries are uncommon. In our series only 4% of injuries were due to vertical compression. Usually there is an asymmetrical vertical compression with lateral flexion (Fig. 4-55). This may result in a compression fracture of one of the lateral masses of C1 or a pillar fracture. Fractures of the uncinate process or a transverse process fracture may also occur (97,98). Flexion compression forces may also lead to burst fractures (91,92).

Summary

A thorough understanding of the mechanism of injury and stability of the injury is imperative in proper management of cervical spine trauma. This discussion has reviewed a more simplified approach to the mechanism of injury (Table 4-6).

In our series of 420 cervical spine fractures and fracture-dislocations, the injuries could be classified into five basic groups. Again, remembering that the mechanisms

of injury are rarely pure, especially in the case of axial compression, hyperextension or hyperflexion injuries occurred in 88% of patients. Flexion-rotation injuries (unilateral locked facets and anterior subluxations) were detected in 12% of patients. Only 4% could be classified as having vertical compressive injuries. Certain patients with undisplaced odontoid or isolated spinous process fractures could not be definitively categorized. No neurologic symptoms were present in the undisplaced odontoid group. Solitary spinous process fractures may be the result of flexion, extension, or direct trauma. These fractures are stable and of little clinical significance.

The above approach, when accompanied with assessment of radiographs for indications of instability (Table 4-7), is simple and reliable in determining the mechanism of injury and proper method of open or closed stability of the fracture.

Cervical Spine Fractures and Fracture-Dislocations

Cervical spine injuries in adults most frequently involve the lower cervical spine (81% in our series of 420 patients). Nineteen percent of injuries involved the upper cervical spine (from the occipital condyles to C2). Multiple injuries are common. The average number of injuries per patient is 2.2 (151,152).

The anatomic relationships of the upper cervical spine are unique, and the mechanisms of injury differ somewhat from those affecting the lower cervical spine. Therefore, in discussing specific cervical spine injuries the upper and lower segments will be presented separately.

Upper Cervical Spine

Atlanto-occipital Region

Injuries involving the occipital condyles and atlanto-occipital articulation are rare (119,156). We noted only 1

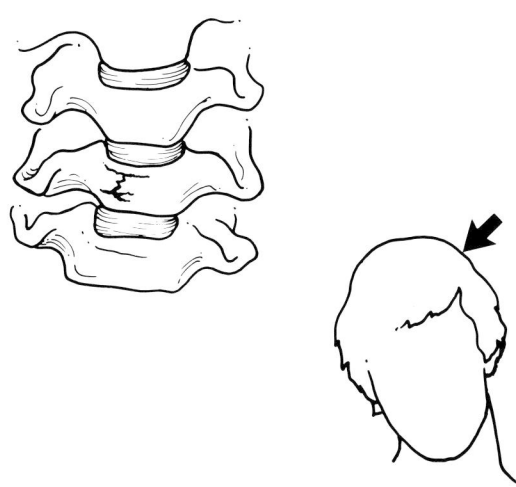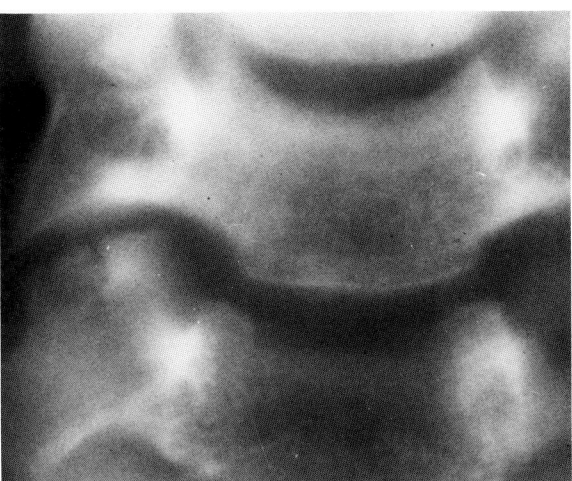

A

B

FIG. 4-55. A: Illustration of vertical compression with lateral flexion resulting in asymmetric fracture. B: Tomogram demonstrating lateral compression injury with compression of C6 (*arrow*).

fracture of the occipital condyles in our series of 420 patients. Fewer than 10 cases have been reported since 1817 (156). Fractures of the condyle may result from shearing or rotary forces and blows to the calvarium from above, similar to the mechanism that results in a Jefferson's fracture (123). These injuries may disrupt the hypoglossal canal, injuring the jugular vein and the 9th, 10th, and 11th cranial nerves. However, often the trauma may seem minor with no neurologic deficit (156). As with other upper cervical spine injuries, tomography (AP and lateral projections) is extremely valuable in demonstrating these injuries. Routine radiographs are often normal and computed tomography may miss this fracture due to partial volume affects (Fig. 4-56) (122).

Atlanto-occipital dislocations are also rare. This injury usually occurs in high-velocity motor vehicle accidents. The lesion is usually the result of shearing forces directed either to the face or to the occipital region. Others have suggested flexion or hyperextension and distraction as the mechanism of injury (114,206). Death is due to brainstem injury. Two cases of atlanto-occipital dislocation were noted in our series. Both patients were in their teens. Atlanto-occipital dislocation is more common in children owing to their smaller condyles and the more horizontal articular relationship of the condyles with the lateral masses of the atlas (209). Although the injury is almost always fatal, 15 survivors have been reported in the literature (206).

Radiographically, the diagnosis is usually obvious on the lateral view of the skull or cervical spine (Fig. 4-57).

The occipital condyles lose their normal articular relationship with the atlas, and a large hematoma is present in the retropharyngeal space. Powers devised a ratio that may be helpful in diagnosing anterior dislocations on routine lateral views (177). The distance from the basion to the spinolaminar line of C1 (BC) divided by the distance from the posterior margin of the anterior arch of C1 to the posterior margin of the foramen magnum (DA) should be less than 1 (Fig. 4-58). If this ratio is greater than 1, a dislocation is present. Since the measurement is a ratio, the technique does not require standardization of target-film distance. Odontoid fractures have been described in association with atlanto-occipital dislocations and should be carefully checked on radiographic examinations (141).

Atlas (C1)

In our experience fractures of the atlas account for approximately 4% of all spinal injuries. Others report a similar incidence (141,151,152,163). Five types of fractures have been described based on the anatomic region affected. They include fractures of the anterior arch, posterior arch and lateral mass, transverse process and Jefferson's fracture (130,188,190). Fractures most commonly involve the lateral masses and the posterior arch (Fig. 4-59 and 4-60). Sherk and Nicholson reported that posterior arch fractures account for 67% of fractures of the atlas. Posterior arch fractures are the result of hyper-

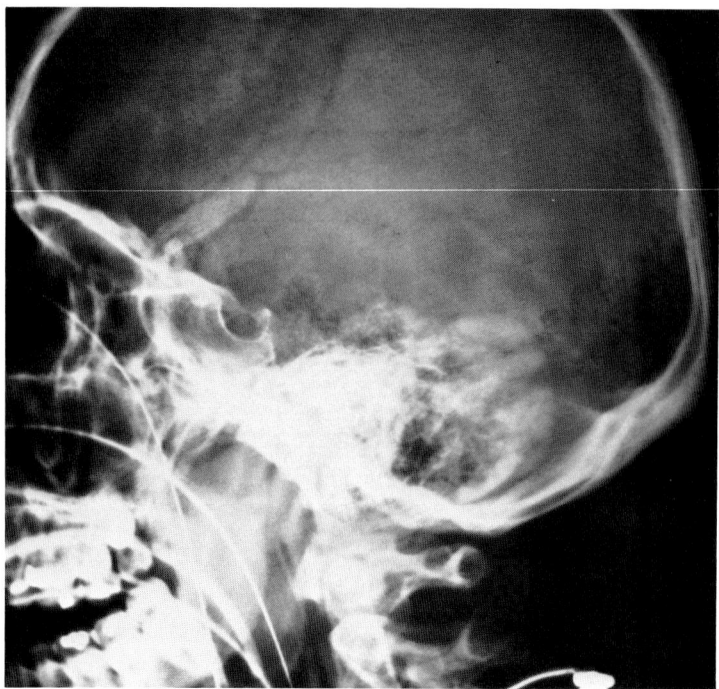
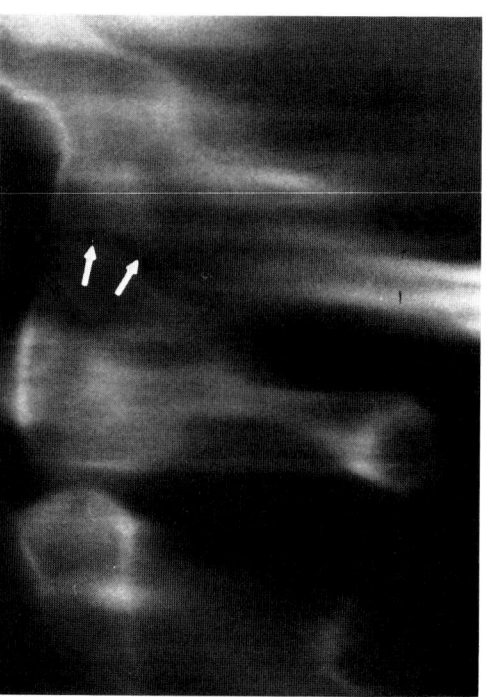

FIG. 4–56. A: Lateral view of the skull is normal. CT images were also normal. Lateral tomogram (**B**) demonstrates a horizontal fracture of the occipital condyle.

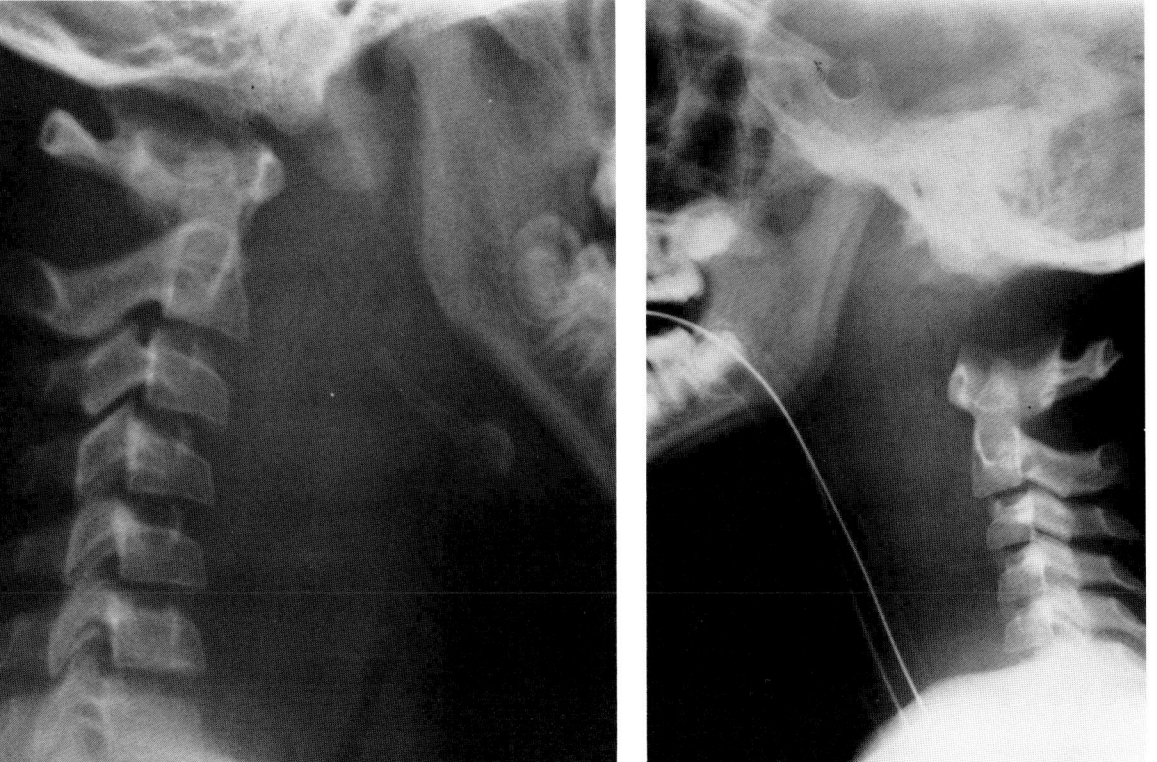

A   B

FIG. 4–57. Two patients with atlanto-occipital dislocations. **A:** Lateral view of the cervical spine demonstrating a huge prevertebral hematoma and anterior subluxation of the occipital condyles on C1. **B:** Lateral view demonstrates a huge prevertebral hematoma with distraction of the occipital condyles from C1.

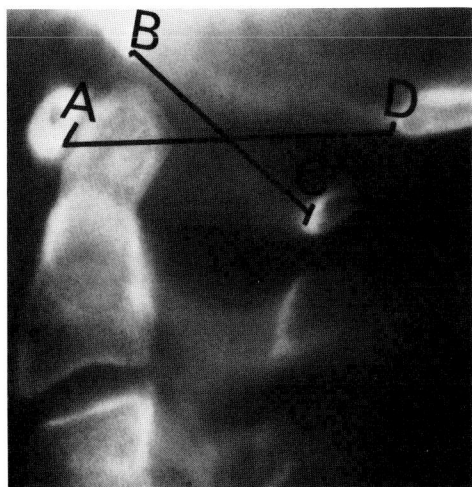

FIG. 4–58. Radiograph of the upper cervical spine demonstrating the normal occipito-atlantal relationship.

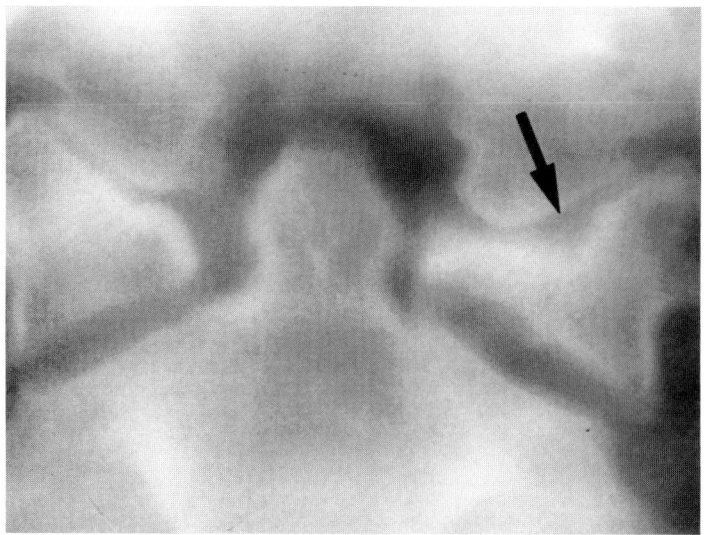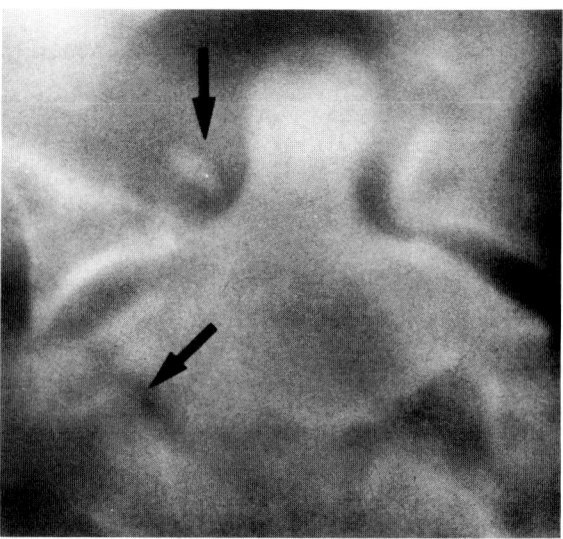

A   B

FIG. 4–59. AP tomograms demonstrating lateral mass fractures in C1. **A**: Compression fracture of the left lateral mass (*arrow*). **B**: Avulsed tubercle (*upper arrow*) and displacement of the lateral mass with a verticle fracture in C2 (*lower arrow*).

extension injuries in which the arch is compressed be-tween the occiput and spinous process of the axis (151,152). Associated injuries are common (Table 4-8). Hangman's fractures were noted in 15% of these pa-tients. Spinous process fractures of C7 were evident in 25% of patients with posterior arch fractures of C1. Our experience is similar to Segal et al. (188) who reported lower cervical spine fractures in 22% of patients with C1 fractures. Other skeletal fractures were noted in 18% of patients, frequently in the upper thoracic spine. As this is a hyperextension injury, one should not be surprised by the frequently associated facial injuries. Care must be taken not to mistake a normal congenital cleft (2–4% of the normal population) for a fracture (Fig. 4-61) (151).

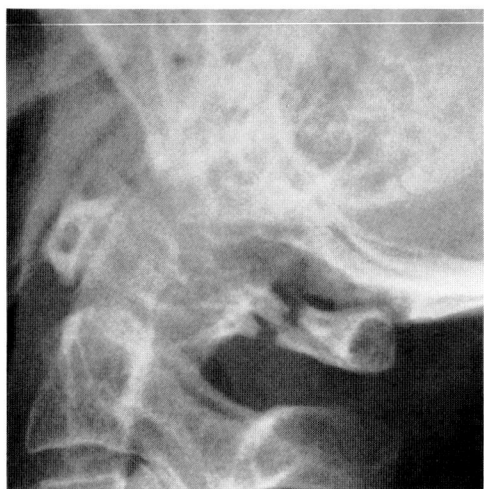

FIG. 4–60. Lateral view of the upper cervical spine demon-strating a posterior arch fracture. There is no swelling near the anterior arch.

Transverse process fractures due to lateral flexion forces have been described (123,151).

Pure Jefferson fractures result from a force directed vertically to the skull (160). The force is transmitted to the occipital condyles, which leads to lateral displace-ment of the lateral masses of the atlas (Fig. 4-62A). The lateral displacement is a result of the anatomic configura-tion of these articulations, and fractures occur in the ante-rior and posterior arches (Fig. 4-62B). The anterior and, more specifically, the posterior arch are the weak points in the ring of the atlas. In our experience asymmetrical compression of the lateral mass with an associated ring fracture is more common than double breaks in the ante-rior and posterior arch. This is due to some degree of lateral or rotary motion along with the vertical force (Fig. 4-63). Pure vertical compression with the neck in neutral position is required for the symmetric four-part break in the ring. In either situation, the cord is protected owing to the outward displacement of the fracture fragments. Less commonly, horizontal fractures of the anterior arch occur (Fig. 4-64). This injury also results from hyperex-tension and avulsion at the insertion of the longus colli (152,179). To date, only 13 cases have been reported. It

TABLE 4–8. Hangman's fractures (6% of 420 cases)

Associated findings	Incidence (%)
Spinal injuries	
C1	15%
T1-T4	10%
Neurologic symptoms	
Complete	0
Transient	10%

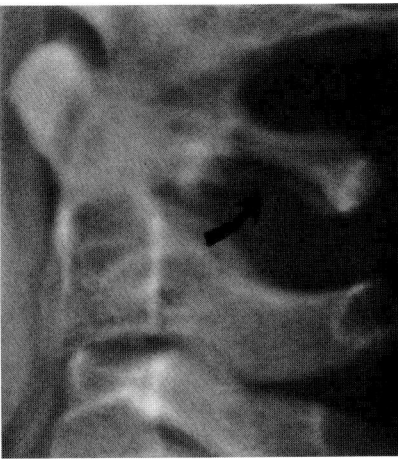

FIG. 4–61. Normal congenital cleft in the posterior ring of C1. Note the sharp sclerotic images.

is essential to exclude other associated hyperextension injuries (161).

Neurologic complications with atlas fractures are rare (141,151,152,155,160). However, significant retropharyngeal hemorrhage resulting in difficulty in breathing has been reported (155). Delayed basilar invagination may also occur if proper treatment is not instituted (137).

Radiographically, most injuries of C1 can be detected on the AP odontoid view or on the lateral view of the cervical spine or skull (Fig. 4-62A). Several significant features noted on the AP odontoid view or AP tomograms should be stressed (Fig. 4-62B). Outward displacement of the lateral masses of the atlas of greater than 6.9 mm indicates a tear or avulsion of the transverse ligament (195). However, normal features such as the insertion of the transverse ligament and bipartite superior fac-

ets should not be confused with fractures (162). Subtle changes may require conventional or computed tomography for complete evaluation (Fig. 4-63). Computed tomography is especially useful in evaluating the ring of the atlas (see Fig. 4-65) (163).

Atlantoaxial Dislocations

Traumatic dislocations of the atlas on the axis are rare. The transverse ligament will normally maintain the relationship of the odontoid with C1 unless the dens is fractured or the ligament is avulsed from its insertion (Figs. 4-65 and 4-66). Subluxations of the atlas on the axis are most often related to inflammatory conditions such as rheumatoid arthritis, Behçet's syndrome, retropharyngeal infection, and congenital abnormalities (137,

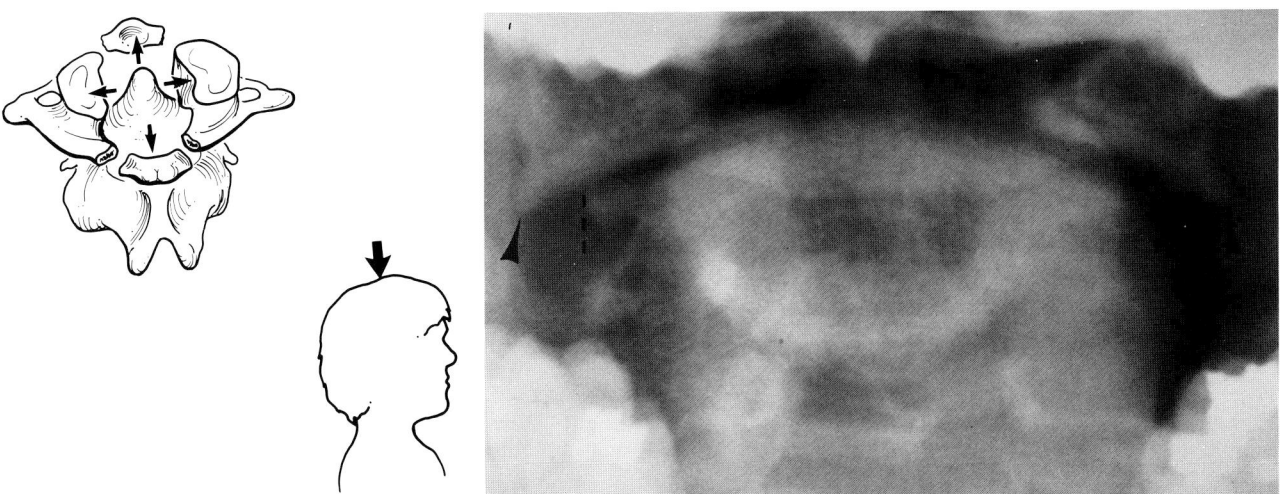

A   B

FIG. 4–62. A: Illustration of mechanism of injury for Jeffersons fracture. **B:** Open mouth odontoid view demonstrating lateral displacement of the lateral masses (*arrows*). Vertical lines mark the margins of C2.

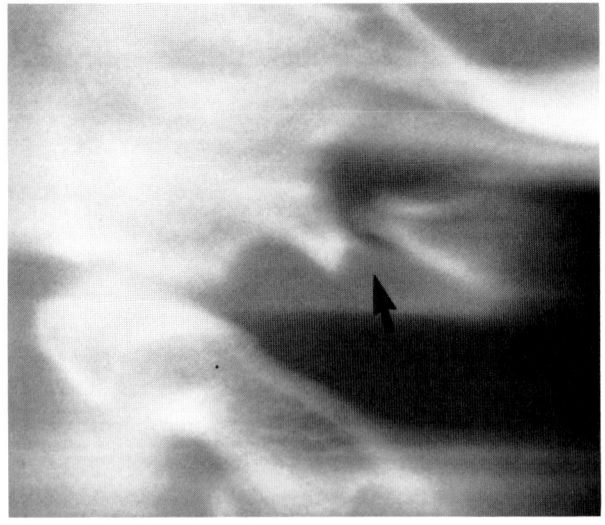

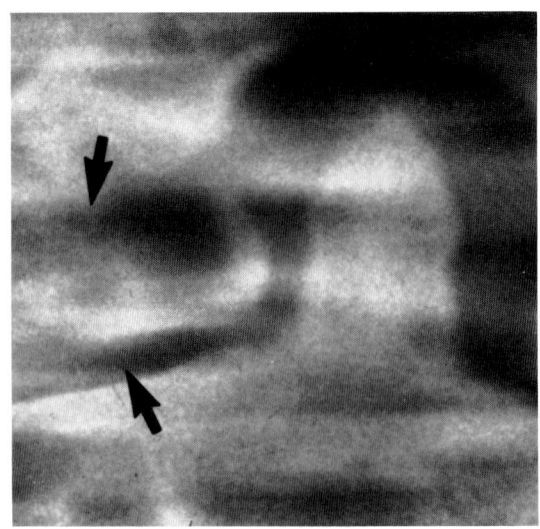

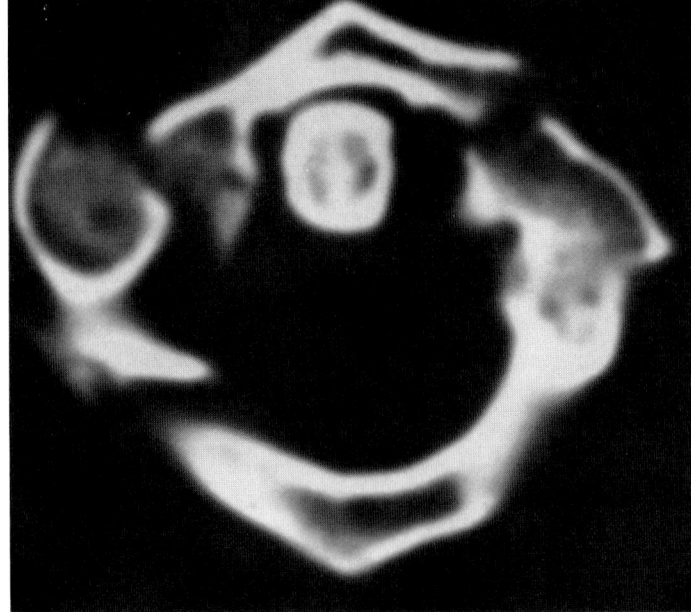

FIG. 4-63. Lateral (A) and AP (B) tomograms of a Jeffersons fracture with asymmetrical involvement (*arrows*). CT scan (C) demonstrates the fracture more clearly.

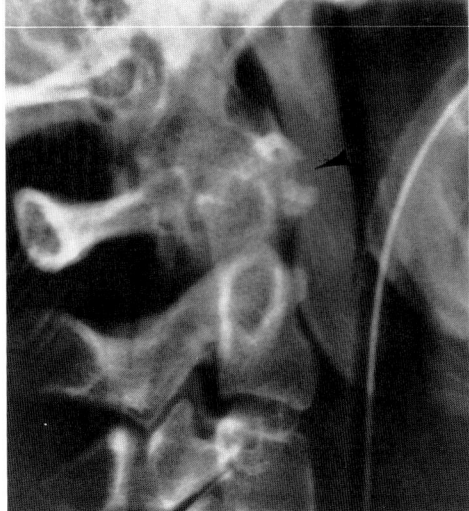

FIG. 4-64. Lateral view of the upper cervical region demonstrating an avulsion fracture of the anterior ring of C1 (*arrow*).

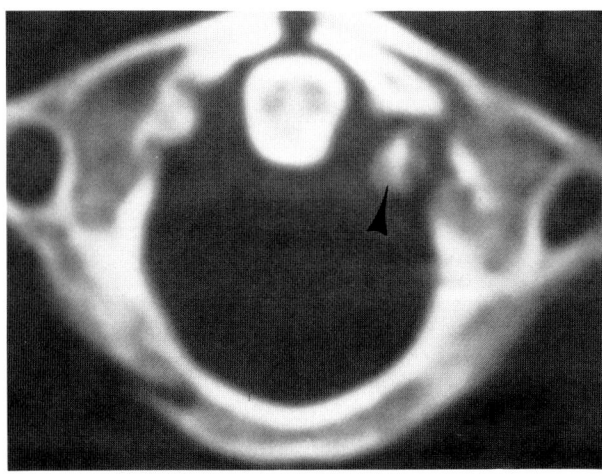

FIG. 4-65. CT scan demonstrating multiple fractures of C1 and avulsion of the transverse ligament attachment (*arrow*).

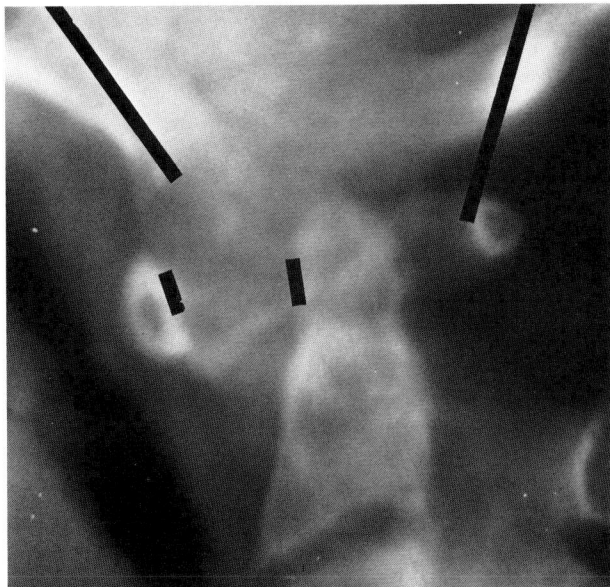

FIG. 4-66. Lateral tomogram of the upper cervical spine demonstrating disruption of the transverse ligament with marked subluxation of C1 on the odontoid. Note the clivus and laminar lines.

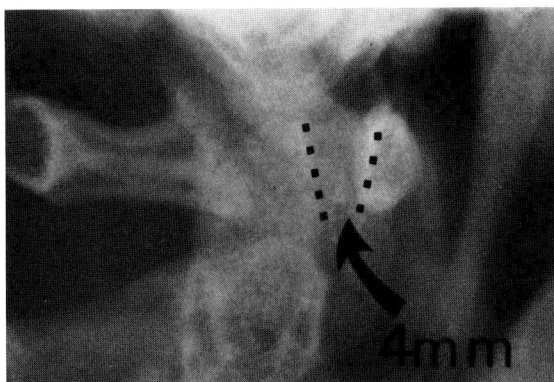

FIG. 4-67. Lateral view of the upper cervical spine. C1 subluxation on the odontoid measuring 4 mm.

155,162,166,179,189,195). Traumatic dislocations may be anterior, posterior, or rotary in nature. The lesion is uncommon, accounting for only 1% (4 of 420) of cervical spine injuries in our series. The transverse ligament was intact in all cases. In each instance the trauma resulted in an avulsion fracture at the insertion of the ligament from the lateral mass of the atlas. Measurement of the C1-odontoid distance exceeded 3 mm in the neutral position in all cases (Fig. 4-67). Associated fractures of the lateral mass of the atlas and the upper facet of the axis were present in 25% of the cases (Fig. 4-59B). This confirmed the asymmetrical vertical compression as the

mechanism of injury. If the lateral radiograph is normal, carefully performed flexion and extension fluoroscopic studies may be necessary to demonstrate the lesion (Fig. 4-68). Also, measurement of the AP diameter of the spinal canal is helpful. If the distance from the posterior aspect of the odontoid to the spinolaminal line of the atlas is less than 18 mm, neurologic symptoms are more likely to occur (152).

Posterior and rotary dislocations are even more uncommon than anterior dislocations (115,124,159). Rotary dislocation requires 45° of rotation of C1 on the axis for locking to occur (152). This condition differs from the rotary fixation described by Fielding and Hawkins (145). Sixty-five degrees of rotation is required for fixation to occur if the transverse ligament and odontoid are anatomically normal (145). If the ligament is interrupted, less rotation is required (144). Cord injury and vertebral artery injury have been reported with rotary fixation. In describing 17 cases of rotary fixation, Fielding and Hawkins defined the following four types of injuries (Fig. 4-69) (145).

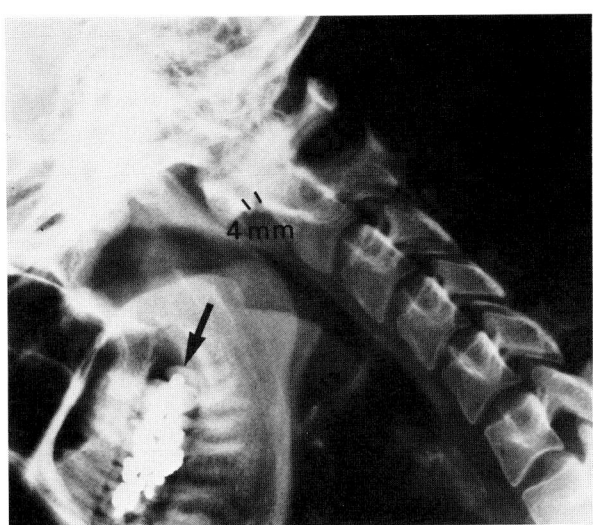
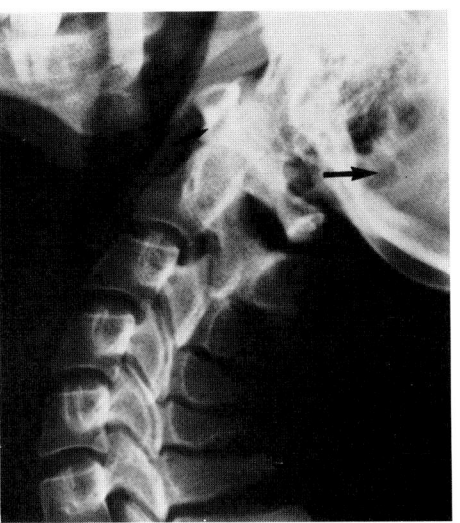

FIG. 4-68. Anterior subluxation of C1 on C2 during flexion (A) that reduced with extension (B).

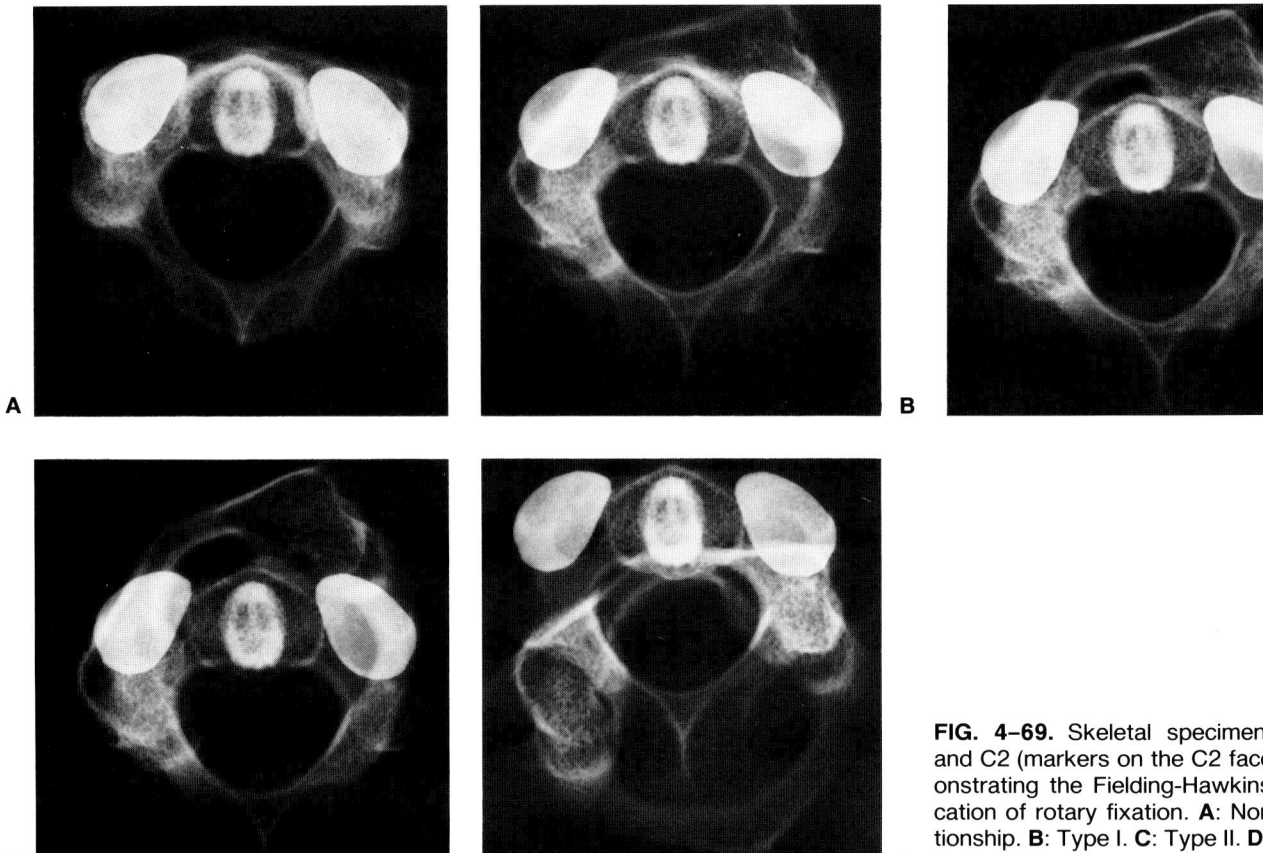

FIG. 4–69. Skeletal specimens of C1 and C2 (markers on the C2 facets) demonstrating the Fielding-Hawkins classification of rotary fixation. **A**: Normal relationship. **B**: Type I. **C**: Type II. **D**: Type III. **E**: Type IV.

Type I

Rotary fixation without anterior subluxation of the atlas on the axis (transverse ligament intact).

Type II

Rotary fixation with 3–5 mm of atlantoaxial subluxation.

Type III

Rotary fixation with greater than 5 mm of atlantoaxial subluxation.

Type IV

Rotary fixation with posterior atlantoaxial subluxation (deficient dens required).

Type I is the most common lesion reported (145). Clinically, these lesions have been noted following trauma and dental procedures and associated with retropharyngeal infections. The patient usually presents with the head rotated to the side. Neurologic deficits are rare.

The exact etiology is unclear, but fixation may be related to capsular entrapment in the atlantoaxial facets (145).

Radiographically, the AP and lateral odontoid views may be sufficient for diagnosis (Fig. 4-70). However, 15°-rotation AP odontoid views are more definitive. Normally the motion of C1 and C2 is independent on rotation-AP views. If rotary fixation is present, C1 and C2 maintain a constant relationship when rotated. Computed tomography is most accurate for evaluation and allows differentiation from torticollis or simple rotation more readily than routine radiographs (Fig. 4-71).

Axis

Fractures of the axis are common, accounting for 15% of cervical spine injuries. Others report the incidence of fracture of the axis to be as high as 27% (152). Fractures of the odontoid and pedicles account for 80% of the injuries to the axis (125). The vertebral body is involved in about 15% of cases, usually through an anterior inferior chip fracture. The facets, lamina, and spinous processes are less frequently involved (125,152,193).

Odontoid fractures may result from anterior shearing (hyperextension), posterior shearing (hyperflexion), or lateral flexion injuries. Odontoid fractures account for

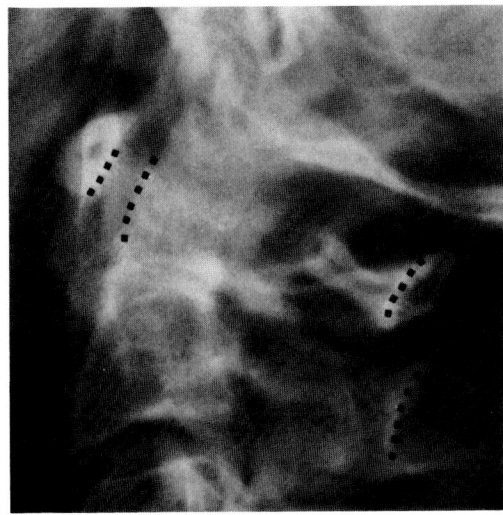

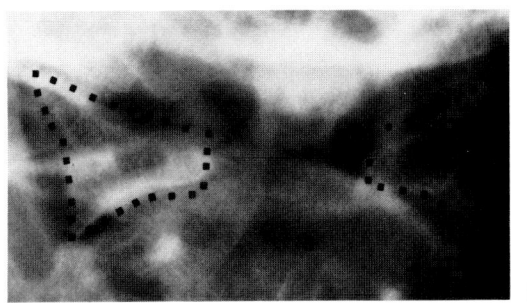

FIG. 4-70. Lateral (**A**) and AP (**B**) views demonstrating Type II rotary fixation.

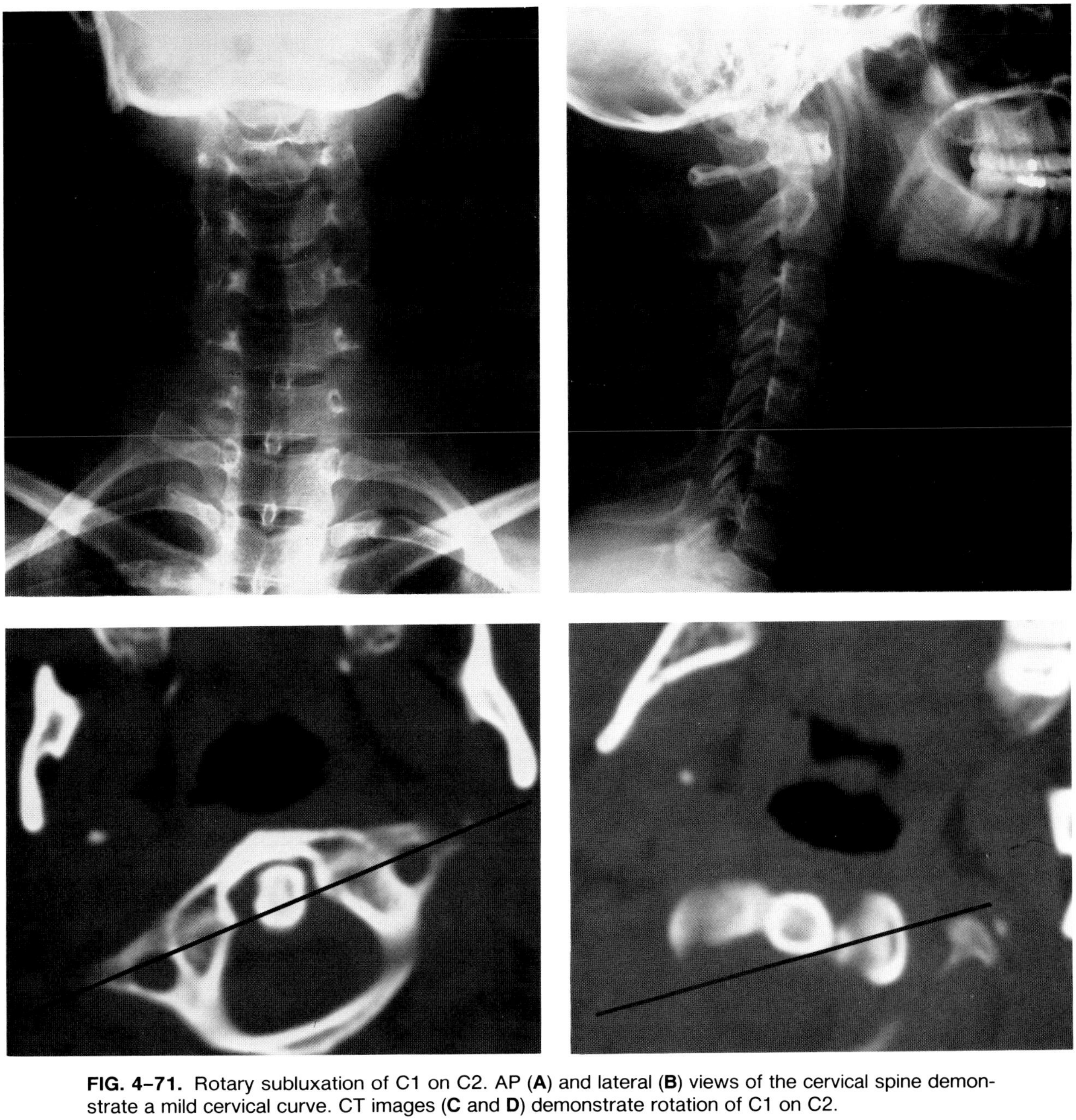

FIG. 4-71. Rotary subluxation of C1 on C2. AP (**A**) and lateral (**B**) views of the cervical spine demonstrate a mild cervical curve. CT images (**C** and **D**) demonstrate rotation of C1 on C2.

11–13% of all cervical spine fractures (125). Patients with odontoid fractures usually present with neck pain and rarely have neurologic symptoms (182). Even if there is displacement of the fractures, there is usually sufficient space to prevent cord injury. Although mortality in such cases has been reported to be as high as 30%, associated head injuries make exact mortality figures difficult to interpret (181). Associated fractures of the atlas are not uncommon (8% in our series). Forty-one percent of our patients sustained associated head, facial, and extraspinal injuries.

In a significant number of cases, odontoid fractures are undisplaced and subtle, requiring tomography for definitive diagnosis and classification (Fig. 4-72). The mechanism of injury in these cases is often difficult to determine. If the fracture is slightly displaced, the mechanism of injury is more easily established. When the fracture is displaced, the lateral view of the skull or cervical spine and the open-mouth odontoid view are usually adequate for diagnosis.

Radiographically, one should check carefully for retropharyngeal soft tissue swelling, which may be the only clue to an odontoid fracture (Fig. 4-72) (56). Tomography is frequently required for diagnosis and classification of the fractures. Anderson and D'Alonzo's classifica-

tion is commonly utilized and is helpful in determining proper management and prognosis of the fracture (Fig. 4-73) (116,151,207). The classification divides odontoid fractures into three types: Type I, oblique fracture of the tip of the odontoid; Type II, fracture of the base of the odontoid; Type III, fracture enters the body of the axis (116,129,194).

Type I fractures may be due to avulsion of the alar ligament. These are the least common odontoid fractures (Table 4-9) and usually require tomography for diagnosis (Figs. 4-74 thru 4-76). Because of the different clinical picture and rarity of this lesion, some authors have excluded it from the odontoid fracture classification. Burke et al. (125) prefer to simplify odontoid fractures into high (Type II) and low (Type III) categories.

Type II fractures usually occur above the insertion of the accessory ligament, which provides at least a portion of the blood supply to the odontoid (Fig. 4-77). This may explain the high incidence of non-union with this fracture. Type II fractures are the most common type of odontoid fracture, accounting for 59–67% of odontoid fractures (129). The majority of Type II fractures are due to motor vehicle accidents or falls. Neurological involvement may include upper extremity monoplegia, occipital neuralgia, Brown-Séquard syndrome, hemiparesis,

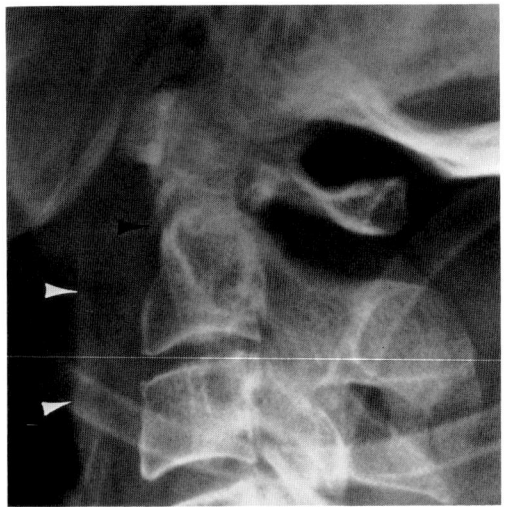

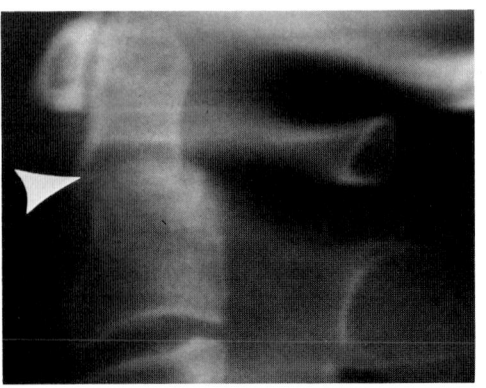

FIG. 4–72. A: Lateral view of the upper cervical spine demonstrates prevertebral swelling (*white arrows*) and cortical irregularity at the anterior odontoid base (*black arrow*). AP (**B**) and lateral (**C**) tomograms demonstrate a fracture with slight anterior displacement (*arrows*). The AP tomogram is less helpful— both views should be obtained.

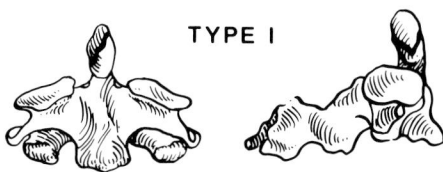

TYPE I

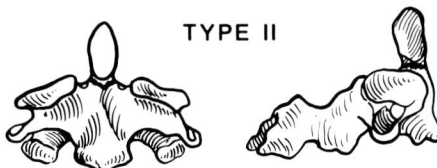

TYPE II

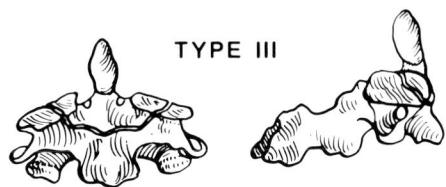

TYPE III

FIG. 4–73. Classification of odontoid fractures. Type I, upper odontoid; Type II, base of odontoid; Type III, involves the body of C2.

TABLE 4–9. *Odontoid fractures*

Type	Incidence (%)
I	8
II	59 (54% non-union)
III	33

grams should be considered whenever symptoms are present even if routine views are normal. Both AP and lateral are necessary for these injuries may be very subtle (Fig. 4-80).

Type III fractures account for about 33% of odontoid fractures (see Fig. 4-81). These fractures are frequently impacted anteriorly, and anterior displacement can be identified in up to 90% of patients. Undisplaced type III fractures almost always unite with proper treatment (Fig. 4-82) (116,181,194,207). Neurological involvement is slightly less common than with type II fractures (129). Non-union is common (40%) if anterior displacement exceeds 5 mm.

Identification of type III fractures frequently requires tomography. Undisplaced fractures can be very subtle (Figs. 4-83 and 4-84). Computed tomography is not as useful in these patients.

Care must be taken not to mistake normal variants or overlying structure for a fracture. Normally, the cortex of the odontoid is contiguous vertically with the body of the axis. The odontoid may deviate posteriorly, resulting in a convex anterior margin (Fig. 4-85). This is normal. Anterior bowing of the odontoid is not normal, and in this case one should suspect a Type III fracture (Fig. 4-85B). On the open-mouth odontoid view, overlying structures may be confused with fracture lines. These include the posterior arch of the atlas, the occiput, the base of the tongue, and clefts in the teeth (132). The os odontoideum (Fig. 4-86) is well-marginated and should

and quadraparesis. Clark and White (129) noted one or more of these changes in approximately 20% of type II fractures. Non-union with these injuries may be as high as 72% if displacement is present (Fig. 4-78) (181). Posterior displacement appears to indicate a poorer prognosis (182,194).

A significant number of type II odontoid fractures will be overlooked on routine radiographs. Also, CT may miss this injury as the fracture line may lie entirely within the image plane (Fig. 4-79). Therefore, AP and lateral tomograms may be the best technique. Tomo-

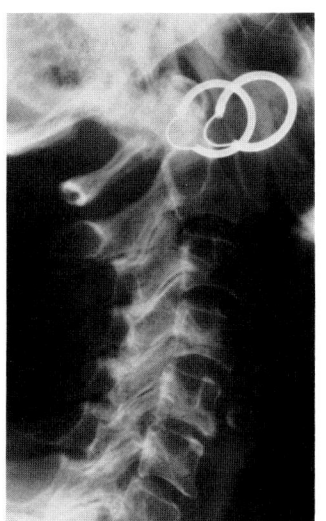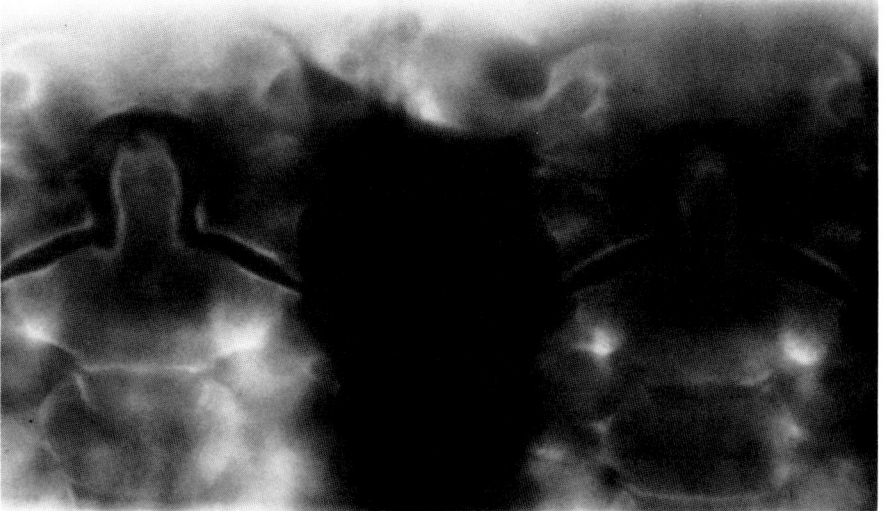

FIG. 4–74. A: Lateral radiograph is normal. **B:** AP tomograms demonstrate a Type I odontoid fracture.

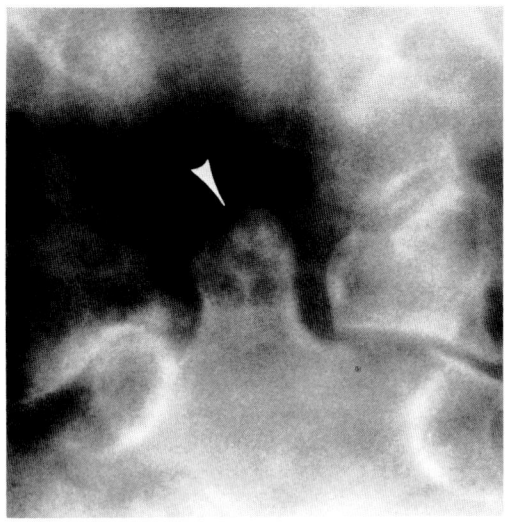

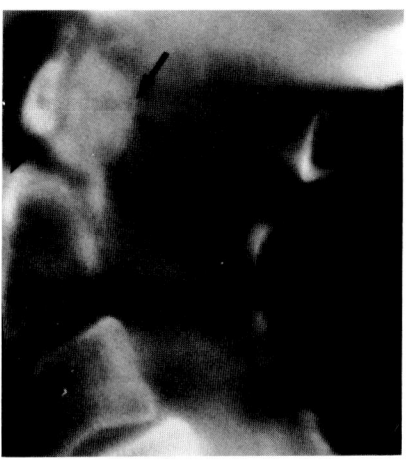

FIG. 4-76. Lateral tomogram demonstrating Type I (*black arrow*) and Type II fractures (*open arrow*).

FIG. 4-75. Angled open mouth odontoid view with rotary subluxation of C1 on C2 and a Type I odontoid fracture (*arrow*).

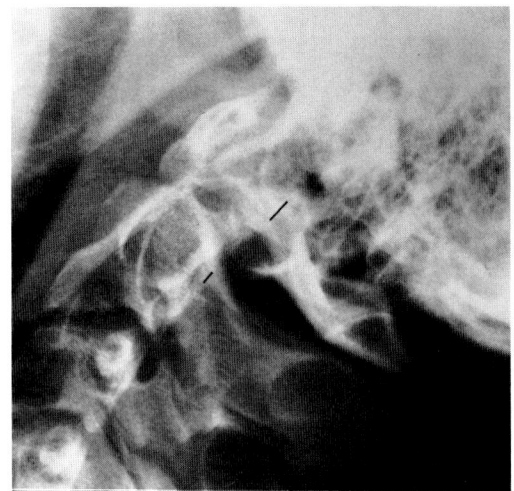

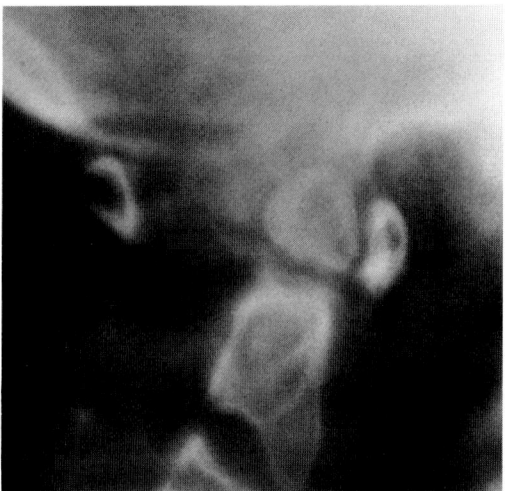

A   B

FIG. 4-77. Normal lateral radiograph (**A**) and tomogram (**B**). The tomogram clearly demonstrates the Type II fracture.

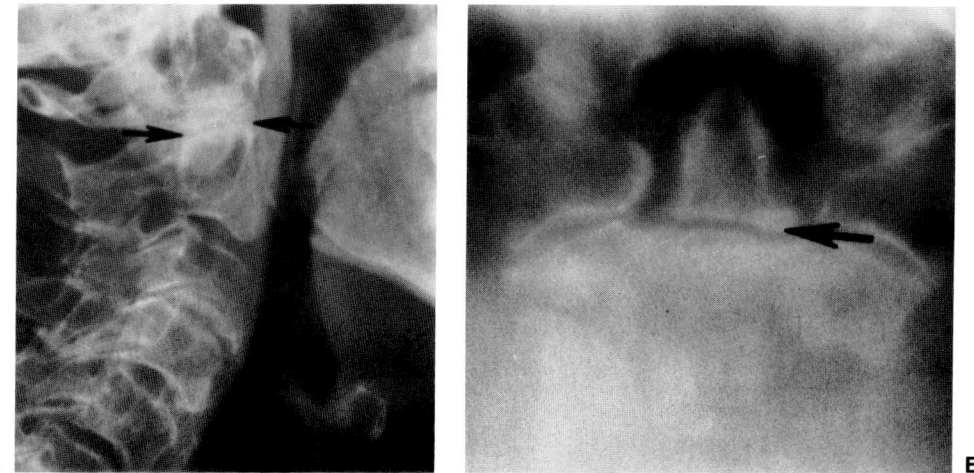

FIG. 4–78. A: Lateral view of the cervical spine shows sclerosis (*arrows*) at the base of the odontoid. **B**: AP tomogram demonstrates an ununited Type II odontoid fracture (*arrow*) with sclerotic margins.

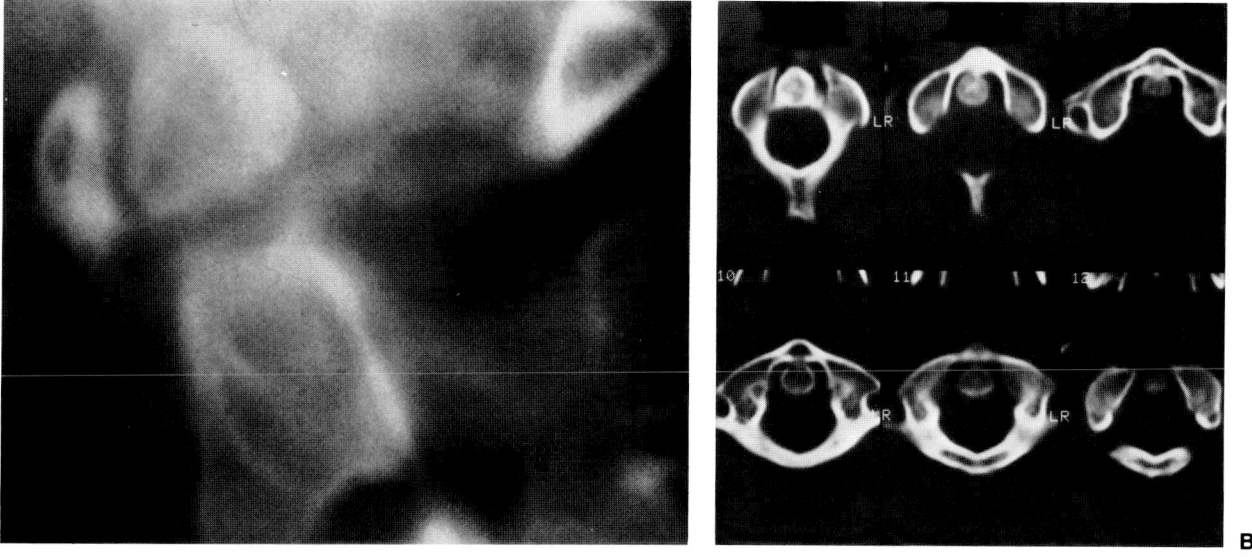

FIG. 4–79. CT images (**A**) are normal. Lateral tomogram (**B**) clearly demonstrates the Type II odontoid fracture.

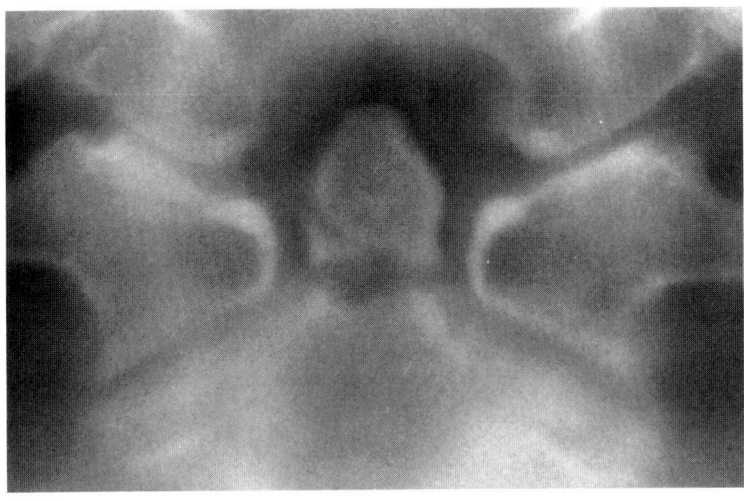
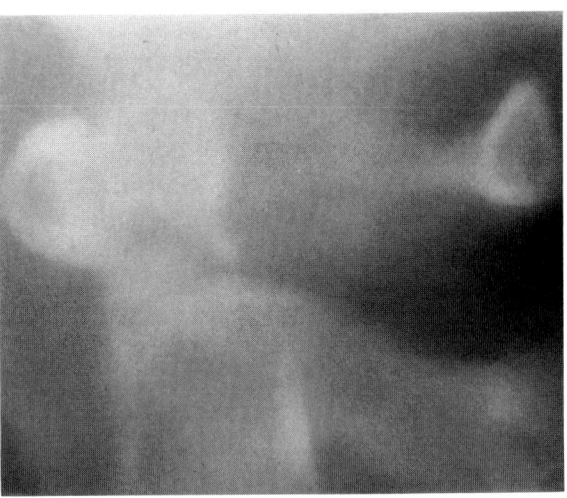

A

B

FIG. 4–80. AP (**A**) and lateral (**B**) tomograms of a comminuted Type II odontoid fractures. The fracture is much more easily seen on the AP tomogram in this case.

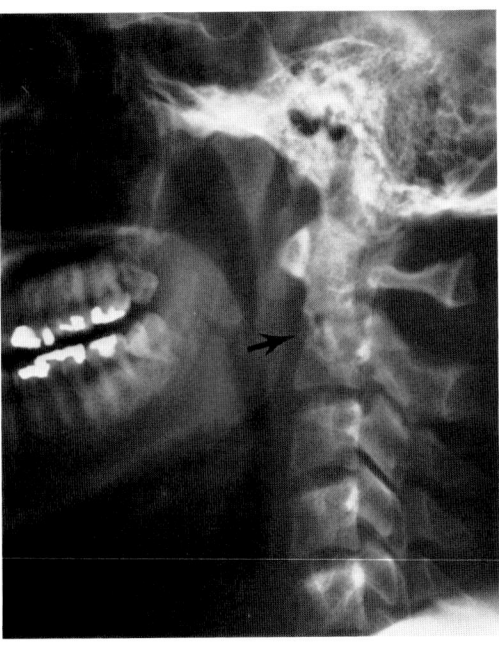

FIG. 4–81. Lateral view of the upper cervical spine with Halo in place. There is a Type III odontoid fracture with anterior impaction (*arrow*). There is also prevertebral soft tissue swelling.

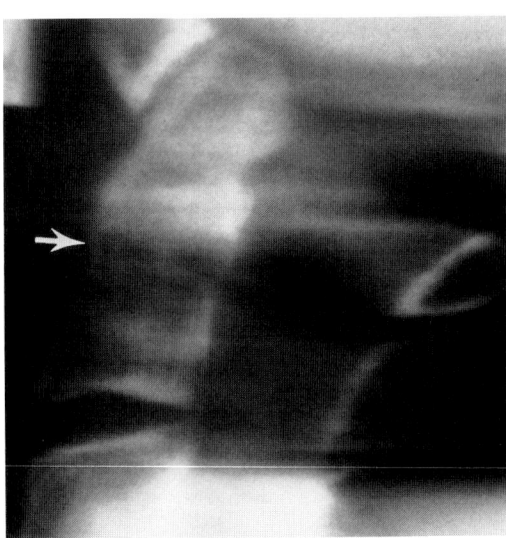

FIG. 4–82. Lateral tomogram of an undisplaced Type III odontoid fracture.

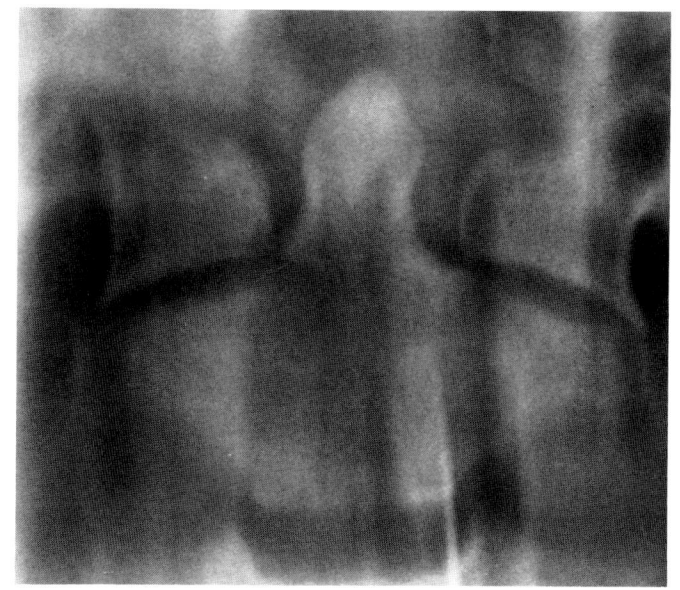

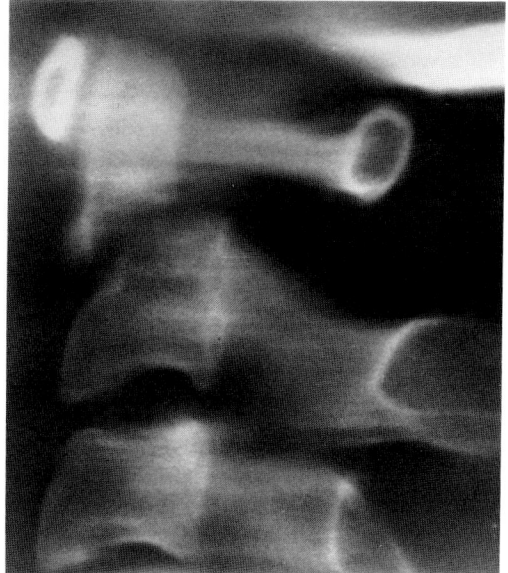

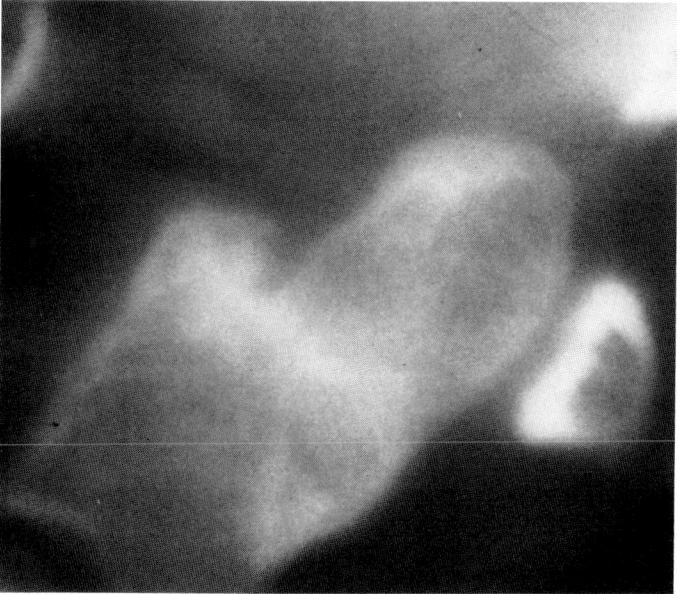

FIG. 4–83. AP (**A**) and lateral (**B**) tomograms of an anteriorly displaced Type III odontoid fracture. After treatment the fracture is healed, but there is increased angulation (**C**).

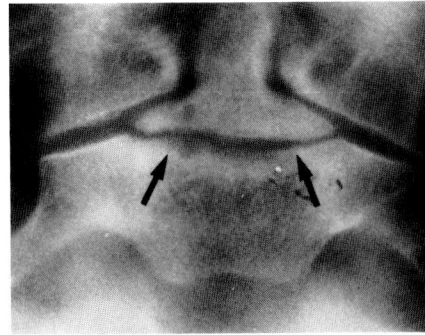

FIG. 4–84. AP tomogram of an ununited (*arrows*) Type III fracture.

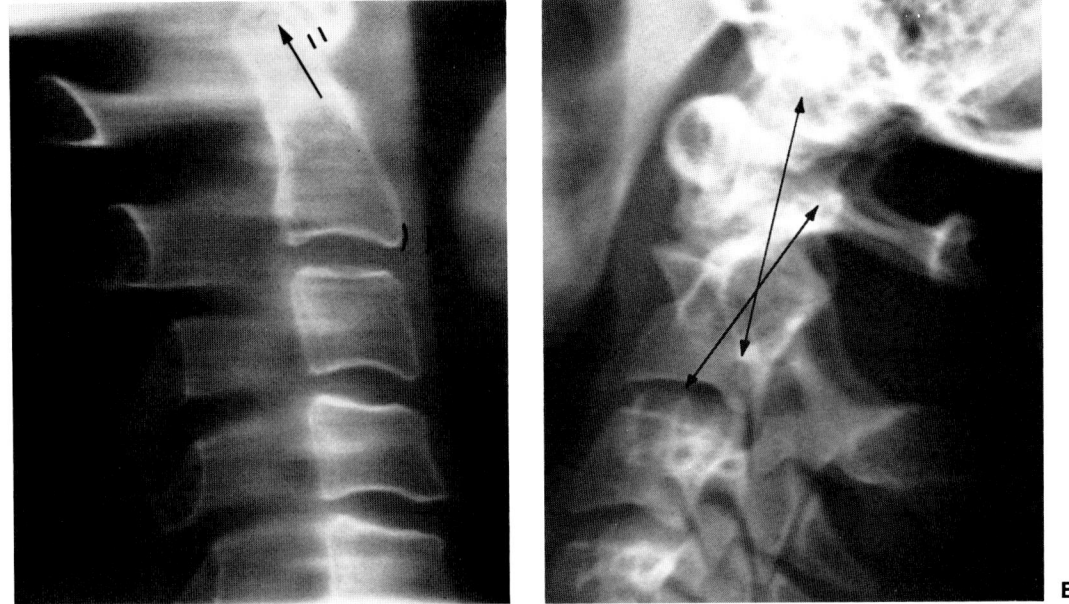

FIG. 4–85. **A**: Lateral tomogram of C2 showing the normal configuration of the odontoid. Slight posterior (*arrow*) positioning is normal. **B**: Lateral view of the upper cervical spine with anterior angulation of the odontoid due to an old fracture.

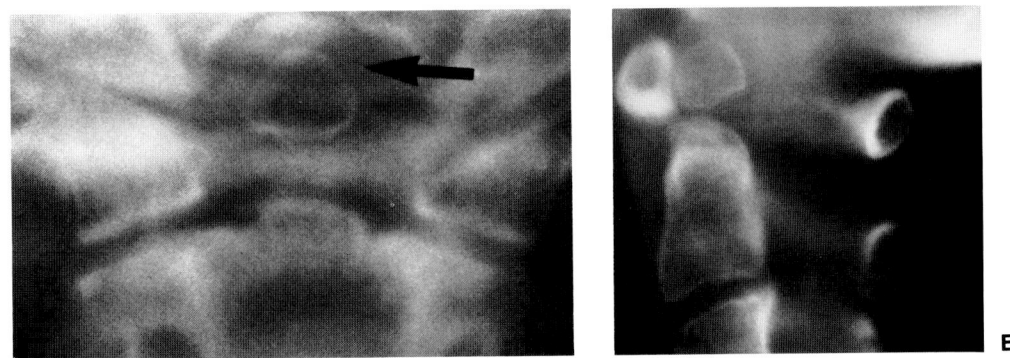

FIG. 4–86. AP (**A**) and lateral (**B**) tomograms in a patient with an os odontoideum. Note the increased cortical thickness in **B** compared to Fig. 4-76.

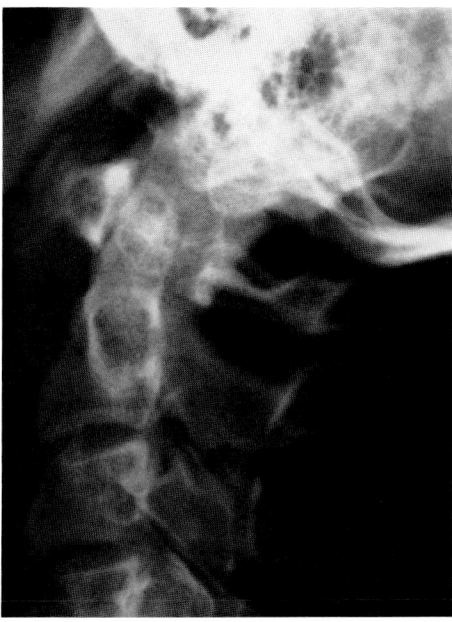

FIG. 4-87. Lateral view of the upper cervical spine with heterotopic ossification along the anterior margin of C1.

not be mistaken for an acute fracture. This odontoid change may be a congenital variant, but many believe this represents an old non-united Type II fracture (152). Chronic changes in the odontoid (os odontoideum, rheumatoid arthritis, or degenerative arthritis) can be differentiated from an acute process when hypertrophy of the anterior arch of C1 is identified. Holt et al. (158) demonstrated increased cortical thickness (Fig. 4-86B) and hypertrophy of the anterior arch of C1 in patients with chronic changes. However, degenerative changes in older patients (Fig. 4-87) may be present prior to acute injury. Therefore, the usefulness of this sign is questionable (see Figs. 4-82 and 4-85B).

Variations in odontoid fractures may also occur (Figs. 4-88 and 4-89). In general, if the fracture occurs below the base of the odontoid and there is less than 5 mm displacement, one can expect healing to occur.

Combination fractures also need to be considered. Associated skull fractures (Fig. 4-90) and adjacent cervical spine fractures are not uncommon. More important, up to 20–25% of patients will have associated lower cervical spine fractures (Fig. 4-91).

Fractures of the neural arch of the axis (hangman's fractures) occur as frequently as odontoid fractures (54,125,174). The injury results from hyperextension, and usually anterior subluxation of C2 on C3 is evident

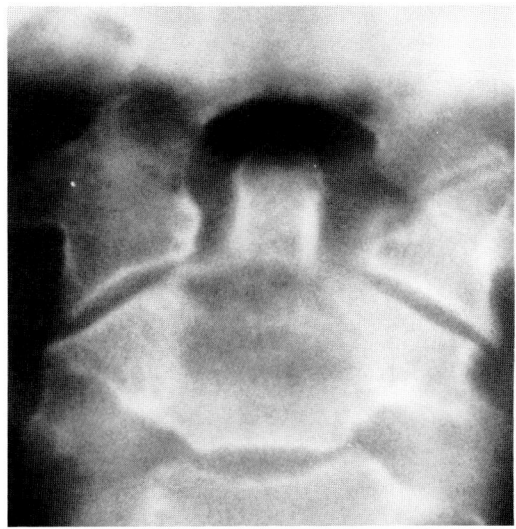
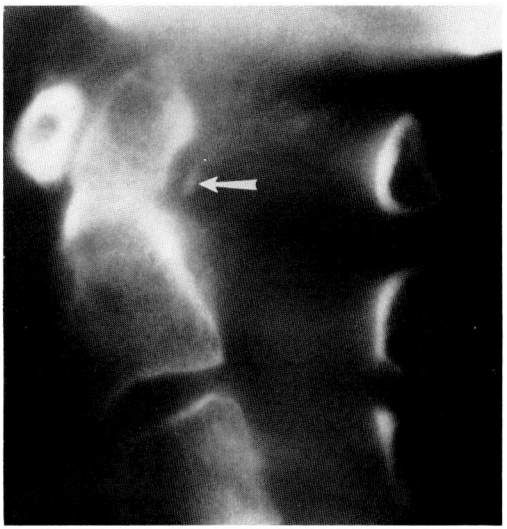

A   B

FIG. 4-88. AP (A) and lateral (B) tomograms of a posterior odontoid chip fracture (arrow). This is of little clinical significance but associated injuries need to be excluded.

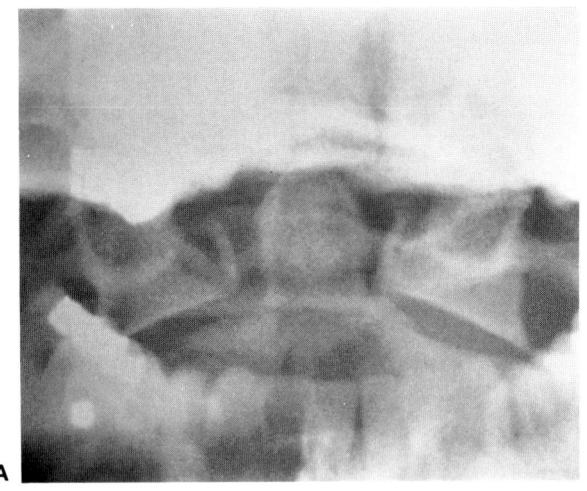

A

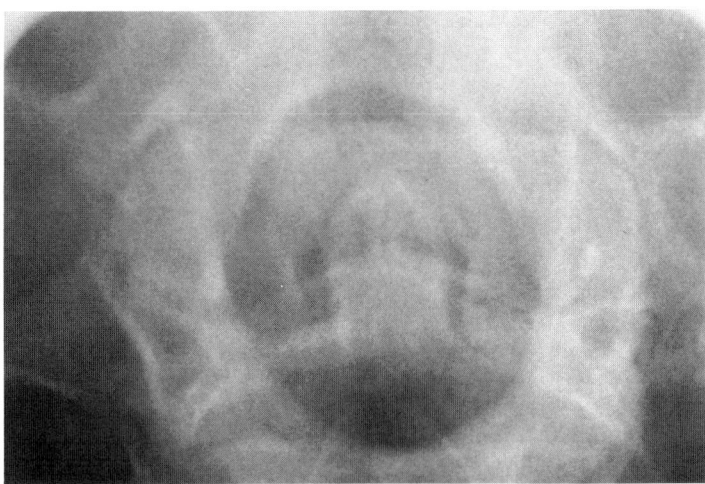

B

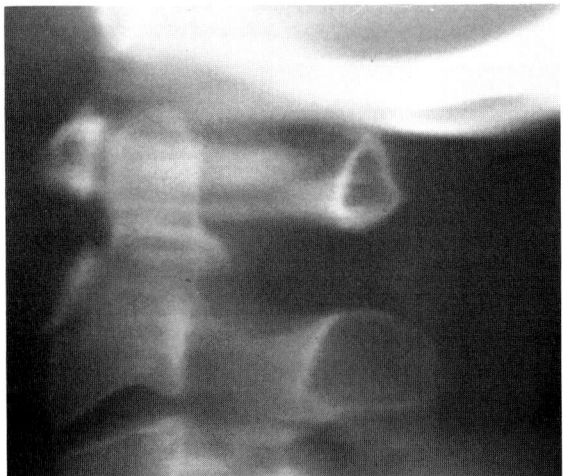

C

FIG. 4–89. Open mouth routine (**A**) and angled (**B**) views of the odontoid. The lateral tomogram (**C**) demonstrates the comminuted fracture involving the body of C2 and the base of the odontoid. There is minimal displacement.

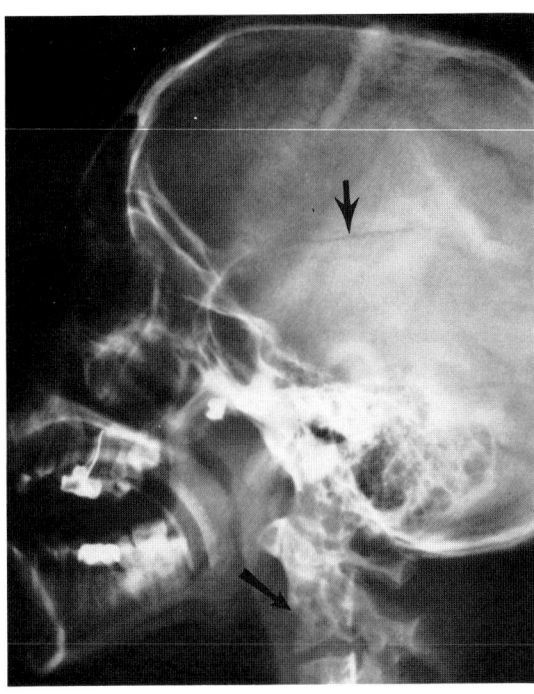

FIG. 4–90. Lateral view of the skull demonstrating a linear skull fracture (*upper arrow*) and an anteriorly impacted Type III odontoid fracture (*lower arrow*).

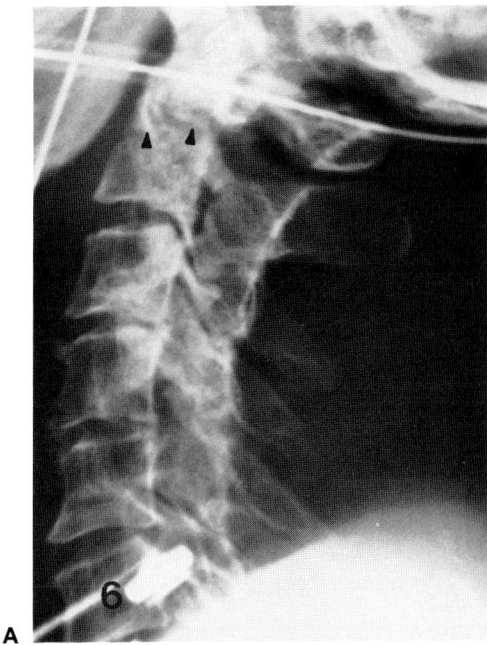

A

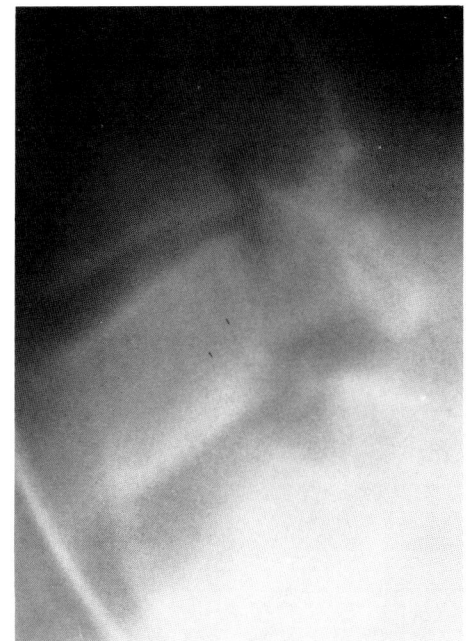

B

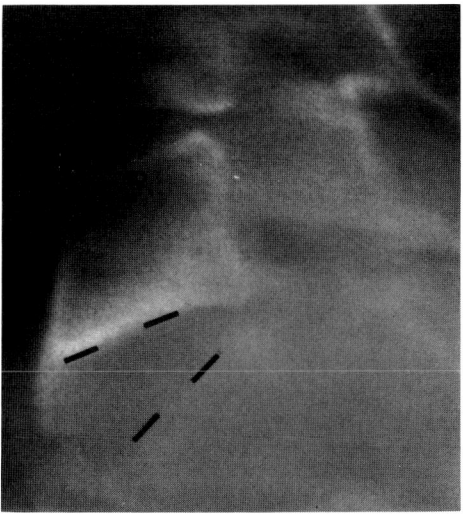

C

FIG. 4–91. Lateral view of the cervical spine with an undisplaced Type III odontoid fracture (**A**) (*arrows*). C7 is not seen. Lateral tomograms of the lower cervical spine (**B, C**) demonstrate an unstable hyperextension injury with anterior fanning (*lines*) of the interspace.

on the lateral radiograph (Fig. 4-92). The lesion, as originally described, occurred as a result of judicial hanging (204). This mechanism of hyperextension and sustained distraction resulted in death. Flexion-compression and flexion-distraction have also been implicated in hangman's fracture (140,147). Most of these injuries today are the result of motor vehicle accidents with transient hyperextension, and therefore neurologic damage is not common. In our series, 10% of patients experienced transient neurologic deficits, but no permanent damage occurred. Other authors have reported a higher incidence of neurologic complication (30–35%) (142, 146,170).

Although hangman's fractures have been considered pedicle fractures, this may be anatomically incorrect. Burke et al. (125) prefer the term *traumatic spondylolisthesis* of C2, as by definition C2 does not have true

pedicles. This may be true, but the terminology will not change quickly and I suspect the term *pedicle fracture* will continue to be used.

Effendi et al. (140) have classified hangman's fractures into three categories (Fig. 4-93). Basically, the fractures are classified according to the relationship of C2 to C3. If there is no forward displacement of C2 on C3 (no damage to the C2 disk and anterior longitudinal ligament), the damage is confined to the posterior elements—Type I (Fig. 4-94). With anterior displacement of C2 on C3 (Fig. 4-95), the lesion becomes a Type II injury. When both the posterior and anterior fragments are anteriorly displaced, it is a type III injury (Fig. 4-93C and 4-96). Type II and III lesions are unstable and require halo immoblization (140).

Associated cervical and distal spinal fractures are also not uncommon (Fig. 4-97). Fifteen percent of our pa-

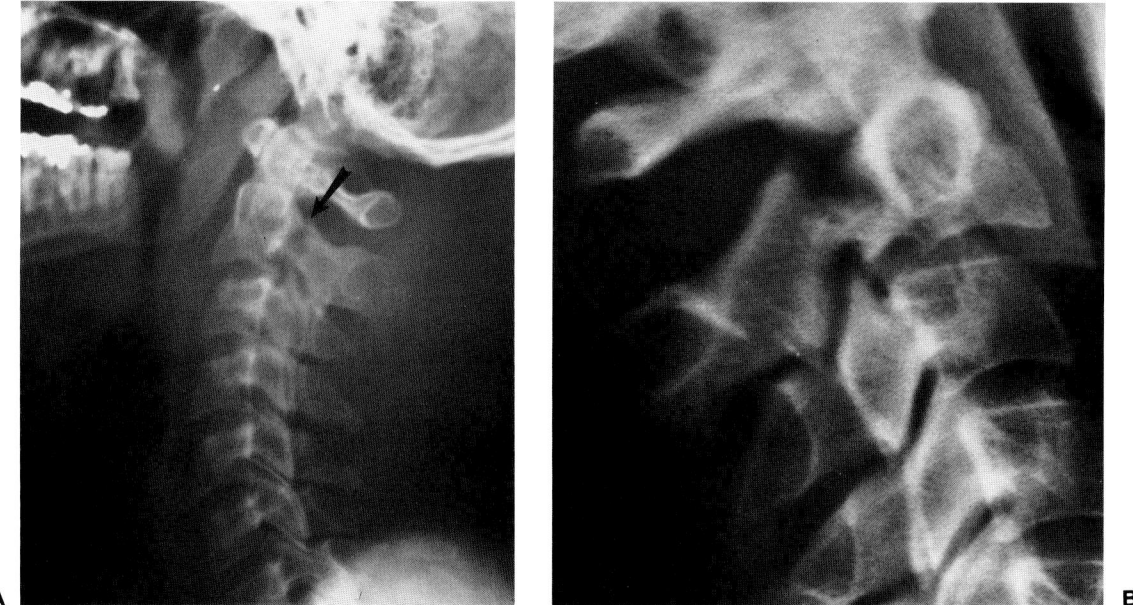

FIG. 4-92. Hangman's fractures. **A:** Lateral view showing a minimally displaced fracture of C2 neural arch (*arrows*). **B:** Displaced hangman's fracture.

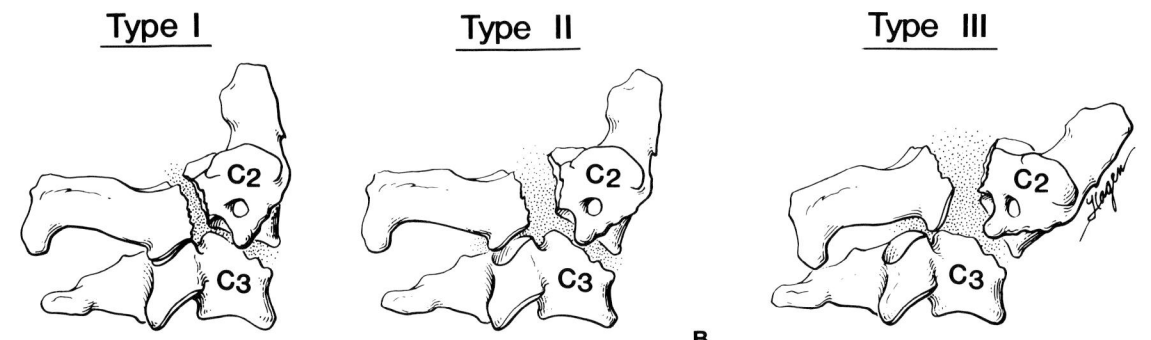

FIG. 4-93. Hangman's fracture as classified by Effendi et al. (140). **A:** Type I: traumatic spondylolisthesis with no displacement. **B:** Type II: the anterior fragment is displaced but the posterior fragment maintains its normal position. **C:** Type III: fracture dislocation with both fragments displaced.

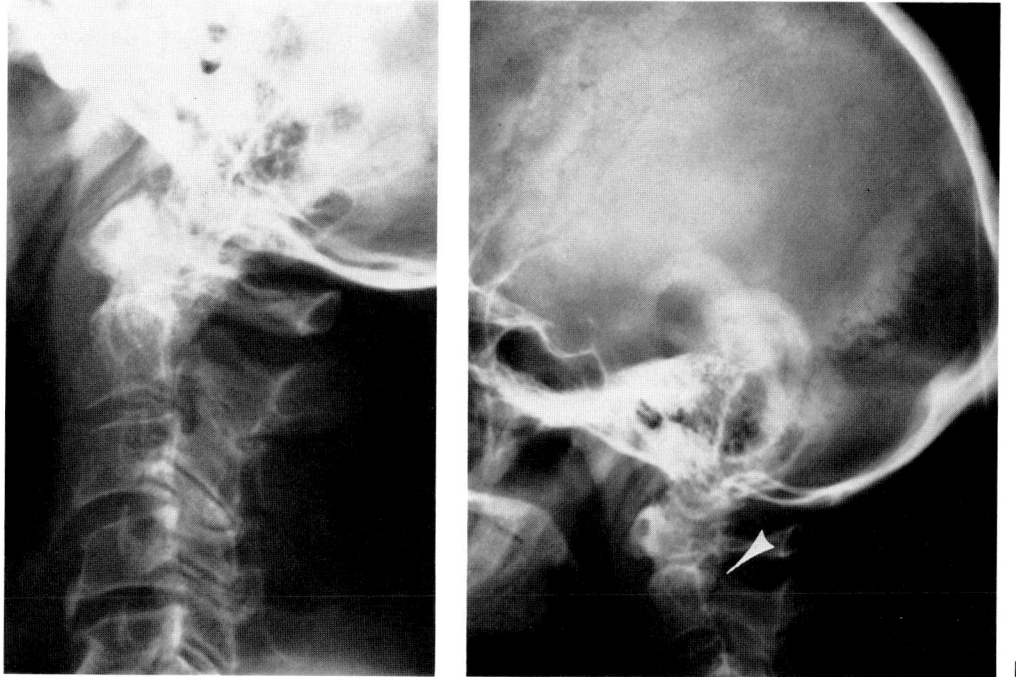

A   B

FIG. 4–94. Effendi Type I traumatic spondylolisthesis. **A**: Lateral view of the cervical spine suggests an undisplaced fracture. **B**: Lateral view of the skull shows the fracture (*arrow*) more clearly due to tube centering and improved geometry.

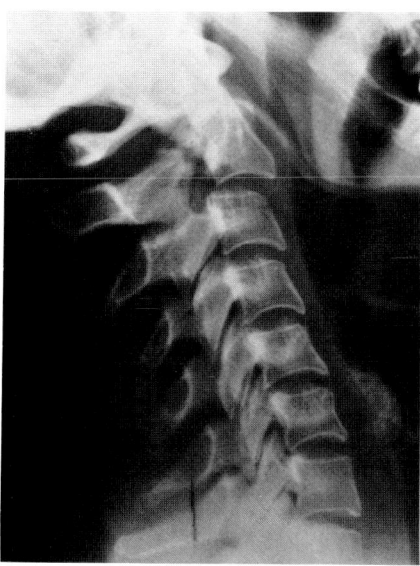

FIG. 4–95. Lateral view of the cervical spine demonstrating a hangman's fracture with anterior displacement of C2 on C3 (Type II).

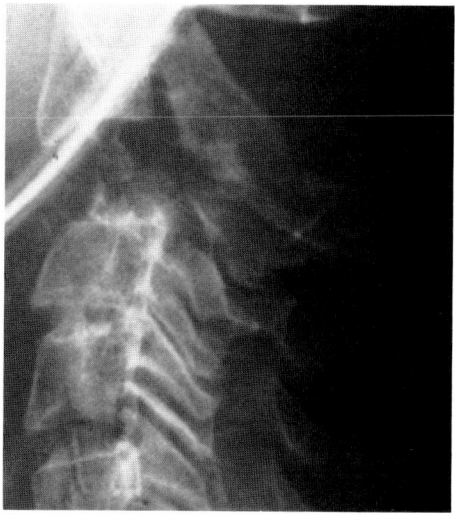

FIG. 4–96. Type III hangman's fracture with displacement of both fracture fragments of C2 on C3.

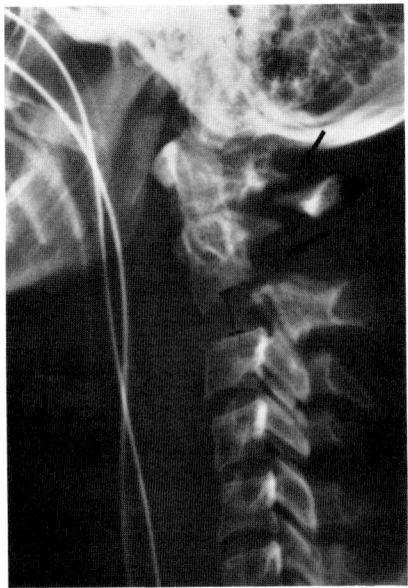
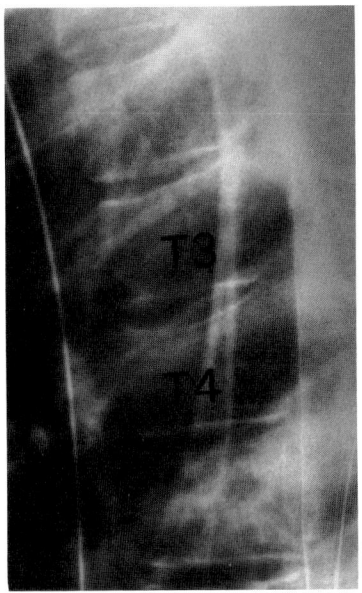
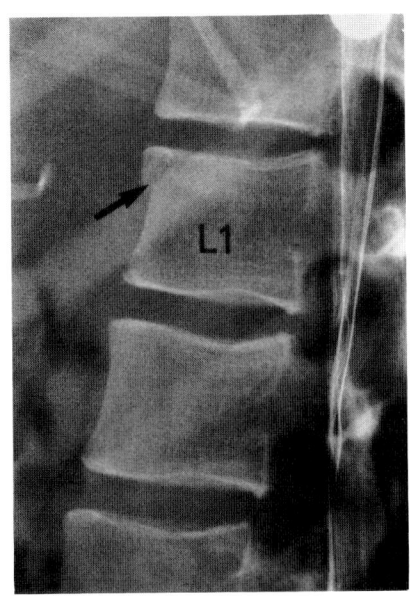

FIG. 4–97. Multiple spinal injuries following a motor vehicle accident. **A**: Lateral view of the cervical spine with fractures of C1 and a Type III traumatic spondylolisthesis (*arrows*). Lateral views of the thoracic (**B**) and lumbar (**C**) spine show associated compression of T3, T4 and L1.

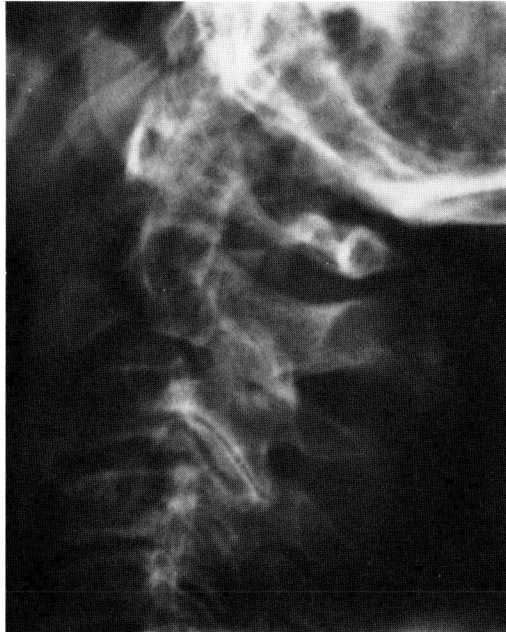

FIG. 4–98. Hyperextension injury of the cervical spine with an anterior inferior body fracture of C2 and a less obvious C2 pedicle fracture.

tients sustained associated C1 arch fractures (see Table 4-8). In one case the posterior arch fracture was more obvious than the pedicle fracture of the axis. Knowledge of the C1 hyperextension injury should make one search more diligently for traumatic spondylolisthesis of the axis. Fractures of the upper thoracic spine were noted in 10% of patients with hangman's fractures (Fig. 4-97). Fractures in this region are more likely to be associated with neurologic injury and should not be overlooked.

Fractures of the body of the axis occurred in 13–15% of patients (125). These fractures were all the result of hyperextension injuries and usually involved the anterior inferior margin of the vertebral body (Fig. 4-98). Soft tissue swelling was common and often marked. The injury is more common in elderly, osteopenic patients (125). No neurologic symptoms were present.

Isolated fractures of the lamina, spinous process, and facets of the axis are uncommon. Facet fractures of the axis are often associated with compression-rotation or

TABLE 4–10. *C2 Fractures (165 patients)[a]*

Location	No. of cases	Percent
Odontoid	68	41
Hangman's	62	38
Hyperextension	21	13
Teardrop (anterior		
inferior body C2)	10	6
Hyperextension dislocation		
Lamina	2	1
Spinous process	2	1

[a] (125).

TABLE 4–11. *Cervical spine: Location of injury in 420 patients[a]*

Location	Incidence
Vertebral arch	42
Vertebral body	31
Disk	27
Posterior ligaments	22
Anterior ligaments	4

[a] Multiple injuries result in total > 100%.

lateral compression injuries, which result in associated lateral mass fractures of the atlas (112). Odontoid fractures have also been reported with articular fractures of the axis (170). Table 4-10 summarizes the incidence of C2 fractures reported by Burke et al. (125).

Lower Cervical Spine (C3-C7)

In adults, lower cervical spine injuries occur four times more frequently than upper cervical spine fractures. In our experience, 81% of 420 injuries were located at the C3-C7 level. Fractures of the posterior arch were most common, occurring in 42% of patients (Table 4-11). Vertebral body fractures were the second most common, occurring in 31% of patients. The average number of injuries was 2.2 per patient (94,97).

Vertebral Arch Fractures

Vertebral arch fractures have been well discussed by other authors (152,186). Our experience differs slightly from the distribution of fractures described by Gehweiler (152). Fractures observed in our series are set out in Table 4-12.

Fractures of the lamina were the most common in our series. The mechanism of injury was almost always hyperextension (Fig. 4-99). Spinous process fractures were commonly associated with these fractures. The majority of the laminar fractures occur in the C5-C7 region. Pillar views and tomography (conventional or computed) are often necessary to detect laminar fractures (Fig. 4-100). CT may also be helpful; however, several cases of undisplaced fractures not evident on CT were easily demonstrated with conventional tomography. This is true of any undisplaced fracture in which the fracture is aligned

TABLE 4–12. *Vertebral arch fractures[a]*

Location	Incidence
Lamina	28
Pedicle	25
Spinous process	22
Pillar	16
Facet	9
Transverse process	2

[a] Multiple injuries result in total > 100%.

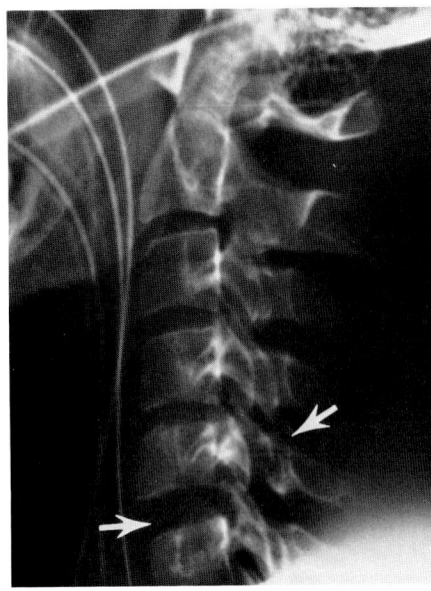

FIG. 4–99. Hyperextension injury with widening of the C5 disc space and a chip fracture anteriorly (*arrow*). The lamina of C5 is fractured (*posterior arrow*).

parallel to the slice. The increased utilization of tomography in our practice may be at least partially responsible for the higher incidence of laminar fractures in our series. Fractures of the lamina frequently extend into the base of the spinous process, resulting in displaced spinous process. This should not be confused with the more benign clay shoveler's fracture. Laminar fractures with spinous process involvement have been reported frequently with hyperextension injuries of the Type V classification (comminuted vertebral arch fracture with hyperextension fracture-dislocation (152,154).

Pedicle fractures were present in 25% of vertebral arch injuries (Table 4-12). Most pedicle fractures were noted with hangman's fractures (C2). However, pedicle fractures were also noted at the lower cervical spine with hyperextension injuries. Thus pedicle fractures are rarely noted unless a hyperextension injury is present (121,122,133). These injuries may be visible on the lateral or oblique views (Fig. 4-101). Conventional or computed tomography is frequently necessary for diagnosis (122,176). Acheson et al. (113) reported 82% of pedicle fractures were overlooked on plain films but detected with CT.

Spinous process fractures account for 22% of vertebral arch injuries (Fig. 4-102). Most spinous process fractures occur at the C5-T1 level. This fracture may result from direct trauma, hyperextension, or hyperflexion; and it is only through careful evaluation of the remaining vertebral units that the mechanism of injury may be established (122,133). Solitary spinous process fractures may be difficult to classify (Fig. 4-103) (127,138,152,157). On the AP view, a double spinous process may be the only clue to an unsuspected spinous process fracture (see Fig. 4-28E and F) (127). In other cases the lateral view is usually most useful.

Fractures of the articular pillars have been reported to be the most common arch fracture (122,152). These injuries usually occur at the C6 level. In our series pillar fractures occurred in 16% of vertebral arch fractures (Table 4-12). The mechanism of injury is usually hyperextension (hyperextension fracture-dislocation of Type IV or Type V) or lateral flexion (133,152,154). Occasionally, the AP view will demonstrate the lesion. These fractures are best demonstrated with pillar views or computed tomography (Fig. 4-104). Up to 60% will be overlooked on plain film examinations (113). There is usually no cord injury with a pillar fracture, but radiculopathy may result, especially if proper treatment is not instituted.

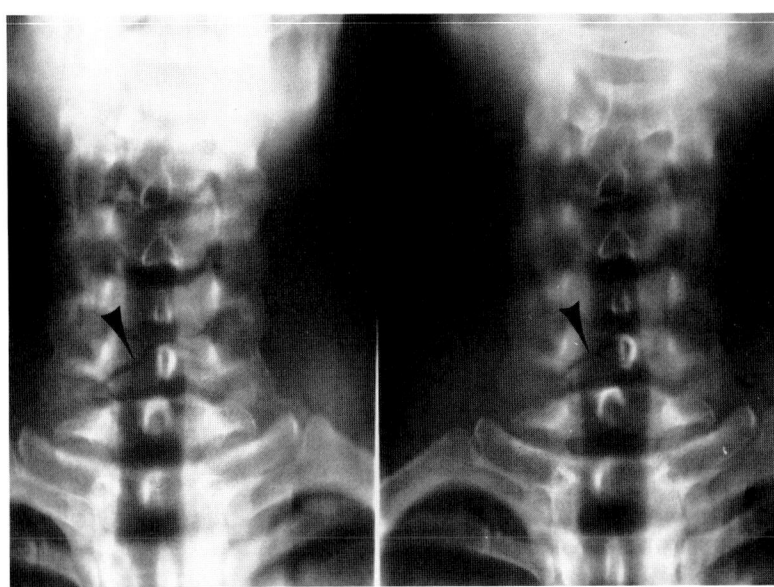

FIG. 4–100. AP tomogram demonstrating an undisplaced fracture of the lamina at C6 (*arrows*).

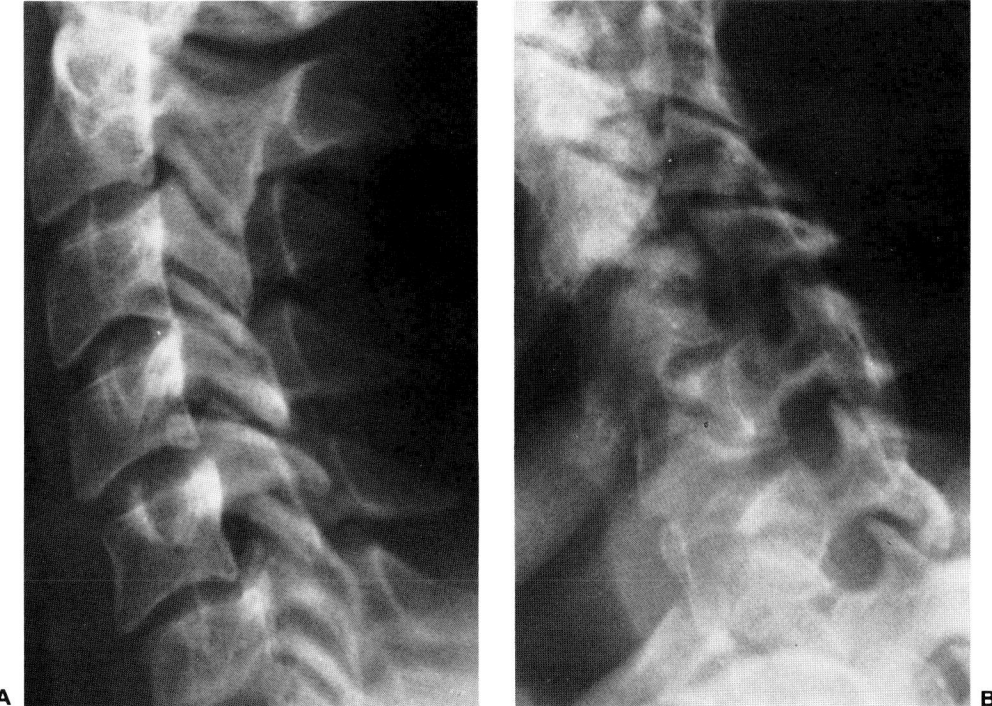

FIG. 4–101. Lateral (**A**) and oblique (**B**) views demonstrating a unilateral C5 pedicle fracture. The facet is rotated anteriorly. Note the slight subluxation of C5 on C6.

Several types of pillar fractures have been described. The most common is the easily overlooked simple compression fracture (Fig. 4-104) (192,199). Smith (192) has described several signs that may be of value in detecting pillar fractures; these are presented in Table 4-13. Foraminal narrowing was the most common sign detected. This radiographic feature was present in 31% of patients (192). Asymmetry of the pillars of greater than 2 mm in vertical height has also been described with pillar fractures (Fig. 4-104B) (197). Asymmetry and degenerative

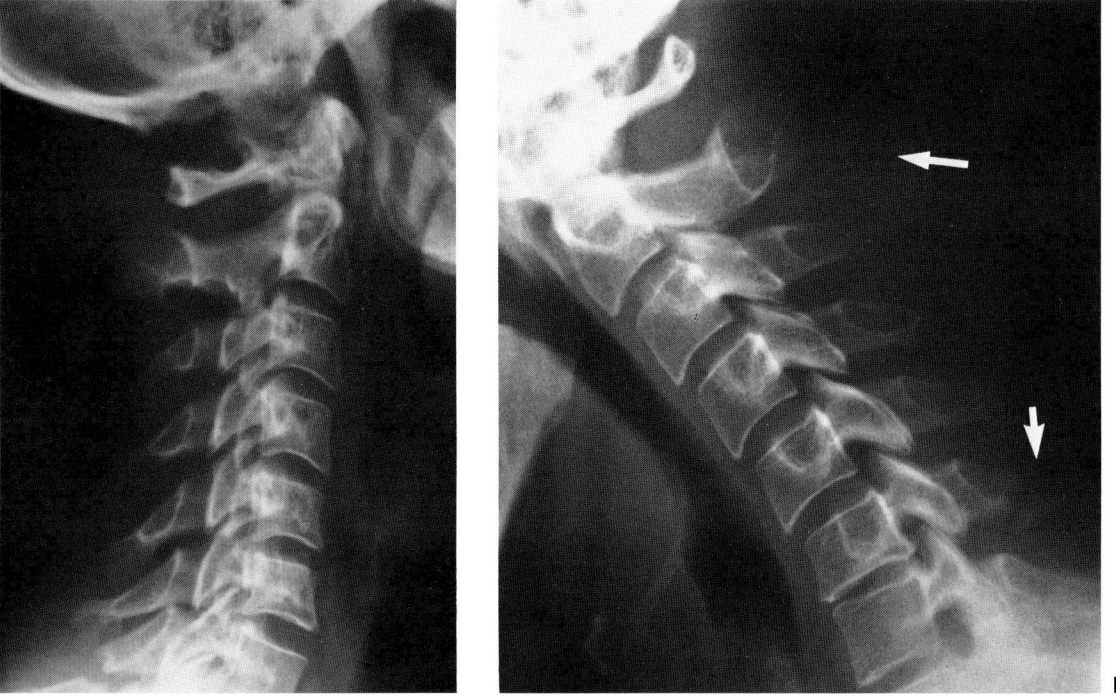

FIG. 4–102. Spinous process fractures. **A:** Solitary spinous process fracture at C7. **B:** Flexion views of C6 spinous fracture (*lower arrow*). There is no instability.

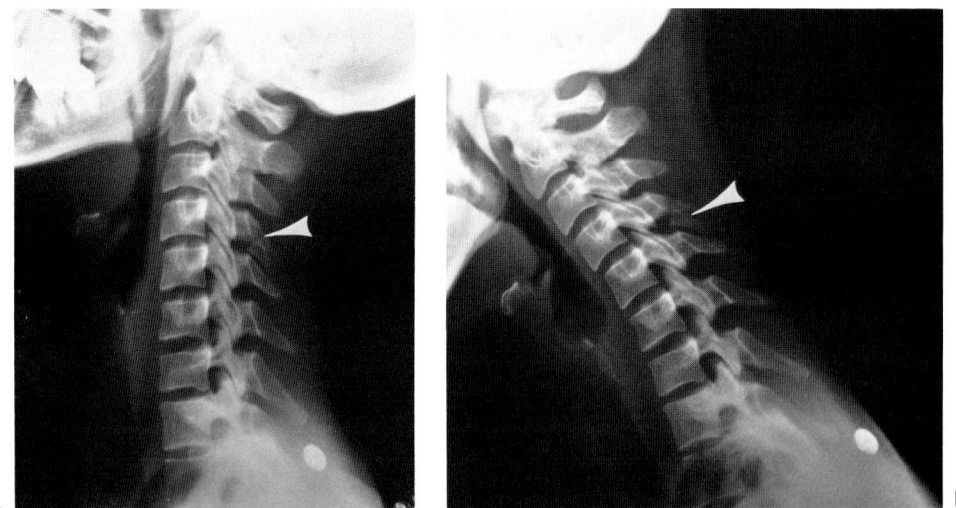

FIG. 4–103. Bifid spinous process at C4 with fracture of one segment (*arrow*). The fracture is evident on the lateral view (**A**) but displaces and is easily seen on the flexion view (**B**).

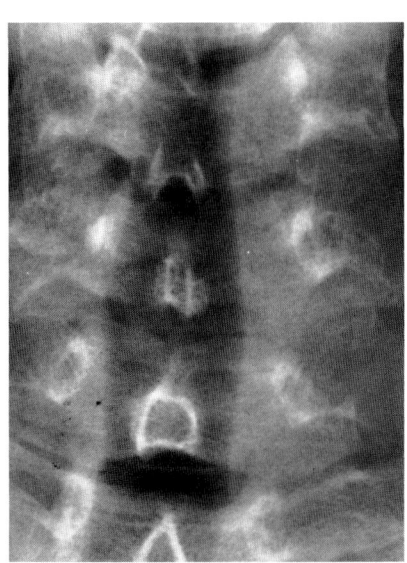

FIG. 4–104. A: AP view in a patient with a pillar fracture of C6 on the right. The only clue to the abnormality is a subtle change in the configuration of articular pillars. **B**: Pillar view demonstrating a compression fracture of right C6 articular pillar. **C**: Myelogram in the same patient demonstrates an extradural defect at C6 on the right due to a traumatic disc protrusion.

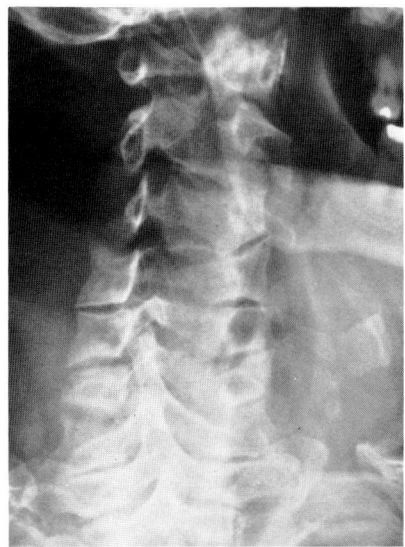

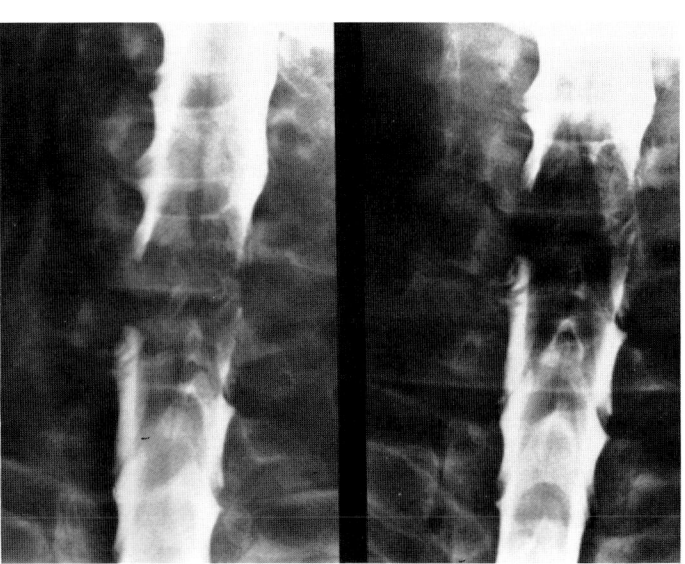

TABLE 4–13. *Radiographic signs of pillar fracture*

Feature	View on which feature is identified
Foraminal narrowing	Oblique
Triangular articular process	Oblique
Unilateral displacement	Oblique
Double lateral mass	Lateral
Subluxation	Lateral

ᵃ (192).

changes in the pillars are common in older patients, which adds to the confusion. These patients are usually totally asymptomatic. Computed tomography or AP and lateral tomograms should be obtained if plain film signs suggest a pillar fracture (113,122).

Facet fractures comprised 9% of vertebral arch fractures. These were most common with hyperflexion and flexion-rotation injuries (122,133). Oblique and lateral views may demonstrate this lesion, but conventional or computed tomography is usually required (Fig. 4-105). Radicular symptoms are common with solitary facet fractures (205). Facet fractures are usually detected with

multiple injuries, including injuries of the posterior ligaments and disk (152).

Finally, transverse process fractures are uncommon, occurring in only 2% of our patients (Fig. 4-106). The injury results from lateral flexion or direct trauma, such as from the chest strap of a seatbelt (117). Associated upper rib fractures are common with seatbelt injuries. Hyperextension injuries in the lower cervical spine, odontoid fractures, and hangman's fractures have also been reported in relation to seatbelt injuries (198).

Vertebral Body Fractures

Thirty-one percent of cervical spine injuries involved the vertebral body. Seventy-five percent of the fractures were in the C5-C7 region (Table 4-14). Fractures were demonstrated on the AP and lateral views, with oblique views adding additional information. Tomography and CT are less frequently required for detection of vertebral body fractures. However, evaluation of fragment position and classification is aided with CT (113,118,213).

Vertebral body fractures have several radiographic pre-

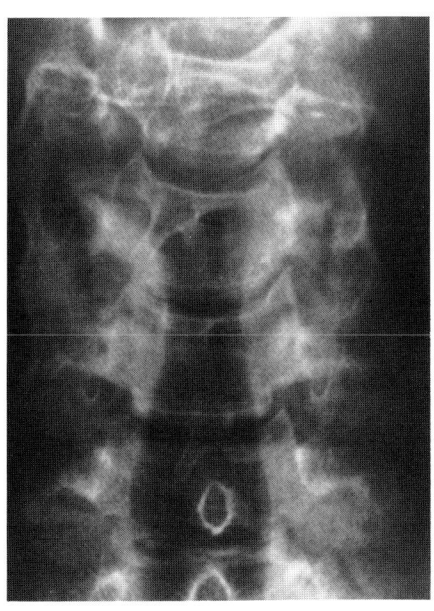

A

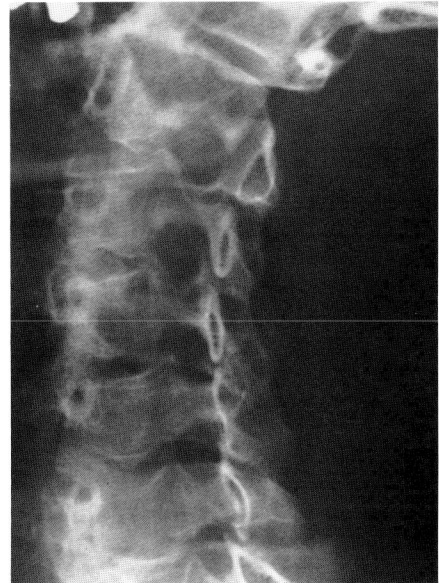

B

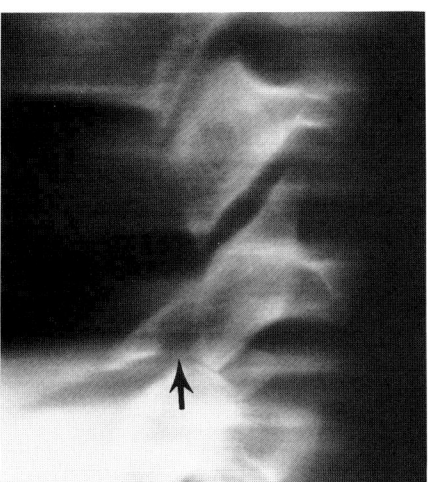

C

FIG. 4–105. AP (**A**) and oblique (**B**) views following flexion rotation injury. Note the malalignment of the spinous process on the AP view, and the oblique view (**B**) suggests perching at C4-C5. The tomogram (**C**) demonstrates the inferior facet fracture at C4 (*arrow*).

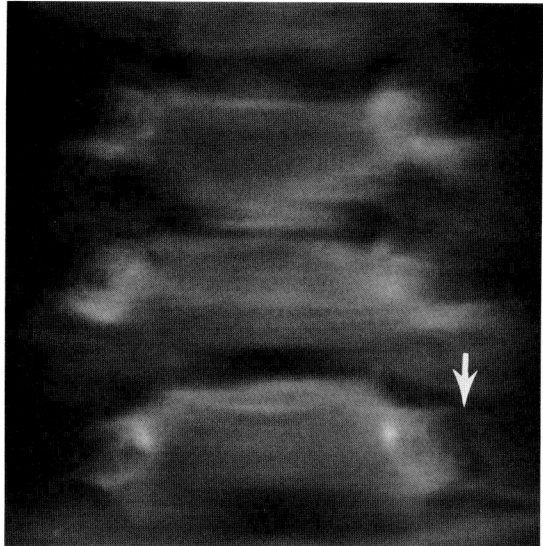

FIG. 4-106. AP tomogram demonstrating a fracture of the left transverse process of C7 (*arrow*).

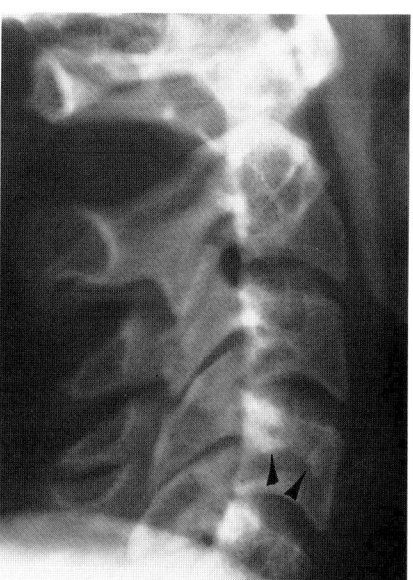

FIG. 4-107. Overlapping transverse process (*arrows*) should not be confused with a fracture.

sentations: (1) chip fractures, usually of the anterior superior or anterior inferior margin; (2) triangular fractures; (3) burst fractures; (4) wedge fractures, usually anterior but also lateral; (5) uncinate process fractures; and (6) sagittal fractures. Care must be taken not to mistake overlying structures for vertebral body fractures (Fig. 4-107) (134).

Chip fractures are commonly due to hyperflexion injuries (anterior superior margin) and hyperextension injuries (anterior inferior margin). Following hyperextension injury, the fracture fragment is avulsed with the anterior longitudinal ligament and in most instances enters the disk space (Fig. 4-108) (95,138,152,187). Hyperflexion injuries are often associated with posterior ligament disruption and are therefore unstable (Fig. 4-109). Hyperextension injuries are usually stable unless the fracture of the body is associated with a posterior arch fracture, in which case the lesion is unstable (157).

Larger triangular or teardrop fractures of the vertebral body are more significant. Lee et al. (168) reviewed 109 patients with triangular fractures. Seventy-two percent involved the anterior inferior body and 16% the anterior superior margin of the body. The anterior inferior fracture is the typical teardrop fracture defined by Schneider and Kahn (Fig. 4-110) (187). The majority of triangular

fractures involved the lower cervical spine (67%). Neurologic involvement, usually quadriplegia, was present in 87% of patients (103,168).

Simple compression fractures are most often anterior and result from flexion-compression injuries (Fig. 4-111). The posterior ligaments may be intact, depending upon the degree of associated posterior element distraction. The posterior ligaments must be evaluated at some point in the stage of treatment to be certain that the lesion is stable. This requires fluoroscopically controlled flexion and extension views.

Lateral wedge fractures and uncinate fractures are the

TABLE 4-14. *Fractures of the cervical vertebral body in 420 patients*

Location	Incidence	
C2	8	
C3	7	
C4	10	
C5	20	
C6	22	75% C5-C7
C7	23	

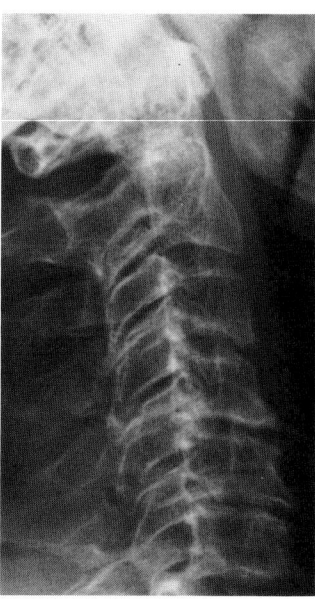

FIG. 4-108. Hyperextension injury with widening of the anterior interspace and a "flake" fracture from the inferior body of C6.

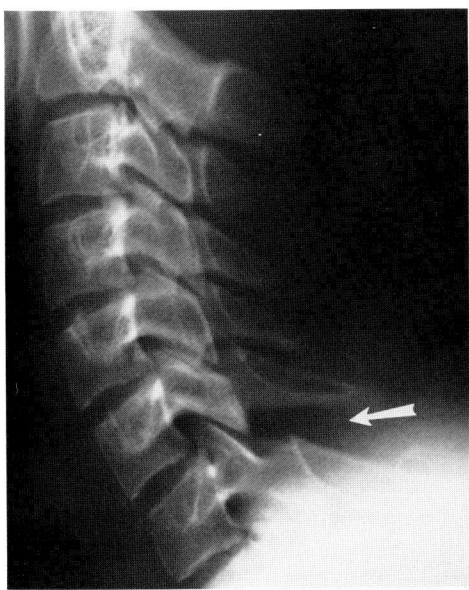

FIG. 4–109. Lateral view of the cervical spine demonstrating a chip fracture and mild compression of C7. The interspinous distance (arrow) at C6-C7 is increased indicating an unstable lesion.

result of asymmetric vertical compression or lateral flexion injuries. These fractures are rare (152).

Burst fractures in the cervical spine result from vertical compression forces with the spine in neutral position. These injuries are much more common in the lumbar (76%) and thoracic (20%) region. Only about 4% occur in the cervical spine (118). The ligaments are intact and the lesions are usually stable. However, fragments in the spinal canal result in neurologic deficits (152,187). Compression of the vertebral body is often obvious with burst

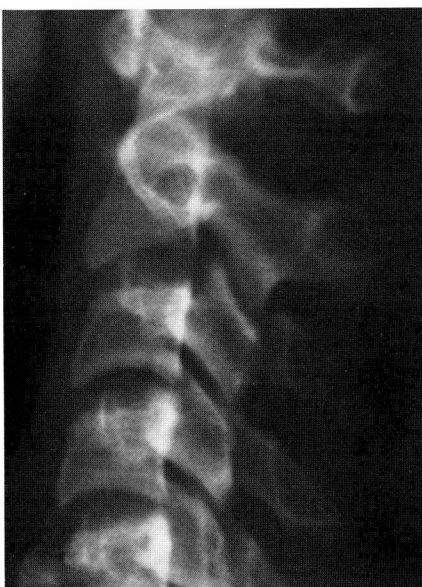

FIG. 4–110. Triangular fracture of the anterior inferior body of C5. The major fragment is displaced posteriorly into the spinal canal.

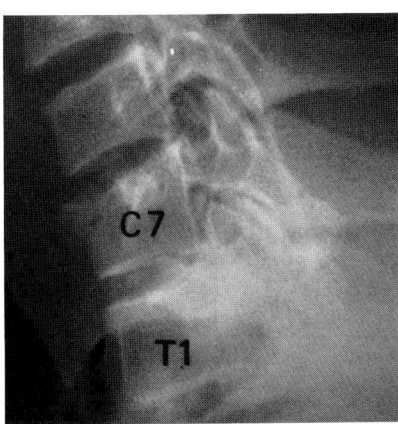

FIG. 4–111. Lateral view of the cervical spine demonstrating compression fractures of C7 and T1 (arrow).

fractures. However, subtle changes such as disruption of the posterior vertebral line is a useful indicator of a burst fracture. Normally, the posterior vertebral margin is concave or straight. If this line becomes convex, a burst fracture is almost always present (135). CT is extremely helpful in evaluating these injuries and in localizing the number and size of intraspinal fragments and epidural hematomas (203).

Sagittal fractures (Fig. 4-112) of the vertebral bodies may be associated with triangular fractures (168). The diagnosis may be difficult on the AP and lateral views. Tomography and, more important, CT are usually required. There is almost always an associated posterior arch fracture (191). These fractures are uncommon (171,191), but neurologic damage is usually severe, resulting in quadriplegia (148). Sagittal fractures are also unstable and may require surgical stabilization (171). CT is particularly valuable in differentiating burst fractures with fragments in the spinal canal from sagittal fractures (131).

Subluxations and Fracture-Dislocation

Most significant ligament injuries involve the posterior complex. In our series, 73% of these injuries occurred at the C5-C7 level. Anterior ligament injuries are most common in the C2-C4 and the C6-C7 intervals. Often the changes noted radiographically (body fractures, disk space narrowing or widening, widening of the interspinous distance, and subluxation) will aid in determining whether ligament injury has occurred. Posterior ligament injuries are unstable if complete disruption has occurred, and one must guard against overlooking the often subtle changes associated with this injury (Fig. 4-113) (67,136,173,175).

Posterior ligament injuries may occur without associated fracture (hyperflexion sprain) and may result in widened interspinous distance, disk space narrowing, and subluxation (Fig. 4-114). These findings may be evident on the upright lateral view but obscured on the su-

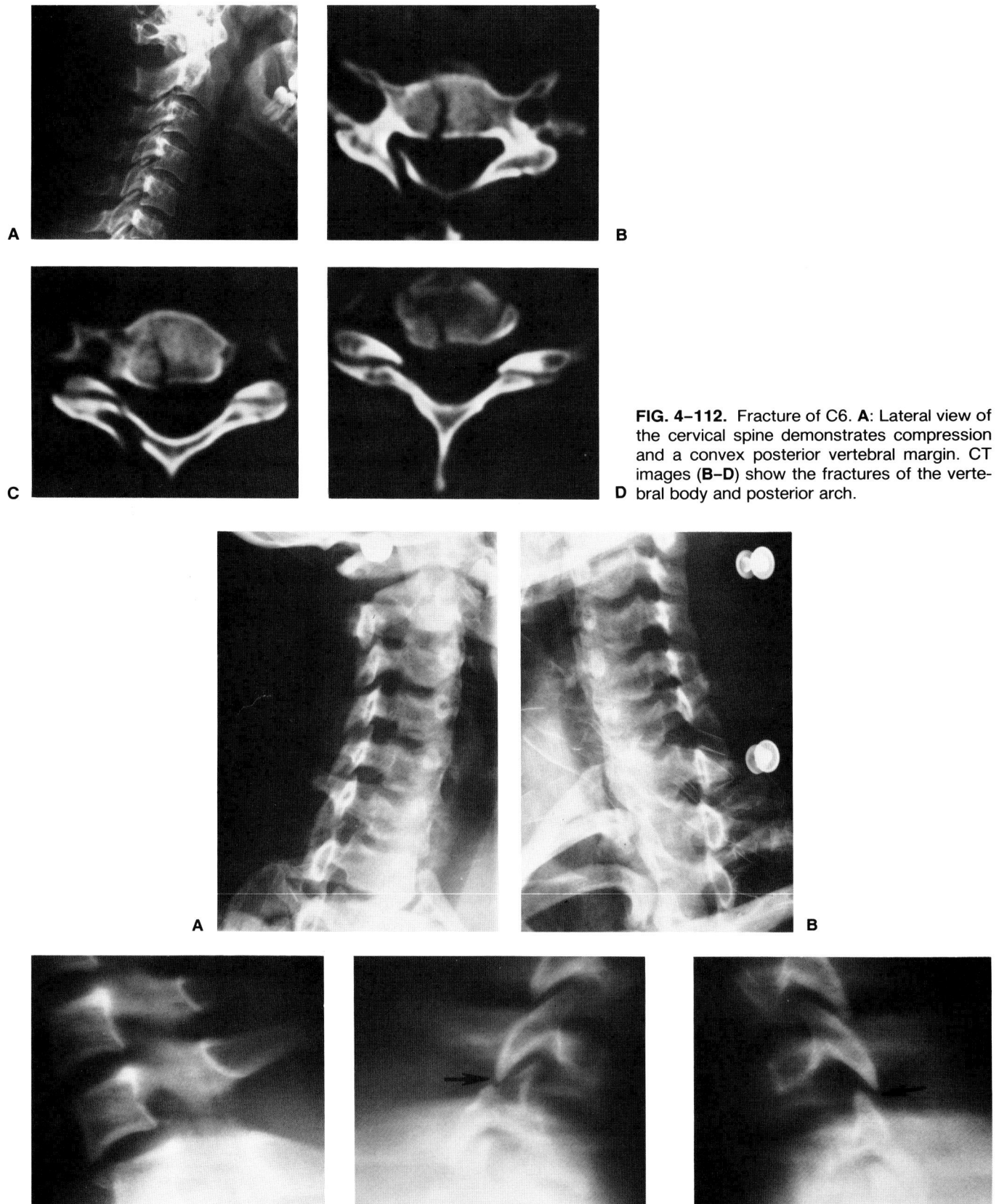

FIG. 4-112. Fracture of C6. **A:** Lateral view of the cervical spine demonstrates compression and a convex posterior vertebral margin. CT images (**B-D**) show the fractures of the vertebral body and posterior arch.

FIG. 4-113. Flexion compression injury. The oblique views (**A, B**) demonstrate widening of the C6-C7 facet joints with slight subluxation. The lateral tomograms (**C**) demonstrate compression of C7 with widening of the interspinous distance. The superior facet of C7 on the right (**D**) is fractured and ligaments and capsules torn with near perching of the facets on the left (**E**).

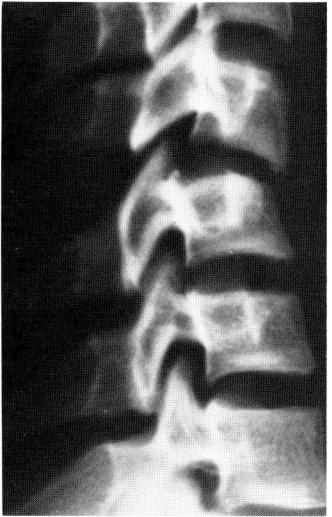 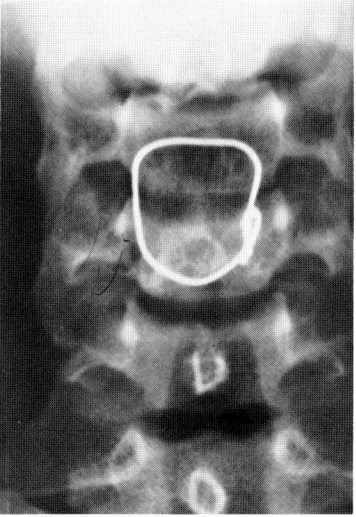 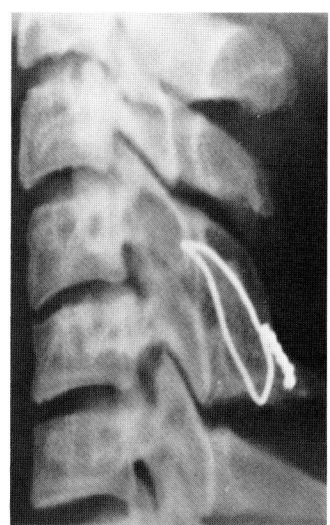

A   B   C

FIG. 4–114. A: Lateral roentgenogram of the cervical spine in a 17-year-old boy who sustained a flexion injury in a diving accident. Note the increased distance between the spinous processes of C4 and C5, the kyphotic angulation at this level and the subluxation of the facet joints. No neurological deficit. Anterior (**B**) and lateral (**C**) roentgenograms of the cervical spine of the same patient one year after posterior interspinous wiring and fusion. The patient is asymptomatic.

pine lateral. For this reason, if the supine views are negative, it has been suggested that an upright lateral be obtained in patients with suspected flexion injuries (133,152). The ligament disruptions result from either flexion-rotation or disruptive hyperflexion injuries (124,143,152,164,185,200). These injuries are easily overlooked. Delay in diagnosis may result in cervical deformity and neurologic deficits (143,164,175,185,200). Cheshire noted persistent instability in 21% of patients with subluxation when the instability was treated conservatively (128). Signs of instability (angulation of greater than 11° and subluxation greater than 3 mm) must be kept in mind. Flexion and extension views may be re-

quired for diagnosis (Fig. 4-115). This technique should not be performed acutely, as spasm often results in a false-negative study.

The same forces that result in isolated ligament disruption, if continued, may lead to unilateral or bilateral facet dislocation or locking. In our experience actual locking is less common than perching of the facets. This phenomenon is due to partial reduction of the hyperflexion process combined with osteochondral impaction of the inferior facet into the superior facet of the vertebra below. This is especially common with bilateral facet dislocation.

Unilateral locking or perching of the facets is com-

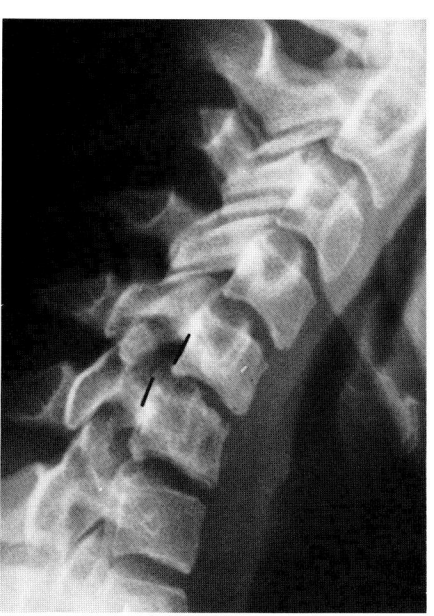 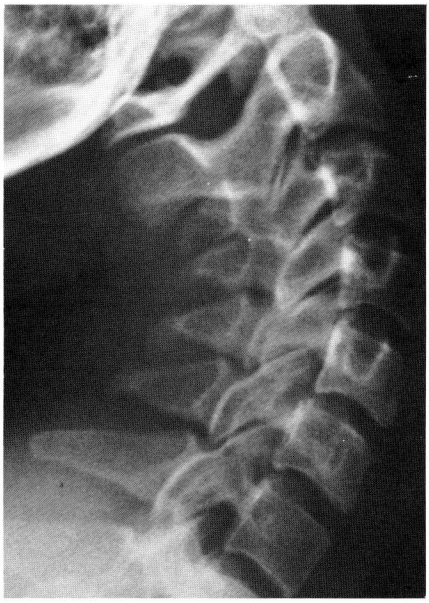

A   B

FIG. 4–115. Ligament injury with chronic mild instability. Flexion (**A**) and extension (**B**) views show slight widening of the C4-C5 interspinous distance with 3 mm of anterior subluxation. Note the partially ossified ligaments (*arrow*).

mon. This injury was noted in 12% of our patients (420 cases). Scher reported unilateral facet locking in 16% of 525 spinal injuries (183). The injury occurs most frequently at the C4-C6 levels. Associated fractures have been reported in 35% of patients (183). There is often only minimal subluxation, and, if only the lateral view is obtained, this lesion may be easily missed. The oblique view is most helpful in detecting facet dislocations (Fig. 4-116). Radiographically the AP view will demonstrate lateral displacement of the spinous process at the level of the lesion, with the spinous process rotated to the side of the involved facets. On the lateral view there will appear to be a true lateral appearance below the lesion and an oblique view above. This results in the "bow tie" sign (153) (see Fig. 4-48). Variation in the distance between the spinolaminar line and articular pillars may also be useful in detecting subtle unilateral facet injuries (Fig. 4-117) (208). As mentioned earlier, the oblique view is most helpful, but tomography is usually necessary to evaluate the degree of locking or perching and to exclude an associated facet fracture (Fig. 4-118). Radiculopathy is common with this lesion. The injury results from

disruption of the capsule and interspinous ligaments, with minor involvement of the disk and posterior longitudinal ligament (120,180).

Bilateral facet locking has been reported to be twice as common as unilateral facet locking (150). In our experience, however, the two lesions occurred with equal frequency. This may be due to the patient population or to increased awareness of the subtle changes present with unilateral facet locking (120,152,153,180). With bilateral facet locking or perching, there is no significant rotary component. The degree of subluxation, as noted on the lateral radiograph, is usually more than 50% of the AP diameter of the vertebral body below (Fig. 4-119). There is also marked widening of the interspinous distance, widening of the apophyseal joints, and narrowing of the disk space. On the AP view there is widening of the interspinous distance at the level of the injury. Oblique views offer the most diagnostic information, revealing either locking or perching of both facets. Bilateral locked facets are associated with a high incidence of cord damage (72% quadriplegic), and the injury is unstable (157).

The flexion teardrop (hyperflexion fracture-disloca-

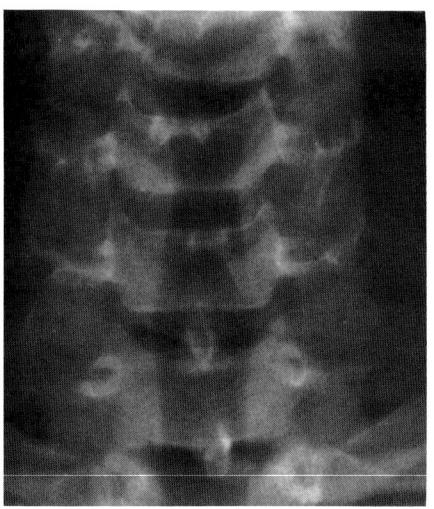

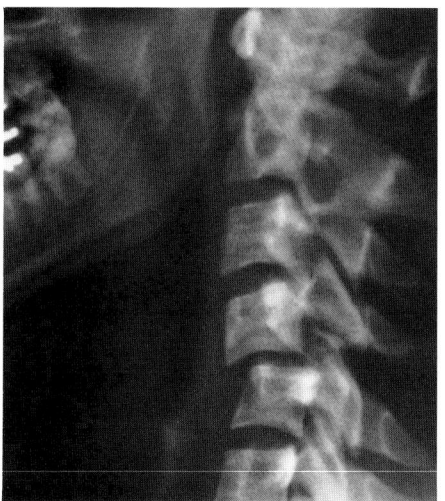

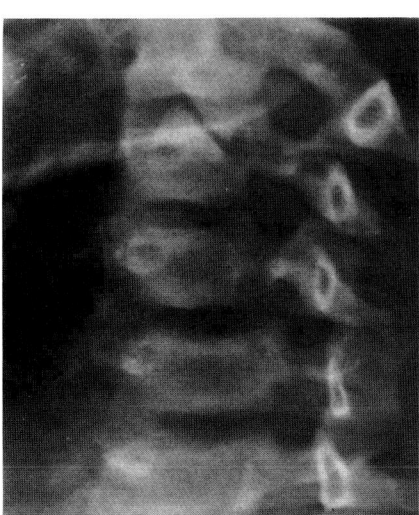

FIG. 4-116. Unilateral locked facet. A: AP view demonstrating rotation of the spinous process at C4-C5. B: Lateral view shows anterior subluxation with rotation at the C4-C5 level. C: The locking is clearly demonstrated at C4-C5 on the oblique view.

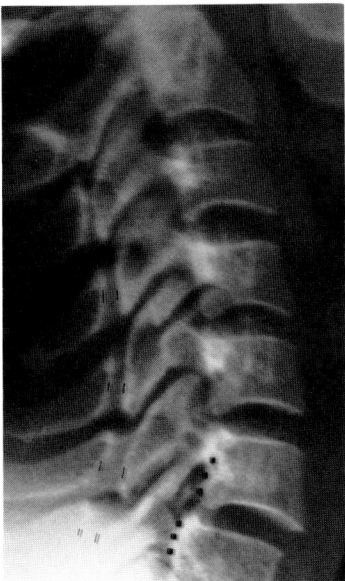

FIG. 4–117. Lateral view of the cervical spine with slight subluxation of C6 on C7. Note the variation in distance between the spinolaminar line and pillars (*lines*) changes at the level of the injury.

tion) is uncommon but is one of the most unstable cervical spine injuries (152,157,165). The injury results from a flexion-compression force with an anterior triangular fracture and posterior displacement of the major body fragment into the spinal canal (Fig. 4-120). This injury should not be confused with other anterior triangular vertebral body fractures (Table 4-15). Both anterior and posterior ligament complexes are interrupted making the lesion truly unstable (165). Anterior cord syndrome (quadriplegia, loss of pain, temperature, and touch) is characteristic of this injury. The injury occurs most frequently at the C5 level (165).

Anterior ligament injuries are often associated with anterior inferior chip fractures of the vertebral body (Fig. 4-51). The mechanism of injury is disruptive hyperextension. These injuries are most common at the C2-C4 and C6-C7 levels. Changes may be subtle, with hematoma or displacement of the prevertebral fat stripe being the only indication of injury (137). Facial fractures and central cord syndrome are frequently present. MRI is useful in this setting (167). Edeiken-Monroe et al. (139) noted these features in all 20 patients with hyperextension fracture dislocation. As noted previously, on the

TABLE 4-15. *Flexion teardrop fracture: Radiographic features on the lateral view*

Triangular anterior vertebral fragment
Displacement of posterior fragment into the spinal canal
Widened facet joints
Widened interspinous distance
Angular deformity

lateral view hyperextension injuries may be difficult to differentiate from hyperflexion injuries. Oblique views may indicate that the mechanism of injury is hyperextension when neural arch fractures are identified, or hyperflexion with facet locking or perching and facet joint widening and interspinous distance changes.

Differentiation of degenerative subluxation from acute trauma can be difficult in the elderly patient with degenerative changes in the spine (169). It is not uncommon for these patients to have cord symptoms due to spondylosis. MRI or myelography may be needed to identify the lesions in these patients (178). However, plain film findings may also be useful in differentiating acute injury from degenerative subluxation. Degenerative subluxation typically leads to anterior or posterior subluxation without asymmetric widening of either the disk space or facet joint (Fig. 4-121). Acute trauma leads to anterior or posterior disk space widening or narrowing and asymmetric facet joint widening (see Fig. 4-118A).

Cervical Spine Trauma—Associated Injuries

Cervical spine injuries are frequently associated with fractures of the thoracic and lumbar spine (15%) (Table 4-16). Head injuries (18%), facial injuries (4%), and other extraskeletal injuries are also common and may be helpful in determining the mechanism of cervical injury.

The possibility of overlooking a second distal spine injury may result in significant risk to the patient and improper management. Examination of the entire spine has been advocated and should be carried out in patients with significant cervical spine injury (126,184). Calenoff reported that in 30 patients with multiple level injuries, 80% sustained two separate lesions while in 20% there were injuries at three or more levels (126) (see Fig. 4-97).

In examining the distribution of cervical spine lesions related to injuries in the thoracic and lumbar spine, certain patterns evolved. Of the 420 patients with cervical spine fractures, 12% (50 patients) sustained associated thoracic fractures and 3% (13 patients), associated lumbar fractures. Table 4-17 describes the pattern noted in these patients. Patients with upper cervical lesions (C2 and above) tended to have associated fractures in the

TABLE 4-16. *Cervical spine trauma: Associated injuries*

Location	Incidence (%)
Head	18
Thoracolumbar spine	15
Thoracic—12	
Lumbar—3	
Extremities	13
Chest	5
Facial bones	4
Abdomen	3
Pelvis	2

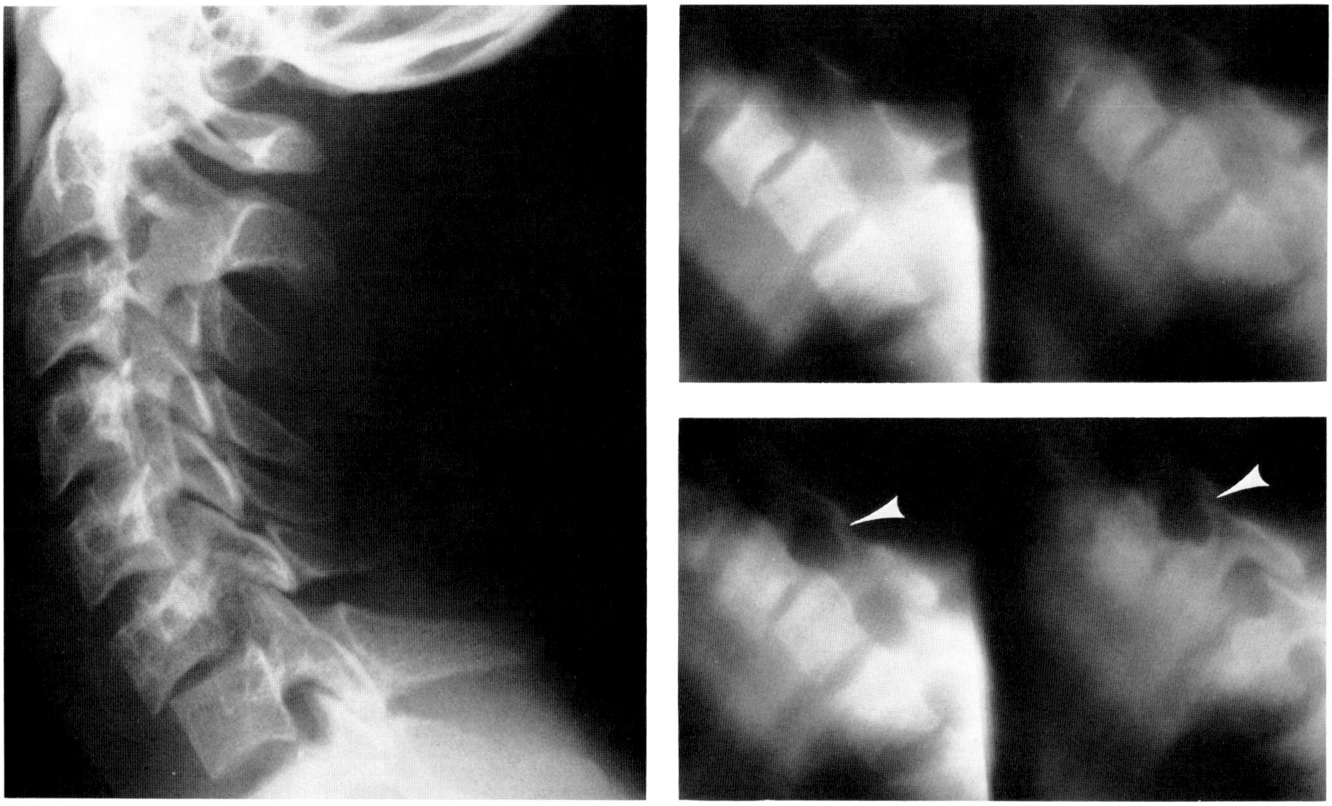

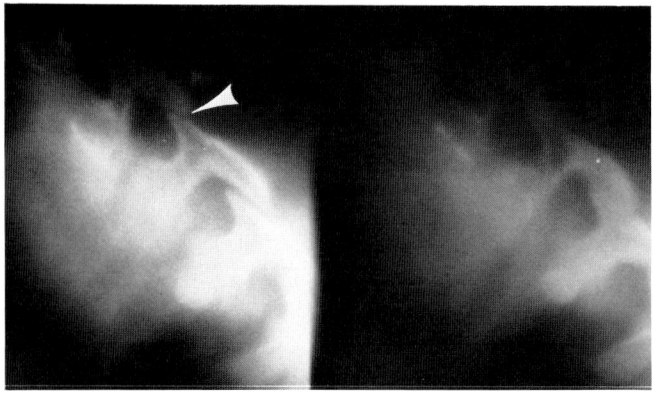

FIG. 4–118. A: Lateral view of the cervical spine demonstrates anterior subluxation of C6 on C7. Lateral tomograms (**B–D**) show subluxation of the facet joints (*arrows*) but no locking or perching.

TABLE 4–17. *Distribution of cervical spine injuries related to thoracolumbar fractures*

Extracervical location	Incidence (%)
With C1-C2	
T1-T4	0
T5-T8	67
T9-T12	33
L1-L3	100
L4-L5	0
With C3-C7	
T1-T4	27
T4-T8	46
T9-T12	77
L1-L3	57
L4-L5	43

upper thoracic and upper lumbar region. The upper thoracic lesions are easily overlooked owing to the soft tissues of the shoulders. Significant neurologic deficit is often present with these fractures. There was also a high incidence of upper and lower cervical spine injuries. Patients with lower cervical spine injuries sustained a more uniform distribution of thoracic and lumbar fractures but tended to have mid-thoracic and upper lumbar fractures.

In patients with spinal trauma, especially if they are comatose or uncooperative, radiographs of the entire spine are essential. Tomography may be necessary to evaluate the lower cervical and upper thoracic region as well as other questionable areas that are not clearly dem-

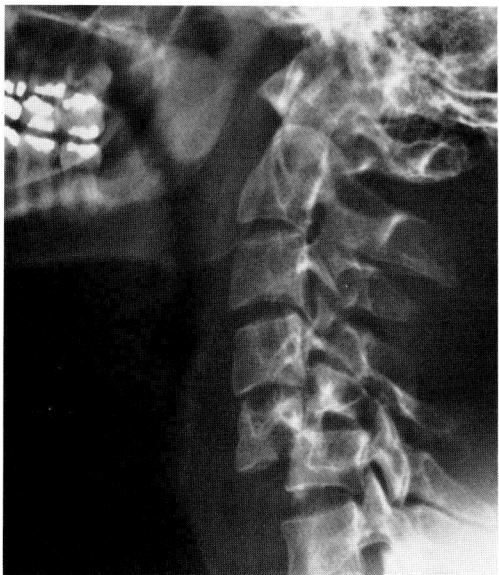

FIG. 4-119. Bilateral locked facets with greater than 50% subluxation of C5 on C6.

onstrated with routine views. Unsuspected neurologically significant lesions can be overlooked if the entire spine is not evaluated in the acutely injured patient.

Cervical Spine Injuries—Essentials of Management

Injuries to the Atlas and the Axis

Because of the unique anatomy of the first two cervical vertebrae, their injuries have characteristics that set them apart from injuries to the rest of the cervical spine. If fatality does not occur, proper diagnosis and treatment usually produces good results with relatively few se-

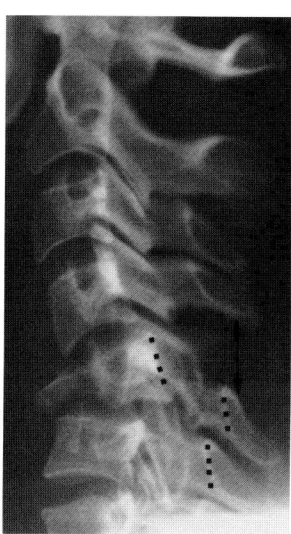

FIG. 4-120. Lateral view of the cervical spine with a flexion teardrop fracture dislocation at C5.

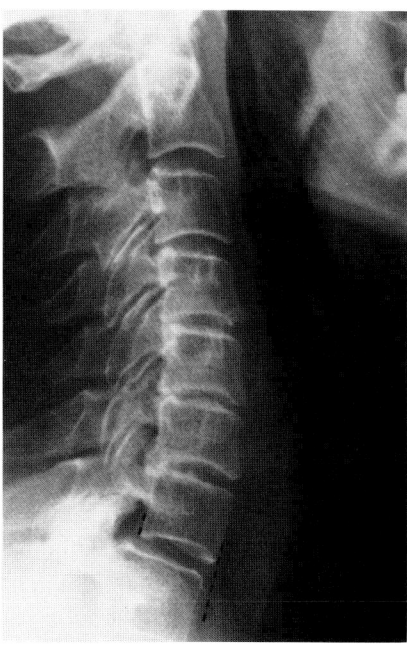

FIG. 4-121. Lateral view of the cervical spine with anterior subluxation of C7 on T1. There is degenerative narrowing of the C4 and C5 interspaces. The C7 interspace is symmetrical (no widening anteriorly or posteriorly) and the facet joints are uniformly narrow and sclerotic at C7-T1.

quelae. We will discuss briefly the management of the most important and frequent lesions in this area.

Occipitocervical Dislocations

A few cases of survival have been reported after this usually fatal injury. The treatment of choice is surgical stabilization by occipito-C2 arthrodesis followed by halothoracic immobilization for a minimum of 12 weeks.

Injuries to the Atlas

These consist of fractures of the posterior or anterior arch and transverse ligament tears.

Injuries to the Posterior and Anterior Arches

Fractures through the posterior arch of the atlas are the most common lesions of these vertebrae. If fractures through the anterior arch can be ruled out by computed tomography, simple immobilization with a collar will suffice. If, however, fractures have occurred through both posterior and anterior arches of the atlas (Jefferson's injury), halothoracic immobilization for 8–12 weeks will be necessary to ensure proper healing. As previously discussed, this injury is the result of an axially directed force that squeezes the lateral masses of the atlas between the occipital condyles and the lateral masses of the axis; the resulting effect is an explosion failure of the atlas with separation of its lateral masses. An uncommonly associated injury that needs to be ruled out is a tear through the transverse ligament of the axis. Spence has noted that a pathognomonic sign of this tear is a separation of the lateral masses of the atlas from the odontoid greater than 6.9 mm in the open-mouth odontoid view (195). If this lesion is present, a two-stage treatment is mandatory: first, a halothoracic device for 8–12 weeks to allow the fracture to heal; second, a posterior atlantoaxial fusion to treat the ligament injury.

Transverse Ligament Tears

The potential for cord compression in this injury is high. The diagnosis is usually made by flexion-extension lateral x-rays obtained under fluoroscopy. If the distance between the odontoid and the anterior arch of C1 is greater than 5 mm, insufficiency of the transverse ligament is present and operative stabilization by C1-C2 posterior arthrodesis is the treatment of choice.

Injuries to the Odontoid

These are probably the most commonly missed injuries of the cervical spine in the emergency evaluation of neck injuries.

Type I fractures are uncommon and usually are the result of an avulsion force that does not place the stability of the atlantoaxial area in jeopardy; therefore, simple collar immobilization suffices.

Type II fractures, or fractures through the base of the odontoid, can be difficult to diagnose. Usually the open-mouth view and the lateral cervical spine x-rays will suf-

fice to procure the diagnosis. But if the fracture is undisplaced, tomography may be necessary. These fractures, particularly if displaced, have a high incidence of nonunion (194,196,197). The high mechanical stresses in this area, the small surface area of the fracture, and the partial interruption of the blood supply to the odontoid may all play a role in the failure to heal. If the fracture is undisplaced, or if anterior displacement of less than 4 mm can be reduced by gentle manipulation, halothoracic immobilization of 12 weeks produces satisfactory healing in the majority of the cases, especially if the patient is under 40 years of age. If, however, anterior displacement cannot be reduced, or if posterior displacement of the odontoid has occurred (Fig. 4-122), early atlantoaxial fusion should be the treatment of choice. Posteriorly displaced odontoid fractures are relatively rare, but when they are seen in elderly patients, they carry a particularly bad prognosis, primarily related to the often associated respiratory complications. If surgery is contraindicated because of the general condition of the patient, application of a halo-vest and early mobilization of the patient offers the best possible means to avoid the commonly seen respiratory complications.

Type III odontoid fractures occur through the body of the axis. As a rule, these are stable injuries through cancellous bone, and they heal promptly with halothoracic immobilization (129,197).

Injuries to the Axis (140,146)

The most common injury is the so-called "hangman's fracture," or fracture through the pedicles of the axis. Today, this injury is most commonly seen in multiple-system trauma victims and is usually the result of an extension force. These injuries have been classified by

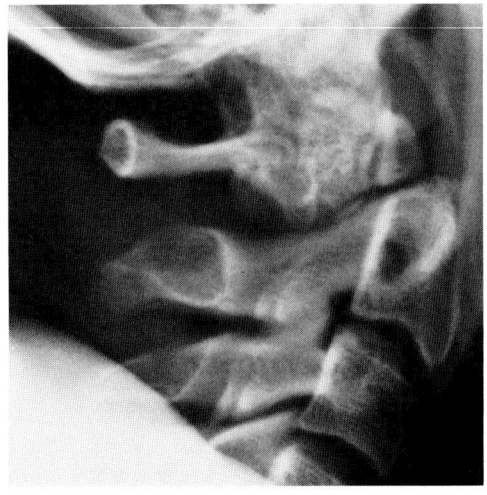
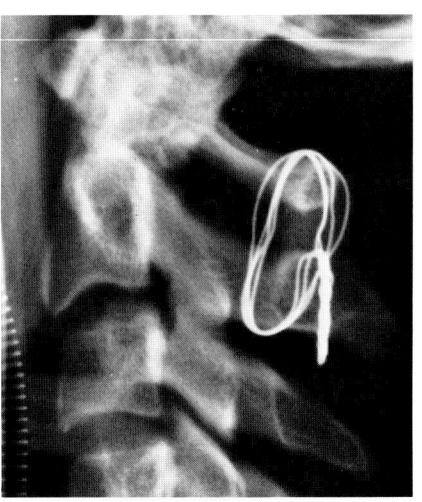

A   B

FIG. 4-122. A: Lateral x-ray of cervical spine in a 20-year-old male involved in a motorcycle accident. No neurological deficit. Note one hundred percent posterior displacement of the odontoid. B: Same patient after early posterior atlantoaxial fusion.

Effendi and colleagues (Fig. 4-123) (140). Basically, injuries can be classified according to whether there is displacement of C2 on C3. If no forward displacement of the body of the axis on the third cervical vertebra is noted—that is, if there is no damage to the C2-C3 disk and anterior longitudinal ligament (Type I)—then the damage is confined to the posterior elements of the axis and simple immobilization with a collar will suffice. However, if significant displacement of the body of C2 on C3 is present (Type II), or, if in addition C2-C3 facet dislocation has occurred (Type III), then the injury is unstable and in this instance halothoracic immobilization is indicated until healing occurs. Type III injuries are very rare and require reduction of the dislocated facets. Non-union of this injury is uncommon (Fig. 4-124), and, if it occurs, it is best treated with anterior C2-C3 arthrodesis (196). Posterior C1-C3 arthrodesis, the obvious alternative, unnecessarily restricts the rotation available at the C1-C2 level and is not advisable.

Injuries to the Lower Cervical Spine

The management of injuries to the lower cervical spine is based on the clinical assessment of the integrity of the neurologic structures and on the radiologic assessment of stability (197,201). The goals of treatment are to decompress the neurologic structures and to stabilize the spine. Decompression is usually achieved by realignment, but it may at times require removal of bony fragments from the canal (most commonly from the anterior aspect of the canal). In general, stable lesions without neurologic deficit require only the minimal support provided by a collar. Unstable or potentially unstable lesions require more aggressive treatment. When the injury involves primarily ligamentous structures, early surgical stabilization is preferred, since conservative treatment often produces late instability. However, if the

injury is predominantly bony, more conservative treatment with halothoracic immobilization followed by a late stability assessment is justified.

Sprains

Posterior ligamentous injuries can have very serious consequences. They are the result of a flexion mechanism, commonly occur between the ages of 14 and 22, and usually involve a single interspace between C4 and T1. They have been named "hidden" injuries because they often are not recognized (200). The pathologic lesion consists of tears of the ligamentum nuchae, the interspinous ligament, and often the ligamenta flava. The characteristic radiologic features of these injuries include (1) an increase in the distance between the spinous process of the two involved vertebrae, (2) a small compression fracture of the superior and anterior corner of the inferior vertebra, (3) an often subtle intervertebral subluxation, and (4) a loss of the normal cervical lordosis (see Fig. 4-114). If the ligament damage is small, simple collar immobilization usually suffices. However, if the subluxation shows a tendency to increase in a controlled flexion lateral x-ray of the cervical spine, wiring of the spinous process and posterior arthrodesis is the treatment of choice (see Fig. 4-114). Failure to recognize these injuries early may have disastrous consequences, as cases of late dislocation have occurred with subsequent neurologic compromise (Fig. 4-125).

Dislocations and Fracture-Dislocations

In the cervical spine, pure flexion or flexion associated with rotation can produce either a unilateral or a bilateral dislocation of the facets. The radiographic features of these two injuries have been described. Beatson (120)

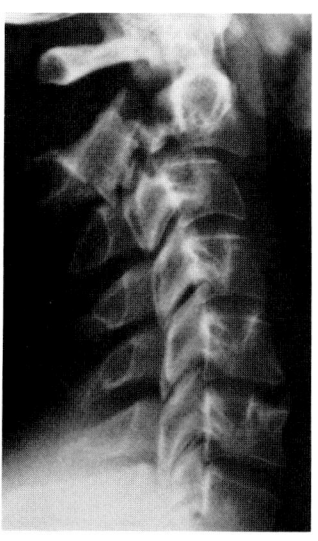
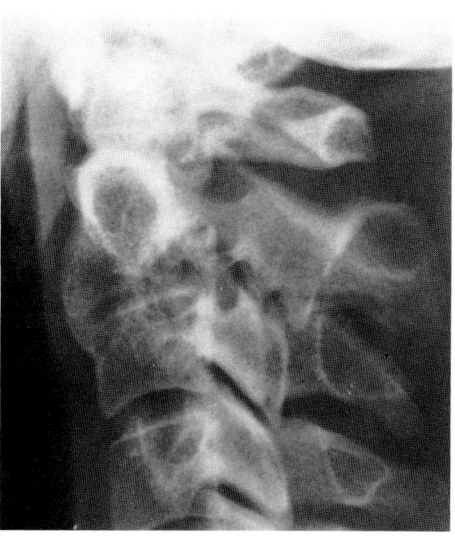

A

B **FIG. 4-123. A**: Lateral roentgenogram of cervical spine in a 27-year-old male involved in an automobile accident. No neurological deficit. Note significant forward subluxation of C2 on C3, indicating damage to the anterior ligamentous and disk structures. **B**: Healed fracture.

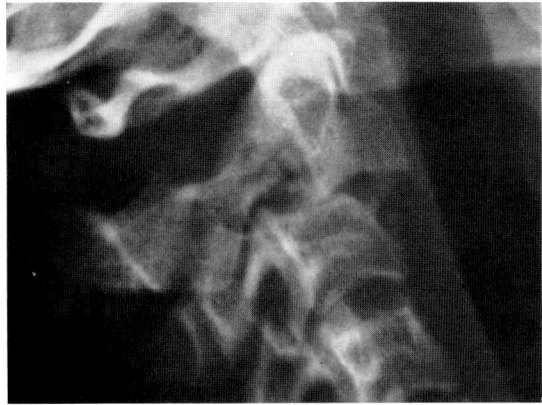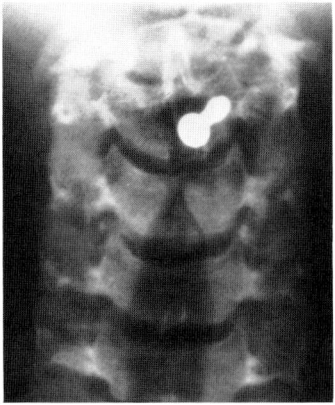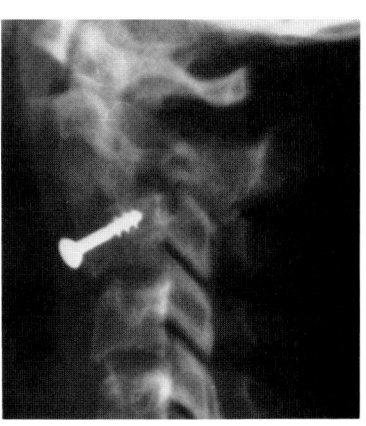

A
B
C

FIG. 4-124. **A**: Lateral roentgenograms of the cervical spine of a 23-year-old female involved in an automobile accident. Film obtained three months after injury. Patient has been treated with a collar and is still symptomatic. Cineradiography confirmed motion at the fracture site, indicating nonunion. Anteroposterior (**B**) and lateral (**C**) roentgenograms of the cervical spine of the same patient three months after anterior interbody fusion C2-C3. The patient is asymptomatic.

has clearly shown in his cadaver experiments that, if forward displacement encompasses less than 50% of the anteroposterior diameter of the vertebral body, the lesion is a unilateral facet dislocation, whereas, if the displacement is 50% or more of the anteroposterior diameter of the body, the lesion is always a bilateral dislocation (Fig. 4-126).

Management in this case should be no different from that of dislocations of any other joint in the body. Whether neurologic deficit is present, reduction of the dislocation should be undertaken if the diagnosis is made early (172,196,197). This is accomplished usually by directed traction through cranial tongs or a halo (Fig.

4-126C). Since these injuries encompass primarily ligamentous disruptions, it is now believed that healing with stability seldom is achieved, and this explains the current tendency to stabilize these injuries surgically with early interspinous wiring and fusion of the dislocated vertebral segment (Fig. 4-126D and E) (197,202).

If closed reduction cannot be achieved, as frequently occurs in the case of unilateral facet dislocations, open reduction followed by stabilization is recommended. The technique of closed manipulation (172) of the dislocated facet has been popular elsewhere but is not frequently practiced in the United States.

When subluxation or dislocation is associated with

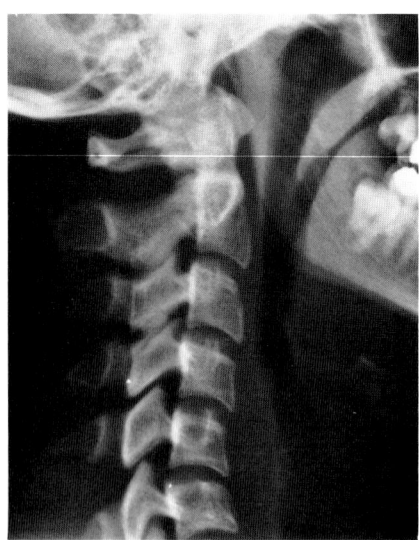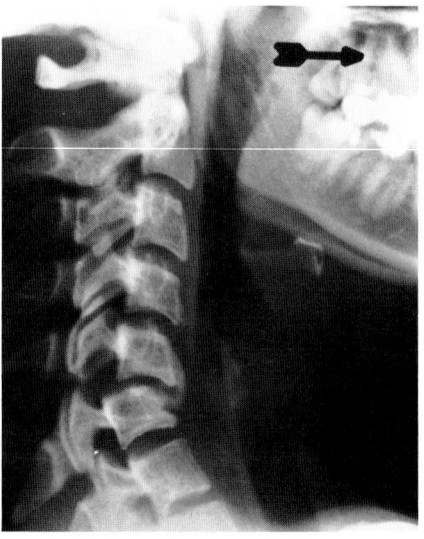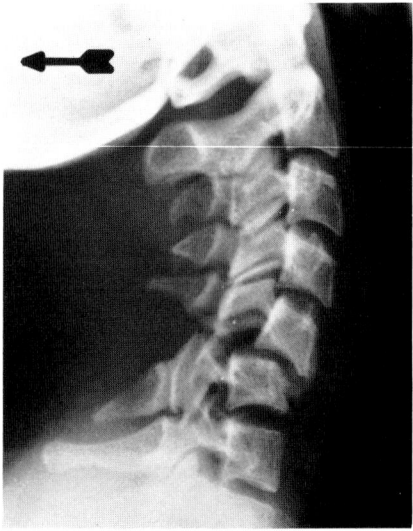

A
B
C

FIG. 4-125. **A**: Lateral roentgenogram obtained immediately after this 25-year-old female was involved in an automobile accident. The obvious ligamentous injury at the C5-C6 interspace was missed. The patient was not treated. Flexion (**B**) and extension (**C**) lateral roentgenograms of the same patient obtained six months after injury. The patient has now developed neurological symptoms (Lhermitte's sign) and has significant neck pain. Note the perching of the facet joints that has occurred as well as the precarious stability achieved by calcification and ossification of the anterior longitudinal ligament.

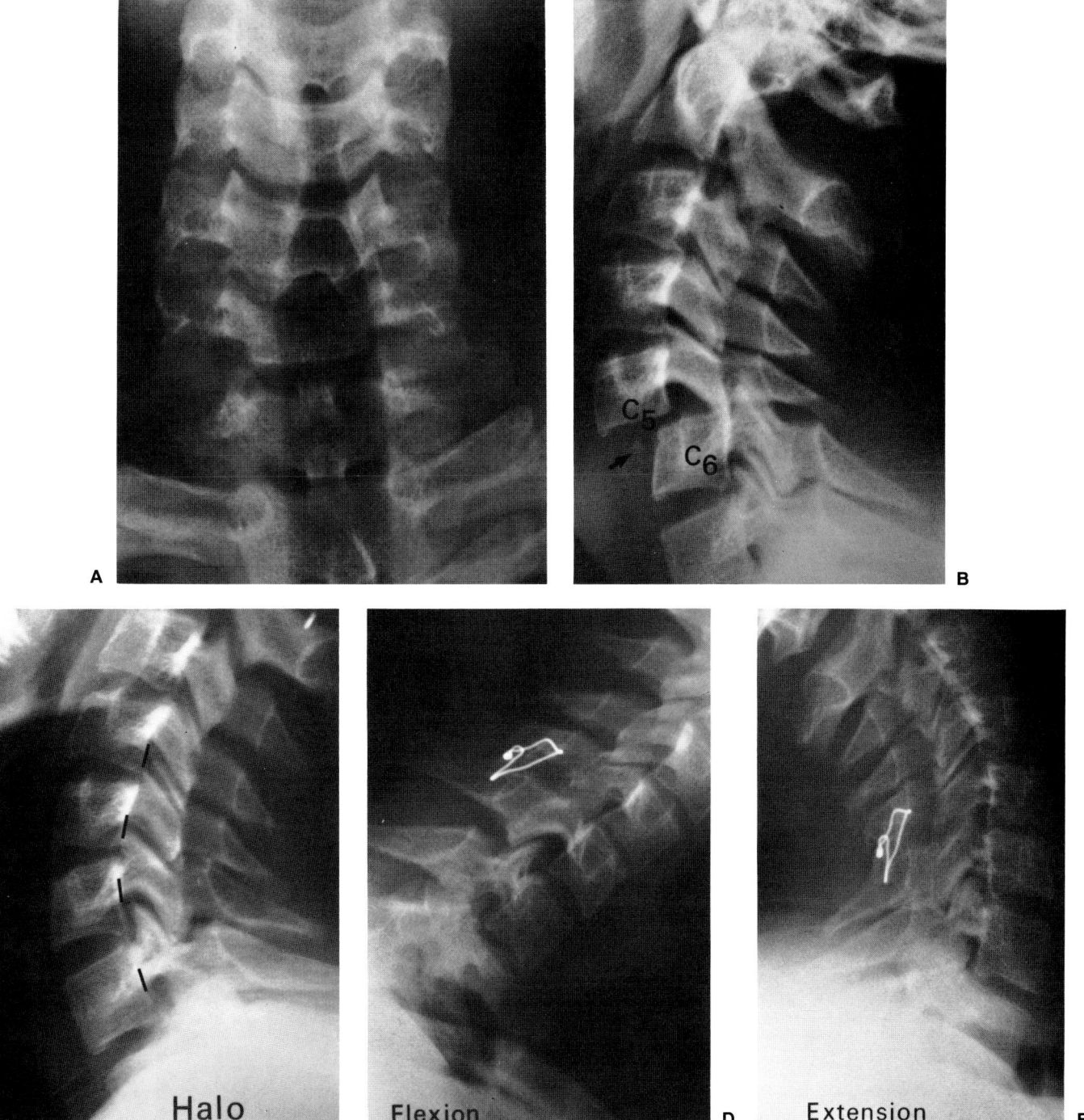

FIG. 4–126. Anteroposterior (**A**) and lateral (**B**) roentgenogram of the cervical spine of a 17-year-old boy who sustained a massive flexion injury during a wrestling match. Profound paraparesis is present. This is clearly a bilateral facet dislocation. Lateral roentgenogram (**C**) of the same patient obtained two hours after admission and immediately after reduction has been achieved by halo traction. The alignment of the cervical spine has been restored. Flexion-extension lateral roentgenograms (**D, E**) of the cervical spine of the same patient obtained three months after posterior interspinous wiring and fusion. One year after injury the patient has returned neurologically to normal and leads a very active life in sports. Early realignment of the spine has been essential in achieving this recovery.

fractures of the tip of the inferior facet (Fig. 4-127A), a rather common occurrence resulting in isolated root deficits, reduction is difficult to achieve and even more difficult to maintain (Fig. 4-127B). The root deficit often lingers with conservative management, but early decompression of the involved root by removal of the loose facet fragment followed by surgical stabilization has produced very satisfactory results in our hands (Fig. 4-127C and D).

When dislocations or fracture-dislocations have occurred in patients with pre-existing cervical spondylosis and reduction has been achieved, late instability after conservative management with halothoracic immobilization for a period of 8–12 weeks has produced very satisfactory results. Thus when these lesions occur in patients afflicted with cervical spondylosis, conservative rather than surgical management is justified.

Extension Injuries

These are relatively common injuries, resulting frequently from falls or automobile accidents. Often these patients are of middle or advanced age and are afflicted

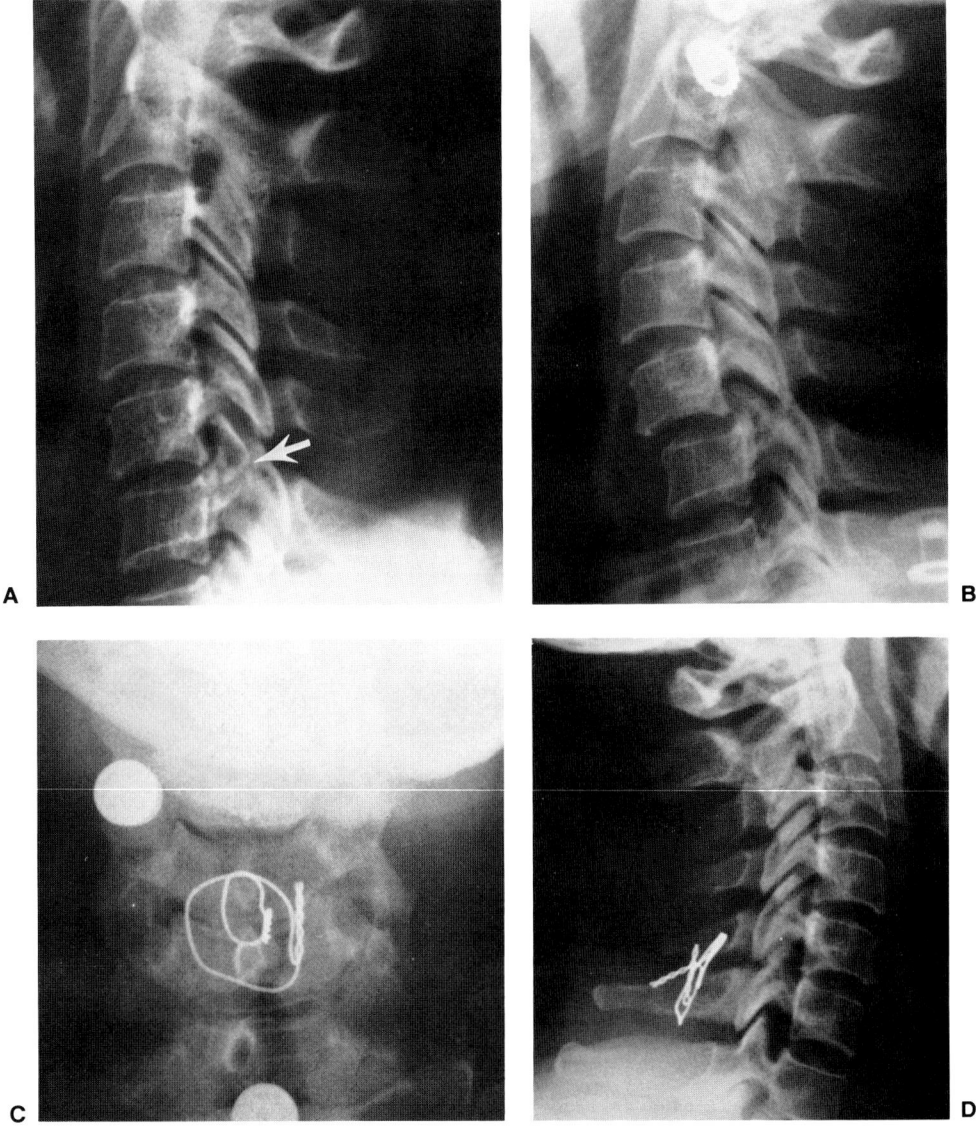

FIG. 4–127. A: Lateral roentgenogram of the cervical spine of a 52-year-old female involved in a single car accident. The patient presents with an acute left C6 radiculopathy. Note fracture of the superior facet of C6 (*arrow*). **B**: Lateral roentgenogram obtained two days after admission of the same patient who has been treated with halo vest immobilization. Note the forward subluxation of C5 on C6. The patient remains very symptomatic and her root deficit has not improved. Anteroposterior (**C**) and lateral (**D**) roentgenograms of the same patient shortly after removal of the facet fragment and posterior interspinous wiring and fusion. Two months postoperatively, the patient was free of symptoms and her neurologic deficit has recovered fully.

with cervical spondylosis and often no evidence of skeletal damage can be encountered. Typically, these patients will present with a central cord syndrome. It is well known that the anteroposterior diameter of the spinal canal decreases significantly in extension, and it is postulated that an anteroposterior compression of the cord either by osteophytes or by the hypertrophic ligamenta flava causes a temporary interruption of the blood supply to the central part of the cord, resulting in edema or infarction of this area. The treatment of these injuries should be conservative with support by a collar for a period of 6 weeks. If there is no improvement, or if deterioration occurs, an MRI or myelography should be considered (Fig. 4-128).

Vertebral Body Fractures

Most vertebral body fractures can be treated conservatively and will heal with support by a cervical orthosis. This applies to chip fractures, minor wedge fractures, uncinate process fractures, and triangular fractures.

However, the comminuted vertebral body fracture resulting from a flexion-compression mechanism, and also known as the flexion teardrop fracture-dislocation, is a very unstable injury (Fig. 4-129). The vertebral body is usually split into two portions—the anterior one is displaced forward like a teardrop, and the posterior portion protrudes into the spinal canal and impacts the cord. In addition, there is usually a fracture through the posterior arch and widening of the interspinous distance. As a rule, the neurologic deficit is profound, but often it involves only the anterior part of the cord. In this injury,

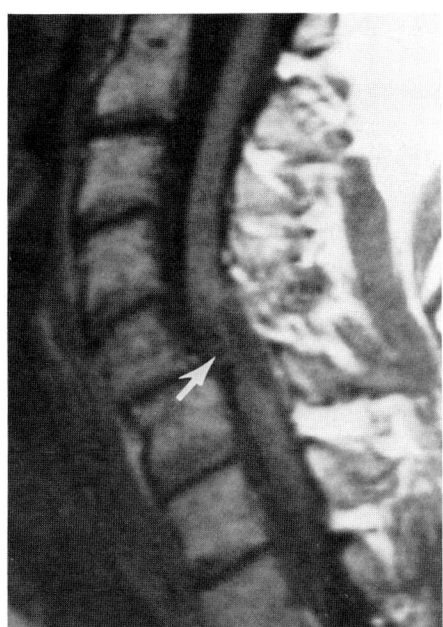

FIG. 4–128. Sagittal SE 500/20 MR image with cord disruption (*arrow*) after trauma.

traction through cranial tongs or a halo can often realign the spinal canal and decrease the pressure on the anterior spinal cord. However, maintaining this reduction requires prolonged traction in the recumbent position for a period of 12–16 weeks. Thus the current trend is to effect surgical removal of the comminuted vertebral body through an anterior approach and replacement with a bone graft with or without internal fixation (Fig. 4-129B and C) (150,196).

Summary

The current philosophy of management of cervical injury is based upon a careful assessment of the neurologic deficit and a careful study of x-rays. Early decompression of the neural elements, achieved most often by realignment of the spinal canal and occasionally by removal of bone fragments, followed by early stabilization provides the best chance for recovery of the neural elements, assures stability, facilitates rehabilitation, and minimizes late sequelae.

Follow-up imaging with routine films, tomography, and CT or MRI is indicated to be certain that fixation is maintained and fragments are stable. Complications of internal and halo fixation such as pin loosening and infection also need to be documented (149). MRI is particularly useful for evaluation of the spinal cord. However, if plate and screw fixation devices are too near the cord, the artifact may be too severe for optimal evaluation.

THORACIC AND LUMBAR SPINE TRAUMA

Anatomic differences in the cervical, thoracic, and lumbar spine must be considered in any discussion of trauma to these regions. Thus the cervical spine is more prone to injury than the thoracic and lumbar spine by virtue of its increased range of motion and fewer supporting structures.

In the thoracic spine, a slight kyphotic curve is normally present. This is in contrast to the lordotic curves evident in the cervical and lumbar regions. Also, the spinal canal in the thoracic region is circular and smaller in diameter than the cervical or lumbar portions of the spine. As one progresses inferiorly, the vertebral bodies increase in size and the disks increase in height, resulting in an increasing resistance to vertical compression forces.

The lumbar segment is similar to the cervical segment in that both contain a greater potential for motion than the thoracic segment. However, the large paraspinal muscles in the lumbar region provide more stability than the cervical musculature (239). Owing to differences in range of motion, transition in the facet joints, and other anatomic factors, the thoracolumbar junction is the area most susceptible to injury. Thus the majority of injuries

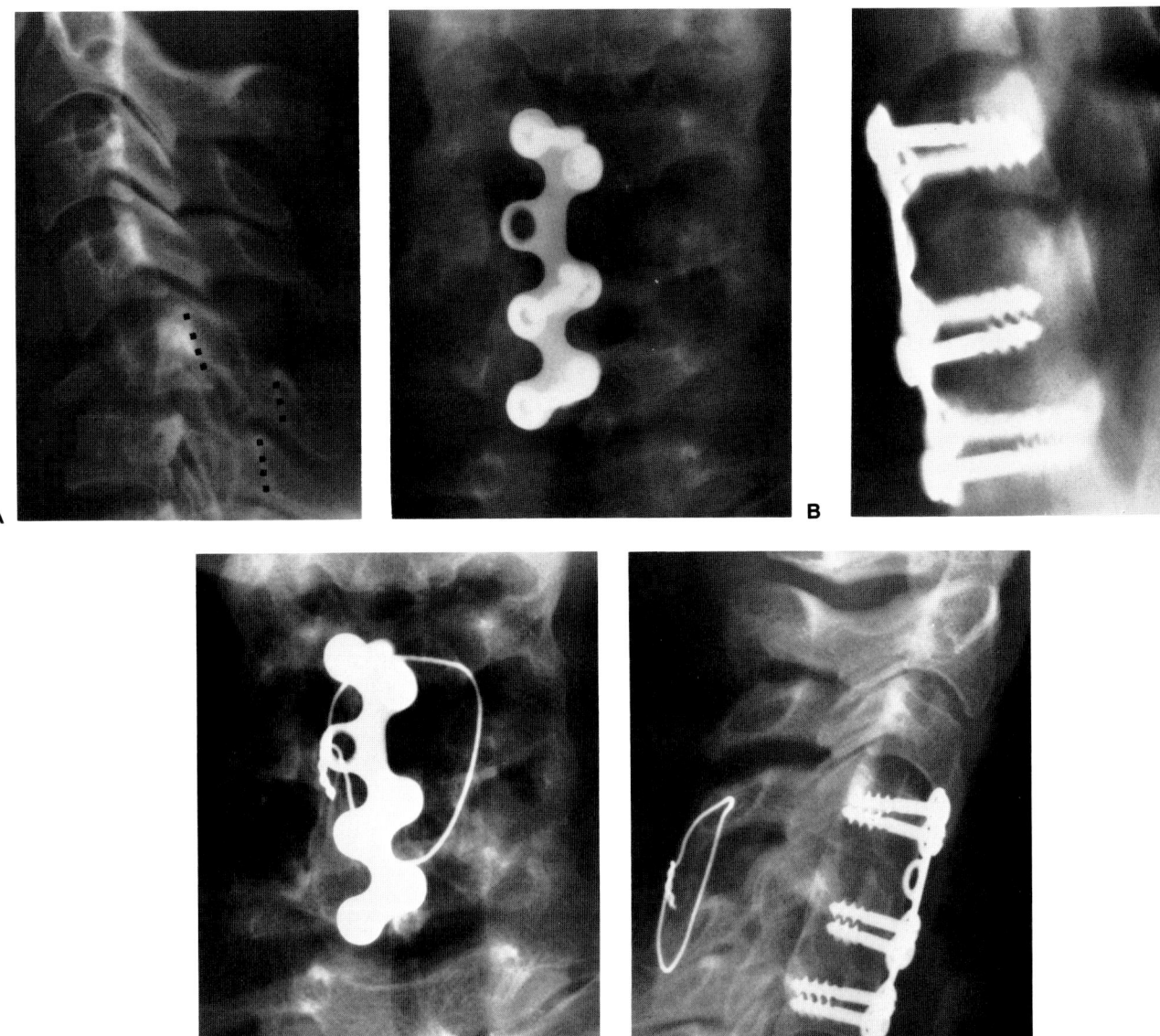

FIG. 4-129. A: Lateral roentgenogram of the cervical spine of a 22-year-old female involved in a motor vehicle accident. The patient presents with a profound anterior cord syndrome. Note the coronal fracture of the vertebral body, the posterior displacement of the body of C5 into the canal, as well as the posterior element fracture and interspinous widening. Anteroposterior (**B**) and lateral (**C**) roentgenogram of the same patient treated immediately after admission with anterior decompression of the spinal canal by removal of the comminuted vertebral body and replacement with a bone graft with internal fixation. Anteroposterior (**D**) and lateral (**E**) roentgenogram of the same patient six months after injury. Because of significant posterior disruption, a delayed posterior wiring and bone grafting was carried out on this patient. Neurologic recovery was very satisfactory to the point where the patient is now walking three years after injury, although with some residual deficit in the lower extremity.

occur at this level. Nicoll reported that 66% of the thoracolumbar fractures occurred between T12 and L2 (264).

Mechanism of Injury

Discussion of thoracolumbar trauma can best be accomplished by utilizing a mechanism of injury approach (231,239,250). The majority of fractures and fracture-dislocations are due to hyperflexion, flexion-rotation, vertical compression, hyperextension, and shearing forces (Table 4-18) (217,221,232,239,248,264).

The mechanisms of injury in the thoracolumbar spine are similar to those in the cervical spine, but because of significant anatomic differences the results and presentation may vary. Holdsworth established his classification of spinal injury based on two columns, the anterior and posterior (248). More recently, Denis described a three-

TABLE 4-18. *Thoracolumbar spine trauma: Mechanisms of injury*

Hyperflexion
 Flexion-compression
 Lateral flexion
 Flexion-rotation
 Flexion-distraction
 Seatbelt injuries
Vertical compression
Hyperextension
Shearing

column approach to evaluating spinal injury (Fig. 4-130) (230). The anterior column includes the anterior longitudinal ligament, anterior annulus and disk, and the ventral half of the vertebral body. The middle column includes the posterior vertebral body, disk, annulus, and posterior longitudinal ligament. The posterior column includes the neural arch and posterior ligament complex. It has been demonstrated that rupture of the posterior longitudinal ligament and annulus is necessary for instability to occur (231). Involvement of two columns leads to an unstable injury.

Hyperflexion Injuries

Hyperflexion injuries are by far the most common injury in the thoracic and lumbar spine. Most often the injury is due to flexion-compression forces that result in a simple anterior wedge fracture of the vertebral body. The posterior complex is almost always intact; therefore, this is a stable injury.

The axis of the force in hyperflexion injuries is centered in the nucleus pulposus or in the midportion of the intervertebral disk. Thus the appearance of the injury may vary, depending upon the spinal level involved. In the upper thoracic region the disks are narrower and the fracture is more typically a true anterior wedge fracture (Fig. 4-131). In the thoracic region, especially the upper thoracic spine, the anterior height of the vertebral bodies is normally 1.5 mm less than the posterior height (226). In the lower thoracic and lumbar region the disks are larger and more effective as shock absorbers. Thus herniation into the cartilaginous end-plates is more likely to occur in the lower thoracic and lumbar regions (Fig. 4-132). If the flexion force continues, the anterior body is more likely to be compressed (239).

The degree of compression and changes in the disk space are important in wedge fractures of the vertebral bodies. If compression is greater than 50% and if the disk space is narrowed, the prognosis is less favorable (227). These findings along with multiple contiguous wedge fractures may lead to delayed instability. Multiple contiguous wedge fractures in the upper thoracic region may lead to cord deficits (Fig. 4-133) (217).

Anterior wedge fractures can almost always be detected on AP and lateral projections of the involved areas (Table 4-19). On the AP view, one should check for evidence of paraspinal soft tissue swelling, which is often present with anterior compression fractures (Fig. 4-134). Paraspinal swelling in the upper and mid-thoracic regions can mimic traumatic aortic rupture (229). The interpedicular distance and posterior elements are normal with a simple wedge fracture. The same force that results in a wedge fracture may disrupt the posterior ligaments or bony structures if the magnitude of the force is sufficient. Occasionally, the loss of height and trabecular

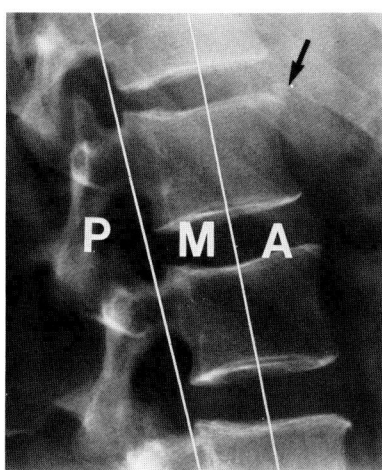

FIG. 4-130. Lateral view of the thoracolumbar junction demonstrating the 3 columns. A, anterior; M, middle; P, posterior. Note the normal variant (*arrow*) in L1. This should not be confused with a fracture.

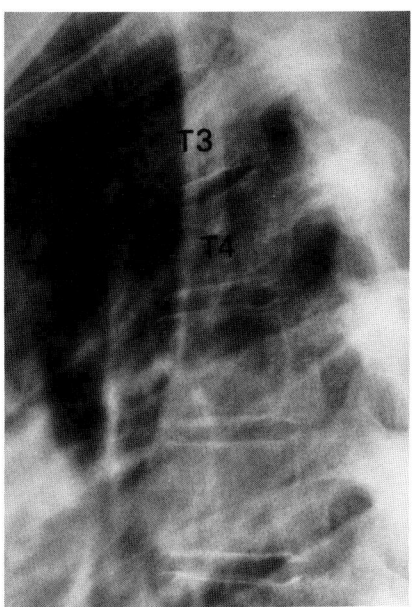

FIG. 4-131. Anterior compression fractures of T3 and T4. Compression fractures are frequently multiple.

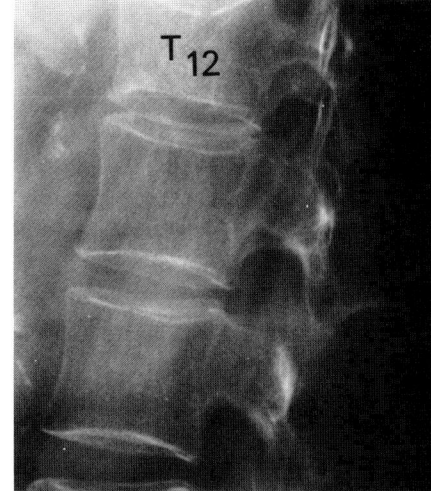

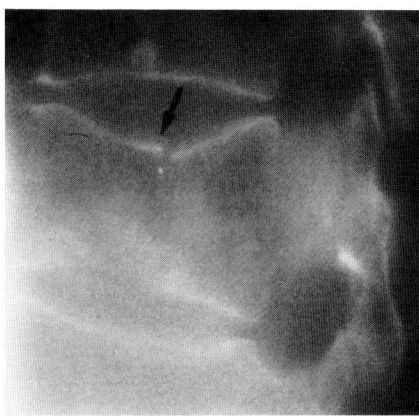

FIG. 4-132. Elderly female with osteoporosis and pain following a fall. **A**: There is loss of height at T12. ? acute vs. senile osteoporosis. **B**: Lateral tomogram clearly demonstrates an acute fracture (*arrow*) with end plate involvement.

TABLE 4-19. *Radiographic fractures of anterior wedge (compression) fractures*

Soft tissue swelling
Anterior superior cortical impaction
Loss of height anteriorly
Buckling of the anterior cortex
Trabecular condensation
End-plate fracture
Disk space narrowing

compression can be detected on the AP view (Fig. 4-135), but diagnosis is better accomplished on the lateral view (Fig. 4-136). Compression or buckling of the anterior superior cortex of the vertebral body is the most common feature. Disk-space narrowing and vertebral end-plate fracture may be present. The latter is more common in osteoporotic vertebral bodies (Fig. 4-132) (233). However, these features are more commonly noted with burst fractures. Occasionally tomography (Fig. 4-132) is required to detect a subtle compression fracture or to visualize a suspicious area. Lateral tomograms are especially important in the upper thoracic region, where penetration of the shoulders is often difficult (Fig. 4-133) (226). This can easily be accomplished with the Versigraph without moving the patient. AP tomograms should also be obtained to exclude vertebral arch injury, which may result in instability and quite different management of the patient. With simple anterior wedge fractures computed tomography is rarely necessary.

The list of differential diagnostic possibilities that may be confused with anterior wedge fractures is extensive (Table 4-20). Diagnostic problems are common in elderly patients with osteopenia (Fig. 4-137), in pathologic

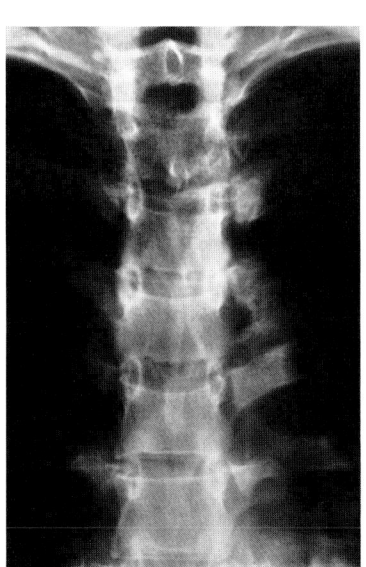

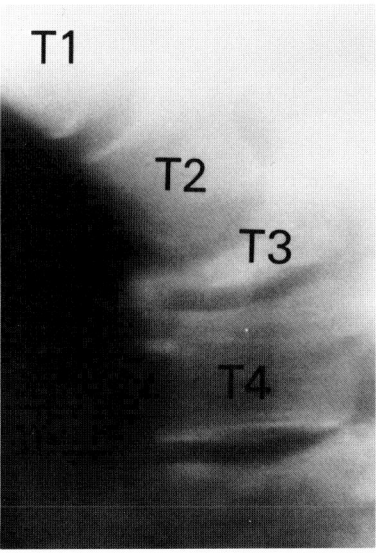

FIG. 4-133. Patient with upper thoracic pain and neurologic deficit in the lower extremities. Routine AP view (**A**) was thought to be normal. The upper thoracic region could not be evaluated on routine lateral views. Tomograms (**B**) demonstrate 75° compression of T3, mild compression of T4, and marked kyphotic deformity.

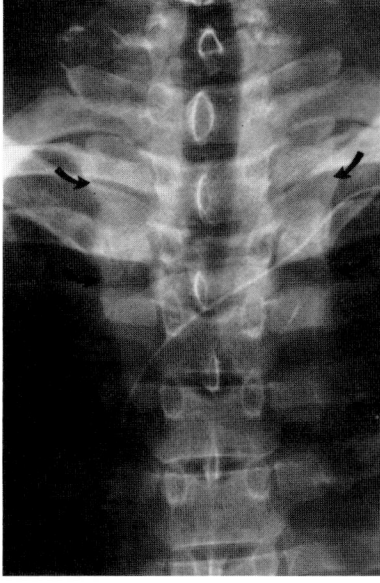
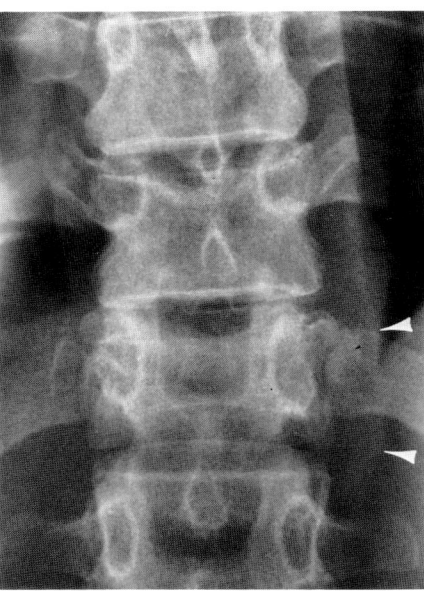

A

B

FIG. 4-134. Thoracic compression fractures. **A:** Marked soft tissue swelling (*arrows*) due to multiple upper thoracic compression fractures. This is a particularly useful sign as the lateral view is often underinterpreted in this region. **B:** More subtle paraspinal swelling (*arrows*) due to mild compression of T12.

conditions that are difficult to differentiate from simple traumatic lesions, and occasionally in infectious conditions or cases of nuclear herniation.

Lateral flexion injuries may result in lateral vertebral wedge fractures. This injury is stable (217), although it has been reported to result in a somewhat poorer prognosis than a simple anterior wedge fracture (264). Radiographically there is almost always some degree of paraspinal soft tissue swelling, especially in the thoracic region. The asymmetric compression is best appreciated on the AP view (Fig. 4-138).

The same forces responsible for anterior wedge fractures, if continued, result in distraction of the posterior complex. Ligament disruption or vertebral arch frac-

tures may occur, resulting in an unstable fracture-dislocation (267,270). Although it is common in the cervical spine, locking of the facets is rare in the thoracic and lumbar spine (240,248). The facets and large paraspinal muscles in the lumbar region, and the costal elements and chest in the thoracic region, provide more stability (239). Radiographically the appearance of locked facets is similar to that described in the cervical spine. The overriding of facets is easily seen on lateral views and tomograms. The facet appears "naked" on axial CT images for the inferior facets no longer articulate with the superior facets of the vertebra below (240).

The majority of flexion-distraction injuries occur at the thoracolumbar junction. Usually the compression force is centered in the midportion of the body and nucleus pulposus with distraction posteriorly. The incidence of neurologic complications may be as high as 70% (239). Flexion-distraction injuries with disruption of the posterior ligament complex or fractures of the arch are unstable (Fig. 4-137) (273,278). The degree of compression may be minimal; and therefore not only the

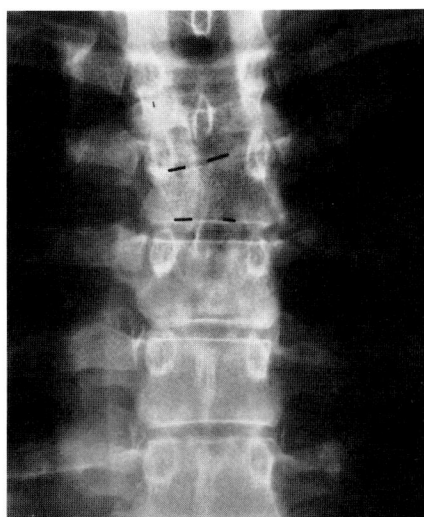

FIG. 4-135. Lateral wedge fracture of T4 (*dotted lines*). The degree of wedging is best demonstrated on the AP view or AP tomography.

TABLE 4-20. Anterior wedge fractures: Differential diagnosis[a]

Congenital
Hemivertebra
Pathologic
Infection
Neoplasm
Primary
Metastatic
Metabolic
Scheuermann's disease
Kümmell's disease
Schmorl's nodes

[a] (239).

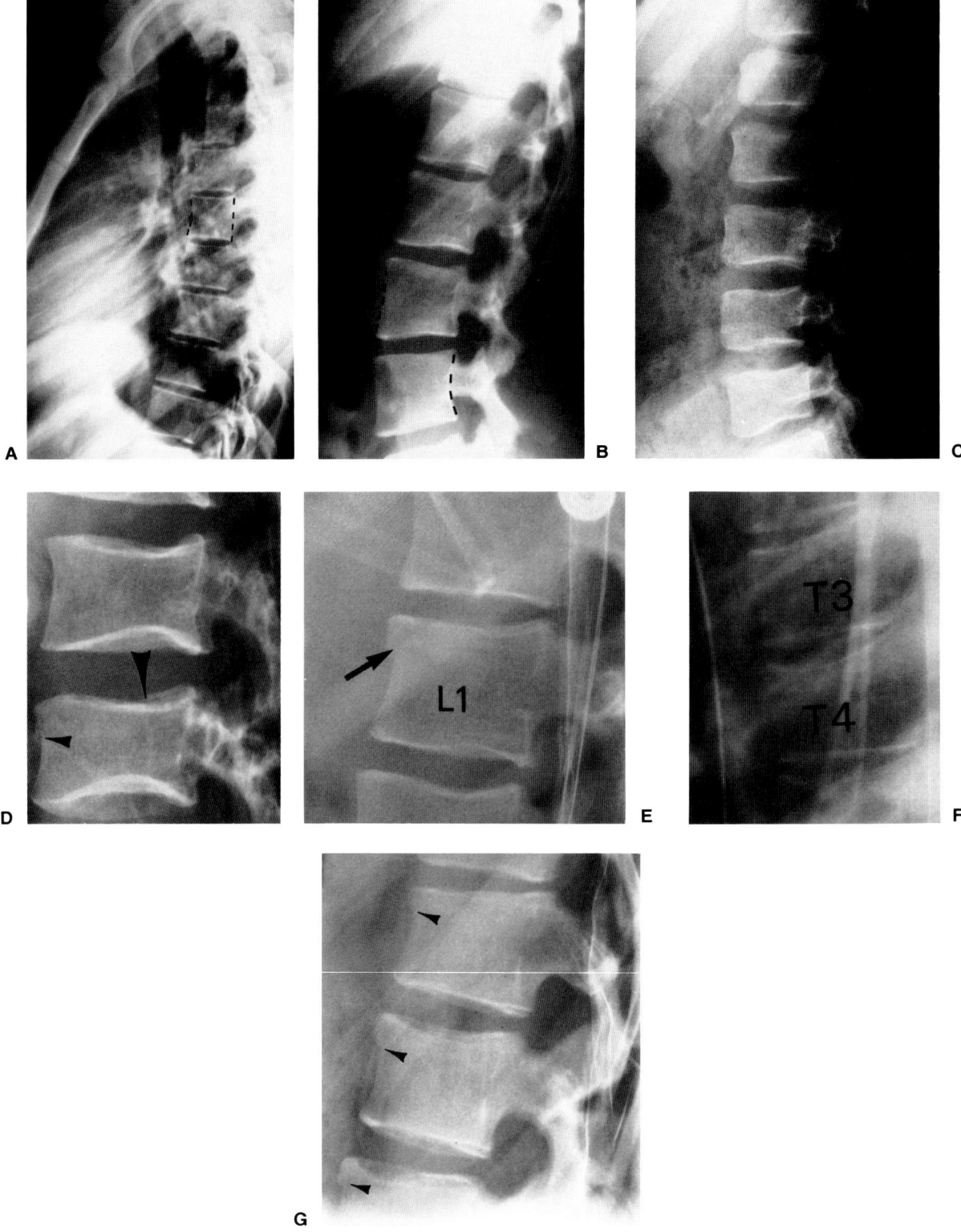

FIG. 4–136. Anterior compression injuries. **A, B**: Normal lateral views of the adult thoracic (**A**) and lumbar (**B**) spine. Note the normal concave appearance of the anterior and posterior vertebral bodies in the lumbar region (*broken lines*). The posterior margin of the thoracic vertebrae is nearly straight (*broken lines*). **C**: Normal lateral view of the lumbar spine in a young teenager with incompletely ossified ring epiphysis in the upper lumbar region. **D**: Subtle end-plate compression of L4 (*arrow*) with buckling (*arrow*) of the anterior cortex. **E**: Anterior cortex buckle (*arrow*) due to compression fracture of L1. **F**: Lateral view of the upper thoracic spine with loss of height of T3 and T4 due to compression fractures. **G**: Subtle anterior cortical buckling in three contiguous vertebrae (*arrows*) at the thoracolumbar junction.

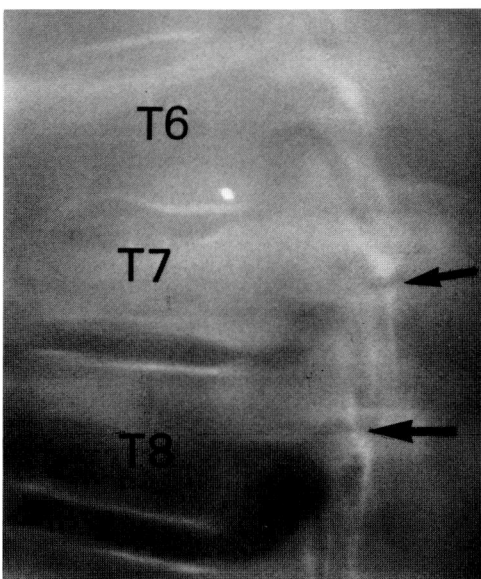

FIG. 4-137. Flexion/distraction injury with compression of T7 and posterior arch fractures at T7 and T8 (*arrows*). The posterior element fractures were not seen on CT or routine views. CT slices were in the plane of the fracture and overlooked due to partial volume effect.

compression but, more important, the posterior injury may be overlooked. Tomography in the AP and lateral projections can be accomplished with ease in the acutely injured patient. Computed tomography is also of value but may require more patient manipulation than can be tolerated during the early assessment period. If the patient can be moved to the CT gantry, valuable information regarding the status of the spinal canal can be ob-

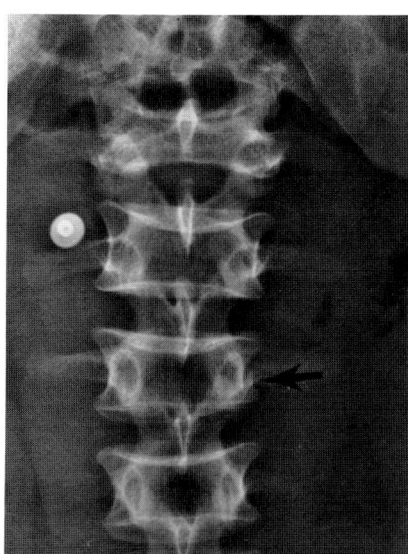

FIG. 4-138. AP view of the lumbar spine with compression of L3 on the right (*arrow*) due to a lateral flexion (compression) injury.

tained (Fig. 4-139). Other authors have also noted CT to be of value in examining the facet joint (266), but in our experience tomography is preferred for undisplaced horizontal fractures and facet evaluation. Myelography is occasionally required to determine the level of obstruction due to the fractures.

Seatbelt injuries (due to use of a lap belt) result from a mechanism similar to flexion-distraction trauma except for the fact that the fulcrum is located more anteriorly at the abdominal wall and the injuries more commonly involve the midlumbar region (L1-L3) (220,239,272). This injury was initially described by Chance in 1948. Rogers (272) has described three different patterns of fulcrum injury:

1. Disruption of the posterior ligaments, facets, and disks occur with the spinous process, transverse processes, and pedicles intact.

2. A transverse fracture of the posterior arch occurs and may involve the posterior superior body.

3. Transverse fractures are present in the posterior arch and body. The lamina, transverse processes, and pedicles are usually involved (Fig. 4-140).

The location (L1-L3), lack of significant vertebral compression, and increased incidence of abdominal injury are the major differences between the seatbelt injury and the flexion-distraction injury previously discussed. Several large series have discussed the complications associated with seatbelt or anterior fulcrum injuries (223,230,238,251,272). Abdominal wall hematomas as well as intra-abdominal pathology may result. Lacerations in the bowel, especially the ileum, duodenum, and antimesenteric border of the jejunum are common. Lacerations of the liver, spleen, and pancreas may also occur (229,239,272). The incidence of neurologic involvement is lower (less than 20%) than in the case of flexion-distraction injuries, in which the fulcrum is at the midvertebral body level (239). The degree of vertebral compression may be minimal and occasionally no anterior injury is detectable (Fig. 4-141). Evaluation of the arch on the AP views should be performed with great care (Fig. 4-142). In our experience, 25% of seatbelt injuries were not detected on the lateral view. This is the result of the absence of significant compression. Also, the posterior elements are often not entirely included on the supine lateral projection. The AP view may provide the only clue to this significant unstable injury. Radiographic evaluation frequently requires tomography or CT to determine the extent of injury (211,259).

The change in configuration of seatbelts has caused some changes in injury patterns. The use of a shoulder support in addition to or instead of the waist restraint has caused different upper thoracic, lower cervical injuries. These include transverse process fractures and upper thoracic fractures (247).

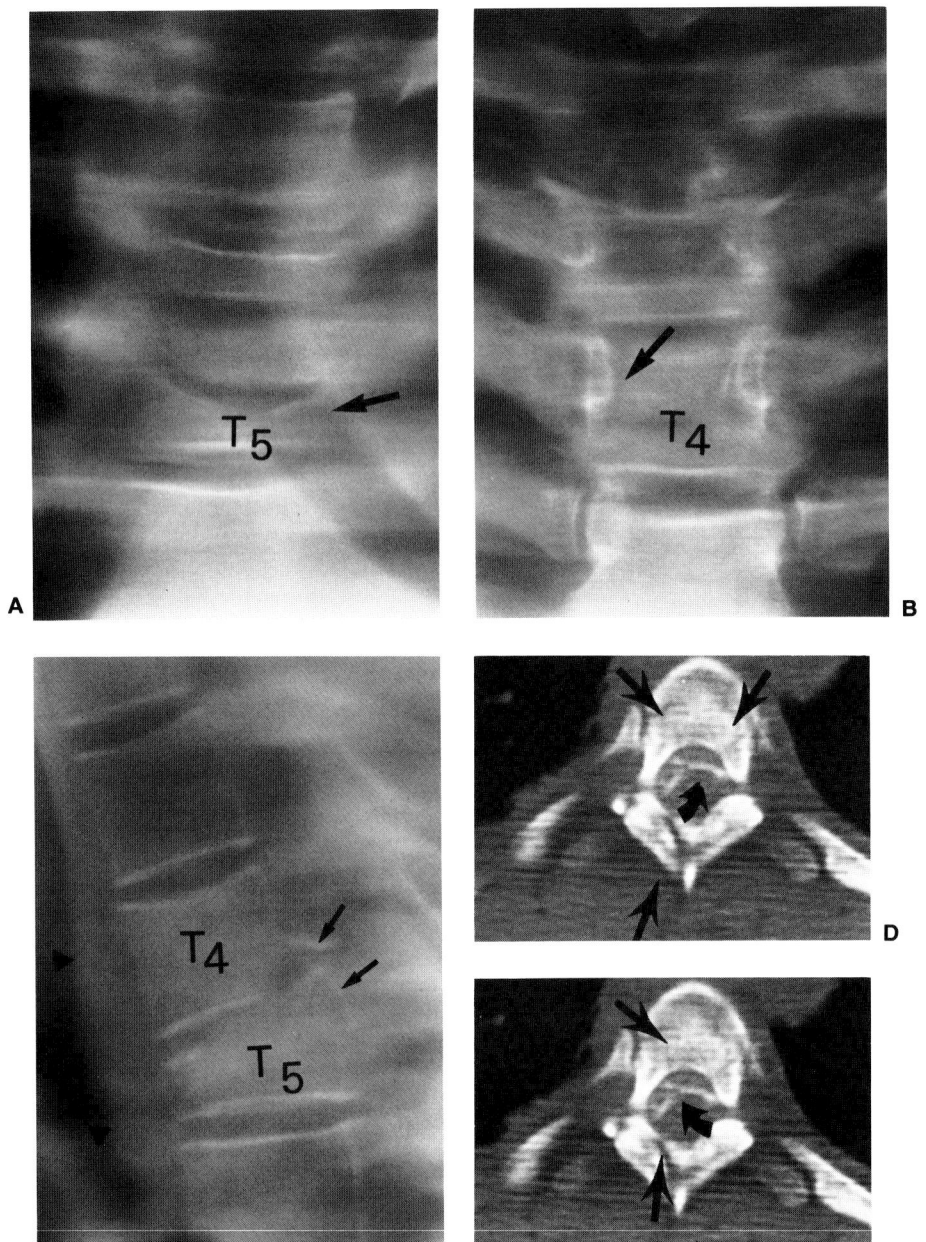

FIG. 4–139. Upper thoracic spine fracture. The AP (**A, B**) and lateral (**C**) tomograms demonstrate the fractures at T4-T5. There is also soft tissue swelling. CT scans (**D, E**) clearly demonstrate the bony fragments in the spinal canal.

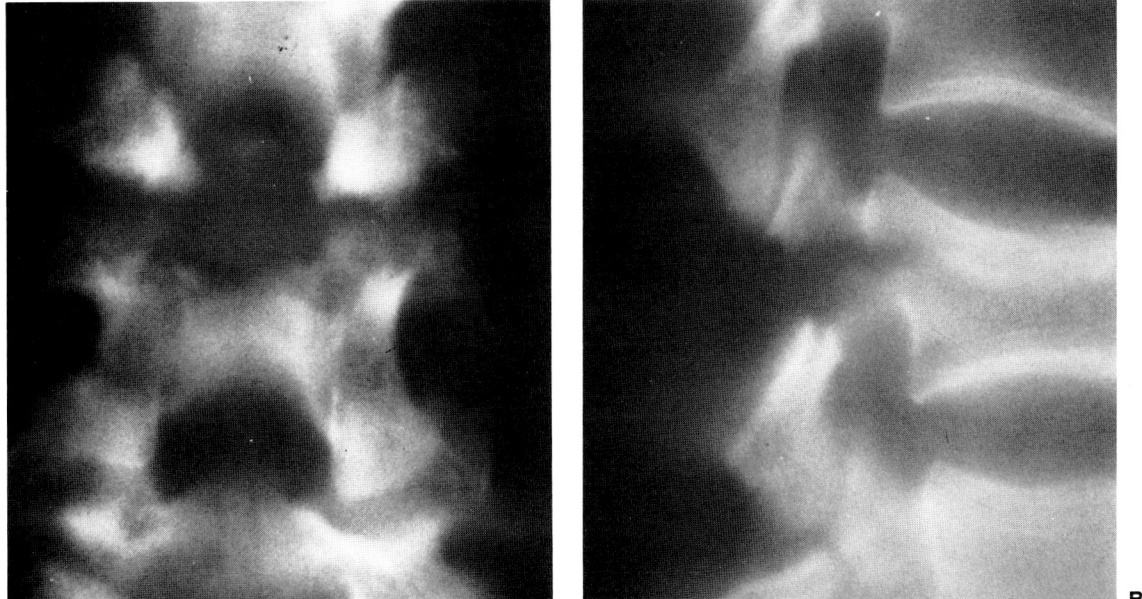

FIG. 4–140. AP (**A**) and lateral (**B**) tomograms demonstrate a transverse fracture of the pedicle and lamina of L2 with compression of the vertebral body.

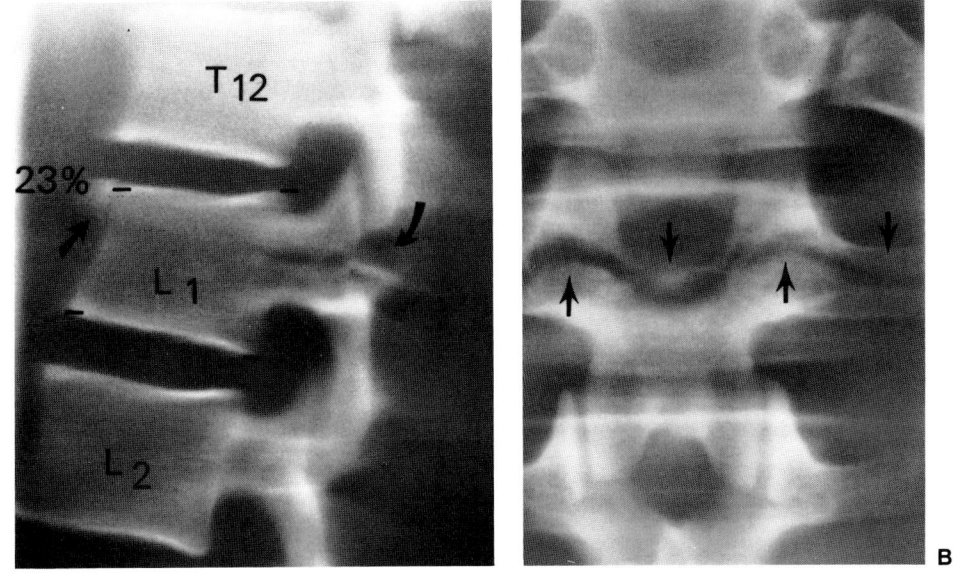

FIG. 4–141. A: Lateral tomogram of the upper lumbar spine with a seat belt fracture. Note the minimal compression of L1 with obvious posterior distraction (*curved arrow*). **B:** Lateral lumbar spine with posterior arch fracture of L2 (*arrow*) and minimal vertebral compression.

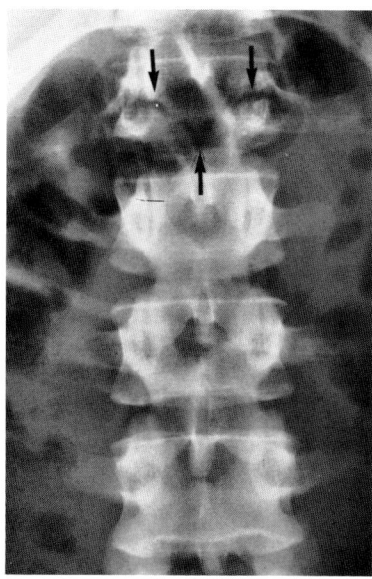 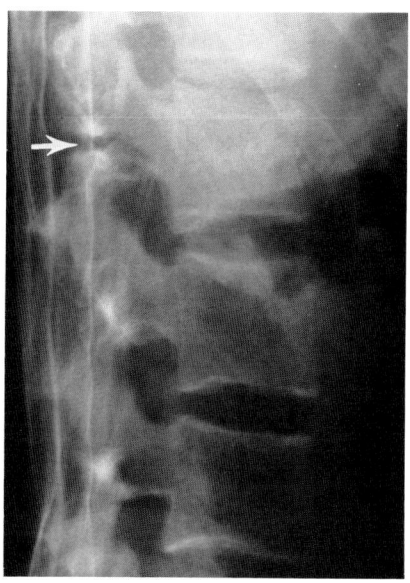

FIG. 4-142. Subtle L1 posterior arch fracture (*arrows*) seen only on the AP (**A**) view. The fracture (*arrows*) is obvious on the AP tomogram (**B**).

Flexion-Rotation Injuries

Fortunately, flexion-rotation injuries of the thoracolumbar spine are uncommon (225,256,258,262,288). When it occurs, the lesion is among the most unstable of spinal injuries (217,248). The injury usually occurs at the thoracolumbar junction owing to the transition in the facet joints (217). The incidence of neurologic deficit approaches 70% (217). This injury is easily overlooked, because it is uncommon, and, more important, reduction of the dislocation tends to occur in the supine position (248).

Radiographic features of the injury are similar to a unilateral locked facet in the cervical spine. On the AP view, the spinous process may be rotated to the side of the involvement, and a fracture through the upper endplate may be present. The disk space may appear asymmetric or tilted to one side. On the lateral view, the disk space is often narrowed and the interspinous distance increased. A "slice fracture" (248) of the upper vertebral body is usually more obvious on the lateral view. Fractures of the articular processes and lamina frequently require tomography or CT for detection (Fig. 4-143 and 4-144) (258). Computed tomography is most useful in evaluating the degree of involvement of the spinal canal (Fig. 4-145).

Vertical Compression Injury

Vertical compression injuries (axial loading with or without associated flexion) result in burst fractures of the vertebral bodies with outward displacement of fracture fragments, herniation of the disk into the end-plates, and posterior extension of the disk and fracture fragments into the spinal canal. Burst fractures are uncommon accounting for only 1.5% of spinal injuries (260). This injury may be stable if the posterior ligaments remain intact (217,236,239,248,277). Most injuries occur at the T12-L2 level. Although potentially stable, the incidence of neurologic involvement is high owing to displacement of bone fragments into the spinal canal (236,254,277). Since at least two columns are involved and it may be difficult to evaluate the posterior ligament, we recommend these fractures be considered unstable.

Denis (230) classified burst fractures based upon their radiographic appearance (Fig. 4-146). Type A burst fractures comprised 22.7% of cases in Atlas et al. (212) series. These fractures have superior and inferior posterior vertebral fragments with multiple small fragments. Axial loading is the typical mechanism of injury (230). Type B fractures are most common accounting for 54.7% of injuries (212). This injury involves the superior posterior end plate, and it frequently has a single fracture line extending into the inferior end plate. Axial loading combined with flexion forces are the most likely mechanism of injury with this fracture pattern. Type C burst fractures involve the posterior inferior end plate and are rare (212,230,282).

Injuries associated with translation (Type D) were subdivided into two categories that together comprise 20% of burst fractures (212,230). Lateral translation is more common than sagittal translation (Fig. 4-146) (212). Asymmetric axial loading can cause unilateral burst injuries (Type E), which are also rare (212).

Takata et al. (282) reviewed an uncommon variant of the burst injury: the posterior vertebral margin fracture. This injury is more subtle than the typical burst fracture and has been associated with strenuous sports activities. Both flexion and extension have been implicated as mechanisms of injury. Three categories of fracture have

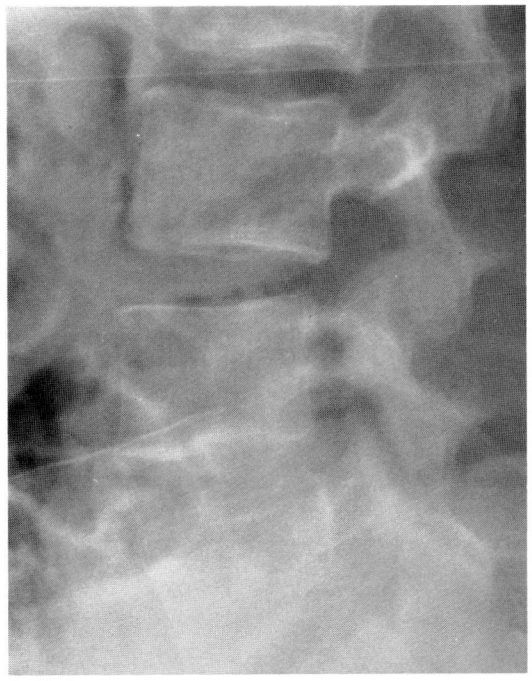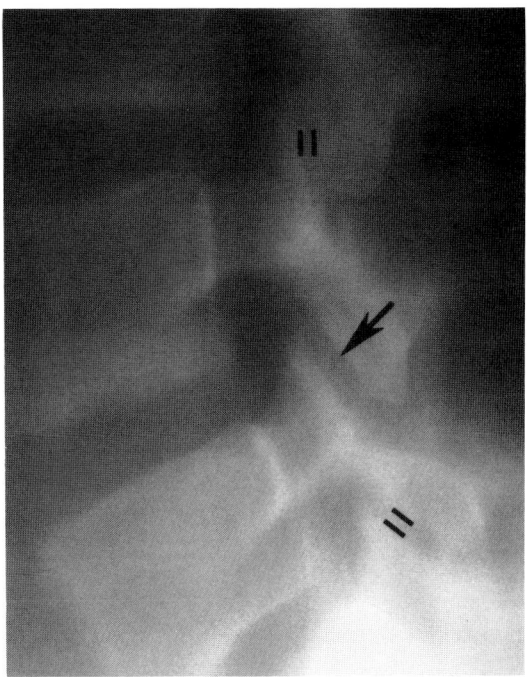

A   B

FIG. 4-143. Subtle flexion rotation injury in the lower lumbar spine. The lateral view (**A**) shows apparent widening of the L4-L5 facet joints. Lateral tomogram (**B**) clearly demonstrates the widened facet joint (*arrow*) on the left.

been described (Fig. 4-147). Type I (33% of cases) is a posterior vertebral rim fracture. Type II (29% of fractures) is a larger posterior rim fracture (Fig. 4-148). Type II (38%) is a smaller localized fracture (Fig. 4-147).

Burst fractures can usually be seen on the AP and lateral views (Fig. 4-149). Such fractures involve multiple bony fragments and compression of the body and disk space. The interpedicular distance is increased on the AP view, and, if tomograms are obtained, arch fractures are

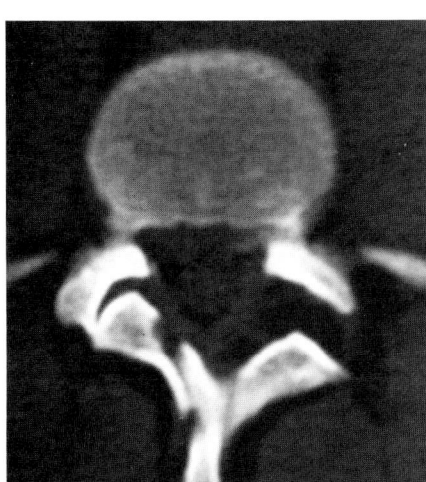

FIG. 4-144. CT image following a flexion-rotation injury demonstrates separation of the facet joint on the left with a laminar fracture and mild subluxation on the right.

also commonly seen. The posterior vertebral line is usually abnormal (Fig. 4-150) on the lateral view (224). Although the degree of spinal canal involvement can often be appreciated on the lateral view or lateral tomogram, CT is the technique of choice for the best evaluation of the spinal canal (Figs. 4-149 and 4-150) (216,260,276,281,282,286). Bony fragments, dural tears (Fig. 4-151), and epidural hematomas may be detected with this modality (215,218,222,246,255,265,284). The incidence of separate associated spinal injuries is greater than 40% (212). Therefore, radiographs of the entire spine should be obtained when a burst fracture is detected.

Hyperextension Injury

Hyperextension injuries in the thoracolumbar spine are rare. Roaf demonstrated posterior arch fractures but could not disrupt the strong anterior longitudinal ligament with pure hyperextension (Fig. 4-152) (271). He believed that rotary motion was required for ligament disruption. The forces applied result in posterior compression and anterior distraction, the opposite of hyperflexion injuries. The incidence of neurologic complications with this injury is also high (219,245,261). De Oliveira described ten patients with dorsal blows to the back that resulted in hyperextension of the segment above the level of the injury (232). The majority of the injuries occurred in the midlumbar region. Lateral ra-

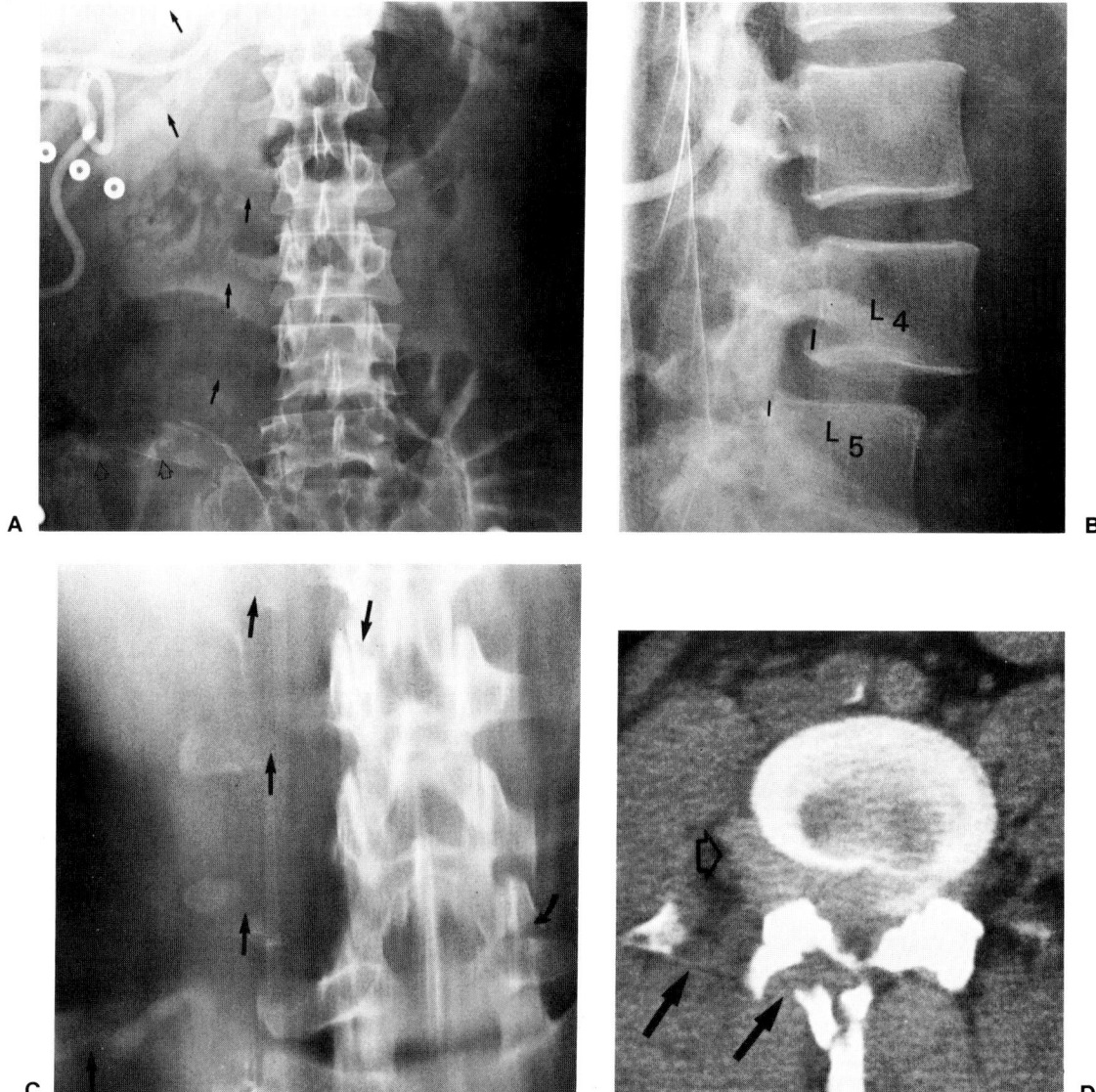

FIG. 4–145. Complex rotary injury of the lower lumbar spine. **A**: AP view demonstrates multiple transverse process and rib fractures (*arrows*) with displacement of L4 on L5 to the left. **B**: Lateral view shows anterior subluxation of L4 on L5 with slight disc space narrowing. **C**: AP tomogram demonstrates the transverse process fractures and right iliac crest fracture (*vertical arrows*). There are also facet fractures at L5 on the left (*curved arrow*) and L2 on the right (*upper arrows*). **D**: CT scan more clearly demonstrates the canal and hemorrhage around the intervertebral foramina (*open arrow*).

forces. Computed tomography is useful in evaluation of the spinal canal and subtle fractures. Mild subluxation or position changes can be difficult to evaluate on axial images (215).

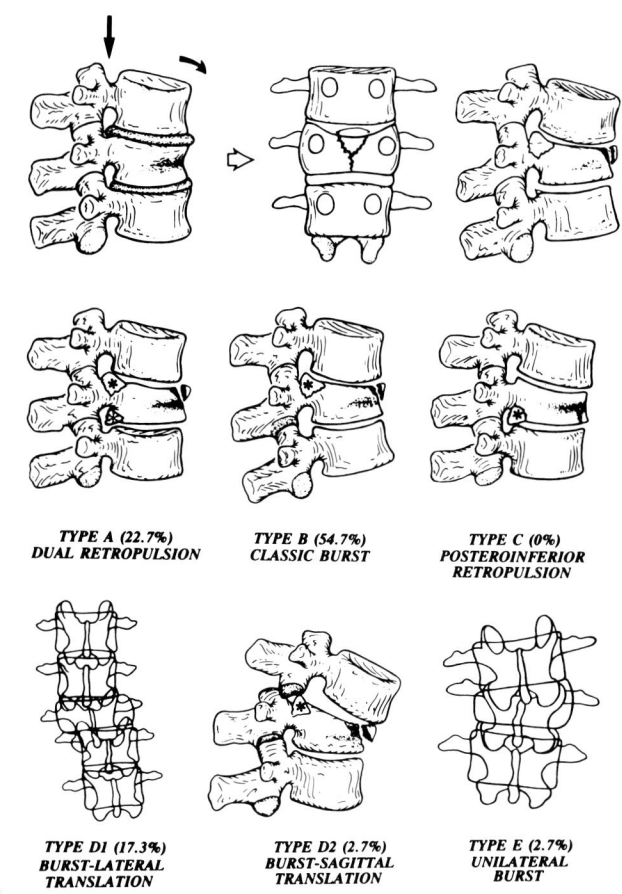

TYPE A (22.7%)
DUAL RETROPULSION

TYPE B (54.7%)
CLASSIC BURST

TYPE C (0%)
POSTEROINFERIOR RETROPULSION

TYPE D1 (17.3%)
BURST-LATERAL TRANSLATION

TYPE D2 (2.7%)
BURST-SAGITTAL TRANSLATION

TYPE E (2.7%)
UNILATERAL BURST

FIG. 4–146. Illustrations of the mechanism of injury (**A**) and classification of burst fractures (**B**) (118).

diographs revealed posterior subluxation of the vertebral body above the level at which the trauma occurred. The incidence of neurologic injury in these patients was not significant and healing occurred without residual pain.

Radiographic findings with hyperextension injuries are similar to those noted in the cervical spine. The features are best detected on the lateral view (Fig. 4-152). The disk space may be widened anteriorly, and the posterior structures may be fractured owing to compression

Shearing Injury

Shearing forces result in anterior dislocation of the vertebra at the level of the injury onto the vertebra below (217,239,248,252,253). In our experience this injury is more common in the thoracic region. The posterior complex is usually disrupted, resulting in a very unstable lesion (217,241,248). Neurologic injury is common. Lateral views and tomography are most helpful in evaluation of this injury (Fig. 4-153). Often the patient's condition is such that movement to the CT gantry is not wise or essential in the acute situation.

Minor Fractures

Fractures of the posterior arch without an associated fracture-dislocation are uncommon (210,213,241,244, 249,251,261,267–269,278). Fractures of the articular processes may result from twisting injuries and have been described in skiers (267). Smith described posterior arch fractures involving the lamina and pars following jumping injuries; all patients presented with neurologic deficits (278). Murray has determined that pars interarticularis fractures may actually be stress fractures (263,268,269). Fractures of the transverse processes are most common in the lumbar region and are usually due to direct trauma or muscle contraction (Fig. 4-154) (216). These fractures are usually not significant by themselves, but associated retroperitoneal hematoma and renal injury may result. Fractures of the spinous processes may be due to flexion, extension, or direct trauma. The most common location is the lower cervical and upper thoracic region. This injury is rare in the lumbar spine.

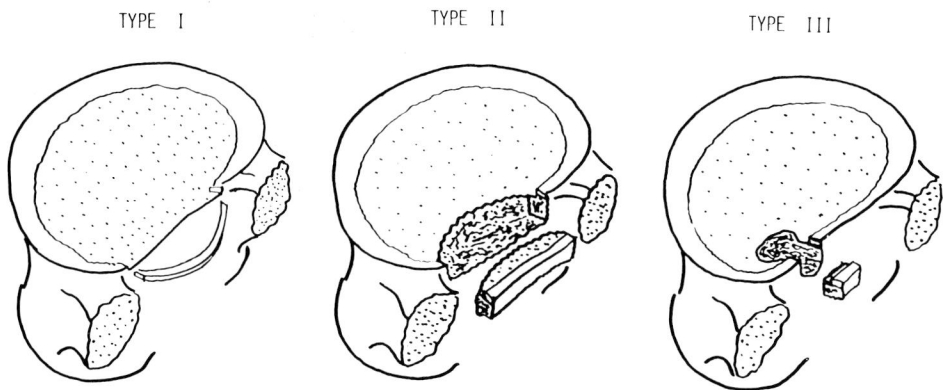

TYPE I TYPE II TYPE III

FIG. 4–147. Illustration of the classification for posterior margin fractures (282).

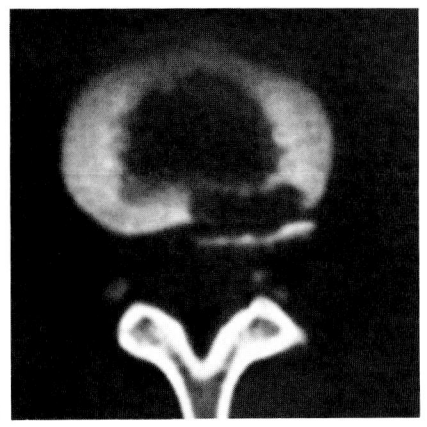
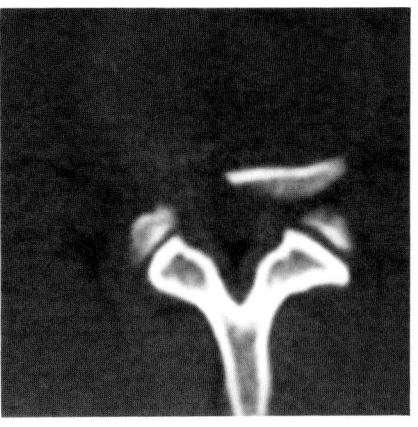

FIG. 4-148. Type II posterior vertebral margin fracture. CT images (**A, B**) show a rim fracture that has rotated so the cortex is directed anteriorly.

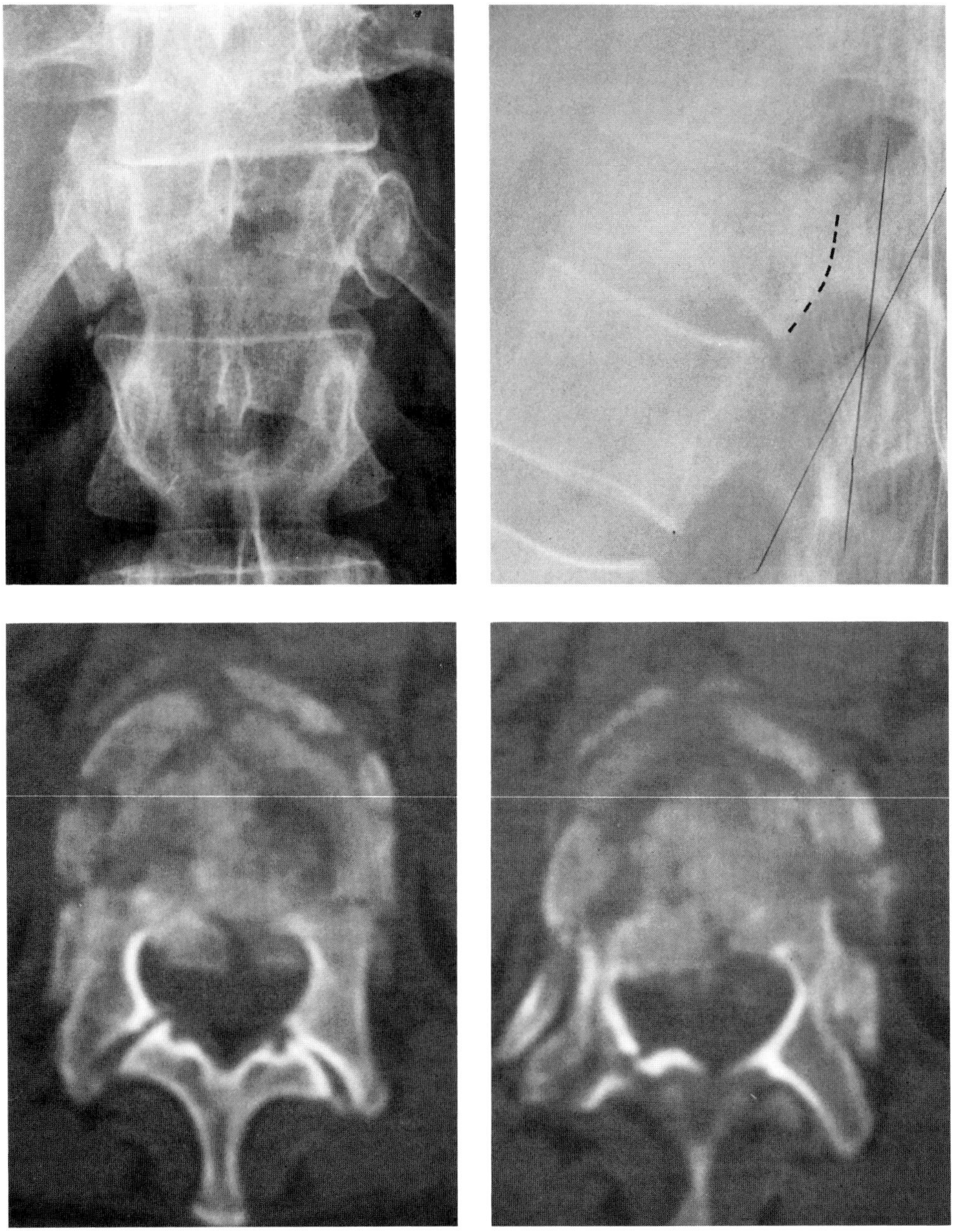

FIG. 4-149. Burst fracture (Type A) with multiple small fragments. **A:** AP view of the spine shows spreading of the T12 pedicles indicating a burst fracture. There are associated rib fractures. **B:** Lateral view shows compression with bulging of the posterior spinal line (*broken lines*). There is kyphotic angulation (*lines*). **C, D:** Axial CT images at the upper and lower level of the vertebral body show marked fragmentation with narrowing of the spinal canal.

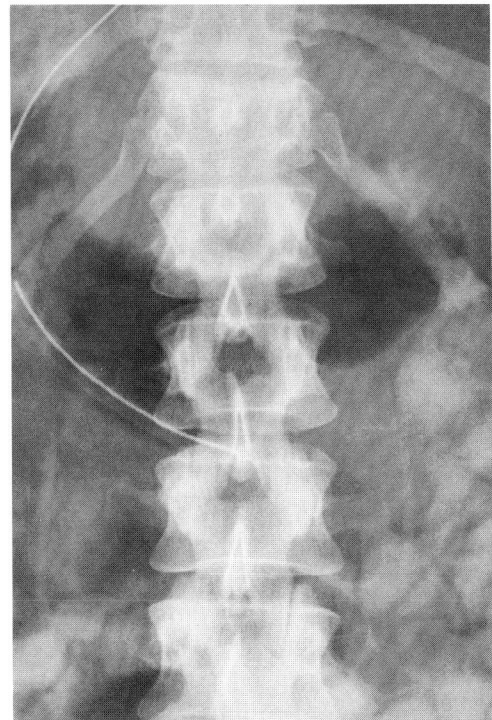

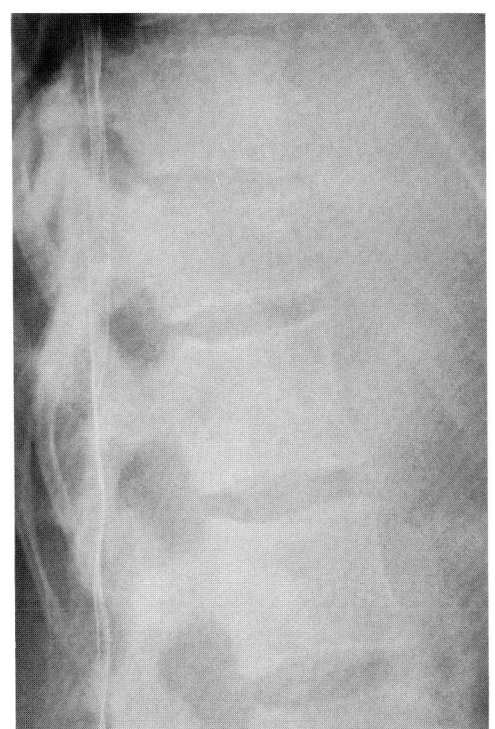

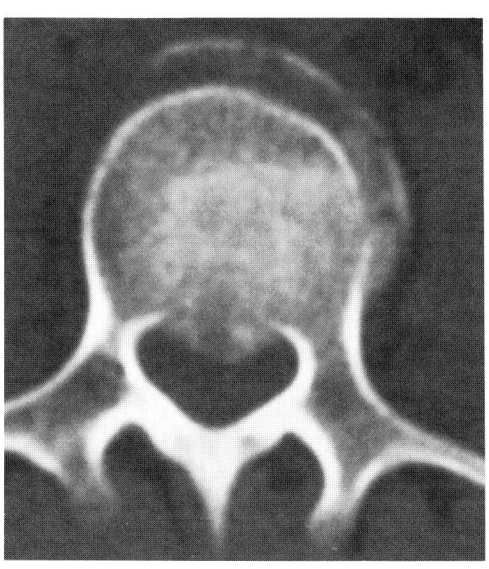

FIG. 4–150. **A**: AP view of the lumbar spine shows apparent compression of T12 with slight widening of the interpedicular distance. **B**: Lateral view shows compression of T12. **C**: CT image shows anterior fragmentation with bulging of the posterior cortex reducing the spinal canal diameter.

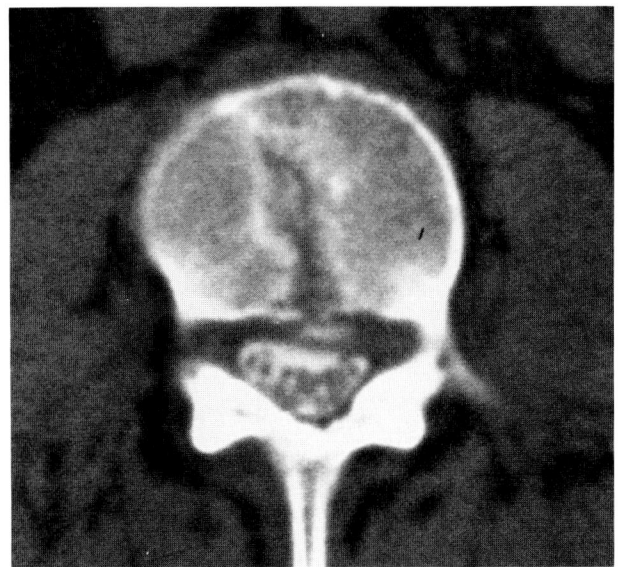

FIG. 4–151. Subtle burst fracture. CT with metrizamide demonstrates the fracture with a fragment displacing the dural sac posteriorly. There is no dural tear.

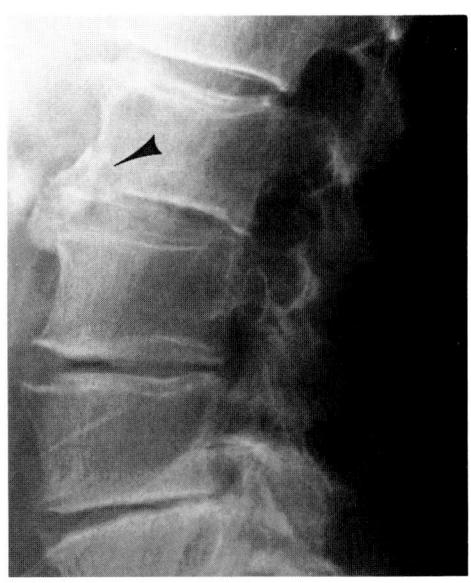

FIG. 4–152. Lateral view of the lumbar spine demonstrating a subtle oblique fracture of the inferior aspect of L2 (*arrow*) due to hyperextension.

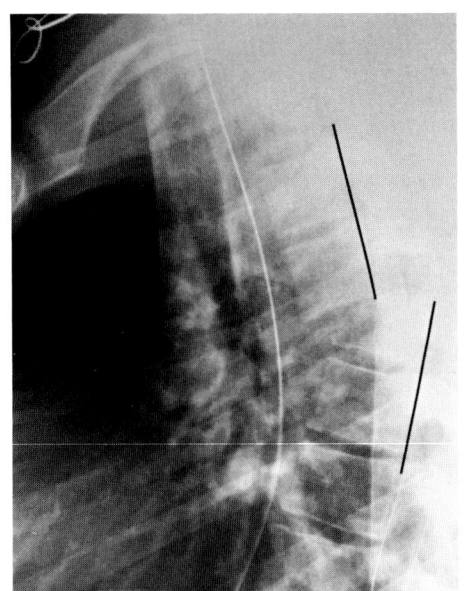

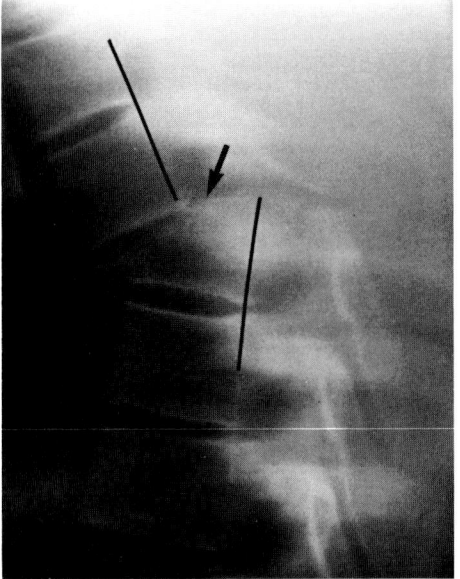

A

B

FIG. 4–153. Thoracic dislocation seen on the lateral view (**A**) and lateral tomogram (**B**).

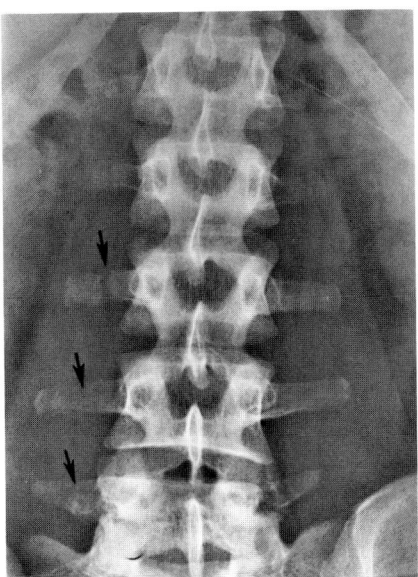

FIG. 4–154. Multiple transverse process fractures (*arrows*). These are best seen on the AP view.

The most difficult problem in isolated arch fractures is differentiating these findings from congenital clefts and spondylolysis (213). Clinical history, previous films, and tomography are essential for proper evaluation of these injuries (Fig. 4-155). Congenital clefts and old non-united fractures have well-defined sclerotic margins. Acute fractures have irregular nonsclerotic margins.

Thoracic and Lumbar Injuries— Essentials of Management

About one-third of these spinal injuries will result in neurologic deficit. At least in the United States the inci-

dence of incomplete injuries is on the increase—perhaps owing to improvement in the emergency medical system. Proper early evaluation and treatment can have a vast impact on the future of the patient—not only from the point of view of ultimate function but also from that of lifetime cost of follow-up treatment (235,260,280).

Initially, the critical questions are again those of the extent of neurologic deficit and spinal instability. The answer to the first question is based on careful clinical evaluation. Complete neurologic deficit at the level of T10 or above will be the result of cord injury and is therefore irreversible. However, deficit below the skeletal level of T10 would necessarily involve the conus medullaris and/or the roots of the cauda equina. Cauda equina lesions behave like peripheral nerves, and therefore they have a better prognosis for neurologic recovery. This justifies a more aggressive approach to management of injuries at the thoracolumbar junction and below.

Evaluation of spinal instability is based on a careful study of radiographs. In general, lesions that involve the anterior and posterior elements of the spine, whether they are associated with neurologic deficits, should be considered unstable, particularly if significant displacement or significant angulation is present at the injury site. On the other hand, injuries that involve only the anterior or the posterior elements alone are generally considered stable. In addition, late instability can occur as a result of late kyphotic angulation, which is more common after multiple compression fractures or after bursting injuries treated with inadequate external support for an insufficient period of time. Late progressive angulation can result in progressive neurologic deterioration related to tethering of the cord around the kyphotic deformity. Computed tomography and MRI are very

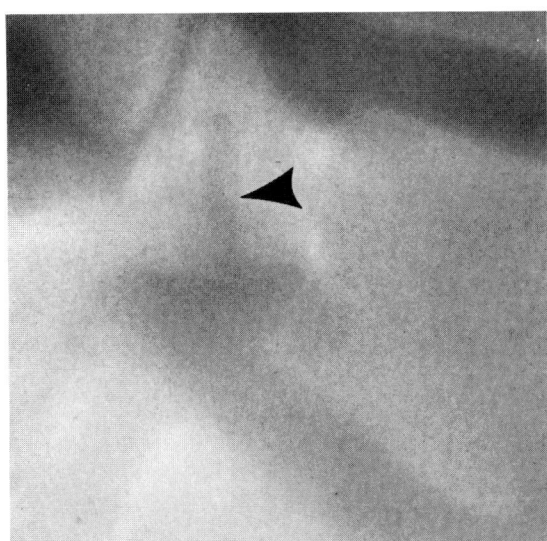

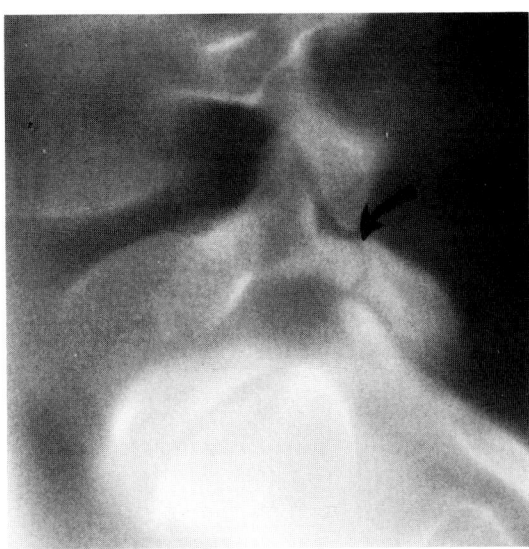

A

B

FIG. 4–155. A: Tomogram demonstrating an acute pedicle fracture entering the L5 facet (*arrow*). **B**: Tomogram with sclerosis of the pars at L5 due to a stress fracture (*curved arrow*).

useful for evaluating the bony structures and spinal cord (237,243,275,283).

Management of injuries to the thoracic and lumbar spine remains controversial. The goals of treatment are decompression of the neural elements and stabilization of the spine. Decompression can usually be achieved by realignment of the spinal canal. Postural realignment followed by prolonged recumbency has been favored by European spinal cord injury centers (214). In the United States, on the other hand, early surgical intervention (234,260,279,280) and spinal instrumentation have been preferred. Although no hard data are yet available comparing the results of nonoperative and operative treatment methods, evidence is accumulating that shows superior results with properly executed operative techniques that achieve decompression and stabilization simultaneously.

Decompression is often achieved by simple realignment using Harrington rod instrumentation, but with specific injuries such realignment may require removal of bony fragments from the spinal canal. Preoperative assessment of the spinal canal compromise can be accomplished using computed tomography with intrathecal contrast medium or with MRI (Fig. 4-156). Decompression can be carried out through a posterolateral approach or, more commonly, through an anterior approach. In either instance, it needs to be combined with stabilization and bone grafting.

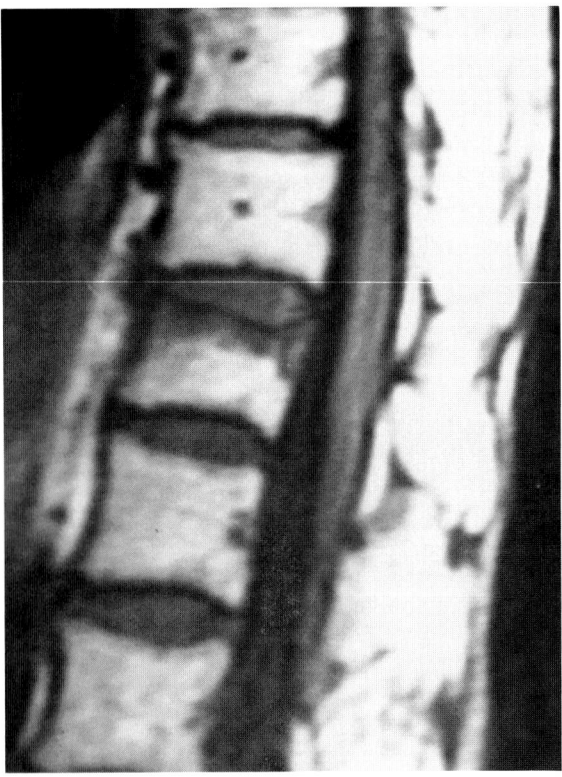

FIG. 4-156. Sagittal SE 500/20 MR image shows a lower thoracic fracture with normal spinal cord.

It is now well established that decompressive laminectomies for spinal trauma are seldom indicated (231,274). Neurologic deterioration and laminar fractures have been reported after laminectomy. Also, an increased incidence of kyphosis following laminectomy has been reported, along with chronic spinal instability. Laminectomy for trauma offers no advantages and many risks.

There are many questions at the moment that require answers. For example, the correlation between neural canal compromise as seen on CT scan and its effects on neurologic recovery is not clear (277). There is emerging evidence, however, that indicates that canal decompression correlates with neurologic recovery. Other questions that need answers concern the type of instrumentation to be utilized, the length of the instrumentation, the length of bony fusion necessary in healing, and the need for urgent (as opposed to delayed) surgical intervention. These questions are a focus of current research efforts that may offer answers in the near future.

Management of Specific Injuries

Flexion Injuries

Compression Fractures

Simple compression fractures require little treatment. Usually they are stable injuries, since the posterior elements are intact, and there is no neurologic deficit. In the elderly osteoporotic patient, the use of a corset or other similar orthosis is advisable.

Severe compression fractures involving more than 50% of the vertical dimension of the vertebral body or multiple contiguous compression fractures should be managed in a hyperextension cast or orthosis for a prolonged period of time. If significant kyphosis is present, Harrington distraction instrumentation and a spinal fusion might be the treatment of choice. Neglected injuries of this type can often be very painful and may require combined anterior and posterior procedures for treatment (Fig. 4-157).

Flexion-Distraction Injuries

These injuries occur more commonly in the thoracolumbar junction or in the upper lumbar spine. If the injury has occurred through the bony elements (Chance fracture), management with a hyperextension body cast usually suffices. However, if a fracture-dislocation has occurred that primarily involves the disk and posterior ligamentous complex (Fig. 4-158A and B), open reduction and internal fixation of the level involved combined with bone grafting are necessary (Fig. 4-154C and D).

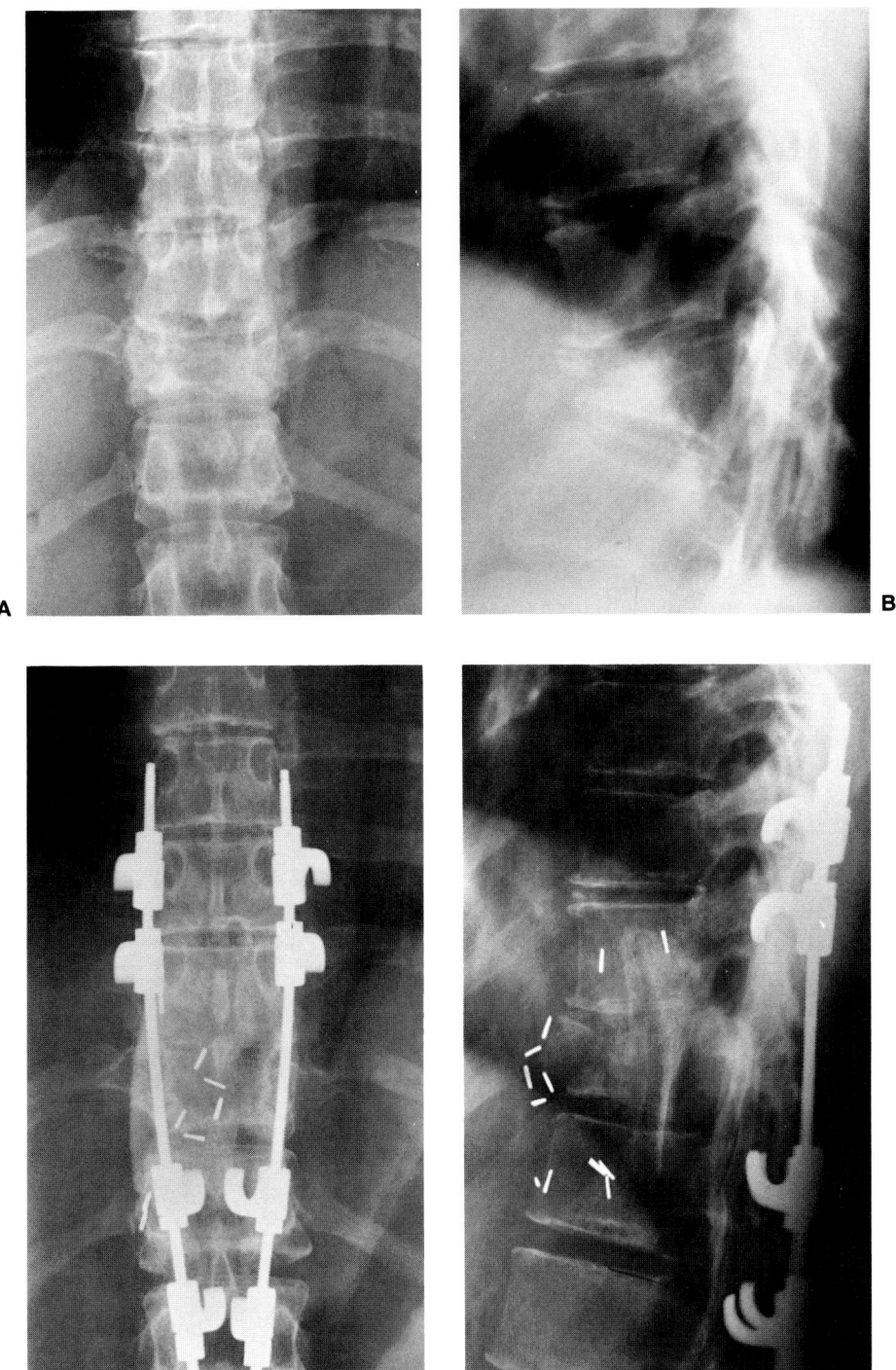

FIG. 4–157. Anteroposterior (**A**) and lateral (**B**) roentgenograms of the thoracic spine of a 33-year-old female involved in a motor vehicle accident. Injury is now five months old. The patient is having significant pain, but no neurologic deficits. Because of significant pain, the patient required surgical management. As a first stage an anterior correction of the kyphosis with anterior interbody fusion was undertaken. This was followed by a second stage of posterior decompression, Harrington rod instrumentation and fusion. Anteroposterior (**C**) and lateral (**D**) roentgenograms obtained three months after injury. The patient has minimal symptoms.

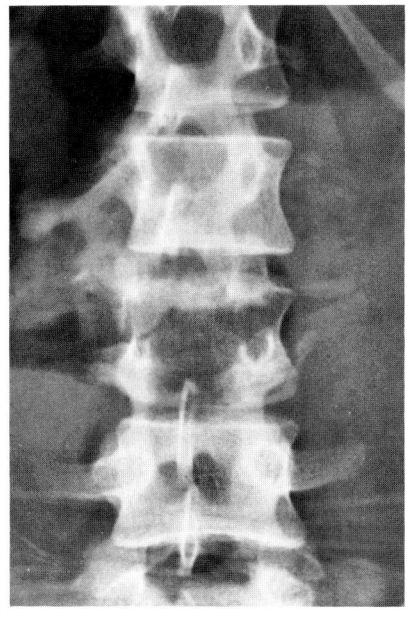
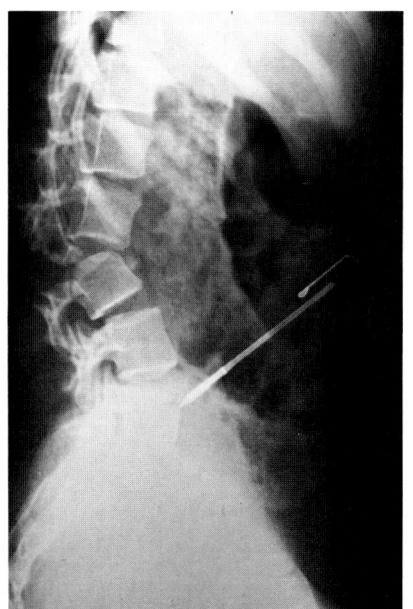
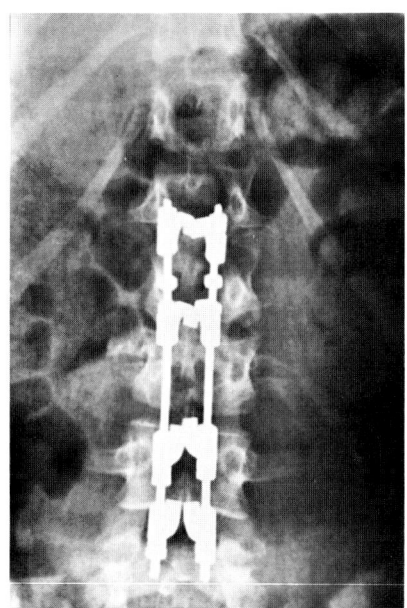
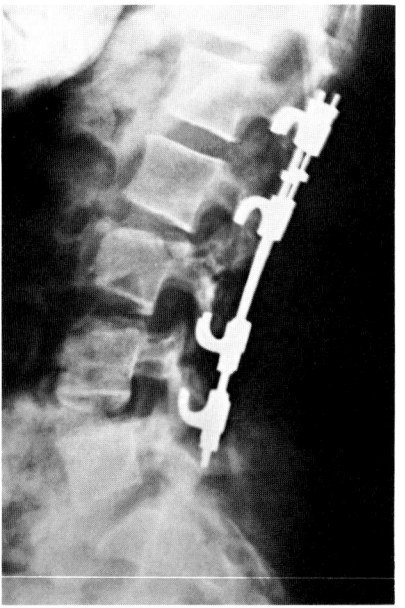

FIG. 4-158. Anteroposterior (**A**) and lateral (**B**) roentgenograms of the lumbar spine of a 14-year-old girl involved in a motor vehicle accident. Note the complete ligamentous disruption both anteriorly and posteriorly with significant separation of the spinous processes and disruption of both columns of the spine. No neurological deficit. Anteroposterior (**C**) and lateral (**D**) roentgenograms obtained one month after open reduction and internal fixation of the previous lesion, utilizing compression Harrington instrumentation. The patient has remained asymptomatic.

Flexion-Rotation Injuries

These very unstable lesions occur almost exclusively at the thoracolumbar junction—a transitional area between the fixed thoracic spine and the more mobile lumbar segments (Fig. 4-159A and D). The typical, very unstable slice fracture-dislocation often associated with neurologic deficit requires spinal instrumentation and spinal fusion (Fig. 4-159E and F). Surgery here may not assist neurologic recovery but serves to stabilize the spine and allow early rehabilitation.

The quality of the reduction should be assessed both by conventional radiographs and CT (Fig. 4-159G and H) (255,286). Recent evidence indicates that the reduc-

tion of the spinal canal improves significantly with early surgical intervention (260,285).

Bursting Fractures

The results of a vertical compression mechanism, bursting fractures can be stable if no damage to the posterior elements occurs. However, quite often an associated element of rotation produces fractures through the laminae, rendering these injuries unstable (Fig. 4-160). Neurologic compromise occurs frequently, and even in those injuries that do not initially produce neurologic deficits, late neurologic changes have been reported with a fre-

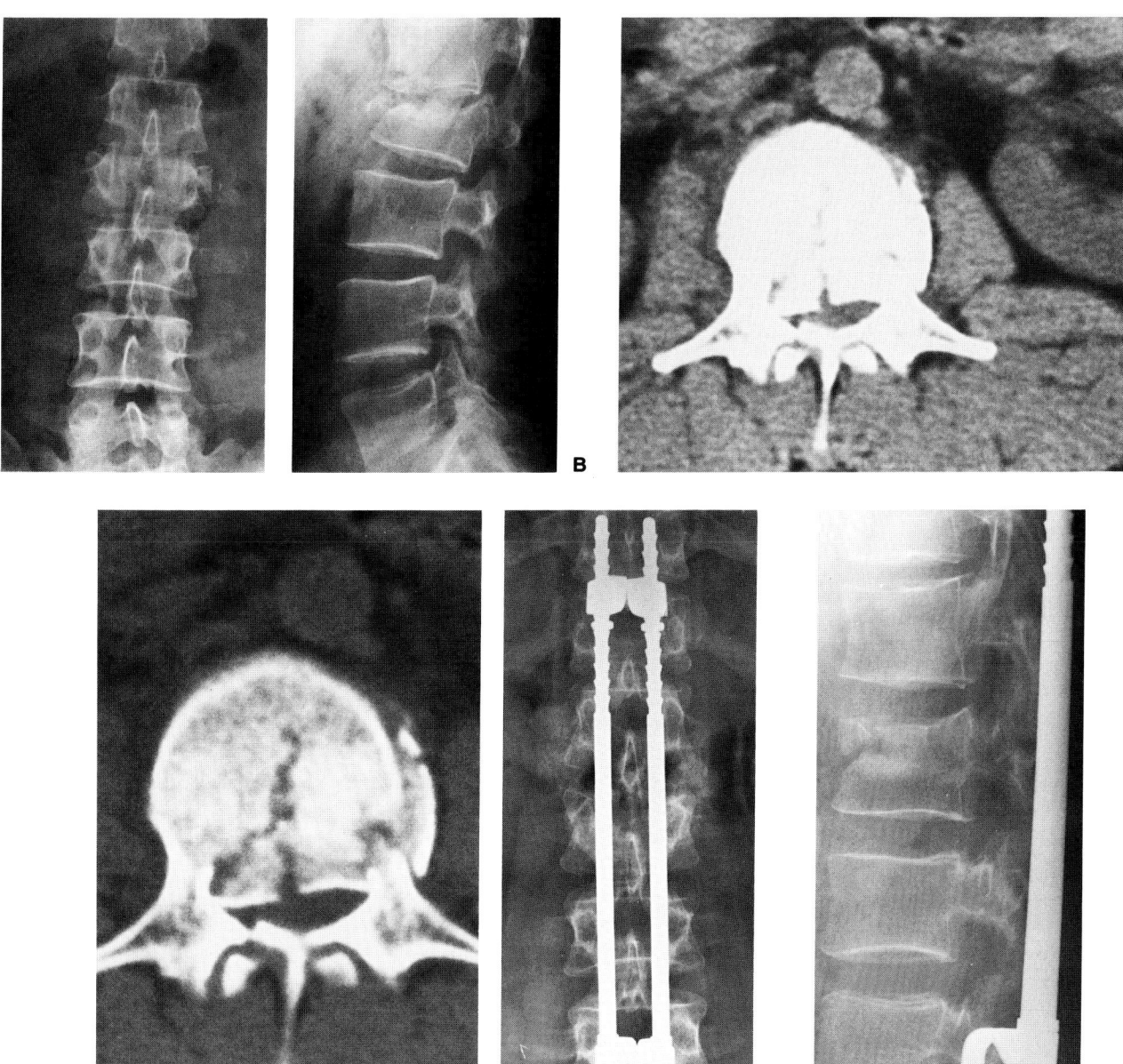

FIG. 4–159. Anteroposterior (**A**) and lateral (**B**) roentgenograms of the lumbar spine of a 38-year-old male with a typical slice fracture-dislocation of L1 on L2. Preoperative CT scans (**C, D**) at the level of the injury on the same patient. Note the significant compromise of the spinal canal. Anteroposterior (**E**) and lateral (**F**) roentgenograms of the same patient after realignment of the spinal canal and reduction of the fracture-dislocation with Harrington distraction instrumentation. Minimal neurological deficit present pre-operatively has recovered. Postoperative CT scan (**G, H**), confirming the quality of the decompression of the canal.

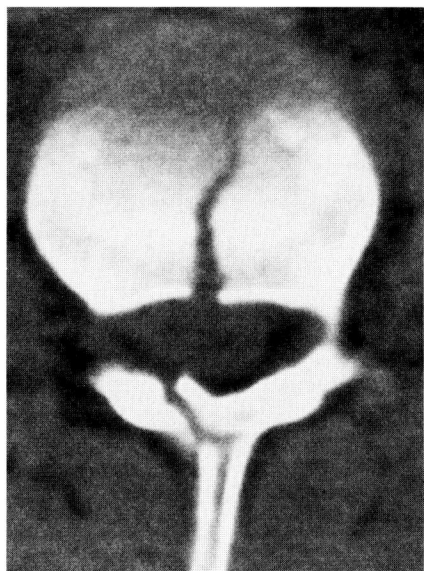

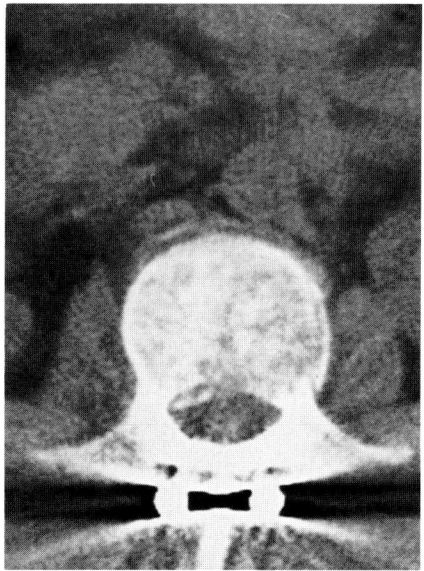

(FIG. 4-159. *Continued.*)

quency of about 20%. CT scanning is the technique of choice both to evaluate the initial degree of spinal canal compromise (Fig. 4-160C and D) and to assess the degree of canal decompression achieved by treatment (Fig. 4-160E). Metal artifact can be significant (Fig. 4-160E), and in these situations MRI may be more useful than CT. In our experience, artifacts from nonferromagnetic materials occur less often with MRI than with CT, especially at lower field strengths.

The treatment of these injuries remains controversial. If no neurologic deficit is present, and, if the degree of canal compromise is moderate, conservative treatment with external immobilization (a body cast) is justified (231). Careful follow up, however, is essential. For those injuries that have significant canal compromise or are associated with neurologic deficit, surgical decompression is the treatment of choice. Some authors prefer anterior decompression followed by anterior interbody fusion (287). Others prefer posterior instrumentation utilizing Harrington distraction rods (Fig. 4-160F and G) followed by postoperative assessment of the decompression achieved and, if necessary, a late anterior decompression and fusion (231). Regardless, postoperative support with a body cast or a thoracolumbosacral orthosis is necessary until evidence of bony healing is present radiologically.

Shear Injuries

These injuries occur primarily in the thoracic spine and usually result in complete disruption of both anterior and posterior elements. Also, severe neurologic deficit is usually present (Fig. 4-161). In addition, associated injury to the intrathoracic structures (for example, aorta, vena cava, esophagus) is common, and the treatment of the associated injuries can delay treatment of the spine and spinal cord injury.

Because of the stabilizing effect of the rib cage, some of these injuries can be treated conservatively; healing will occur even with rather marked translational deformities (Fig. 4-161B). The tendency, however, is to stabilize these injuries with rigid internal fixation by means of Harrington rod instrumentation and sublaminar wires (Fig. 4-162).

The object of treatment in thoracic and lumbar injuries, as in the case of cervical injuries, is to restore the dimensions of the spinal canal in order to achieve neural decompression and to stabilize the spine. It appears evident today that this can be achieved more expeditiously utilizing surgical means. This technique allows the added advantages of a shortened hospital stay and a more prompt and easier rehabilitation.

Radiographic Evaluation of Fusion Complications

Imaging of the postoperative spine has been attempted with routine radiographs, tomography, CT, MRI, and radionuclide studies (235,237,275,283). Problems occur due to metal and its adverse affect on image quality. However, one should be aware of the common complications and attempt to use the imaging technique best suited for evaluation (Table 4-21) (235,260,274).

One should always have routine radiographs initially to determine whether the appliances are the actual cause of the patient's symptoms (Fig. 4-163). CT and MRI are especially useful for evaluating the spinal cord and canal.

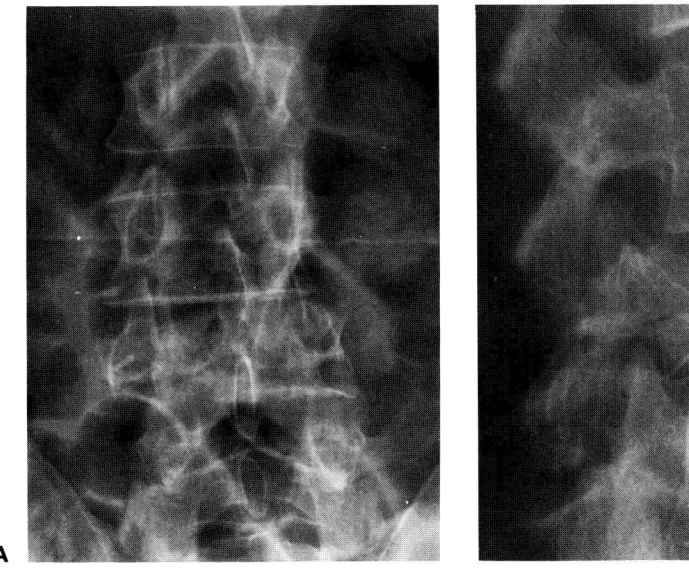

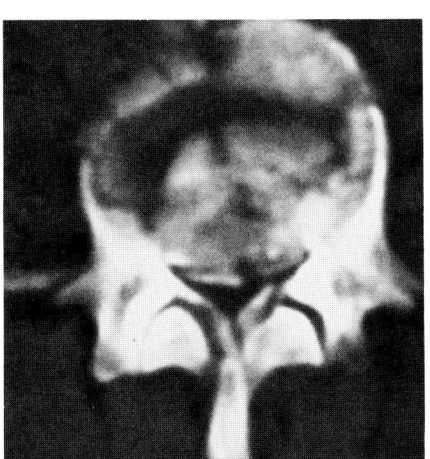

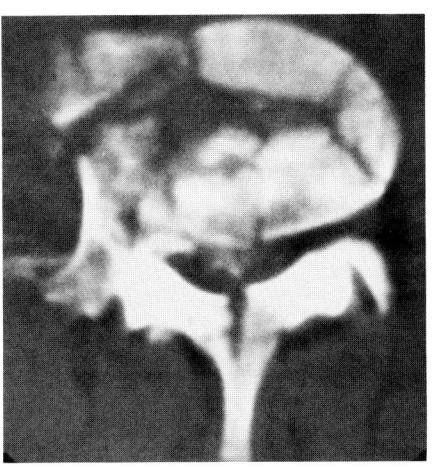

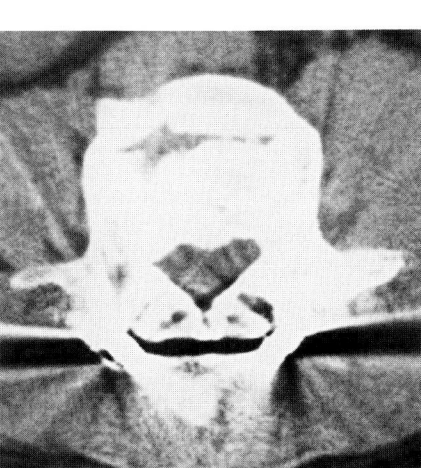

FIG. 4–160. Anteroposterior (**A**) and lateral (**B**) roentgenograms of the lumbar spine of a 40-year-old male who sustained this burst fracture of L4 in a parachuting accident. The patient has significant cauda equina compression. CT images (**C, D**) of the same patient, confirming both the canal compromise as well as the fracture through the posterior elements that render this injury unstable. Postoperative CT image (**E**) obtained one year after posterior instrumentation on the same patient. Note the quality of the decompression achieved of the spinal canal. One year postoperative roentgenograms of the lumbar spine (**F, G**) of the same patient after distraction Harrington instrumentation achieved realignment of the spinal and decompression of the spinal canal. Patient has had a satisfactory clinical recovery. Lateral tomograms of the same patient obtained one year after injury: (**H**) is obtained through the right of the vertebral body; (**I**) is through the left of the vertebral body. When comparing these with the CT image (**E**), one can see that union has not occurred on the right of the vertebral body but is firm on the left. Anteroposterior (**J**) and lateral (**K**) radiographs of the same patient obtained one-and-a-half years after injury after removal of the Harrington instrumentation. Note the posterolateral bone grafting that accompanied the decompression.

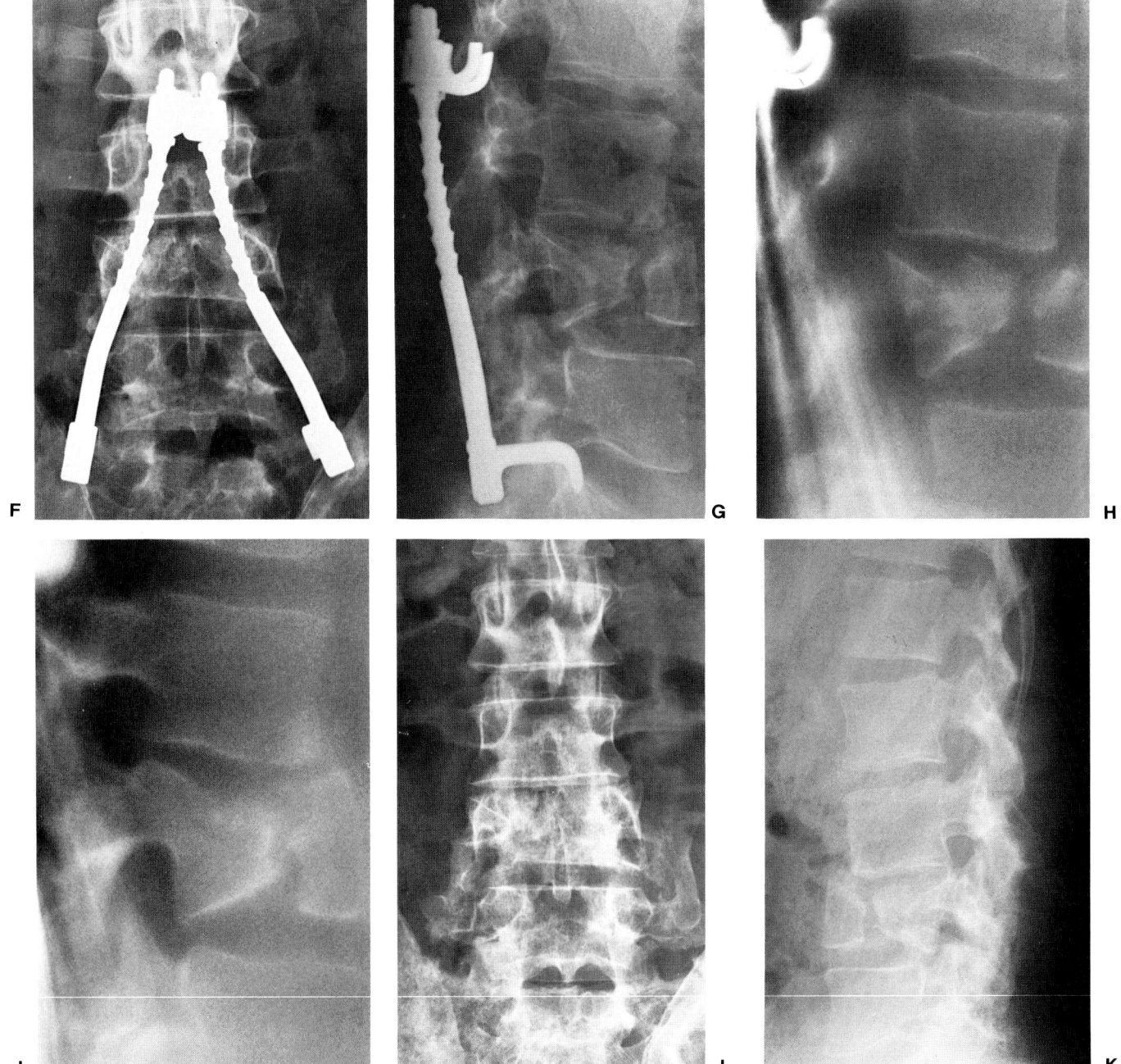

F

G

H

I

J

K

(**FIG. 4–160.** *Continued.*)

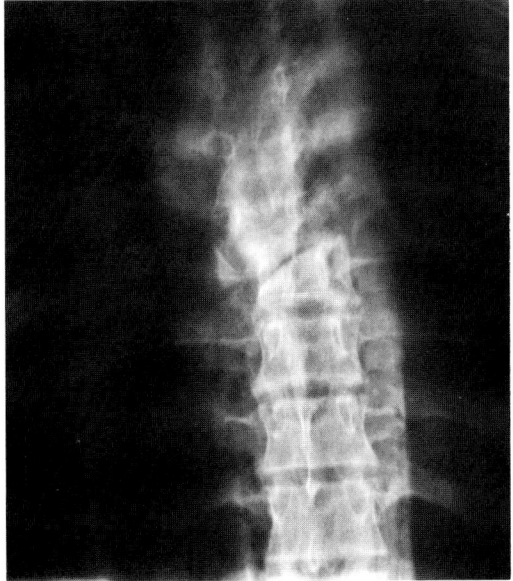
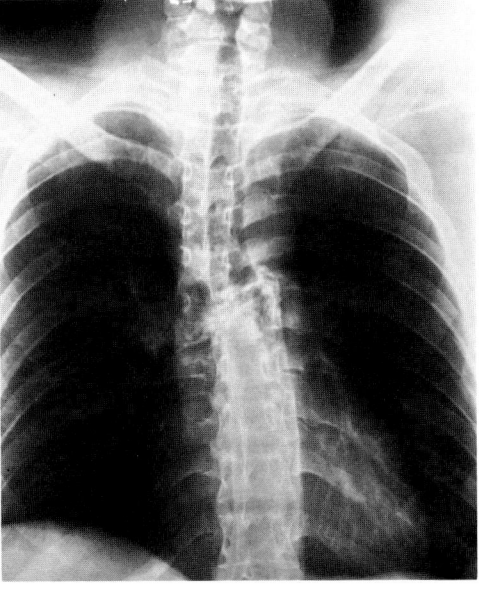

FIG. 4–161. A: AP radiograph of the thoracic spine of a 22-year-old male involved in a car-train collision. Complete neurological deficit is present at the level of T9. In addition there was an associated tear of the thoracic aorta. **B**: Radiograph of the thoracic spine of the same patient three months after admission. The patient had been treated with recumbency for six weeks followed by simple immobilization with a brace. Note complete healing of the injury with significant deformity, which causes no discomfort.

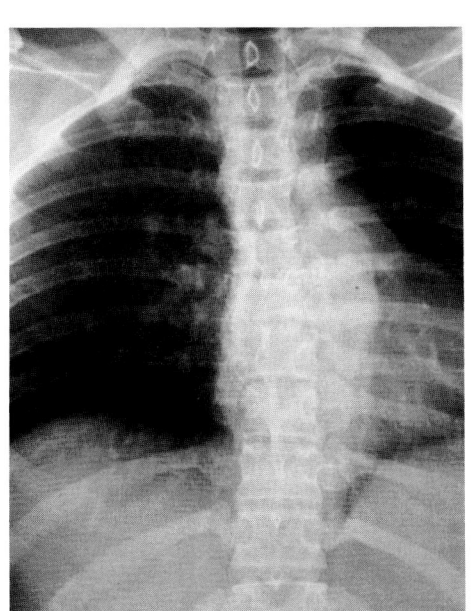
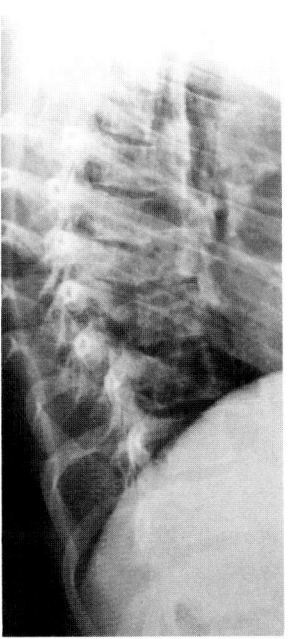
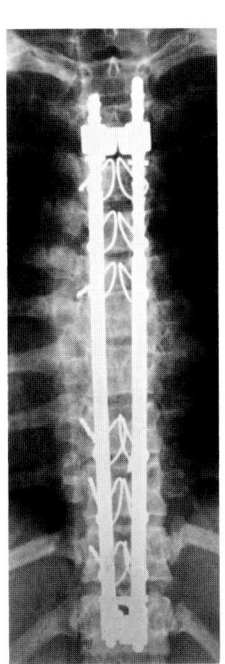
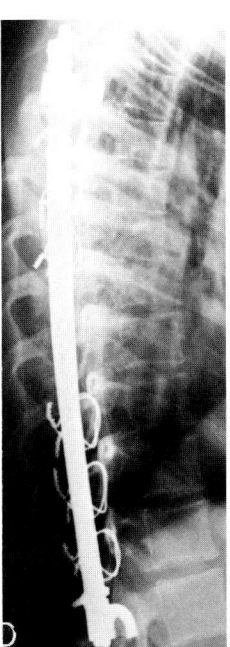

FIG. 4–162. Anteroposterior (**A**) and lateral (**B**) radiographs of the thoracic spine of a 27-year-old female involved in an automobile accident. Complete paraplegia at the level of T6 is present. Note complete dislocation of T6 on T7. AP (**C**) and lateral (**D**) views after internal fixation.

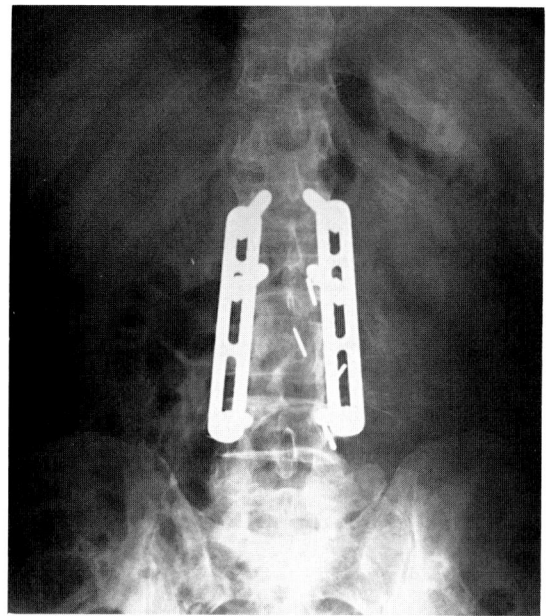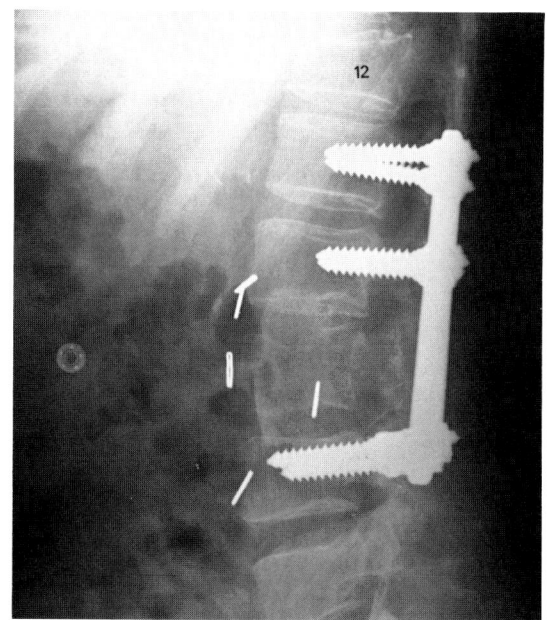

A   B

FIG. 4-163. AP (**A**) and lateral (**B**) views follow Steffee Plate and screw fixation of an L3 burst fracture. The appliances are in good position and the alignment is normal. However, a compression fracture of T12 has developed since the surgery.

Although artifact due to metal may be significant (Fig. 4-160E), on occasion it does not effect the area being evaluated (Fig. 4-159H). Theoretically, MRI should be useful in evaluating bony, versus fibrous, or non-union. High signal intensity should be evident on T2-weighted images if a non-union or pseudarthrosis is present. Conventional AP and lateral tomograms may be sufficient in more obvious cases (Fig. 4-164).

SPONDYLOLYSIS AND SPONDYLOLISTHESIS

Spondylolysis is a defect in the pars interarticularis. The defect is usually bilateral (74%) and occurs in 5–7.2% of the general population (302,312). In patients with low back pain, the incidence is increased to approximately 10% (302). The incidence of spondylolysis increases with age and is more common in whites than in blacks. There is also a strong familial tendency (312).

TABLE 4-21. *Imaging of the spine: Complications following treatment*[a]

Complication	Imaging technique
Infection	Gallium-67 or Indium-111 MRI[b]
Loss of fixation	Routine radiographs
Rod fracture	Fluoroscopy
Hook dislodgment	Fluoroscopy
Pseudarthrosis	MRI, tomography, CT
Neurologic deterioration	CT, MRI
Kyphotic deformity	Lateral tomograms, MRI
Vertebral distraction	Lateral tomograms

[a] (235,260).
[b] Metal may interfere with image quality.

Individuals in certain professions, such as football linemen and weight lifters, also demonstrate an increased incidence of spondylolysis (290,297,302). The defect is most commonly noted at the L5 (67%) and L4 (10%) levels. Congenital spinous process defects are encountered 5 to 10 times more commonly in patients with spondylolysis (290).

Spondylolisthesis is anterior slippage or subluxation of the vertebral body. This is most commonly related to spondylolysis but may also be present without a true interruption of the pars interarticularis.

Many theories have been formulated in an attempt to define the etiology of spondylolysis (Table 4-22). The suggestion that this may be congenital has been widely disputed and most clearly discussed by Newman and Stone (305). Evidence against the congenital theory includes the following: (1) the defect has never been found in a fetus or stillborn, (2) the incidence increases with age and is rarely noted in infants prior to walking, and (3) the defect occasionally heals (291,304). Others have suggested various acquired etiologies (Table 4-22) (303,306,

TABLE 4-22. *Spondylolysis: Etiologic theories*

Separate ossification centers
Postnatal fractures
Exaggerated lordosis
Weak supporting structures
Dysplasia
Birth fracture
Stress fracture
Articular facet impingement
Pathologic fractures

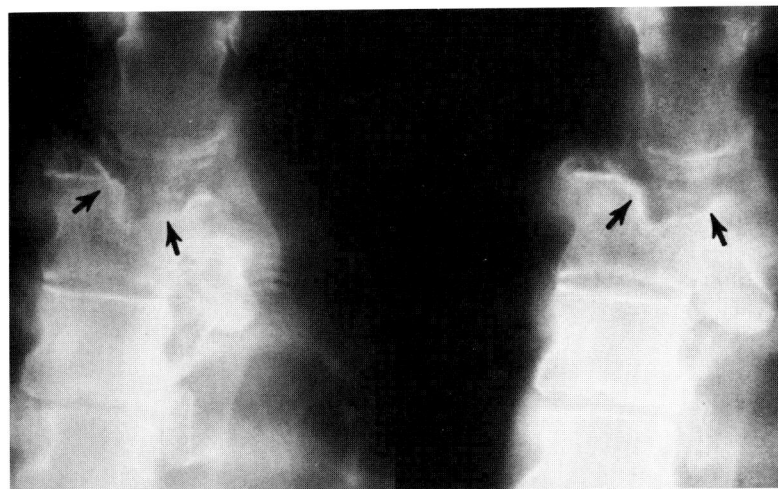

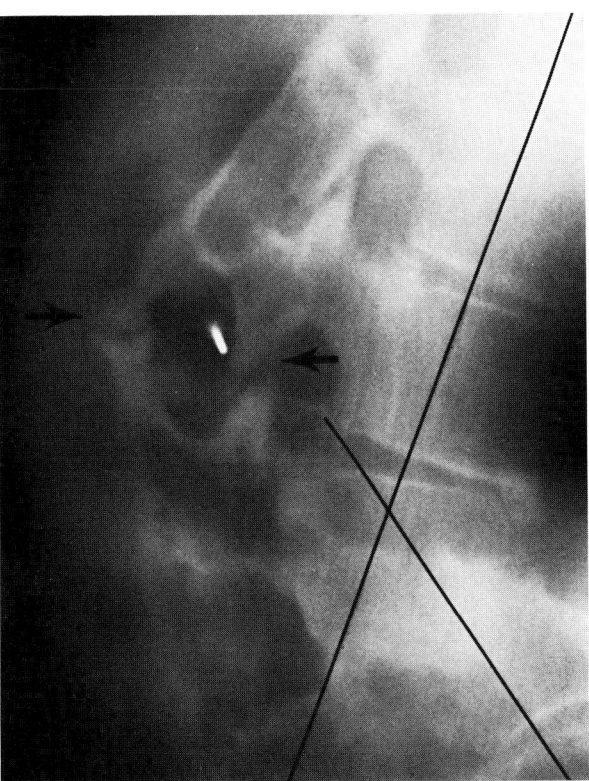

FIG. 4-164. AP (**A**) and lateral (**B**) tomograms after thoracic fusion. There is considerable kyphotic deformity with pseudarthrosis (*arrow*).

308,309). Most authors agree, however, that the defect is due to a combination of (1) an hereditary defect in the cartilage model of the arch and (2) the strain placed on the lower back due to upright posture and lumbar lordosis (290,310,312).

Spondylolisthesis may result from causes other than spondylolysis, such as degenerative facet disease, changes in the facet angles, or degenerative disk disease (293,305,310). Table 4-23, based on the work of Wiltse, Newman, and MacNab (299) summarizes the possible etiologies of spondylolisthesis. Spondylolisthesis of the nonspondylolytic variety usually occurs in patients over 50 years of age and is five times more common in females than in males. The location of the level also differs,

being more common at the L4-5 level (80%). Multiple levels are involved in 5% of patients, with the degree of slippage rarely exceeding 30% (290,309). The incidence of neurologic involvement in degenerative spondylo-

TABLE 4-23. *Spondylolisthesis: Etiology*

Upper sacral dysplasia
Degenerative changes
Pathologic fractures
Pars defects
Acute fractures
Stress fractures
Elongated pars
Posterior arch fractures

listhesis is also higher than in spondylolytic spondylo-listhesis. Rosenberg noted neurologic complications in 30% of patients in this category (307).

Patients with spondylolysis and spondylolisthesis may be asymptomatic. This is especially common in children, where up to 50% of cases are noted incidentally (298). Symptomatic patients usually present with a low back pain that may radiate into the legs or buttock. On physical examination an exaggerated lumbar lordotic curve and occasionally a dimple may be evident, if the changes are advanced (290).

Radiographic evaluation is usually complete with the AP, lateral, coned-down lateral, and oblique views (289,290). Angling the tube 30° to the head on the AP view may also assist in demonstrating the pars defect (290). Motion views are also useful in evaluating stability (294). Findings on the AP view include sclerosis of the opposite pedicle if the lesion is unilateral (296), and foreshortening of the spine in cases of advanced spondylolisthesis (Figs. 4-165 and 4-166). The lateral view is usually best for detection of the pars defects, adjacent sclerosis, and the often associated degenerative disk disease (Fig. 4-167). The degree of subluxation is usually graded according to the system established by Meyerding (301). The vertical body is divided into four equal segments from anterior to posterior, and the degree of slippage is graded I through IV according to these measurements (Fig. 4-168). In nonspondylolytic spondylolisthesis the defect is most commonly at the L4-L5 level, and the degree of associated degenerative change is obvious on the lateral view (Fig. 4-168). The lumbosacral angle is also decreased in these patients compared with patients with spondylolytic spondylolisthesis. In normal patients, this angle measures approximately 34°. In patients with nonspondylolytic spondylolisthesis, the angle is about 20°, and if spondylolysis is present the angle is increased to about 60° (290). Oblique views are often confirmatory and increase one's confidence in detecting pars defects (Fig. 4-166). The facet joints are also seen to better advantage (Fig. 4-166).

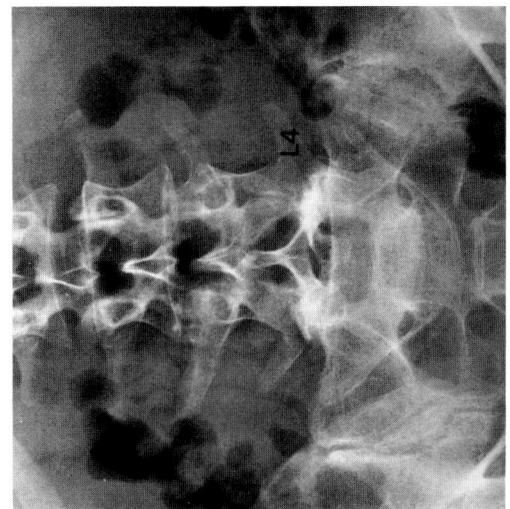

A

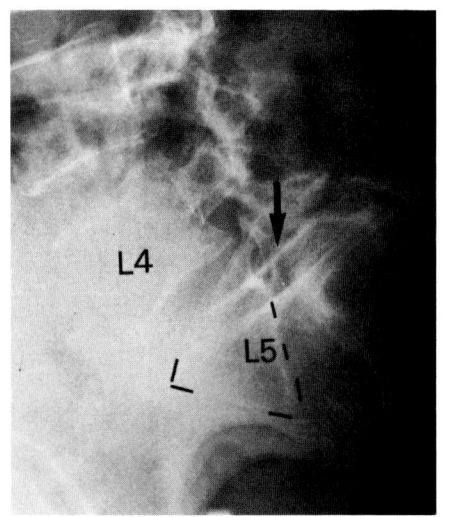

B

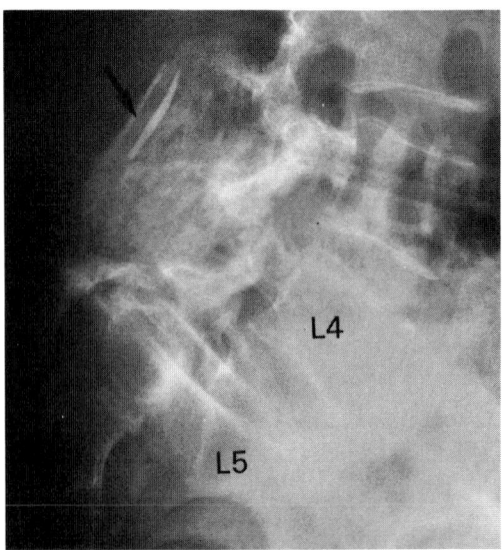

C

FIG. 4–165. Spondylolysis with complete dislocation of L5 on S1. There is foreshortening of the lumbar spine on the AP view (A). Only 4 lumbar vertebrae are seen. The degree of displacement is best seen on the lateral view (B). The patient was treated with bone graft fusion from L3 to the sacrum (C).

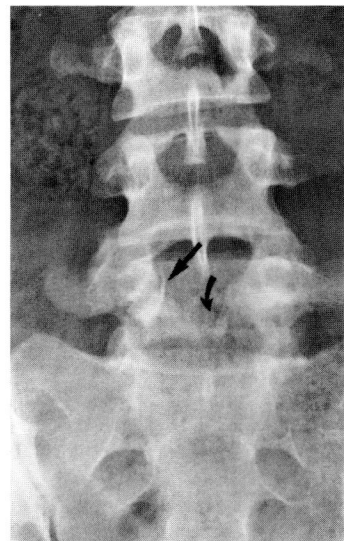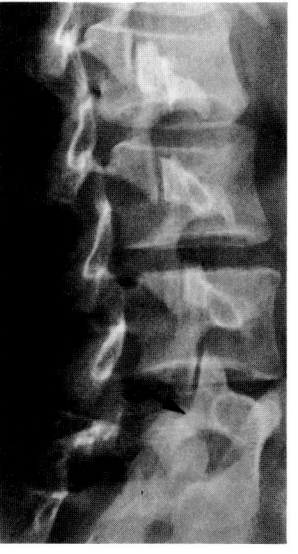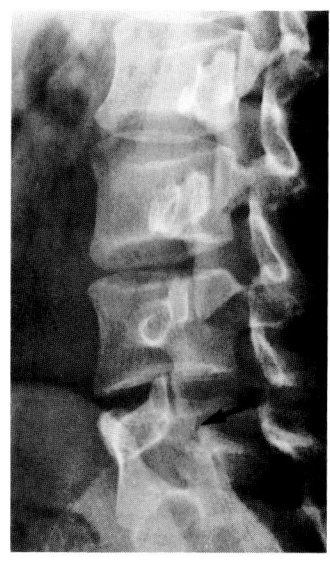

A   B   C

FIG. 4–166. Pars defect at L5 on the right. The AP view (**A**) demonstrates spina bifida at L5 with sclerosis of the right pedicle. The left oblique (**B**) shows sclerosis and elongation of the pars. The right oblique (**C**) demonstrates that the L5-S1 facet "steps back" due to a pars defect at L5.

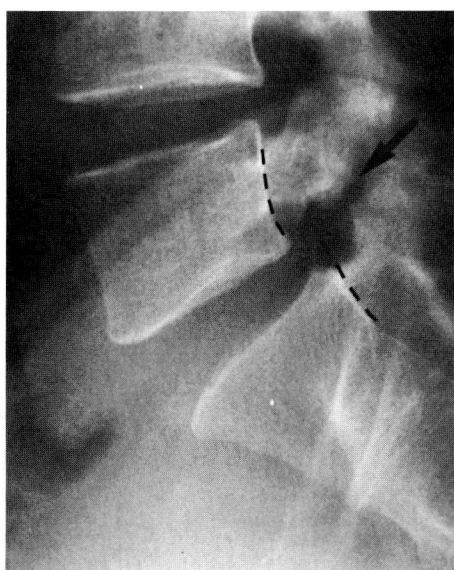

FIG. 4–167. Coned lateral view of the lumbar spine demonstrating a pars defect at L5 (*arrow*) with slight subluxation of L5 on S1.

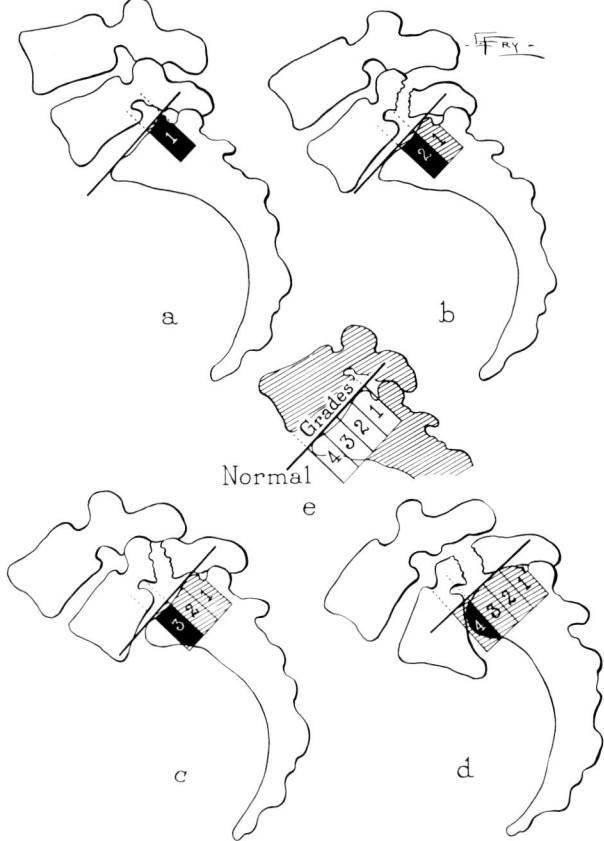

FIG. 4–168. Illustration of grading system for spondylolisthesis. a, Grade 1; b, Grade 2; c, Grade 3; d, Grade 4; e, Normal. (From Meyerding HW. Spondylolisthesis. *Surg Gyn Obst* 1932;54:371–377, with permission.)

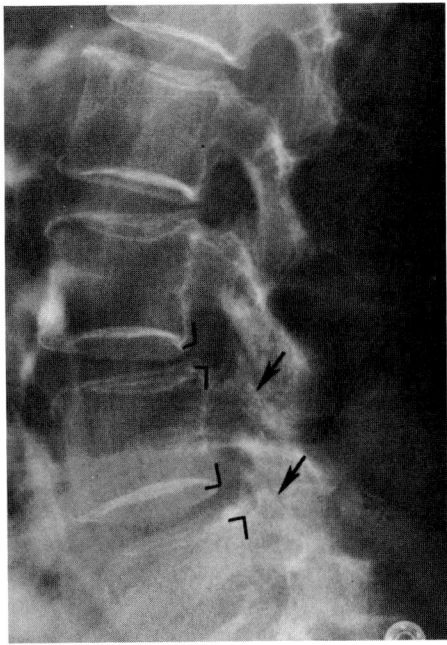

FIG. 4-169. Lateral view of the lumbar spine. There are degenerative changes in the facet joints (*arrows*) with subluxation of L4 on L5 and L3 on L4. No pars defects.

Tomography is frequently of value in studying spondylolysis and other defects in the posterior arch (Fig. 4-170). Computed tomography may be helpful in selected cases but can also present a confusing picture. Because of their alignment, the facet joints may be confused with a pars defect. A vacuum sign has been described in the facet joints in patients with degenerative spondylolisthesis (292). Conventional myelography or CT studies with metrizamide may be useful in patients with evidence of neurologic involvement (290,302).

Posterior displacement of the vertebral body may also occur (retrolisthesis) (290,302). This entity is commonly seen with degenerative disk disease (291). The incidence in the general population is 4.7%, which is about the same as that of spondylolysis (300). There is a tendency for retrolisthesis to occur in the upper lumbar region, especially L2, as well as in the cervical spine. Most of the features are evident on the lateral view and have been well summarized by Melamed (300). Degenerative disk changes, abnormal lordosis, narrowing of the intervertebral foramina, prominent spinous processes, and facet joint abnormalities are usually present (300).

Treatment of Spondylolysis and Spondylolisthesis

Most patients with spondylolysis have few or no symptoms and require only conservative treatment.

If symptoms are significant and especially if they are associated with neurologic signs of root irritation or cauda equina claudication, surgical treatment is justified. Spondylolysis of L5 or grades I and II spondylolisthesis can be managed successfully with posterolateral L5-S1 fusion when low back pain is the only presenting complaint, or with removal of the posterior loose element of L5 and posterolateral fusion when leg pain is also a problem; in the latter instance, decompression of the involved root (usually the L5 or S1 root) may require a rather extensive bony removal on the involved side.

Grades III and IV spondylolisthesis require more extensive surgical procedures. Posterior decompression combined with L4-S1 lateral mass fusion is the procedure of choice. Attempts to effect reduction of the spondylolisthesis have, by and large, been unsuccessful, but in severe spondylolisthesis anterior and posterior procedures may be necessary.

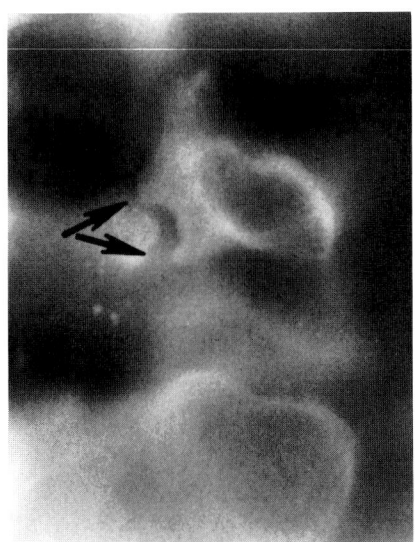

A

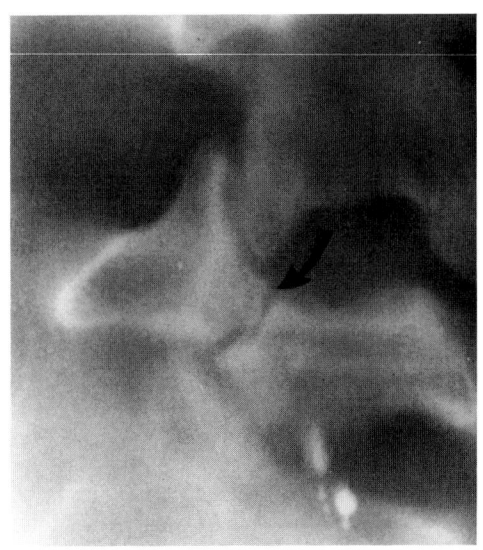

B

FIG. 4-170. Oblique tomograms (**A, B**) demonstrating bilateral pars defects at L5. CT scans demonstrating bilateral pars defects at L5.

Evaluation of the mechanical success of the fusion procedure requires flexion and extension lateral radiographs of the lower lumbar spine. Right and left side-bending views have also been utilized but are difficult to interpret.

Degenerative spondylolisthesis occurs more commonly, as noted, at the L4-L5 interspace. If associated with symptoms of spinal stenosis, posterior decompression and lateral mass fusion of the L4-L5 space is indicated. If posterior decompression alone is carried out, further spondylolisthesis commonly will be observed.

Even when a lateral mass fusion follows the decompression, further forward displacement occurs in the early postoperative period before the fusion becomes solid.

ANKYLOSING SPONDYLITIS

The radiographic and clinical features of ankylosing spondylitis are well described in the literature (314). The disease is most common in young males and typically effects the sacroiliac joints, thoracolumbar spine and

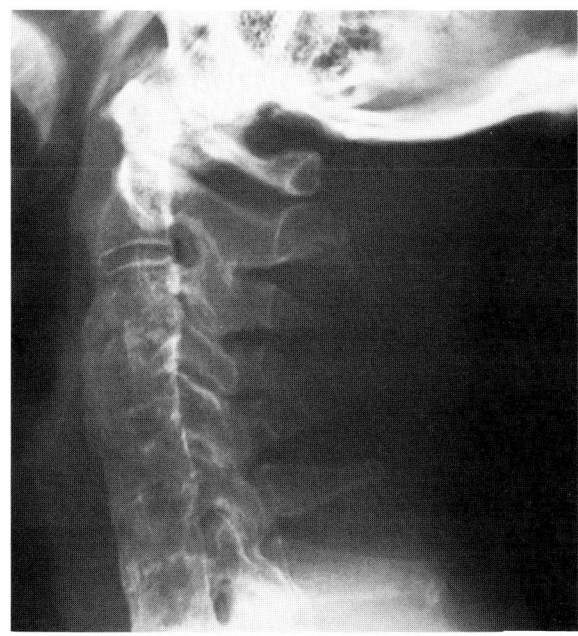
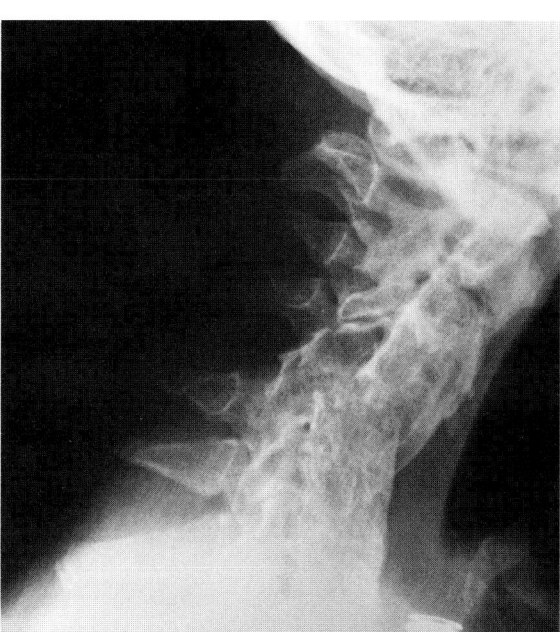
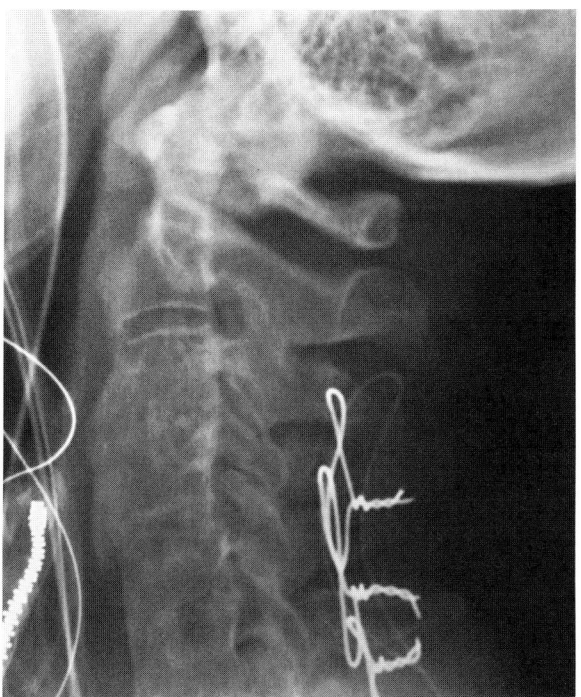

FIG. 4-171. Patient with longstanding ankylosing spondylitis. Lateral radiograph (A) demonstrates a slight defect at the C4-C5 interspace (arrow) anteriorly. The patient had experienced a minor fall. Several days later (B) the untreated injury is completed and obvious. Posterior fusion (C) reduced the angular deformity but not the quadriplegia.

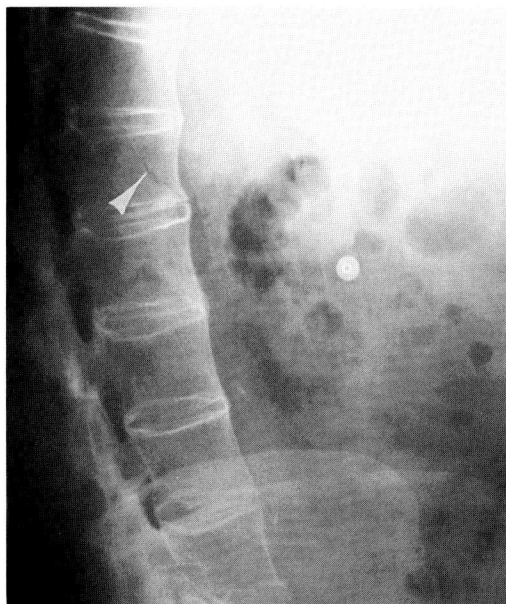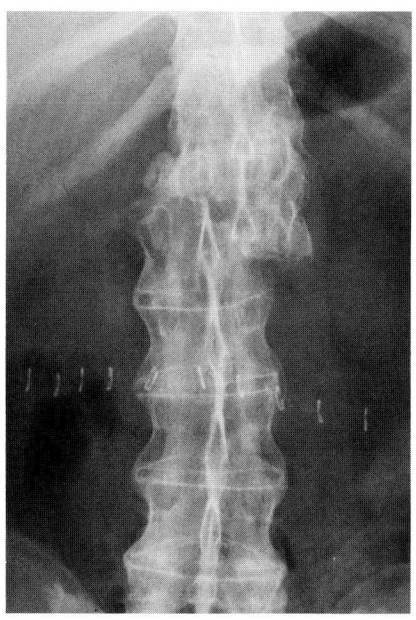

FIG. 4–172. Lateral view of the lumbar spine. The subtle fracture in L1 (*arrow*) was overlooked. Two weeks later (**B**) after minor trauma there is an obvious fracture dislocation at this level.

cervical spine in that order. This condition is mentioned here due to the frequency of overlooked fractures and the significant morbidity and mortality that result (313–316).

In our experience, over 50% of spine fractures are missed initially in this patient population. This is because of several factors. The main problem is that these fractures are often subtle (Figs. 4-171 and 4-172). Trauma is usually minor. In addition, the injuries are usually at the disk space level, which may be difficult to

evaluate when ligament ossification is segmental or incomplete.

Fractures occur most frequently in the lower cervical spine (Fig. 4-173). Patients with minor symptoms should be carefully evaluated to be certain that injuries are not overlooked. Simple tomography, in the lateral projection, is often more useful than CT in detecting these subtle injuries. In addition, the entire spine should be evaluated as multiple injuries are not uncommon.

When injuries are overlooked, significant neurologic

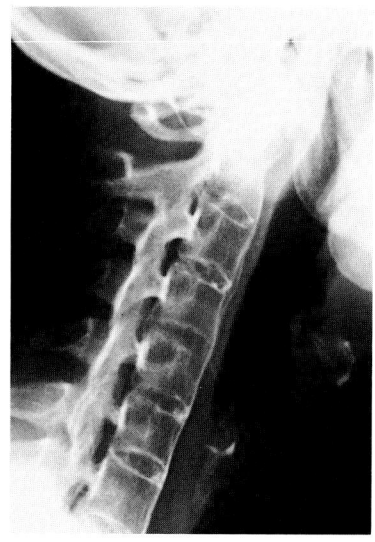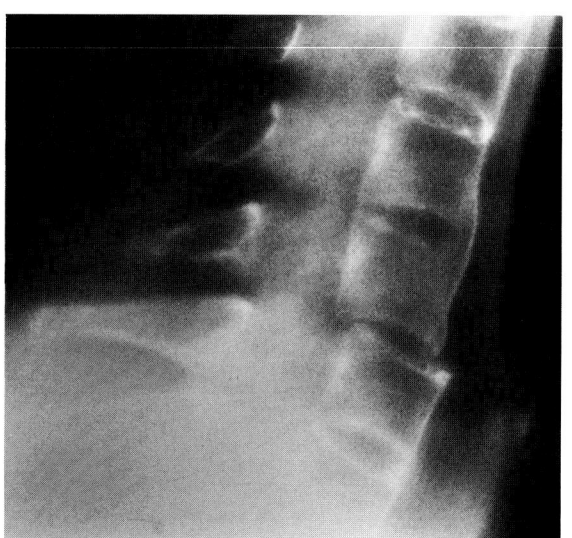

FIG. 4–173. Ankylosing spondylitis with normal alignment on the lateral view (**A**). Lateral tomogram (**B**) shows disruption through the C6-C7 interspace.

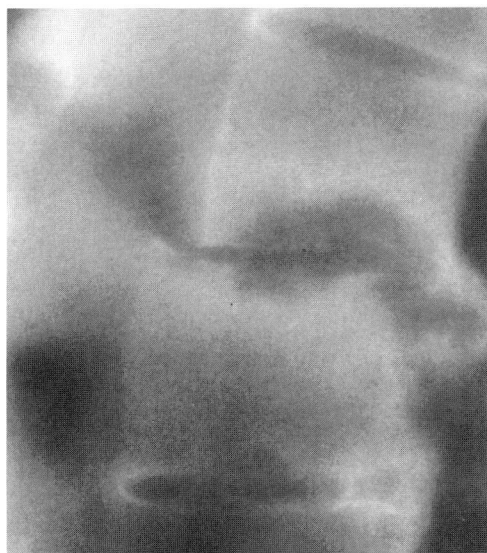

FIG. 4-174. Lateral tomogram demonstrating pseudarthrosis after fracture in a patient with ankylosing spondylitis.

damage can occur (314–316). Pseudarthrosis (Fig. 4-174) is not an uncommon complication of fractures in patients with ankylosing spondylitis.

REFERENCES

Anatomy

1. Christenson PC. The radiologic study of the normal spine. *Radiol Clin North Am* 1977;15:133–154.
2. Chusid JG. *Correlative neuroanatomy and functional neurology.* Los Altos, CA: Lange Publishers, 1970.
3. Gehweiler JA, Osborne RL, Becker RF. *The radiology of vertebral trauma.* Philadelphia: W. B. Saunders Co., 1980, pp. 3–88.
4. Goss CM. *Gray's anatomy of the human body.* Philadelphia: Lea and Febiger, 1973.
5. Hollinshead WH. *Anatomy for surgeons.* Vol. 3: *The back and the limbs,* 3rd ed. Philadelphia: Harper and Row Publishers, 1982.
6. Jablecki CK, Aguilo JJ, Piepgras DG, Zincke H, Goldstein NP. Paraparesis after renal transplantation. *Ann Neurol* 1977;2:154–155.
7. Janes JM, Hooshmand H. Severe extension-flexion injuries of the cervical spine. *Mayo Clin Proc* 1965;40:353–369.
8. Lee BCP, Kazam E, Newman AD. Computed tomography of the spine and spinal cord. *Radiology* 1978;128:95–102.
9. Vakili H. *The spinal cord.* New York: Intercontinental Medical Book Corp., 1967.
10. Wicke L. *Atlas of radiologic anatomy,* 3rd ed. Baltimore: Urban and Schwarzenberg, 1982.

Radiographic Evaluation of the Spinal Trauma

11. Abel MS. The exaggerated supine oblique view of the cervical spine. *Skel Radiol* 1982;8:213–219.
12. Abel MS, Teague JH. Unilateral lateral mass compression fractures of the axis. *Skel Radiol* 1979;4:92–98.
13. Acheson MB, Livingston RR, Richardson ML, Stimach GK. High-resolution CT scanning in the evaluation of cervical spine fractures: Comparison with plain film examinations. *AJR* 1987;148:1179–1185.
14. Angtieaco EJC, Binet EF. Radiology of thoracic and lumbar fractures. *Clin Orthop* 1984;189:43–57.
15. Axel L, Costantini J, Listerud J. Intensity correction in surface-coil MR imaging. *AJR* 1987;148:418–420.
16. Ballinger PW. *Merrill's atlas of radiographic positions and radiologic procedures,* 5th ed. St. Louis: C. V. Mosby Co., 1982.
17. Beers GJ, Raque GH, Wagner GG, et al. MR imaging in acute cervical spine trauma. *J Comput Assist Tomogr* 1988;12:755–761.
18. Bernau A, Berquist TH. *Orthopedic positioning in diagnostic radiology.* Baltimore: Urban and Schwartzenberg, 1983.
19. Berquist TH. Imaging of adult cervical spine trauma. *Radiographics* 1988;8:667–694.
20. Binet FF, Moro JJ, Marangola JP, Hodge CT. Cervical spine tomography in trauma. *Spine* 1977;2:163–172.
21. Brandt-Zawadzki M, Jeffrey RB, Minagi H, et al. High resolution CT of the thoracolumbar fractures. *Am J Neuroradiol* 1982;3:69–74.
22. Brandt-Zawadzki M, Miller EM, Federle MP. CT in evaluation of spine trauma. *AJR* 1981;136:369–375.
23. Cancelmo JJ. Clay shoveler's fracture. A helpful diagnostic sign. *AJR* 1972;115:540–543.
24. Cheshire DJE. The stability of the cervical spine following conservative treatment of fractures and fracture-dislocations. *Paraplegia* 1969;7:193–203.
25. Christenson PC. Radiographic study of the normal spine. *Radiol Clin North Am* 1977;15:133–154.
26. Daffner RH. *Imaging of vertebral trauma.* Rockville: Aspen Press, 1988.
27. Daffner RH, Deeb ZL, Goldberg AL, Kardabarow A, Rothfus WE. The radiologic assessment of post-traumatic vertebral instability. *Skel Radiol* 1990;19:103–108.
28. Daffner RH, Deeb ZL, Rothfus WE. The posterior vertebral line: Importance in detection of burst fractures. *AJR* 1987;148:93–96.
29. Daniels DL, Grogan JP, Johansen JE, Meyer GA, Williams AL, Haughton VM. Cervical radiculopathy: Computed tomography and myelography compared. *Radiology* 1984;151:109–113.
30. Dennis LN, Rogers LF. Superior mediastinal widening from spine fractures mimicking aortic rupture on chest radiographs. *AJR* 1989;152:27–30.
31. Dowart RH. Computed tomography of the lumbar spine: Techniques, normal anatomy, pitfalls, and clinical applications. *CRC-Gut Rev Diag Imag* 1984;22:1–42.
32. England AC, Shippel AH, Ray MJ. A simple view for demonstration of fractures of the anterior arch of C1. *AJR* 1985;144:763–764.
33. Engmann DR, Rubin JB. Cervical spine: MR imaging with a partial flip angle, gradient-refocused pulse sequence. *Radiology* 1988;166:467–472.
34. Fielding JW. Cineroentgenography of the normal cervical spine. *J Bone Joint Surg* 1957;39A:1280–1288.
35. Fielding JW, Stillwell WT, Chynn KY, et al. Use of CT for diagnosis of atlanto-axial rotary fixation. *J Bone Joint Surg* 1978;60B:1102–1104.
36. Flannigan BD, Lofkin RB, McGlade C, et al. MR imaging of the cervical spine: Neurovascular anatomy. *AJR* 1987;148:785–790.
37. Forsyth HF. Extension injuries of the cervical spine. *J Bone Joint Surg* 1964;46A:1792–1797.
38. Fuchs AW. Thoracic vertebrae. *Radiol Clin Photo* 1941;17:2.
39. Gebarrhi SS, Maynard FW, Gabrielson TO, Knake JE, Latack JT, Hoff JT. Post traumatic progressive myelopathy. *Radiology* 1985;157:379–385.
40. Gehweiler JA, Osborne RL, Becker RF. *The radiology of vertebral trauma.* Philadelphia: W. B. Saunders Co., 1980.
41. Gerlock AJ, Kirchner SG, Heller RM, et al. *The cervical spine in trauma.* Philadelphia: W. B. Saunders Co., 1978.
42. Goldberg AL, Rothfus WE, Deeb ZL, Frankel DG, Welberger JE, Daffner RH. Hyperextension injuries of the cervical spine. *Skel Radiol* 1989;18:283–288.
43. Goldberg AL, Rothfus WE, Deeb ZL, et al. The impact of magnetic resonance on the diagnostic evaluation of cervicothoracic trauma. *Skel Radiol* 1988;67:89–95.
44. Harris JH. Radiographic evaluation of spinal trauma. *Orthop Clin North Am* 1986;17:75–86.

45. Haughton VM. MR imaging of the spine. *Radiology* 1988;166:291–301.
46. Hohl M. Normal motions in the upper portion of the cervical spine. *J Bone Joint Surg* 1964;46A:1777–1779.
47. Karnaze MG, Gado MA, Sartor KJ, Hodges FJ, III: Comparison of MR and CT myelography in imaging the cervical and thoracic spine. *AJR* 1988;150:397–403.
48. Kaufman HH, Harris JH, Spencer JA, et al. Danger of traction radiography for cervical trauma. Letter to the editor. *JAMA* 1982;247:2369.
49. Keene JS, Goletz TH, Lilleas F, et al. Diagnosis of vertebral fracture: A comparison of conventional tomography, and computed-axial tomography. *J Bone Joint Surg* 1982;64A:586–594.
50. Kulkarni MV, Bondurant FJ, Rose SL, Narayama PA. 1.5 Tesla magnetic resonance imaging of the cervical spine. *Radiographics* 1988;8:1059–1082.
51. Kulkarni MV, McArdle CB, Kopanicky D, et al. Acute spinal cord injury: MR imaging at 1.5 T. *Radiology* 1987;164:837–843.
52. Lauridsen KN, DeCarvalho A, Andersen AH. Degree of vertebral wedging of the dorsolumbar spine. *Acta Radiol Diagn* 1984;25:29–32.
53. Lewis CA, Castillo M, Hudgins PA. Cervical prevertebral fat stripe: A normal variant simulating prevertebral hemorrhage. *AJR* 1990;155:559–560.
54. Marar BC. Fracture of the axis arch: Hangman's fracture. *Clin Orthop* 1975;106:155–165.
55. McAff PC, Yuan HA, Fredricksson BE, Lulicky JP. The value of computed tomography in thoracolumbar fractures. *J Bone Joint Surg* 1983;65A:461–473.
56. Miles KA, Mairaris C, Finlay D, Barnes MR. The incidence and prognostic significance of radiologic abnormalities in soft tissue injuries to the cervical spine. *Skel Radiol* 1988;17:493–496.
57. Miller MD, Gehweiler JA, Martinez S, et al. Significant new observations in cervical spine trauma. *AJR* 1978;130:659–663.
58. Mirvis SE, Geisler FH, Jelinek JJ, Joslyn JN, Gellad F. Acute cervical spine trauma: Evaluation with 1.5 T MR imaging. *Radiology* 1988;166:807–816.
59. Mirvis SE, Diaconus JN, Chirico PA, Reiner BI, Joslyn JN, Militello P. Protocol driven radiographic evaluation of suspected cervical spine injury: Efficacy study. *Radiology* 1989;170:831–834.
60. Morris RE, Hasso AN, Thompson JR, Hinshaw DB, Vu LH. Traumatic dural tears: CT diagnosis using matrizamide. *Radiology* 1984;152:443–446.
61. Naidich JB, Naidich TP, Garfein C, et al. The widened intraspinous distance. A useful sign of anterior cervical dislocation in the supine frontal projection. *Radiology* 1977;123:113–116.
62. Papanicolaou N, Wilkinson RH, Emans JB, Treves S, Micheli LJ. Bone scintigraphy and radiology in young athletes with low back pain. *AJR* 1985;145:1039–1044.
63. Pech P, Kilgore DP, Pojunas KW, Haughton VM. Cervical spine fractures: CT detection. *Radiology* 1985;157:117–120.
64. Roub LW, Drayer BP. Spinal computed tomography: Limitations and applications. *AJR* 1979;133:267–273.
65. Roush RD, Salciccioli GG. Fracture of the anterior tubercle of the atlas. *J Bone Joint Surg* 1982;64A:626–627.
66. Scher AT. Unilateral locked facet in cervical spine injuries. *AJR* 1977;129:45–48.
67. Scher AT. Anterior cervical subluxation: An unstable position. *AJR* 1979;133:275–280.
68. Sköld G. Sagittal fractures of the cervical spine. *Injury* 1978;9:294–296.
69. Smith GR, Beckly DE, Abel MS. Articular mass fracture: A neglected cause of post-traumatic neck pain? *Clin Radiol* 1976;27:335–340.
70. Tadmor R, Davis KR, Roberson GH, et al. Computed tomography in evaluation of traumatic spinal injuries. *Radiology* 1978;127:825–827.
71. Templeton PA, Young JWR, Mirvis SE, Buddemeyer EU. The value of retropharyngeal soft tissue measurements in trauma of the adult cervical spine. *Skel Radiol* 1987;16:98–104.
72. Vandemark RM. Radiology of the cervical spine in trauma patients: Practice, pitfalls and recommendations for improving efficacy and communication. *AJR* 1990;155:465–472.
73. VanSchark JJP, Verbiest H, VanSchark FDJ. Morphometry of

the lower lumbar vertebrae as soon on CT scans: Newly recognized characteristics. *AJR* 1985;143:327–335.
74. Vines FS. The significance of "occult" fractures of the cervical spine. *AJR* 1969;107:473–504.
75. Wales LR, Knopp R, Streetwieser DR. Acute cervical spine trauma: Efficacy of supine oblique and pillar (vertebral arch) views. Presentation, ARRS meeting, Atlanta, April 1983.
76. Whalen JP, Woodruff CL. The cervical prevertebral fat stripe. *AJR* 1970;109:445–451.
77. White AA. Biomechanical analysis of clinical stabilization of the cervical spine. *Clin Orthop* 1975;109:85–96.
78. White RR, Newberg A, Seligson D. Computerized tomographic assessment of the traumatized dorsolumbar spine before and after Harrington instrumentation. *Clin Orthop* 1980;146:150–156.
79. Wojcik WG, Edeiken-Monroe BS, Harris JH. Three-dimensional computed tomography in acute cervical spine trauma: A preliminary report. *Skel Radiol* 1987;16:261–269.
80. Woodring JH, Goldstein SJ. Fractures of the articular process of the spine. *AJR* 1982;139:341–344.
81. Young JWR, Resnik CS, DeCandido P, Mirvis SE. The laminar space in the diagnosis of rotational flexion injuries of the spine. *AJR* 1989;152:103–107.

Cervical Spine Trauma—Mechanisms of Injury

82. Atlas SW, Regenbogen V, Rogers LF, Kim KS. The radiographic characterization of burst fractures of the spine. *AJR* 1986;147:575–582.
83. Babcock JL. Cervical spine injuries: Diagnosis and classifications. *Arch Surg* 1976;116:646–651.
84. Barquet A, Pereyra D. An unusual hyperextension injury to the cervical spine. *J Bone Joint Surg* 1988;70A:1393–1395.
85. Bedbrook GM. Spinal injuries with tetraplegia and paraplegia. *J Bone Joint Surg* 1979;61B:267–284.
86. Bedbrook GM. Stability of spinal fractures and fracture dislocations. *Paraplegia* 1971;9:23–32.
87. Brackman R, Penning L. *Injuries of the cervical spine.* Amsterdam: Excerpta Medica, 1971.
88. Bradford DS, Thompson RC. Fractures and dislocations of the spine. *Minn Med* 1976;59:711–720.
89. Cheshire DJE. The stability of the cervical spine following the conservative treatment of fractures and fracture-dislocations. *Paraplegia* 1969;7:193–203.
90. Cintron E, Gilula LA, Murphy WA, Gehweiler JA. The widened disk space: A sign of cervical hyperextension injury. *Radiology* 1981;141:639–644.
91. Daffner RH. *Imaging of vertebral trauma.* Rockville: Aspen Press, 1988.
92. Daffner RH, Deeb ZL, Rothfus WE. "Fingerprints" of vertebral trauma—a unifying concept based on mechanisms. *Skel Radiol* 1986;15:518–525.
93. Denis F. Spinal stability as defined by the three column spine concept in acute spinal trauma. *Clin Orthop* 1984;189:65–76.
94. Dolan KD. Cervical spine injuries below the axis. *Radiol Clin North Am* 1977;15:247–259.
95. Edeiken-Monroe B, Wagner LK, Harris JH. Hyperextension dislocation of the cervical spine. *AJR* 1986;146:803–808.
96. Forsyth HF. Extension injury of the cervical spine. *J Bone Joint Surg* 1964;46A:1792–1799.
97. Gehweiler JA, Osborne RL, Becker RF. *The radiology of vertebral trauma.* Philadelphia: W. B. Saunders Co., 1980.
98. Gehweiler JA, Clark WM, Schaaf RE, Powers B, Miller MD. Cervical spinal trauma: The common combined conditions. *Radiology* 1979;130:77–86.
99. Gerlock AJ, Kirchner SG, Heller RM, et al. *The cervical spine in trauma.* Philadelphia: W. B. Saunders Co., 1978.
100. Harris JH. Acute injuries of the spine. *Semin Roentgenol* 1978;13:53–68.
101. Holdsworth F. Fractures, dislocations and fracture-dislocations of the spine. *J Bone Joint Surg* 1970;52A:1534–1551.

102. Jacobs B. Cervical fractures and dislocations (C3-C7). *Clin Orthop* 1975;109:18–32.

103. Kim KS, Chen HH, Russell EJ, Rogers LF. Flexion teardrop fracture of the cervical spine: Radiographic characteristics. *AJR* 1989;152:319–326.

104. Marar BC. Hyperextension injuries of the cervical spine. *J Bone Joint Surg* 1974;56A:1655–1662.

105. Scher AT. Unilateral locked facet on cervical spine injuries. *AJR* 1977;129:45–48.

106. Scher AT. Anterior cervical subluxation: An unstable position. *AJR* 1979;133:275–280.

107. Selecki BR, Williams HBL. Injury to the cervical spine and cord in man. *Aust Med Assoc* 1970.

108. Webb JK, Broughton RBK, McSweeney T, Pork W. Hidden flexion injury of the cervical spine. *J Bone Joint Surg* 1976;58B:322–327.

109. Whalen JD, Woodruff CL. The cervical prevertebral fat stripe. *AJR* 1970;109:445–451.

110. White AA. Biomechanical analysis of clinical stability in the cervical spine. *Clin Orthop* 1975;109:85–96.

111. Whitley JE, Forsyth HF. The classification of cervical spine injuries. *AJR* 1960;83:633–644.

Cervical Spine Fractures and Fracture-Dislocations

112. Abel MS. Unilateral mass compression fracture of the axis. *Skel Radiol* 1979;4:92–98.

113. Acheson MB, Livingston RR, Richardson ML, Stimac GK. High-resolution CT scanning in the evaluation of cervical spine fractures: Comparison with plain film examinations. *AJR* 1987;148:1179–1185.

114. Alker JJ, Young OS, Leslie EV. High cervical spine and craniocervical junction injuries in fatal traffic accidents: A radiologic study. *Orthop Clin North Am* 1978;9:1003–1010.

115. Altongy JF, Fielding JW. Combined atlanto-axial and occipito-atlantal rotary subluxation. *J Bone Joint Surg* 1990;72A:923–926.

116. Anderson LD, D'Alonzo RT. Fractures of the odontoid process of the axis. *J Bone Joint Surg* 1978;56A:1663–1674.

117. Arndt RD. Cervical transverse process fractures: Further observations of the seat belt syndrome. *J Trauma* 1975;15:600–602.

118. Atlas SW, Regenbogen V, Rogers LF, Kina KS. The radiographic characterization of burst fractures of the spine. *AJR* 1986;147:575–582.

119. Banna M, Stevenson GW, Tumel A. Unilateral atlanto-occipital dislocation complicating an anomalic of the atlas. *J Bone Joint Surg* 1983;65A:685–687.

120. Beatson RT. Fractures and dislocations of the cervical spine. *J Bone Joint Surg* 1963;45B:21–35.

121. Barquet A, Pereyra D. An unusual extension injury of the cervical spine. *J Bone Joint Surg* 1988;70A:1393–1395.

122. Berquist TH. Imaging of adult cervical spine trauma. *Radiographics* 1988;8:667–694.

123. Bolender N, Cromwell LD, Wendling L. Fracture of the occipital condyle. *AJR* 1978;131:729–731.

124. Brackman R, Penning L. *Injury of the cervical spine.* London: Excerpta Medica, 1970.

125. Burke JT, Harris JH. Acute injuries of the axis vertebra. *Skel Radiol* 1989;18:335–446.

126. Calenoff L, Chessare JW, Rogers LF, et al. Multiple level spinal injuries: Importance of early recognition. *AJR* 1978;130:665–669.

127. Cancelmo JJ. Clay shoveler's fracture. A helpful diagnostic sign. *AJR* 1972;115:540–543.

128. Cheshire DJE. The stability of the cervical spine following the conservative treatment of fractures and fracture-dislocations. *Paraplegia* 1969;7:193–203.

129. Clarke CR, White AA. Fractures of the dens. *J Bone Joint Surg* 1985;67A:1340–1348.

130. Clyburn TA, Lionberger DR, Tullos HS. Bilateral fracture of the transverse process of the atlas. *J Bone Joint Surg* 1982;64A:948.

131. Coin CG, Pennink M, Ahmad WD, Keranen VJ. Diving type injury to the cervical spine. Contribution of CT to management. *J Comput Assist Tomogr* 1979;3:362–372.

132. Daffner RH. Pseudo-fracture of the dens: Mach bands. *AJR* 1977;128:607–612.

133. Daffner RH, Deeb ZL, Rothfus WE. "Fingerprints" of vertebral trauma—a unifying concept based on mechanisms. *Skel Radiol* 1986;15:518–525.

134. Daffner RH, Deeb ZL, Rothfus WE. Pseudofractures of the cervical vertebral body. *Skel Radiol* 1986;15:295–298.

135. Daffner RH, Deeb ZL, Rothfus WE. The posterior vertebral line: Importance in the detection of burst fractures. *AJR* 1987;148:93–96.

136. Daffner RH, Deeb ZL, Goldberg AL, Kandabarow A, Rothfus WE. The radiologic assessment of post-traumatic vertebral instability. *Skel Radiol* 1990;19:103–108.

137. Day GL, Jacoby CG, Dolan KD. Basilar invagination resulting from untreated Jefferson fracture. *AJR* 1979;133:529–531.

138. Dolan KD. Cervical spine injuries below the axis. *Radiol Clin North Am* 1977;15:247–259.

139. Edeiken-Monroe B, Wagner LK, Harris JH Jr. Hyperextension dislocation of the cervical spine. *AJR* 1986;146:803–808.

140. Effendi B, Roy D, Cornish B, Dussault RG, Laurin CA. Fractures of the ring of the axis. *J Bone Joint Surg* 1981;63B:319–327.

141. Eismont FJ, Bohlman HH. Posterior atlanto-occipital dislocation with fracture of the atlas and odontoid process. *J Bone Joint Surg* 1978;60A:397–399.

142. Elliot JM, Rogers LF, Wissinger JP, Lee JF. The hangman's fracture. *Radiology* 1972;104:303–307.

143. Evans DK. Anterior cervical subluxation. *J Bone Joint Surg* 1976;58B:318–321.

144. Fielding JW, Cochran GV, Lawsing JF III, Hohl M. Tears of the transverse ligaments of the atlas. *J Bone Joint Surg* 1974;56A:1683–1691.

145. Fielding JW, Hawkins RJ. Atlanto-axial rotary fixation. *J Bone Joint Surg* 1977;59A:37–44.

146. Francis WR, Fielding JW. Traumatic spondylolysis of axis. *Orthop Clin North Am* 1978;9:1011–1027.

147. Francis WR, Fielding JW, Hawkins RJ, Pepin J, Hensinger R. Traumatic spondylolisthesis of the axis. *J Bone Joint Surg* 1981;63B:313–318.

148. Friedman RS. Vertical fractures of the cervical vertebral bodies. *Radiology* 1954;62:536–542.

149. Garfin SR, Botte MJ, Waters RL, Nickel VL. Complications in use of the Halo fixation device. *J Bone Joint Surg* 1986;68A:320–325.

150. Gassman J, Selingson D. The anterior cervical plate. *Spine* 1983;8:700–707.

151. Gehweiler JH, Duff DE, Martinez S, et al. Fractures of the atlas vertebra. *Skel Radiol* 1976;1:97–102.

152. Gehweiler JH, Osborne RL, Becker RF. *The radiology of vertebral trauma.* Philadelphia: W. B. Saunders Co., 1980.

153. Gerlock AJ, Kirchner SG, Heller RM, et al. *The cervical spine in trauma.* Philadelphia: W. B. Saunders Co., 1978.

154. Goldberg AL, Rothfus WE, Deeb ZL, Frankel DG, Wilberger JE, Daffner RH. Hyperextension injuries of the cervical spine. *Skel Radiol* 1989;18:283–288.

155. Hanj SY, Witten DM, Musselman JP. Jefferson fracture of the atlas. *J Neurosurg* 1976;44:368–371.

156. Harding-Smith J, MacIntosh PK, Sherbon KJ. Fracture of the occipital condyle. *J Bone Joint Surg* 1981;63A:1170–1171.

157. Harris JH. Acute injury of the spine. *Semin Roentgenol* 1978;13:11–26.

158. Holt GR, Helms CA, Mark PL, Gillespy T III. Hypertrophy of C-1 anterior arch: Useful sign to distinguish os odontoideum from acute dens fracture. *Radiology* 1989;173:207–209.

159. Jackson RH. Simple uncomplicated rotary dislocations of the atlas. *Surg Gynecol Obstet* 1927;45:156–164.

160. Jefferson G. Fracture of the atlas vertebra. *J Bone Joint Surg* 1920;7B:407–422.

161. Jevtich V. Horizontal fracture of the anterior arch of the atlas. *J Bone Joint Surg* 1986;68A:1094–1095.

162. Kattan KR. Two features of the atlas vertebra simulating fracture by tomography. *AJR* 1979;132:963–965.

163. Kershner MS, Goodman CA, Perlmutler GS. CT in diagnosis of an atlas fracture. *AJR* 1977;128:688–689.
164. Kessler LA. Delayed traumatic dislocation of the cervical spine. *JAMA* 1973;224:124–125.
165. Kim KS, Chen HH, Russell EJ, Rogers LF. Flexion teardrop fracture of the cervical spine: Radiographic characteristics. *AJR* 1989;152:319–326.
166. Koss JC, Dalinka MA. Atlanto-axial subluxation in Bechet's syndrome. *AJR* 1980;134:392–393.
167. Kulkarni MV, Bondurant FJ, Rose SL, Narayama PA. 1.5 Tesla magnetic resonance imaging of acute spinal trauma. *Radiographics* 1988;8:1059–1082.
168. Lee C, Kim KS, Rogers LF. Triangular cervical vertebral body fractures. Diagnostic significance. *AJR* 1982;138:1123–1132.
169. Lee C, Woodring JH, Rogers LF, Kim KS. The radiographic destruction of degenerative slippage (spondylolisthesis and retrolisthesis) from traumatized slippage of the cervical spine. *Skel Radiol* 1986;15:439–443.
170. Marar BC. Fracture of the axis arch. *Clin Orthop* 1975;106:155–165.
171. McCoy SH, Johnson KA. Sagittal fractures of the cervical spine. *J Trauma* 1976;16:310–312.
172. McSweeney T. Fractures, fracture-dislocations, and dislocations of the cervical spine. In Jeffreys TE et al. *Disorders of the cervical spine.* London: Butterworths, 1980, pp. 48–80.
173. Miles KA, Maimaris C, Finlay D, Barnes MR. The incidence and prognostic significance of soft tissue injuries to the cervical spine. *Skel Radiol* 1988;17:493–496.
174. Mirvis SE, Young JWR, Lim C, Greenberg J. Hangman's fracture: Radiologic assessment in 27 cases. *Radiology* 1987; 163:713–717.
175. Nash CL. Acute cervical soft tissue injury and late deformity. *J Bone Joint Surg* 1979;61A:305–307.
176. Pech P, Kilgore SP, Pojunas KW, Haughton UM. Cervical spine fractures. CT detection. *Radiology* 1985;157:117–120.
177. Powers B, Miller MD, Kramer RS, Martinez S, Gehweiler JA. Traumatic anterior atlanto-occipital dislocation. *Neurosurg* 1979;4:12–17.
178. Regenbogen VS, Rogers LF, Atlas SW, Kim KS. Cervical spinal cord injuries in patients with cervical spondylosis. *AJR* 1986;146:277–284.
179. Roush RD, Salciccioli GG. Fracture of the anterior tubercle of the atlas. *J Bone Joint Surg* 1982;64A:626–627.
180. Roaf R. A study of the mechanics of spinal injuries. *J Bone Joint Surg* 1960;42B:810–823.
181. Roberts A, Wickstrom J. Prognosis of odontoid fractures. *Acta Orthop Scand* 1973;44:21–30.
182. Schatzker J, Rorabeck CH, Waddell JP. Fracture of the dens (odontoid process). *J Bone Joint Surg* 1971;53B:392–405.
183. Scher AT. Unilateral locked facet in cervical spine injuries. *AJR* 1977;129:45–48.
184. Scher AT. Double fractures of the spine: An indication for routine radiographic examination of the entire spine after injury. *S Afr Med J* 1978;53:411–413.
185. Scher AT. Anterior cervical subluxation: An unstable position. *AJR* 1979;133:275–280.
186. Scher AT. Cervical lamina fractures. Radiological identification. *S Afr Med J* 1981;58:76–78.
187. Schneider RC, Kahn EA. Chronic neurologic sequelae of acute trauma to the spine and spinal cord: The sign of acute flexion or tear drop fracture dislocation of the cervical spine. *J Bone Joint Surg* 1956;38A:985–997.
188. Segal LS, Grimm JO, Stauffer ES. Non-union of fractures of the atlas. *J Bone Joint Surg* 1987;69A:1423–1434.
189. Sherk HH. Lesions of the atlas and axis. *Clin Orthop* 1975;109:33–41.
190. Sherk HH, Nicholson JT. Fracture of the atlas. *J Bone Joint Surg* 1970;52A:1017–1024.
191. Sköld G. Sagittal fractures of the cervical spine. *Injury* 1978;9:294–296.
192. Smith GR, Beckly DE, Abel MS. Articular mass fracture: A neglected cause of post-traumatic neck pain? *Clin Radiol* 1976;27:335–340.

193. Smoker WRK, Dolan KD. The "fat" C2: A sign of fracture. *AJR* 1987;148:609–614.
194. Southwick WO. Management of fractures of the dens. *J Bone Joint Surg* 1980;62A:482–486.
195. Spencer KF, Decker S, Sell KW. Bursting atlantal fracture associated with rupture of the transverse ligament. *J Bone Joint Surg* 1970;52A:543–549.
196. Stauffer ES. Cervical spine trauma. In: *Orthopaedic knowledge update I. Home study syllabus.* Chicago: American Academy of Orthopaedic Surgeons, 1984, pp. 199–208.
197. Stauffer ES, Kaufer H, Kling TF. Fractures and dislocations of the spine. In: Rockwood CA and Green DP: *Fractures in adults,* Vol. 2, 2nd ed. Philadelphia: J.B. Lippincott, 1984, pp. 987–1092.
198. Taylor TK, Nade S, Bannister JH. Seat belt fractures of the cervical spine. *J Bone Joint Surg* 1976;58B:328–331.
199. Vines FS. The significance of "occult" fractures of the cervical spine. *AJR* 1969;107:473–504.
200. Webb JK, Broughton BK, McSweeney T, Pork W. Hidden flexion injury of the cervical spine. *J Bone Joint Surg* 1976;58B:322–327.
201. White AA, Southwick WO, Panjabi MM. Clinical stability in the lower cervical spine. A review of past and present concepts. *Spine* 1976;1:15–27.
202. Whitehill R, Richman JA, Glazer JA. Failure of immobilization of the cervical spine by halo vest. *J Bone Joint Surg* 1986;68A:326–332.
203. Wojcik WG, Edeiken-Monroe B, Harris JH. Three-dimensional computed tomography in acute cervical spine trauma. *Skel Radiol* 1987;16:261–269.
204. Wood-Jones F. The ideal lesion produced by judicial hanging. *Lancet* 1913;1:53.
205. Woodring JH, Goldstein SJ. Fractures of the articular process of the spine. *AJR* 1982;139:341–344.
206. Woodring JH, Selke AC, Duff DE. Traumatic atlanto-occipital dislocation with survival. *AJR* 1991;137:21–24.
207. Yates A. Odontoid fracture. *Semin Roentgenol* 1977;173:233–235.
208. Young JWR, Resnick CS, DeCandido P, Mirvis SE. The laminar space in the diagnosis of rotational flexion injuries of the cervical spine. *AJR* 1989;152:103–107.
209. Zilch H. Traumatische atlantooccipital Verrenkung. *Chirurg* 1977;48:417–422.

Thoracic and Lumbar Spine Trauma

210. Abel MS. Jogger's fracture and other fractures of the lumbosacral spine. *Skel Radiol* 1985;13:221–227.
211. Angtuaco EJC, Binet EF. Radiology of thoracic and lumbar fractures. *Clin Orthop* 1984;189:43–57.
212. Atlas RW, Regenbogen V, Rogers LF, Kim KS. The radiologic characterization of burst fractures of the spine. *AJR* 1986;147:575–582.
213. Bailey W. Anomalies of fractures of the vertebral articular process. *JAMA* 1973;108:266–270.
214. Bedbrook GM. Fracture dislocations of the spine with and without paralysis. The case for conservatism and against operative techniques. In: Leach RE, et al, eds. *Controversies in orthopedic surgery.* Philadelphia: W. B. Saunders Co., 1982, pp. 423–445.
215. Boechat MI. Spinal deformities and pseudo fractures. *AJR* 1987;149:97–98.
216. Bowerman JW, McDonnell EJ. Radiology of athletic injuries: Football. *Radiology* 1985;117:33.
217. Bradford DS, Thompson RC. Fractures and dislocations of the spine. Indications for surgical intervention. *Minn Med* 1976;59:711–720.
218. Brandt-Zawadzki M, Jeffrey RB, Minagi H, et al. High resolution CT of thoracolumbar fractures. *AJR* 1982;138:699–704.
219. Burke DC. Hyperextension injuries of the spine. *J Bone Joint Surg* 1971;53B:3–12.
220. Burke DC. Spinal cord injuries and seat belts. *Med J Aust* 1973;2:801–806.

221. Calenoff L, Chessare JW, Rogers LF, et al. Multiple level spinal injuries. Importance of early recognition. *AJR* 1978;130:665–669.
222. Cammesa FP, Eismont FJ, Green BA. Dural laceration occurring with burst fractures and associated laminar fractures. *J Bone Joint Surg* 1989;71A:1044–1052.
223. Chance GQ. Note on a type of flexion fracture of the spine. *Brit J Radiol* 1948;21:452–453.
224. Daffner RH, Deeb ZL, Rothfus WE. The posterior vertebral line: Importance in detection of burst fractures. *AJR* 1987;148:93–96.
225. Daffner RH. Case report 570. *Skel Radiol* 1989;18:489–490.
226. Daffner RH, Deeb ZL, Rothfus WE. Thoracic fractures and dislocations in motorcyclists. *Skel Radiol* 1987;16:280–284.
227. Day B, Kokan P. Compression fractures of the thoracic and lumbar spine from compressor injuries. *Clin Orthop* 1977;124:173.
228. Dehner JR. Seat belt injuries of spine and abdomen. *AJR* 1971;111:833–843.
229. Dennis LN, Rogers LF. Superior mediastinal widening from spine fractures mimicking aortic ruptures on chest radiographs. *AJR* 1989;152:27–30.
230. Denis F. The three column spine and its significance in classification of acute thoracolumbar spinal injuries. *Spine* 1983;8:817–831.
231. Denis F. Thoracolumbar spine trauma. In: *Orthopedic knowledge update I: Home study syllabus.* Chicago: American Academy of Orthopaedic Surgeons, 1984, pp. 227–236.
232. De Oliveira JC. A new type of fracture-dislocation of the thoracolumbar spine. *J Bone Joint Surg* 1978;60:481–488.
233. DeSmet AA, Robinson RG, Johnson BE, Luhert BP. Spinal compression fractures in osteoporotic women: Patterns and relationship to kyphosis. *Radiology* 1988;166:497–500.
234. Flesh JR, Leider LL, Erickson DL, Chon SN, Bradford DS. Harrington instrumentation and spine fusion for unstable fractures and fracture dislocations of the thoracic and lumbar spine. *J Bone Joint Surg* 1977;59A:143–153.
235. Foley WJ, Calenoff L, Hendrix RW, Schafer MF. Thoracic and lumbar spine fusion: Postoperative radiologic evaluation. *AJR* 1983;141:373–380.
236. Frederickson BE, Yaun HA, Miller H. Burst fracture of the 5th lumbar vertebra. *J Bone Joint Surg* 1982;64A:1088–1094.
237. Freedy MR, Midler KD, Eick JJ, Granke DS. Traumatic lumbosacral nerve root avulsion: Evaluation with MR imaging. *J Comput Assist Tomogr* 1989;13:1052–1057.
238. Garrett JW, Braunstein PW. Seat belt syndrome. *J Trauma* 1962;2:220–238.
239. Gehweiler JA, Osborne RL, Becker RF. *The radiology of vertebral trauma.* Philadelphia: W. B. Saunders Co., 1980.
240. Gellad FE, Lavine AM, Joslyn JN, Edwards CC, Bosse M. Pure thoracolumbar facet dislocation: Clinical features and CT appearance. *Radiology* 1986;161:505–508.
241. Gertzbein SD, Offierski C. Complete fracture-dislocation of the thoracic spine without spinal cord injury. *J Bone Joint Surg* 1979;61A:449–451.
242. Ghormley RK, Hoffman HOE. Fracture of the vertebral process. *Proc Staff Meetings, Mayo Clinic* 1962;17:17–19.
243. Goldberg AL, Rothfus WE, Deeb ZL, et al. The impact of magnetic resonance on diagnostic evaluation of acute thoracolumbar trauma. *Skel Radiol* 1988;17:89–95.
244. Golimbu C, Firoozinia H, Rafii M, et al. Computed tomography of thoracic and lumbar spine fractures that have been treated with Harrington instrumentation. *Radiology* 1984;151:731.
245. Griffin JB, Sutherland GH. Traumatic posterior fracture-dislocation of the lumbosacral joint. *J Trauma* 1980;20:426–428.
246. Guerra J, Garfin SR, Resnick D. Vertebral burst fractures: CT analysis of the retropulsed fragment. *Radiology* 1984;153:769–772.
247. Hampson S, Coombs R, Hemingway H. Fractures of the upper thoracic spine—an additional "seatbelt" syndrome. *Brit J Radiol* 1984;57:1033–1034.
248. Holdsworth F. Fracture and fracture-dislocations of the spine. *J Bone Joint Surg* 1970;52A:1534–1551.
249. Horne J, Cockshott WP, Shannon HS. Spinal column damage from water ski jumping. *Skel Radiol* 1987;16:612–616.
250. Hubbard DD. Fractures of the dorsal and lumbar spine. *Orthop Clin North Am* 1976;7:605–614.
251. Ireland ML, Micheli LJ. Bilateral stress fracture of the lumbar pedicles in a ballet dancer. *J Bone Joint Surg* 1987;69A:140–142.
252. Jacobs RR. Bilateral fracture of pedicles through the fourth and fifth lumbar vertebrae with anterior displacement of the vertebral bodies. *J Bone Joint Surg* 1977;59A:409–410.
253. Kälebo P, Kadzcolka R, Sward L, Zachrisson BE. Stress views in the comparative assessment of spondylolytic spondylolisthesis. *Skel Radiol* 1989;17:570–575.
254. Kaplan PA, Orton DF, Asleson RJ. Osteoporosis with vertebral compression fractures, retropulsed fragments, and neurologic compromise. *Radiology* 1987;165:533–535.
255. Keene JS, Goletz TH, Lilleas F, et al. Diagnosis of vertebral fractures: A comparison of conventional radiography, conventional tomography, and computerized axial tomography. *J Bone Joint Surg* 1982;64A:586–594.
256. Kramer KM, Levine AM. Unilateral facet dislocation of the lumbosacral junction. *J Bone Joint Surg* 1989;71A:1258–1261.
257. MacLeod JH, Nicholson DM. Seat belt trauma to the abdomen. *Can J Surg* 1969;12:202–206.
258. Manaster BJ, Osborn AG. CT patterns of facet dislocation in the thoracolumbar region. *AJR* 1987;148:335–340.
259. McAfee PC, Yaun HA, Frederickson BE, Lubicky JP. The value of computed tomography on thoracolumbar fractures. *J Bone Joint Surg* 1983;65A:461–473.
260. McAfee PC, Bohlman HH. Complications following Harrington instrumentation for fractures of the thoracolumbar spine. *J Bone Joint Surg* 1985;67A:672–686.
261. Mitchell LC. Isolated fracture of the articular process of the lumbar vertebra. *J Bone Joint Surg* 1933;15:608–614.
262. Morris BA. Unilateral dislocation of a lumbosacral facet. *J Bone Joint Surg* 1981;63A:164–165.
263. Murray RO, Colwill MR. Stress fractures of the pars interarticularis. *Proc Roy Soc Med* 1968;61:555–557.
264. Nicoll EA. Fractures of the dorso-lumbar spine. *J Bone Joint Surg* 1949;31B:376–394.
265. Nykamp PW, Levy JM, Christenson F, Dunn R, Hubbard J. Computed tomography for bursting fractures of the lumbar spine. *J Bone Joint Surg* 1978;60:1108–1109.
266. O'Callahan PJ, Ulrich CG, Hansen AY, Kieffer SA. CT of facet distraction in flexion injuries of the thoraco-lumbar spine: The "naked" facet. *AJR* 1980;134:563–568.
267. Omar MM, Levinsohn EM. An unusual fracture of the vertebral process in a skier. *J Trauma* 1979;19:212–213.
268. Papanicolaou N, Wilkinson RH, Emans JB, Treves S, Micheli LJ. Bone scintigraphy and radiography in young athletes with low back pain. *AJR* 1985;145:1039–1044.
269. Pennell RG, Maurer AH, Banakdapour A. Stress injuries of the pars interarticularis: Radiologic classification and indications for scintigraphy. *AJR* 1985;145:763–766.
270. Rennie W, Mitchell N. Flexion distraction fractures of the thoracolumbar spine. *J Bone Joint Surg* 1973;55A:386–390.
271. Roaf R. A study of the mechanism of spinal injuries. *J Bone Joint Surg* 1960;42B:810–823.
272. Rogers LF. The roentgenographic appearance of transverse or Chance fractures of the spine: The seat belt fracture. *AJR* 1971;111:844–849.
273. Rogers LF, Thayer C, Weinberg PE, Kim KS. Acute injuries of the upper thoracic spine with associated paraplegia. *AJR* 1980;134:67–73.
274. Rothman SLG, Glenn WV, Kerber CW. Postoperative fractures of lumbar articular facets. *AJR* 1985;145:779–784.
275. Rothman SLG, Glenn WV. CT evaluation of interbody fusion. *Clin Orthop* 1985;193:47–56.
276. Roub LW, Drayer BP. Spinal computed tomography: Limitations and applications. *AJR* 1979;133:267–273.
277. Shuman WP, Rogers JV, Sickler ME, et al. Thoracolumbar burst fractures: CT dimensions of the signal canal relative to postsurgical improvement. *AJR* 1985;145:337–341.
278. Smith ER, Northrup CH, Loop JW. Jumper's fractures: Pattern of thoracolumbar injuries associated with vertical plunges. *Radiology* 1977;122:657–663.

279. Stauffer ES. Open reduction and internal fixation of unstable thoracolumbar fractures and dislocations. In: Leach RE, et al., eds. *Controversies in orthopaedic surgery.* Philadelphia: W. B. Saunders Co., 1982, pp. 446–454.
280. Stauffer ES, Neil JL: Biomechanical analysis of structural stability of internal fixation in fractures of the thoracic lumbar spine. *Clin Orthop* 1975;112:159–164.
281. Tadmor R, Davis KR, Roberson GH, et al. Computed tomography in evaluation of traumatic spinal injuries. *Radiology* 1978;127:825–827.
282. Takata K, Insue S, Takahashi K, Ohtsuka Y. Fracture of the posterior margin of a lumbar vertebra. *J Bone Joint Surg* 1988;70A:589–594.
283. Teplick JG, Haskin ME. Computed tomography of the postoperative lumbar spine. *AJR* 1983;141:865–884.
284. Thoen DD, Huggins IG. Diagnostic subtleties in CT evaluation of the LS spine: Insights in digital imaging. 1982;1:14–20.
285. Villem J, Lindahl S, Irstam L, Nordwall A. Unstable thoracolumbar fractures: A study by CT and conventional roentgenology of the reduction effect of Harrington instrumentation. *Spine* 1984;9:214–219.
286. White RR, Newberg A, Seligson D. Computerized tomographic assessment of the traumatized dorsolumbar spine before and after Harrington instrumentation. *Clin Orthop* 1980;146:150–156.
287. Whitesides TE, Shah SGA. On the management of unstable fractures of the thoracolumbar spine. Rationale for anterior decompression and fusion and posterior stabilization. *Spine* 1976;1:99–107.
288. Zoltan JD, Gilula LA, Murphy WA. Unilateral facet dislocation between the fifth lumbar and first sacral vertebrae. *J Bone Joint Surg* 1979;61A:767–769.

Spondylolysis and Spondylolisthesis

289. Amato M, Totty WG, Gilala LA. Spondylolysis of the lumbar spine: Demonstration of defects and laminal fragmentation. *Radiology* 1984;153:627–629.
290. Gehweiler JA, Osborne RL, Becker RF. *The radiology of vertebral trauma.* Philadelphia: W. B. Saunders Co., 1980.
291. Gillespie HW. Vertebral retroposition (reversed spondylolisthesis). *Brit J Radiol* 1951;24:193–197.
292. Grogan JP, Hemminghytt S, Williams AL, Carrera GF, Haughton VM. Spondylolysis studied with computed tomography. *Radiology* 1982;145:737–742.
293. Junghanns H. Spondylolisthesis. *Beitr Klin Chir* 1930;148:554.
294. Kälebo P, Kadziolka R, Swärd L, Zachrisson BE. Stress views in the comparative assessment of spondylolytic spondylolisthesis. *Skel Radiol* 1989;17:570–575.
295. Lekbowitz DM, Quencer RM. Vacuum facet phenomenon: A computed tomographic sign of degenerative spondylolisthesis. *Radiology* 1982;144:562.

296. Maldague BE, Malghem JJ. Unilateral arch hypertrophy with spinous process tilt: A sign of arch deficiency. *Radiology* 1976;121:576–574.
297. McCarroll JR, Miller JM, Ritter MA. Lumbar spondylolysis and spondylolisthesis in college football players. *Am J Sports Med* 1986;14:404–406.
298. McKee BW, Alexander WJ, Dunbar JS. Spondylolysis and spondylolisthesis in children: A review. *J Can Assoc Radiol* 1971;22:100–109.
299. MacNab I. Spondylolisthesis with an intact neural arch—the so-called pseudo-spondylolisthesis. *J Bone Joint Surg* 1950; 32B:325–333.
300. Melamed A, Ansfield DJ. Posterior displacement of lumbar vertebra. *AJR* 1947;58:307–328.
301. Meyerding HW. Spondylolisthesis as an etiologic factor in backache. *JAMA* 1938;111:1971–1976.
302. Moreton RD. Spondylolysis. *JAMA* 1966;195:671–674.
303. Nathan H. Spondylolysis. Its anatomy and mechanism of development. *J Bone Joint Surg* 1959;41A:303–320.
304. Newman PH, Stone KH. The etiology of spondylolisthesis. *J Bone Joint Surg* 1963;45B:39–59.
305. Newman PH. Spondylolisthesis. Its cause and effect. *Ann R Coll Surg Engl* 1955;16:305–323.
306. Roberts RA. *Chronic low back ache due to lumbar structural derangements.* London: H.K. Lewis, 1947.
307. Rosenberg NJ. Degenerative spondylolisthesis. *J Bone Joint Surg* 1975;57A:467–474.
308. Rower GG, Roche MB. The etiology of separate neural arch. *J Bone Joint Surg* 1953;35A:102–110.
309. Sullivan CR, Bickel WH. The problem of traumatic spondylolysis. A report of 3 cases. *Am J Surg* 1960;100:698–708.
310. Taillard WF. Etiology of spondylolisthesis. *Clin Orthop* 1976;117:30.
311. Wiltse LL, Newman DH, MacNab I. Classification of spondylolysis and spondylolisthesis. *Clin Orthop* 1976;117:23–29.
312. Wiltse LL. The etiology of spondylolisthesis. *J Bone Joint Surg* 1962;44A:539–560.

Ankylosing Spondylitis

313. Kewalramani LS, Taylor RG, Albrand OW. Cervical spine injury in patients with ankylosing spondylitis. *J Trauma* 1975;15:931–934.
314. Resnick D, Niwayama G. Ankylosing spondylitis. In: Resnick D, Niwayama G. *Diagnosis of bone and joint disorders,* vol. 2. Philadelphia: W. B. Saunders, 1988, pp. 1103–1170.
315. Surin VV. Fractures of the cervical spine in patients with ankylosing spondylitis. *Acta Orthop Scand* 1980;51:79–84.
316. Woodruff FB, Dewing SB. Fracture of the cervical spine in patients with ankylosing spondylitis. *Radiology* 1963;80:17–21.

Imaging of Orthopedic Trauma,
Second Edition, edited by T.H. Berquist,
Mayo Clinic © 1992. Published
by Raven Press, Ltd., New York.

CHAPTER 5

The Pelvis and Hips

Thomas H. Berquist and Mark B. Coventry

Anatomy, 207
  Skeletal Anatomy, 207
  Ligaments and Articulations, 210
  Vascular Anatomy, 213
  Neuroanatomy, 216
  Genitourinary and Gastrointestinal Anatomy, 216
Imaging of the Pelvis and Hips, 216
  Routine Radiography, 216
  Pelvis, 216
  Hip, 222
Pelvic Fractures, 227
  Classification of Pelvic Fractures, 228
  Treatment of Pelvic Fractures, 244
  Complications Associated with Pelvic Fractures, 252
Dislocations and Fracture-Dislocations of the Hip, 260
  Classifications of Dislocations and Fracture-Dislocations of the Hip, 261
  Radiographic Evaluation of Dislocations and Fracture-Dislocations of the Hip, 264

Treatment of Dislocations and Fracture-Dislocations of the Hip, 267
Complications of Dislocations and Fracture-Dislocations of the Hip, 268
Femoral Neck Fractures, 269
  Classification of Femoral Neck Fractures, 269
  Radiographic Evaluation of Femoral Neck Fractures, 270
  Treatment of Femoral Neck Fractures, 272
  Complications of Femoral Neck Fractures, 278
Trochanteric Fractures, 284
  Classification of Trochanteric Fractures, 284
  Treatment of Trochanteric Fractures, 289
Evaluating Soft Tissue Trauma, 294
  Arthrography, 294
  MRI, CT, and Ultrasonography, 305
References, 305

ANATOMY

The pelvis is a weight-bearing structure for the trunk and lower extremities and also serves to protect the lower abdominal viscera. The pelvic ring consists of two innominate bones that articulate at the pubic symphysis. The pelvis is divided by the iliopectineal line into an upper false and a lower true pelvis. The false pelvis contains the organs of reproduction, the lower urinary and digestive tracts, and the vessels and nerves to the lower extremities (1,7,9,13,25).

The weight-bearing function of the pelvis is particu-

larly important in orthopedic practice. In the erect position, the weight-bearing forces are directed from the femurs to the acetabula and then to the spinal column via the iliac wings, the sacroiliac joints, and the sacrum, respectively (13,25). This forms the major, or femorosacral, arch. Secondary support is derived from the tie arch formed by the horizontal pubic rami (Fig. 5-1A). In the sitting position, the weight is distributed from the spine to the sacroiliac joints and then through the ilia to the ischial tuberosities, forming the ischiosacral arch. Again, a secondary tie arch is formed by the ischial rami and the inferior pubic rami (Fig. 5-1B). Following trauma, the tie arches usually fracture prior to the major arches (13).

Skeletal Anatomy

The innominate bone is composed of the ilium, ischium, and pubis (Fig. 5-2), which during childhood are separated by the triradiate cartilage. During the second

T. H. Berquist: Department of Diagnostic Radiology, Mayo Medical School, Mayo Clinic Jacksonville, Jacksonville, Florida 32224.

M. B. Coventry: Department of Orthopedic Surgery, Mayo Medical School and Mayo Clinic, Rochester, Minnesota 55905.

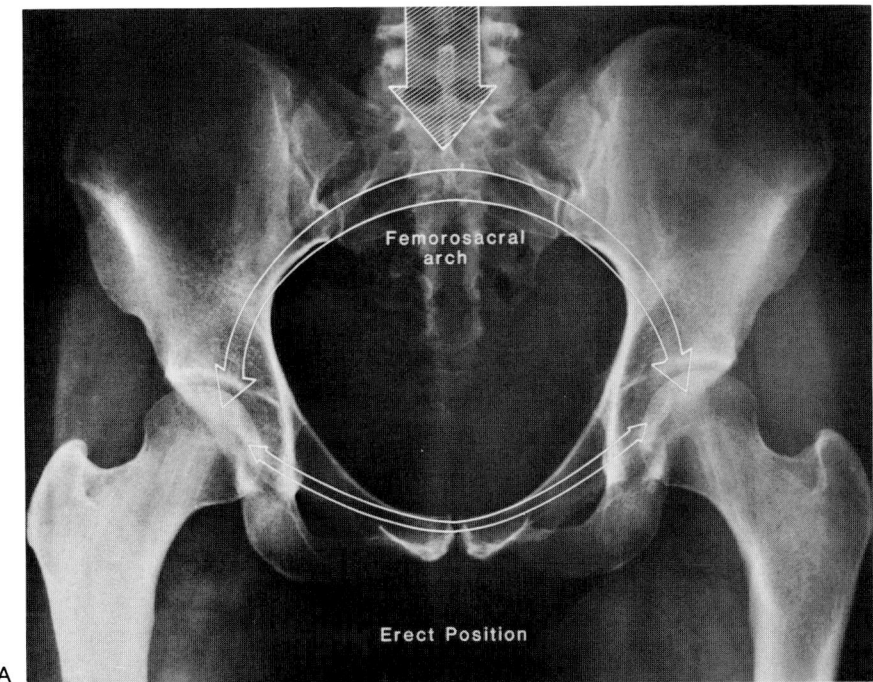

Erect Position

A

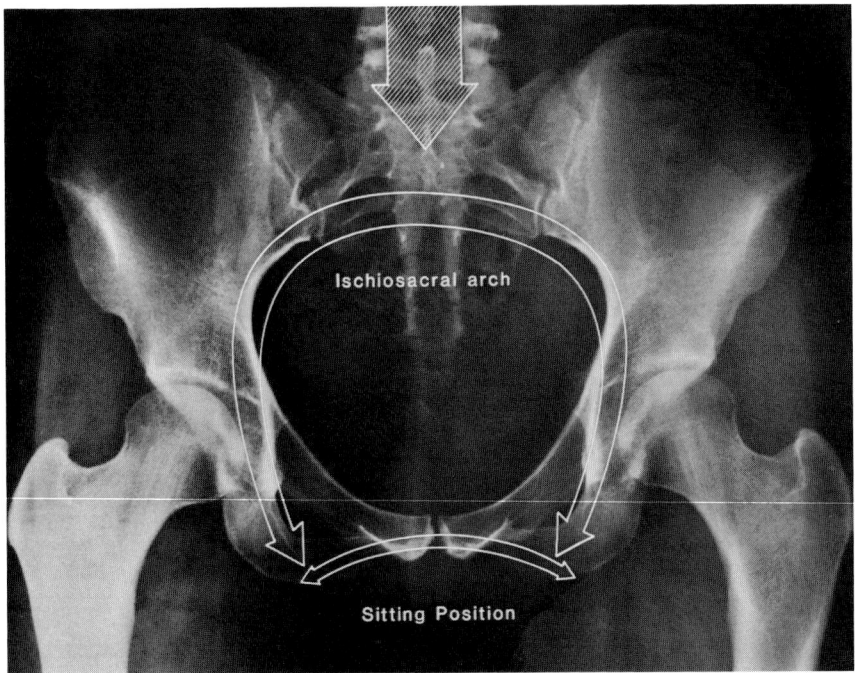

Sitting Position

B

FIG. 5–1. Weight bearing forces of the pelvis. **A:** Erect position: The forces are transmitted from the femoral heads to the spine via the ilia. The secondary arch is formed by the pubic rami. **B:** Sitting position: The forces are directed from the spine to the ischial tuberosities via the sacroiliac joints. A secondary arch is formed by the ischial and inferior pubic rami. (Modified from 13, with permission).

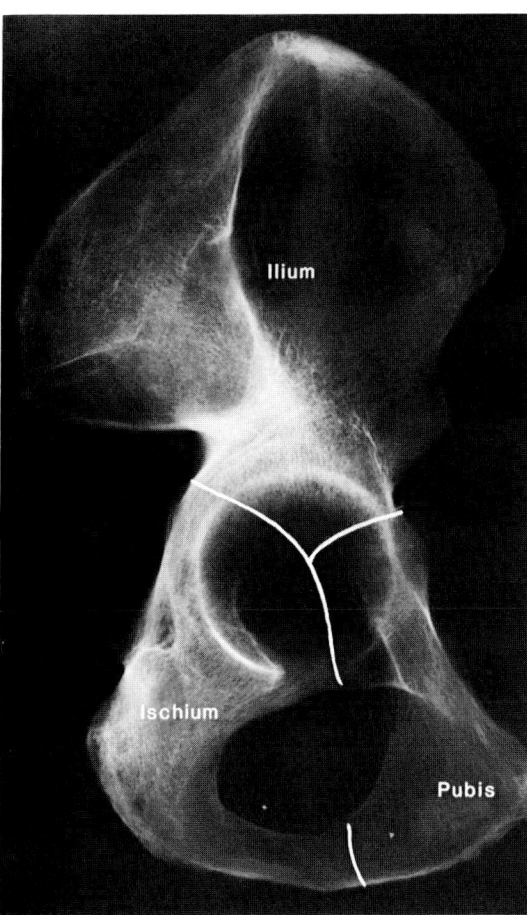

FIG. 5-2. Specimen radiograph of the innominate bone demonstrating the three components (ilium, ischium, pubis).

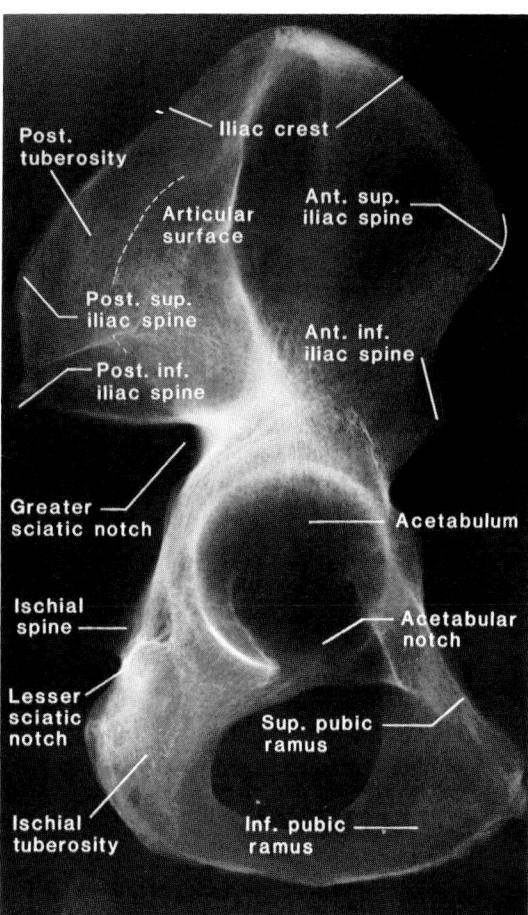

FIG. 5-3. Lateral specimen radiograph of the innominate bone with anatomic labels.

decade, these three bones fuse, forming the acetabulum (2,13,25).

The ilium is composed of a wing and body. The wing is large, with three palpable structures that are helpful in clinical evaluation and radiographic positioning. These structures are the anterior superior iliac spine, the iliac crest (which extends from the anterior superior iliac spine to the posterior superior iliac spine), and the posterior superior iliac spine (Fig. 5-3). The iliac wing is covered by muscles medially and laterally. Medially, the wing serves as the origin of the iliacus, the quadratus lumborum, the erector spinae, and the transversus abdominis (7,13,25). The gluteal muscles originate from the lateral aspect of the ilium, the sartorius from the anterior superior iliac spine, the rectus femoris from the anterior inferior iliac spine, and the tensor fascia lata from the anterior iliac crest (7,13,25). The posterior superior aspect of the ilium contains a large rough area for attachment of the posterior sacroiliac ligaments (Fig. 5-3). This area is termed the *iliac tuberosity.* Anterior to the tuberosity is the cartilage-covered surface that articulates with the sacrum, forming the sacroiliac joint. Immediately inferior to the articular surface of the ilium is the greater sciatic notch.

The body of the pubic bone articulates with its mate via the pubic symphysis. The superior pubic ramus extends superolaterally to the acetabulum and forms the upper margin of the obturator foramen. The inferior pubic ramus courses posteriorly and laterally and is contiguous with the ischium. The inferior pubic ramus forms the lower margin of the obturator foramen (Fig. 5-3). The bodies of the pubic bones have small projections anteriorly and superiorly (pubic tubercles), which along with the symphysis are palpable in most patients and are valuable as anatomic landmarks for radiographic positioning. Multiple muscle groups originate from the inferior pubic ramus near the pubic symphysis. These include the muscles of the pelvic floor (deep transversus perinei, levator ani, and sphincter urethrae), the adductor longus, adductor brevis, gracilis, adductor magnus and obturators internus and externus. The pectineus and rectus abdominis are attached to the superior pubic ramus (1,7,8,11,13).

The ischium (Figs. 5-2 and 5-3) consists of a large body that forms the posterior inferior portion of the acetabulum, a tuberosity (directed inferiorly), and a ramus, which is contiguous with the inferior pubic ramus. The ischial spine projects posteromedially and forms the lower margin of the greater sciatic notch. The coccygeus and levator ani attach to the ischial spine. The large ischial tuberosity serves as the origin of the semimembranosus, semitendinosus, biceps femoris, quadratus femoris, and a portion of the adductor magnus (1,7,11).

The sacrum consists of five fused vertebral segments, which decrease in size inferiorly. The sacrum articulates with the coccyx inferiorly and with the ilia laterally. Superiorly, the sacrum articulates with the body of L5 via the lumbosacral disk. Posteriorly, it articulates with the apophyseal joints of L5. The surface of the sacrum is concave ventrally and convex dorsally. Four pairs of sacral foramina allow passage of the dorsal and ventral rami of the spinal nerves. The large lateral mass of the sacrum is formed by the fused lateral articular processes of the first three sacral segments (1,7,9,11,12).

The coccyx consists of four to five rudimentary segments that articulate with the last sacral segment. Four muscles attach to the coccyx. These include a portion of the gluteus maximus, the coccygeus, levator ani, and the sphinctor ani (11). (See Chapter 4 for more detail on the anatomy of the sacral and coccygeal vertebrae.)

Ligaments and Articulations

The articulations of the pelvis and hips are summarized in Table 5-1 (11,18). The sacroiliac joint is supported by strong posterior sacroiliac ligaments (short and long fibers). The anterior sacroiliac ligaments provide much less support and serve as little more than a capsule for the sacroiliac joint. The sacrotuberous and sacrospinous ligaments connect the lower lateral aspects of the sacrum to the ischial tuberosity and ischial spine, respectively. These ligaments prevent posterior displacement of the sacrum (4,5,9). The articular anatomy and surrounding ligaments combine to produce minimal motion at the sacroiliac joints (4,5,9,13). The iliolumbar and sacrolumbar ligaments restrict the rotary and ventral motion of the lower lumbar spine (Fig. 5-4).

The articulation of the pubic bones is separated by a fibrocartilaginous disk that is contiguous with the superior and inferior pubic ligaments. The superior and inferior ligaments blend with the stronger anterior pubic ligament. These ligaments allow only slight motion at the pubic symphysis. Although minimal, such motion at the

pubic symphysis and sacroiliac joints allows single undisplaced fractures to occur near these structures. Displaced fractures are usually multiple, as one would expect with the ring configuration of the pelvis (1,7,11,13,23).

The femoral head articulates with the acetabulum, forming a spheroidea (ball and socket) joint. The acetabulum is formed by the ischium (45%) the ilium (35%), and the pubic bone (20%) and is directed in an anterior, laterocaudad direction (3,18,22). The bony acetabular rim is incomplete inferiorly (the acetabular notch) and is bridged in this region by the transverse ligament. The transverse ligament is contiguous with the cartilaginous acetabular labrum, which forms a supporting lip around the remainder of the acetabular margin. The synovial-lined capsule is supported by several ligaments as well as by the surrounding muscle groups. The iliofemoral ligament (Fig. 5-5) is shaped like an inverted Y and lies anterior to the pubofemoral ligament and just inferior to the rectus femoris (1,7,10). A weak area may be present at the crossing point of these two ligaments. This weak area allows communication between the iliopsoas bursa and the hip joint, and arthrography demonstrates such communication in up to 20% of patients (10). The iliofemoral and ischiofemoral ligaments (Fig. 5-5) are thicker posteriorly and cross inferiorly, creating the zona orbicularis. The fibers of the capsule and capsular ligaments attach 5–6 cm beyond the acetabular labrum posteriorly as compared with the perilabral attachment anteriorly. More detailed articular anatomy will be discussed in the section on hip arthrography in this chapter.

The periarticular anatomy of the hip is important to the clinician and radiologist (Fig. 5-6). Knowledge of the various muscle groups and their fat planes and recognition of the relationship between the neurovascular anatomy and the hip joint are of great clinical significance. For example, four fat planes have been identified radiographically, and displacement of these fat planes may indicate intra-articular or periarticular disease (10,17,18) (Fig. 5-7).

The fat plane of the obturator internus lies medial to this muscle in the bony pelvis. The iliopsoas fat plane is medial and parallel to the iliopsoas muscle as it inserts into the lesser trochanter. The two other fat planes lie lateral to the hip. The more medial of the two was origi-

TABLE 5-1. *Articulations of pelvis and hips*

Articulation	Type	Motion
Lumbosacral		
Facet joints	Diarthrodial	Gliding
Disk space	Amphiarthrosis	Minimal
Sacroiliac	Diarthrodial	Gliding minimal
Sacro-coccygeal	Amphiarthrosis	Minimal motion
Pubic symphysis	Amphiarthrosis	Minimal motion
Hip	Spheroidea (ball and socket)	Motion around central axis

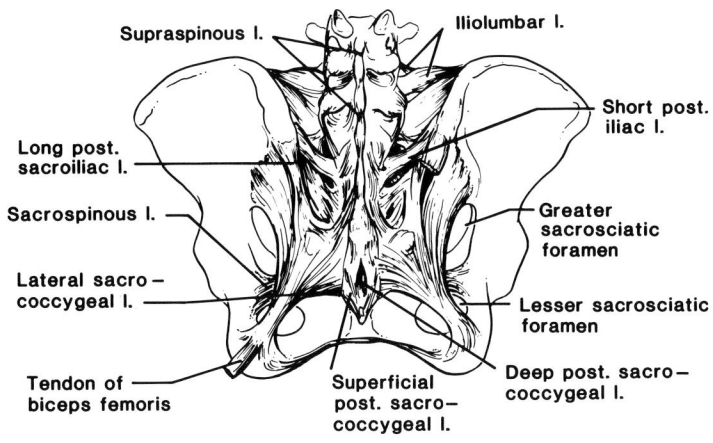

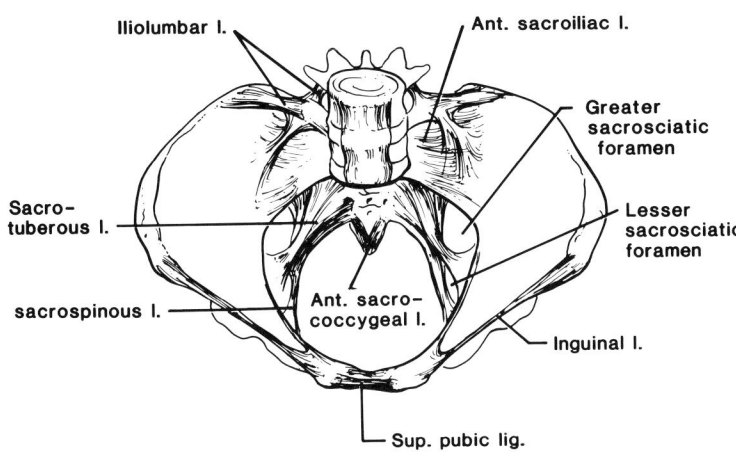

FIG. 5-4. Posterior ligaments (*upper illustration*) and anterior ligaments (*lower illustration*) of the pelvis.

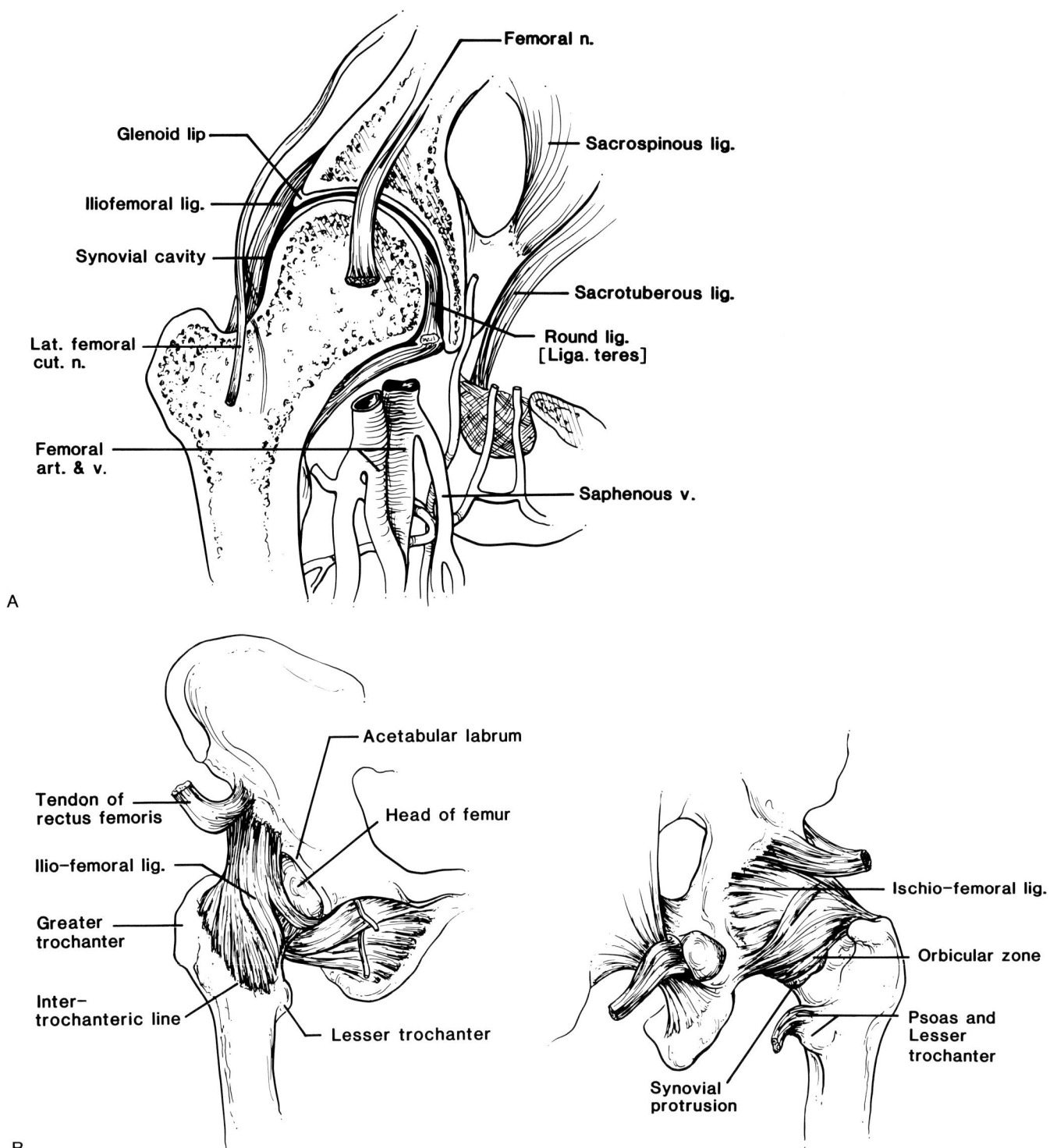

FIG. 5–5. Anatomy of the hip: **A:** Coronal section demonstrating articular surface, ligaments, arteries, and nerves. **B:** Anterior ligaments of the hip. **C:** Posterior ligaments of the hip.

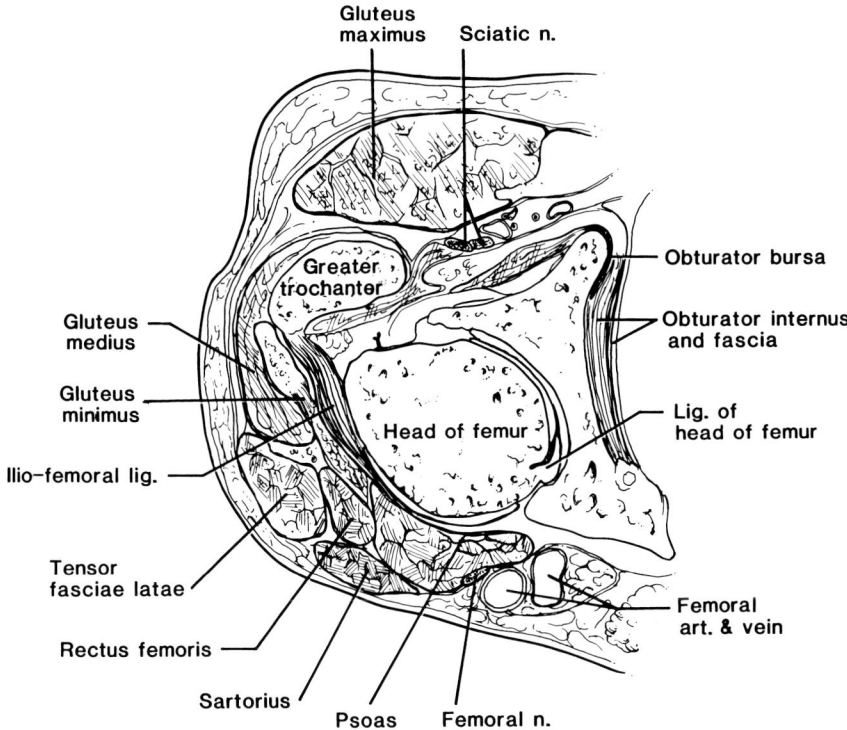

Gluteus maximus
Sciatic n.
Greater trochanter
Obturator bursa
Obturator internus and fascia
Gluteus medius
Gluteus minimus
Head of femur
Lig. of head of femur
Ilio-femoral lig.
Tensor fasciae latae
Femoral art. & vein
Rectus femoris
Sartorius
Psoas bursa
Femoral n.

FIG. 5-6. Axial illustration of periarticular anatomy of the hip.

nally thought to be adjacent to the capsule and therefore of great value in detecting joint pathology. However, Guerra (10) demonstrated that the largest portion of this fat plane (the portion demonstrated on the AP radiograph) is between the rectus femoris and the tensor fasciae latae and is, in fact, anterior to the capsule of the hip.

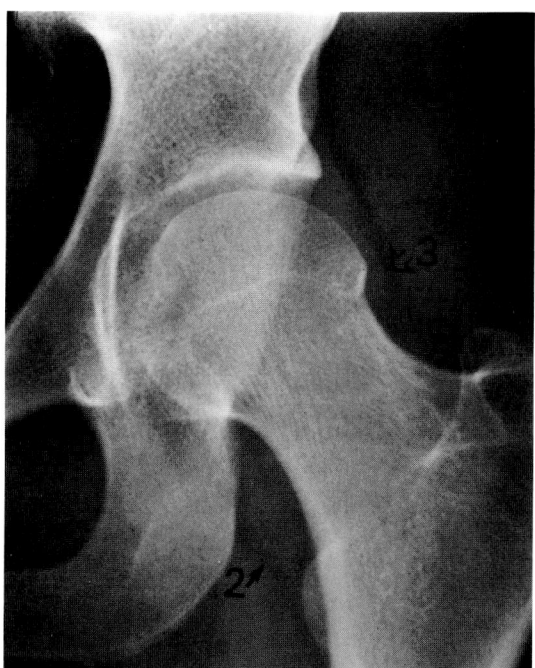

FIG. 5-7. Fat planes of the hip. 1: obturator internus, 2: iliopsoas, 3: pericapsular, 4: gluteal.

It is this portion of the fat plane that is visible on the AP radiograph of the hip. The small juxtacapsular portion of this fat plane, on the other hand, is not visible radiographically. The more lateral of the two fat planes lies between the gluteus medius and gluteus minimus. According to Guerra (10), the two fat planes nearest the hip (Fig. 5-7) are seen in 75% of patients. Our experience indicates that the iliopsoas and pericapsular fat planes are visible in 95% of patients, the obturator internus in 79%, and the gluteal in 53%. Thus significant joint pathology must be present before distortion of the fat planes will be detectable radiographically.

Muscle insertions related to the hip (Fig. 5-6) include the following: (1) The iliopsoas inserts in the lesser trochanter; (2) the gluteus maximus inserts into the tensor fasciae latae over the greater trochanter and into the linea aspera of the upper femur; (3) the gluteus medius, gluteus minimus and the piriformis insert into the greater trochanter; and (4) the quadratus femoris inserts just below the posterior aspect of the greater trochanter (1,7,11).

Finally, the sciatic nerve courses posterior to the femoral head (Fig. 5-6), and the femoral artery and veins lie just medial and anterior to the femoral head (1,7,11).

Vascular Anatomy

The rich vascular supply of the pelvis is partly responsible for the fact that the most frequent and most significant complication of pelvic trauma is hemorrhage (14,19–21,24). The relationship of certain vessels to the

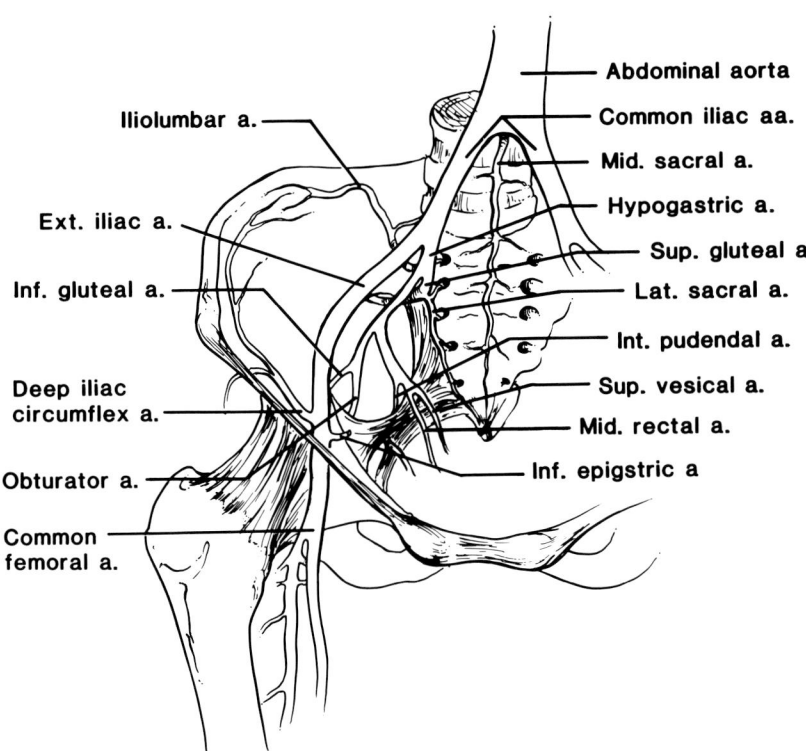

FIG. 5-8. Illustration demonstrating the blood supply to the pelvis and hips.

bones and joints of the pelvis and hips are particularly important for the angiographer and surgeon.

Typically the abdominal aorta bifurcates at the L4 level, forming the common iliac arteries (Fig. 5-8). The common iliac arteries divide again to form the internal iliac (hypogastric) and external iliac. This division occurs just anterior to the sacroiliac joints (1,7,11).

The external iliac passes inferiorly to the inguinal ligament, forming the common femoral artery. The common femoral then divides once again, forming the superficial and deep femoral (profunda) arteries. The deep femoral provides the major source of blood supply to the hip through the medial and lateral femoral circumflex branches. The femoral head receives a lesser portion of

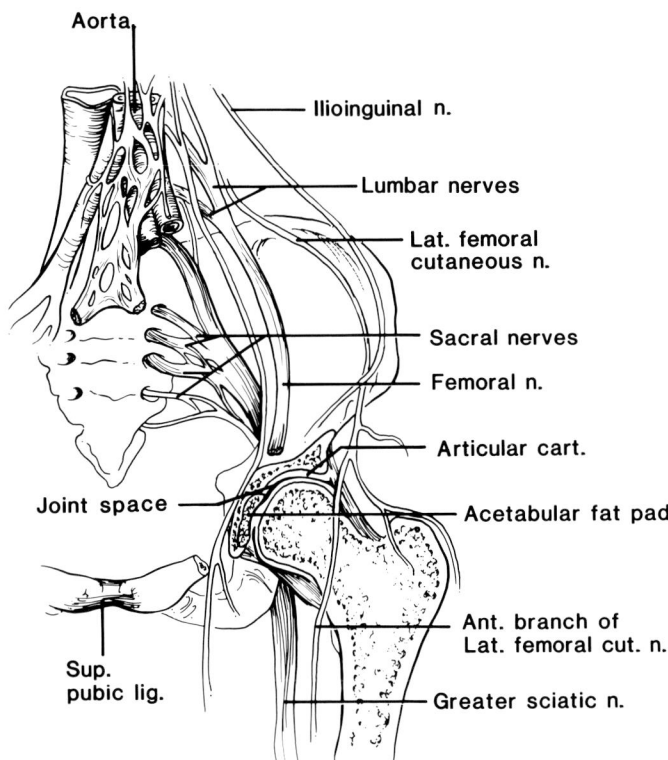

FIG. 5-9. Illustration of pelvic neuroanatomy.

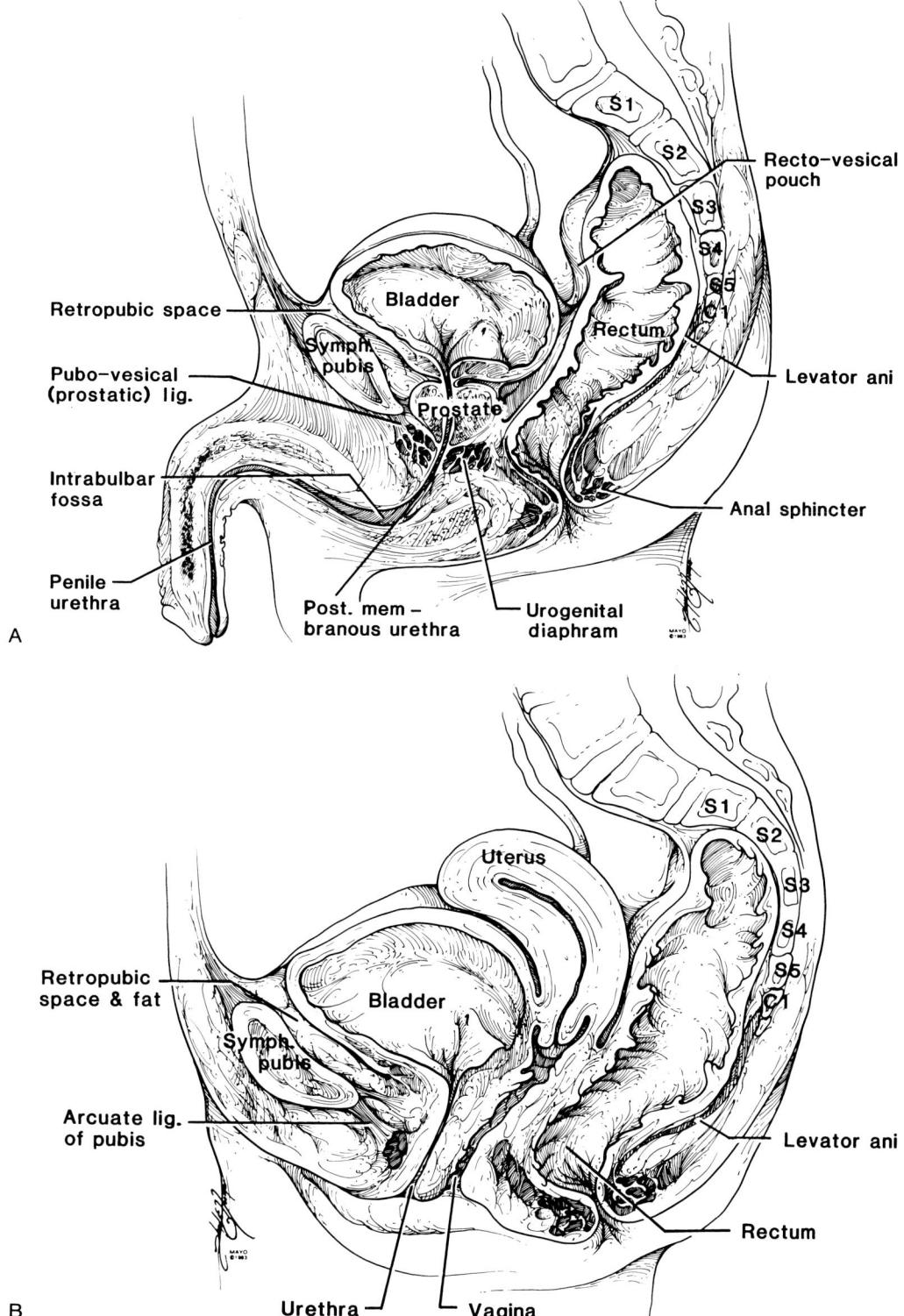

FIG. 5–10. Illustrations of the genitourinary (GU) tract: **A:** Sagittal section of the male genitourinary tract. **B:** Sagittal section of the female GU tract.

its vascular supply from the branches of the obturator internus. These smaller branch vessels follow the ligamentum teres femoris to the femoral head (1,7,11,19).

The internal iliac artery supplies the major portion of the pelvis. Knowledge of the anatomic distribution of its branches is important for proper angiographic diagnosis and treatment of pelvic hemorrhage (13,14,21,24). The first major branch of the internal iliac is the iliolumbar artery, which follows the wing of the ilium superiorly. The superior gluteal artery runs posteriorly just inferior to the sacroiliac joint. Because of its location and course, it is susceptible to injury with sacroiliac fracture-dislocations (15). The lateral sacral arteries and their branches are at risk with sacral or sacroiliac trauma (24). The anterior pelvic branches of the internal iliac are more frequently injured in cases of displaced fractures of the obturator ring. These vessels include the obturator, internal and external pudendals, and the rectal and vesical branches.

The vessels of the pelvis have a rich anastomotic network with vessels from the contralateral hemipelvis. Venous hemorrhage may also result in significant blood loss following pelvic trauma (16).

Neuroanatomy

The nerve supply of the pelvis and hips is derived from the lumbosacral plexus (Fig. 5-9). The lumbosacral plexus in turn is formed by the ventral rami of L1-S2. Portions of the ventral rami of T12 and S3 also contribute to this plexus. Certain neuroanatomic relationships become clinically significant in dealing with trauma to the pelvis and hips. The sacral branches exit through the ventral sacral foramina and may be injured with sacral trauma, as sacral fractures frequently involve these foramina. The largest branch of the sacral plexus, the sciatic nerve (L4-S3), exits the bony pelvis and passes just posterior to the femoral head (Figs. 5-6 and 5-9). This nerve is thus susceptible to injury in patients with posterior dislocations of the hip. Injury to the branches supplying the genitourinary tract (S2-S4) may result in bladder and bowel incontinence and impotence in males. These aspects will be discussed further in the section dealing with complications of pelvic fractures (1,11,26).

Genitourinary and Gastrointestinal Anatomy

The bladder lies immediately dorsal to the pubic symphysis in both males and females. The peritoneum is reflected over the dome of the bladder and then takes a caudad course, forming the vesicorectal pouch (Fig. 5-10).

In the male (Fig. 5-10A), the urethra passes through the prostate (prostatic urethra). The prostatic urethra is continuous with the membranous urethra just above the urogenital diaphragm. This area has been classically described as the part of the urethra most susceptible to injury (17). The membranous urethra is the shortest portion of the posterior urethra and lies within the urogenital diaphragm. The anterior portions of the urethra (bulbus and cavernous) lie below the urogenital diaphragm. Both the bladder and the prostate are fixed anteriorly by the pubovesicle and puboprostatic ligaments. The ligamentous attachments of the prostate allow less motion inferiorly (i.e., near the urogenital diaphragm) than superiorly (6). The urogenital diaphragm is stronger in males than in females and is suspended between the ischial rami to form the anterior floor of the pelvis.

In the female (Fig. 5-10B), the urethra is 3–5 cm in length and fixed to the vagina posteriorly and to the urogenital diaphragm inferiorly. The female urethra is not as immobile as the male urethra and is therefore less frequently injured following pelvic trauma.

The rectum and a short segment of the distal sigmoid colon are located in the true pelvis. The rectum occupies the presacral space approximately 1 cm ventral to the sacrum. The sigmoid colon is situated near the psoas muscle. Because of its well-developed mesentery, the sigmoid colon is mobile and is rarely injured following pelvic fracture. The rectum has no mesentery and is more rigidly fixed. However, in our experience, injury to the rectosigmoid is rare.

More specific anatomic data will be provided with specific clinical problems in later sections of this chapter.

IMAGING OF THE PELVIS AND HIPS

Routine Radiography

Newer imaging modalities, especially computed tomography (CT), have greatly influenced the radiographic approach to diagnostic problems of the pelvis and hips. However, routine radiography remains the major technique for initial evaluation. Radiographic assessment of these patients should enable the physician to identify the area of injury and also provide sufficient anatomic information for the institution of proper therapy, at least in the period immediately following the injury. In most cases, fulfillment of these goals requires that more than one radiographic projection be obtained. This section will discuss the commonly employed routine radiographic procedures used in evaluation of acute trauma.

Pelvis

AP View

Prior to positioning the patient for any view of the pelvis or hips, certain palpable landmarks must be considered. These anatomic landmarks include (1) the anterior superior iliac spine, (2) the iliac crest, (3) the pubic

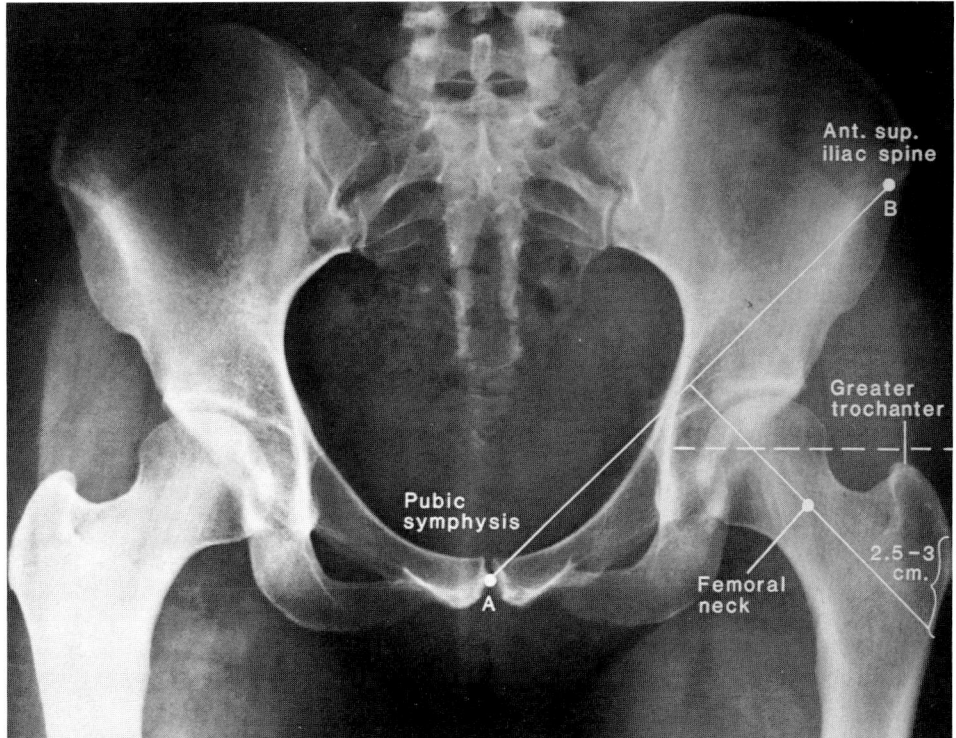

FIG. 5–11. AP radiograph of the pelvis. Note the palpable anterior superior iliac spine (**B**), pubic symphysis (**A**), and greater trochanter. These landmarks are useful in localizing the femoral head and neck.

symphysis, and (4) the greater trochanter (Fig. 5-11) (28,38).

The AP view of the pelvis and hips should be the initial examination in patients with suspected trauma. It provides sufficient information for detection of most pelvic fractures. The findings of the AP view can then be applied to decisions regarding further views. The AP view is obtained with the patient in the supine position on the radiographic table (Fig. 5-12A). The feet should be internally rotated 15°, so that the medial borders of the great toes are approximated. In certain cases, such as a hip fracture, this may not be possible for the patient. This positioning is important and should be used when possible, for it overcomes the natural anteversion of the femoral necks and allows visualization of the neck and greater trochanter (Fig. 5-12B). Improper positioning of the feet (Fig. 5-12C) results in the greater trochanter obscuring the femoral neck and the clear demonstration of the lesser trochanter alone. Proper positioning may be facilitated by the use of sand bags.

A 14 × 17 inch cassette (crosswise) is positioned in the Bucky tray with the top of the cassette 1.5 inches above the iliac crest (palpable). The central beam is centered on the cassette and aligned perpendicular to the cassette (Fig. 5-12A). Gonadal shielding should be used only if it will not obscure possible pathology. Thus it is rarely used in patients with suspected pelvic fractures. Gonadal shields may obscure the sacrum in females and the anterior arch in males.

The AP view of the pelvis and hips provides a significant amount of bone and soft tissue information, and the radiograph should be systematically reviewed. When this view is properly obtained, the entire pelvis, sacrum, and proximal fourth of the femurs are included on the film (Fig. 5-12D). The integrity of the pubic symphysis and obturator rings (formed by the pubic and ischial rami) should be studied, and any displaced anterior fracture should alert the physician to the possibility of a second fracture (usually posterior and near the sacroiliac joint or sacrum). The joint space of both hips can also be assessed. The distance from the teardrop (inferomedial acetabular wall) to the medial edge of the femoral head should be symmetrical. An increase in distance of ≥1 mm suggests an effusion, subluxation, or intra-articular fragment (64). The sacroiliac joints should be compared for symmetry, and the arcuate lines of the sacrum should be carefully compared to exclude subtle fractures of the sacrum. The lower lumbar spine is usually also visible on this view, and any transverse process fracture should alert one to the need for more careful study of the anatomy immediately above and below the fracture (27,31).

Soft tissue structures may be extremely helpful in detecting subtle fractures (47). Slight displacement of the obturator fat plane may be the only clue to an adjacent fracture (Fig. 5-13). Views of the other fat planes about the hip (iliopsoas, lateral pericapsular, and gluteal fat stripes) may be helpful, but usually a large amount of fluid must be present in the hip joint before these struc-

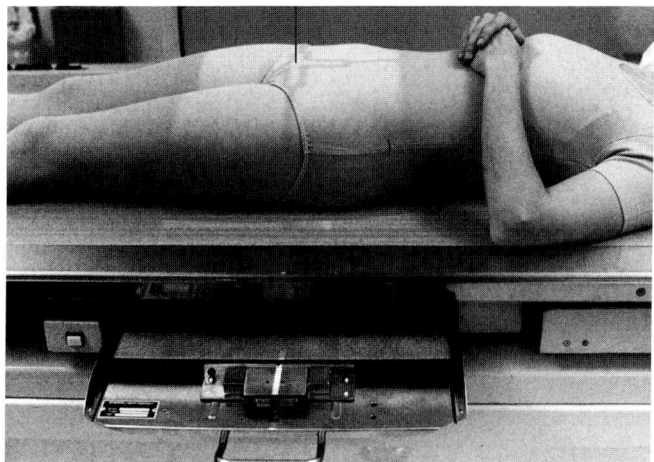

A

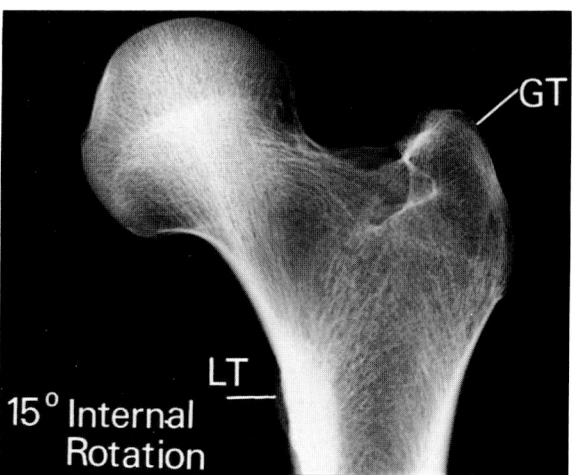

GT

LT

15° Internal
Rotation

B

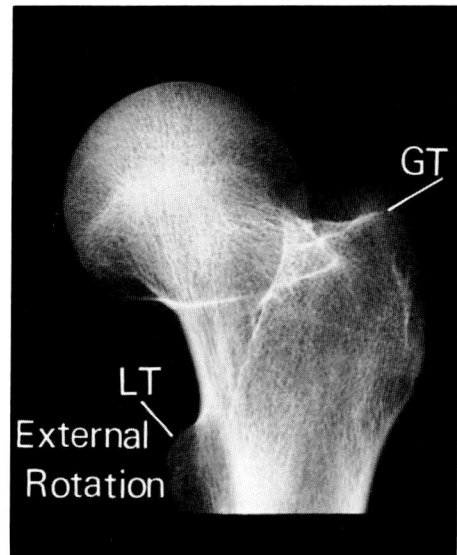

GT

LT
External
Rotation

C

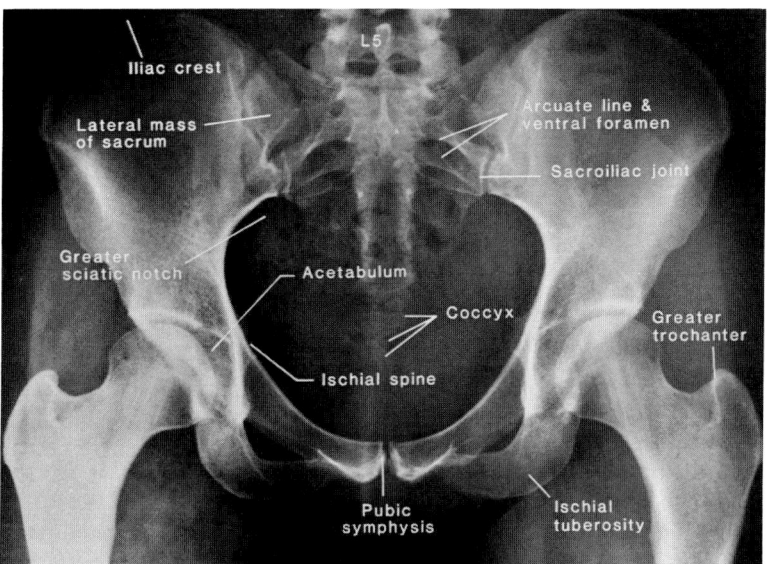

Iliac crest

L5

Lateral mass
of sacrum

Arcuate line &
ventral foramen

Sacroiliac joint

Greater
sciatic notch

Acetabulum

Coccyx

Greater
trochanter

Ischial spine

Ischial
tuberosity

Pubic
symphysis

D

FIG. 5–12. A: Patient positioned for AP view of the pelvis. The elbows are flexed with the hands resting on the abdomen. The upper margin of the 14 × 17 cassette is 1 to 1.5 inches above the iliac crest with the beam (*vertical line*) perpendicular to the center of the cassette. **B:** Specimen radiograph with proper amount of internal rotation (15°). Note the position of the greater and lesser trochanter. **C:** Specimen radiograph in external rotation changes the treater and lesser trochanteric appearance and obscures the femoral neck. **D:** Normal AP radiograph of the pelvis with anatomic labels.

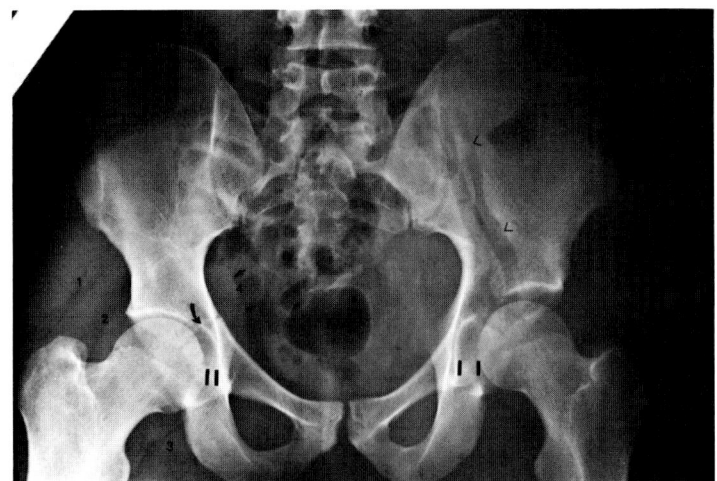

FIG. 5–13. AP view of the pelvis. There is an obvious displaced fracture of the left ilium (*open arrows*). The fat planes are all visible (gluteal, 1; pericapsular, 2; iliopsoas, 3; obturator internus, 4) on the right. The obturator internus is displaced medially providing a clue to assist in detection of the central acetabular fracture (*curved arrow*). Note the joint asymmetry due to hemarthrosis on the left (*lines*).

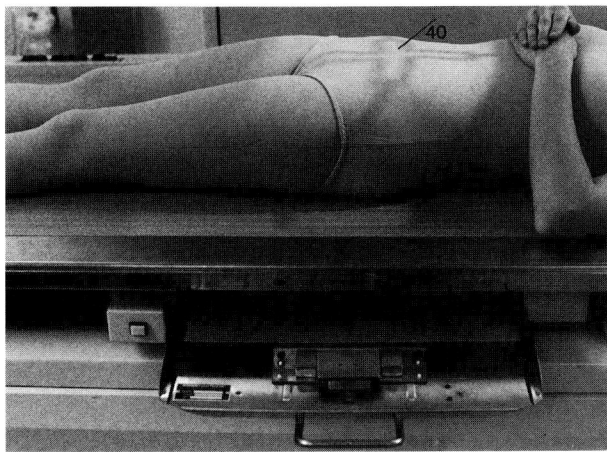

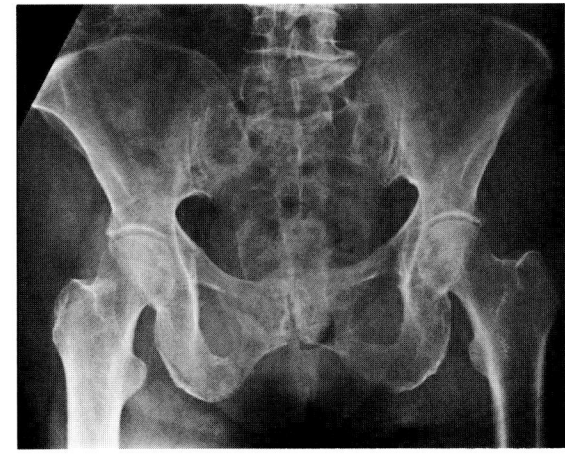

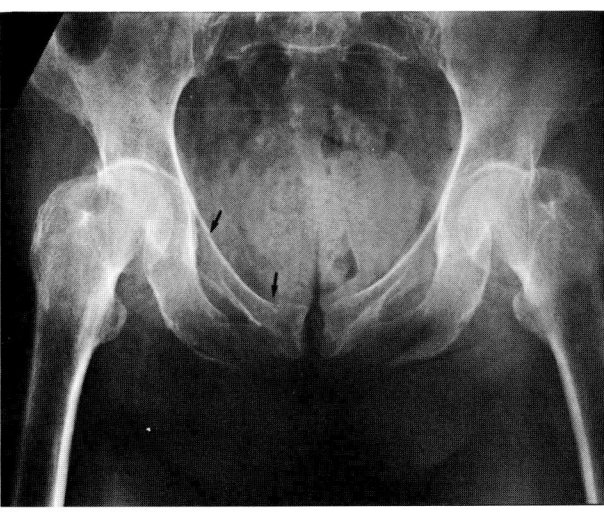

FIG. 5-14. **A:** Patient positioned for the inlet view. The tube is angled 40° to the feet. **B:** AP view of the pelvis: Patient sustained trauma to the pelvis with pain anteriorly. **C:** Inlet view: There are two minimally displaced fractures of the pubic ramus on the right (*arrows*). These were not evident on the AP view.

tures are altered on the AP radiograph. The bladder is often visible in the midpelvis near the symphysis (41), and elevation or deviation of the soft tissue shadow of the bladder may be present with pelvic hematoma or posterior urethral rupture. In complex pelvic fractures, large hematomas may obscure the bladder and perivesical fat entirely.

AP Angled Views

Clarification of findings on the AP view of the pelvis may be accomplished with inlet and tangential projections (28,54,67). The inlet projection is obtained with the patient in the supine position (as in the AP projection). The tube is angled 40° toward the feet (Fig. 5-14A). The midpoint of the 14 × 17 cassette should be centered with the central beam. This view assists in evaluation of the internal architecture of the pelvic ring (Fig. 5-14B, C). Displaced fracture fragments are more easily assessed with this view.

The tangential view is taken with the patient supine and the tube angled 25° (males) or 40° (females) toward the head (Fig. 5-15A). The cassette is positioned with its

center at the midpoint of the x-ray beam (54,65,67). This view allows better evaluation of the anterior pelvis, ventral foramina, and margins of the sacrum (Fig. 5-15B). Superior or inferior displacement of fracture fragments is evident on this view (67). An additional advantage of the AP angled views is that they are obtained without moving the patient. This is especially important in evaluating the severely injured patient (69,70).

Lateral View

The inlet and tangential views essentially fulfill the necessary requirement of obtaining two views at 90° angles. However, occasionally a lateral view of the pelvis is necessary for evaluation of the acetabulum or femoral head (30). This view can be obtained in several ways. The patient can be positioned on the side, although this may not be possible following trauma. In this situation, the lateral view can be obtained using the cross-table technique (Fig. 5-16A). When possible, a support cushion should be placed under the hip to assure that the

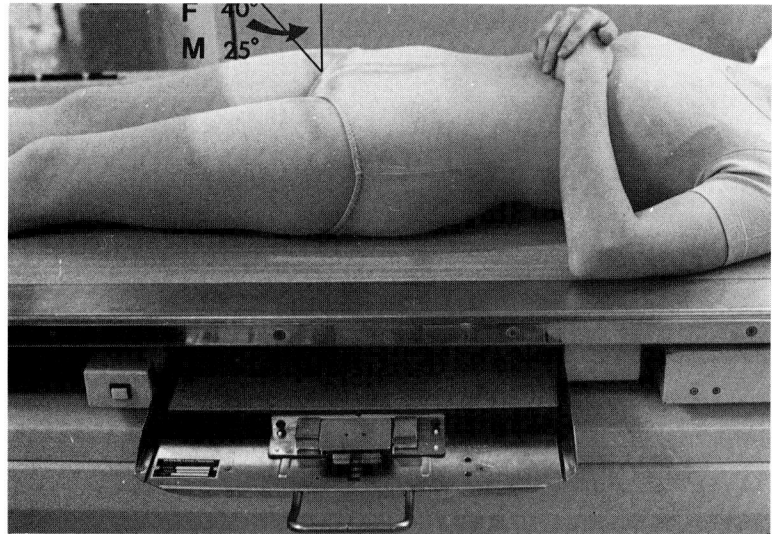

A

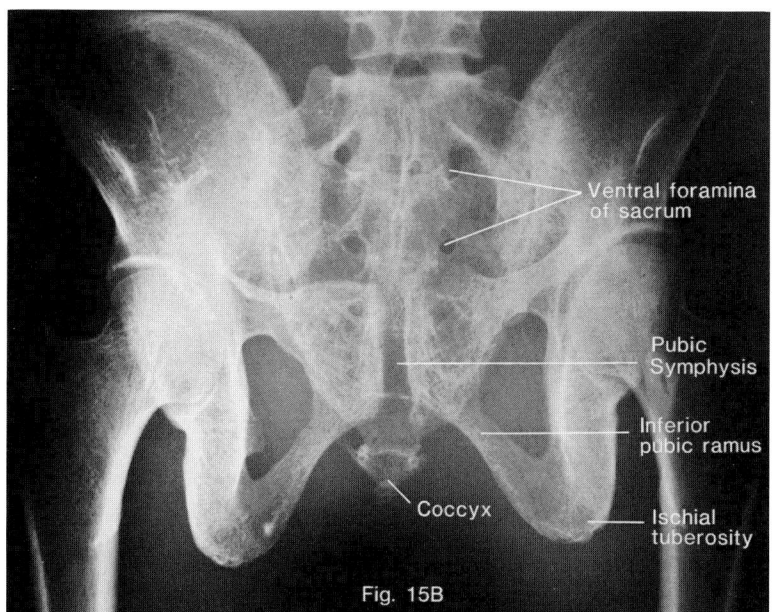

B

FIG. 5–15. A: Patient positioned for tangential view. The tube is angled to the head (25° for males, 40° for females) and centered just below the pubic symphysis. B: Note the radiograph improved visualization of the anterior pelvis (anatomy labeled).

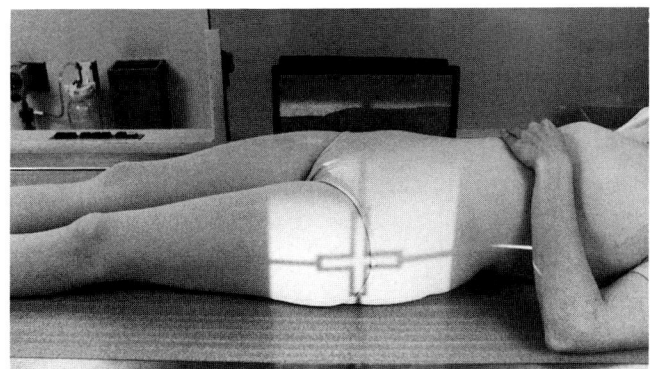

A

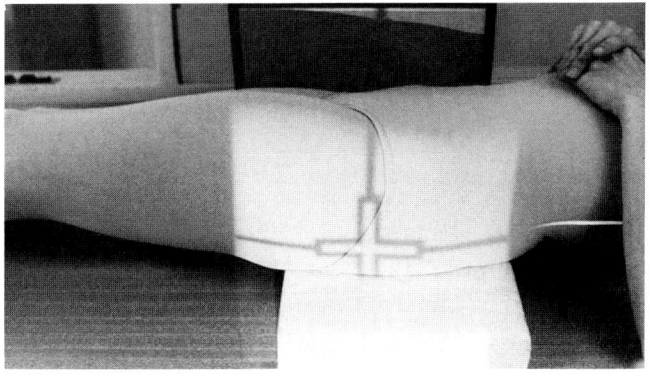

B

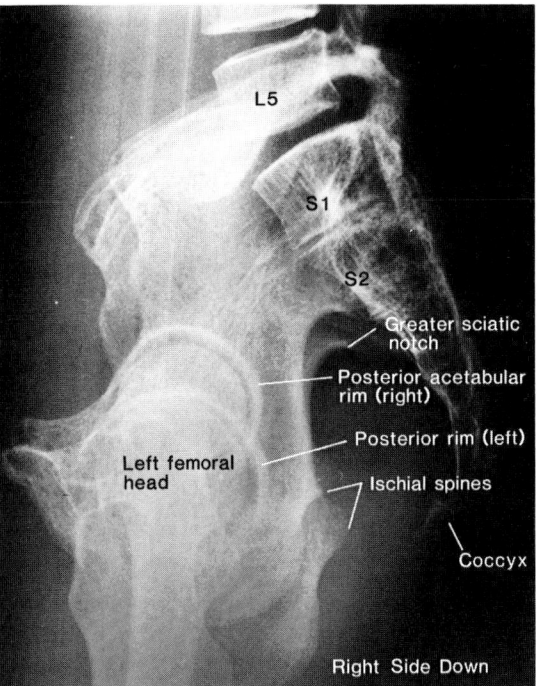

C

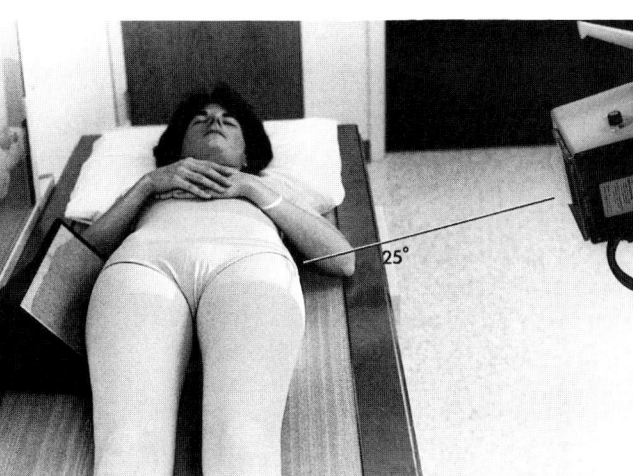

D

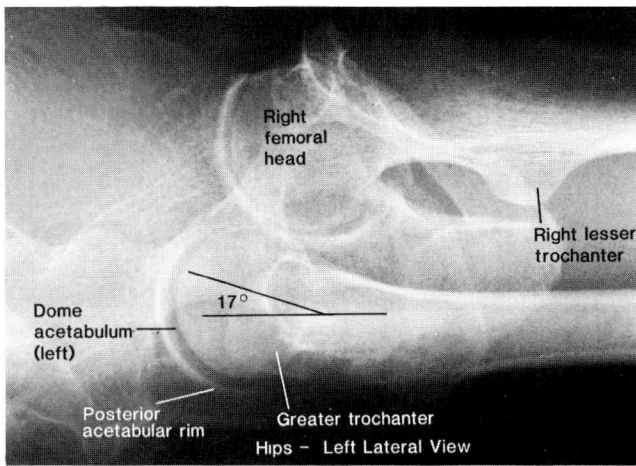

E

FIG. 5-16. A: Patient positioned for cross-table lateral view of the pelvis and hips. The beam is perpendicular to the center of the upright cassette. The beam is centered just above the palpable greater trochanter. **B:** Patient positioned for cross-table lateral with cushion in place to optimize posterior structural detail. Centering is the same as Fig. 5-16A. **C:** Lateral view of the pelvis with right side closest to the film. Note the magnification of the left femoral head. **D:** The patient is supine with the tube angled 25° off the horizontal. Centering is just above the GT with the cassette angled to be perpendicular to the beam. **E:** Both hips are visualized with this angled technique.

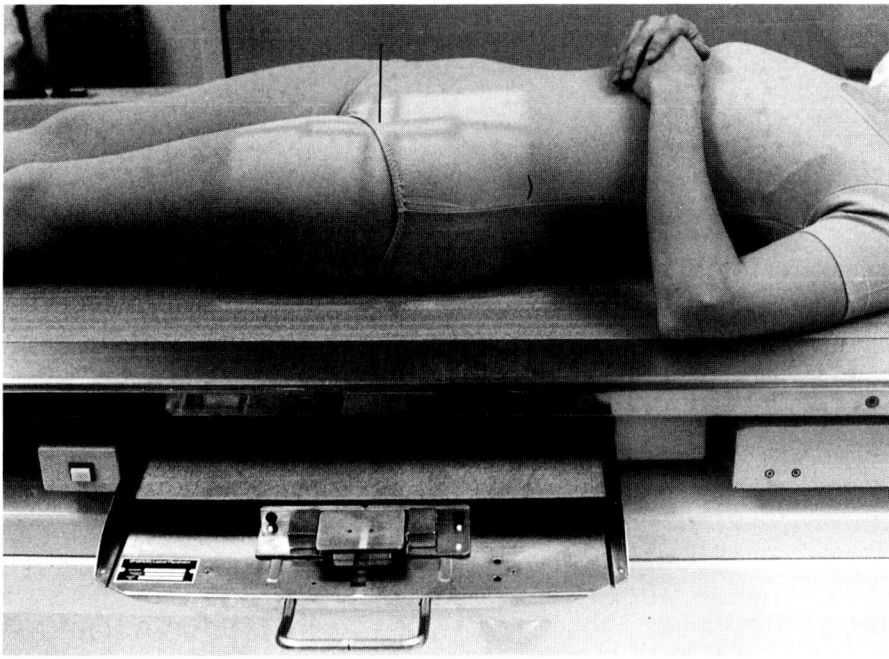
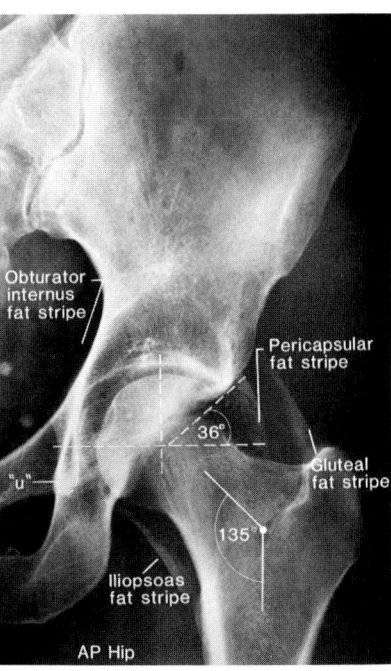

A

B

FIG. 5–17. A: Patient positioned for the AP view of the hip. The beam is perpendicular to the 10 × 12 inch cassette and centered 2 inches medial to the anterior superior iliac spine (palpable) and just above the greater trochanter (palpable). B: AP view of the hip with radiographic data illustrated. See Table 5-2.

posterior structures are included on the film (Fig. 5-16B). The central beam is centered just above the greater trochanter (palpable) and aligned perpendicularly to the cassette. The image obtained is demonstrated in Fig. 5-15C.

An important alternative technique is performed by angling the tube and cassette (Fig. 5-16D) (28,30,45). This is a modification of the technique described by Johnson (45). The tube is angled 25° to the table with the

patient supine. The beam is centered just above the greater trochanter, with the cassette angled so that it is perpendicular to the beam. This results in an excellent view of the hips and acetabular domes (Fig. 5-16E). The patient's condition and the prior results of the AP view dictate which of the above views will be most useful.

Hip

AP View

The patient is supine on the radiographic table. The sagittal plane of the central beam should be centered 2 inches medial to a line longitudinal to the anterior superior iliac spine (palpable). Transverse centering should be at the level of the greater trochanter (palpable) (28,31). A 10 × 12 inch cassette is placed in the Bucky tray with the center perpendicular to the central beam (Fig. 5-17A). This view provides better visualization of the hip and surrounding structures than the AP view of the pelvis. Table 5-2 lists the skeletal, soft tissue, and radiographic angles that should be evaluated on the AP view of the hip (Fig. 5-17) (27,59). A single AP view of the hip is inadequate for complete evaluation. This is especially true if a complete evaluation of the acetabulum and anterior and posterior columns is required (52,68). Oblique views of the hip are particularly helpful in this regard. These projections were popularized by Judet (46).

TABLE 5-2. *Radiographic evaluation of the hip*

AP View

Skeletal Anatomy

1. Iliopubic line
2. Ilioischial line
3. Radiographic "U" (teardrop)
4. Dome of acetabulum
5. Post rim
6. Anterior rim

Angles

1. CE angle of Wibert (normal 20–40°, average 36°)
2. Neck shaft angle (135° normal, >135° = coxa valga, <135° = coxa vara)

Fat Planes

1. Obturator internus
2. Iliopsoas
3. Pericapsular
4. Gluteal

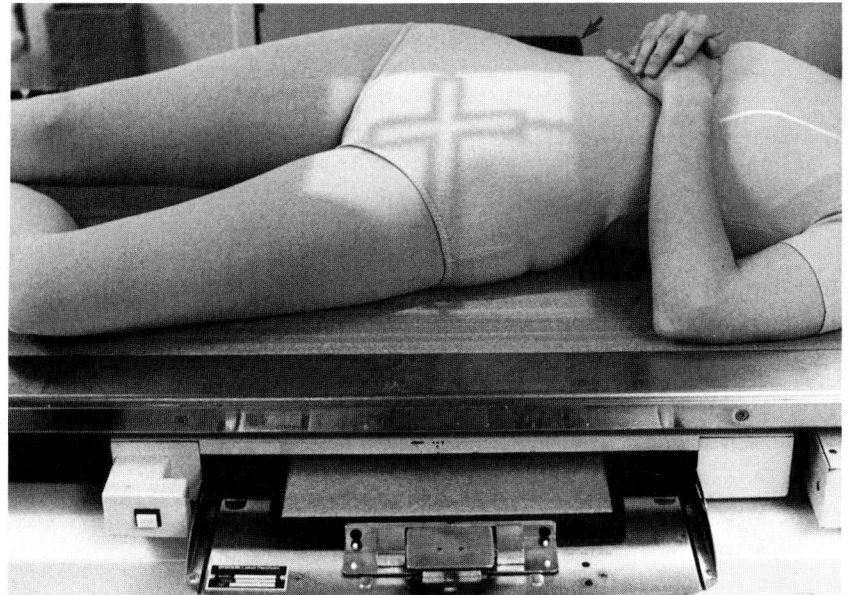

A

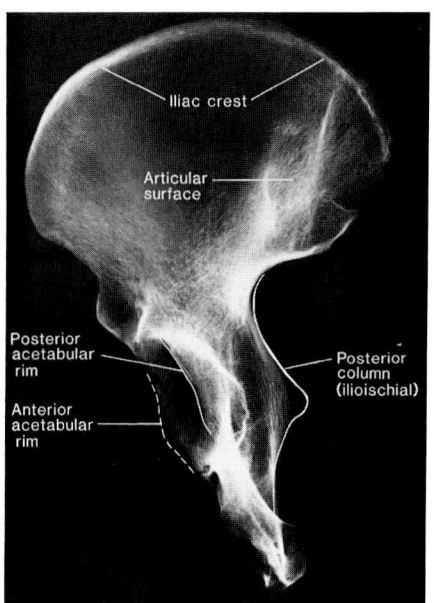

Iliac crest

Articular
surface

Posterior
acetabular
rim

Anterior
acetabular
rim

Posterior
column
(ilioischial)

B

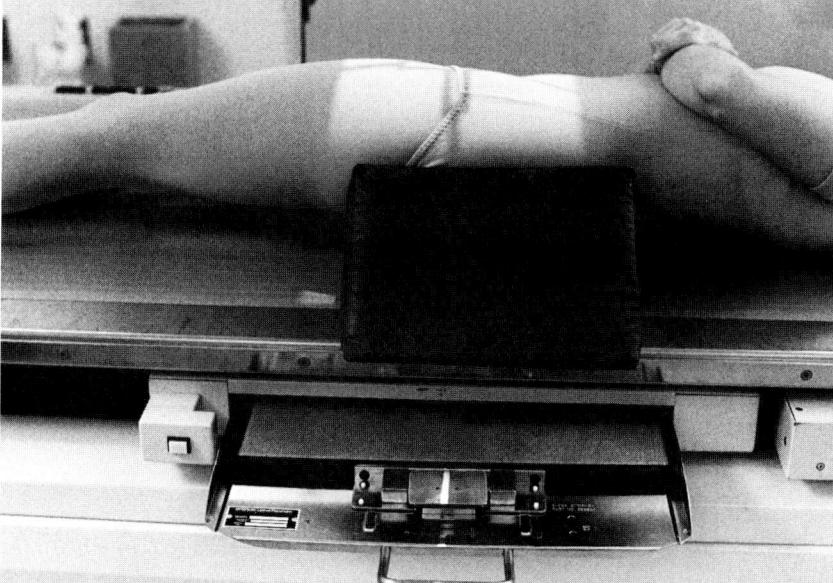

C

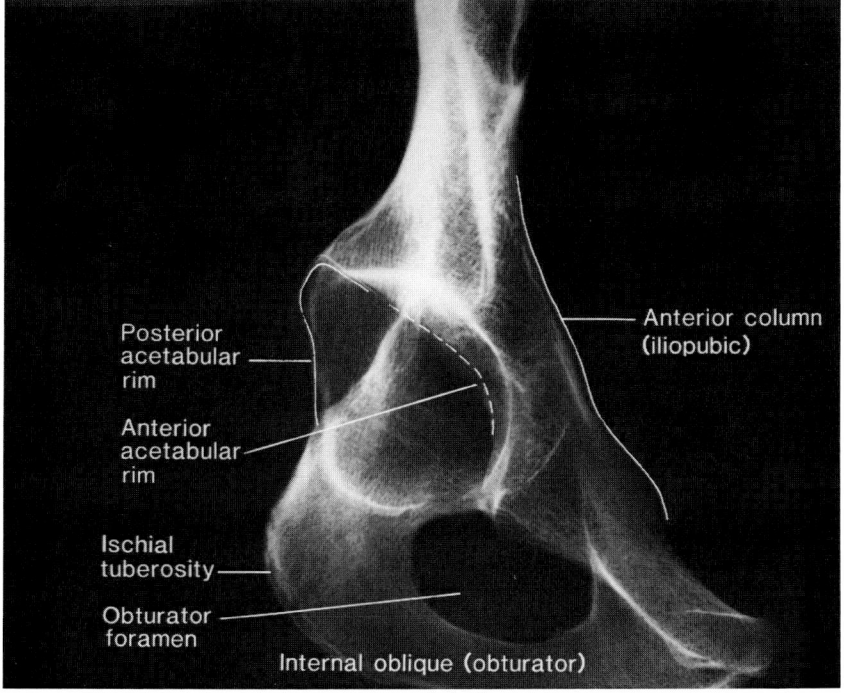

Posterior
acetabular
rim

Anterior
acetabular
rim

Ischial
tuberosity

Obturator
foramen

Anterior column
(iliopubic)

Internal oblique (obturator)

D

FIG. 5–18. A: Patient positioned for posterior oblique view. The involved hip is closest to the film with the opposite hip elevated 45° (45° wedge under hip [*arrow*]). **B:** Specimen radiograph of the innominate bone demonstrating the anatomy (*labeled*) depicted with the posterior oblique view. **C:** Patient positioned for anterior oblique views. The involved hip is rotated 45° away from the film. **D:** Specimen radiograph of anterior oblique view. Note the anterior column is clearly demonstrated. The posterior acetabular rim is projected laterally free of overlying structures. The obturator foramen is clearly seen.

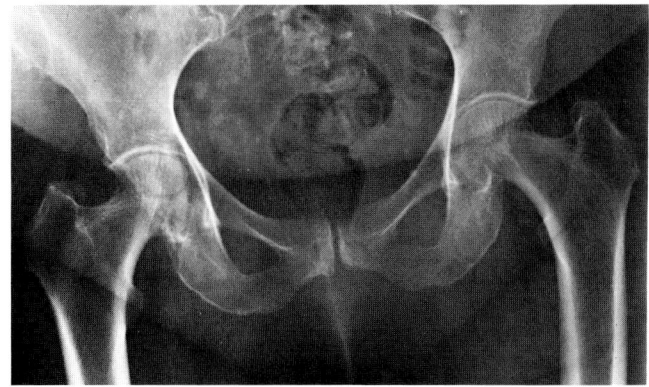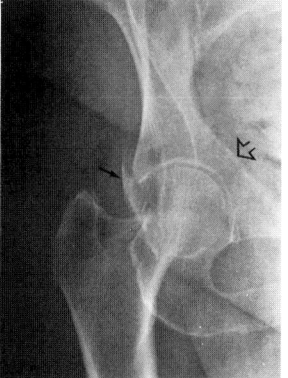

A   B

FIG. 5–19. A: AP view of the pelvis in a patient with right hip pain following trauma. No definite fracture is visible. **B:** Anterior oblique view clearly demonstrating the posterior acetabular rim fracture (*arrow*). The central acetabular region and anterior column are intact (*open arrow*).

Judet Views

The first of two Judet views (posterior oblique) is obtained with the involved hip rotated posteriorly 45° toward the film (Fig. 5-18A). This view clearly demonstrates the iliac wing (iliac view). The anterior rim of the acetabulum is projected laterally to the posterior rim. The posterior column is also seen to better advantage. The anterior oblique view is obtained with the involved hip rotated 45° away from the film (46) (Fig. 5-18C). The anterior oblique view clearly demonstrates the posterior rim of the acetabulum and the anterior column. The obturator foramen is clearly seen. Therefore, this view is often referred to as the obturator oblique (Fig. 5-18D).

Both views begin with the patient in the supine position. To obtain consistency in position, 45° wedges should be placed under the patient's hip and back (Figs. 5-18A and C). The central beam is perpendicular to the

cassette and centered on the hip. The oblique views are particularly useful in detecting subtle fractures of the acetabulum (especially the central acetabulum) and pelvic columns (Fig. 5-19) (46,68).

Lateral View

Evaluation of the upper femur often requires a lateral view to provide a second view at an angle of 90° to the AP view. The commonly used technique for obtaining a lateral view of the hip is demonstrated in Fig. 5-20 (35,53). The patient is supine with the uninvolved hip flexed 90° and the ankle supported to assist in positioning. The foot on the injured side is internally rotated 15° if possible (patients with acute fractures of the femoral neck may be unable to maintain this position). The cassette (10 × 12 inch) is positioned perpendicularly both to the table and to the central beam (Fig. 5-20A). The cassette should be aligned perpendicularly to a line from the

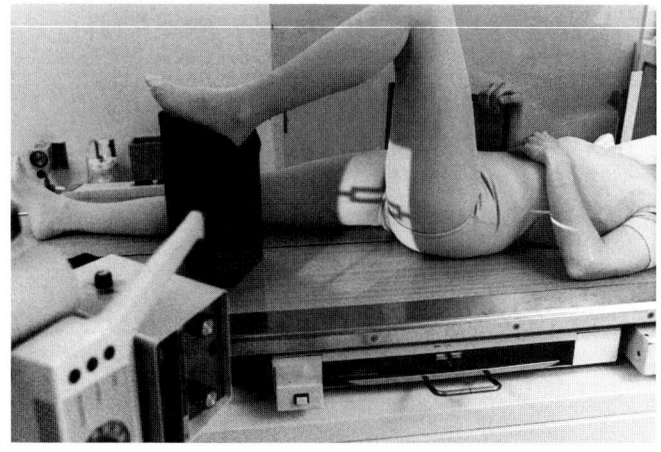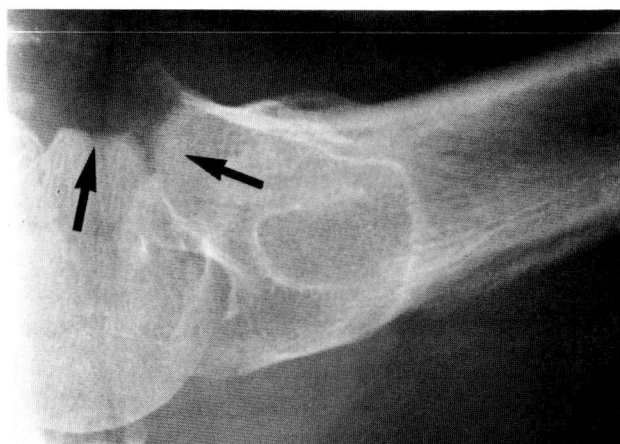

A   B

FIG. 5–20. A: Patient positioned for lateral view of the right hip. The left knee is flexed 90° and supported by a cushion. The central beam is centered just below the greater trochanter (palpate) with the cassette and beam perpendicular to a line from the anterior superior iliac spine to the symphysis (see Fig. 5-11). **B:** Lateral view of the hip. Subcapital fracture with rotation of the head (*left arrow*) and position of the neck (*right arrow*). This view is particularly useful for position and evaluation of the posterior cortex.

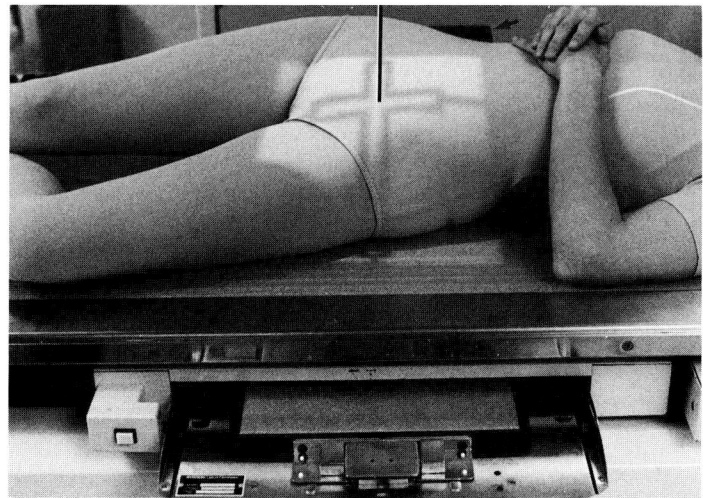

A

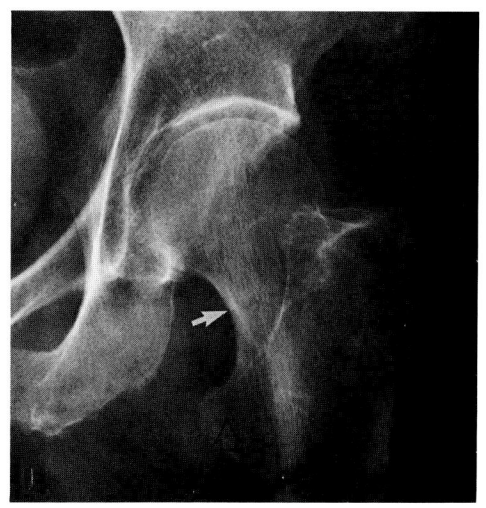

B

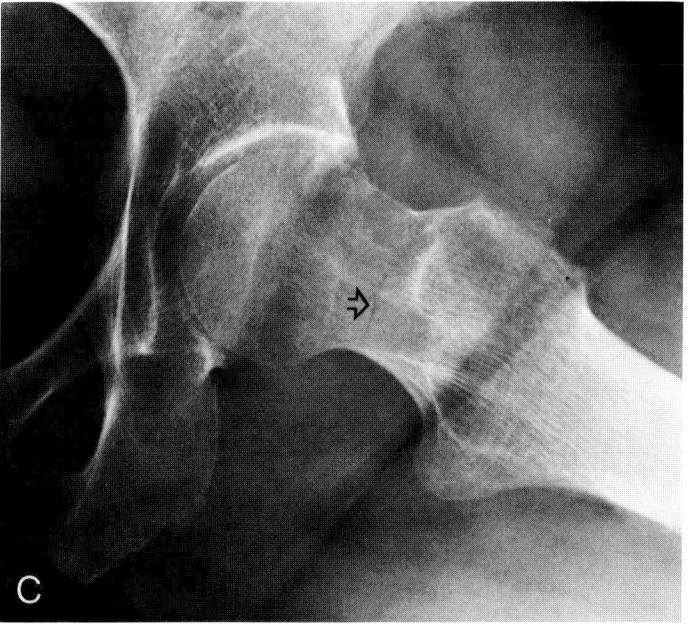

C

FIG. 5–21. A: Patient positioned for oblique view of the hip. The patient's opposite hip is elevated and supported by a cushion wedge (*arrow*). The knee is flexed and the thigh slightly raised toward the head. The beam is perpendicular to the cassette and centered between the symphysis and anterior superior iliac spine. AP view (**B**) demonstrates the hip is externally rotated with the lesser trochanter (*open arrow*) totally seen. There may be a subtle fracture (*white arrow*). The oblique view (**C**) demonstrates an undisplaced fracture of the femoral neck (*open arrow*).

pubic symphysis to the anterior superior iliac spine (palpable). The central beam is centered just below the greater trochanter (palpable). The radiograph demonstrates the hip joint, femoral neck, and trochanters (Fig. 5-20B). An alternative method is to position a curved cassette medial to the involved hip, with the tube lateral to the patient and angled toward the feet (28,51).

In severely injured patients these techniques may be impossible. In this situation the Johnson method (45) is often very helpful. The cassette (10 × 12) is placed next to the hip to be examined, forming a 65° angle with the radiographic table. Angling the tube 25° to the table and perpendicularly to the cassette results in a lateral view of both hips (similar to Fig. 5-16D). If the tube is also angled toward the head 25°, only the hip next to the film is obtained. An alternative to these methods is to position the patient at an oblique angle of 20°–25° oblique to the table, with the cassette perpendicular to the table and the

tube perpendicular to the film (Fig. 5-16). The resulting radiograph is similar to that produced by the other techniques. The hip closest to the film will be less magnified, and the radiographic detail will be sharper.

Oblique View

The patient is positioned with the affected side of the hip toward the 10 × 12 inch cassette. The opposite hip is supported by a cushion wedge (Fig. 5-21A). The knee should be flexed and the thigh raised about 45°. The beam is centered between the symphysis and anterior superior iliac spine (Figs. 5-11 and 5-21A) (28,50). This view allows improved visualization of the femoral neck, acetabulum, and lesser trochanter. It is also often helpful in detecting subtle femoral neck fractures (Fig. 5-21B and C).

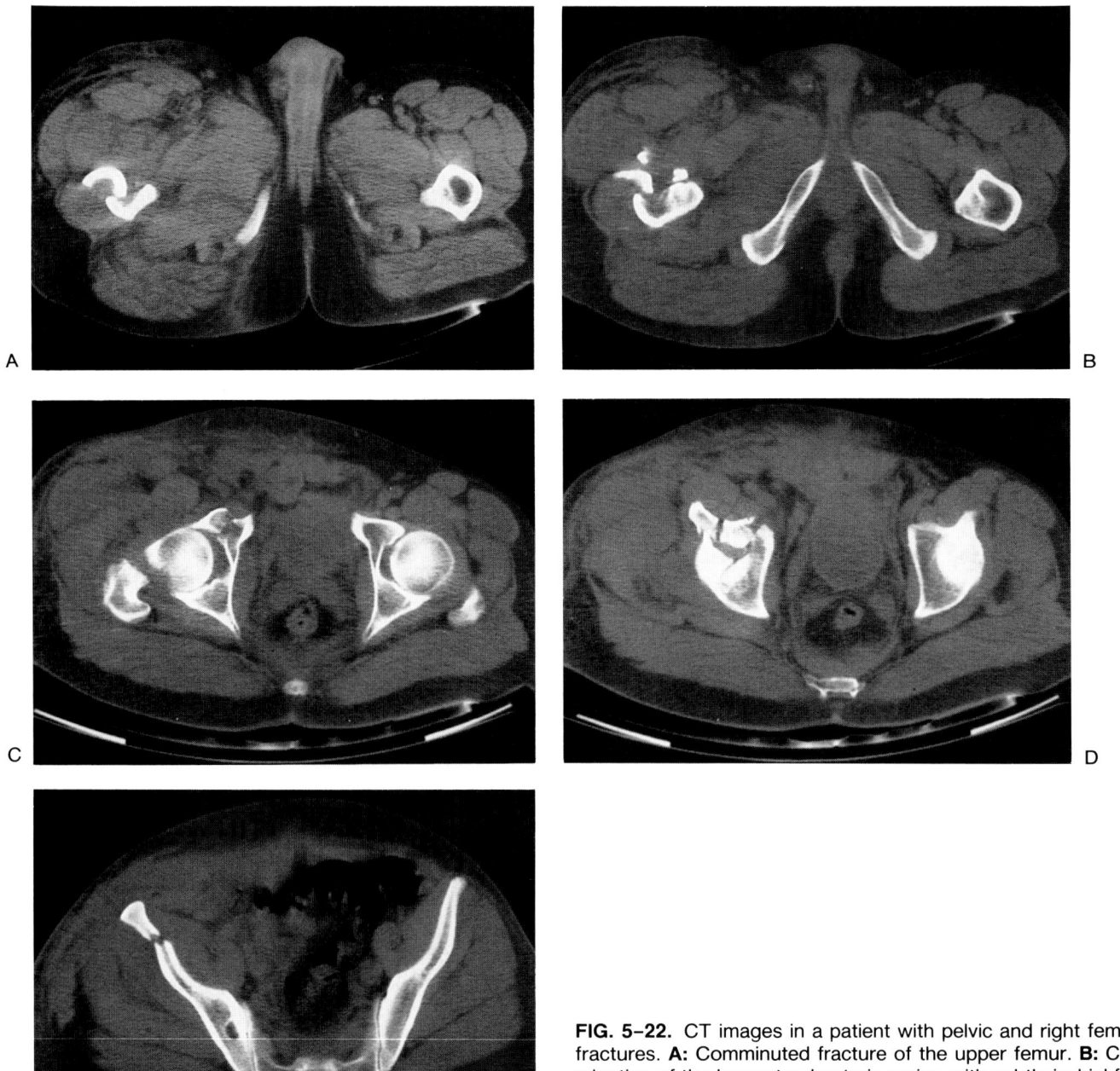

FIG. 5-22. CT images in a patient with pelvic and right femoral fractures. **A:** Comminuted fracture of the upper femur. **B:** Comminution of the lesser trochanteric region with subtle ischial fractures. **C:** Fractures of the right femoral neck and anterior acetabulum. **D:** Comminuted fracture of the right acetabular dome. **E:** Fracture of the anterior right ilium with hematoma.

Computed Tomography

There are many other techniques available for study of the pelvis and hips (28,31,37,39,43,44,50,55,66). In addition to routine radiography, tomography, radionuclide scans, and specifically computed tomography (CT) are often of value in complete evaluation of trauma to the pelvis and hips. CT is the technique of choice for evaluation of fracture fragments, their position and orientation, soft tissue hematoma, and intra-articular fragments (Fig. 5-22) (36,40,56,58,69). In some cases, CT can be performed immediately after an AP view of the pelvis. This, of course, depends on the patient's condition (69). Prior to obtaining the CT scans, certain decisions should be considered. Are three-dimensional reconstructions necessary? Will angiography be required? If acetabular fractures are evident, three dimensional reconstruction can provide valuable information for surgical planning (33,34,38,48,60). Thin slices (1.5 mm or 3 mm overlapping) are needed for best results (Fig. 5-23). Normally, 5 mm slice thicknesses are used. If significant hemorrhage is evident and angiography (diagnostic or therapeutic)

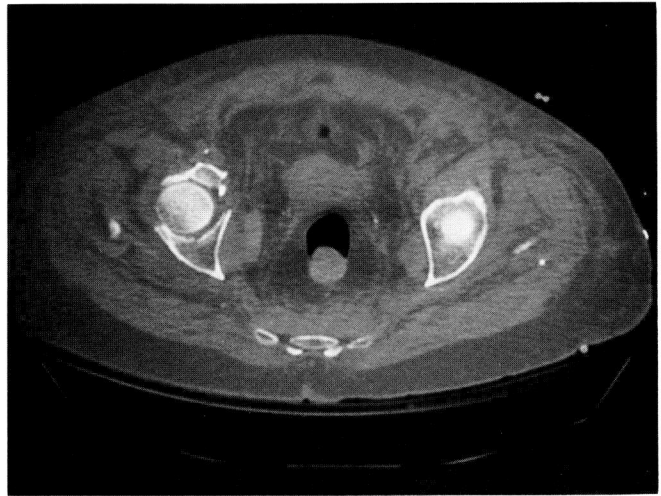

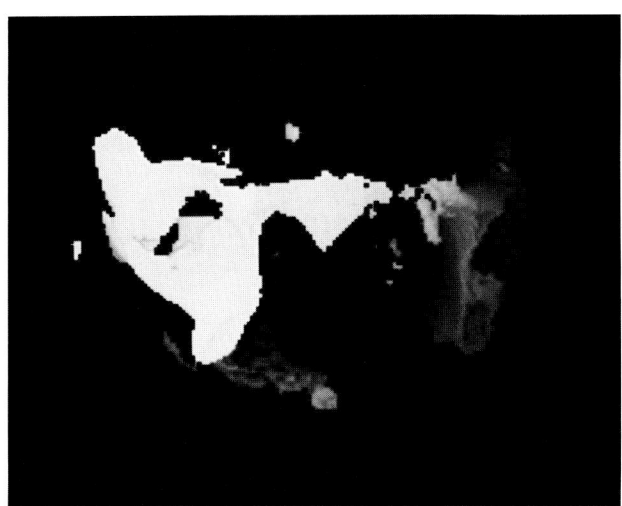

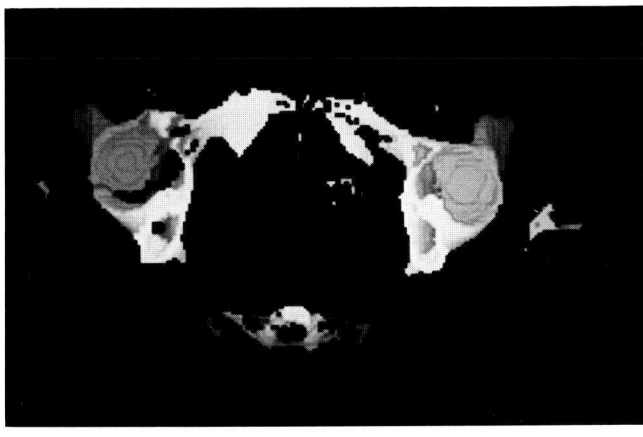

FIG. 5-23. Conventional (**A**) and three-dimensional reconstructions (**B, C**) of a complex acetabular fracture.

may be indicated, it is useful to avoid contrast in the bladder or extravasate in the pelvis due to IV contrast that is usually given with CT imaging.

Magnetic resonance imaging (MRI), arthrography, ultrasonography, and other diagnostic techniques are also useful in selected situations (29,32,42,49,57,61–63,71). These techniques will be discussed more completely later.

PELVIC FRACTURES

Pelvic fractures represent a small percentage (2–3%) of all skeletal fractures (74,132). The severity of the fracture depends upon the mechanism of injury. Minor pelvic fractures (fractures of individual bones or single breaks in the pelvic ring) are fairly common in older individuals following simple falls. Severe pelvic injury is usually the result of high-velocity motor vehicle accidents, industrial accidents, or falls of a significant distance. Table 5-3 summarizes the etiology and associated mortality rate of severe pelvic injury in patients treated in our department. Complex pelvic fractures tend to occur in younger individuals (50% under 30 and 77% under 50 years of

age), with males outnumbering females 3:1 (Table 5-4) (137). In our series of over 100 patients with complex pelvic fractures (Key and Conwell Class III), the overall mortality rate was 22%. Massive hemorrhage was the most common and potentially life-threatening complication.

The proper management of pelvic fractures requires complete radiographic assessment of the pelvic ring (72,73). This requires multiple radiographic views and, in certain cases, CT and angiography. Detection of posterior fractures is particularly important, as complications (hemorrhage, instability, etc.) increased significantly with double breaks in the pelvic ring (116,129,134, 137,152).

TABLE 5-3. *Complex pelvic fractures*

Etiology	% Patients	Mortality rate
MVA	43	26%
Farm accident	18	0%
Pedestrian accident	17	41%
Motorcycle accident	8	38%
Falls	6	17%
Other	8	0%

TABLE 5-4. *Complex pelvic fractures: Age distribution*

Age (yrs.)	% Patients	
	Male	Female
15–20	13	13
21–30	16	8
31–40	8	2
41–50	15	2
51–60	5	1
61–70	7	0
>70	4	4

Classification of Pelvic Fractures

A thorough understanding of the classification of pelvic fractures is essential for effective communication between the orthopedist or examining physician and the radiologist (155,161). Multiple classifications of pelvic fractures have been developed, each of which is designed to help the physician determine the proper management and prognosis of the pelvic fracture (Table 5-5).

Tile (152) proposed a classification based on Pennal's study of 354 pelvic fractures (Table 5-5). This classification is based on the forces that result in pelvic fracture. Such forces include anteroposterior compression, lateral compression, vertical shearing, and combined force injuries (158,159). Connally and Hedberg proposed that pelvic fractures be considered major if the weight-bearing surface of the acetabulum is involved or if both obturator rings are fractured (84). Watson-Jones (154) divided pelvic fractures into three categories, with Type II being the most significant (Table 5-5).

The above mechanisms produce certain radiographic patterns that are useful in planning therapy (89,157–160). Lateral compression injuries comprise nearly half

TABLE 5-5. *Pelvic fracture classifications*

Tile-Pennal[a]
  1. Anteroposterior compression
      Open book
      Straddle fractures
  2. Lateral compression
      Ipsilateral double fractures
      Bucket handle fractures
      Straddle fractures with posterior disruption
  3. Vertical shearing fractures

Connally-Hedberg[b]
  Major
    Bilateral rami fractures
    Acetabular dome fractures
  Minor

Watson-Jones[c]
  Type I: Avulsion fractures
  Type II: Fracture and dislocation of the pelvic ring
  Type III: Sacrococcygeal fractures

[a] (151), [b](84), [c](151).

of major pelvic fractures (159). Young et al. (159) described three patterns of injury due to a lateral blow to the pelvis. Type I injuries are due to forces directed to the posterior pelvis and minimal distortion of the pelvic ring is noted (Fig. 5-24A). Unilateral or bilateral pubic rami are always present. These fractures are typically oblique or horizontally oriented. There is an associated crush injury of the sacrum or sacroiliac joint. Since the ligaments are intact, the injury is stable (89,159). Central acetabular fractures occured in 19% of cases. Type II injuries occur when the lateral force is applied to the anterior pelvis resulting in medial displacement of the innominate bone on the side of the injury. Rotation of the anterior innominate bone leads to either rupture of the ipsilateral sacroiliac joint (Type IIA) or fracture of the iliac wing (Type IIB) (Fig. 5-24B and C) (157). Both configurations are unstable. Type III injuries are the most severe and result in bilateral posterior instability (157,159). The force is directed more anteriorly resulting in internal rotation of the innominate bone on the injured side and lateral displacement of the contralateral side. Type III injuries involve the sacroiliac joint and posterior ligament complex (Type IIIA) or the ipsilateral iliac wing (Type IIIB) (Fig. 5-24D and E) (89,159). Pubic rami fractures associated with lateral compression injuries differ from anterior compression injuries. Fractures are typically oblique or horizontal or buckling in appearance (Fig. 5-25) (157). Daffner (89) described six radiographic and CT features of lateral compression injuries. These included horizontal obturator ring fractures, vertical sacral buckle fracture (best seen on CT), horizontal iliac fractures, bilateral sacroiliac diastasis, central acetabular fractures, and evidence of rotation on CT images.

Anterior compression injuries account for 21% of major pelvic fractures (157,159,160). Pubic rami fractures, or diastasis of the symphysis with associated posterior injury to the sacroiliac joints, sacrum, or iliac wings occurs. Pubic rami fractures tend to be vertically oriented with anterior compression injuries. Diastasis of the pubic symphysis may reach 2.5 cm without disruption of the sacroiliac ligaments. Three fracture patterns have been described (Fig. 5-26). Type I injuries have vertical pubic rami fractures or mild diastasis of the pubic symphysis. The anterior sacroiliac ligaments may be involved (Fig. 5-26A). Type II injuries result when continued force causes further anterior separation (>2.5 cm) (Fig. 5-26B) with disruption of the anterior sacroiliac, sacrospinous, and sacrotuberous ligaments. Further widening of both the symphysis and sacroiliac joint occurs with Type III injuries (Fig. 5-26C) due to further ligament injury. Common findings of anterior compression injuries include diastasis of the symphysis and sacroiliac joints and vertical pubic rami fractures (89).

Vertical shear injuries account for 6% of pelvic frac-

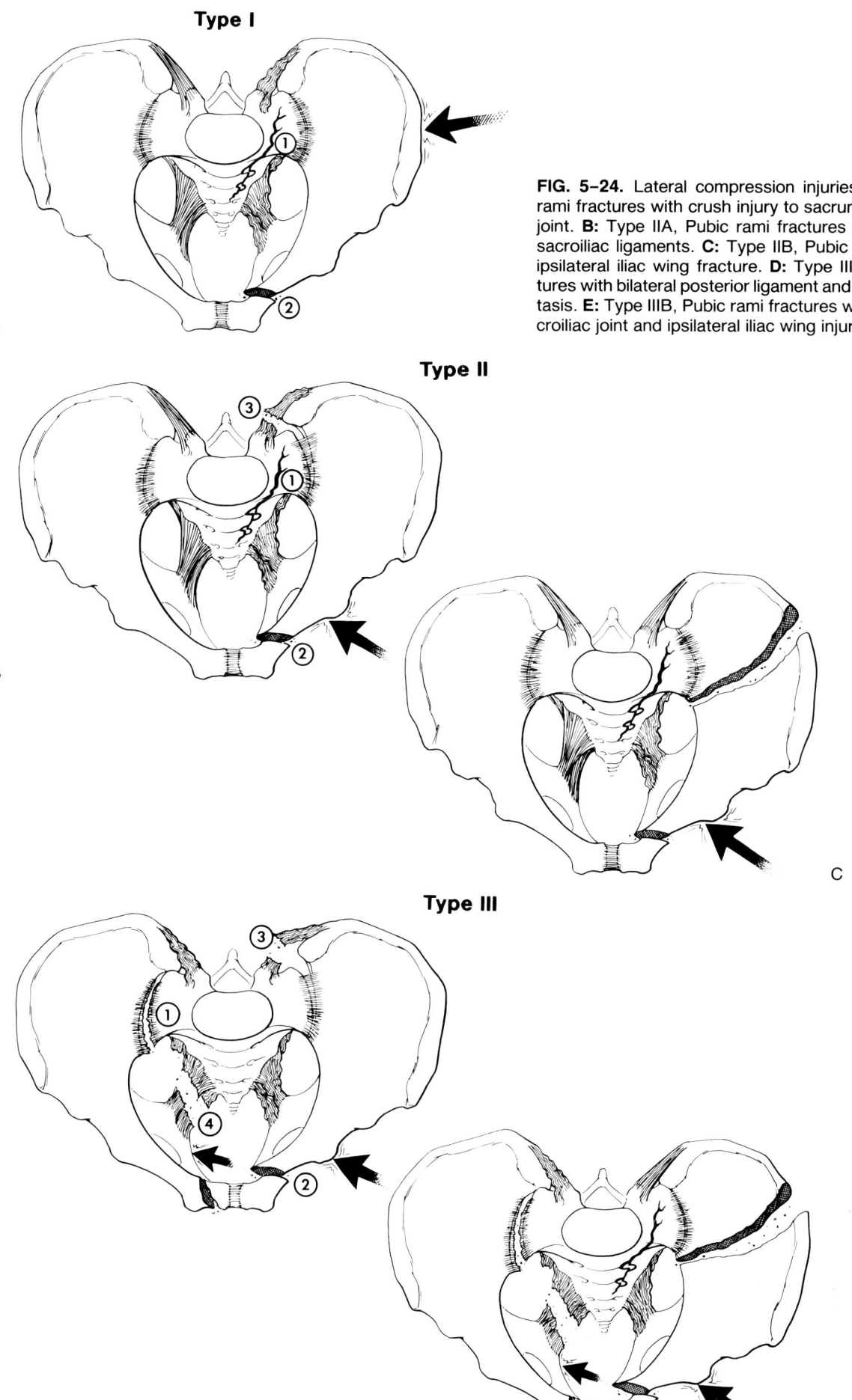

FIG. 5-24. Lateral compression injuries. **A:** Type I, Pubic rami fractures with crush injury to sacrum, ilium or sacroiliac joint. **B:** Type IIA, Pubic rami fractures with rupture of the sacroiliac ligaments. **C:** Type IIB, Pubic rami fractures with ipsilateral iliac wing fracture. **D:** Type IIIA, Pubic rami fractures with bilateral posterior ligament and sacroiliac joint diastasis. **E:** Type IIIB, Pubic rami fractures with contralateral sacroiliac joint and ipsilateral iliac wing injuries.

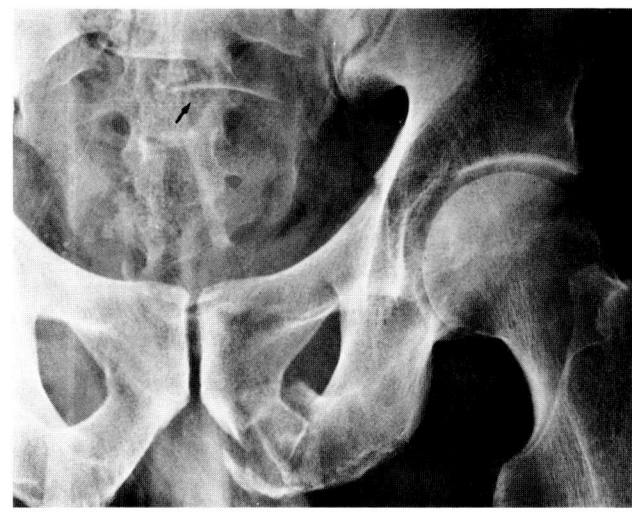

FIG. 5–25. Lateral compression injury with fractures (*arrows*) of the left acetabulum, sacrum, and pubic ramus.

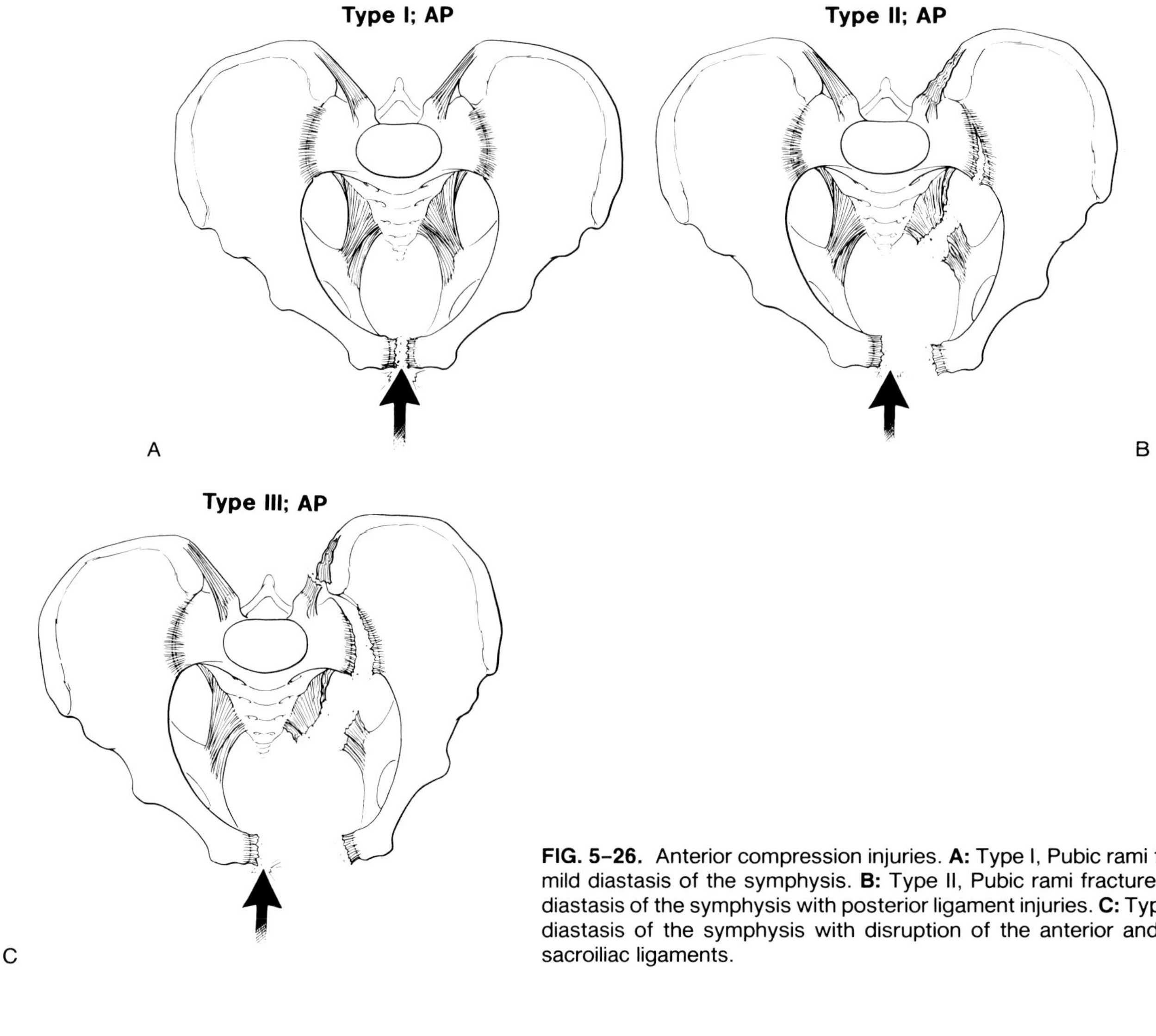

Type I; AP

A

Type II; AP

B

Type III; AP

C

FIG. 5–26. Anterior compression injuries. **A:** Type I, Pubic rami fracture or mild diastasis of the symphysis. **B:** Type II, Pubic rami fractures or wider diastasis of the symphysis with posterior ligament injuries. **C:** Type III, Wide diastasis of the symphysis with disruption of the anterior and posterior sacroiliac ligaments.

Vertical Shear

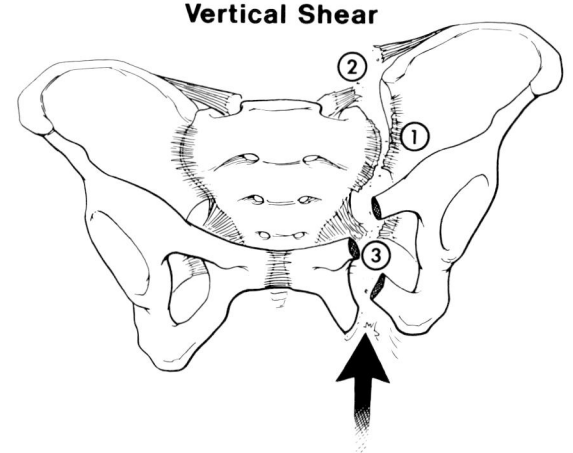

FIG. 5–27. Vertical shearing injury with disruption of the anterior and posterior ring.

tures (157). These injuries result from vertical forces directed through the femur or lateral to the midline (Fig. 5-27). Disruption of the hemipelvis via the symphysis and sacroiliac joint or iliac and pubic rami fractures result in a definite step off on AP radiographs.

Complex or combined forces account for 14% of pelvic fractures. Lateral compression with either anterior or shearing forces are most common (89,157–159).

These fracture patterns are useful in determining the mechanism of injury and, therefore, the method of reduction.

We prefer to use the classification proposed by Key and Conwell (104) and modified by Kane (103). This classification, shown in Table 5-6, will be applied to facilitate the following discussion of pelvic fractures. The incidence of each fracture class is included in Table 5-6.

These numbers are based on a review of 750 pelvic fractures over a 14-year period at Mayo Clinic (137).

Class I Fractures

Class I fractures include breaks in individual bones without interruption of the pelvic ring (Fig. 5-28). This type of fracture occurred in 25% of patients in our series (Table 5-6). Several types of fractures fall within this category, including avulsion fractures. These fractures (Fig. 5-29) commonly occur in young athletes. Avulsion fractures result from sudden muscle contraction, with the break occurring at the origin or insertion of the muscle. Common locations for avulsion fractures include the following areas (Fig. 5-29): (1) anterior superior iliac spine by the sartorius (Fig. 5-30), (2) anterior inferior iliac spine by the rectus femoris (Fig. 5-31), (3) ischial tuberosity by the hamstrings, (4) greater trochanter by the gluteal muscles, and (5) lesser trochanter by the iliopsoas muscle. These fractures usually heal satisfactorily unless displacement exceeds 2 cm. Sciatic nerve injury has been reported with avulsion fractures of the ischium (117). Other avulsion injuries can also occur. Differentiation of certain injuries from normal ossification centers may be difficult (Fig. 5-32). The os acetabuli marginalis superior may persist in adults but typically fuses by 20 years of age (81).

Fractures of the individual bones of the obturator ring (ischium and pubic rami) (Fig. 5-28) are usually caused by minor falls in elderly patients, but they may also occur with the stress of overactivity in the osteopenic patient (Fig. 5-33) (86,87). Insufficiency fractures are discussed more completely in Chapter 16. Rankin reported that these fractures of the individual bones were the most

TABLE 5–6. *Key and Conwell classification: Kane modification, 750 patients, Mayo Clinic*[a]

Class	% Patients	Description
I	25	Fractures of individual bones without interruption of the pelvic ring Single ramus fracture Avulsion fracture Duverney fracture Transverse sacral fracture Coccyx fracture
II	36	Single break in the pelvic ring Fracture of two ipsilateral rami Fracture near or subluxation of pelvic symphysis or SI joint
III	16	Double breaks in the pelvic ring Straddle fracture Sprung pelvis Malgaigne fracture Bucket handle fracture Complex fracture
IV	24	Acetabular fractures Undisplaced Displaced

[a] (103).

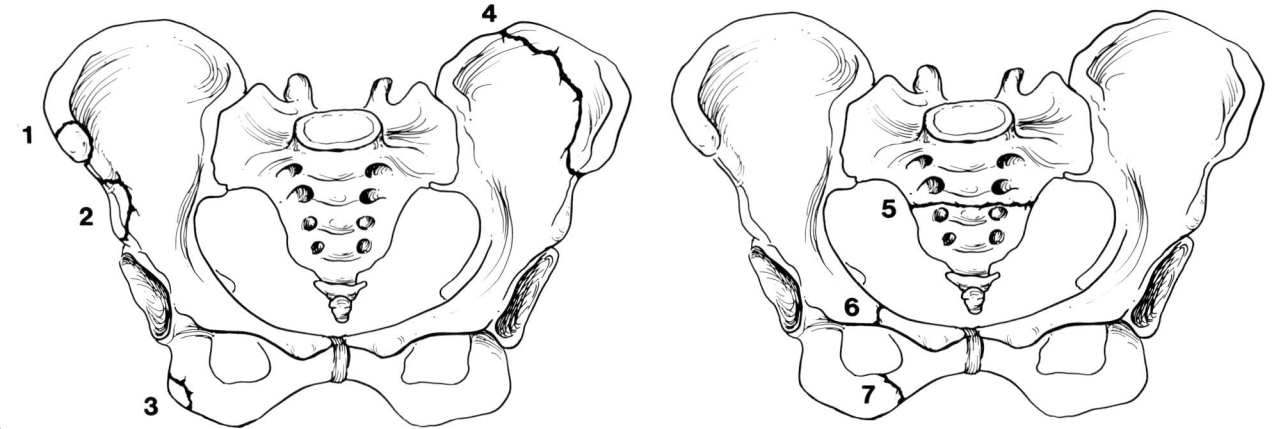

FIG. 5–28. Illustrations of Class I fractures: Individual breaks without interruption of the pelvic ring. **A:** Avulsion fractures of the anterior superior iliac spine (1), anterior inferior iliac spine (2), ischial tuberosity (3), and ilium (4) (Durverney Fracture). **B:** Transverse fracture of the sacrum (5), superior pubic ramus (6) or inferior pubic ramus (7). If both rami are fractured the ring is interrupted—a Class II fracture.

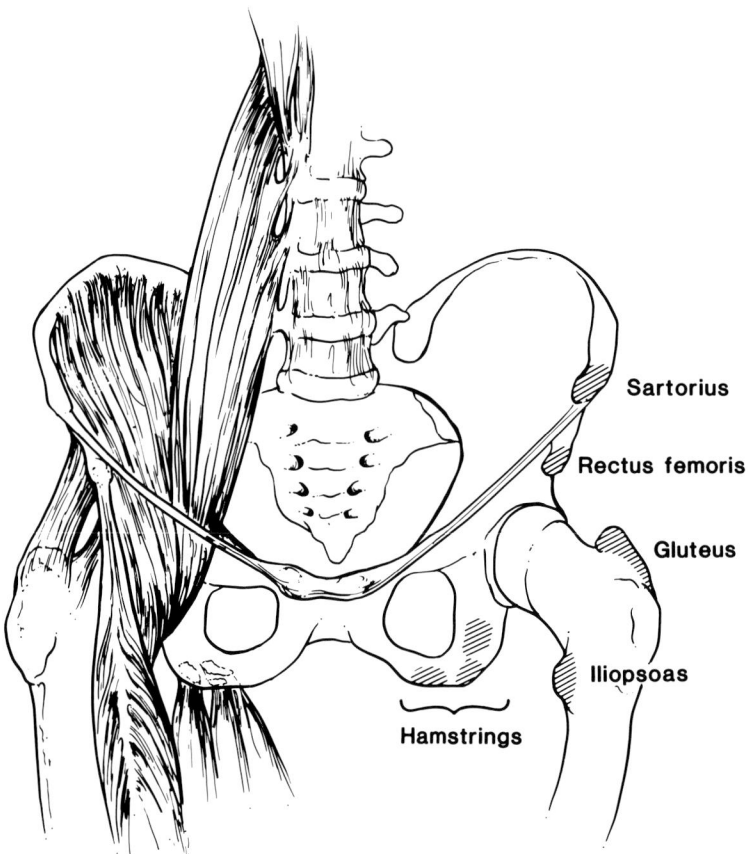

Sartorius

Rectus femoris

Gluteus

Iliopsoas

Hamstrings

FIG. 5–29. Common avulsion fractures of the pelvis and hips. Illustration of the muscle insertions and origins.

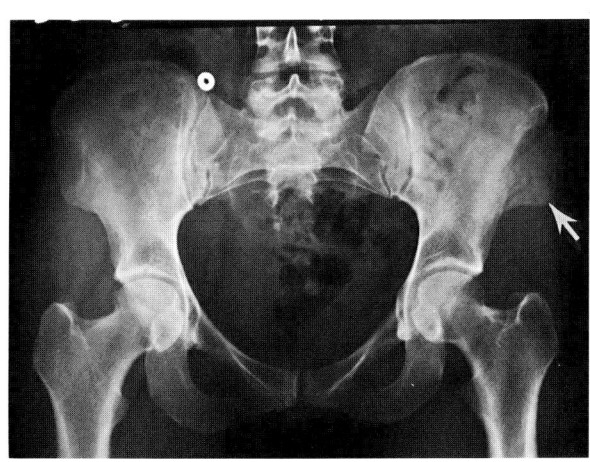

FIG. 5–30. Avulsion fracture of the left anterior superior iliac spine with a large ilial fragment (*arrow*).

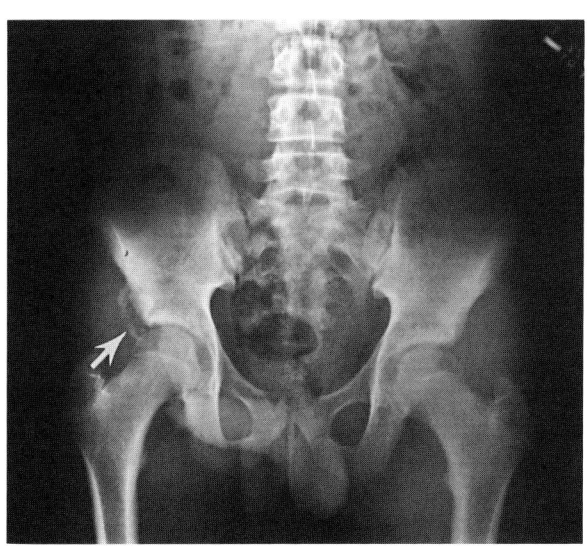

FIG. 5–31. Avulsion of the right anterior inferior iliac spine (*arrow*).

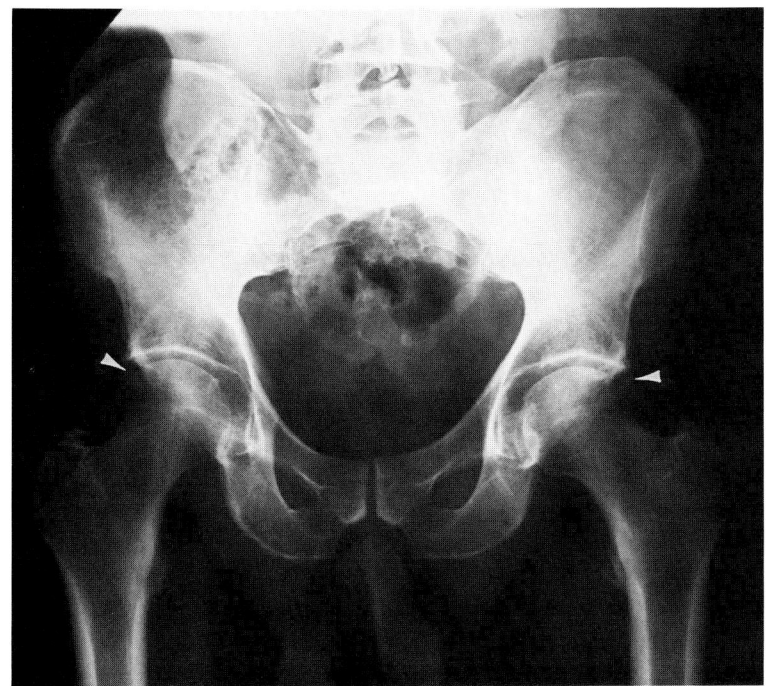

FIG. 5–32. AP view of the pelvis demonstrating normal ossicles along the supra-acetabular margins (*arrows*).

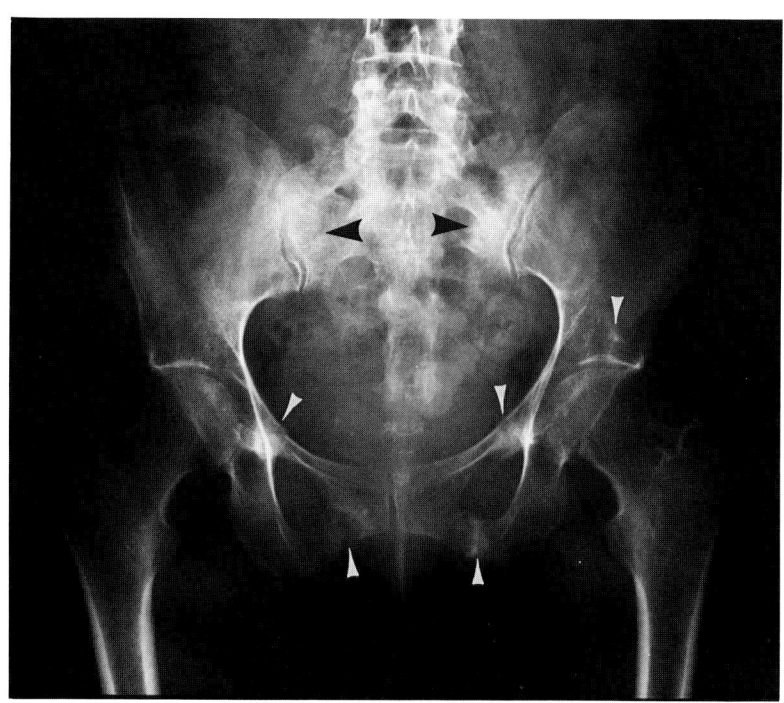

FIG. 5–33. AP view of the pelvis demonstrating multiple insufficiency fractures (*arrows*) involving the sacrum, pubic rami, and left acetabulum.

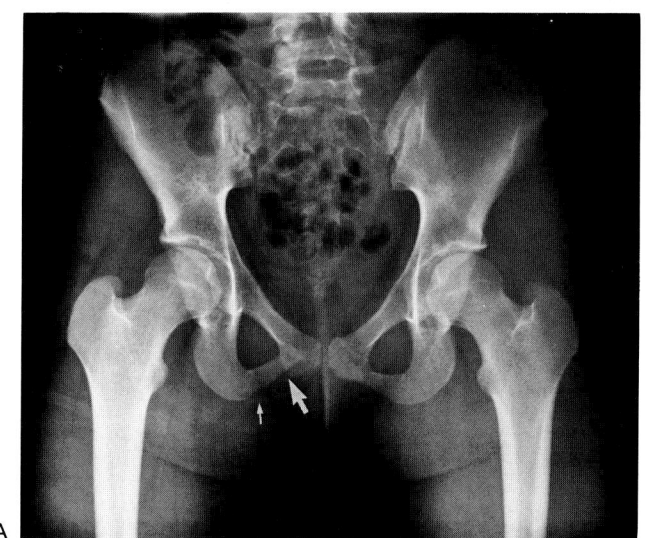

A

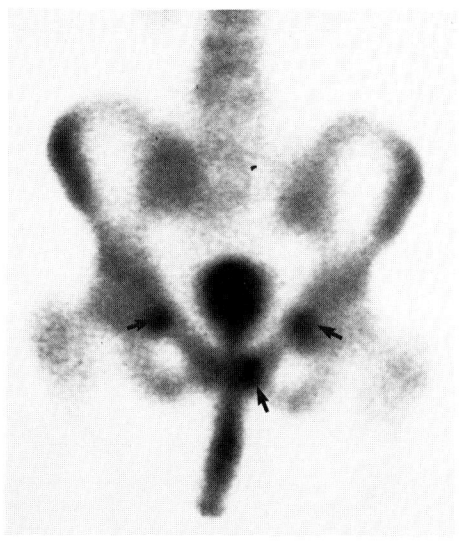

B

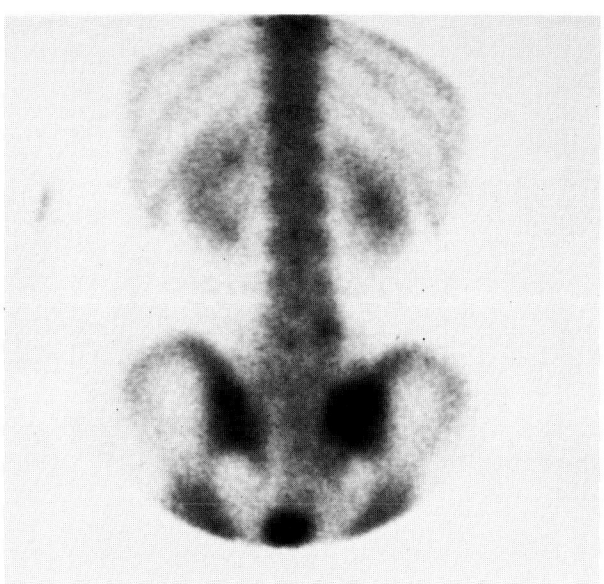

C

FIG. 5–34. Patient with anterior pelvic pain following a motor vehicle accident (MVA). **A:** AP view of the pelvis shows a subtle fracture of the inferior pubic ramus (*large white arrow*) with avulsion of the ischial epiphysis (*small arrow*). **B:** Anterior radioisotope scan (technetium) demonstrates undisplaced superior rami fractures bilaterally, and the posterior scan (**C**) diastasis of the SI joint. This is really a class III fracture. Complications are much more common with Class III fractures.

common type of fracture in his series of 449 patients (130). Such fractures may be overlooked, as the patient usually presents with hip pain, and the history leads one to search for a subcapital fracture of the femur or an intertrochanteric fracture. Fractures of the ischial ramus are particularly troublesome, as they are often associated with subtle central acetabular fractures (133). In these situations, careful examination of the acetabulum with Judet (oblique) views, isotope scans, or tomography should be performed (Figs. 5-34 and 5-35). This type of subtle fracture may be difficult to detect with computed tomography.

Fractures of the iliac wing without involvement of the acetabulum or sacroiliac joint (Fig. 5-28A) were described by Duverney in 1751 (92). This fracture occurs following a direct blow to the ilium or with lateral compressive forces (90,132,152). As in the case of avulsion fractures and fractures of the rami, Duverney fractures are usually evident on the AP radiograph of the pelvis. In subtle cases, further views, tomography, or radioisotope studies may be required.

Isolated transverse fractures of the sacrum and coccyx are due to direct trauma (Fig. 5-36). These fractures have

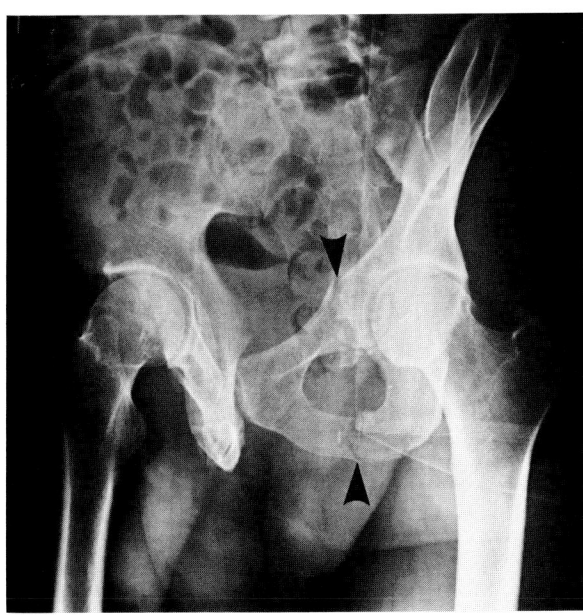

FIG. 5-35. The anterior oblique view of the hip is also very useful in evaluating the obturator ring for double fractures (*arrows*).

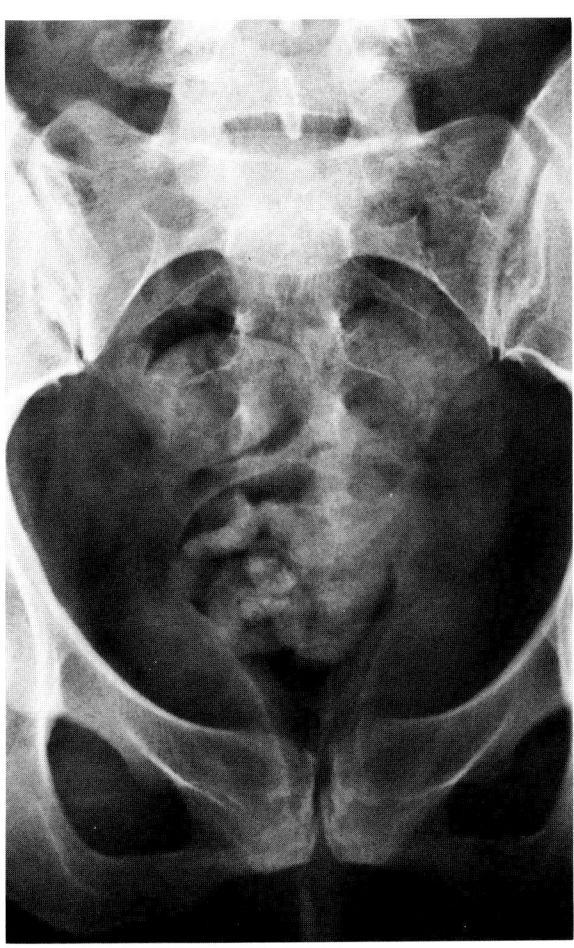
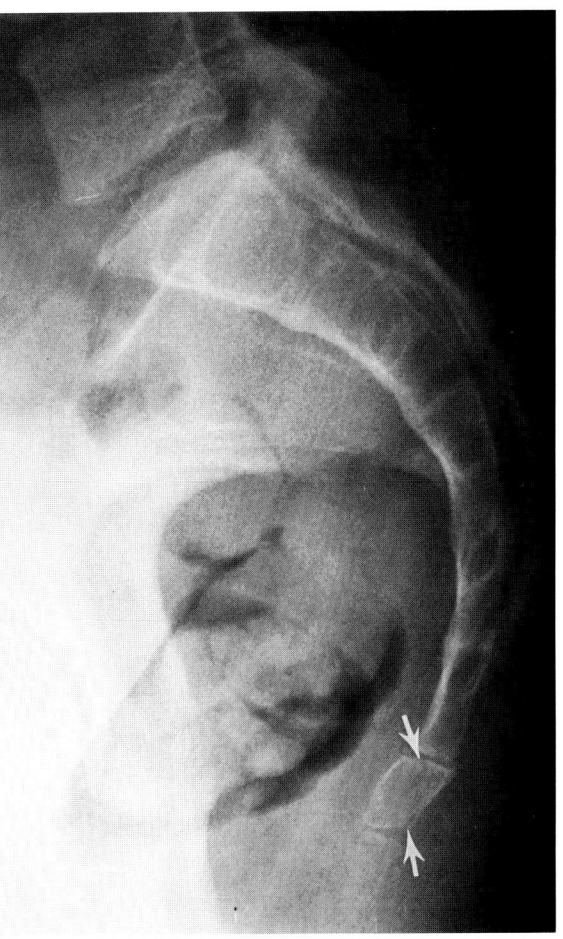

A   B

FIG. 5-36. Isolated fracture of the coccyx is not detectable on the AP view (**A**). The lateral view (**B**) shows a subtle vertical fracture (*arrows*) of the first coccygeal segment.

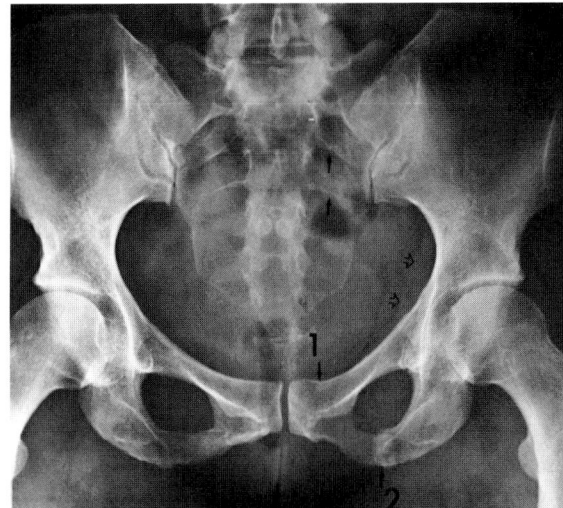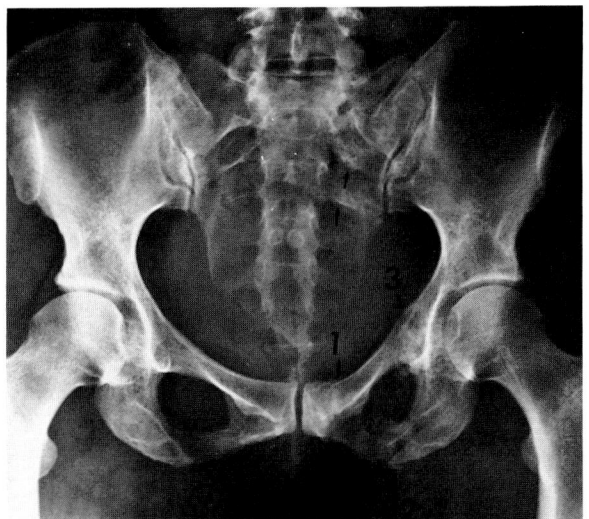

A   B

FIG. 5-37. Patient with pelvic pain and blood loss following pelvic trauma. **A:** There are subtle fractures of the obturator ring on the left (*lower black arrows*) with displacement of the obturator fat stripe due to hematoma (*open arrows*). Subtle torus fractures of the arcuate lines (*upper arrows*) were missed on this examination. **B:** Follow-up examination three months later. The sacral fractures (*black arrows*) more obvious due to callus formation.

not been commonly reported in the literature. Furey (94) reported an incidence of 8% and Connally and Hedberg (84) reported an incidence of 7% in their reviews of pelvic fractures. Identification of transverse sacral fractures on the AP view of the pelvis is often difficult owing to overlying bowel content or bladder distention. Careful attention must be given to the lateral cortical margins and the arcuate lines so that subtle fractures are not overlooked (Fig. 5-37) (101). Jackson reported that up to 70% of sacral fractures were overlooked on initial examination (101). In our experience, 50% of sacral fractures

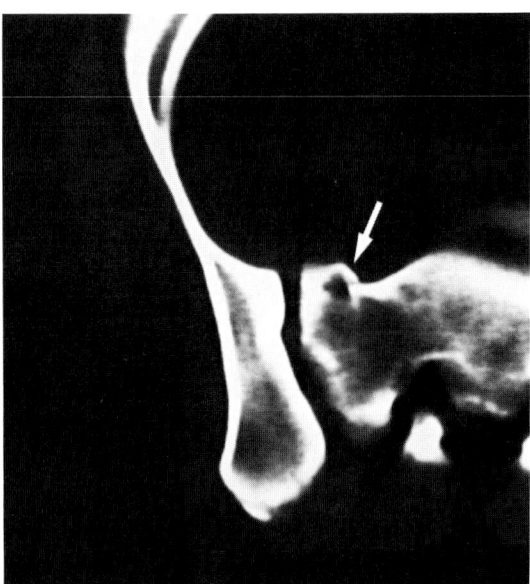

FIG. 5-38. CT scan of the right sacroiliac area. Note the buckle fracture of the sacrum near the SI joint (*white arrow*).

were missed in more severe pelvic injury (Class III fractures) (137). Lateral views may be helpful, especially if slight displacement is present. Computed tomography is the technique of choice for evaluating posterior pelvic fractures (Fig. 5-38) (141).

Fractures and fracture-dislocations of the coccyx occur with falls to the sitting position and are more common in females. The fracture site is extremely tender. Pain may be exaggerated on rising from the sitting position as a result of gluteal muscle contraction (132). Lateral radiographs are most useful for identification of coccygeal fractures and dislocations (Fig. 5-36).

Class II Fractures

Class II fractures, characterized by a single break in the pelvic ring, are the most common type of pelvic fracture in our series (36% of 750 pelvic fractures) (137). Single breaks in the pelvic ring usually occur near the pubic symphysis (Fig. 5-39), or, more rarely, near the sacroiliac joint (152). The minimal motion in these articulations allows a single break to occur. According to Taylor, normal motion at the pubic symphysis is 1 mm in males and 1.5 mm in females (148). In Rankin's series, fractures of the left obturator ring were more common than fractures of the right (130). Class II fractures may be due to direct blows, crush injury, or indirect trauma through the femur (132).

Radiographically, identification of anterior Class II fractures is usually accomplished on AP or AP-angled views of the pelvis. Unfortunately, many Class III fractures (anterior and posterior fractures) remain undiagnosed because of the examiner's focus on this obvious

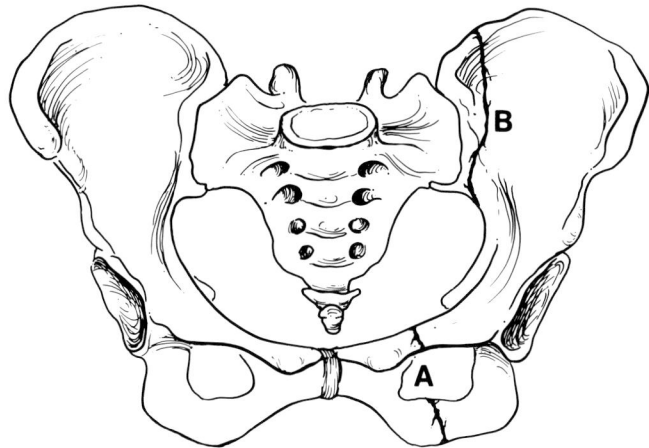

FIG. 5–39. Class II pelvic fracture with a single break in the pelvic ring usually occurs near the symphysis (**A**) or the sacroiliac joint (**B**).

anterior injury. If the posterior fracture goes undiagnosed, a stable and relatively uncomplicated Class II fracture will be treated when the patient may actually have a much more serious Class III fracture. Class III fractures (lateral compression Type II and III, anterior compression II and III, vertical shear) are unstable and

are more likely to lead to serious complications (111,116,129,132,137).

In our review of pelvic fractures, we noted that 33% of posterior fractures were overlooked on the initial interpretation of the radiographs (usually only an AP view of the pelvis) (137). A careful review of these cases and all Class III fractures resulted in an approach that assists in locating potential posterior fractures. Fractures of the anterior rami were graded according to the degree of displacement. A Grade 1 fracture is an anterior ramus fracture with no displacement (Fig. 5-40A). None of these patients had posterior fractures, even in retrospect. A Grade 2 fracture is a ramus fracture with displacement of one-half, or less than one-half, of the width of the ramus (Fig. 5-40B). In these patients, only 20% had fractures posteriorly, and all these fractures involved the ipsilateral sacroiliac joint or ilium near the sacroiliac joint. These fractures were due to lateral compression or vertical shearing forces. A Grade 3 fracture is an anterior ramus fracture with displacement greater than one-half the width of the ramus (Fig. 5-40C). In patients with Grade 3 fractures, there was always a second fracture, and about 80% were on the ipsilateral side. If both obturator rings are fractured, the fracture is by definition already an instance of the Class III type. However, symmet-

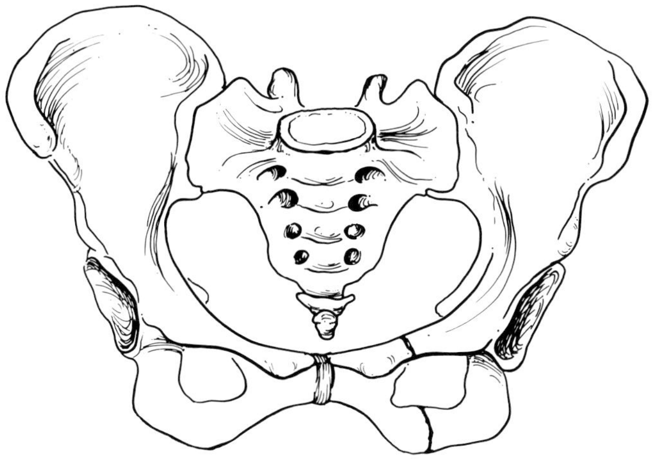

A

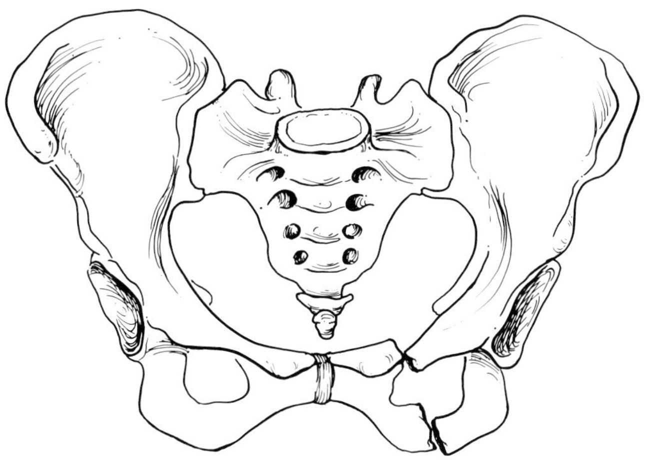

B

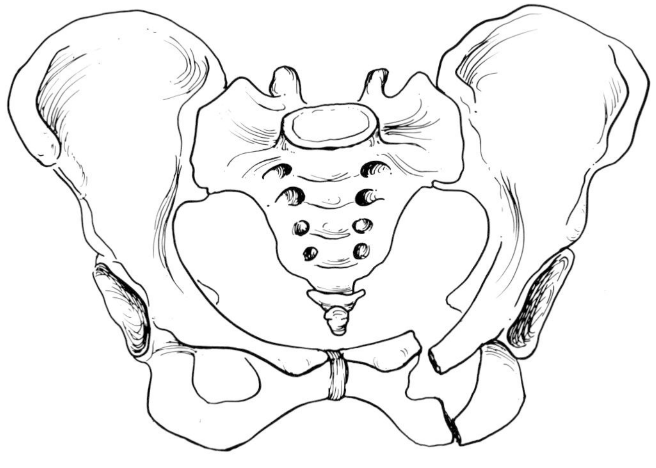

C

FIG. 5–40. Classification of anterior ring fractures to assist in detection of the posterior fracture. **A:** Grade 1 fracture, no displacement. **B:** Grade 2 fracture, displaced one-half the width of the superior ramus. **C:** Grade 3 fracture displaced the full width of the upper ramus or more.

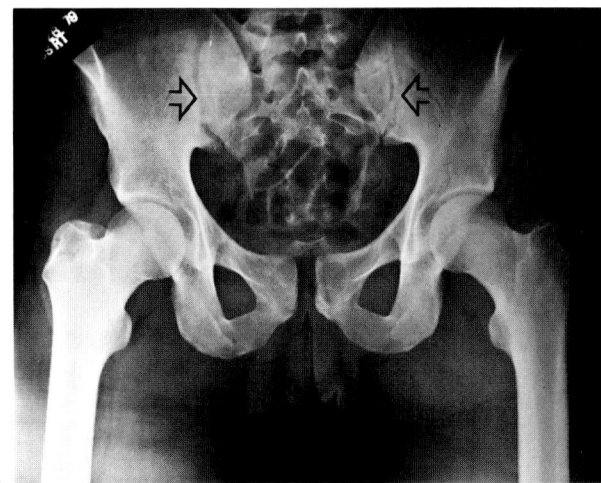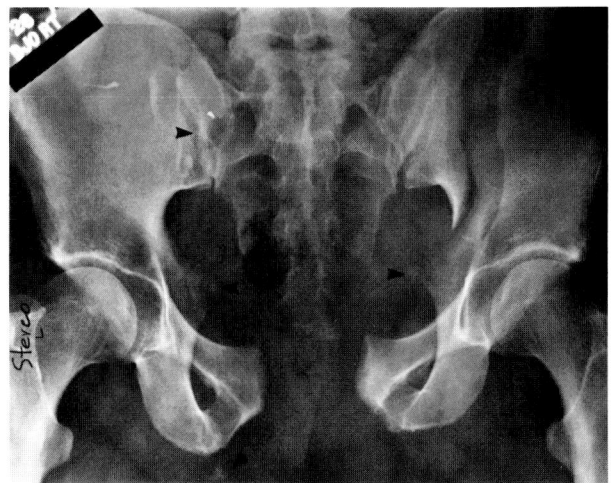

A   B

FIG. 5-41. Diastasis of the pubic symphysis with bilateral posterior injuries. **A:** Slight diastasis of the pubic symphysis with no articular step-off (*black arrow*). There is diastasis of both SI joints (*open arrows*). **B:** Wide separation of the pubic symphysis resulted in avulsion of the ischial spines (*arrows*) (Anterior Compression Type III), ischial tuberosity on the right (*arrow*); separation of the right sacroiliac joint (*arrow*) and a displaced iliac fracture on the left near the SI joint.

rical sacroiliac joint diastasis or adjacent fractures were found in 40% of the patients with Grade 3 fractures. Diastasis of the pubic symphysis with no vertical displacement usually results in bilateral posterior fractures or sacroiliac separations (anterior compression Type III) (Fig. 5-41). If the diastasis includes a vertical displacement, the posterior injury is usually on the elevated side.

The above categories may not be entirely adequate, but they help point the way to detection of posterior injuries. Therefore, if an anterior fracture is identified and falls within Grades 2 or 3, one must search diligently for a posterior fracture. For this task, CT is the procedure of choice at our institution. This modality can successfully identify unsuspected fractures as well as provide valuable information regarding soft tissue injury.

Class III Fractures

Class III fractures result in two or more breaks in the pelvic ring. Of 750 patients, 15% were included in this category (137). These injuries are usually unstable compared with the stable Class I and Class II fractures. Significant morbidity and mortality also result from Class III fractures. In our series, the mortality rate in patients with Class III fractures was 22% (137).

Class III fractures tend to occur in younger individuals (52% less than 30 years of age) and are more common in males than females by a 3:1 ratio. The etiology is most often a high-velocity motor vehicle accident, farm accident, or pedestrian accident.

Multiple fracture patterns occur with Class III fracture. Straddle fractures, i.e., bilateral fractures of both pubic rami (Fig. 5-42), occurred in 33% of patients with

unstable fractures in Dunn and Morris's series (90). This fracture occurs with direct trauma to the region of the pubic symphysis or with lateral compression (132).

Malgaigne fractures, first described in 1859, are double vertical breaks in the pelvic ring (Fig. 5-42B). By definition this type of fracture requires an anterior disruption of the pubic ring with a second fracture posterior to the acetabulum. The posterior fracture may involve the ilium adjacent to the sacroiliac joint, or diastasis of the sacroiliac joint may be present. Anteriorly, there may be fractures of the rami or diastasis of the pubic symphysis (79). Malgaigne fractures have been reported to be the most common of Class III fractures (149). In our series, 38% of Class III fractures were Malgaigne fractures (137). This fracture may be caused by lateral compression, anteroposterior compression, vertical shearing, or combined forces. A variant of the Malgaigne fracture, the bucket-handle fracture, is the result of an oblique force. The result in this case is an anterior fracture with the posterior fracture or dislocation on the contralateral side of the pelvis (Fig. 5-42C).

Severe multiple fractures are very unstable, and significant complications almost always result (Fig. 5-43) (132,137). In our group of over 100 Class III fractures, three subgroups of fractures could be distinguished. The largest subgroup was characterized by severe multiple fractures and consisted of 46% of the patients. The two other subgroups were characterized by straddle fractures, occurring in 16% of the patients, and Malgaigne fractures, occurring in 38% of the patients. Also of importance was the high incidence of associated sacral fractures (Fig. 5-43B), evident in 23% of the patients with Class III fractures, and the unfortunate fact that 50% of

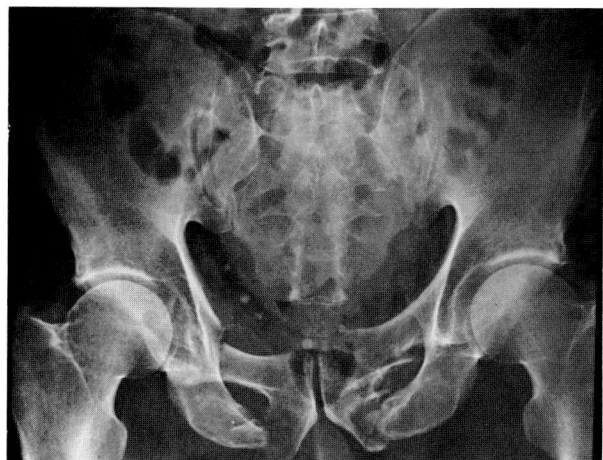

A

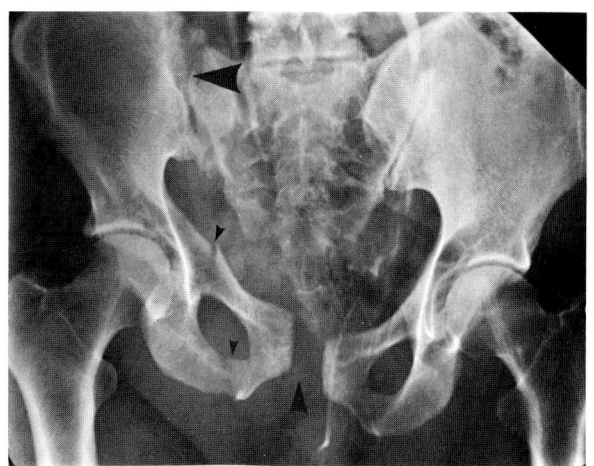

B

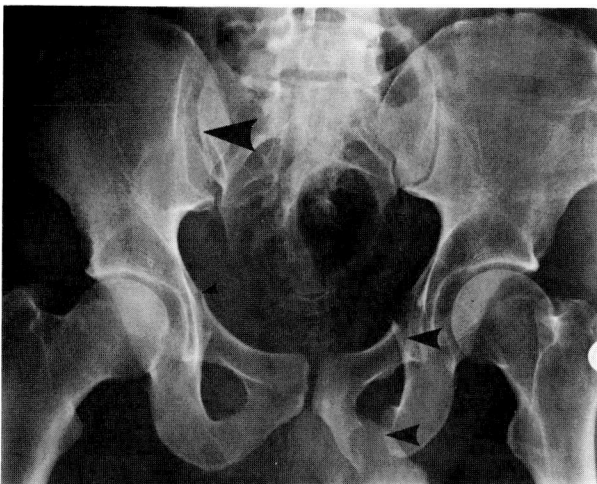

C

FIG. 5-42. Class III fractures. **A:** Straddle fracture with fractures of both pubic rami bilaterally. **B:** Malgaigne fracture (vertical shearing injury) with disruption of the pubic symphysis (*large arrow*) elevation of the right hemipelvis and fracture dislocation of the right sacroiliac joint (*large upper arrow*). There are also minimally displaced fractures (*small arrows*) of the right pubic rami. The bladder and Foley catheter are deviated to the left by a large pelvic hematoma. **C:** Bucket handle fracture with fracture of the left obturator ring (*lower large black arrows*) and separation of the contra-lateral SI joint (*upper large arrow*). Bialteral pelvic hematomas with a central acetabular fracture (*small arrow*) on the right.

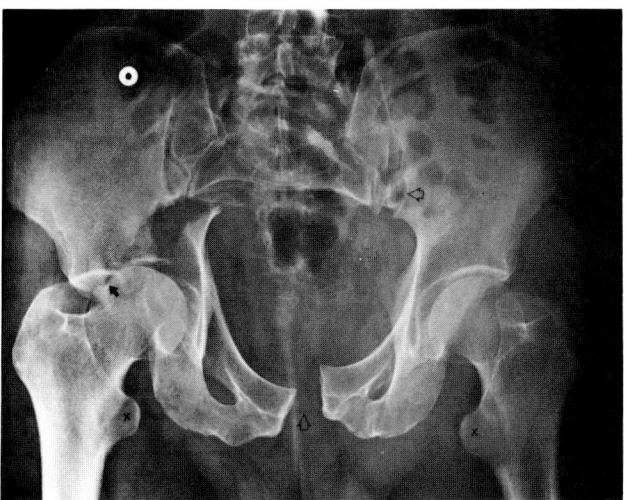

A

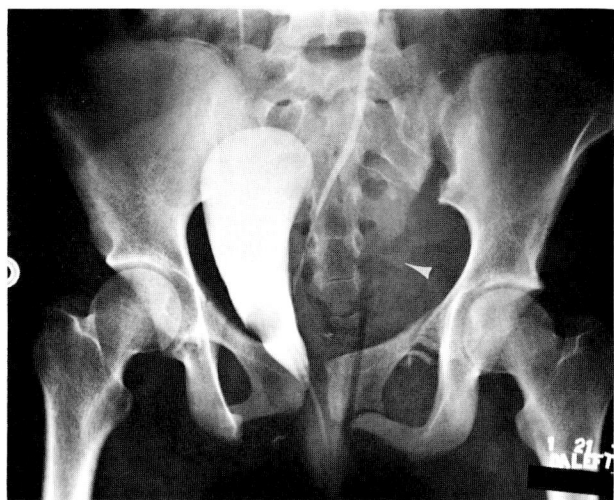

B

FIG. 5-43. Complex pelvic fractures. **A:** There is separation of the pubic symphysis and left SI joint (*open arrows*). In addition there is a displaced acetabular fracture on the right with an osteochondral fracture on the right femoral head (*black arrow*). Both hips are externally rotated (X) on lesser trochanter. **B:** Bilateral obturator ring fractures with separation of the left SI joint. There is comminution of the lower sacrum (*white arrow*) and the bladder is deviated to the right by the large pelvic hematoma.

these fractures were missed on initial radiographic evaluation. Solitary sacral fractures are much less common.

Routine radiographic evaluation is often all that is required to identify complex displaced fractures. Initial management decisions can be made with AP and oblique or angled views. CT is useful for complete evaluation of Class III fractures or to differentiate Class II from Class III.

Class IV Fractures

Class IV fractures are fractures of the acetabulum. Acetabular fractures have been described with increasing frequency in recent years (91,93,102,107,126,127,137,147, 153). In our experience, acetabular fractures make up about 24% of all pelvic fractures. Key and Conwell divided these fractures into undisplaced and displaced. However, a more complex and accurate approach is required for the proper evaluation and management of acetabular fractures. We will therefore deviate from the Key and Conwell classification at this point.

Multiple approaches to the classification of acetabular fractures have been proposed. Certain authors have clas-

TABLE 5-7. Acetabular fracture classification based on position of femoral head

1. Stewart and Milford,[a] 1954
   - Grade I: Linear or stellate fracture of the acetabular floor with no displacement of the femoral head
   - Grade II: Comminuted fracture with mild to moderate central displacement of the femoral head and acetabular fragments
   - Grade III: Marked displacement of the fracture fragments and protrusion of the femoral head into the pelvis. With or without comminution of the superior acetabulum
   - Grade IV: Central dislocation with associated fracture of the head or neck of femur
2. Rowe and Lowell,[b] 1961
   - Group I: Linear undisplaced acetabular fracture with single or multiple lines
   - Group II: Posterior fracture with small or large posterior fragment
   - Group III: Central acetabular fracture with displacement of femoral head
   - Group IV: Superior or burst fracture with disruption of the acetabulum
3. Eichenholtz and Stark[c]
   - Type IA: Little or no central displacement of the femoral head
   - Type IB: Little or no central displacement of the femoral head and anterior pelvic fracture
   - Type IIA: Central head displacement with no anterior pelvic fracture
   - Type IIB: Central head displacement and anterior pelvic fracture
   - Type III: Head dislocated centrally without anterior fracture

[a] (147), [b] (135), [c] (93).

TABLE 5-8. Acetabular fracture classification based on anterior and posterior column

Judet, Judet, Letournel,[a] 1964
- Elementary fractures
  - Posterior acetabular rim
  - Ilioischial (posterior) column
  - Iliopubic (anterior) column
  - Transverse fractures
- Complex fractures
  - Fracture with femoral head dislocation
  - Both columns disrupted

Tile,[b] 1980
- Simple
  - Anterior column
  - Posterior column
  - Transverse
- Complex
  - T fractures
  - Dome fractures
  - Acetabulum and iliac wing
  - Acetabulum and adjacent sacroiliac joint

[a] (102), [b] (151).

sified acetabular fractures according to the position of the femoral head (Table 5-7) (91,93,105,147). Judet and colleagues (102) classified fractures according to the involvement of the anterior and posterior columns (Table 5-8). Tile (151) describing the experience of Pennal, Davidson, and Plewes found that the prognosis of acetabular fractures depends upon the degree of involvement of the weight-bearing surface, the degree of displacement, and the presence or absence of anterior pelvic ring fractures. This classification (Table 5-8) distinguishes simple fractures from more complex fractures, with the latter characterized by involvement of the dome, T fractures, iliac wing fractures, and disruption of the adjacent sacroiliac joint. The Judet approach will be used in the following discussion of acetabular fractures.

Elementary or single acetabular fractures (Table 5-8) were the most common in Judet's series (111 of 173 patients) (102). However, Tile (151) reported complex fractures to be more common, a finding confirmed in our series of cases. Acetabular fractures result from force transmitted to the femoral head via the greater trochanter or lower extremity (102). Radiographic evaluation of acetabular fractures requires high-quality AP and Judet views, at a minimum. CT is especially helpful in evaluating complex fractures. This technique allows more accurate assessment of the size, relationship, and degree of displacement of the fracture fragments. Three-dimensional CT images are particularly useful in operative planning (112,113,136,143).

Elementary Acetabular Fractures

Posterior acetabular fractures may involve a single fragment or multiple fragments and, on occasion, may result in impaction of the acetabular articular surface (102). These fractures are easily seen on the anterior oblique view, as the posterior acetabulum is more clearly visualized. With large or multiple fragments, CT is the technique of choice for more complete evaluation (Fig. 5-22D) (96,112,113). The fracture usually results from lower extremity trauma (usually at the knee) with the hip flexed approximately 90° (Fig. 5-44). The size of the fragment is also related to the degree of femoral abduction. The greater the abduction, the larger the fragment (Fig. 5-45) (102).

Fractures of the posterior (ilioischial) column usually begin above the acetabulum, extend through the posterior aspect of the acetabulum, and include the ischial ramus (Fig. 5-46). The iliopubic line and radiographic U remain intact on the AP radiograph, allowing one to attribute the fracture to the posterior column. The dome of the acetabulum remains intact (102,109,151). This fracture results from a blow to the knee with the hip flexed 90° and abducted about 20° (102). Posterior dislocation or subluxation of the hip is frequently associated with this fracture, and sciatic nerve injury may result (102,109,136,151).

Transverse fractures involve both the anterior and posterior column and frequently the ischial spine (Fig. 5-47). The mechanism of injury is a blow to the lateral aspect of the greater trochanter or the posterior aspect of the pelvis, with the hip flexed and abducted (102). Radiographically these fractures are easily missed on the AP view, especially when no displacement is present. Judet (oblique) views (Fig. 5-48) are required and occa-

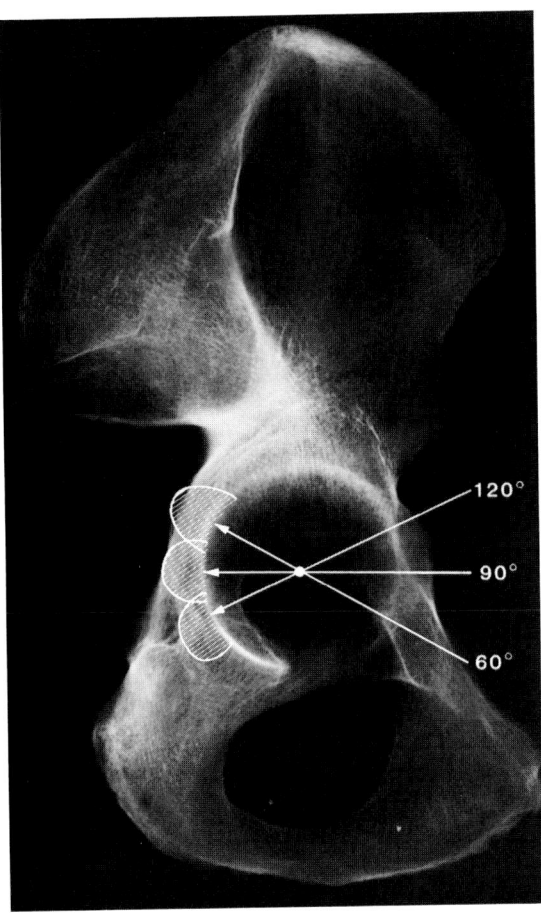

FIG. 5–44. Lateral view of the innominate bone demonstrating how the position of the femur (120°–60° flexion) results in posterior acetabular fractures.

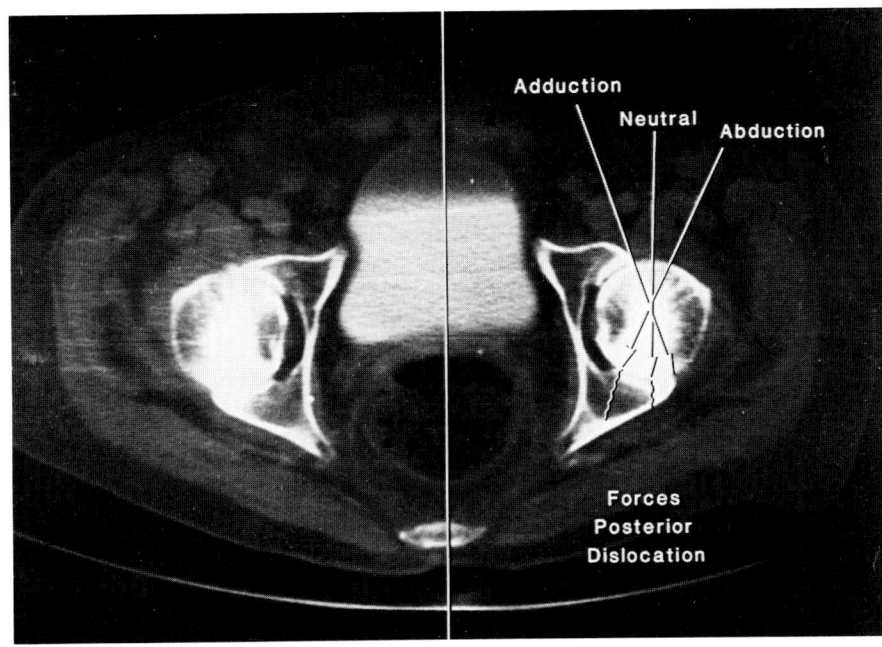

FIG. 5–45. CT scan of the pelvis through the femoral heads. The degree of adduction or abduction of the femur also affects the size of posterior acetabular fragments.

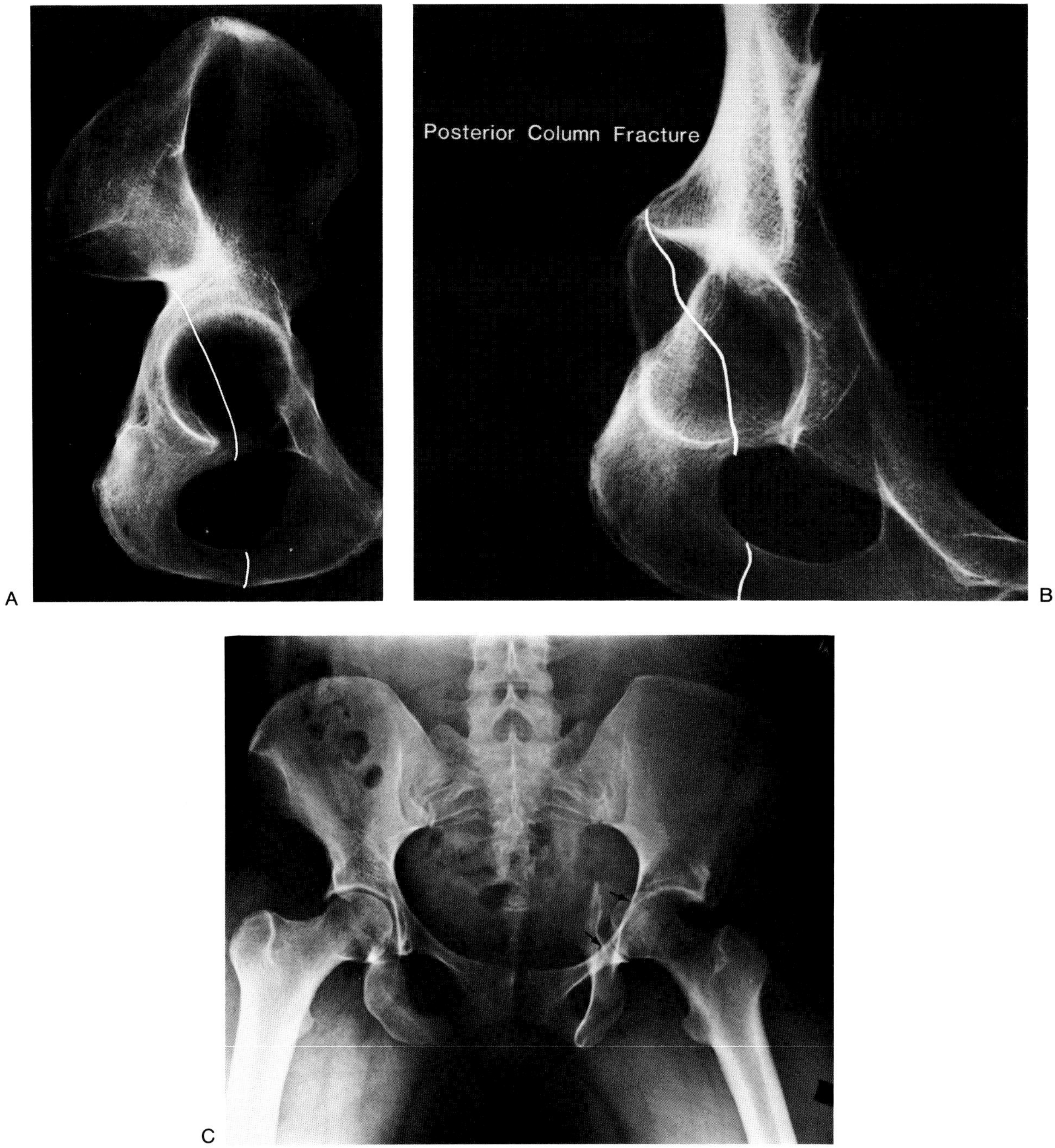

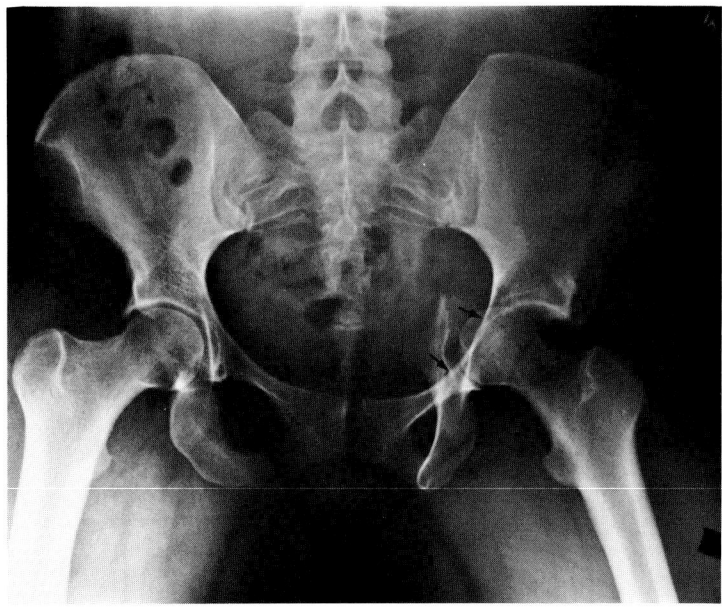

FIG. 5–46. Specimen radiograph in the lateral (**A**) and anterior oblique projections (**B**) demonstrating the course of a posterior column fracture. Note that the anterior (iliopubic) column is intact. **C:** AP view of the pelvis with displaced posterior column fracture. The anterior column (*arrow*) is intact.

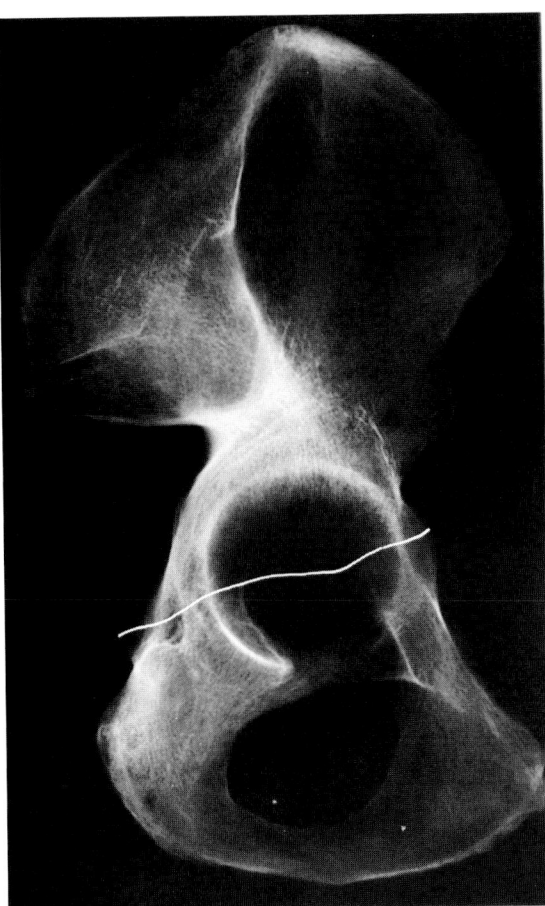

FIG. 5–47. Transverse acetabular fractures typically involve both columns and the ischial spine (*white line*).

sionally conventional tomography or radioisotope scans as well. CT may miss this type of fracture if the fracture line is parallel to the slice. This may be the one situation in which CT is not the technique of choice in evaluation of the pelvis.

Fractures of the anterior column (iliopubic column) are less common than posterior column fractures (151). The prognosis with these injuries is reportedly better compared with posterior column fractures (151). These fractures usually begin just above the anterior inferior iliac spine and extend inferiorly to involve the inferior pubic ramus near the junction with the ischium (Fig. 5-49). The iliopubic line is disrupted on the AP radiograph, and once again the oblique views will clearly demonstrate the disruption of the anterior column and intact posterior column. The injury is thought to be the result of a blow to the greater trochanter with the hip externally rotated, an uncommon situation indeed (102,151).

Complex Acetabular Fractures

Complex acetabular fractures result in multiple fracture lines and increased morbidity. Fractures with significant central displacement of the femoral head and acetabular fragments lead to complications similar to those of Class III pelvic fractures (Fig. 5-50). The complications will be discussed in detail later in this chapter.

Comminution of the acetabulum may result in a *T* pattern, with splitting of the anterior and posterior columns as well as a transverse fracture. Recognition of the

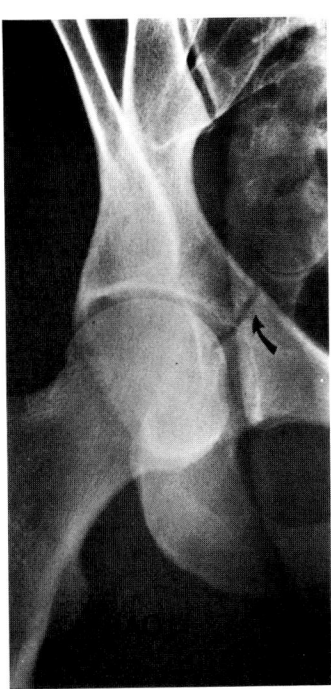
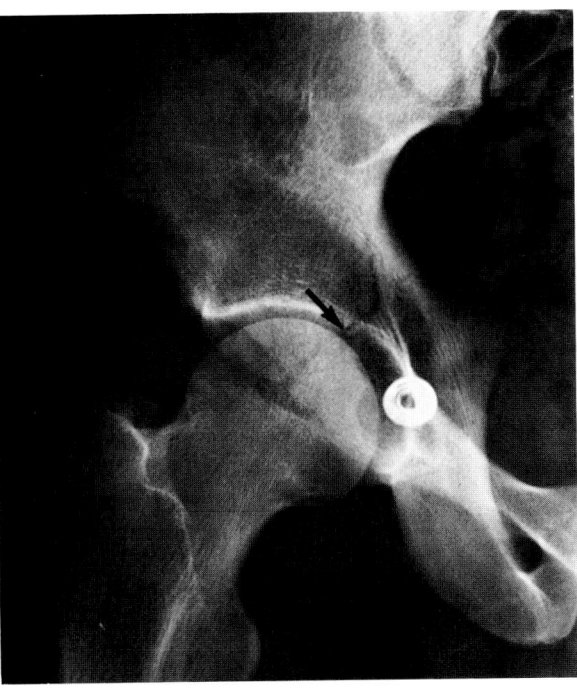

FIG. 5–48. Transverse undisplaced acetabular fracture demonstrated with the anterior (**A**) and posterior (**B**) oblique views.

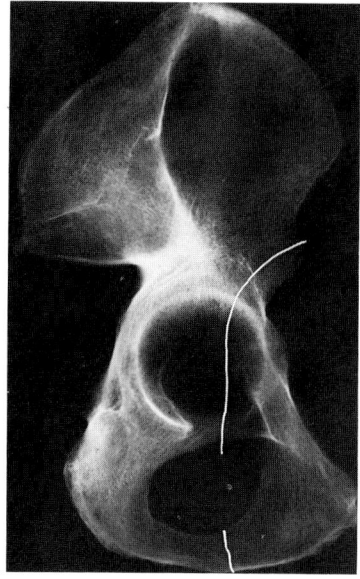 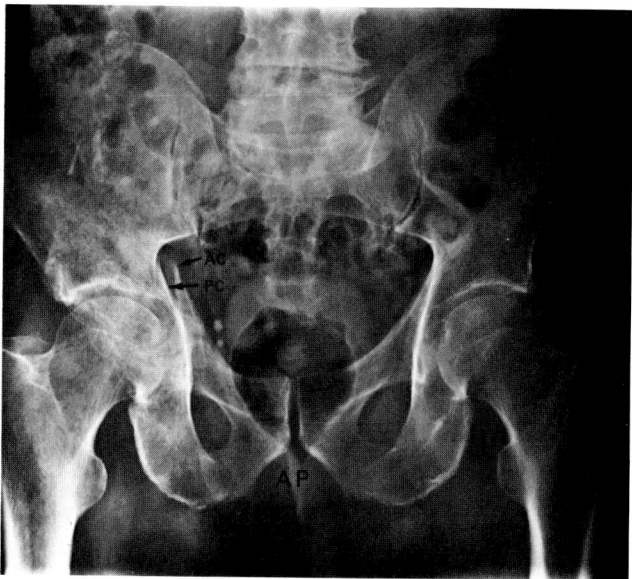

A   B

FIG. 5–49. A: Specimen radiograph demonstrating the typical course (*white line*) of the anterior column fracture. **B:** AP radiograph demonstrating an anterior column (AC) fracture. Note the posterior column (PC) or ilioischial line is intact.

division of the columns is important, as surgical correction of one column alone will not result in anatomic reduction of the acetabulum (151). Vertical cleft fractures that separate the anterior and posterior columns are particularly well demonstrated with CT. The plane of the fracture is almost perpendicular to the scan slice (Fig. 5-51).

Fragmentation or displacement of the weight-bearing surface of the acetabulum is of particular importance (Fig. 5-51). Any malrotation or comminution of the

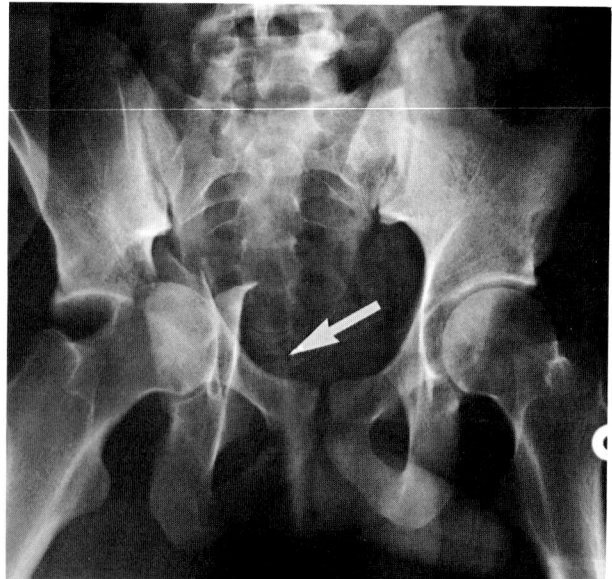

FIG. 5–50. Acetabular fracture with disruption of both columns and central displacement of the femoral head. Note the dislocation of the 1st and 2nd coccygeal segments (*white arrow*).

dome of the acetabulum must be corrected. This may be the most important indication for surgical intervention (102,109,151). Complex fractures with involvement of the iliac wing or adjacent sacroiliac joint also result in a poorer prognosis. The sacroiliac joint involvement may be subtle and difficult to detect even with comparison of the joints. CT is particularly valuable in these situations (Fig. 5-52). Evaluation of the sacrum, sacroiliac joint, acetabular dome, and the joint space is better accomplished with CT than with routine films or conventional tomography (96,136,137). The evaluation of the position of the acetabular fragments (Fig. 5-52) and intra-articular fragments is particularly effective with CT (96).

Treatment of Pelvic Fractures

Detailed radiographic examination, as outlined in this chapter, is essential for the orthopedic treatment of pelvic fractures. Proper radiographic definition of the injury is a prerequisite to effective treatment. The four classes of pelvic fractures lend themselves to a number of generalizations regarding treatment. These will be discussed in this section.

Class I Fractures

In the acute phase of the Class I fracture, there is really no treatment indicated. These fractures heal and usually do not involve residual deficits. Occasionally crutches or a cane may be necessary as an aid while pain is present. An exception to this would be the fracture-dislocation of the coccyx, which needs immediate reduction. This can be performed through rectal manipulation of the

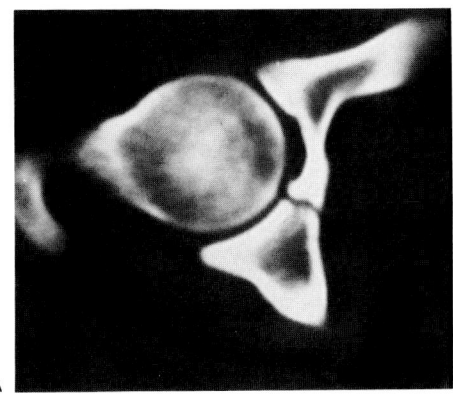
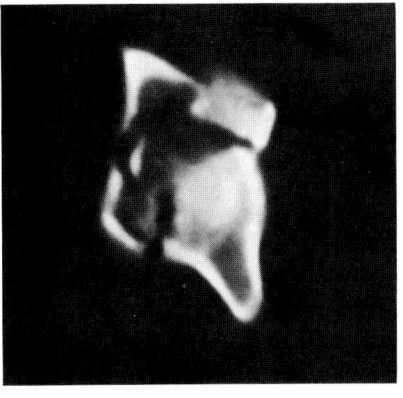
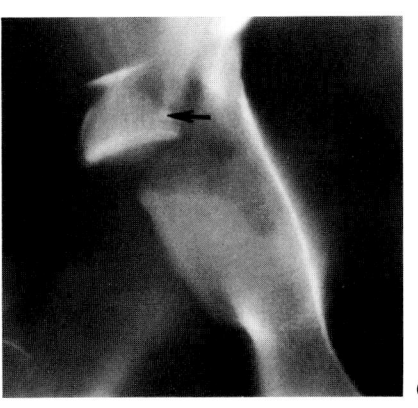

FIG. 5-51. CT scan of vertical cleft fracture (**A**) with associated hematoma, a higher section (**B**) demonstrates comminution of the dome of the acetabulum with a rotated fragment. **C:** AP tomogram demonstrates the large fragment seen in **B** but is much less useful in treatment planning and exact positioning of the fragments.

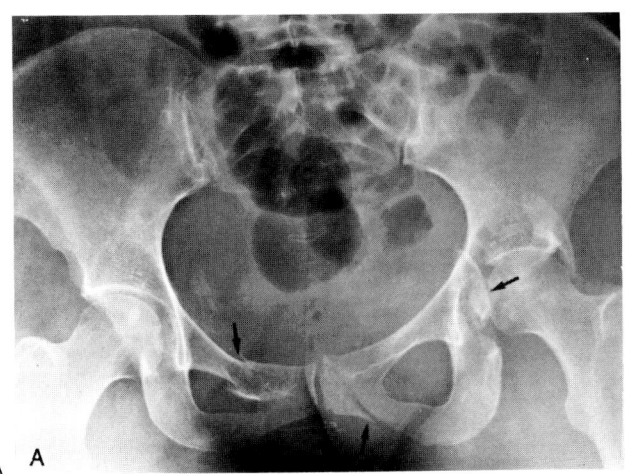
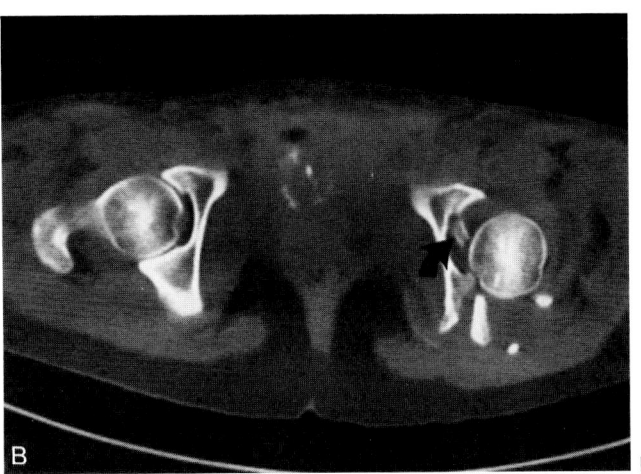

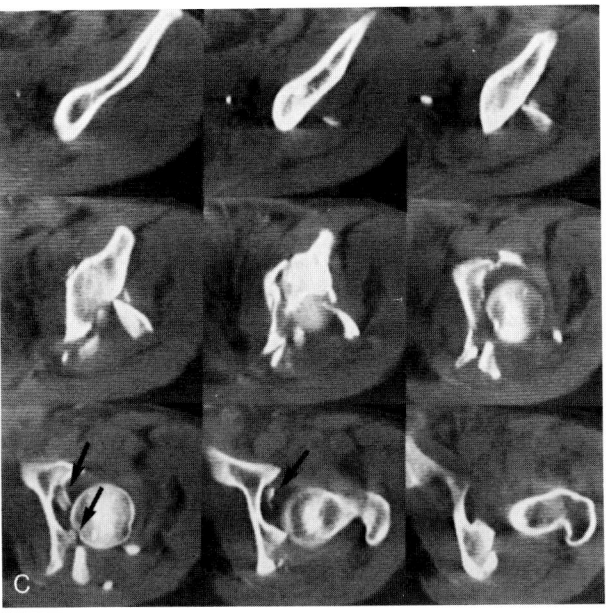

FIG. 5-52. Patient with a complex pelvic fracture following a high velocity motor vehicle accident (MVA). **A:** AP view of the pelvis demonstrating bilateral pubic rami fractures (*arrows*) and fracture dislocation of the left hip. **B:** CT scan through the joint spaces demonstrates multiple acetabular fragments with a large anterior fragment in the joint space (*arrow*), posterior subluxation of the femoral head, and an impaction fracture of the head posteriorly. **C:** Collage of CT sections from the ilium to below the joint (moves top L to R).

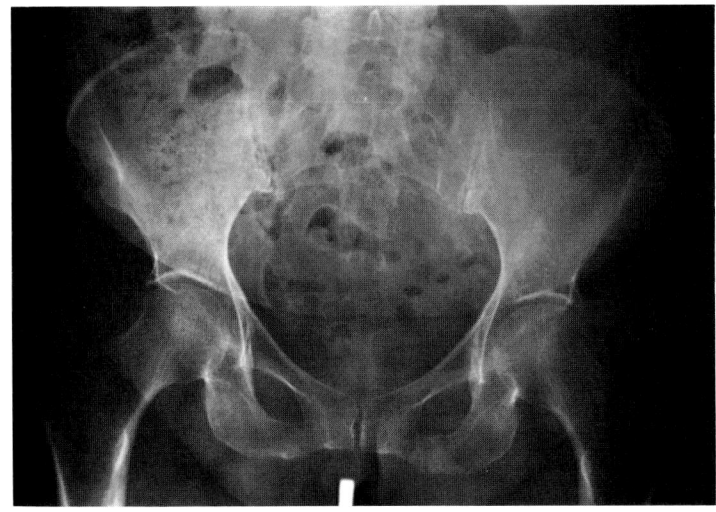 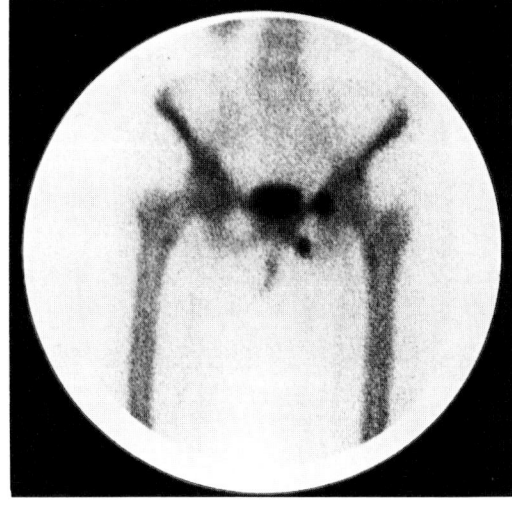

FIG. 5–53. A 76-year-old woman with six weeks of pain in left groin and hip region. No history of injury. Osteoporosis. **A:** Questionable stress fracture in the superior and inferior pubic rami on the left. **B:** Confirmation with technetium scanning. Healing was uneventful.

fragment, usually best done with the patient under anesthesia.

Often not diagnosed is the stress fracture of the pelvis. This is most commonly seen in elderly patients with osteopenia (Fig. 5-53). A long spell of walking or a fall or even a slight twist may result in a fracture of the pubic ramus, usually the inferior element, or a fracture of both pubic rami. No radiographic findings are present. The symptoms are sometimes diffuse, and the diagnosis may be confirmed only with Tc-99m scanning. This should be positive within 2–3 days of the injury and certainly by 1 week. The management of the patient and the prognosis depend on the diagnosis. While these patients will usually recover fully, union may be delayed for up to 2 years if tension forces instead of the usual compressive forces act on the fracture.

Residual deficits in Class I fractures are usually minimal. However, fracture of the coccyx may result in continued discomfort and may even, in extreme cases, require coccygectomy. Fractures through the sacrum are notorious also for residual nerve injuries. The initial fracture may even be undiagnosed until the patient presents with sacral nerve deficits.

Class II Fractures

Treatment is usually minimal for a single break in the pelvic ring, a fracture that is basically stable. The most common Class II fracture involves both the superior and inferior pubic ramus. Treatment in this case is symptomatic, with rest, often crutches, and sometimes a pelvic support if the sacroiliac joints appear involved.

Residual deficits of Class II fractures typically relate to the sacroiliac joint. Although the joint will usually stabilize, it may remain unstable and produce symptoms. Radiographic visualization of the joint is difficult. Films taken with the patient standing and with alternate weight bearing will often demonstrate instability if both the pubic symphysis and sacroiliac joint are involved. Oblique views may show sclerosis. Isotope scans will demonstrate increased uptake in the sacroiliac joint. CT scans are most useful in the demonstration of sacroiliac joint incongruity. Local injection of anesthetic agents into the joint will often localize the source of pain to the joint. Ultimately, if other methods fail, fusion of the joint may be necessary.

Class III Fractures

These are unstable fractures and require a vigorous approach by the orthopedist. The first consideration is always the accompanying visceral and vascular complications that may be present, and these take priority over the skeletal treatment. If, however, the bladder or urethra requires surgical repair, the orthopedist can concurrently stabilize the pubis and occasionally remove or stabilize comminuted fractures in the region of the lower urinary tract. The above injuries will be discussed more fully in the section on complications of pelvic fractures.

The use of external fixation is a fairly recent innovation that has made the handling of unstable pelvic fractures less difficult (Fig. 5-54). As soon as the patient's general condition allows, fixation is applied. This will stabilize the fragments and lessen hemorrhage and other visceral trauma. In a recent review of 45 patients with fractures of the pelvis, the Baylor group reduced the time from injury to application of the Hoffman apparatus to 2.2 days in their previous 25 patients (156). Use of external fixation provides comfort to the patient and allows more rapid mobilization. It must be emphasized, however, that external fixation will do very little in the way of reduction, and closed reduction must precede or accom-

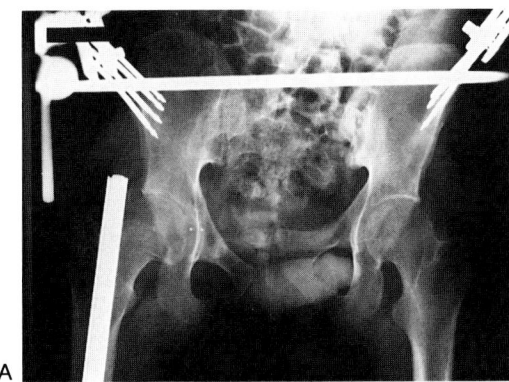
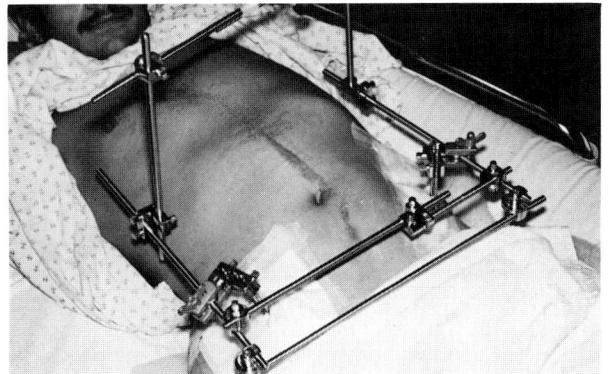

FIG. 5–54. (Hoffman apparatus as external fixateur). A 19-year-old male, motor vehicle accident. Unstable vertical fracture left side of pelvis. Fracture shaft of right femur. Preliminary traction followed by application of Hoffmann-Vidal apparatus. **A:** Pins in place in iliac crest and apparatus applied. **B:** The patient in bed with the external fixateur in place.

pany its application. Lower extremity traction alone or as an adjunct is indicated in vertical shear (Malgaigne) fractures. If possible, the fixation device is left in place for 8 weeks. Walking may be allowed, depending on the type of fracture. If the injury is primarily unilateral, the opposite extremity can bear weight with the aid of crutches after 3 weeks. Bilateral unstable shear fractures, on the other hand, are best treated in recumbency for 8 weeks following stabilization with external fixation (106,146).

Other methods of partially stabilizing and reducing these unstable fractures have in the past included manipulation and spica casting, traction, and the pelvic compression sling. While the sling can reduce the diastasis of the pelvis, pressure against the bony prominences creates skin problems. If used, the sling must be padded with thick layers of foam, and the patient must be carefully monitored.

Residual deficits of Class III fractures are common. Continued pain due to instability, especially in the sacroiliac joint and low back, is often present. Leg length discrepancy may also occur (Fig. 5-55).

Class IV Fractures

These fractures primarily involve the acetabulum, although frequently other pelvic fractures accompany such fractures. Similarly, Class III fractures may have acetabular involvement, making them merge with the Class IV type.

The same principles apply here as in other fractures involving a joint: namely, the normal anatomic configuration must be restored. Fractures that result in intrapelvic protrusion of the femoral head have been treated in the past with lateral and distal traction combined with pins in the femur and greater trochanter area. This treatment may reduce some of these fractures; and, if the dome of the acetabulum is intact, this may be all that is necessary. Traction may also be used as a preliminary to open reduction under anesthesia. Stability must then be

assessed. If the hip is unstable in flexion, open reduction and fixation of the posterior fragment is indicated (Fig. 5-56). The next stage resulting from forces in the anteroposterior direction is the posterior column fracture. These are the most common of the severe acetabular fractures. They must be opened, reduced, secured by plate and screws, and bent to conform. If this is done during the first 10 days to 3 weeks, a satisfactory result should occur; but the ultimate course depends in part on how badly the femoral head is damaged (Figs. 5-57 and 5-58).

Transverse fractures are more complex, making internal fixation more difficult. But, again, it is essential to restore the acetabulum to its normal configuration if possible. Anterior column fractures are fortunately rare. They require an anterior surgical approach and internal fixation.

Treatment of the complex central fracture-dislocation and the comminuted dome fracture does not always result in anatomic reduction. Thus, lateral-distal traction seems about all one can do initially, and the hip is then reconstructed at a later date through total hip replacement (Fig. 5-59).

The pioneer work of Judet and Letournel has shown that restoration of the acetabulum should be carried out if at all possible by open reduction and internal fixation (108). Careful evaluation of the anatomic aspects of the fracture must be carried out prior to any surgery. Routine radiographs and Judet views should always be obtained (Fig. 5-60). These can be complemented with CT scans. If the patient's general status does not permit surgery, it can be delayed. Letournel, for example, has described the surgical repair of acetabular fractures more than 3 weeks after injury (108).

Incongruence between the femoral head and the acetabular crescent is a strict indication for open reduction and internal fixation. One must use a fracture table that allows adequate positioning and traction of the limb. The transverse fractures pose the more difficult aspects of the operation. Complete reconstruction of the hip

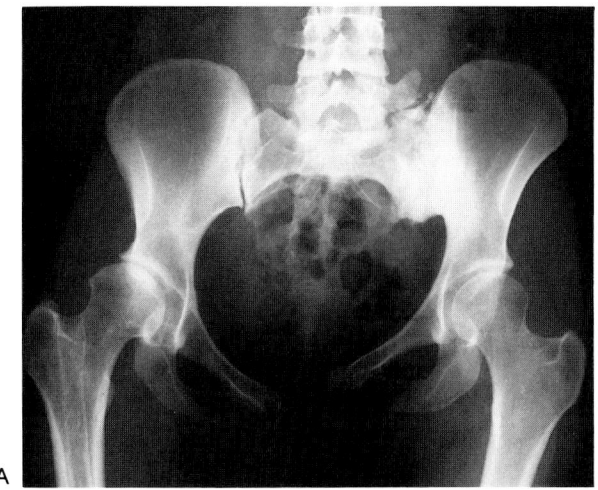

A

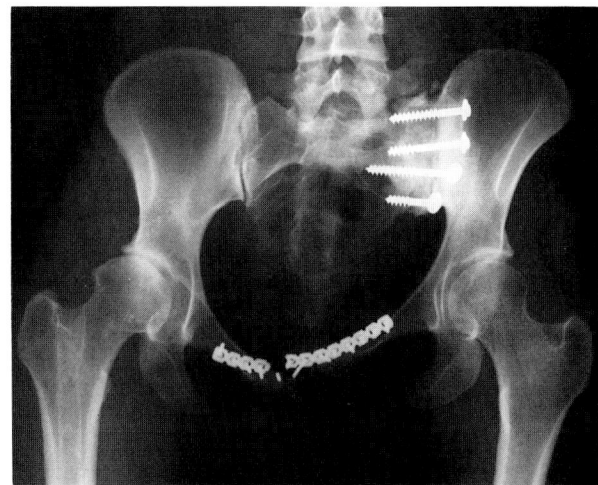

B

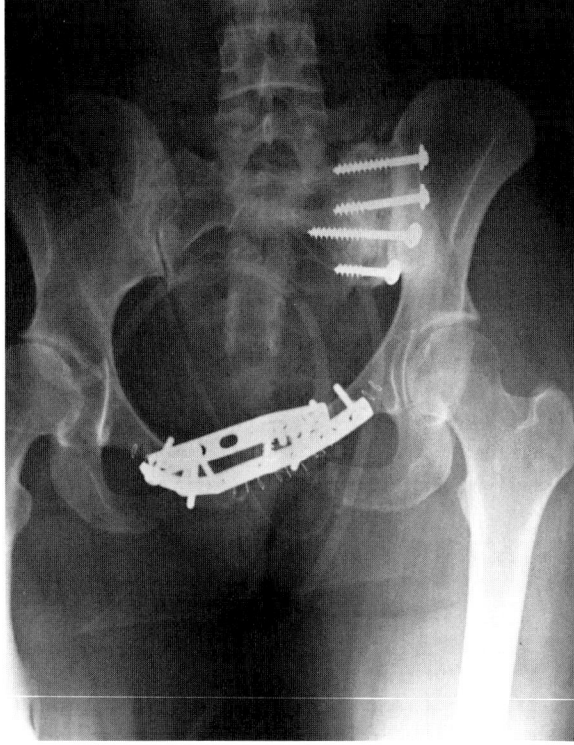

C

FIG. 5–55. Complex pelvic fracture. **A:** Diastasis of the pubic symphysis with chronic changes in the left sacroiliac joint and instability. **B:** The left sacroiliac joint and symphysis were reduced with internal fixation. **C:** Failure to maintain reduction of the symphysis required a second procedure to achieve stability.

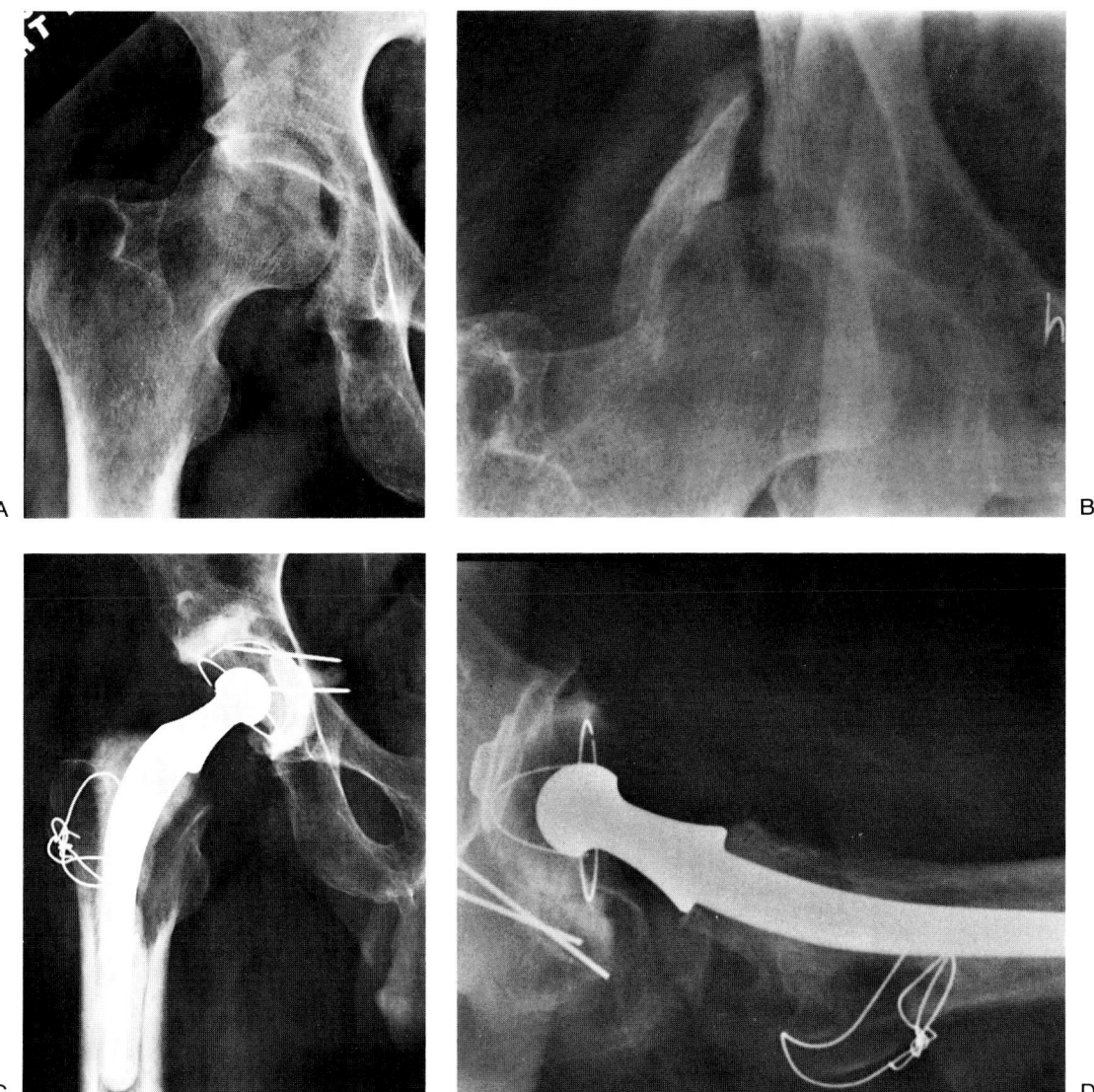

FIG. 5–56. A 45-year-old male, motor vehicle accident. Original x-rays interpreted in local emergency room as being negative. Returned two days later and x-rays still called negative. Put on crutches. After nine weeks the diagnosis was made. **A:** Anterior posterior view of the right hip. **B:** Oblique view showing the posterior fragment. **C:** Following open reduction and internal fixation of the fractured fragment. The dome of the acetabulum posteriorly showed damage of the cartilage as did the head of the femur and a primary total hip arthroplasty was done. **D:** Lateral x-ray one year post surgery.

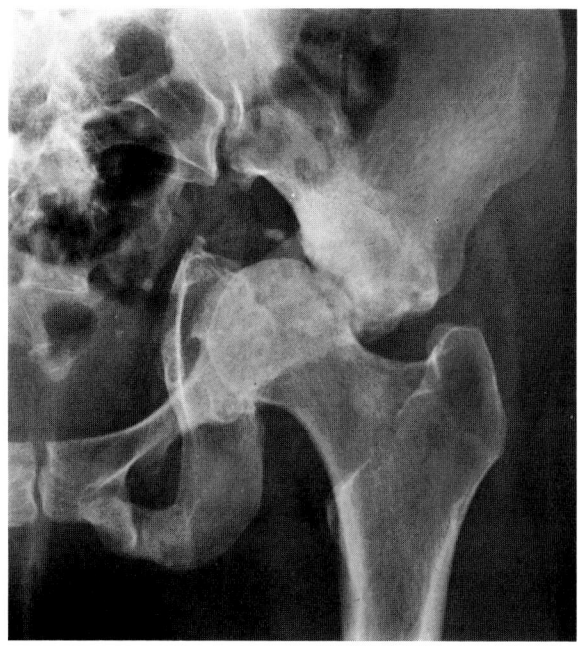

FIG. 5–57. A 28-year-old woman, motor vehicle accident. Patient treated in traction for six weeks. Union failed to occur. This is the appearance one year later with frank nonunion of the posterior pillar and traumatic arthritis of the head and acetabulum. Early open reduction and internal fixation of the posterior pillar would probably have obviated the need for subsequent total hip arthroplasty.

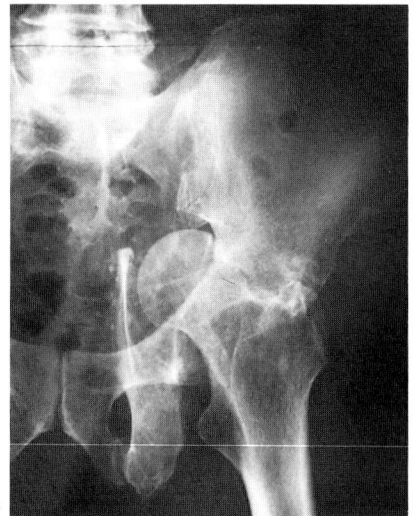

A

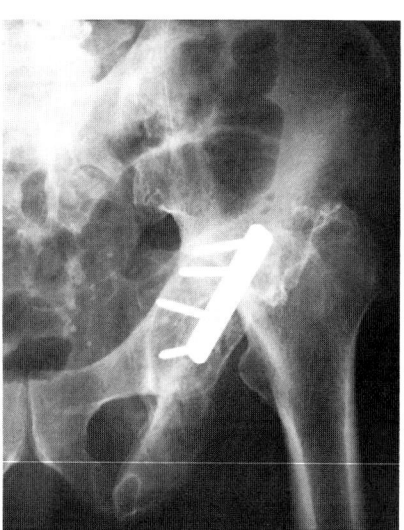

B

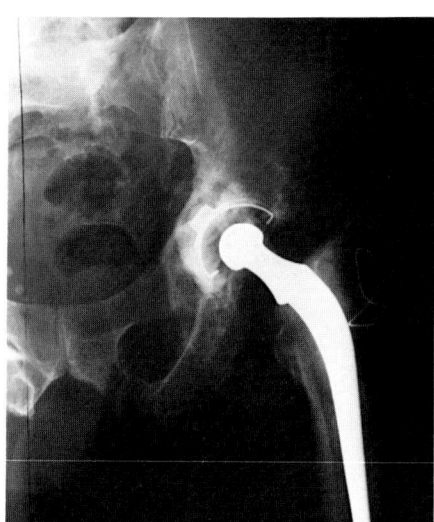

C

FIG. 5–58. A 68-year-old male, untreated fracture of the left pelvis with nonunion of the posterior pillar. A: Seven months post injury. B: Open reduction, internal fixation of acetabular fracture, removal of head and neck of femur and pin traction in distal femur. C: Six weeks after internal fixation hip explored and fracture found to be united, plate removed, and total hip arthroplasty done. Appearance eight weeks following total hip arthroplasty.

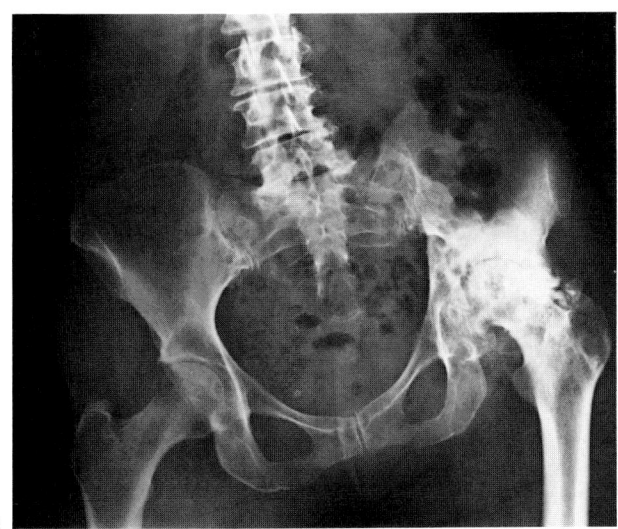
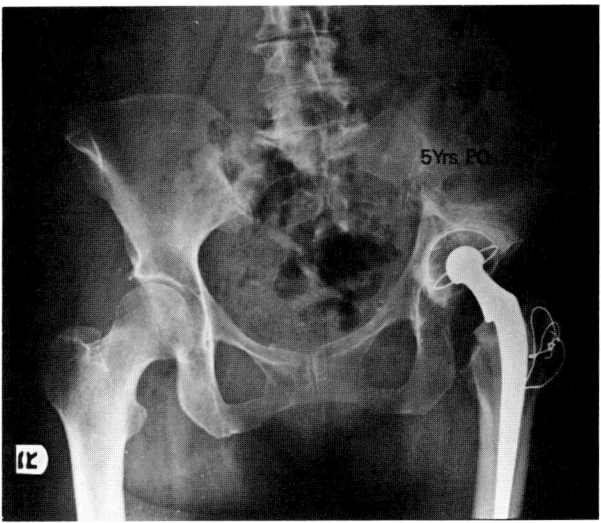

A

B

FIG. 5–59. A 54-year-old woman, 21 years prior in motor vehicle accident, fracture of femoral neck and acetabulum. Femoral neck fracture "pinned". Now pain, deformity, and very limited motion. **A:** Appearance of the left hip and pelvis. **B:** Total hip arthroplasty done; appearance five years later.

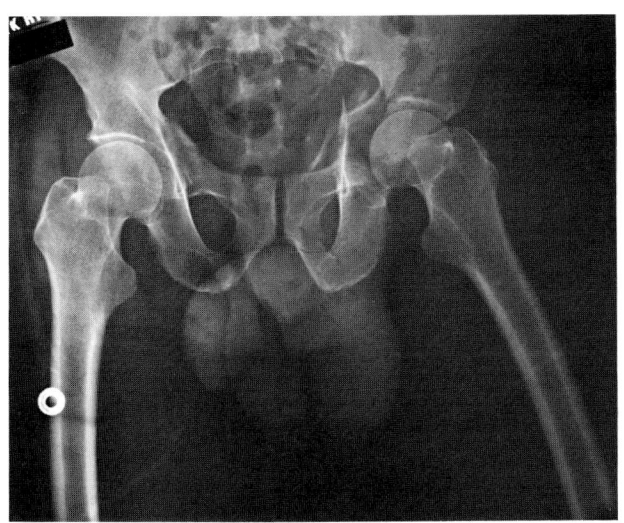
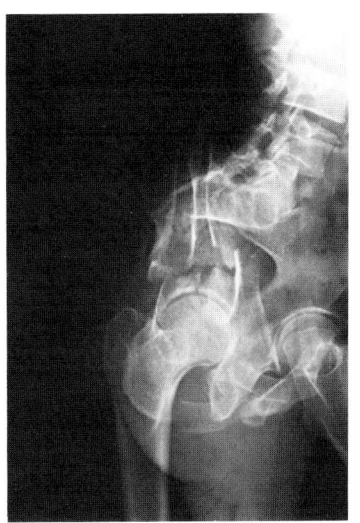

A

B

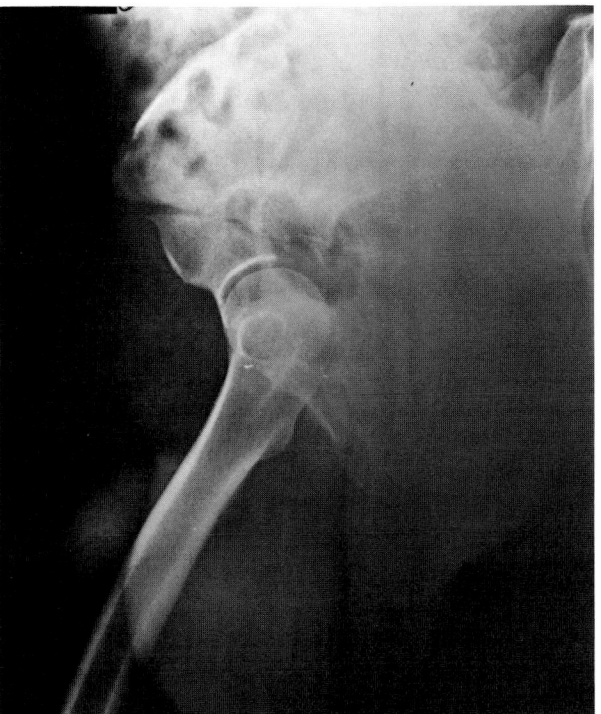

C

FIG. 5–60. A 49-year-old male, motorcycle accident. **A:** Appearance of pelvic fractures (anterior-posterior x-ray). Note the dome of the acetabulum appears intact. **B:** Obturator oblique view. Fracture into dome of acetabulum now evident. **C:** Iliac oblique view. Dome of acetabulum appears basically intact.

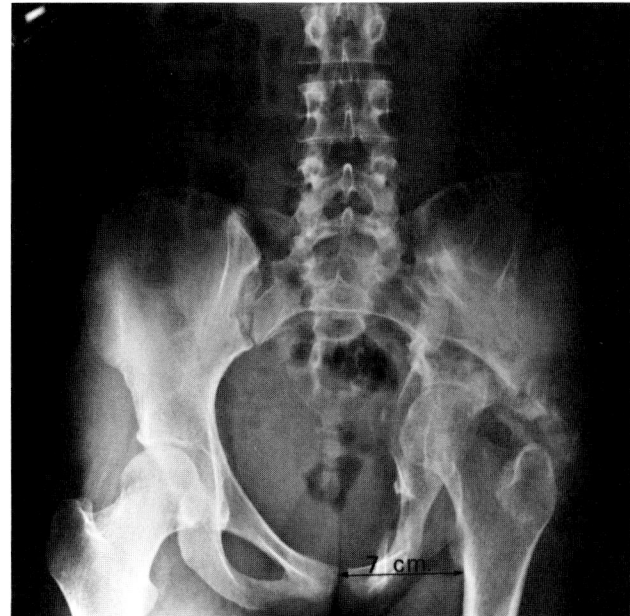
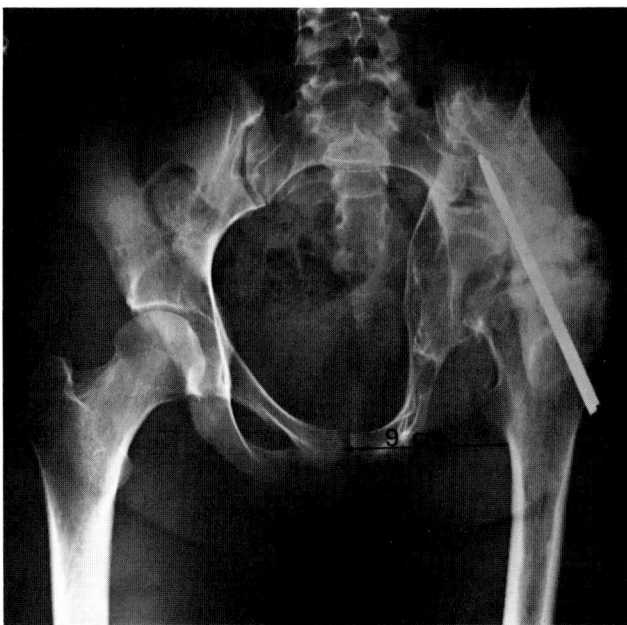

A   B

FIG. 5-61. A 19-year-old woman, motor vehicle accident. Severe compound fracture of pelvis untreated. Four months following injury, severe pain, on crutches, 45° flexion contracture, minimal motion. **A:** Anterior-posterior view of pelvis. **B:** Eight months following arthrodesis. Hip solid, extremity in neutral position, pain relieved, femur lateralized by 2 cm, 1 and 1.5 cm added length, full activity without walking aid.

could be achieved with good clinical and radiographic results in 50% of these cases. Twenty percent showed some lateral arthritic changes radiographically. It seems preferable when possible to reduce and internally fix these fractures rather than to proceed with a primary total hip arthroplasty.

The residual deficits of Class IV pelvic fractures include fractures that remain unreduced as well as fractures that result in traumatic arthritis. As mentioned, unreduced fractures can often be reduced at a later date. This is especially true of ununited posterior column fractures. These of necessity will require total hip arthroplasty in conjunction with reduction, usually as a second stage. As we have emphasized elsewhere, total hip arthroplasty in the presence of an unstable acetabulum is doomed to failure (88). Stable, secure foundation for placement of the acetabular prosthesis is imperative. This will often require not only open reduction but bone grafting as well, and once union is obtained the reconstruction can be done.

Occasionally the fracture is impossible to reduce, so that total hip arthroplasty cannot be performed. In such cases, fusion will be necessary (Fig. 5-61).

Complications Associated with Pelvic Fractures

The complications associated with pelvic fractures are directly related to the degree of trauma (98,99). There-

fore, the classification presented here assists in determining prognosis. Complications associated with Class I and Class II pelvic fractures are usually minor. Hematoma formation adjacent to the fracture site is usually the only abnormality noted. This is a very helpful finding that may lead one to identify an undisplaced fracture. With Class I and Class II fractures more significant injuries may occur to other areas, but the pelvic injury in these situations is usually not a significant clinical problem. The most severe complications result from Class III fractures (double breaks in the pelvic ring) and displaced Class IV (acetabular) fractures. Table 5-9 summarizes the incidence of immediate complications in these fracture categories at the Mayo Clinic (137).

Pelvic Hemorrhage

The most common and significant complication is pelvic hemorrhage. All patients with Class III fractures

TABLE 5-9. *Complex pelvic fractures:
Immediate complications*

Hemorrhage	71% (required transfusion)
Associated fractures	65% (average 2.2/pt)
Neurological	21%
Genitourinary	19%
Head	11%
Chest	11%
Abdomen	11%

demonstrated a significant drop in their hemoglobin. Seventy-one percent of patients with Class III or displaced Class IV fractures required over 10 units of blood (137). The overall mortality rate was 22%, but in patients requiring more than 5 units of blood the mortality rate increased to 45%. Renal failure is commonly related to the shock resulting from massive hemorrhage, and this adds significant morbidity and mortality (111,116,137). A less common but significant complication is infected hematoma, which occurred in 3% of our patients with complex pelvic fractures. Infection is more common with open pelvic fractures, but it has also been reported with closed fractures (122). The mortality rate is as high as 50% in these patients (134).

Hemodynamically unstable patients must be managed aggressively prior to complete radiographic evaluation. Anti-shock garments and external fixation devices can be employed. Mucha (118-122) employs antishock garments and suggests diagnostic and therapeutic angiography when bleeding is not controlled. Hemodynamically stabilized patients have a mortality rate of 3.4% compared to 42% in hemodynamically unstable patients (121).

The radiographic evaluation should be performed with as little movement of the patient as possible. Patient motion may increase the hemorrhage (133). Fortunately, with complex pelvic injuries, the classification and significance of the injury can almost always be determined with the AP view of the pelvis. Occasionally angled views (with the tube angled caudad or cephalad) are helpful and can be obtained without moving the patient.

In Mucha's series, angiography was required to control bleeding in only 3% of patients (118). Indications for angiographic intervention include (1) failure of anti-shock garments to control bleeding or loss of >4 units of blood in 24 hours or >6 units in 48 hours, (2) expanding hematomas, (3) open pelvic fractures, and (4) when angiography is required to evaluate the aorta or other regions of potential vascular injury (118). Angiography will usually identify multiple bleeding sites (Fig. 5-62). The sites can also be somewhat localized by assessing the fracture sites and the degree of displacement. The superior gluteal artery and anterior branches of the internal iliac artery are most commonly involved (160). Once the bleeding sites have been identified, embolization with autogenous clotting material or Gelfoam will usually control the bleeding (114,115,131,150). In larger vessels, occlusion with inflated balloon catheters may be required (124,144). In patients with sacral fractures, posterior bleeding sites may present a granular appearance rather than the more easily identifiable extravasation that is usually seen. This must be kept in mind for optimum control of all bleeding sites (142).

In experienced hands, angiographic embolization is 85-95% successful in controlling hemorrhage. Failures may be caused by severe vessel disease that prevents successful catheterization or coagulopathy that prevents normal clot formation (118).

Adjacent or Distant Fractures

The frequency with which additional adjacent or distant fractures occur with pelvic fractures is not surprising. Sixty-five percent of patients with complex pelvic fractures sustained other fractures. The average number of fractures was 2.2 per patient (Table 5-10). As would be expected, lower extremity fractures were especially common (Fig. 5-63).

Neurologic Complications

Neurologic complications are also common (Table 5-11), occurring in 21% of patients with complex pelvic injury. Injury to the lumbosacral plexus is especially common if the sacrum is fractured (Fig. 5-64) (75,95, 125). Sacral fractures were involved in 23% of our Class III pelvic fractures. The diagnosis is usually not made initially; rather, the injury is detected during the convalescent period. Leg weakness, incontinence, and impotence may result. Sciatic nerve injuries occurred in 4% of our patients (137).

Genitourinary Injuries

Injuries to the genitourinary system have been reported to occur in 4–22% of patients with pelvic fractures (110,116,127,137). Combined series report an average injury rate of 13% (103). Hartmann reported an incidence of 15.5% with unilateral pubic rami fractures, but the incidence increased to 41% with double anterior fractures (straddle) (100). There is no doubt that the incidence of lower urinary tract injury (urethra and bladder) is much higher with displaced fractures of both obturator rings or diastasis of the pubic symphysis. However, evaluation of the genitourinary system is warranted in almost any patient with a pelvic fracture (133).

Damage to the urethra is the most common injury (83,110,116,127). The anatomy of the male genitourinary system results in the male urethra being more prone to injury than the female (Fig. 5-10). The prostatic urethra is fixed in the prostate and extends from the bladder neck to the urogenital diaphragm. The membranous urethra lies within the urogenital diaphragm. These two portions of the urethra make up the posterior urethra. The short segment between the prostate and the urogenital diaphragm has been described as the area most susceptible to injury (83,139). The anterior urethra (bulbous and cavernous portions) is located below the urogenital diaphragm and is less likely to be injured. The female urethra is short and the urogenital diaphragm less well

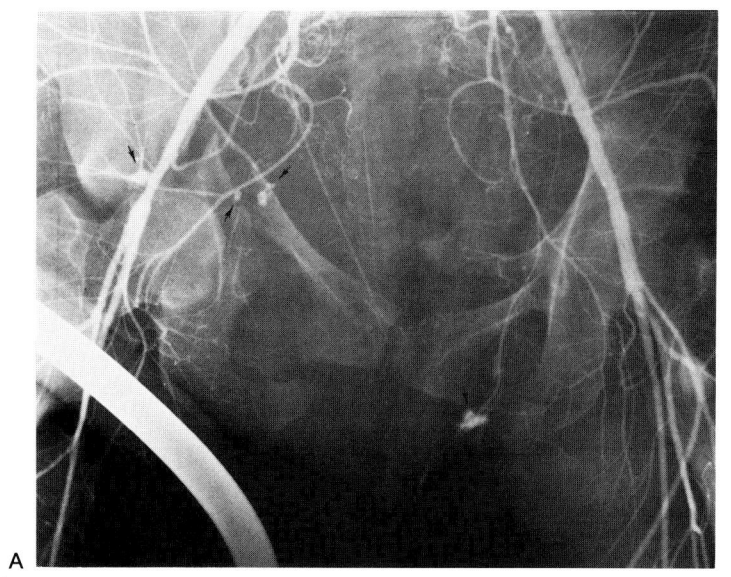

A

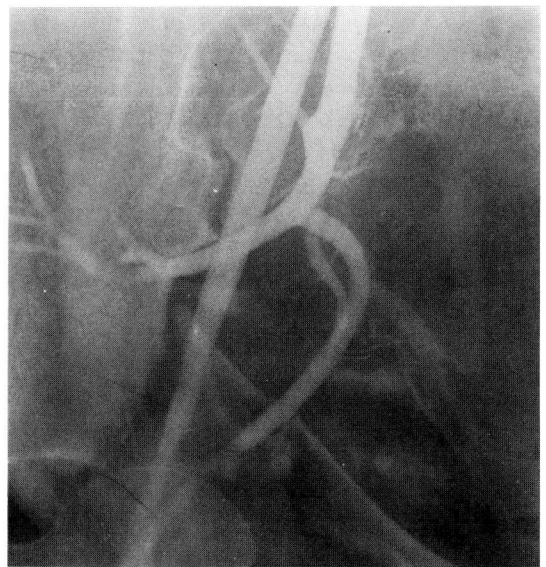

B

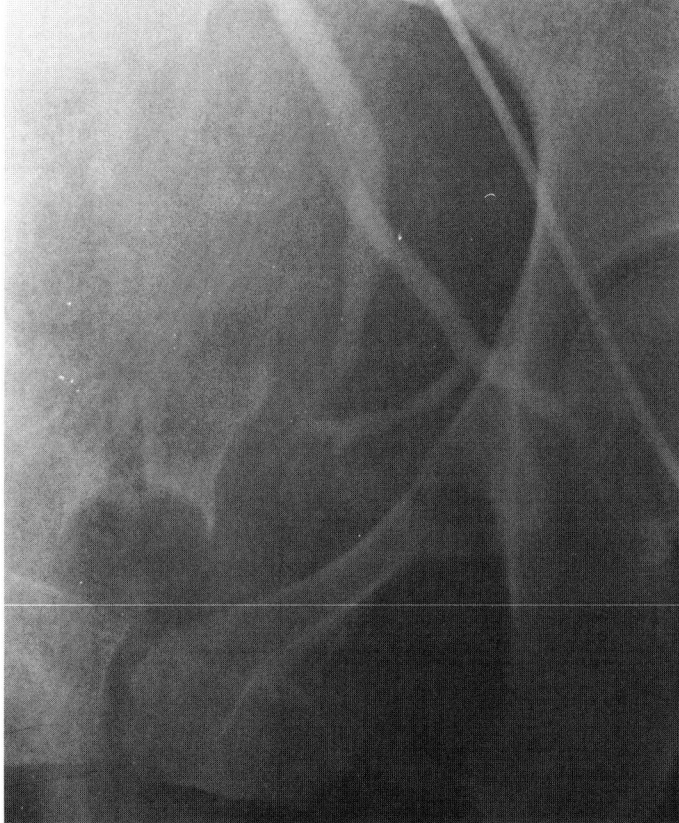

C

FIG. 5–62. Complex pelvic fracture with active pelvic arterial bleeding. A: Contrast extravasates from the bleeding vessels (*arrows*). Repeat angiograms on the right (B) and left (C) following gel foam embolization; the bleeding is now controlled.

TABLE 5–10. *Complex pelvic fractures: Associated skeletal injuries*

Location	Fractures	Location	Fractures
Skull	8	Chest	24
Facial bones	8	Rib	22	
Upper extremity	32	Sternum	2	
Clavicle	4	Spine	14
Scapula	2	Lower extremity	60
Humerus	9	Femur	24	
Forearm	15	Tibia-fibula	30	
Wrist	2	Foot	6	

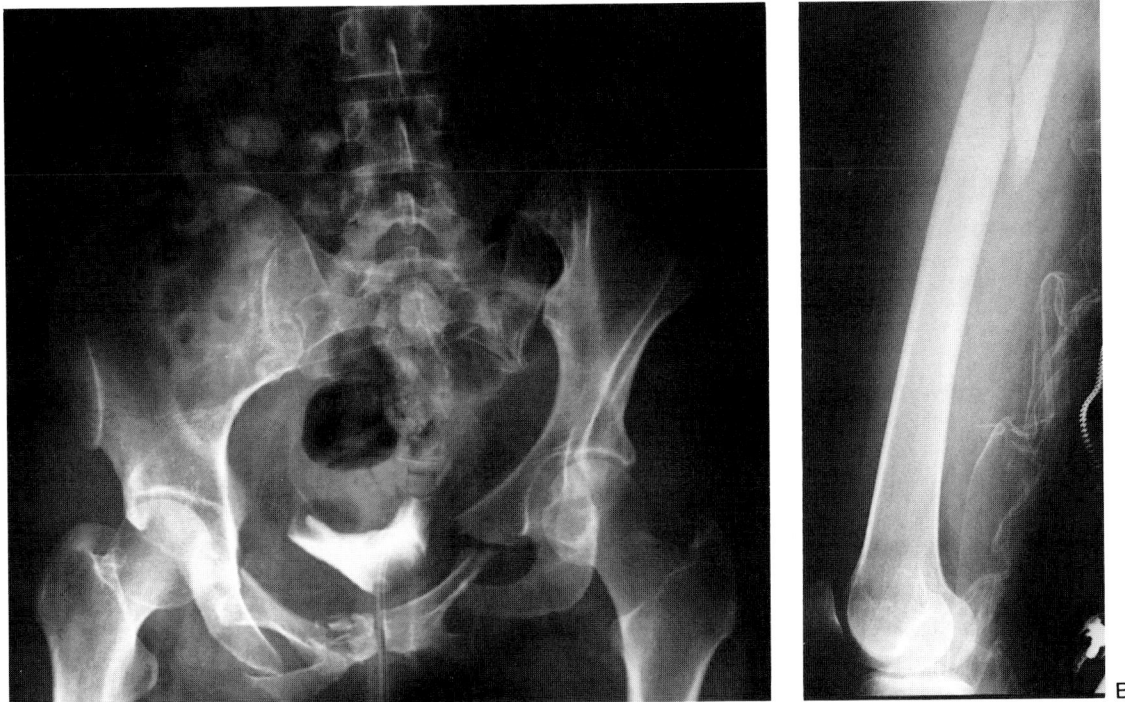

A B

FIG. 5–63. Complex pelvic fracture due to vertical shearing forces. AP view of the pelvis (**A**) demonstrates a Class III fracture with hematoma elevating the bladder. Lateral view of the right femur (**B**) shows a comminuted femoral fracture.

TABLE 5–11. *Complex pelvic fractures: Neurological complications (21% of patients)*

Quadriceps (femoral nerve)	6%
Gluteal (superior and inferior gluteal nerve)	6%
Sciatic nerve	4%
Dorsiflexors of foot (peroneal nerve)	2%
Cord injury	2%
Hamstring	1%

developed, allowing greater mobility and less susceptibility to injury.

Clinical evaluation of the urethra with rectal examination and assessment of the classic triad of blood at the urethral meatus, inability to void, and bladder distention are useful in proper management of the patient. The radiographic evaluation is essential for complete evaluation of the entire urinary tract. If angiography is necessary (diagnosis and treatment of massive hemorrhage), it should be performed prior to retrograde studies of the urethra and bladder. Contrast medium in the bladder or extravasate in the pelvis will obscure bleeding sites on the angiogram (140). In patients in whom urethral injury is suspected because of clinical history or from radiographic features of the fracture, a retrograde urethrogram must be performed prior to urethral catheterization. This procedure is easily accomplished by placing a Foley catheter in the distal urethra and gently injecting contrast material into the urethra. The procedure should be performed with fluoroscopic guidance. If no defect in the urethra is evident, a Foley catheter can be placed in the bladder and a cystogram performed to exclude the possibility of bladder rupture. It is too difficult to fill the bladder during the urethrogram, and distention with 200-300 ml of contrast is required to assess the bladder (97,133,138). Radiographs of the urethra and bladder

should be obtained in the AP and oblique positions. Following completion of filming with the bladder distended, the contrast medium should be allowed to drain. This prevents overlooking small tears. At this stage in the examination, the excretory urogram can be performed to evaluate the upper urinary tract.

Sandler and colleagues have proposed a classification for urethral injuries based on the patterns of extravasation during retrograde urethrography (Fig. 5-65) (139). Type I injuries cause stretching of the posterior urethra due to hematoma with no actual tear. Type II injuries result from rupture of the posterior urethra just above the urogenital diaphragm (previously considered the most common injury). In Type III injuries, the urethra and urogenital diaphragm are ruptured, resulting in extravasation of contrast medium below the urogenital diaphragm. Sandler's results indicate that the Type III injury was in fact the most common and occurred four times as frequently as the Type II injury (139). This has also been our experience. The incidence of urethral rupture in our cases was 9%, with only 1 case of disruption of the female urethra. Additional complications involving these injuries included impotence in 78% of males and stricture formation requiring dilatation in 89% of male patients. Fistula formation occurred as a late complication of urethral rupture in 1 patient (Fig. 5-66) (137).

Anterior urethral injuries are rare. We did not encounter any in our review of 750 cases. Since that study, several anterior urethral ruptures have been detected. Both were due to soft tissue trauma (Fig. 5-67). There was no associated pelvic fracture.

Bladder injuries have been reported to be the most common injury of the genitourinary system following pelvic fracture. Injuries include contusions, extraperitoneal rupture, intraperitoneal rupture, and both intra- and extraperitoneal tears (77). A rupture must be present

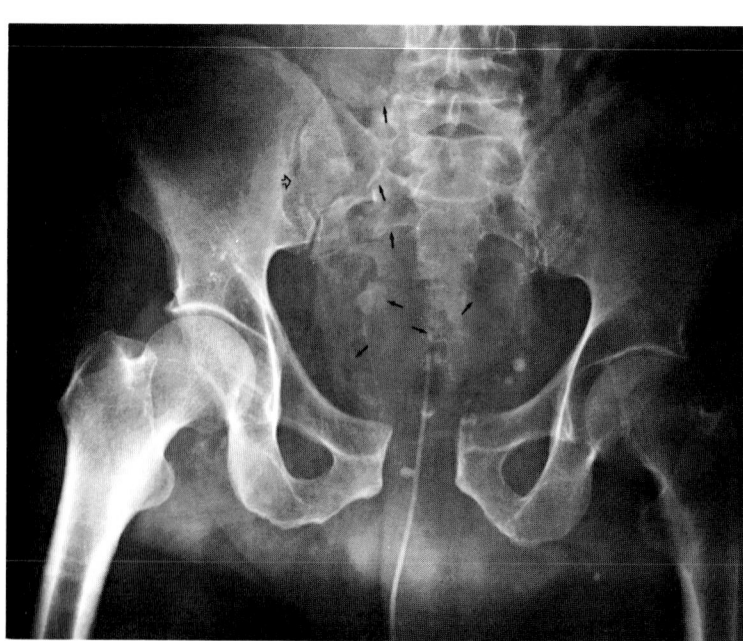

FIG. 5–64. Complex pelvic fracture with a comminuted sacral fracture (*black arrows*). There is also separation of the right SI joint (*open arrow*) and a fracture of the right transverse process of L5.

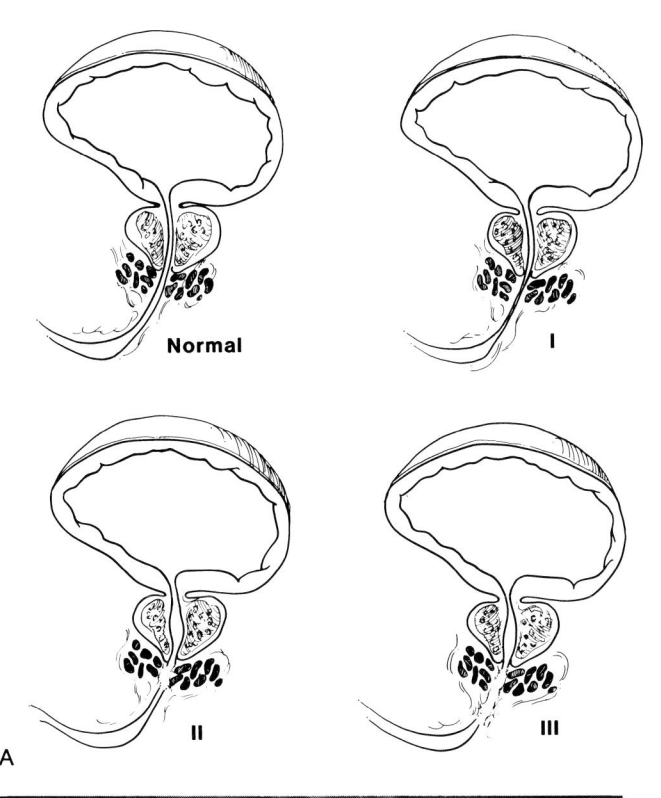

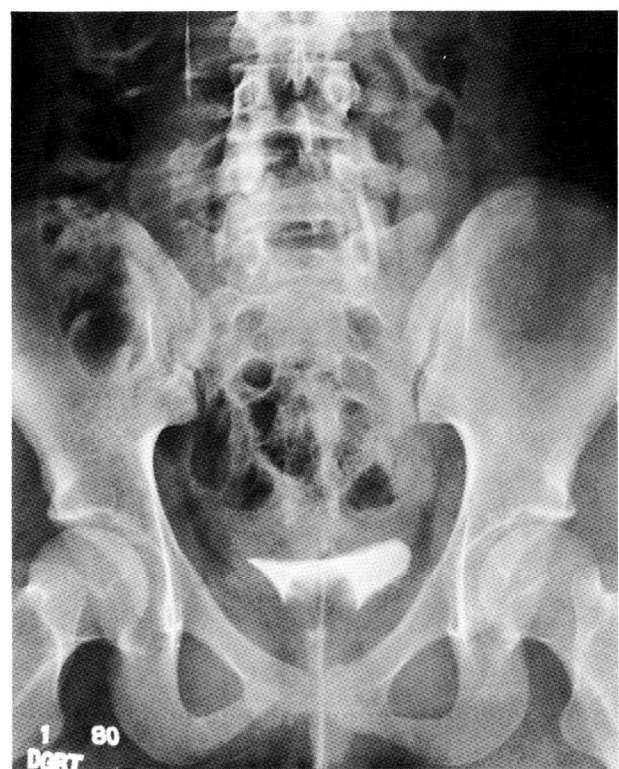

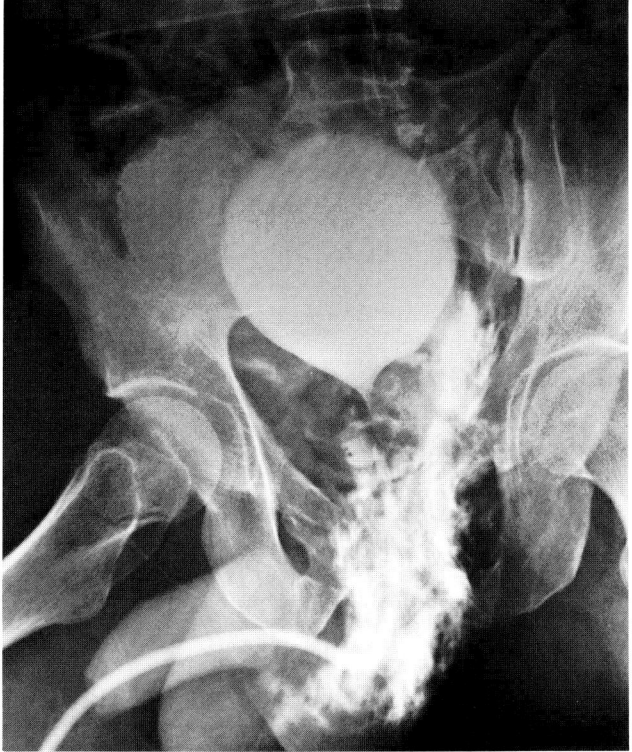

FIG. 5-65. A: Classification of urethra injuries. Type I, stretching of the posterior urethra due to hematoma. Type II, rupture of the posterior urethra with extravasation above the urogenital diaphragm. Type III, rupture with extravasation below the urogenital diaphragm. B: Anterior pelvic fracture with elevation of the bladder, stretching the posterior urethra (Type I). Foley catheter in the bladder. C: Type III rupture of the posterior urethra with extravasation of contrast above and below the urogenital diaphragm. There is marked elevation of the bladder due to hematoma.

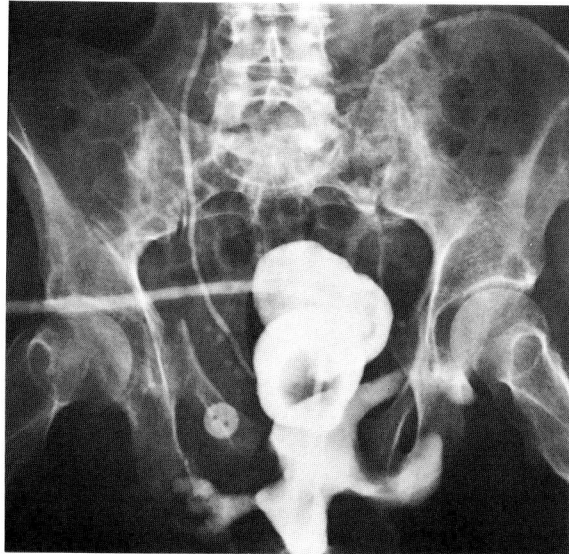

FIG. 5-66. Old pelvic fracture. Fistulas have developed around the area of the ruptured urethra. Suprapubic tube in place.

TABLE 5-12. *Complex pelvic fractures: Genitourinary complications (19% of patients)*

Kidney	3%
Laceration	
Contusion	
AVM	
Bladder rupture	4%
Extraperitoneal	
Intraperitoneal	
Urethral rupture	9%
Impotence (78% of urethral ruptures)	
Urethral stricture (89% of urethral ruptures)	
Vaginal laceration	2%
Neurogenic bladder	1%

marizes the genitourinary complications that occurred in patients with complex pelvic fractures.

Injuries to the Head, Chest, and Abdomen

Injuries to the head, chest and abdomen were associated with pelvic fractures in 33% of patients, 11% in each category (Table 5-9). Significant chest injuries included pneumothorax and rupture of the diaphragm. Ruptured diaphragms have been reported to occur more frequently with Malgaigne fractures (110).

Abdominal injuries included ruptured liver, spleen, small bowel, and colon, all occurring with an incidence of 2%. Intrapelvic rupture of the rectum and anus occurred in 3 patients. This is significant in that infection of the pelvic hematoma and an abscess may result. Actual entrapment of the bowel by pelvic fracture fragments has also been reported (78). The small bowel is most frequently involved. Injury to the pelvic viscera

for bladder injury to be visible on the radiograph. Contusions are more difficult to detect. Rupture of the bladder occurred in only 4% of our patients, but Sandler et al. (138) reported an incidence of 10%. The incidence of extraperitoneal rupture is usually 56-80% (Fig. 5-68) (82,138). Extraperitoneal rupture is the result of penetration of the bladder by fracture fragments or shearing of the pubovesical ligaments. Intraperitoneal rupture usually results from blunt trauma to the abdomen with a distended bladder (Fig. 5-69). Significant renal trauma (laceration) was noted in 3% of patients. Table 5-12 sum-

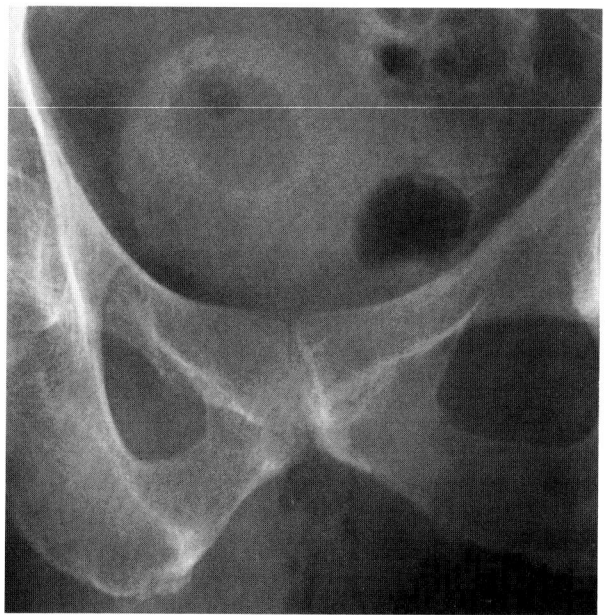

A

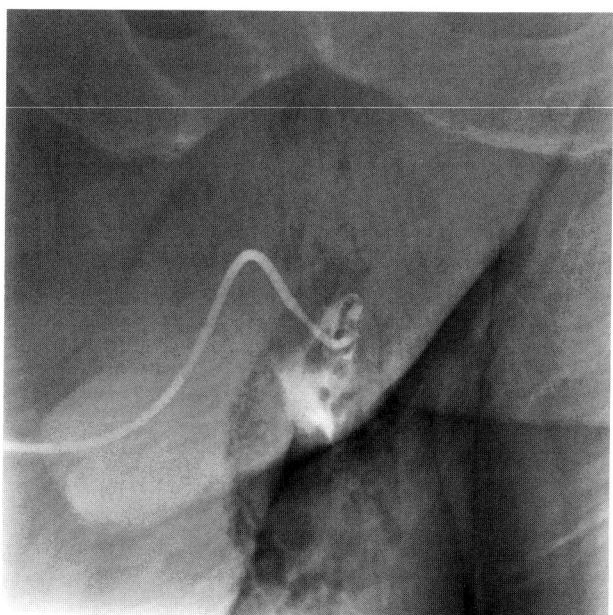

B

FIG. 5-67. Anterior urethral rupture. AP (**A**) view of the pelvis shows air in the soft tissues below the symphysis. There is no anterior fracture. Carefully performed retrograde urethrogram (**B**) shows rupture in the proximal membranous urethra.

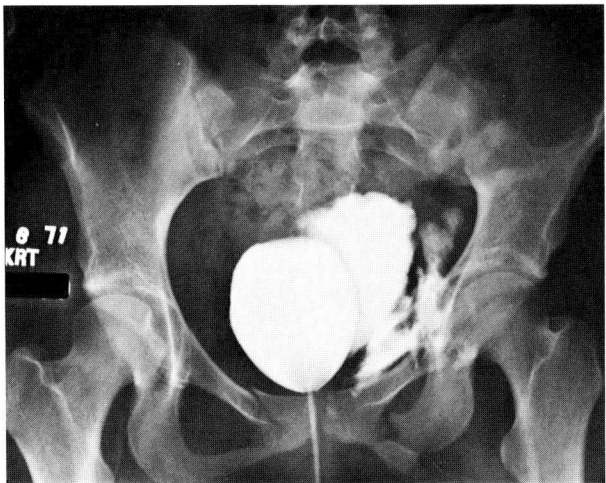

FIG. 5–68. Pelvic fracture with extra peritoneal bladder rupture. There is extravasation of contrast material from the left side of the bladder. Contrast remains in the pelvis.

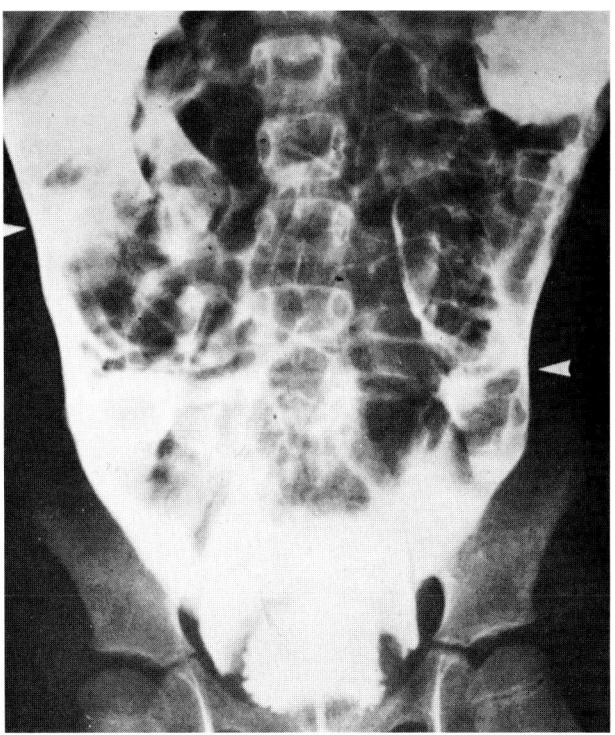

FIG. 5–69. Intraperitoneal rupture with contrast outlining loops of bowel.

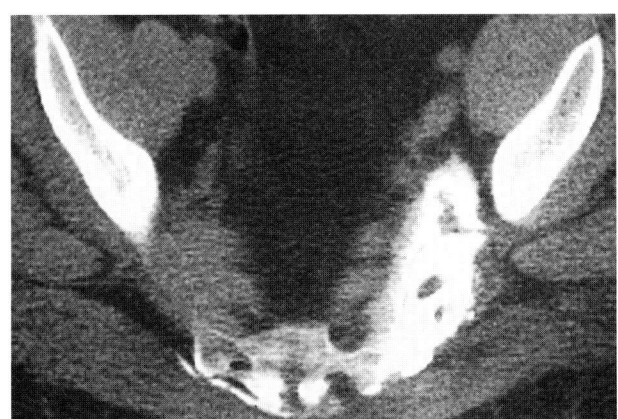 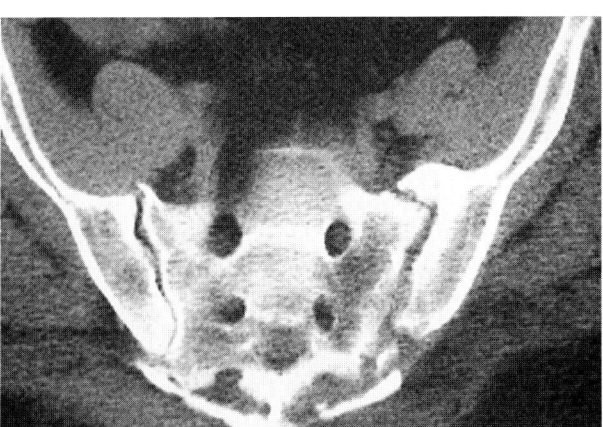

A   B

FIG. 5–70. CT images in a patient with an old Class III fracture. **A:** There is considerable ossification around the sciatic nerve on the left. **B:** Ossification posterior to both sacroiliac joints.

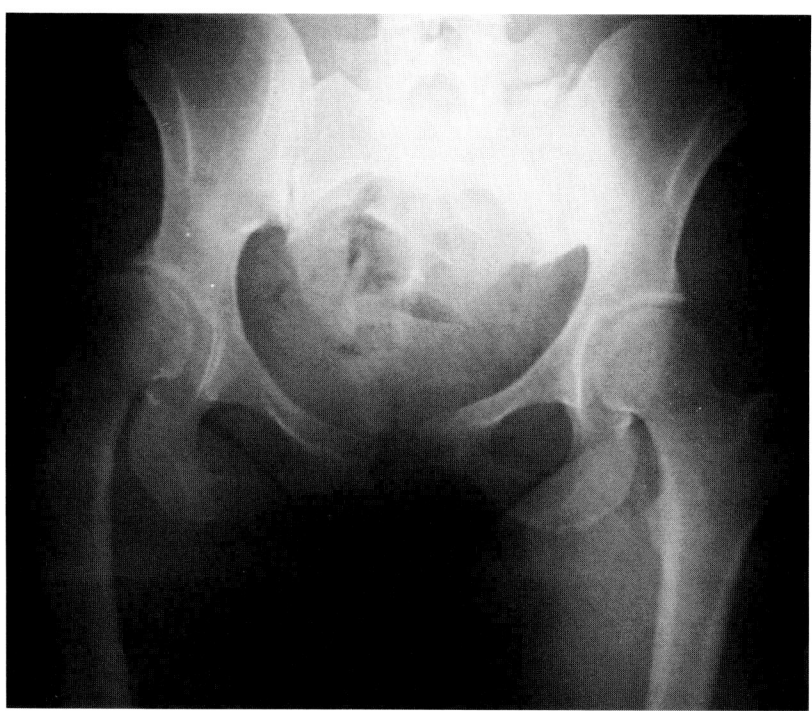

FIG. 5-71. Unstable fracture with symphysis diastasis.

and open pelvic fractures deserve further discussion owing to the severity of this complication. Perry defines an open fracture as a fracture that communicates with the vagina, rectum, or perineum, or with a cutaneous laceration (129). Postoperative sites with surgical drains in place should be included in this category. Patients with open pelvic fractures have severe pelvic and extrapelvic injuries, and the mortality rate may be as high as 42% (129). Mechanism of injury also differs somewhat in that the majority of open fractures are the result of motorcycle or pedestrian accidents rather than motor vehicle accidents. Open pelvic fractures have more significant hemorrhage owing to the lack of tamponade normally seen with close injuries. The incidence of sepsis and renal failure is also significantly increased (83).

Delayed Complications

Delayed complications are also a significant problem in patients with pelvic fractures (Table 5-13). Such complications occurred in 47% of patients with complex pelvic fractures. Adult respiratory distress syndrome (ARDS), pulmonary emboli, and myocardial infarcts were not uncommon (Table 5-13). However, no deaths occurred in our group of patients as a result of these complications (137).

Long-term orthopedic complications can also occur. For example, leg length discrepancy was evident in 10% of our patients with Class III pelvic fractures. These were all patients with double vertical or shearing fracture-dislocations of the Malgaigne type. Other orthopedic problems include instability of the sacroiliac joint and pubic symphysis (Fig. 5-71), avascular necrosis of the femoral head, malunion, non-union, and myositis ossificans.

DISLOCATIONS AND FRACTURE-DISLOCATIONS OF THE HIP

Dislocations of the hip account for only about 5% of all skeletal dislocations (182). Motor vehicle accidents, motorcycle accidents, and falls from significant heights are responsible for the majority of hip dislocations (180). These injuries are most frequent in young adults (average age, 31 years in Reigstad's study [180]), with males outnumbering females 3:1. Because of the degree of trauma necessary to cause this injury, severe multiple injuries are found in up to 75% of patients (183). Thus, there is significant economic impact associated with dislocation of the hip.

Dislocations may occur centrally (Fig. 5-57), posteriorly (Fig. 5-72), or anteriorly (Fig. 5-73). Central disloca-

TABLE 5-13. *Complex pelvic fractures: Delayed complications (47% of 120 Patients)*

Complications		% Patients
Adult respiratory distress syndrome (ARDS)		8
Pulmonary embolus		10
Myocardial infarct		1
Stress ulcers		4
Incontinence		3
Infection		9
Pelvic hematoma	3	
Other	6	
Orthopedic		12
Leg length discrepancy	10	
Avascular necrosis femoral head	2	

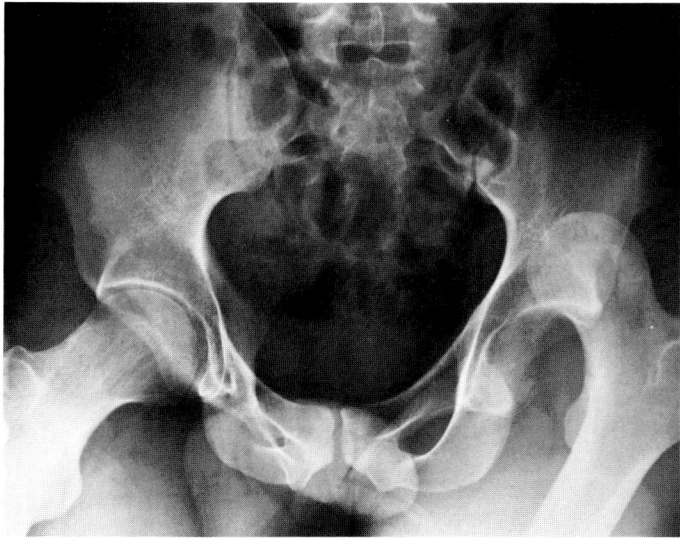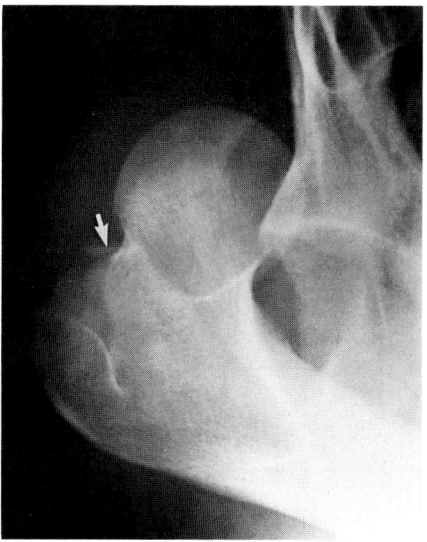

A   B

FIG. 5-72. Posterior dislocation of the left hip. The AP view (**A**) demonstrates the empty acetabular fossa with the femoral head projected superiorly. The anterior oblique (**B**) view clearly demonstrates the posterior dislocation. There is a small fracture fragment (*arrow*) near the greater trochanter.

tions have already been discussed in the section of this chapter dealing with pelvic and acetabular fractures. Of the other two types, posterior dislocations are much more common than anterior dislocations (166,182,189). Fractures of the femoral head and acetabulum may be associated with either type of dislocation (171).

Classification of Dislocations and Fracture-Dislocations of the Hip

Posterior Dislocations

Posterior dislocations occur seven to ten times more frequently than anterior dislocations (166,182,189).

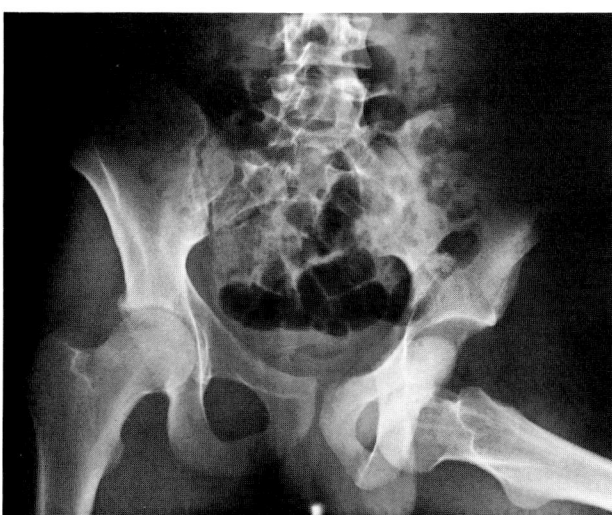

FIG. 5-73. Anterior dislocation of the left hip seen on the AP view of the pelvis. The femoral head typically lies over the ischium or obturator foramen.

This injury results when a compressive force is applied to the knee or foot with the hip in the flexed position (for example, striking the knee against a dashboard of a car in a motor vehicle accident) (166). Fractures of the posterior acetabulum are frequently associated with posterior dislocations of the hip. The size of the fragment is dependent upon the position of the femur at the time of injury (Fig. 5-45). If the hip is flexed in a neutral position, a posterior rim fracture may result. With the hip abducted, a larger posterior fragment or comminution is more likely to occur. Adduction may result in a tiny chip fracture or pure dislocation of the hip.

Clinically, patients with posterior dislocations usually present with four findings: (1) the hip flexed and externally rotated; (2) elevation of the trochanter; (3) a palpable prominence in the gluteal region; (4) bruising of the buttock (175).

Classifications of posterior dislocations have been devised by Stewart and Milford (187) and Thompson and Epstein (Table 5-14) (172,190). These classifications are

TABLE 5-14. *Classification[a]: Posterior dislocation of the hip*

Type	Definition
I	Posterior dislocation with no or only a minor acetabular fracture (Figs. 5-72 and 5-74)
II	Posterior dislocation with a single large acetabular fracture (Fig. 5-75)
III	Posterior dislocation with comminution of the acetabular rim with or without a major fragment
IV	Posterior dislocation with fracture of the acetabular floor
V	Posterior dislocation with fracture of the femoral head

[a] (166,172,173,190).

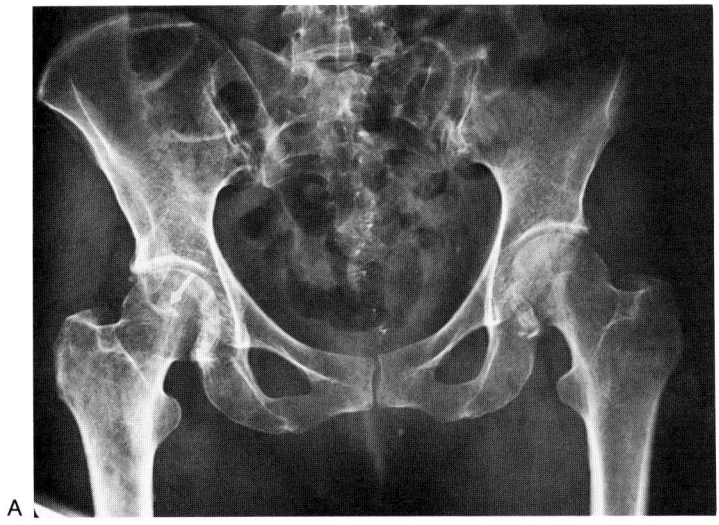
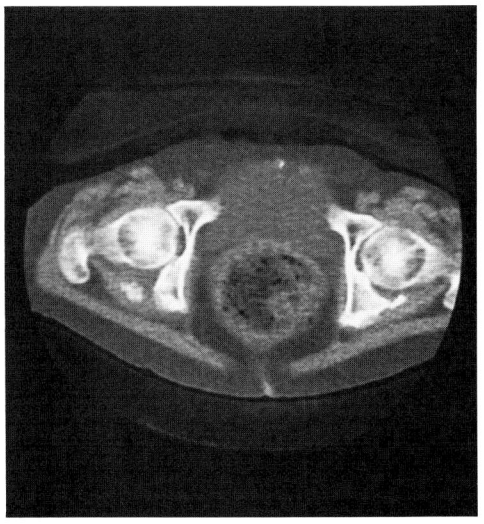

FIG. 5-74. An elderly patient with continued pain several days following reduction of a posterior dislocation of the right hip. This was felt to be uncomplicated at the time of reduction. **A:** AP pelvis with no evidence of joint widening. There is a density projected over the femoral head. **B:** CT scans revealed small acetabular fragments bilaterally, larger on the right. Thus, this would be classified as a Thompson-Epstein Type I.

quite similar in many respects. They are both based upon the associated fractures of the acetabulum and femur, and both correlate closely with clinical results and prognoses (Figs. 5-74 and 5-75). Dislocations with more complex acetabular fractures or femoral head fractures carry a more guarded prognosis compared with simple dislocations or dislocations with minimal acetabular involvement (Fig. 5-76).

Femoral head fractures with posterior dislocations of

the hip were once considered rare (164). Recent advances in imaging techniques and increased awareness of this association, however, have resulted in improved detection of femoral head injuries (172,174,176,179,181, 186,188). The incidence of femoral head fractures with posterior dislocations is reported to be up to 63% (Fig. 5-77) (174,181,188). Fracture of the femoral head occurs more frequently if the hip is flexed less than 90° (especially at about 60°). This forces the femoral head against

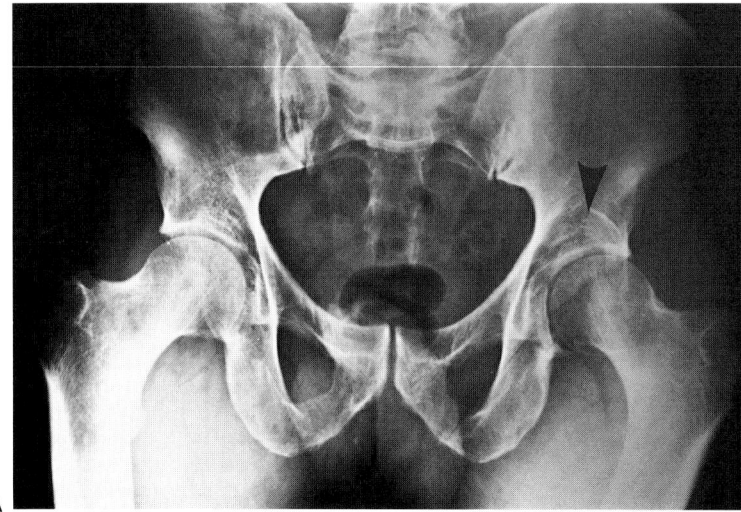
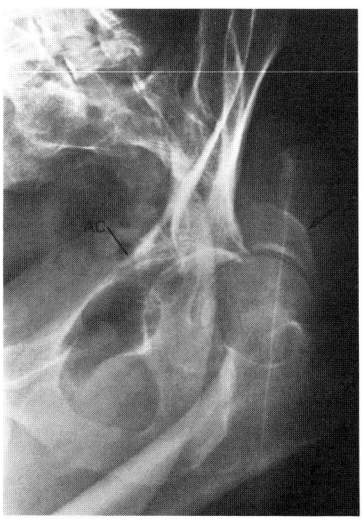

FIG. 5-75. Patient with hip pain following a motor vehicle accident (MVA). **A:** The AP pelvis shows widening of the joint space on the left with a white cortical line in the region of the acetabulum (*arrow*). **B:** Judet (anterior oblique) view demonstrates the posterior dislocation with a large posterior acetabular fragment (*arrow*). The femoral head appears intact. This represents a Type II dislocation.

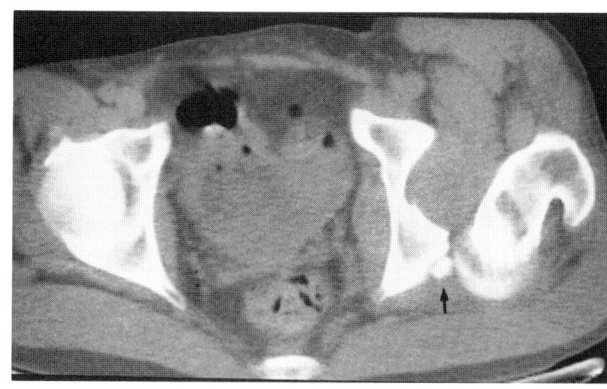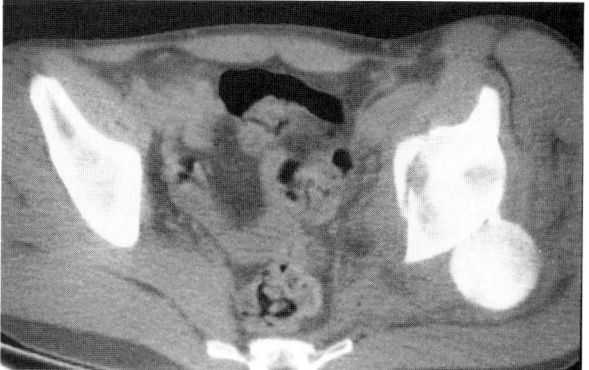

FIG. 5–76. CT images (**A, B**) demonstrate a posterior dislocation with comminution of the acetabular dome and posterior rim.

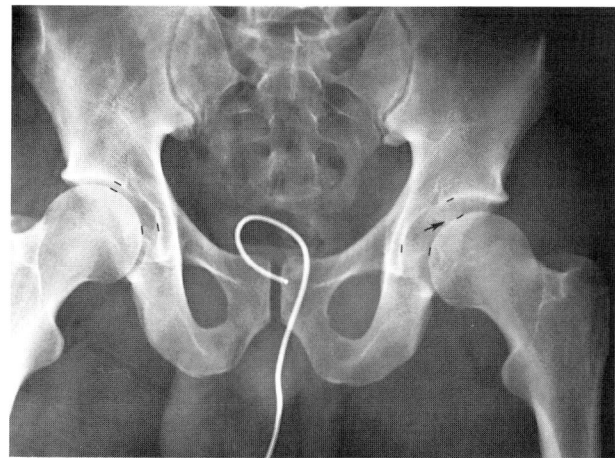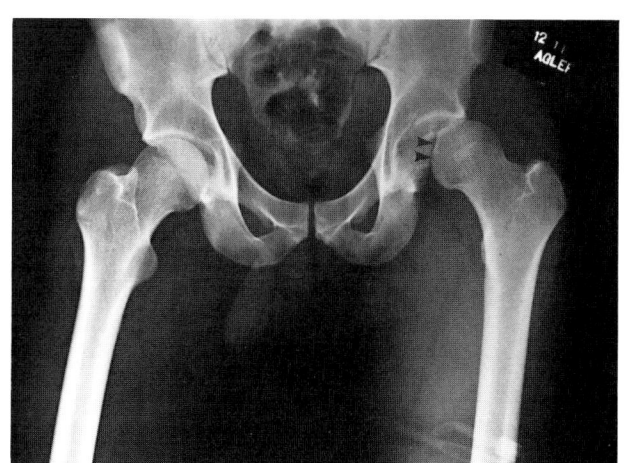

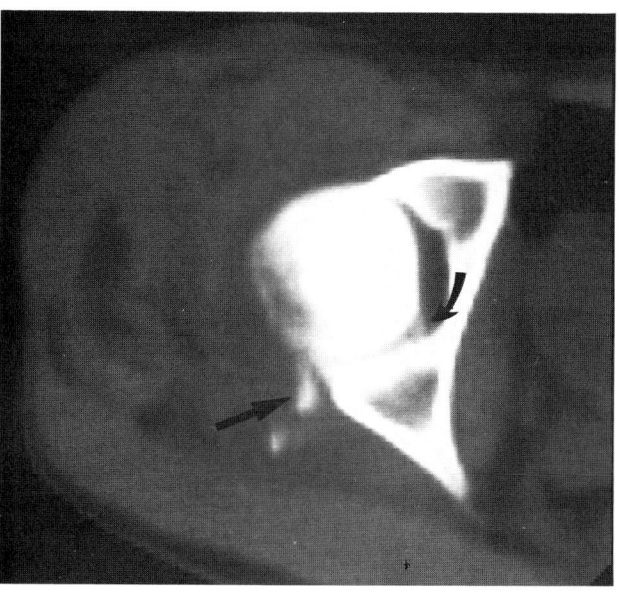

FIG. 5–77. Posterior dislocation with intra-articular fragment. **A:** Post-reduction AP film following dislocation of the left hip. The joint space is widened indicating an intra-articular fragment. Subtle density (*arrow*), but the origin is not clear. **B:** Dislocation with small fragments in the joint space that appear to arise from the flattened area on the femoral head (*arrows*), Thompson-Epstein, Type V. **C:** CT scan following reduction of what was thought to be an uncomplicated dislocation. Note the small head fragment in the joint space (*curved arrow*) and small posterior acetabular fragments (*arrow*). In this situation, what was considered a Type I dislocation was actually a Thompson-Epstein Type V.

the stronger posterior superior margin of the acetabulum and may result in an osteochondral shearing or impacted fracture (181).

Identification of intra-articular fragments from the femoral head or the acetabulum is essential in determining the method of treatment. The size, location, and degree of involvement of the weight-bearing surface of the femoral head and acetabulum must be clarified (Fig. 5-78). Pipkin (178) based his classification of femoral head fractures on the relationship of the fracture to the fovea and the presence or absence of associated acetabular or femoral neck fractures (Table 5-15) (Fig. 5-79). Femoral neck fractures associated with posterior dislocations are particularly troublesome and may interefere with reduction (178).

Anterior Dislocations

Anterior dislocations (Fig. 5-73) account for 13–18% of hip dislocations (166,167,173,182,184,189). This injury results from forced abduction and external rotation of the hip. The neck or greater trochanter impinges on the acetabulum and forces the femoral head to dislocate in an anterior inferior direction (166). This type of dislocation is often described by the position of the femoral head on the AP radiograph of the pelvis and hips. With the hip in extension, the head may overlie the pubis or ilium. In flexion, the head is seen over the obturator foramen. This is the most common presentation (167,169). Table 5-16 summarizes the Epstein Classification for anterior dislocations (173).

Fractures of the femoral head occur frequently with anterior dislocations of the hip (Fig. 5-80) (185). Dussault (169) reported femoral head fractures in 8 of 11 anterior dislocations, and DeLee (167) noted associated femoral head fractures in 17 of 22. Shearing fractures of the femoral head may result as the femoral head passes the inferior acetabulum. Impaction fractures of the posterior superior and lateral aspect of the head have an ap-

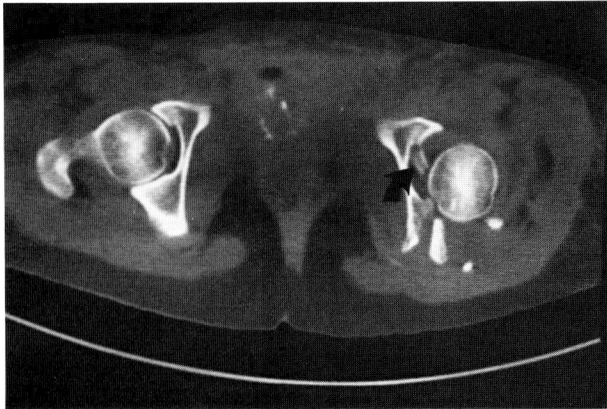

FIG. 5–78. CT image after posterior fracture dislocation with fragments in the joint space (*curved arrow*) and posterior impaction of the femoral head.

TABLE 5-15. *Posterior dislocations with associated femoral head fractures: Pipkin classification[a]*

Type I	Fracture of the femoral head inferior to the fovea
Type II	Fracture of the femoral head cephalad to the fovea
Type III	Either Type I or Type II with an associated femoral neck fracture
Type IV	Types I, II, or III with an associated acetabular fracture

[a] (178).

pearance similar to a Hill-Sachs defect (Fig. 5-81). This defect may be seen on the AP view if the hip is properly positioned (15° of internal rotation) (169). The lesion occurs when the head impinges on the anterior inferior acetabulum during the dislocation (169). The degree of impaction is significant. DeLee reported an increased incidence of osteoarthritis if the depression exceeded 4 mm (167). Tomography may be helpful in evaluating the degree of impaction of these fractures (Fig. 5-81C). Fractures of the anterior inferior margin of the acetabulum have also been described (3 of 11 cases in Dussault's series) (169).

Radiographic Evaluation of Dislocations and Fracture-Dislocations of the Hip

In the severely injured patient, the AP view of the pelvis and hips may be all that is possible. The patient's condition and the urgency of attending to severe hemorrhage or head injuries may also result in inadequate examination of the hips. Despite these difficulties, a thorough examination of this single view can yield significant information and assist in determining which additional studies may be most helpful.

Most complete dislocations are obvious on the AP view. The femoral head lies superior and lateral to the acetabulum following posterior dislocation (Fig. 5-72). The femoral head is usually projected over the obturator foramen when anterior dislocation has occurred (Fig. 5-73). Careful attention to detail is necessary in more subtle injuries and in evaluation of associated injury. Shenton's line may be interrupted on the involved side

TABLE 5-16. *Classification of anterior hip dislocation: Epstein[a]*

Type	Definition
IA	Superior dislocations with head in pubic or supraspinous location
IB	IA plus associated femoral head fracture
IC	IA plus associated acetabular fracture
IIA	Inferior location with head over obturator foramen or perineum
IIB	IIA plus femoral head fracture
IIC	IIA plus associated acetabular fracture

[a] (166,173).

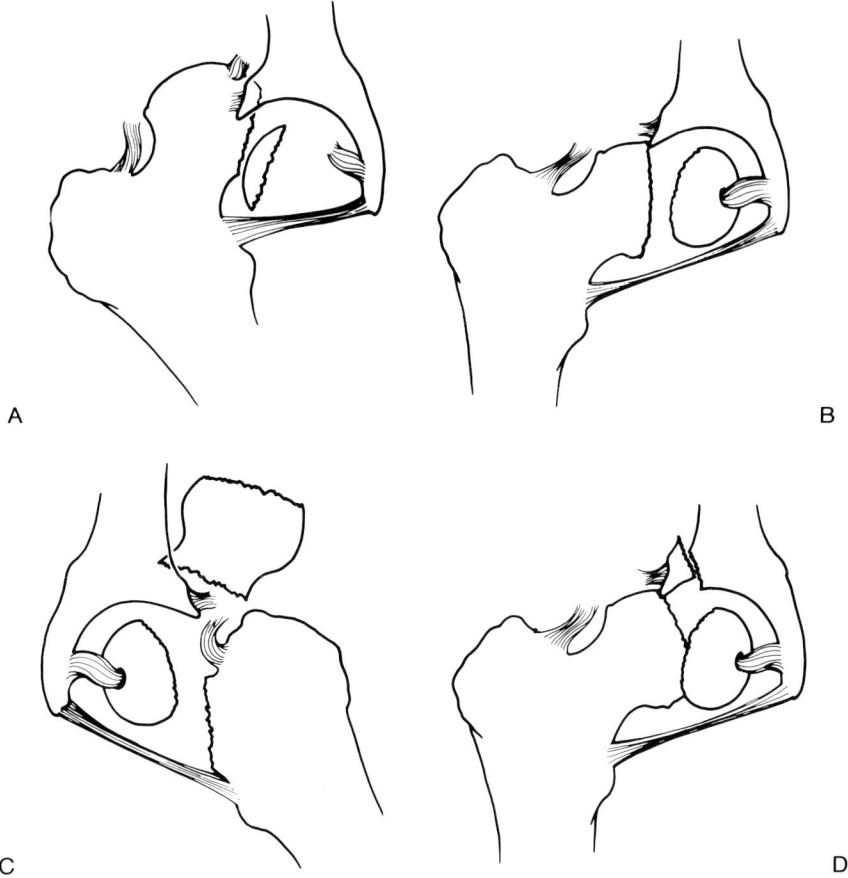

FIG. 5–79. Pipkin classification of femoral head fractures. **A:** Type I, posterior dislocation of femoral head fractures inferior to the fovea. **B:** Type II, posterior dislocation with femoral head fracture above the fovea. **C:** Type I or II with associated femoral neck fracture. **D:** Type I, II, or III with an associated acetabular fracture (from 181, with permission).

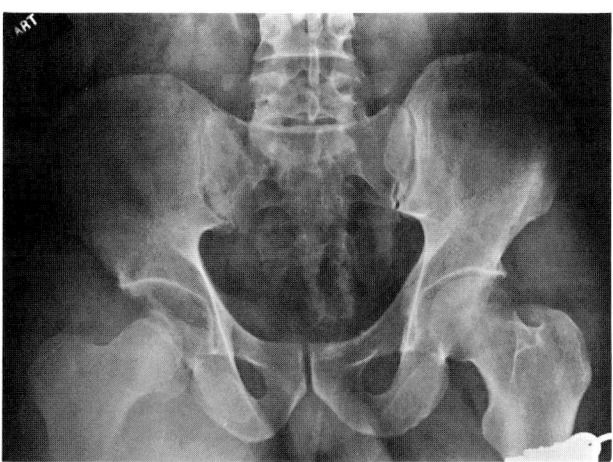

FIG. 5–80. AP view of the pelvis following anterior fracture-dislocation of the right hip. There are multiple femoral head fragments.

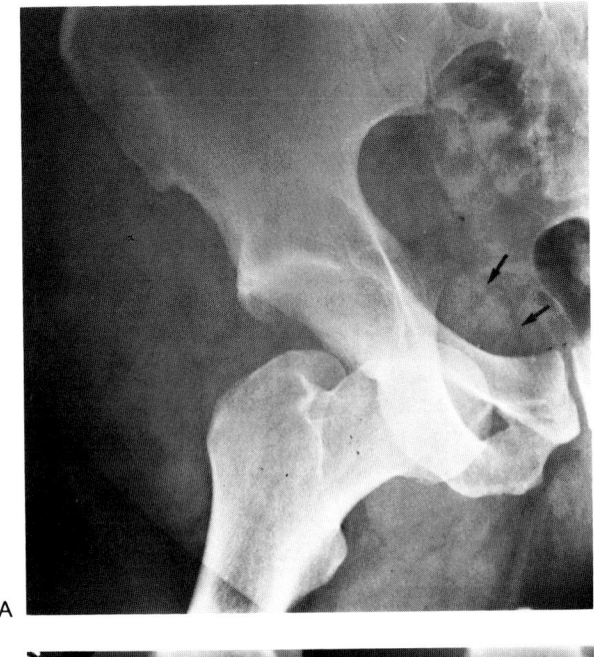

A

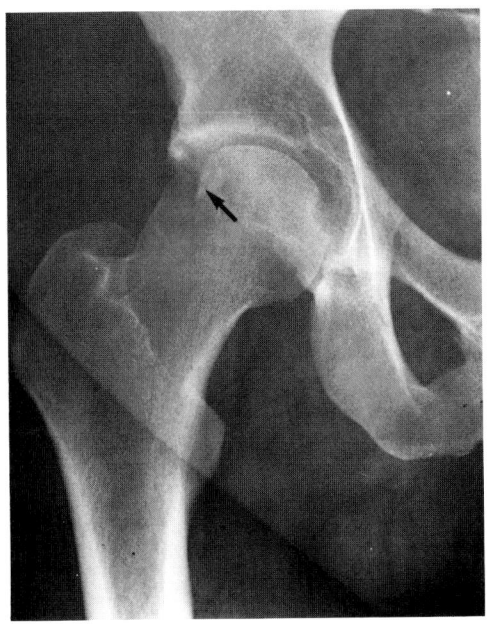

B

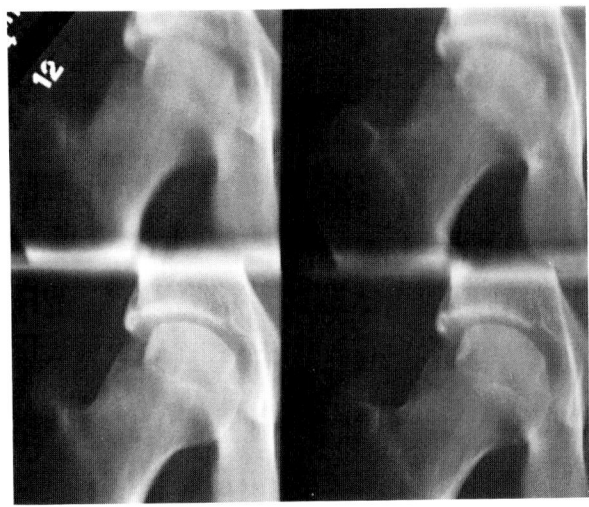

C

FIG. 5-81. Anterior dislocation of the right hip. **A:** Iliac oblique view demonstrating anterior dislocation with displacement of the obturator fat stripe (*arrows*). **B:** AP view of the right hip after reduction. There is an osteochondral impaction on the superior lateral aspect of the femoral head. **C:** AP tomogram demonstrates the defect in the head more clearly.

and may be one of the only clues for detection of subluxation or a subtle dislocation. The joint spaces should be compared. An increase in the joint space of more than 2 mm compared with the normal side should indicate the possibility of intra-articular fracture fragments or soft tissue interposition (Fig. 5-77). This is particularly important following reduction of a dislocation (186). With the hip removed from the acetabulum, bone fragments may be evident in the region of the joint space. These should be carefully evaluated for position changes following reduction. The femoral head should maintain its normal smooth configuration with uniform density. Impacted or displaced osteochondral fractures will alter the surface configuration (Figs. 5-77 and 5-81). Density differences may indicate an overlying fracture fragment (Fig. 5-74). Fractures of the femoral neck may also be associated with anterior dislocations (Fig. 5-82).

Ideally, oblique views of the hip (Judet views) should always be obtained (Fig. 5-83). Also, because of the mechanism of injury, it is essential that the femur and knee on the involved side be examined to exclude associated fractures. Unfortunately, fractures of the ipsilateral knee and femur, although uncommon, often mask the hip dislocation. As a result, the pelvis is not radiographed or is less than thoroughly evaluated (165,170).

Femoral head fractures are often seen on the AP view when associated with anterior dislocations. They appear as depressed defects on the superior lateral margin (169). However, identification of fragments in the joint space and evaluation of both the acetabular margins and the weight-bearing surface of the femoral head are best accomplished with tomography or computed tomography. In certain cases, moving the patient to the CT scanner is not desirable, and in these cases we have used conventional tomography on the Versigraph. Axial tomograms can also be obtained with the Versigraph. Although the

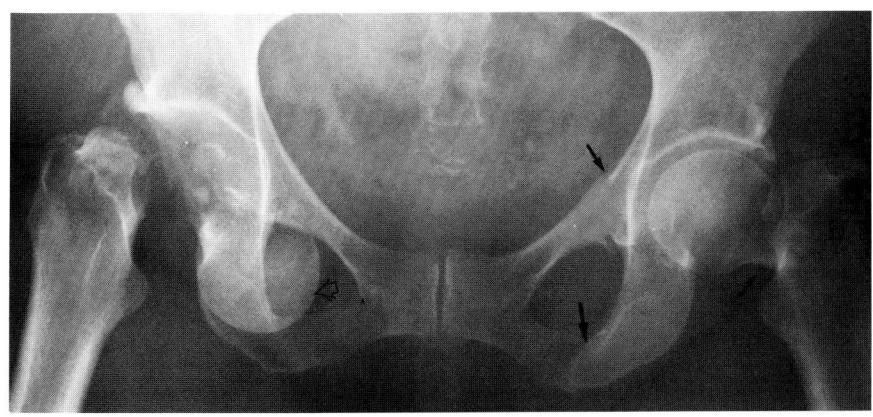

FIG. 5-82. AP view of the pelvis following a high velocity motor vehicle accident (MVA) demonstrates bilateral femoral neck fractures with anterior dislocation of the right femoral head (*open arrow*). Pubic rami fractures on the left (*arrows*).

detail does not match that obtained with CT, the information gained can be of great value. Complete evaluation is essential to proper treatment. Smith and Loop have shown that over 70% of their initial classifications were incorrect when based on initial radiographic studies (186). Tomography and computed tomography greatly reduce these errors. Detection of unsuspected intra-articular fragments is especially important, as open reduction is often indicated. Table 5-17 summarizes the radiographic approach to fracture-dislocations of the hip.

Treatment of Dislocations and Fracture-Dislocations of the Hip

If the hip dislocates and no fracture is detected through careful radiographic study, including analysis of oblique views, then the matter is relatively simple. Reduction should be accomplished as soon as possible. The incidence of avascular necrosis is high if the hip remains dislocated for more than 12 hours. Reduction usually requires an anesthetic. The reduction should be checked

for stability, with the hip in 90° of flexion and posterior forces placed on the femur. If it is stable, the patient can be put in traction. After the acute pain subsides, mobilization can begin with partial weight bearing. There seems to be little evidence to justify a long period on crutches. Crutches should be used only until the pain subsides. Then gradual resumption of normal activities should begin. Subsequent degenerative arthritis is rare if there has been no fracture of either the head or the acetabulum.

If the dislocated femoral head is accompanied by a fracture, the fracture may involve the head itself, the acetabulum, or the femoral neck. The femoral head is usually involved in a shear type of fracture (Fig. 5-84). Open reduction is indicated if more than one-third of the head is involved or if a fragment is interposed between the head and acetabulum. If the fracture fragment is relatively small and lies inferiorly in the "axilla" of the hip, traction and early ambulation is all that need be done. These small fragments need not be removed if they do not lie between the femoral head and acetabulum. Larger fragments can be returned to their bed in the femoral head and held with a screw. If this is not possible, they must be removed.

If the fracture accompanying the dislocation involves the acetabulum and not the head, small posterior fragments can be neglected, provided that the hip is stable. If there is instability, which implies a larger posterior fragment, then open reduction and internal fixation of the fragment is necessary (see Fig. 5-75). The head can be inspected at this time for obvious injury to the cartilage, but primary arthroplasty is seldom necessary with these types of fractures. If the acetabular fragment is large or central, it should be treated with open reduction and internal fixation, as described for Class IV pelvic fractures. As in fractures of the femoral head, acetabular fractures accompanied by dislocation may lead to degenerative arthritis at a later date. Sciatic nerve palsy may accompany the fracture-dislocation. The nerve should be inspected if open reduction is performed.

If the fracture-dislocation is accompanied by a fracture of the femoral neck, treatment is a much more complicated problem (Fig. 5-82). All acetabular fragments

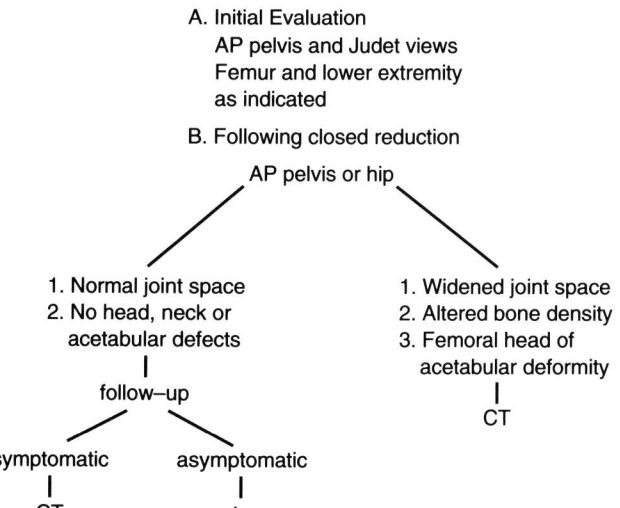

A. Initial Evaluation
  AP pelvis and Judet views
  Femur and lower extremity
  as indicated

B. Following closed reduction

AP pelvis or hip

1. Normal joint space
2. No head, neck or
   acetabular defects
      |
   follow–up

symptomatic   asymptomatic
    | |
   CT   stop

1. Widened joint space
2. Altered bone density
3. Femoral head of
   acetabular deformity
      |
     CT

FIG. 5-83. Fracture-dislocation of the hip: pre- and post-reduction radiographic evaluation.

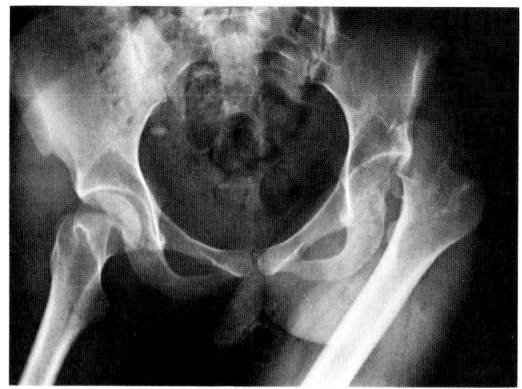
A

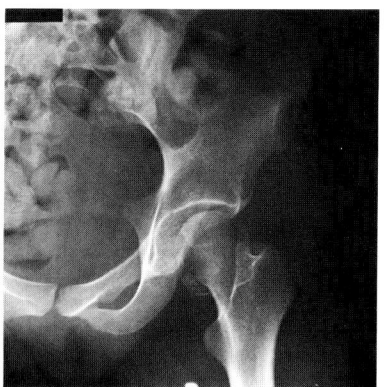
B

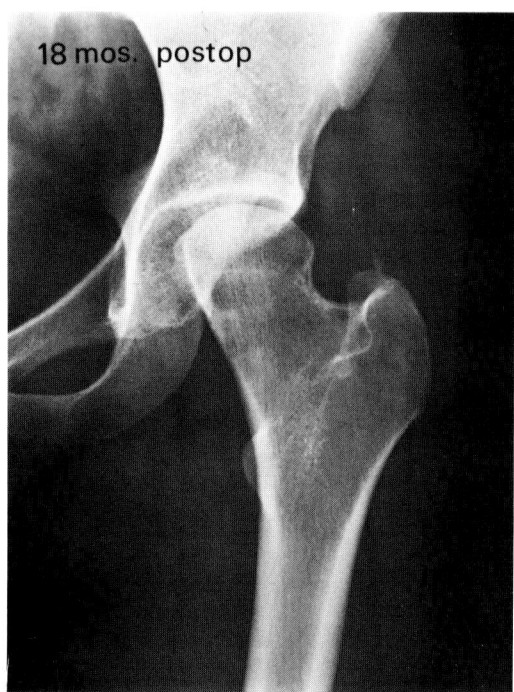
C

FIG. 5-84. A 23-year-old female with multiple lacerations and head injury following a motor vehicle accident. **A:** AP view of the pelvis with shearing fracture of the femoral head and posterior dislocation of the hip. **B:** Following reduction, the femoral fragments are inferior. The head is slightly lateral in the acetabulum. **C:** Eighteen months following open reduction and removal of three osteochondral fragments. There is deformity of the head and early avascular necrosis.

must be reduced and internally secured; in addition, the femoral neck fracture must be reduced and secured by primary internal fixation. If reduction and stable fixation is not possible, then a primary endoprosthesis (either one-piece or bipolar) should be inserted at the time of the open reduction.

TABLE 5-17. Complications: Fracture/dislocations of the hip

Common complications
Osteoarthritis
Avascular necrosis of the femoral head
Sciatic nerve injury
Associated fractures
Uncommon complications
Infection
Myositis ossificans
Redislocation
Thrombophlebitis
Pulmonary embolus

Complications of Dislocations and Fracture-Dislocations of the Hip

Regardless of the type of dislocation, it is important to obtain early reduction (i.e., within 24 hours) (166,182). Delay in reduction leads to an increase in the complication rate, particularly with regard to avascular necrosis (Table 5-17). The incidence of avascular necrosis is reported to be 5–26% (166,182). Results are uniformly poor if reduction is delayed beyond 48 hours (163). Although the incidence of avascular necrosis is highest in more severe injuries, avascular necrosis occurs in children even with Grade I dislocations (Stewart and Milford classification) (181). The incidence is reported to be lower (8%) in patients with anterior dislocations (163). Incidence also varies with the method of treatment. The incidence of avascular necrosis is 15.5% of patients following closed reduction and 40% of patients following open reduction (166). One must keep in mind that patients requiring open reduction usually have more significant injuries. The average time of appearance for avascular necrosis is 17 months following injury; however, it may develop even later (166,181).

The sciatic nerve (especially the peroneal portion) is susceptible to injury with posterior dislocations owing to its relationship to the posterior acetabulum and femoral head. The incidence of injury with posterior dislocations is reported to be 10–17% (166,167,182). Significant sciatic nerve injury usually indicates prompt surgical reduction of the dislocation (162,171). Epstein indicated that the internal rotation of the hip normally associated with posterior dislocation caused stretching of the sciatic nerve and was an important factor in producing the injury (173).

Fractures associated with dislocations of the hip are common owing to the severity of trauma necessary to cause the primary lesion. Associated fractures of the adjacent femur are of particular importance, as they may result in the dislocation being overlooked (165,170). Femoral shaft fractures mask the clinical signs of dislocation. Rosenthal reported ipsilateral fractures of the femur (4%) and patella (4%) (183). The hip injury was unrecognized initially in all patients with femoral shaft fractures. Roeder reported major associated injuries in over 75% of the patients in his study (181). These injuries included (1) lower extremity fractures, (2) craniofacial trauma, (3) upper extremity trauma, (4) chest injury.

Rosenthal also reported an 11% incidence of abdominal injury (ruptured spleen and liver laceration) requiring laparotomy (183).

Arthritis may be the most common complication and may develop as late as 15 years after the injury (164,166, 173,181). Epstein reported post-traumatic arthritis in 23% of patients (173). The incidence of arthritis increased to 35% in patients with closed reductions compared with 17% in the case of open reductions. The incidence of arthritic complications also strongly depends on the patient's weight and activity. The complication is more common in patients with acetabular fractures or fractures involving the weight-bearing surface of the femoral head (181,191).

Less common complications include infection, myositis ossificans, and redislocation (177,181,183). Thrombophlebitis and pulmonary embolus have also been noted during the initial hospitalization phase (166, 168,183).

FEMORAL NECK FRACTURES

Femoral neck fractures occur predominantly in the elderly and are more common in females than in males (201,203). The femoral neck is frequently demineralized in this patient population. Thus, neck fractures have been considered pathologic (227). Bone mineral analysis clearly demonstrates decreased mineralization in females over 65 years of age (204). Spontaneous fatigue fractures have also been described (212).

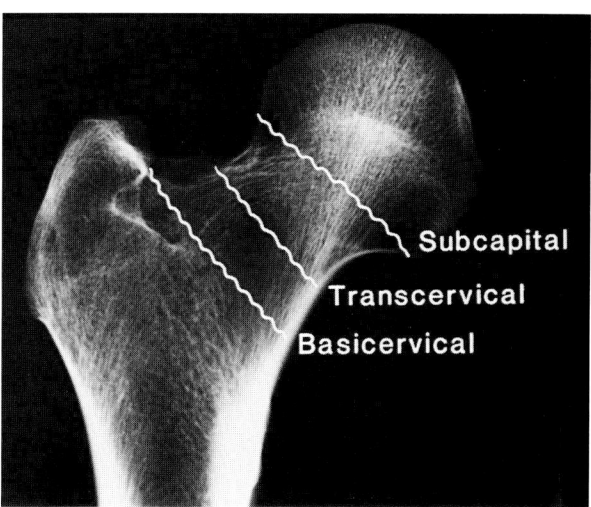

FIG. 5–85. Femoral specimen demonstrating the location of common femoral neck fractures.

The fracture usually occurs following minimal trauma. The following theories have been proposed to explain how this fracture occurs: (1) it may follow direct trauma from a fall; (2) a microfracture may become complete with minor trauma (microfractures are present in osteoporotic bone and result from chronic stress); (3) the fracture may derive from rotational forces during a fall (208,227).

Classification of Femoral Neck Fractures

Fractures of the femoral neck may be subcapital (most common), transcervical, or basilar (Fig. 5-85). Fractures may be complete or incomplete. Stress fractures are

TABLE 5–18. *Classifications: Femoral neck fractures*[a]

Pauwel's Classification	
Type I	Femoral neck fracture with an angle of 30° or less
Type II	Femoral neck fracture with an angle of between 30° and 70°
Type III	Femoral neck fracture with an angle greater than 70°
Garden's Classification	
Stage I	Incomplete or impacted fracture of the femoral neck with no displacement of the medial trabeculae
Stage II	Complete fracture of the femoral neck with no displacement of the medial trabeculae
Stage III	Complete fracture of the femoral neck with varus angulation and displacement of the medial trabeculae
Stage IV	Complete fracture with the femoral neck with total displacement of the fragments

[a] (206,217).

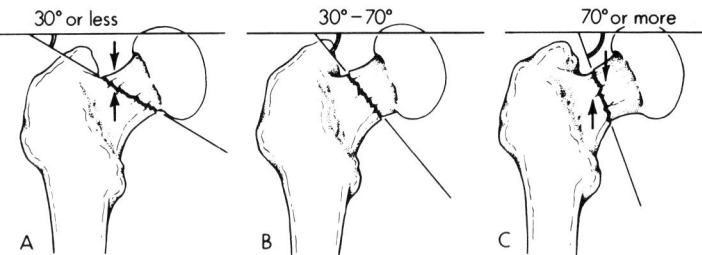

FIG. 5–86. Illustration of femoral neck fractures based on Pauwel's classification. **A:** Fracture line is 30° or less from vertical—Class I. **B:** Fracture line is between 30° and 70°—Class II; **C:** Fracture line is >70°—Class III (from 233, with permission).

common in young athletes and in patients with metabolic bone disease. These will be discussed in Chapter 16.

Various classifications have been established for femoral neck fractures (Table 5-18). Pauwel's classification (217,223) was based on the angle of the fracture (Fig. 5-86). Type 1 fractures formed an angle of 30° or less; Type 2 fractures formed an angle of between 30° and 70°; and Type 3 fractures formed an angle of greater than 70°. Fractures that are more horizontal (Type 1) tend to impact, which imparts some degree of stability and enhances healing. If the fracture is more vertical (Type 3), the weight-bearing forces will tend to cause varus shearing, and instability will result (206,223). Garden stated that the angle described by Pauwell is based on the radiographic angle of the fracture (208). The angle is more applicable following reduction.

Garden's classification is more commonly used (Table 5-18). This classification is based upon whether stable reduction can be achieved or whether instability will occur following reduction (206). Four stages of fracture were described, with nonunion and instability confined to Stage III and IV fractures. Stage I fractures are incomplete, with valgus positioning of the femoral neck (Fig. 5-87). Stage II fractures are complete, but the medial trabecular pattern is not displaced (Fig. 5-88). Stage III fractures are complete with varus angulation, and the medial trabeculae are also displaced (Fig. 5-89). Stage IV fractures are completely displaced, and the femoral head fragment returns to its normal position in the acetabulum (Fig. 5-82). The medial trabeculae are disrupted and displaced but may maintain their normal angulation.

Radiographic Evaluation of Femoral Neck Fractures

The trabecular pattern should be carefully evaluated on the AP view. The margins of the femoral neck and

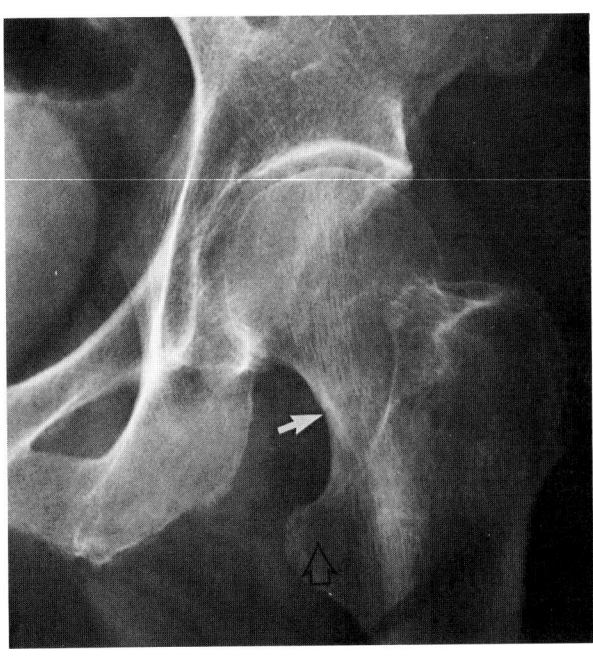

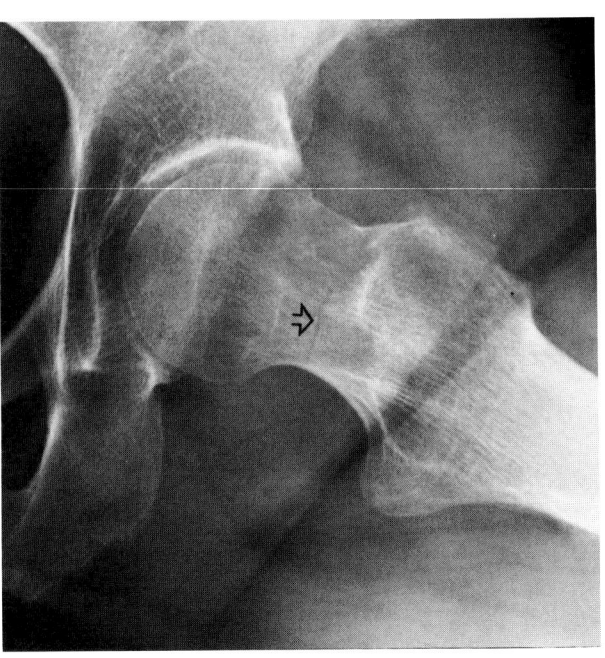

FIG. 5–87. Elderly female with left hip pain. **A:** AP view demonstrates subtle lucent line through the medial trabeculae (*white arrow*) slight external rotation (*open arrow* on lesser trochanter). **B:** The oblique view clearly demonstrates the undisplaced fracture (Garden Stage I).

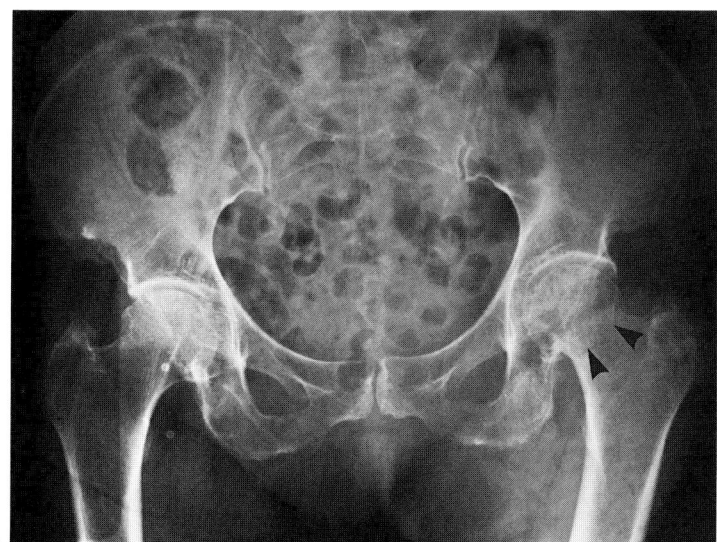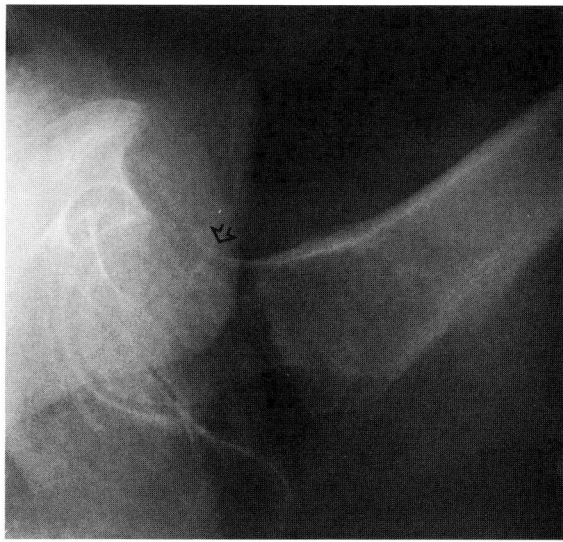

A   B

FIG. 5–88. Elderly female with Garden Stage II fracture. **A:** AP view demonstrates a complete fracture (*arrows*) with no change in the medial trabeculae. **B:** The lateral view demonstrates a subtle fracture (*open arrow*).

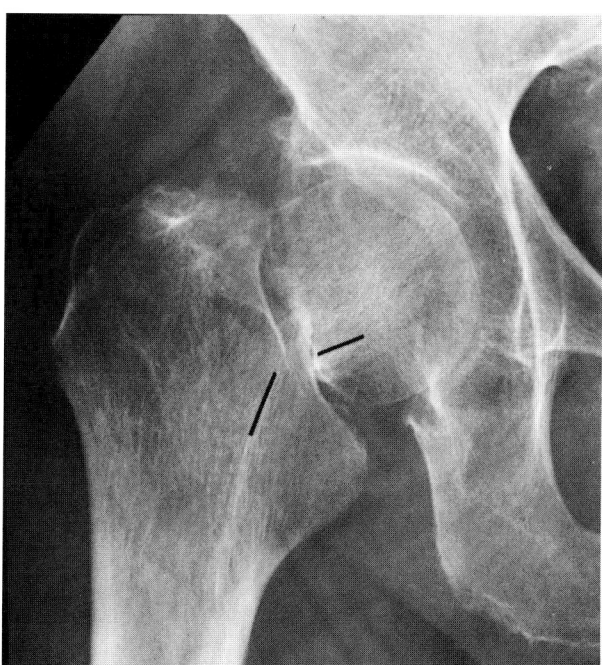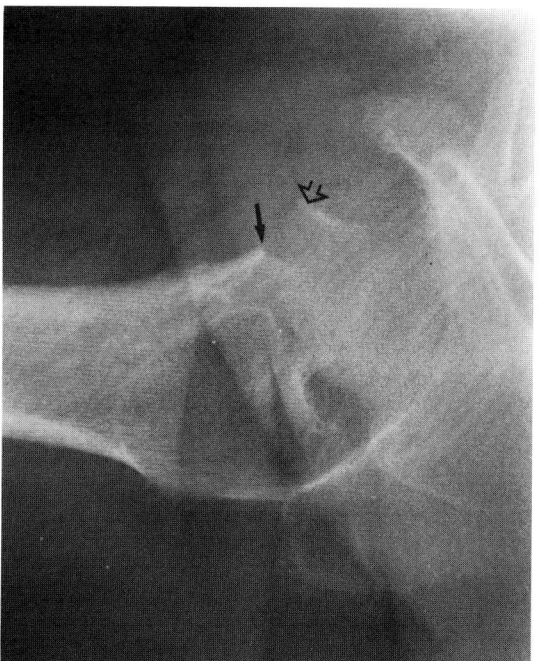

A   B

FIG. 5–89. Garden Stage III fracture of the femoral neck. **A:** AP view demonstrates a displaced femoral neck fracture. The femoral head is rotated and the trabecular pattern (*black lines*) malaligned. **B:** The lateral view demonstrates the position of the distal (*black arrow*) and proximal (*open arrow*) cortical margin.

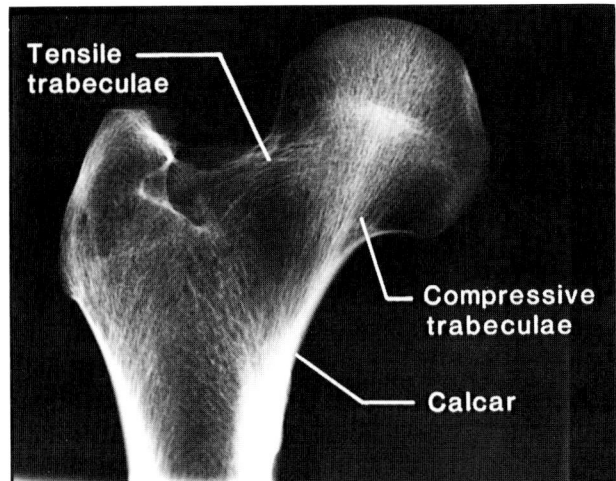

FIG. 5–90. Specimen radiograph of the upper femur demonstrating the trabeculae in the femoral neck.

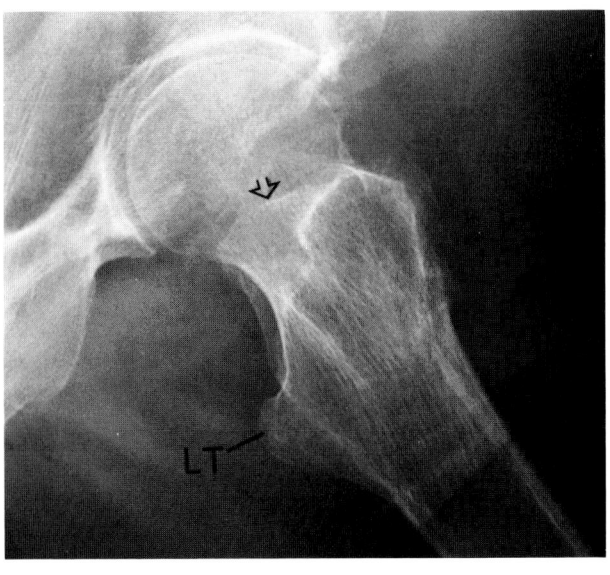

FIG. 5–91. Oblique view of the hip. The greater trochanter (*open arrow*) overlies the femoral neck and should not be mistaken for a fracture. LT, lesser trochanter.

junction with the head are also important (Fig. 5-90). If degenerative lipping is present, a line may project over the neck, mimicking a fracture. On examining the oblique view (Fig. 5-91), one must take care not to mistake the cortical margin of the greater trochanter for a fracture.

Incomplete fractures (Garden Stage I, Fig. 5-87), stress fractures, and subtle undisplaced fractures (Garden Stage II, Fig. 5-88) require multiple views, tomography, and occasionally isotope studies (Fig. 5-92) for diagnosis and accurate classification. Isotope scans are positive in 95% after 72 hours. Isotope studies provide a means for earlier detection of stress fractures than routine radiographs (see Skeletal Scintigraphy section in Chapter 1). Computed tomography is of little value in undisplaced horizontal fractures. This type of fracture may be missed with CT, and in any case the above modalities are adequate. The more complex fractures (Garden Stages III and IV) can be classified on the AP view, but at least one additional view (preferably the lateral view) is required for complete evaluation (Fig. 5-89).

Treatment of Femoral Neck Fractures

The treatment of femoral neck fractures depends on many factors, the most important being whether the fracture is stable or unstable (195,207). An initially stable fracture would include stress or fatigue fractures and Garden Stage I and most Garden Stage II fractures. Unstable fractures include Garden Stages III and IV fractures. This division into stable or unstable fractures classifies the fracture at the time of its occurrence or at least at the time of its treatment; it does not classify the fracture after treatment. Unless an unstable fracture is stabilized in the course of treatment, it will remain unstable and thus require a form of treatment different from that applied to the stable fracture. The stable fracture will either remain stable after injury or will tend to become unstable because of stresses placed upon it.

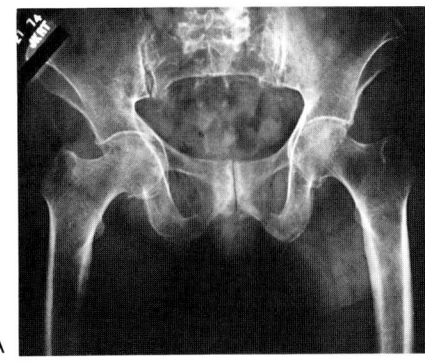
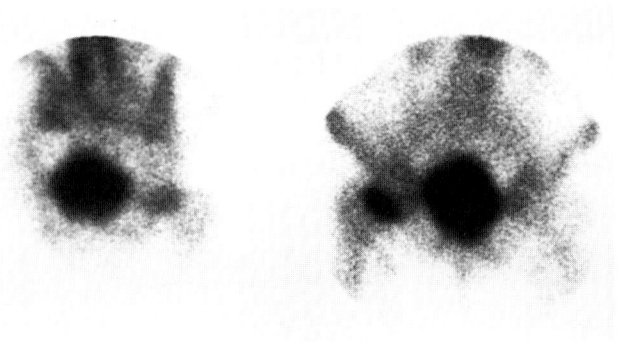

A
B

FIG. 5–92. Elderly female with hip pain following a fall. **A:** AP view of the pelvis and hip is negative. Tomogram and oblique views were also normal. **B:** Tc-99m scan demonstrates a femoral neck fracture on the right.

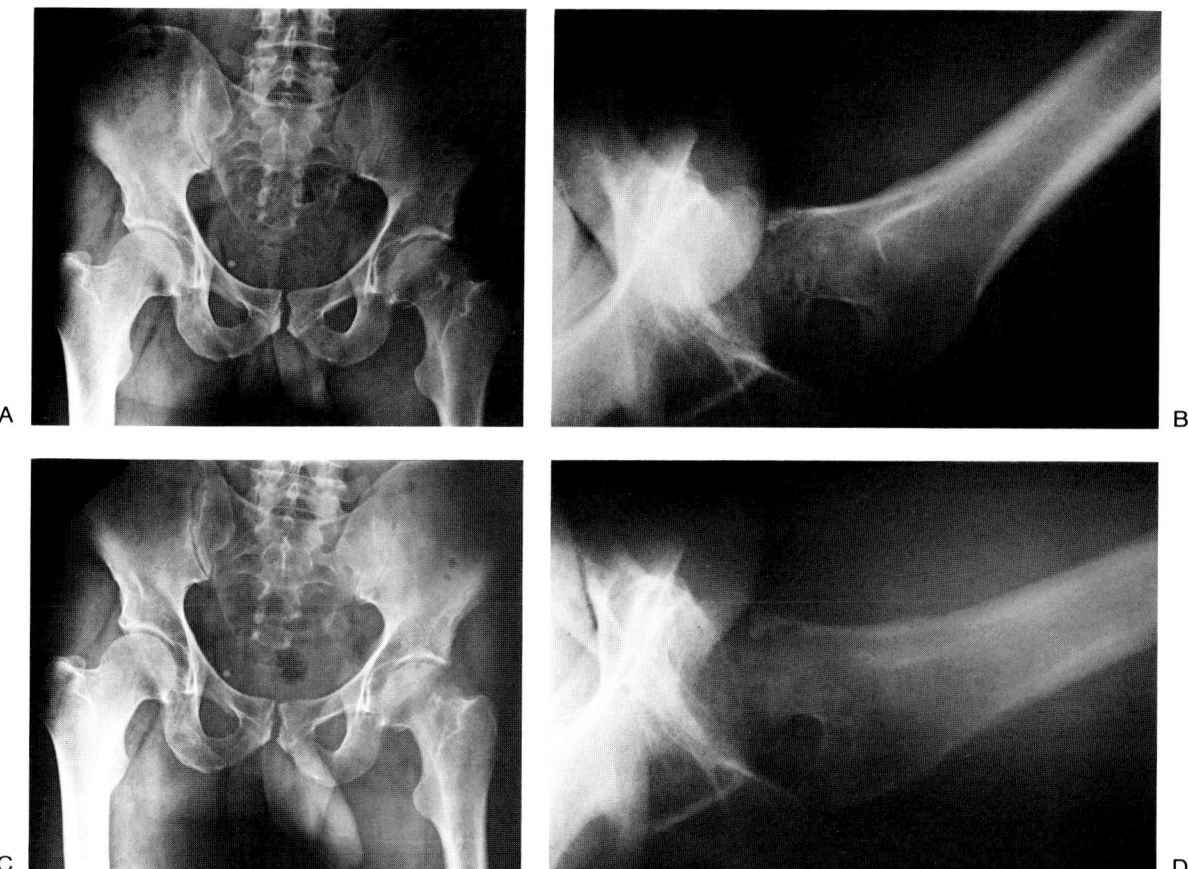

FIG. 5–93. A 44-year-old farmer who fell off a haybaler onto his hip. The patient was able to walk but with pain. X-rays initially (**A, B**) read negative but subsequently showed impacted subcapital fracture of the left femoral neck. AP (**C**) and lateral (**D**) radiographs four months later after nonsurgical treatment show a healed fracture.

Over the years, controversy has centered on whether an impacted fracture, or even a stress fracture, should be internally fixed or whether it can be treated without surgery. The definition of exactly what constitutes an impacted fracture has further confused the issue. A strict definition would make the impacted fracture one that is undisplaced but complete, which allows the patient to walk and to raise the limb unaided while lying in the supine position (Figs. 5-93 and 5-94). Hanson and Solgaard used a slightly more liberal definition (209). Their definition of impacted fractures included both subcapital and transverse cervical fractures that showed some displacement but which were still basically impacted. They further defined the fracture as one in which the patient could raise the straight leg 2 days after injury. They found that 80% of these healed without any intervention. They allowed walking with aids from the onset. Eight of their 42 patients did show some secondary displacement, and most of these required operation. Meyers (215) on the other hand, believes, as do most orthopedists, that all fractures should be secured with pins to insure against such impacting. These two views represent the present thinking among orthopedists. How-

ever, if the impacted fracture disimpacts and loses position, it can be treated with an endoprosthesis or even with reduction and internal fixation. Thus, perhaps internal fixation of this fracture is not truly necessary. In our series of 23 impacted fractures, defined according to the more strict criteria, only one became disimpacted. These patients were not given a general anesthetic or subjected to an open operation with its minimal but definite risks. Nor is there any advantage in treating an impacted fracture with prolonged bed rest, as advocated by some. If the fracture is truly impacted, the patient should be able to move about with partial weight-bearing any time after the injury, taking care only to avoid rotational forces or a subsequent fall (which is not likely in this group of patients).

Controversy also surrounds treatment of unstable femoral neck fractures, as in the case of Garden Stages III and IV fractures. Debate centers on whether these fractures should be reduced and internally fixed or whether the femoral head should be replaced with an endoprosthesis. Many series have been reported comparing the two methods. All agree that a well-reduced, united femoral head is better for the patient than a prosthesis. How-

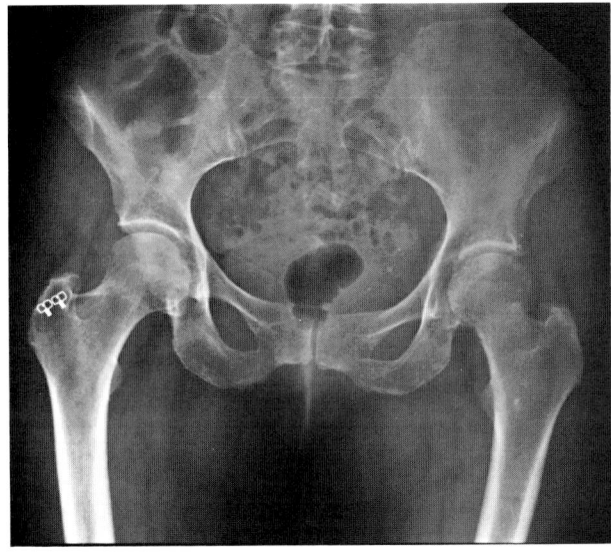

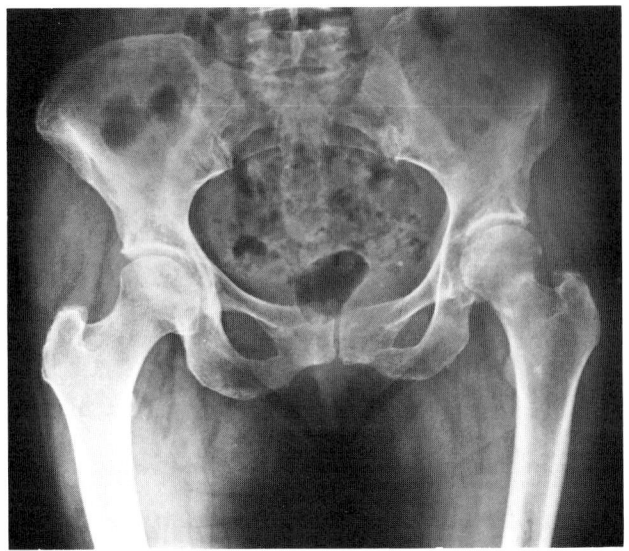

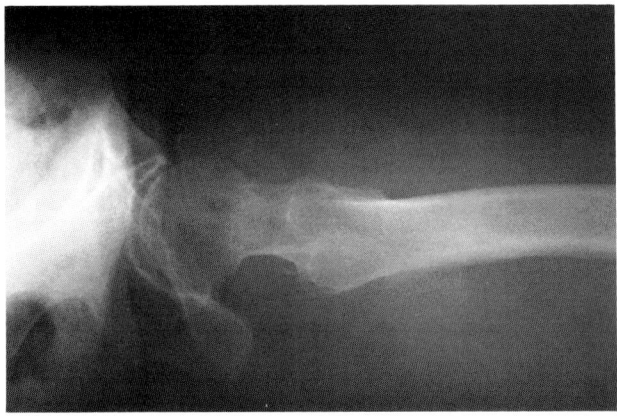

FIG. 5-94. An 85-year-old female fell at home. Able to walk but with pain. Severe medical problems prevented surgery. Patient allowed to ambulate with walker, partial weight bear. **A:** Appearance after injury with impacted Garden II fracture, left femoral neck. **B:** Anterior posterior appearance six weeks later with healing. **C:** Lateral.

ever, a stable, anatomic reduction with secure internal fixation is not easily obtained, especially in Garden Stage IV types or in the patient with osteoporosis. In the old person who is less active (with age 70 as a criterion), primary femoral head replacement continues to be the more commonly used method for unstable fractures. Söreide and colleagues found that patients who had endoprosthetic replacement fared better at 1 year than those treated with internal fixation (226).

Sikorski and Barrington compared the Thompson prosthesis with closed reduction and internal fixation achieved by two crossed Garden screws (224). They, too, found that the results were better with the use of endoprostheses, with less overall complications. Their patients, however, were all over 70. Our present belief is that unstable fractures in this older, less-active age group are better treated with the endoprosthetic replacement, both in the immediate and long-term time frame. But in the younger patient, or at least in the more physically active patient, pin fixation is preferable if it can secure stable anatomic reduction (221).

In addition, there are certain patients who might profit from primary total hip arthroplasty rather than endoprosthetic replacement. Coats and Armour have out-

lined their limited indications for total hip replacement in the patient with a femoral neck fracture (202). One candidate is the rare patient who has degenerative arthritis prior to the fracture of the femoral neck. In this case total hip arthroplasty is indicated if stable reduction and internal fixation cannot be obtained. Coats and Armour believe that the more active, younger patient may be a candidate for total hip arthroplasty rather than endoprosthesis if operative intervention is necessary because stable reduction cannot be obtained.

If internal fixation is used, multiple parallel pins (at least four in number, which are threaded into the proximal fragment, and with a smooth shaft distally) is preferred today rather than heavy screws, Smith-Petersen nails, and so forth (Figs. 5-95 and 5-96). Rubin and colleagues found pins to be fully effective in their laboratory studies. Their next preference was a sliding screw-plate. The sliding screw-plate will securely hold the fracture, does not cause undue trauma during insertion, supplies compression, and allows for slight absorption at the fracture site without holding the fracture apart (Fig. 5-96) (219,228).

Types of endoprosthesis are also controversial at this time. Should a prosthesis be cemented or not? The

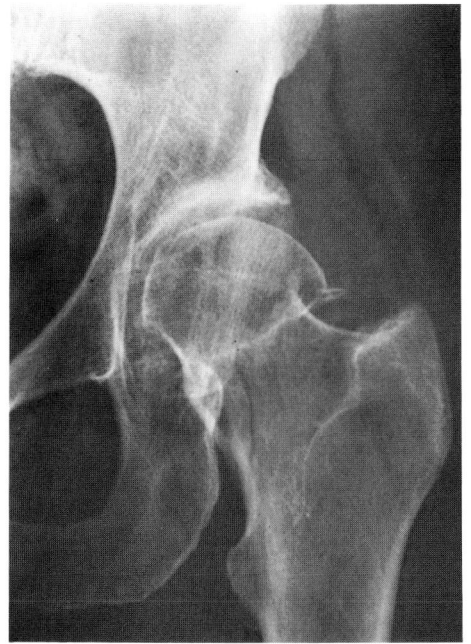

A

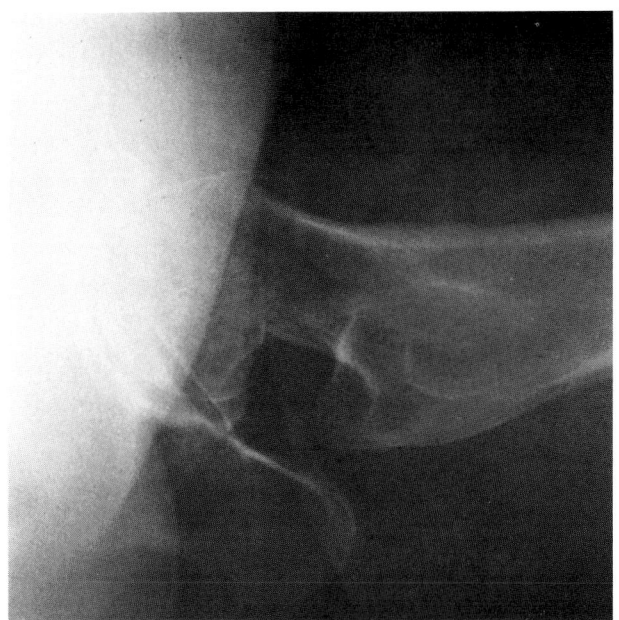

B

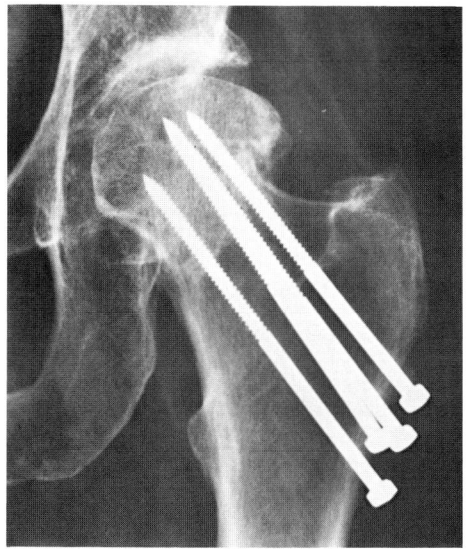

C

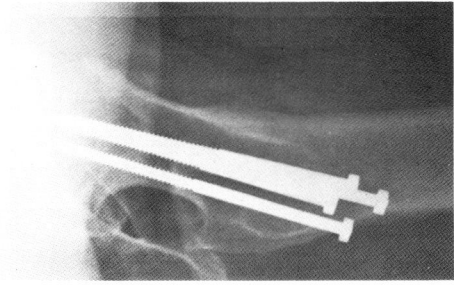

D

FIG. 5–95. A 62-year-old female fell at home. AP (**A**) and lateral (**B**) radiographs show a comminuted fracture. Nine months following closed reduction and internal fixation with four Knowles pins (**C, D**), the fracture has healed in excellent position.

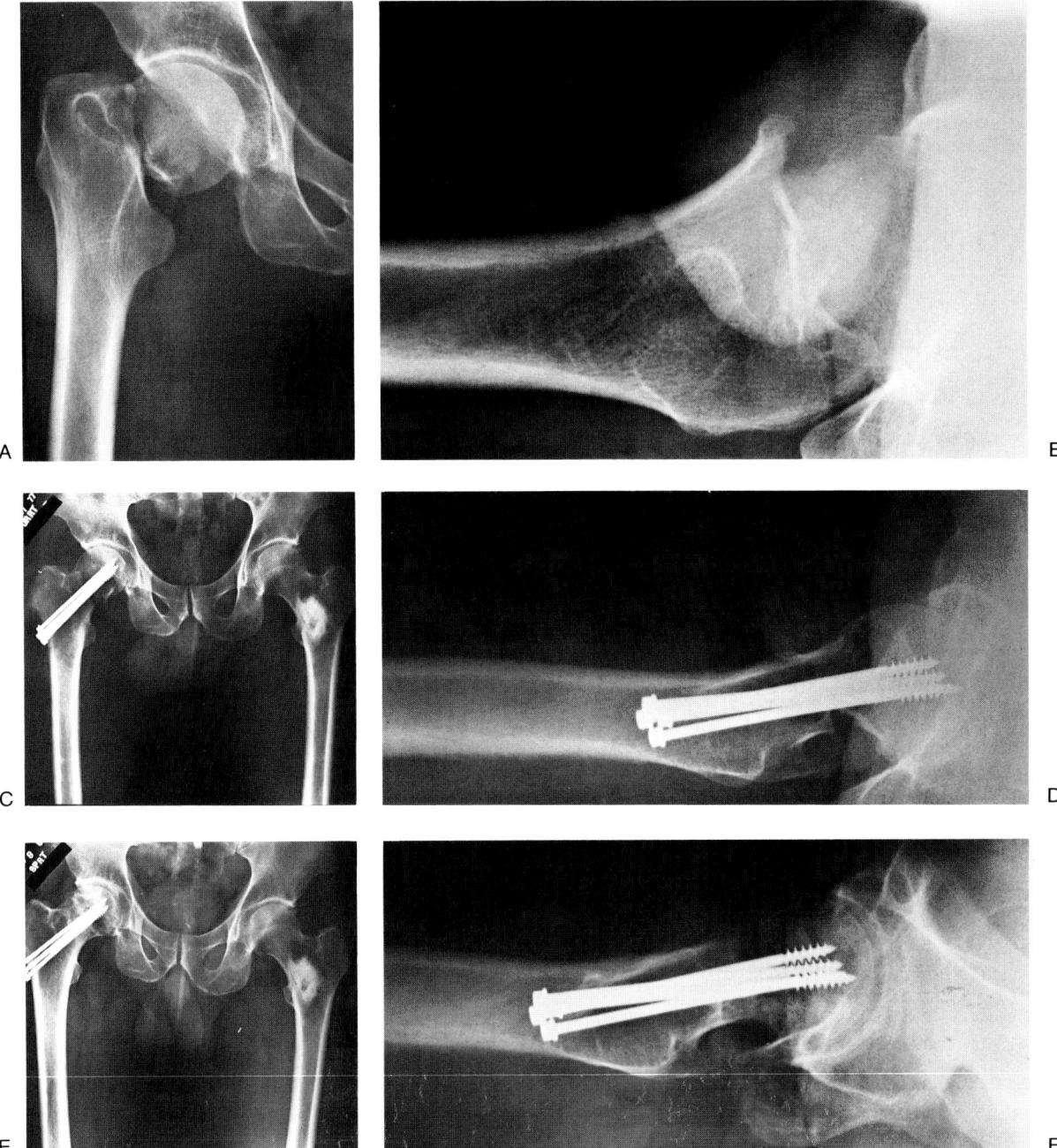

FIG. 5-96. A 49-year-old male fell fifteen feet while working on a scaffold and sustained Garden Stage III fracture of the right femoral neck. AP (**A**) and lateral (**B**) radiographs at the time of injury. Closed reduction and internal fixation with four Knowles pins as noted on AP (**C**) and lateral (**D**) radiographs. Six years following fracture, the AP (**E**) and lateral (**F**) radiographs show minimal early degenerative changes and avascular necrosis. The osteoblastic lesion in the left intertrochanteric area has remained unchanged and is symptomless. It probably represents an ossified chondroma.

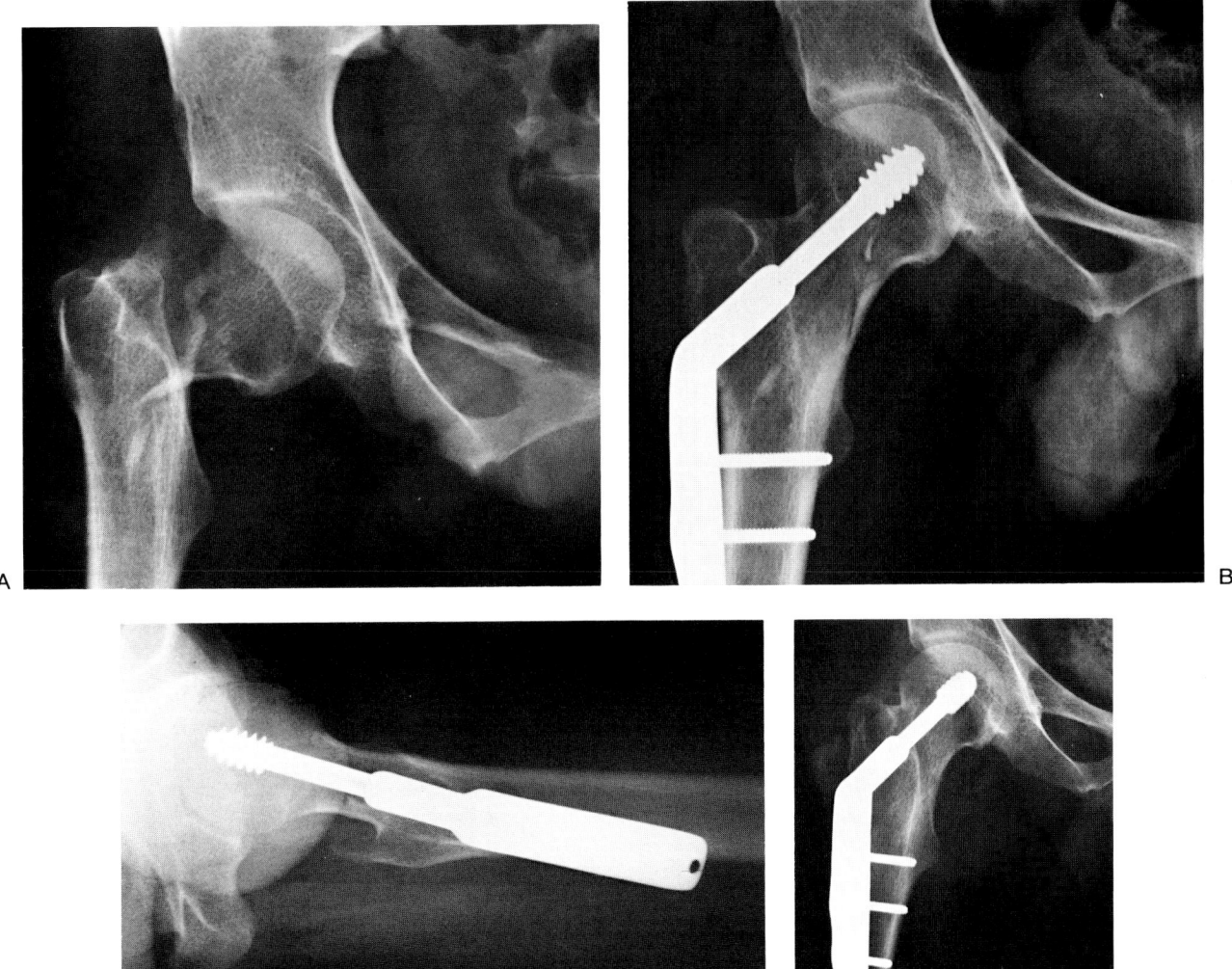

FIG. 5–97. A 28-year-old male with severe poliomyelitis. AP (**A**) radiograph showed a comminuted femoral neck fracture with complete displacement following a fall. AP view (**B**) eight weeks following open reduction and internal fixation with a compression screw-plate. Lateral (**C**) and AP (**D**) views four months following internal fixation. Healing in anatomic position has occurred.

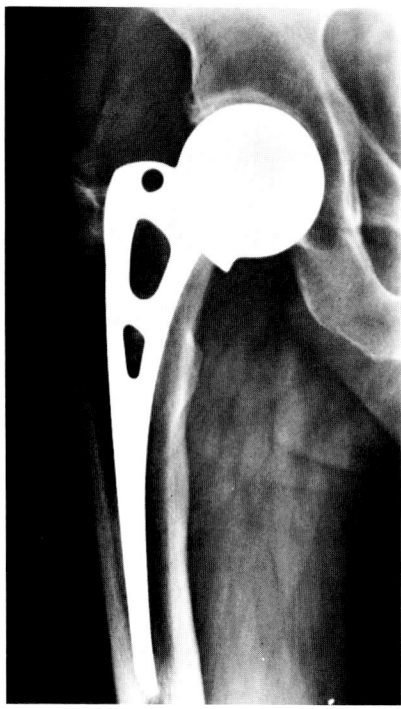

FIG. 5–98. A 43-year-old male with alcoholic avascular necrosis. Original Moore prosthesis eleven years after insertion. Note sclerosis (stress concentration) at tip of prosthesis. Patient symptomless and there is no sign of motion.

Thompson prosthesis is usually cemented. The classic Moore type should not be cemented because of its fine fenestrations. Recent Moore prostheses are available without fenestrations, however, and various stem sizes are available to fit the intramedullary canal better if a press-fit rather than cementing is desired (Figs. 5-98 and 5-99). Again, should a prosthesis be bipolar (the so-called *articulated endoprosthesis* (Fig. 5-100) to decrease wear and load stresses on the acetabular cartilage? These matters have not been completely resolved. Finally, porous-coated prostheses are appealing in that they allow bony ingrowth. What will their place be in the management of femoral neck fractures?

Complications of Femoral Neck Fractures

Complications of femoral neck fractures depend in part on whether they are intracapsular or extracapsular, whether they are comminuted, whether they are stable or unstable, and, of course, very important, whether the circulation to the femoral head has been impaired. There are significant mortality rates (~21.6%) in the first year after fracture (229).

Avascular necrosis is the most significant problem following subcapital fractures. The incidence approaches 24% (198). Barnes reported a higher incidence in females

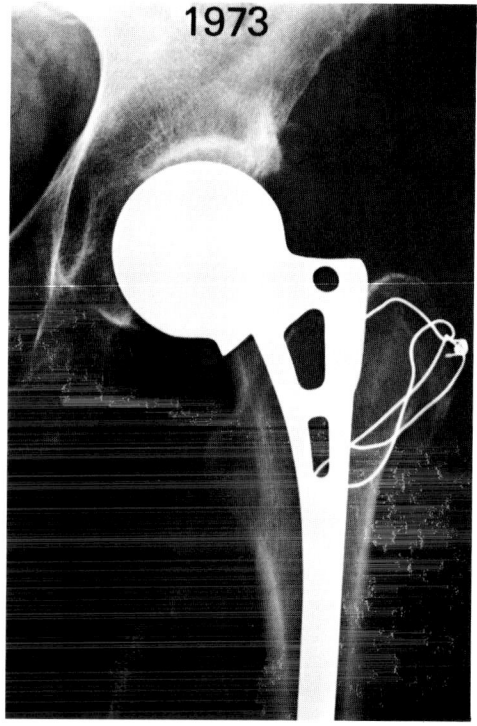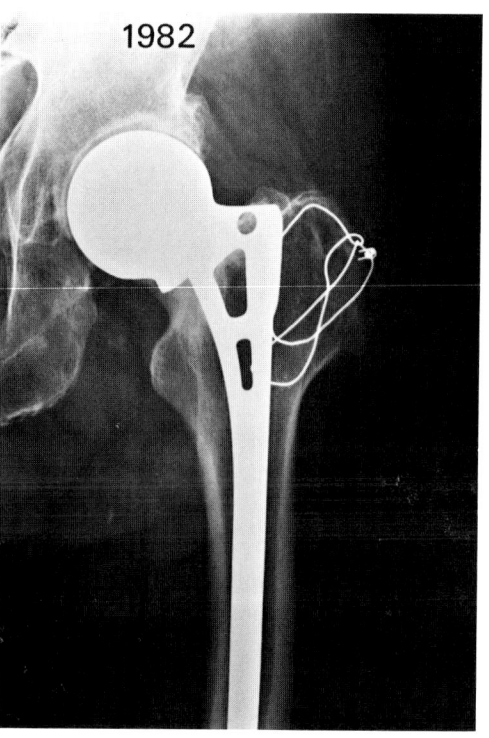

FIG. 5–99. A 62-year-old male. Straight stem Moore prosthesis for avascular necrosis. **A:** AP radiographic appearance eight weeks after insertion of endoprosthesis. AP radiograph (**B**) eleven years post surgery shows there has been some adaptive sclerosis at the medial femoral neck and calcar. There has been some thinning of the acetabular cartilage. No evidence of loosening. No pain.

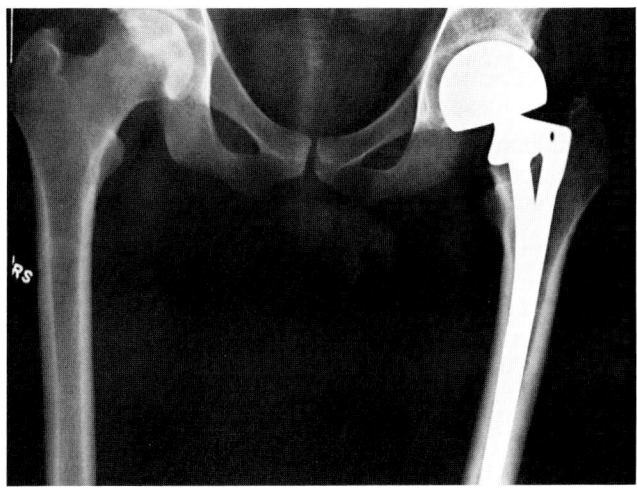

FIG. 5-100. A 48-year-old male with a Bateman-type bipolar endoprosthesis.

(24%) than in males (15%) (196). This complication most commonly occurs following Garden Stages III and IV fractures (192).

Blood is supplied to the femoral head through the retinacular artery, which ends as the lateral epiphyseal artery (Fig. 5-101). Further vascular supply is derived from the medial epiphyseal artery, a branch of the inferior retinacular artery. Arterial damage is increased with rotation and displacement of the fracture fragments (196). Poor contact, unstable reduction, and disruption of the retinacular vessels are the most significant factors leading to avascular necrosis. Arnoldi noted sufficient vascular supply to the femoral head from the foveal artery in only 4% of patients (193). The average onset is 9–12 months following the fracture (198). Changes may occur in 3–5 months or as late as 3 years following the injury. Meyers has taken the important step of performing technetium scans on all femoral neck fractures and has re-

ported 34 undisplaced or impacted fractures with technetium scans performed within 48 hours of admission (215). He concluded that, if the scan shows an absence of circulation in the femoral head (as it did in 3 of his patients), then a primary muscle pedicle graft should be used in addition to an *in situ* pinning of the fracture. With this limited experience, he has so far been able to prevent late segmental collapse. Certainly scanning is helpful in diagnosing avascular necrosis.

Ficat (205) has defined the stages of avascular necrosis (Table 5-19). Initially the radiograph is negative and the technetium scan may be positive. The earliest radiographic finding is increased density of the femoral head (Stage II) (196). This may occur as early as 3 months or as late as 36 months, with the average time of appearance 10 months. With early ambulation and more aggressive therapy, the density difference may be less obvious. Previously the density of the head was thought to result

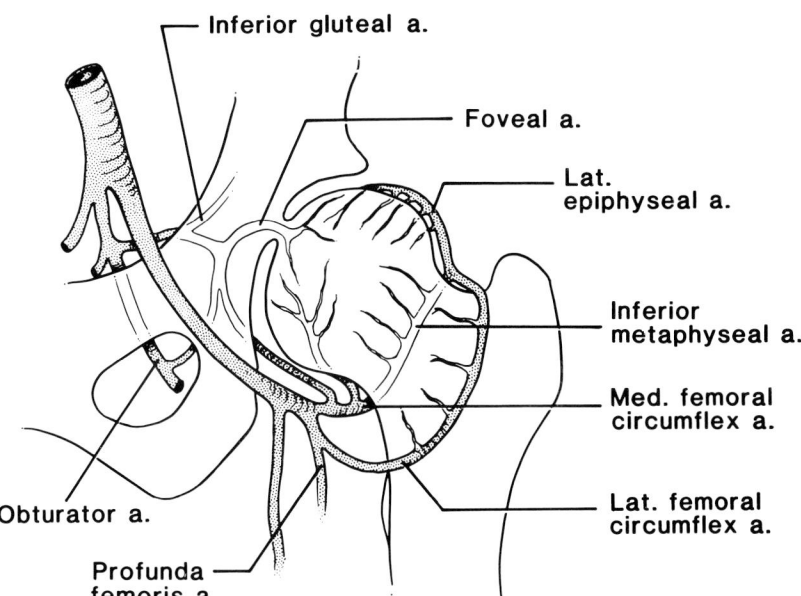

Inferior gluteal a.

Foveal a.

Lat. epiphyseal a.

Inferior metaphyseal a.

Med. femoral circumflex a.

Lat. femoral circumflex a.

Obturator a.

Profunda femoris a.

FIG. 5-101. Illustration of blood supply to the femoral head.

TABLE 5–19. *Staging of avascular necrosis of the hip*

Stage	Clinical	Radiograph	Isotope	MRI	Pathology
0	No symptoms	Normal	±	?	Hematopoietic cell necrosis after several days; fat cell necrosis after 48 hours
I	May have symptoms	Normal or may have patchy osteoporosis	Uniform uptake	↓ Signal intensity T1 (Fig. 5–102) inhomogeneous signal intensity	Sinus congestion, fibroblasts, hypoplastic marrow, empty lacunae
II	Pain, stiffness	Osteoporosis, mixed osteoporosis and sclerosis, cystic changes (may require tomography)	Nonuniform uptake	Wedge-shaped crescent sign (x-ray stage III)	Necrotic central tissue, margin fibrous with revasculation and new bone on dead trabeculae
III	Stiffness, groin and knee pain	Crescent sign sequestra, cortical collapse, joint preserved	Photon deficient (cold spot)	Crescent sign sequestra, cortical collapse, joint preserved	Necrosis surrounded by granulation tissue
IV	Pain and limp may be severe	Stage III plus degenerative changes with narrowed joint space		Stage III plus degenerative changes with narrowed joint space	Changes of stage III exaggerated

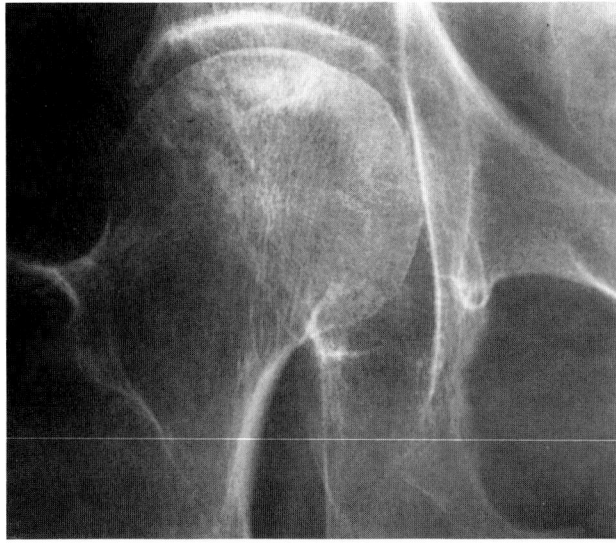

FIG. 5–102. A: AP radiograph demonstrating subchondral lucency and sclerosis due to avascular necrosis.

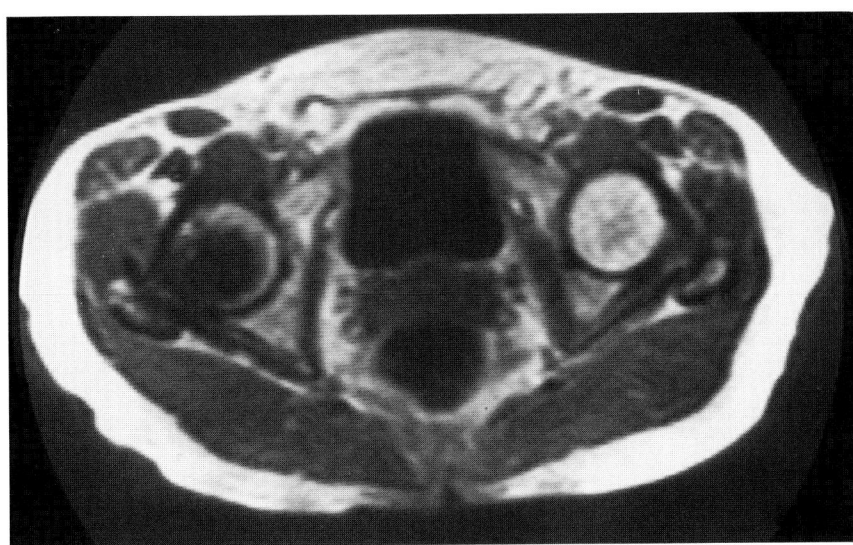

FIG. 5-103. Axial SE 500/20 image of the hips. There is loss of signal intensity in the right femoral head due to early avascular necrosis.

from disuse osteoporosis, which caused the neck to appear less dense than the femoral head (196,200). However, the frequent use of a prosthesis in patients with femoral neck fractures has provided a greater pathologic correlation with the radiographic changes. De Haas (204) and Phemister (219) stated that the increased density of the femoral head is due to appositional new bone formation on the necrotic trabeculae. If necrotic bone does not lose calcium, the addition of new bone would increase the density. Bobechko studied pathologic changes in rabbit femurs and correlated them with the radiographic appearance (200). His findings confirmed the statements of De Haas and Phemister. The increased density of the femoral head is due to reossification and not to increasing necrosis.

Structural collapse of the femoral head (Stage III) results in irregularity of the head. This occurs as early as 5 months and as late as 24 months following the injury. This is the most common sign of avascular necrosis (198). Early radiographic changes consist of a subchondral lucency (the crescent sign, Fig. 5-102) (216). This is often best seen on the oblique view of the hip.

Early diagnosis and prereduction prediction of avascular necrosis would be helpful in determining which patients may require total hip arthroplasty. Isotope studies have met with some success, but magnetic resonance imaging is the most sensitive technique for early detection of avascular necrosis (194,197,199,213–215).

The earliest features of avascular necrosis may be difficult to separate from edema or transient osteoporosis of the hip with magnetic resonance imaging (199,214). Although in theory signal intensity changes may be noted within a matter of hours, the hemopoeitic elements do not become necrotic for several days. Therefore, in Stage 0 or Stage I disease (Table 5-19), only a uniform loss of

signal intensity in the femoral head may be evident on MR images (Fig. 5-103). More typical geographic changes of avascular necrosis occur after this (Fig. 5-104). At this time radiographs, tomograms, and even isotope scans may be normal. By the time the crescent sign (Stage III) or collapse of the femoral head has occurred, the MR features are more similar to what is seen on conventional radiographs. Subtle changes in articular cartilage and head configuration are best appreciated when both coronal and sagittal images are obtained (Fig. 5-104). Once joint space narrowing begins to occur, the MR features are usually not much more useful than conventional radiographs (Table 5-19) (199).

Treatment of Stages I and II fractures has traditionally relied upon a watch and wait approach. Not all cases progress, but most do; and Ficat (205) and Hungerford (211) have encouraged core decompression in this group. Bonfiglio continues to treat these patients with drilling and bone grafting (225). Owing to shear fractures of the bone underlying the cartilage, replacement becomes necessary in the case of Stage III fractures. These will not heal, and pain persists because of the synovitis caused by this intra-articular fracture. Finally, the treatment of Stage IV fractures (Table 5-19) is either endoprosthesis or total hip arthroplasty (Fig. 5-105).

Other complications include malunion, non-union, and later degenerative arthritis. Careful radiographic follow-up of fragment position and fixation device changes is important (210,219,228). Non-union can be defined as failure to demonstrate bony growth across the fracture site 4 months after injury. Non-union may result from inadequate fixation or interruption of blood supply. In this case, synovial fluid interferes with callus formation at the fracture site. The incidence of non-union is lower if proper fixation is obtained and the fractures are im-

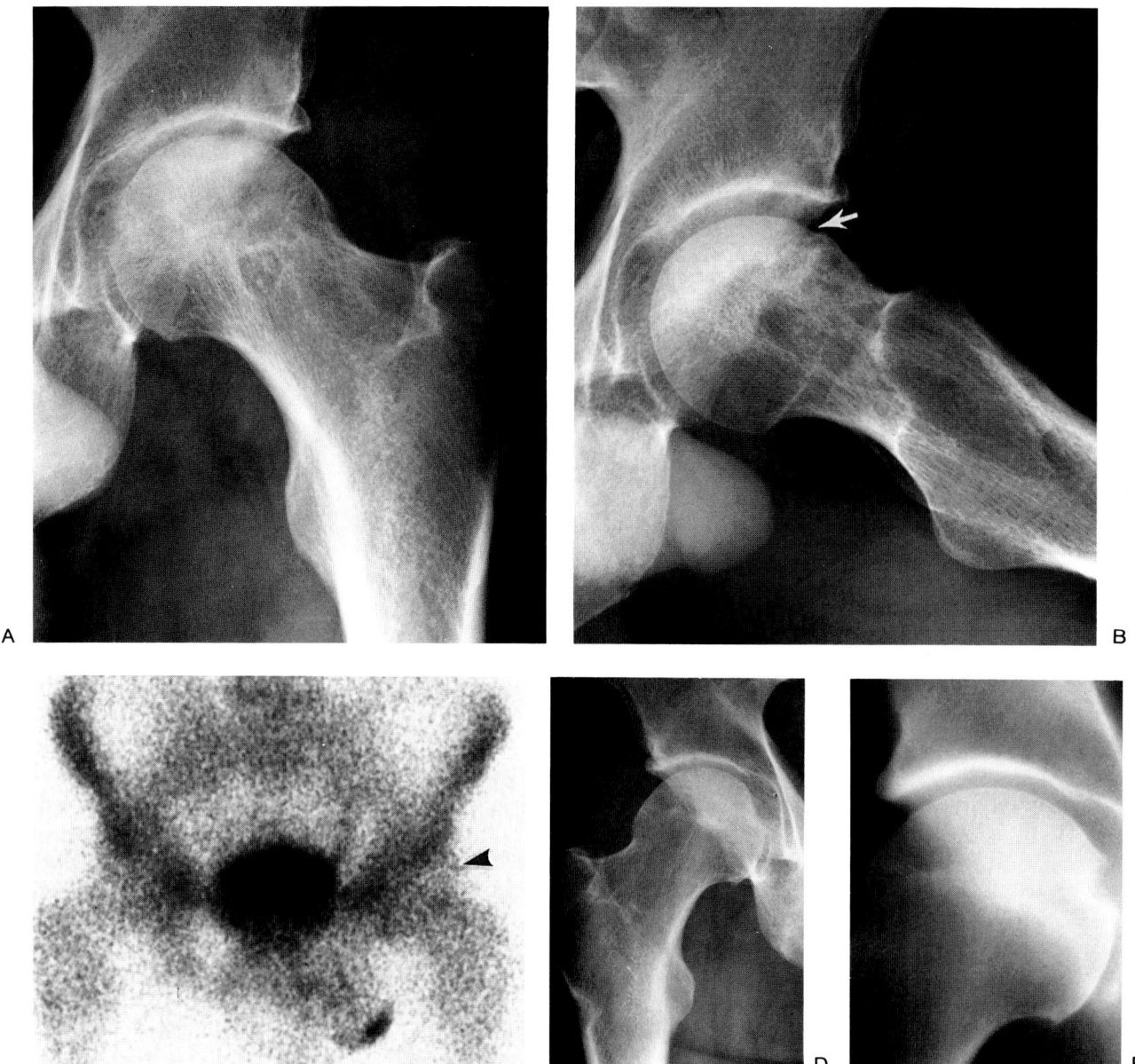

FIG. 5–104. Patient with avascular necrosis on the left demonstrated on AP (**A**) and oblique (**B**) views of the hip. Note the articular deformity (*arrow* in **B**). Isotope scan (**C**) shows a subtle photopenic area (*arrow*) on the left. AP view (**D**) and tomogram (**E**) of the right hip were negative.

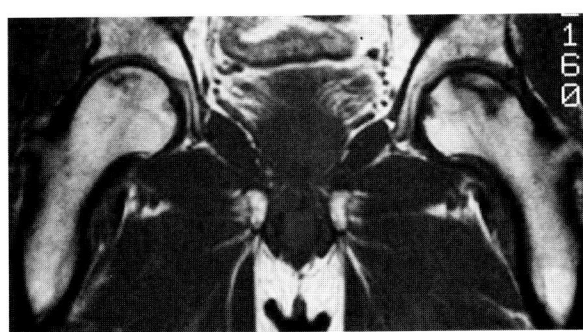
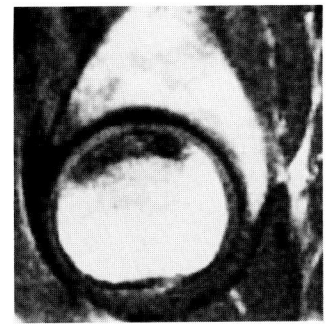
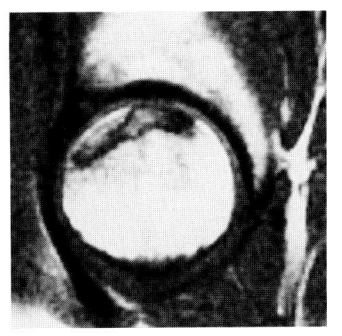

FIG. 5-104. (*Continued.*) Coronal SE 500/20 MR image (**F**) shows bilateral avascular necrosis, more marked on the left. Sagittal images (**G, H**) show the intact cartilage over the defect.

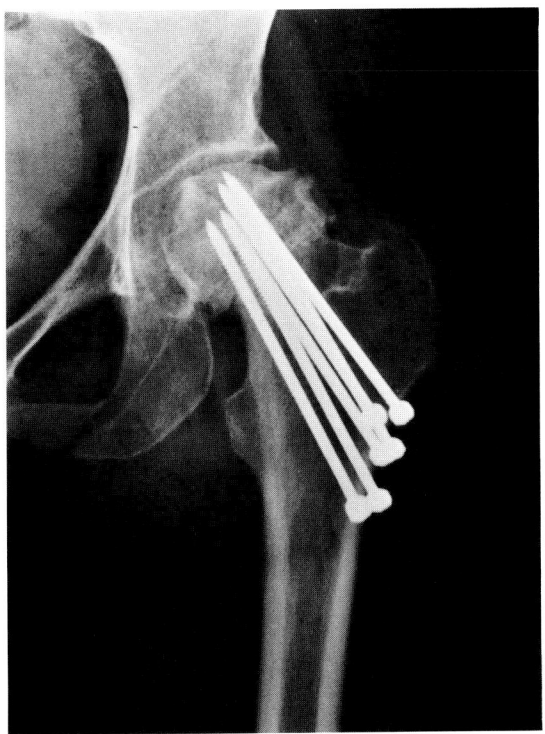
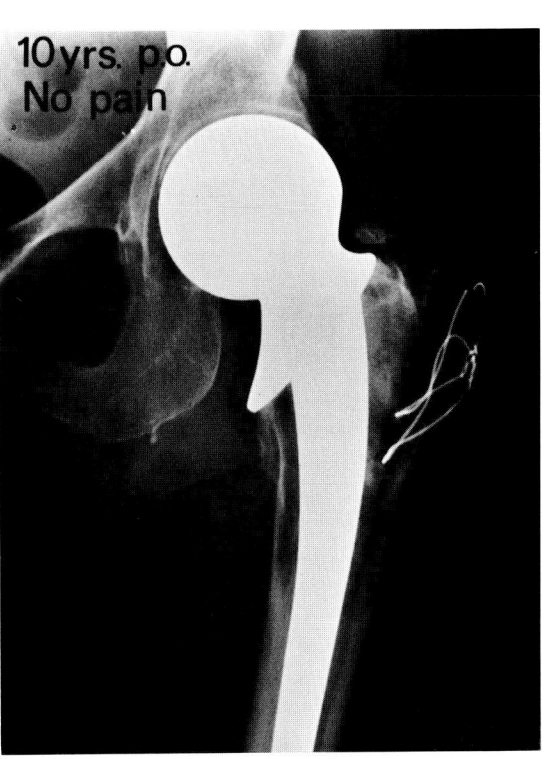

FIG. 5-105. A 49-year-old female with avascular necrosis. Patient fell from a horse two years previously and had closed reduction and internal fixation with multiple pins. **A:** Appearance two years following fracture and pinning. Avascular necrosis. At this time the head was replaced with a cemented Thompson prosthesis. **B:** Ten years following Thompson prosthesis with no evidence of loosening or acetabular migration, and no pain.

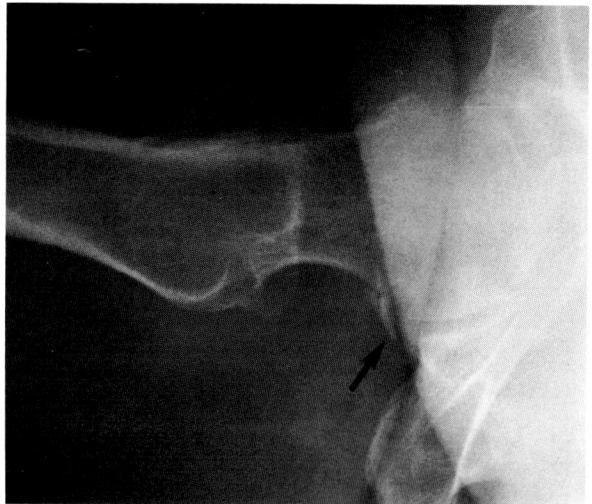

FIG. 5-106. Lateral view of the hip demonstrating fragmentation of the posterior cortex (*arrow*).

pacted. In displaced fractures, non-union may occur in 25–33% of patients (192,198). Factors increasing the degree of instability include the obliquity of the fracture line (Pauwel's Type III) and the degree of comminution of the posterior cortex (222). The lateral view is most useful in assessing the degree of posterior cortical involvement (Fig. 5-106).

Careful radiographic assessment of the fracture line will demonstrate widening and irregularity in early non-union. This progresses to sclerosis of the fracture margins during the later stages. Comparison views from the time of initial injury are extremely helpful in evaluation of potential non-union. Tomography, isotope scans, and magnetic resonance imaging may also be useful.

In the past, subtrochanteric valgus osteotomy was per-

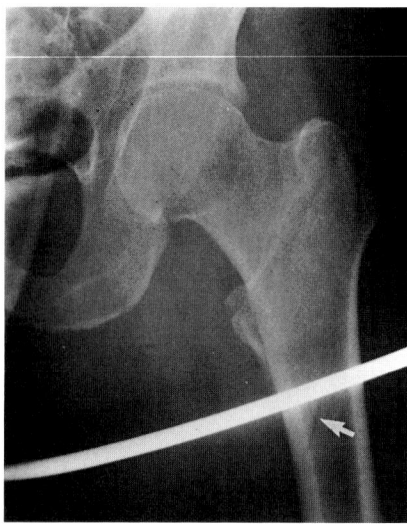

FIG. 5-107. AP view of the left hip with traction device in place. There is an undisplaced intertrochanteric fracture with subtrochanteric involvement (*arrow*).

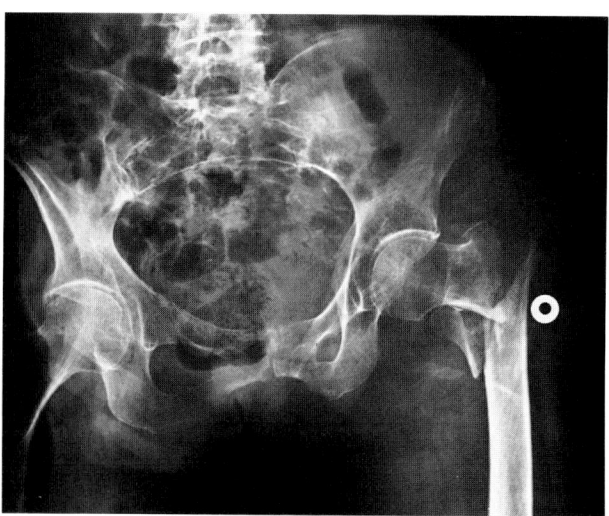

FIG. 5-108. AP view of the pelvis. There is a four-part intertrochanteric fracture. Varus angulation is present. The vertical orientation of the major fracture line increases instability.

formed to create compressive rather than shear forces at the fracture site. Non-union has also been treated with bone grafting. Currently, replacement with an endoprosthesis or total hip arthroplasty is considered most effective.

TROCHANTERIC FRACTURES

Trochanteric fractures generally follow the trochanteric line. These fractures may extend into the subtrochanteric region. Avulsion fractures of the greater and lesser trochanter may occur separately or in association with intertrochanteric and subtrochanteric fractures. For purposes of discussion, three categories can be distinguished: (1) intertrochanteric fractures, (2) subtrochanteric fractures, and (3) avulsion fractures.

Classification of Trochanteric Fractures

Intertrochanteric Fractures

Unlike subcapital fractures, intertrochanteric fractures are extracapsular. The vascular supply is rarely at risk. Thus, non-union and avascular necrosis are uncommon complications (231,234). Intertrochanteric fractures also occur most commonly in elderly patients with an almost equal incidence in males and females (235,247).

The fracture line usually extends between the greater and lesser trochanters (Fig. 5-107). In certain cases, an intertrochanteric fracture may be difficult to differentiate from a basicervical fracture. Comminution of the fracture with detachment of the greater and lesser trochanters (four-part fracture) is common (Fig. 5-108). Al-

TABLE 5–20. *Intertrochanteric fracture classifications*

Ender Classification[a]
  Type 1: Eversion fracture
  Type 2: Impaction fracture
  Type 3: Diatrochanteric fracture
Tronzo Classification[b]
  Type 1: Fracture involving one of the trochanters
  Type 2: Simple trochanteric fracture with or without minimal displacement. Posterior neck intact.
  Type 3: Comminution of the posterior wall with a calcar spike. Large lesser trochanteric fragment.
  Type 4: Same as Type 3 with associated displacement of the greater trochanter
  Type 5: Comminution of the posterior cortex with a telescoping fragment
Evans Classification[c]
  Type 1: Undisplaced two-part fracture
  Type 2: Displaced two-part fracture
  Type 3: Three-part fracture with greater trochanter displaced
  Type 4: Three-part fracture with displaced calcar and lesser trochanter
  Type 5: Four-part fracture with medial and posterior lateral cortex fractures (combined 3 and 4)

[a] (236), [b](243,244), [c](237).

though a single fracture in the region of the calcar is usually stable, comminution of the calcar or displacement with the lesser trochanter is unstable. Fractures with a nearly vertical orientation also tend to be unstable.

The fracture usually results from a fall, with direct trauma and the muscle forces about the hip both playing a part in the mechanism of injury. The external rotators tend to remain with the proximal fragment and the internal rotators with the distal fragment (234).

Table 5-20 summarizes the commonly used classifications of intertrochanteric fractures. Fractures may be simply classified as displaced or undisplaced (240,254, 263). DeLee (234) considered an intertrochanteric fracture stable if, when reduced, there was cortical contact medially and posteriorly. The medial cortex is not comminuted and the lesser trochanter is intact (Fig. 5-107). Comminution of the medial cortex and more vertically oriented fractures were considered unstable. Dimon and Hughston stressed these two factors along with the presence of a large posterior fragment as indicators of instability (235). Ender's classification was based on the mechanism of injury (236). However, the most commonly used classification is the Evans' system, as modified by Jensen and Michaelsen in 1975 (243,244). This classification is based on the prognosis for anatomic reduction and the likelihood of post-reduction instability (Fig. 5-109) (244). The primary considerations are the degree of comminution of the calcar region and the greater trochanter. Involvement of these structures increases the chances of instability following reduction. The direction of the fracture line is also important. Stable fractures follow the

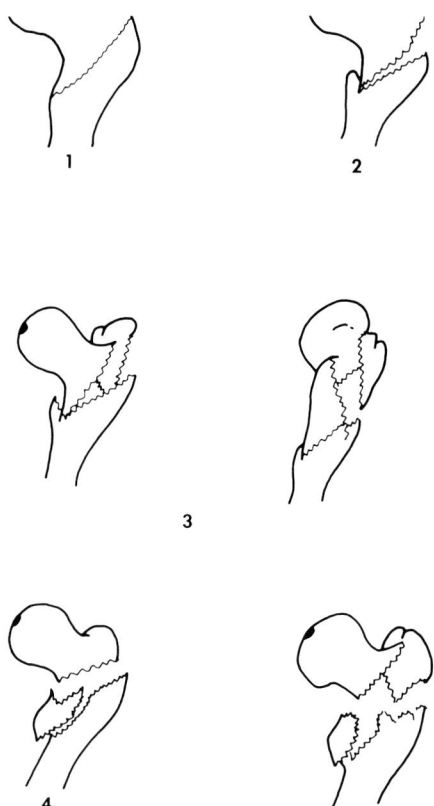

FIG. 5–109. Classification of trochanteric fractures by Evans modified by Jensen and Michaelson (243,244). Type I: undisplaced 2-fragment fracture. Type 2: displaced 2-fragment fracture. Type 3: 3-part fracture with dislocated greater trochanter. Type 4: 3-fragment fracture with loss of medial support due to loss of the lesser trochanter or calcar fragment. Type 5: 4-part fracture with loss of medial and posterolateral support. Types 1 and 2 are stable. Types 3–5 are unstable (from 243).

intertrochanteric line. Instability occurs when the obliquity is reversed (234). Using this classification, Type 1 and 2 fractures are stable fractures that can be reduced in 94% of cases (243). The remaining types are unstable. When the greater trochanter was detached (Type 3), only 33% could be reduced. If the calcar was involved (Type 4), only 21% could be reduced. Also following reduction, stable Type 1 and 2 fractures dislocated in only 9% of cases compared with 58–90% for Types 3, 4, and 5 (243).

Radiographic evaluation requires high-quality AP and lateral views. This allows evaluation of the calcar and posterior and medial cortex. Subtle undisplaced fractures may require further evaluation with tomography and radioisotope scans.

Significant mortality and morbidity may occur with intertrochanteric fractures unless early reduction and immobilization are obtained. Boyd and Griffin reported mortality rates of 18% in 300 patients with trochanteric fractures (231). Most patients are elderly, and prolonged bed rest may result in such complications as pulmonary

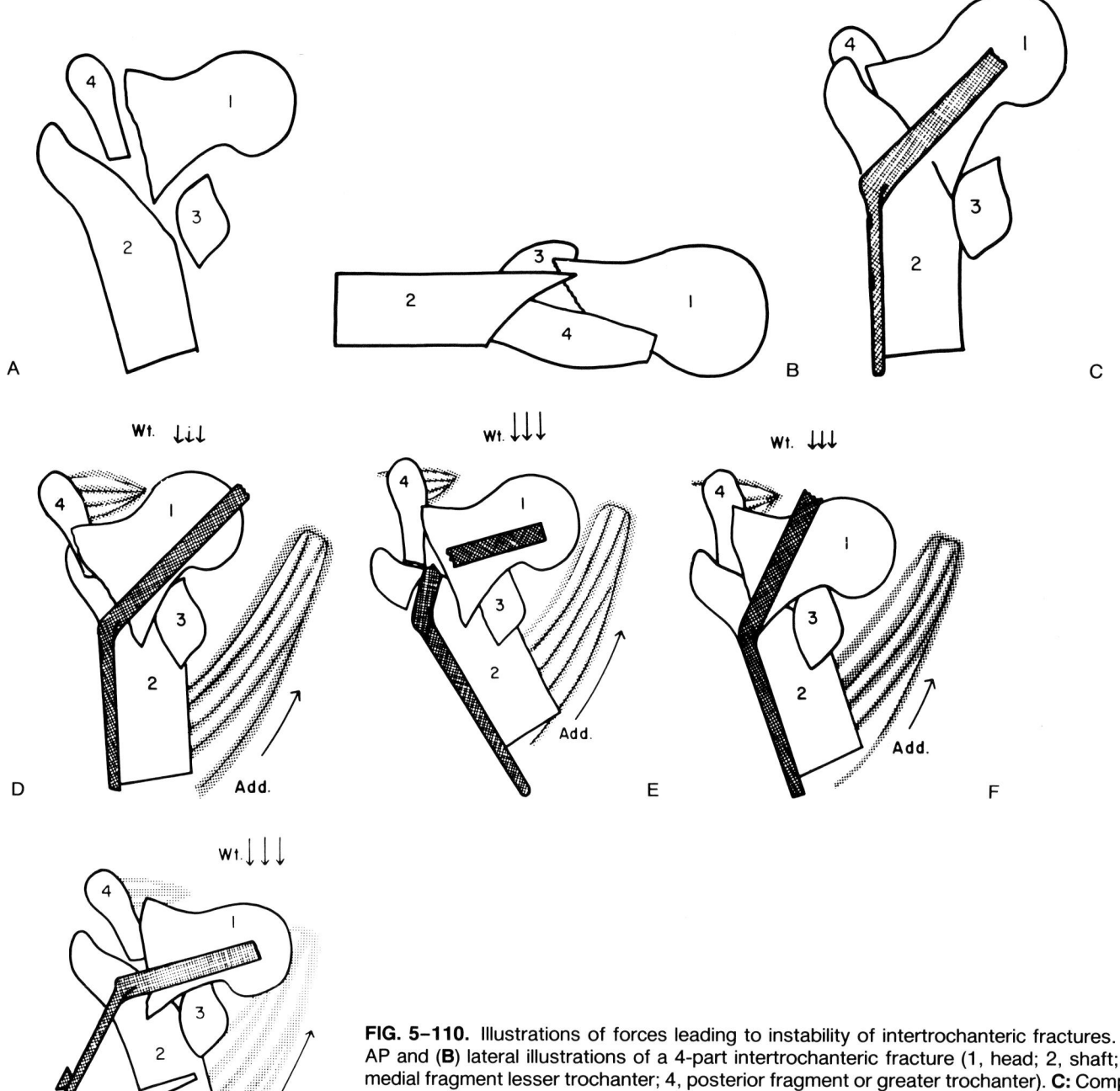

FIG. 5–110. Illustrations of forces leading to instability of intertrochanteric fractures. **A:** AP and (**B**) lateral illustrations of a 4-part intertrochanteric fracture (1, head; 2, shaft; 3, medial fragment lesser trochanter; 4, posterior fragment or greater trochanter). **C:** Complications resulting from weight bearing and muscle forces. **D:** Nail penetrating femoral head. **E:** Nail fracture. **F:** Nail penetrates the femoral neck. **G:** Screw fracture with varus collapse (from 235, with permission).

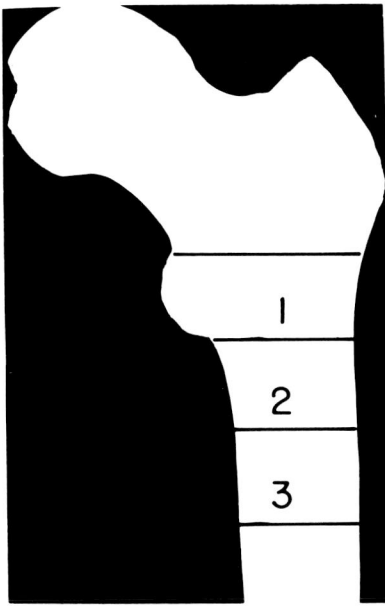

FIG. 5-111. Illustration of Fielding Classification of subtrochanteric fractures. (From Fielding JW, et al. Classification of subtrochanteric fractures. *Surg Obst Gyn* 1966;122:555.)

emboli, phlebitis, and infection. Even when healing occurs, many patients may be unable to return to normal full activity (251).

Non-union and avascular necrosis are uncommon complications of intertrochanteric fractures. These com-

TABLE 5-21. *Subtrochanteric fracture classifications*

Fielding Classification[a]
   Zone 1: Fracture includes the lesser trochanteric region
   Zone 2: Fracture 1–2 inches distal to the lesser trochanter
   Zone 3: Fracture 2–3 inches distal to the lesser trochanter
Boyd and Griffin Classification[b]
   Type I: Linear intertrochanteric fracture
   Type II: Comminuted fracture with the main fracture along the intertrochanteric line
   Type III: Subtrochanteric fracture with at least one fracture line passing through or just below the lesser trochanter
   Type IV: Comminuted trochanteric fracture extending into the shaft. Fracture lines in at least two planes.
Seinsheimer Classification[c]
   Group I: Undisplaced fracture (less than 2 mm displacement)
   Group II: Two-part fracture
         A. Transverse fracture
         B. Spiral fracture
         C. Spiral fracture with lesser trochanter involvement
   Group III: Three-part fractures
         A. Spiral fracture with lesser trochanter involvement
         B. Spiral fracture with butterfly fragment
   Group IV: Four part fractures
   Group V: Subchanteric fractures with extension into the intertrochanteric region and involvement of the greater trochanter

[a] (238), [b](231).

plications are more frequent with femoral neck fractures. Post-reduction instability, however, occurs commonly with complex fractures (Evans' Types 3 to 5) (243). Figure 5-110 demonstrates the forces responsible for failure to maintain reduction following internal fixation. Location of the fracture (calcar and posterior cortex involvement) and muscle forces play a significant role in this post-reduction instability (235).

Subtrochanteric Fractures

Subtrochanteric fractures involve the cortical bone below the lesser trochanter. Associated involvement of the shaft and intertrochanteric region is common. Boyd and Griffin reviewed 300 patients with trochanteric fractures, excluding avulsion fractures (231). Thirty-three percent of the fractures involved the subtrochanteric region. Fractures tend to occur in younger patients following significant trauma (motor vehicle accidents), in elderly patients with intertrochanteric involvement, and in patients with underlying pathology. Pathologic fractures tend to be transverse. Rogers suggests that any transverse subtrochanteric fracture be studied carefully for underlying pathology (256). Evaluation may require tomography or isotope scans.

Fielding divided subtrochanteric fractures into three zones (Fig. 5-111) (238). Zone 1 included the lesser trochanter, Zone 2, the 1–2 inches distal to the lesser trochanter, and Zone 3, the 2–3 inches below the lesser trochanter (Table 5-21). The significant factor is the involvement of the diaphysis (cortical bone). Cortical bone heals more slowly. Also biomechanical studies have demonstrated that the subtrochanteric region is a high-stress area, which makes treatment difficult (245,257).

The Boyd and Griffin classification was based upon the prognosis and ease of obtaining and maintaining re-

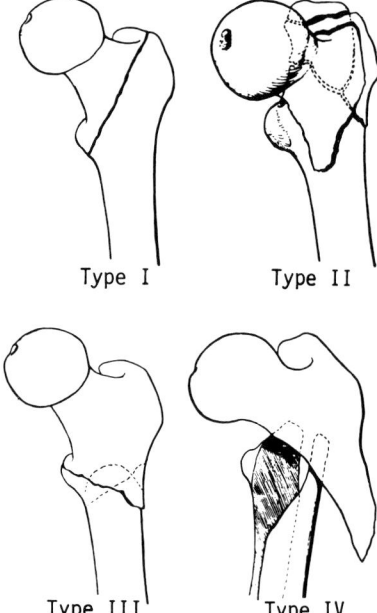

Type I   Type II

Type III   Type IV

FIG. 5–112. Illustration of Boyd and Griffin Classification (from 231).

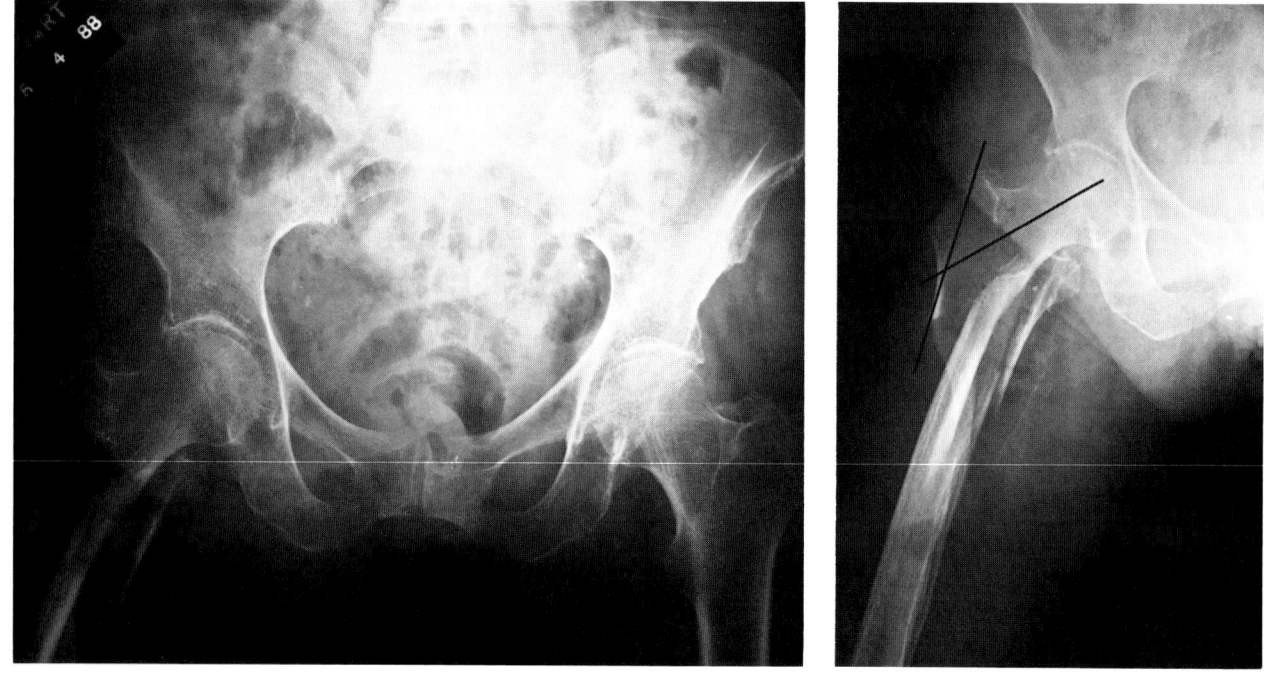

A   B

FIG. 5–113. AP view of the pelvis (**A**) and femur (**B**) in a comminuted subtrochanteric fracture with a long oblique-spiral fracture line and lesser trochanteric involvement.

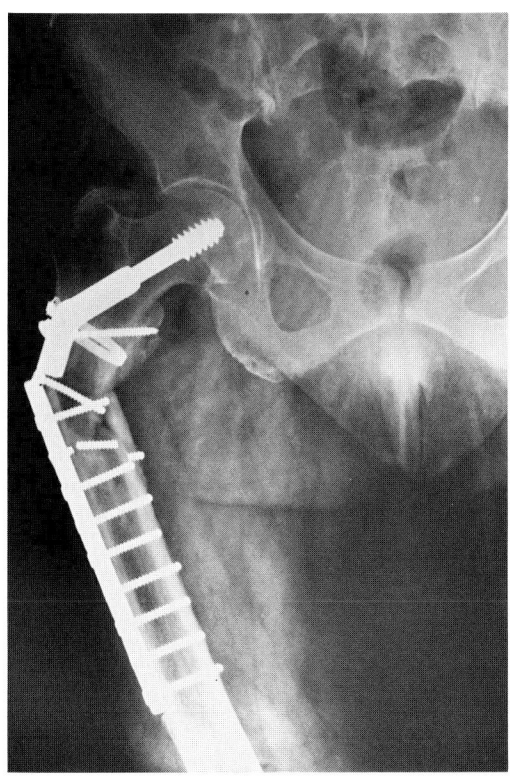

FIG. 5–114. Subtrochanteric fracture with sliding screw and long side plate. The plate and screws have fractured with loss of reduction.

duction (Table 5-21) (231). In the case of Type I fractures, which are characterized by linear breaks in the intertrochanteric region (Figs. 5-107 and 5-112), reduction was least difficult. Types III and IV fractures were subtrochanteric, and in these cases loss of reduction was common. Medial migration of the distal fragment as a result of adductor muscle forces was a significant factor in reduction failures.

Seinsheimer (261) divided subtrochanteric fractures into eight categories (Table 5-21). If bone-to-bone contact can be established medially, the fracture is considered stable. Most treatment failures involved Group III fractures. These are three-part fractures with involvement of the lesser trochanter or an associated butterfly fragment. The longer the spiral (greater than 8 cm), the poorer the prognosis (Fig. 5-113) (261).

Radiographic evaluation requires AP and lateral views. Both projections (see section on Routine Radiography of the Pelvis and Hips) can be obtained without moving the patient. Thus, risk of further displacement of the fracture fragments is not of concern. If transverse fractures are present, tomography may be required to exclude pathologic fractures.

Complications associated with subtrochanteric fractures are essentially the same as those seen with intertrochanteric fractures. The significant difference is an increased incidence of treatment failures in the case of subtrochanteric fractures. Fractures (Fig. 5-114) and dis-

placement of fixation devices are not unusual (232,255,261).

Avulsion Fractures

Greater trochanter avulsions are due to abrupt contractions of those muscles attaching to the greater trochanter. This fracture occurs in the elderly patient but is uncommon unless associated with an intertrochanteric fracture (234). Undisplaced fractures may be difficult to detect on the AP view. Oblique views and, occasionally, tomography may be necessary to demonstrate the fracture.

Lesser trochanteric avulsions are due to iliopsoas contractions and more commonly occur in young athletes (173). Rogers stated that avulsion fractures of the lesser trochanter in adults are uncommon unless there is underlying pathology (256). Metastasis is especially common in the older age group (230).

Treatment of Trochanteric Fractures

As in femoral neck fractures, the treatment of trochanteric fractures also depends on their stability. Types 1 and 2 intertrochanteric fractures are reasonably stable, with good cortical support medially acting as a buttress. Thus, they can be treated in a variety of ways and simply

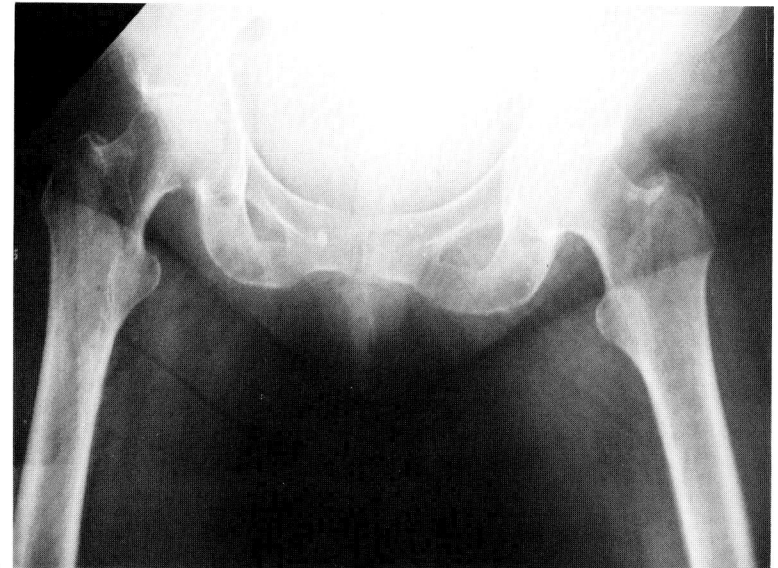

A

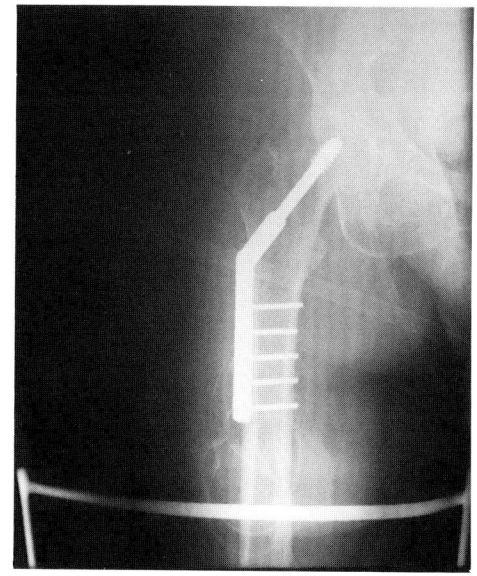

B

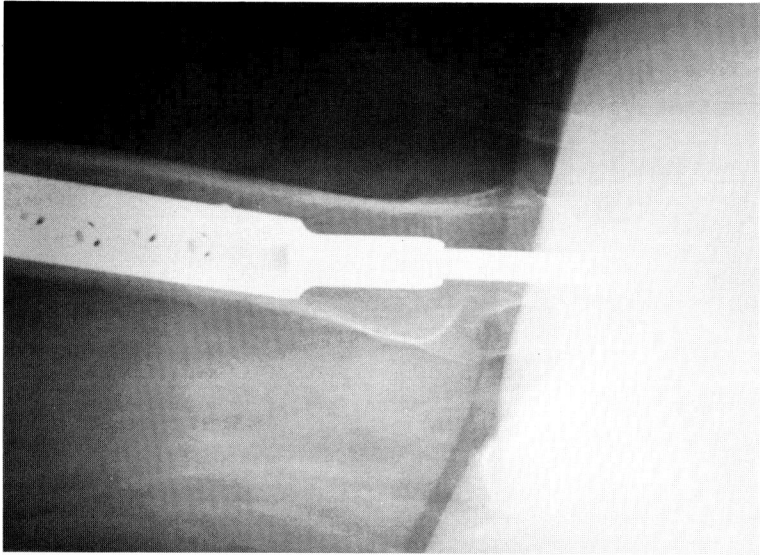

C

FIG. 5–115. A 63-year-old female involved in a motor vehicle accident. Type I intertrochanteric fracture (A). Appearance on admission. The fracture was internally fixed with a Richard's sliding nail-plate (B, C).

held by internal fixation until union occurs. The sliding nail-plate or screw-plate is quite sufficient for most of these fractures (Fig. 5-115). Fixed nail-plates without the sliding component should not be used (Fig. 5-110), for stresses at the angle of the nail plate are considerable, especially if some absorption occurs at the fracture site. Heyse-Moore and colleagues compared the Richards screw-plate with the Jewett nail-plate in a large series of intertrochanteric fractures and found the Richards screw-plate superior, as it resulted in considerably fewer complications (242). Ender pinning is also excellent and diminishes surgical time, blood loss, and the incidence of infection (236).

In the more unstable fracture (usually four-part fractures with no medial stability), one must be especially cautious in selecting the type of internal fixation (249,252,262). The ordinary nail-plate will invariably

fail. A sliding screw-plate can be successful provided that the distal fragment is displaced medially. This method has been demonstrated by Dimon and Hughston (235). In this case, medial displacement will relieve the lateral tension forces. A valgus position of the proximal fragment will act in the same way and can be achieved by an additional osteotomy. The latter was recommended by Sarmiento and Williams (258).

Ender nailing can also be used in the unstable intertrochanteric fracture if a reduction of the fracture in valgus is first obtained (Fig. 5-116). Often an additional pin in the greater trochanter is helpful for control of position (246,253,277). Significant complications may occur, however, and the operation is not an easy one. Experience leads to skill in placing Ender rods, and careful monitoring with an image intensifier in two planes will minimize the risk of complications. Ender nails seldom

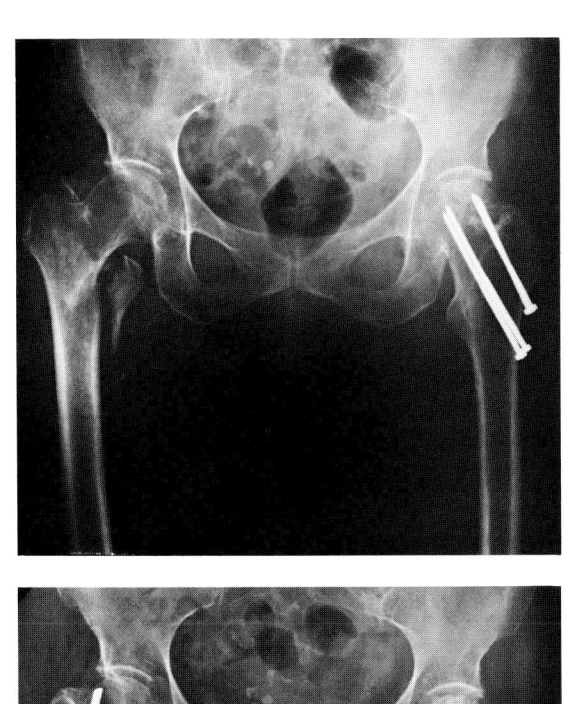

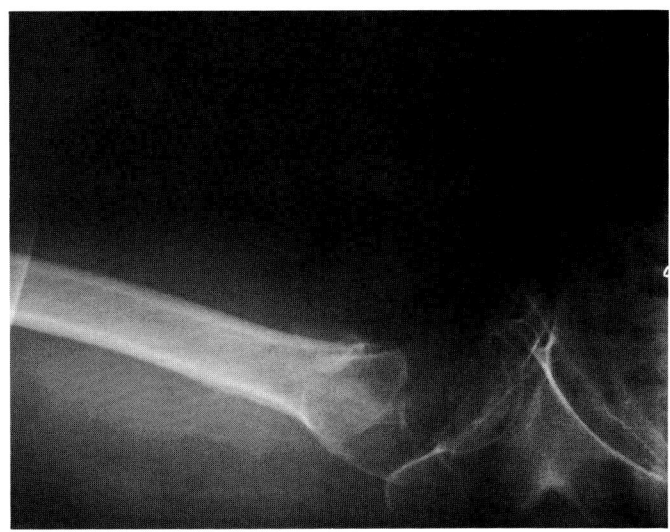

A

B

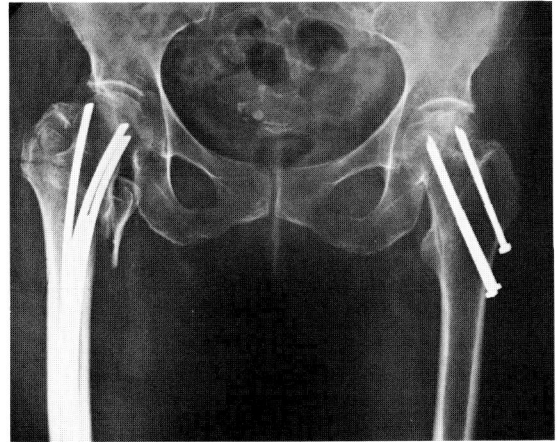

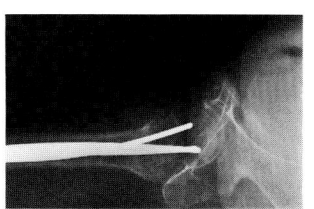

C

D

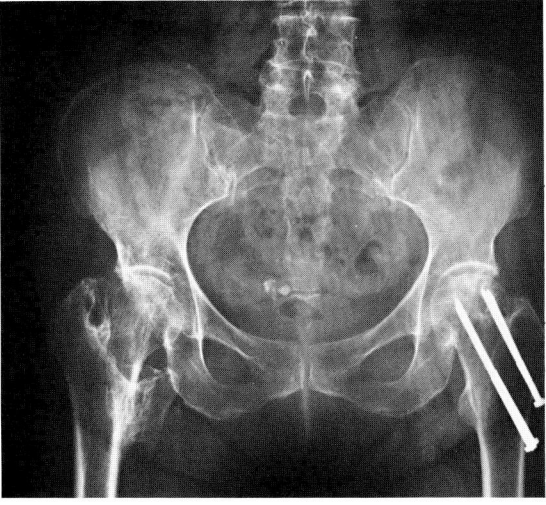

E

FIG. 5-116. An 81-year-old female, intertrochanteric fracture on the right following a fall. Unstable. AP (**A**) and lateral (**B**) radiographs prior to internal fixation. Note result of previous femoral neck fracture on left secured by four Knowles pins with good result. AP (**C**) and lateral (**D**) views following closed reduction and fixation with four Ender nails. AP view (**E**) three years following Ender nailing of right hip. Because of some protrusion at the knee the pins were removed one year after insertion. Fractures healed in almost anatomic position.

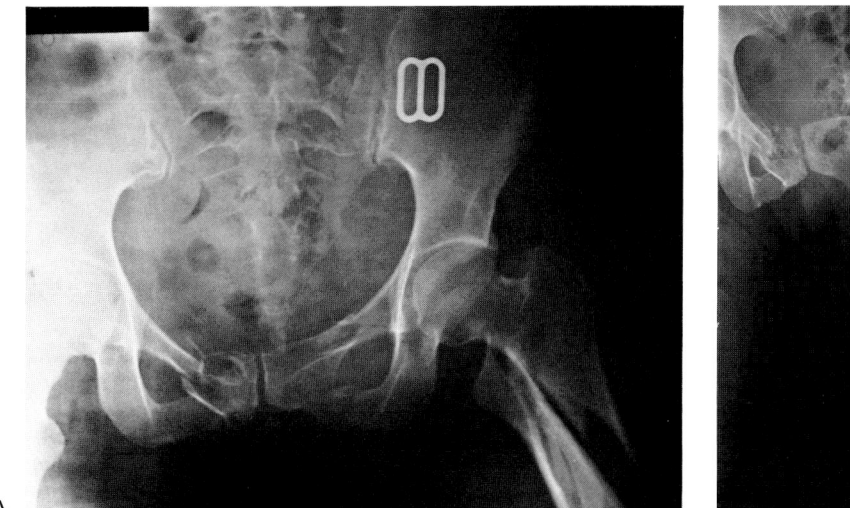

A

B

FIG. 5-117. A 45-year-old female involved in a motor vehicle accident with multiple fractures, including pelvis, forearm, ankle and tibia and fibula on the ipsilateral side. A long Richard's screw-plate with interfragmentary fixation with two screws was elected for the femur. **A:** Appearance of the upper femur following fracture. **B:** Three months following internal fixation. Union eventuated in excellent position.

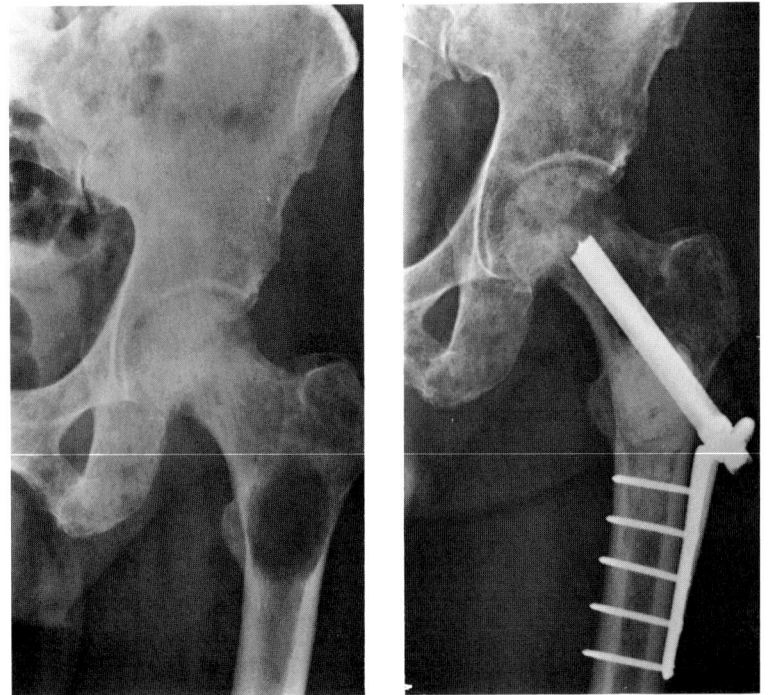

A

B

FIG. 5-118. A 66-year-old male, multiple myeloma. Lytic lesions throughout the skeleton, but especially in the intertrochanteric area where fractures are imminent. **A:** Appearance at time of internal fixation. **B:** Methacrylate placed into the large cavity opposite the lesser trochanter followed by McLaughlin nail-plate. This provided adequate stability with the addition of the methacrylate.

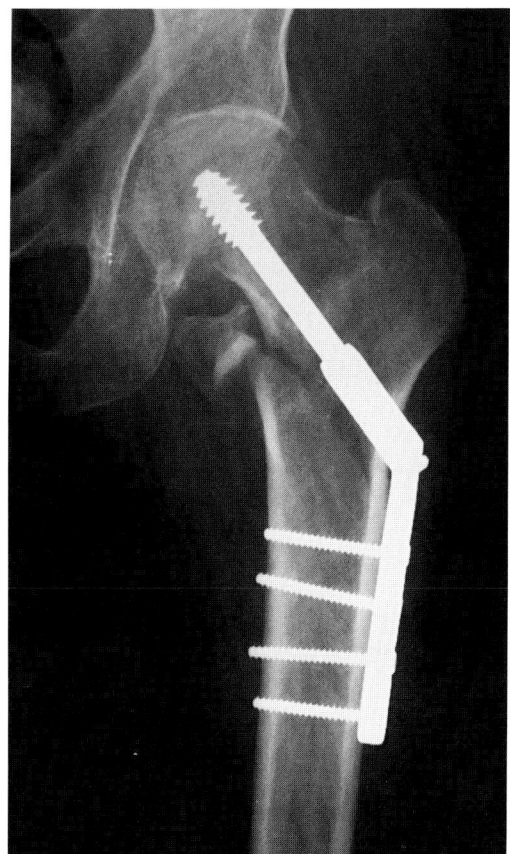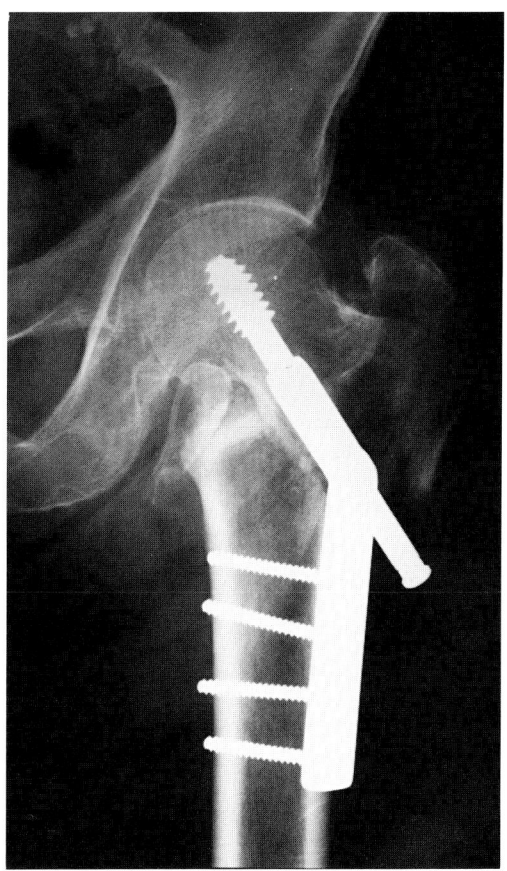

A   B

FIG. 5-119. A: Unstable subtrochanteric fracture with sliding-screw plate fixation. **B:** One month following surgery the fragments have collapsed and the screw protrudes into the soft tissues.

migrate proximally. If they do, they can be extracted from their entrance point above the knee. Pain about the knee is more common and may occur from distal migration of the nails. It can be relieved by removing them. Union is usually obtained with Ender fixation. An external rotation deformity may occur; it can be minimized by reduction and nailing with the distal fragment in relative internal rotation. Although useful in some patients, the incidence of failure or reoperation may be higher if Ender nailing is not used in carefully selected patients (232,233).

A badly comminuted intertrochanteric fracture in an older, debilitated patient who must be rapidly mobilized may be treated with a primary trochanteric prosthesis of the Leinbach type. The indications are quite limited, but, in the octogenarian with a comminuted fracture and marked osteoporosis, an endoprosthesis may be the proper choice (248). For these unstable four-part fractures in the osteoporotic patient, even methyl methacrylate reinforcement can be used in conjunction with some type of blade or nail-plate fixation (260).

The subtrochanteric fracture requires different treatment (234,241). Because of the differences in stress at this level, lateral nail plating or sliding screw plating is seldom indicated. An exception is the very long comminuted fracture with a high degree of instability. Here a long ASIF nail-plate with additional bone grafting and cerclage wires or transfixion screws may salvage this type of fracture (Fig. 5-117).

Most subtrochanteric fractures are ideally treated with the Zickel nail (264). While mastering the technique of the Zickel nail is difficult, its superiority for this purpose has been proved with time and use (265,266). Ender nails are a useful alternative, especially in the patient who is a poor operative risk.

Pathologic fractures occur rather frequently in the area of the trochanter and should receive special attention (250,267). The addition of methyl methacrylate as an adjunct in the management of pathologic fractures was reported in a combined study from several orthopedic centers (241). The acrylic is used, of course, in conjunction with internal fixation, the type depending on the lesion and its level (Fig. 5-118). Included in this study were 63 patients who were treated for fractures of the femoral head and neck and 109 patients treated for trochanteric and subtrochanteric fractures. Bony union after irradiation is actually enhanced by the use of acrylic.

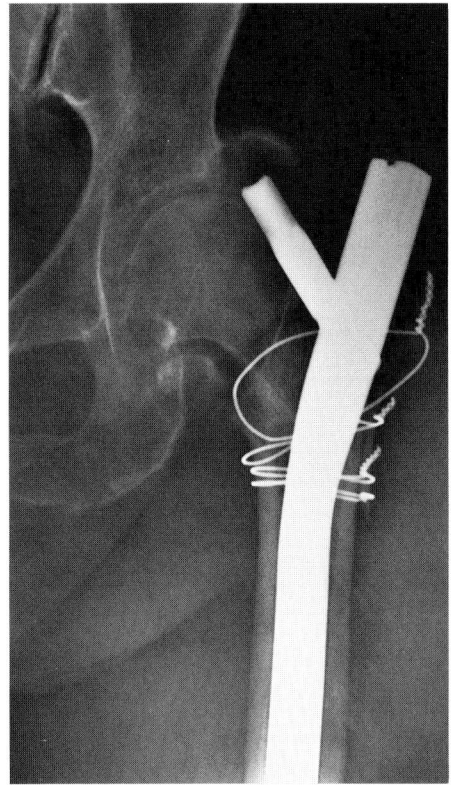
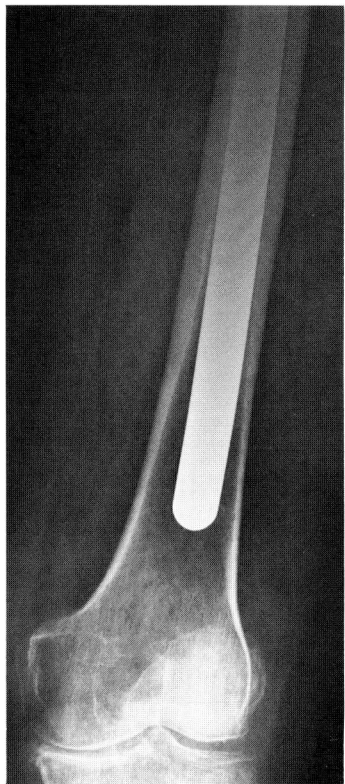
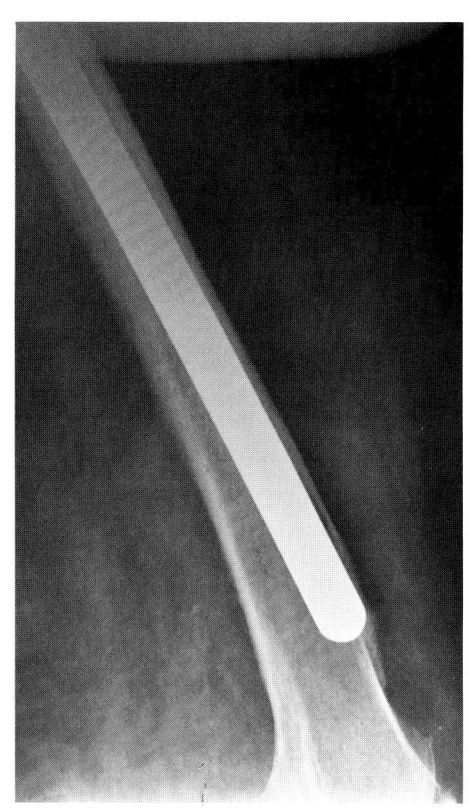

A

B

C

FIG. 5-120. Old left subtrochanteric fracture. AP view of the pelvis (**A**) and AP (**B**) and lateral (**C**) views of the femur show the medullary nail has protruded through the anterior femoral cortex and the upper portion of the fixateur through the femoral neck.

Treatment of avulsion fractures is usually conservative. Surgical intervention is not indicated unless the fragment is displaced more than 2 cm (234).

Routine radiography is generally sufficient to follow patients following reduction of trochanteric and subtrochanteric fractures. The presence of metal can hinder conventional field MRI. Examinations should begin with at least two radiographic views, typically AP and lateral (255,259). Serial images are most useful in evaluating changes in fragment or fixation position (Fig. 5-119). Tomography is still useful for evaluation of fracture union.

Common complications can be identified on radiographs. These include fracture of fixation devices, loss of reduction, and migration of fixation devices through the femur (Fig. 5-120), femoral head, or even into the pelvis (232,255,259).

EVALUATING SOFT TISSUE TRAUMA

There are numerous techniques for evaluating trauma and/or trauma-related soft tissue disorders in the pelvis and hips. Ultrasonography, CT, and MRI have provided valuable information in this regard (268,269,291). However, arthrography and diagnostic and therapeutic injections remain important tools for evaluation of intra and extra-articular hip disorders (271,272). MRI has not replaced these techniques in imaging the hip to the degree that it has in imaging the knee and shoulder (269).

Arthrography

Arthrography provides valuable information in patients with pain, instability, clicking, locking, and other symptoms related to the pelvis and hips. The study should be tailored to the clinical symptoms of each patient. Variable imaging techniques such as tomography, CT, single versus double contrast, and injection of anesthetic and/or anesthetic-steroid combinations must be considered to obtain optimum information. When properly performed, the articular cartilage, capsule, and synovium can be accurately assessed and pain localized (272,273,281,282).

Indications for hip arthrography vary with the age of the patient. In children, arthrography is most frequently performed to evaluate septic arthritis, congenital hip dysplasia, and Legg-Calvé-Perthes disease (271,273, 282). Arthrography in adults is usually performed to evaluate arthritides (e.g., rheumatoid arthritis, pigmented villonodular synovitis, osteoarthritis), infection, and intra-articular loose bodies (271). In this section we will concentrate on trauma-related disorders in the hip, sacro-

TABLE 5-22. *Adult hip arthrography:*
Indications and techniques

Indication	Technique
Arthritis	Routine
Osteoarthritis	
Rheumatoid arthritis	
Septic arthritis	
Pigmented villonodular synovitis	Tomography
Loose bodies	Tomography
Osteoarthritis	
Trauma	
Synovial chondromatosis	Tomography plus double contrast
Osteonecrosis	Tomography
Acetabular labral tears	Routine (multiple obliques)
	CT with air alone or double contrast
Iliopsoas bursal enlargement	Routine

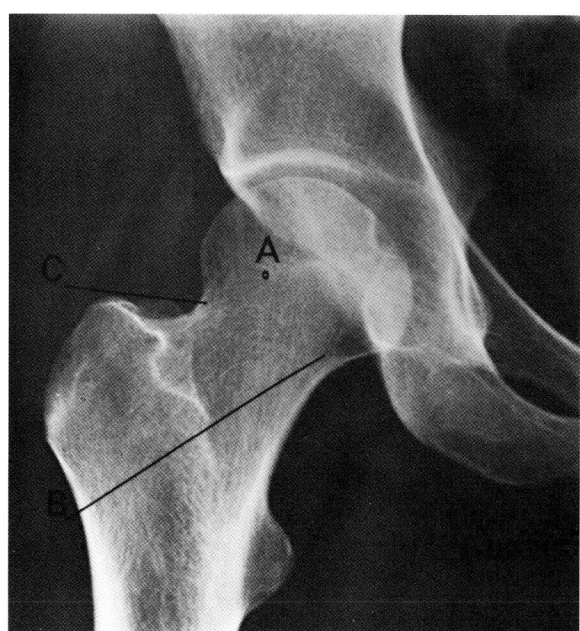

FIG. 5-121. AP view of the hip demonstrating injection approaches. A, vertical, B, anterolateral, C, lateral.

iliac joint, and pubic symphysis. The study is frequently performed to evaluate acetabular labral tears. A less common indication is evaluation of enlarged iliopsoas bursae (283,287,290). Table 5-22 summarizes the indications for conventional arthrography at the Mayo Clinic.

Arthrographic Technique

Prior to performing arthrography, all radiographic studies (routine films, isotope scans, CT scans, etc.) should be thoroughly reviewed and the clinical findings discussed with the referring physician. These steps assist in determining the proper method of injection, appropriate contrast material, and the filming technique that will best demonstrate the suspected pathology. Although allergic reactions during arthrography are rare (271), a history of significant allergy to a contrast medium may require a difficult approach to the examination. If previous reactions were mild (i.e., hives, with no respiratory or vascular symptoms), premedication with diphenhydramine (Benadryl) or chlorpheniramine (Chlor-Trimeton) may be all that is necessary. If a severe reaction occurred, the examination should not be performed. If necessary, injection of air followed with CT or tomography may be useful in patients with significant histories of allergic reaction. Bleeding is rarely reported with arthrography. Gelman stated that patients with clotting disorders or with platelet counts of less than 50,000 per ml may have bleeding problems during the procedure (271).

Arthrography requires high-quality fluoroscopic equipment with easy access to the patient (see Introduction to Arthrography in Chapter 1). The hip and pubic symphysis are approached with the patient supine. The injection site is prepared using sterile technique. AP scout film is routinely obtained prior to injection. Scout films prior to the injection help prevent unnecessary re-

peat injections, which is significant in that repeating films will often result in a suboptimal study.

The injection site for the hip is determined by the fluoroscopic appearance of the hip and the location of the femoral artery. The femoral artery, which must be palpated prior to injection, generally runs medial to the femoral neck. However, in patients with significant deformities of the hip as a result of previous surgery or trauma, the relationship of the neck to the femoral artery may vary. In making the injection we generally use an anterior approach, with the needle directed vertically just lateral to the midline at the junction of the head and neck (Fig. 5-121). The anesthetic needle is positioned over the area, and the skin is infiltrated to form a wheal. After anesthetizing the superficial soft tissues, a 22-gauge, 3.5-inch needle is advanced vertically until it makes contact with the femoral neck. The patient is then instructed to flex the hip slightly. This assures that the bevel of the needle is within the joint capsule. Larger needles (18 gauge) may be required in patients with suspected pyogenic arthritis. This will make aspiration of purulent material less difficult. Alternate approaches, such as the anterolateral (Fig. 5-121B) and lateral (Fig. 5-121C), may be used if the clinical situation dictates (273).

Needle position can be confirmed by (1) aspiration of synovial fluid, (2) injection of a small amount of contrast medium (0.5 ml), (3) injection of air, or (4) injection of 5–10 ml of sterile saline and reaspiration of the fluid. In the latter situation, unaspirated saline may dilute the contrast medium. Although the incidence is rare, air embolism has been reported with air arthrography (276). Therefore, we prefer to use a small, test injection if no synovial fluid can be aspirated. Aspiration of the joint or saline flush with aspiration is usually performed if synovial fluid analysis for crystals, rheumatoid factor, immunoglobulins, or infection is indicated. Care must be taken not to inject large amounts of contrast medium prior to aspiration for culture purposes, as the contrast medium is a bacteriostatic agent.

The choice of contrast agent and filming technique varies with the clinical situation (Table 5-22). In routine situations, 6 ml or more of contrast medium (meglumine such as Hypaque-M-60) is injected. If too much contrast medium is injected, subtle changes will be obscured. Epinephrine is occasionally mixed with the contrast medium if tomography is contemplated. Use of epinephrine allows the contrast medium to remain in the joint for longer periods, resulting in improved film quality (285). In certain cases, double contrast technique (4 ml of contrast material plus 10 ml or more of air) is used. Other cases call for use of air alone.

Following the injection of the contrast agent or agents, the hip is exercised and observed fluoroscopically. Any painful motions, clicking, or position changes of intra-articular bodies can be observed. Patients are positioned fluoroscopically for filming. This technique provides added information and ensures proper positioning. Films are taken in internal and external rotation and in lateral and oblique projections. Depending upon the information obtained fluoroscopically, further views following exercise or additional oblique views are also obtained. If necessary, computed tomography or tomography may be obtained. This requires additional planning on the part of the arthrographer. If tomography is contemplated, the injection is usually made on the tomography table to reduce the time required to obtain the films.

Following the arthrogram, bupivacaine (Marcaine) or a combination of bupivacaine and betamethasone (Celestone) is often injected. This is helpful in patients without definitive arthrographic findings. The injection helps determine whether the pain is intra-articular and in this way facilitates treatment programs in many cases. Betamethasone is not used if surgery is contemplated or if infection is suspected.

Arthrographic Demonstration of Normal Anatomy

The normal arthrogram demonstrates the articular cartilage, labrum, capsular configuration, and synovial characteristics of the hip joint (Fig. 5-121) (271,273,281, 282). The margins of the capsule extend from the acetabular rim to the base of the femoral neck. There are four recesses (Fig. 5-122). Proximally, the superior articular recess extends above the cartilaginous labrum. Inferiorly, the inferior recess outlines the inferior labrum. The superior recess colli lies above the femoral neck, and the inferior recess colli is found at the lower margin of the neck (282). The distal insertion of the capsule is irregular and should not be mistaken for synovial inflammation. The acetabular labrum is difficult to visualize in its entirety. Oblique views demonstrate the labrum to best advantage (Fig. 5-122B). A constant extrinsic defect is seen below the femoral head owing to the transverse ligament. With the patient in the supine position, the posterior labrum may be seen as a straight line along the upper portion of the neck. Inferior to the labral line is the orbicular zone, which is caused by thickened ligamentous fibers encircling the capsule. The articular cartilage on the femoral head is well demonstrated and is usually thicker than the acetabular articular surface (273). Medially, the acetabular fossa is well demonstrated, but in normal patients the ligamentum teres is usually not visualized (272). Communication of the capsule with the iliopsoas bursa occurs in 15–20% of patients owing to a defect between the iliofemoral and pubofemoral ligaments (272,290).

Indications for Hip Arthrography

Arthritis

Arthrographic evaluation of patients with post-traumatic and inflammatory joint diseases allows one to obtain anatomic and laboratory information. Synovial fluid should always be aspirated. If no fluid can be obtained, a saline flush (nonbacteriostatic sterile saline) with reaspiration can provide information regarding infection. Fluid analysis will vary depending upon the clinical situation (crystals in suspected gout or pseudogout; rheumatoid factor, differential count, and Gram stain in cases of suspected infection; immunoglobulins in chondrolysis). Grossly bloody fluid may indicate pigmented villonodular synovitis (277,281).

Evaluation of the articular cartilage is usually adequate with conventional film techniques. Tomography is useful in patients with abnormal routine radiographs or when subtle findings are suspected. For example, in patients with chondrolysis, tomography will assist in detection of the subtle erosions in the articular cartilage (277). Double-contrast technique may provide additional anatomic information.

The configuration of the capsule (Fig. 5-122) is also easily defined arthrographically. The normal hip should accommodate at least 10 ml of fluid (213). In patients with long-standing inflammatory arthritis or restricted motion for long periods following injury, the capsule may decrease in size with loss of the normal recesses (Fig. 5-123). Symptoms similar to adhesive capsulitis in the shoulder may develop. Injection of contrast material may be very difficult in patients with advanced capsulitis. Identification of communicating sinus tracts or abcess cavities is also important. This finding may be present in infectious arthritis.

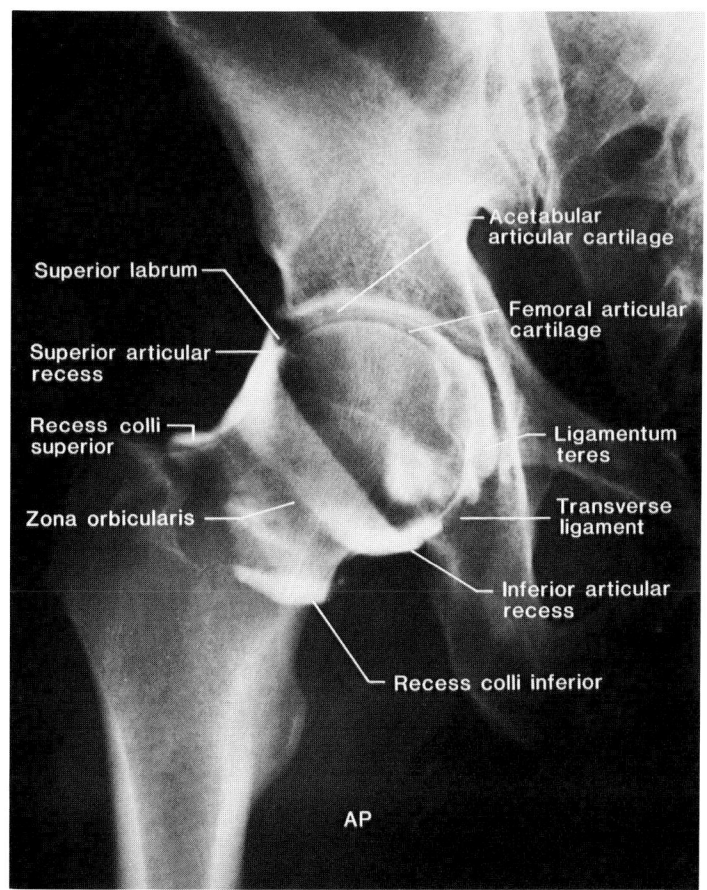

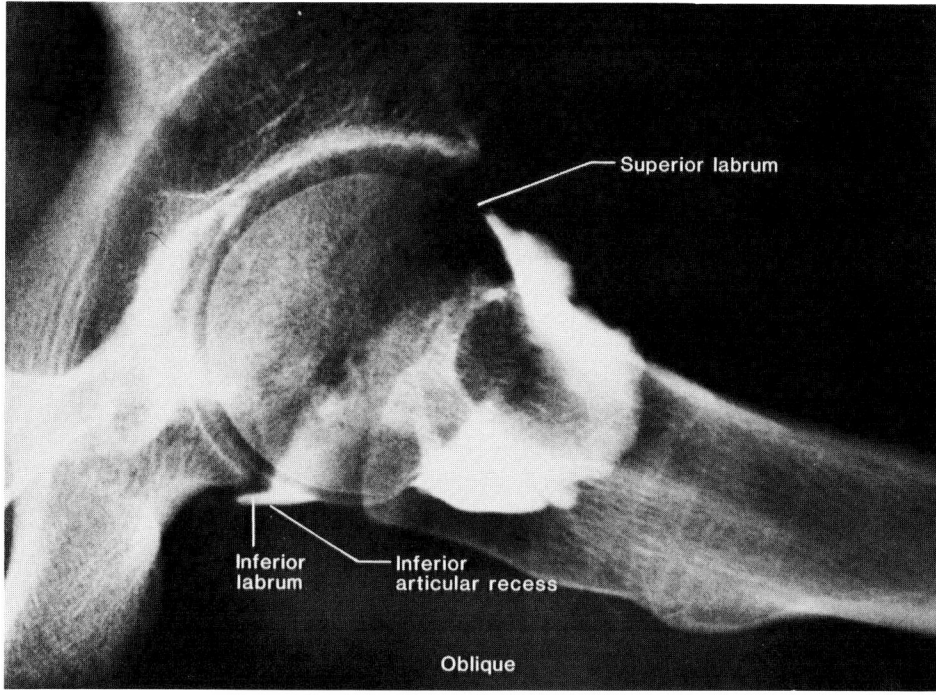

FIG. 5-122. Normal hip arthrogram. Anatomy labeled (**A**) AP view, (**B**) oblique view.

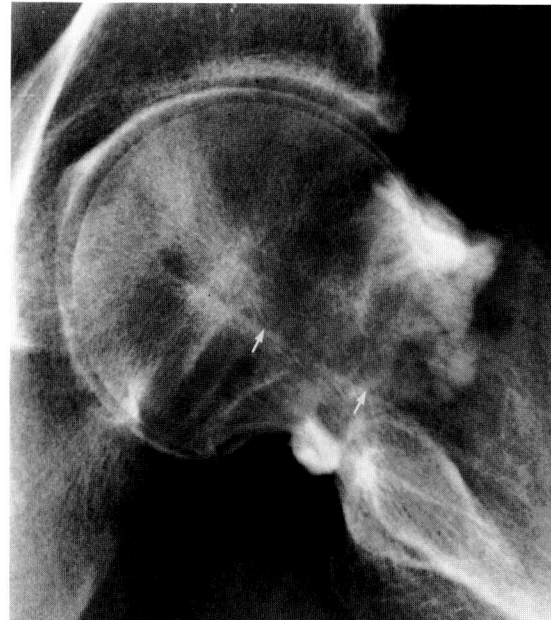

FIG. 5–123. Painful hip with decreased range of motion following previous fracture and surgery. The femoral screw had been removed (*white arrows*). The oblique view demonstrates reduction in the size of the recesses due to early capsulitis. Small bony spur on the inferior margin of the head (*arrow*). Capsular volume 5 cc's.

Synovial evaluation is usually adequate with routine arthrographic techniques (274). In patients with suspected pigmented villonodular synovitis, double-contrast technique, with or without tomography, may be necessary to detect subtle granular changes in the synovium. In later stages, large lucent defects may be difficult

to differentiate from synovial chondromatosis. A bloody synovial aspirate and erosive changes in the femur or acetabulum may be present with pigmented villonodular synovitis. Large areas of synovial proliferation may also be evident in rheumatoid arthritis and chronic infections. Lymphatic filling may be present with any chronic inflammatory arthritis.

Loose Bodies

Arthrography is frequently useful in identification of intra-articular osteocartilaginous bodies. On occasion, subtle areas of calcification or more obvious calcifications may be evident on the plain films (Fig. 5-124). Arthrography will confirm the location of these densities. The most common cause of intra-articular loose bodies is degenerative arthritis (282). Fragments of cartilage are nourished by synovial fluid and may actually increase in size over a period of time (282).

Patients with osteonecrosis, Legg-Calvé-Perthes disease, osteochondritis dissecans, and previous fracture-dislocations of the hip may require arthrography to evaluate the articular surface. The position of the fragment (loose or covered by articular cartilage) can be assessed. Tomography is often necessary in these patients (Fig. 5-125).

A less common condition, synovial chondromatosis, may also cause loose bodies within the joint space (Fig. 5-126). This condition is due to synovial metaplasia and results in fine synovial irregularity. These areas of proliferation are released into the joint space and usually grow

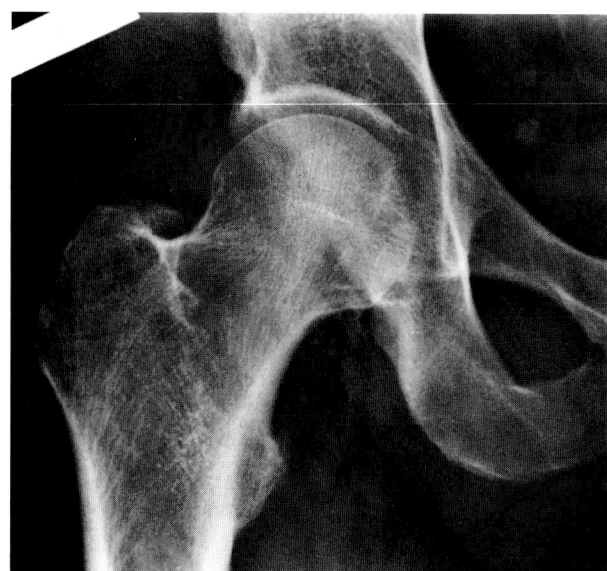

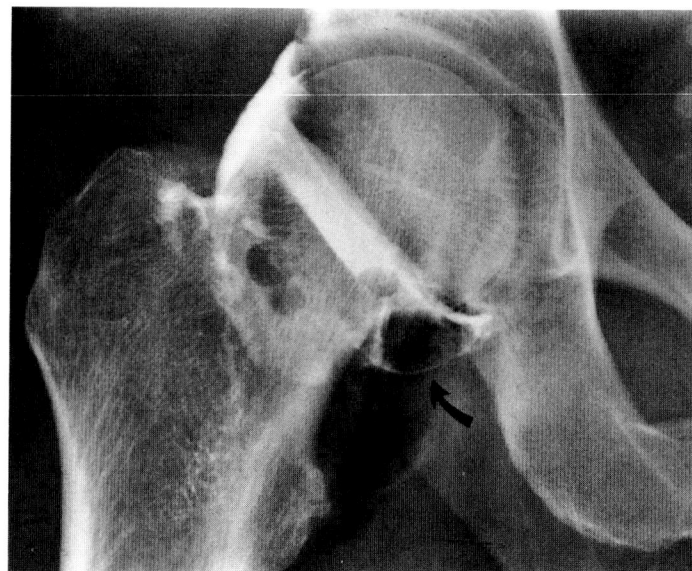

FIG. 5–124. Male patient with right hip pain and clicking. The AP (**A**) view demonstrates a faint density inferior to the femoral head (*curved arrow*). The arthrogram (**B**) confirms the intra-articular location of this loose body.

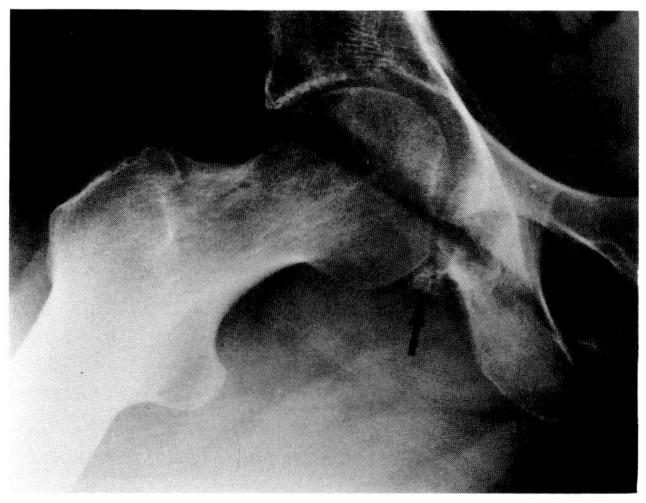

A

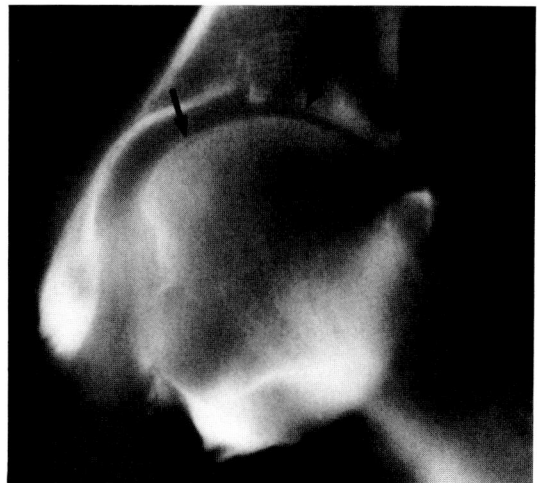

B

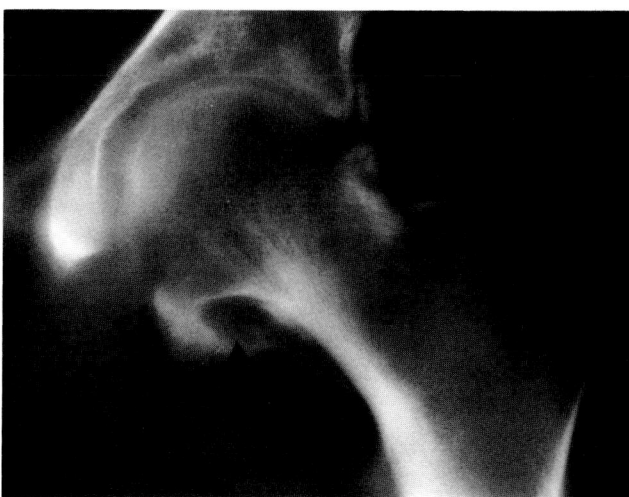

C

FIG. 5-125. Patient with chronic hip pain following a motor vehicle accident. The oblique view of the hip **(A)** demonstrates joint space narrowing superiorly with bony densities inferior to the head. Arthrotomogram demonstrates the following: **B:** thinning of the articular cartilage with subchondral lucency (*arrows*) and irregularity of the femoral head below the fovea. The capsular volume is also reduced **(C).** Cartilaginous body inferior to the femoral head (*arrow*). This may have originated from the femoral head defect.

to significant size before symptoms develop. Calcification of these chondral bodies may occur (282).

Acetabular Labral Tears

Evaluation of suspected acetabular labral tears is one of the most frequent indications for hip arthrography in our practice. Patients with tears in the labrum present with pain, clicking (especially with flexion and external rotation of the hip), and decreased range of motion (278). Routine radiographs are of little value. Conventional arthrography (Fig. 5-127) allows partial evaluation of the labrum, although the anterior and posterior portions are difficult to visualize. In this case, fluoroscopically positioned oblique views in the frog-leg position allow evaluation of a large portion of the labrum. Tomography is also useful in studying the inferior portions. However, early experience indicates that these methods are not sufficiently accurate and that CT (Fig. 5-128) with air or double-contrast technique or MRI may prove to be the most valuable methods for evaluation of the labrum (Fig. 5-129) (269,270).

Enlarged Iliopsoas Bursa

As mentioned earlier, the joint capsule communicates with the iliopsoas bursa in 15–20% of patients (269,270,286). In long-standing inflammatory arthritis, this communication may enlarge, resulting in an inguinal mass (Fig. 5-130) (279,280,282,283). If the bursa extends cephalad, compression of the femoral vessels, bladder, and colon may occur (219). A triad of findings may suggest the diagnosis. These features include (1) a mass in the inguinal region, (2) pressure effects on the bladder, colon, or femoral vessels, and (3) radiographic evidence of arthritic changes in the hip. Associated arthritic conditions include osteoarthritis, rheumatoid arthritis, pigmented villonodular synovitis, and synovial chondromatosis (280).

Snapping Tendon Syndromes

There are several causes of pain and snapping in the hip. Labral tears, snapping of the iliotibial band over the greater tuberosity, and snapping of the iliopsoas tendon

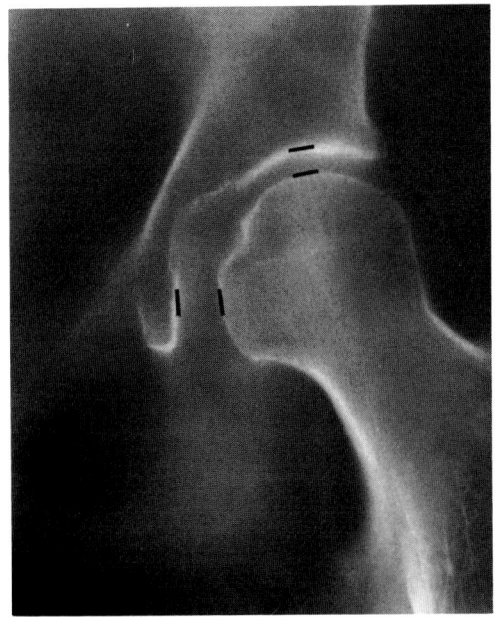

A

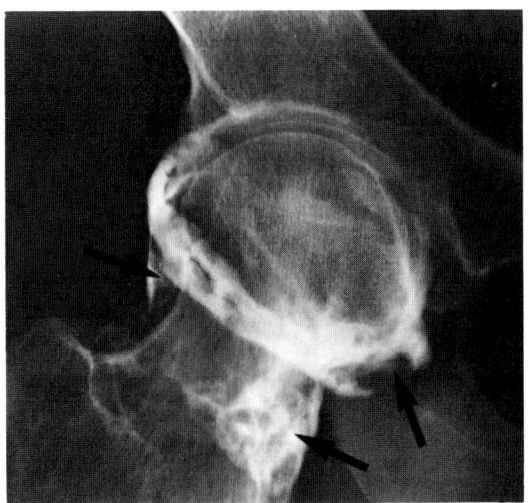

B

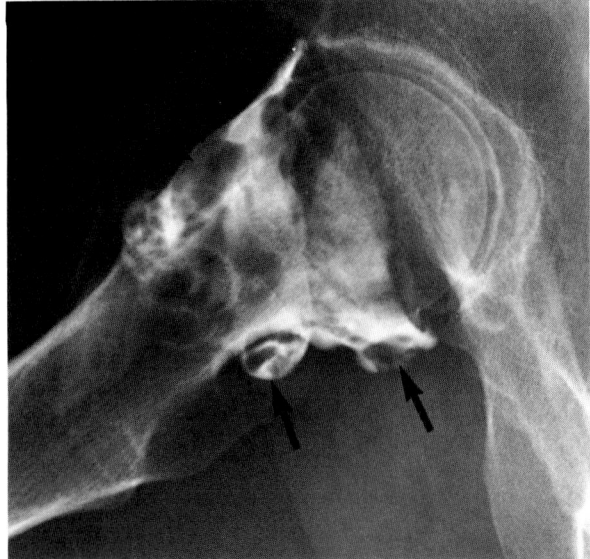

C

FIG. 5-126. Female patient with chronic hip pain and snapping after jogging for several years. **A:** AP tomogram of the hip is normal. Note the joint spaces superiorly and medially. The AP (**B**) and oblique (**C**) views of the arthrogram demonstrate multiple large lucent filling defects (*arrows*). Surgically proved synovial chondromatosis.

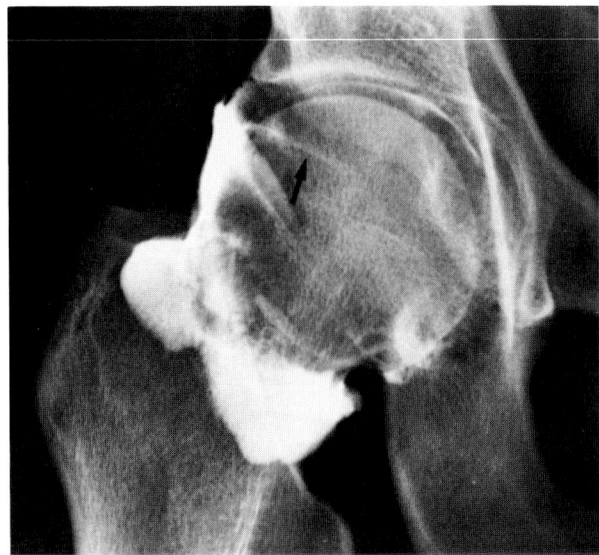

A

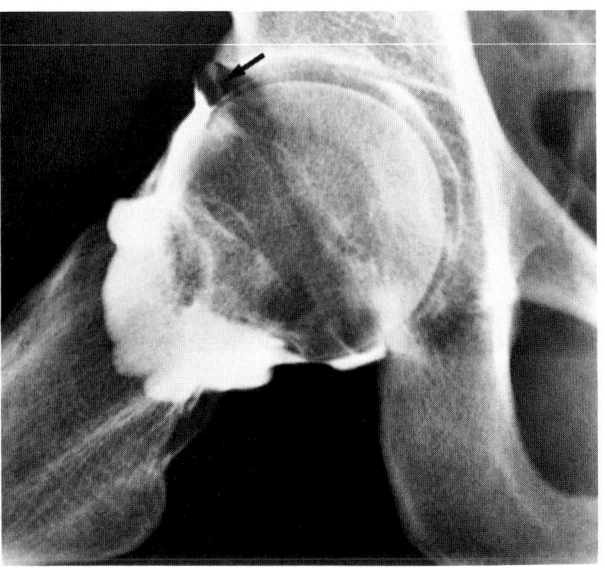

B

FIG. 5-127. Patient with suspected acetabular labral tear. The AP view (**A**) demonstrates a faint area of contrast in the superior labrum (*curved arrow*) with a linear cleft of contrast (*arrow*) over the upper femoral head. The oblique view (**B**) clearly demonstrates the tear (*arrow*).

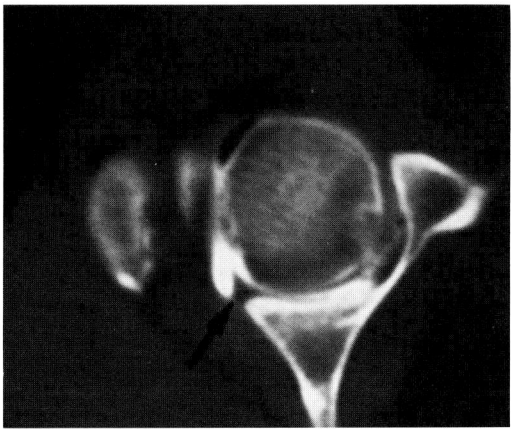

FIG. 5-128. CT scan in the anterior oblique position demonstrating the posterior acetabular labrum (*arrow*).

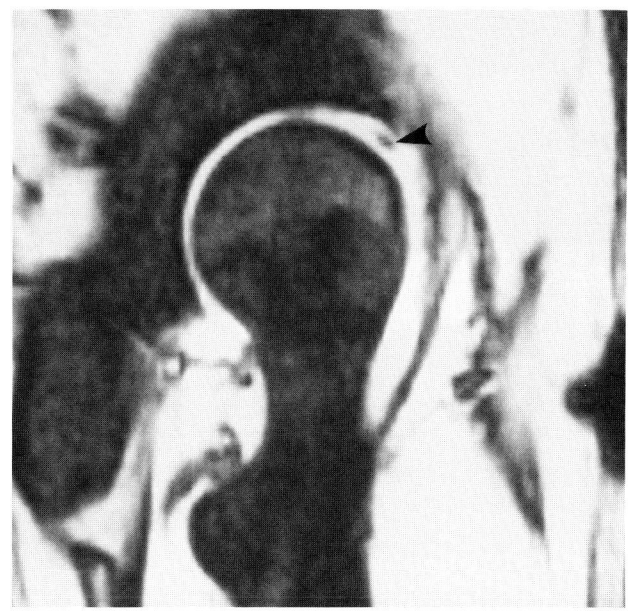

FIG. 5-129. Oblique gradient echo (MRGR) image of the hip demonstrating a tear (*arrow*) in the acetabular labrum.

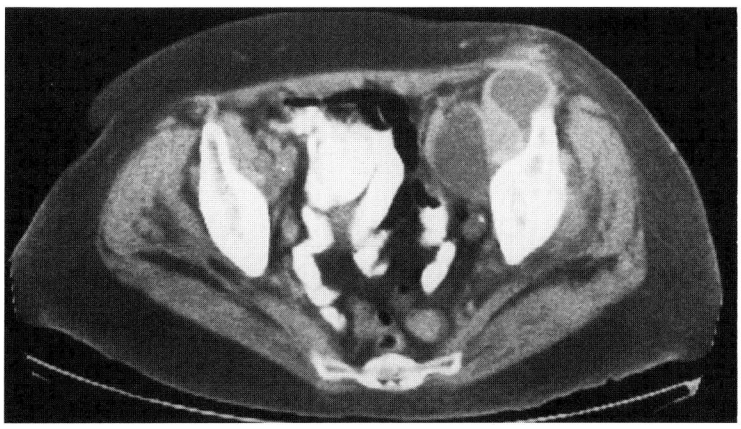

A

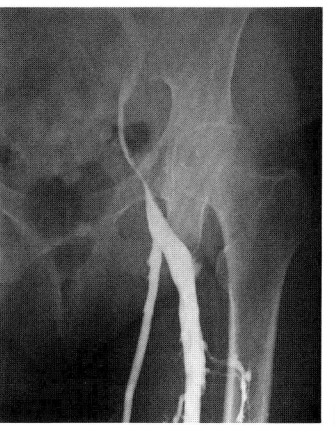

B

FIG. 5-130. A: Axial CT image demonstrates an enlarged iliopsoas bursa. **B:** Venogram demonstrating compression of the femoral vein with low-grade obstruction.

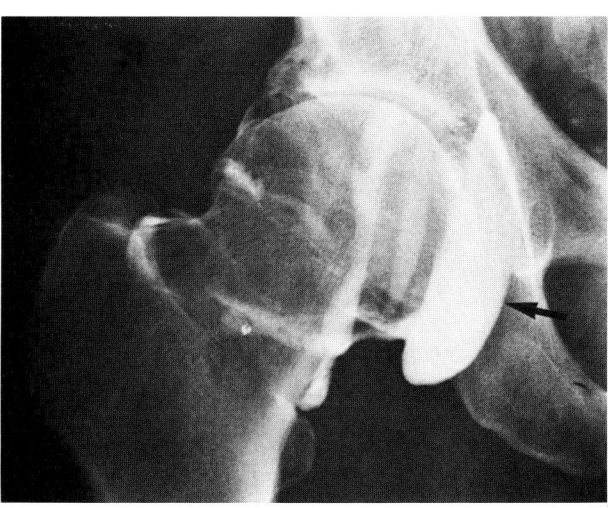

FIG. 5-131. AP view of the right hip following arthrogram demonstrating an enlarged iliopsoas bursa (*arrow*).

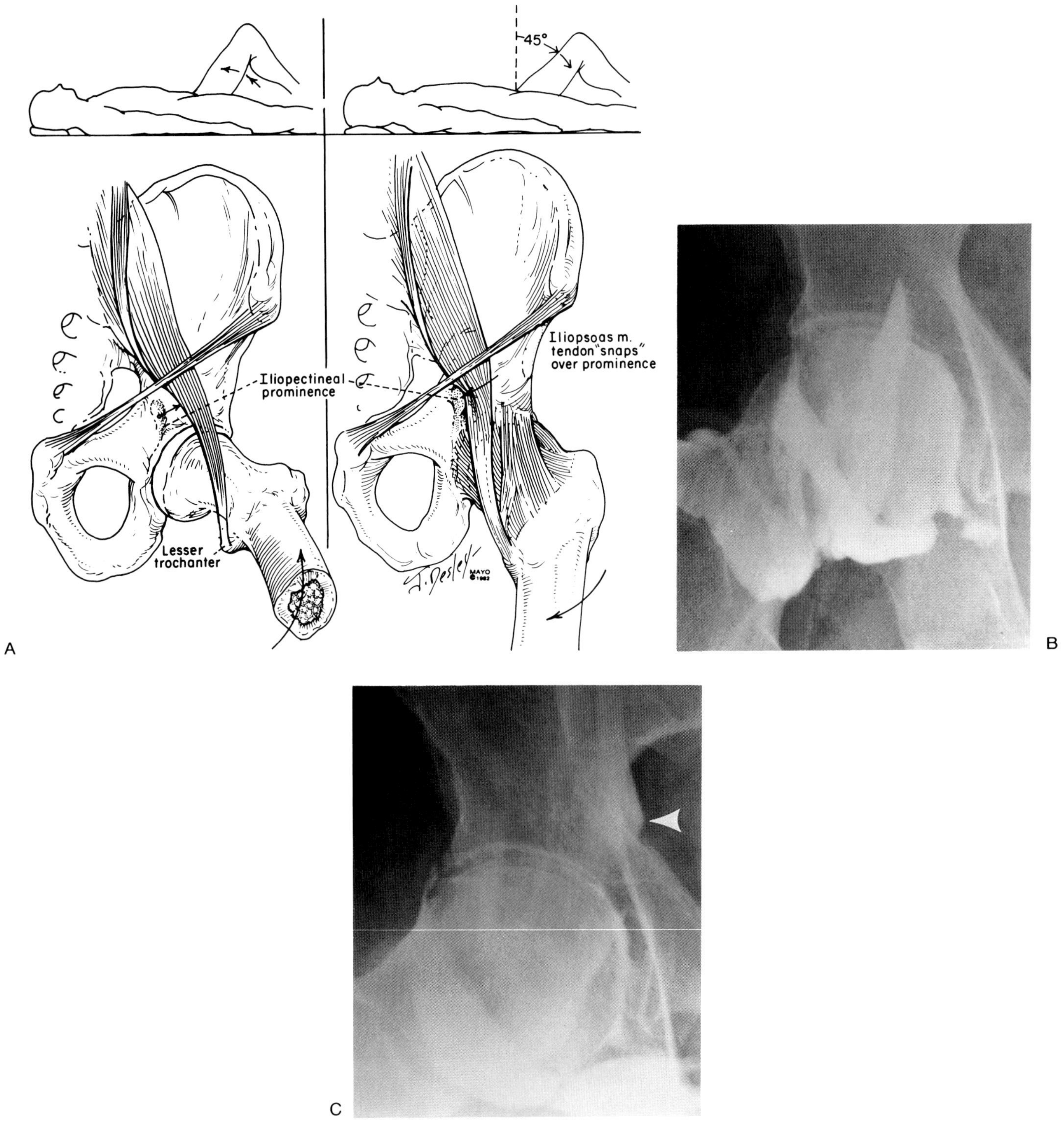

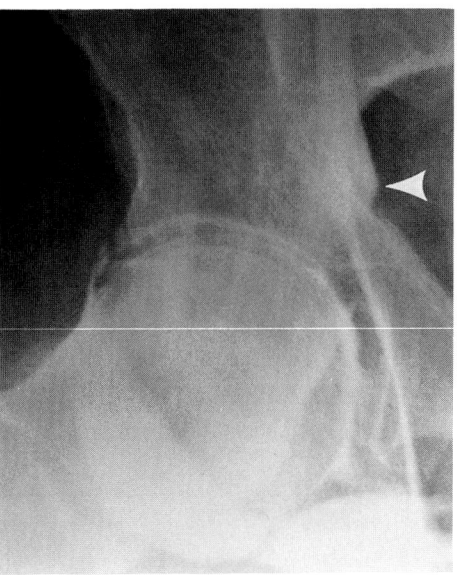

FIG. 5-132. Snapping iliopsoas tendon. **A:** Illustration of leg motion and tendon anatomy resulting in snapping of the tendon over the iliopectineal eminence. **B** and **C:** Post iliopsoas injection showing medial displacement of the tendon (*arrow*) in (**C**) due to tendon entrapment as it moves over the eminence. In this patient the iliopsoas bursa communicated with the hip. When this occurs, the amount of contrast should be limited so the hip capsule is not distended (from 275, with permission).

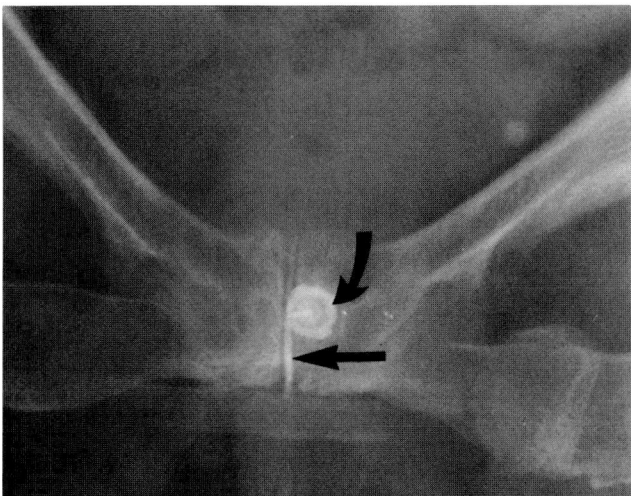

FIG. 5-133. AP view of the pelvis taken during injection of the pubic symphysis. Note the linear configuration of the joint seen with contrast medium injection. The patient had mild instability following pelvic fracture. Symptoms improved after injection of anesthetic.

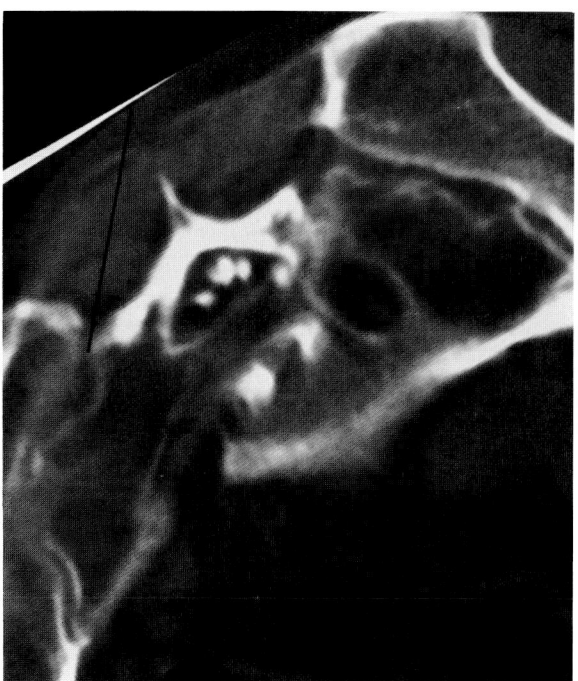

FIG. 5-134. Oblique CT image of the sacroiliac joint demonstrating the injection technique.

over the iliopectineal eminence or lesser trochanteric ridge have all been implicated (275,278,284,288). Imaging with diagnostic or therapeutic injection is most commonly employed with snapping the iliopsoas tendon. Arthrograms may demonstrate an enlarged iliopsoas bursa (Fig. 5-131). Changes in the bursa can be observed or videotaped as the patient flexes and extends the hip. There are two problems with using arthrography to make this diagnosis. First, the iliopsoas bursa communicates with the hip in only 15–20% of patients (290). Second, distention of the hip capsule with contrast can displace the tendon enough to reduce the snapping. Therefore, direct injection of the tendon is most useful. The tendon passes over the medial aspect of the femoral head (Fig. 5-132A). The needle can be advanced vertically onto the femoral head and contrast material gently

injected as the needle is slowly edged back (Fig. 5-132B,C). Contrast will flow along the tendon or may enter the iliopsoas bursa (275). We typically inject Marcaine and Celestone with the contrast medium to assist in diagnosis and treatment. Low osmolality contrast media is most useful because it is less irritating. The patient is asked to flex and extend the hip (Fig. 5-132A) while the tendon movement is documented fluoroscopically or with videotape. The tendon will snap over the iliopectoneal eminence or lesser trochanteric ridge when symptoms are related to the iliopsoas tendon. Surgical transfer may be required in patients who do not respond to injection (275).

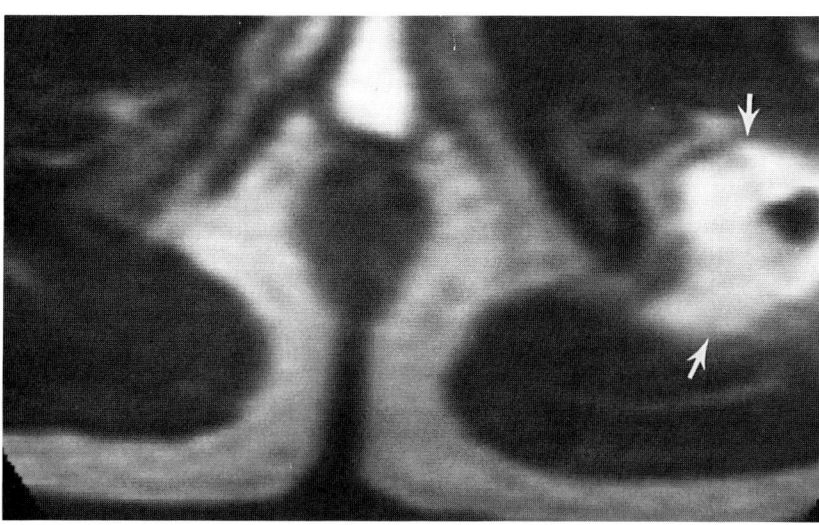

FIG. 5-135. Axial SE 2000/60 image demonstrating a tear of the hamstring tendons at the ischial origins (arrows).

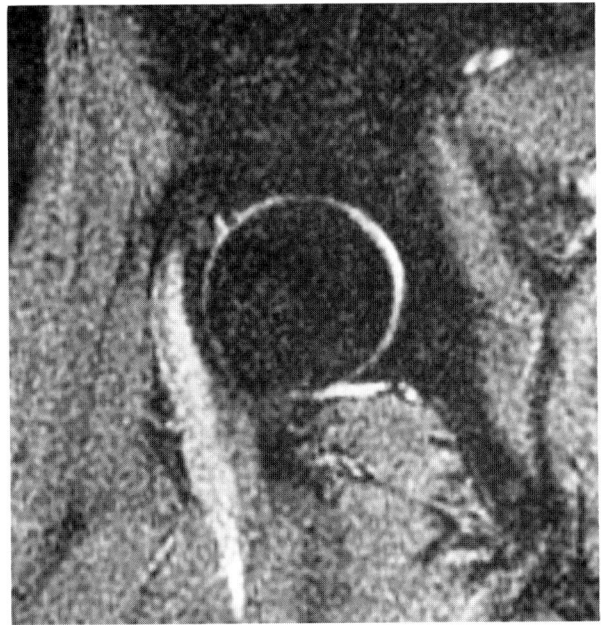 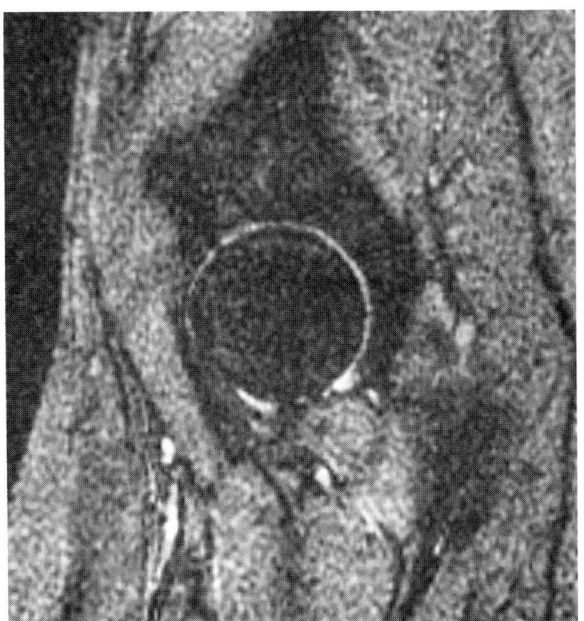

FIG. 5–136. Acute bleeding into the iliopsoas muscle (**A**) with normal side (**B**) for comparison on oblique gradient echo (MPGR) images.

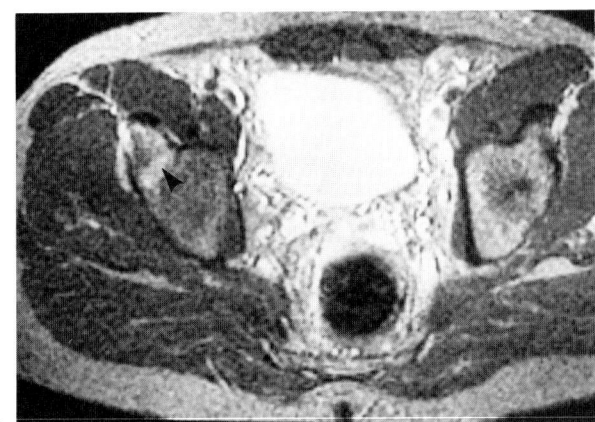 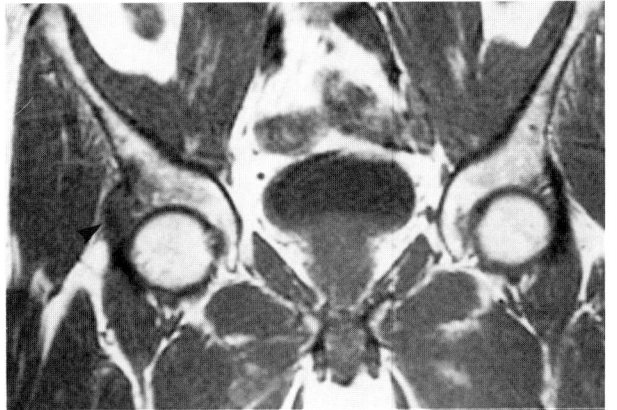

FIG. 5–137. Jogger with right hip pain. Radiographs were normal. Axial SE 2000/60 (**A**) and coronal SE 500/20 (**B**) images demonstrate a subtle stress fracture of the anterior inferior iliac spine (*arrows*) (from 269, with permission).

Pubic Symphysis and Sacroiliac Joint

Arthrography and injection of the pubic symphysis and sacroiliac joints is usually performed to document the sight of pain in patients with post-traumatic instability. The arthrogram is performed mainly to document proper needle position.

The pubic symphysis is easily entered via direct anterior vertical approach. The patient is supine and the joint usually optimally visualized without rotating the patient. After usual sterile preparation, a small amount of anesthetic (1% Xylocaine) is injected into the skin over the joint. A 1.5-inch, 22-gauge needle can be directed into

the joint with fluoroscopic guidance and the position confirmed with 0.5–1 cc of contrast material (Fig. 5-133). Alternating upright weight-bearing views are useful in demonstrating subtle instability during the arthrogram.

The sacroiliac joint is entered posteriorly with the patient obliqued with the involved side down (Fig. 5-134). The thick sacroiliac ligaments must be transversed by the needle to enter the joint. Contrast medium can be used to confirm needle position prior to injection of Marcaine and Celestone for both the pubic symphysis and sacroiliac joints. Approximately 2 cc is all that can be injected into the sacroiliac joint. In patients with suspected instability, it is useful to obtain upright views of the sacroiliac joint with weight alternated on the right and left to check for excessive motion. The lower margins of both sacroiliac joints should remain uniform with no step off in normal patients. A change of greater than 2 mm on the involved side indicates laxity. Following significant trauma, the CT images should be reviewed or a new scan performed to evaluate the joints and to be certain that heterotopic bone has not covered the joint posteriorly. This will prevent successful injection (see Fig. 5-70).

MRI, CT, and Ultrasonography

Evaluation of all soft tissue injuries and sequalae can be difficult. However, proper use of newer techniques can provide valuable information concerning muscle, ligament, and nerve injury as well as subtle osseous injury that may be overlooked (269).

Computed tomography can provide valuable information concerning the articular structures of the hip. However, contrast injection is useful to optimize this data and, therefore, it is usually invasive (see Fig. 5-128) (270,272,289). Although arthrography and tenography are valuable, MRI is being used with more frequency to evaluate subtle injuries in the pelvis and hips. Muscle, ligament, and tendon tears (Fig. 5-135 and 5-136), nerve injuries, and subtle osseous injuries (Fig. 5-137) can be detected and followed using MRI (269,280,286).

Ultrasonography is less frequently used in our practice. However, superficial tendon injuries and hip effusions can be evaluated with this imaging technique (268,290).

REFERENCES

Anatomy

1. Anderson JE. *Grants atlas of anatomy.* 8th ed. Baltimore: Williams and Wilkins, 1983.
2. Armbuster TG, Guerra J, Resnick D, et al. The adult hip: An anatomic study. *Radiology* 1978;128:1–10.
3. Bowerman JW, Sena JM, Chang R. The teardrop shadow of the pelvis. Anatomy and clinical significance. *Radiology* 1982; 143:659–662.
4. Brooke R. The sacroiliac joint. *J Anat* 1924;58:299.
5. Bucholz RW. The pathologic anatomy of Malgaigne fracture-dislocations of the pelvis. *J Bone Joint Surg* 1981;63A:400–404.
6. Clark SS, Prudencio RF. Lower urinary tract injury associated with pelvic fracture: Diagnosis and management. *Surg Clin North Am* 1972;52:183–201.
7. Clements CD. *Gray's anatomy of the human body,* 13th ed. Philadelphia: Lea and Febiger, 1985.
8. Fisher MR, Kricun ME. *Imaging of the pelvis.* Aspen Press, 1989.
9. Francis CC. The human pelvis. St. Louis: C. V. Mosby Co., 1952.
10. Guerra J, Armbruster TG, Resnick D, et al. The adult hip: An anatomic study. Part II: Soft tissue landmarks. *Radiology* 1978;128:11–20.
11. Hollinshead WH. *Anatomy for surgeons.* 3rd ed. Philadelphia: Lea and Febiger, 1982.
12. Jackson H, Barke JT. Sacral foramina. *Skel Radiol* 1984;11:282–288.
13. Kane WJ. Fractures of the pelvis. In: Rockwood CA, Green DP. *Fractures in adults,* 2nd ed. vol. 2. Philadelphia: J.B. Lippincott, 1984;1093–1209.
14. Lang EK. Transcatheter embolization of pelvic vessels for control of intractable hemorrhage. *Radiology* 1981;140:331–339.
15. Miller WE. Massive hemorrhage in fractures of the pelvis. *South Med J* 1963;56:933–938.
16. Motsay GJ, Manlove C, Perry JF. Major venous injury in pelvic fractures. *J Trauma* 1969;9:343–346.
17. Reichman S. Roentgen soft tissue appearances in hip disease. *Acta Radiol Diagn* 1967;6:167.
18. Resnick D, Niwayama G. Anatomy of the individual joints. vol. 2. In: Resnick D, Niwayama G. *Diagnosis of bone and joint disorders,* 2nd ed. Philadelphia: W. B. Saunders Co., 1988.
19. Reuter SR, Redman HC. Gastrointestinal angiography. Philadelphia: W. B. Saunders Co., 1977.
20. Ring EJ, Athanasoulis C, Waltman AC, Margolies VM, Baum S. Arteriographic management of hemorrhage following pelvic trauma. *Radiology* 1973;109:65–70.
21. Ring EJ, Waltman AC, Athanasoulis C. Angiography in pelvic trauma. *Surg Gynecol Obstet* 1974;139:375–380.
22. Rowe CR, Lowell JD. Prognosis of fractures of the acetabulum. *J Bone Joint Surg* 1961;43A:30–59.
23. Sacs BJ. Normal acetabular anatomy for acetabular fracture assessment: CT and plain film correlation. *Radiology* 1986; 159:139–145.
24. Sclafani SJR, Becker JA. Traumatic presacral hemorrhage: Angiographic diagnosis and therapy. *AJR* 1982;138:123–126.
25. Thaggard A III, Harle TS, Carlson V. Fractures and dislocations of the bony pelvis and hips. *Semin Roentgenol* 1978;13:117–134.
26. Truex RC, Carpenter MB. *Strong and Elwyns human neuroanatomy.* Baltimore: Williams and Wilkins, 1964.

Imaging of the Pelvis and Hips

27. Armbuster TG, Guerra J, Resnick D, et al. The adult hip: An anatomic study. *Radiology* 1978;128:1–10.
28. Ballinger PW. *Merrill's atlas of radiographic positions and radiologic procedures.* 5th ed. St. Louis: C. V. Mosby Co., 1982.
29. Berman L, Catterall A, Meiere HB. Ultrasound of the hip: A review of the applications of a new technique. *Brit J Radiol* 1986;59:13–17.
30. Berkebile RD, Fisher DL, Albrecht LF. The gull-wing sign: Value of the lateral view of the pelvis in fracture-dislocations of the acetabular rim and posterior dislocation of the femoral head. *Radiology* 1965;84:937–939.
31. Bernau A, Berquist TH. *Orthopaedic positioning in diagnostic radiology.* Baltimore: Urban and Schwarzenberg, 1983.
32. Berquist TH. *Magnetic resonance of the musculoskeletal system.* New York: Raven Press, 1990.
33. Burk DL, Mears DC, Herbert DL, Straub WH, Cooperstein LA, Beck EA. Pelvic and acetabular fractures: Examined by angled CT scanning. *Radiology* 1984;153:548.
34. Burk DL, Mears DC, Kennedy WH, Cooperstein LA, Herbert DL. Three dimensional computed tomography of acetabular fractures. *Radiology* 1985;155:183–186.
35. Danielius G, Miller L. Lateral view of the hip. *X-ray Technol* 1938;9:176.
36. Dihlmann W, Nebel G. Computed tomography of the hip joint capsule. *J Compt Assist Tomogr* 1983;7:278–285.
37. Dodig D, Ugarkovic B, Orlic D. Bone scintigraphy in idiopathic asceptic femoral head necrosis. *Eur J Nucl Med* 1983;8:23–25.
38. Fishman EK, Drebin B, Magid D, et al. Volumetric rendering techniques: Applications for three dimensional imaging of the hip. *Radiology* 1987;163:737–738.
39. Friedman LJ. Lateral roentgen ray study of the hip joint. *Radiology* 1936;27:240.
40. Glynn TP, Kreipke DL, DeRosa GP. Computed tomography arthrography in traumatic hip dislocation. *Skel Radiol* 1989;18:29–31.

41. Harris JH, Loh CK, Perlman HC, et al. The roentgen diagnosis of pelvic extraperitoneal effusion. *Radiology* 1977;125:343.
42. Hencke A, Reiser M, Schmucher F, et al. Selective digital subtraction arteriography in necrosis of the femoral head. *Skel Radiol* 1987;16:270–274.
43. Hickey PM. Value of the lateral view of the hip. *AJR* 1916;3:308–309.
44. Janes L. Lateral roentgenography of the neck of the femur. *AJR* 1935;33:504.
45. Johnson CR. A new method for roentgen examination of the upper femur. *J Bone Joint Surg* 1932;30:859–866.
46. Judet R, Judet J, Letournel E. Fractures of the acetabulum: Classification and surgical approaches to open reduction. *J Bone Joint Surg* 1964;46A:1615–1646.
47. Kalman MA. Radiology of soft tissue shadows in the pelvis: Another look. *AJR* 1978;130:493–498.
48. Knapp RH, Vannier MW, Marsh JL. Generation of three dimensional images from CT scans: Technological perspective. *Radiol Tech* 1985;56:391–398.
49. Lancaster SJ, Cummings RJ. Hip aspiration: Verification of needle position by air arthrography. *J Ped Orthop* 1987;7:91–92.
50. Lauenstein C. Das Rontgenbild einer Luxatio femores infraglenoidales. *Fortschr Roentgenstr* 1900;3:186.
51. Leonard RD, George AW. Cassette with a convex curve. *AJR* 1932;28:261–263.
52. Letournel E. Acetabular fractures: Classification and management. *Clin Orthop* 1980;151:81–106.
53. Lorenz: Die rontgenographische Darstellung des subskapularen Raumes und des Schenkelhalses im Querschnitt. *Forschr Roentgenstr* 1918;25:342.
54. Pennal GF, Tile M, Waddell JP, Garside H. Pelvis disruption: Assessment and classification. *Clin Orthop* 1980;151:12–21.
55. Phillips HB. New roentgen demonstration of the neck of the femur. *Am J Surg* 1928;5:392–393.
56. Pritchard RS, Shah HR, Nelson CL, FitzRandolph RL. MR and CT appearance of iliopsoas bursal distension secondary to diseased hips. *J Compt Assist Tomogr* 1990;14:797–800.
57. Robinson HJ, Hartleben DD, Lund G, Schreman J. Evaluation of magnetic resonance imaging in the diagnosis of osteonecrosis of the femoral head. *J Bone Joint Surg* 1989;71A:650–663.
58. Saks BJ. Normal acetabular anatomy for acetabular fracture assessment: CT and plain film correlation. *Radiology* 1986;159:139–145.
59. Schultz RJ. *The language of fractures.* Baltimore: Williams and Wilkins, 1972.
60. Scott WW, Fishman EK, Magid D. Acetabular fractures: Optimal imaging. *Radiology* 1987;165:537–539.
61. Speer KP, Spritzer CE, Harrelson JM, Nunley JA. Magnetic resonance imaging of the femoral head after acute intracapsular fracture of the femoral neck. *J Bone Joint Surg* 1990;72A:98–103.
62. Staple TW, Jung D, Mork A. Snapping tendon syndrome: Hip tenography with fluoroscopic monitoring. *Radiology* 1988;166:873–874.
63. Staple TW. Arthrographic demonstration of iliopsoas bursa extension of the hip joint. *Radiology* 1972;102:515–516.
64. Sweeney JP, Helms CA, Minagi H, Louie KW. The widened teardrop distance: A plain film indicator of hip joint effusion in adults. *AJR* 1987;149:117–119.
65. Taylor R. Modified AP projection of the anterior bones of the pelvis. *Radiogr Clin Photo* 1941;17:67.
66. Teufel S. Eine gezielte Aufsichtsaufnahme der Hüftgelenkspfanne. *Röntgenpraxis* 1938;10:398.
67. Tile M. Pelvic fractures: Open vs non-operative treatment. *Orthop Clin North Am* 1980;11:423–464.
68. Tile M. Fractures of the acetabulum. *Orthop Clin North Am* 1980;11:481–506.
69. Young JWR, Burgess AR, Brumback RJ, Poka A. Pelvic fractures: Value of plain radiography or early assessment and management. *Radiology* 1986;160:445–451.
70. Young JWR, Burgess AR, Brumback RJ, Poka A. Lateral compression fractures of the pelvis: The importance of plain radiographs in the diagnosis and surgical management. *Skel Radiol* 1986;15:103–109.
71. Zieger MM, Dorr U, Schulz RD. Ultrasonography of hip joint effusions. *Skel Radiol* 1987;16:607–611.

Pelvic Fractures

72. Bassett LW, Gold RH, Epstein HC. Anterior hip dislocation: Atypical superolateral displacement of the femoral head. *AJR* 1983;141:385–386.
73. Bavendam FA, Nedelman SH. Some considerations in roentgenology of fractures and dislocations. *Semin Roentgenol* 1966;1:407–436.
74. Berquist TH. *Imaging of the acutely injured patient.* Baltimore: Urban & Schwartzenburg, 1985.
75. Bonnin JG. Sacral fractures and injury to the cauda equina. *J Bone Joint Surg* 1945;27:113–127.
76. Bowerman JW. *Radiology and injury in sport.* New York: Appleton-Century-Crofts, 1977.
77. Brosman SA, Paul JG. Trauma of the bladder. *Surg Gynecol Obstet* 1976;143:605–608.
78. Buchanan TI. Bowel entrapment by pelvic fracture fragments: A case report and review of the literature. *Clin Orthop* 1980;147:164–166.
79. Bucholz RW. The pathologic anatomy of Malgaigne fracture-dislocations of the pelvis. *J Bone Joint Surg* 1981;63A:400–404.
80. Caudle RJ, Crawford AH. Avulsion fracture of the acetabular margin. *J Bone Joint Surg* 1988;78A:1568–1570.
81. Clark SS, Prudencio RF. Lower urinary tract injury associated with pelvic fractures. *Surg Clin North Am* 1972;52:183–201.
82. Colapinto V. Trauma of the pelvis: Urethral injury. *Clin Orthop* 1980;151:46–55.
83. Colapinto V, McCallum RW. Injury to the male posterior urethra in fractures of the pelvis: A new classification. *J Urol* 1977;118:575–580.
84. Connally WB, Hedberg EA. Fractures and dislocations of the pelvis. *J Trauma* 1969;9:104–111.
85. Cooke CP, Levinsohn EM, Baker BE. Septic hip in pelvic fracture with urologic injury. *Clin Orthop* 1980;147:253–257.
86. Cooper KL, Beabout JW, Swee RG. Insufficiency fractures of the sacrum. *Radiology* 1985;156:15–20.
87. Cooper KL, Beabout JW, McLeod RA. Supra-acetabular insufficiency fracture. *Radiology* 1985;157:15–17.
88. Coventry MB. The treatment of fracture-dislocations of the hip by total hip arthroplasty. *J Bone Joint Surg* 1974;56A:1128–1134.
89. Daffner RH. Pelvic trauma. In: McCort JJ, ed. *Trauma radiology* New York: Churchill Livingstone, 1990.
90. Dunn W, Morris HD. Fractures and dislocations of the pelvis. *J Bone Joint Surg* 1968;50A:1634–1648.
91. Dunn WA, Russo CL. Central acetabular fractures. *J Trauma* 1973;13:695–705.
92. Duverney JG. Traite des maladies des os, vol. 1. Paris: De Bure l'Aine, 1751.
93. Eichenholtz SN, Stark RM. Central acetabular fractures: A review of 35 cases. *J Bone Joint Surg* 1964;46A:695–714.
94. Furey WW. Fractures of the pelvis with special reference to associated fractures of the sacrum. *AJR* 1942;47:89–96.
95. Goodell CL. Neurologic deficits associated with pelvic fractures. *J Neurosurg* 1966;24:837–842.
96. Harley JD, Mack LA, Winquist RA. CT of acetabular fractures: Comparison with conventional radiography. *AJR* 1982;138:413–417.
97. Harris JJ, Harris WH. *The radiology of emergency medicine.* Baltimore: Williams and Wilkins, 1975.
98. Hartmann K. Blasen- und Harnröhrenverletzungen bei Beckenbrüchen. *Arch klin Chir* 1955;282:943.
99. Holdsworth EW. Dislocations and fracture-dislocations of the pelvis. *J Bone Joint Surg* 1948;30B:461–466.
100. Howard FM, Meaney RP. Stress fractures of the pelvis during pregnancy. *J Bone Joint Surg* 1961;43A:538–540.
101. Jackson H, Kam J, Harris JH, et al. The sacral arcuate lines in upper sacral fractures. *Radiology* 1982;145:35–39.
102. Judet R, Judet J, Letournel E. Fractures of the acetabulum: Classification and surgical approaches to reduction. *J Bone Joint Surg* 1964;46A:1615–1646.
103. Kane WJ. Fractures of the pelvis. In: Rockwood CA, Green DP.

Fractures in adults, 2nd ed. Philadelphia: J.B. Lippincott, 1984;1073–1209.
104. Key JA, Conwell HE. Management of fractures, dislocations, and sprains. St. Louis: C. V. Mosby Co., 1951.
105. Knight RA, Smith H. Central acetabular fractures. *J Bone Joint Surg* 1958;49A:1–16.
106. Kvarstein B, Riska EB, Slatis P. Pelvic fractures. *Ann Chir Gynaecol* 1981;70:256–263.
107. Lansinger O. Fractures of the acetabulum: A clinical, radiological, and experimental study. *Acta Orthop Scand* 1977;165:1–94.
108. Letournel E. Surgical repair of acetabular fractures more than three weeks after injury, apart from total hip arthroplasty. *Int Orthop* 1979;2:305–313.
109. Letournel E. Acetabular fractures: Classification and management. *Clin Orthop* 1980;151:81–106.
110. Levine JI, Crampton RS. Major abdominal injury associated with pelvic fractures. *Surg Gynecol Obstet* 1963;116:223.
111. Looser KJ, Crombie HD. Pelvic fracture: An anatomic guide to the severity of injury. A review of 100 cases. *Am J Surg* 1976;132:638–641.
112. Mack LA, Harley D, Winquist RA. CT of acetabular fractures: Analysis of fracture patterns. *AJR* 1982;138:407–412.
113. Mack LA, Duesdieker GA, Harley JD, Bach AW, Winquist RA. CT of acetabular fractures: Postoperative appearances. *AJR* 1983;141:891–894.
114. Margolies MN, Ring EJ, Waltman AC, et al. Arteriography in the management of hemorrhage from pelvic fractures. *N Engl J Med* 1972;287:317–321.
115. McAvoy JM, Cook JH. A treatment plan for rapid assessment of the patient with massive blood loss and pelvic fractures. *Arch Surg* 1978;113:986–990.
116. McMurtry R, Walton D, Dickinson D, et al. Pelvic disruption in the polytraumatized patient. A management protocol. *Clin Orthop* 1980;151:22–30.
117. Miller A, Stedman GH, Beisaw NE, Gross PT. Sciatica caused by avulsion fracture of the ischial tuberosity. *J Bone Joint Surg* 1987;69A:143–144.
118. Mucha P, Welch TJ. Hemorrhage in major pelvic fractures. *Surg Clin North Am* 1988;68:757–773.
119. Mucha P, Farnell MB. Analysis of pelvic fracture management. *J Trauma* 1984;24:379–386.
120. Mucha P. Pelvic fractures. *Probl Gen Surg* 1984;1:154–170.
121. Mucha P, McGanity PLJ. Recognizing and avoiding complications with pelvic fractures. *Inf in Surg Jan* 1985;53–62.
122. Mucha P, Farnell MB. Analysis of pelvic fracture management. *J Trauma* 1984;24:379–386.
123. O'Keefe TJ. Retroperitoneal abscess: A potentially fatal complication of closed fracture of the pelvis. *J Bone Joint Surg* 1978;60A:1117–1121.
124. Paster SB, Van Houten FX, Adams DF. Percutaneous balloon catheter. A technique for control of arterial hemorrhage caused by pelvic fractures. *JAMA* 1974;230:573–575.
125. Patterson FP, Morton KS. Neurological complications of fractures and dislocations of the pelvis. *Surg Gynecol Obstet* 1961;112:702.
126. Pearson JR, Hagedorn EJ. Fractures of the pelvis involving the floor of the acetabulum. *J Bone Joint Surg* 1962;44B:550–561.
127. Peltier LF. Complications associated with fractures of the pelvis. *J Bone Joint Surg* 1965;47A:1060–1064.
128. Pennal GF, Tile M, Waddell JP, Garside H. Pelvic disruption: Assessment and classification. *Clin Orthop* 1980;151:12–21.
129. Perry JF. Pelvic open fractures. *Clin Orthop* 1980;151:41–45.
130. Rankin LM. Fractures of the pelvis. *Ann Surg* 1937;106:226–277.
131. Ring EJ, Athanasoulis C, Waltman AC, et al. Arteriography in management of hemorrhage from pelvic fractures. *Radiology* 1973;109:65–70.
132. Rockwood CA, Green CP. *Fractures in adults.* Philadelphia: J.B. Lippincott Co., 1984.
133. Rogers LF. *Radiology of skeletal trauma.* New York: Churchill Livingstone, 1982.
134. Rothenberger DA, Kellam J, McGonigal D. Open pelvic fractures: A lethal injury. *J Trauma* 1978;18:184–187.
135. Rowe CR, Lowell JD. Prognosis of fractures of the acetabulum. *J Bone Joint Surg* 1961;43A:30–59.
136. Saks BJ. Normal acetabular anatomy for acetabular fracture assessment: CT and plain film correlation. *Radiology* 1986;159:139–145.
137. Sampson J, Berquist TH. Pelvic fractures: A review of 750 cases. Presentation, American Roentgen Ray Society, Las Vegas, NV, 1981.
138. Sandler CM, Hall JT, Rodriguez MB, Corsure JN. Bladder injury in blunt pelvic trauma. *Radiology* 1986;156:633–638.
139. Sandler CM, Harris JH, Corriere JN, et al. Posterior urethral injury after pelvic fracture. *AJR* 1981;137:1233–1237.
140. Sandler CM, Phillips JM, Harris JD, et al. Radiology of the bladder and urethra in blunt pelvic trauma. *Radiol Clin North Am* 1981;19:195.
141. Sauser DD, Billemoria PE, Rouse GA, et al. CT evaluation of hip trauma. *AJR* 1980;138:269–274.
142. Sclafani SJA, Becker JA. Traumatic presacral hemorrhage: Angiographic diagnosis and therapy. *AJR* 1982;138:123–126.
143. Scott WW, Fishman EK, Magid D. Acetabular fractures: Optimal imaging. *Radiology* 1987;165:537–539.
144. Sheldon GF, Winestock DP. Hemorrhage from open pelvic fracture controlled intraoperatively with balloon catheter. *J Trauma* 1978;18:68–70.
145. Silakovich W, Love L. Stress fracture of the pubic ramus. *J Bone Joint Surg* 1954;36A:573–576.
146. Slatis P, Karaharju E. External fixation of unstable pelvic fractures. *Clin Orthop* 1980;171:75–80.
147. Stewart MJ, Milford LW. Fracture-dislocation of the hip. An end result study. *J Bone Joint Surg* 1954;36A:315–341.
148. Taylor RG. Pelvic dislocation. *Brit J Surg* 1942;39:126–132.
149. Thaggard A III, Harle TS, Carlson V. Fractures and dislocations of the bony pelvis and hip. *Semin Roentgenol* 1978;13:117–134.
150. Thompson KR, Goldin AR. Angiographic technique in interventional radiology. *Radiol Clin North Am* 1980;17:375–391.
151. Tile M. Fractures of the acetabulum. *Orthop Clin North Am* 1980;11:481–506.
152. Tile M. Pelvic fractures: Operative vs. non-operative treatment. *Orthop Clin North Am* 1980;11:423–464.
153. Urist MR. Fractures of the acetabulum: The nature of traumatic lesions. Treatment and 2-year end results. *Ann Surg* 1948;127:1150–1164.
154. Watson-Jones R. Dislocations and fracture-dislocations of the pelvis. *Brit J Surg* 1938;25:773–781.
155. Weil GC, Price EM, Rusbridge HW. The diagnosis and treatment of fractures of the pelvis and their complications. *Am J Surg* 1939;44:108–116.
156. Wild JJ, Hanson GJ Jr, Tullos HL. Unstable fractures of the pelvis treated by external fixation. *J Bone Joint Surg* 1982;64A:1010–1019.
157. Young JWR, Burgess AR, Brumback RJ, Poka A. Pelvic fractures: Value of plain radiography in early assessment and management. *Radiology* 1986;160:445–451.
158. Young JWR, Burgess AR. *Radiologic management of pelvic ring fractures.* Baltimore: Urban and Schwarzenberg, 1987.
159. Young JWR, Burgess AR, Brumback RJ, Poka A. Lateral compression fractures of the pelvis: Importance of plain radiographs in diagnosis and surgical management. *Skel Radiol* 1986;15:103–109.
160. Young JWR, Resnick CS. Fractures of the pelvis: Current concepts of classification. *AJR* 1990;155:1169–1175.
161. Zorn G. Beckenbrüche mit Harnröhrenverletzungen ihre Behandlung und Ergebnisse. *Beitr klin Chir* 1960;201:147.

Dislocations and Fracture-Dislocations of the Hip

162. Armstrong JR. Traumatic dislocation of the hip joint. *J Bone Joint Surg* 1948;30B:430–445.
163. Brav EA. Traumatic dislocation of the hip. Army experience and results over a 12-year period. *J Bone Joint Surg* 1962;44A:1115–1134.
164. Chakraborti S, Miller IM. Dislocation of the hip associated with fracture of the femoral head. *Injury* 1975;7:134–142.
165. Dehne E, Immerman EW. Dislocation of the hip combined with

fracture of the shaft of the femur on the same side. *J Bone Joint Surg* 1951;33A:731–745.

166. DeLee JC. Fractures and dislocations of the hip. In: Rockwood CA, Green DP. *Fractures in adults,* vol. 2. Philadelphia: J.B. Lippincott Co., 1984, pp. 1211–1356.

167. DeLee JC, Evans JA, Thomas J. Anterior dislocation of the hip associated with femoral head fractures. *J Bone Joint Surg* 1980;62A:960–964.

168. Dorfman GS, Froelich JA, Groman JJ, Urbanek PJ, Herndon JH. Lower extremity venous thrombosis in patients with acute hip fractures. *AJR* 1990;154:851–855.

169. Dussault RG, Beauregard G, Fauteaux P, Lauren C, Boisjoly A. Femoral head fracture following anterior hip dislocation. *Radiology* 1980;135:627–629.

170. Ehtisham SMA. Traumatic dislocation of the hip joint with fracture of the femoral shaft on the same side. *J Trauma* 1976;16:196–205.

171. Epstein HC. Posterior fracture-dislocation of the hip—comparison of open and closed methods of treatment in certain types. *J Bone Joint Surg* 1961;43A:1079–1098.

172. Epstein HC. Posterior fracture-dislocation of the hip. *J Bone Joint Surg* 1974;56A:1103–1127.

173. Epstein HC. Traumatic dislocation of the hip. *Clin Orthop* 1973;92:116–142.

174. Ghormley RK, Sullivan R. Traumatic dislocation of the hip. *Am J Surg* 1953;85:298–301.

175. Helal B, Skevis X. Concealed traumatic dislocation of the hip. *Proc Roy Soc Med* (Orthop Sec) 1966;59:119.

176. Hougaard K, Thomsen PB. Traumatic posterior fracture dislocation of the hip with fracture of the femoral head, neck or both. *J Bone Joint Surg* 1988;70A:233–238.

177. Keigh JE, Brashear HR, Giulford WB. Stability of posterior fracture-dislocations of the hip. *J Bone Joint Surg* 1988;70A:711–714.

178. Pipkin G. Treatment of Grade IV fracture-dislocations of the hip. *J Bone Joint Surg* 1957;39A:1027–1042.

179. Richardson P, Young JWR, Porter D. CT detection of cortical fracture of the femoral head associated with posterior hip dislocation. *AJR* 1990;155:93–94.

180. Reigstad A. Traumatic dislocation of the hip. *J Trauma* 1980;20:603–606.

181. Roeder LF, DeLee JC. Femoral head fractures associated with posterior hip dislocation. *Clin Orthop* 1980;147:121–130.

182. Rogers LF. *Radiology of skeletal trauma.* New York: Churchhill Livingstone, 1982.

183. Rosenthal RE, Coker WL. Fracture-dislocations of the hip: An epidermiological review. *J Trauma* 1979;19:572–581.

184. Scadden WJ, Dennyson WG. Unreduced obturator dislocation of the hip: A case report. *S Afr Med J* 1978;53:601–602.

185. Scham SM, Fry LR. Traumatic anterior dislocation of the hip with fracture of the femoral head. A case report. *Clin Orthop* 1969;62:133–135.

186. Smith GR, Loop JW. Radiological classification of posterior hip dislocation. *Radiology* 1976;119:569–574.

187. Stewart MJ, Milford LW. Fracture-dislocations of the hip. *J Bone Joint Surg* 1954;36A:315–342.

188. Tehranzadeh J, Vanarthos W, Pais MJ. Osteochondral impaction of the femoral head with associated hip dislocation: CT study in 35 patients. *AJR* 1990;155:1049–1052.

189. Thaggard A III, Harle TS, Carlson V. Fractures and dislocations of the bony pelvis and hips. *Semin Roentgenol* 1978;13:117–134.

190. Thompson VP, Epstein HC. Traumatic dislocation of the hip. *J Bone Joint Surg* 1951;33A:747–778.

191. Urist MR. Fracture-dislocation of the hip joint. *J Bone Joint Surg* 1948;30A:699–727.

Femoral Neck Fractures

192. Ambrose GB, Garcia A, Neer CS. Displaced intracapsular fractures of the neck of the femur. *J Trauma* 1963;3:361–369.

193. Arnoldi CC, Lemperg RK. Fractures of the femoral neck. *Clin Orthop* 1977;129:217–222.

194. Asnis SE, Shoji H, Bohne WHO. Scintimetric evaluation of complications of femoral neck fractures. *Clin Orthop* 1976;121:149–156.

195. Banks HH. Factors influencing the results in fractures of the femoral neck. *J Bone Joint Surg* 1962;44A:931–964.

196. Barnes R, Brown J, Garden RS, Nicoll EA. Subcapital fractures of the femur. A prospective review. *J Bone Joint Surg* 1976;58B:2–24.

197. Bassett LW, Mirra JM, Craccholo A, Gold RH. Ischemic necrosis of the femoral head. Correlation of magnetic resonance imaging and histologic sections. *Clin Orthop* 1987;233:181–187.

198. Bayliss AP, Davidson JK. Traumatic osteonecrosis of the head of the femur following intracapsular fractures: Incidence and earliest radiographic features. *Clin Radiol* 1977;28:407–414.

199. Berquist TH. *Magnetic resonance of the musculoskeletal system.* New York: Raven Press, 1990.

200. Bobechko WP, Harris WR. The radiographic density of avascular bone. *J Bone Joint Surg* 1960;42B:626–632.

201. Bowerman J. *Radiology and injury in sports.* New York: Appleton Century-Crofts, 1977.

202. Coats RL, Armour P. Treatment of subcapital femoral fractures by total hip replacement. *Injury* 1979;11:132–135.

203. De Haas W, Macnab I. Fractures of the neck of the femur. *S Afr Med J* 1956;30:1005–1010.

204. Dunn WL, Wahner HW, Riggs BL. Measurement of bone minimal content in human vertebra and hip by dual-photon absorptiometry. *Radiology* 1980;136:485–487.

205. Ficat P, Arlet J. Diagnostic de l'ostéo-necrose fémorocapitale primitive au stade I (stade pré-radiologique). *Rev Chir Orthop* 1968;54:637.

206. Garden RS. Stability and union of subcapital fractures of the femur. *J Bone Joint Surg* 1964;46B:630–712.

207. Garden RS. Reduction and fixation of subcapital fractures of the femur. *Orthop Clin North Am* 1974;5:683–712.

208. Griffiths WEG, Swanson SA, Freeman MAR. Experimental fatigue fractures of the femoral neck. *J Bone Joint Surg* 1971;54B:136–143.

209. Hanson BA, Solgaard S. Impacted fractures of the femoral neck treated by early mobilization and weight-bearing. *Acta Orthop Scand* 1978;49:180–185.

210. Harper M, Neustorf J. Fractures of the femoral neck associated with technical errors in closed medullary nailing of the femur. *J Bone Joint Surg* 1986;68A:624–626.

211. Hungerford DS. Pathogenic consideration in ischemic necrosis of bone. *Can J Surg* 1981;24:583–586.

212. Jeffrey CC. Spontaneous fracture of the femoral neck. *Orthop Clin North Am* 1974;5:713–727.

213. Markisz JA, Knowles RJR, Altchek DW, Schneider R, Whalen JP, Cahill PT. Segmental patterns of avascular necrosis of the femoral heads: Early detection with MR imaging. *Radiology* 1987;162:717–720.

214. Mitchell DG, Kressel HY, Arger PH, Dalinka M, Spritzer CE, Steinberg ME. Avascular necrosis of the femoral head: Morphologic assessment by MR imaging with CT correlation. *Radiology* 1986;161:739–742.

215. Meyers MH. Impacted and undisplaced femoral neck fractures. The hip. *Proceedings of the Tenth Open Scientific Meeting of the Hip Society.* St. Louis: C. V. Mosby Co., 1982.

216. Norman A, Bullough P. The radiolucent crescent sign. An early diagnostic sign of necrosis of the femoral head. *Bull Hosp Jt Dis Orthop Inst* 1963;24:99–104.

217. Pauwel F. Der Schenkelausbruch: ein mechanishes Problem. Grundlagen des heilungsvorganges Prognose und kausale Therapie. Stuttgart: Ferdinande Enke, 1935.

218. Phemister DB. Bone growth and repair. *Ann Surg* 1935;102:261.

219. Richardson ML, Kilcoyne RF, Mayo RA, Lamont JG, Hastrup W. Radiographic evaluation of modern fixation devices. *Radiographics* 1987;7:685–701.

220. Rubin R, Trent P, Arnold W, et al. Knowles pinning of experimental femoral neck fractures: Biomechanical study. *J Trauma* 1981;21:1036–1039.

221. Salvati EA, Wilson PD. Long-term results of the femoral-head replacement. *J Bone Joint Surg* 1972;55A:1355–1356.

222. Scheck M. Intracapsular fractures of the femoral neck. Commin-

ution of the posterior cortex as a cause of unstable fracture. *J Bone Joint Surg* 1959;41A:1187–1200.
223. Schultz RJ. *The language of fractures.* Baltimore: Williams and Wilkins, 1972.
224. Sikorski JM, Barrington R. Internal fixation versus hemiarthroplasty for the displaced subcapital fracture of the femur: A prospective, randomized study. *J Bone Joint Surg* 1981;63B:356–361.
225. Smith K, Bonfiglio M, Montgomery W. Nontraumatic necrosis of the femoral head treated with tibial bone grafting: Follow-up note. *J Bone Joint Surg* 1980;62A:845–847.
226. Söreide O, Mölster A, Raugstad TS. Internal fixation versus primary prosthetic replacement in acute femoral neck fractures: A prospective, randomized clinical study. *Br J Surg* 1979;66:56–60.
227. Stevens J, Freeman PA, Nordin BEC, et al. The incidence of osteoporosis in patients with femoral neck fractures. *J Bone Joint Surg* 1962;44B:520–527.
228. Turner A, Taylor JF, Casty H, Owen R. The radiographic evaluation of multiple pin fixation of the femoral head. *Br J Radiol* 1984;57:887–890.
229. White BL, Fisher WD, Laurin CA. Rate of mortality for elderly patients after fracture of the hip in the 1980s. *J Bone Joint Surg* 1987;69A:1335–1340.

Trochanteric Fractures

230. Bertin KC, Horstman J, Coleman SS. Isolated fracture of the lesser trochanter in adults: An initial manifestation of metastatic disease. *J Bone Joint Surg* 1984;66A:770–773.
231. Boyd HB, Griffin LL. Classification and treatment of trochanteric fractures. *Arch Surg* 1949;58:853–866.
232. Brodell JD, Leve AR. Disengagement and intrapelvic protrusion of the screw from a sliding screw-plate device. *J Bone Joint Surg* 1983;65A:697–700.
233. Chapman MW, Bowman WE, Csongradi JJ, Day LJ, Trafton PG, Bovidl EG. The use of Ender's pins in extracapsular fractures of the hip. *J Bone Joint Surg* 1981;63A:14–28.
234. DeLee JC. Fractures and dislocations of the hip. In: Rockwood CA, Green DP. *Fractures in Adults,* vol. 2. Philadelphia: J.B. Lippincott, 1984, pp. 1211–1356.
235. Dimon JH, Hughston JC. Unstable intertrochanteric fractures of the hip. *J Bone Joint Surg* 1967;49A:440–450.
236. Ender HG. Treatment of trochanteric and subtrochanteric fractures of the femur with Ender pins. The hip. *Proceedings of the Sixth Open Scientific Meeting of the Hip Society.* St. Louis: C. V. Mosby Co., 1978.
237. Evans EM. The treatment of trochanteric fractures of the femur. *J Bone Joint Surg* 1949;31B:190–203.
238. Fielding JW. Subtrochanteric fractures. *Clin Orthop* 1973;92:86–99.
239. Haentjens P, Castileyn PP, DeBoeck H, Handelberg F, Opdecain P. Treatment of unstable intertrochanteric and subtrochanteric fractures in elderly patients. *J Bone Joint Surg* 1989;71A:1214–1224.
240. Hafner RHV. Trochanteric fractures of the femur. *J Bone Joint Surg* 1951;33B:513–516.
241. Harrington K, Sim FH, Enis JE, et al. Methyl methacrylate as adjunct in internal fixation of pathologic fractures: Experience in 375 cases. *J Bone Joint Surg* 1976;58A:1047.
242. Heyse-Moore GH, MacEachern AG, Evans DC. Treatment of intertrochanteric fractures of the femur. A comparison of the Richards screw-plate with the Jewett nail-plate. *J Bone Joint Surg* 1983;65B:262–267.
243. Jensen JS. Classification of trochanteric fractures. *Acta Orthop Scand* 1980;51:803–810.
244. Jensen JS, Michaelsen M. Trochanteric fractures treated with McLaughlin osteosynthesis. *Acta Orthop Scand* 1975;46:795–803.
245. Kock JC. The laws of bone architecture. *Am J Anat* 1917;21:177–298.
246. Kuderna H, Böhler N, Collon DJ. Treatment of intertrochanteric and subtrochanteric fractures of the femur by the Ender method. *J Bone Joint Surg* 1976;58A:604–611.

247. Kyle RF, Gustilo RB, Premer RF. Analysis of 622 intertrochanteric hip fractures. *J Bone Joint Surg* 1979;61A:216–221.
248. Lord G, Marotte JH, Blantard JP, et al. Head and neck arthroplasty in treatment of intertrochanteric fractures after age 70. *Rev Chir Orthop* 1977;63:135–148.
249. May JMB, Chacha PB. Displacement of trochanteric fractures and their influence on reduction. *J Bone Joint Surg* 1968;50B:318–323.
250. Mickelson MR, Bonfiglio M. Pathologic fractures of the proximal part of the femur treated by Zickel nail fixation. *J Bone Joint Surg* 1976;58A:1067–1070.
251. Mulholland RC, Gunn DR. Sliding screw-plate fixation of intertrochanteric femoral fractures. *J Trauma* 1975;12:581–591.
252. Naimark A, Kossoff J, Schepsis A. Intertrochanteric fractures: Current concepts on an old subject. *AJR* 1979;133:889–894.
253. Pankovich AM, Tarabishy I. Ender nailing of intertrochanteric and subtrochanteric femoral fractures. *J Bone Joint Surg* 1980;62A:635–645.
254. Rasmussen K. McLaughlin osteosynthesis in trochanteric fractures. *Acta Chir Scand* 1953;108:246.
255. Richardson ML, Kilcoyne RF, Mayo KA, Lamont JG, Hastrup W. Radiographic evaluation of modern fixation devices. *Radiographics* 1987;7:685–701.
256. Rogers LF. *Radiology of skeletal trauma.* New York: Churchill Livingstone, 1982.
257. Rybicki EF, Simonen FA, Weis EG Jr. On the mathematical analysis of stress in the human femur. *J Biomech* 1972;5:203–215.
258. Sarmiento A, Williams EM. Unstable trochanteric fracture: Treatment with valgus osteotomy and I-beam nail-plate: Preliminary report of 100 cases. *J Bone Joint Surg* 1970;52A:1309–1318.
259. Sartoris DJ, Kerr R, Goergen T, Resnick D. Sliding-screw plate fixation of proximal femoral fractures. *Skel Radiol* 1985;14:104–110.
260. Schatzker J. Methyl methacrylate as adjunct in internal fixation of intertrochanteric fractures of the femur. *Can J Surg* 1979; 22:179–182.
261. Seinsheimer F. Subtrochanteric fractures of the femur. *J Bone Joint Surg* 1978;60A:300–306.
262. Sernbo I, Johnell O, Gentz C, Nelsson J. Unstable intertrochanteric fractures of the hip. *J Bone Joint Surg* 1988;70A:1297–1303.
263. Wade PA, Campbell RD, Kerin RJ. Management of intertrochanteric fractures of the femur. *Am J Surg* 1959;97:634–643.
264. Whatley JR, Garland DE, Whitecloud T III, et al. Subtrochanteric fracture of the femur: Treatment with ASIF blade-plate fixation. *South Med J* 1978;71:1372–1375.
265. Yelton C, Low W. Ictrogenic subtrochanteric fracture: A complication of Zickel nails. *J Bone Joint Surg* 1986;68A:1237–1240.
266. Zickel RE, Bercik MJ, Licciardi LM. A continuing study on the use of the Zickel intramedullary appliances in fractures and lesions of the proximal femur. The hip. *Proceedings of the Sixth Open Scientific Meeting of the Hip Society.* St. Louis: C. V. Mosby Co., 1978.
267. Zickel RE, Mouradin WH. Intramedullary fixation of pathologic fractures in lesions of the subtrochanteric region of the femur. *J Bone Joint Surg* 1976;58A:1061–1066.

Evaluating Soft Tissue Trauma

268. Berman L, Catterall A, Meire HB. Ultrasound of the hip: A review of applications of a new technique. *Br J Radiol* 1986;59:13–17.
269. Berquist TH. *Magnetic resonance of the musculoskeletal system.* Raven Press: New York, 1990.
270. Dihlmann W, Nebel G. Computed tomography of the hip joint capsule. *J Compt Assist Tomogr* 1983;7:278–285.
271. Ghelman B, Freiberger RH. The adult hip. In: Freiberger RH, Kaye JJ, eds. *Arthrography.* New York: Appleton-Century-Crofts, 1979.
272. Glynn TP, Kreiphe DL, DeRosa GP. Computed tomography arthrography in traumatic hip dislocation. *Skel Radiol* 1989;18:29–31.

273. Kevin A, Levine J. A technique for arthrography. *Skeletal Radiol* 1981;6:11.
274. Lequesne M, Becker J, Bard M, et al. Capsular constriction of the hip: Arthrographic and clinical considerations. *Skeletal Radiol* 1981;6:1–10.
275. Lyons JC, Peterson LFA. The snapping iliopsoas tendon. *Mayo Clin Proc* 1984;59:327–329.
276. McCauley RGK, Wunderlich BK, Zimbler S. Air embolism as a complication of hip arthrography. *Skeletal Radiol* 1981;6:11–13.
277. Moule NJ, Golding JR. Idiopathic chondrolysis of the hip. *Clin Radiol* 1974;25:247–251.
278. Patterson I. Torn acetabular labrum. *J Bone Joint Surg* 1957;39B:306–309.
279. Penkava RR. Iliopsoas bursitis demonstrated by computed tomography. *AJR* 1980;135:175–176.
280. Pritchard RS, Shah HR, Nelson CL, FitzRandolph RL. MR and CT appearance of iliopsoas bursal distension secondary to diseased hips. *J Comp Assist Tomogr* 1990;14:797–808.
281. Razzano CD, Nelson CL, Wilds AH. Arthrography of the adult hip. *Clin Orthop* 1974;99:86–93.
282. Resnick D, Niwayama G. *Diagnosis of bone and joint disorders.* Philadelphia: W. B. Saunders Co., 1988.
283. Sartoris DJ, Danzig L, Gilula L, Greenway G, Resnick D. Synovial cysts of the hip joint and iliopsoas bursitis. *Skel Radiol* 1985;14:85–94.
284. Silver SF, Connell DG, Duncan CP. Case report 550. *Skel Radiol* 1989;18:327–328.
285. Spataro RF, Katsberg RW, Burgeron FA, et al. Epinephrine enhanced knee arthrography. *Invest Radiol* 1978;13:286.
286. Speer KP, Spritzer CE, Harrelson JM, Nunley JA. Magnetic resonance imaging of the femoral head after acute intracapsular fracture of the femoral neck. *J Bone Joint Surg* 1990;72A:98–103.
287. Staple TW. Arthrographic demonstration of iliopsoas bursa extension of the hip joint. *Radiology* 1972;102:515–516.
288. Staple TW, Jung D, Mork A. Snapping tendon syndrome: Hip tenography with fluoroscopic monitoring. *Radiology* 1988;166:873–874.
289. Sweeney JP, Helms CA, Minagi H, Louie KW. The widened teardrop distance: A plain film indicator of hip joint effusion in adults. *AJR* 1987;149:117–119.
290. Warren R, Kaye JJ, Salvati EA. Arthrographic demonstration of an enlarged iliopsoas bursa complicating osteoarthritis of the hip. *J Bone Joint Surg* 1975;57A:413–415.
291. Zieger MM, Dörr U, Schultz RD. Ultrasonography of hip joint effusions. *Skel Radiol* 1987;16:607–611.

Imaging of Orthopedic Trauma,
Second Edition, edited by T.H. Berquist,
Mayo Clinic © 1992. Published
by Raven Press, Ltd., New York.

CHAPTER 6

The Femur and Thigh

Claire E. Bender, Donald C. Campbell II, and Thomas H. Berquist

Anatomy, 311
Femoral Shaft Fractures, 314
   Mechanism of Injury, 314
   Classifications of Femoral Shaft Injuries, 315
   Radiographic Evaluation, 317

Treatment Methods, 318
Complications, 326
Soft Tissue Injuries, 329
References, 332

The femur is the longest, largest, and strongest bone in the body. Because of its length, width, and role as a primary weight-bearing bone, it must tolerate the extremes of axial loading and angulatory stresses. Massive musculature envelops the femur. This musculature provides abundant blood supply to the bone, which also allows great potential for healing. Thus, the most significant problem relating to femoral shaft fractures is not healing, but restoration of bone length and alignment so that the femoral shaft will tolerate the functional stresses demanded of it (33).

The soft tissue compartments of the thigh are large and accommodate significant hemorrhage and edema. However, isolated soft tissue injury or injury in association with fracture or fracture treatment are not uncommon in the thigh (1,2,20,26,27).

ANATOMY

The shaft of the femur is tubular in shape (Fig. 6-1). It is generally smooth, except for the linea aspera, which is a prominent posterior longitudinal ridge extending from the intertrochanteric crest inferiorly to the middle half of the femur, where it diverges into a medial and lateral lip to become the respective supracondylar lines. The pectineal line extends from the lesser trochanter between the gluteal tuberosity and upper medial lip of linea aspera

inferiorly to blend with this lip or the middle part of the linea (21). The body of the femoral shaft is slightly bowed anteriorly (Fig. 6-1C). In standing position, the femoral shaft normally inclines medially about 10°. Structurally, the femur can resist angulating forces. But, as a tubular structure, its design is not the best for resisting torsional forces (21,33).

Multiple muscle groups surround the femoral shaft (Fig. 6-2). Hip flexors, extensors, and abductors and knee flexor and extensor groups provide a bulk of soft tissue protection. The muscles of the thigh are divided into three fascial compartments (35,39). The anterior compartment includes the quadriceps femoris, sartorius, iliopsoas, and pectineal muscles. Neurovascular structures include the femoral artery, vein, and nerve (Fig. 6-3) (21,35). The medial compartment contains the gracilis, adductor group, and obturator externus. The deep femoral artery and vein are also included in the medial compartment. The posterior compartment (Fig. 6-3) contains the sciatic nerve and hamstring muscles. The three compartments are separated by the lateral and medial septa (Fig. 6-3) (21,35,39).

Blood supply to the femoral shaft is through metaphyseal, periosteal, and endosteal vessels. The very rich periosteal blood supply is from the large surrounding muscles and is interrupted only in injuries in which extensive stripping has occurred. The nutrient arteries are perforating vessels that originate from the profunda femoris artery. The perforating branches encircle the femur posteriorly and perforate the muscle attachments adjacent to the linea aspera. Usually, there are four perforating branches. The lower part of the femur is supplied by a long, descending branch of the nutrient artery in the in-

   C. E. Bender, D. C. Campbell II: Departments of Diagnostic Radiology and Orthopedic Surgery, Mayo Medical School, Mayo Clinic, Rochester, Minnesota 55905.
   T. H. Berquist: Department of Diagnostic Radiology, Mayo Medical School, Mayo Clinic Jacksonville, Jacksonville, Florida 32224.

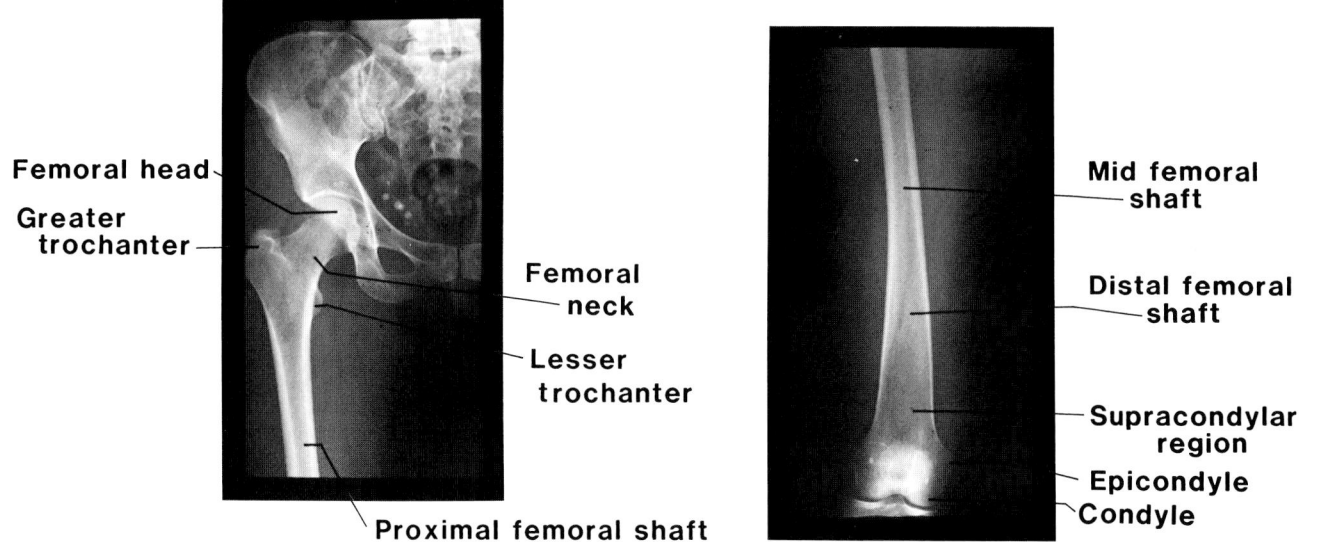

Femoral head
Greater trochanter
Femoral neck
Lesser trochanter
Proximal femoral shaft

A

Mid femoral shaft
Distal femoral shaft
Supracondylar region
Epicondyle
Condyle

B

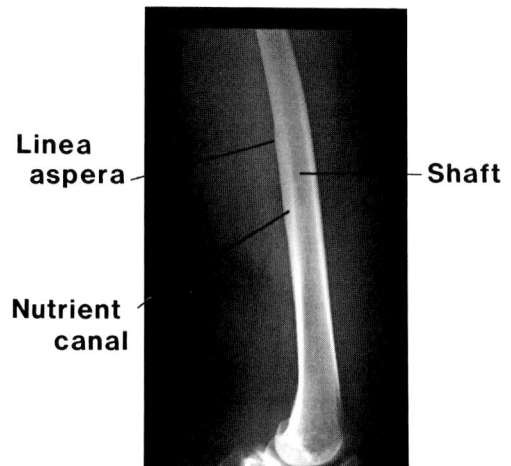

Linea aspera
Shaft
Nutrient canal

C

FIG. 6-1. Normal AP (**A, B**) and lateral (**C**) views of the femur.

THE FEMUR AND THIGH / 313

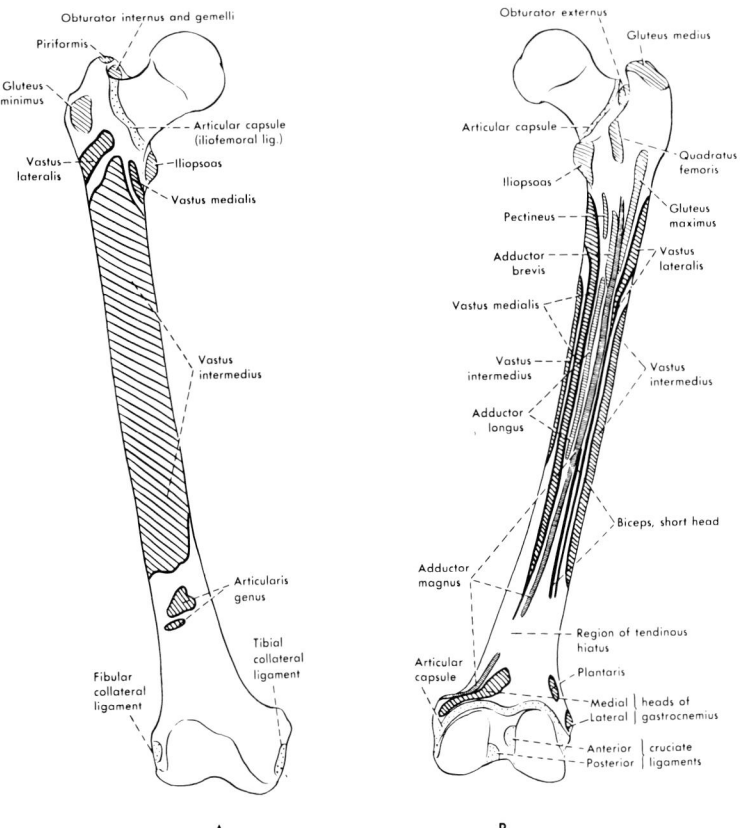

FIG. 6-2. A: Anterior muscle attachments of femur. **B:** Posterior muscle attachments of femur (from 21, with permission).

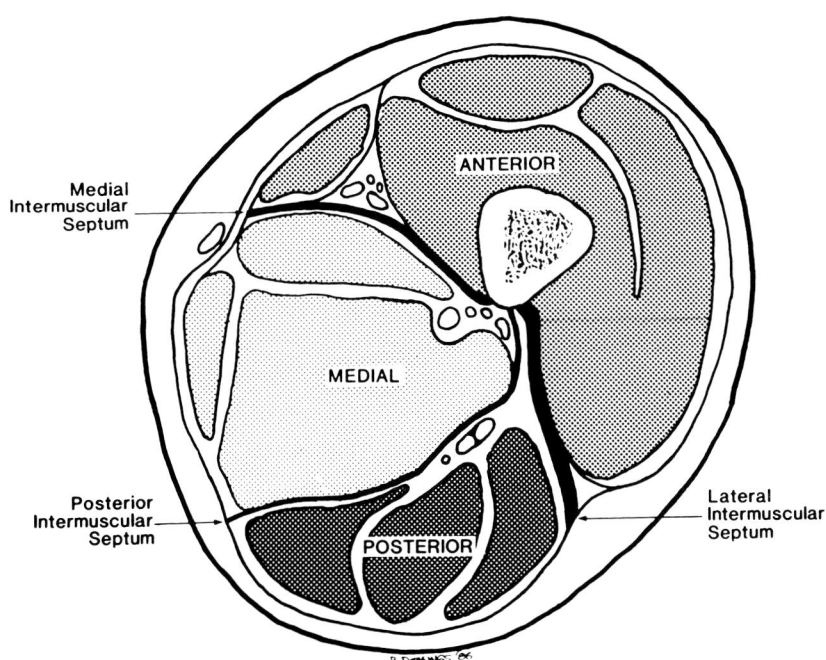

FIG. 6-3. Illustration of the fascial compartments of the thigh (from 39, with permission).

tramedullary canal (21). The main femoral artery, which is located medially to the shaft, perforates the adductor hiatus. With distal skeletal injury, this may be the site of vascular injury.

The sciatic nerve, well-cushioned medially and posteriorly in the thigh, is rarely injured at the shaft level.

FEMORAL SHAFT FRACTURES

Mechanism of Injury

Major external violence, as encountered in trauma from motor vehicle accidents, is the usual mechanism of injury. Young adults and children are predominantly injured. The metaphyseal areas in the younger population are wider and dissipate stress better than the diaphysis. Thus, fracture of the femoral shaft is more likely to occur. However, in aging bones or in patients with metabolic bone disease, the metaphyseal areas are more brittle and more susceptible to fracture than the diaphysis. Fractures in patients with upper femoral fixation devices or arthroplasty of the hip or knee tend to fracture at the edge of the component (11,22,28). Because severe violence is often involved in the production of femoral shaft fractures, significant soft tissue damage usually occurs as well.

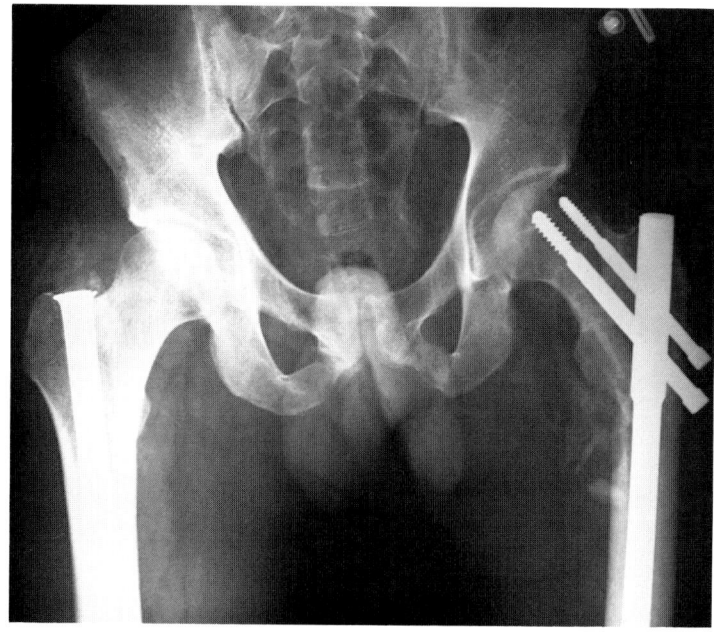

A

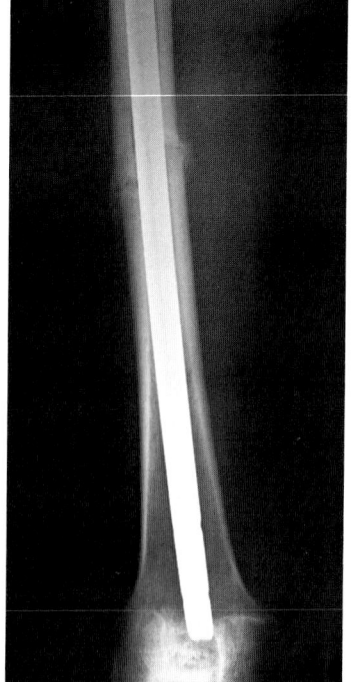

B

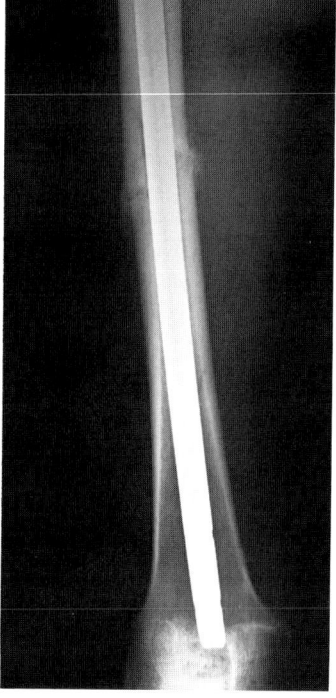

C

FIG. 6-4. AP views of the pelvis and upper femurs (**A**), right femoral shaft (**B**), and lateral views (**C**) demonstrate a healing Winquist Type I fracture with medullary nail fixation. There is an associated comminuted subtrochanteric fracture on the left with two interlocking pins in position.

Classifications of Femoral Shaft Injuries

Fractures may be either open or closed. Open fractures suggest greater injury to both bone and soft tissues. Open fractures may result from external damage to the soft tissues or from extrusion of fracture fragments from the inside outward.

Soft tissue injury classification is difficult on routine radiographs but it is important to be familiar with these orthopedic categorizations because of their implications for treatment. Grade I and II open fractures have less tissue distraction and wound contamination. Grade IIIA and IIIB open fractures have extensive soft tissue, periosteal, and bone involvement. This results in higher risk of infection with any method of fixation (6).

Simple fractures may be transverse, oblique, or spiral. With greater injury force, segmental or comminuted fractures may occur. Occasionally, subtle linear fractures along the shaft may be present that are not visible radiographically. These are important to recognize if internal fixation is contemplated (23). If these fractures go undetected, the simple fracture may be converted to a comminuted type secondary to shattering of bone during attempts at fixation. Winquist and Hansen (45,46) devised a commonly used classification system for femoral shaft fractures. The classification is based on circumferential

cortical contact. Type I fractures have a small comminuted fragment with greater than 50% cortical contact (Fig. 6-4). Type II fractures are more comminuted but maintain a greater than 50% cortical apposition (Fig. 6-5). With Type III fractures, there is less than 50% cortical contact resulting in less stability and increased rotation, shortening, and translation (Fig. 6-6). Type IV fractures are severely comminuted with no cortical contact at the fracture site (7,8,45,46).

Fractures of the femoral shaft may also be classified according to the type of force that produced the fracture. Angulation forces produce transverse fractures, transverse fractures with butterfly fragments, and segmental fractures; torsional forces produce oblique and spiral oblique fractures; impaction forces produce comminuted or segmental fractures; and penetrating forces may result in bone loss (40).

Finally, fractures may be classified according to location. Fractures of the middle third of the shaft are most common. At this level, overriding of fracture fragments and shortening of the limb usually result (45,46). The displacement of the fracture may be the result of muscle pull. The proximal fragment may be rotated outward because of the forces of gravity and external rotator muscles (21,25). In fractures of the upper third, the proximal fragment tends to be flexed by the iliopsoas, abducted by

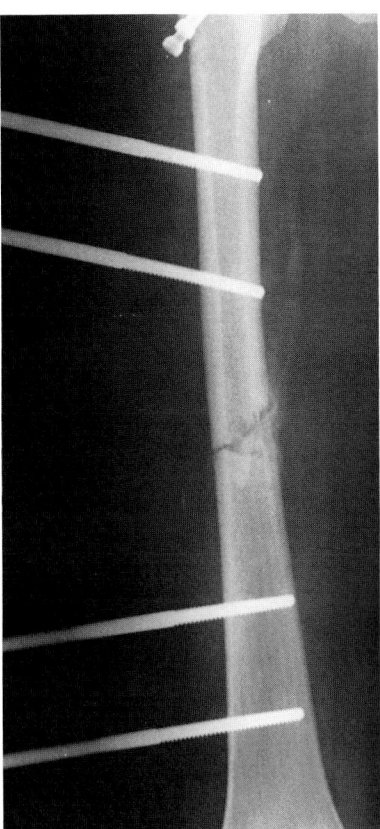 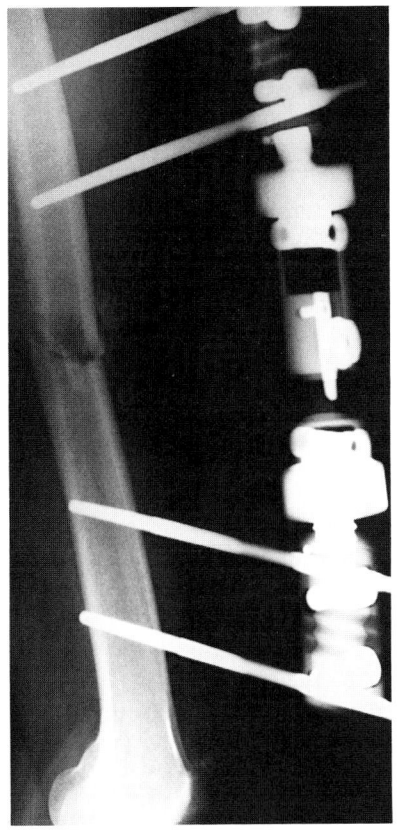

A   B

FIG. 6-5. Combined femoral neck and Type II femoral shaft fractures on the right. AP view of the femur with three canulated pins fixing the femoral neck fracture. There is comminution of the midshaft femoral fracture with normal alignment and cortical contact. External fixation pins are in position above and below the fracture site. Lateral view (**B**) after attachment of the external fixateur shows only slight posterior angulation.

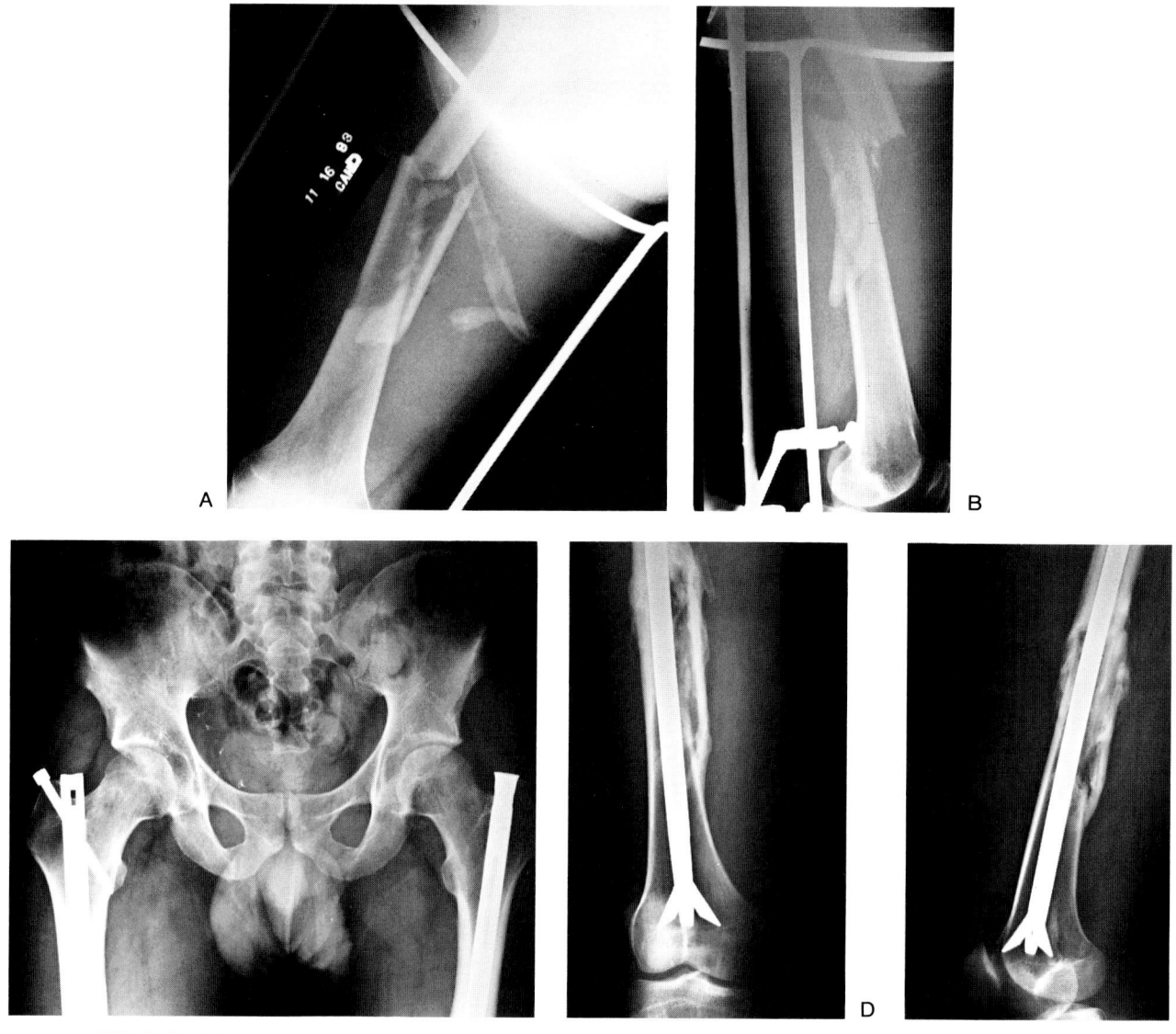

FIG. 6–6. AP (**A**) and lateral (**B**) views of a comminuted, overriding fracture of the midshaft of the right femur (Type III). Six months following treatment with a Brooker-Wills locking medullary nail the AP pelvis (**C**) and AP (**D**) and lateral femur (**E**) show the fracture has healed. Note there is also a medullary rod on the left from an earlier fracture.

the gluteus medius and gluteus maximus, and externally rotated by the short rotators and the forces of gravity. The distal fragment may be adducted by the pull of the adductor muscles. In fractures of the lower third of the shaft, shortening and displacement can occur. Posterior displacement of the distal fragment occurs because of the action of the gastrocnemius, popliteus, and plantaris muscles. Injury to the popliteal vessels may occur (21,33).

Combination injuries involving the ipsilateral femoral neck and tibia are not uncommon (38,42). Associated femoral neck fractures may be very subtle. Swiontkowski et al. (38) reviewed 83 patients with femoral shaft fractures. Sixty-two patients had associated femoral neck fractures and one-third were initially overlooked (Fig. 6-5). Combined femoral shaft and tibial fractures are frequently open injuries (58%) requiring extensive surgical reconstruction. In addition, life threatening injuries to the head, chest, and abdomen are common (10–20%), and mortality rates may reach 15% (42).

Radiographic Evaluation

The clinical diagnosis of femoral shaft fractures is usually quite easy. Angular deformity, shortening, and pain are readily apparent. An expanding thigh is a sign of hemorrhage and should alert physicians to the possibility of shock and/or compartment syndrome (12,35,37,39).

Standardized views of the femoral shaft include AP and lateral projections (Fig. 6-7; see Fig. 6-1), using the Potter-Bucky technique. It is mandatory that the adjacent hip and knee joints be included on the films because of the significant incidence of associated ipsilateral injuries. The tibia, fibula, and foot and ankle should also be examined carefully and radiographs obtained if necessary.

The AP view of the femur (Fig. 6-7A) is obtained with the patient supine, legs extended. The unaffected leg should be slightly abducted. The foot is internally rotated approximately 15° in order to position the patella anteriorly and to minimize anteversion of the femoral

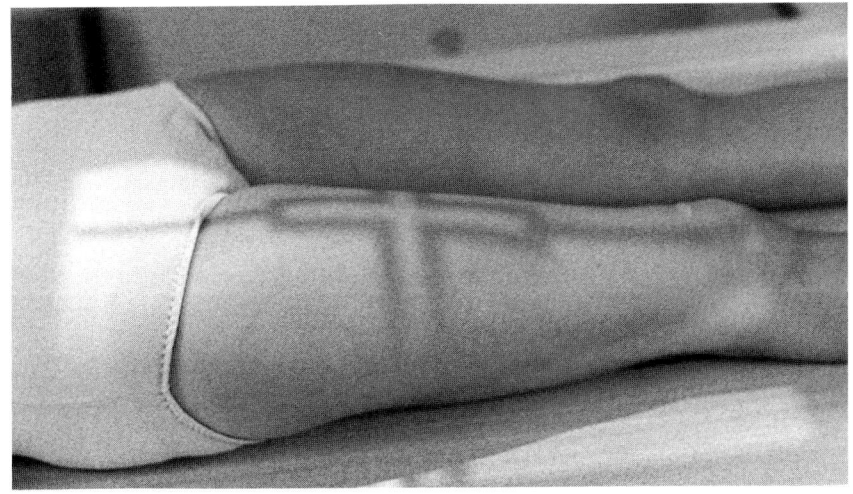

A

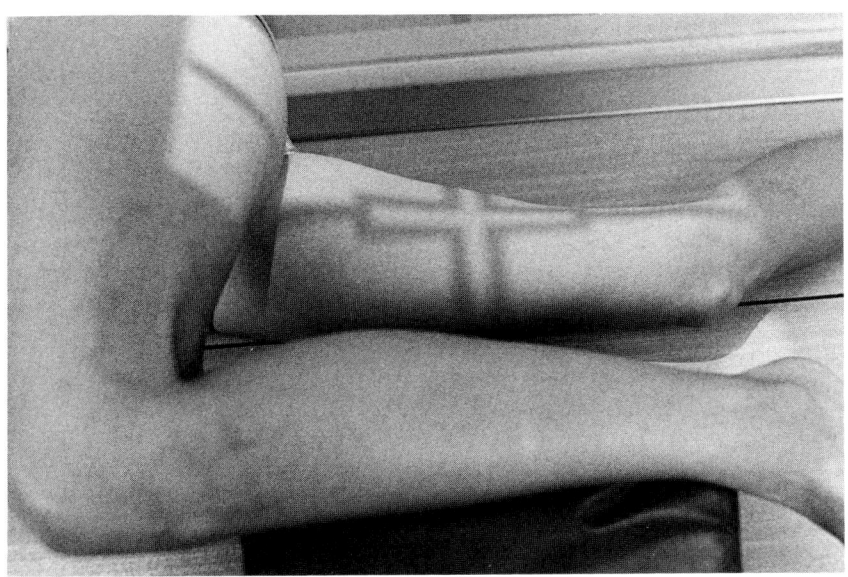

B

FIG. 6–7. Patient positioned for AP (A) and lateral (B) views of the femur.

neck. The central x-ray beam is directed vertically to the midpoint of the cassette. Soft tissues of the thigh must be included on the film. In this way, subcutaneous air or hematomas are readily detected. With larger patients, it is necessary to radiograph the upper and lower femurs separately. The central beam is directed perpendicularly to the film in each case.

The lateral view is obtained with the patient turned onto the affected side. The uppermost knee is flexed and placed on a large pad in front of the involved extremity. The pelvis is then adjusted for a true lateral position. The involved dependent knee is slightly flexed. The central beam is directed perpendicularly to the midpoint of the film. A severely injured patient is not moved because of the danger of fracture displacement. A grid-front cassette is then placed along the medial or lateral aspect of the thigh and knee, with the central beam directed horizontally and perpendicularly to the cassette. Only the knee is usually included on this film. Proximal femur evaluation is performed with lateral hip views. X-ray examination of the hip is essential; femoral neck fracture, dislocation and acetabular fractures may be present. A lead apron is used for gonadal shielding.

Because of the severity of injury or its association with multiple skeletal injuries, true AP and lateral views often cannot be obtained. Careful attention to the position of the bony landmarks of the hip and knee and width of the cortex of the opposing fracture fragments will alert the physician to rotational deformity. Additional techniques such as tomography, computerized tomography (CT), and magnetic resonance imaging (MRI) are not generally required in the acute setting.

Treatment Methods

Fracture of the femoral shaft is often the result of major violence. Additional bony injuries to the patient often occur and must also be treated. Any patient with a fracture of the femoral shaft is a potential candidate for shock. Immediate treatment of this complication must be carried out as the clinical situation indicates. Prompt splinting will reduce bleeding, additional soft tissue injury, and pain.

The basic principles in treatment of femoral shaft fractures are restoration of position and alignment, maintenance of length, immobilization until bone union occurs, and restoration of normal function after union. Apposition of bone fragments is required for union and acceptable alignment is necessary to minimize disabling deformities. Shortening of one-quarter inch is well tolerated without hip or knee disability; shortening of greater than 1.5 inches should be considered unacceptable (5–8,38,42).

While all agree that definitive treatment should begin as soon as possible for bone union to occur, the manage-

ment of femoral shaft fractures is complex and remains controversial. Historically, in the first three decades of the century, fracture management has evolved from traction, body casts, and bracing to the wide use of internal fixation and back again to nonoperative management of cases in which operative complications present significant risk (5,18,24,47). Moreover, no single treatment applies to all fractures at the same anatomic level. Important considerations before institution of therapy include severity or comminution of fracture, soft tissue damage, and the patient's age, medical and physical condition, occupation, and associated injuries (femoral neck and tibial fractures). In this survey various methods of treatment of femoral shaft fractures will be discussed.

Traction and Casting

Over 500 years ago, skin traction was used as the primary treatment method. During the Civil War in the United States, adhesive plaster was used for traction, which became known as *Buck's extension*. Today, traction splinting is best used in the emergency treatment of femoral shaft fractures. The current application consists of traction applied to the foot and ankle with countertraction in the groin.

Skeletal traction is useful for the primary immobilization of a fracture of the femoral shaft when an operation must be delayed because of severity of injury and additional trauma (40). This is the method of choice for highly comminuted fractures in which the surgeon cannot obtain good fixation and immobilization. Usually, a traction pin is placed either through the proximal tibia about 2 inches below the joint line or through the distal femur at the level of the adductor tubercle (Fig. 6-8). Suspension of the involved extremity with the knee flexed demands careful consideration and care. The position with the knee flexed is a more comfortable position and more adequately reduces muscle forces, allowing easier alignment of the fracture (1). Skeletal traction is indicated for oblique and transverse fractures when conditions preclude operation.

There are many disadvantages to skeletal traction. Prolonged bedrest and convalescence are required (5). With excessive traction, distraction may contribute to delayed union or non-union. With traction, the incidence of malunion, delayed union, and non-union is greater than with internal fixation. Pin tract infections may occur. Decubitus ulcers and other complications related to the immobilization of the patient also often occur. Hospitalization is usually prolonged when compared with treatments using cast bracing or internal fixation (5,40).

Treatment of femoral shaft fractures with skeletal traction requires periodic radiographic evaluation. Careful portable AP and lateral films should be obtained fre-

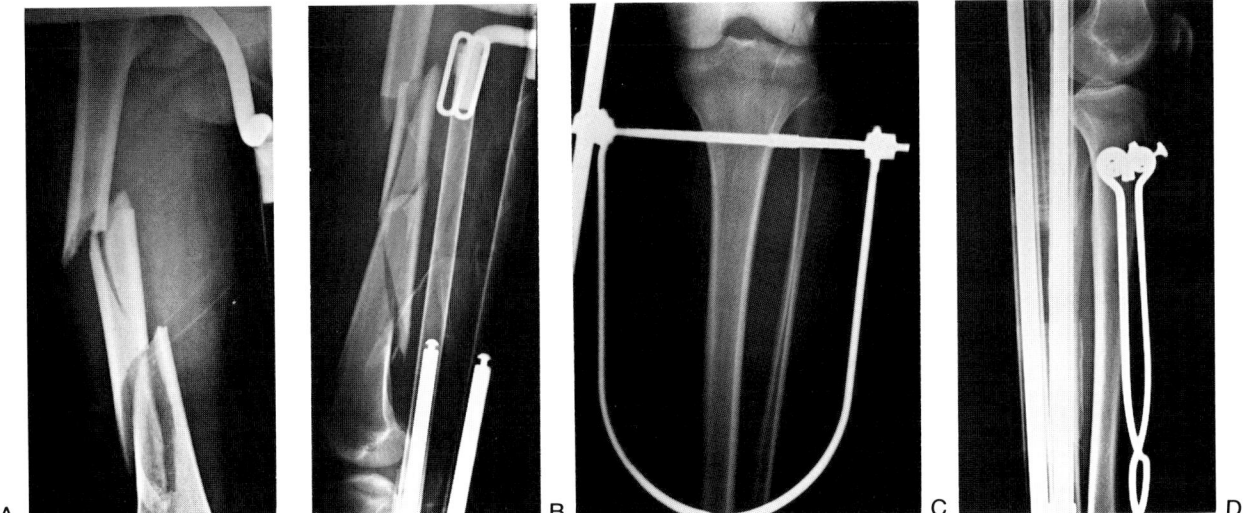

FIG. 6–8. AP (**A**) and lateral (**B**) views of a comminuted femoral shaft fracture. AP (**C**) and lateral (**D**) views with traction pin in proximal tibia.

quently during the early course of treatment. Angulation, rotation, distraction, and overriding of fracture fragments must be corrected. Errors can be avoided by standardizing the AP and lateral views with each patient.

Treatment of fractures of the femoral shaft by casting is one of the oldest forms of therapy. In certain patients, it is even mandatory and probably lifesaving. Immobilization in a cast is indicated in uncontrollable patients (i.e., patients with head injury) and in patients with severe wounds and severe infections of the back and buttock (40).

Disadvantages of cast treatment include discomfort, prolonged immobilization and convalescence, joint stiffness, muscle atrophy, and increased possibility of delayed union, non-union, and malunion (18).

The cast brace technique (Fig. 6-9) avoids some of these disadvantages. Although favored by many orthopedists, its use remains controversial. Advantages of this treatment include early knee motion and ambulation and avoidance of surgical complications. Frequent radiographic follow up is necessary in order to avoid unacceptable results. Preliminary skeletal traction is also controversial, but it is generally recommended for unstable fractures. Cast brace treatment is most useful for fractures at or distal to the midshaft level. The purpose of the cast brace is to provide a total contact capsule about the thigh, allowing the muscles to exert a hydrodynamic stabilizing effect on the fracture (33). Suspension of the cast brace is obtained by casting the foot and leg and incorporating polycentric joints at the level of the knee. A skele-

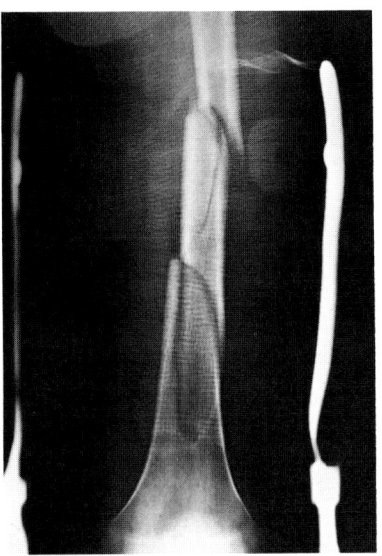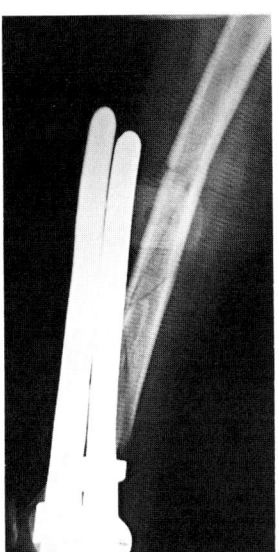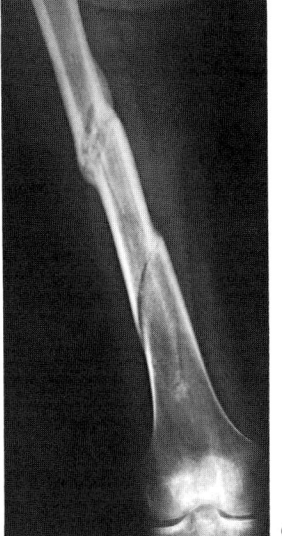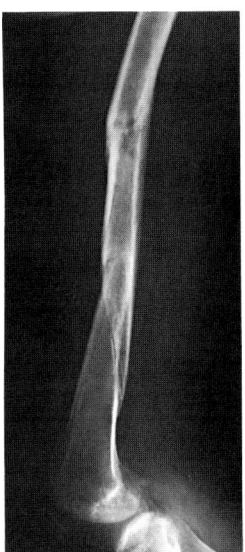

FIG. 6–9. Cast-bracing seen on AP (**A**) and lateral (**B**) views (same patient as in Fig. 6-8). AP (**C**) and lateral (**D**) views four months after injury demonstrated healing.

tal traction pin inserted for preliminary traction may be incorporated into the cast during the early period. Correction of angular malalignment can be obtained by wedging the cast in the early period. The length of time required in the cast brace is usually 8–10 weeks.

Internal Fixation

Internal fixation is also a primary means of treatment of femoral shaft fractures. Various methods of internal fixation include use of intramedullary nail, occasionally supplemented with wires, screws, or, rarely, plates; use of dual plates placed at right angles to each other on the femoral shaft; and bone grafting. Occasionally, a bone graft may be fixed to the femoral shaft with screws or wire. When considering internal fixation, the orthopedic surgeon must evaluate the geometry of the fracture and then choose a method appropriate for that particular fracture.

The Küntscher intramedullary nail (Fig. 6-10) is best designed for fractures of the middle shaft. With this device, stresses are shared by both the appliance and the bone. The cross-sectional design of the Küntscher nail is a hollow cloverleaf pattern. This allows the nail to be compressed in the narrowest portion of the intramedullary canal. Other rods are available with cross-sectional shapes of diamonds, flanges, or squares and are thought to have improved mechanical qualities and to provide better control of rotation (47). These devices have also been experimentally shown not to engage and compress the entire endosteal ring, thus allowing endosteal revascularization (32). The interlocking nail is a modification of the hollow intramedullary nail and is becoming popular. It permits fixation of the proximal or distal fracture fragment, or both at once, by placing a transverse screw through the bone and through the nail itself (Fig. 6-11). This technique reduces rotation at the fracture site and also controls shortening. Both static and dynamic methods are employed. Radiographic assessment of the cortex (Winquist classification) is important in choosing the proper technique. Static interlocking nails are used with more comminuted injuries with little cortical opposition (Fig. 6-11 and 6-12). When cortical contact is able to support a portion of the stress (Winquist Types I and II) screws are used on only one side of the fracture (Fig. 6-4). This allows impaction of the cortical portion of the fracture (7,24). It is possible, therefore, to use the technique of intramedullary nail fixation in fractures that would otherwise be too comminuted for this method (3,5–8,19,38,42).

Other intramedullary devices include flexible round Rush pins and Ender nails (Fig. 6-13). These devices are inserted without reaming and therefore produce less endosteal damage. Ender nailing is typically reserved for patients with simple transverse or short oblique fractures with general cortical opposition (Fig. 6-15D–H) (29).

Each method has its advantages and drawbacks. Intramedullary nailing is the procedure of choice in certain fractures of the middle three-fifths of the femoral shaft. This is especially true in closed fractures with fracture surfaces that permit interlocking of the fracture fragments, thus preventing rotation following reduction (Winquist Type I and II). Often these fractures can be reduced closed, and the intramedullary rod can be inserted through a small incision at the greater trochanter. Fractures of the proximal or distal femoral shaft may require additional postoperative external immobilization. Comminution and obliquity of the fracture are relative contraindications to intramedullary nail fixation. Additional fixation with wire (Fig. 6-14), screws, or plates may be necessary to attain rigid immobilization. Wire fixation has limitations; it affords limited stability and may loosen in the postoperative period. Also, if the type of metal used in the wire differs from that used in the nail, electrolysis may occur. Interfragmentary fixation with screws may increase stability. Although plates can be added to attempt further stabilization, the combination of intramedullary rodding and plating will disrupt both periosteal and endosteal circulation, increasing the risk of delayed union or non-union (30).

The advantages of intramedullary nailing, especially with closed technique, include the relatively small incision, preservation of the soft tissue envelope, early periosteal callus, early weight-bearing and ambulation, decreased joint stiffness, reduced risk of infection, and shorter hospitalization (6–8,19,24).

Plate fixation (Fig. 6-15) as a primary method of femoral shaft fracture treatment remains controversial (33). Most advocates include unusual comminution or location of fractures as indications for its use, making intramedullary nailing impractical. Plating does permit anatomic reconstruction of bone, but at the same time a large operative wound is necessary. Bone fragments may be devitalized, increasing the risk of infection and delayed healing. The plate also functions as a load-bearing device and is thus susceptible to fatigue and fracture (Fig. 6-15D, E). Intramedullary fixation, a load-bearing system, allows maximal bone impact and minimal stress on the device (44,45). In rare cases, it may be judged that plate fixation is the best method of treatment but that a single plate will be inadequate. In such a case, double plates may be utilized, positioned parallel to one another. These plates are oriented approximately 90° apart on the circumference of the femoral shaft. If double plates are used, they should not be of the same length in order to avoid stress concentration at the ends of the plates. In some patients, bone quality may be so poor that the purchase of the screws in the bone is inadequate. In these cases it may be helpful to utilize methyl methac-

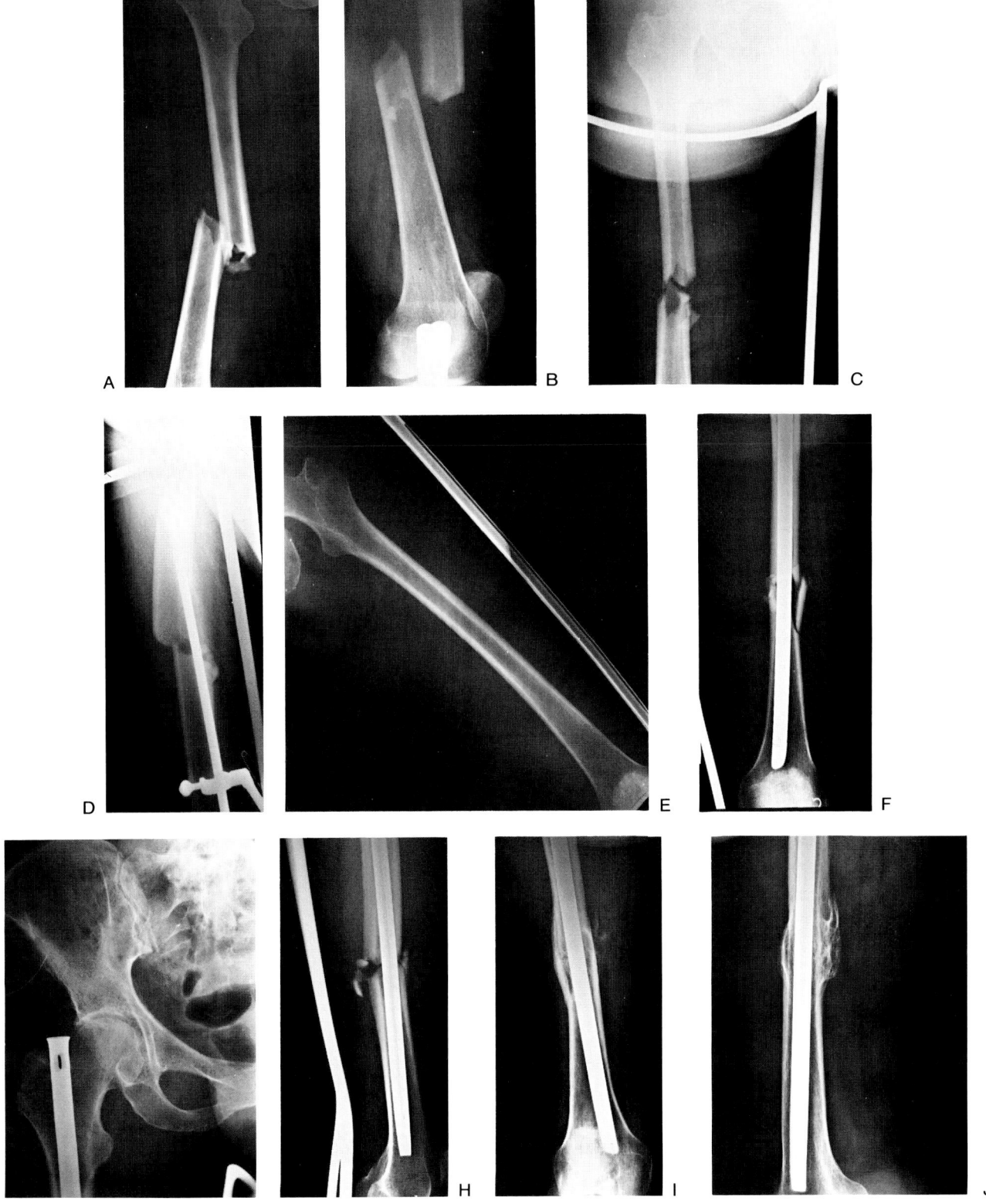

FIG. 6–10. Comminuted fracture (Winquist Type IV): AP (**A**) and lateral (**B**) views of a midshaft with overriding and rotation of fracture. Skeletal traction (**C** and **D**) shows improved alignment but a gap between the fragments. **E:** Preoperative film measuring IM rod with normal intramedullary canal. Immediate postop films to check rod placement (**F, G, H**). **I** and **J:** 20 months following surgery, the fracture is united.

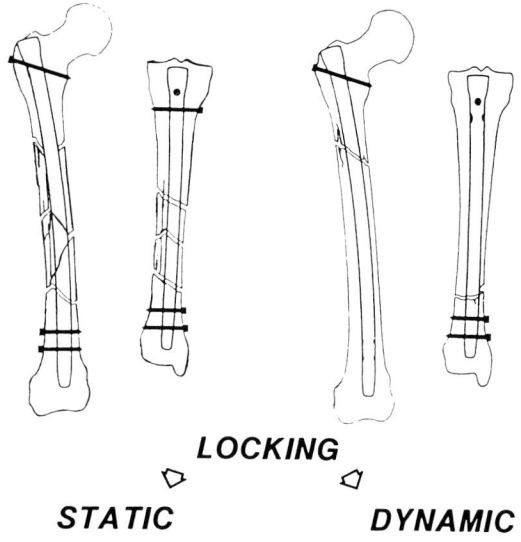

LOCKING

◁   ◁

STATIC   DYNAMIC

FIG. 6–11. Illustration of static and dynamic interlocking medullary nailing. Static locking places screws above and below the fracture preventing rotation and axial sliding. Dynamic locking places screws on one side of the fracture, which prevents rotation but allows compression of fragments with weight-bearing (from 24, with permission).

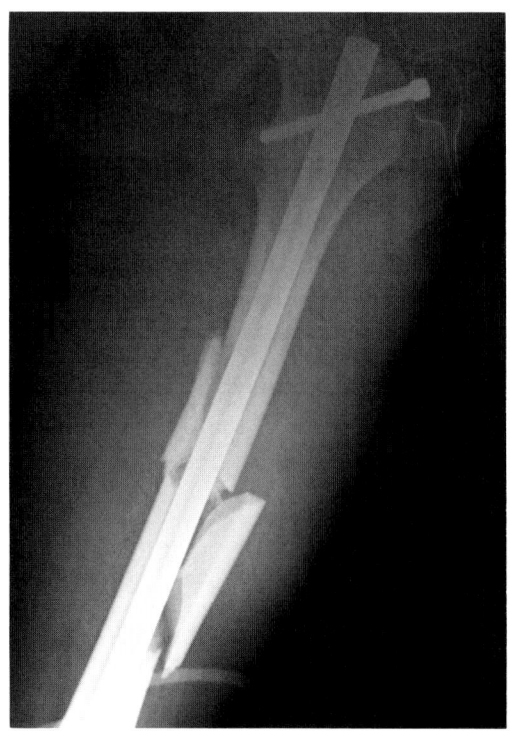

A

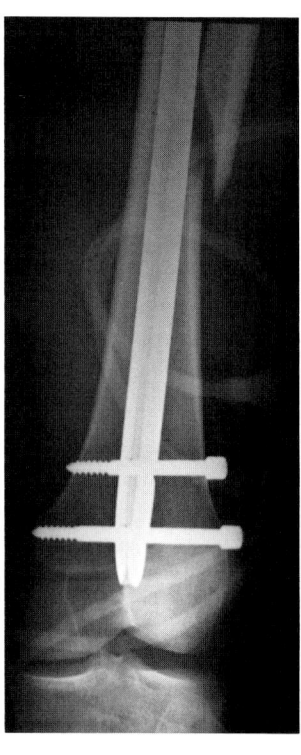

B

FIG. 6–12. High velocity comminuted fracture of the mid-femur (Type IV) with static interlocking nail fixation. AP views of the upper (**A**) and lower (**B**) femur show displaced fragments with good alignment of the femur and interlocking screws above and below the fracture.

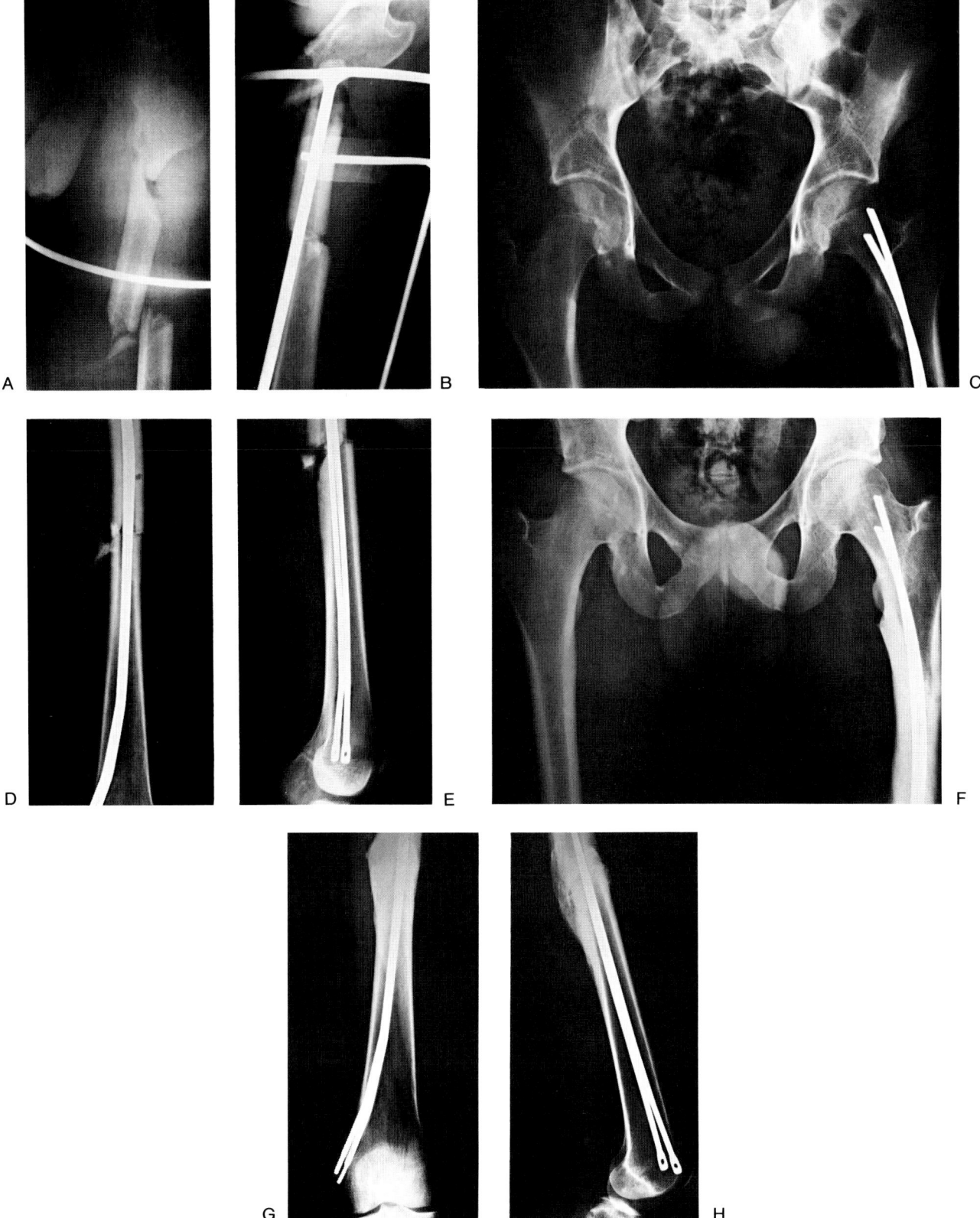

FIG. 6-13. AP (**A**) and lateral (**B**) views of a comminuted fracture of the proximal femur in traction. AP (**C,** **D**) and lateral (**E**) views following Ender rodding. AP (**F, G**) and lateral (**H**) views one year following surgery show the fracture has healed.

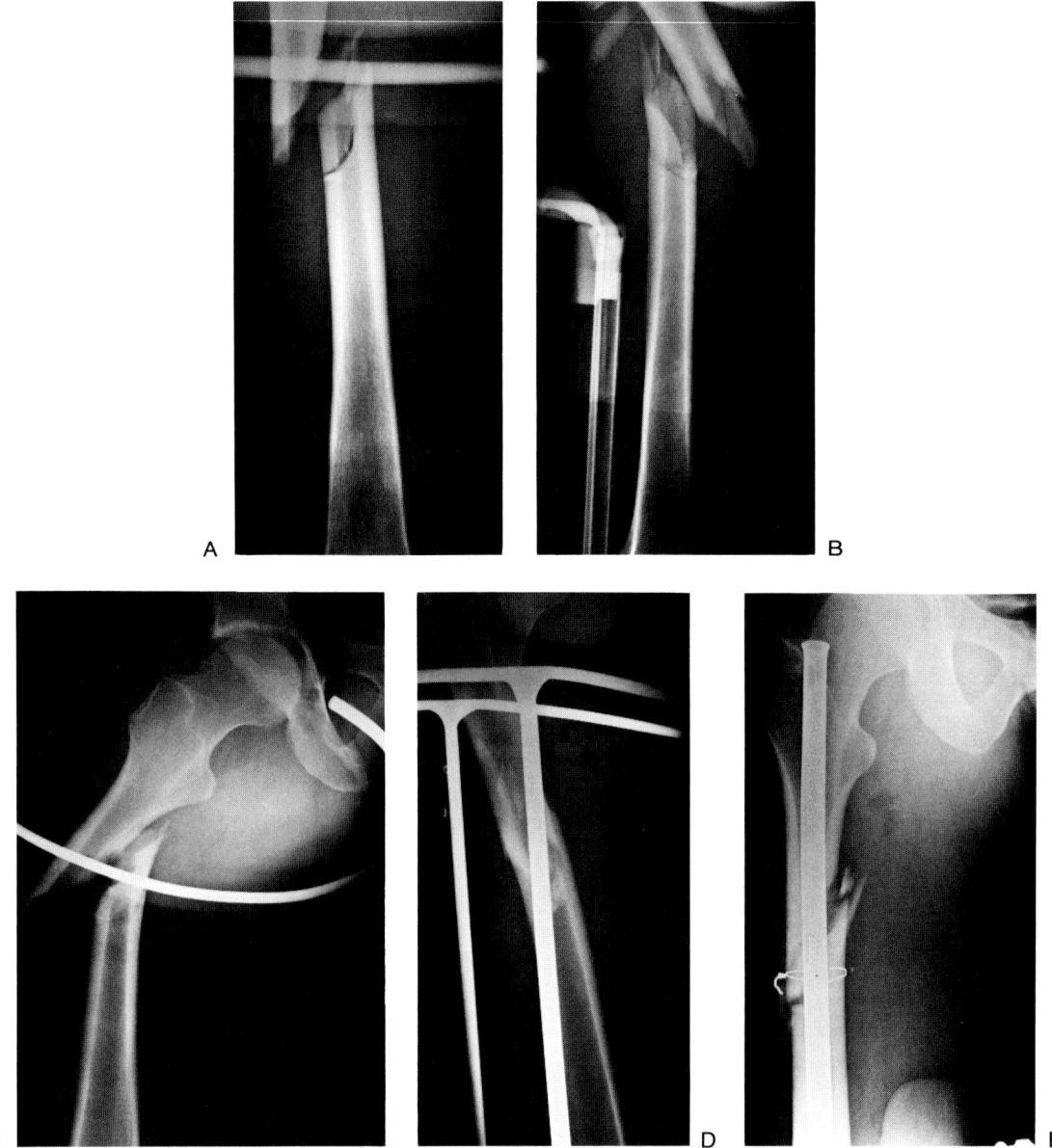

FIG. 6–14. Initial AP (**A**) and lateral (**B**) views of an oblique fracture proximal femoral shaft with angulation and displacement. Three days later AP (**C**) and lateral (**D**) views show lack of reduction with abduction of the proximal fragment. The fracture was reduced with an intramedullary rod and cerclage wire (**E**).

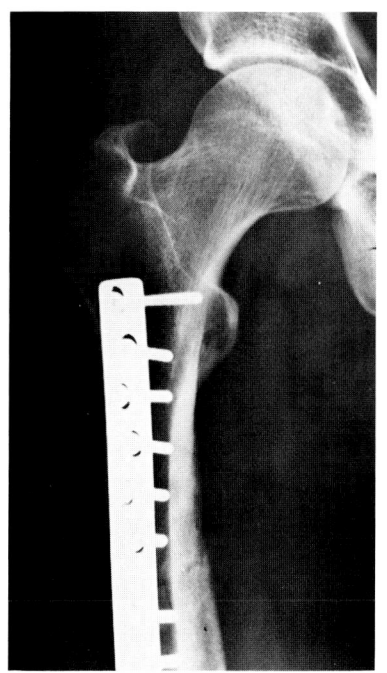

A

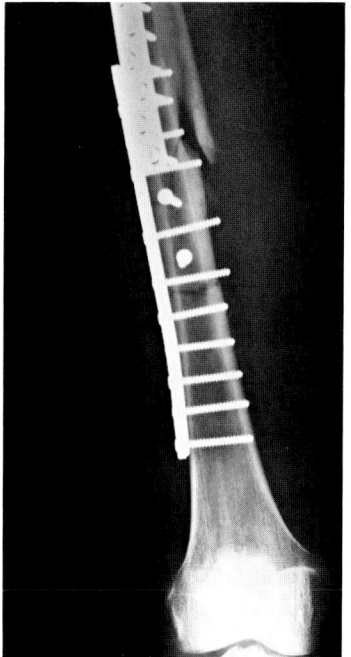

B

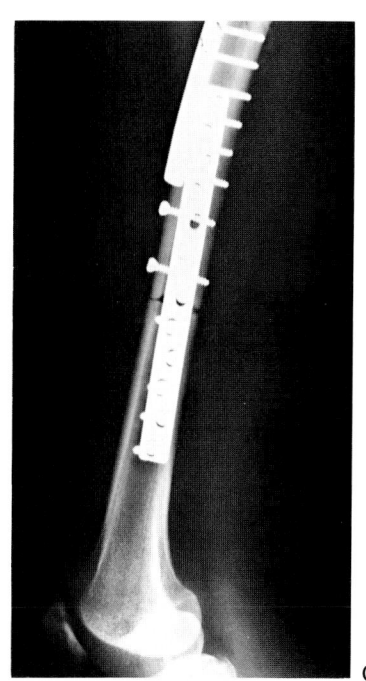

C

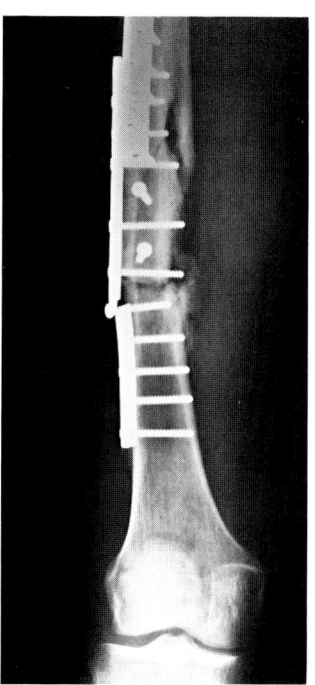

D

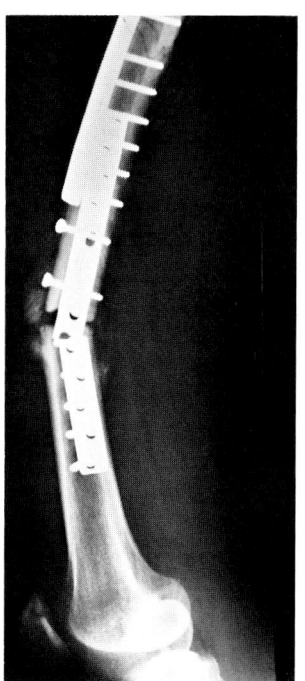

E

FIG. 6–15. Comminuted fracture of the femoral shaft with two plates and segmental screws demonstrated on the AP (**A, B**) and lateral (**C**) views of the femur. AP (**D**) and lateral (**E**) views three months after surgery demonstrate fracture of the lower plate with anterior angulation of the lower fracture.

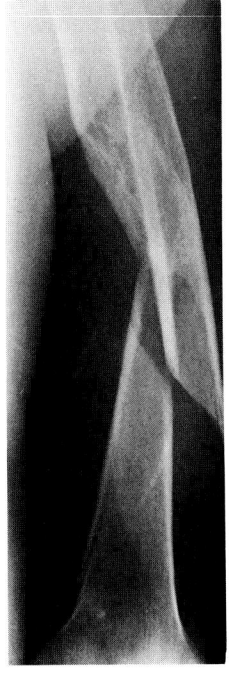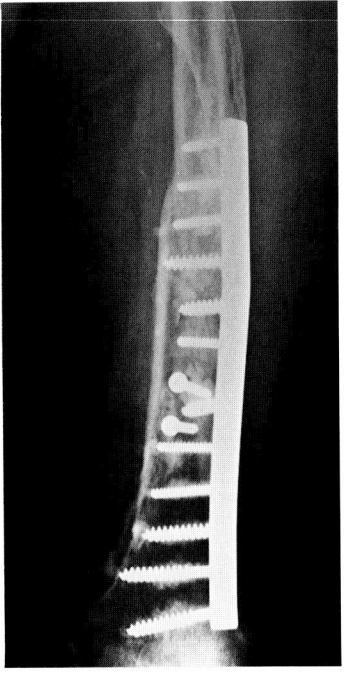

A B

FIG. 6–16. A: Spiral fracture of the distal femoral shaft with an old fracture deformity proximally. **B:** Fixation with interfragmentary lag screws and plate screws. Methyl methacrylate cement was used to enhance fixation.

rylate bone cement, which is injected into the screw holes, to better anchor the screws (Fig. 6-16). Femoral fractures treated by plating usually require special protective measures following surgery. These may consist of casts, braces, and restricted weight-bearing.

Bone grafts play a role in fracture treatment. The goal of bone grafting is to expedite union and to decrease the incidence of non-union. Autogenous bone grafts are more desirable than homogeneous grafts. Autogenous corticocancellous bone may be particularly useful. Vascularized fibular grafts (Fig. 6-17) are useful when reconstruction of bone defects is necessary.

Complications

All methods of treatment of femoral shaft fractures carry the risk of major complications (Table 6-1). These include infection and refracture (6). Refracture occurs in approximately 6% of femoral fractures treated by closed methods and in 1% of those treated by open methods. Such fractures usually consist of simple stress fractures without displacement. Treatment with protected weight-bearing and support using a cast brace or other device is usually sufficient. In addition, fixation devices may undergo bending, migration, or breakage.

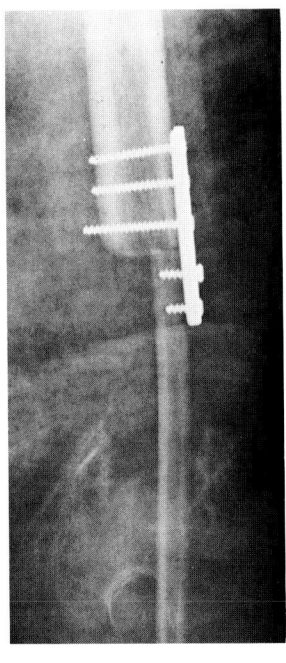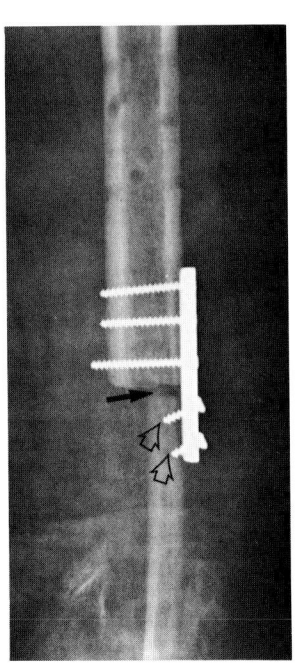

A B

FIG. 6–17. A: High velocity injury resulted in distal femoral shaft loss. Lower extremity length is maintained by fibular graft with proximal internal fixation. **B:** Five days later separation of proximal graft occurred (*black arrow*). Note shift of distal two plate screws (*open arrows*).

TABLE 6-1. *Femoral shaft fractures*

Complications

Local
    Osseous
        Refracture
        Fracture of fixation devices
        Non-union
        Mal-union
        Delayed union
        Associated fractures
        Infection
        Avascular necrosis (AVN) of femoral head
        Leg length discrepancy
    Soft Tissue
        Compartment syndrome
        Venous thrombosis
        Arterial injury
        Neural injury
Systemic
    Distant fractures
    Fat emboli
    Pulmonary emboli
    Acute respiratory distress syndrome (ARDS)
    Pneumonia
    Head injury
    Abdominal injury

[a] (5–8,15,17,28,29,35,38).

Vascular injuries may occur at the time of fracture or during treatment. Thrombosis, laceration, false aneurysm formation, and arteriovenous fistula formation are potential complications. Arterial injuries are more common in fractures of the distal third of the shaft and in the supracondylar region (12,35).

Nerve injury is quite rare at the time of initial injury because of the protective role that the large muscle mass provides. Most frequently, the peroneal nerve is injured as a result of prolonged or poorly monitored traction. Damage may occur to this nerve at the head of the fibula.

Rarely, nerve injury occurs due to surgical trauma or improperly placed fixation devices (Fig. 6-18).

Other soft tissue complications such as compartment syndrome may also occur (12,35). On occasion, pain presenting as bursitis, or snapping of the iliotibial band may develop due to the prominent heads on interlocking screws (Fig. 6-12). Removal of screws, preferably after fracture healing is complete, may be necessary. Brumback et al. (8) reported that screw removal was necessary in 7% of 85 patients treated with static or dynamic interlocking medullary nails.

Non-union of the femoral shaft occurs in 1% of cases (10). Factors influencing non-union include inadequate fixation, insufficient immobilization, excessive traction with distraction, and wound infection following internal fixation (33). Treatment requires proper immobilization and therefore consists of intramedullary rodding or plating, often with bone grafting (Fig. 6-19). Electrical stimulation is a controversial but increasingly common adjunct to treatment of fracture non-unions. Loss of reduction can potentially occur with any treatment method. This complication is less frequent with interlocking intramedullary nailing (5–8).

Malunion is more common than non-union. Because of unequal muscle forces, there is a tendency for angulation. Malunion is often associated with skeletal traction and plaster cast treatment of these fractures (33,38).

Delayed union is not uncommon in uncomplicated fracture management. Persistent bone pain and tenderness are the mainstay of clinical diagnosis. Radiographically, the diagnosis is usually obvious. Treatment usually consists of improved external support and ambulatory care.

A serious complication of femoral shaft fractures is the unrecognized injury to the ipsilateral hip (Fig. 6-20), knee, tibia, and fibula. These injuries are not uncommon, and early detection and treatment are important.

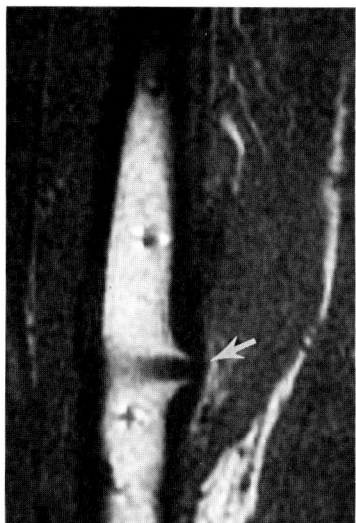
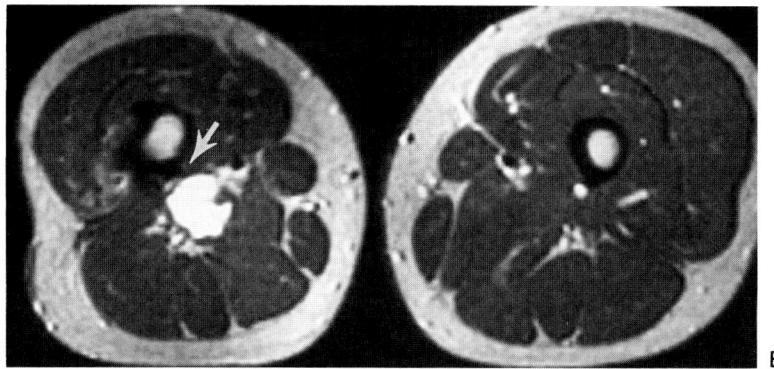

FIG. 6-18. Patient with chronic thigh pain after plate and screw fixation of a femoral fracture. The fixation devices were removed. Sagittal SE 500/20 image (**A**) shows old pin tracts with cortical deformity (*arrow*) posteriorly. Axial SE 2000/60 image (**B**) demonstrates a post traumatic neuroma in the same region as the cortical defect (*arrow*).

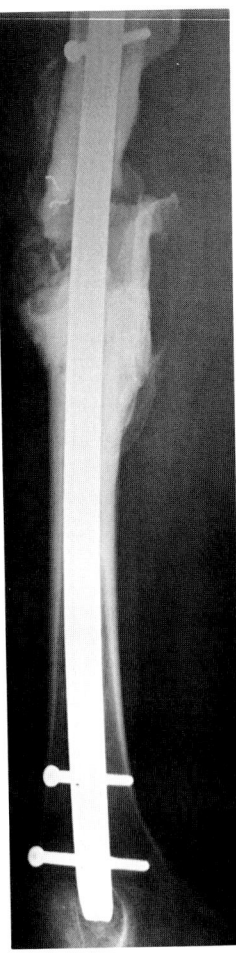

FIG. 6-19. Ununited upper femoral fracture. Treatment with a static interlocking medullary nail and bone grafting was instituted.

They are usually associated with severe trauma, such as in motor vehicle accidents. Ipsilateral hip dislocation is usually posterior. This may be accompanied by acetabular fracture as well. Early recognition favors reduction and decreases the incidence of avascular necrosis of the femoral head.

Concomitant fracture of the ipsilateral hip and leg can also occur without femoral shaft fractures and can easily be overlooked at the time of injury. Separate AP and lateral radiographs of the hip, knee, and leg should be obtained in any patient who has localized pain as well as in the critically injured patient. Thorough repeated examination of the entire patient is the best method for detecting associated injuries.

The incidence of bilateral femoral fractures is 7% (3). Treatment is controversial and more difficult than for isolated femoral shaft fractures. In general, intramedullary fixation is more strongly indicated in such cases.

Systemic complications also occur. These problems may be related to the acute injury, treatment, or prolonged hospitalization (Table 6-1) (5,34,35,38,41–43). Local complications are more commonly related to the extent of injury and treatment (fixation) method. Delayed treatment and prolonged hospitalization increase the incidence of venous thrombosis and pulmonary complications (5).

Radiographic evaluation of healing and complications of femoral fractures is usually accomplished with routine radiographs (Figs. 6-10 and 6-13). Metal fixation devices limit the use of CT and MRI. Radionuclide studies (see Chapter 15, Infection) are useful for detection of subtle infection.

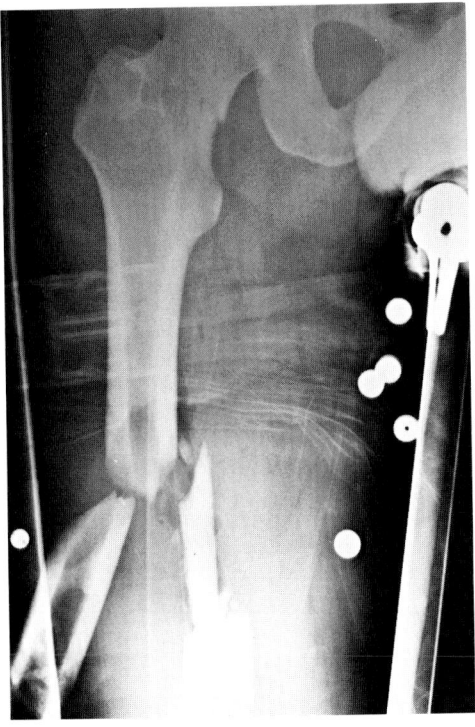

FIG. 6-20. AP view of the femur with a comminuted midshaft fracture. Note the minimally displaced femoral neck fracture.

SOFT TISSUE INJURIES

Soft tissue injuries in the thigh may occur alone or in association with fractures as described above. Injuries include contusion, hematoma, and disruption of the muscle and/or tendon units (2,26,27). Clinical evaluation of these injuries may be sufficient. Imaging techniques such as ultrasonography, CT, and MRI can provide valuable information on the exact type and extent of injury. MRI is particularly useful for evaluating muscle and neurovascular injuries in the thigh (4,14).

Hamstring injuries are common in sprinters and most are first or second degree (see Chapter 3, Soft Tissue Injuries) (Fig. 6-21) (2). These injuries are common (33% of runners), heal slowly, and reinjury is frequent (1,20). MRI is most useful for detection and for following the healing process (4,31).

Injuries to the quadriceps mechanism are common in contact sports. Contusion, hematoma (Fig. 6-22), and significant hemorrhage can occur. If not properly managed, myositis ossificans can develop (2).

Adductor muscle injuries occur most frequently with running and cutting (change in direction while running). The origins of the muscles (Fig. 6-23) are most commonly involved (2,4).

Compartment syndrome is less frequent in the thigh than in the forearm and lower leg. The compartments of the thigh are large (Fig. 6-3) and can accommodate up to 4 liters of blood before significant elevations in pressure develop (12,37,39). Compartment syndromes in the thigh have been reported following crush injuries, femoral fractures (Fig. 6-24), with overuse syndromes (Fig. 6-25), arterial ischemia, burns, and following external compression for treatment of femoral and pelvic frac-

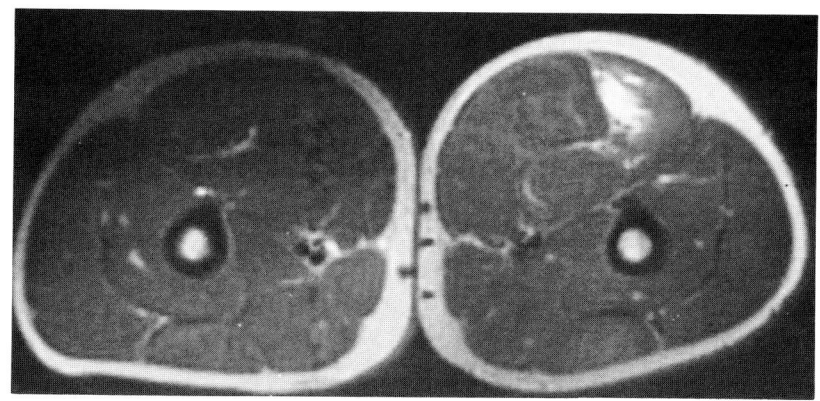

A

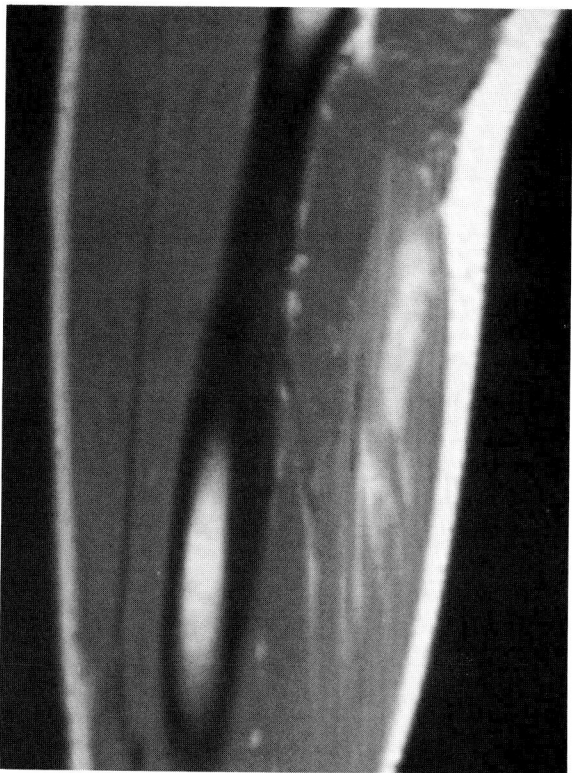

B

FIG. 6-21. Axial (**A**) and sagittal (**B**) images of a first degree hamstring muscle tear. There is infiltrative high signal in the muscle.

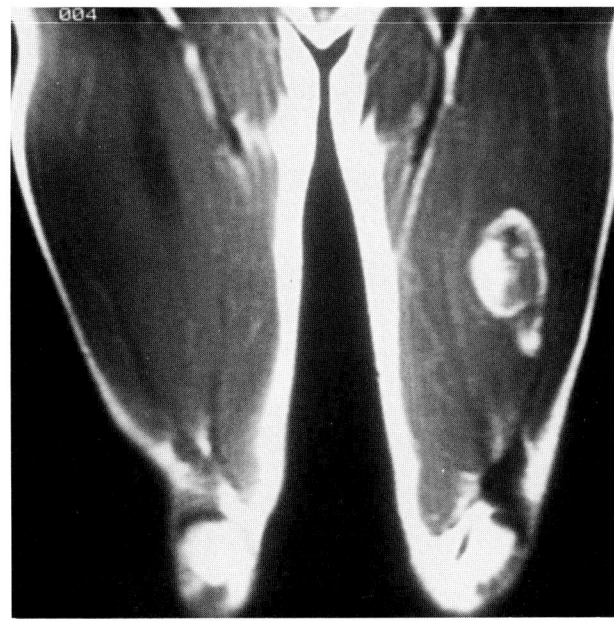

FIG. 6–22. Coronal MR image of the anterior compartment demonstrating a large hematoma.

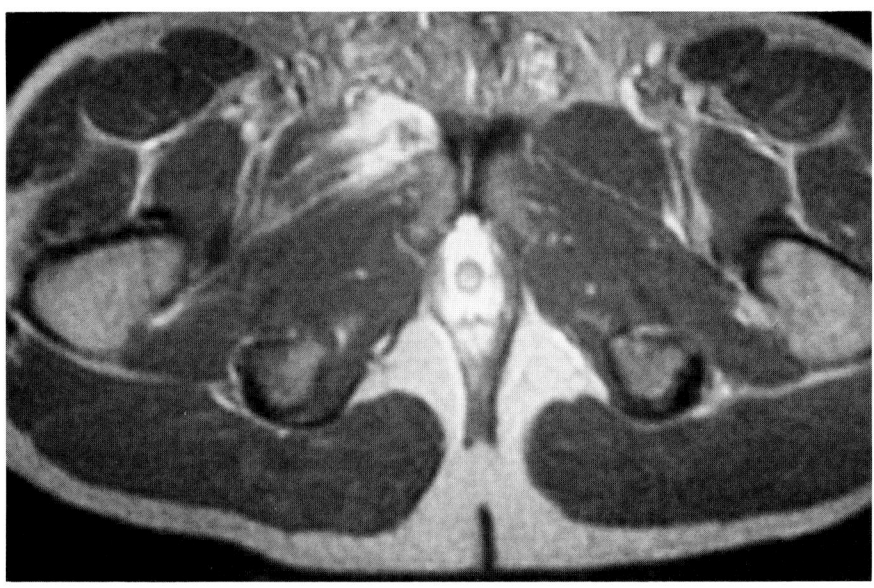

A

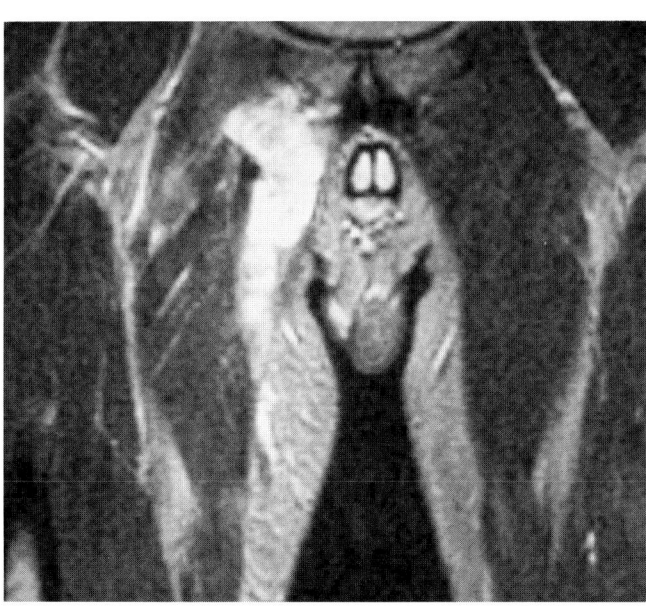

B

FIG. 6–23. Axial (**A**) and coronal (**B**) SE 2000/60 images demonstrate a muscle tear at the adductor origin with hematoma formation.

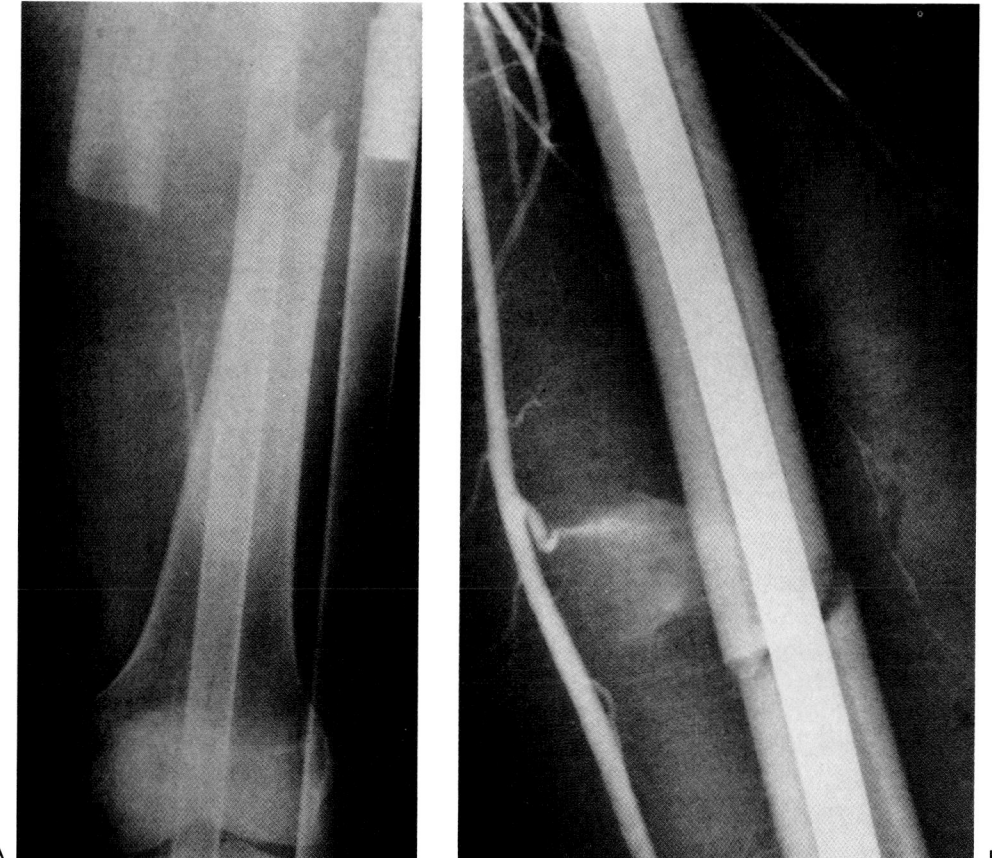

A   B

FIG. 6-24. Femoral fracture demonstrated on an AP radiograph (A). After internal fixation with medullary nailing, compartment syndrome developed. Angiogram (B) shows hemorrhage from a large branch of the superficial femoral artery (from 39, with permission).

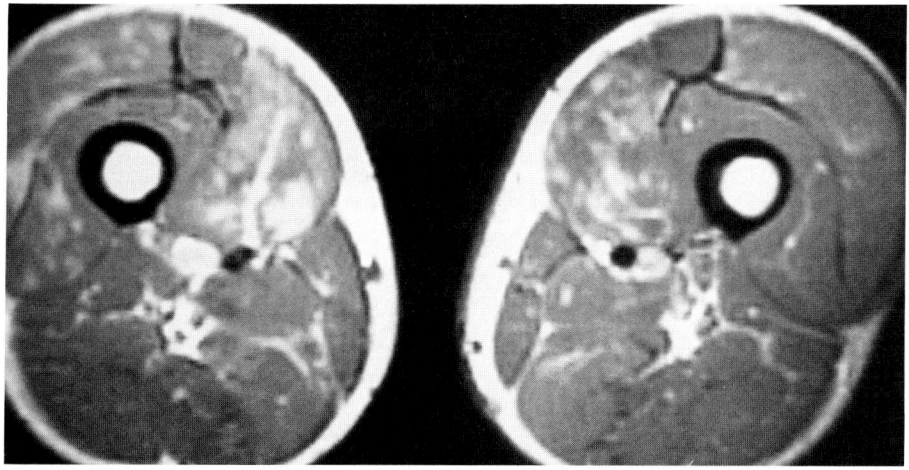

FIG. 6-25. Axial SE 2000/30 MR images of the thigh demonstrating areas of increased signal intensity in both thighs due to overuse syndrome.

tures (12,39). The pressure required to cause muscle ischemia is not clearly defined, but most reports suggest intracompartment pressures should exceed 30 mm Hg (35,39).

Patients with compartment syndrome have pain, swelling and, on physical examination, a tense thigh. Imaging may not be indicated and, in fact, may delay treatment when symptoms are obvious and pressures elevated. Fascectomy should be accomplished as soon as possible when the diagnosis is established. Delays in treatment can result in significant muscle necrosis (35,39).

REFERENCES

1. Agre JC. Hamstring injuries: Proposed etiological factors, prevention, and treatment. *Sports Med* 1985;2:21–33.
2. Baker BE. Current concepts in the diagnosis and treatment of musculotendinous injuries. *Med Sci Sports Exer* 1984;16:323–327.
3. Beam HP Jr, Seligson D. Nine cases of bilateral femoral shaft fractures. A composite view. *J Trauma* 1980;20:399.
4. Berquist TH. *Magnetic resonance of the musculoskeletal system.* New York: Raven Press, 1990.
5. Bone LB, Johnson KD, Weigel PJ, Scheinberg R. Early versus delayed stabilization of femoral fractures. *J Bone Joint Surg* 1989;71A:336–341.
6. Brumback RJ, Ellison PS, Poka A, Bathon H, Burgess AR. Intramedullary nailing of open femoral fractures of the femoral shaft. *J Bone Joint Surg* 1989;71A:1324–1330.
7. Brumback RJ, Reilley JP, Poka A, Lakatos RP, Bathon H, Burgess AR. Intramedullary nailing of femoral shaft fractures. Part I: Decision making errors with interlocking fixation. *J Bone Joint Surg* 1988;70A:1441–1425.
8. Brumback RJ, Uwagie-Ero S, Lakatos RP, Poka A, Bathon GH, Burgess AR. Intramedullary nailing of femoral shaft fractures. Part II: Fracture-healing with static interlocking fixation. *J Bone Joint Surg* 1988;70A:1453–1462.
9. Bucholz RW, Ross SE, Lawrence KL. Fatigue fractures of interlocking nail in the treatment of fracture of the distal part of the femoral shaft. *J Bone Joint Surg* 1987;69A:1391–1399.
10. Carr CR, Wingo CH. Fractures of the femoral diaphysis. A retrospective study of the results and costs of treatment by intramedullary nailing and by traction and a spica cast. *J Bone Joint Surg* 1973;55A:690–700.
11. Clancey GJ, Smith RF, Madenwald MB. Fracture of the distal end of the fracture below hip implants in elderly patients. *J Bone Joint Surg* 1983;65A:491–494.
12. Clancey GJ. Acute posterior compartment syndrome in the thigh. *J Bone Joint Surg* 1985;67A:1278–1280.
13. Eriksson E, Hovelius L. Ender nailing in fractures of the diaphysis of the femur. *J Bone Joint Surg* 1979;61A:1175–1181.
14. Fleckestein JL, Weatherall PT, Parkey RW, Payne JA, Peshock RM. Sports-related muscle injuries. Evaluation with MR imaging. *Radiology* 1989;172:793–798.
15. Franklin JL, Winquist RA, Benirsehke SK, Hansen ST. Broken intramedullary nails. *J Bone Joint Surg* 1988;70A:1463–1471.
16. Green SA. Complications of external skeletal fixation. *Clin Orthop* 1983;180:109–115.
17. Hanks GA, Handal JA, Evarts CM. Deep venous thrombosis after trauma to the lower extremity in patients who had a previous arthrodesis of the hip. *J Bone Joint Surg* 1989;71A:1414–1417.
18. Hardy AE. The treatment of femoral fractures by cast-brace application and early ambulation. *J Bone Joint Surg* 1981;65A:56–64.
19. Harper MC. Fractures of the femur treated by open and closed intramedullary nailing using the fluted rod. *J Bone Joint Surg* 1985;67A:699–708.
20. Heiser TM, Weber J, Sullivan G, Clare P, Jacobs RR. Prophylaxis and management of hamstring injuries in intercollegiate football players. *Am J Sports Med* 1984;12:368–370.
21. Hollinshead WH. *Anatomy for surgeons, vol. 3: The Back and Limbs. 3rd ed.* New York: Harper & Row, 1982.
22. Johansson JE, McGroom R, Barrington TW, Hunter GA. Fracture of the ipsilateral femur in patients with total hip replacement. *J Bone Joint Surg* 1981;63A:1435–1442.
23. Jupiter JB, Bour CJ, May JW. The reconstruction of defects in the femoral shaft with vascularized transfers of fibular bone. *J Bone Joint Surg* 1987;69A:365–374.
24. Kempf I, Grosse A, Beck G. Closed locked intramedullary nailing. *J Bone Joint Surg* 1985;67A:709–720.
25. Luchini MA, Sarakhan AJ, Mitcheli LJ. Acute displaced femoral-shaft fractures in long-distance runners. *J Bone Joint Surg* 1983;65A:689–691.
26. McKeag DB. The concept of overuse. *Primary Care* 1984;11:43–59.
27. McMaster PE. Tendon and muscle ruptures. *J Bone Joint Surg* 1933;15:705–722.
28. Merkel KD, Johnson EW. Supracondylar fractures of the femur after total knee arthroplasty. *J Bone Joint Surg* 1986;68A:29–43.
29. Pankovich AM, Goldflies ML, Pearson RC. Closed under nailing of femoral shaft fractures. *J Bone Joint Surg* 1979;61A:222–232.
30. Rand JA, An KN, Chau EYS, et al. A comparison of the effect of open intramedullary nailing and compression-plate fixation on fracture-site blood flow and fracture union. *J Bone Joint Surg* 1981;63A:427–442.
31. Renstrom P. Swedish research in sports traumatology. *Clin Orthop* 1984;191:144–158.
32. Rhinelander FW. Effect of medullary nailing on normal blood supply of the diaphyseal cortex. *Instr Course Lect* 1973;22:161.
33. Rockwood CA, Green DP. *Fractures.* Philadelphia: J. B. Lippincott Co., 1984.
34. Sartoris DJ, Kerr R, Goergen T, Resnick D. Sliding-screw plate fixation of proximal femoral fractures: Radiographic assessment. *Skel Radiol* 1985;14:104–110.
35. Schwartz JT, Brumback RJ, Lakatos R, Poka A, Bathon H, Burgess AR. Acute compartment syndrome of the thigh. *J Bone Joint Surg* 1989;71A:392–400.
36. Star AM, Whittaker RP, Shuster HM, Duda J, Menkowitz E. Difficulties during removal of fluted femoral intramedullary rods. *J Bone Joint Surg* 1989;71A:341–344.
37. Styf JR, Korner LM. Chronic anterior compartment syndrome of the leg. *J Bone Joint Surg* 1986;68A:1338–1352.
38. Swiontkowski MF, Hansen ST, Kellam J. Ipsilateral fractures of the femoral neck and shaft. *J Bone Joint Surg* 1984;66A:260–268.
39. Tarlow SD, Achterman CA, Hayhurst J, Ovadia DN. Acute compartment syndrome in the thigh complicating fracture of the femur. *J Bone Joint Surg* 1986;68A:1439–1443.
40. Taylor LW. Principles of treatment of fracture and non-union of the shaft of the femur. *J Bone Joint Surg* 1963;45A:191.
41. Thoresen BO, Alho A, Eheland A, Stromsoe K, Folleras G, Haukebo A. Interlocking intramedullary nailing in femoral shaft fractures. *J Bone Joint Surg* 1985;67A:1313–1320.
42. Veith RG, Winquist RA, Hansen ST. Ipsilateral fractures of the femur and tibia. *J Bone Joint Surg* 1984;66A:991–1002.
43. White GM, Healy WL, Brumback RJ, Burgess AR, Brooker AF. The treatment of fractures of the femoral shaft with the Brokker-Wills distal locking intramedullary nail. *J Bone Joint Surg* 1986;68A:865–876.
44. Winquist RA, Hansen ST. Segmental fractures of the femur treated by closed intramedullary nailing. *J Bone Joint Surg* 1978;60A:934–938.
45. Winquist RA, Hansen ST Jr. Comminuted fractures of the femoral shaft treated by intramedullary nailing. *Orthop Clin North Am* 1980;1:633–648.
46. Winquist RA, Hansen ST Jr, Clawson DK. Closed intramedullary nailing of femoral fractures. A report of 520 cases. *J Bone Joint Surg* 1984;66A:529–539.
47. Zickel RE. Fractures of the adult femur excluding femoral head and neck. *Clin Orthop* 1980;147:93–114.

*Imaging of Orthopedic Trauma,
Second Edition*, edited by T.H. Berquist,
Mayo Clinic © 1992. Published
by Raven Press, Ltd., New York.

CHAPTER 7

The Knee

James A. Rand and Thomas H. Berquist

Anatomy and Biomechanics of the Knee, 333
  Osseous Anatomy, 333
  Meniscus, 334
  Ligaments, 335
  Muscles, 340
  Vascular Supply, 341
  Biomechanics, 341
Routine Radiographic Techniques, 344
  AP View, 344
  Lateral View, 344
  Oblique Views, 346
  Notch View, 350
  Patellar Views, 350
  Stress Views, 350
Patellar Disorders, 352
  Anatomy, 353
  Biomechanics, 353
  Examination, 355
  Patellofemoral Pain Syndromes, 359
  Patellar Instability, 362

Fractures about the Knee, 363
  Osteochondral Fractures, 363
  Patellar Fractures, 364
  Supracondylar Fractures of the Femur, 367
  Fractures of the Tibial Condyles, 370
  Ipsilateral Fractures of the Femur and Tibia, 377
Soft Tissue and Articular Disorders, 379
  Ligamentous Injuries of the Knee, 379
  Natural History, 379
  Diagnosis, 380
  Types of Instability, 381
  Treatment, 387
Knee Arthroscopy and Imaging Techniques for
    Articular and Periarticular Disorders, 389
  Arthrographic Technique, 389
  MRI Techniques, 399
  Computed Tomography and Ultrasonography, 401
  Arthroscopy, 417
References, 425

The knee is anatomically and functionally complex and subjected to tremendous forces during normal activity. The ability of the knee to continue to function satisfactorily as a stable, pain-free, mobile support depends upon the integrity of its dynamic and static restraints. The complex kinematics of the knee are still incompletely understood. A knowledge of the anatomy and mechanics of the knee is essential for an understanding of the response of the knee to soft tissue or bony injury and prosthetic replacement.

ANATOMY AND BIOMECHANICS OF THE KNEE

The anatomy of the knee may be divided into static and dynamic anatomic restraints that guide normal mo-

tion and prevent abnormal motion (Table 7-1). The static restraints consist of the bony architecture, menisci, and ligaments. The dynamic restraints include the musculotendinous units and the stabilizing effect of joint load.

Osseous Anatomy

The bony architecture of the knee is unique and accounts for some of the complexity of knee motion. The anterior aspect of the femoral condyles is oval, providing increased stability in extension, while the posterior aspect is spherical, providing increased motion and rotation in flexion. The surface area of the medial femoral condyle is greater than that of the lateral condyle, reflecting the importance of the medial femoral condyle in load transmission across the knee. In the sagittal plane, the femoral condyle is eccentric, producing a cam-like mechanism that aids in maintaining collateral ligament tight-

J. A. Rand: Department of Orthopedic Surgery, Mayo Medical School, Mayo Clinic, Rochester, Minnesota 55905.
T. H. Berquist: Department of Diagnostic Radiology, Mayo Medical School, Mayo Clinic Jacksonville, Jacksonville, Florida 32224.

TABLE 7-1. *Restraints of knee motion*

Static	Dynamic
Bony architecture	Musculotendinous units
Menisci	Joint Load
Ligaments	

ness in extension and laxity in flexion. The tibial plateaus vary in shape, with the medial plateau being concave on its weight-bearing surface and the lateral tibial plateau slightly convex. This anatomic difference is important for the so-called "screw-home" mechanism of knee motion. The intercondylar eminence between the tibial plateaus provides both a mechanical block to translation and a place for cruciate ligament attachment. The degree of conformity between the tibia and femur is not exact and is improved considerably by the presence of the menisci. The patella is a sesamoid bone in the extensor mechanism (5,27). It is roughly triangular and ends in a rounded point on its anteroinferior margins, so that its anterior height exceeds its posterior height (54). The articular surface is divided into medial and lateral facets by a vertical ridge. A second vertical ridge near the medial border isolates the odd facet. The patella may be divided into Wiberg types (72). Type I has equal-sized medial and lateral facets. Type II has a smaller medial facet. Type III has a very small medial facet that is convex with a broad concave lateral facet. Type II is the most frequent type, occurring in 57% of knees (54).

The degree of conformity between the patella and femur is poor, especially when the multiple anatomic variations of the patella are considered. The patella functions to improve the lever arm of the extensor mechanism and helps to protect the femoral articular surface from direct trauma (5,27).

Meniscus

The importance of the menisci in joint function and the adverse consequences of meniscal excision are now well recognized (62). The lateral meniscus is small in diameter, circular, and wider and thicker than the medial meniscus (6). The medial meniscus is thinner, narrower, and more semicircular and transcribes a larger circle than the lateral meniscus. The medial meniscus is firmly attached to the capsule of the knee by fibrous tissue. The lateral meniscus has a less firm attachment and is separated from the fibular collateral ligament and posterolateral capsule by the popliteus tendon. A ligament of Wrisberg may attach the lateral meniscus to the medial condyle of the femur but is sometimes absent. In fact, a ligament of Wrisberg (posterior meniscofemoral) or Humphry (anterior meniscofemoral) is absent in 30% of knees (21).

The medial meniscus is attached anteriorly to the anterior intercondylar fossa of the tibia and is anterior to the anterior cruciate ligament (27). The posterior attachment of the medial meniscus is fixed to the posterior intercondylar fossa of the tibia. The anterior attachment of the lateral meniscus is to the intercondylar eminence of the tibia and is lateral and posterior to the anterior cruciate ligament. The posterior attachment of the lateral meniscus is posterior to the intercondylar eminence of the tibia. The transverse ligament may connect the anterior margin of the two menisci. Abnormal menisci may be present, such as a discoid lateral meniscus. The vascular supply to the menisci is from branches of the middle genicular and the medial and lateral genicular arteries (56). Only the outer 30% of the meniscus has a vascular supply and is capable of a healing response. The remainder of the meniscus relies upon diffusion from the synovial fluid. Both menisci slide posteriorly with knee flexion (6).

The functions of the menisci include lubrication, force transmission, stability, articular cartilage nutrition, and shock absorption. In 1936, King showed that the extent of degeneration of articular cartilage in the canine knee correlated with the segment of the meniscus removed and was greatest following complete meniscectomy (37). Claims have also been made for the menisci as important guides for the rotation of the tibia on the femur (25). Thus meniscal injuries may affect the synchronous motion between the tibia and femur, leading to areas of articular cartilage erosion.

The menisci also aid in the distribution of load across the knee (35). The area of load bearing in the knee is increased from 2 cm^2 on each condyle in the absence of the menisci to 6 cm^2 in the presence of menisci (68). At a 1,000 N load the menisci transmit 45% of the load across the knee (61). The medial meniscus may carry 50% and the lateral meniscus 70% of the joint load (58). At a 1,000 N load the menisci occupy 70% of the total contact area, and excision of the menisci doubles peak pressure from 3 MPa to 6 MPa (18). The lateral meniscus contributes more to weight bearing in the lateral compartment than does the medial meniscus in the medial compartment (18). Meniscal excision decreases the area for load transmission by approximately 50% (43). Meniscectomy may result in a threefold increase in stress across the joint (38). The effect of partial meniscectomy on load bearing of the meniscus has been studied by Burke and colleagues (8). Partial meniscectomy does not affect load-bearing function in the peripheral rim of the meniscus and allows a more normal pressure distribution than total meniscectomy (8).

The medial meniscus contributes to anteroposterior stability of the knee. The importance of the medial meniscus for this stability has been investigated by Levy and colleagues (39). If the anterior cruciate is intact, medial meniscectomy does not affect the anteroposterior displacement of the knee or its coupled rotation. However, if the anterior cruciate is sectioned, loss of the medial meniscus significantly increases anteroposterior knee laxity and results in a loss of the coupled internal rotation associated with anterior tibial displacement (39). Removal of both menisci with all ligaments intact results in 2 mm of increased laxity in the anteroposterior plane a 45°–90° of flexion (45).

The clinical correlation of this biomechanical information has been well documented. In 1948, Fairbank presented the classical roentgenographic findings following a meniscectomy: (1) an anteroposterior ridge, (2) generalized flattening of the femoral condyle, (3) narrowing of the joint space, and (4) squaring of the tibial margin (14) (Fig. 7-1). Thirty years following meniscectomy, only 38% of the patients had a normal, symptom-free knee (65). The best long-term result occurs after a partial meniscectomy for a bucket-handle tear, with 67% having excellent results (65). At 17.5 years following meniscectomy, 39.4% of the knees were found to have degenerative arthritis (32). Therefore, meniscectomy is not an innocuous procedure and should be performed only when necessary. When feasible, partial meniscectomy is preferable to total meniscectomy.

Ligaments

The ligamentous restraints for the knee may be considered with respect to their anatomic location. Thus, they can be classified as either medial or posteromedial, lateral or posterolateral, anterior, or central (27,63).

Medial Ligamentous Structures

The medial ligamentous structures are complex, and their functional importance is controversial. Warren and Marshall have divided the medial capsular structures into three layers, from superficial to deep (69). Layer I consists of the deep fascia. Layer II is composed of the superficial medial collateral ligament. Layer III consists of the joint capsule deep to the medial ligament. Layer I, the deep fascia, serves as a support for the muscle bellies and neurovascular structures. The sartorius muscle inserts into this layer. Layer I merges with Layer II 1–2 cm anterior to the superficial medial ligament (Fig. 7-2) (69). The tendons of the gracilis and semitendinosus lie between Layers I and II.

The superficial medial ligament lies in Layer II and is composed of two parts. The anterior portion of this ligament consists of long, parallel fibers 11 cm × 1.5 cm (70). The anterior fibers are attached to the medial femoral condyle just distal to the adductor tubercle and are located around the axis of flexion of the knee. The tibial insertion of these fibers is in the anteromedial aspect of the tibia 4.6 cm distal to the joint line (6). The posterior oblique fibers of the superficial medial ligament have the same femoral attachment as the anterior parallel fibers but are triangular in shape, with the apex extending posteriorly along the joint line (6,70). Other authors have believed that these posterior oblique fibers are part of the deeper posterior oblique ligament (28,30). The maximum length of the superficial medial ligament is seen at 45° of flexion, when it is increased 1.75 mm over its

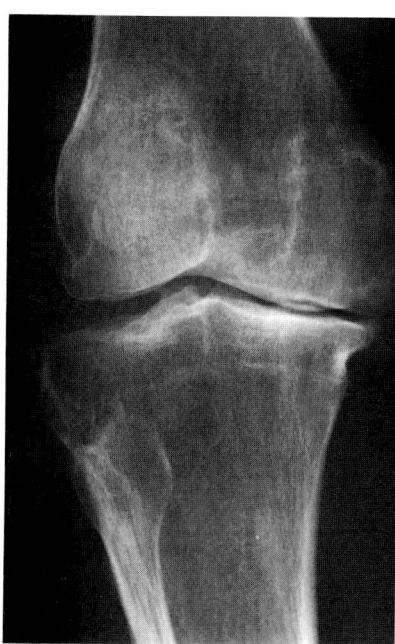

FIG. 7–1. Fairbanks changes affecting the medial compartment of the right knee of a 40-year-old man 15 years following medial meniscectomy.

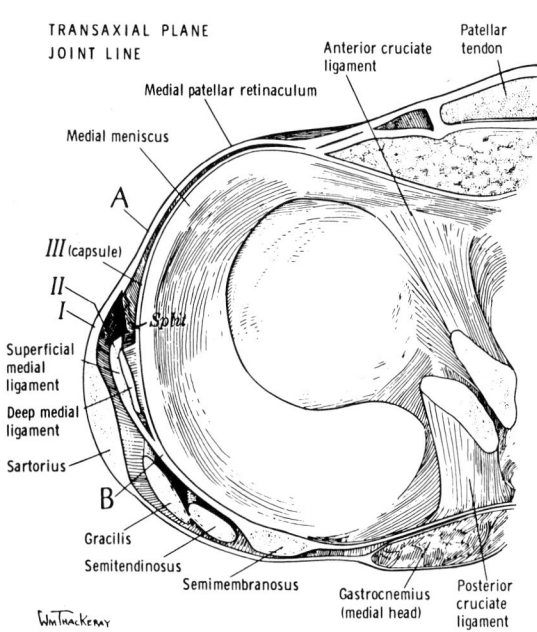

FIG. 7–2. Layers of the medial aspect of the knee (from 69, with permission.)

resting length (3,70). During extension, the superficial medial ligament moves anteriorly, while in flexion it moves posteriorly (6). The posterior border of the superficial medial ligament is tightest in extension and becomes slack at 30° of flexion, allowing normal rotation of the tibia on the femur (3,64). In extreme flexion, the posterior border of the ligament slips under the anterior border near its femoral attachment (3).

Layers II and III join posteriorly to form the posteromedial capsule and are joined by the tendon sheath of the semimembranosus (69). Layer II splits at the anterior margin of the superficial medial ligament. The anterior fibers of the split join with Layer I, forming the parapatellar retinacular fibers (69). Layer II, on the other hand, is the true capsule of the knee (70). The anterior portion of the capsule is thin but may be important in preventing lateral patellar subluxation and anteromedial rotatory instability (64). Layer III is thickened beneath the superficial medial ligament and has been referred to as the deep medial ligament or middle capsular ligament (69). The deep medial ligament is attached to the medial femoral epicondyle anterior to the superficial ligament and is strongly attached to the outer margin of the medial meniscus (64). It extends distally as the coronary ligament to attach to the tibia just below the articular margin.

The posteromedial capsule has been termed the *posterior oblique ligament*. It extends from the posterior margin of the superficial medial ligament anteriorly to the insertion of the direct head of the semimembranosus posteriorly (28,30,64) and from the adductor tubercle proximally to the tibia distally (30). The posterior oblique ligament has a firm attachment to the medial meniscus and the posteromedial corner of the knee (30,55). The distal attachment consists of three arms: (1) the central, or tibial, arm, which attaches to the margin of the articular surface and is central to the upper edge of the semimembranous tendon; (2) the superior, or capsular, arm, which is continuous with the posterior capsule and the proximal part of the oblique popliteal ligament; and (3) the inferior, or distal, arm, which attaches distally to the sheath of the semimembranosus and tibia (Fig. 7-3) (30). The posterior oblique ligament is relaxed at 60° of flexion. This ligament has been felt to be essential for static medial capsular stability.

The parallel anterior fibers of the superficial medial ligament are the primary stabilizers of the medial side of the knee to valgus stress (70). Isolated section of the deep medial capsular ligament and posterior oblique ligament alone does not allow medial joint space opening (70). Division of the superficial medial ligament results in a 2° increase in external rotation in extension and a twofold increase in external rotation at 90° of flexion. The superficial medial ligament provides 57.4% of the restraint to valgus stress at 5° of flexion and 78.2% at 25° of flexion (23). The anterior and middle parts of the medial capsule

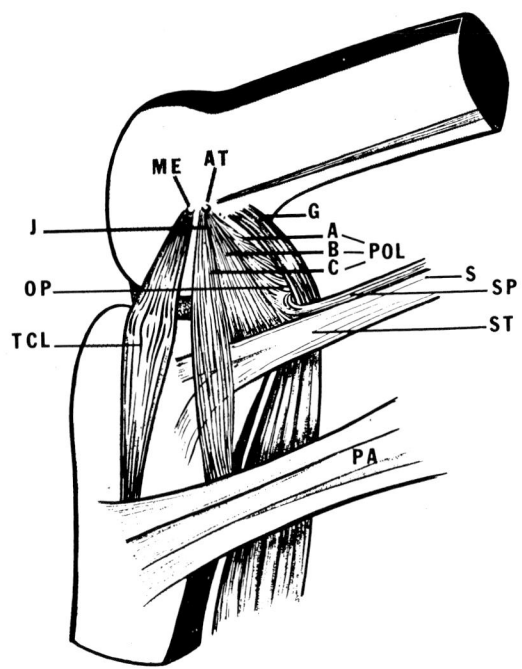

FIG. 7–3. The three arms of the posterior-oblique alignment (POL) (from 30, with permission.)

provide only 4–8% of the restraint to valgus stress. The posteromedial capsule provides 17.5% of the restraint to valgus stress.

Lateral Ligamentous Structures

The lateral aspect of the knee contains many important stabilizing structures. These structures may be considered from anterior to posterior or from superficial to deep layers. The anterior third consists of the capsular ligament, which extends posteriorly from the lateral border of the patellar tendon and patella to the anterior border of the iliotibial band, and is reinforced by the lateral retinaculum from the quadriceps mechanism (29). The middle third is composed of the iliotibial band and the capsular ligament deep to it and extends posteriorly as far as the fibular collateral ligament (29). Both the iliotibial tract (which provides static support) and the iliotibial band (which provides dynamic support) reinforce the middle-third capsular ligament (29). The middle third of the lateral capsule extends from the lateral epicondyle of the femur to the tibial joint line, providing static support at 30° of flexion. Finally, the posterior third consists of the capsular and noncapsular ligaments that compose the arcuate complex (29). The arcuate complex is composed of the fibular collateral ligament, the arcuate ligament, and the aponeurosis of the popliteus muscle.

The lateral aspect of the knee consists of three layers (Figs. 7-4 and 7-5) (57). The superficial layer, or Layer I, consists of the iliotibial tract and its expansion anteriorly

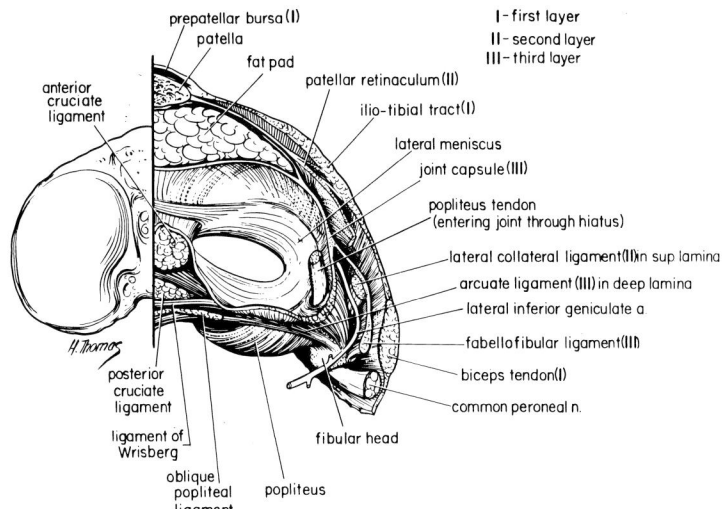

FIG. 7–4. The three layers of the lateral aspect of the knee (from 57, with permission.)

and the superficial portion of the biceps and its expansion posteriorly. The peroneal nerve lies on the posterior aspect of the biceps tendon.

Layer II is formed by the retinaculum of the quadriceps and is incomplete (57). It is composed of two patellofemoral ligaments. The proximal ligament joins the terminal fibers of the lateral intramuscular system. The distal ligament ends posteriorly on the fibula or posterolateral capsular reinforcements provided by the lateral head of the gastrocnemius on the femoral condyle (57). The proximal patellofemoral ligament travels in Layer II

obliquely from the patella, attaching to the margin of the lateral meniscus, and terminates on Gerdy's tubercle. The fibular collateral ligament lies in Layer II and extends from the posterior lateral femoral condyle proximal to the groove of the popliteus to the lateral side of the head of the fibula anterior to the styloid process (27,57).

Layer III is the lateral joint capsule (57). The capsular attachment to the outer edge of the lateral meniscus is the coronary ligament and contains a hiatus for the popliteus tendon. Posterior to the overlying iliotibial tract, the capsule divides into two laminae (57). The superfi-

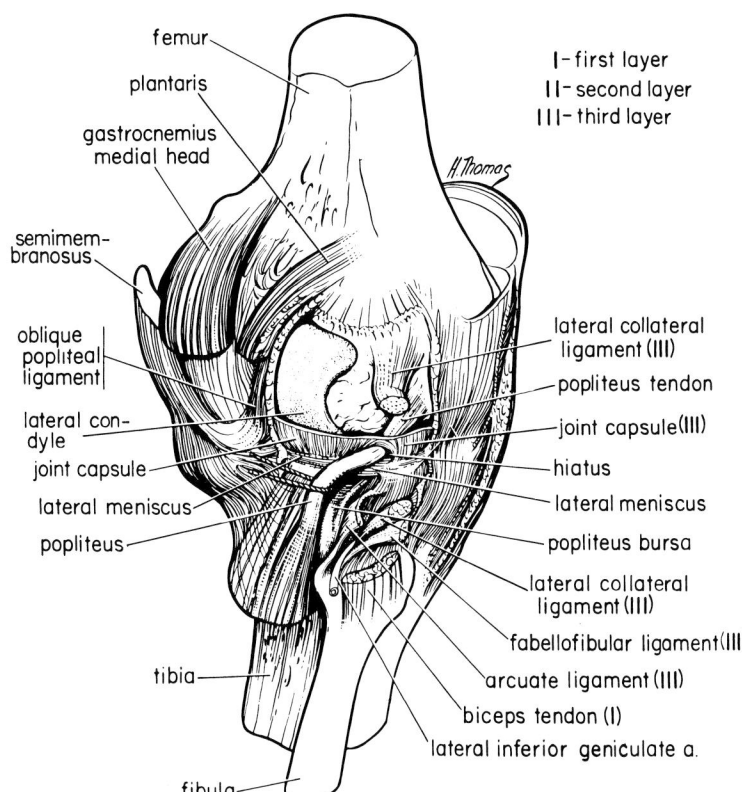

FIG. 7–5. The structure of the posterolateral aspect of the knee (from 57, with permission.)

cial lamina encompasses the fibular collateral ligament and ends posteriorly at the fabellofibular ligament. The deep lamina forms the coronary ligament and terminates posteriorly at the arcuate ligament. The Y-shaped arcuate ligament spans the junction between the popliteus muscle and its tendon and extends from the fibula to the femur (57). The inferior lateral genicular vessels pass between these two laminae. The arcuate and fabellofibular ligaments insert on the apex of the fibular styloid process. They ascend to the lateral head of the gastrocnemius, where they join the posterior termination of the oblique popliteal ligament. The arcuate ligament fans out over the musculotendinous portion of the popliteus muscle and adheres to it (57).

Three anatomic variations in the posterolateral aspect of the knee have been identified (57). In 13% of knees, the arcuate ligament alone reinforces the capsule. In 20% of knees, the fabellofibular ligament alone reinforces the capsule. In 67% of knees, both the arcuate and fabellofibular ligaments reinforce the posterolateral capsule. Seebacher and colleagues noted that the size of the fabella correlated with these anatomic variations (57). If the fabella was large, there was no arcuate ligament, but the fabellofibular ligament was also large. Conversely, when the fabella was absent, only the arcuate ligament was present.

Biomechanical studies of the importance of the lateral stabilizers have been performed (23). The lateral collateral ligament is the primary restraint to varus stress, providing 55–69% of the restraint. The entire lateral capsule provides only 8–17% of the restraint to varus stress.

Cruciate Ligaments

The cruciate ligaments are one of the key aspects of the functional anatomy of the knee. Injuries to the cruciate ligaments are frequent clinical problems resulting in significant morbidity. The anterior cruciate ligament has its femoral attachment on the posterior aspect of the medial surface of the lateral femoral condyle (2,21). The tibial attachment of the anterior cruciate ligament is to a fossa anterior and lateral to the anterior tibial spine. Fascicles from the anterior cruciate ligament may blend with the anterior and posterior attachments of the lateral meniscus (2,21). The anterior cruciate ligament does not attach to the tip or upper part of the anterior surface of the anterior tibial spine (21). The tibial attachment is wider and stronger than the femoral attachment (2, 11,12,16,21,27).

The fascicles of the anterior cruciate ligament create a slight outward spiral as they cross the joint. These fascicles have been divided into an anteromedial band and a posterolateral bulk (2,21). The anteromedial band originates at the proximal aspect of the femoral attachment and inserts at the anteromedial aspect of the tibial attachment. The anteromedial band becomes tense in flexion as the anterior cruciate ligament twists on itself, while the posterolateral bulk becomes loose (Fig. 7-6) (2,20,21). In extension, the posterolateral bulk becomes tight while the anteromedial band becomes lax (2,20). A positive anterior drawer test indicates a tear of the anteromedial band (20). The posterolateral band is a secondary restraint and the medial collateral ligament a tertiary restraint to the anterior drawer test (20). The anterior cruciate ligament limits external and internal rotation in extension. It is usually a continuum of fascicles, a different portion of which is taut throughout the range of motion (2).

The posterior cruciate ligament is attached to the anterior portion of the intercondylar aspect of the medial femoral condyle. The tibial attachment of the posterior cruciate ligament is to a depression behind the intra-articular upper surface of the tibia (21). The posterior cruciate ligament sends a slip to blend with the posterior horn of the lateral meniscus. The fibers of the posterior cruciate ligament are attached in a lateromedial direction on the tibia and in an anteroposterior direction on the femur (21). The posterior cruciate ligament may be divided into an anterior portion that forms the bulk of the ligament and a smaller posterior part (21). The posterior fibers are loose in flexion while the bulk is taut (Fig. 7-7). In extension, the posterior fibers become taut while the anterior fibers relax.

The transitional zone between cruciate ligament and bone is mediated by a transitional zone of fibrocartilage and mineralized fibrocartilage that allows for a graduated change in stiffness and stress concentration at the attachment site (2,50). The femoral attachment of both cruciate ligaments and the tibial attachment of the posterior cruciate ligament are behind the axis of flexion of the knee (21). The location of the cruciate attachment

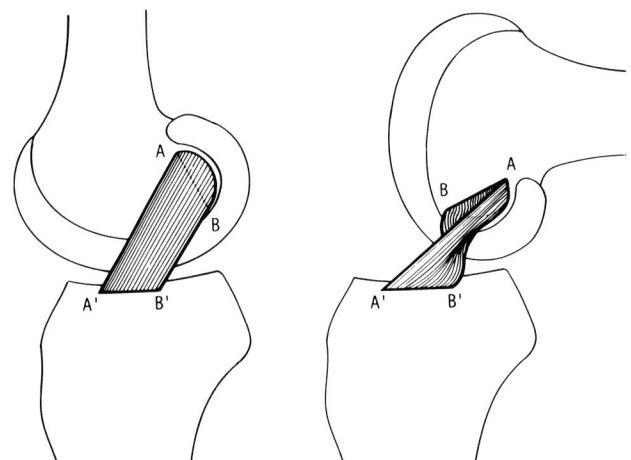

FIG. 7-6. The two bands of the anterior cruciate ligament and their differential tensions during flexion and extension of the knee (from 21, with permission.)

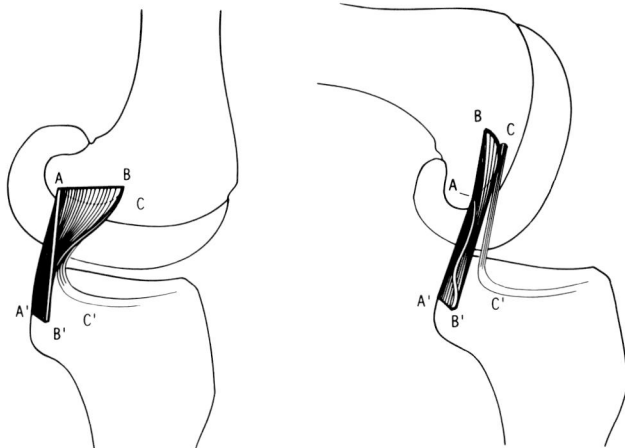

FIG. 7–7. The two bands of the posterior cruciate ligament and their differential tensions during flexion and extension of the knee (from 21, with permission.)

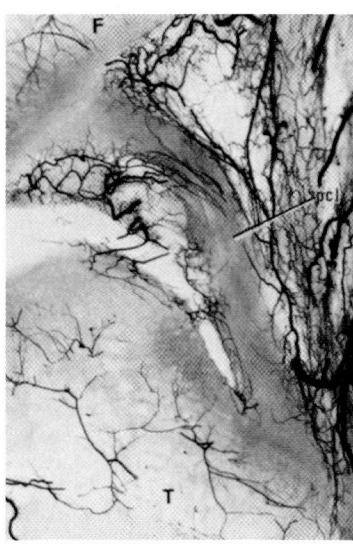

FIG. 7–9. The vascular supply to the posterior cruciate ligament (from 56, with permission.)

sites combined with the cam-shaped femoral condyle results in the differential tightening of portions of each cruciate ligament with flexion-extension motion (21). The eccentric cruciate ligament attachments result in their being wound in flexion and unwound in extension with respect to each other (33).

The vascular supply to the cruciate ligaments is derived from branches of the middle genicular artery, which also supplies the synovial membrane and posterior capsule (56). The largest branch is the tibial intercondylar artery (Figs. 7-8 and 7-9) (34,56). The anterior cruciate ligament is covered by a synovial fold, the ligamentum mucosum, which contains many of the small vascular branches (2). A few small branches from the lateral inferior genicular artery may contribute to this vascular plexus. The vessels are oriented in a longitudinal manner parallel to the fibers of the ligament. The vascular supply to the anterior cruciate ligament is predominantly of soft tissue origin without a significant contribution from the osseous junctions (2,56). The posterior cruciate ligament receives arteries originating

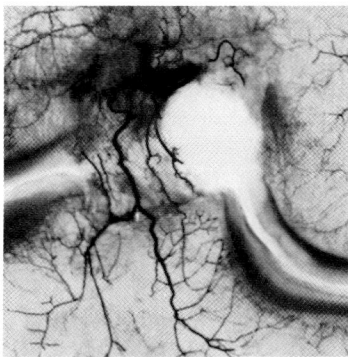

FIG. 7–8. The vascular supply to the anterior cruciate ligaments (from 56, with permission.)

from the infrapatellar fat pad entering along the anterior synovial fold (1). A few vessels enter the proximal part of the ligament from a posterior direction along the intercondylar notch. The posterior cruciate ligament has a greater number of intrinsic vessels than the anterior cruciate ligament (1). The central portion of the cruciate ligaments is less well vascularized than the proximal and distal parts (1). Although the vasculature appears important for cruciate ligament nutrition, diffusion of nutrients may also play a role, especially if the vasculature is disrupted (71).

The nerve supply to the anterior cruciate ligament derives from branches of the tibial nerve that penetrate the joint capsule posteriorly (2). Most of the fibers are related to vasomotor control, but some may have a proprioceptive function (2,34).

The cruciate ligaments together provide 13–14% of the restraining moment to valgus stress (23). At 25° of flexion, the posterior cruciate ligament provides 75% of the restraint to valgus stress provided by the two cruciate ligaments (23). The cruciates provide 12–22% of the restraint to varus stress (23). Therefore, the cruciate ligaments are secondary restraints to medial and lateral opening of the knee upon stress. The tensile strength of the anterior cruciate ligament is 600 ± 132 N, while that of the posterior cruciate ligament is 450 ± 12 N (10). Other authors have suggested that the anterior cruciate ligament can withstand loads of 1,000 to 1,730 N prior to microscopic failure (9,10,22,50). The tensile strength of the human anterior cruciate ligament decreases with age (50). Since ligaments are viscoelastic, the rate of loading determines the mode of failure. Under high loading rates for the anterior cruciate ligament, primary ligamentous disruption occurs; under low loading rates, tibial avulsion fractures are more frequent (49). The strain to maximum load for the anterior cruciate ligament is 20–30% (34). When ligamentous failure occurs, the ligament undergoes 57–100% elongation prior to loss of continuity (49). Ligament failure results in serial failure throughout the entire ligament prior to final separation, giving a "mop-end" appearance (34).

Functionally, the cruciate ligaments in conjunction with the collateral ligaments help control lateral rotation of the tibia on the femur (6). The anterior cruciate ligament acts as a check against external rotation in flexion but does not limit internal rotation (21). The anterior cruciate ligament prevents anterior displacement of the tibia on the femur, especially in extension (6). Severance of the anterior cruciate ligament results in hyperextension, increased external rotation of 6°–12°, increased internal rotation of 2°–8°, and increased anterior drawer in extension and, to a lesser extent, in flexion as well (21). Loss of the posterior cruciate ligament results in instability in flexion, with a 3° increase in medial and an 8° increase in lateral rotation, as well as posterior displacement of the tibia on the femur in flexion (21).

Anterior Ligamentous Structures

The anterior aspect of the knee consists primarily of the extensor mechanism of the knee. The four-part structure of the quadriceps is well known. The rectus femoris becomes tendinous 5–8 cm proximal to the patella (54). The rectus fibers fan out over the patella and are continuous with the patellar tendon. The vastus medialis has two components (54). The proximal fibers are long while the distal fibers are oblique in orientation. Some of the fibers insert into the patella while others contribute to the medial retinaculum. The vastus lateralis becomes tendinous 2.8 cm proximal to the patella (54). The medial fibers of the vastus lateralis insert into the patella, while the lateral fibers contribute to the lateral retinaculum. The vastus intermedius lies deep to the other muscle groups and sends fibers into the superior border of the patella (54). There is a blending of the tendinous fibers at the insertion of the various muscle groups into the patella, creating a complex structure.

The fascia lata spreads to create a superficial interlocking layer with the quadriceps complex, contributing to the patellar retinacula (54). The patellofemoral ligaments are thickenings of the joint capsule that connect the patella to the femoral epicondyles. The most common is the lateral epicondylopatellar ligament of Kaplan. Actually two lateral patellofemoral ligaments are frequently present (54). The proximal ligament terminates on the lateral intermuscular system. The distal one ends on the fabella and posterolateral capsule. On the medial side, a patellofemoral ligament runs deep to the vastus medialis and attaches near the femoral attachment of the medial superficial ligament (69).

The patellar ligament is flat and receives fibers from the central portion of the rectus femoris (54). The closer the patellar profile to that of Wiberg Type III, the broader was the lateral patellofemoral ligament. The larger the patellar ligament, the smaller the size of the medial patellofemoral ligament. These findings on radiographs may be helpful in assessing the potential for lateral patellar subluxation.

Muscles

The quadriceps mechanism is an important dynamic stabilizer of the knee, and its anatomy has been described. Other important dynamic stabilizers exist. On the lateral aspect of the knee, the iliotibial tract, as described earlier, provides passive ligament tension and also transmits active muscle forces. The popliteus muscle is important in the screw-home mechanism of the knee. Activity in the popliteus muscle coincides with internal rotation of the tibia on the femur (41). The popliteus muscle extends from the lateral femoral epicondyle to the proximal posterior medial tibia proximal to the popliteal line (27). The biceps femoris, which attaches to the fibular head, is an important dynamic restraint on the lateral aspect of the knee (28,29). Studies of the contributions of these dynamic stabilizers to lateral knee stability in cadavers have shown minimal restraint but probably do not reflect the in vivo situation.

On the medial aspect of the knee, the semimembranosus is an important dynamic stabilizer (69). There are five sites of attachment of the semimembranosus (Fig. 7-10) (69). The semimembranosus inserts into the posteromedial corner of the tibia below the joint line. A second bony insertion lies anteriorly on the medial aspect of the tibia below the joint line deep to the superficial medial ligament. The semimembranosus tendon sheath sends an extension into the posterior capsule, which forms the oblique popliteal ligament. The oblique popliteal ligament supports the posterior aspect of the knee and inserts into the medial aspect of the lateral femoral condyle. Two additional insertions include one in the posteromedial capsule and another distal to the tibia posterior to the oblique portion of the superficial medial ligament. Through its multiple sites of attachment, the semimembranosus provides a dynamic reinforcement for the posterior medial aspect of the knee (28,30,64). It is an internal rotator of the tibia and supports the knee against valgus thrust as well as anteromedial tibial displacement (64). The medial and lateral heads of the gastrocnemius reinforce their respective corners of the knee (28).

The pes anserinus muscles, the sartorius, gracilis, and semitendinosus muscles flex the knee and hold the tibia within a normal range of external rotation on the femur (17,64). These muscles attach to the anteromedial tibia

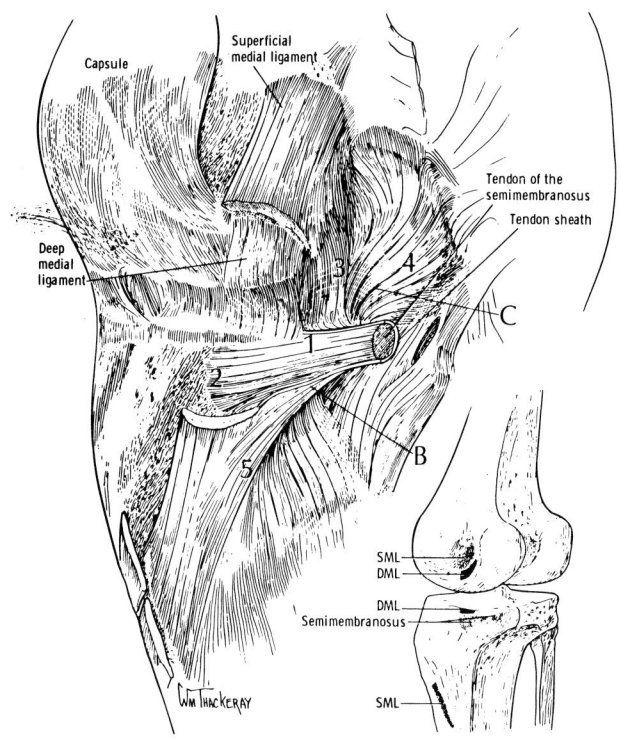

Capsule

Superficial
medial ligament

Tendon of the
semimembranosus

Tendon sheath

Deep
medial
ligament

3
4
1
2
C
B
5

SML
DML

DML
Semimembranosus

SML

Wm Thackeray

FIG. 7–10. The five sites of attachment of the semi-membranous muscle on the posteromedial aspect of the knee (from 69, with permission.)

below the joint line and the fascia of the leg. Even after transplantation, the pes muscles continue to function primarily as flexors, although their rotational activity is increased (17,51). The contribution to rotational force provided by the pes muscles is 34% for the sartorius, 40% for the gracilis, and 26% for the semitendinosus (51). However, the long-term effectiveness of pes transfer is questionable when done as the sole treatment of antero-medial instability (17).

Few studies have been performed on the *in vivo* effect of the musculature as dynamic stabilizers. The effective stiffness of the medial ligamentous complex may be increased by 108% by the pes anserinus and by 164% by the quadriceps femoris muscle groups (53). The maximum amount of tibial torque that can be sustained without injury to the knee ligaments may be effectively doubled by maximum muscle resistance (60).

Vascular Supply

The vascular supply about the knee is provided by five major groups of vessels: the supreme genicular, the medial and lateral superior genicular, the medial and lateral inferior genicular, the middle genicular, and the anterior and posterior tibial recurrent arteries (56). The supreme

genicular arises from the femoral artery and divides into three branches: the saphenous, the muscular articular, and the deep oblique. The saphenous branch is subcutaneous. The muscular branch supplies part of the vastus medialis and contributes to the parapatellar plexus. The deep oblique branch supplies muscles along the medial aspect of the femoral shaft and the anterior and medial aspects of the distal femur. The medial and lateral superior genicular arteries are branches from the popliteal artery and contribute to the *rete articulare genu* and the epiphyseal circulation. The medial and lateral inferior genicular arteries arise from the popliteal artery and lie deep to the collateral ligaments. The middle genicular arises from the popliteal artery and supplies the cruciate ligaments, the distal femoral, and the proximal tibial epiphyses. The anterior and posterior tibial recurrent arteries arise from the anterior tibial artery and supply the anterior aspect of the knee, the superior tibiofibular joint, and the lateral condyle of the tibia. The patella is supplied by midpatellar vessels penetrating the middle third of its anterior surface and by polar vessels entering the apex behind the patellar ligament. Therefore, the majority of the vascular supply to the patella is in its inferior half, making the proximal half of the patella susceptible to ischemia following fracture (57).

Biomechanics

The complexity of knee motion and the extent of force transmission across the knee underscore the importance of a thorough understanding of knee mechanics for appropriate management of knee disorders (48). The functional importance of the various static stabilizers is summarized in Table 7-2.

The forces acting across the knee during normal walking include a direct compression force, a mediolateral shear force, and an anteroposterior shear force that is resisted by the cruciate ligaments (46). These forces are generated by the effect of gravity and muscular action. The joint forces occurring during normal walking are 2–4 times body weight, with a mean of 3.03 times body weight (46,47). There are three peaks of loading during the gait cycle. These correspond to muscle activity in the hamstrings, quadriceps femoris, and gastrocnemius (46). The peak force is during the late-stance phase associated with contraction of the gastrocnemius (15). A force equal to body weight is present in the late swing phase, corresponding to contraction of the hamstrings as they decelerate the knee (15). The maximum forces developed in the quadriceps are 167 lb, in the hamstrings, 270 lb, and in the gastrocnemius, 234 lb (47).

Forces acting on the cruciate ligaments range as high as 112 lb, with the posterior cruciate ligament carrying two-thirds of the load (40,42,47). Forces acting in the medial collateral ligament are small, with a maximum

TABLE 7–2. *Ligamentous restraints*

Author	Stress	Primary stabilizer	Secondary stabilizer
Butler (9,10)	Anterior	ACL 85–87%	ITB 25% Middle medial capsule 22% Middle lateral capsule 21% MCL 16% LCL 12%
Markolf (45)	Anterior	ACL	ACL + PCL Menisci MCL + LCL
Fukubayashi (19)	Anterior	ACL	
Crowninshield (12)	Anterior	ACL	Middle medial capsule MCL + LCL Posteromedial capsule
Butler (9,10)	Posterior	PCL 90–94%	Posterolateral capsule + popliteus 58% MCL 16% Posterior medial capsule 7% LCL 6% Middle medial capsule 6%
Markolf (45)	Posterior	PCL	ACL + PCL Menisci MCL + LCL
Fukubayashi (19)	Posterior	PCL	
Crowninshield (12)	Posterior	PCL	MCL + LCL Posteromedial capsule Middle medial capsule
Grood (23)	Valgus	MCL 57–58%	ACL + PCL 13–15% Anterior + middle Medial capsule 4–8% Posteromedial capsule 4–17%
Warren (69,70)	Valgus	MCL	Middle medial capsule
Markolf (45)	Valgus	MCL	ACL + PCL Menisci
Crowninshield (12)	Valgus	MCL	Middle medial capsule Posterior medial capsule
Lipke (40)	Internal rotation	ACL	Posterolateral capsule LCL

value of 29 lb. However, forces carried by the lateral collateral ligament are as high as 148 lb and act to prevent adduction of the knee during stance phase. The maximum shear force developed during walking is 0.26 times body weight (47). In stance phase, during normal walking with the knee between 0° and 30° of flexion, the femorotibial force peaks at 3 times body weight (7). Upon arising from a chair or ascending or descending a slope or stairs, forces of several times body weight occur with knee flexion angles of 60° or more. Patellofemoral forces are also quite high with increasing knee flexion. During stance phase, the greater part of the load is transmitted by the medial condyles, while in swing phase the load acts mainly on the lateral condyles (47).

The stress (force per unit area) depends upon the load and the contact area for force transmission. The medial compartment contact area is 1.6 times greater than the lateral compartment contact area and is present through the first 35° of flexion (36). The mean area of contact on the medial plateau is 4.68 cm². With increasing knee flexion, these contact areas decrease in area and move posteriorly on the tibial plateaus (36). The menisci appear to contribute to the static loading (36). At small loads, contact occurs on the lateral and posterior borders of the menisci and on a small area of the medial aspect of the tibial spine (7). With increasing loads, the contact area spreads to both meniscal surfaces and exposed articular cartilage. With no applied load, the area of contact is 50% of the lateral meniscus, 55% of the medial meniscus, and 12% of the exposed cartilage on the medial tibial plateau (7). With 150 kg of applied load, the average area of contact is 65% of the lateral meniscus, 67% of the medial meniscus, 38% of the lateral exposed cartilage, and 43% of the medial exposed cartilage (7). Excision of the menisci decreases the areas of contact by approximately 50% (43).

The effects of joint deformities on the force transmission across the knee have been studied. Perry examined the effect of knee flexion on the quadriceps force required to stabilize the knee (52). She concluded that the quadriceps force required to stabilize the flexed knee is proportional to the load on the femoral head and the angle of knee flexion. For each degree of flexion, the required force increased an average of 6% of the load on the femoral head. For a 70 kg man, quadriceps tension rises from 187 N at 5° of flexion to 1,375 N at 30° (52). The compression forces on the patella also depend on the angle of knee flexion.

Any change in the direction of the patellofemoral reaction force carried by an abnormal patellar position will provide abnormal stresses in the joint (13). In knee flexion, the patellofemoral reaction force can exceed the tibiofemoral reaction force. The patella displaces the extensor tendon forward away from the point of contact between the tibia and femur. Patellectomy may result in a 14% increase in tibiofemoral reaction force and a 250% increase in tangential force in the tibiofemoral joint (13). These findings emphasize the functional impairment induced by a knee flexion contracture or loss of the patella.

The effects of varus and valgus changes in axial alignment of the knee on force transmission have also been investigated. The normal angle between the femur and tibia on AP radiographs is 7° ± 2° (13). This angle is the anatomic axis. The mechanical axis of the knee is a line drawn from the center of the femoral head to the center of the ankle. The mechanical axis normally falls within the center of the knee on weight-bearing stance. A variation of 4° in the anatomic axis can change the line of force transmission across the joint to the outer one-third of a compartment, and a variation of 10° can place the line of force transmission beyond the articular surface (13). A high correlation exists between the mechanical and anatomic axis when the mechanical axis falls within the knee (31). However, when the mechanical axis falls outside the joint, there is a wide range of tibiofemoral angles (31). The line of action of the resultant force across the knee varies during gait (43). The resultant force depends upon the power of the lateral muscles, body weight, varus or valgus deformity, and the center of gravity of the body (43). The line of action of the resultant force may be displaced medially by weakening of the lateral muscles, by an increase in body weight, by a varus deformity, or by permanent displacement of the center of gravity of the body to the side opposite the loaded knee (43).

Comparative evaluation of static radiographs and dynamic gait analysis has revealed a discrepancy in calculating force transmission across the knee (31). For varus deformities, the load on the medial tibial plateau rapidly approaches 100% of the total load on the joint. However, for valgus deformities, there is no significant correlation between the mechanical axis and the dynamic force transmission across the joint. The discrepancy can be explained by the normal horizontally directed medial shear force that develops on weight bearing (31). A similar lack of correlation between the angular deformity of the knee and the force distribution across the joint upon gait analysis has been noted by Harrington (24). The center of pressure in the knee varies with the gait cycle and is not directly related to the magnitude of angulation of the joint. The inclination of the tibia in the coronal plane also affects the magnitude of the abducting-adducting moments on the knee (24).

Joint load is an important mechanism for knee stability. Application of a tibiofemoral contact force increases anteroposterior, mediolateral, varus-valgus, and torsional stiffness with a corresponding laxity (44). Joint load is an important protective mechanism that avoids ligament strain (44). The compression load is generated by body weight and muscle action (26,44). These findings emphasize the importance of the dynamic stabilizers in maintaining joint stability. The most important factor in reducing laxity under load is the conformity of the condylar surfaces (26).

The complex kinematics of knee motion are continually being studied. During knee flexion-extension, rotation in a horizontal plane occurs, ranging from 4°–13°. External rotation of the tibia occurs during knee extension and reaches a peak value just before heel strike (15). The rotatory motion of the knee with flexion and extension has been termed the *screw-home* mechanism. The rotatory motion is synchronous with a coupling of extension and lateral tibial rotation or flexion and medial rotation (25). The axis of rotation for this rotatory motion is the medial intercondylar tubercle of the tibial plateau (59). Integrity of the anterior cruciate ligament is essential for control of this rotatory motion. Pathologic lesions, such as meniscus tears, disrupt the normal synchronous movement (25,60).

A coupled motion of tibial rotation and anteroposterior motion of the knee also exists. Upon anterior displacement of the tibia, there is a coupled internal rotation, while on posterior displacement there is an associated external rotation (19,66,67). The rotation averages 7° (66). Sectioning of the anterior cruciate ligament eliminates the coupled internal rotation, while sectioning of the posterior cruciate ligament eliminates the coupled external rotation (19). These findings emphasize the importance of the cruciate ligaments for normal knee kinematics.

The axis of rotation of the knee for flexion-extension is not static but changes on knee motion. In the normal knee, the instant center of rotation lies within the femoral condyle, indicating a sliding mechanism for knee motion (4). The total translational movement of the instantaneous center axis is about 10 mm (4). The cruciate ligaments have little effect on the location of the instantaneous center of rotation, which depends more upon the geometry of the bones and perhaps the collateral ligaments (4).

The kinematics of the knee are complex and require the coordinated function of the bony architecture, ligamentous guides, and muscular function for satisfactory synchronous movement. Derangements in knee mechanics may lead to articular surface damage and degenerative arthritis.

ROUTINE RADIOGRAPHIC TECHNIQUES

Routine radiography will be discussed here. Other techniques, including computed tomography (CT) magnetic resonance imaging (MRI), and arthrography will be discussed in anatomic sections as they apply to specific clinical problems. AP and lateral radiographs fulfill the minimum requirement for examination of the knee following trauma. In addition, we routinely obtain both oblique views.

AP View

The AP view is obtained with the patient supine, the leg extended, and the patella positioned anteriorly (74,75). The cassette should be centered about 1 cm below the apex of the patella (palpable) (Fig. 7-11A). The central beam may be angled slightly to the head (5°) or perpendicular to the cassette. This view (Fig. 7-11B) demonstrates the medial and lateral compartments. The patella can be seen extending just above the intercondylar area of the femur. The tibial spines are clearly demonstrated.

Upright standing views are required to accurately access the femorotibial joint. Several techniques can be used in patients who are able to bear weight for this procedure. Typically, a 14 × 17 cassette is positioned posterior to the knee so that the lower femurs and upper tibia and fibulas are included on the film. The tube is parallel to the floor or angled slightly (tibial plateau 10° caudad posteriorly) toward the feet (74,75). More recently, a 45° weight-bearing view has been described by Rosenberg et al. (89). The knees are flexed 45° and the tube angled 10° off the horizontal (Fig. 7-12A). The tube is positioned 40 inches from the cassette. This method was more accurate than conventional extension weight-bearing views in evaluating cartilage lesions (89).

Lateral View

The lateral view may be obtained using routine positioning or with the cross-table technique (74,75,91). In most situations, the lateral projection is obtained by po-

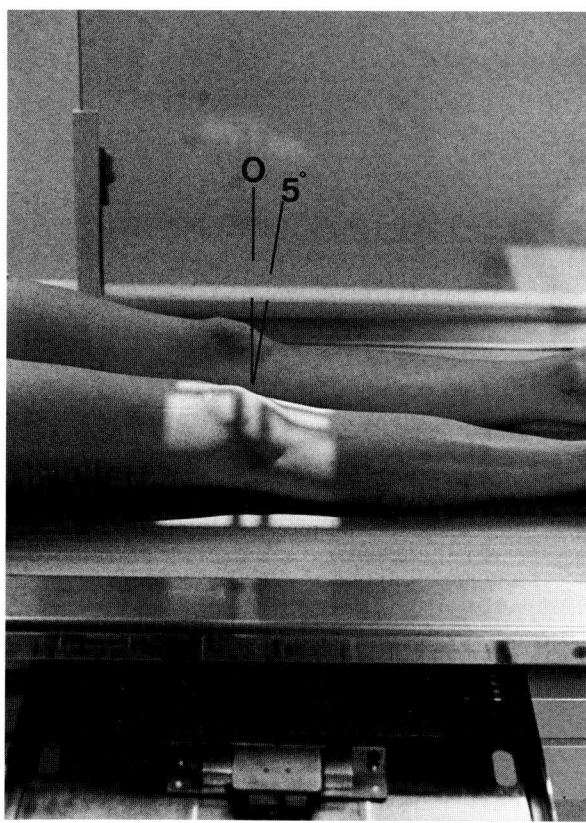

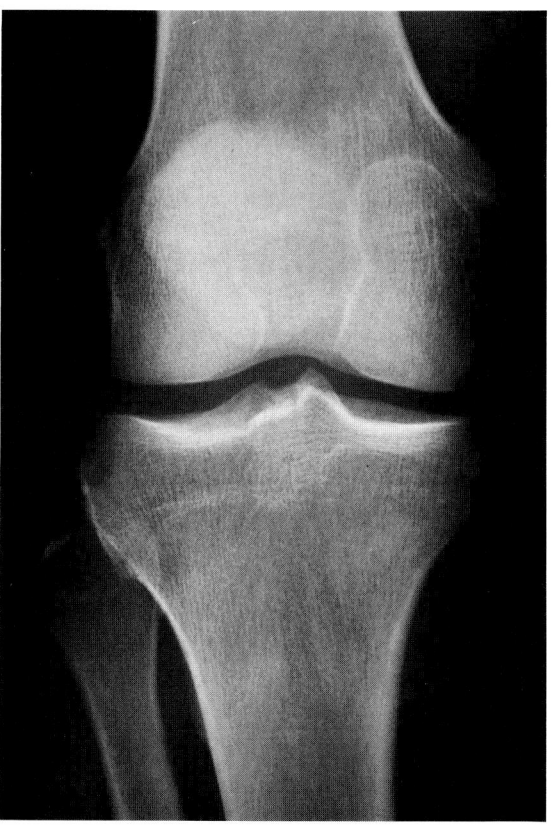

A   B

FIG. 7–11. A: Patient positioned for AP view of the knee. The central beam (*broken line*) is centered 1 cm below the apex of the patella and is perpendicular (0) or angled (5°) to the head. **B:** Normal AP view of the knee demonstrating the distal femur and upper tibia and fibula.

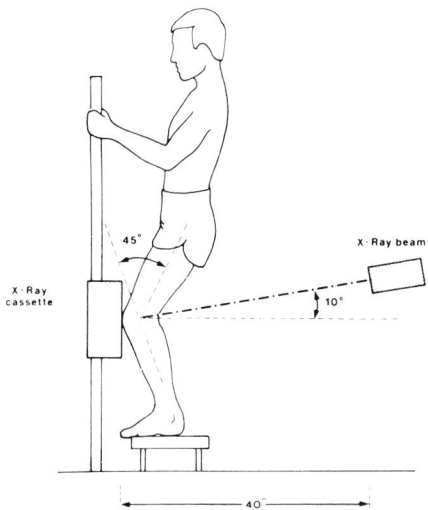

A

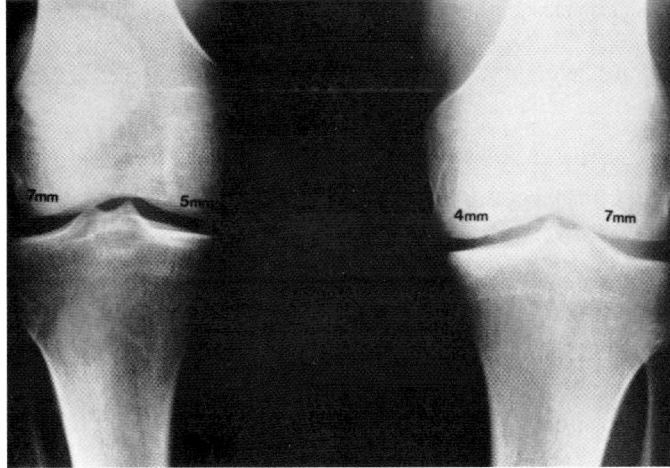

B

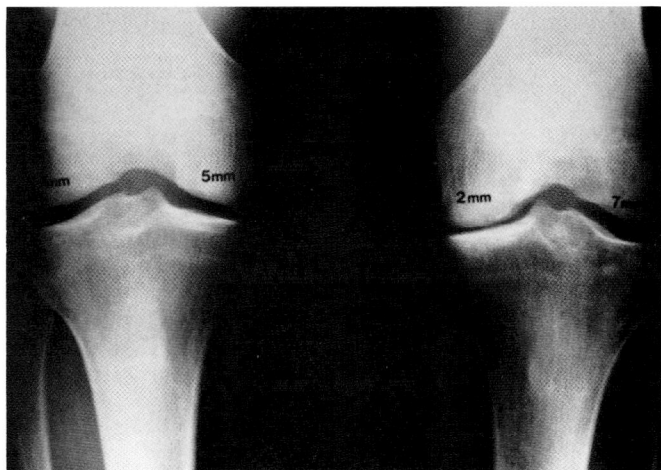

C

FIG. 7–12. A: Illustration of patient positioned for 45° PA flexion weight-bearing view. Standing PA (**B**) and 45° flexion views (**C**) in the same patient. Note that the narrowing is more impressive on the latter (from 89, with permission.)

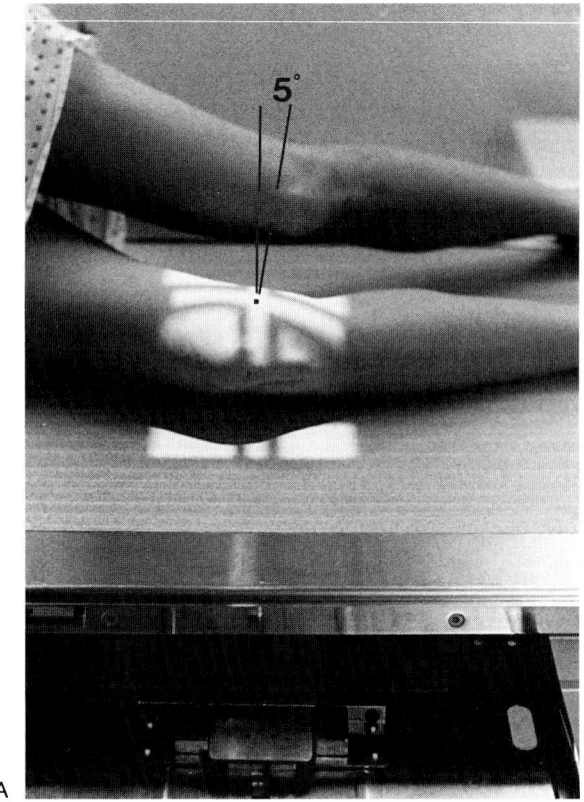
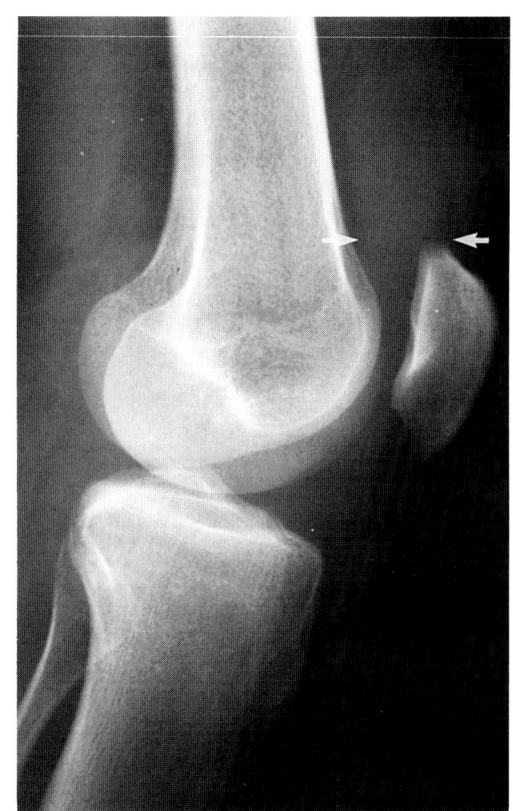

A   B

FIG. 7–13. A: Patient positioned for routine lateral view of the right knee. The knee is flexed about 30°. The central beam (*broken line*) is angled 5° toward the head and centered on the joint space that is just inferior to the apex of the patella. **B:** Lateral view of the knee demonstrating an effusion in the suprapatellar bursa (*arrows*).

sitioning the patient on the side with the involved knee adjacent to the table top (Fig. 7-13A). The knee should be flexed about 30°. This permits more accurate assessment of the patellofemoral space and patellar position. The 8- × 10-inch cassette is centered under the joint with the beam angled 5° to the head (75). This prevents the magnified medial condyle from obscuring the joint space (74).

This view (Fig. 7-13B) allows one to assess the patella, patellofemoral space, tibial plateau, and upper fibula. Effusions may also be detected on the lateral view. Detection of effusions on the lateral view is approximately 77% accurate (79). In the presence of an effusion, the posterior quadriceps tendon may be indistinct, the suprapatellar and prefemoral fat pads may be separated by 5 mm or more (Fig. 7-13B), or a suprapatellar soft tissue density larger than 10 mm may appear (79,80). The patella may also be displaced more anteriorly in relationship to the femur. An uncommon sign is displacement of the fabella. This displacement requires a large effusion (79).

An alternative method for the lateral view, the cross-table technique (Fig. 7-14A), is useful in patients who cannot be moved or in patients with subtle fractures. The cassette is positioned perpendicularly to the table and may be held between the knees for support. A small

cushion under the knee will ensure that the entire structure is included in the film. The beam is centered on the joint and directed perpendicularly to the cassette. This view will demonstrate a lipohemarthrosis, which may be the only indication of an intra-articular fracture (Fig. 7-14B).

Oblique Views

Both oblique views can be obtained with the patient supine. For the internal oblique view, the leg is internally rotated about 45° (Fig. 7-15A). The cassette is centered under the joint space with the central beam perpendicular to the cassette. This view provides excellent detail of the upper fibula and tibiofibular articulation. The lateral femoral condyle is also seen to better advantage (Fig. 7-15B).

The external oblique is obtained using the same parameters but with the leg rotated externally 45° (Fig. 7-16A). The fibula is projected behind the upper tibia. The medial tibial plateau and femoral condyle are clearly demonstrated (Fig. 7-16B).

An alternate method for oblique views is available for patients who cannot be moved. The tube can be angled 45° medially and laterally with the cassette positioned flat on the table and opposite the tube (77).

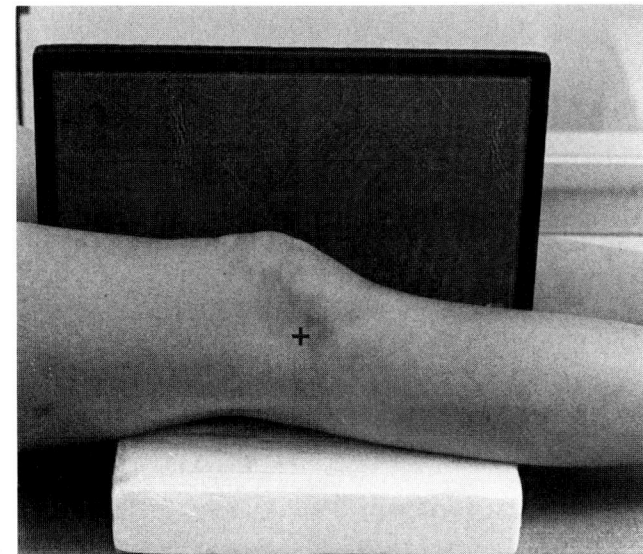

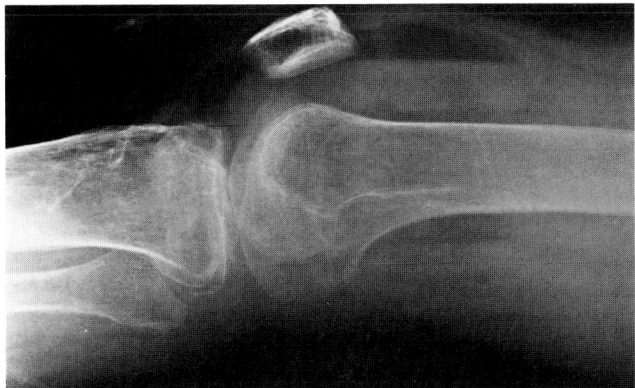

FIG. 7-14. A: Patient positioned for cross-table lateral of the knee. A small cushion under the knee will assure that the entire structure is included on the film. The beam is centered on the joint (+) and perpendicular to the cassette. B: Cross-table lateral view of the knee demonstrating a lipohemarthrosis due to a subtle intra-articular fracture.

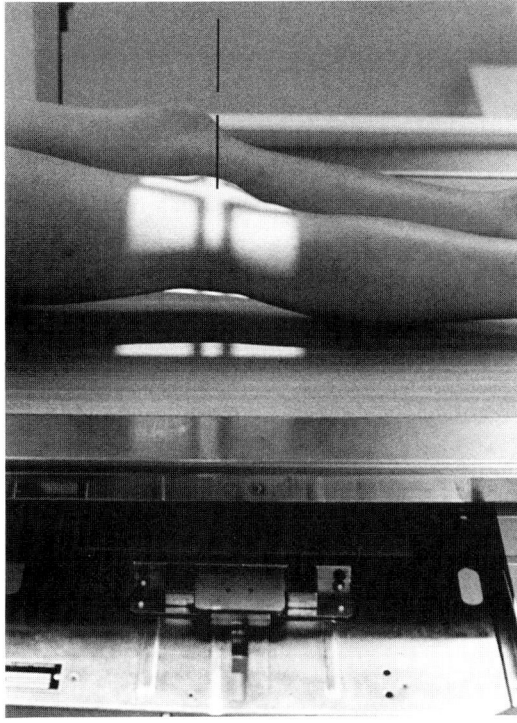

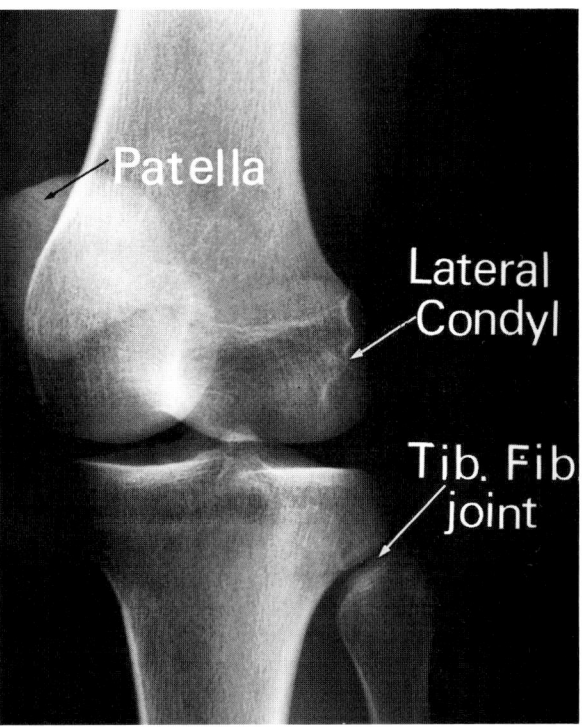

FIG. 7-15. A: Patient positioned for the internal oblique view. The leg is internally rotated about 45°. The beam is perpendicular to the joint. B: Internal oblique view demonstrating the tibiofibular articulation and lateral femoral condyle.

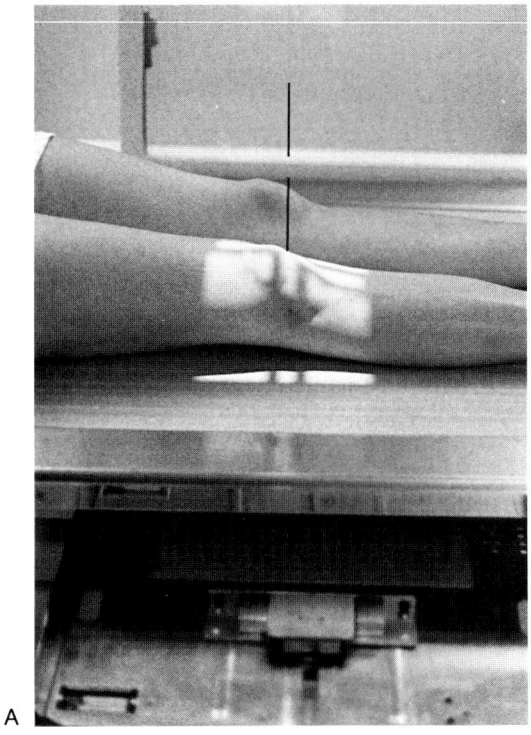
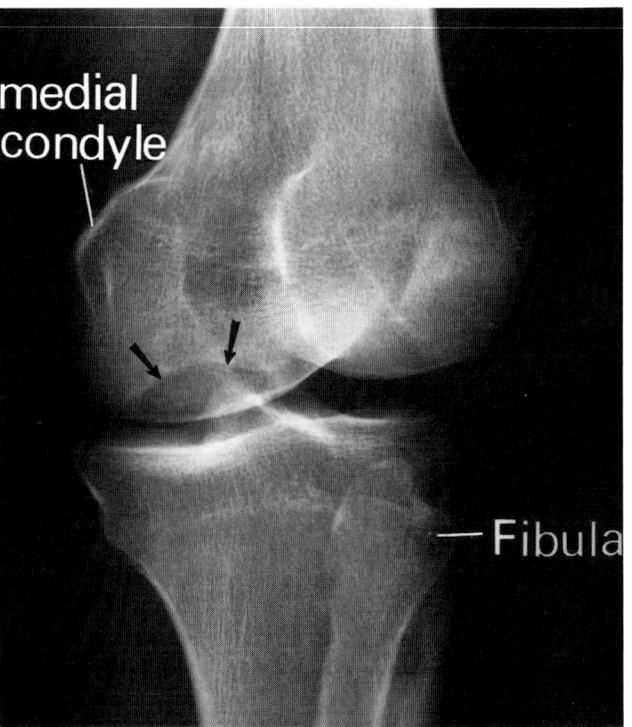

A

B

FIG. 7-16. A: Patient positioned for the external oblique. The leg is externally rotated about 45°. **B:** The radiograph demonstrates the medial structures more clearly. Note the large osteochondral defect in the medial condyle (*arrows*).

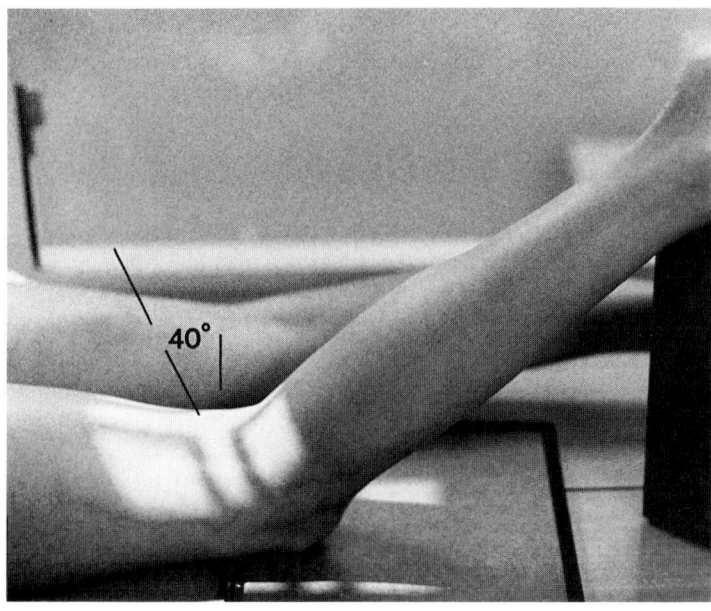
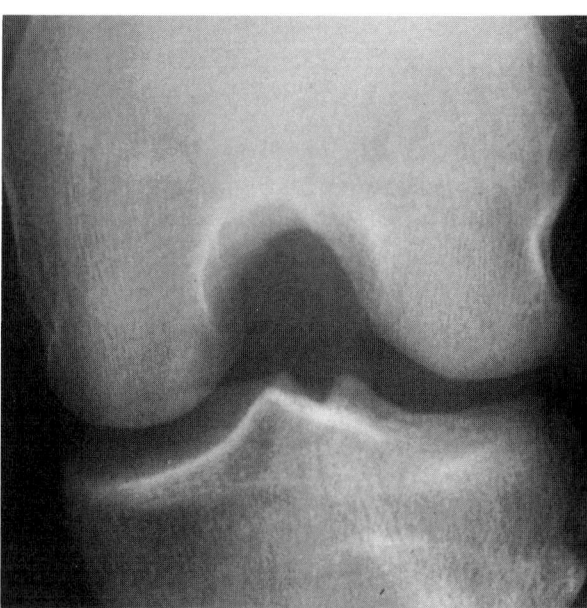

A

B

FIG. 7-17. A: Patient positioned for notch view of the knee. The lower leg is supported by a cushioned prop. The tube is angled 40° toward the feet. **B:** Normal notch view of the knee. Patient positioned for the patella views.

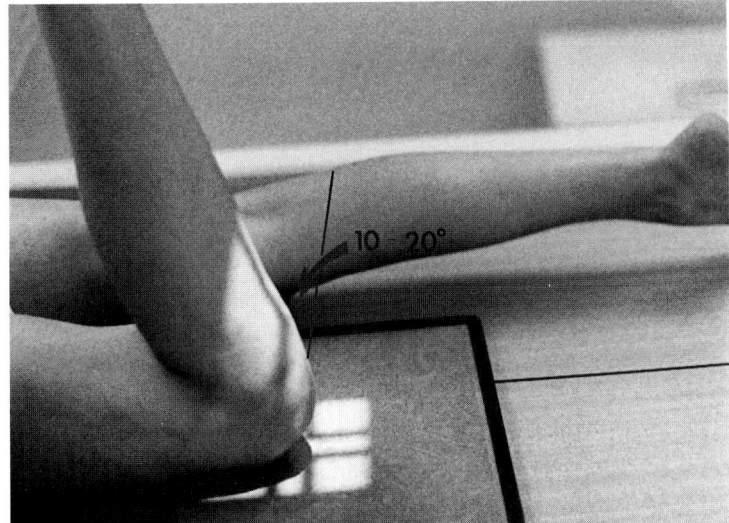

A

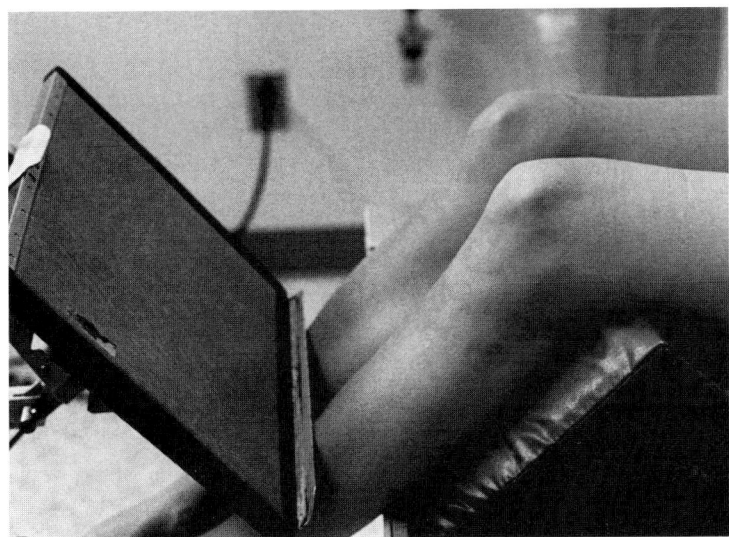

B

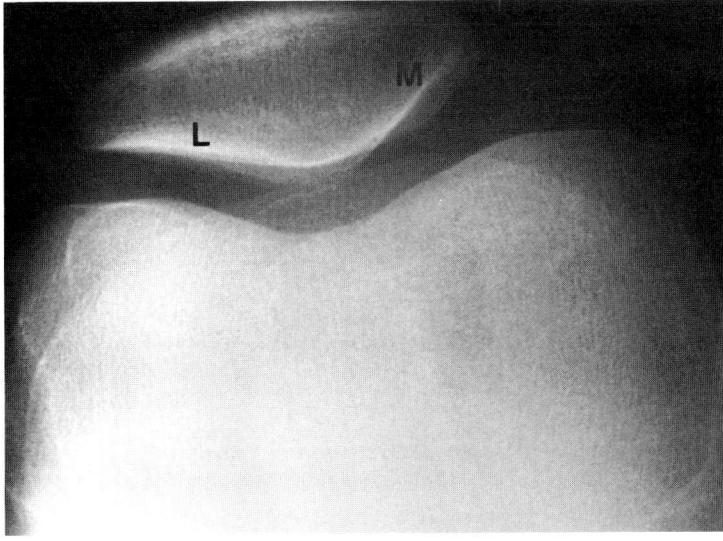

C

FIG. 7-18. A: Settegast technique with the patient prone and the knee flexed. The tube is angled 10–20° to the head and centered on the anterior aspect of the knee. **B:** Merchant view with the legs flexed 45° and the beam centered on the cassette and angled 30° to the horizontal. **C:** Patellar view demonstrating the medial (M) and lateral (L) facets and relationship to the femoral condyles.

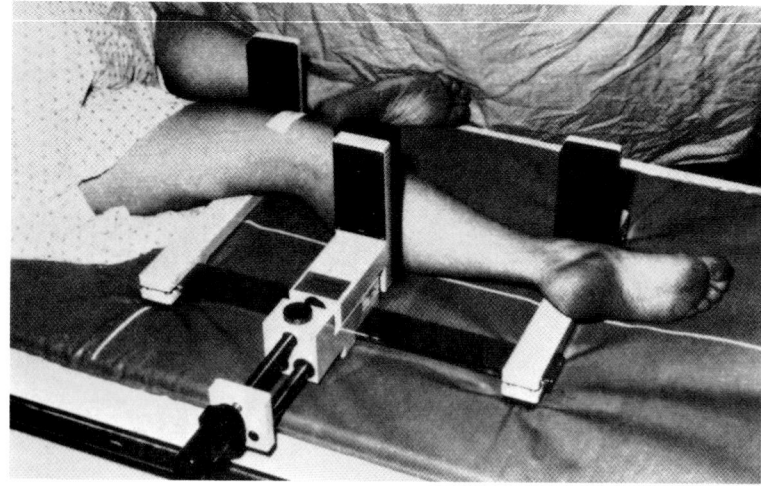

A

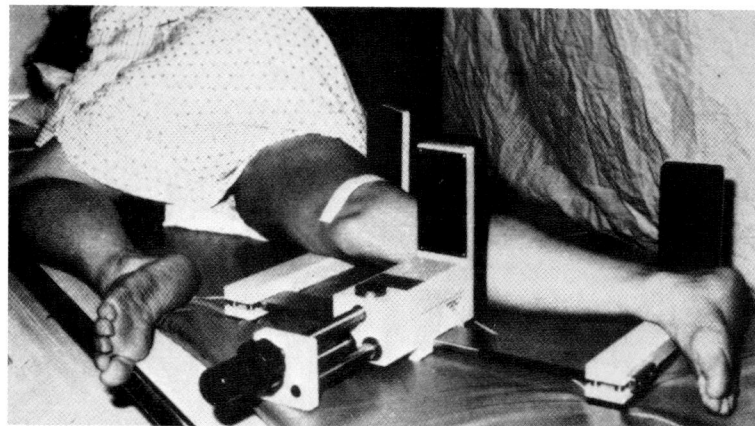

B

FIG. 7-19. Devices for AP stress views (**A, B**) (from 88, with permission.)

These four views (AP, lateral, and both obliques) are usually sufficient for evaluation of the acutely injured patient. However, the clinical setting may dictate that views of the patella or intercondylar notch be obtained.

Notch View

This view is obtained with the patient prone on the table. The knee is flexed 40° and supported on a bolster (Fig. 7-17A). The 8 × 10 cassette is placed under the knee with the tube centered on the cassette and angled 40° toward the feet. Simultaneous views of both knees can also be obtained.

This view is particularly useful in evaluating patients with osteochondritis dissecans, in visualizing the tibial spines, and in detecting osteochondral fragments in the joint space (Fig. 7-17B) (74,76). An alternative method has been described by Holmblad (81).

Patellar Views

Tangential views of the patella are frequently required to evaluate position, fractures, and the patellofemoral joint space (Fig. 7-18C). Numerous techniques have been described for patellar evaluation (74,75,78,82,

85,86). These will be discussed more fully later in this chapter. The two most commonly used techniques at our institution are the Merchant (87) and Settegast (90) methods.

The Settegast technique is performed with the patient prone. The involved knee is flexed 90° with the cassette centered under the knee. The beam is angled about 10°–20°, so that it is perpendicular to the patellofemoral joint (Fig. 7-18A).

Consistency is obtained more readily with the Merchant view (Fig. 7-18B). The knees are flexed 45° over the table with the cassette perpendicular to the legs. The beam is angled 30° to the horizontal and centered on the cassette (74,75,87). The resulting view clearly demonstrates the patella and patellofemoral relationship.

Stress Views

Initial assessment of suspected ligament injury can be accomplished with stress views. Accuracy of stress views depends upon the experience of the examining physician and the patient's symptoms. Pain and swelling make it difficult to perform this technique in the acutely injured knee. MRI is valuable in this setting and will be discussed more fully in the section on soft tissue injuries. Stress views in patients with acute injuries usually re-

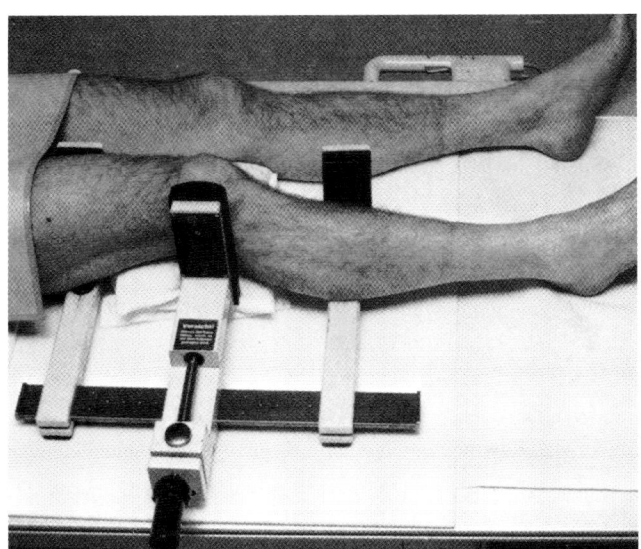

FIG. 7-20. Device for varus and valgus stress views with electronic pressure indicator (from 92, with permission.)

quire anesthetic injection, general anesthesia, or spinal anesthesia. The examination is most commonly performed manually by fixing the extremity with a bolster or strap and applying force in the opposite direction. Jacobsen (83,84) has devised an instrument (agonylaxometer) to obtain more accurate measurements. Commercial devices are now available to obtain more consistency for both AP and varus-valgus stress views (Fig. 7-19 and 7-20) (88,92).

Positioning of the joint for both mediolateral and AP instability is best done fluoroscopically. This allows proper angulation of the tube to ensure that the beam is tangential to the joint surfaces.

The measurement can be calculated from the films using the normal knee for comparison. In the normal knee, minimal motion is possible with stress. On the AP view, lines are constructed along the inferior margin of the femoral condyles and lower cortical margins of the tibial plateaus. The angle formed by these lines, as well as the vertical distance in the joint space, is then measured during varus and valgus stress (Fig. 7-21) (84). The femoral line is not difficult to evaluate; however, variation in the tibial plateaus can create confusion (83,84). The most inferior cortical line should be used (83).

Measuring AP instability is much more difficult using radiographic techniques. Positioning is more difficult, and consistency in measurement is difficult to obtain (84,88). Clinical examination is probably as accurate in most situations of suspected capsular or cruciate ligament injury. If AP stress views are to be performed, the knee is flexed 90° with anterior and posterior forces applied to the tibia just below the knee. Lateral views should be obtained on both the injured and uninvolved knee during these maneuvers. Jacobsen (84) has described this technique in detail. The most important factor is consistency in noting anatomic landmarks. We choose to use the posterior tibial margin (Fig. 7-22) and anterior condylar margin for measuring. The posterior tibial margin can also be used (88). The point at which the condylar line is perpendicular to the tibial line is used for the anterior measurement. Measurement differences that are greater than 3 mm between the normal and abnormal knee suggest ligament injury (see Fig. 7-21).

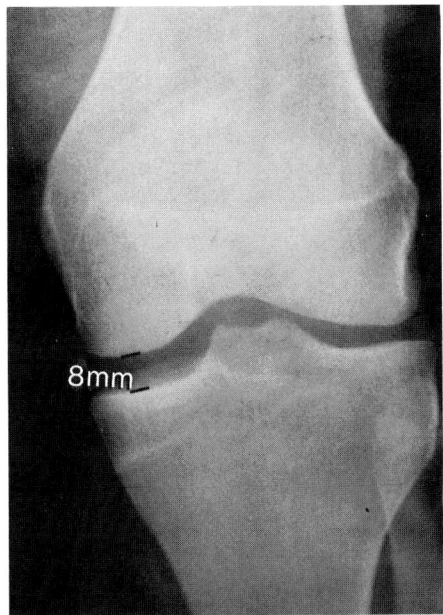
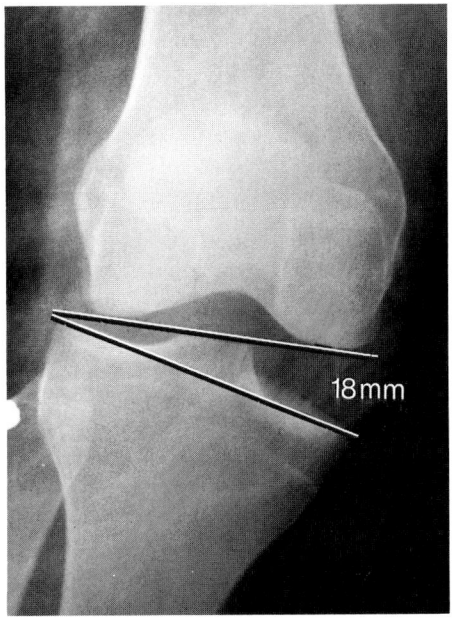

A   B

FIG. 7-21. Young athlete with suspected medial collateral ligament tear and internal derangement. **A:** Stress view of the normal left knee demonstrates joint space of 8 mm. Note the double line of the tibial plateau medially. The lower cortical margin (*line*) was chosen. **B:** Stress view on the right demonstrates a joint space opening of 18 mm confirming the suspected ligament damage. The angle formed by the tibial and condylar lines could also be used.

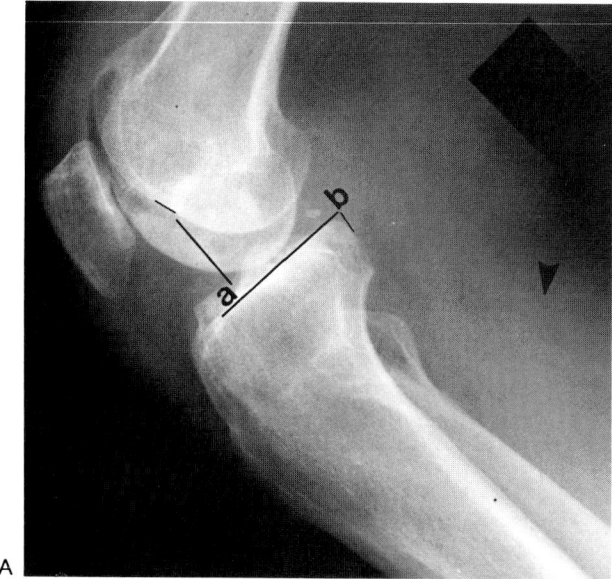
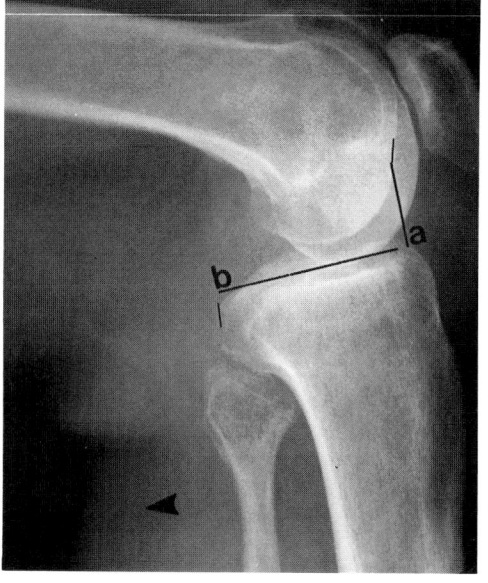

FIG. 7–22. Patient with suspected ligament instability. The anterior and posterior stress views were performed. **A:** Anterior stress on the tibia. The knee is not in a true lateral position. Note the overlap of the medial and lateral (*line*) femoral condyles. This reduces measurement accuracy. The tibial surface (*line*) and posterior margin are labeled and the distance (a–b) can be calculated and compared with the neutral radiograph. **B:** Posterior stress view. Again there is not true alignment.

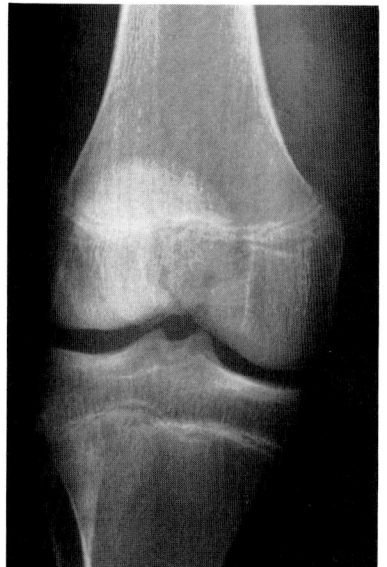
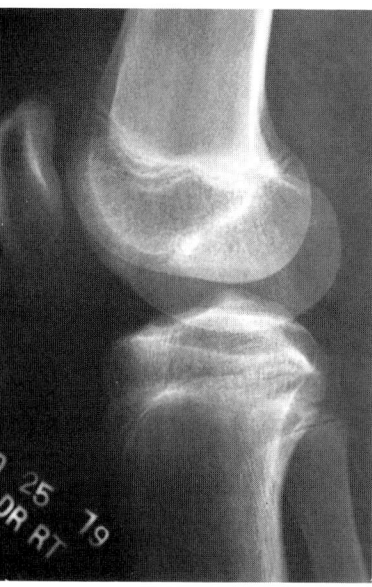
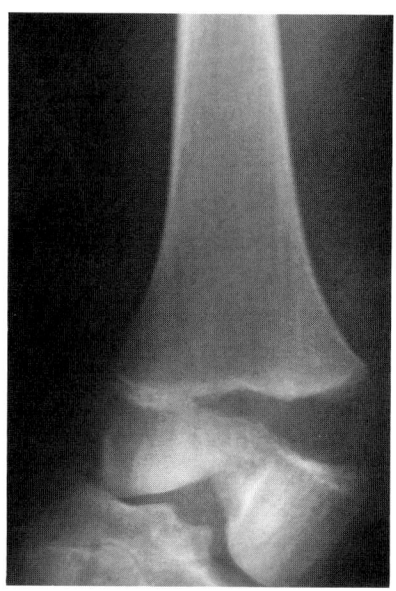

FIG. 7–23. AP (**A**) and lateral views (**B**) in a 16-year-old with knee pain following trauma. The subtle Salter-Harris fracture was overlooked. Lateral stress view (**C**) displaces the epiphysis demonstrating the fracture at risk of further vascular injury.

Stress views must be performed with care in patients with open growth plates. MRI may be preferred for detection of ligament and growth plate injuries (Fig. 7-23).

There are numerous routine views that have not been discussed. Some of these will be discussed later in this chapter as they apply to specific clinical situations. Other radiographic techniques (tomography, CT, MRI, etc.) will also be included (73,74,75).

PATELLAR DISORDERS

Disorders of the patellofemoral joint are frequent clinical problems. Patellofemoral arthralgia, instability, and fractures are frequent. A knowledge of the anatomy, biomechanics, and techniques of radiographic study of the patellofemoral joint is necessary to diagnose and treat these problems.

Anatomy

Although the anatomy of the patellofemoral joint has been discussed earlier in this chapter, a review of some of the pertinent aspects of anatomy is essential in order to comprehend many patellar problems. The triangular patella is divided on its articular surface by a vertical median ridge into medial and lateral facets. A small vertical ridge divides the medial facet from the most medial odd facet. The medial facet is convex while the lateral facet is concave. The thickest articular cartilage, which may measure up to 4–5 mm in thickness, is present on the median ridge (107). The trochlear surface of the femur may be divided into convex medial and lateral facets. The lateral trochlear facet is larger and extends more proximally than the medial facet (159). The superior aspect of the lateral trochlear facet has a smooth transition with the anterior femoral cortex, while the superior medial trochlear facet has a prominent bony and cartilaginous ridge from 3–8 mm in height (147).

The stabilizers of the patella are both static and dynamic. The static stabilizers on the medial side are the patellofemoral ligament superiorly and the meniscopatellar ligament inferiorly (107). The lateral static stabilizers are the patellofemoral ligament superiorly and the meniscopatellar ligament inferiorly. The fascia lata also has an attachment laterally to the patella. As the lateral stabilizers are denser than the medial stabilizers, there is greater strength on the lateral side. The dynamic stabilizers consist of the four components of the quadriceps muscle. The patellar ligament extends from the inferior part of the patella to the tibial tubercle and has a slight lateral orientation.

The vascular supply to the patella is extensive. An anastomotic circle of vessels surrounds the patella. The main vessels contributing to the anastomosis are the supreme genicular, medial superior genicular, medial inferior genicular, lateral superior genicular, lateral inferior genicular, and anterior tibial recurrent arteries. The intra-osseous arteries are composed of two main systems (155). One system is the midpatellar vessels, which enter vascular foramina on the middle anterior surface. The second system enters from the infrapatellar anastomosis behind the patellar ligament. Therefore, the proximal part of the patella may be susceptible to ischemic changes following fracture.

A variety of patellar shapes may be present as well as varying configurations of the trochlea (Fig. 7-24). The dysplasias may be a potential source of confusion to the examining physician and in some instances may be pathologic (Fig. 7-25). Wiberg reported on the major patellar types (159). In Type I, the medial and lateral patellar facets are equal in size. In Type II, the medial facet is slightly smaller than the lateral facet. In Type III, the medial patellar facet is very small, and there may be hypoplasia of the medial trochlear facet of the femur. A Wiberg Type II patella is the most frequent type (108). Aplasia and hypoplasia (patella parva) of the patella may occur but are usually associated with other lesions or systemic syndromes (108). The flattened patella or hemipatella with one facet (alpine hunter's cap) is frequently associated with symptoms of patellar instability (108). Patellar fragmentation (Fig. 7-26) is a common finding, with a bipartite patella being present in 0.05–1.66% of knees (108). A bipartite patella may be distinguished from a fracture by (1) a clearly defined radiolucency with rounded margins separating the fragments, (2) sclerosis of the margins, and (3) bilaterality of the lesion.

Biomechanics

In the extended position, the patella lies above the trochlear surface of the femur and rests on a layer of subsynovial fat (159). In this position, the patella lies laterally in 87% of knees, with contact being made between the crest of the patella or lateral facet and lateral trochlear facet (104). Contact between the patella and trochlea occurs at 10°–20° of flexion and involves the inferior aspect of the patella (Fig. 7-27) (113,119). In 20°–30° of flexion, only 29% of patellas are centered in the trochlear groove (104). With increasing flexion, the area of contact moves proximally on the patella, and only the articular surface of the patella contacts the trochlea between 30° and 80° of flexion (113,119). With increasing flexion, the patella also becomes more centered in the trochlear groove, and 96% of the patella is centered with 90° of flexion (104). Beyond 80°–90° of knee flexion, the patellar tendon begins to articulate with

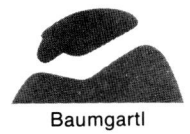
Baumgartl

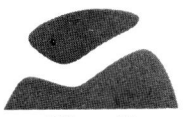
Wiberg III

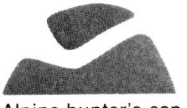
Alpine hunter's cap

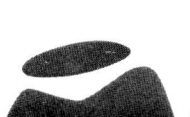
Pebble

Half-moon

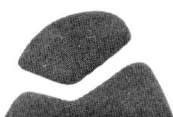
Patella magna

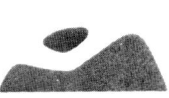
Patella parva

FIG. 7–24. Variations in patellar shape (from 107, with permission.)

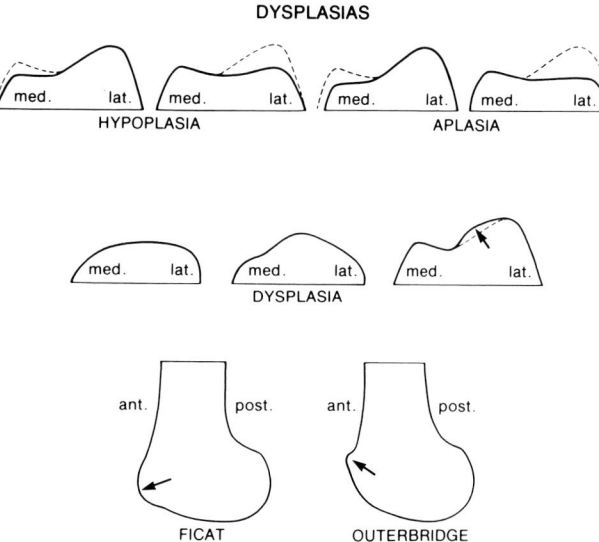

DYSPLASIAS

HYPOPLASIA   APLASIA

DYSPLASIA

FICAT   OUTERBRIDGE

FIG. 7–25. Variations in trochlear appearance. (from 107, with permission.)

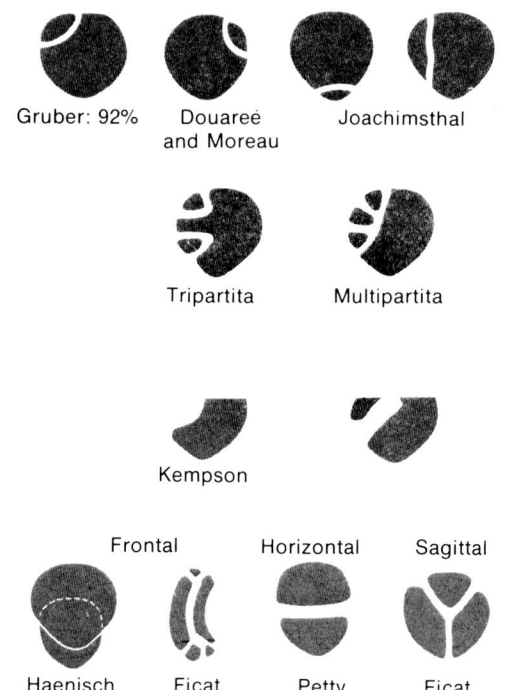

Gruber: 92%   Douareé and Moreau   Joachimsthal

Tripartita   Multipartita

Kempson

Frontal   Horizontal   Sagittal

Haenisch   Ficat   Petty   Ficat

FIG. 7–26. Fragmentation of the patella (from 107, with permission.)

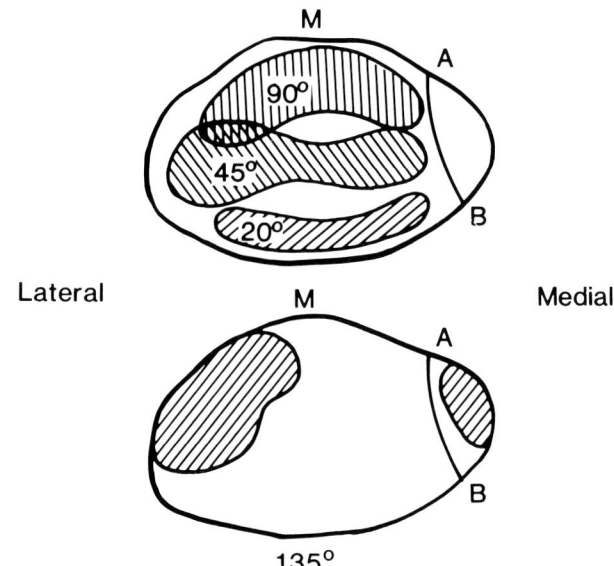

Lateral   Medial

135°

FIG. 7–27. Patellofemoral contact apex in different degrees of knee flexion (from 107, with permission.)

the femur (113,119). Beyond 90° of flexion, the medial patellar facet lies within the intercondylar notch of the femur (113,119). At 135° of flexion, the odd facet begins to articulate with the medial femoral condyle (113). The lack of contact on the odd facet except at maximal knee flexion may account for areas of chondromalacia frequently seen in this location (112,113). Osteochondritis dissecans of the medial femoral condyle may be related to trauma from contact of the patella in this area upon maximal knee flexion (112). The size of the contact area between the patella and femur ranges from a low of 2

cm^2 at 30° to 3.5–6.0 cm^2 at 90° of knee flexion (107,119). The greater contact area with increased flexion aids in the distribution of patellofemoral forces over a broad area (119).

The screw-home mechanism of the knee with external rotation of the tibia in the terminal 30° of extension rotates the tibia laterally. This external rotation produces a valgus vector between the quadriceps tendon and the patellar ligament, the Q-angle (119). This valgus vector tends toward lateral displacement of the patella and must be resisted by the static and dynamic medial stabilizers, which consist of the vastus medialis, medial retinaculum, and the bony architecture of the femur and patella (119). As knee flexion progresses, the patella is drawn from its superior lateral position onto the trochlear surface of the femur and gradually into the intercondylar notch, resulting in a C-shaped tracking that is open laterally (119).

The patella facilitates knee extension by increasing the distance between the extensor mechanism and the rotational axis of the femur (107,119). The patella also centralizes the action of the quadriceps muscle, allowing transmission of its force around an angle during knee flexion with minimal loss due to friction (119). Additionally, the patella protects the underlying surfaces of the femoral condyles (119). The viscoelastic articular cartilage allows some deformation under load, which in turn allows better force distribution to a larger area (119).

In full extension, the patella is responsible for almost 30% of the quadriceps moment arm (126). Following patellectomy, a 15–30% increase in quadriceps force is necessary to obtain full extension (126). Loss of the patella lever arm results in increased compression forces between the femur and tibia (138). Patellectomy results in a decrease in stance-phase flexion and decreased flexion with ascending or descending stairs (127). An alteration in the path of the instant center also occurs following patellectomy (127). Patellofemoral compression forces are substantial and result from muscle activity about the knee during knee flexion. Two factors increase these forces with increasing knee flexion: (1) an increase in the moment arm of the flexor, and (2) an increase in the resultant normal vector to the patellofemoral contact surface (107,119,132). The patellofemoral reaction force is approximately 0.5 times body weight for level walking and 3.3 times body weight during stair climbing (152). Patellofemoral forces increase from near 0 in full extension to 2.0 times body weight at 60° of knee flexion (151). The increased patellofemoral forces correspond to an increase in the quadriceps force needed to stabilize the knee with increasing knee flexion (151). During deep knee bends, a patellofemoral reaction force of up to 7.8 times body weight may be generated (141). Contact stresses of up to 35–40 psi have been measured on the patellofemoral joint (106). Between 13% and 30% of the patellar surface bears joint loads of between 421 and 3,420 N, resulting in stress values equal to or in excess of tibiofemoral stresses (141).

Elevation of the tibial tuberosity has been utilized as a technique to increase the moment arm for the extensor mechanism and thus decrease patellofemoral stress (106,126,138). An anterior displacement of 2 cm reduces patellar compression forces by 50% (137,138). Experimentally, an elevation of the tibial tuberosity by 1.3 cm results in an 83.5% reduction in average stress (106). Following patellectomy, a 1.5 cm elevation of the tibial tuberosity will restore the normal extensor moment arm (126).

Examination

Evaluation of the patellofemoral joint must include both a careful physical examination and approximate radiographs. The problems to be detected are those of instability and degeneration of the articular cartilage. Therefore, examination must be directed at associated abnormal anatomy, patellar position, stability, motion, crepitus, and effusion. Alignment of the patella in extension and flexion should be evaluated as well as the pattern of patellar tracking during motion. A lateral subluxing patella often may be seen to lie more laterally than normal in the flexed position (118,135). The Q-angle (Fig. 7-28) may also reveal significant information. It is measured clinically by drawing a line from the tibial tuberosity to the center of the patella and a second line along the direction of the quadriceps mechanism. The normal Q-angle is 14°, with greater than 20° considered abnormal (93,122). An increased Q-angle has been associated with patellar instability and degenerative changes. Evaluation of the hip for excess femoral anteversion and the tibia for external torsion should also be performed, as

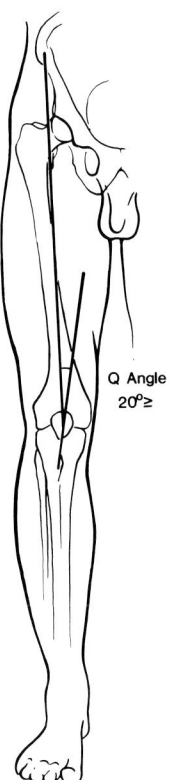

FIG. 7-28. Method of measurement of the "Q-angle".

both these anatomic changes will lead to an increase in the Q-angle (93,124).

Other anatomic problems that have been associated with instability include a deficient or high-riding vastus medialis obliquus, contracted iliotibial band, excess valgus alignment of the knee, and a deficient lateral femoral condyle (93). The "apprehension test" consists of lateral displacement of the patella in both extension and in 20°–30° of flexion with the quadriceps relaxed (118,119,121). If there is laxity of the medial restraints and subluxation of the patella, the patient's symptoms of instability are reproduced. Patellofemoral crepitation should be sought as evidence of degenerative changes in the articular cartilage. Palpation of the patella during active flexion and extension of the knee may reveal crepitus. Passive proximal distal and medial lateral movement of the patella while a compression force is applied may reveal crepitation (118). Subluxation of the patella in a medial and lateral direction with palpation of the facets for tenderness is also helpful but not specific, as synovial tissue is also examined. Atrophy of the vastus medialis may be seen on visual examination with the quadriceps contracted and should be compared with the contralateral limb (118,124). Measurements of the thigh circumference of both limbs should be performed at a fixed distance above the adductor tubercle. The presence or absence of knee effusion and especially a hemarthrosis following an acute injury should also be evaluated.

Radiographs taken of the patellofemoral joint must include AP, lateral, and axial patellar views. The lateral radiograph should be taken in 30° of flexion to place the patellar tendon under tension (see Fig. 7-13) (107). Additional lateral views in 60° and 90° of flexion may be useful to evaluate the patellofemoral joint space at different areas of contact (107). The lateral radiograph is also useful in assessing the height of the patella relative to the joint line. A high-riding patella, or patella alta, is associated with recurrent lateral subluxation, dislocation, and chondromalacia (107,122,123,154). A low-riding patella, or patella infra (patella baja), is usually seen postoperatively following excessive distal transfer of the tibial tuberosity, but it may also be seen in achondroplasia (107).

Patella alta may be assessed according to three measurements: the Insall-Salvati index, the Blackburne index, or Blumensaat's line (97,123,150). In Blumensaat's method, the lower pole of the patella should lie superior to a line projected along the ventral aspect of the intercondylar notch. This technique is usually unreliable (97,123,150). The Insall-Salvati index (Fig. 7-29C) is determined by the ratio of the length of the patellar tendon to the length of the patella (123). The value for this ratio is 1.02 ± 0.13 (mean and standard deviation) (93,123). Any deviation of more than 20% is abnormal (123). In Blackburne's technique, the ratio of the articular length of the patella to the height of the lower pole of the articular cartilage above the tibial plateau is measured (97). The normal value is defined as 0.8 (0.54–1.06, 0.95 ± 0.13), and patella alta is present when the ratio is greater than 1.0 (85). There is little correlation between the techniques for measuring patella alta (150). The most widely used technique is that of Insall and Salvati.

Axial views of the patellofemoral joint are used to view the joint line without distortion, to assess the configuration of the patella and trochlea, and to indicate the relationship of the patella to the femur (105,118,136). A variety of techniques have been utilized with varying degrees of knee flexion (Fig. 7-30). The traditional "skyline"

view as described by Settegast has the knee in acute flexion, but this view does not visualize patellofemoral relationships in the area where patellar subluxation and dislocation most frequently occur (Fig. 7-30A). Since instability of the patella occurs close to full extension, other radiographic techniques have been advocated. The Jaroschy or Hughston view is taken with the knee in 50° to 60° of flexion and with the x-ray tube angled 45° from the vertical (Fig. 7-30B) (118). Wiberg recommended 40° of knee flexion and Brattstrom 90° (100,159). Ficat recommended views in 30°, 60°, and 90° of knee flexion to evaluate subluxation as well as successive areas of patellofemoral contact at the inferior, middle, and superior thirds (Figs. 7-30C and 7-31) (107,108). Malghem and Maldague (136), recommend lateral rotation with the knee flexed 30° to improve detection of subluxation. Egund (105) suggested a standing technique with the knee flexed 15°. The two most useful techniques currently being used are those of Merchant and Laurin (134,144). In the Merchant technique, the knee is flexed 45°, and the x-ray beam is oriented 30° from the horizontal, providing a beam-to-femur angle of 30° (Fig. 7-30D) (144). In the Laurin technique, the knees are flexed 20°–30°, and the x-ray beam is directed cephalad from below parallel to the anterior surface of the tibia (Fig. 7-30E) (134).

Using these special axial views, a variety of measurements of the trochlea, patella, and patellofemoral congruence may be made. The sulcus angle (Fig. 7-32) is defined as the angle formed by the highest point on the medial and lateral femoral condyles and the lowest point in the intercondylar sulcus. The normal sulcus angle is 141°–142° (100), 138° ± 6° (144), or 137° (93). A higher value for the sulcus angle is indicative of dysplasia and a tendency to sublux (128). The congruence angle (Fig. 7-32) is formed by a line bisecting the sulcus angle and a second line projected from the apex of the sulcus angle through the lowest point on the articular ridge of

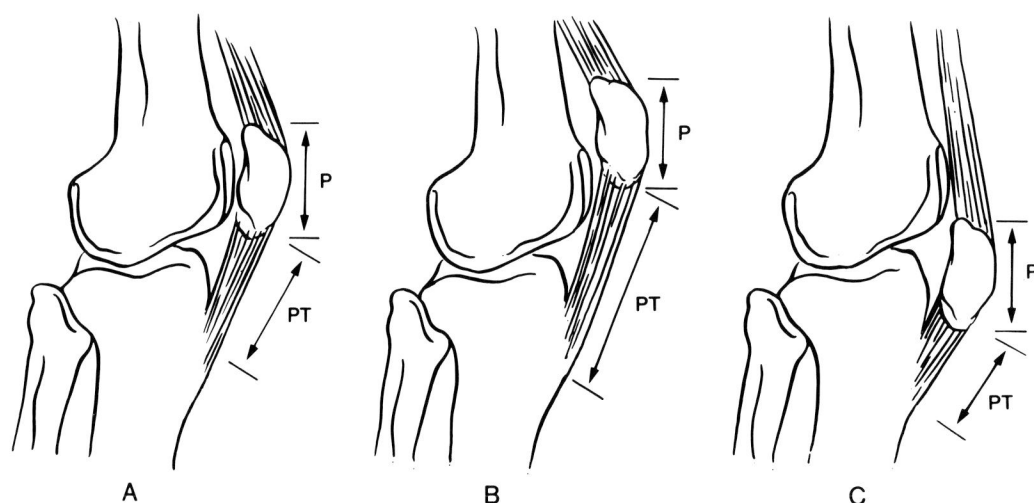

FIG. 7–29. A: Normal patellofemoral relationship. B: Patella alta. C: Patella infra as measured by Insall-Salvati technique.

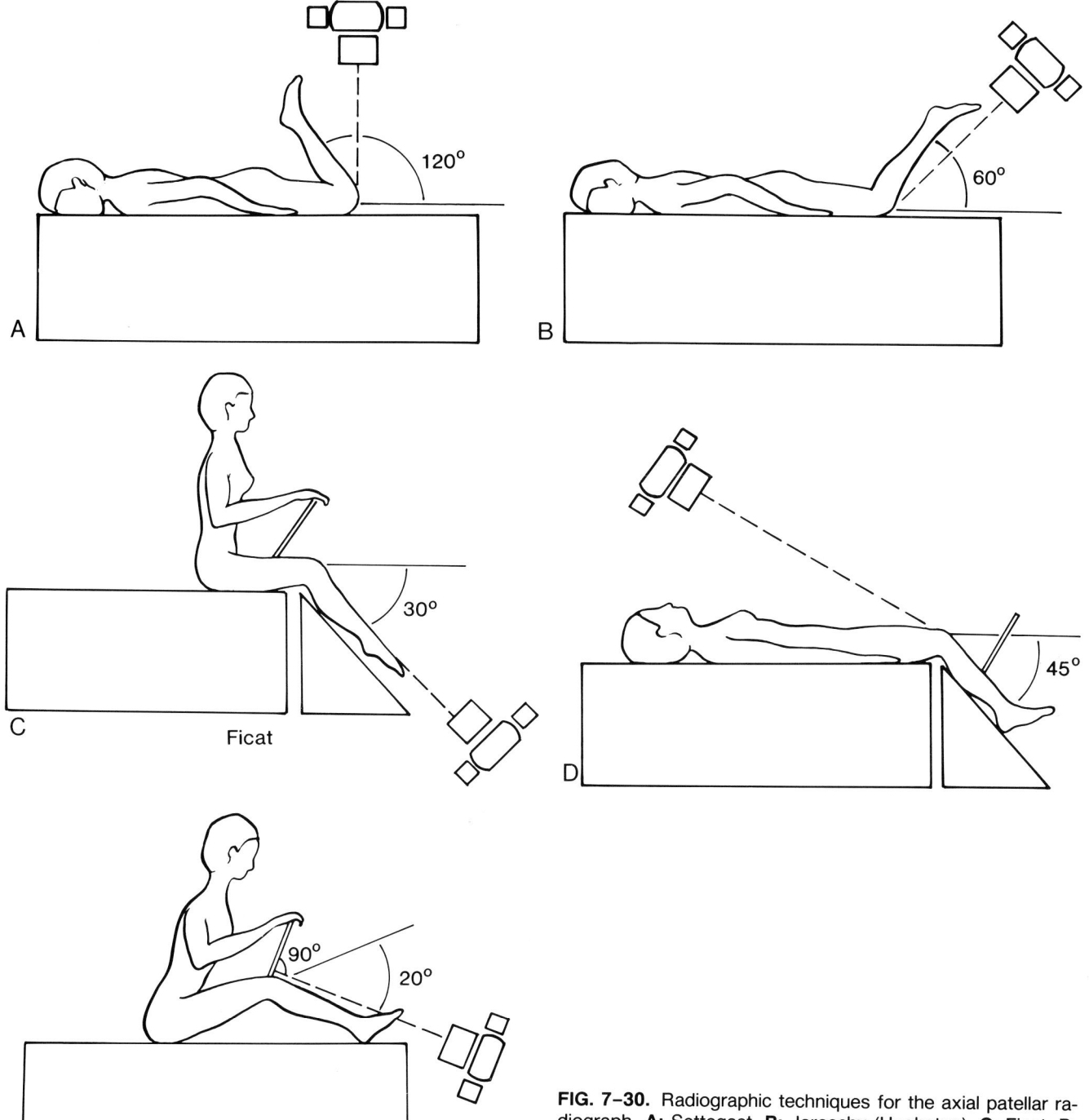

FIG. 7–30. Radiographic techniques for the axial patellar radiograph. **A:** Settegast. **B:** Jaroschy (Hughston). **C:** Ficat. **D:** Merchant. **E:** Laurin.

the patella (144). If the apex of the patellar articular ridge is lateral to the zero line it is positive, and if medial it is negative. The normal congruence angle is −6° (124), or −8° ± 6° (93). It is 23° in knees with recurrent dislocation (144). The lateral patellofemoral angle is defined by two lines: (1) a line joining the summits of the femoral condyles, which is a function of the femoral sulcus and is related to the stabilizing role of the lateral femoral condyle, and (2) a line through the limits of the lateral patellar facet (Fig. 7-33) (133,134). The lateral patellofemoral angle is open laterally in 97% of normal knees, while it is

parallel in 80% and open medially in 20% of knees with subluxation of the patella (134). The patellofemoral index is the ratio between the thickness of the medial patellofemoral interspace and that of the lateral patellofemoral interspace (Fig. 7-34) (133). The lateral patellofemoral interspace corresponds to the shortest distance between the lateral patellar facet and the articular surface of the lateral femoral condyle. The medial patellofemoral interspace is measured by calculating the shortest distance between the lateral limit of the medial patellar facet and the medial femoral condyle. The nor-

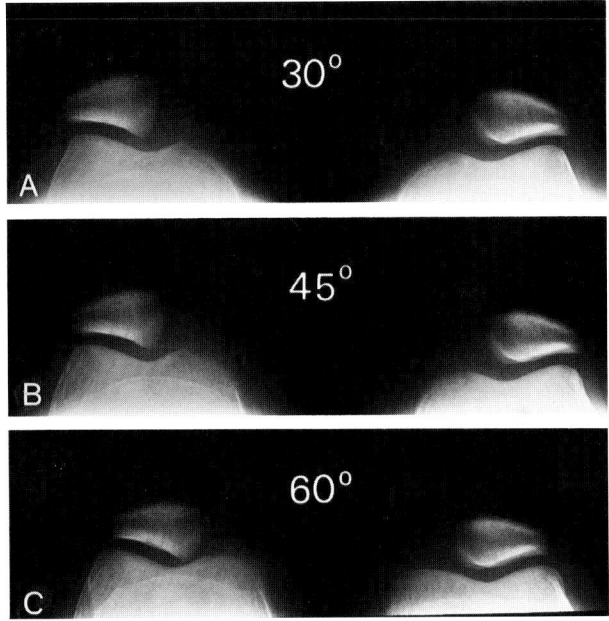

FIG. 7–31. Axial views of the patella in varying degrees of knee flexion in the same patient. **A:** 30°; **B:** 45°; **C:** 60°.

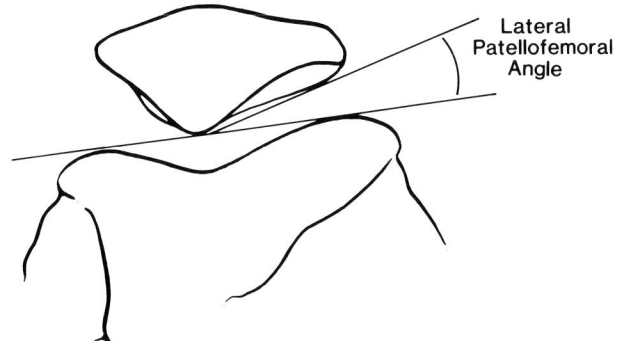

FIG. 7–33. Lateral patellofemoral angle.

mal patellofemoral index is 1.6 or less (133). An increased patellofemoral index is present in 97% of patients with chondromalacia patellae (133).

Lateral patellar displacement may be assessed by drawing a line perpendicular to the line joining the summits of the femoral condyles. The perpendicular line originates at the margin of the articular cartilage of the medial femoral condyle (Fig. 7-35) (133). In 97% of normal cases, the medial edge of the patella is medial to this line and, in 3%, it is lateral to the line by only 1 mm (133). In subluxing patellae, the medial edge of the patella touches or is lateral to this line in 53% (134). In the case of lateral subluxation, the importance of a relaxed extensor mecha-

nism during the axial radiograph has been emphasized by Laurin (133), but Sikorski (156) has recommended a vigorous quadriceps contraction to visualize lateral subluxation more effectively. Some variation in the measured parameters of patellar position also exists based upon sex (93) and should not be confused with subluxation. Lateral patellar rotation with quadriceps contraction may be estimated from the ratio of the lateral to medial patellar facets. An increased patellar rotation may correlate with chondromalacia (156).

Axial radiographs of the patella will visualize osteochondral fractures of the lateral femoral condyle associated with recurrent patellar dislocation as well as marginal fractures of the medial aspect of the patella (110). Calcification in the medial patellar retinaculum without a fracture is also indicative of a previous patellar dislocation with tearing of the medial retinaculum (Fig. 7-36).

Other techniques have also been used for the evaluation of the patella. Computed tomography (CT) has been

PATELLO FEMORAL INDEX

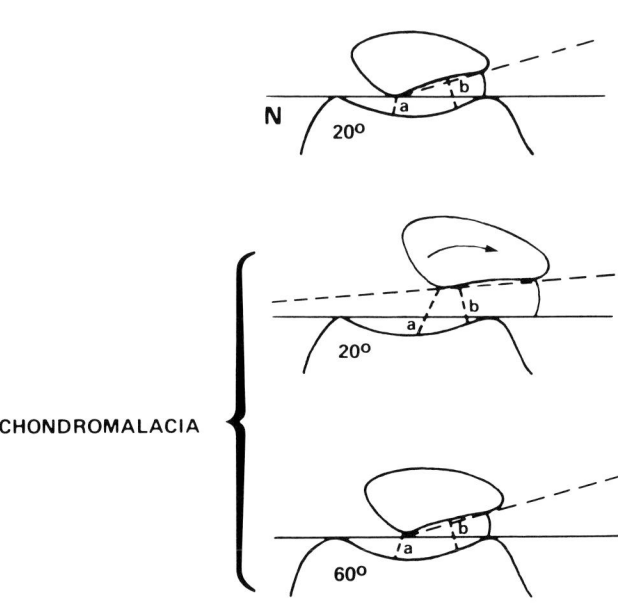

FIG. 7–34. Patellofemoral index (from 133, with permission.)

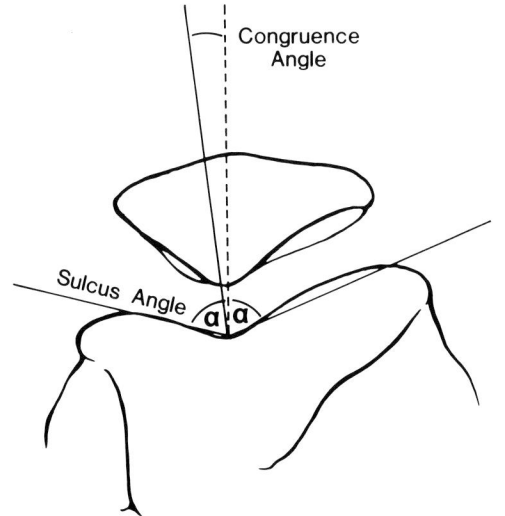

FIG. 7–32. Sulcus angle is formed by a line drawn from the highest point on the medial and lateral femoral condyle and the longest point in the intercondylar sulcus-congruence angle (see text).

LATERAL PATELLAR DISPLACEMENT

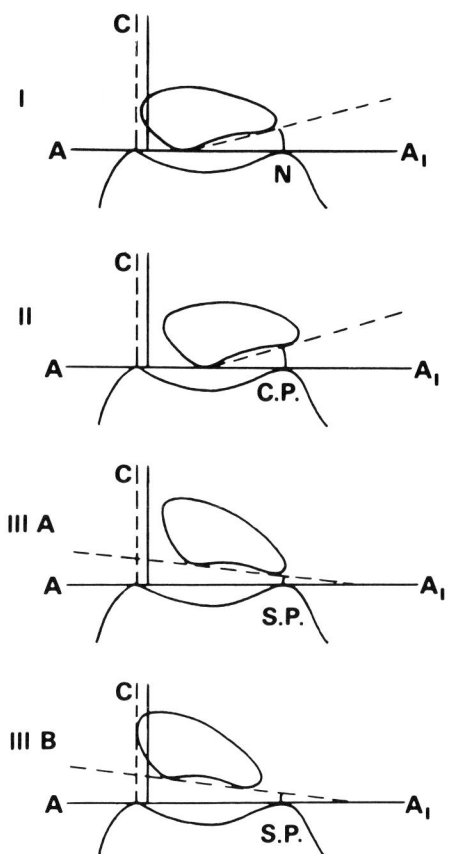

FIG. 7-35. Technique of assessment of lateral patellar displacement (from 133, with permission.)

FIG. 7-36. Axial view revealing severe subluxation of the right patella.

used to evaluate patellar subluxation (120,129,140,157). Axial images can be obtained at 0°, 20°, and 45° with and without quadriceps contraction. Conventional axial CT techniques using 5-mm-thick slices provide adequate patellar images (140). Patellar tracking disorders are more effectively imaged using fast CT with multiple rapid images during flexion and extension (157). Arthrography has been advocated as an additional diagnostic modality for evaluation of the patellofemoral joint (107,108). Injection of contrast material can be used to evaluate the integrity of the articular cartilage of the patella when combined with axial radiographs or CT images obtained at 30°, 45°, 60°, and 90° of flexion (107,158). The diagnosis of chondromalacia of the patella using arthrography has been reported to be as high as 90% (117). MRI, using T1 (SE 500/20) and gradient echo T2* sequences is a valuable technique for evaluating patellar articular cartilage. Motion studies are also possible using the latter technique (98,115). However, arthroscopy has been stated to be a more efficient technique for evaluation of small areas of chondromalacia on the medial facet of the patella (107).

Patellofemoral Pain Syndromes

The clinical syndromes related to the patellofemoral joint are those related to pain and instability. The term *chondromalacia patellae* was initially used by Aleman in 1928 to describe episodes of crepitus and synovitis associated with softening and fissuring of the articular surface of the patella (94). Aleman recognized that, in a series of 220 patients undergoing arthrotomy, one-third of the knees had abnormal articular cartilage on the patella without symptoms referable to the patellofemoral joint. Unfortunately, the term *chondromalacia patellae* has been used for a variety of disorders varying from pathologic studies to reviews of clinical symptomatology without any pathologic confirmation. To avoid this confusion, the term *patellofemoral pain syndrome,* as recommended by other authors (107,108,112,128), is best utilized for the description of the patient with patellofemoral pain without instability. The term *chondromalacia* is best restricted to cases involving description of a pathologic entity.

Patellofemoral arthralgia or pain in the anterior aspect of the knee presents with retropatellar pain associated with sitting and ascending or descending stairs and with crepitation (107,125). Symptoms of giving way, pseudolocking, and swelling are frequent (111,125). On physical examination, there is patellofemoral crepitation, pain on compression of the patella, facet tenderness, effusion, and perhaps abnormal patellar tracking (107,125). The differential diagnosis includes prepatellar bursitis, painful retropatellar fat pad, pes anserinus bursitis, plica syndrome, meniscal lesions, generalized synovitis, and ligamentous instability (107,114). The "excessive lateral pressure syndrome" is a clinical radiologic entity characterized by pain and radiographic evidence of tilting of the patella laterally without lateral subluxation (107). Physical examination reveals a tight lateral retinaculum. Radiographs reveal (1) narrowing of cartilage, (2) increased density in the subchondral bone layer, with a change in alignment of the trabeculae from their normal orientation perpendicular to the equator of the patella to a position perpendicular to the lateral facet, and (3) a tight and thickened lateral retinaculum (107).

The pathologic changes of chondromalacia patellae frequently accompany the clinical syndromes of anterior knee pain. The pathologic changes may be classified in several manners. Outerbridge classified the changes in the articular cartilage into four grades: (1) softening and swelling of the articular cartilage, (2) fragmentation and fissuring in an area 0.5 inch or less, (3) fragmentation and fissuring in an area greater than 0.5 inch in diameter, and (4) erosion of cartilage down to bone (Fig. 7-37) (147). An arthroscopic grading system for chondromalacia has also been suggested (125). These arthroscopic grades include (1) early fibrillation or softening of the articular cartilage, involving one or more facets of the patella without involvement of the femur; (2) fragmentation or erosion of the articular surface that is limited to the patella; and (3) articular cartilage changes involving the femur as well as the patella. Goodfellow and colleagues have suggested that there are two distinct pathologic processes affecting the patella: basal degeneration and surface degeneration (112). Surface degeneration is present in youth, becomes more frequent with age, and primarily affects the odd facet (112). This process is not associated with patellofemoral pain in youth but may lead to degenerative arthritis in later years. Basal degeneration is a fasciculation of collagen in the middle and deep zones of cartilage that later affects the surface (112). Basal degeneration affects the ridge separating the medial from the odd fact and is associated with patellofemoral pain in the young individual (112). It may be divided into three stages: (1) fasciculation of the deep collagen layers with an intact surface, (2) blister formation, and (3) fasciculation extending through the surface of the articular cartilage. Basal degeneration may be the result of excessive pressure and trauma to the patella in this area (112).

Chondromalacia may also be classified by its anatomical location. Five groups have been established (108).

Group 1 involves the lateral patellar facet, usually just lateral to the median ridge. Group 2 involves the medial facet, usually the odd facet. Group 3 is central chondromalacia affecting the median ridge and extending onto both facets. Group 4 is bipolar chondromalacia involving the central portion of the two facets separated by a normal median ridge. Group 5 is global or total chondromalacia involving the totality of both facets.

The etiology of chondromalacia and patellofemoral pain has remained controversial. Chondromalacia patellae may be related to biomechanical or biochemical causes (125). Biomechanical causes can be divided into acute and chronic problems. Acute problems include dislocation, direct trauma, and fracture. Chronic problems include recurrent subluxation, patellar malalignment, excessive lateral pressure syndromes, and meniscal injury leading to loss of synchronous joint motion (125). Biochemical causes include (1) diseases affecting articular cartilage, such as rheumatoid arthritis, recurrent hemarthrosis, alkaptonuria, crystal synovitis, sepsis, and adhesions; (2) iatrogenic factors resulting from intra-articular steroids or prolonged immobilization; and (3) degenerative factors, such as primary osteoarthritis (125). Another etiologic classification system has established six major categories: (1) trauma; (2) dislocation; (3) malalignment with patellar subluxation; (4) normal alignment with osteochondral ridge; (5) increased cartilage vulnerability, as is typical following surgery or immobilization; and (6) occupational hazards (149). The importance of a prominent osteochondral ridge on the medial aspect of the trochlear surface of the femur, which results in shearing forces on the patella at 15°–30° of flexion, has been emphasized by Outerbridge (147–149) but not by other authors. Ficat and colleagues have

FOUR STAGES OF CHONDROMALCIA

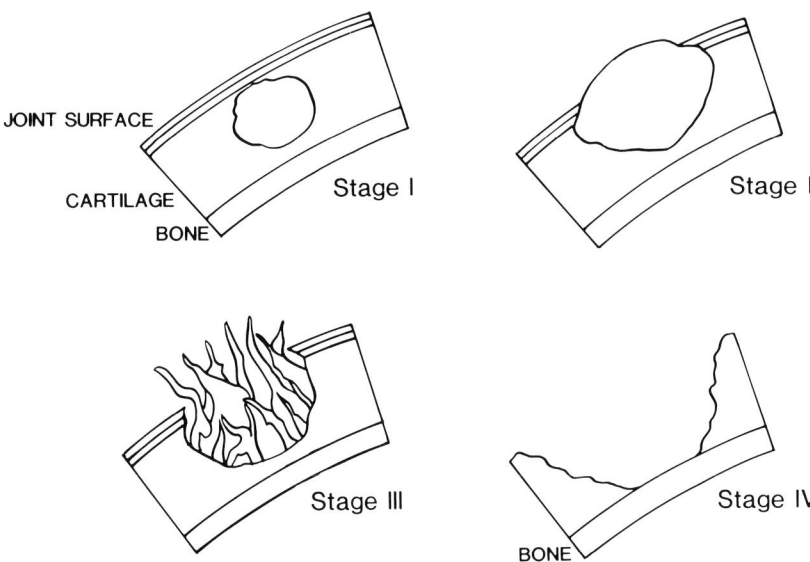

FIG. 7-37. Outerbridge classification of chondromalacia.

suggested that chondromalacia involving the lateral facet of the patella is a manifestation of the excessive lateral pressure syndrome (108). Central chondromalacia may be a manifestation of excessive pressure related to anatomic abnormalities (107). Chondromalacia of the medial patellar facet may relate to incongruity in the trochlea or patellar facets, leading to increased stress (118,147–149,159). Laurin and colleagues have stated that chondromalacia patellae results from malalignment leading to excessive pressure on the lateral facet and that hypopressure on the medial facet results in chondromalacia in that area (Fig. 7-38) (134).

Radiologic evaluation of patients with patellofemoral pain and chondromalacia has been performed by several investigators. In one series of 83 knees, only 40 showed an abnormal Q-angle and only 24 showed patella alta (122). In a series of 71 knees with chondromalacia, patella alta was seen in 38% and Haglund's excavation in 56% (150). Compared with control knees, the findings were statistically significant (150). Other radiologic changes such as subchondral sclerosis, osteophytes, lateralization of trabeculae, internal decalcification, or Wiberg patella type were not significantly different (150). The lateral patellofemoral angle opens laterally in 90% of knees with chondromalacia patellae and in 97% of normal knees (133). In 53 patients, the Q-angle was increased to 20°, patella alta measured 1.08, and the congruence angle was −2°, all of which were statistically significant when compared with control values (93). When axial radiographs are nondiagnostic, one should consider MRI or CT to more clearly define the articular cartilage and evaluate position changes during flexion and extension (157).

Treatment of the patient with patellofemoral pain depends upon the recognition of the etiologic factor or factors responsible for the disorder. A nonoperative regimen may be utilized initially. This consists of modification in activity to avoid repetitive knee flexion, especially under load, and may also include isometric quadriceps strengthening, salicylates, and crutches with immobilization for acute episodes of synovitis (103,128, 149,160). In a series of 100 knees with patellofemoral pain, arthroscopic visualization of the articular surface of the patella, and nonoperative treatment, all patients

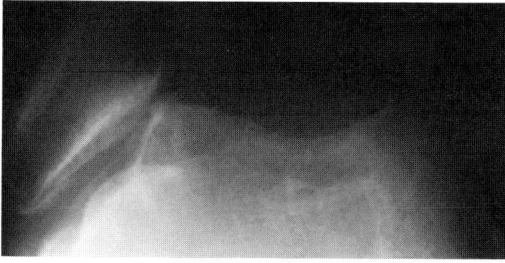

FIG. 7–38. Chronic recurrent lateral patellar dislocation occurring with repetitive knee flexion over a one-year period resulting in severe chondromalacia.

with a normal articular surface became asymptomatic. Of the patients with synovitis and fibrillation of the patella but without femoral changes, 75% became asymptomatic. However, only 18% of patients with changes involving the patella and femur became asymptomatic (160).

These results indicate that the presence of pathologic changes on the joint surface correlates with a less satisfactory prognosis and that caution should be used in applying pathological terms such as chondromalacia to the patellofemoral pain syndrome. In a series of 75 athletes with a clinical diagnosis of patellofemoral pain, 66% were able to return to unrestricted activity and 23% to restricted athletics when treated with a four-phase program consisting of (1) symptomatic control, (2) isometric quadriceps and hamstring exercises, (3) a graduated running program, and (4) a maintenance program (103). Therefore, a nonoperative treatment regimen should be the initial form of therapy for the patient with patellofemoral pain.

Surgical treatment of the patient with patellofemoral pain should be considered only after a failure of at least 6 months of nonoperative treatment. The operative treatment options include lateral retinacular release, proximal realignment, distal realignment, tibial tubercle elevation, chondrectomy (shaving), facetectomy, medial ridge excision from the trochlear surface of the femur, and patellectomy (128,149). Lateral retinacular release has a minimum morbidity and may be performed arthroscopically. The best results with this technique correlate with absence of patella alta, a normal sulcus angle, and a Q-angle of 20° or less (128). In a series of 60 knees with Outerbridge Grades 1 or 2 chondromalacia treated by lateral retinacular release, 87% satisfactory results were present at 1 year but decreased to 37% at 3 years (146). In a short-term follow up of 6 months, 76% of 174 knees with a patellar compression syndrome were improved following lateral retinacular release (107). In a series of patients with patellar compression syndrome treated by lateral retinacular release, 28 of 31 were improved at an average of 18 months following surgery (130). Although localized excision of areas of abnormal cartilage to subchondral bone has been found to result in pain relief in 18 of 23 knees (112), longer follow up is needed to assess this mode of therapy. Shaving of the patella is unreliable, leading to only 43% satisfactory results (96). In a series of 184 knees with chondromalacia patellae treated by a variety of techniques and monitored with a 4-year follow up, satisfactory results were obtained in 67% of 71 knees treated by trephine combined with drilling, in 61% of 57 treated by facetectomy, in 57% of 35 treated by shaving, and in only 19% of 12 treated by a combined procedure (142). Worse results have been reported with en bloc excision of articular cartilage when compared with knees in which the articular cartilage is intact and has been treated with realignment procedures (122). An 83% satisfactory result has been obtained in 53 knees treated by proximal realignment compared with 56% of 34 knees treated by distal realignment procedures (122). Relief of patellofemoral pain following proximal realignment correlates with correction of the congruence angle more than with the grades of chondromalacia (121). Satisfactory results have been obtained in 37 of 39 knees treated by elevation of the tibial tuberosity at 4.7 years of follow up (137). Patellectomy remains the ultimate salvage technique for the knee in which other modes of therapy have failed. Patellectomy will provide 83% satisfactory results but will result in significant quadriceps weakness (96,153).

Patellar Instability

Patellar subluxation and dislocation represent problems related to more extensive extensor malalignment than that present with chondromalacia. Subluxation and dislocation may follow a significant traumatic incident, or malalignment and trauma may both be etiologic factors. Many authors have stated that recurrent patellar subluxation and dislocation have predisposing congenital components (95,100,118,131). In one series, 73% of the knees with subluxation of the patella had at least one congenital deficiency (118). The importance of superimposed trauma has been debated. Heywood found a history of major trauma in only 5% of 90 knees (116). In a series of athletes, 72% reported a traumatic onset of symptoms (118). Although the patella may be dislocated by a direct blow to the medial aspect of the knee, an indirect mechanism of injury is more frequent (95,118). The normal Q-angle results in a lateral vector to the extensor mechanism that tends to displace the patella laterally (107). The patella subluxes or dislocates when a strong quadriceps contraction is combined with external rotation of the tibia, genu valgum, and slight knee flexion, such as during the acceleration phase of activity, when the quadriceps is contracting and the extremity is weight bearing (95).

Recurrent patellar subluxation may be considered to be of two types, major or minor (107). In a major subluxation, the patella tracks laterally over the trochlear facet and returns to the patellofemoral groove with an audible snap on the beginning of knee flexion (107). In a minor subluxation, the patella deviates laterally without clinically apparent relocation (107). Acute patellar dislocation is usually lateral but may be medial, intra-articular, or superior (131).

The pathologic changes associated with recurrent dislocation or subluxation include damage to the articular cartilage and the soft tissues. Tearing of the medial retinaculum either from damage to the medial border of the patella or from rupture of the origin of the vastus medialis obliquus may occur (95). Tears of the medial capsule of the knee, the cruciate ligaments, and the menisci may also occur and must be carefully sought (95). A hemar-

throsis is a frequent finding. The pathologic changes that appear in the articular cartilage are a result of trauma to the medial patellar facet and lateral trochlear facet during relocation of the patella (116). Trauma may lead to such pathologic changes as chondromalacia, osteochondritis dissecans, osteochondral fracture, loose bodies, and late patellofemoral arthritis (116).

A variety of factors predisposing to chondromalacia and the patellar pain syndrome have been reviewed. These same anatomic abnormalities have been implicated in the pathogenesis of recurrent subluxation and dislocation (95,107,118,130,131). The physical examination and history of symptoms are critical in the recognition of these abnormalities and have been reviewed earlier. An electromyographic study of recurrent patellar subluxation has revealed diminished activity in the vastus medialis muscle, especially at 30° of flexion. This diminished activity is felt to be secondary to static alterations of the extensor mechanism (139). Radiographic findings are useful in diagnosis and merit review. In Hughston's experience, the more frequent abnormalities visualized include tilting or subluxation of the patella and a relatively low lateral femoral condyle visualized on the axial view (118). Femoral dysplasia with a shallow sulcus was a frequent finding in another series (100). A lateral patellofemoral angle that opened medially (40%) or in which the lines were parallel (60%) was found in a series of recurrent patellar subluxations compared with the normal angle, which is open laterally in 97% of knees (134). A radiographic study of recurrent patellar dislocations revealed an abnormal sulcus angle in 60%, Wiberg type III patella in 45%, patellar subluxation in the axial view in 100%, patella alta in 49%, and an abnormal Q-angle in 52% of knees (130). However, no single factor or combination of factors leads to an increased frequency of redislocation when compared with other knees that present only one abnormality (130). In a series of 37 knees with recurrent lateral subluxation, the Q-angle was not significantly different from controls, but patella alta (1.23), sulcus angle (147°30′), and congruence angle (16°) were different from controls (93). Soft tissue calcification along the medial border of the patella related to ossification of the torn medial retinaculum also often indicates previous dislocation (107,143).

The natural history of the untreated patellar subluxation or dislocation is controversial. In Heywood's series, 15% had complete cessation of symptoms after physical therapy with development of the quadriceps (116). Crosby and Insall found that dislocation became less frequent with advancing age (102). There was little evidence of osteoarthritis, with 65% of patients having satisfactory results after nonoperative treatment. The risk of recurrent dislocation is significantly less in patients older than 20 years of age compared with those less than 20 years of age at the time of the initial dislocation (130). In a series of 50 knees with a single patellar dislocation followed for 5 years, 44% developed at least one recurrent dislocation, and 27% had symptoms severe enough to merit late reconstruction (101). In contrast, other authors have felt that all recurrent subluxation will proceed to cartilage damage and patellofemoral arthritis as well as possible dislocation (107). Therefore, operative treatment may be indicated.

A multitude of operative procedures have been described for patellar subluxation and dislocation. These can be divided into seven major types: (1) capsulorrhaphy, (2) fascioplasty, (3) osteotomy, (4) patellectomy, (5) patellar ligament procedures, (6) myotendinous procedures, and (7) combined procedures (107,153). In deciding which procedure or procedures are indicated, the possible components of the malalignment must be evaluated and treatment directed at the abnormal components (128). The four components to be evaluated are right lateral structures, lax medial structures, an increased Q-angle, and patella alta (128). The extent of damage to the articular surface must also be assessed. Acute surgical repair of a dislocation with correction of any underlying pathology has been advocated (99). Of 17 knees treated by acute repair, there were no recurrent dislocations, but 12 knees remained painful (99). Lateral retinacular release has the lowest morbidity of all the surgical options. Arthroscopic lateral release has given 86% satisfactory results at 1 year and 74% satisfactory results at 40–58 months (145). Poor results with this technique correlate with failure to maintain quadriceps strength (145). Proximal realignment of the extensor mechanism yields 75% satisfactory results, with no evidence of osteoarthritis at 8 years of follow up (102). In contrast, distal realignment yields 59% satisfactory results, with evidence of degenerative changes in 22 of 31 knees (102).

In summary, patellar problems are a frequent clinical problem. A careful distinction between clinical symptoms and pathologic changes in the articular cartilage must be made. A detailed history, physical examination, and radiologic study is necessary to define the problem. Treatment must be directed at any underlying anatomic abnormalities.

FRACTURES ABOUT THE KNEE

Fractures about the knee have a variable presentation. Injury may occur to the distal femur, proximal tibia, or patella. Fracture may be extensive or may involve only small osteocartilaginous fragments. A recognition of the fracture types and assessment of the results of treatment are essential to obtain satisfactory results.

Osteochondral Fractures

Fractures involving the joint surface may result from direct blows or indirect injuries. Recognition of these lesions may be difficult, and careful interpretation of the clinical presentation and high-quality radiographs are essential to define the lesion. One of the most frequent areas of injury involves the patella and is associated with patellar dislocation. As the patella dislocates laterally, damage to the lateral patellar facet and lateral trochlear facet of the femur may occur from shearing forces (197). Upon reduction of the dislocation, the patella strikes the prominent edge of the lateral femoral condyle, resulting in cartilaginous injury or osteocartilaginous fractures of the medial patellar facet as well as the trochlear surface of the femur (Fig. 7-39) (197). Fractures complicate 5–28% of all acute patellar dislocations. Treatment of these injuries is by excision or replacement of the articular fragments depending upon size, combined with repair of the acute dislocation (215).

Fractures involving the weight-bearing surface of the joint may be exogenous, resulting from direct injury, or endogenous. The latter involve combined rotatory and compression forces (190). In the case of exogenous fractures, the applied forces include compaction, due to direct force applied vertically; shearing, due to rotatory or translational forces; or avulsion, due to the pull of ligamentous attachment (172,179,204). Exogenous shearing forces result in peripheral chondral fractures, while endogenous forces result in centrally located lesions (190). The clinical diagnosis of these injuries is difficult, with the lesion remaining unsuspected in one-third of knees (190). The clinical presentation is usually a rotatory stress accompanied by a snap and an acute onset of swelling with hemarthrosis (190,195,203). The differential diagnosis must include meniscal and/or ligamentous injury.

Radiographically, the displaced fragment may be difficult to visualize. High-quality radiographs are required, including AP, lateral, tunnel, and axial views (190,195). The defect in the femoral condyle is difficult to visualize initially but becomes sclerotic with the passage of time (195). Early treatment is indicated. Replacement of the fragment and fixation are indicated if it is large, on the weight-bearing surface, and accessible (190,195,203). Either Smillie nails or bone pegs may be utilized for fixation (187). If the fragment is small (Fig. 7-40) or only cartilaginous, the fragment may be removed and the bed trephined (203). Early active motion is essential for nourishment of the articular cartilage (195,203).

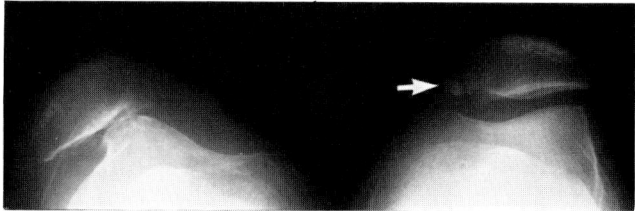

FIG. 7–39. Osteochondral fracture of the medial patella (*arrow*) on the right with dislocation of the left patella.

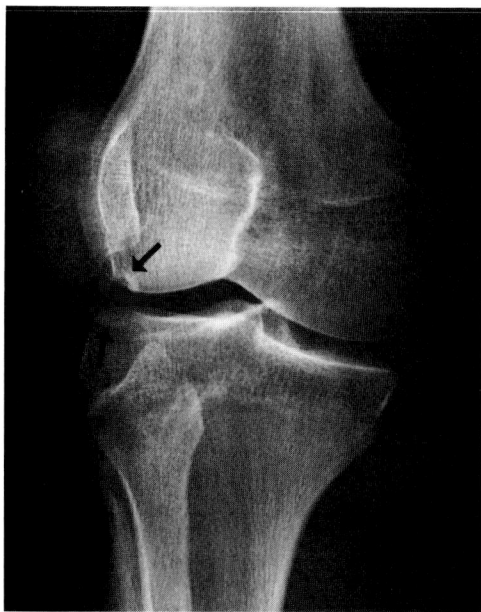

FIG. 7–40. Osteochondral fracture of the lateral femoral condyle.

Patellar Fractures

Fractures of the patella are frequent injuries, comprising 1% of all injuries (167). The subcutaneous position of the patella at the anterior aspect of the knee places it in a vulnerable position for direct trauma. The most frequent modes of injury in a series of 422 patellar fractures were

motor vehicle accidents in 28%, falls on level ground in 54%, falls from a height in 14%, and other means of direct trauma in 4% (167). Indirect violence owing to quadriceps force on a semiflexed knee may also result in a patellar fracture (167). Considerable separation of the fracture fragments most frequently accompanies indirect violence (Fig. 7-41) (167).

Patellar fractures may be classified into several types: transverse or oblique, which comprise 34%; comminuted or stellate, which comprise 16%; longitudinal fractures, which comprise 28%; apical and basal fractures, which comprise 28%; and frontal plane fractures (167). The position of the knee at the time of injury as well as the mechanism of injury influences the type of fracture that occurs. Indirect violence results in a transverse fracture, while direct violence usually results in a comminuted fracture but may also result in other fracture types as well (Fig. 7-42) (167). Careful attention should be directed to assessment of the degree of fracture surface separation, as wide separation indicates significant tearing of the patellar retinacula.

Patellar fractures affect all age groups, and a slight male predominance has been noted. In addition to a history of the mechanism or injury, a careful physical examination is essential. Palpation for separation of the patellar fragments and the extent of hemarthrosis should be performed. Recognition of the extent of injury to the soft tissues is important, whether the fracture is open or closed. Active extension of the knee to 0° by the patient is the most useful technique for assessment of associated

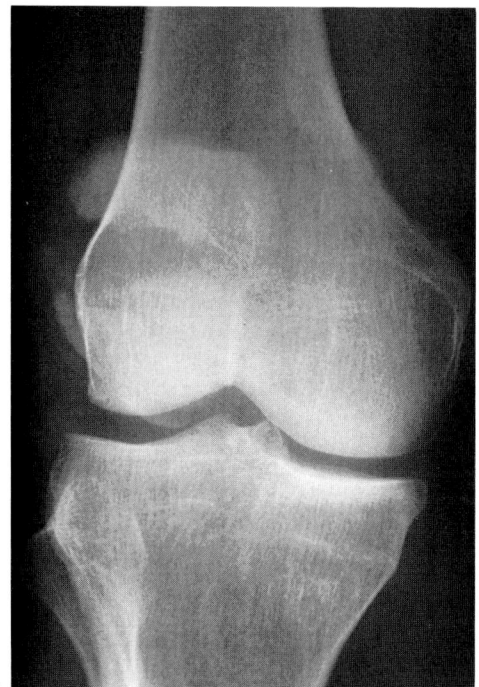
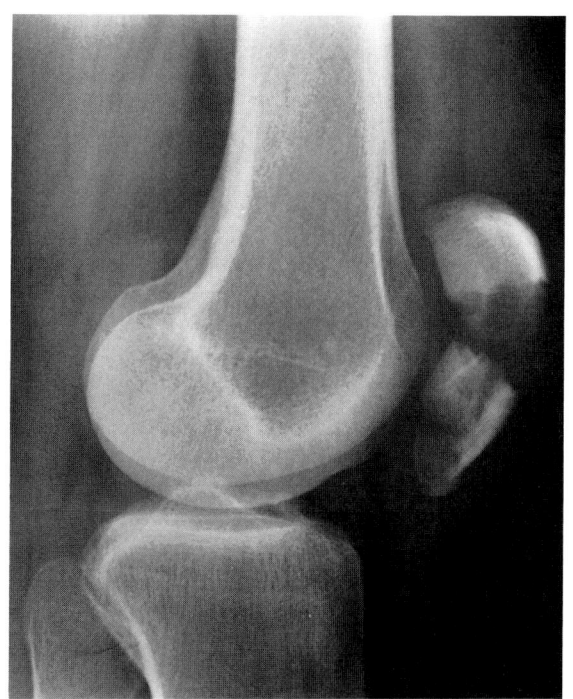

FIG. 7–41. AP (**A**) and lateral (**B**) views of a displaced transverse patellar fracture resulting from indirect violence.

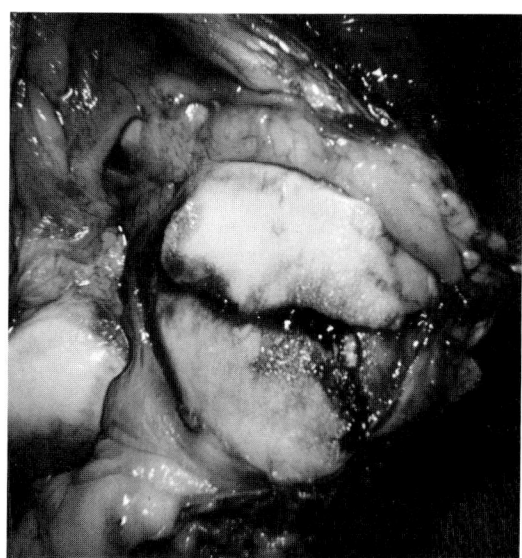

FIG. 7-42. Operative appearance of a comminuted patellar fracture following direct violence.

damage to the retinacula. Complete knee extension is not possible in the presence of a complete tear of the retinacula (167). Concomitant injuries are frequent and are present in at least 15% of patients (167).

Accurate assessment of the patella requires excellent-quality radiographs including AP, lateral, and axial views. The bipartate patella is a normal variant (Fig. 7-43) that involves the upper outer quadrant of the patella. This is frequently bilateral and should not be confused with a fracture. When assessing patellar fractures, the axial view is important in determining the degree of incongruence of the articular surface, which is the key to decisions regarding the mode of treatment. These same views are essential in the evaluation of treatment (Fig. 7-44). Particular attention must be given to the degree of fracture fragment separation, the accuracy of restoration of articular surface congruency, and the extent of comminution.

The principles of treatment include (1) anatomic fracture reduction, (2) maintenance of reduction until union, (3) repair of the soft tissues, and (4) restoration of the functional integrity of the joint (167). The options for treatment are nonoperative or operative. Operative treatment may consist of reduction and internal fixation of all fragments, partial patellectomy with repair of the extensor mechanism, or total patellectomy. The generally accepted criterion for nonoperative treatment is a fracture separation of not greater than 2–3 mm with minimal incongruency of the articular surface (167). For nonoperative treatment to be successful, the patellar retinacula must be intact. The preservation of extension capability is present in 39% of fractures (167). Once the

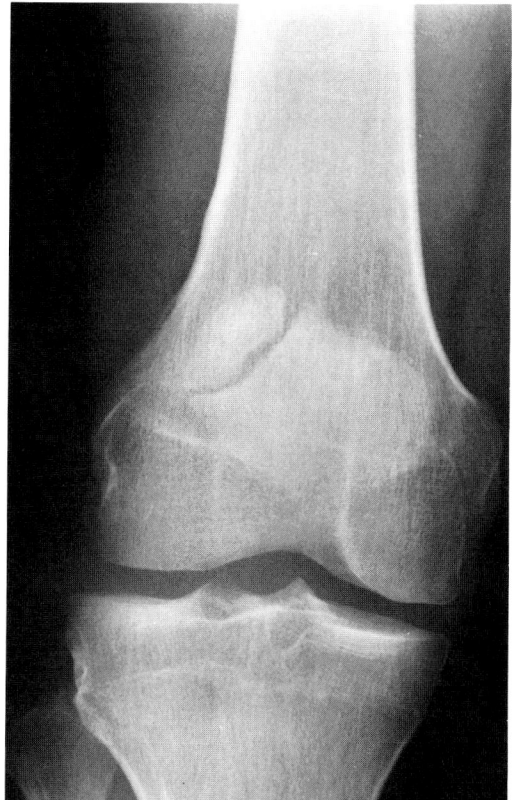

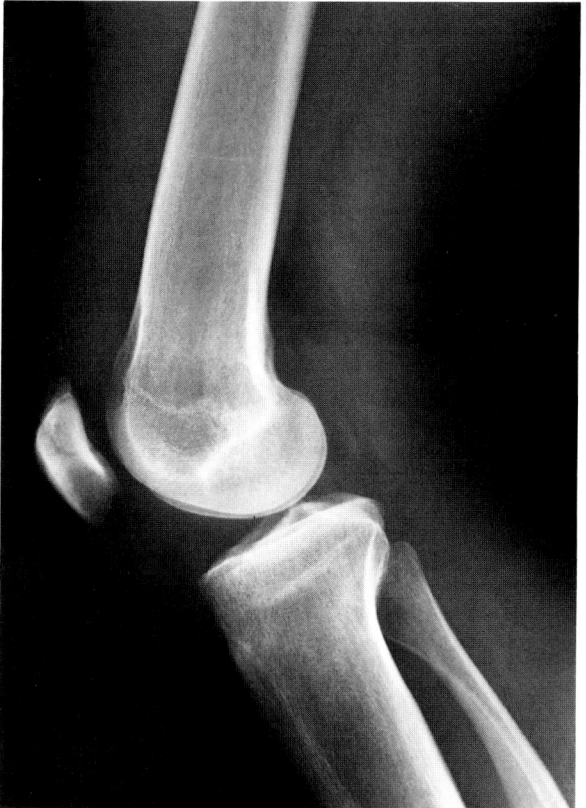

A

B

FIG. 7-43. AP (A) and lateral (B) views of a bipartate patella.

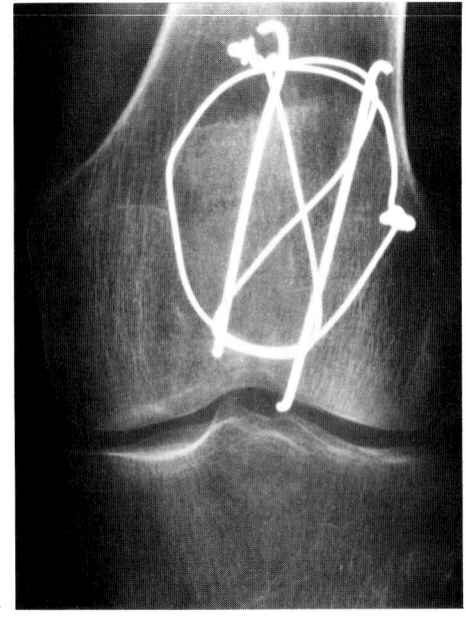
A

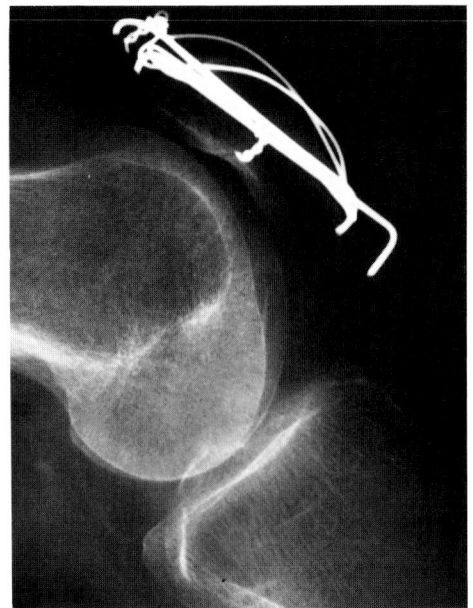
B

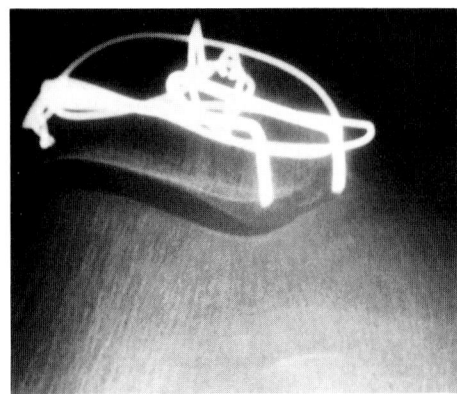
C

FIG. 7–44. AP (A), lateral (B) and axial (C) view of the patella in Fig. 7-45 following internal fixation with a modified tension band technique and circlage wire.

fracture surface separation reaches 4 mm, loss of active quadriceps function occurs.

In one study, nonoperative treatment of 287 fractures in 282 patients was utilized for fractures with less than 3-mm articular surface displacement and less than 4-mm diastasis (167). Treatment consisted of a cylinder cast for 4 weeks. Nonunion occurred in 4 fractures. At a mean follow up of 8.9 years, the result was satisfactory in 99% (167). Boström recommends nonoperative treatment for fractures in which extension capacity is preserved, the diastasis is 3–4 mm or less, and the step in the articular surface is 2–3 mm or less (167).

Accordingly, operative treatment is recommended for fractures with loss of active extension of the knee, a diastasis of more than 3–4 mm, and a step in the articular surface of more than 2–3 mm (167). Operative treatment that included osteosynthesis (75 cases), partial patellectomy (28 cases), or total patellectomy (5 cases) in 108 knees achieved 79% satisfactory results at 8.9 years of follow up (167). In the case of the most severe frac-

tures, satisfactory results were obtained in 81% following osteosynthesis and in 82% following partial patellectomy, but in only one of five treated by total patellectomy (167).

The results of treatment correlate with the degree of separation of fracture fragments. Satisfactory results were obtained in 98% of cases if only slight diastasis was present. Results were satisfactory in only 80%, however, with diastasis greater than 4 mm and tears of the patellar retinacula (167). Osteoarthritis of the patellofemoral articulation did not correlate with enlargement of the patella or with a step in the articular surface of greater than 1 mm (167). In a 10–30-year follow up, patellar enlargement did correlate, but the extent of the step in the articular surface did not correlate with osteoarthritis (226). Osteoarthritis of the patellofemoral joint was present in 70% of the fractured joints and in only 31% of contralateral uninjured knees (226). Osteoarthritis of the patellofemoral joint was observed in 22% of the knees at 8.9 years of follow up (167). Osteoarthritis correlated with the severity of injury, as it was present in 42% of comminuted fractures and in only 19% of the other fracture types (167).

The technique of internal fixation of the patella and the mechanical stability of the repair have been studied (228). A comparison between circumferential wiring, Magnusson wiring, and modified tension-band wiring revealed improved stability with the Magnusson or modified tension-band techniques (Fig. 7-44) (228). The retinacular repair also contributed to the stability of the repair.

Partial patellectomy with retention of one major fragment has been advocated for comminuted patellar fractures (162). The adverse consequences of total patellectomy from a biomechanical standpoint have already been reviewed in the section of this chapter on the patella. The decision regarding the portion of the patella to be removed is based upon the degree of comminution and location of the major fragment. Frequently, the comminution is distal and fragments can be removed with preservation of the proximal fragment (162). In this case, the patellar ligament is repaired and attached to the articular edge of the patella to prevent tilting or instability of the patella. In a series of 58 displaced fractures of the patella treated by partial patellectomy, none required subsequent patellectomy or chondroplasty of the patella at a 4-year follow up (162). Partial patellectomy has also been advocated for displaced longitudinal fractures of the patella (162).

In considering partial patellectomy, a knowledge of the blood supply to the patella is important. The two sources of intra-osseous arterial supply are through midpatellar vessels entering anteriorly and polar vessels entering inferiorly behind the patellar ligament (218). In traverse fractures of the midpatella, the superior fragment is easily isolated from the blood supply. This accounts for the 25% incidence of partial avascular necrosis seen in a series of 162 of these fractures (Fig. 7-45) (218). These findings have led to the recommendation that the distal one-half of the patella should be preserved (218).

Total patellectomy has been utilized in the management of severe comminuted fractures. A long-term follow up (4–13 years) of 31 patients treated by patellectomy for fractures revealed 22% excellent, 39% good, and 39% poor results (229). In this series of 31 patients, no evidence of osteoarthritis was found, and there was no correlation between symptoms and calcification in the patellar tendon. Maximal recovery of knee function following patellectomy required up to 3 years (229).

Supracondylar Fractures of the Femur

A supracondylar fracture of the femur is a fracture involving the distal 9 cm of the femur measured from the

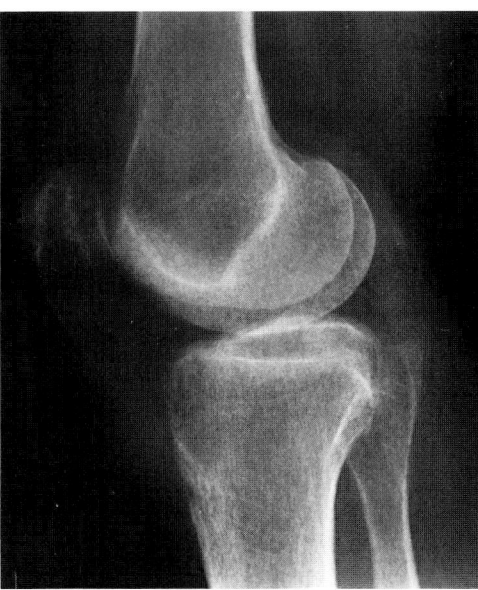

FIG. 7-45. Avascular necrosis of the proximal pole of the patella following a transverse fracture. Note the difference in density of the upper and lower poles.

articular surface of the femoral condyles (177). An intraarticular fracture of the femoral condyle may accompany the diaphyseal or metaphyseal component (177). Other authors have stated that a supracondylar fracture may involve up to the distal 15 cm of the femur (220).

The average age of the patient affected by supracondylar fractures is variable but has been taken to be 40 years (227), 54 (220), 47 (198), and 54 (181), with a range from 16–101 cases in various series (196). There is no sex predilection. The extent of trauma necessary to induce a fracture decreases with age, as the frequency of osteoporosis increases (196). Associated local injuries are frequent. In a series of 83 supracondylar femur fractures, there were 2 ipsilateral tibial plateau fractures and 5 major knee ligamentous injuries that comprised the results of fracture treatment (220).

A variety of classification schemes have been utilized for supracondylar femur fractures. Schatzker and colleagues have divided the fractures into three types: Type I, simple; Type II, comminution without joint involvement; and Type III, fracture with involvement of the articular surface (220). Healy and Brooker suggested four groups: (1) simple intra-articular, (2) simple extraarticular, (3) complex intra-articular, and (4) complex extra-articular (181). A simple fracture was defined as nondisplaced, while a complex fracture was defined as having a displacement greater than 1–2 mm, angulation, comminution, or a combination of these factors.

The most widely utilized classification is that of Neer and colleagues, with Type I defined as minimal displacement (31%), Type IIA as medial displacement of the condyles (29%), Type IIB as lateral displacement of the condyles (21%), and Type III as conjoined supracondy-

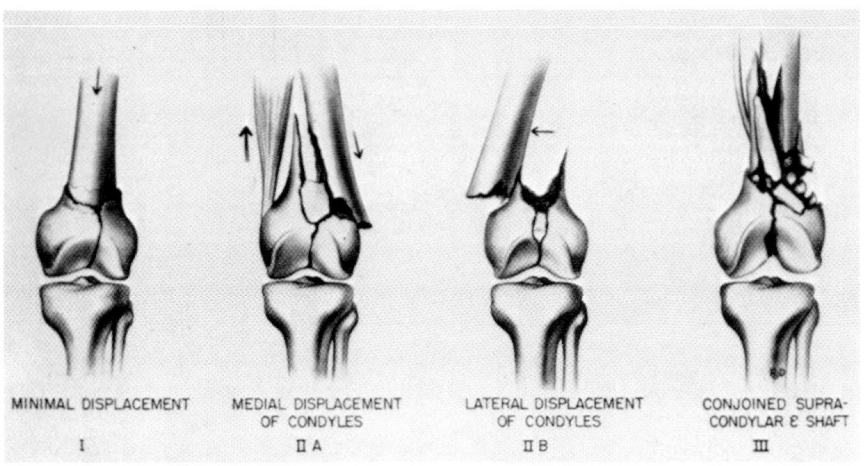

FIG. 7-46. Classification of supracondylar femur fractures (from 202, with permission.)

lar and shaft fractures (19%) (Fig. 7-46) (202). The mechanism of injury was trivial trauma in 45% and included all Type I and 15% of 25 Type IIA injuries (202). Type I fractures result from trauma to the flexed knee with osteoporotic bone. Type IIA fractures result from a violent force applied to the anterolateral side of the flexed knee, while Type IIB result from a force to the lateral side of the extended knee or the medial side of a flexed knee. Type III fractures result from extensive violence to the anterior aspect of the flexed knee.

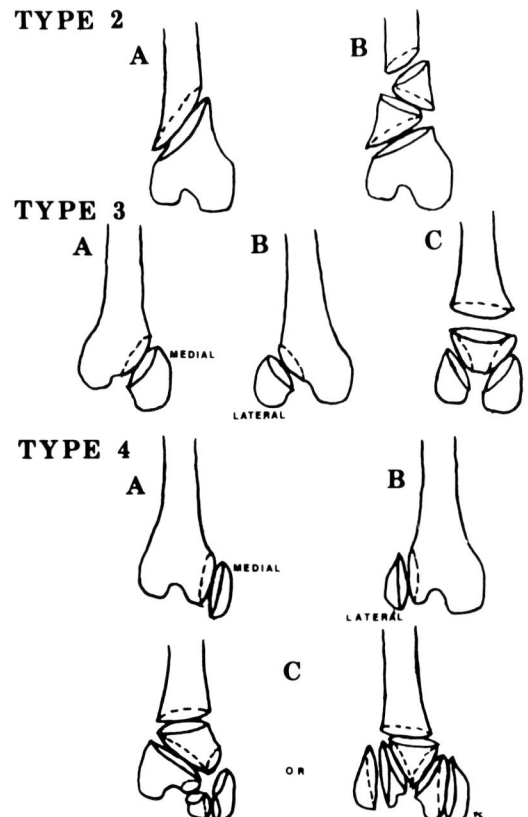

FIG. 7-47. Classification of supracondylar femur fractures (from 224, with permission.)

A more recent classification is that of Seinsheimer, with 4 types recognized (Fig. 7-47) (224). Type I is nondisplaced with less than 2 mm displacement of the fragments. Type II involves the distal metaphysis without extension into the intercondylar notch or femoral condyles and has two subtypes: (a) two-part fractures and (b) comminuted fractures (Fig. 7-48B). Type III involves the intercondylar notch, in which one or both condyles are separate fragments, and has three subtypes: (a) the medial condyle is separated, (b) the lateral condyle is separated, and (c) both condyles are separated. Type IV involves the articular surface of the femoral condyle and has two subtypes: (a) a fracture through the lateral condyle (two-part or comminuted) and (b) more complex comminuted fractures involving one femoral condyle and the intercondylar notch, both femoral condyles, or all three.

Treatment of supracondylar fractures of the femur may be nonoperative, involving combinations of traction and cast immobilization, or operative. Treatment may be complicated by the fact that the adductors, quadriceps, hamstrings, and gastrocnemius muscles pull the distal fragment into flexion, adduction, and shortening, while the hip externally rotates and may lead to a fracture deformity of varus and internal rotation (202,227). Nonoperative treatment with traction thus encounters four major problems. These include excessive flexion of the knee, varus and internal rotation of the distal fragment relative to the external rotation of the hip, inconsistent radiographs that are not corrected for the rotated position of the limb in traction, and prolonged immobilization of the knee (202). In a series of 77 fractures followed for a mean of 5.6 years, satisfactory results were obtained in 15 of 29 treated operatively compared with 43 of 48 nonoperatively (202). Inadequate fixation in osteoporotic bone, which necessitated prolonged immobilization, was the major reason for poor results in the operatively treated group. In a series of fractures followed for at least 1 year, satisfactory results were obtained in 67% of 144 nonoperatively compared with 54%

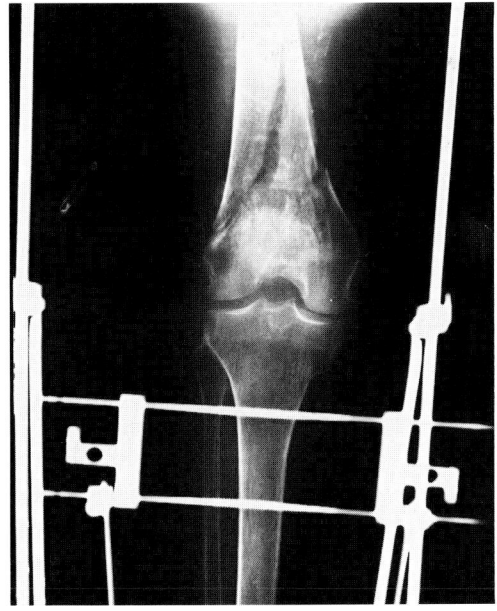
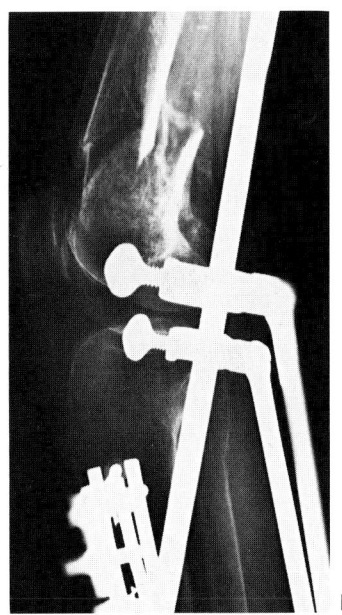

A

B

FIG. 7-48. AP (**A**) and lateral (**B**) radiograph of comminuted supracondylar femur fracture in traction. There is residual flexion of the distal fragment due to the pull of the gastrocnemius muscle. This would be a Type IIB of Seisheimer.

of 69 treated by open reduction and internal fixation (227). Delayed union or non-union occurred in 20 of the 69 fractures treated operatively compared with 14 of 144 treated nonoperatively (227). A survey of orthopedic surgeons in 1972 suggested that 61% favored closed over open treatment (214). The major reason that closed treatment gave preferable results in early series was that inadequate implants and techniques allowed early motion of the knee. Traction followed by a cast brace has been utilized in 150 distal femoral fractures, with union occurring within 15 weeks and no non-unions (199). However, 30% of these patients had less than 90° of knee flexion. A recent comparative study of open and closed treatment of 98 fractures, however, revealed satisfactory results in 38 of 47 treated operatively compared with 18 of 51 treated nonoperatively (181). Satisfactory results were obtained with closed treatment in the nondisplaced fractures, while superior results were obtained by internal fixation compared with nonoperative treatment in the case of complex fractures.

Part of the recent success of open methods is due to a variety of newer implants developed for the internal fixation of supracondylar fractures of the femur. One of these involves an intramedullary device with screw fixation of the condyles (188,232). Using the Zickel supracondylar device in 15 patients, union occurred by 14 weeks, with one non-union (232). However, 6 patients required a cast brace for additional support following surgery. In a series of 27 fractures treated with the Zickel device, union occurred in 16 weeks, with 88% satisfactory results (188). However, complications occurred in 31%, and 50% required additional operative procedures, usually for removal of the fixation device (195). Another implant, the angled blade plate, was used in 15 fractures, none of which were comminuted, and union occurred in

14 (204). However, there were 4 infections, and 5 knees had less than 90° of knee flexion. In another series of 71 fractures, in which 49 were available for follow-up, 24 were treated with a supracondylar blade plate. This method achieved a satisfactory result in 75.5% compared with 12 of 25 treated nonoperatively (219). In another series, 49 of 83 fractures treated with a blade plate were available for follow-up. Of 17 fractures treated without technical error, 71% had satisfactory results; satisfactory results were seen in only 21% of 18 fractures with technical errors of fixation (220). Fourteen fractures were treated nonoperatively, but the results of treatment were not analyzed (220). Eighty percent satisfactory results have been obtained in 30 fractures treated with a blade plate, with union at 16 weeks and a 6.6% incidence of infection (198). In another series of 26 supracondylar femur fractures treated with a blade plate, union was obtained within 16 weeks; these showed no infection and an average knee motion of 120° (177).

The technical errors related to internal fixation that may lead to poor results include incomplete reduction, failure to achieve interfragmental compression, failure to use bone grafts to correct defects, incorrect use of acrylic cement, too long an implant, and incorrect implant positioning (221).

Indications for open reduction and internal fixation of supracondylar femoral fractures include open intra-articular fractures with displacement, associated neurovascular injuries, associated ipsilateral fractures of the tibia or tibial plateau, multiple trauma (198,221), and a fractured patella in which rigid fixation will allow early knee motion. Relative contraindications to internal fixation include a severely comminuted fracture or osteoporotic bone in an elderly patient (221).

Therefore, well-performed internal fixation of supracondylar fractures of the femur with careful restoration of the articular surface and early knee motion will provide excellent results. However, internal fixation is technically difficult; and, if poorly performed, it will lead to worse results than nonoperative treatment. In addition, it carries the risk of infection.

Fractures of the Tibial Condyles

Fractures of the tibial condyles represent problems in management. Treatment is controversial. The objective of treatment is to obtain a stable, painless, mobile joint and to delay the onset of arthrosis. The etiology of these injuries is variable, but they are frequently related to motor vehicle accidents (54%) and falls (46%). Any age group may be affected, but these fractures occur most frequently in the sixth decade. The sexes are affected equally.

The diagnosis of the fracture is based upon the history of injury and a physical examination of the knee effusion, tenderness, range of motion, and stability (192). Routine radiographs in an AP plane will demonstrate the fracture, but these are inadequate to determine the extent of displacement of all fragments. Moore has recommended a tibial plateau radiograph, which allows more accurate estimation of the extent of condylar depression (200). The normal articular surface of the tibia forms an angle of 76° with the line of the tibial crest (i.e., posterior slope). Therefore, in the tibial plateau view, the radiographic beam must be angled at 105° to the tibial crest to be parallel to the articular surface of the tibia (200). Tomography has been recommended to evaluate the amount of articular surface depression or displacement, the site of the fracture, and the extent of comminution (175,221). Tomography is especially useful in differentiating split-depression fractures from fractures in which depression of the articular surface alone is present (Fig. 7-49) (175). Tomography led to more accurate reclassification of 13 of 21 such fractures when compared with classification drawn from plain radiographs (175). The amount of depression is quantitated by measuring the distance from the remaining intact articular surface or an extension of the other tibial condyle to the point of maximum depression (221). Arthrotomography using double-contrast techniques is also useful in assessing the degree of incongruity of the articular surface following fracture union (161). Computed tomography is useful in demonstrating the axial orientation of fracture fragments (207). Therefore, radiography should be utilized to assess the extent of the fracture, the degree of comminution, the depth of articular surface depression, and the extent of lateral displacement or condylar widening.

Patients with a tibial condylar fracture should be evaluated for associated injuries as well. Neurovascular injuries may accompany these fractures. Peroneal palsy was present in 6 of 260 fractures in one study (211) and has been found to occur in 1–5% of all cases (170). One contusion of the popliteal artery leading to a compartment syndrome occurred in a series of 260 fractures (211). The possibility of other fractures, such as a fracture of the femoral condyle, should also be considered.

The most frequent associated injuries are to the menisci and ligaments of the knee. In a series of 291 tibial condylar fractures, ligamentous insufficiency was the primary reason for an unacceptable result in 4.5% (165). In a series of 91 fractures treated operatively, 33 ligamentous injuries were repaired (231). Tears of the medial collateral ligament were the most frequent (13 of 16) and occurred in conjunction with fractures of the lateral condyle (231). Repair of the cruciate ligaments was performed in 13 of 24 knees (231). Enlargement of the medial joint space on valgus stress roentgenograms is a sign of collateral ligament insufficiency (225,231). The presence of a capsular rupture on an arthrogram or MRI has been helpful in identifying ligamentous injuries (225). In a follow-up study of 196 knees, 20% were noted to be unstable as a result of ligamentous insufficiency (231). In one series, a rupture of the medial collateral ligament always accompanied a fracture of the lateral tibial plateau and proximal fibula (225). In another series of 260 fractures, rupture of the anterior cruciate ligament was present in 5.4%, rupture of the medial collateral ligament in 3.8%, and rupture of the posterior cruciate or lateral collateral ligament in 0.4%. In contrast to other authors, Rasmussen stated that, although ligamentous injuries may contribute to instability, they are of minor consequence compared with the fracture and may be ignored (211). He believes that stress roentgenograms are of little therapeutic benefit. In contrast, Schatzker and colleagues believe that stress views are valuable in determining whether instability is due to fracture or ligamentous tear (221). In another series of 208 fractures, ligamentous calcification was noted in 16% at follow-up (201). Comparison for laxity between the injured and noninjured knee on stress radiographs at follow-up revealed no significant differences in laxity.

Meniscus tears, the other most frequent injury associated with tibial condylar fractures, were present in 19 of 110 fractures, of which 7 were peripheral and could be repaired (168). In another series, 14 peripheral meniscus tears were repaired in a series of 94 fractures (221). A torn meniscus was seen in 44 of 91 fractures (165). Meniscus injuries have been reported in up to 50% of fractures at arthrotomy (213). The results of 35 meniscectomies associated with 200 fractures revealed worse results in the knees treated with meniscectomy (173).

A variety of classification schemes have been suggested for tibial condylar fractures. These various classifications make comparison between series difficult. Porter chose to classify fractures as either split, bicondylar, or crush types (206). Burri suggests a classification includ-

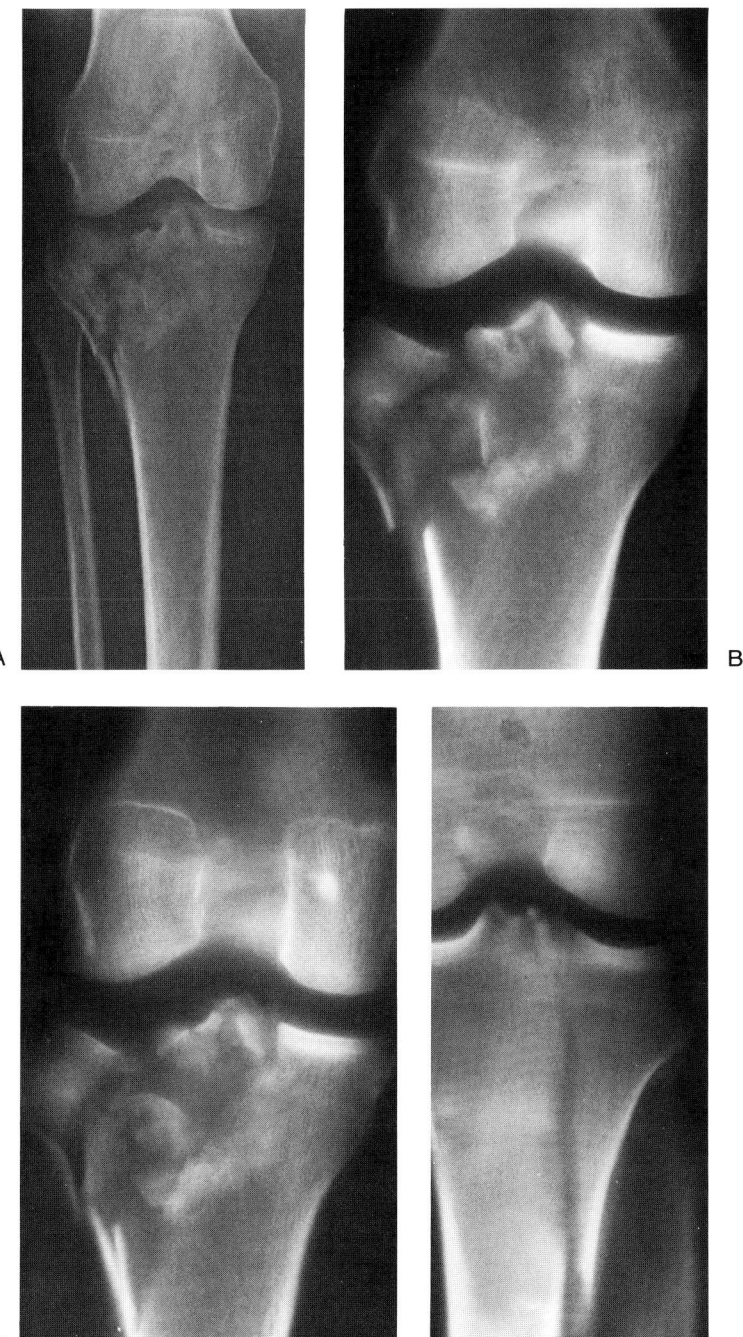

FIG. 7–49. AP (**A**) and AP tomograms (**B, C**) of a split depression lateral tibial plateau fracture. Compare to the pure split type without displacement in **D**.

ing nondisplaced fractures of the condyles, mono- and bicondylar displaced-depression fractures, fractures with impaction, combination fractures, and comminuted fractures (170). Schatzker and colleagues suggest that Type I include pure cleavage fractures; Type 2, cleavage fractures combined with depression; Type 3, pure central depression fractures; Type 4, fractures of the medial condyle; Type 5, bicondylar fractures; and Type 6, tibial plateau fractures with dissociation of the tibial metaphysis and diaphysis (221). Schulak and Gunn suggest an alternative classification, with Type I including mini-

mally displaced fractures; Type II, displaced lateral plateau fractures; Type III, displaced medial plateau fractures; and Type IV, displaced bicondylar fractures (222). Type II divides into three categories: local or total depression, split, and mixed. Type III also divides into total and split depression categories. The most widely utilized classification, however, is that of Hohl and Luck as modified by Hohl (Fig. 7-50) (184,185). Type I is undisplaced and constitutes 24%; Type II is central depression and constitutes 26%; Type IV is total depression and constitutes 11%; Type V is split and constitutes 3%; Type

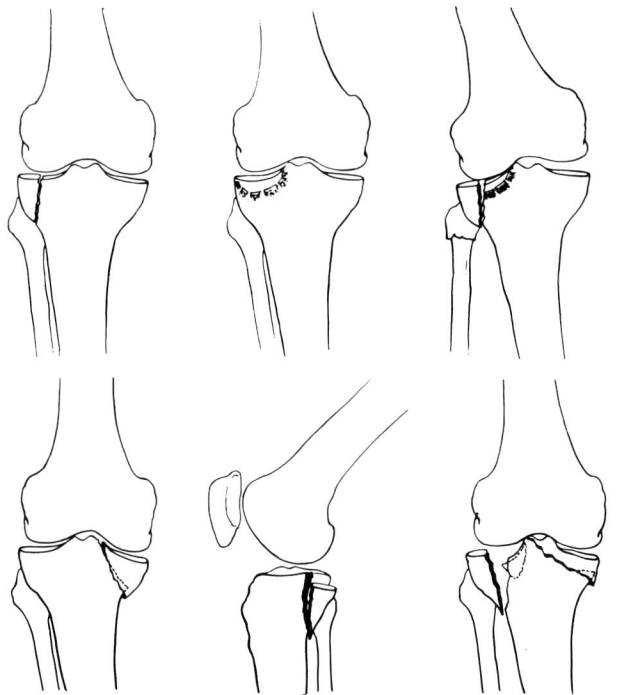

FIG. 7–50. Classification of tibial plateau fractures (from 184, with permission.)

VI is comminuted and constitutes 10%. The frequency of the various types is outlined in Table 7-3.

The mechanism of injury of the various fracture types has been reviewed by several authors. Schulak and Gunn have provided an excellent review (Fig. 7-51) (222). One factor affecting the type of fracture is the point of the impact; this in turn determines the size of the fragment (211). The extent of crushing depends upon the age of the patient, the resistance of the subchondral bone, the amount of knee flexion, and the magnitude of the axial force (211). The majority of these fractures are produced by the prominent anterior part of the lateral femoral condyle being driven like a wedge into the underlying tibial plateau (211). The frequent lateral plateau fractures result from combined abduction and compression forces (163).

A wide variety of the therapeutic modalities have been utilized in the management of these injuries. Two philosophies of treatment have emerged: (1) nonoperative treatment with early knee motion to mold the displaced fragments into acceptable positions, and (2) operative reduction of the fracture with various types of internal fixation. The objective of any treatment method is to provide a mobile, painless, stable, well-aligned knee with function as close to normal as possible. The choice of treatment will be influenced by the age, general health, and ambulatory status of the patient as well as by associated injuries, the extent of fracture displacement, and the experience of the surgeon.

Nonoperative treatment generally consists of an initial period of traction followed by cast immobilization. Apley has advocated closed reduction followed by early motion of the knee in skeletal traction (163). In a 5-year follow-up study of 27 of 48 tibial condylar fractures treated by traction (69% of which were displaced fractures), satisfactory results were obtained in 21 knees (163). Early motion serves to restore movement and power, molds the fractured tibial condyle to the shape of the femoral condyle, and promotes healing (163,164). Mobilization in a cast brace following an early period in traction has resulted in a decreased hospitalization time and satisfactory results. In the case of unstable fractures, internal fixation should be utilized prior to application of the cast brace (169,223). In a series of 29 fractures treated with a cast brace (of which 7 received some internal fixation), 26 had satisfactory results, with progression of deformity in only 1 knee (223). In a series of 30 fractures of which 5 received internal fixation treated by a cast brace, there was no progression of deformity (169). However, an experimental study of tibial condylar fractures fixed with a cast brace revealed that fractures with an associated fracture of the fibular head or with concurrent medial condylar fractures were not suitable for this technique, because collapse will occur (216). Cast-brace treatment should be reserved for fractures with minimal displacement involving the lateral plateau and in which the fibular head is intact; alternatively, it may be used as a supplementary treatment following internal fixation (169,216,223). Closed reduction followed by a hip spica cast has been utilized in the management of 61 displaced fractures of the tibial plateau (174). At 3.8 years of follow-up, 85% satisfactory results were achieved. The initial displacement correlated inversely with the end result, and the poorest results were seen in the split depression fractures (174). Nonoperative treatment has also been recommended for management of central compression fractures in which the knee in extension is stable under stress (212). A 4- to 9-year follow-up of 40

TABLE 7-3. Frequency of tibial condylar fractures

Author	No.	Type I	Type II	Type III	Type IV	Type V	Type VI
Hohl	805	24	26	26	11	3	10
Dovey	261	18	14	40	5	2	21
Lucht	109	28	23	17	11	4	17
Bakalim	197	18	45	45	11	10	16
Bowes	110	48	12	13	5	2	20

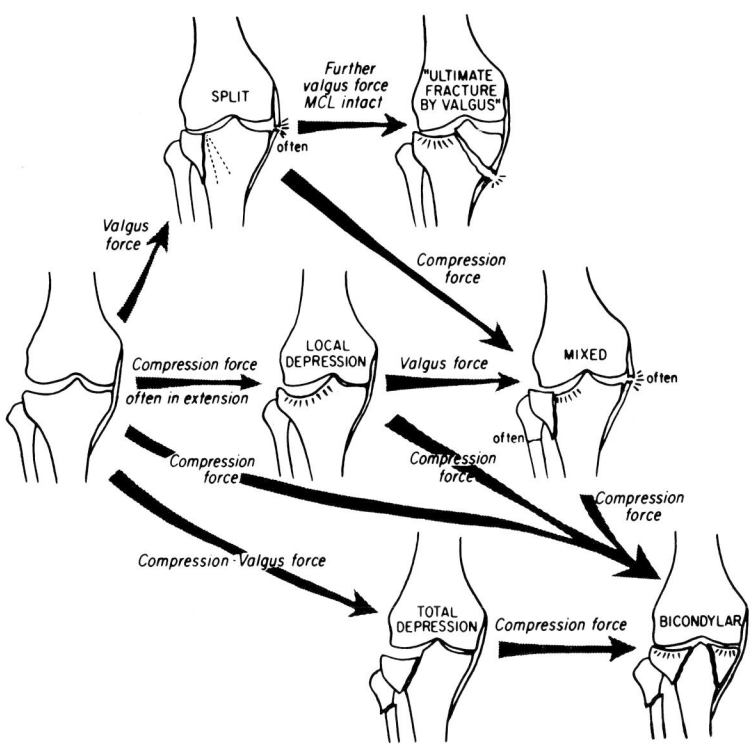

FIG. 7–51. Mechanisms of injury producing the various types of fractures of the tibial plateau (from 222).

displaced fractures treated by cast immobilization revealed satisfactory results in 30 of 32 knees (212). Roentgenographic evidence of moderate arthrosis was noted in only 2 knees. Closed reduction followed by limited fixation with a wire loop combined with cast immobilization has been utilized for bicondylar plateau fractures (180). In a 6- to 12-year follow-up of 12 knees, satisfactory results were present in 10 knees with no loss of fracture reduction.

The decision regarding operative treatment and the factors affecting the long-term results have been reviewed by many authors. However, data on operative vs. nonoperative treatment of comparable groups of patients with similar fractures is not available. Generally, the more severe the injury, the more frequently surgical treatment is utilized (191). A review of various authors' indications for operative treatment and their results will aid in evaluation of these treatment modalities.

The factors that result in permanent disability after fracture are limited motion, instability, angular deformity, lack of full extension, pain, traumatic arthritis, and muscle weakness (184). Limited motion relates to prolonged immobilization. Instability results from either residual depression of the articular surface, ligamentous laxity, degenerative changes, or a combination of these factors. Angular deformity results from incomplete fracture reduction, collapse of the fracture during healing, or degenerative change. Lack of full extension follows from prolonged immobilization with the knee held in flexion or from the posterior capsular contracture associated

with fractures involving the posterior tibial condyles. Traumatic arthritis relates to the degree of malalignment, the accuracy of reduction, and the extent of articular cartilage damage.

Rasmussen has stated that the presence of lateral instability in extension is an indication for operative treatment (209–211). Instability depends more upon the localization and extent of compression than upon its depth (209–211). Anteriorly located compression makes the knee unstable in full extension, while posterior compression results in instability in slight flexion (209). Only the fractures that produce instability in extension require operative treatment (209–211).

In a series of 192 fractures, Rasmussen found that instability in extension was present in 46% (210). A 10° increase in lateral deviation upon clinical testing compared with the normal side was taken as a sign of instability requiring surgical treatment (211). The frequency of instability according to fracture type in 260 fractures was 70% of 66 split depression fractures, 24% of 80 local compression fractures, 45% of 29 medial condyle fractures, and 52% of 48 bicondylar fractures (211). Of 260 fractures in which 44% were treated operatively, follow-up was obtained in 78% at a mean of 7.3 years following fracture (211). Using instability as the criterion for surgery, 87% had satisfactory results at follow-up. There was a lack of correlation between the functional and anatomic results. Of the 202 patients followed, 21% had roentgenographic evidence of arthrosis. Arthrosis was present in 42% of the bicondylar fractures compared with 16% of the lateral and 21% of the medial condyle fractures (210,211). Arthrosis also correlated with axial alignment. It was present in 79% of the patients with varus alignment and in 31% with excess valgus alignment greater than 10°, but arthrosis was found in only 13% of the knees with normal alignment (210,211). Arthrosis was found in 46% of the knees with instability in extension compared with 14% with instability in 20° of flexion or the 18% associated with normal stability (210,211). Condylar widening greater than 5 mm appeared to correlate with osteoarthritis (210). The presence of osteoarthritis correlated with a poor clinical result (211).

In a series of 200 fractures followed for 1.5–10 years of which 62 were treated surgically, the split depression fractures had better results with nonoperative care, while the bicondylar fractures had similar results regardless of the method of treatment (173). In local compression fractures, the result correlated with the amount of depression. Acceptable results were present in 94% of the fractures with less than 3 mm of depression but in only 50% of fractures with more than 10 mm of depression (173,191). A residual valgus deformity of greater than 10° was present in 4% and correlated with a poor result. Instability in full extension was present in 7.5% of the knees but did not influence the clinical result. Although the radiographs may reveal significant bony depression, fibrocartilage was found to fill the defect in 2 knees.

A comparative study of operative reduction versus nonoperative treatment with either traction or cast immobilization was performed in 39 patients who had local depression fractures exceeding 10 mm (206). At 6 years of follow-up, 10 of 10 treated by nonoperative means compared with 4 of 20 treated operatively had unacceptable results (206). Therefore, operative treatment was recommended for fractures with greater than 10 mm of depression.

Another study assessed treatment modalities in a series of 109 fractures in which 53% were treated and followed for an average of 5.75 years (193). Nonoperative treatment provided satisfactory results for fractures that were depressed less than 10 mm. All patients with depression greater than 10 mm were treated operatively, with 79% satisfactory functional results but only 58% acceptable anatomic results. Improved results were seen with knee motion begun prior to the eighth week. Acceptable results were seen in 90% of these knees compared with 71% in which motion was begun at a later date (193).

The results of treatment correlate with the fracture type. One study established this correlation in a series of 197 fractures followed for a mean of 4.5 years (165). Nonoperative treatment provided satisfactory results in 35 of 36 undisplaced fractures. In local depression fractures, satisfactory results were obtained in 30 of 39 treated nonoperatively compared with 29 of 50 treated

operatively. The results correlated with the accuracy of reduction. Results were acceptable in 47 of 62 fractures with less than 5 mm of residual depression compared with 13 of 27 with more than 5 mm of residual depression. A satisfactory result was obtained in 12 of 18 total depression fractures with less than 5 mm of depression compared with 1 of 3 with depression greater than 5 mm. Of 19 split fractures, all had acceptable results, and the result did not correlate with the extent of residual widening. Finally, of 31 bicondylar fractures, acceptable results were obtained in 21 and correlated with the accuracy of reduction.

Hohl has reported on an extensive series of 917 tibial plateau fractures and has suggested a treatment regimen based upon fracture types (182–185). For undisplaced fractures, a soft dressing followed by protected weight bearing until bone union occurs gives generally satisfactory results. Immobilization should not exceed 3 weeks to avoid adhesion formation. Local depression fractures with less than 5 mm of depression may be treated nonoperatively, while depression of greater than 5–8 mm requires operative reduction to avoid valgus deformity and instability. The prognosis for local depression fractures depends upon the accuracy of reduction and the maintenance of the articular surface as well as the integrity of the soft tissues (184). The results for split depression fractures correlate with the quality of reduction. Poor results are obtained if more than 11 mm of residual depression is present (182–185). Although split fractures often lead to poor results, the best results are obtained with operative treatment. Comminuted fractures appear best treated by manipulation and traction, possibly aided by limited open reduction (Fig. 7-52) (182–185). The results following treatment utilizing this approach correlated with several factors. Fractures with less than 4 mm of depression had better results than those with greater depression (183). Residual condylar widening of greater than 4 mm was associated with less satisfactory results. Instability was present in 30% of knees with less than 7 mm of depression compared with 46% of knees with greater amounts of depression. The frequency of degenerative change increased with the extent of angular deformity. Degenerative change appeared in 46% with no deformity and in 84% if the deformity was greater than 15° (183). Early motion within 2 weeks of injury provides improved results compared with later mobilization of the knee (183).

Utilizing the principles of restoration of articular congruity, limb alignment, and early motion, acceptable results were obtained in 84% of 110 fractures (168). Anatomic reduction did not always lead to an acceptable result if knee motion was delayed (168).

Operative methods of treatment are being more widely utilized as surgical techniques and implants improve (170,221). In one study, satisfactory results at 28 months of follow-up were present in 78% of surgically

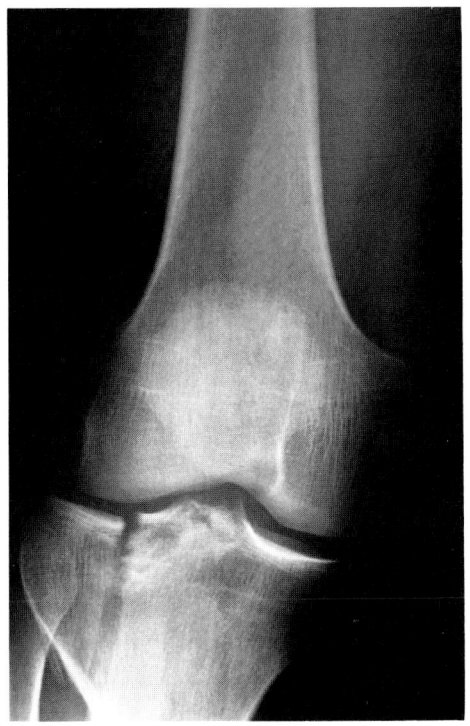

A

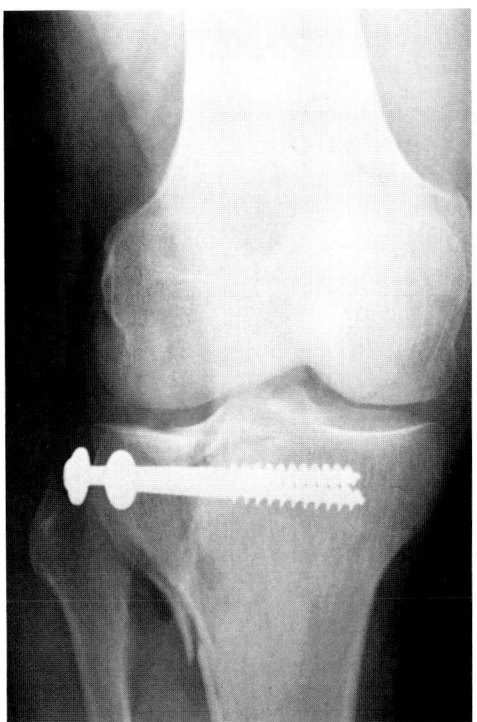

B

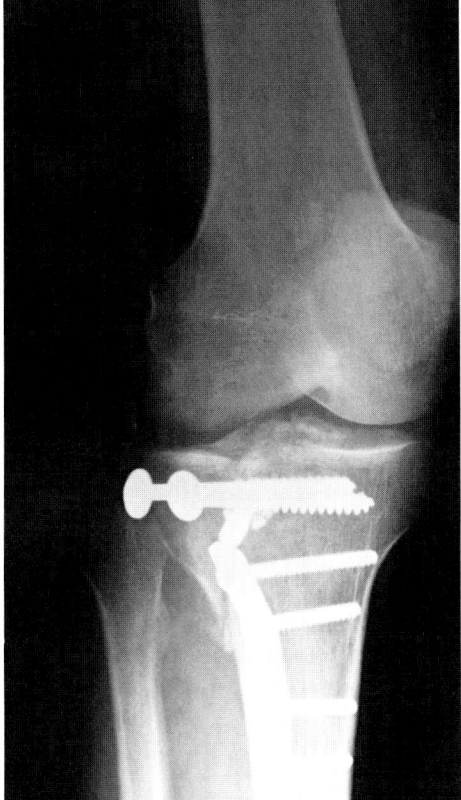

C

FIG. 7-52. **A:** AP view of the knee demonstrating a lateral plateau fracture with less than 4 mm of depression. Initial treatment (**B**) with two cancellous screws did not maintain reduction. A third posterior screw and side plate were added one month later (**C**).

treated fractures compared with 58% of the nonoperative group (221). Schatzker and colleagues recommended anatomic reduction, bone grafting as necessary, and internal fixation followed by early motion as the most appropriate form of management for displaced fractures (221). They stated that the articular defect does not fill with articular cartilage and remains incongruous. Surgical experience is also relatively important in the operative management of tibial plateau fractures. In a series of 278 fractures treated operatively, good results

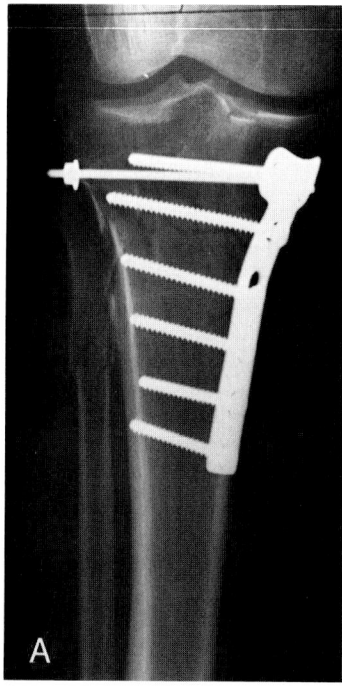
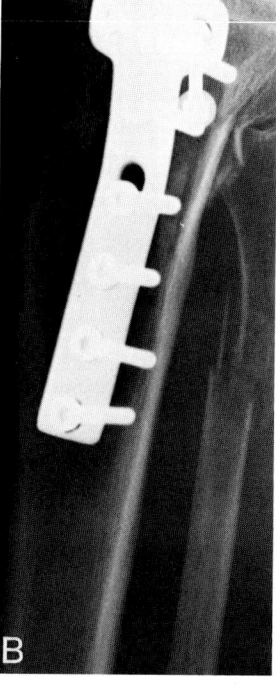

FIG. 7–53. AP (A) and lateral (B) radiographs of a local condylar depression type fracture of the lateral tibial plateau treated with a buttress plate. There is still an area of residual depression of the articular surface.

were obtained in 66% of cases by less experienced surgeons compared with 76% by more experienced surgeons (170). Burri and colleagues recommended operative treatment for all fractures with depression, displacement, or impaction and suggested use of a buttress plate (Fig. 7-53) (170).

Fractures of the tibial plateau merit careful evaluation to determine the fracture type, mechanism of injury, and extent of articular surface displacement. Associated injuries of the soft tissues, especially ligaments and menisci, must be sought and treated. The best results correlate with reduction of the fracture and correction of articular surface incongruity, instability, and axial alignment of the knee. The treatment choice should allow early knee motion.

Avulsion and stress fractures of the upper tibia also deserve mention here. The Segond fracture (Fig. 7-54) is a small vertical fracture of the lateral aspect of the tibia

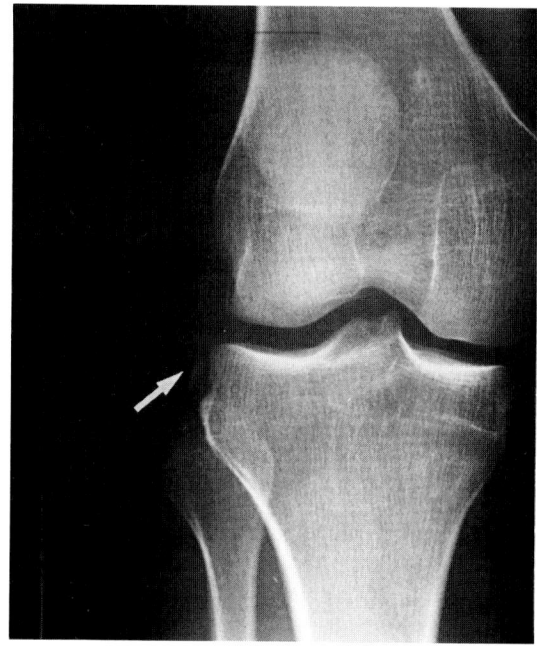
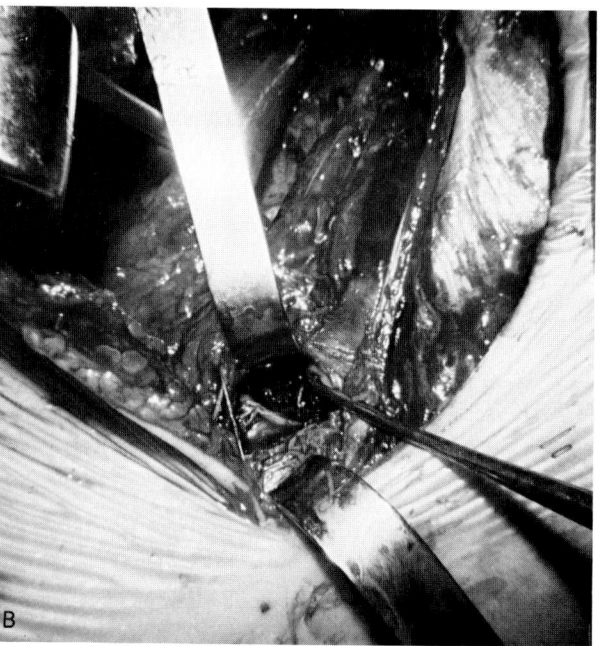

FIG. 7–54. A: AP radiograph of the lateral capsular avulsion sign and (B) operative appearance of disruption of the middle-third lateral capsular ligament at the tip of the probe.

just distal to the plateau (172,179). The injury is usually the result of external rotation in association with varus stress. Detection of the fracture can usually be accomplished with routine AP, oblique, or tunnel views. There is a high incidence of associated anterior cruciate ligament and meniscal injuries. Therefore, MRI is often indicated to fully evaluate the bone and soft tissue injury.

Stress fractures of the upper tibia are not uncommon (208,217). Fractures can occur in young runners and are usually diagnosed with routine radiographs or radionuclide scans. Older patients present a more complex problem. Symptoms are often attributed to other knee disorders and delayed or missed diagnosis is not unusual (194,217). Routine radiographs and radionuclide scans may not be as specific in this setting. MRI (Fig. 7-55) is often more definitive in diagnosing stress fracture and differentiating stress fractures from early osteonecrosis and other knee disorders.

Ipsilateral Fractures of the Femur and Tibia

Ipsilateral fractures of the femur and tibia present problems in management related to loss of stabilization of the knee and difficulty in rehabilitation. This injury has been termed the *floating knee* (166). High-velocity trauma is required to inflict these injuries, and floating knee occurs most frequently in motor vehicle accidents (166,178,186,189,205). Associated injuries frequently involve other organ systems and additional skeletal trauma, both of which should be carefully sought (166,178,186,189,205). Severe abdominal and thoracic injuries are present in 20% of cases (178,186,205). The mortality rate in these patients is 4–13% (176,178). The fractures are frequently open (59% in a series of 222 fractures) (176). Neurovascular injuries are present in 7% and knee ligamentous injuries in 8% (176). Ligament injuries about the knee are frequently difficult to diagnose initially because of the instability of the fractures; accordingly, they are seen five times more frequently at follow-up than at the time of injury (176). Men are affected more frequently than women, and the patients are generally in the second to fourth decades of life (163,176,178,186,189,205).

Two classifications have been utilized for these fractures. Blake and McBryde classified Type 1 as the case in which the knee is isolated completely from either shaft fracture (166). In type 2A, the injury extends into the knee joint, while in Type 2B the injury involves the hip or ankle joints. Fraser and colleagues classified 222 cases as follows: Type 1, 71%, a shaft fracture of the tibia and femur without extension into the knee; Type 2A, 16.5%, fracture into the tibial plateau; Type 2B, 4.5%, fracture intra-articularly in the distal femur; and Type 2C, 8%, articular fractures on both sides of the knee (Fig. 7-56) (176).

Treatment of these fractures may consist of nonoperative management of both fractures, operative treatment of one fracture, or operative treatment of both fractures. In one study, nonoperative management of both fractures consisting of traction for the femur and a cast for the tibia was utilized in 24 cases (230). Delayed union of the tibia occurred in 6 fractures and non-union in 2, while delayed union of the femur occurred in 3 fractures. Only 9 of 24 cases obtained full knee motion. A selected series of 15 cases treated initially in traction followed by a cast brace revealed healing of the femoral fracture by 15 weeks in all fractures, but 6 tibial fractures required secondary procedures for delayed union (171).

In a report of 20 ipsilateral fractures of the femur and tibia, 9 femoral fractures and 2 tibial fractures received internal fixation (205). The average healing time for both fractures when the femur was treated operatively but the tibia nonoperatively was 14 weeks; the average healing time was 22.5 weeks when both fractures were treated nonoperatively. In a series of 37 cases, 11 femoral and 0 tibial fractures were treated operatively, while 26 cases with combined femoral and tibial fractures were treated nonoperatively (166). Delayed union or non-union occurred in 13 femurs and 20 tibias. Of the 26 cases with both fractures, 13 required delayed surgical procedures. Knee motion of 90° or more was obtained in 20 knees. Significant functional disability was present at follow-up in 60–70% of the patients. In a series of 52 cases, 26 femoral fractures and 29 tibial fractures received nonoperative treatment (178). Three femoral fractures developed non-union (1 with nonoperative treatment), and 10 tibias had delayed union (8 with nonoperative treatment). Infection occurred in 5 tibial and 1 femoral fracture, 3 of which had operative treatment. Gillquist and colleagues thus recommended internal fixation of both fractures (178). In a later series of 21 cases using internal fixation for 16 femoral and 13 tibial fractures, there were no problems with femoral union and 2 cases of delayed union of the tibia (186). Excellent results were obtained in 16 femoral and 17 tibial fractures (186).

A comparison of operative treatment of both fractures in 14 cases, operative treatment of only 1 fracture in 3 cases, and nonoperative treatment of both fractures in 15 cases was performed (189). Clinical union was obtained by 25 weeks in the first group, by 23 weeks in the second group, and by 34.8 weeks in the third group. Satisfactory results were obtained in 12 of 14 treated operatively, 0 of 3 treated by fixation of one fracture, and 4 of 10 treated nonoperatively. In a series of 222 cases, 35% required late operation for delayed union, non-union, osteomyelitis, refracture, or malunion regardless of treatment type (176). The 222 cases were divided into three treatment groups: Group I included 27 cases in which both fractures were internally fixed, Group II included 92 cases in which only one fracture was fixed, and Group III included 91 cases in which both fractures were

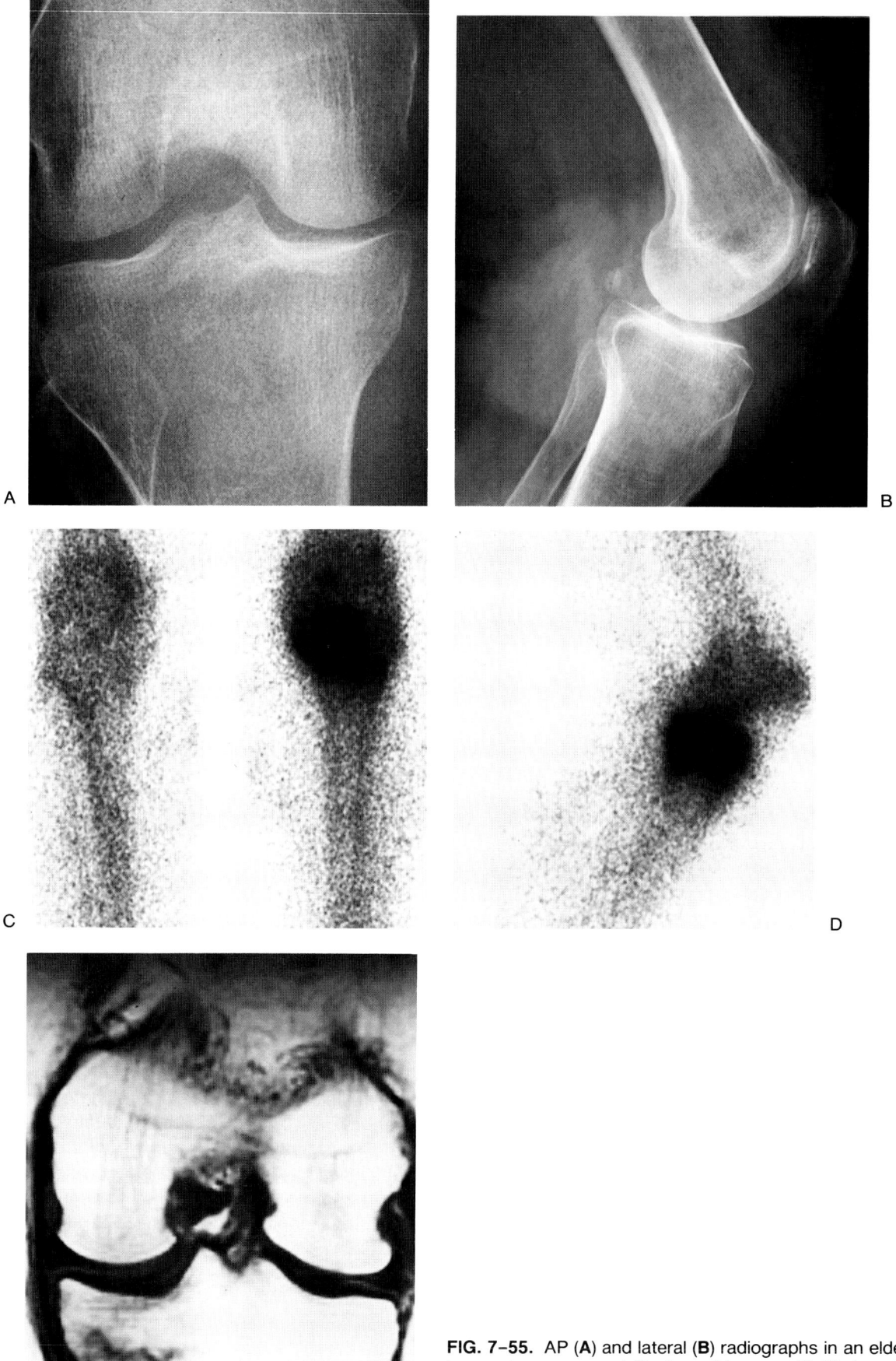

FIG. 7–55. AP (**A**) and lateral (**B**) radiographs in an elderly female with knee pain were normal. Radionuclide scans (**C, D**) show increased tracer in the upper tibia. Coronal SE 500/20 MRI (**E**) shows a stress fracture.

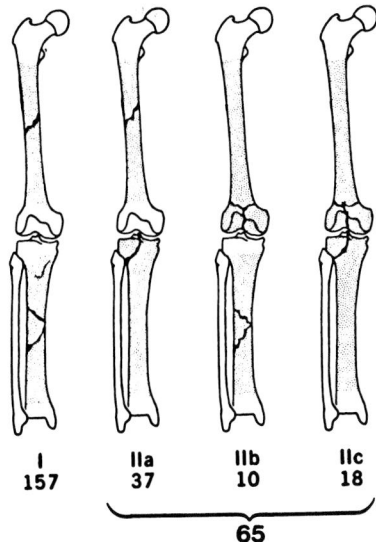

I
157

IIa
37

IIb
10

IIc
18

65

FIG. 7–56. Classification of ipsilateral fracture of the femur and tibia (from 176, with permission.)

treated nonoperatively. Satisfactory results were obtained in 30% of Group I, 36% of Group II, and 23% of Group III. Infection occurred in 30% of Group I compared with 11% in Group II, and 8% in Group III. Fraser and colleagues recommended internal fixation of the femur followed by cast-brace treatment of the tibial fracture (152).

In conclusion, careful attention to the types of fracture, the degree of displacement, and the adequacy of reduction is essential in treating fractures about the knee. A treatment program should be directed toward early mobilization of the knee, accurate reduction of the articular surface, and axial alignment of the limb. A treatment modality that meets these objectives with the lowest complication rate, whether operative, nonoperative, or some combination of the two, should be selected.

SOFT TISSUE AND ARTICULAR DISORDERS

Ligamentous Injuries of the Knee

Injuries to the ligaments of the knee are frequent clinical problems. Injuries may occur by direct trauma but most frequently result from indirect mechanisms. The early diagnosis of these injuries requires a high index of suspicion. The morbidity following injury is variable and relates to the extent of the initial injury, the mode of treatment, the functional demands of the patient, and any subsequent injuries. A knowledge of the natural history of ligamentous injuries, the techniques of diagnosis, and the classification of these injuries is essential before deciding upon treatment. A large number of reconstructive techniques are currently being utilized for chronic and, in some instances acute, injuries. Long-term results

of these techniques will need to be obtained prior to assessment of their efficacy, especially in the prevention of arthrosis. Therefore, a detailed review of these reconstructive techniques will not be included in this discussion.

Natural History

Injury to the anterior cruciate ligament is one of the most frequent knee ligamentous injuries and is present in 70% of the knees with an acute hemarthrosis (see the discussion of arthroscopy later in this chapter). Unfortunately, few studies have focused upon the natural history of these lesions. Other associated knee ligamentous injuries are variable. In addition, methods of treatment and the functional demands of different patients also vary. Thus a homogeneous group of patients is difficult to obtain (259).

Feagin and colleagues have presented the results obtained in primary repair of acute tears of the anterior cruciate ligament (239–241). Primary repair of the torn anterior cruciate ligament was performed in 64 cases (240). At a 2-year follow-up of 30 patients, 25 had satisfactory results (239,240). However, at 5 years (32 cases), 71% had pain, 66% stiffness, 94% instability, and 53% a significant reinjury (239,241). The conclusion from these studies was that "incompetence of the anterior cruciate ligament leads to progressive deterioration of function of the knee" (240). McDaniel and Dameron studied 53 knees with documented anterior cruciate ligament tears at an average of 10 years after injury (267). Seventy-two percent of the patients returned to sports, and 47% felt that they had no restrictions because of the knee. Factors associated with improved results were adequate muscle rehabilitation, stability with anterior and rotatory stress, and return to unrestricted sports. Poorer results were associated with medial and lateral meniscectomy, thigh atrophy, restricted sports, and instability with anterior and rotatory stresses. Twenty-eight of the 53 knees showed evidence of arthrosis with Fairbank's signs, but 9 knees had not had a meniscectomy.

Noyes and colleagues studied 103 patients with chronic laxity of the anterior cruciate ligament without other associated major ligamentous injuries at a mean of 5.5 years of follow-up (274). Subjective disability was noted by 31% for walking, 44% for activities of daily living, and 74% for sports activities (273). If a meniscectomy had been performed, there was a two- to fourfold increase in symptoms of pain and swelling (274). At 5.5 years, 21% of the knees, and, at 11.2 years, 44%, had roentgenographic evidence of arthrosis—even those without meniscectomy (275). Kennedy reported on 31 untreated tears of the anterior cruciate ligament followed at 44 months and found that 77% had a satisfactory result (258). The greater the anterior instability, the poorer the result (258). In 10 of 50 knees with a documented anterior cruciate ligament tear, a meniscectomy was performed, but no poor results occurred, and there was no progressive instability (258). Fetto and Marshall reported 223 knees with anterior cruciate ligament insufficiency with 2–3 years of follow-up (243). Of 176 knees that did not undergo early surgery, there were 68 isolated anterior cruciate ligament injuries and 108 with lesions of other ligaments, frequently the medial collateral ligament. There was significant deterioration in function over time for both isolated anterior cruciate ligament and mixed ligamentous lesions. At 2 years, only 15% of the knees were minimally symptomatic. Sixty-six of 78 knees had evidence of arthrosis on roentgenograms. At 5 years of follow-up, only 15% of untreated knees were rated as better than poor. Arnold and colleagues reported 105 untreated tears of the anterior cruciate ligament followed at 4.3 years (233). On a rating scale of 100 points, the mean score of these patients was 55. Radiographic evidence of arthrosis was present in 29% of the knees. Balkfors studied 383 knees with a variety of ligamentous injuries at a minimum of 5 years after injury (235). The most frequent injury was an isolated anterior cruciate ligament tear (39%) or an anterior cruciate plus medial collateral ligament tear (30%). Of 183 anterior cruciate ligament injuries of which 86 had primary repair, 30% had subjective symptoms, 40% noted instability, and 35% avoided athletics. There were no differences between the repair and nonrepair groups. Of 165 injuries of the anterior cruciate ligament of which 125 were complete and 40 partial tears, gonarthrosis was seen in 15 complete tears but in 0 partial tears. A roentgenographic review of 368 knees revealed osteophytes in 33% and gonarthrosis in 7% (235). Twenty-two of the 26 knees with gonarthrosis had had a meniscectomy (235). Balkfors concluded that gonarthrosis is increased by a factor of 10 in patients with knee ligament injuries (235).

Diagnosis

The diagnosis of acute knee ligamentous injuries may be difficult but must be carefully sought. The most frequent injury involves the anterior cruciate ligament, but a variety of ligamentous injuries may occur (Table 7-4). Even with a careful search, ligamentous stretching and a change in the biomechanical function of a ligament may occur without obvious visual signs or failure, making diagnosis difficult. Following failure of a primary ligamentous stabilizer of the knee, progressive stretching and failure with time may occur in the secondary stabilizers, changing the pattern of knee instability.

Assessment of an acute knee injury requires a careful history and physical examination. The acute anterior cruciate ligament injury presents with a characteristic history and physical examination. The most common

TABLE 7–4. *Frequency of ligamentous injuries in 389 knees (235)* *

Ligament	No.	Percent of Total Knee Injuries
ACL	151	39
ACL and MCL	118	30
ACL and PCL	1	0
Medial capsule MCL	47	12
Posterior medial, capsule	12	3
ACL and LCL	7	2
LCL	2	1
PCL	19	5
MCL and PCL	8	2
MCL, ACL, and PCL	17	4
MCL, ACL, PCL, and LCL	1	0
MCL, PCL, and LCL	1	0
ACL and PCL	2	1
ACL, PCL, and LCL	3	1
Total	389	100

* ACL, anterior cruciate ligament; PCL, posterior cruciate ligament, MCL, medial collateral ligament, LCL, lateral collateral ligament.

mechanism of injury is indirect (78%), with deceleration and a rapid change in direction ("cutting") being frequent (242,274). Two common mechanisms of indirect injury have been reported. One is a sudden external rotation of the tibia on the femur combined with knee flexion and a valgus force (241,243,258). Injury to the medial collateral ligament and medial meniscus are common in this type (243). The other frequent indirect mechanism is hyperextension of the knee with the leg in internal rotation (233,243,258). A less common mechanism is hyperflexion (243). Finally, forced internal rotation of the tibia on the femur may also tear the anterior cruciate ligament, as will an anteriorly directed force applied to the posterior surface of the tibia while in 90° of flexion (258).

Other characteristic aspects of the history of the injury have been reported. The sites of anterior cruciate injury were midsubstance in 72%, proximal end in 18%, distal end in 4%, and unrecorded in 6% in a series of 50 knees (258). Patients report hearing or feeling a "pop" at the moment of injury with a frequency of 34% (243) 65% (274), or 86.7% (233). Inability to bear weight on the affected knee immediately following injury is frequent, reaching 77% in one series (233). Acute knee swelling within 12 hours is common and represents a hemarthrosis (242,274). The combination of a pop at the time of injury, the inability to continue participation in athletics, and gross swelling of the knee that is maximal within 12 hours of injury gives a diagnostic accuracy of 85% for an acute tear of the anterior cruciate ligament (241).

The physical examination at the time of the initial injury may be difficult because of pain and guarding by the patient. In one series, only 6.8% of the anterior cruciate ligament tears were diagnosed at the time of the original injury (274). The physical examination reveals evidence of increased anterior laxity on drawer examination in 93.7% (Fig. 7-57) (242). However, other authors have found the anterior drawer sign without anesthesia to be present in only 10% (238). The Lachman test performed in 20°–30° of flexion is more reliable than the anterior drawer; it is positive without anesthesia in 85% and with anesthesia in 100% (238). Associated injuries to the medial and lateral ligamentous structures as well as to the meniscus should be sought. Examination under general anesthesia to eliminate muscle spasm and guarding is necessary if a hemarthrosis has accumulated by the time the patient is seen.

Arthroscopy is an essential part of evaluation of the acutely injured knee and is discussed in more detail later in the section on knee arthroscopy and imaging techniques. Arthrography, once frequently used, has been largely replaced by MRI for the evaluation of the acutely injured knee. Both techniques will detect capsular tears, meniscal injuries, and may aid in the definition of anterior cruciate ligament tears (261,278).

Routine radiography remains important in the evaluation of knee ligamentous injuries. A joint effusion on the lateral view appears as an ovoid soft tissue density in the retropatellar region (see Fig. 7-13B) (278). Avulsion fractures of either end of the anterior cruciate ligament may be seen on the lateral or tunnel view (Figs. 7-54, 7-58, and 7-59). An avulsed fragment from the lateral tibial plateau, the lateral capsular sign or Segond fracture, has a high correlation with injury to the anterior cruciate ligament (Fig. 7-54) (265,278,284). The lateral capsular sign represents an avulsion of the tibial attachment of the middle one-third of the lateral capsule and a tear of the

anterior cruciate (284). This sign is infrequent, however, being present in only 3 of 50 knees with tears of the anterior cruciate ligament (265). Notches may be present on the lateral femoral condyle seen on the lateral or internal oblique roentgenogram (Fig. 7-60; see also Fig. 7-15). These result from chronic anterior subluxation of the lateral femoral condyle into the tibia, leading to impingement (233,265). Stress roentgenograms are also helpful (Figs. 7-61 and 7-62; see also Figs. 7-21 and 7-22).

Types of Instability

An understanding of the types of instabilities of the knee and the specific tests for each instability is essential for patient management. Instability may be either straight or single-plane, rotatory, or combined (254). One-plane instability may be either medial, lateral, anterior, or posterior (244). Rotatory instability may be anteromedial, anterolateral, posteromedial, or posterolateral (244). The presence of posteromedial rotatory instability is controversial (251). Combined instabilities may be anteromedial-anterolateral, anterolateral-posterolateral, or anteromedial-posteromedial (244). The instabilities are classified by the direction of movement of the tibia relative to the femur upon a specific stress. A single-plane instability means that the posterior cruciate ligament is torn and, therefore, that the axis of rotation has been lost (251). Upon stress, the tibia does not rotate but the knee joint opens in a way similar to a door (254). In contrast, in a rotatory instability, the posterior cruciate ligament is intact and provides an axis for rotatory movement (254).

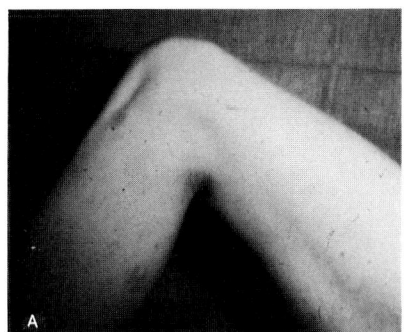 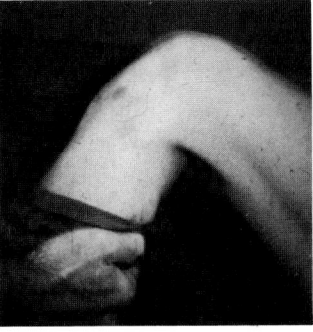 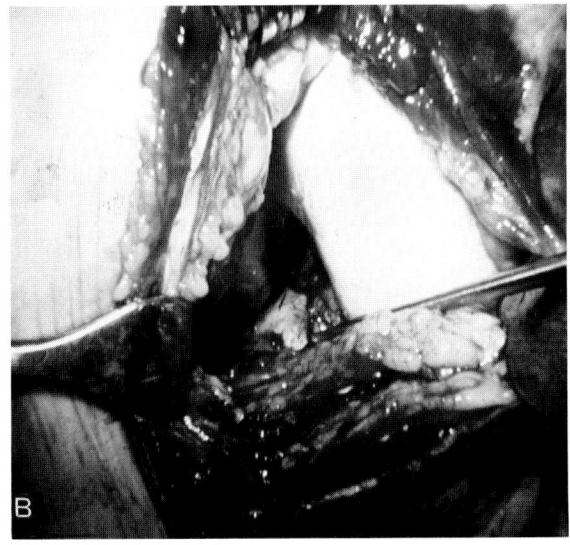

FIG. 7–57. A: Positive anterior drawer sign and (B) operative photograph of a tear of the anterior cruciate.

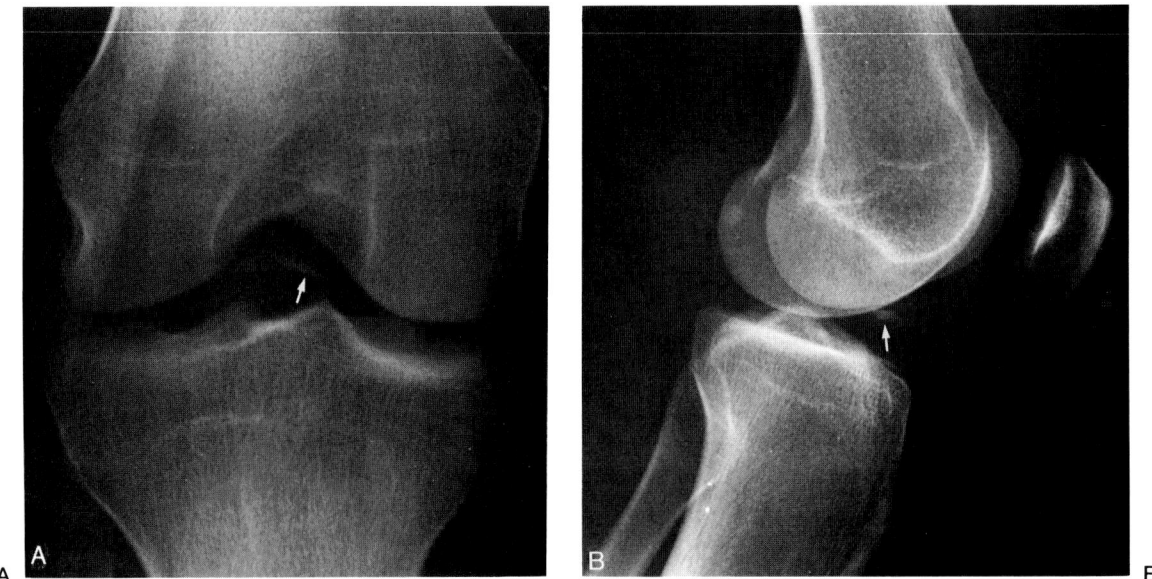

FIG. 7-58. AP (**A**) and lateral (**B**) radiographs revealing an avulsion fracture indicative of a tear of the anterior cruciate ligament.

The magnitude of the force, the position of the knee, the state of muscle tone, the quality of the bone, the degree of fixation of the foot, and the extent of body load all affect the magnitude and type of injury. The extent of ligamentous tearing or sprain may be classified (251). An injury with a minimum number of fibers torn and localized tenderness but no instability is a Grade 1 sprain. A disruption of more fibers associated with tenderness but no instability is a Grade 2 sprain. Complete disruption of the ligament with resultant instability is a Grade 3

sprain. The degree of instability may also be classified by the amount of joint surface separation upon stress (251). A 1+ instability involves up to 5 mm of opening, a 2+ instability involves 5–10 mm of opening, and a 3+ instability involves 10 mm or more opening upon stress. Since individuals vary in their extent of ligamentous laxity, so it is essential to compare the injured to the noninjured side.

A variety of clinical signs and tests are utilized in the evaluation of individuals with knee instabilities. A re-

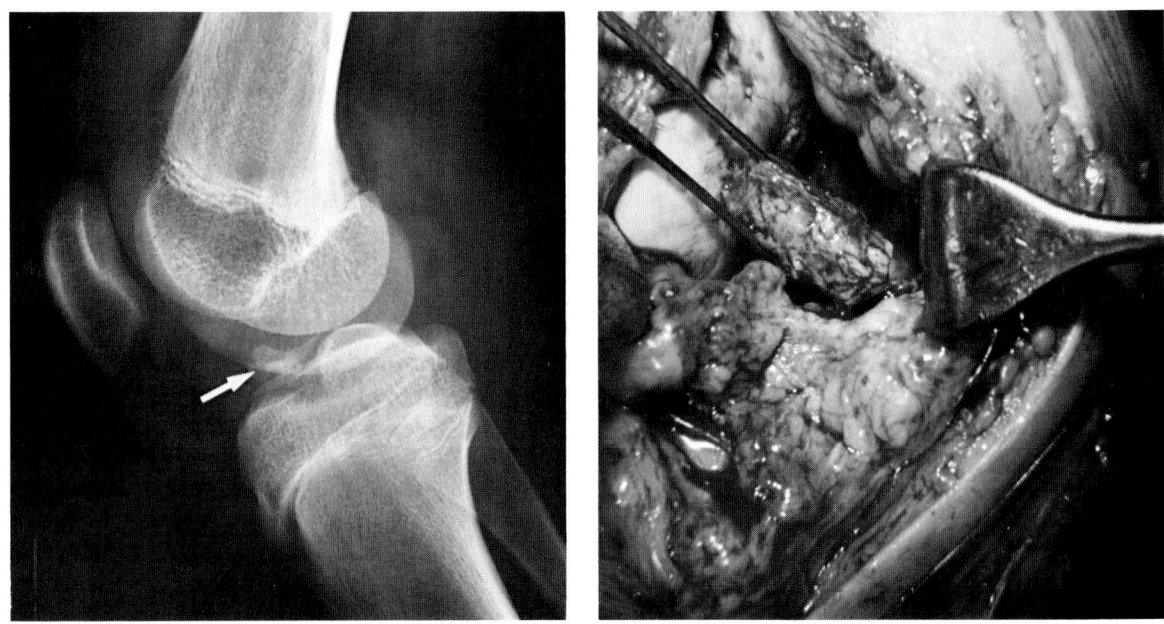

FIG. 7-59. A: Lateral radiograph and (**B**) operative photograph of a large tibial avulsion fracture that had occurred three years previously. The anterior cruciate ligament was lastly attached to this fragment.

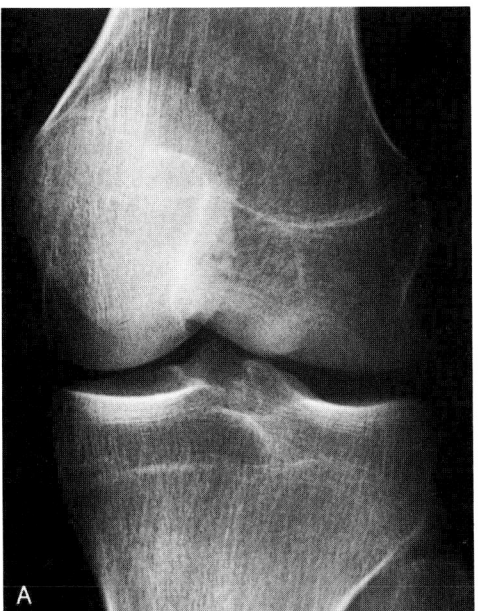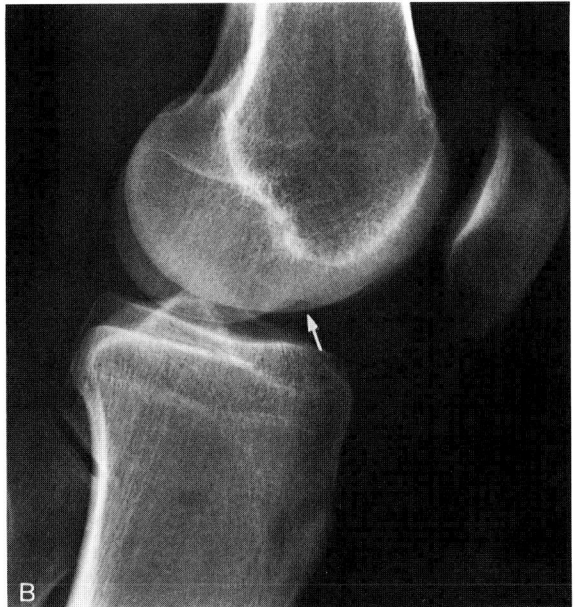

FIG. 7–60. AP (**A**) and lateral (**B**) radiographs displaying the impression defect on the lateral femoral condyle associated with chronic anterolateral rotatory instability.

view of the injured structures and the findings associated with each pattern of instability will aid in the comprehension of both the examination and the instability.

Straight or Single-Plane Instability

A straight or single-plane medial instability indicates a tear of the medial compartment ligaments combined with a tear of the posterior cruciate ligament. The injured structures may include the middle-third medial capsular ligament, the superficial medial ligament, the posteromedial capsular ligament, and both cruciate ligaments (244,251). An opening of the knee medially upon valgus stress with the knee in full extension will occur (Fig. 7-61) (251). A Grade 1 or 2 sprain of the middle-third capsular ligament and superficial medial ligament will be stable to valgus stress in extension but may show

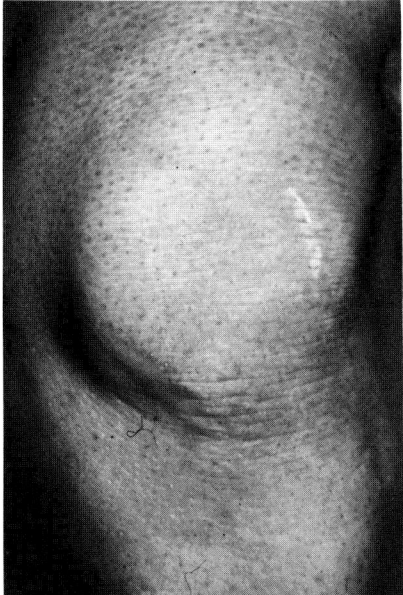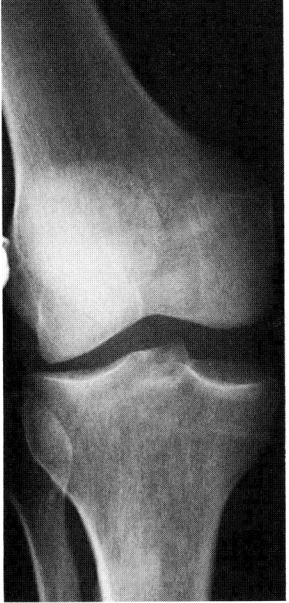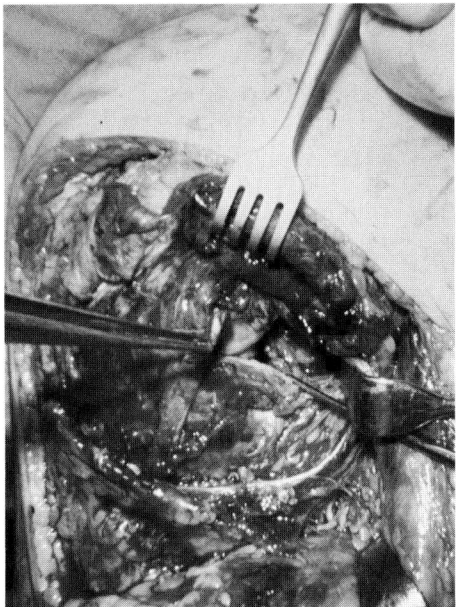

FIG. 7–61. A: Clinical appearance under stress. **B:** AP stress radiograph and (**C**) operative photograph of a complete medial capsular disruption. The superficial medial ligament is illustrated by the forceps and the tear of the posteromedial capsule by the probe.

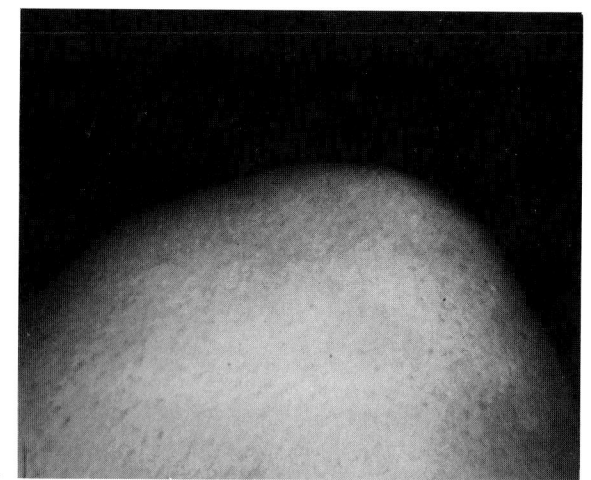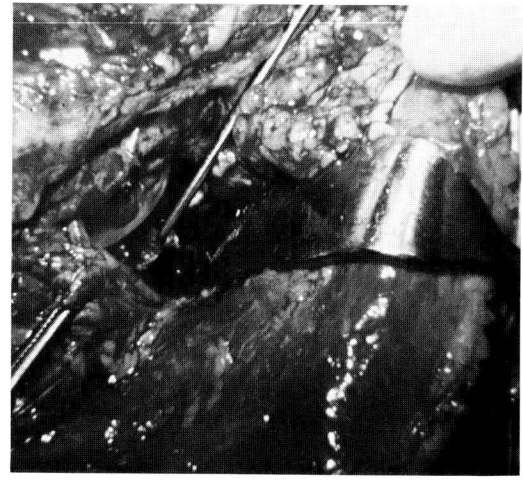

FIG. 7-62. A: Posterior sag of the tibia on the femur associated with an acute tear of the posterior cruciate ligament. **B:** Operative photograph of acute posterior cruciate ligament tear indicated by probe.

severe instability in 30° of flexion (244). A straight lateral instability results from a tear of the lateral compartment ligaments combined with a tear of the posterior cruciate ligament (252). The injured structures may include the middle-third lateral capsular ligament, the fibular collateral ligament, the arcuate-popliteus complex, both cruciates, the biceps tendon, the iliotibial tract, and the peroneal nerve (244).

Physical examination reveals instability upon varus stress with the knee in full extension (252). Instability to varus stress at 30° but stability at 0° indicates a sprain of the middle-third lateral capsular ligament (244). A straight anterior instability results from a tear of both cruciate ligaments (251). An apparent straight anterior drawer test may occur in the presence of a combined anteromedial and anterolateral rotatory instability (251). A straight posterior instability results from a tear of the posterior cruciate combined with the posteromedial (posterior oblique) capsular ligament and the arcuate complex (251). A positive posterior drawer sign is evident when the tibial condyles subluxate equal amounts posteriorly (251). A combined posterolateral and posteromedial rotatory instability may give a similar drawer sign (244).

Rotatory Instability

An anteromedial rotatory instability demonstrates medial laxity and anterior displacement of the medial tibial condyle on the femur upon anterior drawer testing (244). Injury may involve the medial compartment ligaments, including the middle-third medial capsular ligament, superficial medial ligament, posteromedial capsule (posterior oblique), anterior cruciate ligament, and frequently peripheral detachment of the medial meniscus (251,280).

The basic lesion necessary for an anteromedial rotatory instability is a rupture of the medial capsular ligament; this rupture allows abnormal external rotation of the tibia (256,280). The mechanism of injury that results in an isolated lesion of the medial capsular ligament is a valgus external rotation stress applied to the knee in a position of 90° of flexion (280). The anterior medial capsule is most frequently injured with the knee flexed 90°, the middle portion with the knee flexed between 30° and 90°, and the posterior portion with the knee close to full extension (280). The sequence of injury begins with the rupture of the superficial medial ligament, and ends with rupture of the anterior cruciate ligament (280). Peripheral tears of the medial meniscus are frequently present in fresh injuries, while posterior horn tears of the medial meniscus are present in chronic injuries related to repetitive impingement (280). In a series of 24 acute injuries, the middle portion of the medial capsule was torn in 24, a peripheral tear of the medial meniscus was present in 23, and an anterior cruciate ligament tear appeared in only 5 knees (280). In a series of 45 knees, the same authors found a deficient anterior cruciate ligament in all knees and laxity of the arcuate ligament complex and injury to the lateral meniscus in 44 knees.

Physical findings include a positive valgus stress test at 30° of flexion and a positive anterior drawer test performed with the tibia in 15°–30° of external rotation (280). An abduction or valgus stress test that is negative at 0° but positive at 30° of flexion indicates a tear of the medial compartment ligaments (251). The extent of displacement during the anterior drawer test correlates with the extent of injury, with a positive 1+ test indicating injury to the capsule alone and a positive 3+ test indicating capsular, collateral, and anterior cruciate ligament injury (280).

An anterolateral rotatory instability of the knee reveals anterior and lateral subluxation of the tibia on the femur as the knee approaches extension (244). Injury may involve the middle-third lateral capsular ligament, arcuate ligament, anterior cruciate ligament, and frequently the posterior horn of the lateral meniscus (251,252).

A biomechanical study of knee ligamentous structures revealed increases in external rotation and anterior drawer testing with injury to the anterior cruciate ligament alone (262). The internal rotation was increased by sectioning of the lateral collateral ligament or posterolateral complex. If the anterior cruciate was intact, sectioning of the posterolateral ligament alone did not increase internal rotation. In contrast, Hughston believes that the key element for anterolateral rotatory instability is a tear of the middle-third lateral capsular ligament (252). In chronic anterolateral rotatory instability, laxity of the posterolateral capsule was combined with a tear of the anterior cruciate in 45 of 45 knees (236). The lateral meniscus invariably had peripheral detachment or a posterior horn tear related to chronic impingement during subluxation of the tibia. In a series of 36 knees with acute anterolateral rotatory instability, the middle-third lateral capsular ligament was torn in 21 cases; the lateral capsule in 16; the anterior cruciate ligament in 4; the anterior cruciate ligament, lateral capsule, and iliotibial tract in 3; and the anterior cruciate combined with iliotibial tract in 2 (235). The mechanism of injury is usually indirect, with rotation without contact in 10 of 14 cases. Direct trauma was noted in 4 of 14 acute injuries. Deceleration with cutting away from the supporting foot combined with knee flexion has been felt to be the most frequent mechanism of injury (257).

Physical examination reveals a positive anterior drawer test, with the tibia in neutral or slight internal rotation showing increased forward displacement of the lateral tibial condyle (252). A variety of specialized tests have been devised to reproduce the anterior subluxation of the lateral tibial plateau or its reduction. The tests for anterolateral rotatory instability include the pivot shift, jerk, flexion-rotation drawer, Slocum, and Losee tests (Table 7-5) (246,247,252,264,265,271). All of these tests are designed to identify anterior subluxation of the lateral tibial plateau on the lateral femoral condyle with the knee in mild flexion and reduction of the subluxation at 30°–40° of flexion (246,247,264,265,279). The iliotibial tract causes the subluxation of the tibia to reduce upon flexion (248).

An experimental study was performed to determine the structural defects and mechanics of the pivot shift (242). Sectioning of the anterior cruciate ligament alone induced a positive pivot shift in 89% of the knees tested. Sectioning of this ligament alone induced both components of the pivot shift, the increased anterior displacement of the tibia and the increased internal rotation. Sectioning of the iliotibial band, lateral collateral ligament, or popliteus singly or in combination will not induce a pivot shift in the presence of an intact anterior cruciate ligament. Lateral meniscectomy will eliminate the pivot shift. The pivot shift results in the lateral meniscus being forced posteriorly, followed by a sudden anterior subluxation of the tibia and lateral meniscus beneath the lateral femoral condyle, resulting in widening of the lateral compartment. When the knee is in 0°–20° of flexion, the instant center of rotation is displaced anteriorly (281). At 20°–40° of flexion the instant center of rotation suddenly displaces posteriorly. The "crossover" test consists of immobilization of the foot of the affected extremity with the patient instructed to rotate his body, crossing the unaffected leg over the fixed foot (233). A sensation that the knee will give way is a positive sign of pivot shift.

In addition to the physical examination and history of the knee's giving way, especially on cutting, radiographs are valuable in diagnosis. The lateral capsular sign was

TABLE 7-5. *Tests for anterolateral rotatory instability*

Test	Author	Technique	Mechanics
Pivot Shift	Galway and McIntosh	Supine, valgus stress, foot in internal rotation, knee in extension	Sudden reduction at 30° during flexion
Jerk	Hughston	Supine valgus stress foot in internal rotation, knee in 90° flexion	Subluxation maximal at 30° during extension then reduction upon further extension
Flexion rotation drawer	Noyes	Supine, knee in 20°–30° of flexion, downward drawer, free femoral rotation	Reduction with further knee flexion
A.L.R.I. test	Slocum	Lateral decubitus position on opposite side, 30°–50° posterior rotation of pelvis, knee in 10° of flexion, foot supported on table	Reduction at 25°–45° upon knee flexion
Losee	Losee	Supine knee and hip in 45° flexion, external rotation valgus stress	Subluxation followed by reduction upon extension

present in 3 of 36 knees in one series (236) and in 3 of 50 knees in another (270). A notch in the lateral femoral condyle is frequently visible (233) and was present in 14 of 15 knees in another series (264). Arthrography may diagnose tears of the lateral meniscus as well as tears of the anterior cruciate ligament (236,278).

Posterolateral rotatory instability is present when there is increased external rotation of the tibia in a posterolateral direction. This instability results from a tear of the arcuate complex (252). Biomechanical studies have shown that sectioning of the posterolateral complex and the lateral collateral ligament results in significantly increased external rotation (262). Additional sectioning of the anterior cruciate ligament results in only a small increase in external rotation. The injured structures include the arcuate-popliteus complex (arcuate ligament, fibular collateral ligament, popliteus muscle, and gastrocnemius muscle), the biceps femoris, the lateral capsular ligament, and perhaps the posterior cruciate ligament (234,244). In a series of 17 knees, the popliteus musculotendinous unit was torn in 16, the arcuate ligament in 17, the fibular collateral ligament in 10, the gastrocnemius in 4, the biceps femoris in 8, and the iliotibial tract in 2 (234). The peroneal nerve was injured in 2, the anterior cruciate ligament in 11, and the lateral meniscus in 4 of the 17 knees.

The mechanism of injury in posterolateral rotatory instability is direct trauma to the proximal medial tibia, resulting in hyperextension or an indirect mechanism of hyperextension and external rotation (234). The physical findings in acute injuries include tenderness and induration over the arcuate complex and positive results in several specific tests. The adduction of varus stress test performed at 30° of flexion is frequently positive (11 of 12) but is not diagnostic (234). A positive posterolateral drawer test or external rotation recurvatum test, on the other hand, is diagnostic of posterolateral rotatory instability (234,252,260). The external rotation recurvatum test is produced by holding the leg by the toes with the knee extended. Recurvatum and apparent varus occurs as the tibia rotates posteriorly (251,252,255). The posterolateral drawer test is a posterior drawer test performed with the tibia in neutral, internal, and external rotation (255). The posterior drawer test in internal rotation must be negative to indicate a functioning posterior cruciate ligament (255). An increased posterior drawer in 15° of external rotation compared with neutral rotation with further posterior displacement of the lateral rather than medial tibial plateau is considered positive (255). In the reverse pivot shift, the posterior subluxation of the lateral tibial plateau reduces as the flexed knee is extended and the tibia is externally rotated (257).

Posteromedial rotatory instability is controversial. Hughston and colleagues claim that posteromedial rotatory instability does not exist, because an intact posterior cruciate ligament would prevent posteromedial subluxa-

tion of the tibia, and an absent posterior cruciate ligament would in any case eliminate the rotatory component, making a straight posterior instability (251). A posteromedial instability results from tears of the superficial medial ligament, the medial capsular ligament, the posterior oblique ligament, and the anterior cruciate ligament (260). Disruption of these ligaments allows a posteromedial sag. The mechanism of injury is hyperextension and valgus force (260). Physical examination reveals the posteromedial sag of the tibia, minor hyperextension, and medial opening of the joint space on valgus stress of the extended knee (260).

Combined Instability

Combined rotatory instabilities may occur, the most frequent being a combined anterolateral and posterolateral or anteromedial and anterolateral (251). A longstanding anteromedial rotatory instability may progress to combined anteromedial-anterolateral instability from repetitive stress to the secondary stabilizers. In this combined instability, the anterior drawer sign performed in neutral may appear to displace directly forward, indicating a straight anterior instability (251). However, specific tests for each type of instability will be present and tests for the posterior cruciate ligament will indicate its integrity. Combined anterolateral-posterolateral rotatory instability may result from the same injury, with severe damage to the lateral joint ligaments and anterior cruciate ligament. Physical examination will reveal positive tests for both types of instability. In a series of 17 knees with posterolateral rotatory instability, 6 had a combined anterolateral-posterolateral, 3 a combined anteromedial-anterolateral-posterolateral, and 1 a combined anteromedial-posterolateral rotatory instability (234).

Posterior cruciate ligament injuries leading to a straight posterior instability are less frequent lesions than those involving the anterior cruciate ligament. In the presence of a posterior cruciate ligament tear, all instabilities become straight because the tibia no longer rotates on the femur about a central axis (254). Gallie and LeMesurier in 1927 stated that, with a torn posterior cruciate ligament, "the patient is almost invariably left with a knee in which the femur dislocates violently and painfully forward, whenever weight is borne on the flexed limb" (245).

The mechanism of injury to the posterior cruciate ligament is violent trauma, with either posterior displacement of the tiba on the femur when the knee is in flexion or hyperextension (258,268). Motor vehicle accidents, falls, and sports injuries are the most frequent etiologies (254,268,282). Associated ligamentous injuries are frequent. In a series of 32 acute injuries, 26 had injury to the medial compartment, 2 to the lateral compartment, and 1 to both the medial and lateral compartments

(254). Other frequent injuries are to the anterior cruciate ligament and posterior horn of the medial or lateral meniscus (254,282). Physical examination may reveal abrasions or lacerations over the proximal tibia (13 of 21 knees) (282). Additional physical findings include tenderness in the popliteal fossa and hemarthrosis (282). The posterior drawer sign with the tibia in internal rotation is positive in the knee with a chronic deficiency in the posterior cruciate ligament, but it may be negative in an acute injury if the arcuate complex is not injured (see Fig. 7-62) (251). The posterior drawer test was negative in 20 of 29 knees with an acute posterior cruciate ligament tear (254). A positive abduction or adduction stress with the knee in 0° is a reliable sign of a tear of the posterior cruciate ligament (251). In 26 knees with acute injuries of the posterior cruciate ligament and medial compartment, the abduction stress test in full extension was negative in only one knee under anesthesia (254). In contrast, the adduction stress test at 0° was negative in all patients with a torn posterior cruciate except for the 3 knees with lateral compartmental injury (254). The anterior drawer test with the knee in full internal rotation was negative in only 4 of 30 acute posterior cruciate ligament tears (254). In 7 knees with an intact anterior cruciate but torn posterior cruciate ligament, a positive anterior drawer test was present in external rotation. Genu recurvatum may accompany this injury (282). Radiographic findings may or may not be present. Failure of the ligament may occur at either its femoral or tibial attachment or its midsubstance. In 29 knees, the location of the tear was at the femoral attachment in 16, at the tibial attachment in 8, and midsubstance in 5 (254). An avulsion fracture frequently accompanies only avulsion of the tibial attachment and may present as only a small flake of bone in the intracondylar notch (258,268,282,283).

Treatment of the torn posterior cruciate ligament may be operative or nonoperative with cast immobilization. Nonoperative treatment of 5 knees with avulsion fractures of the tibial end of the posterior cruciate ligament resulted in 2 non-unions with poor results (282). In another series of 6 tibial avulsions, 4 of 5 displaced fractures progressed to non-union and functional disability (268). Therefore, surgical repair of the torn posterior cruciate ligament and repair of associated injuries is recommended by most authors (254,258,268,282,283). Open reduction and internal fixation is indicated for fractures with 0.3 cm separation or 0.5 cm upward displacement with or without rotation from the tibial base (282). Surgery is also indicated for comminuted fractures with large, rotated fragments (282). Internal fixation of 6 fractures resulted in union in 5, with satisfactory results in these cases (268). In a series of 26 acute posterior cruciate ligament tears followed for an average of 9 years following repair, patients reported 25 good and 1 fair result (254). Objective examination of 20 of the 25 knees revealed 13 good, 4 fair, and 3 poor results (254). There-

fore, early diagnosis and treatment of injuries of the posterior cruciate give satisfactory results.

Treatment

The treatment of injuries to the major ligamentous structures of the knee is controversial. The options include nonoperative treatment with later reconstruction if needed or early surgical repair. Early surgical repair may be combined with reconstructive techniques to augment the strength of severely injured ligamentous structures (237,263).

In 1917, Hey Groves stated that "ruptures of the crucial ligaments are now much more frequently recognized than formerly . . . [an injury] which produces permanent total disablement for active pursuits . . ." (250) Hey Groves recognized the phenomenon of the pivot shift and described a reconstructive technique for the cruciate ligaments using the iliotibial band (249). Palmer contributed much to the diagnosis and function of the knee ligaments and recommended early repair (277). O'Donoghue recommended early surgical repair within 2 weeks of injury and claimed that better results would be obtained with early repair than with late reconstruction (276). Although these and many other reports have recommended early treatment, some selected lesions continue to receive nonoperative management.

Nonoperative care must be considered in view of the natural history of the lesions being treated, the extent of instability, and the activity level and goals of the patient. Primary repair of an "isolated" midsubstance tear of the anterior cruciate ligament has revealed a high incidence of instability at 5 years (241). Therefore, many surgeons consider this lesion to be unsuitable for primary repair and recommend either nonoperative care or primary reconstruction (274). Nonoperative treatment consisting of a vigorous physical therapy program has been utilized in 24 knees with an anterior cruciate ligament tear (275). Although 59% of the patients returned to sports, 13 of 22 knees showed some degenerative changes on radiographs, and 42% required a meniscectomy. The best results were obtained with a hamstring-quadriceps strength ratio that was equal (248). In a series of 84 knees with chronic anterior cruciate ligament laxity treated with a vigorous rehabilitation program and followed for 3 years, one-third of the knees improved but remained somewhat symptomatic, one-third became worse with increasing symptoms, and 18 of the knees required reconstruction (273). Therefore, 43% of the 84 knees benefited from the rehabilitation program. However, it was not possible to predict which knee would or would not improve with physical therapy (273). Therefore, Noyes and colleagues recommended an initial nonoperative approach to the knee with a chronic anterior cruciate ligament deficiency.

Bracing may be combined with a muscle rehabilitation program to control rotatory stresses (Fig. 7-63). A brace will aid in the control of rotatory instabilities of the knee (269). Nonoperative treatment with a cast brace has been utilized in highly selected patients for medial collateral ligament injuries. In a prospective randomized study of isolated complete medial collateral ligament injuries treated either by surgery or a cast brace, the results at 2–3 years of follow-up were similar. Therefore, selected patients with either acute ligament injuries or chronic instabilities may be treated nonsurgically with satisfactory results, but extreme care in patient selection appears essential.

The long-term results of acute repair for rotatory instabilities have been reported by few authors. Hughston and colleagues reported on a series of 93 of 154 knees treated with primary repair of acute anteromedial rotatory instability with a follow-up of 7.9 years (253). Satisfactory results were obtained in 89% subjectively but in only 73% objectively (253). Nine knees required subsequent reconstructive surgery. Meniscectomy had an adverse effect; no knee with a meniscectomy revealed excellent results, and the overall results were decreased 5% by a meniscectomy (253). There were no significant differences among the knees with or without a functioning anterior cruciate ligament (253). Hughston and colleagues concluded that the key to a satisfactory result was

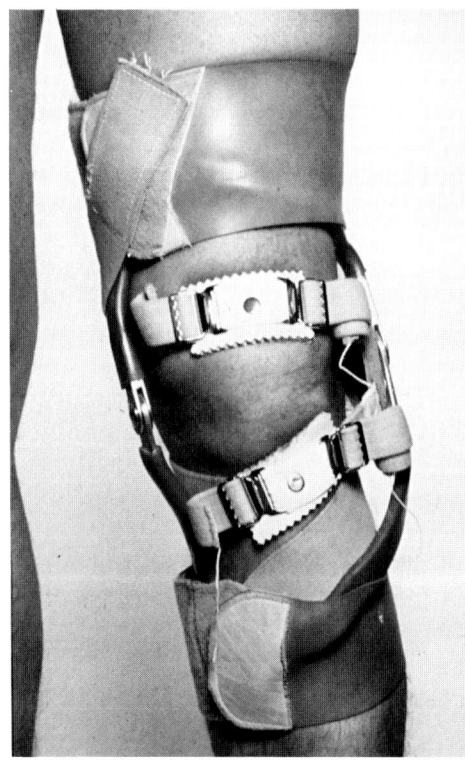

FIG. 7–63. Lennox-Hill brace utilized for chronic ligamentous instability.

preservation of the medial meniscus and repair of the posterior oblique ligament. Norwood and colleagues reported the results of acute repair of 21 of 36 knees with acute anterolateral rotatory instability followed at 5.4 years (270). Satisfactory results were obtained in 16 of the 21 knees. Resection of the anterior cruciate ligament did not adversely affect the results. Finally, Baker and colleagues reported results obtained with 17 knees treated for acute posterolateral rotatory instability followed at 4.5 years (234). Satisfactory results were obtained in 85% subjectively and in 77% objectively.

Although early surgical repair of all injured structures may give a high proportion of satisfactory results, some individuals will present late with chronic instability. A multitude of reconstructive procedures have been advocated for each of the various instabilities. However, a detailed description of these reconstructive procedures and their results is beyond the scope of this review. The indication for anterior cruciate ligament reconstruction has been aptly stated by O'Donoghue: ". . . instability sufficiently severe to interfere with the person's normal everyday living" (276). The reconstructive procedures may be considered extra-articular, intra-articular, or combined. The extra-articular reconstruction attempts to reinforce the secondary stabilizers of the knee and partially to substitute their function for that of the anterior cruciate ligament. In contrast, the intra-articular reconstruction attempts to reproduce normal anterior cruciate ligament function but does not address the problem of the damaged secondary stabilizers. With either of these approaches, the reconstruction is forced to bear the load that is normally shared by the anterior cruciate ligament and secondary stabilizers. In contrast, the combined procedure attempts to reinforce the secondary stabilizers as well as to reconstruct the function of the anterior cruciate ligament, allowing load sharing among the reconstructed structures. Although some extra-articular reconstructions have been found to fail with time, the long-term results of many of the reconstructive procedures are not yet available. Many important factors go into patient selection and choice of a reconstruction. The demands of the individual, the ability to cooperate in a prolonged rehabilitation program, and the patient's comprehension of long-term limitations are essential. The surgical technique must consider the strength of the graft utilized, its vascularity, the time of beginning rehabilitation and motion, and the duration of time needed for obtaining maximal strength and integrity of the graft (272).

In summary, the early diagnosis and treatment of injuries to the ligaments of the knee will optimize the treatment options available. In the presence of significant instability in the active individual, early repair of all injured structures will give satisfactory results. Late reconstructions may provide an alternative mode of salvage in those individuals for whom a late diagnosis is made, but further data are necessary to determine optimal techniques.

KNEE ARTHROSCOPY AND IMAGING TECHNIQUES FOR ARTICULAR AND PERIARTICULAR DISORDERS

The evaluation and management of articular and periarticular disorders has been greatly aided by the development of arthroscopy. Arthrography, computed tomography (CT), ultrasonography, and specifically MRI have greatly improved imaging capability in these conditions. These techniques are useful in the evaluation of menisci, cruciate ligaments, articular cartilage, synovial diseases, loose bodies, intra-articular fractures, patellar alignment, and periarticular soft tissue disorders (316,321, 357,421). A review of the role of these modalities and their accuracy is valuable for the attending physician.

The complexity of examining the extrameniscal portions of the knee (cruciate ligaments, collateral ligaments, plicae, etc.) necessitates good communication between the referring physician and the radiologist. MRI has largely replaced other techniques for imaging purposes. However, in a given clinical setting each imaging technique may play a role. Therefore, we will discuss techniques and applications as they apply to MRI, arthrography, CT, and ultrasonography.

Arthrographic Technique

As demonstrated in Table 7-6, the approach to knee arthrography varies considerably with the clinical indication. Review of the clinical data, radiographs, isotope scans, and CT studies should be accomplished prior to the arthrogram. This will allow proper planning of the arthrographic technique.

The equipment and arthrogram tray are important and have been discussed in Chapter 1, Diagnostic Techniques. The most frequently used positive contrast agents are diatrizoate meglumine (Hypaque-M-60 and Renografin-M-60) (309,333). Contrast material is rapidly absorbed and diluted, which necessitates rapid film-

ing. Delays of 5–10 minutes may result in suboptimal studies. Metrizamide (Amipaque) and Dimer-X have been investigated as potential arthrographic contrast media. Recently non-ionic agents such as Iotrolan and Hexabrix have also been employed (288,398). They provide the advantage of prolonged concentration in the joint, allowing more time for filming (333,370). Nonionic agents allow adequate images to be obtained for up to 30 minutes following injection. Epinephrine (0.3 ml of 1:1000) may also be added to the contrast material. This results in reduced fluid accumulation in the joint, higher iodine concentrations, and more time for filming (309,333,347,425). This is especially helpful if additional special views, tomography, or CT will be performed with the arthrogram. However, increased reactive changes in the synovium occur when epinephrine is used with ionic agents (305).

Air or CO_2 may be used alone or in conjunction with positive contrast material (341,363,390,413). Air is more readily available than CO_2 and causes less pain following the arthrogram (341). However, CO_2 is more rapidly absorbed and consequently reduces the chance of air embolus (413). But air embolism is extremely rare (309); we have not experienced air embolism or infection using room air. Room air will remain in the joint for several days and patients should be informed that the joint may be "noisy" until the air is absorbed.

When the contrast medium and film techniques have been chosen, the patient is positioned on the radiography table. The patient should be supine with the involved knee closest to the examiner. The knee is prepared using sterile technique (334,348). A cushion may be positioned under the knee for comfort and to assist with aspiration (375). The injection may be performed using a medial or lateral approach (334). This decision depends on the site of the suspected lesion and the skin condition. Areas of cutaneous inflammation should obviously be avoided. Although the medial patellofemoral joint is slightly wider than the lateral, the lateral approach is more frequently chosen (309,333,348). There is less soft tissue laterally, and in our practice the lesion is usually on the medial side.

Numerous injection techniques have been described both with and without local anesthetic (309,347,348, 350,432). The injection depends on the clinical setting. In the acutely injured or painful knee, aspiration and anesthetic injection may be required prior to the arthrogram. This will allow adequate stressing of the joint during the arthrogram. In the usual situation, local anesthetic with a single-syringe injection technique is used. The patient's leg is internally rotated. This allows free movement of the patella and permits a superior angle for the needle as it enters the joint. The needle should enter the joint at the midpoint of the patella. The local anesthetic is injected in the skin inferior to the point at which the needle will enter the joint (Fig. 7-64). The soft tissues

TABLE 7–6. *Indications and approach to knee arthrography*

Indication	Technique
Meniscal tears	Single or double contrast (D/C)
Cruciate ligament	D/C (tomo, xero), CT
Articular cartilage	D/C ± tomo, CT
Synovitis	D/C
Loose bodies	Single ± tomo
Chondromalacia	D/C, axial views, CT
Popliteal cysts	Single or D/C
Plicae	D/C + CT, tomography, special views
Extra-articular	D/C ± CT

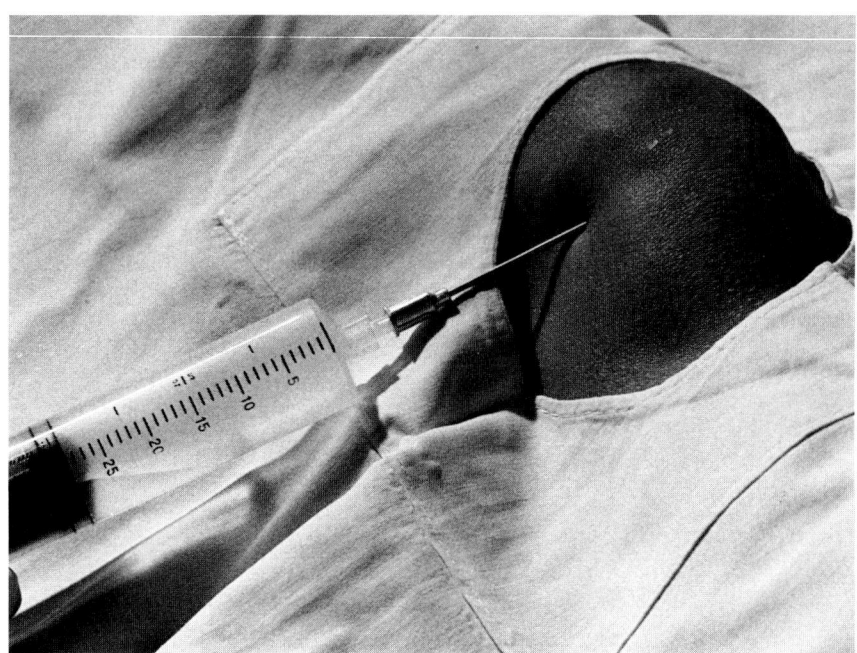

FIG. 7-64. Needle placement for knee arthrography. The needle is angled superiorly to enter the joint inferior to the mid patella. This position keeps the air in the distal portion of the syringe allowing the intra-articular position to be easily checked.

are infiltrated slightly as the needle is advanced into the joint. Proper needle position is noted if the anesthetic meets no resistance or if fluid can be aspirated from the joint. If fluid is present, it should be aspirated as completely as possible. This is facilitated by the knee pad. In some cases gravity will allow better evacuation, as aspiration may be hindered by synovium drawn against the needle tip. A catheter with side holes has also been used for more complete aspiration (375). Examination of the fluid may be very helpful. Microscopic analysis for crystals, Gram stain, culture, etc. may be indicated. Wear particles, for example, have been described in patients with osteoarthritis, chondromalacia, and meniscal tears (420). The presence of blood in the fluid may indicate a ligament tear, peripheral meniscal separation, or, rarely, synovial hemangioma (309,333,380,407).

The presence or absence of fluid in the joint has some bearing on the amount of contrast material injected. If the joint is "dry", 3–5 ml of contrast material is used with about 20–40 ml of air. If a large effusion is evacuated, 5–7 ml of contrast material or even slightly more may be used. In certain cases, single-contrast may be used instead of the preferred double-contrast technique. If significant allergy to iodine is present, air alone may be injected (Table 7-6).

With the standard double-contrast technique, the anesthetic needle is left in position and a 20–25 ml syringe, with 5 ml of contrast material and 20 ml of air, is attached to the needle. The upward angle of the needle results in the air filling the distal portion of the syringe. Gentle pressure on the barrel of the syringe will meet no resistance if the needle is within the joint capsule. Once this is confirmed, the contents of the syringe can be injected with one gentle motion. The syringe can be re-

filled with air and an additional 20+ ml injected. Following removal of the needle the joint is slowly exercised with the patient on the table. By rotating the patient to the right and left the contrast can be uniformly distributed in the medial and lateral compartments. The patient may also be exercised in the upright position (walking, etc.), but this may result in excess air bubble formation. The possibility of syncopal episodes can also be avoided by exercising the knee on the table (309,348).

Filming of the medial and lateral menisci should be performed fluoroscopically using a stress device (Fig. 7-65). Nine to twelve images of each meniscus should be obtained. We routinely examine the medial meniscus in both the prone and supine position (double-contrast technique), as subtle tears are more easily detected (416). If indicated, the lateral meniscus may be similarly studied. Following fluoroscopic filming, overhead films are obtained in the AP and lateral projections. A stress lateral should be obtained for evaluation of the anterior cruciate ligament (Fig. 7-66) (317,332,333,356,408, 414,417). Notch views and patellar views may also be indicated. If indicated (Table 7-6), CT or tomography may be required for complete evaluation.

We do not routinely reaspirate the joint following the procedure. If significant discomfort is present, reaspiration may be useful. Patient activity following the examination may be restricted for 24 hours (348). However, in most cases normal activity is allowed.

Normal Arthrographic Anatomy

The anatomy of the knee has been described earlier in this chapter. Certain points bear repeating in describing

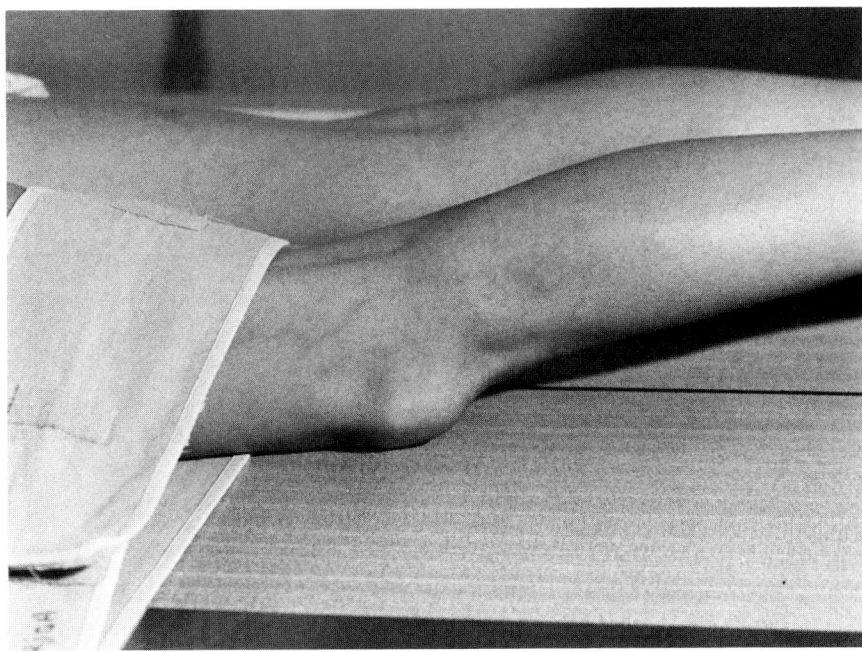

FIG. 7-65. Patient positioned for examination of the medial meniscus. Adjustable strap allows the knee to be easily stressed.

the normal arthrographic anatomy. The normal medial meniscus is C-shaped (Fig. 7-67C). The transverse length is greater posteriorly (average 14 mm) than anteriorly (average 6 mm) (404). The meniscus is firmly attached to the capsule and deep portion of the medial collateral ligament. This reduces mobility and results in an increased incidence of tears compared with the lateral meniscus (309,333). Anteriorly, the medial meniscus is attached to the tibia anterior to the anterior cruciate ligament attachment. Posteriorly the medial meniscus attaches to the tibia midway between the lateral meniscus and the posterior cruciate ligament attachment.

The lateral meniscus is smaller, more circular, and more equal in width (Fig. 7-67C) than the medial meniscus. The anterior two-thirds of the meniscus is attached to the coronary ligament. Posteriorly, the popliteus tendon with its synovial sheath passes through the joint capsule. This results in incomplete attachment of the meniscus posteriorly. In some cases, the popliteus muscle may partially attach to the lateral meniscus posteriorly (355). The lateral wall of the tendon is attached to the joint capsule in most cases. Therefore, contrast medium will not completely surround the tendon (438). The meniscus maintains superior and inferior attachments except

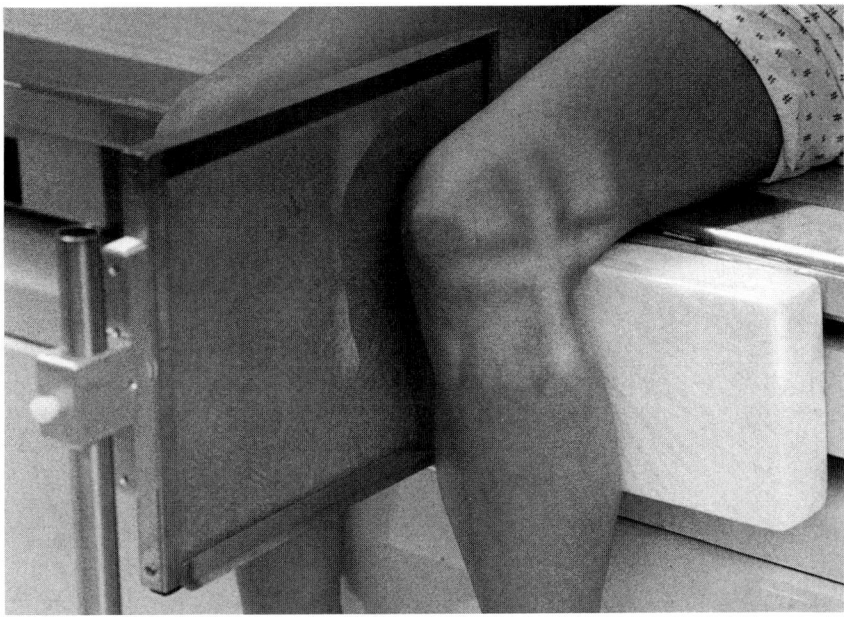

FIG. 7-66. Patient positioned for the stress lateral view. The knee is flexed over the bolster. Cassette position is maintained by the patient. This permits consistency for examination of the cruciate ligaments (334,408).

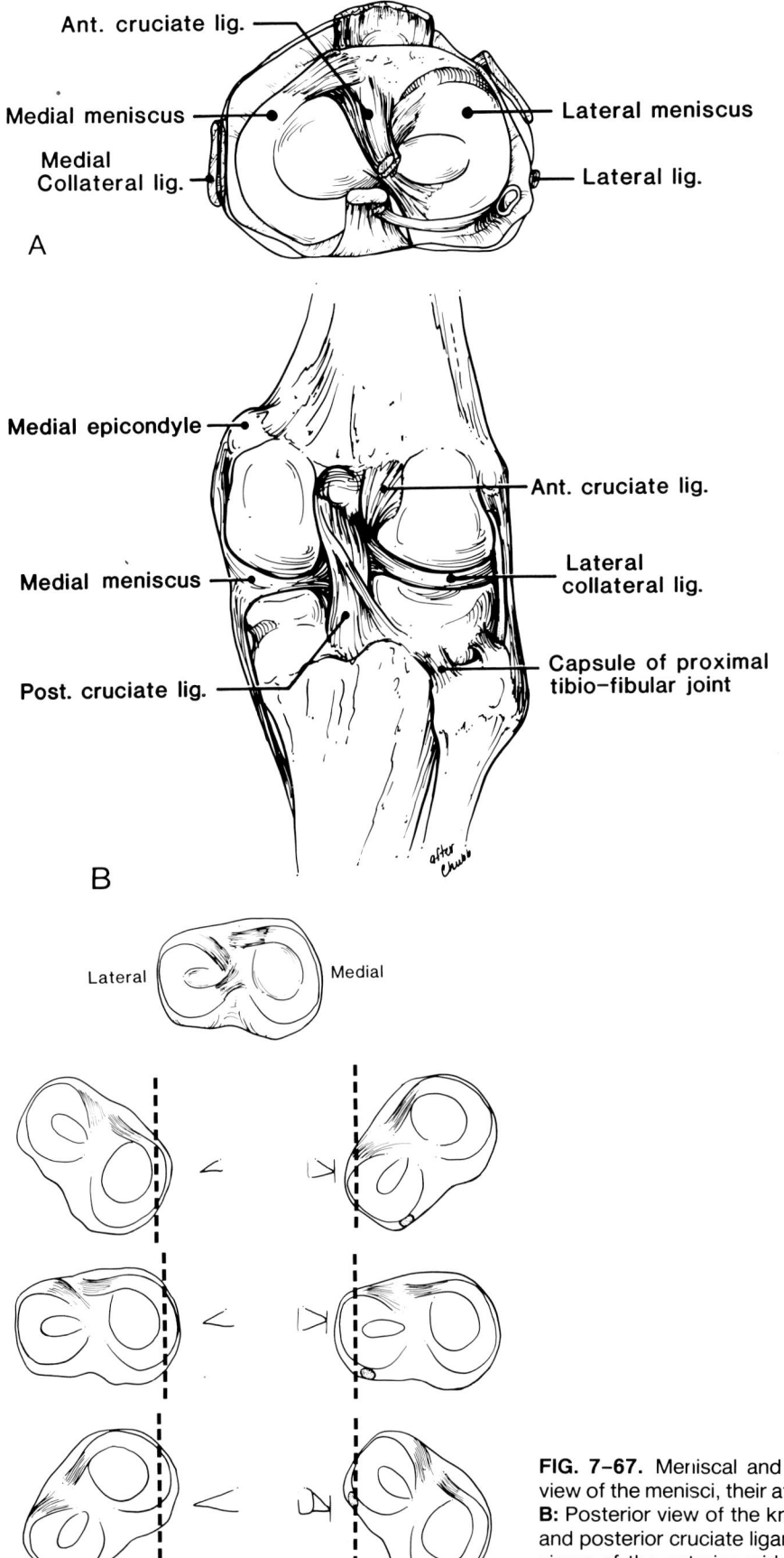

FIG. 7-67. Meniscal and ligament anatomy of the knee. A: Axial
view of the menisci, their attachments and ligamentous relationships.
B: Posterior view of the knee demonstrating the collateral ligaments
and posterior cruciate ligament. C: Illustration of axial and tangential
views of the anterior mid and posterior portions of the medial and
lateral meniscus.

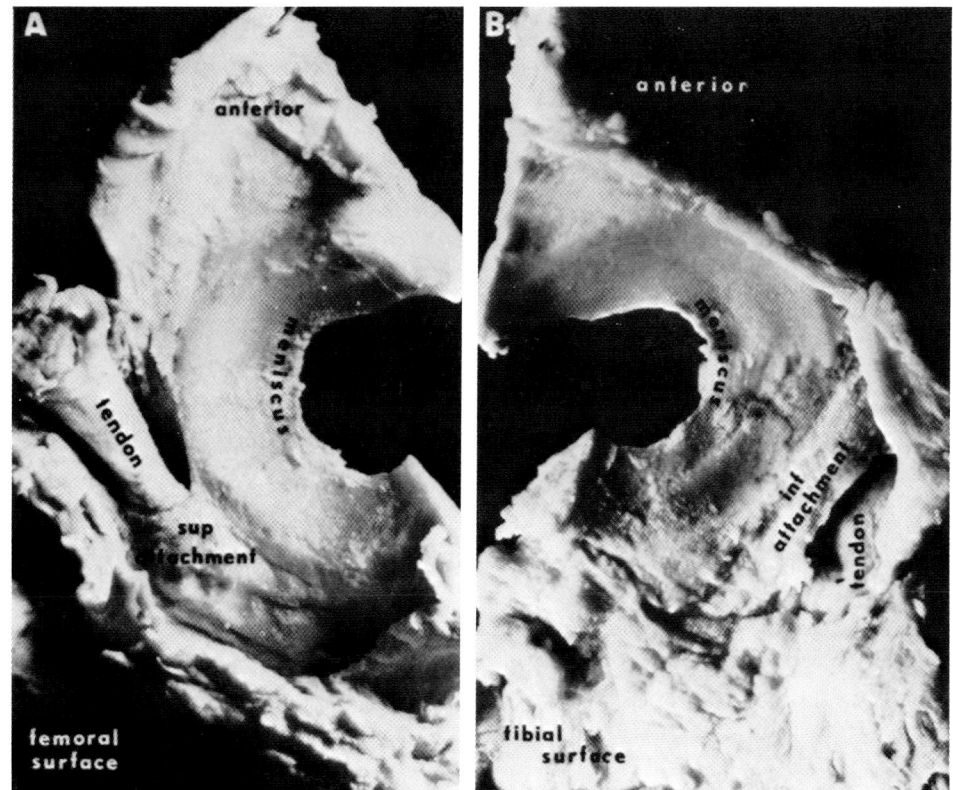

FIG. 7-68. Anatomy of the posterior horn of the lateral meniscus. **A:** Lateral meniscus viewed from the femoral surface. The superior attachment covers the tendon except where it exits the tunnel superiorly. **B:** Tibial surface of the lateral meniscus. The inferior attachment is interrupted where the popliteus tendon enters the tunnel (from 438, with permission.)

where the tendon enters the joint inferiorly and exits superiorly (Fig. 7-68) (437). Failure to visualize these attachments or changes in the normal configuration of the tunnel may be associated with meniscal tears (Fig. 7-69) (333,368,438).

The cruciate ligaments are extrasynovial and intracapsular. They are best demonstrated on the stressed lateral view and notch views (see Figs. 7-70 and 7-71B). The anterior cruciate ligament arises between the anterior horns of the menisci in the anterior intercondylar fossa. The ligament angles superiorly to insert into the medial aspect of the lateral femoral condyle (310). The posterior cruciate ligament attaches to the posterior intercondylar portion of the tibia and courses anteriorly to insert into the lateral aspect of the medial femoral condyle. Brody and colleagues studied the cruciate ligaments in 167 patients (295). The apical angle formed by the cruciate ligaments and the fact that the anterior cruciate inserts into the tibia approximately 8 mm posterior to the anterior tibial margin assist in differentiating the anterior cruciate ligament from the infrapatellar plica. The normal infrapatellar plica inserts more anteriorly than the anterior cruciate ligament. The angle formed with the posterior cruciate ligament was 90° or more in 76% of cases.

The normal apical angle formed by the cruciate ligaments is never greater than 90° (295).

As mentioned above, the deep fibers of the medial collateral ligaments are attached to the capsule and medial meniscus. The superficial fibers arise below the adductor tubercle and insert near the upper tibial metaphysis. The lateral collateral ligament is not associated with the joint capsule in the manner of the medial collateral ligament. Its origin is the lateral femoral condyle, and it inserts into the superior aspect of the fibular head (Figs. 7-67 and 7-72) (301,333).

The articular cartilage on the femoral condyles, tibia, and patella is well demonstrated in the double-contrast technique (Figs. 7-73 and 7-74). The cartilage should be smooth and 2–4 mm thick (309). Subtle changes in the articular cartilage or menisci may be overlooked if too much contrast material is injected.

The joint capsule is large and normally freely communicates with the suprapatellar (quadriceps) bursa (Fig. 7-72B). The gastrocnemio-semimembranous bursa communicates with the joint in 50% of patients. The proximal tibiofibular joint may communicate with the joint capsule in up to 10% of patients. The normal arthrographic views are demonstrated in Figs. 7-73 through 7-75.

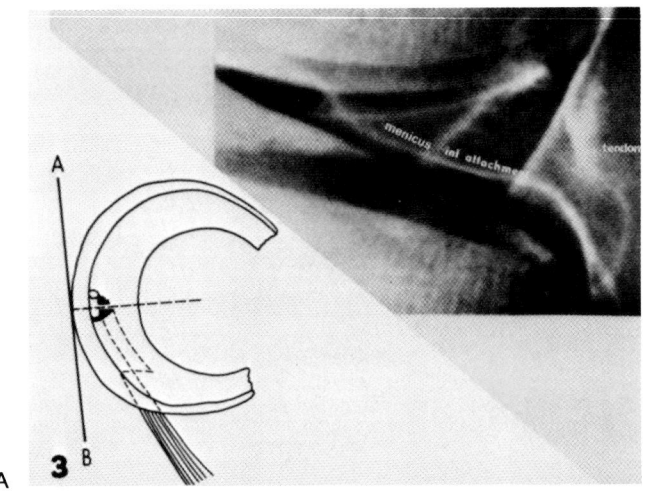

A

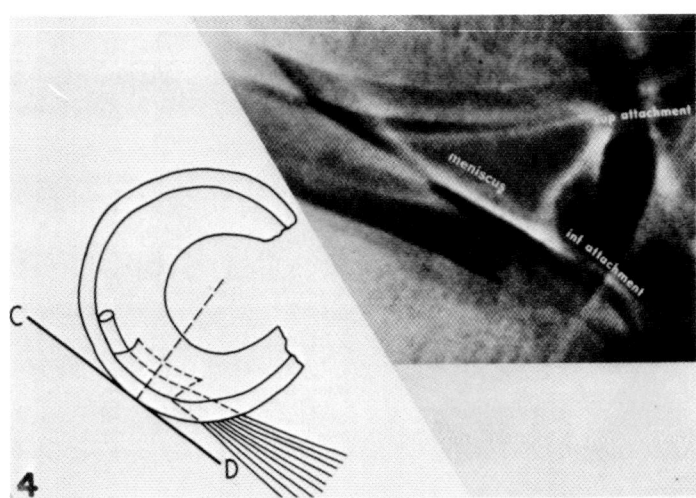

B

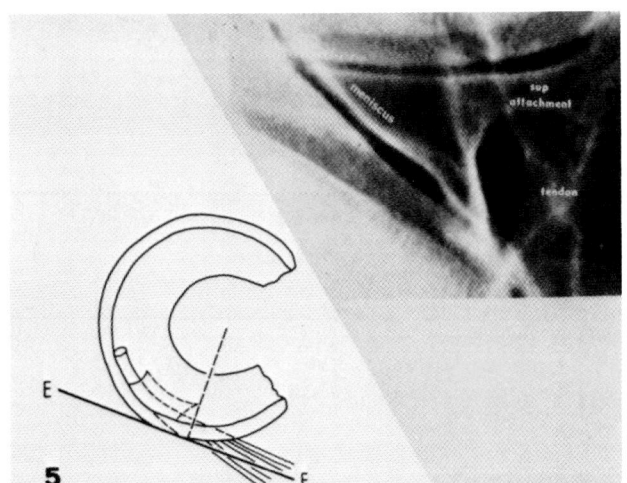

C

FIG. 7-69. Radiographic anatomy of the posterior horn of the lateral meniscus. **A:** Arthrogram with the beam (AB) tangential to the mid portion of the meniscus where the popliteal tendon exits the tunnel. The arthrogram shows the inferior attachment but no superior attachment. **B:** Arthrogram with the beam (CD) tangential to the mid portion of the tunnel. Both the superior and inferior attachments are evident. **C:** Arthrogram with the beam (EF) tangential to the point where the tendon enters the tunnel. The superior attachment is present but the inferior attachment is absent (from 438, with permission.)

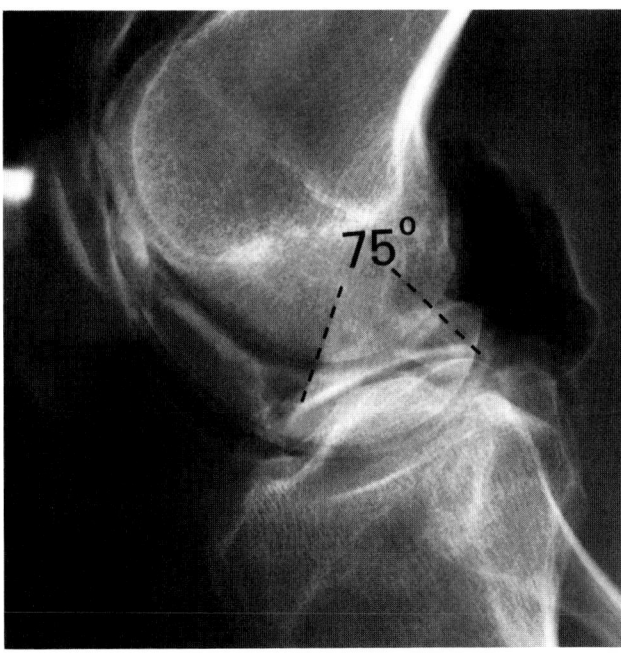

FIG. 7-70. Double contrast lateral view. The angle formed by the anterior and posterior cruciates is 75°. Note the distance from the anterior insertion to the anterior tibial margin.

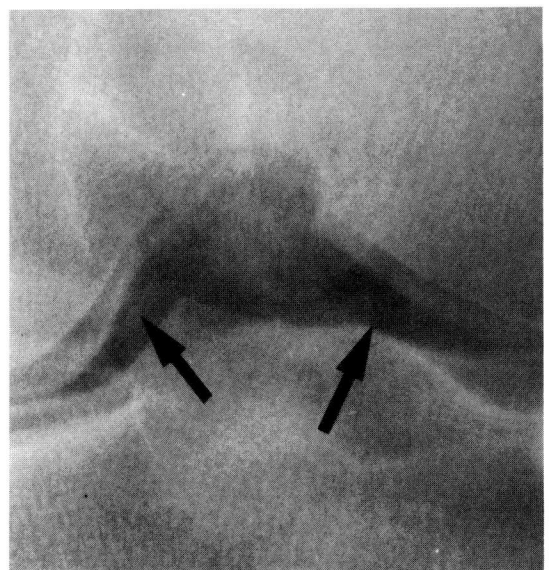 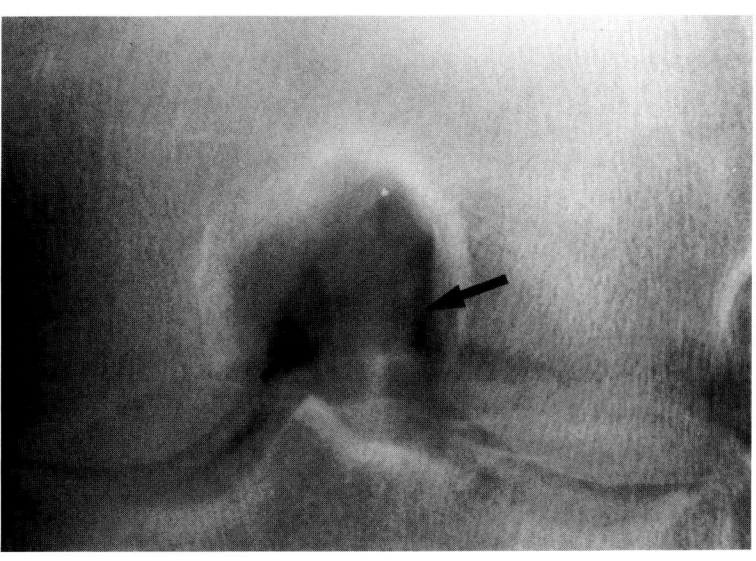

A   B

FIG. 7–71. Notch views taken following double contrast arthrogram. **A:** Normal articular cartilage on the femoral condyles (*arrows*). **B:** Changing the angle slightly results in visualization of the cruciate ligaments (*arrows*).

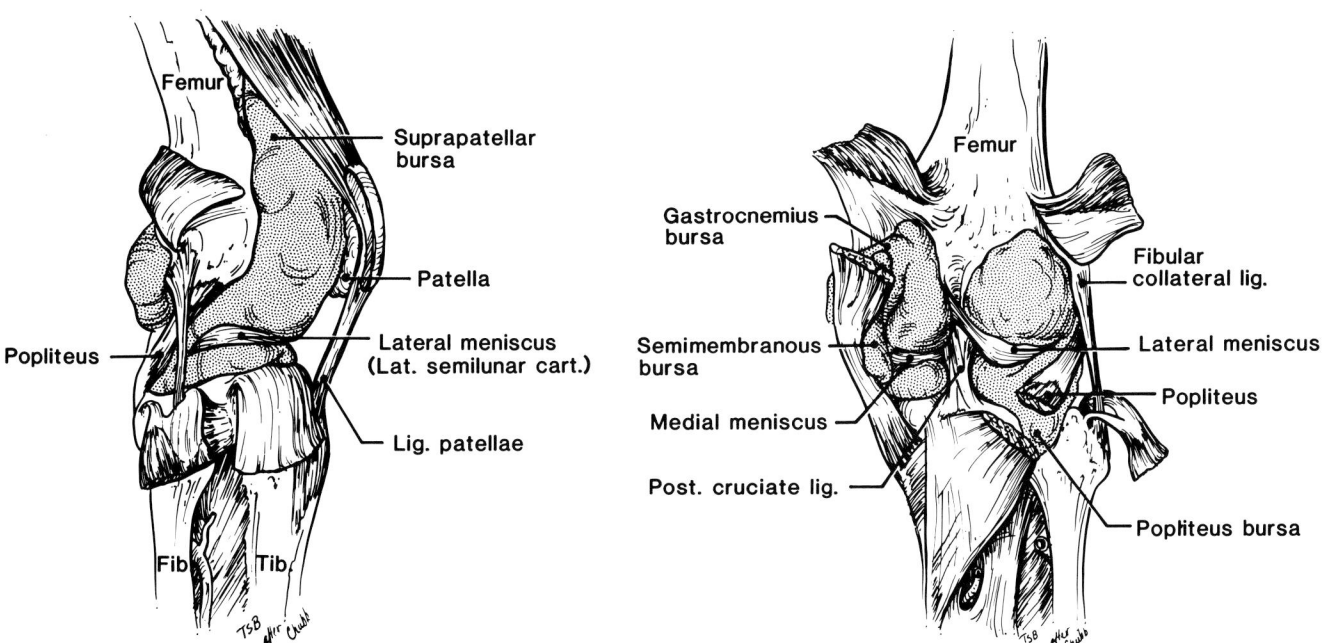

A   B

FIG. 7–72. Illustrations of the distended knee joint. **A:** Lateral view demonstrating the suprapatellar (quadriceps) bursa, posterior recess, and popliteus tendon. **B:** Posterior view demonstrating the semimembranous bursa and popliteus bursa.

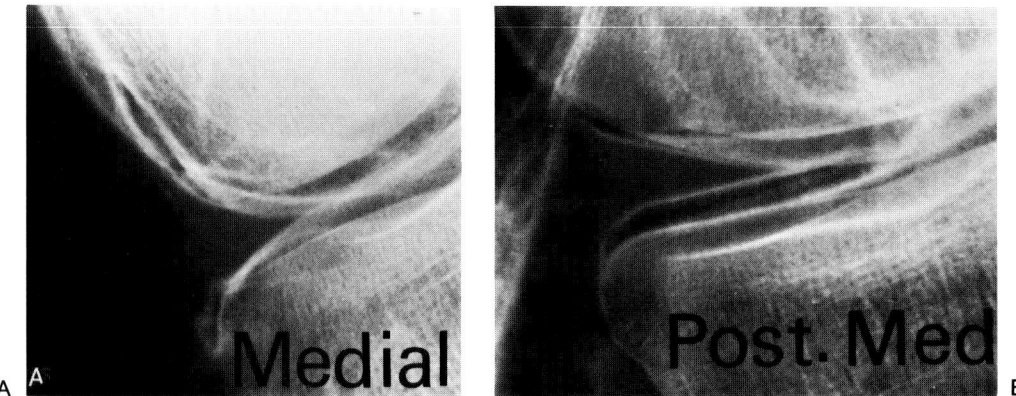

FIG. 7–73. Normal medial meniscus with double contrast technique. **A:** Anterior horn of the medial meniscus. Note the normal inferior recess. **B:** Posterior medial meniscus. Note the size difference between the anterior and posterior horns. There is contrast in the semi-membranous bursa posteriorly but the meniscus is not obscured.

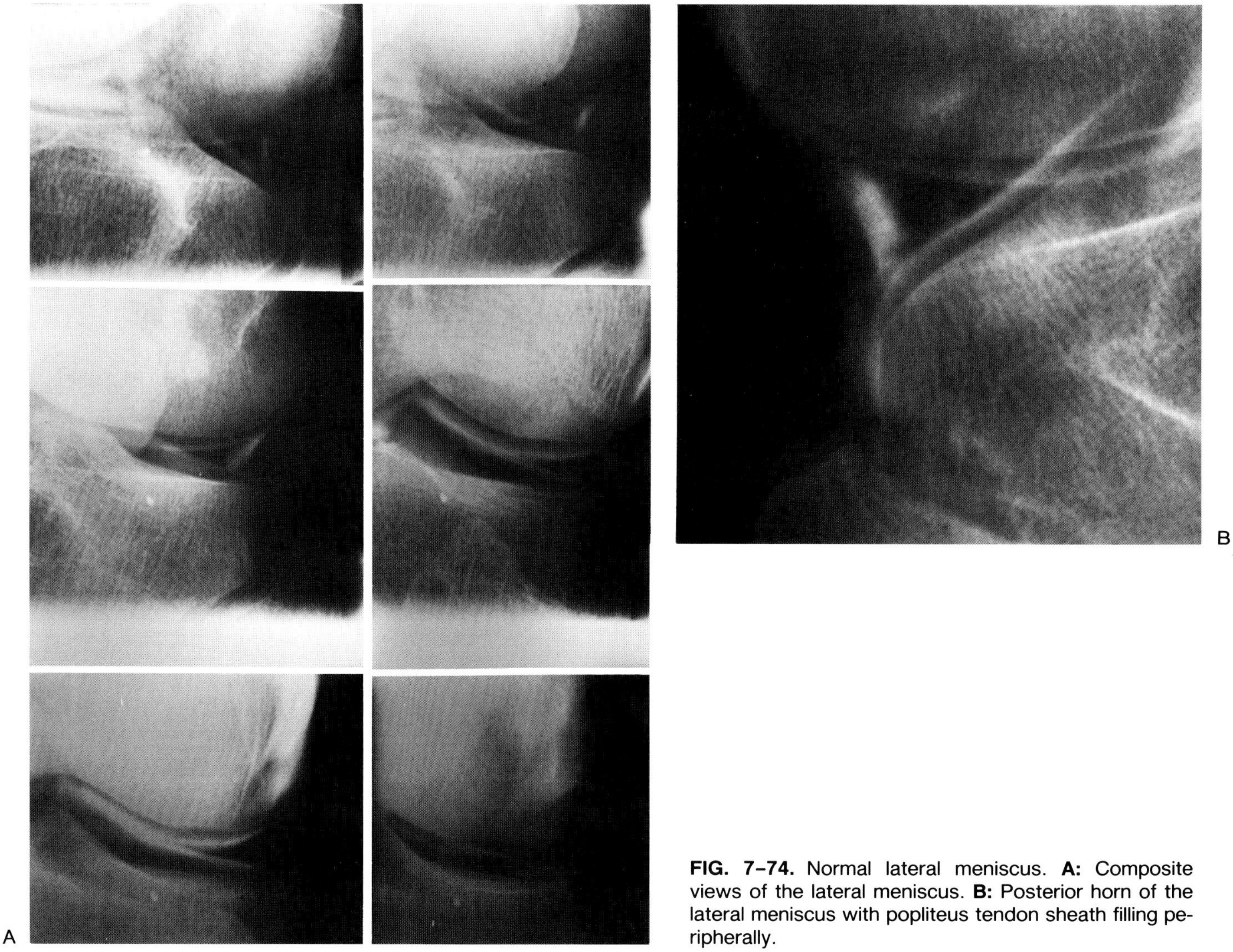

FIG. 7–74. Normal lateral meniscus. **A:** Composite views of the lateral meniscus. **B:** Posterior horn of the lateral meniscus with popliteus tendon sheath filling peripherally.

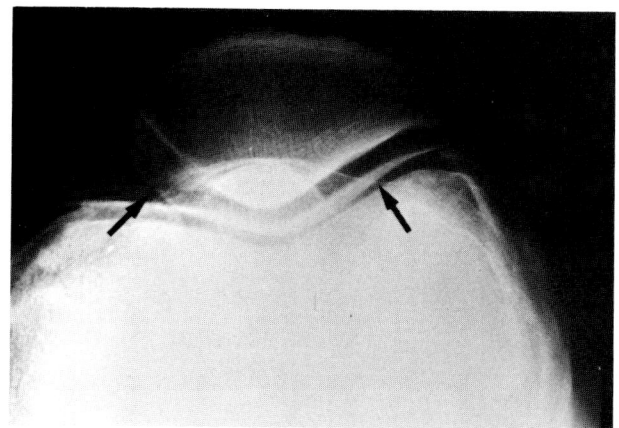

FIG. 7-75. Axial view of the patella following double contrast arthrogram. The articular cartilage on the femoral condyles and patella is clearly demonstrated.

Pitfalls in Knee Arthrography

Most errors in knee arthrography are related to misinterpretation of normal structures or faulty technique. Complications with the technique are rare.

Proper injection technique is critical. Contrast medium should not be injected in the region of the suspected pathology. Extravasation may lead to findings simulating collateral ligament tears or obscure the anatomy of interest. Too much contrast material can obscure subtle changes or pool in the inner condylar region, simulating a loose body (349).

With double-contrast technique, the patient must be exercised slowly to avoid excess air bubble formation.

Air bubbles may simulate chondral bodies. Exercise must be sufficient to coat the menisci. If the undersurface of the menisci is not thoroughly coated, the area should be reexamined. Freiberger noted lack of inferior coating in association with meniscal tears (333).

Errors in positioning are common if one is not an experienced arthrographer. Tangential positioning of the menisci may be difficult, especially in the case of the lateral meniscus. Also, improper distraction of the joint may cause buckling of the meniscus or anatomic distortion, mimicking a tear (Fig. 7-76) (346). An overlying semimembranous bursa may obscure the midportion of the medial meniscus, making evaluation more difficult (Fig. 7-77).

Normal anatomy may also be confused with pathology. The anterior portions of the menisci lose their normal triangular configuration near the insertion. If films are taken in this position, the meniscus may appear torn (Fig. 7-78). Synovial folds and fat may also be superimposed on the anterior menisci, mimicking tears (349).

Meniscal recesses are common inferiorly in the anterior lateral meniscus and superiorly in the posterior medial meniscus (350). Recesses in other locations most likely represent partial peripheral tears (Fig. 7-79) (349,350). These tears may heal with conservative treatment, as reepithelialization can occur peripherally (350).

Errors in interpretation due to the above problems or misinterpretation are not uncommon. Watt found a 50% reporting error rate in patients in whom the arthrographic and surgical findings did not correlate (435). For example, oblique bucket-handle tears may look normal if the central fragment is totally detached (347).

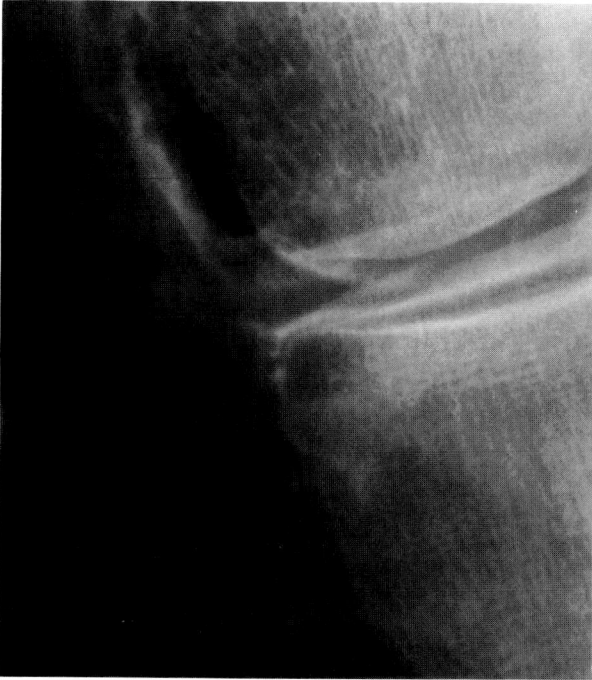
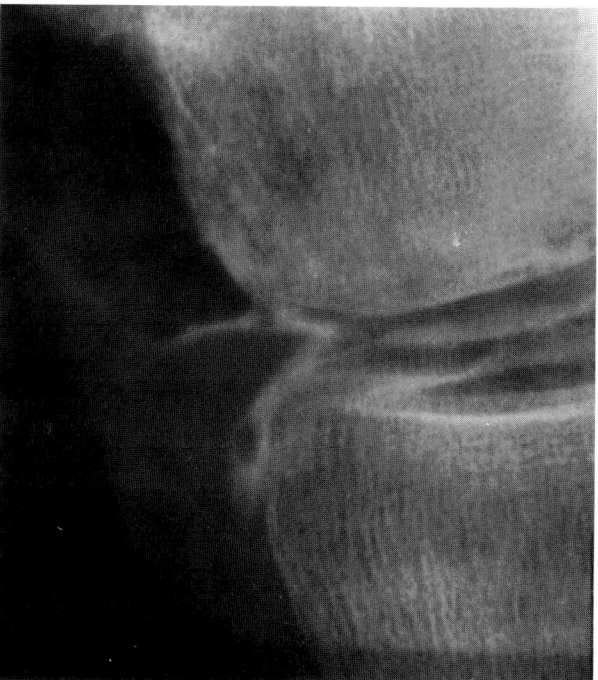

A   B

FIG. 7-76. Anterior horn of the medial meniscus. **A:** Initial view appears abnormal due to insufficient distraction of the joint and improper positioning. **B:** Repositioning demonstrates a normal meniscus.

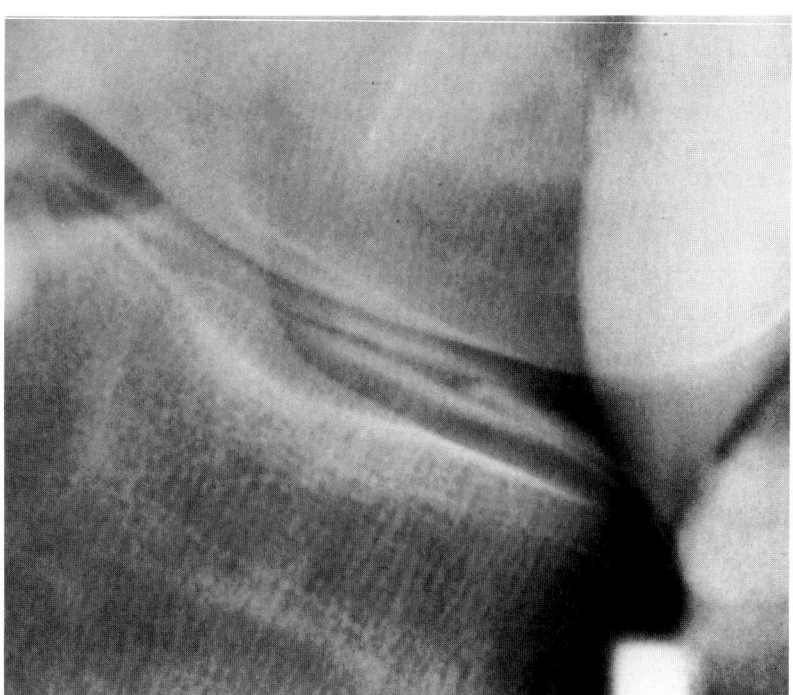

FIG. 7-77. Arthrogram of the mid portion of the medial meniscus. An enlarged semimembranous bursa obscures the peripheral portion of the meniscus.

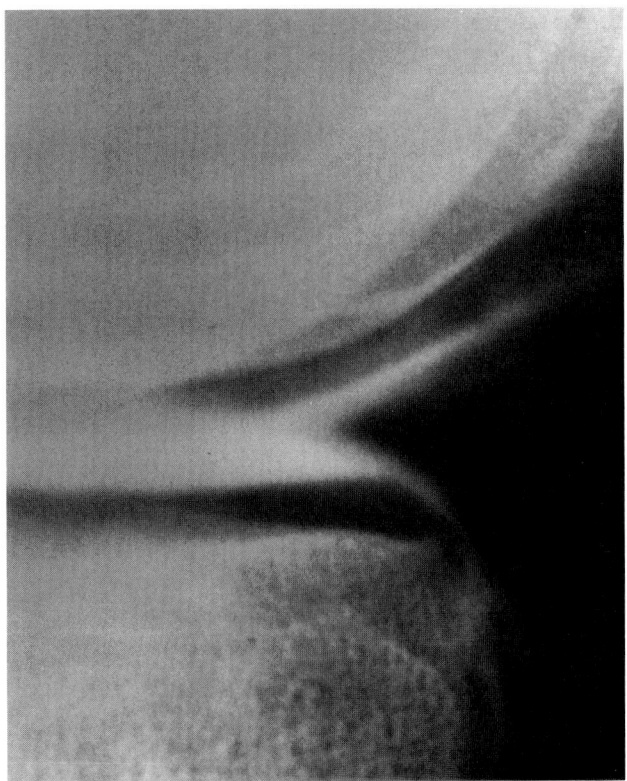

FIG. 7-78. Film taken of the anterior horn of the medial meniscus in an almost lateral position. The inner margin is not sharp. The triangular appearance is lost near the insertion of the meniscus anteriorly. This is not abnormal.

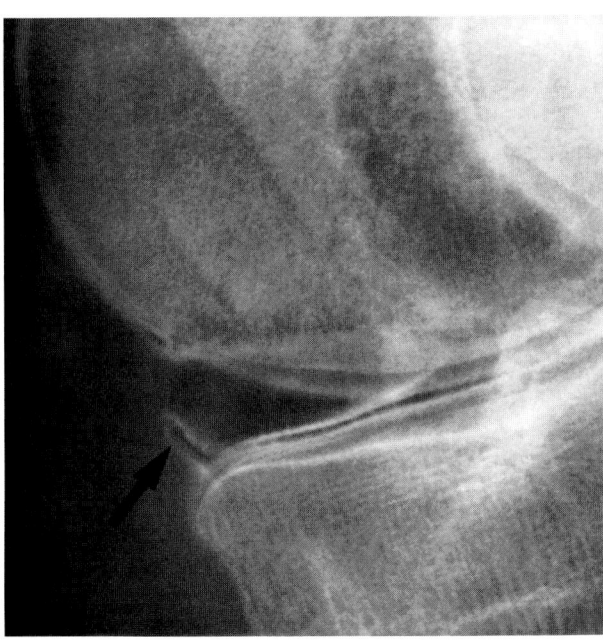

FIG. 7-79. Partial peripheral tear in the posterior medial meniscus. There is a long densely coated cleft in the inferior posterior portion of the medial meniscus due to a partial tear (*arrow*).

Significant complications following knee arthrography, on the other hand, are rare. Contrast medium reactions (usually urticaria) occur in 1–2% of patients (309,333). Occasionally, painful synovitis with effusion may occur within 24 hours of the injection. This occurs in about 1% of patients (286). More rarely this may require removal of the fluid.

Infections are also rare (412). In a combined series of 33,000 cases only 2 infections were reported (309, 333,393).

Air embolism (1 case) and pneumomediastinum (1 case) have been reported following double-contrast technique (309).

MRI Techniques

Techniques utilized for magnetic resonance imaging (MRI) of the knee will vary depending upon the clinical indication and imaging system employed. Although many techniques and image planes can be used, the discussion here will be oriented toward the routine screening examination that can be employed for most articular and periarticular disorders. Specific changes when required will be discussed in the next sections on specific indications.

Typically, the patient is placed in the magnet gantry in the supine position. The knee is usually examined with a closely coupled coil and externally rotated 15°–20° in order to facilitate visualization of the anterior cruciate ligament on sagittal images (Fig. 7-80) (290,291,324, 424,428). In certain cases when motion studies or different knee positions such as the flexed position are required, flat coils or the larger body coil may be necessary (300).

Selection of pulse sequences may be at first confusing, however, typically T1- and T2-weighted spin-echo sequences or gradient-echo sequences are all that are required for examination of the knee. Spin-echo sequences most typically employed are short TR, TE sequences and long TR, multi-echo sequences. The latter are most useful, because the first echo provides intermediate contrast that is excellent for identifying meniscal lesions and anatomy. The second echo provides T2-weighted contrast that is critical for evaluation of the cruciate ligaments and other structures (290,291).

Some institutions examine the knee using sagittal and coronal spin-echo acquisitions. The exact approach depends upon the imaging hardware and software available. We find that using a T2-weighted multi-echo sequence with a TE of 20/60 and a TR of 2000 with one nex, 192 views, and 3-mm slices with 1.5-mm gaps and a 16-cm field of view is optimal. This acquisition requires only 7.3 minutes in each of the two planes.

More recently, we have begun to use the above T2-weighted spin-echo sequence in the sagittal plane with multi-slice gradient-echo acquisitions performed in the radial plane (Fig. 7-81). This interleaved radial (GRIL) technique provides meniscal images similar to those provided by typical arthrographic examinations. This improves the tangential geometry for evaluating menisci. The pulse sequence used for the radial GRIL technique is a TR of 700 and TE of 31 and 12 with a flip angle of 25°. Five-millimeter thick slices are used with 18° of separation (Fig. 7-81) (291).

These long TR and medium TE gradient echos provide excellent contrast for delineation of meniscal tears and ligament injuries. Long TR gradient-echo images seem to have special capabilities for depicting chondral and osteochondral lesions as well.

Newer techniques such as three-dimensional acquisitions and the use of gadolinium have also been explored. To date, these types of examinations are not frequently used on a routine basis, however, they may be of value in selected clinical situations (291).

Pitfalls in MRI

A normal anatomy of the knee has been reviewed previously in this chapter and will not be repeated here. However, it is important to recall certain factors in the evaluation of MR images. The normal appearance of muscle, ligament, tendon, and cartilaginous tissue has been well documented in the literature. The menisci of the knee as well as the ligaments and tendons have low signal intensity on both T1- and T2-weighted pulse sequences. Articular cartilage, because of its increased water content compared to menisci, has a somewhat gray appearance and slightly higher signal intensity than muscle on typical MR pulse sequences. Fat and marrow have high signal intensity and neural structures are slightly lower in intensity than normal muscle.

Most mistakes in the interpretation of MR images are related to improper selection of pulse sequences for the disease process being studied or are due to normal anatomic variants. Figure 7-82A shows axial images of the knee in a patient being evaluated for synovial disease. The T1-weighted image shows the synovial fluid to be low in signal intensity, which obscures the synovitis and articular cartilage compared to the T2-weighted image in Fig. 7-82B.

Normal anatomic variants such as the transverse ligament that lies in the anterior joint space and the ligaments of Humphrey and Wrisberg that accompany the posterior cruciate ligament should not be confused with meniscal or ligament injuries (Fig. 7-83) (291). Other

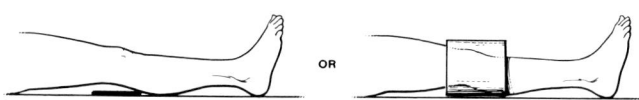

FIG. 7-80. Illustration of a patient positioned for MR examination of the knee (from 291, with permission.)

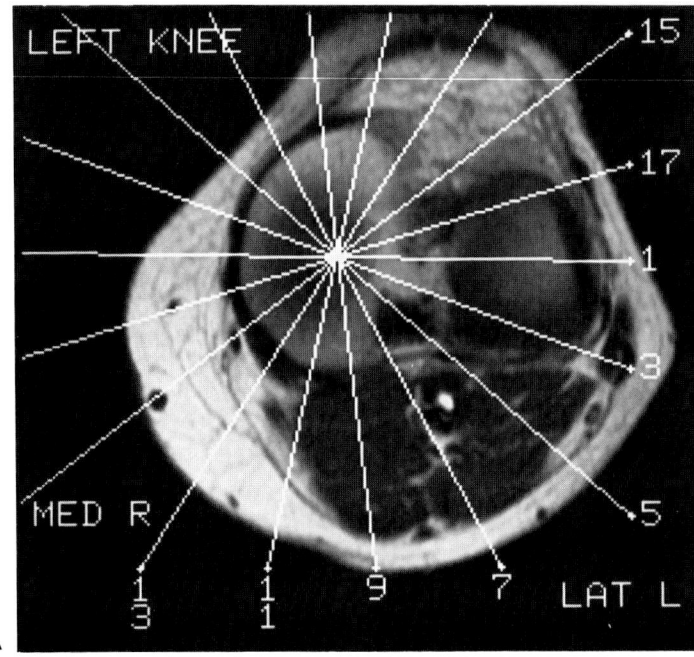

A

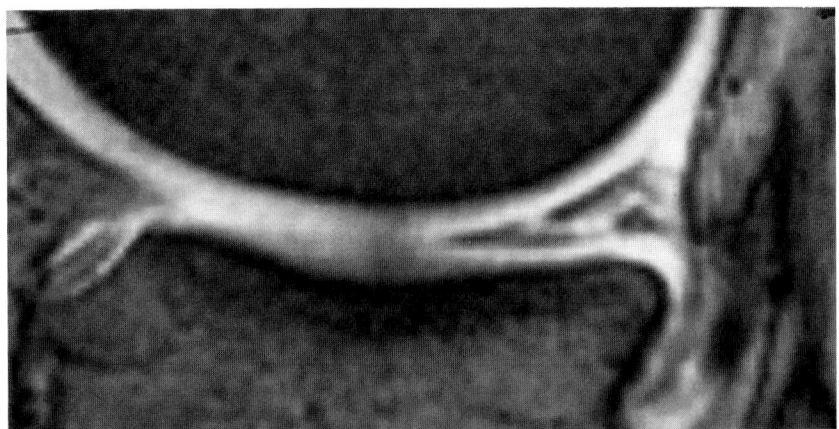

B

FIG. 7–81. A: Axial scout MR image with program for radial GRIL imaging. **B:** GRIL images corresponding to image 13 in **A** demonstrating a posterior medial meniscus tear.

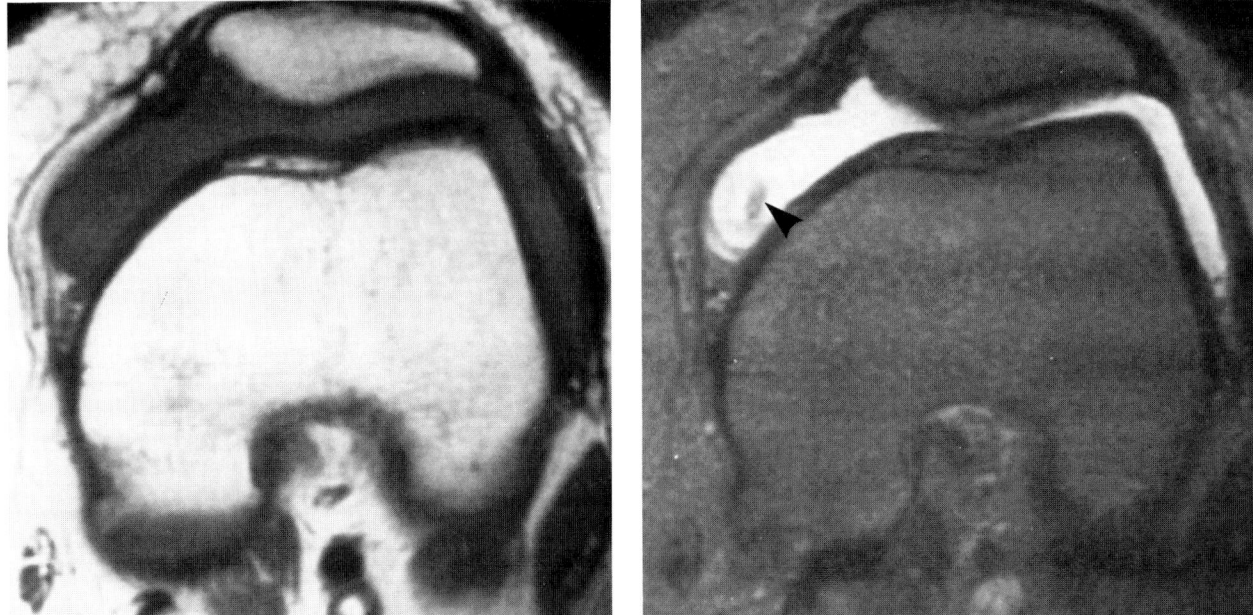

A

B

FIG. 7–82. Axial SE 500/20 (**A**) and SE 2000/60 (**B**) images of the knee in a patient with synovial proliferation. The synovial disease (*arrow*) is visible only on the T2-weighted image (**B**).

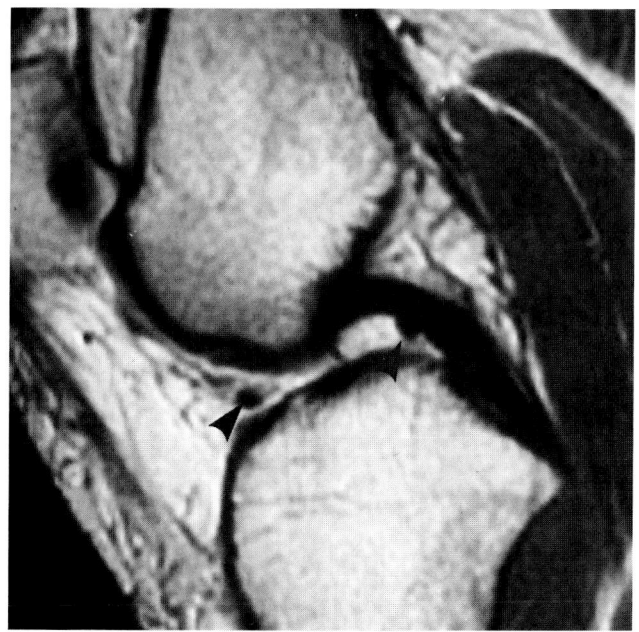

FIG. 7–83. Sagittal SE 2000/60 image of the knee. The transverse ligament (*anterior arrow*) and ligament of Humphrey (*posterior arrow*) should not be confused with meniscal or ligament injury.

anatomic variants and technical changes that may cause confusion will be discussed more specifically later in the sections dealing with specific applications for MRI and arthrography of the knee.

Computed Tomography and Ultrasonography

Both computed tomography (CT) and ultrasonography can be used in certain situations to evaluate articular

and periarticular disorders of the knee (383). Neither of these techniques are used as frequently as MRI or arthrography. Computed tomography in combination with arthrography (see Table 7-6) is more commonly employed but both techniques are used less frequently since the advent of MRI.

CT, when used to evaluate the knee, is accomplished usually with only one leg in the CT gantry. The limb being examined is immobilized with the knee flexed 8°–10°. Two- to five-millimeter-thick slices with 256 × 256 matrix and a 13-cm field of view are commonly employed. Axial examination takes approximately 30–40 minutes. Reconstructions can be performed if necessary (403). Coronal and sagittal reconstructions are particularly useful for examination of the menisci and cruciate ligaments (336,402,403). As noted above, the use of contrast agents and/or air in combination with CT may enhance the accuracy of these studies.

Ultrasonography of the knee is particularly useful for the evaluation of popliteal cysts and the superficial tendon and ligamentous structures, but it is also used to evaluate the articular cartilage (285,330).

Meniscal Abnormalities

Knee arthrography, although often replaced by MRI, is most commonly performed to evaluate the menisci. Tegtmeyer evaluated double- and single-contrast technique in 951 patients and felt that both were equally effective in detecting meniscal tears (432). Double-contrast technique, however, offers better anatomic detail of the menisci, articular cartilage, and cruciate ligaments (432). Therefore a more complete examination is usually obtained. Also, prone and supine films with

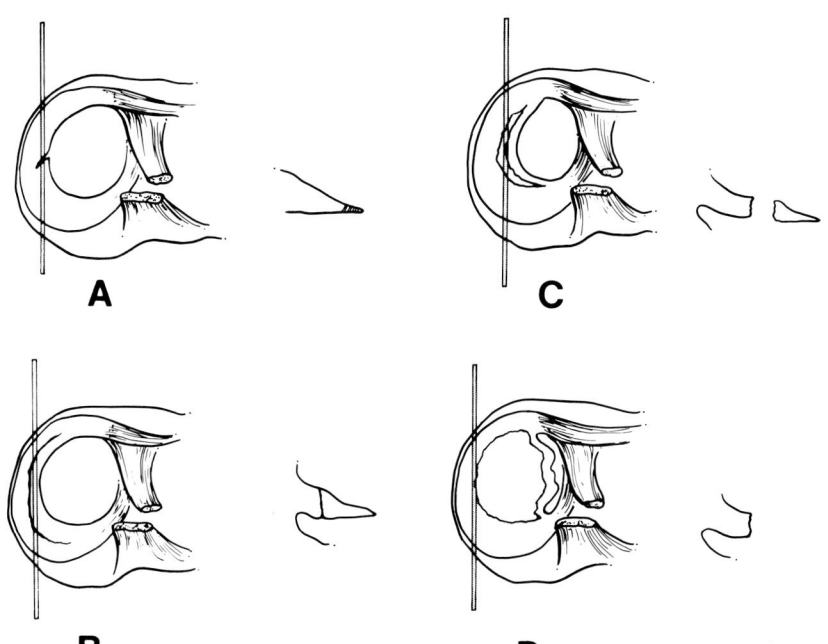

FIG. 7–84. Illustration demonstrating the appearance of the meniscus from above and tangentially as seen by the fluoroscopist. **A:** Radial tear in the body of the meniscus. **B:** Undisplaced vertical tear. **C, D:** Bucket handle tears with varying degrees of separation.

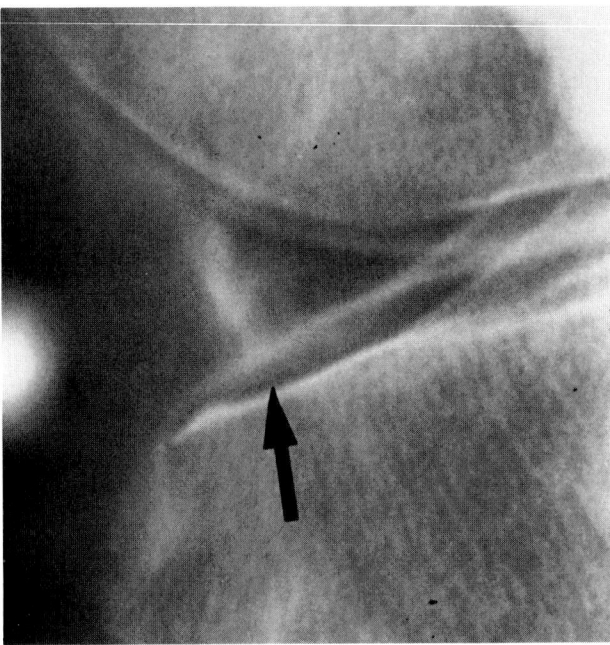

FIG. 7-85. Vertical tear of the meniscus. There is a vertical contrast collection (*arrow*) in the medial meniscus.

double-contrast techniques increase the detection rate of subtle tears (416).

Meniscal Tears

Arthrography is extremely accurate in detecting meniscal tears. Most tears occur medially owing to the lack of mobility of the medial meniscus. Brown reported lateral meniscal tears in 37% of patients and tears in both me-

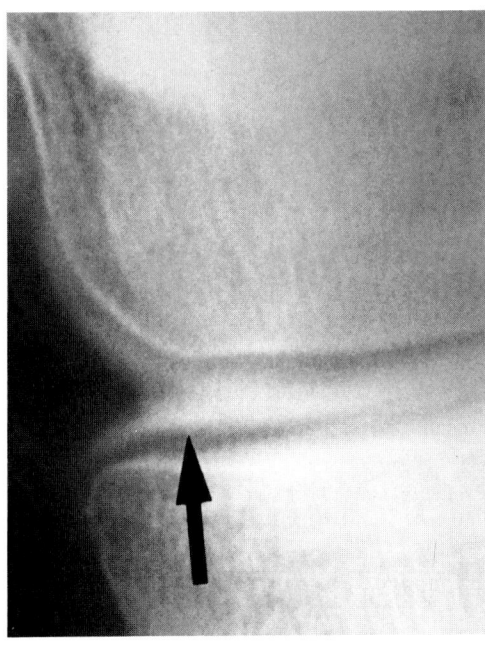

FIG. 7-86. Central (radial) meniscal tear. There is enhanced contrast appearance at the inner apex of the meniscus with loss of the normal triangular configuration.

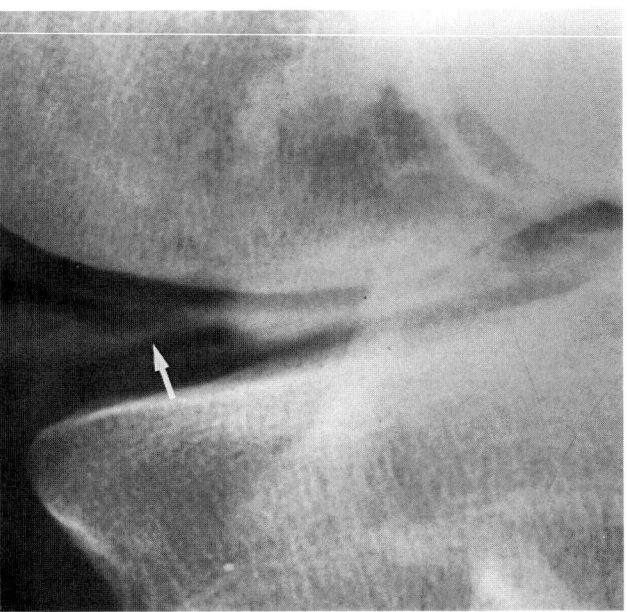

FIG. 7-87. Arthrogram demonstrating a horizontal tear (*white arrow*) in the posterior horn of the medial meniscus.

nisci in 9% of cases (297). Nicholas reported 99.7% accuracy in detection of medial meniscal tears and 93% accuracy for lateral tears using double-contrast technique (393). The accuracy is definitely related to the experience of the examiner.

Arthrography is accurate in defining the location of the tear. This is the most important factor for the orthopedic surgeon. However, exact description of the tear is often difficult arthrographically, although certain descriptive terms are well accepted. Tears are commonly described as vertical, horizontal, radial, complex, and partial or complete. The appearance of the tear depends upon the positioning of the meniscus in the radiographic beam (Fig. 7-84). A vertical tear divides the triangular meniscus into central and peripheral segments (Fig.

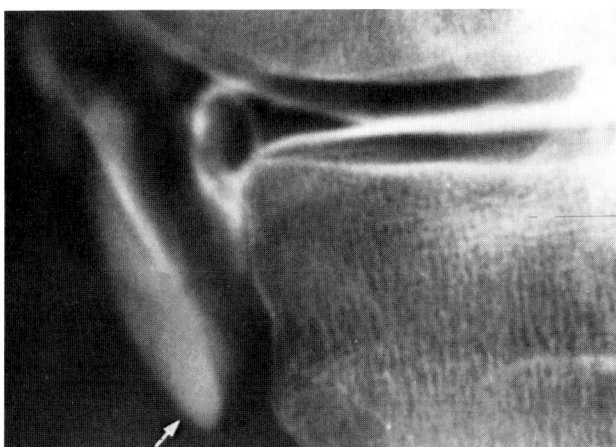

FIG. 7-88. Complex peripheral tear in the medial meniscus. Note the collection of contrast material medially (*arrow*) due to an associated medial collateral ligament tear.

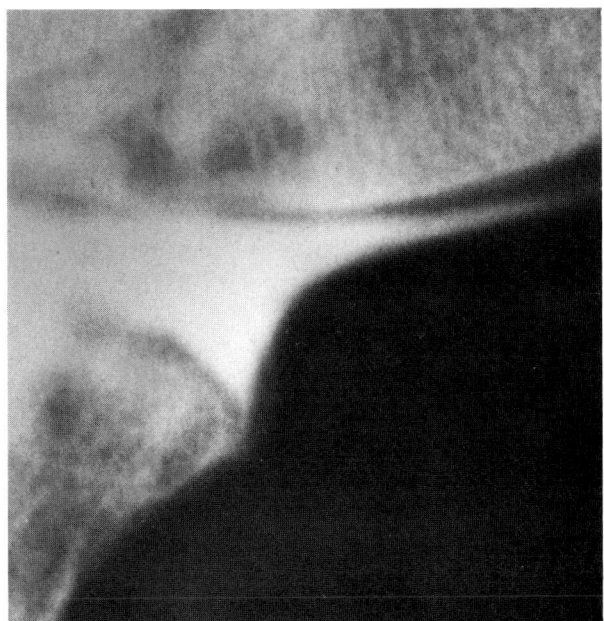
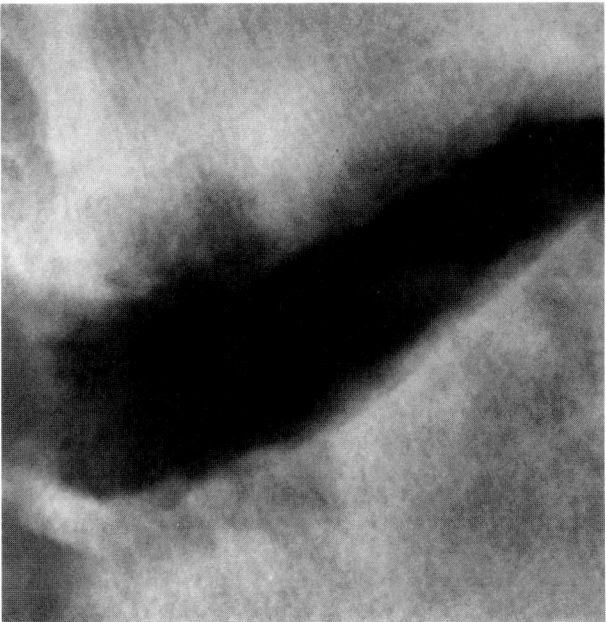

FIG. 7–89. Post meniscectomy arthrograms. **A:** Patient with recent medial meniscectomy and persistent pain. The arthrograms show no remaining meniscus anteriorly. **B:** Later changes may result in extensive cartilage loss, synovitis, and subchondral bony erosion.

7-85). If the anterior and posterior horn remain intact, this tear is termed a bucket-handle tear. With bucket-handle tears, the inner fragment may be displaced into the intercondylar region. Radial tears are vertical tears in the inner margin of the meniscus. Arthrographically, these are often subtle and usually present with an area of contrast density on the inner margin of the meniscus (Fig. 7-86). Horizontal tears begin medially and usually do not extend to the periphery of the meniscus (Fig. 7-87). Peripheral meniscal cysts may be associated with these tears.

Peripheral tears usually originate from the inferior tibial surface (309). These tears may be partial or complete. The outer one-third of the meniscus has a rich blood supply and therefore healing may occur. The medial two-thirds of the meniscus relies on the synovial fluid for nourishment. Complex tears are demonstrated by extensive involvement and multidirection disruption (Fig. 7-88).

Detection of lateral meniscal tears is somewhat more difficult than detection of medial tears. The posterior anatomy (Figs. 7-68 and 7-69) and the slightly increased difficulty in obtaining true tangential positioning is responsible. Subtle changes in the popliteus tendon sheath may be useful. If the normal oval or rectangular shape is not present, a lateral meniscus tear should be suspected (335). Pavlov and Goldman noted changes in the popliteus tendon in 58 patients. In 47 patients, the bursa was narrowed or compressed. Forty-five patients (78%) had torn menisci. Discoid menisci were present in 4 patients (7%). When the popliteus bursa was absent, the lateral meniscus was torn in 64% of cases (405).

Postoperative evaluation of the menisci may be difficult. One cannot be certain if tears are new or represent posterior horn remnants not completely removed at the time of surgery. Degenerative changes in the articular cartilage are common following meniscectomy (Fig. 7-89) (309,313).

Meniscal Tears: MRI Findings

Although MRI has largely replaced arthrography in detection of meniscal tears, the above discussion is useful in that arthrography is still a valuable technique and also the appearance of MR images is similar to that described with arthrography (Fig. 7-90). However, there are several important differences and classifications that are important and bear further discussion.

The appearance of meniscal tears on MR images has been well documented (290,291,307,324,325). Increased signal intensity has been noted within the menisci on T1, T2, and gradient-echo sequences. These changes can be seen with mucoid degeneration as well as meniscal tears. Grading systems for meniscal tears have been described and are useful in improving the accuracy of MR imaging. The most common system with some modifications was initiated by Crues et al. (307). A Grade 1 meniscal lesion is globular in nature and does not communicate with the articular surface (Fig. 7-90B). Grade 2 signal intensity is linear in nature and remains within the substance of the meniscus. We believe that Stage II lesions are precursors for complete tears (307,325,424,428). With Grade 3 tears, there is increased signal intensity within the meniscus that extends

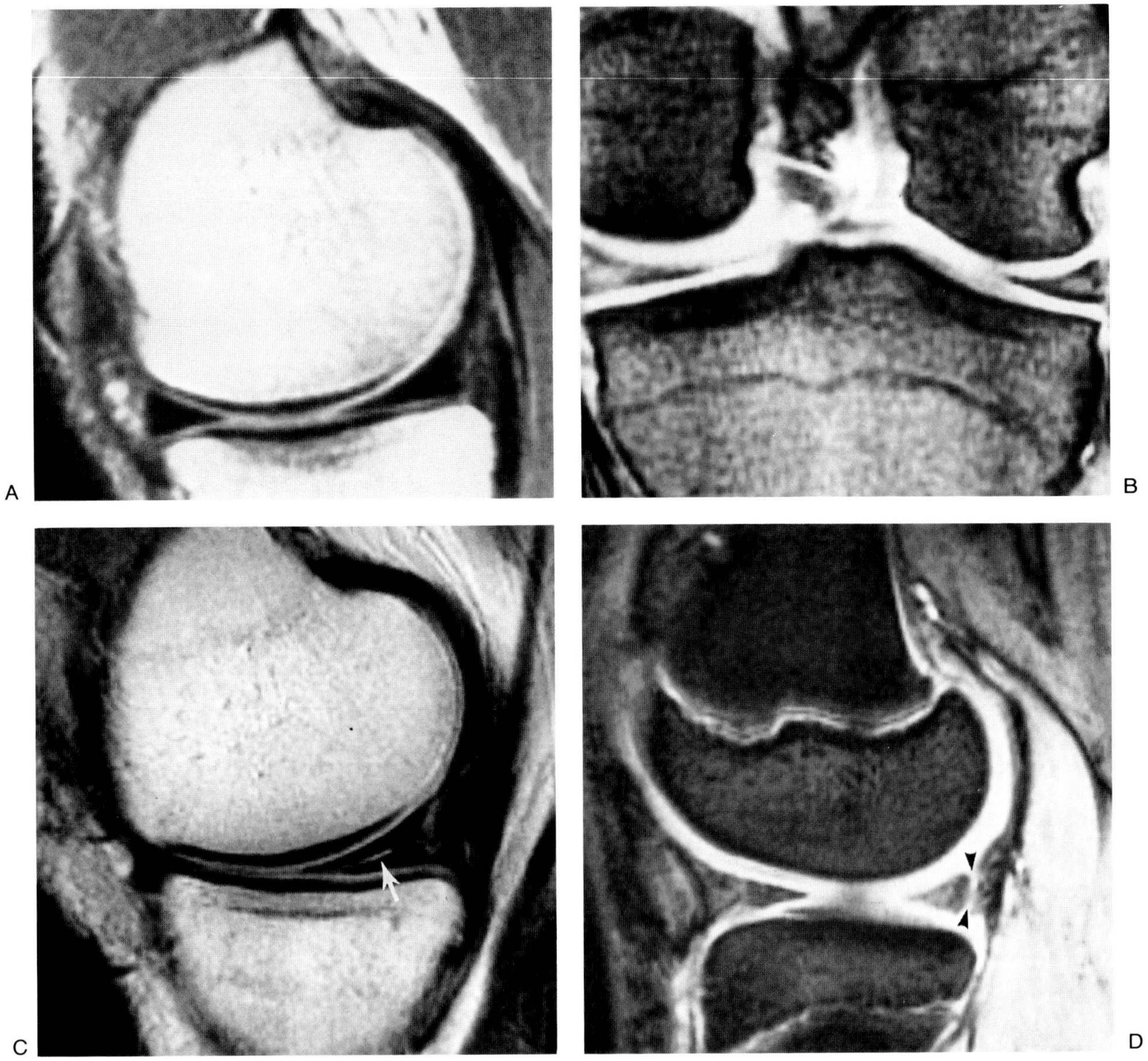

FIG. 7-90. MRI of meniscal tears. **A:** Sagittal SE 500/20 image of a normal medial meniscus. **B:** Coronal GRIL image demonstrates increased signal in the meniscus (Grade 1) that does not communicate with the articular surface. **C:** Sagittal SE 2000/30 image of the medial meniscus demonstrating a horizontal tear (*arrow*) (Grade 3) in the posterior horn. **D:** GRIL sagittal image with high signal in the meniscal recesses (*arrows*) that should not be confused with a tear.

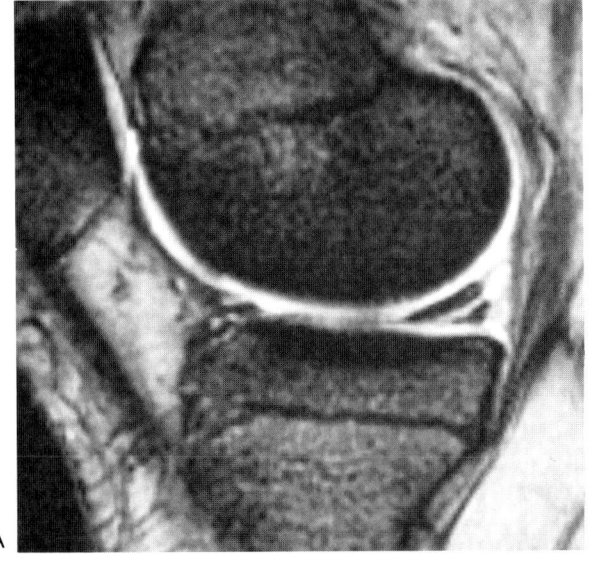

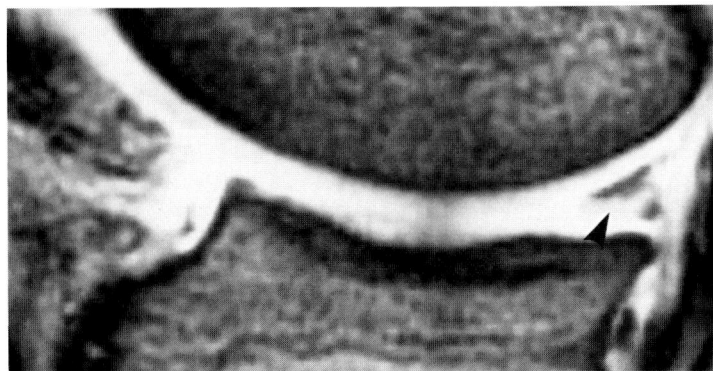

FIG. 7-91. Meniscal tears. **A:** Grade 3A tear that communicates with the inferior articular surface of the posterior horn of the medial meniscus. **B:** Grade 3B tear with marked irregularity (*arrow*) of the inferior meniscal margin.

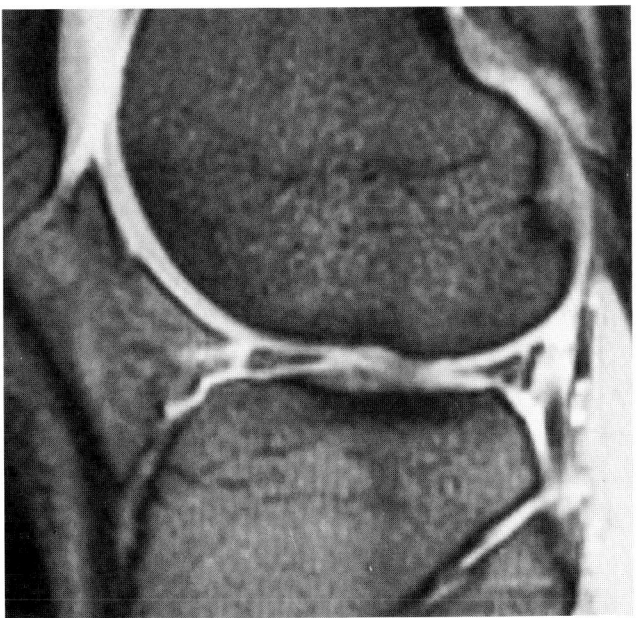

FIG. 7-92. Sagittal GRIL image of a complex tear in the posterior horn of the lateral meniscus.

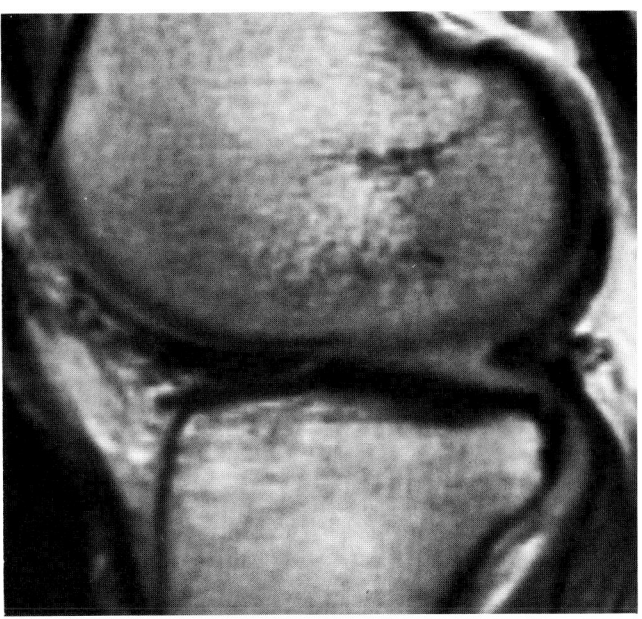

FIG. 7-93. Sagittal MR image demonstrating rounding and hazy irregularity of the posterior medial meniscus due to a radial tear.

to the articular surface (Fig. 7-90C). This can be further subdivided into Grades 3A and 3B. Grade 3A signal intensity is a linear intermeniscal signal that abuts the articular margin. Grade 3B has a more irregular area of signal intensity adjacent to the articular surface. The latter are more often associated with extensive degenerative change in adjacent areas of the meniscus (Fig. 7-91) (291,307). Grade 4 menisci are more distorted and have more complex tears (Fig. 7-92) (291,307).

Other tears such as radial tears (Fig. 7-93) and bucket handle tears (Fig. 7-94) can also be characterized with MRI.

As noted above, the accuracy of arthrography exceeds 90% in detection of meniscal tears. This is especially true when evaluating the medial meniscus. Data with MRI indicate an accuracy of 90–98% for the medial meniscus and 91–94% for the lateral meniscus (291,307). Sensitivity and specificity for the medial meniscus are 99% and 90% respectively and 97% for both sensitivity and specificity of the lateral meniscus in our experience (291).

Discoid Menisci

Discoid menisci are abnormally broad and disk shaped. The lateral meniscus is more commonly involved than the medial meniscus. Because of their configuration, the meniscus extends further between the femoral condyle and tibial plateau and is more susceptible to tearing (Fig. 7-95) (309,333,345). The etiology is uncertain. Some authors believe this to be a congenital defect; however, the consensus is that the presence of discoid menisci is a developmental defect due to abnormal peripheral attachments (291,309,333,373).

The majority of discoid menisci produce symptoms during childhood. Thus, the condition should be suspected in children with symptoms of internal derangement (333).

Hall detected 27 discoid lateral menisci in reviewing 985 knee arthrograms (incidence 2.7%) (345). The majority (19 of 27, or 70%) were typical disk-shaped menisci. The remaining menisci presented different shapes. Hall

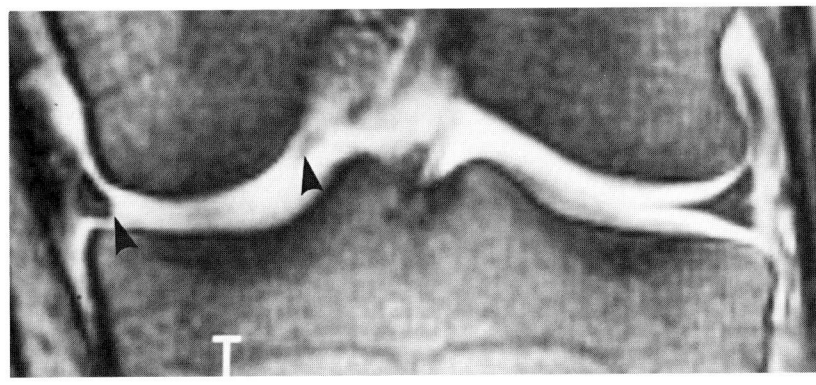

FIG. 7-94. Coronal GRIL image demonstrating a bucket handle tear of the medial meniscus (arrow). The inner remnant is in the mid joint space (arrow).

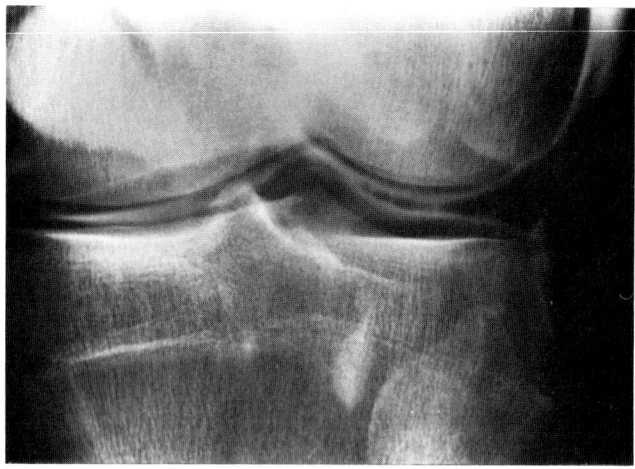

FIG. 7-95. Discoid lateral meniscus with multiple vertical tears.

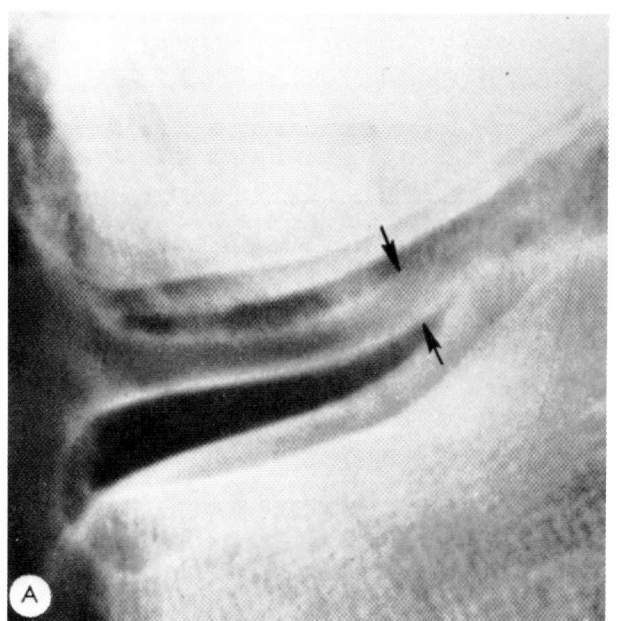

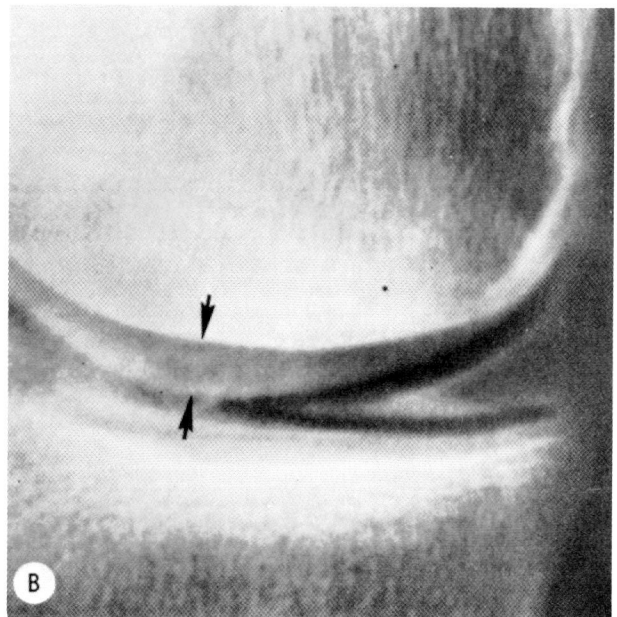

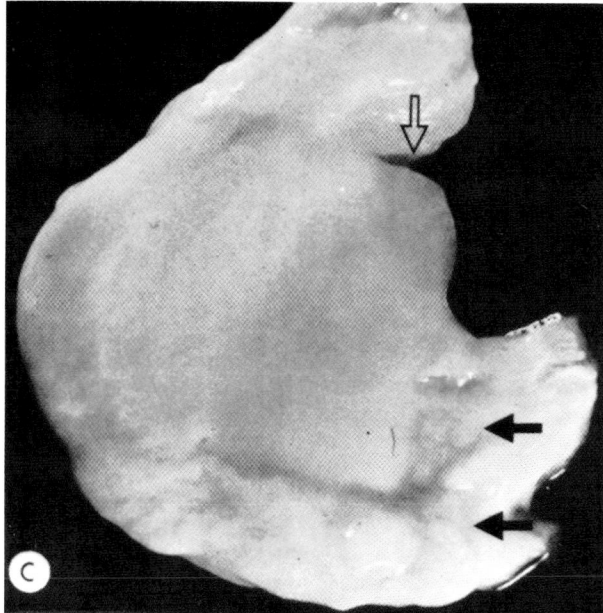

FIG. 7-96. Slab type of discoid lateral menisci. **A:** The meniscus extends farther into the joint space and has fairly uniform width. The medial margins (*arrows*) are often indistinct. **B:** The articular cartilage on the medial femoral condyle is thicker than the lateral condyle (**A**). **C:** Specimen of slab-type meniscus. Surgical markers (*lower arrows*). The tear (*open arrow*) was not detected arthrographically (from 345, with permission.)

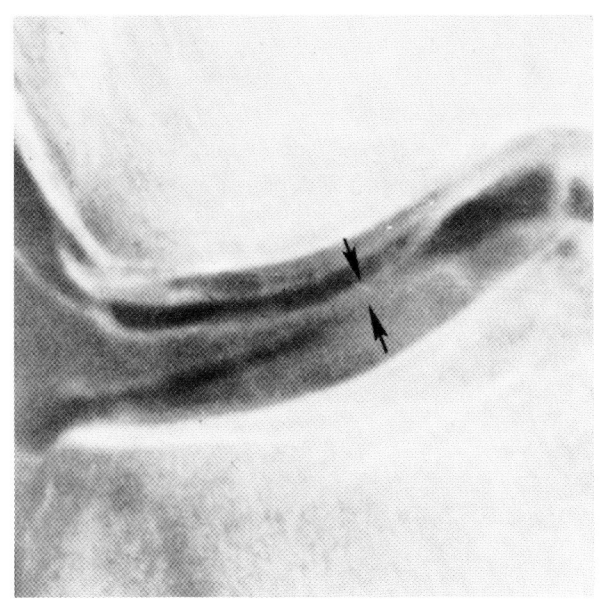

FIG. 7-97. Biconcave type of discoid lateral meniscus with central thickening (*arrows*) (from 345, with permission.)

classified discoid lateral menisci into six types (345). These menisci had the following characteristics:

Type 1, slab type. Thick rounded slab with parallel superior and inferior surfaces (Fig. 7-96).
Type 2, biconcave type. Slab-like with a thin central portion (Fig. 7-97).
Type 3, wedge type. Often smaller than the slab type. Appearance is that of an elongated triangular meniscus.

Type 4, asymmetric. Anterior horn larger than the posterior horn (Fig. 7-98).
Type 5, forme fruste. Between normal and slab-type.
Type 6, grossly torn. Menisci fall into one of the first five types but with extensive tears.

No discoid medial menisci were noted in Hall's series of 985 arthrograms (345).

MRI features are similar to those seen with arthrography. Changes in shape are easily appreciated on coronal and sagittal images (291). There have been no studies to compare the accuracy of arthrography and MRI in detection of discoid menisci.

Degenerative Meniscal Lesions

The menisci are composed of fibrocartilage made up of collagen and noncollagen proteins. With age, the ratio of collagen to noncollagen protein decreases. This occurs more commonly in the medial meniscus, resulting in less degenerative change in the lateral menisci (362). Noble and Hambleim noted degenerative tears in 60% of the menisci in 100 cadavers (394). The average age was 65 years.

The arthrographic findings include fraying, increased contrast coating due to the irregular surface, and partial horizontal tears (Fig. 7-99). Similar features are noted on MR images. T2-weighted images demonstrate irregularity with increased signal in and along the margins of the meniscus (Fig. 7-100).

Ossicles in the menisci have also been reported (292,419). Patients usually present with a painful knee.

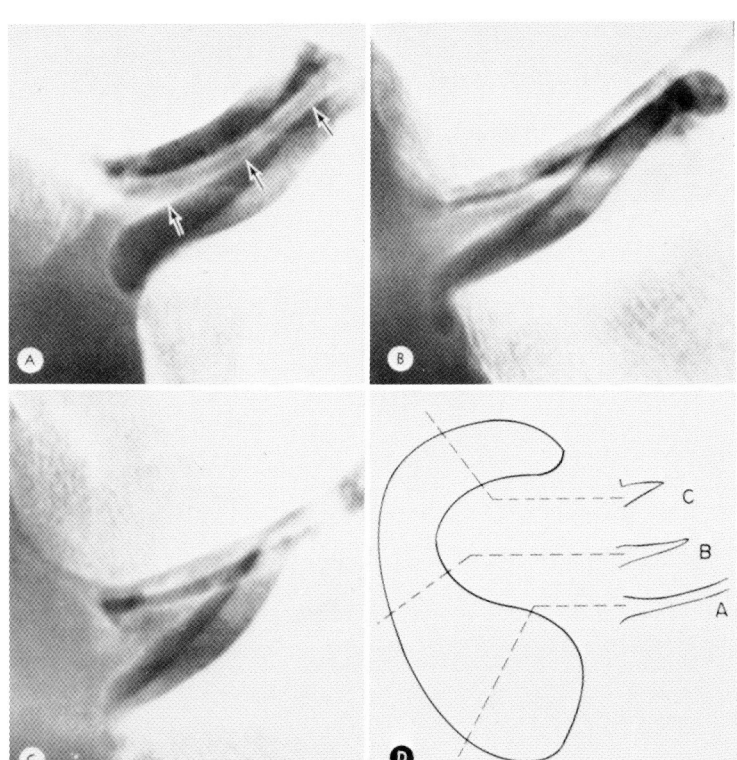

FIG. 7-98. Discoid meniscus with asymmetric anterior horn enlargement. **A:** Enlarged anterior horn (*arrows*) that extends into the joint space. **B:** The mid portion of the meniscus is only minimally elongated. **C:** The posterior horn is more normal appearing except for failure to visualize the popliteal tendon. **D:** Diagram of the meniscus seen from above. Tangential views: anterior, A; mid body, B; and posteriorly, C. (From 345, with permission.)

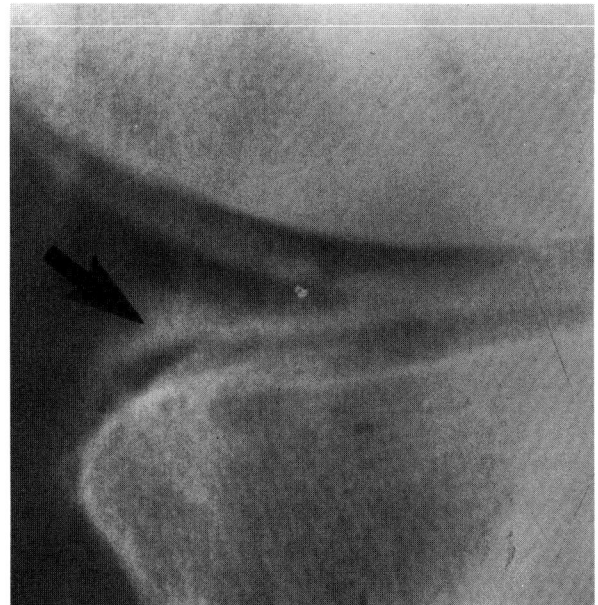
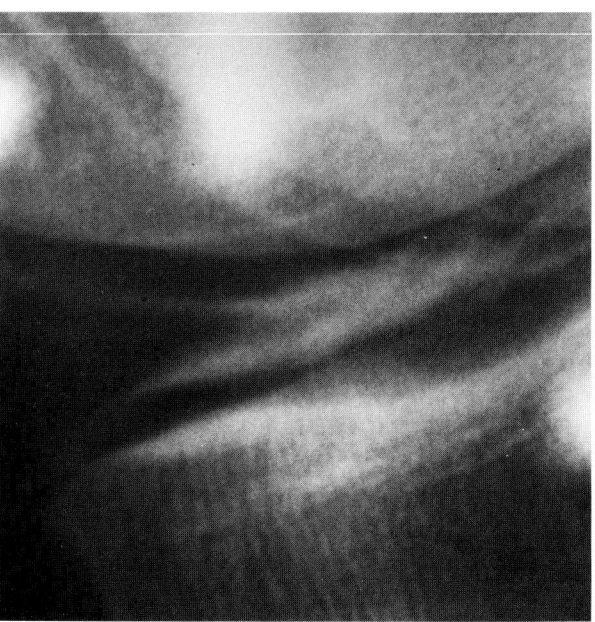

A

B

FIG. 7–99. Degenerative changes in the menisci. **A:** Early degenerative change in the medial meniscus with increased contrast absorption inferiorly (*arrow*). **B:** Enhanced absorption along the central margins of the meniscus with a subtle horizontal tear.

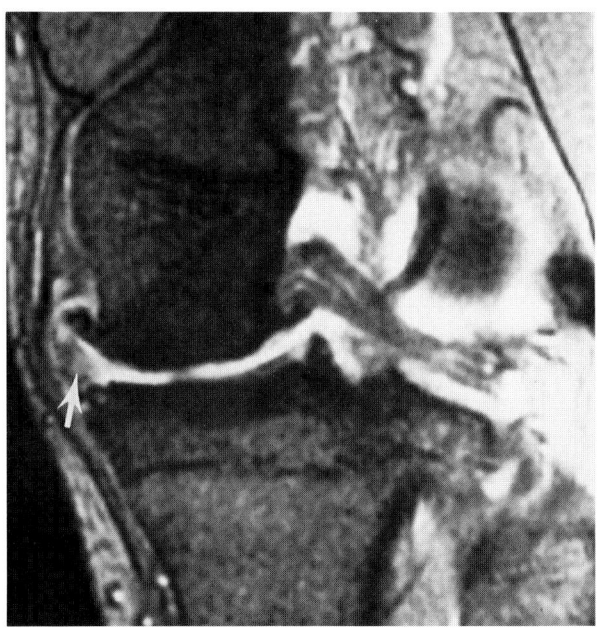

FIG. 7–100. Oblique coronal gradient-echo image of the knee in a patient with osteoarthritis. The margins of the meniscus (*arrow*) are indistinct. Articular cartilage is eroded with joint space narrowing.

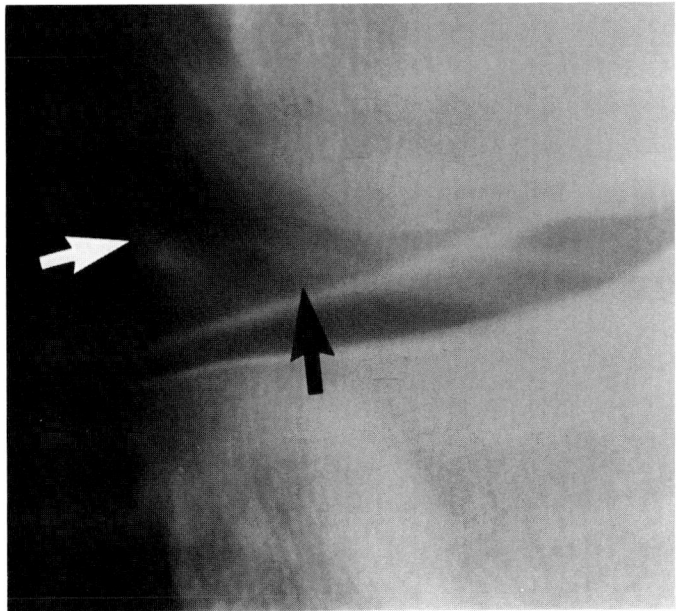
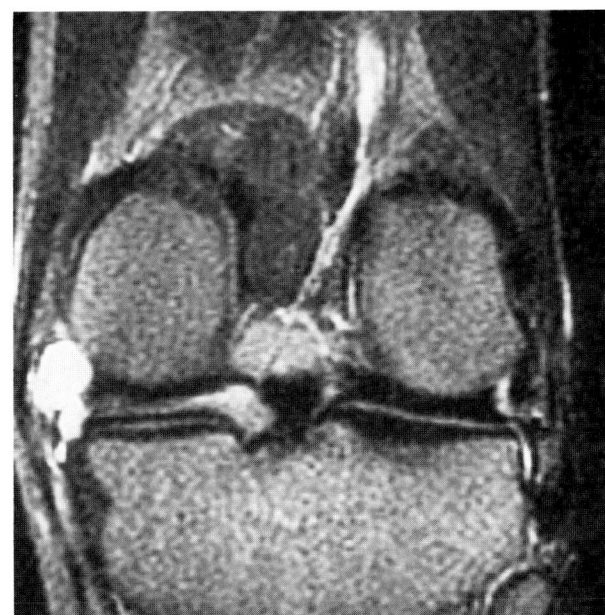

FIG. 7–101. Meniscal cysts: **A:** Arthrogram demonstrates a horizontal tear (*black arrow*) filling a cystic structure peripherally (*white arrow*). **B:** Coronal MR image demonstrating a typical high signal intensity meniscal cyst.

The etiology is unclear but may be due to recurrent trauma or heterotopic bone formation (292). Ossicles can be differentiated from loose bodies by their intrameniscal location. This finding may occur in either meniscus, and an associated tear is often present.

Meniscal cysts have been reported in about 1% of patients (291). Schuldt and Wolfe noted meniscal cysts in 50 of 2,522 arthrograms (419). The lateral meniscus was involved twice as frequently as the medial meniscus. Patients presented with a palpable mass in most cases. In all cases, horizontal tears were present that allowed arthro-

graphic communication with the cyst (Fig. 7-101). Arthrography will not demonstrate the cyst if a communicating tear is not present (333). However, MRI (Fig. 7-101B) can identify both meniscal cysts and ganglia along the joint easily (291).

Ligament Abnormalities

Tears of the anterior cruciate ligament are much more common than posterior cruciate ligament tears (309,333). Associated meniscal tears and collateral ligament tears are common (333). Pavlov reported medial meniscal tears in 63% of anterior cruciate ligament tears (408).

Multiple techniques are available for evaluation of the cruciate ligaments (Table 7-6) (291,342,378,408,409, 427,440). Pavlov utilizes double-contrast technique with a stressed lateral view (see Fig. 7-66) (408). Lateral tomography is also useful in selected cases (286). Dalinka reports 90% accuracy using this technique (311). Computed tomography may also prove useful for evaluating cruciate ligament injuries (403,406,433). However, MRI is probably the most consistent and specific imaging technique (291).

MRI is capable of detecting normal, partially torn and completely torn cruciate ligaments. The posterior cruciate ligament has a nearly straight midline sagittal course and is easily identified on MR images (Fig. 7-102). Tears in the cruciate ligaments are demonstrated as areas of high signal intensity with separation of the normally dark signal intensity ligament. The anterior cruciate ligament is somewhat more difficult to evaluate due to its variable appearance (Fig. 7-103) and its

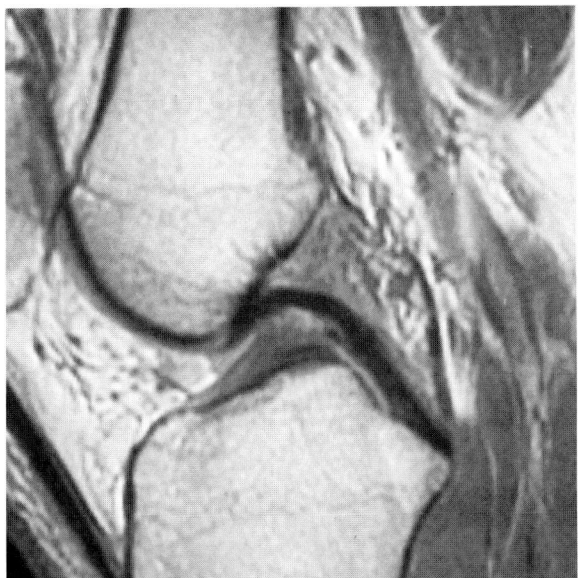

FIG. 7–102. Sagittal MR image demonstrating a normal posterior cruciate ligament.

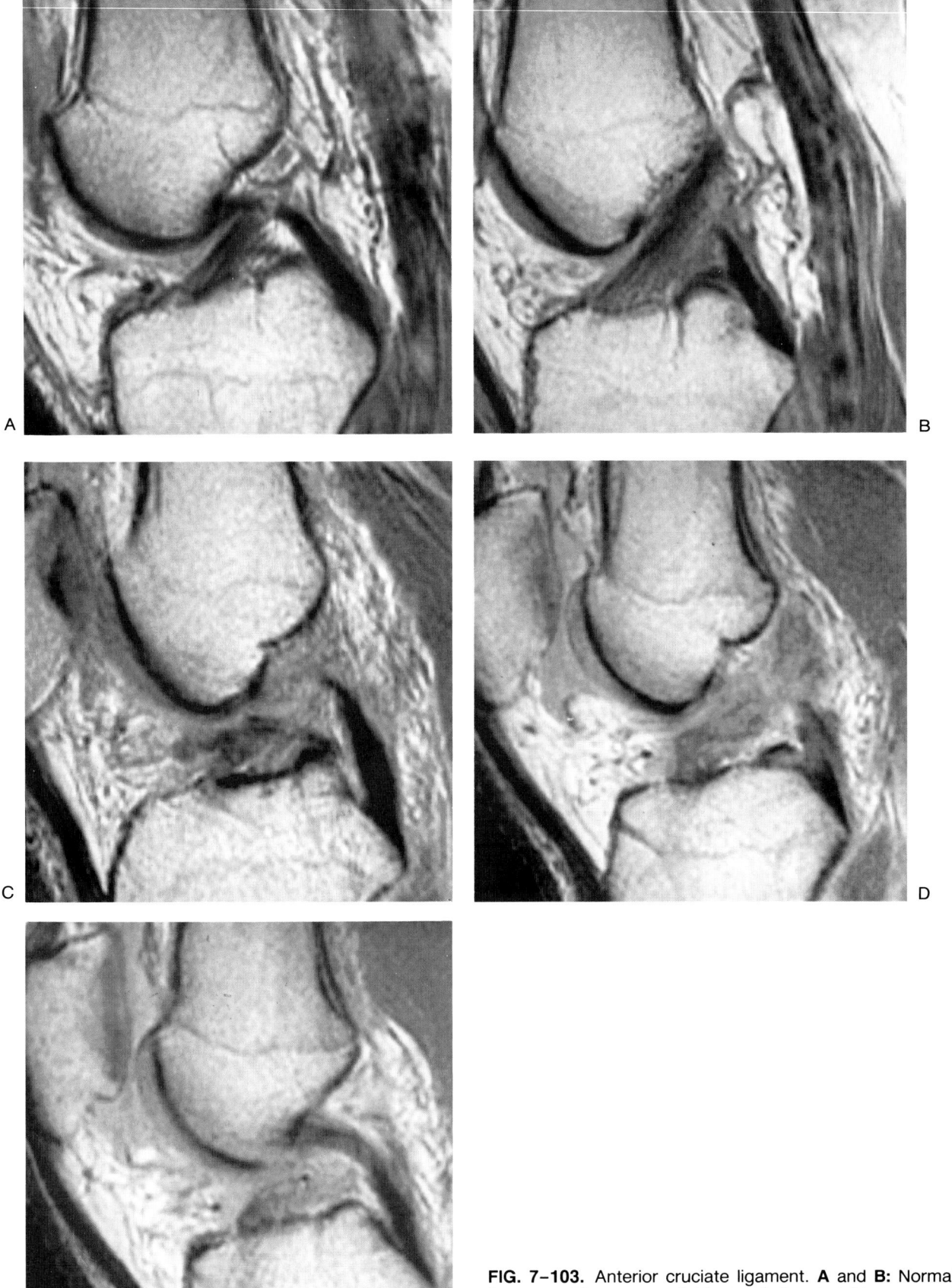

FIG. 7-103. Anterior cruciate ligament. **A** and **B:** Normal cruciate ligaments. The most useful feature is the straight course as the signal intensity varies due to intermixed fatty tissue. Torn anterior cruciate ligaments (**C-E**) show loss of the straight course and signal intensity. Changes are most obvious near the femoral attachments.

TABLE 7-7. *Criteria for anterior cruciate ligament tears*

Acute—Complete
1. Discontinuity with increased signal intensity between segments or at femoral attachment on T2-weighted sequences.
2. Flat or horizontal distal (tibial segment) with high signal intensity near the femoral attachment.
3. Wavy ligament or curved course.
4. Acute angulation of an intact posterior cruciate ligament.

Acute—Incomplete
Areas of increased signal intensity and thickening on T2-weighted sequences.

Chronic
1. Thickening with slight increase in signal intensity that doesn't increase on second echo of T2-weighted (SE 2000/60, 20) sequence.
2. Irregularity and atrophy.

oblique course within the joint. Care must be taken to identify the entire ligament when possible to avoid false-positive examinations because of partial volume effects. Table 7-7 summarizes the MR criteria for diagnosis of anterior cruciate ligament tears.

When arthrography with the stressed lateral view is used, accuracy in detection of cruciate ligament injury approaches 95% (408). Accuracy for CT arthrography approaches 91% for the posterior cruciate ligament but only 50% for the anterior cruciate ligament (291). MRI is more accurate than arthrographic techniques. Our data demonstrated an accuracy of 95%, specificity of 98%, and positive predictive value of 88%. A negative predictive value of 96% was achieved (291).

Imaging is also useful in study of the collateral ligaments (medial and lateral collateral ligaments) about the knee. The deep fibers of the medial collateral ligament

blend with the capsule. Therefore, disruption of this ligament will result in extravasation of contrast medium at the site of the defect on conventional arthrograms. Findings on MR images (Fig. 7-104) are usually more easily appreciated with areas of high signal intensity within the deep and superficial fibers of the medial collateral ligament or complete separation of the ligament. Tears in the medial meniscus and anterior cruciate ligament are often associated.

The lateral collateral ligament cannot be effectively evaluated with arthrography since its fibers do not blend with the capsule. Stress views may demonstrate widening of the lateral joint space (293,333,407). However, again MR imaging appears to be most effective in evaluation of this structure.

Disruption of the quadriceps tendon and patellar ligament cannot be accomplished with arthrography (369). MRI is again more useful in this setting (Fig. 7-105) (291).

Articular Abnormalities

Evaluation of the articular cartilage can be accomplished with double contrast arthrography, CT, MRI, and certain recent articles also indicate ultrasonography may be useful (291,322,392,403,422). Changes in the articular cartilage may be seen with degenerative arthritis and other arthritides, osteochondritis dissecans, chondral fractures, and chondromalacia.

Degenerative changes in the cartilage may be seen with chronic meniscal injury or degenerative arthritis. The articular surface appears irregular and fissured, with increased contrast enhancement due to the increased absorption of contrast medium (Figs. 7-106 and 7-107) (309).

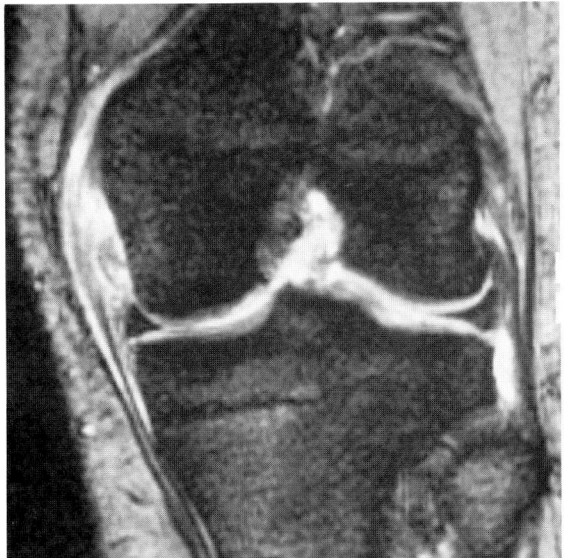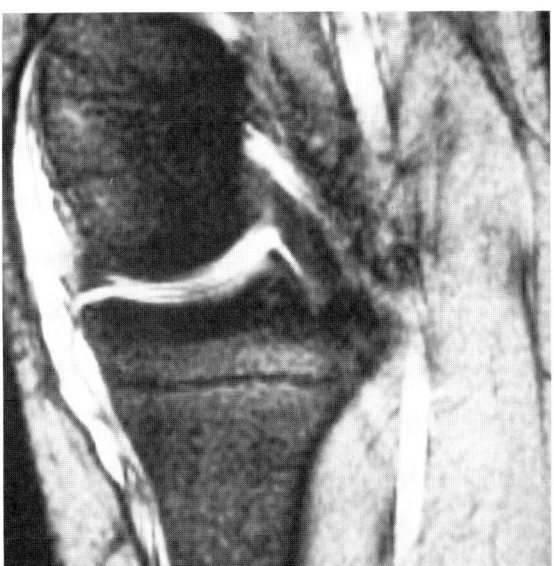

FIG. 7-104. Coronal gradient-echo images demonstrate high signal intensity medially with partial tears **(A)** and complete tears **(B)** in the medial collateral ligament.

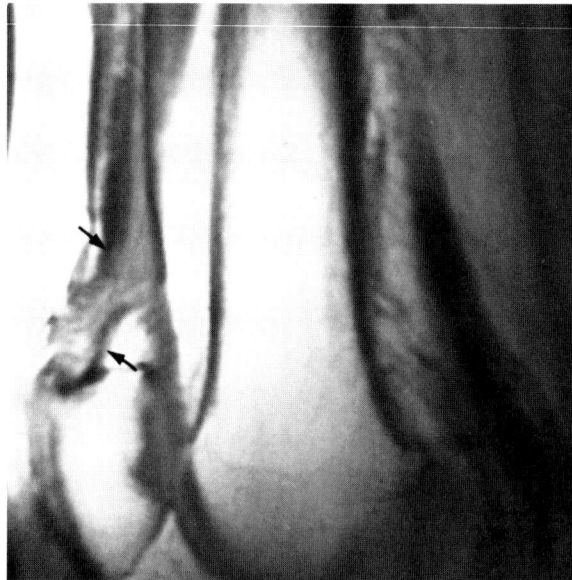

FIG. 7–105. Sagittal SE 500/20 image of the quadriceps tendon demonstrating a tear (*arrows*) just above the patella.

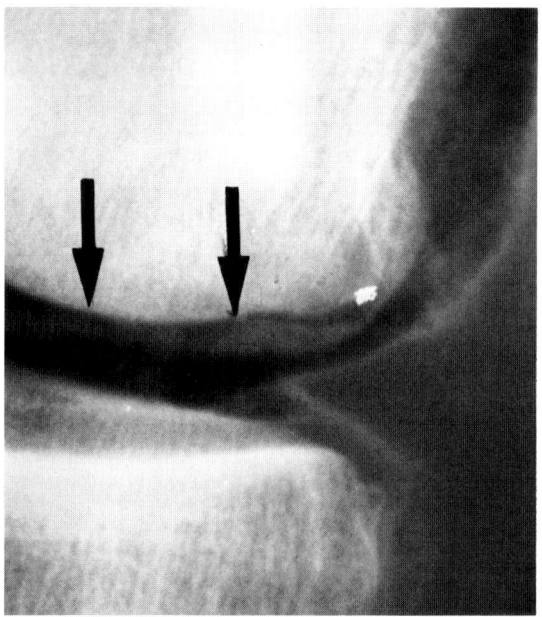

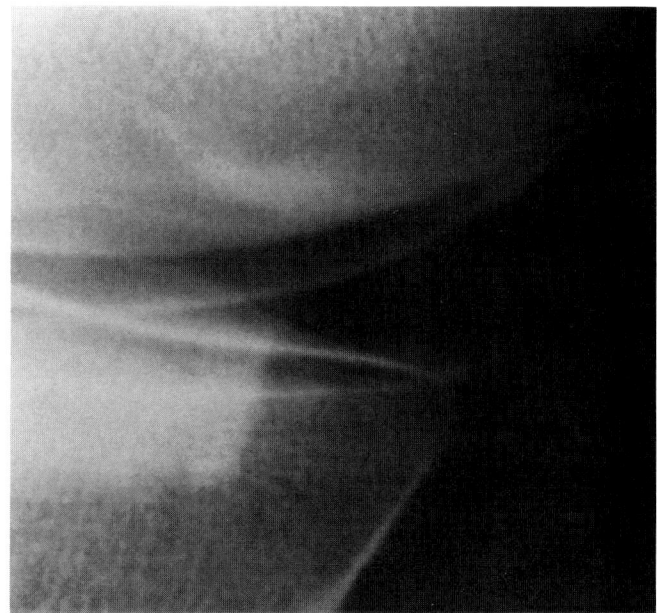

B

FIG. 7–106. Patient with chronic medial compartment pain. **A:** The meniscus is normal. The femoral articular cartilage is thin, irregular, and increased in density. Changes are due to degenerative arthritis. **B:** Normal femoral articular cartilage for comparison. The contrast medium has the normal thin-coated appearance.

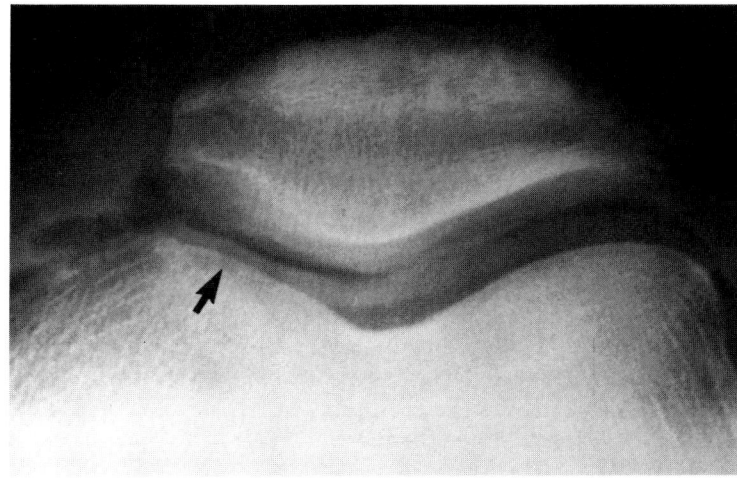

FIG. 7-107. Patient with patellofemoral pain. Axial view of the double contrast arthrogram demonstrates cartilage loss on the medial femoral condyle and patellar facet (*arrow*).

Osteochondritis dissecans is common in young adults. This condition usually involves the lateral surface of the medial femoral condyle. The patella and lateral condyle may also be involved. This condition is thought to occur following acute or chronic trauma (333). Changes may be bilateral and are more common in males (309,333). Arthrography is useful in evaluation of the position of the fragment and the appearance of the articular cartilage. Arthrographic demonstration of intact cartilage over the fragment may lead to conservative management. Similarly, MRI can also demonstrate the same changes. In addition, MRI is capable of detecting abnormalities such as osteochondritis dissecans or osteonecrosis earlier than conventional techniques (Fig. 7-108) (291,322,392).

Chondromalacia of the patella and patellar tracking disorders are common causes of knee pain in young adults. Locking and instability may occasionally be present, causing difficulty in differentiating it from other causes of internal derangement. The exact etiology of chondromalacia is uncertain (309). In the past, arthrography was of little value in evaluation of articular cartilage. However, double contrast arthrography with axial views and lateral views with internal and external rotation may detect these changes (333). Horn described 90% accuracy in detection of chondromalacia arthrographically (360). More important, exclusion of other intra-articular pathology is important. Up to 15% of patients with chondromalacia have associated meniscal tears (363). The combination of arthrography and CT has been used

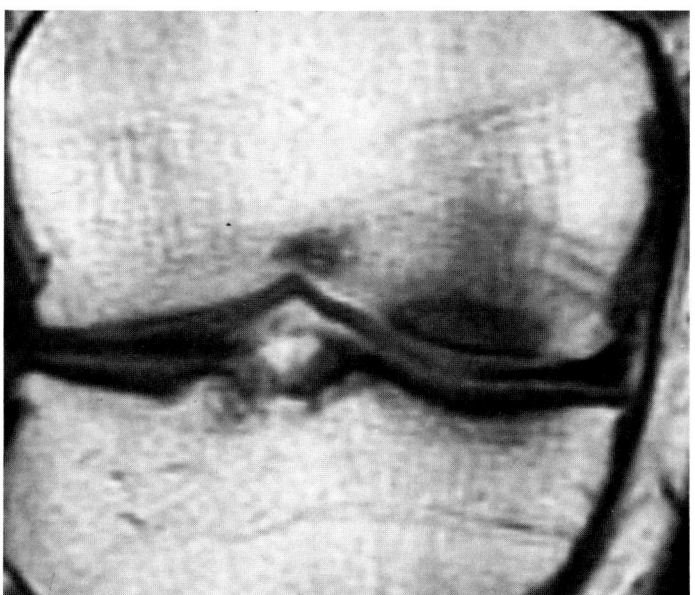

A

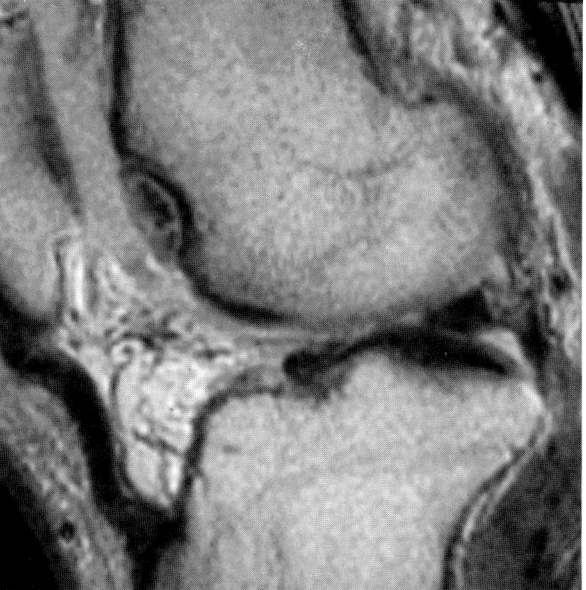

B

FIG. 7-108. Coronal (**A**) and sagittal (**B**) images demonstrating osteochondral defects with intact (**A**) and interrupted (**B**) articular cartilage.

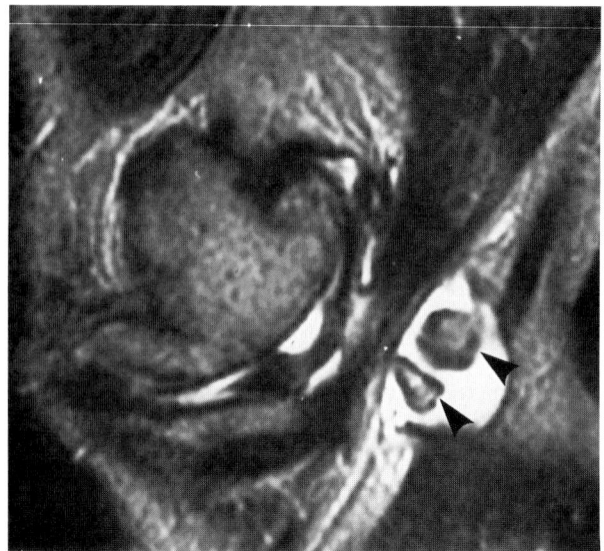

FIG. 7-109. Sagittal T2-weighted (SE 2000/60) image of the knee demonstrating two loose bodies (*arrows*).

to provide the best detail for evaluation of this (293). Currently, MRI is most helpful for it can evaluate not only articular cartilage, but also patellar tracking and all other osseous and soft tissue disorders about the knee (291,422).

Intra-articular loose bodies may result from degenerative disease, trauma, or synovial chondromatosis. Arthrographic detection may be difficult due to the multiple compartments and the size of the capsule. If double contrast technique is used, air bubbles may be mistaken for chondral bodies. In our experience, single contrast technique with tomography or MRI (Fig. 7-109) is most reliable (291).

Synovial Abnormalities

Imaging of synovial abnormalities can be accomplished with arthrography and MRI. Both techniques have been described as useful in detection of changes including synovitis, synovial chondromatosis, neoplasms, cysts, and plicae syndrome (291,309,333,351, 353,380,410,423,426,439).

The significance of the synovial plica was not fully recognized prior to the advent of arthroscopy. These plicae are embryonic remnants that may be present in the normal knee. The most common plica are the suprapatellar, medial patellar, and intrapatellar (Fig. 7-110). These may be present in 20–60% of normal knees (287,294,323). If these plicae become inflamed, they appear white and thick arthroscopically and may be symptomatic. The patients often complain of medial knee pain with exercise (294). The symptoms are usually related to trauma and may be difficult to differentiate from other intra-articular pathology. Plicae may be demonstrated with double contrast technique and tomography using conventional arthrography or with CT (Fig. 7-111 and 7-112) (289,290,353).

Currently, axial CT images after contrast injection or MRI in the sagittal and axial planes are most useful for evaluation of patients with suspected plicae syndrome. History is important in this setting because, typically, MR examinations do not include axial views unless chondromalacia or plica syndrome is suspected (291).

If a plica persists in its entirety, the joint will lose its normal configuration. Persistence of the entire suprapatellar plicae may result in detectable arthrographic or MR changes (Fig. 7-113) (323). In this situation the patient may present with a suprapatellar soft tissue mass (293,294).

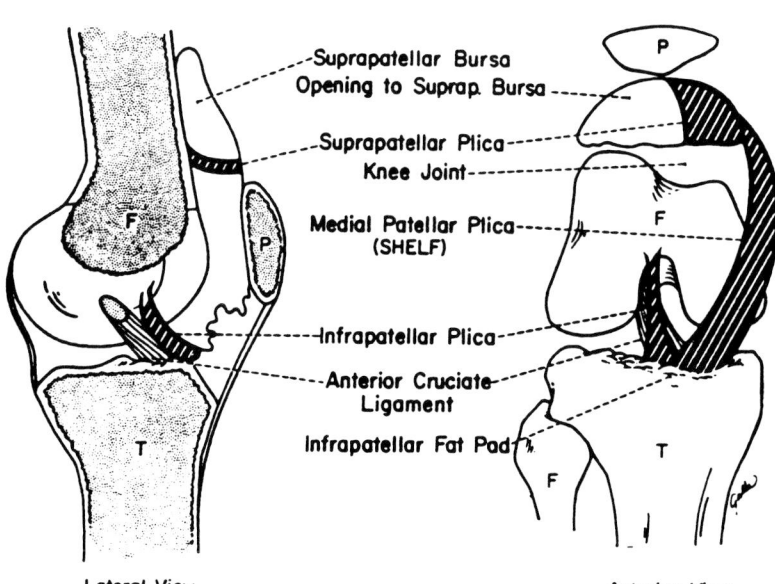

FIG. 7-110. Illustration of synovial plicae of the knee (from 404, with permission.)

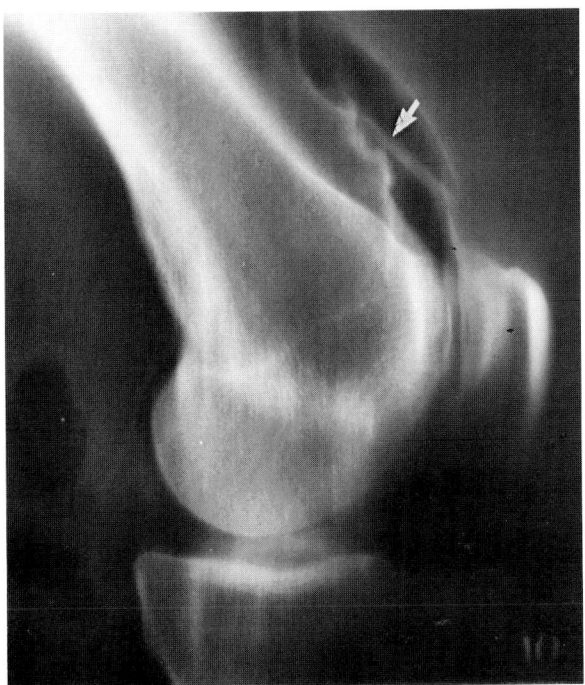

FIG. 7-111. Double contrast arthrotomogram demonstrating the suprapatellar plicae (*arrow*).

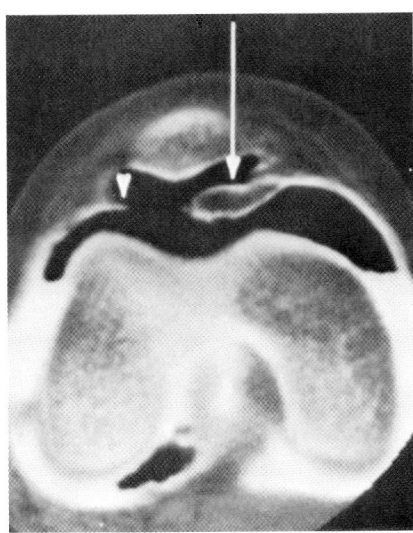

FIG. 7-112. CT scan following double contrast arthrography demonstrating a thickened mediopatellar plicae (*long white arrow*) and small nonthickened lateral plicae (*small arrow*) (from 294, with permission.)

Miscellaneous Conditions

Other syndromes about the knee can also be evaluated with imaging techniques including pes anserine bursitis and snapping syndromes of the periarticular tendons (3,31,381). Inflammatory changes along the pes anserine tendons can be detected with MRI (Fig. 7-114) due to the increased signal intensity caused by inflammatory fluid along the medial tendons (291).

Snapping syndromes have been described in the ankle, hip, shoulder and elbow. More recently, snapping syndromes in the knee have also been described (331,381). The snapping phenomenon is thought to be due to three factors. First, with internal rotation of the tibia, the medial tibial condyle could rotate posteriorly decreasing the angle formed by the tendon and the condyle and increasing the force of displacement. Second, spasm or contrac-

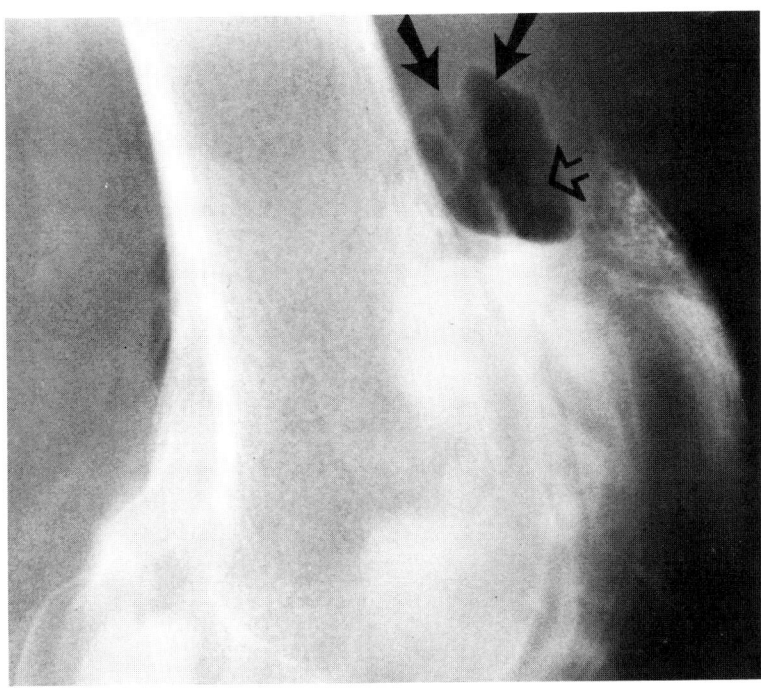

FIG. 7-113. Persistent suprapatellar plicae with synovial thickening (*arrows*) and abnormally short suprapatellar bursa.

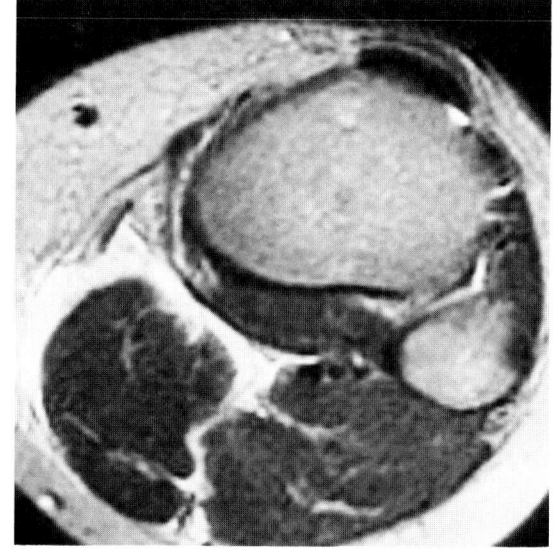

A

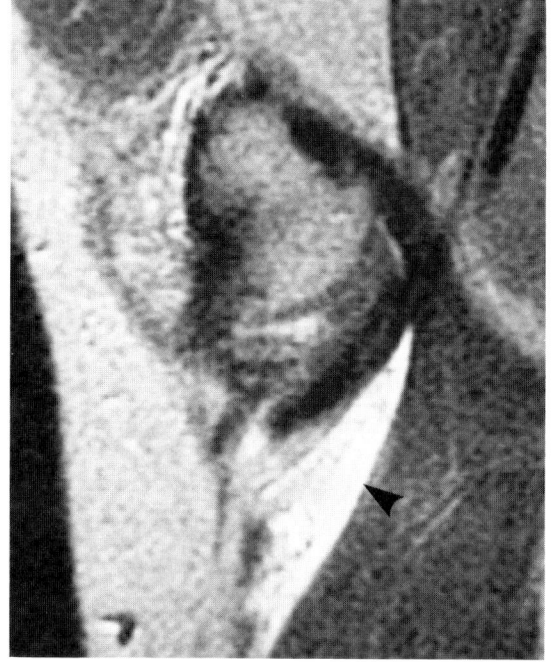

B

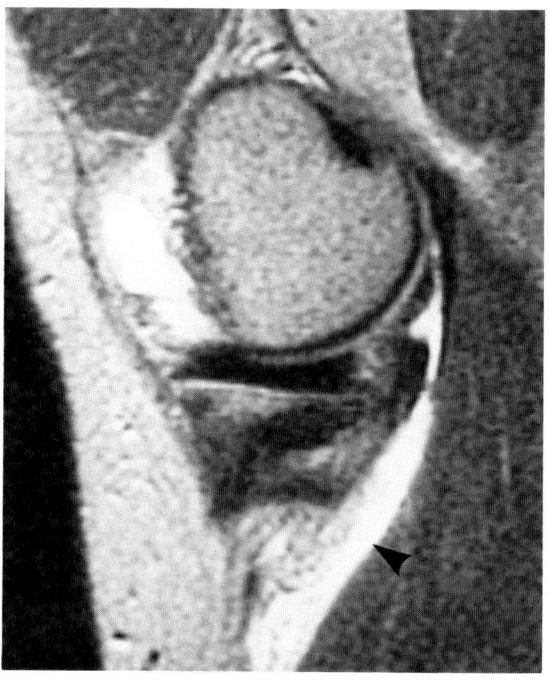

C

FIG. 7–114. SE 2000/60 axial (**A**) and sagittal (**B, C**) images demonstrate increased signal intensity (*arrows*) due to pes anserine bursitis.

ture of the semitendinous muscle could increase the force of displacement. Third, rupture or loosening of the fanned-out fibers could decrease the counter force resisting displacement (381). Peritendinitis, no doubt, also plays a role in this syndrome. Histologic examinations have demonstrated an additional feature, a white fibrocartilaginous cap along the medial femoral condyle that causes friction during flexion and extension of the knee (331).

Identification of this syndrome can be accomplished with flexion and extension MR imaging using T2-weighted sequences with the knee in the lateral position or by injecting the medial tendon sheaths and examining the patient fluoroscopically.

Summary

There are numerous imaging techniques for evaluation of the articular and periarticular disorders of the knee. Conventional arthrography, double contrast arthrography, CT arthrography, arthrotomography, ultrasonography, and MRI have been discussed as they apply to specific clinical situations. Currently, MRI is the technique of choice as a screening examination for the knee because it can evaluate all of the bone and soft tissue structures efficiently. It has largely replaced arthrography for many types of knee conditions. However, arthrography is still valuable in some situations and injection of the knee and proximal tibiofibular articulation (Fig. 7-115) can be very useful both for diagnosis and therapy. Proper communication between the radiologist and clinician is essential so that the most appropriate technique is performed.

Arthroscopy

Arthroscopy of the knee was first performed by Takagi in 1918 (430). Early use of the arthroscope in the United States was primarily related to management of tuberculosis of the knee (298,329). Watanabe developed the first clinically practical arthroscope and published the *Atlas of Arthroscopy* in 1957 (434). Subsequently, much activity has revolved about the development and teaching of diagnostic and arthroscopic surgical techniques (Fig. 7-116).

The initial indications for diagnostic arthroscopy included diagnosis of meniscal lesions or defects of articular cartilage, synovial biopsy, follow-up of surgically treated patients, and visualization of patellofemoral relationships (302,344,384,387,388). Contraindications to arthroscopy included adjacent sepsis and ankylosis of the joint. In an early report on the value of arthroscopy in 60 knees, Casscells found that the arthroscopic diagnosis was correct in 80% of cases, with 6 false-positive and 6 false-negative results (302).

The accuracy of arthroscopy in the diagnosis of intraarticular lesions and especially in comparison to arthrography have been more recently addressed by several authors (Table 7-8) (301,303,306,308,314,337,338,359, 364,366,372,374,385,396). The areas that are difficult to visualize arthroscopically are the posterior horns of the menisci, especially the medial meniscus in a knee with

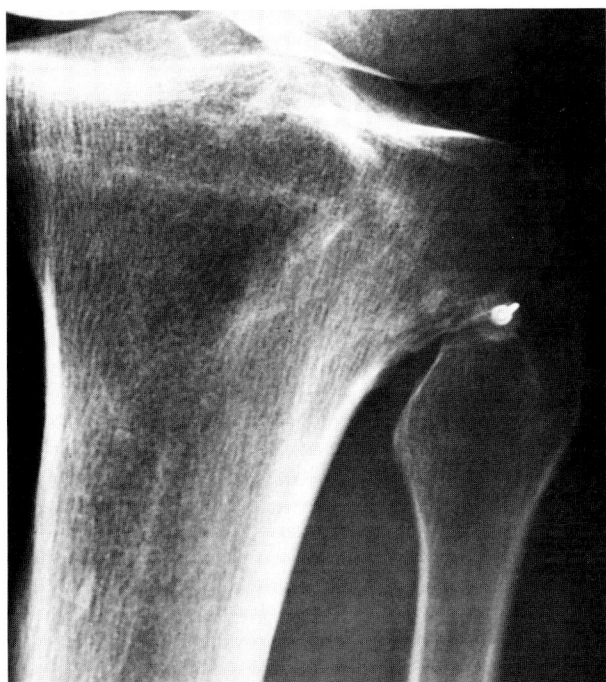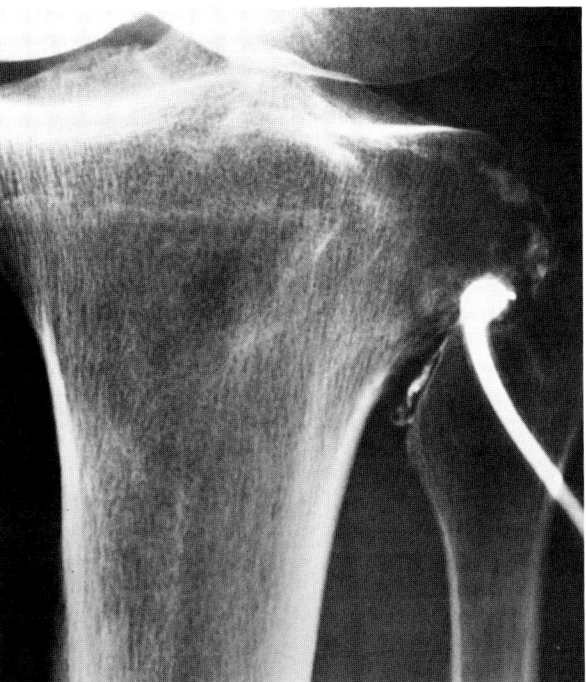

FIG. 7-115. Pain in the proximal tibiofibular joint. Fluoroscopic positioning of the needle (A) and injection of contrast (B) and anesthetic allows the abnormality to be defined.

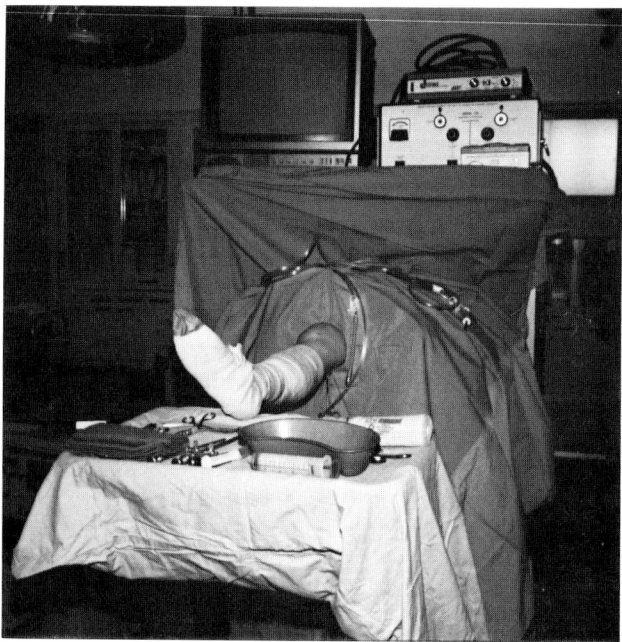

FIG. 7–116. Routine preparation and equipment for arthroscopy.

difficult to evaluate because of the popliteus tendon hiatus (303,374,396). If imaging techniques and arthroscopy are combined, the accuracy of diagnosis increases to 98% (364). Therefore, these two techniques should be considered complementary. Clinical diagnosis is frequently inaccurate because of failure to appreciate associated pathology that may be better defined arthroscopically (372).

Arthroscopic Evaluation

Arthroscopy has proved to be a useful tool in the evaluation of acute knee injuries and should be combined with a careful examination of the ligamentous individual who presents with a history of a valgus, varus, or rotational stress, a rapid deceleration injury to the knee, an audible pop, and the rapid onset of a hemarthrosis, all of which indicate significant injury (318,339,397,399). In such cases, tears of the anterior cruciate ligament (Fig. 7-119) are frequent, appearing in 50–72% of the knees (318,339,397). Other frequent lesions include meniscus injuries, especially at the posterior peripheral detachment (57–62%); osteochondral fractures (6–20%); and posterior cruciate ligament tears (3%) (318,397). Minor ligamentous tears without laxity may be diagnosed in 41% by the presence of capsular hemorrhage (Fig. 7-120) (397). Examination under anesthesia combined with arthroscopy yields useful information in these acute knee injuries in 68% (338), 86% (318), or 94% (396) of the knees. Arthroscopy is not recommended in the evaluation of the patient with severe ligamentous injury and extensive capsular disruption, as saline may extravasate into the calf, leading to a potential compartment syndrome (312). Combined with examination of ligamentous stability under anesthesia, arthroscopy is also useful in the management of knees chronically deficient with regard to the anterior cruciate ligament (312,317). Finally, some patients may benefit from removal of loose bodies or large anterior cruciate stubs that cause im-

tight ligaments (366). The retropatellar fat pad is also difficult to assess arthroscopically. The posteromedial portal (Fig. 7-117), patellar tendon portal (Fig. 7-118), and midpatellar lateral portal have allowed improved visualization of the posterior cruciate ligament, the peripheral attachments of the menisci, and the anterior aspects of the joint. Arthroscopy, on the other hand, appears to be more accurate than arthrography in the diagnosis of patellar problems, tears of the anterior cruciate ligament, and tears of the lateral meniscus (320).

Arthroscopic evaluation of 614 knees resulted in avoidance of open operation in 32%, a change in the planned operation in 27%, and an important change in 41% (315). In some cases, arthroscopy is superior to arthrography and MRI. Tears of the lateral meniscus are

TABLE 7–8. *Accuracy of arthroscopy in diagnosis of intraarticular lesions*

Author	Year	Clinical	Arthroscopy	Arthrography
Nicholas	1970	80	—	97.5
Jackson	1972	68.5	88	68.2[a]
DeHaven	1975	72	94	78
McGinty	1976	—	89.8	50
Hirschowitz	1976	72	94	77
Gillquist	1978	—	91	27*
Gillies	1979	85	68	83
Korn	1979	—	98	94
Carruthers	1980	—	96	—
Ireland	1980	—	84	86
Curran	1980	71	97	52
Casscells	1980	70	95	—
Crabtree	1981	—	93	94

[a] Single contrast.

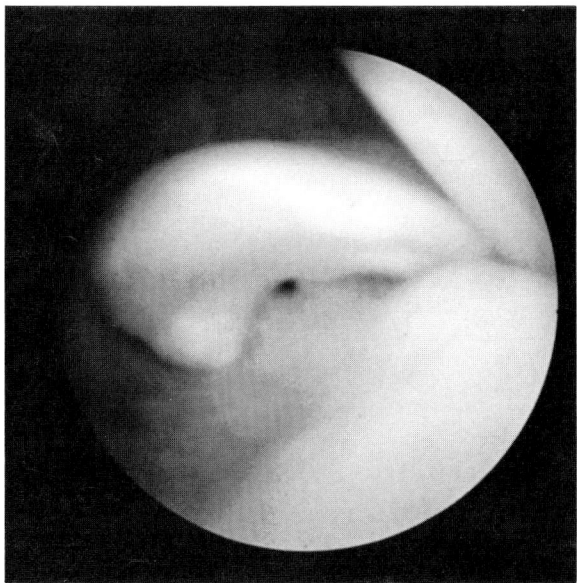

FIG. 7–117. Flap tear of the posterior horn of the medial meniscus that has displaced into the posterior medial compartment as visualized from the posteromedial portal.

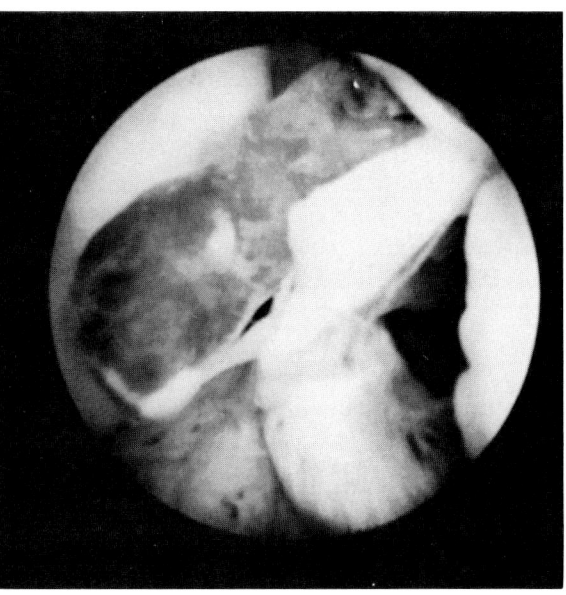

FIG. 7–119. Acute tear of the anterior cruciate ligament in a patient with an acute hemarthrosis. (From Rand JA. The role of arthroscopy in the management of knee injuries in the athlete. *Mayo Clin Proc* 1984;59:77.)

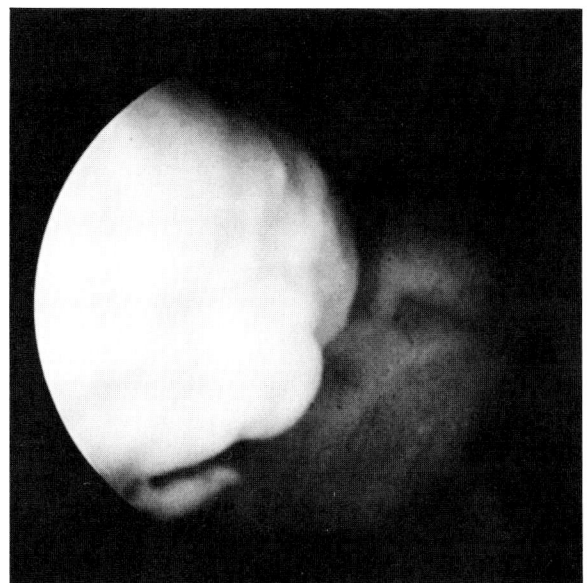

FIG. 7–118. Loose body in the posterolateral compartment as visualized through the intercondylar notch with the arthroscope in the patellar tendon portal.

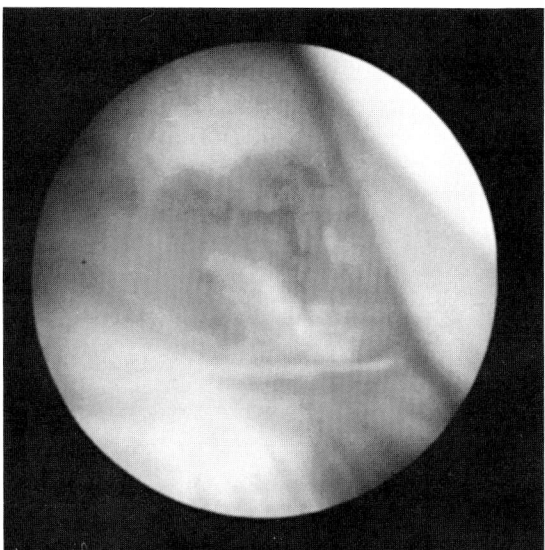

FIG. 7–120. Acute hemorrhage in the medial capsule of the knee following a valgus stress indicating postal capsular tearing. (From Rand JA, Sim FH. The role of arthroscopy in the management of knee injuries in the athlete. *Mayo Clin Proc* 1984;59:77.)

pingement. Partial meniscectomy may also be recommended for meniscal tears in the presence of chronic anterior cruciate ligament insufficiency (312). Following adequate assessment of the degree of instability and correction of intra-articular pathology, a more accurate assessment of the results of a rehabilitation program or the need for ligamentous reconstruction may be made.

The recognition of "new" pathologic lesions that may mimic lesions of menisci have become recognized through arthroscopy. The medial fibrous plica is an example (Fig. 7-121).

Plicae or synovial folds were recognized as early as 1939 by Iino (361). Three synovial folds exist within the knee: the plica synovialis suprapatellaris, the plica synovialis mediopatellaris, and the plica synovialis infrapatellaris (see Fig. 7-110) (404). A lateral plica may also be present (367). The suprapatellar plica is present in 20% of knees and represents a remnant of an embryologic septum that divides the knee (404). The suprapatellar plica is usually asymptomatic. The infrapatellar plica or ligamentum mucosum covers the anterior cruciate ligament (404). This structure may cause confusion in the interpretation of arthrograms that appear similar to the anterior cruciate ligament. The ligamentum mucosum is an asymptomatic structure. The medial synovial plica or shelf is present in 18.9% (404) to 60% (415) of knees.

In some individuals, this latter membrane may become thickened and fibrous, presumably following local trauma. The plica may then impinge on the anteromedial femoral condyle at 30°–45° of knee flexion, resulting in pain and snapping. Patel has noted a 60% incidence of chondromalacia of the medial facet of the patella and a 40% incidence of chondromalacia of the medial femoral condyle adjacent to symptomatic medial plicae (404). A pathologic plica that is symptomatic is present in only 17% of knees that have a medial plica (367). Resection of the plica may be performed arthroscopically, with relief of symptoms in 70–93% of patients (296,367,391).

Arthroscopy has been applied to injuries of the menisci as well as problems associated with meniscal surgery. The functional importance of the menisci has been previously discussed. All menisci regardless of injury or degenerative changes transmit load (354). A partial meniscectomy will decrease load transmission by the meniscus from 85–25% medially or 75–50% laterally (354). Therefore from a mechanical standpoint, partial meniscectomy appears preferable to total meniscectomy. Clinical studies of arthrotomy and partial meniscectomy have found improved results with preservation of a portion of the meniscus (299,386,431). For bucket-handle tears of the meniscus, excellent or good results were obtained in 83% for partial meniscectomy compared with 72% for total meniscectomy (431). Partial meniscectomy results in a shorter rehabilitation time and a fourfold decrease in postoperative complications compared with total meniscectomy (386).

Arthroscopic surgical techniques also allow a selective approach to meniscal lesions. A carefully controlled partial meniscectomy may be performed for a variety of lesions, leaving a stable, contoured, and intact peripheral rim (Fig. 7-122). The long-term results of arthroscopic partial meniscectomy support this technique (377,388, 436). A 6-year follow-up of 208 bucket-handle tears ex-

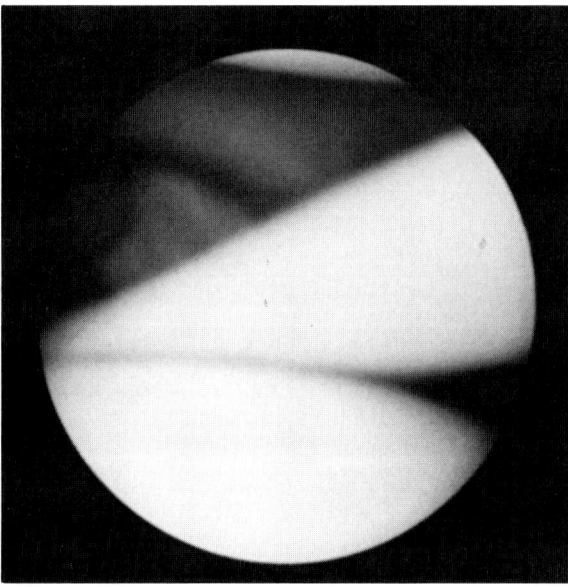

FIG. 7-121. Medial fibrous plica lying between the patella superiorly and medial femoral condyle inferiorly. (From Rand JA, Sim FH. The role of arthroscopy in the management of knee injuries in the athlete. *Mayo Clin Proc* 1984;59:77.)

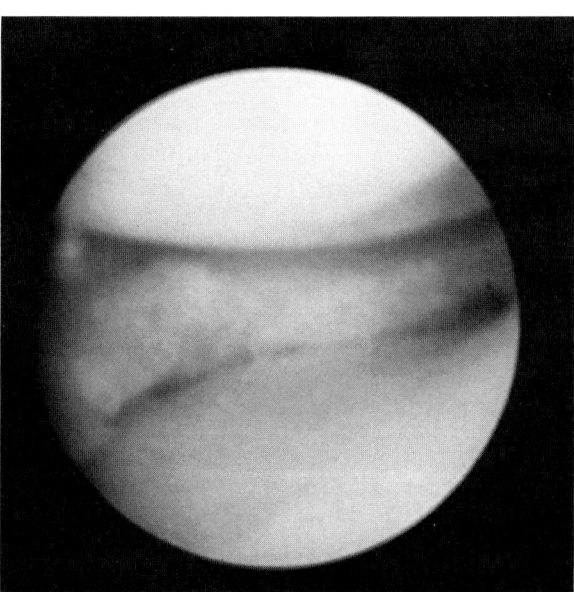

FIG. 7-122. Peripheral rim of the medial meniscus following arthroscopic partial medial meniscectomy. (From Rand JA, Sim FH. The role of arthroscopy in the management of knee injuries in the athlete. *Mayo Clin Proc* 1984;59:77.)

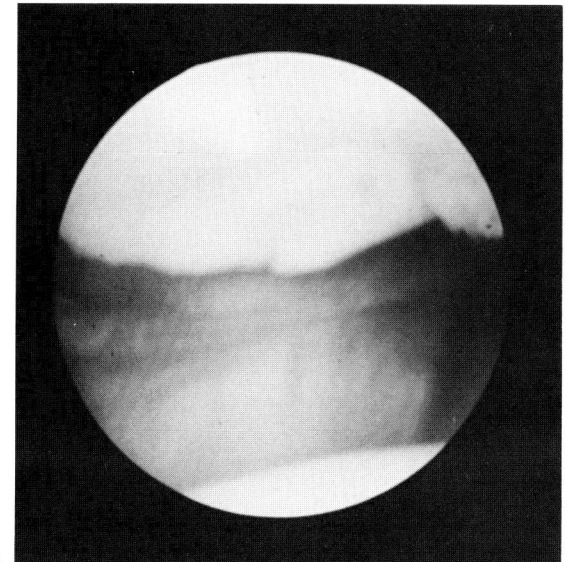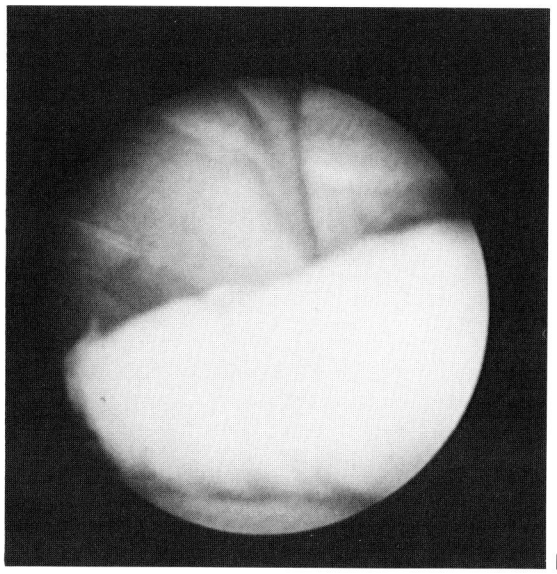

A   B

FIG. 7-123. A: Arthroscopic appearance of an old osteochondral fracture of the patella and **B:** appearance of loose body in the suprapatellar pouch. (From Rand JA, Sim FH. The role of arthroscopy in the management of knee injuries in the athlete. *Mayo Clin Proc* 1984;59:77.)

cised arthroscopically revealed a low morbidity and no evidence of progressive degenerative arthritis (401). A 5-year follow-up of 131 arthroscopic partial meniscectomies revealed 85% good-to-excellent results. Ninety percent excellent or good results in 95 patients with 3 years of follow-up has also been reported (395). Finally, one study reported a success rate of 87% for partial meniscectomy in 125 patients followed for 2 years (340). Arthro-

scopic meniscectomy offers the advantages of selective partial meniscectomy, early rehabilitation, and few complications (365).

Arthroscopic evaluation may also be applied to the identification and management of peripheral tears of the meniscus that may be salvaged by peripheral reattachment. Peripheral detachment of the meniscus most frequently occurs in either an anterior central location or posterior peripheral location. Successful repair has been accomplished in 21 of 22 knees with anterior central detachment (429). Posterior peripheral detachments may be salvaged with only an 8–9% incidence of retear (319). Arthroscopy allows evaluation of the integrity of the body of the meniscus, the extent of the tear, and the possibility of associated lesions, such as a torn anterior cruciate ligament. In some instances, arthroscopic repair of the peripheral tear is feasible.

Arthroscopy has proved valuable in the management of other knee disorders. Loose bodies are a frequent cause of knee symptoms and mimic a torn meniscus (384). Loose bodies may or may not be radio-opaque, making radiographic localization difficult in some cases. In one series, only 38 of 50 loose bodies removed were visible on radiographs (315). Loose bodies may be multiple in 30% of the knees (315). Loose bodies arise from osteochondral fractures (Fig. 7-123), synovial chondromatosis, osteochondritis dissecans, and osteoarthritis (Fig. 7-124). Other lesions that present in a similar manner include foreign bodies, fragments of menisci, and local benign synovial tumors (Fig. 7-125). Common locations for loose bodies include the suprapatellar pouch, especially behind a suprapatellar plica; the intercondylar notch; popliteus tunnel; posteromedial and posterolat-

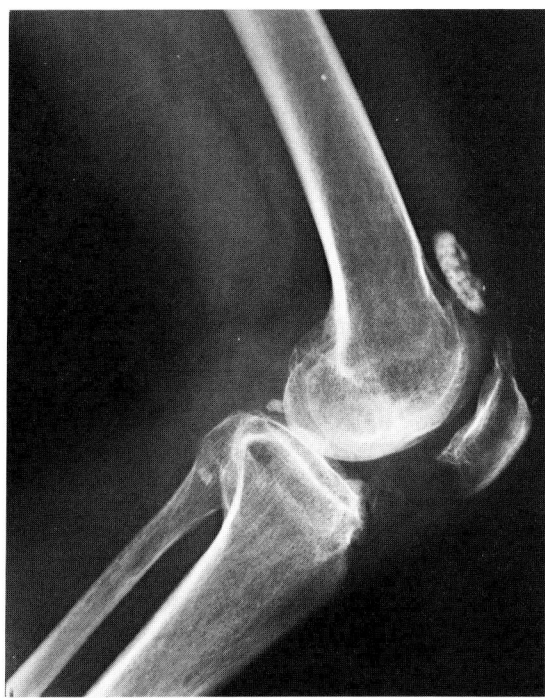

FIG. 7-124. Lateral radiograph showing the typical appearance of loose bodies associated with osteoarthritis.

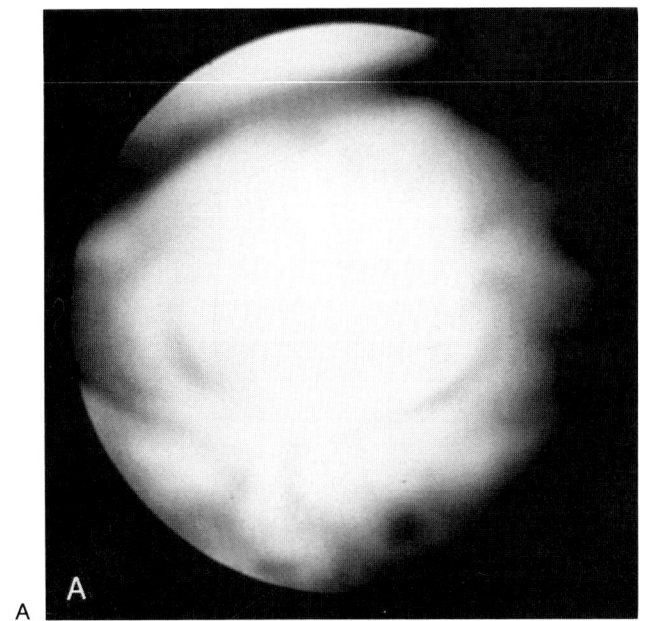

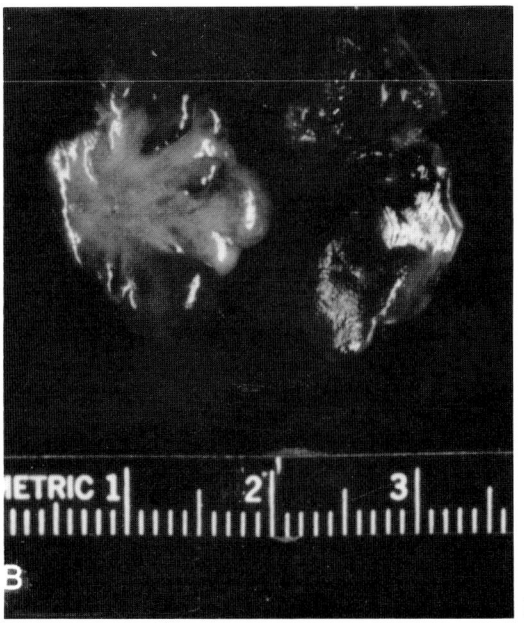

FIG. 7-125. Arthroscopic appearance of a localized pigmental villonodular synovitis attached to the anteromedial joint capsule. **A:** Arthroscopic appearance. **B:** Gross pathology.

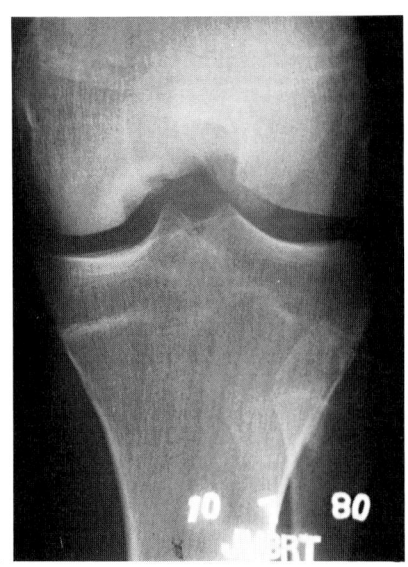

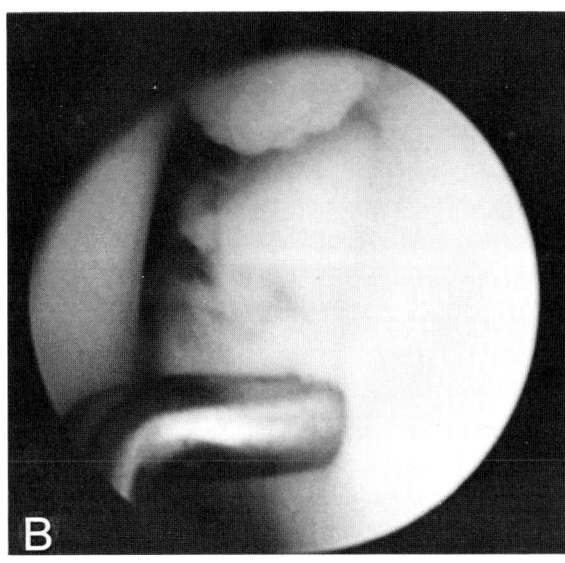

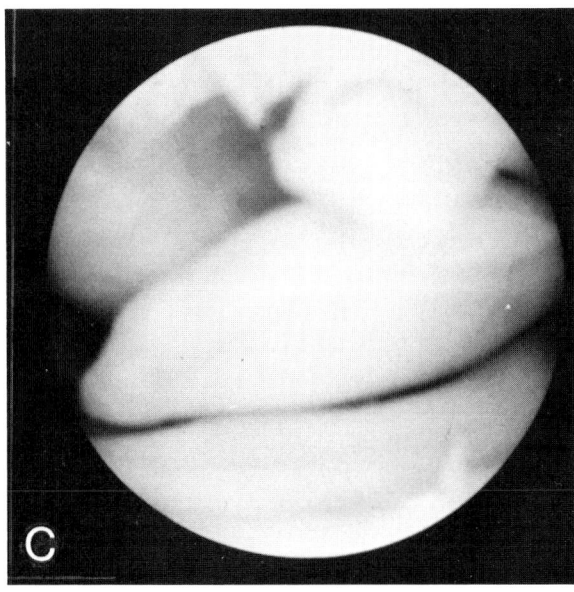

FIG. 7-126. A: Tunnel radiograph of osteochondral dissecans of the medial femoral condyles of a 21-year-old man. **B:** Arthroscopic appearance of fragmentation of the articular cartilage overlying the lesion. **C:** Arthroscopic appearance of lesion with loose body.

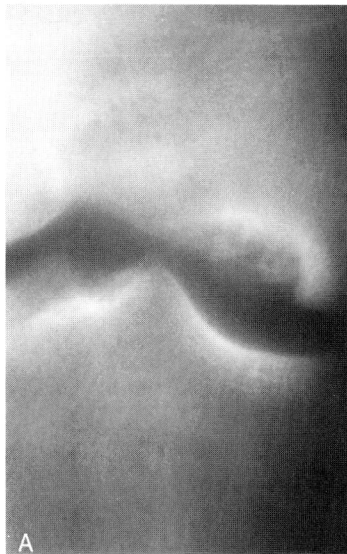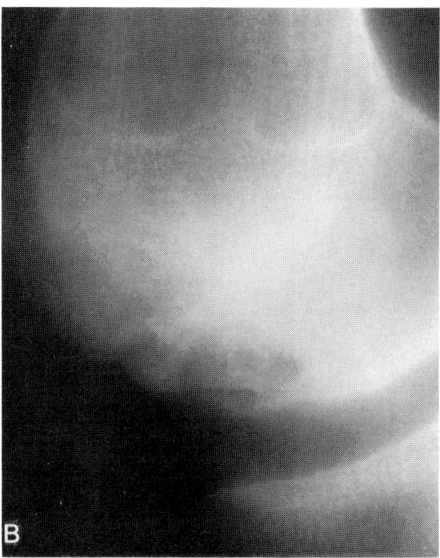

FIG. 7-127. AP (A) and lateral (B) tomogram showing healing osteochondritis dissecans.

eral compartments; and the area beneath the posterior horn of the lateral meniscus (315). The arthroscope allows a thorough evaluation of all of these areas with minimal morbidity. The etiology of the loose bodies may be determined by direct inspection of the joint surface and synovium.

Osteochondritis dissecans in the adult is a difficult lesion to manage (Fig. 7-126). In a long-term study with an average 33-year follow-up, only 10 of 48 patients with adult-onset osteochondritis dissecans did not show evidence of gonarthrosis. In these patients, the gonarthrosis began 10 years earlier than primary gonarthrosis and more commonly involved all three articulations of the knee (379). The etiology of the disorder remains controversial and includes direct or indirect trauma, ischemia, abnormal ossification, and genetic factors (304). Radiographic evaluation should include AP, lateral, and tunnel views for visualization (304,343,344). Tomograms are very useful in the assessment of healing (Fig. 7-127). The classic location is the posterolateral aspect of the medial femoral condyle.

Arthroscopy offers evaluation of the degree of irregularity of the surface, treatment with a decreased rehabilitation time, and fewer complications than open surgery (343). The primary objective of treatment is to save or improve the articular surface with healing of the defect and thus to avoid arthrosis (343). Lesions may be classified on the basis of their arthroscopic appearance into the following types: intact, early separation, partially detached, and crater with loose bodies (343). Lesions should be classified according to location. Lesions of the medial femoral condyle are classified as central, centrolateral, and inferocentral, while those of the lateral femoral condyle are inferocentral, lateral, or anterior (343). Surgical intervention is indicated for patients over the

age of 12 with lesions greater than 1 cm in size located in the weight-bearing area (343). The type of treatment depends upon the stage of the lesion and varies from drilling of intact lesions to trimming the bed and removal of a loose fragment (343). Of 49 knees treated arthroscopically, 44 healed in an average time of 5 months (343).

Arthroscopic techniques have been applied to the management of synovial disorders. Crystalline synovitis associated with chondrocalcinosis may be improved by arthroscopic lavage and debridement (Fig. 7-128) (400). An improvement in symptoms occurred in 16 of 17 knees treated by arthroscopic means (400). Synovectomy of the knee may be performed arthroscopically in the management of the rheumatoid patient who is unresponsive to nonoperative management (289,358). In 33 knees treated with arthroscopic synovectomy with a mean follow-up of 44 months, 70% were symptomatically improved (289).

Arthroscopy has also been applied to the evaluation and management of patellar disorders. The advantages of arthroscopic visualization of patellofemoral relationships include the ability to follow dynamic changes on flexion-extension of the knee. The position of the apex of the patella relative to the intercondylar notch gives valuable information concerning patellar tracking (327,418). A study of incremental patellar tracking with knee flexion revealed slight patellar subluxation of 0°, subluxation with patellofemoral contact at 20°, and centering of the patella in the trochlear groove of the femur by 40°–60° of flexion (327). These arthroscopic findings aid in the interpretation of radiographs of the patellofemoral joint made in varying degrees of knee flexion. Arthroscopy allows visualization of the articular surface of the patella and the extent of chondromalacia (Fig. 7-129). Debridement of the patella may be performed. Lateral

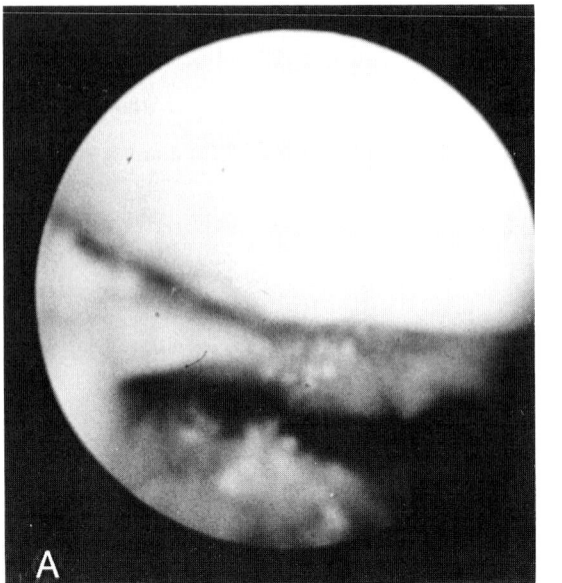 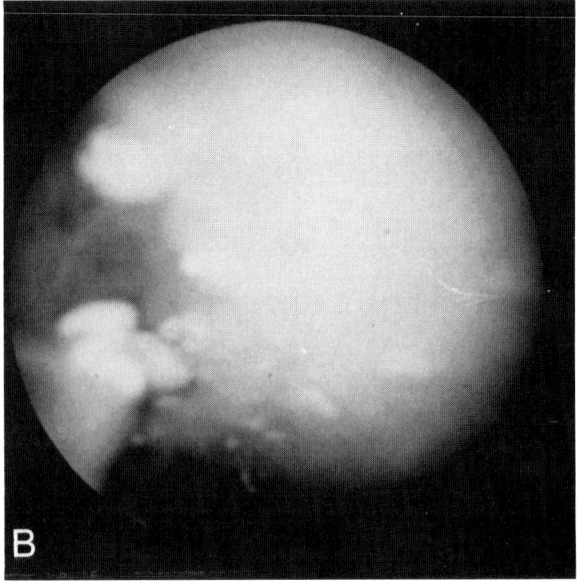

FIG. 7-128. A: Arthroscopic appearance of chondrocalcinosis of the menisci. **B:** Chondrocalcinosis in the articular cartilage.

retinacular release may be performed under arthroscopic control in management of patellar chondromalacia or malalignment (389,418,426).

Arthroscopy is currently being applied to the management of a variety of other knee disorders. Degenerative joint disease may be improved by arthroscopic lavage and debridement (Fig. 7-130). Exposed areas of bone may be drilled to encourage fibrocartilaginous ingrowth. Recently, a technique of abrasion arthroplasty has been applied to areas of exposed bone for this purpose (371).

A superficial debridement of dead and sclerotic bone to a depth of 1 mm is performed until active bleeding is identified. Two-year results have revealed that 75% of the patients improved, with some evidence of an increasing joint space on radiographs (371).

In summary, imaging techniques and arthroscopy are complementary in the evaluation of knee disorders. Arthroscopy allows the surgical management of a variety of lesions with less morbidity than arthrotomy. However, experience is extremely important with either technique in order to obtain optimal information and results.

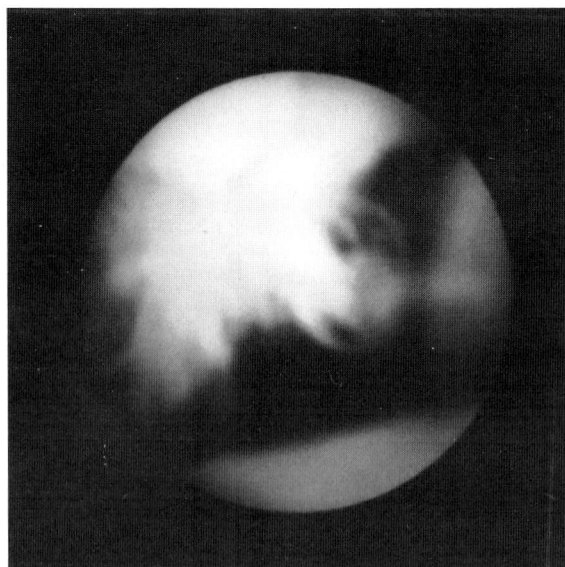

FIG. 7-129. Arthroscopic appearance of chondromalacia of the patella. (From Rand JA, Sim FH. The role of arthroscopy in the management of knee injuries in the athlete. *Mayo Clin Proc* 1984;59:77.)

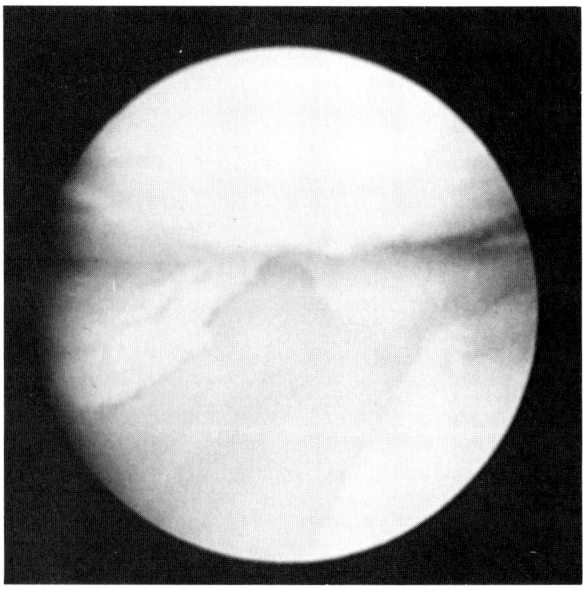

FIG. 7-130. Arthroscopic appearance of an area of exposed bone on the medial tibial plateau and femoral condyle in a patient with osteoarthritis.

REFERENCES

Anatomy and Biomechanics

1. Alm A, Ekstrom H, Gillquist J, Stromberg B. The anterior cruciate ligament. *Acta Chir Scand* (Suppl.) 1974;445:3–49.
2. Arnoczky S. Anatomy of the anterior cruciate ligament. *Clin Orthop* 1983;172:19–25.
3. Bartel DL, Marshall JL, Schieck RA, Wang JB. Surgical repositioning of the medial collateral ligament. *J Bone Joint Surg* 1977;59A:107–116.
4. Blacharski PA, Somerset JH. A three dimensional study of the kinematics of the human knee. *J Biomech* 1975;8:375–384.
5. Bourne MH, Hazel WA, Scott SG, Sim EH. Anterior knee pain. *Mayo Clin Proc* 1988;63:482–491.
6. Brantigan OC, Voshell AF. The mechanics of the ligaments and menisci of the knee joint. *J Bone Joint Surg* 1941;23:44–66.
7. Bullough PG, Walker PS. The distribution of load through the knee joint and its possible significance to the observed patterns of articular cartilage breakdown. *Bull Hosp J Dis* 1976;37:110–123.
8. Burke DL, Ahmed AM, Miller J. A biomechanical study of partial and total medial meniscectomy of the knee. *Orthop Trans* 1977–1978;1:130–131.
9. Butler DL, Noyes FR, Grood ES. Ligamentous restraints to anterior-posterior drawer in the human knee. *J Bone Joint Surg* 1980;62A:259–270.
10. Butler DL, Noyes FR, Grood ES, Miller EH, Malek M. Mechanical properties of transplants for the anterior cruciate ligament. *Orthop Trans* 1979;3:180–181.
11. Clancy WG, Narechania RG, Rosenberg TD, Gmeiner JG, Wisnefske DD, Lange TA. Anterior and posterior cruciate ligament reconstruction in rhesus monkeys. *J Bone Joint Surg* 1981;63A:1270–1283.
12. Crowinshield R, Pope MH, Johnson RJ. An analytical model of the knee. *J Biomech* 1976;9:397–405.
13. Denham RR, Bishop RED. Mechanics of the knee and problems in reconstructive surgery. *J Bone Joint Surg* 1976;60B:345–352.
14. Fairbank TJ. Knee joint changes after meniscectomy. *J Bone Joint Surg* 1948;30B:664–670.
15. Frankel VH. Biomechanics of the knee. *Orthop Clin North Am* 1971;2:175–191.
16. Frankel VH, Burstein AH, Brooks DB. Biomechanics of internal derangement of the knee. *J Bone Joint Surg* 1971;53A:945–962.
17. Freeman BL, Beaty JH, Haynes DB. The pes anserinus transfer. *J Bone Joint Surg* 1982;64A:202–207.
18. Fukubayashi T, Kurosawa H. The contact area and pressure distribution pattern of the knee. *Acta Orthop Scand* 1980;51:871–879.
19. Fukubayashi T, Torzilli P. An in vitro biomechanical evaluation of anterior-posterior motion of the knee. *J Bone Joint Surg* 1982;64A:258–262.
20. Furman W, Marshall J, Girgis FG. The anterior cruciate ligament. *J Bone Joint Surg* 1976;58A:179–185.
21. Girgis FB, Marshall JL, Al Monajem ARS. The cruciate ligaments of the knee joint. *Clin Orthop* 1975;106:216–231.
22. Grood E, Noyes F. Cruciate ligament prosthesis: Strength, creep and fatigue properties. *J Bone Joint Surg* 1976;58A:1083–1088.
23. Grood E, Noyes F, Butler DL, Suntey WJ. Ligamentous and capsular restraints preventing straight medial and lateral laxity in intact human cadaver knees. *J Bone Joint Surg* 1981;63A:1257–1269.
24. Harrington I. Static and dynamic loading patterns in knee joints with deformities. *J Bone Joint Surg* 1983;65A:247–259.
25. Helfet A. Mechanism of derangements of the medial semilunar cartilage and their management. *J Bone Joint Surg* 1959;41B:319–336.
26. Hsieh H, Walker P. Stabilizing mechanisms of the loaded and unloaded knee joint. *J Bone Joint Surg* 1976;58A:87–93.
27. Hollinshead HW. *Anatomy for surgeons*, 3rd ed., vol. 3, *The spine and limbs*. Harper and Row, 1982.
28. Hughston J, Andrews J, Cross M, Moschi A. Classification of knee ligament instabilities. Part I. The medial compartment and cruciate ligaments. *J Bone Joint Surg* 1976;58A:159–172.
29. Hughston J, Andrews J, Cross M, Arnoldo M. Classification of knee ligament instabilities. Part II. The lateral compartment. *J Bone Joint Surg* 1976;58A:173–179.
30. Hughston J, Eilers A. The role of the posterior oblique ligament in repairs of acute medial (collateral) ligament tears of the knee. *J Bone Joint Surg* 1973;55A:923–940.
31. Johnson F, Leitl S, Waugh W. The distribution of load across the knee. *J Bone Joint Surg* 1980;62B:346–349.
32. Johnson R, Kettelkamp D, Clark W, Leaverton P. Factors affecting late results after meniscectomy. *J Bone Joint Surg* 1974;56A:719–729.
33. Kennedy J, Hawkins R, Willis RB, Danylchuk KD. Tension studies of human knee ligaments. *J Bone Joint Surg* 1976;58A:350–355.
34. Kennedy J, Weinberg H, Wilson A. The anatomy and function of the anterior cruciate ligament. *J Bone Joint Surg* 1974;56A:223–235.
35. Kettelkamp D, Chao E. A method for quantitative analysis of medial and lateral compression forces at the knee during standing. *Clin Orthop* 1972;183:202–213.
36. Kettelkamp D, Jacobs A. Tibiofemoral contact area—determination and implications. *J Bone Joint Surg* 1972;54A:349–356.
37. King D. The function of the semilunar cartilages. *J Bone Joint Surg* 1936;18:1069–1076.
38. Krause W, Pope M, Johnson RJ, Wilder DG. Mechanical changes in the knee after meniscectomy. *J Bone Joint Surg* 1976;58A:599–604.
39. Levy M, Torzilli P, Warren R. The effect of medial meniscectomy on anterior-posterior motion of the knee. *J Bone Joint Surg* 1982;64A:883–888.
40. Lipke J, Janecki C, Nelson C, et al. The role of incompetence of the anterior cruciate and lateral ligaments in anterolateral and anteromedial instability. *J Bone Joint Surg* 1981;63A:954–960.
41. Mann RA, Hagy JL. The popliteus muscle. *J Bone Joint Surg* 1977;59A:924–927.
42. Maquet P. The biomechanics of the knee and the surgical possibilities of healing osteoarthritic knee joints. *Clin Orthop* 1980;146:102–110.
43. Maquet P, Van de Berg A, Simonet J. Femorotibial weight-bearing areas. *J Bone Joint Surg* 1975;57A:766–771.
44. Markolf K, Bargar W, Shoemaker SC, Amstutz HC. The role of joint load in knee stability. *J Bone Joint Surg* 1981;63A:570–585.
45. Markolf K, Mensch J, Amstutz H. Stiffness and laxity of the knee—the contributions of the supporting structures. *J Bone Joint Surg* 1976;58A:583–594.
46. Morrison JB. Bioengineering analysis of force actions transmitted to the knee joint. *Biomed Engineering* 1968;3:164–170.
47. Morrison JB. The mechanics of the knee joint in relation to normal walking. *J Biomech* 1970;3:51–61.
48. Noyes FR, Grood ES. The defunction of terms for motion and position of the knee and injuries of the ligaments. *J Bone Joint Surg* 1989;71A:465–472.
49. Noyes FR, DeLucas JL, Torvik PJ. Biomechanics of anterior cruciate ligament failure: An analysis of strain rate sensitivity and mechanism of failure in primates. *J Bone Joint Surg* 1974;56A:236–253.
50. Noyes F, Grood E. The strength of the anterior cruciate ligament in humans and rhesus monkeys. *J Bone Joint Surg* 1976;58A:1074–1082.
51. Noyes F, Sonstegard D. Biomechanical function of the pes anserinus at the knee and the effect of its transplantation. *J Bone Joint Surg* 1973;55A:1225–1241.
52. Perry J, Antonelli D, Ford W. Analysis of knee joint forces during flexed knee stance. *J Bone Joint Surg* 1975;57A:961–967.
53. Pope M, Johnson R, Brown D. The role of the musculature in injuries to the medial collateral ligament. *J Bone Joint Surg* 1979;61A:398–402.
54. Reider B, Marshall J, Koslin B, Ring B, Frazer F. The anterior aspect of the knee joint. *J Bone Joint Surg* 1981;63A:351–356.
55. Richmond J, Sarno RC. Post traumatic intracapsular bone fragments: Association in meniscal tears. *AJR* 1988;150:159–160.
56. Scapinelli R. Studies on the vasculature of the human knee joint. *Acta Anat* 1968;70:305–331.
57. Seebacher J, Inglis A, Marshall J, Warren RF. The structure of

the posterolateral aspect of the knee. *J Bone Joint Surg* 1982;64A:536–541.

58. Seedhom B, Dowson D, Wright V. Functions of the menisci: A preliminary study. *J Bone Joint Surg* 1974;56B:381–382.
59. Shaw J, Murray D. The longitudinal axis of the knee and the role of the cruciate ligaments in controlling transverse rotation. *J Bone Joint Surg* 1976;56A:1603–1609.
60. Shoemaker S, Markolf K. In vivo rotatory knee stability. *J Bone Joint Surg* 1982;64A:208–216.
61. Shrive N, Phil D, O'Connor JJ, Goodfellow JW. Load bearing in the knee joint. *Clin Orthop* 1978;131:279–287.
62. Sim FH. Complications and late results of meniscectomy. AAOS Symp on Athlete's Knee, 1978.
63. Simonet WT, Sim FH. Current concepts in the treatment of ligamentous instability of the knee. *Mayo Clin Proc* 1984;59:67–76.
64. Slocum D, Larson R, James S. Late reconstruction of ligamentous injuries of the medial compartment of the knee. *Clin Orthop* 1974;100:23–55.
65. Tapper E, Hoover N. Late results after meniscectomy. *J Bone Joint Surg* 1969;51A:547–556.
66. Torzilli P, Greenburg R, Insall J. An in vivo biomechanical evaluation of anterior-posterior motion of the knee. *J Bone Joint Surg* 1981;63A:960–968.
67. Trent P, Walker P, Wolf B. Ligament length patterns, strength, and rotation axes of the knee joint. *Clin Orthop* 1976;117:263–270.
68. Walker P, Erkman M. The role of the menisci in force transmission across the knee. *Clin Orthop* 1975;109:184–192.
69. Warren F, Marshall J. The supporting structures and layers on the medial side of the knee. *J Bone Joint Surg* 1979;61A:56–62.
70. Warren F, Marshall J, Girgis F. The prime static stabilizer of the medial side of the knees. *J Bone Joint Surg* 1974;56A:665–674.
71. Whiteside L, Sweeney R. Nutrient pathways of the cruciate ligaments. *J Bone Joint Surg* 1980;62A:1176–1180.
72. Wiberg G. Roentgenographic and anatomic studies on the femoropatellar joint, with special reference to chondromalacia patellae. *Acta Orthop Scand* 1941;12:319–410.

Routine Radiographic Techniques

73. Apple JS, Martinez S, Allen NB, Caldwell DS, Rice JR. Occult fractures of the knee: Tomographic evaluation. *Radiology* 1985;148:383–387.
74. Ballinger PW. *Merrill's atlas of roentgenographic positions and standard radiologic procedures.* 5th ed. St. Louis: C. V. Mosby, 1982.
75. Bernau A, Berquist TH. *Orthopedic positioning in diagnostic radiology.* Baltimore: Urban & Schwarzenberg, 1983.
76. Camp JD, Coventry MB. Use of special views in roentgenography of the knee joint. *US Naval Med Bull* 1944;42:56.
77. Daffner RH, Tabas JH. Trauma oblique radiographs of the knee. *J Bone Joint Surg* 1987;69A:568–572.
78. Egund N. The axial view of the patellofemoral joint. *Acta Radiol Diag* 1986;27:101–104.
79. Englestad BL, Friedman EM, Murphy WA. Diagnosis of joint effusion on lateral and axial projections of the knee. *Invest Radiol* 1981;16:188.
80. Hall FM. Radiographic diagnosis and accuracy in knee joint effusions. *Radiology* 1975;115:49–54.
81. Holmblad EC. Postero-anterior x-ray view of the knee in flexion. *JAMA* 1937;109:1196–1197.
82. Hughston JC. Subluxation of the patella. *J Bone Joint Surg* 1968;50A:1003.
83. Jacobsen K. Radiologic technique for measuring instability in the knee joint. *Acta Radiol (Diagn)* 1977;18:113–125.
84. Jacobsen K. Stress radiographical assessment of antero-posterior, medial, and lateral instability of the knee joint. *Acta Orthop Scand* 1976;47:335–344.
85. Kimberlin GE. Radiological assessment of the patellofemoral articulation and subluxation of the patella. *Radiol Technol* 1975;45:129–137.
86. Malghem J, Maldague B. Patellofemoral joint: 30° axial radiograph with lateral rotation of the leg. *Radiology* 1989;170:566–567.
87. Merchant AC, Mercar RL, Jacobsen RH, Cool CR. Roentgenographic analysis of the patellofemoral congruence. *J Bone Joint Surg* 1974;56:1391–1396.
88. Rijke AM, Tegtmeyer CJ, Weiland DJ, McCue FC III. Stress examination of the cruciate ligaments: A radiographic Lachman test. *Radiology* 1987;165:867–869.
89. Rosenberg TD, Paulos LE, Parter RD, Coward DB, Scott SM. The 45° posteroanterior flexion weight bearing radiograph of the knee. *J Bone Joint Surg* 1988;70A:1479–1482.
90. Settegast H. Typische Roentgenobilder von normalen menschen. *Lehmanns Med Atlanton* 1921;5:211.
91. Suger AM, Naemark A, Felson D, Shapiro JH. Comparison of overhead and cross-table lateral views for detection of knee joint effusions. *AJR* 1985;144:973–975.
92. Tallroth K, Lundholm TS. Stress radiographs in evaluation of degenerative femerotibial joint disease. *Skel Radiol* 1987;16:617–620.

Patellar Disorders

93. Aglietti P, Insall JN, Cerulli G. Patellar pain and incongruence. I. Measurements of incongruence. *Clin Orthop* 1983;176:217–224.
94. Aleman O. Chondromalacia post-traumatica patellae. *Acta Chir Scand* 1928;63:149–190.
95. Bassett FH III. Acute dislocation of the patella, osteochondral fractures, and injuries of the extensor mechanism of the knee. *Instr Course Lect* 1976;25:40–49.
96. Bentley G. Chondromalacia patellae. *J Bone Joint Surg* 1970;52A:221–232.
97. Blackburne JS, Peel JE. A new method of measuring patella weight. *J Bone Joint Surg* 1977;59B:241–242.
98. Bodne D, Quinn SF, Murry WT, et al. Magnetic resonance images of chronic patellar tendinitis. *Skel Radiol* 1988;17:24–28.
99. Boring TN, O'Donoghue DH. Acute patellar dislocation: Results of immediate surgical repair. *Clin Orthop* 1978;136:182–185.
100. Brattstrom H. Shape of intercondylar groove normally and in dislocation of the patella. *Acta Orthop Scand* (Suppl.) 1964;68:134–148.
101. Cofield RH, Bryan RS. Acute dislocation of the patella: Results of conservative treatment. *J Trauma* 1977;17:526–530.
102. Crosby EB, Insall J. Recurrent dislocation of the patella. *J Bone Joint Surg* 1976;58A:9–13.
103. DeHaven KE, Dolan WA, Mayer PJ. Chondromalacia patellae in athletes: Clinical presentation and conservative management. *Am J Sports Med* 1979;7:5–11.
104. Delgado-Martins H. A study of the position of the patella using computerized tomography. *J Bone Joint Surg* 1976;61B:443–444.
105. Egund N. The axial view of the patellofemoral joint. *Acta Radiol Diag* 1986;27:101–104.
106. Ferguson AB, Brown TD, Fu FH, Rutkowski R. Relief of patellofemoral contact stress by anterior displacement of the tibial tubercle. *J Bone Joint Surg* 1979;61A:159–166.
107. Ficat RP, Hungerford DS. *Disorders of the patellofemoral joint.* Baltimore: Williams and Wilkins, 1977.
108. Ficat RP, Philippe J, Hungerford DS. Chondromalacia patellae: A system of classification. *Clin Orthop* 1979;144:55–62.
109. Fornage BD, Rifkin MD, Touche DH, Segal PM. Sonography of the patellar tendon: Preliminary observations. *AJR* 1984;143:179–182.
110. Freiberger RH, Kozier LM. Fracture of the medial margin of the patella: A finding diagnostic of lateral dislocation. *Radiology* 1967;88:902–904.
111. Fulkerson JP, Shea KP. Disorders of patellofemoral alignment. *J Bone Joint Surg* 1990;72A:1424–1429.
112. Goodfellow JW, Hungerford DS, Woods C. Patellofemoral joint mechanics and pathology. II. Chondromalacia patellae. *J Bone Joint Surg* 1976;58B:291–299.
113. Goodfellow JW, Hungerford DS, Zindel M. Patellofemoral mechanics and pathology: I. Functional anatomy of the patellofemoral joint. *J Bone Joint Surg* 1976;58B:287–290.

114. Gruber MA. The conservative treatment of chondromalacia patellae. *Orthop Clin North Am* 1979;10:105–115.
115. Hayes CW, Sawyer RW, Conway WF. Patellar cartilage: In vitro detection and staging with MR imaging and pathologic correlation. *Radiology* 1990;176:479–483.
116. Heywood AWB. Recurrent dislocation of the patella. *J Bone Joint Surg* 1961;43B:508–517.
117. Horns JW. The diagnosis of chondromalacia by double contrast arthrography of the knee. *J Bone Joint Surg* 1977;59A:119–120.
118. Hughston JC. Subluxation of the patella. *J Bone Joint Surg* 1968;50A:1003–1026.
119. Hungerford DS, Barry M. Biomechanics of the patellofemoral joint. *Clin Orthop* 1979;144:9–15.
120. Inoue M, Shino K, Hirose H, Horibi S, Ono K. Subluxation of the patella: Computed tomography of patellofemoral congruence. *J Bone Joint Surg* 1988;70A:1331–1337.
121. Insall JN, Aglietti P, Tria AJ. Patellar pain and incongruence. II. Clinical application. *Clin Orthop* 1983;176:225–232.
122. Insall JN, Falvo KA, Wise DN. Chondromalacia patellae. *J Bone Joint Surg* 1976;58A:1–8.
123. Insall JN, Salvati E. Patella position in the normal knee joint. *Radiology* 1971;101:101–104.
124. Jackson RW. Examination of the patella. *Instr Course Lect* 1976;25:31–36.
125. Jackson RW. Etiology of chondromalacia patellae. *Instr Course Lect* 1976;25:36–40.
126. Kaufer H. Mechanical function of the patella. *J Bone Joint Surg* 1971;53A:1551–1560.
127. Kaufer H. Patellar biomechanics. *Clin Orthop* 1979;144:51–54.
128. Kettelkamp DB. Management of patellar malalignment. *J Bone Joint Surg* 1981;63A:1334–1347.
129. Kettelkamp DB, DeRosa GP. Biomechanics and functional rehabilitation of the patellofemoral joint. *Instr Course Lect* 1976;25:27–31.
130. Larsen E, Lauridsen F. Conservative treatment of patellar dislocations. Influence of evident factors on the tendency to redislocate and the therapeutic result. *Clin Orthop* 1982;171:131–136.
131. Larson RL. Subluxation-dislocation of the patella. In: Kennedy JC ed. *The injured adolescent knee.* Baltimore: Williams and Wilkins, 1979.
132. Larson RL, Cabaud HE, Slocum DB, James SL, Keenan T, Hutchinson T. The patellar compression syndrome: Surgical treatment by lateral release. *Clin Orthop* 1978;134:158–167.
133. Laurin CA, Dussault R, Levesque HP. The tangential x-ray investigation of the patellofemoral joint: X-ray technique, diagnostic criteria, and interpretation. *Clin Orthop* 1979;144:16–26.
134. Laurin CA, Levesque HP, Dussault R, Labelle H, Peides JP. The abnormal lateral patellofemoral angle. *J Bone Joint Surg* 1978;60A:55–60.
135. Leach RE. Malalignment syndrome of the patella. *Instr Course Lect* 1976;25:49–54.
136. Malghem J, Maldague B. Patellofemoral joint: 30° axial radiograph with lateral rotation of the leg. *Radiology* 1989;170:566–567.
137. Maquet P. Advancement of the tibial tuberosity. *Clin Orthop* 1976;115:225–230.
138. Maquet P. Mechanics and osteoarthritis of the patellofemoral joint. *Clin Orthop* 1979;144:70–73.
139. Mariani PP, Caruso J. Electromyographic investigation of subluxation of the patella. *J Bone Joint Surg* 1979;61B:169–171.
140. Martinez S, Korokken M, Fondren FB, Hedlund LW, Goldner JL. Diagnosis of patellofemoral malalignment by computed tomography. *J Comput Assist Tomogr* 1983;7:1050–1053.
141. Matthews LS, Sonstegard DA, Henke JE. Load bearing characteristics of the patellofemoral joint. *Acta Orthop Scand* 1977;48:511–516.
142. McCarroll JR, O'Donoghue DM, Grana WA. The surgical treatment of chondromalacia of the patella. *Clin Orthop* 1983;175:130–134.
143. McDougall A, Brown D. Radiological sign of recurrent dislocation of the patella. *J Bone Joint Surg* 1968;50B:841–843.
144. Merchant AC, Mercer RL, Jacobsen RM, Cool CR. Roentgenographic analysis of patellofemoral congruence. *J Bone Joint Surg* 1974;56A:1391–1396.
145. Metcalf RW. An arthroscopic method for lateral release of the subluxing or dislocating patella. *Clin Orthop* 1982;167:9–18.
146. Osborne AH, Fulford PC. Lateral release for chondromalacia patellae. *J Bone Joint Surg* 1982;64B:202–205.
147. Outerbridge RE. The etiology of chondromalacia patellae. *J Bone Joint Surg* 1961;43B:752–757.
148. Outerbridge RE. Further studies on the etiology of chondromalacia patellae. *J Bone Joint Surg* 1964;46B:179–190.
149. Outerbridge RE, Dunlop JAY. The problem of chondromalacia patellae. *Clin Orthop* 1975;110:177–197.
150. Perrild C, Hejgaard N, Rosenklint A. Chondromalacia patellae: A radiographic study of the patellofemoral joint. *Acta Orthop Scand* 1982;53:131–134.
151. Perry J, Antonelli D, Ford W. Analysis of knee joint forces during flexed knee stance. *J Bone Joint Surg* 1975;57A:961–967.
152. Reilly DT, Martins M. Experimental analysis of quadriceps muscle force and patellofemoral joint reaction force for various activities. *Acta Orthop Scand* 1972;43:126–137.
153. Saltzman CL, Goulet JA, McClellon RT, Schneider LA, Matthews LS. Results of treatment of displaced patellar fractures by partial patellectomy. *J Bone Joint Surg* 1990;72A:1279–1285.
154. Satku K, Bose K, Seaw M. Habitual subluxation of the patella on extension of the knee. *J Western Pacific Orthop Assn* 1983;19:17–22.
155. Scapinelli R. Blood supply of the human patella. Its relation to ischemic necrosis after fracture. *J Bone Joint Surg* 1967;49B:563–570.
156. Sikorski JM. The importance of femoral rotation in chondromalacia patellae as shown by serial radiography. *J Bone Joint Surg* 1979;61B:435–442.
157. Stanford W, Phelan J, Kathol MH, et al. Patellofemoral joint motion: Evaluation by ultrafast computed tomography. *Skel Radiol* 1988;17:487–492.
158. Thyn CJB, Hiller B. Arthrography and the medial compartment of the patellofemoral joint. *Skel Radiol* 1984;11:183–190.
159. Wiberg G. Roentgenographic and anatomic studies of the femoropatellar joint, with special reference to chondromalacia patellae. *Acta Orthop Scand* 1941;12:319–410.
160. Wissinger HA. Chondromalacia patellae: A nonoperative treatment program. *Orthopedics* 1982;5:315–316.

Fractures about the Knee

161. Anderson PW, Harley JB, Maslin PV. Arthrographic evaluation of problems with united tibial plateau fractures. *Radiology* 1976;119:75–78.
162. Andrews JR, Hughston JC. Treatment of patella fractures by partial patellectomy. *South Med J* 1977;70:809–813.
163. Apley AG. Fractures of the lateral tibial condyle treated by skeletal traction and early mobilization. *J Bone Joint Surg* 1956;38B:699–708.
164. Apley AG. Fractures of the tibial plateau. *Orthop Clin North Am* 1979;10:61–74.
165. Bakalim G, Wilppula F. Fractures of the tibial condyles. *Acta Orthop Scand* 1973;44:311–322.
166. Blake R, McBryde A. The floating knee: Ipsilateral fractures of the tibia and femur. *South Med J* 1975;68:13–16.
167. Boström A. Fracture of the patella. A study of 422 patellar fractures. *Acta Orthop Scand* (Suppl.) 1972;143:1–80.
168. Bowes DN, Hohl M. Tibial condylar fractures. Evaluation of treatment and outcome. *Clin Orthop* 1982;171:104–108.
169. Brown GA, Sprague BL. Cast brace treatment of plateau and bicondylar fractures of the proximal tibia. *Clin Orthop* 1976;119:184–193.
170. Burri C, Bartzke G, Coldewey J, Muggler E. Fractures of the tibial plateau. *Clin Orthop* 1979;138:84–93.
171. DeLee JC. Ipsilateral fracture of the femur and tibia treated in a quadrilateral cast brace. *Clin Orthop* 1979;142:115–122.
172. Dietz GW, Wilcox DM, Montgomery JB. Second tibial condyle fracture: Lateral capsular ligament avulsion. *Radiology* 1986;159:467–469.

173. Dovey H, Heerford J. Tibial condyle fractures: A follow-up of 200 cases. *Acta Chir Scand* 1971;137:521–531.
174. Drennan DB, Locher FC, Maylahn DJ. Fractures of the tibial plateau. Treatment by closed reduction and spica cast. *J Bone Joint Surg* 1979;61A:989–995.
175. Elstrom J, Pankovich AM, Sassoon H, Rodriguez J. The use of tomography in assessment of fractures of the tibial plateau. *J Bone Joint Surg* 1976;58A:551–555.
176. Fraser RD, Hunter GA, Waddel JP. Ipsilateral fracture of the femur and tibia. *J Bone Joint Surg* 1978;60B:510–515.
177. Giles JB, DeLee JC, Heckman JD, Keever JE. Supracondylar-intercondylar fractures of the femur treated with a supracondylar plate and lag screw. *J Bone Joint Surg* 1982;64A:864–870.
178. Gillquist J, Rieger A, Sjodahl R, Bylund P. Multiple fractures of a single leg. *Acta Chir Scand* 1973;139:167–172.
179. Goldman AM, Pavlov H, Rubenstein D. The second fracture of the proximal tibia: A small avulsion fracture that reflects ligamentous damage. *AJR* 1988;151:1163–1167.
180. Gottfries A, Hagert CG, Sorensen SE. T and Y fractures of the tibal condyles. *Injury* 1971;3:56–63.
181. Healy WL, Brooker AF. Distal femoral fractures. Comparison of open and closed methods of treatment. *Clin Orthop* 1983;174:166–171.
182. Hohl M. Treatment methods in tibial condylar fractures. *South Med J* 1975;68:985–991.
183. Hohl M. Tibial condylar fractures: Long-term follow-up. *Tex Med* 1974;70:46–54.
184. Hohl M. Tibial condylar fractures. *J Bone Joint Surg* 1967;49A:1455–1467.
185. Hohl M, Luck JV. Fractures of the tibial condyle. A clinical and experimental study. *J Bone Joint Surg* 1956;38A:1001–1018.
186. Hojer H, Gillquist J, Liljedahl SO. Combined fractures of the femoral and tibial shafts in the same limb. *Injury* 1977;8:206–212.
187. Johnson EW, McLeod JL. Osteochondral fragments of the distal end of the femur fixed with bone pegs. *J Bone Joint Surg* 1977;59A:677–679.
188. Joseph FR. Evaluation of the Zickel supracondylar fixation device. *Clin Orthop* 1982;169:190–196.
189. Karlstrom G, Olerud S. Ipsilateral fracture of the femur and tibia. *J Bone Joint Surg* 1977;59A:240–243.
190. Kennedy JC, Grainger RW, McGraw RW. Osteochondral fractures of the femoral condyle. *J Bone Joint Surg* 1966;48B:436–440.
191. Lansinger O, Bergman B, Korner L, Andersson GBJ. Tibial condylar fractures: A twenty year follow-up. *J Bone Joint Surg* 1986;68A:13–18.
192. Lee J, Weissman B, Nikpoor N, Aliabodi P, Sosman JL. Lipo-hemarthrosis of the knee: A review of recent experiences. *Radiology* 1989;173:181–191.
193. Lucht V, Pilgaard S. Fractures of the tibial condyles. *Acta Orthop Scand* 1971;42:366–376.
194. Manco LG, Schneider R, Pavlov H. Insufficiency fractures of the tibial plateau. *AJR* 1983;140:1211–1215.
195. Mathewson MH, Dandy DJ. Osteochondral fractures of the lateral femoral condyle. A result of indirect violence to the knee. *J Bone Joint Surg* 1978;60B:199–202.
196. Merkel K, Johnson EW. Supracondylar fracture of the femur after total knee arthroplasty. *J Bone Joint Surg* 1986;68A:29–43.
197. Milgram JE. Tangential osteochondral fracture of the patella. *J Bone Joint Surg* 1943;25:271–280.
198. Mize RD, Bucholz RW, Gregor DP. Surgical treatment of displaced comminuted fractures of the distal end of the femur. *J Bone Joint Surg* 1982;64A:871–879.
199. Mooney V, Nickel VL, Harvey JP, Snelson R. Cast-brace treatment for fractures of the distal part of the femur. *J Bone Joint Surg* 1970;52A:1563–1578.
200. Moore TM, Harvey JP. Roentgenographic measurement of tibial plateau depression due to fracture. *J Bone Joint Surg* 1974;56A:155–160.
201. Moore TM, Meyers MH, Harvey JP. Collateral ligament laxity of the knee: Long-term comparison between plateau fractures and normal. *J Bone Joint Surg* 1976;58A:594–598.
202. Neer CS, Grantham A, Sheldon ML. Supracondylar fracture of the adult femur. A study of one hundred and ten cases. *J Bone Joint Surg* 1967;49A:591–613.
203. O'Donoghue DM. Chondral and osteochondral fractures. *J Trauma* 1966;6:469–481.
204. Olerud S. Operative treatment of supracondylar-condylar fractures of the femur. *J Bone Joint Surg* 1972;54A:1015–1032.
205. Omer GE, Moll JH, Bacon WL. Combined fractures of the femur and tibia in a single extremity. *J Trauma* 1968;8:1026–1040.
206. Porter BB. Crush fractures of the lateral tibial table. Factors influencing the prognosis. *J Bone Joint Surg* 1970;52B:676–687.
207. Rofii M, Firooznic H, Golimbu C, Bonamo J. Computed tomography of tibial plateau fractures. *AJR* 1984;142:1181–1186.
208. Rand JA, Coventry MB. Stress fractures after total knee arthroplasty. *J Bone Joint Surg* 1980;62A:226–233.
209. Rasmussen PS. Lateral condylar fracture of the tiba. *Acta Orthop Scand* 1971;42:429–464.
210. Rasmussen PS. Tibial condylar fractures as a cause of degenerative arthritis. *Acta Orthop Scand* 1972;43:566–575.
211. Rasmussen PS. Tibial condylar fractures. Impairment of knee joint stability as an indication for surgical treatment. *J Bone Joint Surg* 1973;55A:1331–1350.
212. Rasmussen PS, Sorensen SE. Tibial condylar fractures. Nonoperative treatment of lateral compression fractures without impairment of knee joint stability. *Injury* 1973;4:265–271.
213. Reibel D, Wade P. Fractures of the tibial plateau. *J Trauma* 1962;2:337–352.
214. Riggins RS, Garrick JG, Lipscomb PR. Supracondylar fractures at the femur. *Clin Orthop* 1972;82:32–36.
215. Rorabeck CH, Bobechko WP. Acute dislocation of the patella with osteochondral fracture. *J Bone Joint Surg* 1976;58B:237–240.
216. Sarminento A, Kinman PB, Latta LL. Fractures of the proximal tibia and tibial condyles: A clinical and laboratory comparative study. *Clin Orthop* 1979;145:136–145.
217. Satkin K, Kumor VP, Chacha PB. Stress fractures around the knee in elderly patients. *J Bone Joint Surg* 1990;72A:918–922.
218. Scapinelli R. Blood supply of the human patella. Its relation to ischemic necrosis after fracture. *J Bone Joint Surg* 1967;49B:563–570.
219. Schatzker J, Horne G, Waddel J. The Toronto experience with the supracondylar fracture of the femur: 1966–1972. *Injury* 1975;6:113–128.
220. Schatzker J, Lambert DC. Supracondylar fractures of the femur. *Clin Orthop* 1979;138:77–83.
221. Schatzker J, McBroom R, Bruce D. The tibial plateau fracture. The Toronto experience: 1968–1975. *Clin Orthop* 1979;138:94–104.
222. Schulak DJ, Gunn DR. Fractures of the tibial plateau. A review of the literature. *Clin Orthop* 1975;109:167–177.
223. Scotland T, Wardlaw D. The use of cast-bracing as treatment for fractures of the tibial plateau. *J Bone Joint Surg* 1981;63B:575–578.
224. Seinsheimer F. Fractures of the distal femur. *Clin Orthop* 1980;153:169–180.
225. Shelton ML, Neer CS, Grantham SA. Occult knee ligament ruptures associated with fractures. *J Trauma* 1971;11:853–856.
226. Sorensen KH. The late prognosis after fracture of the patella. *Acta Orth Scand* 1964;34:198–212.
227. Stewart MJ, Sisk TD, Wallace SL. Fractures of the distal third of the femur. A comparison of methods of treatment. *J Bone Joint Surg* 1966;48A:784–807.
228. Weber MJ, Janecki J, McLeod P, Nelson CL, Thompson JA. Efficacy of various forms of fixation of transverse fractures of the patella. *J Bone Joint Surg* 1980;62A:215–220.
229. Wilkinson J. Fracture of the patella treated by total excision. A long-term follow-up. *J Bone Joint Surg* 1977;59B:352–354.
230. Winston ME. The results of conservative treatment of fractures of the femur and tibia in the same limb. *Surg Gynecol Obstet* 1972;134:985–991.
231. Wilppula E, Bakalim G. Ligamentous tear concomitant with tibial condylar fracture. *Acta Orthop Scand* 1972;43:292–300.
232. Zickel RE, Fieti VG, Lawsing JF, Cochran GVB. A new intramedullary fixation device for the distal third of the femur. *Clin Orthop* 1977;125:185–191.

Soft Tissue and Articular Disorders

Ligamentous Injuries of the Knee

233. Arnold JA, Coker TP, Heaton LM, Park JP, Harris WD. Natural history of anterior cruciate tears. *Am J Sports Med* 1979;7:305–313.
234. Baker CL, Norwood LA, Hughston JC. Acute posterolateral rotatory instability of the knee. *J Bone Joint Surg* 1983;65A:614–618.
235. Balkfors B. The course of knee-ligament injuries. *Acta Orthop Scand* (Suppl.) 1982;198:1–99.
236. Cabaud HE, Slocum DB. The diagnosis of chronic antero-lateral rotatory instability of the knee. *Am J Sports Med* 1977;5:99–104.
237. Clancy WG, Ray M, Zoltan DJ. Acute tears of the anterior cruciate ligament: Surgical vs. conservative treatment. *J Bone Joint Surg* 1988;70A:1483–1488.
238. DeHaven KE. Arthroscopy in the diagnosis and management of anterior cruciate ligament deficient knee. *Clin Orthop* 1983;172:52–56.
239. Feagin JA. The syndrome of the torn anterior cruciate ligament. *Orthop Clin North Am* 1979;10:81–90.
240. Feagin JA, Abbott HG, Rokous JR. The isolated tear of the anterior cruciate ligament. *J Bone Joint Surg* 1972;54A:1340–1341.
241. Feagin JA, Curl WW. Isolated tear of the anterior cruciate ligament: 5-year follow-up study. *Am J Sports Med* 1976;4:95–100.
242. Fetto JF, Marshall JL. Injury to the anterior cruciate ligament producing the pivot-shift sign. *J Bone Joint Surg* 1979;61A:710–714.
243. Fetto JF, Marshall JL. The natural history and diagnosis of anterior cruciate ligament insufficiency. *Clin Orthop* 1980;147:29–38.
244. Fowler PJ. The classification and early diagnosis of knee joint instability. *Clin Orthop* 1980;147:15–21.
245. Gallie WE, LeMesurier AB. The repair of injuries to the posterior cruciate ligament of the knee joint. *Am Surg* 1927;85:592–598.
246. Galway RD, Beaupre A, McIntosh DL. Pivot shift: A clinical sign of symptomatic anterior cruciate insufficiency. *J Bone Joint Surg* 1972;54B:763–764.
247. Galway HR, McIntosh DL. The lateral pivot shift: A symptom and sign of anterior cruciate insufficiency. *Clin Orthop* 1980;147:45–50.
248. Giove TP, Miller SJ, Kent BE, Sanford TL, Garrich JG. Non-operative treatment of the torn anterior cruciate ligament. *J Bone Joint Surg* 1983;56A:184–192.
249. Hey Groves EW. The crucial ligaments of the knee joint: Their function, rupture and the operative treatment of the same. *Br J Surg* 1920;7:505–515.
250. Hey Groves EW. Operation for the repair of the crucial ligaments. *Lancet* 1917;2:674–675.
251. Hughston JC, Andrews JR, Cross MJ, Arnoldo M. Classification of knee ligament instabilities. Part I. The medial compartment and cruciate ligaments. *J Bone Joint Surg* 1976;58A:159–179.
252. Hughston JC, Andrews JR, Cross MJ, Arnoldo M. Classification of knee ligament instabilities. Part II. The lateral compartment. *J Bone Joint Surg* 1976;58A:173–179.
253. Hughston JC, Barret GR. Acute anteromedial rotatory instability. Long-term results of surgical repair. *J Bone Joint Surg* 1983;56A:145–153.
254. Hughston JC, Bowden JA, Andrews JR, Norwood LA. Acute tears of the posterior cruciate ligament. *J Bone Joint Surg* 1980;62A:438–450.
255. Hughston JC, Norwood LA. The posterolateral drawer test and external rotational recurvatum test for posterolateral rotatory instability of the knee. *Clin Orthop* 1980;147:82–87.
256. Indelicato PA. Nonoperative treatment of complete tears of the medial collateral ligament of the knee. *J Bone Joint Surg* 1983;65A:323–329.
257. Jakob RP, Hassler H, Staeubli HV. Observations on rotatory instability of the lateral compartment of the knee. *Acta Orthop Scand* (Suppl.) 1981;191:1–27.
258. Kennedy JD, Grainger RW. The posterior cruciate ligament. *J Trauma* 1967;7:367–377.
259. Kennedy JC, Weinberg H, Wilson A. The anatomy and function of the anterior cruciate ligament. *J Bone Joint Surg* 1974;56A:223–235.
260. Larson RL. Physical examination in the diagnosis of rotatory instability. *Clin Orthop* 1983;172:38–44.
261. Liljedahl S, Lindvall N, Wetterfors J. Early diagnosis and treatment of acute ruptures of the anterior cruciate ligament. *J Bone Joint Surg* 1965;47A:1503–1513.
262. Lipke J, Janecki CJ, Nelson CL, et al. The role of incompetence of the anterior cruciate and lateral ligaments in anterolateral and anteromedial instability. *J Bone Joint Surg* 1981;63A:954–960.
263. Lipscomb AB, Anderson AF. Tears of the anterior cruciate ligament in adolescents. *J Bone Joint Surg* 1986;68A:19–28.
264. Losee RE. Concepts of the pivot shift. *Clin Orthop* 1985;172:45–51.
265. Losee RE, Johnson TR, Southwick WO. Anterior subluxation of the lateral tibial plateau. *J Bone Joint Surg* 1978;60A:1015–1030.
266. Manaster BJ, Remley K, Newman AP, Mann FA. Knee ligament reconstruction: Plain film analysis. *AJR* 1988;150:337–342.
267. McDaniel WJ, Dameron JB. Untreated ruptures of the anterior cruciate ligament. *J Bone Joint Surg* 1980;62A:696–705.
268. Meyers MH. Isolated avulsion of the tibial attachment of the posterior cruciate ligament of the knee. *J Bone Joint Surg* 1975;57A:669–672.
269. Nicholas JA. Bracing the anterior cruciate ligament deficient knee using the Lenox Hill derotation brace. *Clin Orthop* 1983;172:137–142.
270. Norwood LA, Andrews JR, Meisterling RC, Glancy CL. Acute anterolateral rotatory instability of the knee. *J Bone Joint Surg* 1979;61A:704–709.
271. Noyes FR, Bassett RW, Grood ES, et al. Arthroscopy in acute traumatic hemarthrosis of the knee. *J Bone Joint Surg* 1980;62A:687–695.
272. Noyes FR, Butler DL, Paulos LE, Grood ES. Intra-articular cruciate reconstruction. I. Perspectives on graft strength, vascularization, and immediate motion after replacement. *Clin Orthop* 1983;173:71–77.
273. Noyes FR, Matthews DS, Mooar PA, Grood ES. The symptomatic anterior cruciate deficient knee. Part II: The results of rehabilitation, activity modification, and counseling on functional disability. *J Bone Joint Surg* 1983;65A:163–174.
274. Noyes FR, Mooar PA, Matthews DS, Butler DL. The symptomatic anterior cruciate deficient knee. Part I: The long-term functional disability in athletically active individuals. *J Bone Joint Surg* 1983;65A:154–162.
275. O'Donoghue DH. An analysis of end results of surgical treatment of major injuries to the ligaments of the knee. *J Bone Joint Surg* 1955;37A:1–13.
276. O'Donoghue DH. A method for replacement of the anterior cruciate ligament of the knee. *J Bone Joint Surg* 1963;45A:905–924.
277. Palmer I. Injuries to the cruciate ligaments of the knee joint as a surgical problem. *Wiederherstellungschirurgie und Traumatologie* 1957;4:181–196.
278. Pavlov H. The radiographic diagnosis of the anterior cruciate ligament deficient knee. *Clin Orthop* 1983;172:57–64.
279. Slocum DB, James JL, Larson RL, Surger KM. Clinical test for anterolateral rotatory instability of the knee. *Clin Orthop* 1976;118:63–69.
280. Slocum DB, Larson RL. Rotatory instability of the knee. *J Bone Joint Surg* 1968;50A:212–225.
281. Tamea CD, Hening CE. Pathomechanics of the pivot shift maneuver. An instant center analysis. *Am J Sports Med* 1981;9:31–37.
282. Torisu T. Isolated avulsion fracture of the tibial attachment of the posterior cruciate ligament. *J Bone Joint Surg* 1977;59A:68–72.
283. Trickey EL. Rupture of the posterior cruciate ligament of the knee. *J Bone Joint Surg* 1968;50B:334–341.
284. Woods GW, Stanley RF, Tullos HS. Lateral capsular sign: X-ray clue to a significant knee instability. *Am J Sports Med* 1979;7:27–33.

Knee Arthroscopy and Imaging Techniques for Articular and Periarticular Disorders

285. Aisen AM, McCune WJ, MacGuire A, et al. Sonographic evaluation of the cartilage of the knee. *Radiology* 1984;153:781–784.

286. Anderson PW, Harley JD, Mosler RT. Arthrographic evaluation of problems with ununited tibial plateau fractures. *Radiology* 1976;119:75–78.
287. Apple JS, Martinez S, Hardaker WT, Daffner RH, Geweiler JA. Synovial plicae of the knee. *Skeletal Radiol* 1982;7:251–254.
288. Apple JS, Martinez S, Khoury MB, Royster R, Allen S. A comparison of Hexabrix and Renografin-60 in knee arthrography. *AJR* 1985;145:139–142.
289. Aritomi H, Yamamoto M. A method of arthroscopic surgery. Clinical evaluation of synovectomy with the electric resectoscope and removal of loose bodies in the knee joint. *Orthop Clin North Am* 1979;10:565–584.
290. Bassett LW, Grover JS, Seeger LL. Magnetic resonance imaging of knee trauma. *Skel Radiol* 1990;19:401–405.
291. Berquist TH. *Magnetic resonance of the musculoskeletal system,* 2nd ed. New York: Raven Press, 1990.
292. Bernstein RM, Folsson HE, Spitzer RM, Robinson KS, Korn MW. Ossicle of the meniscus. *AJR* 1976;127:785–788.
293. Boven F, Bellemans MA, Geurts J, Potvliege R. A comparative study of the patellofemoral joint on axial roentgenograms, axial arthrogram, and CT following arthrography. *Skeletal Radiol* 1982;8:179–181.
294. Boven F, De Boeck M, Polvliege R. Synovial plicae of the knee on CT. *Radiology* 1983;147:805–809.
295. Brody GA, Pavlov H, Warren RF, Ghelman B. Plica synovialis intrapatellaris: Arthrographic significance of anterior cruciate ligament disruption. *AJR* 1983;140:767–769.
296. Broukhim B, Fox JM, Blazina ME, DelPizzo W, Hirsh L. The synovial shelf syndrome. *Clin Orthop* 1979;142:135–138.
297. Brown EW, Allman FL, Eaton SB. Knee arthrography. A comparison of radiographic and surgical findings in 295 cases. *Am J Sports Med* 1978;6:165–172.
298. Burman MS. Arthroscopy or the direct visualization of joints. An experimental cadaver study. *J Bone Joint Surg* 1931;13:669–695.
299. Cargill AOR, Jackson JP. Bucket-handle tear of the medial meniscus. A case for conservative surgery. *J Bone Joint Surg* 1976;58A:248–251.
300. Carlson JW, Gyori M, Kaufman L. A technique for MR imaging of the knee under large flexing angles. *Mag Res Imaging* 1990;8:407–410.
301. Carruthers CC, Kennedy M. Knee arthroscopy: A follow-up of patients initially not recommended for further surgery. *Clin Orthop* 1980;147:275–277.
302. Casscells SW. Arthroscopy of the knee joint. A review of 150 cases. *J Bone Joint Surg* 1971;53A:287–298.
303. Casscells SW. The place of arthroscopy in the diagnosis and treatment of internal derangement of the knee. *Clin Orthop* 1980;151:135–142.
304. Clanton TO, DeLee JC. Osteochondritis dissecans. History, pathophysiology and current treatment concepts. *Clin Orthop* 1982;167:50–64.
305. Corbetti F, Malatesta V, Composampiero A, et al. Knee arthrography: Effects of various contrast media and epinephrine on synovial fluid. *Radiology* 1986;161:195–198.
306. Crabtree SD, Bedford AF, Edgar MA. The value of arthrography and arthroscopy in association with a sports injury clinic: A prospective and comparative study of 182 patients. *Injury* 1981;13:220–226.
307. Crues JV, Mink J, Levy TL, Lotysch M, Stoller DW. Meniscal tears of the knee: Accuracy of MR imaging. *Radiology* 1987;164:445–448.
308. Curran WP Jr, Woodward P. Arthroscopy: Its role in diagnosis and treatment of athletic knee injuries. *Am J Sports Med* 1980;8:415–418.
309. Dalinka MK. *Arthrography.* New York: Springer-Verlag, 1980.
310. Dalinka MK, Garofola J. The infrapatellar synovial fold: A cause for confusion in the evaluation of the anterior cruciate ligament. *AJR* 1976;127:589–591.
311. Dalinka MK, Gohel VK, Rancer L. Tomography in evaluation of the anterior cruciate ligament. *Radiology* 1973;108:31–33.
312. Dandy DJ, Flanagan JP, Stenmeyer V. Arthroscopy and the management of the ruptured anterior cruciate ligament. *Clin Orthop* 1983;167:43–49.
313. Dandy DJ, Jackson RW. The diagnosis of problems after meniscectomy. *J Bone Joint Surg* 1975;57B:349–352.
314. Dandy DJ, Jackson RW. The impact of arthroscopy on the management of disorders of the knee. *J Bone Joint Surg* 1975;57B:346–348.
315. Dandy DJ, O'Carroll PF. The removal of loose bodies from the knee under arthroscopic control. *J Bone Joint Surg* 1982;64B:473–474.
316. Debnam JW, Staple TW. Arthrography of the knee after meniscectomy. *Radiology* 1974;113:67–71.
317. DeHaven KE. Arthroscopy in the diagnosis and management of the anterior cruciate ligament deficient knee. *Clin Orthop* 1983;172:52–56.
318. DeHaven KE. Diagnosis of acute knee injuries with hemarthrosis. *Am J Sports Med* 1980;8:9–14.
319. DeHaven KE. Peripheral meniscus repair. An alternative to meniscectomy. *Orthop Trans* 1981;5:399.
320. DeHaven KE, Collins HR. Diagnosis of internal derangement of the knee. *J Bone Joint Surg* 1975;57A:802–810.
321. DeSmet AA, Neff JR. Knee arthrography for preoperative evaluation of juxta-articular masses. *Radiology* 1982;143:663.
322. DeSmet AA, Fisher DR, Graf BK, Lange RH. Osteochondritis dissecans of the knee: Value of MR imaging in determining lesion stability and the presence of articular cartilage defects. *AJR* 1990;155:549–553.
323. Deutsch AL, Resnick D, Dalinka MK, et al. Synovial plicae of the knee. *Radiology* 1981;141:627–634.
324. Deutsch AL, Mink JH, Fox JM, et al. Peripheral meniscal tears: MR findings after conservative treatment or arthroscopic repair. *Radiology* 1990;176:485–488.
325. Dillon EH, Pope CF, Jokl P, Lynch K. The clinical significance of stage 2 meniscal abnormalities on magnetic resonance knee images. *Mag Res Imag* 1990;8:411–415.
326. Dumas J, Edde DJ. Prospective correlation of double-contrast arthrography and arthroscopy. *Radiology* 1986;160:453–456.
327. Dunbar WH. Incremental patellar tracking: A simple method of evaluation. Arthroscopy Association of North America. Chicago, 1982.
328. Ficat RP, Philippe J, Hungerford DS. Chondromalacia patellae: A system of classification. *Clin Orthop* 1979;144:55–62.
329. Finkelstein H, Mayer L. The arthroscope: A new method of examining joints. *J Bone Joint Surg* 1931;13:583–588.
330. Flavus LD, Scaghion OP, Nessie R, Albisetti W. Ultrasound in degenerative cystic meniscal disease of the knee. *Skel Radiol* 1990;19:441–445.
331. Fornasier VL, Czitrom AH, Evans JA, Hastings DE. Case report 398: Friction by pes anserinus. *Skel Radiol* 1987;16:57–59.
332. Frede TE, Lee JK. The "overturned" lateral view on arthrography of the knee. *Radiology* 1980;134:249.
333. Frieberger RH, Kaye JJ. *Arthrography.* New York: Appleton-Century-Crofts, 1979.
334. Frieberger RH, Pavlov H. Knee arthrography. *Radiology* 1988;166:489–492.
335. Ghelman MI, Dunn HK. Radiology of the knee in joint replacement. *AJR* 1979;127:447–455.
336. Ghelman B. Meniscal tears of the knee: Evaluation by high-resolution CT combined with arthrography. *Radiology* 1985;157:23–27.
337. Gillies H, Seligson D. Precision in the diagnosis of meniscal lesions: A comparison of clinical evaluation, arthrography, and arthroscopy. *J Bone Joint Surg* 1979;61A:343–346.
338. Gillquist J, Hagberg G. Findings of arthroscopy and arthrography in knee injuries. *Acta Orthop Scand* 1978;49:398–402.
339. Gillquist J, Hagberg G, Oretorp N. Arthroscopy in acute injuries of the knee joint. *Acta Orthop Scand* 1977;48:190–196.
340. Gillquist J, Oretorp N. Arthroscopic partial meniscectomy, technique, and long-term results. *Clin Orthop* 1982;167:29–33.
341. Goldberg RP, Hall FM, Wyshak G. Pain in knee arthrography: Comparison of air vs. CO_2 and reaspiration vs. no reaspiration. *AJR* 1981;136:377–379.
342. Griffiths HJ, D'Orsi CJ. Use of xeroradiography in cruciate ligament injury. *AJR* 1974;121:94–96.
343. Guhl JF. Arthroscopic treatment of osteochondritis dissecans: A preliminary report. *Orthop Clin North Am* 1979;10:617–683.
344. Guhl JF. Arthroscopic treatment of osteochondritis dissecans. *Clin Orthop* 1982;167:65–74.

345. Hall FM. Arthrography of the discoid lateral meniscus. *AJR* 1977;128:993–1002.
346. Hall FM. Buckled meniscus. *Radiology* 1978;126:89–90.
347. Hall FM. Further pitfalls in knee arthrography. *J Can Assoc Radiol* 1978;29:179–184.
348. Hall FM. Methodology in knee arthrography. *Radiol Clin North Am* 1981;19:269–275.
349. Hall FM. Pitfalls in knee arthrography. *Radiology* 1976;118:55–62.
350. Hall FM. Pitfalls in the assessment of menisci by knee arthrography. *Radiol Clin North Am* 1981;19:305–328.
351. Halpern AA, Donovan TL, Horowitz B, et al. Arthrographic demonstration of pigmented villonodular synovitis of the knee. *Clin Orthop* 1978;132:193–195.
352. Hamburg P, Gillquist J, Lysholm J. Suture of new and old peripheral meniscus tears. *J Bone Joint Surg* 1983;65A:193–197.
353. Hardaker WT, Whipple TL, Bassett FH. Diagnosis and treatment of plica syndrome of the knee. *J Bone Joint Surg* 1980;62A:221–225.
354. Hargreaves DJ, Seedhom BB. On the bucket-handle tear: Partial or total meniscectomy? A quantitative study. *J Bone Joint Surg* 1979;61B:381.
355. Harley JD. An anatomic arthrographic study of the relationship of the lateral meniscus and popliteus tendon. *AJR* 1977;128:181–187.
356. Hermann J, Alvarez E, Lavine LS. Value of knee arthrography in non-meniscal damage. *NY State J Med* 1977;77:916–920.
357. Hermann J, Yeh H, Lehr-Janus C, et al. Diagnosis of popliteal cyst: Double-contrast arthrography and sonography. *AJR* 1981;137:369.
358. Highgenboten CL. Arthroscopic synovectomy. *Orthop Clin North Am* 1982;13:399–405.
359. Hirschowitz D. Clinical assessment, arthrography, arthroscopy, and arthrotomy in the diagnosis of internal derangement of the knee. *J Bone Joint Surg* 1976;58B:367.
360. Horn JW. The diagnosis of chondromalacia by double-contrast arthrography of the knee. *J Bone Joint Surg* 1977;59A:119–120.
361. Iino S. Normal arthroscopic findings of the knee in adult cadavers. *J Jap Orthop Assoc* 1939;14:467–523.
362. Ingman AM, Ghosh P, Taylor TKF. Variations of collagenous and non-collagenous proteins of human knee meniscus with age and degeneration. *Gerontology* 1974;20:212–223.
363. Insall J, Falvo KA, Wise DW. Chondromalacia patella. *J Bone Joint Surg* 1976;58A:1–8.
364. Ireland J, Trickey EL, Stoker DJ. Arthroscopy and arthrography of the knee. *J Bone Joint Surg* 1980;62B:3–6.
365. Jackson RW. Current concepts review. Arthroscopic surgery. *J Bone Joint Surg* 1983;65A:416–420.
366. Jackson RW, Abe I. The role of arthroscopy in the management of disorders of the knee. *J Bone Joint Surg* 1972;54B:310–322.
367. Jackson RW, Marshall DJ, Fujisawa Y. The pathologic medial shelf. *Orthop Clin North Am* 1982;13:307–312.
368. Jelaso DV. The fascicles of the lateral meniscus: An anatomic-arthrographic correlation. *Radiology* 1975;114:335–339.
369. Jelaso DV, Morris GA. Rupture of the quadriceps tendon: Diagnosis by arthrography. *Radiology* 1975;116:621–622.
370. Johanson JJ, Lilleas FG, Nordshus T. Arthrography of the knee joint with Amipaque. *Acta Radiol (Diagn.)* 1977;18:523.
371. Johnson LL. Arthroscopic abrasion arthroplasty. 50th Annual Meeting, American Academy of Orthopedic Surgeons. Anaheim, CA, 1983.
372. Johnson LL. Impact of diagnostic arthroscopy on the clinical judgement of an experienced arthroscopist. *Clin Orthop* 1982;167:75–83.
373. Kaplan EB. Discoid lateral meniscus of the knee joint. *J Bone Joint Surg* 1957;39A:77–87.
374. Korn MW, Spitzer RM, Robinson KE. Correlations of arthrography with arthroscopy. *Orthop Clin North Am* 1979;10:535–543.
375. Kyo RL, Bigongiari LR. A modern catheter needle for knee arthrography. *Radiology* 1979;132:743–744.
376. Levinsohn EM, Baker BE. Pre-arthrotomy diagnostic evaluation of the knee. A review of 100 cases diagnosed by arthrography and arthroscopy. *AJR* 1980;134:107–111.
377. Levy MI, Torzilli PA, Dould JD, Warren RP. The effect of lateral meniscectomy on motion of the knee. *J Bone Joint Surg* 1989;71A:401–406.
378. Lindblom K. The arthrographic appearance of the ligaments of the knee joint. *Acta Radiol (Suppl)* 1984;74:1–112.
379. Linden B. Osteochondritis dissecans of the femoral condyle: A long-term follow-up study. *J Bone Joint Surg* 1977;59A:769–776.
380. Linson MA, Posner IF. Synovial hemarthrosis as a cause of recurrent knee effusion. *JAMA* 1979;242:2214–2215.
381. Lyu SR, Wu JJ. Snapping syndrome caused by the semitendinosus tendon. *J Bone Joint Surg* 1989;71A:303–305.
382. Major M, Johnson RP, Carrera E, Hussey C. Arthrographic pseudoloosening of Marmar TKA in hemophilic arthropathy. *Clin Orthop* 1981;160:114–117.
383. Manco LG, Kavanagh JH, Fray JJ, Bilfield BS. Meniscus tears of the knee: Prospective evaluation with CT. *Radiology* 1986;159:147–151.
384. McGinty JB. Arthroscopic removal of loose bodies. *Orthop Clin North Am* 1976;13:173–180.
385. McGinty JB, Freedman PA. Arthroscopy of the knee. *Clin Orthop* 1976;121:173–180.
386. McGinty JB, Geuss LF, Marvin RA. Partial or total meniscectomy: A comparative analysis. *J Bone Joint Surg* 1977;59A:763–766.
387. Metcalf RW. An arthroscopic method for lateral release of the subluxing or dislocating patella. *Clin Orthop* 1982;167:9–18.
388. Metcalf RW, Coward DB, Rosenberg TD. Arthroscopic partial meniscectomy: A five-year follow-up study. 50th Annual Meeting. American Academy of Orthopedic Surgeons. Anaheim, CA, 1983.
389. Miller GK, Dickerson JM, Fox JM, et al. The use of electrosurgery for arthroscopic subcutaneous lateral release. *Orthopedics* 1982;5:309–314.
390. Mink JH, Dickerson R. Air or CO_2 for knee arthrography? *AJR* 1980;134:991–993.
391. Mital MA, Hayden J. Pain in the knee in children: The medial plica shelf syndrome. *Orthop Clin North Am* 1979;10:713–722.
392. Nelson DW, DiPaola J, Colville M, Schmidgall J. Osteochondritis dissecans of the talus and knee: Prospective comparison of MR and arthroscopic classifications. 1990;14:804–808.
393. Nicholas JA, Freiberger RH, Killoran PJ. Double-contrast arthrography of the knee. *J Bone Joint Surg* 1970;52A:203–220.
394. Noble J, Hamblen DL. The pathology of the degenerative meniscus of the knee. *J Bone Joint Surg* 1975;57A:180–186.
395. Northmore-Ball MD, Dandy DJ. Long-term results of arthroscopic partial meniscectomy. *Clin Orthop* 1982;167:34–42.
396. Norwood LA, Shields CL Jr, Russo J, et al. Arthroscopy of the lateral meniscus in knees with normal arthrograms. *Am J Sports Med* 1977;5:271–274.
397. Noyes FR, Bassett RW, Grood ES, Butler DL. Arthroscopy in acute traumatic hemarthrosis of the knee. *J Bone Joint Surg* 1980;62A:687–694.
398. Obermann WR, Bloem JL, Hermans J. Knee arthrography. Comparison of Iotrolan and Ioxaglate sodium meglumine. *Radiology* 1989;173:197–201.
399. O'Connor RL. Arthroscopy in the diagnosis and treatment of acute ligament injuries of the knee. *J Bone Joint Surg* 1974;56A:333–337.
400. O'Connor RL. The arthroscope in the management of crystal induced synovitis of the knee. *J Bone Joint Surg* 1973;55A:1443–1449.
401. O'Connor RL, Shahriaree H, Sprague N, Auerbach B. Six years follow-up on arthroscopic excision of bucket-handle tears. *Orthop Trans* 1981;5:401.
402. Passariello R, Trecco F, deParilis F, Masciocchi C, Bonanni G, Zobel BB. Meniscal lesions of the knee joint. CT diagnoses. *Radiology* 1985;157:29–34.
403. Passariello R, Trecco F, DePaulis F, Bonanni G, Masciocchi C, Zobel BB. Computed tomography of the knee joint: Technique of study and normal anatomy. *J Comput Assist Tomogr* 1983;7:1035–1042.
404. Patel D. Arthroscopy of the plicae-synovial folds and their significance. *Am J Sports Med* 1978;6:217–225.
405. Pavlov H, Goldman AB. The popliteus bursa: An indicator of subtle pathology. *AJR* 1979;134:313–321.

406. Pavlov H, Hirschy JC, Torg JS. CT of the cruciate ligament. *Radiology* 1979;132:389–393.
407. Pavlov H, Schneider R. Extrameniscal abnormalities as diagnosed by knee arthrography. *Radiol Clin North Am* 1981;19:287–304.
408. Pavlov H, Warren RF, Sherman MT, Cayea PD. The accuracy of double-contrast arthrographic evaluation of the anterior cruciate ligament. *J Bone Joint Surg* 1983;65A:175–183.
409. Pavlov H. The radiographic diagnosis of the anterior cruciate ligament deficient knee. *Clin Orthop* 1983;172:57–64.
410. Prager RJ, Mall JC. Arthrographic diagnosis of synovial chondromatosis. *AJR* 1976;127:344–346.
411. Resnick D, Newell JD, Guerra J Jr. Proximal tibiofibular joint: Anatomic pathological-radiographic correlation. *AJR* 1978; 131:133–138.
412. Robinson SC. Bacillus cereus septic arthritis following arthrography. *Clin Orthop* 1979;145:237–238.
413. Roebuck EJ. Double-contrast knee arthrography. Some new points of technology including the use of Dimer X. *Clin Radiol* 1977;28:247–257.
414. Rosenthal DI, Murray WT, Jauernek RR, et al. Stressing the knee joint for arthrography. *Radiology* 1980;134:250–251.
415. Sadler RB, Jigarjian A, Picchione PV, et al. Pseudomasses on the supra-patellar pouch at arthrography. *J Can Assoc Radiol* 1980;31:251–253.
416. Salazar JE, Sebes JI, Scott RL. The supine view in double-contrast knee arthrography. *AJR* 1983;141:585–586.
417. Salazar JE, Duke RA, Winer-Muran HT. Locking and unlocking of the knee: Arthrographic demonstration. *AJR* 1986;146:575–576.
418. Schneider D. Arthroscopy and arthroscopic surgery in patellar problems. *Orthop Clin North Am* 1982;13:407–413.
419. Schuldt DR, Wolfe RD. Clinical and arthrographical findings in meniscal cysts. *Radiology* 1980;134:49–52.
420. Sedwick WJ, Guerra J, Danzig LA, et al. Wear particles: Their value in knee arthrography. *Radiology* 1980;136:11–14.
421. Seidl G, Scherak O, Hofner W. Antefemoral dissecting cysts in rheumatoid arthritis. *Radiology* 1979;133:343–347.
422. Shellock FG, Mink JH, Deutsch AL, Fox JM. Patellar tracking abnormalities: Clinical experience with kinematic MR imaging in 130 patients. *Radiology* 1989;172:799–804.
423. Schwemmer M, Edelstein G, Heiken JP, Gilula LA. Synovial cysts of the knee: CT evaluation. *Radiology* 1985;154:175–177.
424. Singson RD, Feldman F, Staron R, Kierson H. MR imaging of displaced bucket handle tear of the medial meniscus. *AJR* 1991;156:121–124.
425. Spataro RF, Katzberg RW, Burgener FA, et al. Epinephrine enhanced knee arthrography. *Invest Radiol* 1978;13:286.
426. Staple TW. Extrameniscal lesions demonstrated by double-contrast arthrography of the knee. *Radiology* 1972;102:311–319.
427. Stoker DJ, Renston P, Fulton A. The value of arthrography of internal derangement of the knee: The first 1,000 are the worst. *Clin Radiol* 1981;32:557–566.
428. Stoller DW, Martin C, Crues JV, Kaplan L, Mark JH. Meniscal tears: Pathologic correlation with MR imaging. *Radiology* 1987;163:731–735.
429. Stone RG. Peripheral detachment of the menisci of the knee: A preliminary report. *Orthop Clin North Am* 1979;10:643–658.
430. Takagi K. *Arthroscope Clin Orthop* 1982;167:6–9.
431. Tapper EM, Hoover NW. Late results after meniscectomy. *J Bone Joint Surg* 1969;51A:517–526.
432. Tegtmeyer CJ, McCue FC, Higgins SM, et al. Arthrography of the knee: A comparative study of the accuracy of single- and double-contrast techniques. *Radiology* 1979;132:37–42.
433. Trecco F, DePaulis F, Bonanni G, et al. The use of computerized tomography in the study of the cruciate ligaments of the knee. *Ital J Orthop traumatol* 1984;10:109–120.
434. Watanabe M, Takeda S, Ikeuchi H. *Atlas of arthroscopy.* 3d ed. Tokyo: Igaku Shoin, 1978.
435. Watt I, Tasker T. Pitfalls in double-contrast knee arthrography. *Br J Radiol* 1980;53:754–759.
436. Weiss CB, Lundberg M, Hamberg P, Dehaven KE, Gillquist J. Nonoperative treatment of meniscal tears. *J Bone Joint Surg* 1989;71A:811–822.
437. Whipple TL, Bassett FH III. Arthroscopic examination of the knee. Polypuncture technique with percutaneous intra-articular manipulation. *J Bone Joint Surg* 1978;60A:444–453.
438. Wickstrom KT, Spitzer RM, Olsson HE. Roentgen anatomy of the posterior horn of the lateral meniscus. *Radiology* 1975;116:617–619.
439. Wilson AJ, Ford LT, Gilulo LA. Migrating mouse: A sign of dissecting popliteal cyst. *AJR* 1988;150:867–868.
440. Wolfe RD, Dieden JD. Cruciate ligament injury. Diagnostic difficulties in the presence of meniscal injury. *Radiology* 1985;157:19–21.

*Imaging of Orthopedic Trauma,
Second Edition*, edited by T.H. Berquist,
Mayo Clinic © 1992. Published
by Raven Press, Ltd., New York.

CHAPTER 8

The Tibia, Fibula, and Calf

Claire E. Bender, Donald C. Campbell II, and Thomas H. Berquist

Anatomy, 433
Mechanism of Injury and Classification
    of Fractures, 437
Radiographic Evaluation, 438

Management of Fractures, 439
Complications, 447
    Soft Tissue Injuries, 450
References, 451

Fractures of the shafts of the tibia and fibula are the most common long bone fractures. Soft tissue injuries to the calf are also common. Treatment of tibial and fibular fractures is similar and, therefore, reference will primarily be made to the tibia.

ANATOMY

The anatomy of the body or shaft of the tibia (Figs. 8-1 to 8-3) is straightforward. The body has three borders: anterior, medial, and interosseous. It also has three surfaces: medial, posterior, and lateral. The anterior border and medial surface are predominately subcutaneous. Special markings include the tibial tuberosity located on the upper anterior border and the soleal line on the upper posterior surface. The tuberosity is the attachment of the ligamentum patellae. The soleal line is the tibial origin of the soleus muscle. There are no special markings on the medial or lateral surfaces of the tibial body (24,28).

The body of the fibular shaft is long and slender. It also has interosseous, anterior, and posterior borders and medial, lateral, and posterior surfaces. The anatomy is difficult to identify because the borders and surfaces spiral laterally and caudally. In addition, there is a prominent medial crest on the midposterior surface of the bone, thus dividing the bone into four possible surfaces (24).

The tibia and fibula are joined by the tibiofibular synovial joint, the interosseous membrane, and the tibiofibular syndesmosis. The tibiofibular synovial joint is between the head of the fibula and the posterolateral part of the lower surface of the tibial condyle (2,24,28).

The interosseous membrane is composed of strong fibers that pass laterally and caudally from the interosseous crest to the fibular crest. The interosseous ligament is the thickest part of the membrane; it lies between the lower ends of the tibia and fibula. The anterior tibial vessels pass just above the interosseous membrane through a small aperture. Inferiorly there is a smaller aperture for the perforating branch of the peroneal artery.

The tibiofibular syndesmosis is between the lower ends of the tibia and fibula. It may be converted into a synovial joint by a diverticulum from the talocrural joint (11). The tibiofibular syndesmosis, the lower, thickened part of the interosseous membrane, and the anterior and posterior tibiofibular ligaments comprise the inferior transverse ligament.

Muscles of the lower leg are divided into anterolateral and posterior groups (Fig. 8-4). The posterior, or calf muscles, are within two compartments. The transverse crural septum, or deep transverse facia of the leg, separates the superficial and deep compartments. The gastrocnemius,˘ soleus, and plantaris form the superficial group; the popliteus, flexor hallucis longus, flexor digitorum longus, and tibialis posterior occupy the deep compartment and arise in part from the covering fascia (2,24).

The anterolateral muscles of the leg consist of the lateral compartment group—the peroneus longus and peroneus brevis—and the anterior compartment group—

C. E. Bender, D. C. Campbell II: Departments of Diagnostic Radiology and Orthopedic Surgery, Mayo Medical School, Mayo Clinic, Rochester, Minnesota 55905.

T. H. Berquist: Department of Dignostic Radiology, Mayo Medical School, Mayo Clinic Jacksonville, Jacksonville, Florida 32224.

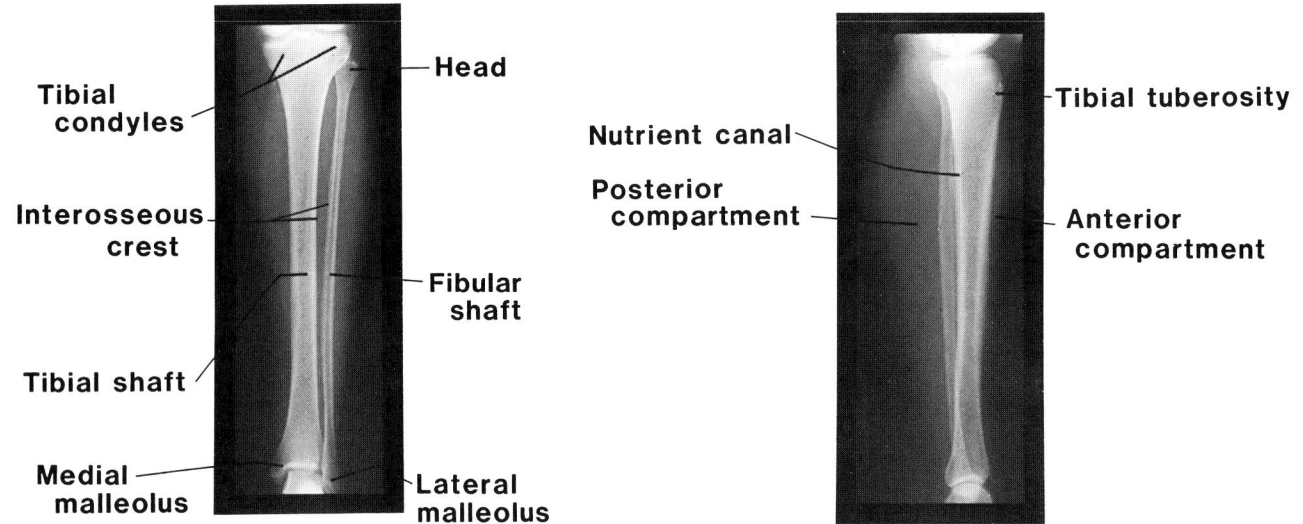

FIG. 8–1. Normal AP (**A**) and lateral (**B**) radiographs of the tibia and fibula.

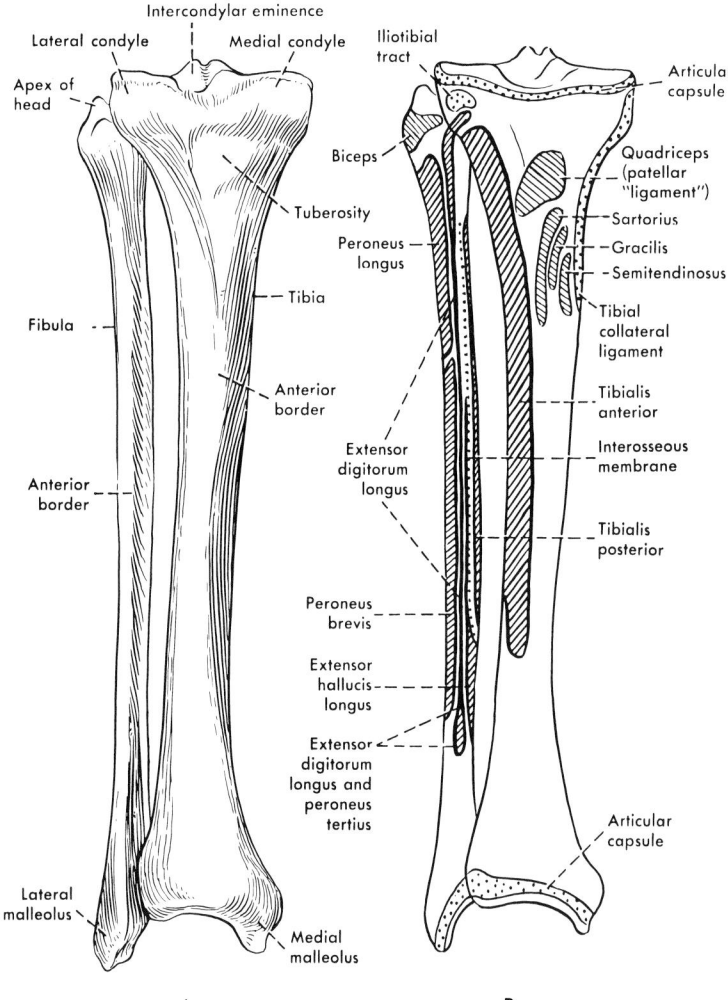

FIG. 8–2. Musculoskeletal anatomy of the tibia and fibula. **A:** Anterior bony anatomy. **B:** Anterior muscle origins and insertions (from 27, with permission.)

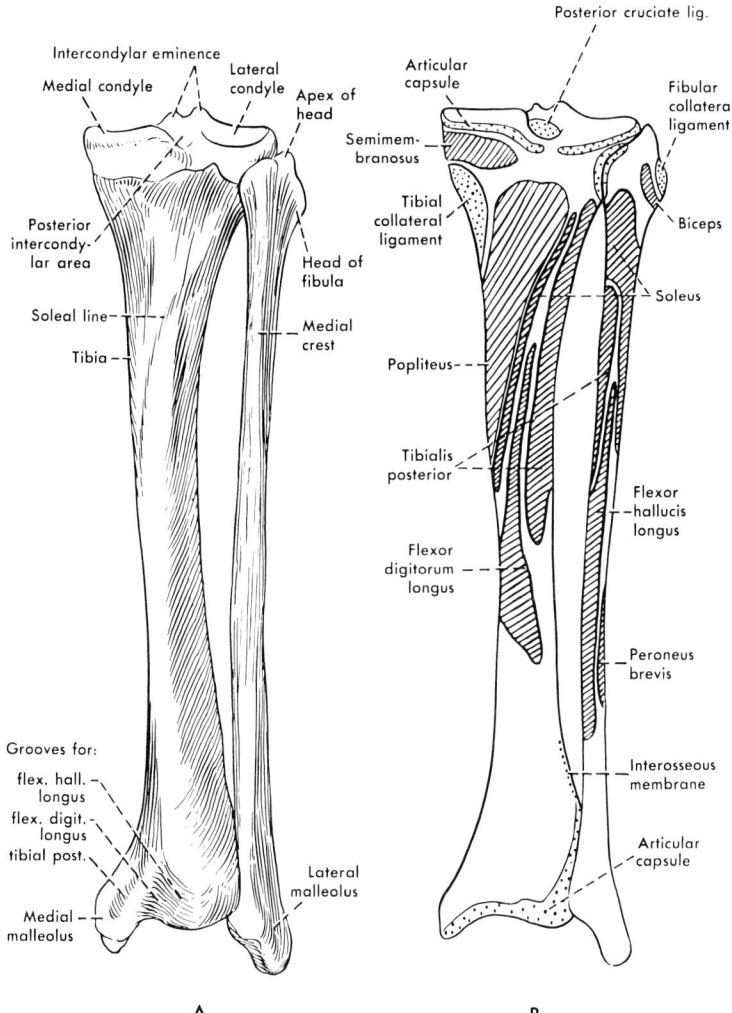

FIG. 8-3. Musculoskeletal anatomy of the tibia and fibula. **A:** Posterior osseous anatomy. **B:** Posterior muscle origins and insertions (from 24, with permission.)

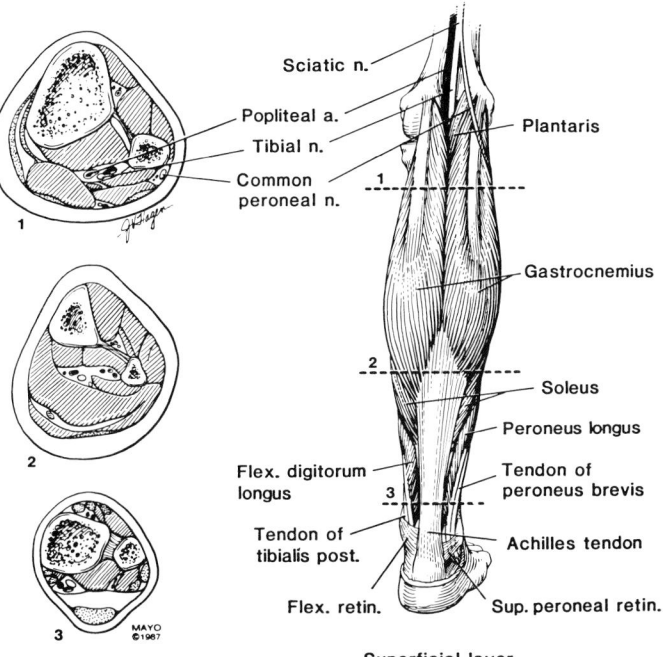

Superficial layer

FIG. 8-4. The muscles of the calf with axial levels demonstrating the anterolateral and posterior compartments (from 2, with permission.)

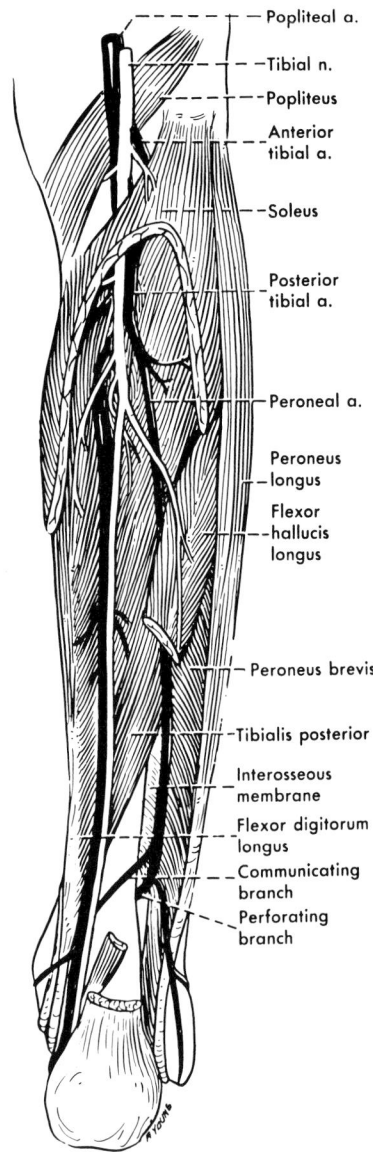

Popliteal a.
Tibial n.
Popliteus
Anterior tibial a.
Soleus
Posterior tibial a.
Peroneal a.
Peroneus longus
Flexor hallucis longus
Peroneus brevis
Tibialis posterior
Interosseous membrane
Flexor digitorum longus
Communicating branch
Perforating branch

FIG. 8–5. The major neurovascular supply to the lower leg (from 2, with permission.)

the tibialis anterior, extensor digitorum longus, and extensor hallucis longus (2,24).

Major vessels (Fig. 8-5) and nerves of the calf arise from parent structures in the popliteal space. Major popliteal arterial branches include the anterior tibial, posterior tibial, and peroneal arteries. A variety of branching patterns are possible. The most common pattern will be described. The origin of the anterior tibial artery is at the level of the popliteus muscle. Accompanied by the anterior tibial vein, it passes laterally and forward between the lower border of the popliteus and the upper border of the tibialis posterior to pass above the upper margin of the interosseous membrane and enters the anterior aspect of the leg (24).

The posterior tibial artery (accompanied by the vein)

continues inferiorly deep to the soleus and then penetrates the deep transverse fascia of the leg. It continues medially downward in a fascial canal with the tibialis posterior and flexor digitorum longus. Most of the posterior tibial artery branches supply the muscles of the posterior compartment (24).

The peroneal artery branches approximately 1 inch below the origin of the posterior tibial artery. Beneath the soleus, it is accompanied by two veins. The peroneal artery passes obliquely downward and laterally across the upper posterior surface of the tibialis muscle and enters a canal formed by the fibula anterolaterally, tibialis posterior anteromedially, and flexor hallucis longus from behind (11). As it passes downward, some of its branches pass through the interosseous membrane to supply the anterior muscle group (24,28).

Three blood-supply systems nourish the tibia: the nutrient artery, the periosteal system, and the epiphyseal-metaphyseal system. The major blood supply to the tibial shaft is the nutrient artery, which arises close to the upper end of the posterior tibial artery at the junction of the upper and middle thirds of the shaft. It enters the tibia posteriorly and has a rather long, oblique intracortical course. When it reaches the intramedullary space, it divides into ascending and descending branches that form a dense network of vessels. These vessels supply approximately two-thirds of the cortex of the tibial shaft (35).

The periosteal vessels originate from the anterior tibial artery or vessels of the interosseous membrane. These vessels run transversely to the long axis of the tibia. Abundant anastomoses exist between these transverse branches and with adjacent muscle arteries (25).

It is the periosteal vessels that are of major importance in fracture healing. Because they run transversely, they are not interrupted as are the nutrient vessels (25,35).

The fibula is similarly supplied by the nutrient artery, periosteal system, and epiphyseal-metaphyseal system. The nutrient artery typically originates from the proximal peroneal artery (24,28,35).

Major nerves in the leg include the tibial and peroneal nerves. The tibal nerve courses through the popliteal fossa lying lateral to the popliteal vessels. It then passes behind them to their medial side as the popliteal vessels enter beneath the soleus muscle. The nerve continues downward with the posterior tibial vessels on the tibialis posterior muscle, then on the posterior aspect of the tibia, prior to entering the neurovascular compartment of the flexor retinaculum.

The common peroneal nerve is located subcutaneously just behind the head of the fibula, where it is extremely vulnerable to injury. It courses laterally and forward around the neck of the fibula deep to the peroneus longus. At this level, it divides into the superficial and deep peroneal nerves. The superficial peroneal nerve runs downward, paralleling the fibula, and supplies the peroneus longus and brevis. The deep peroneal nerve continues forward to penetrate the anterior intermuscular septum to reach the anterior compartment. It courses inferiorly with the tibial vessels.

The leg is divided into three compartments (28). The anterior compartment contains the tibialis anterior, extensor digitorum longus, extensor hallucis longus, and peroneus tertius muscles, the anterior tibial artery, and the deep peroneal nerve. These are enveloped by a relatively tight compartment composed of the tibia medially, fibula laterally, interosseous membrane posteriorly, and the tough anterior fascia. The lateral compartment contains the peroneus longus and brevis muscles. These muscles tend to protect the fibular shaft. The posterior compartment contains the gastrocnemius, soleus, tibialis posterior, flexor hallucis longus and flexor digitorum longus muscles, posterior tibial and peroneal arteries, and posterior tibial nerve. This compartment is larger and more elastic than the anterior compartment (Fig. 8-4) (2,24,28).

MECHANISM OF INJURY AND CLASSIFICATION OF FRACTURES

Direct high-energy forces, such as those associated with motor vehicle accidents or gunshot wounds, can result in severe damage, with open wounds, skin loss, soft tissue damage, and tibial and fibular comminution. Fractures can be transverse, segmental, or comminuted. Indirect injuries usually result from falls or injuries in which the foot is fixed. Fractures of the tibia are usually oblique or spiral. The fibula can remain intact. Generally the greater the injury force, the greater the likelihood that both the tibia and fibula will be fractured (5,28).

Incomplete or simple fractures of the tibia or fibula may occur from a direct blow or fall. The radiographic appearance of these fractures should not be confused with nutrient canals. In the tibia, the vascular grooves have sclerotic margins and run obliquely and inferiorly in the proximal tibia (Fig. 8-1B).

Fractures are more common in the middle and distal thirds of the tibial shaft. Distal shaft fractures may extend into the tibial plafond. These injuries result from a fall from a height or from a blow on the anchored foot that forces the talus up into the tibial plafond (28). Various types of ankle fractures can be associated with these injuries.

Various classification schemes have been developed for tibial fractures. The most useful scheme is one that aids the orthopedic surgeon in fracture management and prognosis. Fractures should be described according to (1) precise anatomic location, (2) pattern of the fracture line, (3) position of the fragments, (4) degree of comminution, and (5) whether the fracture is open or closed.

Ellis (15) proposed a classification of tibial fractures based on severity. A fracture of minor severity is undisplaced, not angulated, and involves only a minor degree of comminution or a minor open wound. Moderate severity is complete displacement or angulation, with a small degree of comminution or a minor open wound. Major severity involves a major comminution or a major open wound with total displacement of the fracture.

Nicoll's (33) classification was based on the most significant factors affecting union: (1) initial displacement, (2) comminution, and (3) associated soft tissue wounds, infections, and distraction. He then graded each of these parameters from moderate to severe or nil to slight. With this system he could reasonably predict the outcome of any type of fracture. In his series of 705 patients (674 treated conservatively), the incidence of delayed union or non-union varied from 9% in the most favorable type to 39% in the least favorable.

Leach (28) prefers a modification of Ellis' classification. Minor fractures should have <50% horizontal displacement. Moderate fractures may have greater than 50% horizontal displacement. Comminution and soft tissue injury must be mild in both groups (Figs. 8-6 and 8-7).

Because of the importance of soft tissues in the healing of open tibial fractures, Müller (32) has classified the severity of soft tissue damage. Grade 1 fractures are compounded from within, with minimal soft tissue damage. Grade II fractures are compounded from without; the soft tissue injury is much less than the degree of bone injury. Grade III fractures are comminuted, and skin and muscle damage is extensive. Gustilio and Anderson

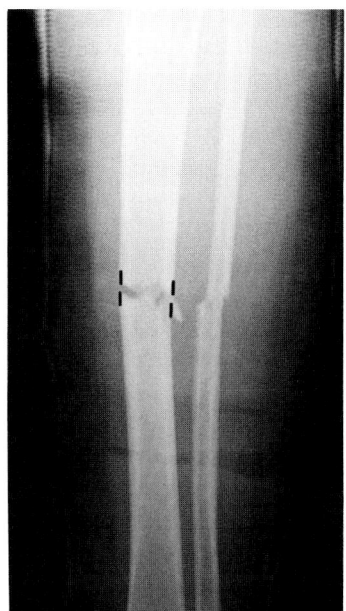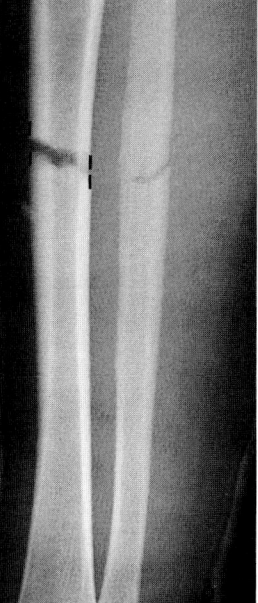

A   B

FIG. 8-6. Minor tibial fracture. Transverse fractures of the mid tibia and fibula with minimal comminution and no soft tissue injury. The AP (**A**) and lateral (**B**) radiographs demonstrate minimal horizontal displacement (*vertical lines*). Cast in place.

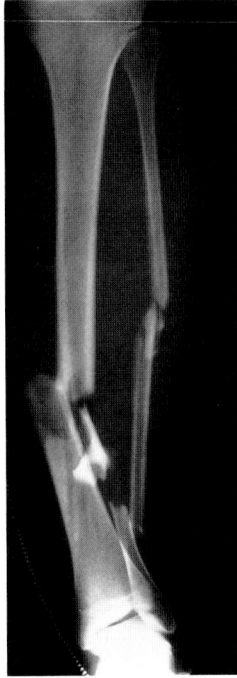

FIG. 8-7. AP view of a major tibial injury with complete horizontal displacement, severe comminution and soft tissue injury. The fibula is also severely comminuted.

provided a similar classification but further subdivided Grade III injuries due to significant differences in prognosis (7,20). Grade IIIA injuries have adequate soft tissue coverage despite laceration or tissue flaps. Grade IIIB injuries are more severe with stripping of the periosteum, exposure of bone, and extensive contamination. Grade IIIC injuries include the above plus arterial injury. The incidence of non-union increases from 27% up to 43% when injury increases from IIIA to IIIB. Amputations may be indicated in up to 25% of patients with IIIB open fractures. Non-union is the rule, infection rates reach

57%, and amputations are eventually required in 78% of Type IIIC open fractures (7).

RADIOGRAPHIC EVALUATION

Standard views of the tibia and fibula include AP and lateral projections, with the patient supine. Adjacent knee and ankle joints must be included on films owing to the possibility of associated injuries (see Fig. 8-1). Unless the lower leg is quite long, the 17-inch long film will include both joints. With longer legs, it is possible to place the film diagonally using opposite corners. However, in some patients two films must be used; the longer film can be placed proximally (including the knee), and a smaller film can be used for the distal leg and ankle. Soft tissues of the leg are included on films in order to exclude injury.

The AP projection (Fig. 8-8) is obtained with the patella anterior and the foot slightly inverted. The central beam is perpendicular to the center of the cassette.

The lateral projection (Fig. 8-9) can be made with the patient turned on the affected side. The knee is slightly flexed. The unaffected side is placed in front of the involved side. If the patient cannot be turned, a cross-table projection is made by placing a nonopaque rigid support under the leg and then placing a cassette along the medial or lateral aspect of the leg.

Oblique projections can give additional information about fracture rotation and alignment.

In all projections, the central ray is directed vertically to the midpoint of the film.

Tomography and other techniques are rarely necessary for diagnosis, although stress fractures are an exception. Stress fractures are thoroughly discussed in Chapter 16. Computed tomography (CT) may be useful in certain spiral fractures (18,27). Magnetic resonance imaging (MRI) may be indicated to evaluate soft tissue injury, soft tissue interposition, or vascular injury (2). In addi-

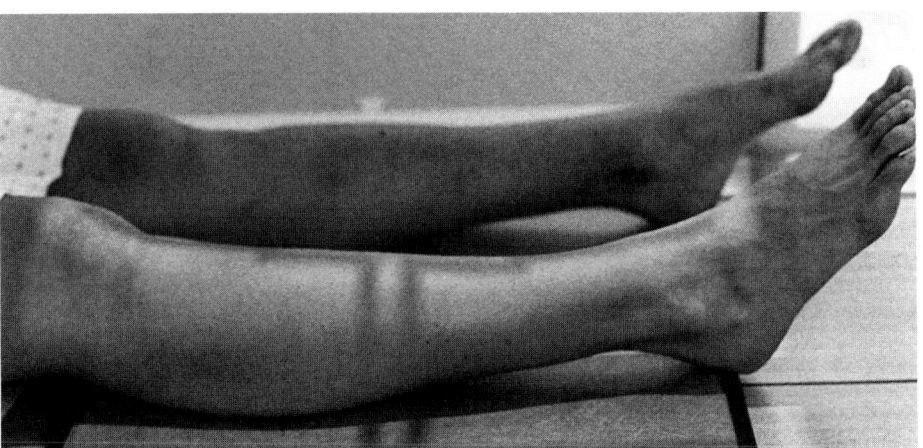

FIG. 8-8. Patient positioned for the AP radiograph of the tibia and fibula.

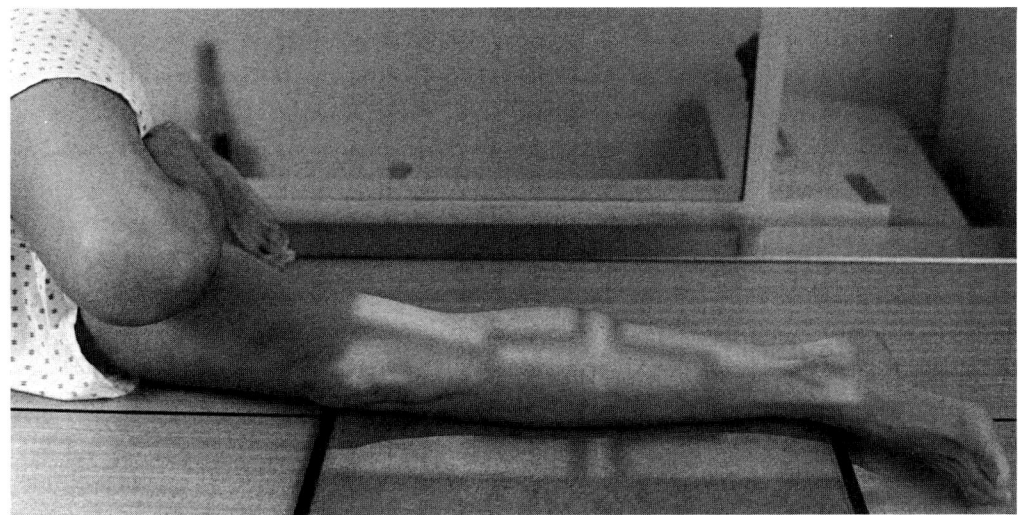

FIG. 8-9. Patient positioned for the lateral view of the tibia and fibula.

tion, MRI is extremely useful for evaluating suspected knee injuries. Up to 22% of patients with tibial fractures have associated ligament injuries in the knee (39).

MANAGEMENT OF FRACTURES

The literature is voluminous with regard to tibial and fibular shaft fracture management. With any fracture, the orthopedic surgeon will use the method of reduction and immobilization that has proved satisfactory in his or her experience (4,13,17,23,31,37).

The methods of fracture treatment are quite varied, and management choices have changed from decade to decade. In the 1930s and 1940s, closed methods were popular. Open reduction was more popular in the 1950s and 1960s. Presently, the method of choice is based upon the experience of the orthopedic surgeon.

Generally, in fractures of both the tibial and fibular shafts, the management is the same. Fracture of the fibula contributes to increased instability of the tibial fracture. With an intact fibula, the displacement of the tibial fracture is usually less, and thus the prognosis is improved.

Basic principles of fracture management include (1) maintenance or restoration of functional length, (2) restoration of normal weight-bearing alignment, (3) preservation of soft tissue, and (4) adjustment of treatment to the fracture (7).

The goal of fracture management is acceptable reduction (28). This means good alignment, no rotation, minimal shortening, and minor angulation in both the AP and lateral planes. Establishing good reduction improves the opportunity for better union. Because of the subcutaneous nature of much of the tibial shaft, only minimal displacement is acceptable. Displacement may be tolerated as long as rotation, shortening, and angulation are

controlled. Rotation must be as nearly perfect as possible in order to maintain a functional extremity. If the opposite limb is normal, assessment of desired rotational position is noted by drawing a line from the normal anterior superior iliac spine through the midpatella down to the foot. This line should normally extend to the space between the first and second toes. In order to maintain normal weight-bearing stresses, the ankle and knee joint surfaces must be parallel.

Acceptable angulation is 5° in the AP and lateral planes (Fig. 8-10). However, with more exact reduction there will be less shortening and a better functional result (28,31).

Shortening of 5–7.5 mm is allowed in most fractures (see Fig. 8-11). In patients with extensive comminuted fractures or bone loss, more shortening may be tolerated. Distraction of fracture fragments is not acceptable. Five mm of distraction can lengthen the healing time of tibial fractures 4–8 months beyond the usual mean healing time of 4 months (40).

Tibial fractures can be managed by closed or open reduction methods (41,43). Choice of method depends upon (1) the type of fracture, (2) the experience of the orthopedic surgeon, and (3) the medical condition of the patient. Most tibial fractures are managed by closed reduction and cast application.

A variety of casting techniques is possible. Long-leg casts are applied with some degree of knee flexion to allow weight-bearing and to relax the pull of the gastrocnemius. The foot is casted in neutral position.

The patellar-tendon-bearing (PTB) below-knee cast for tibial fractures was described by Sarmiento (36). After initial long-leg cast management for several weeks (allowing edema to subside), the carefully molded cast around the tibial condyles and patella is applied. Sarmiento believes that careful molding decreases tibial ro-

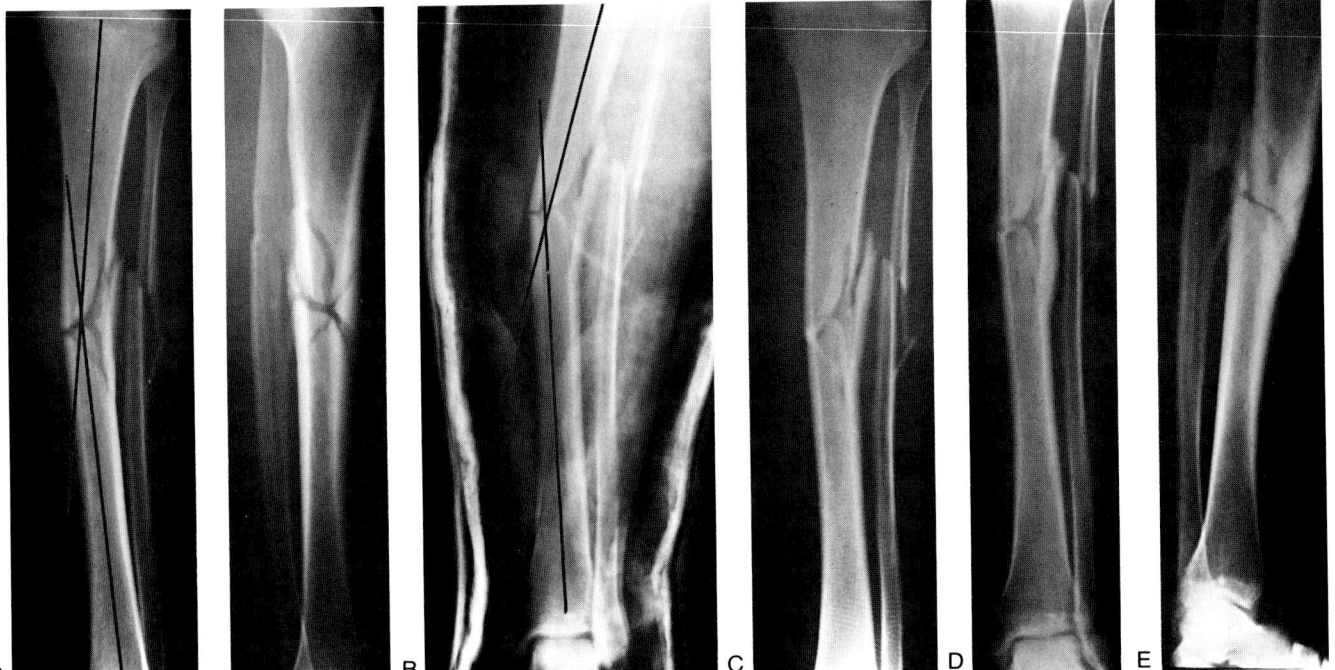

FIG. 8-10. Comminuted fractures of the mid tibia and fibula. There is slight medial angulation of the AP view (**A**) and minimal displacement on the lateral view (**B**). The AP view (**C**) immediately following reduction shows increased angulation (17°). Following remanipulation (**D**) the angulation is reduced to 5°. AP (**E**) and lateral (**F**) views three months after reduction show healing with good callus. There is no significant angulation.

tation and allows progress with weight bearing. Weight-bearing forces are placed on the tibial condyles, but the major distribution is placed on the soft tissues of the leg. With walking, body-weight forces are passed through the soft tissues, under compression, to the cast and then to the ground. Hydrostatic principles are utilized to provide reduced stress at the fracture site. Rigid immobilization is not provided by this cast, but rotation, shortening, and angulation are prevented. The intermittent compression of fracture fragments during weight bearing is a positive factor in healing. The PTB cast also allows easier ambulation and sitting.

Follow up of closed reduction consists of periodic radiographic evaluations to check for change in position of the fracture (Fig. 8-10). If the fracture position has changed since initial treatment, the orthopedic surgeon has several alternatives: (1) reduce the fracture and reapply a new cast, (2) utilize another reduction technique, or (3) wedge the cast. Cast wedging must be done carefully. The site of wedging is the fracture site itself, as performed by Watson-Jones (43), or the intersection of the long axis of the two fragments, as performed by Böhler (3) and Charnley (10). Metal markers can be placed on the cast site and confirmed with radiographs. Opening or closing wedges are used. Open wedging (Fig. 8-11) is preferred because it does not cause pressure on the underlying skin. The major disadvantage of the open wedge is a

tendency toward fracture distraction. Most now prefer application of a new cast to the wedging technique (28).

Insertion of Steinmann pins above and below the fracture site is another method of treatment. With the patient under anesthesia, the pins are placed and the fracture is reduced. Plaster cast is then applied from the toes to the tibial tubercle, incorporating the pins in plaster. The cast is then extended to the thigh level. Pins are removed after 6 weeks. Weight bearing is begun at the appropriate time, depending on the severity of the fracture and the extent of soft tissue injury.

In severe unstable fractures, in which traditional closed reduction techniques do not establish stabilization and where internal fixation is likely to be hazardous, external fixation using the Hoffman apparatus provides a good treatment choice (Fig. 8-12). This device consists of heavy threaded pins carefully placed above and below the fracture with an adjustable frame that has four vertical supports to increase the rigidity of the fixation. The advantages of this device are controlled fracture reduction and accessibility of the wound for debridement and skin grafting. The Fischer apparatus provides similar advantages (Fig. 8-13).

Ender nails have been used with certain fractures, specifically (Type I or II open fractures) short oblique distal tibial fractures (28). Ender nailing is a safe alternative to external fixation in this setting. Holbrook et al. (23) re-

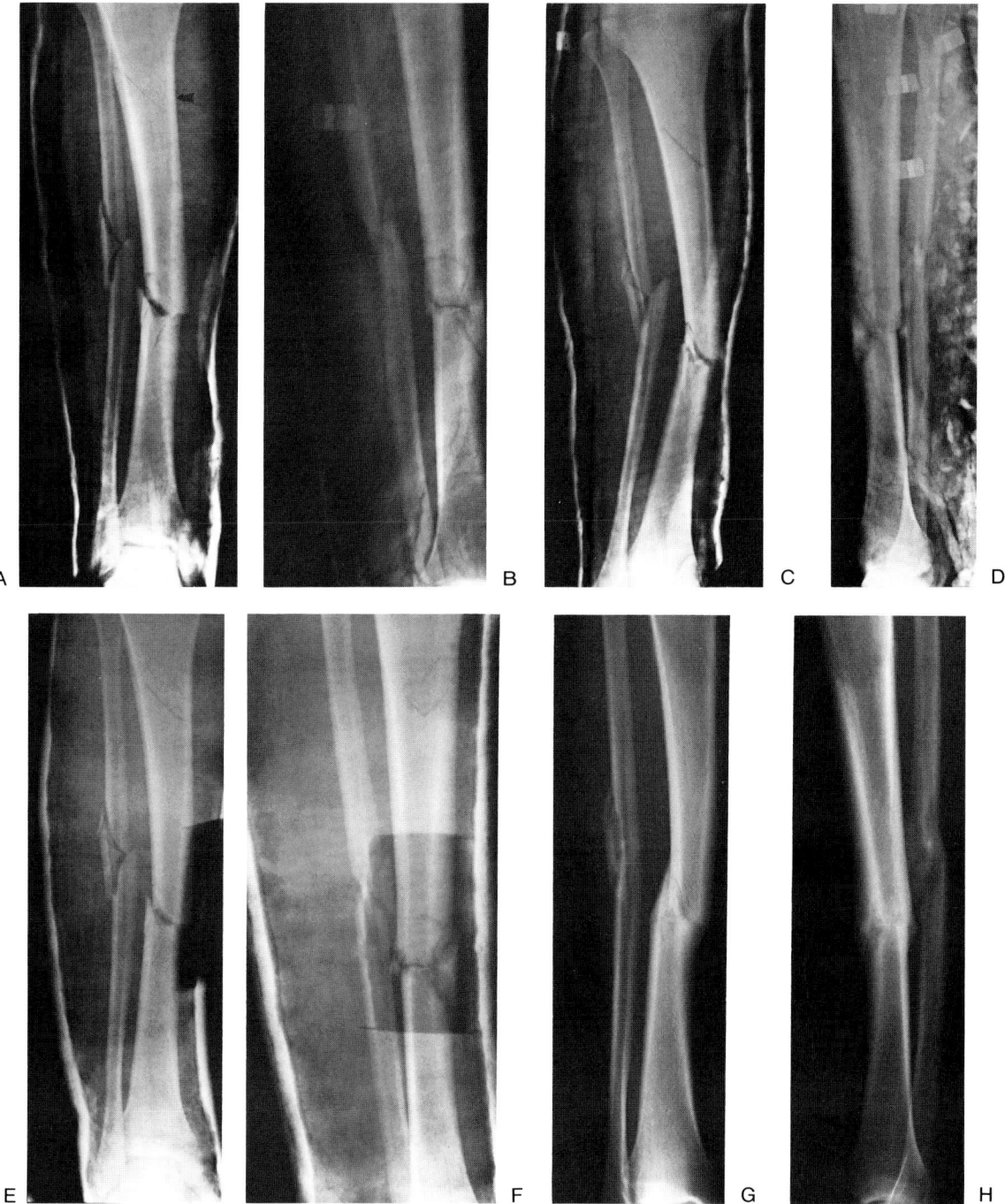

FIG. 8–11. AP (**A**) and lateral (**B**) views of comminuted fractures of the mid tibia and fibula. There is also an undisplaced upper tibial fracture (**A,** arrow). Following casting there is loss of reduction with increased medial angulation (**C**). This is not evident on the lateral view (**D**), which shows no AP angulation. Open wedging was performed and the fracture realigned (**E, F**). AP (**G**) and lateral (**H**) views six months later show the fracture has healed.

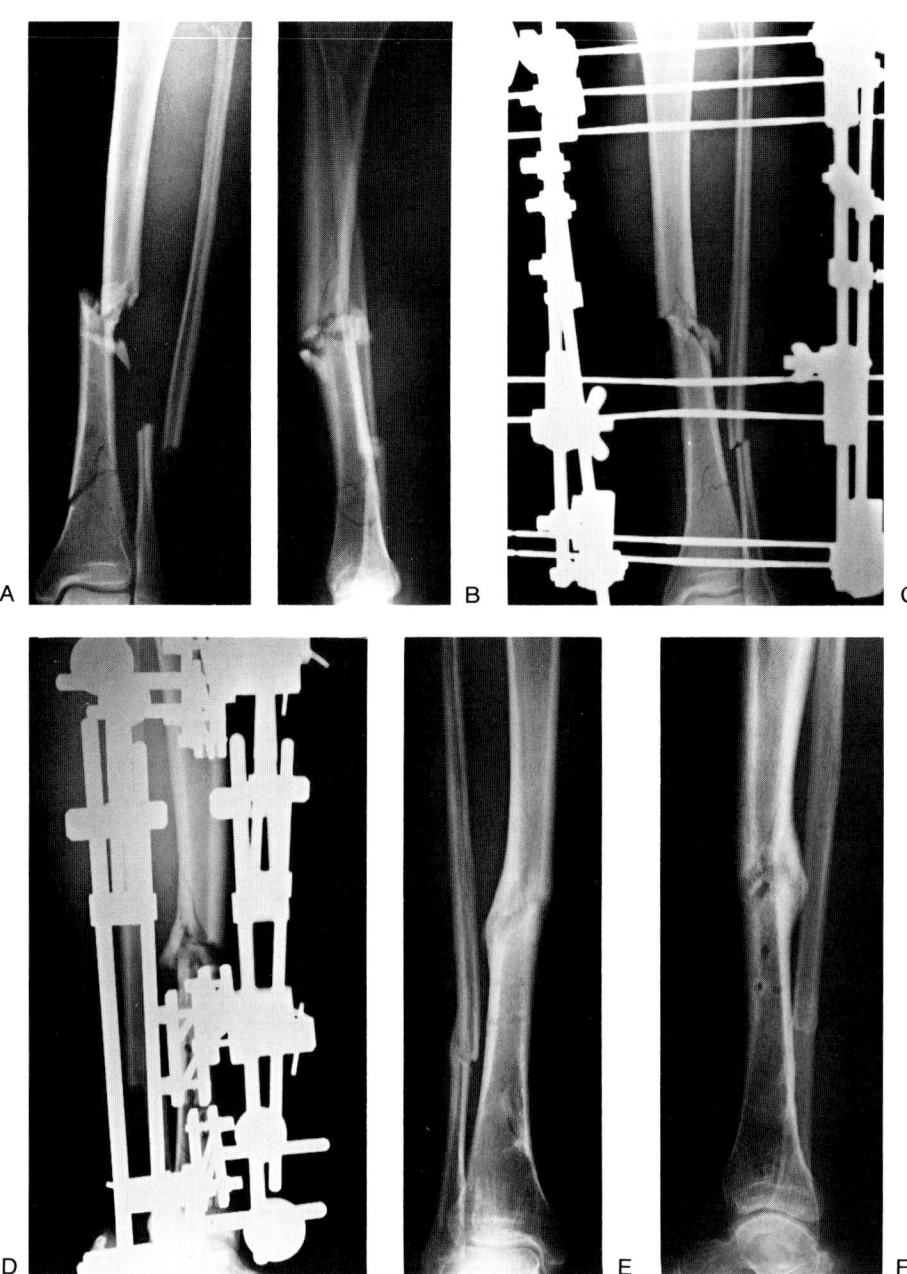

FIG. 8–12. AP (**A**) and lateral (**B**) views of a major fracture of the distal tibia and fibula. There is overriding and rotation of the fragments. Reduction was achieved with Hoffman fixation (**C, D**). The fracture was healed one year later (**E, F**).

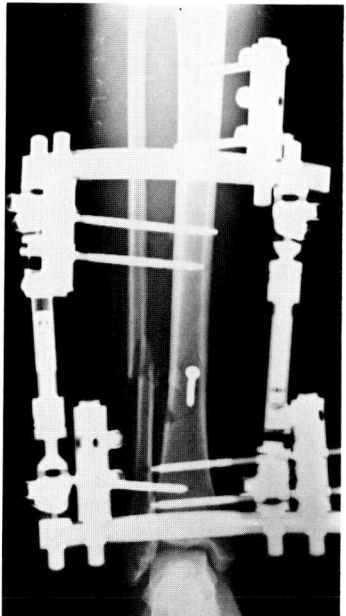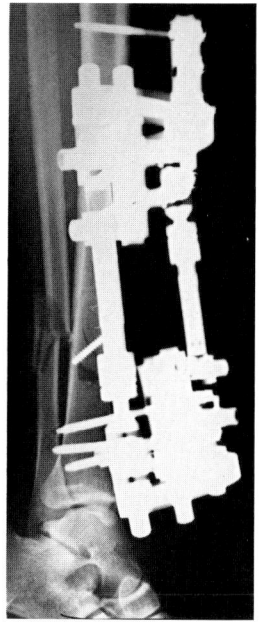

A   B

FIG. 8–13. AP (**A**) and lateral (**B**) views of the distal tibia and fibula with fracture reduction using a Fischer apparatus.

ported equal results using these two methods with regard to time to union, total number of surgical procedures required, range of motion in the knee and ankle, and complications.

Open reduction methods include compression plating, intramedullary nailing, and screw fixation. This has been one of the most controversial subjects in orthopedic surgery. Van der Linden (41) randomized 100 consecutive patients with displaced fractures of the tibial shaft and established two groups, one treated with A0 plate fixation and the other with a conservative method (Fig.

8-14). Caution is emphasized in the use of this technique. Careful attention must be given to maintaining vascular integrity of the bone for good healing. Anatomic results were better and mean healing time was shorter with the A0 plate group, but risk of infection was greater and duration of hospital stay was longer. Van der Linden's conclusions were that A0 plate fixation was suitable for closed longitudinal fractures but not for open fractures. This aspect of tibial fracture treatment remains controversial. Gustilo and Anderson argue strongly against the use of internal fixation in open fractures (20), while Chapman believes it to be a very useful treatment in certain circumstances (9). Other complications include fixation failure, implant failure, delayed union or non-union, and re-fracture.

Intramedullary nailing is used in (1) segmental tibial fractures, (2) angulated or displaced transverse or short oblique fractures of the middle third of the tibial shaft, and (3) non-united fractures (Fig. 8-15). Closed nailing techniques required a short incision at the level of the tibial tubercle. Use of an image intensifier is necessary in order to reduce the fracture properly and to guide the reamers and the intramedullary nail. In this way the periosteal blood supply is not disturbed, and the soft tissue vascularity is maintained. The nail interrupts the endosteal blood supply. Risk of infection is low with this closed technique. Open technique adds an incision at the fracture site. This may be required if closed reduction is not possible—that is, when soft tissues are interposed between the fracture fragments. Some intramedullary devices allow rotation to occur. Therefore, the use of some type of external support such as a brace or cast may be necessary until clinical union has started to progress (17,28).

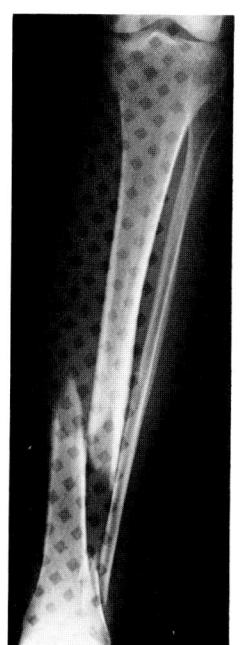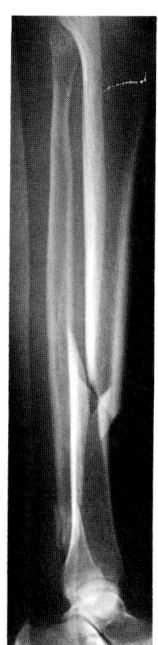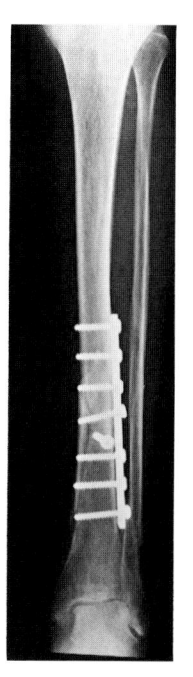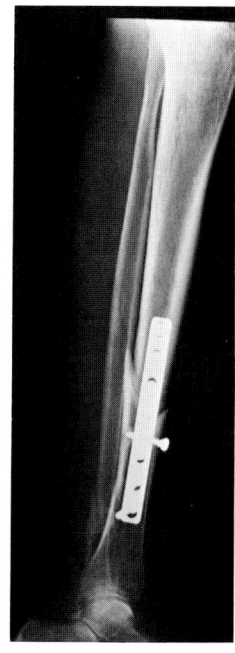

A   B   C   D

FIG. 8–14. AP (**A**) and lateral (**B**) views of overriding fracture of the distal tibia and fibula with several centimeters of shortening. Reduction was accomplished with a 7-hole AO plate and screws (**C, D**).

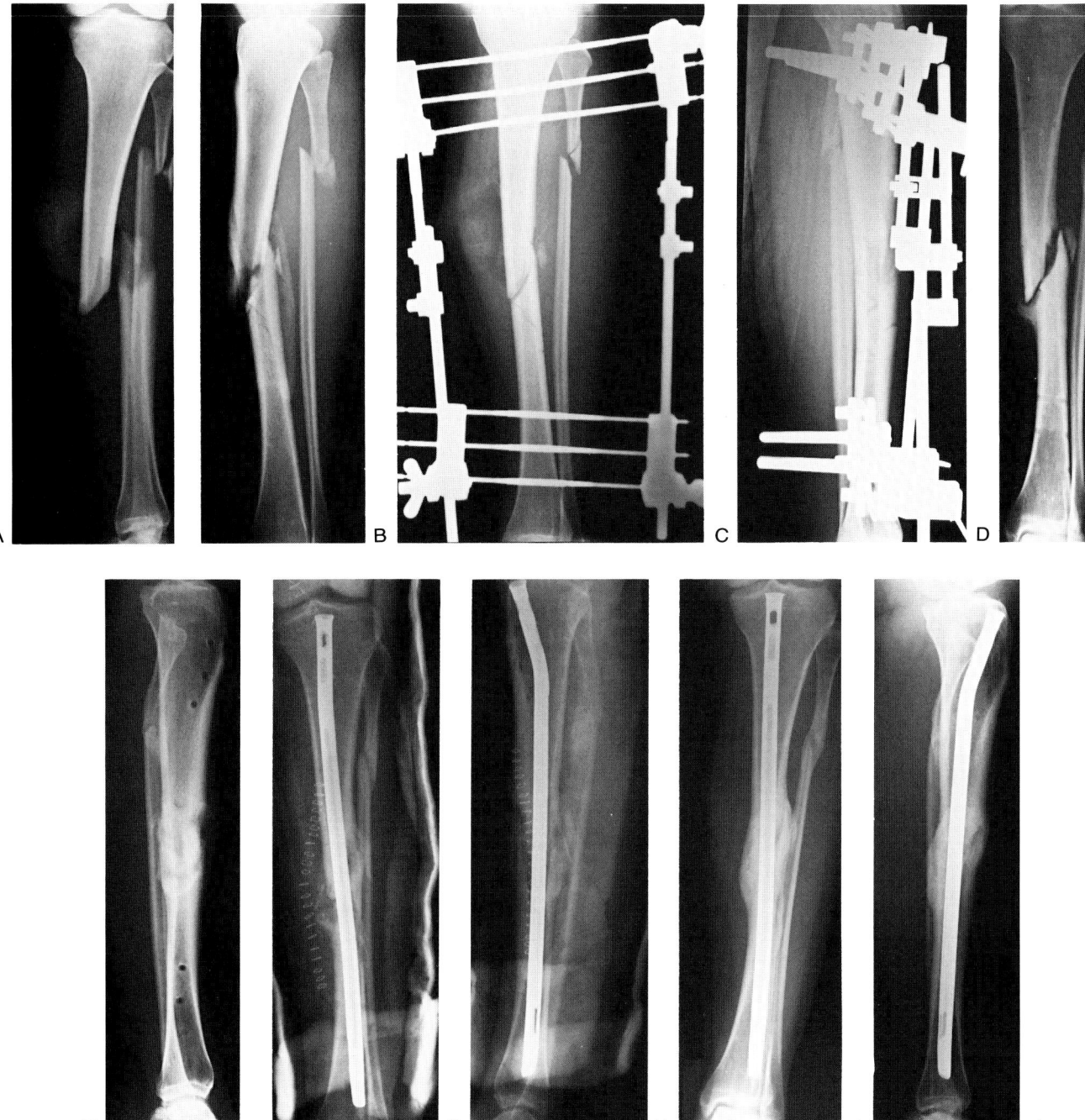

FIG. 8–15. AP (**A**) and lateral (**B**) views of a badly comminuted open tibial fracture. There is 90° rotation of the distal fragment. Initial reduction was accomplished with a Hoffman apparatus (**C, D**). The fracture was not united at four months (**E, F**). An intramedullary rod was used (**G, H**) and healing occurred two months later (**I, J**).

A modification of the Küntscher intramedullary nail allows placement of bone screws transversely through the bone and nail. This can be done at one or both ends of the nail, in this way preventing distraction, overriding, or rotation at the fracture site (Fig. 8-16). Such a device allows the indications for intramedullary nailing to be expanded to include fractures more comminuted or more distal or proximal than was previously the case.

Fixation with multiple screws alone may be achieved in certain oblique fractures. This technique allows anatomic reduction and fixation with minimal soft tissue dissection. Casting or bracing is absolutely necessary

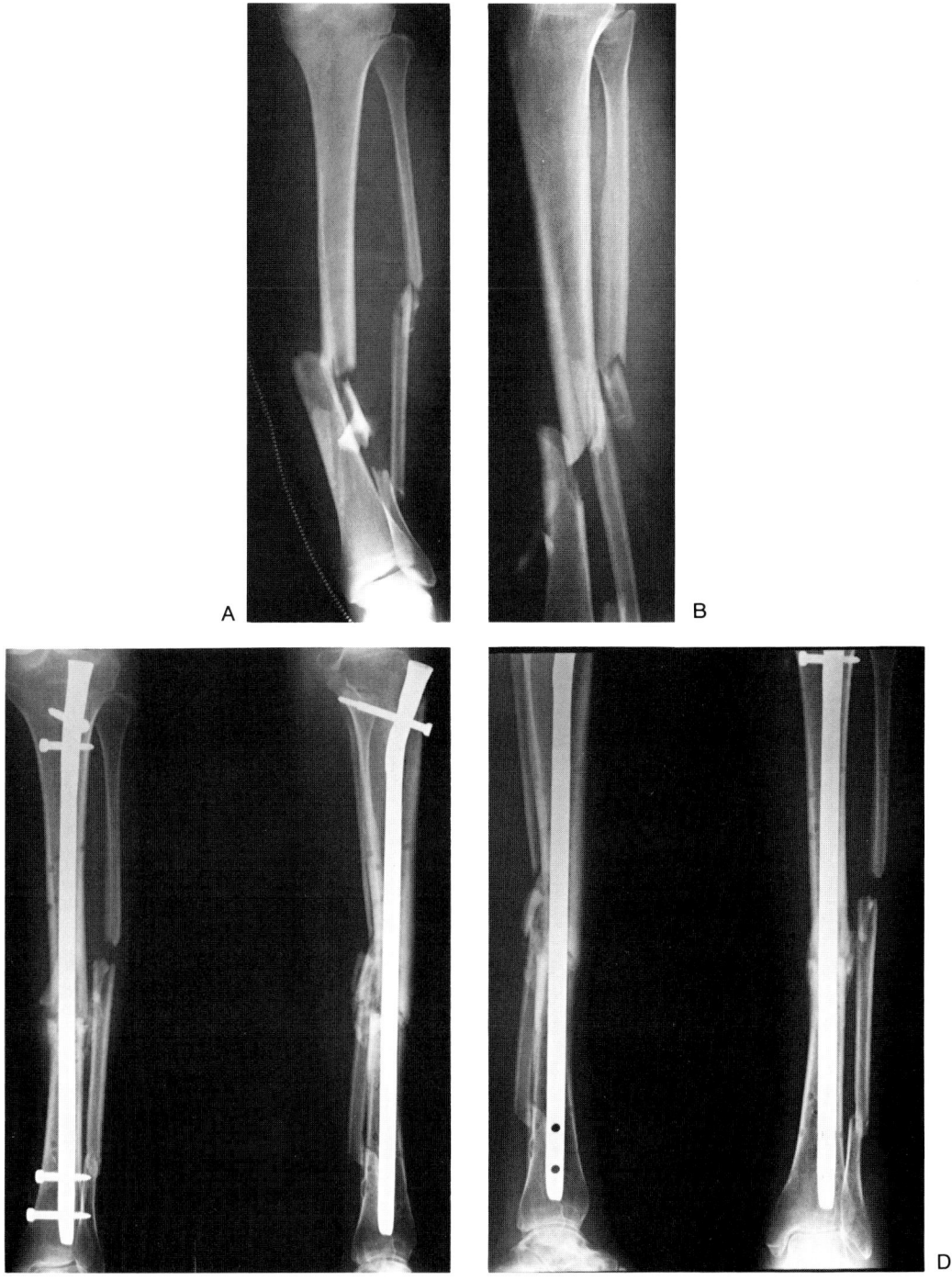

FIG. 8-16. AP (**A**) and lateral (**B**) views of an open comminuted fracture of the tibia with medial angulation. There are displaced mid and distal fibular fractures. The fracture was fixed with a locking medullary rod (**C**). AP (**D**) and lateral (**E**) views after healing of the tibial fracture. The lower locking screws have been removed and weight bearing is permitted.

after such treatment. This technique combined with bone grafting may be useful for treatment of some cases of delayed union (Fig. 8-17) (26,28).

Prognosis for fracture healing is based upon (1) type of fracture, (2) mechanism of injury, (3) soft tissue damage that includes open wounds, (4) infection, and (5) treatment. The treatment method of choice depends upon the orthopedic surgeon's experience and expertise. Generally uncomplicated tibial fractures heal in 10–13 weeks, but open comminuted fractures may take from 16–26 weeks. Delayed union is marked by absence of osseous union radiographically and presence of pain beyond the expected healing time. Non-union is diagnosed clinically by motion across the fracture site and radiographically by a persistent fracture line with sclerosed, flared margins (Fig. 8-18).

Fracture healing time is about the same for the proximal, middle, and distal thirds of the tibia (33,36). The presence or absence of a concomitant fibular fracture affects healing of the tibia. The intact fibula gives strut-like support to the tibia. However, it may also contribute to angular deformity of the tibia, and delayed union or

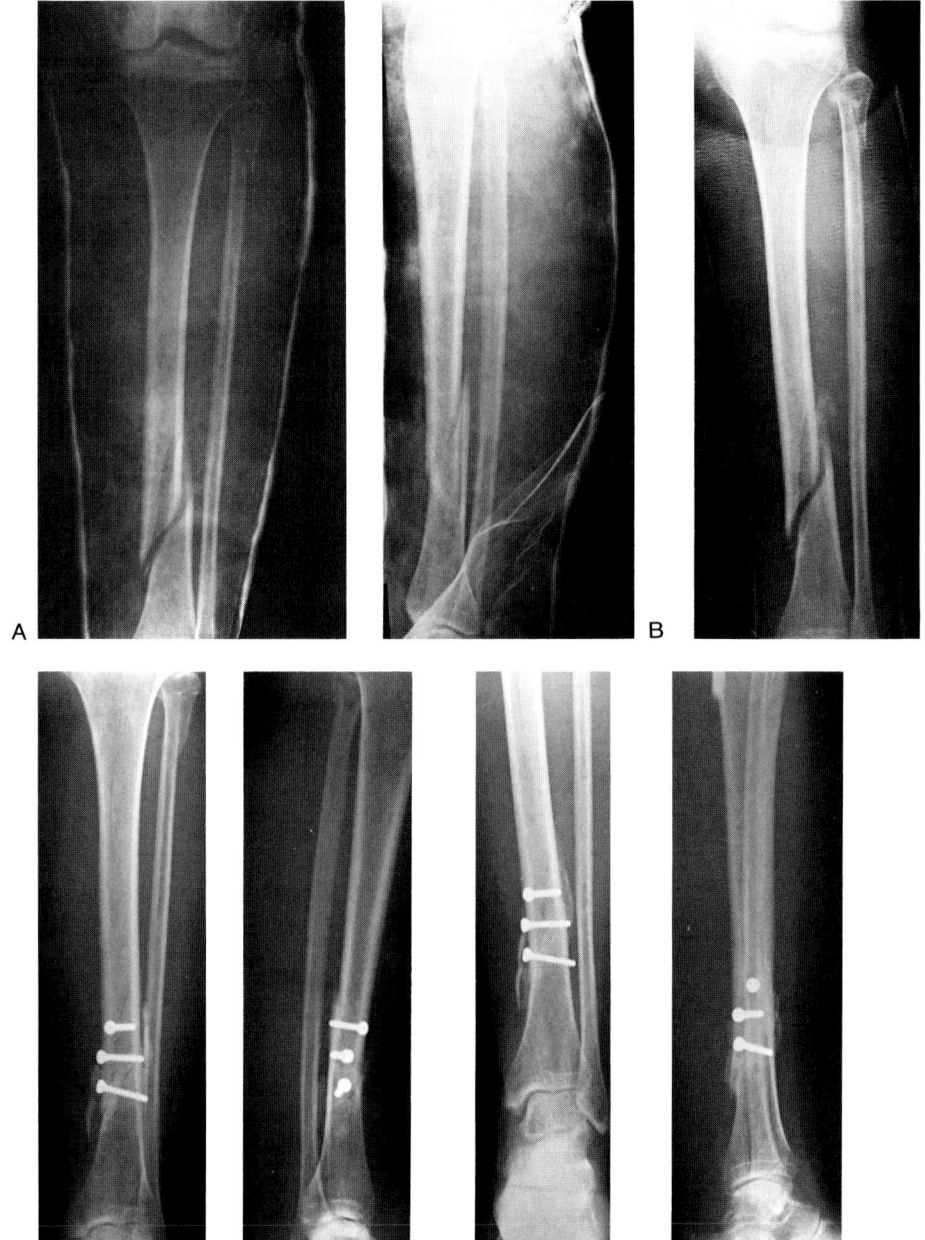

A B C

D E F G

FIG. 8-17. AP (A) and lateral (B) views of the tibia showing a distal spiral fracture of the tibia and proximal fibular fracture. (Both bones must be completely visualized on the radiograph.) Follow-up radiograph in PTB cast at three months (C) shows minimal callus. Bone grafts and leg screws were used (D, E) and healing occurred at five months (F, G).

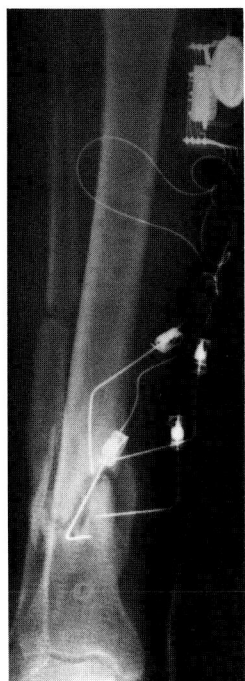
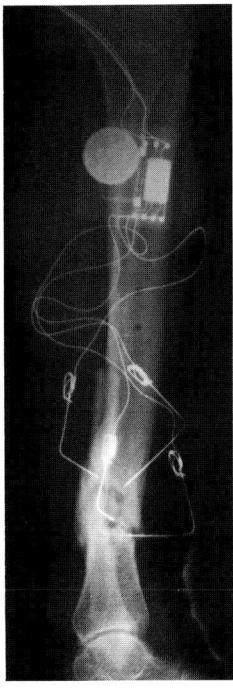

A   B

FIG. 8–18. AP (**A**) and lateral (**B**) views of a distal tibial non-union and percutaneously placed electrodes.

non-union may result. Resection of a small segment of fibula may then be necessary for appropriate tibial healing (13,28,37).

COMPLICATIONS

Delayed union is a common complication of tibial fractures and occurs in up to 15% of patients (28,36). Non-union is most commonly seen in severely displaced comminuted fractures with open wounds but can occur in any type of fracture, especially at the junction of the middle and distal thirds of the shaft. Treatment of non-united fractures includes bone grafts, fibular osteotomy (Fig. 8-18), compression plating, intramedullary nailing, and electrical stimulation.

Electrical stimulation was first used in 1912 for fracture healing, but not until the 1970s did definite interest develop in the use of electrical stimulation (6). Different systems have been developed: (1) constant direct current with percutaneous cathodes (Fig. 8-18), (2) constant direct current with implanted electrodes and power pack, and (3) the inductive coupling device. The success rate is about 80–85% for all three systems. All systems require good basic fracture management. Electricity must be concentrated at the non-union site. Three to six months are required for healing. Ineffective results occur when there is a large gap between fragments or pseudarthrosis. Actively draining osteomyelitis is a contraindication for the percutaneous or implanted electrodes (6,28).

Additional complications include malunion, extremity shortening, infection (Fig. 8-19), skin loss, am-

putation, refracture, and neurovascular injuries (1,4,12, 19,21,29,30).

Direct vascular injuries can be seen in severe, high-energy trauma (Fig. 8-20). The most common injury site is the upper fourth of the tibia, where the anterior tibial artery passes forward through the interosseous membrane. Rare aneurysms of the proximal portion of the anterior and posterior tibial arteries have been described (11,14). Entrapment (Fig. 8-21) of the vessels by fracture fragments has also been described (21).

The anterior compartment syndrome results from increased pressure due to hemorrhage and edema following fracture. Venous flow is impeded, and eventually arterial supply is occluded. Muscle ischemia then occurs. Halpern (22) measured anterior compartment pressures in 20 patients and noted higher pressures when fractures occurred in the proximal third of the tibia, when the fracture was more than 50% displaced, and when the fracture resulted from high-energy trauma. Passive flexion of the toes that elicits pain in the anterior compartment region is the earliest sign. Weakness of the extensor hallucis longus and digitorum longus then occurs, with hypesthesia of the first web space being the last sign. Acutely, the dorsalis pedis pulse may not be absent, but in late stages it is lost. Compartment syndrome can also develop in the posterior and lateral compartments. Treatment involves immediate compartmental fasciotomy and stabilization of the fracture, usually with an external fixator.

Direct nerve injury as a result of fracture is uncommon. Nerve injury is most often due to pressure from the

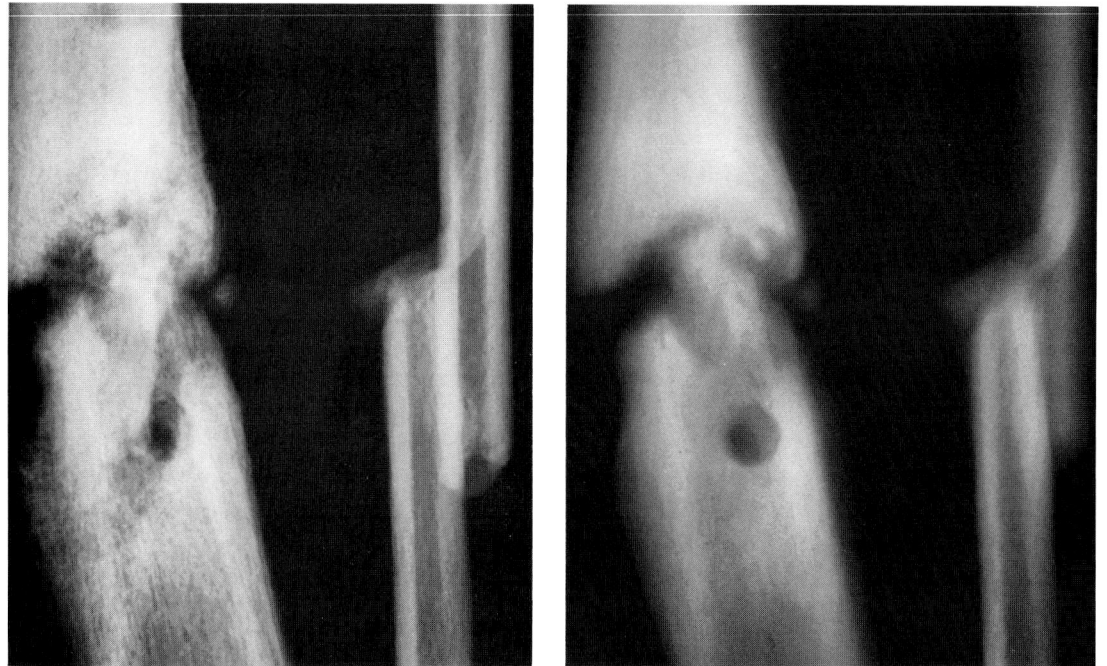

FIG. 8–19. AP view (**A**) of old distal tibial and fibular fractures. Note the cortical thickening and periosteal reaction along the tibia. Tomogram (**B**) shows the abnormalities more clearly including several small sequestra.

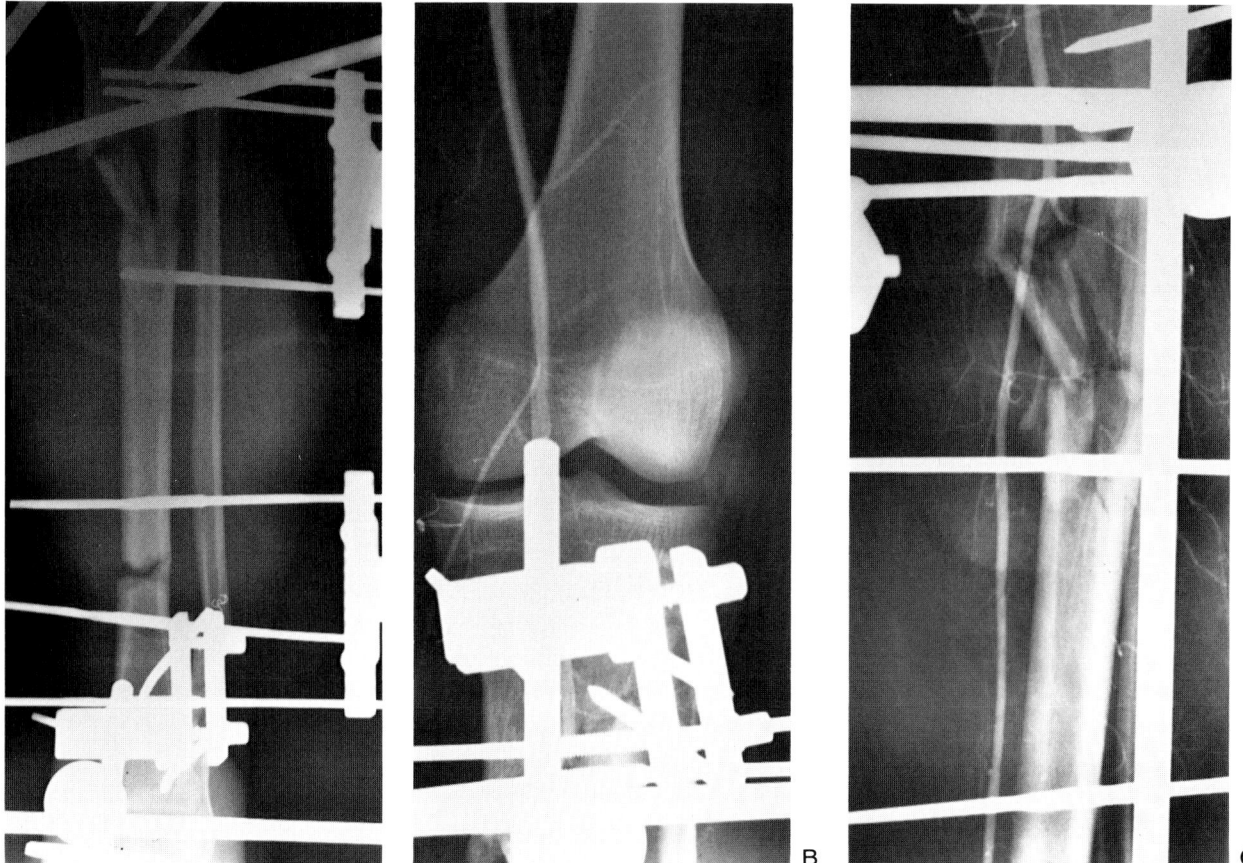

FIG. 8–20. High-velocity comminuted fractures of the upper and distal tibia and fibula. AP radiograph (**A**) shows the fractures and external fixation device. Angiograms of the popliteal region (**B**) and leg (**C**) show occlusion of all but the posterior tibial artery below the trifurcation.

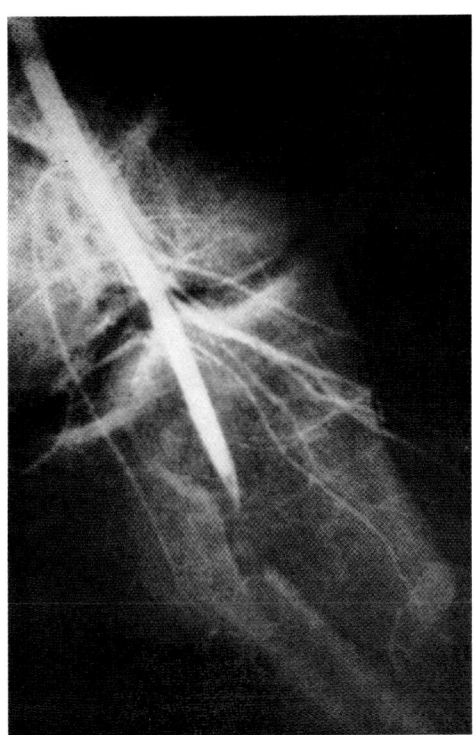

FIG. 8–21. Popliteal artery occlusion due to entrapment by the fibular fragment. Angiogram demonstrates "beak like" appearance of the popliteal artery at the level of entrapment (from 21, with permission.)

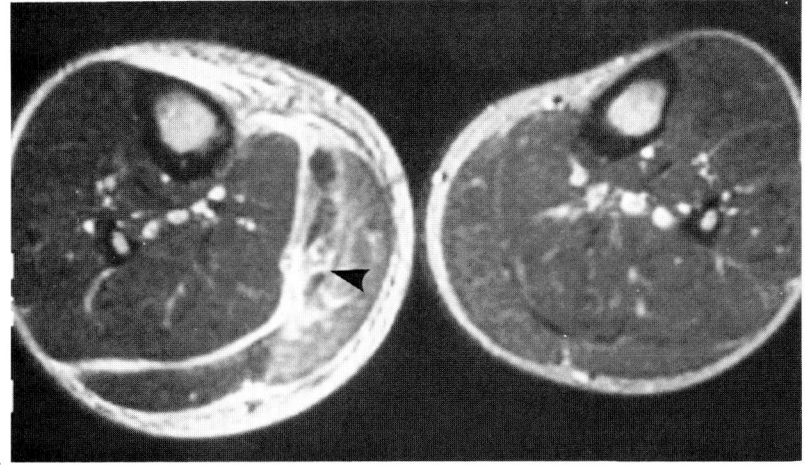

A

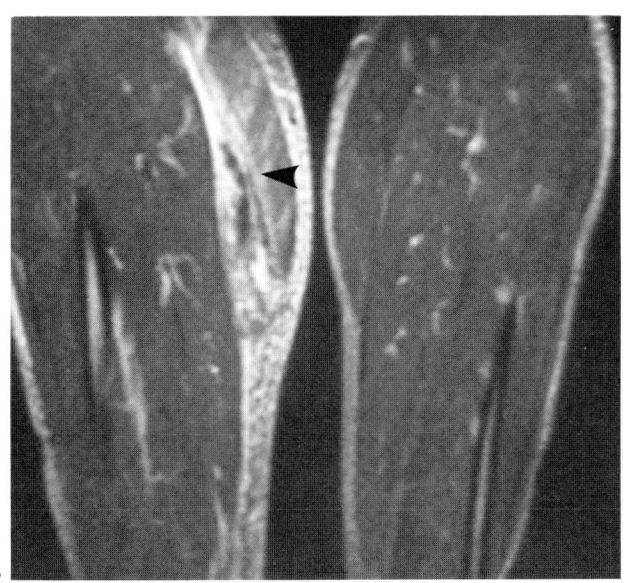

B

FIG. 8–22. Axial (A) and coronal (B) SE 2000/60 images in a hockey player with a medial gastrocnemius tear (arrows) due to direct trauma.

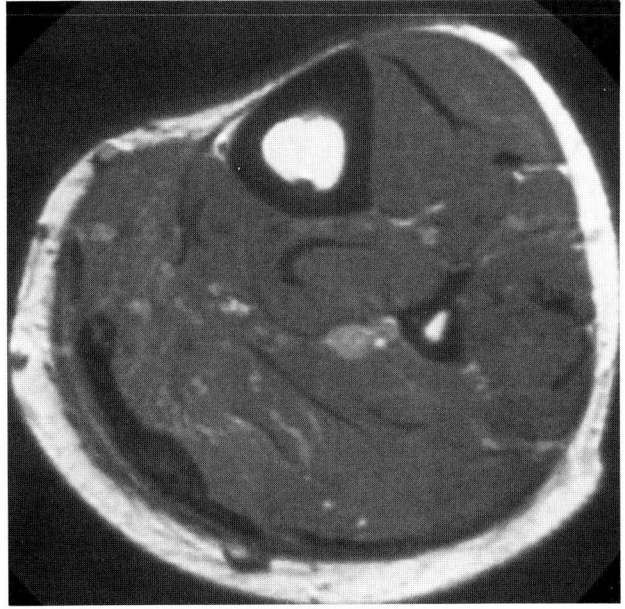

FIG. 8-23. Axial SE 2000/60 image several months after a medial gastrocnemius tear. Scar tissue (low signal) has filled the area in the torn muscle.

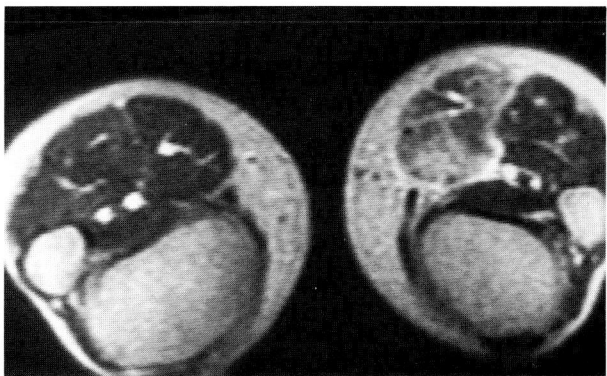

FIG. 8-24. Axial T2-weighted images of the calves demonstrate increased signal intensity in the posterior compartment on the right due to compartment syndrome.

cast or soft tissue swelling where the peroneal nerve crosses the fibular neck (28).

Isolated fractures of the fibular shaft are uncommon; they usually occur from direct violence. Treatment consists of cast application for relief of pain.

Soft Tissue Injuries

Soft tissue injuries may occur in association with fractures or as isolated events. Soft tissue injuries associated with fractures have been described in the previous section. Angiography, venography, and MRI may be useful for evaluating these injuries (2,16,34,38). Computed tomography is generally reserved for identification of osseous abnormalities (1,18,27).

Isolated soft tissue injuries to the calf can result in

contusion, hemorrhage, hematoma, muscle, ligament and tendon tears, and neurovascular injury. Clinical history and physical findings may be adequate for evaluating and treatment planning in minor injuries. However, ultrasonography or MRI are useful to fully evaluate the degree of injury (2,16).

MRI is particularly useful because all soft tissue and osseous structures can be evaluated. MR examinations of the calf are usually performed with the patient prone to avoid compression of the soft tissues in the calf. Axial T1 (SE 500/20) and T2 (SE 2000/60,20) images are usually adequate for detection of most injuries.

Five- to ten-millimeter-thick slices are used most frequently. The head coil or body coil can be used so both legs can be evaluated simultaneously, which allows comparison of the involved extremity with the normal side.

Muscle, ligament, and tendon tears are the most frequent injuries studied with MRI. Hemorrhage and/or edema have high signal intensity on T2-weighted sequences but may be isointense on T1-weighted sequences (Fig. 8-22). With healing, the signal intensity returns to normal over a period of 3–6 months. Reinjury or scar tissue are also easily detected with MRI (Fig.

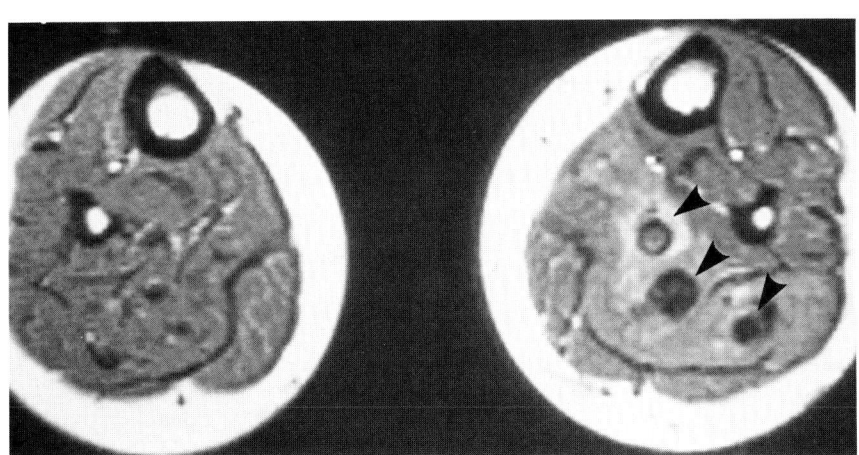

FIG. 8-25. Axial spin-echo (SE 2000/30) images of the calves demonstrate soleal muscle edema with thrombosis and dilatation of three deep veins (*arrows*). Note the normal leg for comparison.

8-23). Scar tissue has low intensity on both T1- and T2-weighted sequences (2,16).

Compartment syndromes can develop in patients without fractures (see above). MR image features are nonspecific. Infiltrative increased signal intensity in the involved compartment with or without fascial distention is evident (Fig. 8-24). Spectroscopy may be useful for detecting ischemic changes. However, compartment pressures are more easily obtained using conventional measurement techniques.

Venous abnormalities, specifically deep venous thrombosis, can be detected with conventional spin-echo sequences (Fig. 8-25). However, because of flow phenomenon, gradient-echo sequences may be easier to interpret. Sequences with a flip angle of 30°, TR of 50 and TE of 12–16 show flow as an area of high signal intensity. Thrombosis will be demonstrated as reduction or absent signal intensity in the vein. Soft tissue edema around the veins is a useful secondary sign (2,34,38).

REFERENCES

1. Aitken AGF, Flodmark O, Newman DE, Kilcoyne RF, Shuman WP, Mack LA. Leg length determination by CT digital radiography. *AJR* 1985;144:613–615.
2. Berquist TH. *Magnetic resonance of the musculoskeletal system.* New York: Raven Press, 1990.
3. Böhler L. *The treatment of fractures,* 5th ed. New York: Grune and Stratton, 1956–1958.
4. Bone LB, Johnson KD. Treatment of tibial fractures by reaming and intramedullary nailing. *J Bone Joint Surg* 1986;68A:877–886.
5. Boyer RS, Jaffe RB, Nixon GW, Condon VR. Trampoline fracture of the proximal tibia in children. *AJR* 1986;146:83–85.
6. Brighton CT. The treatment of non-unions with electricity. *J Bone Joint Surg* 1981;63A:847–851.
7. Carpenter EB. Management of fractures of the shaft of the tibia and fibula. *J Bone Joint Surg* 1966;48A:1640–1646.
8. Caudle RJ, Stern PJ. Severe open fractures of the tibia. *J Bone Joint Surg* 1987;69A:801–806.
9. Chapman MW. Immediate internal fixation in open fractures. *Orthop Clin North Am* 1980;11:579–591.
10. Charnley J. *The closed treatment of common fractures,* 3rd ed. Edinburgh: E. S. Livingstone, 1961.
11. Crellin RO, Tsapogas MJC. Traumatic aneurysm of the anterior tibial artery. Report of a case. *J Bone Joint Surg* 1963;45B:142–144.
12. Daoud A, Saighi-Boaagana A. Treatment of sequestra, pseudarthroses, and defects in the long bones of children who have chronic hematogenous osteomyelitis. *J Bone Joint Surg* 1989;71A:1448–1468.
13. DeLee JC, Hickman JD, Lewis AG. Partial fibulectomy for ununited fractures of the tibia. *J Bone Joint Surg* 1981;63A:1390–1395.
14. Dreyfus U, Fishman J. False aneurysm of the posterior tibial artery complicating fracture of the tibia and fibula. *J Trauma* 1980;20:186–187.
15. Ellis H. Disabilities after tibial shaft fractures. *J Bone Joint Surg* 1958;40B:190–197.
16. Flechenstein JL, Canby RC, Parkey RW, Peschock RM. Acute effects of exercise on MR imaging of skeletal muscle in normal volunteers. *AJR* 1988;151:231–237.
17. Caplin RD, Veith RG, Hansen ST. Treatment of failures after plating of tibial fractures. *J Bone Joint Surg* 1986;68A:1231–1236.
18. Gershuni DH, Shyhar MJ, Thompson B, Resnick D, Donald G, Akeson WH. A comparison of conventional radiography and computed tomography in the evaluation of spiral fractures of the tibia. *J Bone Joint Surg* 1985;67A:1388–1395.
19. Green SA. Complications of external skeletal fixation. *Clin Orthop* 1983;180:109–115.
20. Gustilo RB, Anderson JT. Prevention of infection in the treatment of 1025 open fractures of long bones. *J Bone Joint Surg* 1976;58A:453–458.
21. Hall RF, Gonzales M. Fracture of the proximal part of the tibia and fibula associated with an entrapped popliteal artery. *J Bone Joint Surg* 1986;68A:941–944.
22. Halpern AA, Nagel DA. Anterior compartment pressures in patients with tibial fractures. *J Trauma* 1980;20:786–790.
23. Holbrook JL, Swiontkowski MF, Sanders R. Treatment of open fractures of the tibial shaft: Ender nailing versus external fixation. *J Bone Joint Surg* 1989;71A:1231–1238.
24. Hollinshead WH. *Anatomy for surgeons,* vol. 3: The back and limbs, 3rd ed. Philadelphia: Harper and Row, 1982.
25. Jackson RW, MacNab I. Fractures of the shaft of the tibia. *J Surg* 1959;97:543–557.
26. Johnson EE, Marder RA. Open intramedullary nailing and bone grafting for non-union of tibial diaphyseal fracture. *J Bone Joint Surg* 1987;69A:375–380.
27. Laasonen EM, Jokio P, Lindholm TS. Tibial torsion measured by computed tomography. *Acta Radiol* 1984;25:325–329.
28. Leach RE. Fractures of the tibia and fibula. In: Rockwood CA, Green DP. *Fractures in adults.* vol. 2, 2nd ed. Philadelphia: J. B. Lippincott, 1984;1593–1663.
29. Maurer GJ, Merkow RL, Gustilo RB. Infection after intramedullary nailing of severe open tibial fractures initially treated with external fixation. *J Bone Joint Surg* 1989;71A:835–838.
30. May JW, Jupiter JB, Weiland AJ, Byrd HS. Clinical classification of post-traumatic tibial osteomyelitis. *J Bone Joint Surg* 1989;71A:1422–1428.
31. Merchant TC, Dietz FR. Long-term follow-up after fractures of the tibial and fibular shafts. *J Bone Joint Surg* 1989;71A:599–606.
32. Müller ME, Allgower M, Willenegger H. *Technique of internal fixation of fractures.* Revised for the American Edition by G. Segmuller. New York: Springer-Verlag, 1965.
33. Nicoll EA. Fractures of the tibial shaft. *J Bone Joint Surg* 1964;46B:373–387.
34. Rapoport S, Sastman HD, Dope C, Camputaro CM, Holcomb W, Gore JC. Venous clots: Evaluation with MR imaging. *Radiology* 1987;162:527–530.
35. Rhinelander EW. Tibial blood supply in relation to fracture healing. *Clin Orthop* 1974;105:34.
36. Sarmiento A. A functional below-the-knee cast for tibial fracture. *J Bone Joint Surg* 1967;49A:855–875.
37. Sledge SL, Johnson KD, Henley MB, Watson JT. Intramedullary nailing with reaming to treat non-union of the tibia. *J Bone Joint Surg* 1989;71A:1004–1019.
38. Spritzer CE, Sussman SK, Blunder RA, Saled M, Herfken RJ. Deep venous thrombosis evaluation with limited flip-angle, gradient refocused MR imaging: Preliminary experience. *Radiology* 1988;166:371–375.
39. Templeton DC, Morder RA. Injuries of the knee associated with fractures of the tibial shaft. *J Bone Joint Surg* 1989;71A:1392–1394.
40. Urist MR, Mazet R Jr, McLean FC. The pathogenesis and treatment of delayed union and non-union. A survey of eighty-five un-united fractures of the shaft of the tibia and one hundred control cases with similar injuries. *J Bone Joint Surg* 1954;36A:931–967.
41. van der Linden W, Larsson K. Plate fixation versus conservative treatment of tibial shaft fractures. *J Bone Joint Surg* 1979;61A:873–878.
42. Veith RG, Winquist RA, Hansen ST. Ipsilateral fractures of the femur and tibia. *J Bone Joint Surg* 1984;66A:991–1002.
43. Watson-Jones R. *Fractures and joint injuries,* 5th ed. Baltimore: Churchill Livingstone, London, 1976.

Imaging of Orthopedic Trauma,
Second Edition, edited by T.H. Berquist,
Mayo Clinic © 1992. Published
by Raven Press, Ltd., New York.

CHAPTER 9

The Foot and Ankle

Thomas H. Berquist, Bernard F. Morrey, Joseph R. Cass,
and Kenneth A. Johnson

Soft Tissue Anatomy, 453
   Posterior Musculature, 453
   Anterolateral Musculature, 457
   Foot Musculature, 458
   Osseous and Ligamentous Structures of the
      Ankle, 461
   Osseous and Ligamentous Structures of the Foot, 462
   Common Terms, 465
Imaging Techniques, 468
   Routine Radiographic Techniques, 468
   Clinical Applications, 487
Soft Tissue Trauma, 492

Ligament Injuries, 492
Tendon Injuries, 496
Miscellaneous Soft Tissue Injuries, 505
Fractures, 505
   Ankle Fractures, 509
   Talar Fractures and Dislocations, 525
Mid- and Forefoot Injuries, 557
   Midfoot Fractures and Fracture-Dislocations, 557
   Isolated Tarsal Fractures, 557
   Tarso-metatarsal Fracture-Dislocations, 560
   Metatarsal and Phalangeal Fractures, 568
References, 571

Mastering the anatomy and basic functions of the foot and ankle is equally important to physicians involved in imaging procedures, clinical medicine, and surgery. New radiographic techniques, especially magnetic resonance imaging (MRI), provide more diagnostic information due to improved tissue contrast and the ability to obtain multiple image planes (axial, sagittal, coronal, oblique).

SOFT TISSUE ANATOMY

The lower extremity musculature develops from mesodermal tissues of the lower limb bud (5,8). Functional muscle groups are organized in fascial compartments. To simplify the muscular anatomy of the foot and ankle

we will discuss compartments, or functional groups of muscles, including their origins, insertions, and actions. With this in mind, it is important to review the muscles of the leg that act on the foot and ankle.

The muscles of the leg can be divided into anterior, posterior, and lateral compartments. One of these muscles crosses only the knee, two cross the knee and ankle. The majority arise in the leg and act on both the foot and ankle (1,5,8,9,11,21).

Posterior Musculature

The superficial and deep muscles of the calf are divided into compartments by the crural fascia. The superficial muscle group includes the gastrocnemius, soleus, and plantaris (Fig. 9-1). The gastrocnemius has two heads arising from the medial and lateral femoral condyles. The two heads unite to form the bulk of the muscle in the upper calf. At about the midpoint of the calf, the muscle ends in a wide, flat tendon (Fig. 9-1). The soleus inserts into the anterior aspect of the gastrocnemius tendon. Below this level, the tendon narrows in transverse diameter and thickens forming the Achilles tendon (tendo calcaneous), which inserts on the posterior calcaneous. The gastrocnemius plantar flexes the

T. H. Berquist: Department of Diagnostic Radiology, Mayo Medical School, Mayo Clinic Jacksonville, Jacksonville, Florida 32224.
B. F. Morrey: Department of Orthopedic Surgery, Mayo Medical School, Mayo Clinic, Rochester, Minnesota 55905.
J. R. Cass: Orthopedic Center, Sioux Falls, South Dakota 57105.
K. A. Johnson: Department of Orthopedic Surgery, Mayo Medical School, Mayo Clinic, Scottsdale, Arizona 85259.

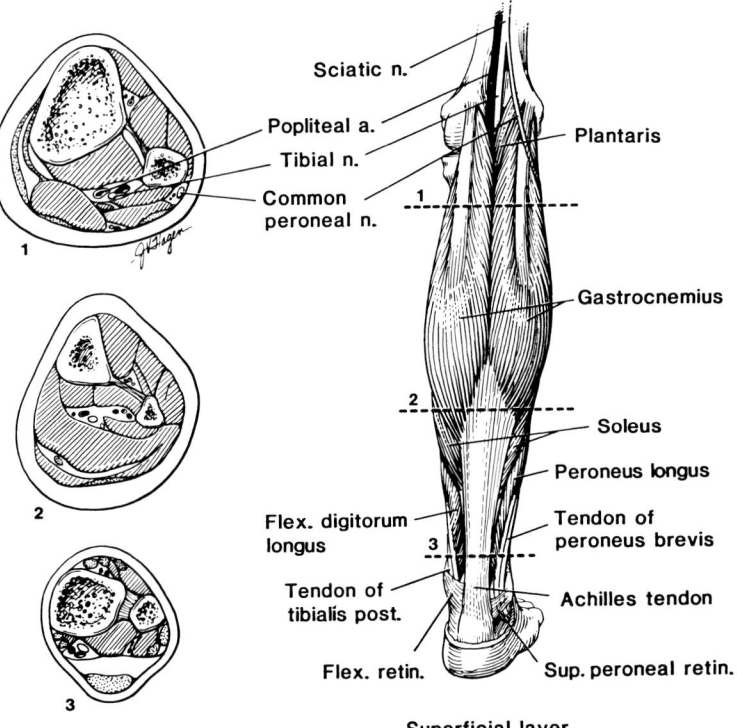

FIG. 9–1. The superficial muscles with axial illustrations at three levels (from 3, with permission.)

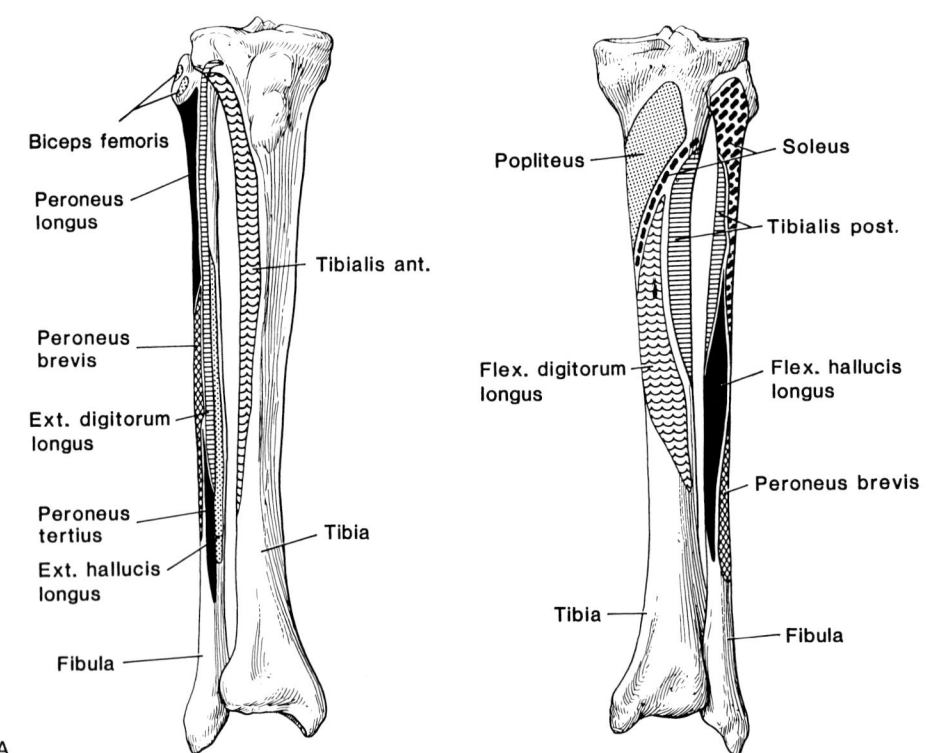

FIG. 9–2. The origins and insertions of muscles to the foot and ankle. **A:** Anterior; **B:** Posterior (from 3, with permission.)

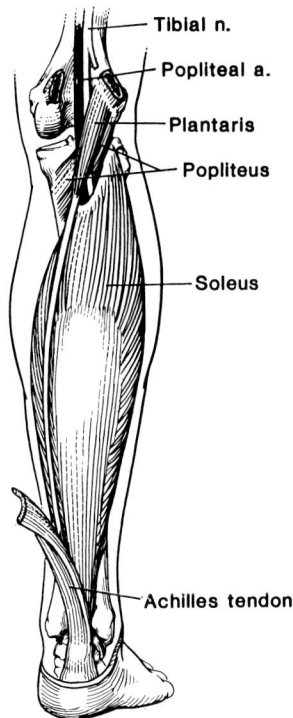

FIG. 9–3. The second muscle layer (from 3, with permission).

foot and also assists in knee flexion during non-weight bearing. Innervation is by the tibial nerve and the vascular supply primarily derived from the posterior tibial artery (5,8,11).

The soleus lies deep to the gastrocnemius (Figs. 9-2 and 9-3) and also has two heads, one arising from the posterior superior fibula and the second from the popliteal line and the posteromedial surface of the proximal tibia. The popliteal vessels and tibial nerve pass deep to the body of the soleus (5,8,9,11). The soleus inserts in the anterior aspect of the gastrocnemius tendon forming the thicker Achilles tendon.

The soleus has no effect on the knee but serves as a

plantar flexor of the foot. Innervation is via the tibial nerve with vascular supply from the posterior tibial artery (1,5,8).

An important, but uncommon variable is the accessory soleus muscle. This accessory muscle bundle extends into Kager's fat triangle anterior to the Achilles tendon and inserts in the anterior aspect of this tendon, the calcaneous, or the flexor retinaculum (Fig. 9-4) (3,6). This muscle may be incidentally noted, but some patients may have clinical symptoms. The most common presenting complaints are soft tissue prominence and/or pain following exercise. Thus, it is important to differentiate this normal variant from a torn muscle remnant or soft tissue tumor.

The plantaris is the third muscle included in the superficial compartment. This small muscle takes its origin from the lateral epicondyle of the femur and the oblique popliteal ligament (5,8). The belly of the muscle is only several inches long and passes between the gastrocnemius and soleus in an oblique direction (Fig. 9-3). The long, thin tendon passes distally along the medial margin of the Achilles to insert in the calcaneous, Achilles, or flexor retinaculum (5,11).

The plantaris functions as a minor flexor of the knee and plantar flexor of the foot. Innervation and blood supply are from the tibial nerve and the posterior tibial artery (5,8).

The deep compartment of the calf contains the popliteus, tibialis posterior, flexor hallucis longus, and flexor digitorum longus. The popliteus is a small triangular muscle forming a portion of the floor of the popliteal fossa (Figs. 9-2 and 9-3) (5,8). Its origin is from the lateral femoral epicondyle, the arcuate popliteal ligament, and capsule of the knee. The insertion is the posterior surface of the upper tibia above the origin of the soleus. The popliteus acts on the knee and leg as a flexor and medial rotator. Neurovascular supply is by the tibial nerve and posterior tibial artery.

The flexor hallucis longus is the most lateral of the

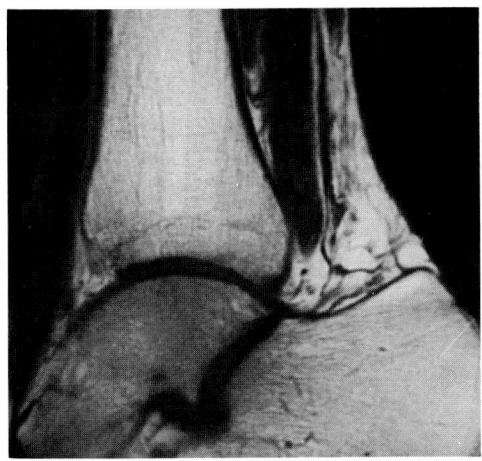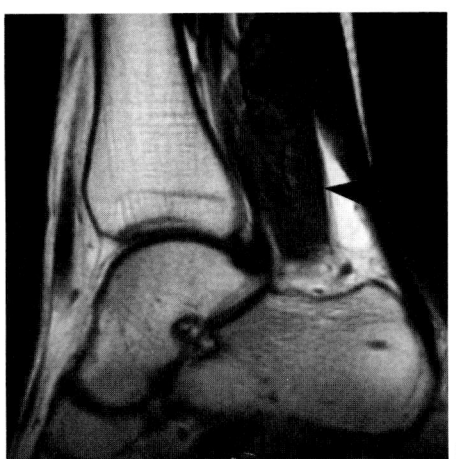

FIG. 9–4. Sagittal SE 500/20 images of a normal ankle (**A**) and a patient with an accessory soleus (**B**, *arrow*).

three remaining deep muscles of the leg (flexor hallucis longus, flexor digitorum longus, and tibialis posterior) (Fig. 9-2). It arises from the lateral aspect of the middle half of the posterior fibula (Fig. 9-2) (5,8,9,11). Its tendon begins above the malleoli of the ankle and courses medially behind the ankle deep to the flexor retinaculum (Fig. 9-5). The tendon is posterior to the tendons of the tibialis posterior and flexor digitorum longus behind the medial malleolus (Fig. 9-5). The tendon passes along the plantar aspect of the foot to insert in the distal phalanx of the great toe (5,8,9,11).

The flexor hallucis longus is a flexor of the great toe and assists in ankle flexion. The muscle is innervated by the tibial nerve and receives its blood supply from the posterior tibial artery (5,8).

The flexor digitorum longus lies medially in the deep compartment of the calf (Fig. 9-5). It arises from the upper half of the posteromedial aspect of the tibia (Fig. 9-2). Along its caudad course, it passes posterior to the tibialis posterior so that at the ankle it lies between the flexor hallucis longus and tibialis posterior (Fig. 9-5). The tendon passes through the flexor retinaculum, posterior to the medial malleolus and then divides into four slips that insert in the distal phalanges of the lateral four digits (5,8). On the plantar aspect of the foot, these four tendon slips are associated with the lumbrical muscles and pass through the divided slips of the flexor digitorum brevis prior to inserting on the distal phalanges (1,5,8).

The flexor digitorum longus flexes the lateral four toes

and also plantar flexes the foot and supinates the ankle (5,8). The muscle is innervated by branches of the tibial nerve and receives its vascular supply from posterior tibial artery branches.

The tibialis posterior is the deepest and most centrally located muscle in the deep posterior compartment (Fig. 9-5). It arises from the upper posterior aspects of the tibia and fibula and the interosseous membrane (Fig. 9-2). Thus it is positioned between the flexor hallucis longus and flexor digitorum longus. The tendon passes medially deep to the flexor retinaculum and flexor digitorum longus. Therefore, it is the most anterior of the three tendons as it passes behind the medial malleolus (Fig. 9-5). The tendon flares to insert in the navicular, tarsal bones, and bases of the 2–4 metatarsals (5,8,9,11).

The tibialis posterior aids in adduction, inversion, and plantar flexion of the foot. The muscle is innervated by branches of the tibial nerve and receives its blood supply from the posterior tibial artery (5,8).

Neurovascular Anatomy of the Calf

The tibial nerve is a continuation of the sciatic nerve at the level of the popliteal fossa. As it passes inferiorly it enters the calf between the heads of the gastrocnemius muscle passing deep to the soleus to lie between the soleus and tibialis posterior in the deep compartment (5,8). The tibial nerve sends branches to all of the superficial

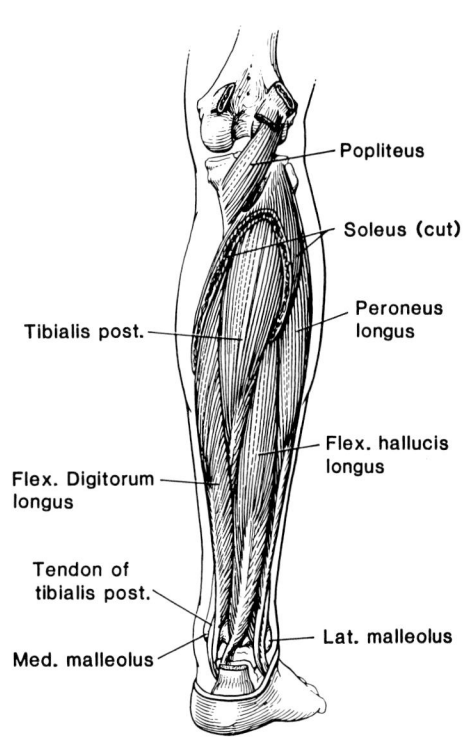

FIG. 9–5. The deep muscles affecting the foot and ankle (from 3, with permission).

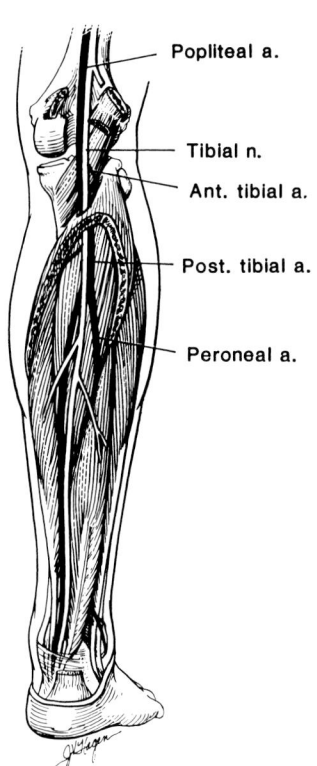

FIG. 9–6. The posterior neurovascular anatomy to the calf and ankle (from 3, with permission).

and deep muscles of the calf (Fig. 9-6). At the ankle level, the nerve generally lies between the flexor hallucis longus and flexor digitorum longus tendons (Fig. 9-6). Distal to the flexor retinaculum it divides forming the medial and lateral plantar nerves (5,8,9,11).

The popliteal artery is a direct continuation of the superficial femoral artery as it passes through the adductor canal. It divides into anterior and posterior tibial branches at the level of the popliteus muscle. The anterior tibial artery enters the anterolateral leg above the upper margin of the interosseous membrane while the posterior tibial artery joins the tibial nerve in the deep compartment of the calf (Fig. 9-6). In the leg, it provides muscular branches to all of the calf muscles and a nutrient artery to the tibia. Its largest branch, the peroneal artery, arises high in the leg and passes deep to the flexor hallucis longus near the interosseous membrane and fibula (Fig. 9-6). At the ankle level it forms anastomotic branches with the posterior tibial artery and perforates the interosseous membrane to supply the dorsal aspect of the foot. Generally paired veins accompany the arteries. These veins are more variable and enter the popliteal vein superiorly (1,2,5,8).

Anterolateral Musculature

The peroneus longus and brevis are the two muscles of the lateral compartment. Both arise from the superior lateral surface of the fibula. The origin of the peroneus longus is more superior with the muscle passing superficial to the peroneus brevis (Fig. 9-2). The muscles pro-

gress caudad in the lateral compartment with their tendons entering a common tendon sheath above the ankle (Fig. 9-7). The tendons pass posterior to the lateral malleolus and deep to the superior and inferior peroneal retinacula. The tendons diverge on the lateral surface of the foot with the peroneus brevis inserting on the base of the 5th metatarsal. The peroneus longus takes an inferior course passing under the lateral aspect of the foot where it inserts on the base of the first metatarsal and medial cuneiform (5,8,9,11).

These muscles serve as evertors of the foot and assist in plantar flexion. Innervation is from the superficial peroneal nerve with branches of the common or deep peroneal nerve supplying a portion of the peroneus longus. Vascular supply is via the peroneal artery (5,8).

Anterior Compartment Musculature

There are four muscles in the anterior compartment. These include the extensor digitorum longus, peroneus tertius, extensor hallucis longus, and tibialis anterior (Fig. 9-8).

The extensor digitorum longus is the most lateral muscle in the anterior compartment (Fig. 9-8) (8). It arises from the lateral tibial condyle, anterior fibula, and interosseous membrane (Fig. 9-2). The tendon passes deep to the superior and inferior extensor retinaculae prior to dividing into four slips that insert and the dorsal aspects

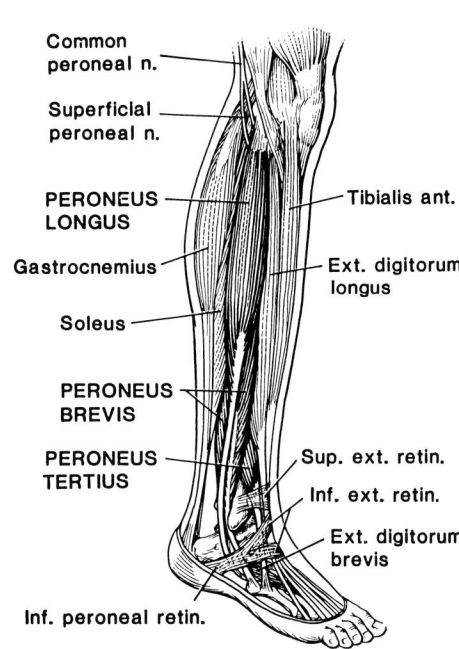

FIG. 9-7. The lateral muscle group (from 3, with permission.)

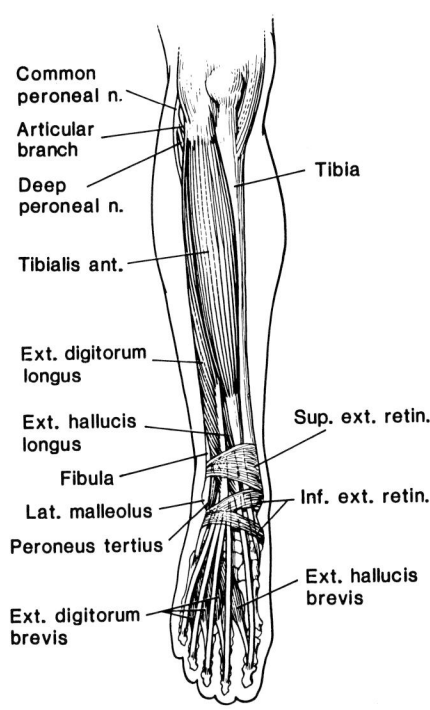

FIG. 9-8. The anterior muscle group (from 3, with permission.)

of the four lateral toes (Fig. 9-8). The insertions are divided such that portions insert in the middle and distal phalanges (5,8).

This muscle dorsiflexes the toes and also assists in eversion of the foot. It is innervated by the deep peroneal nerve and receives its vascular supply from the anterior tibial artery.

The peroneus tertius is closely associated with the extensor digitorum longus, and may be considered a portion of the latter (5). It arises from the distal anterior fibula, interosseous membrane, and membrane of the peroneus brevis (Fig. 9-2). Its tendon passes deep to the extensor retinaculae to insert on the dorsal aspect of the base of the fifth metatarsal (Fig. 9-8). It is supplied by the deep peroneal nerve and anterior tibial artery. This muscle varies in size and may be absent (8).

The extensor hallucis longus lies deep to the extensor digitorum longus and tibialis anterior. It arises from the mid fibula and interosseous membrane and becomes superficial in the lower leg (Fig. 9-2). Its tendon passes deep to the extensor retinaculae to insert on the distal phalanx of the great toe (Fig. 9-8). This muscle extends the great toe and is a weak dorsiflexor and invertor of the foot. It is supplied by the deep peroneal nerve and anterior tibial artery.

The tibialis anterior arises from the lateral tibia surface, deep fascia, and interosseous membrane (Fig. 9-2). It passes inferiorly becoming tendonous in the lower leg. It is the most medial tendon as it passes deep to the extensor retinaculae. It passes along the medial foot to

insert in the medial cuneiform and plantar portion of the first metatarsal (Fig. 9-8) (5,8,9,11).

This muscle is a strong dorsiflexor and inverter of the foot (8). Neurovascular supply is via the deep peroneal nerve and anterior tibial artery.

Neurovascular Anatomy of the Anterolateral Muscles

The common peroneal nerve is a branch of the sciatic nerve and courses laterally in the popliteal fossa. It is subcutaneous and relatively unprotected just below the fibular head (Fig. 9-9). Therefore, it is susceptible to direct trauma in this area (5,8,9,11). As it descends between the fibula and peroneus longus, it divides into two or three branches. These are the superficial, deep, and articular branches of the peroneal nerve (Fig. 9-9). The superficial peroneal nerve lies between the peroneus longus and brevis and supplies these muscles and the subcutaneous tissues. The deep peroneal nerve courses anteriorly, deep to the peroneus longus to supply the anterior muscles of the leg. It joins the anterior tibial artery on the anterior aspect of the interosseous membrane (5,8,9,11).

The anterior tibial artery passes superior to the interosseous membrane in the upper leg and then lies with the deep peroneal nerve along the anterior aspect of the interosseous membrane (Fig. 9-9). It supplies the anterior muscles and continues as the dorsalis pedis artery on the dorsum of the foot (5,8).

Foot Musculature

The muscles of the foot are generally discussed by layer rather than compartments (5–8). The superficial layer of plantar muscles includes the abductor hallucis, flexor digitorum brevis, and abductor digiti minimi (Fig. 9-10).

The abductor hallucis arises from the medial process of tubercle of the calcaneus, the flexor retinaculum, and plantar aponeurosis. Its insertion is the medial side of the flexor surface of the proximal phalanx of the great toe (Fig. 9-10) (5,8). The medial and lateral plantar vessels and nerves pass deep to the proximal position of the muscle as they enter the foot (8). The muscle is supplied by branches of the medial plantar nerve and artery. The abductor hallucis functions weakly as an abductor of the metatarsophalangeal joint of the great toe (5).

The flexor digitorum brevis is the most central of the superficial plantar muscles (Fig. 9-10). It arises from the medial tubercular process of the calcaneus and plantar fascia. Four tendons pass distally and divide into two slips at the level of the proximal phalanx. The tendons of the flexor digitorum longus pass through the divided brevis tendons. The divided tendon slips insert on the middle phalanx (5,8).

The muscle flexes the lateral four toes. It is supplied by the medial plantar nerve and artery, with the lateral

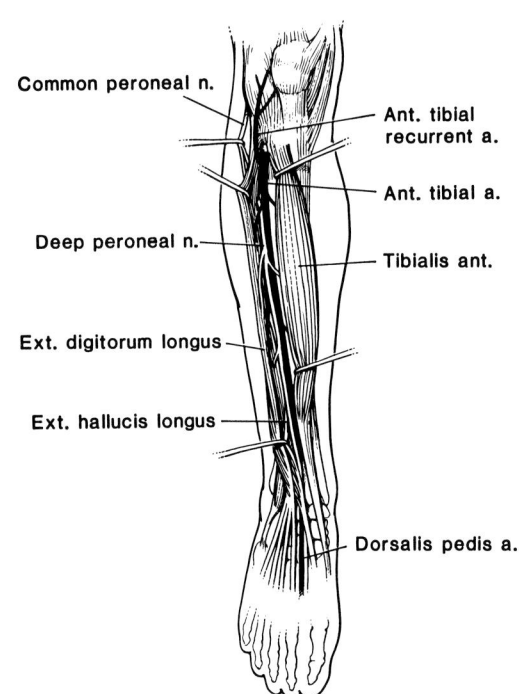

FIG. 9-9. The anterior neurovascular anatomy (from 3, with permission.)

Labels on figure:
- Common peroneal n.
- Ant. tibial recurrent a.
- Ant. tibial a.
- Deep peroneal n.
- Tibialis ant.
- Ext. digitorum longus
- Ext. hallucis longus
- Dorsalis pedis a.

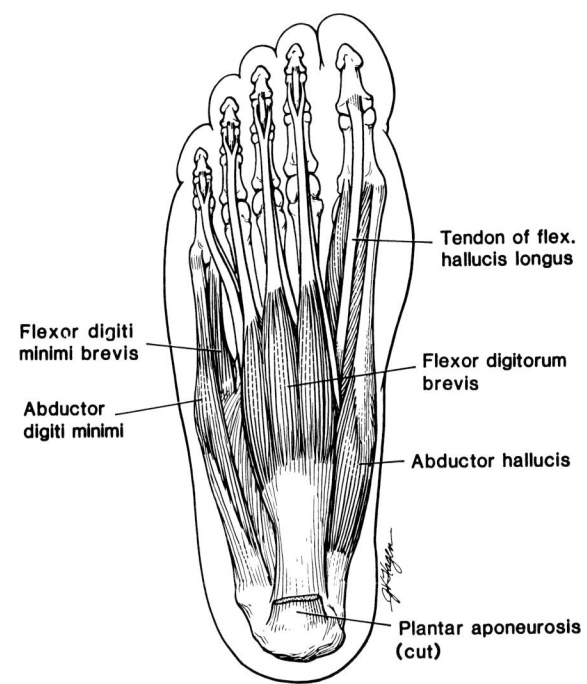

FIG. 9-10. Superficial plantar muscles of the foot (from 3, with permission.)

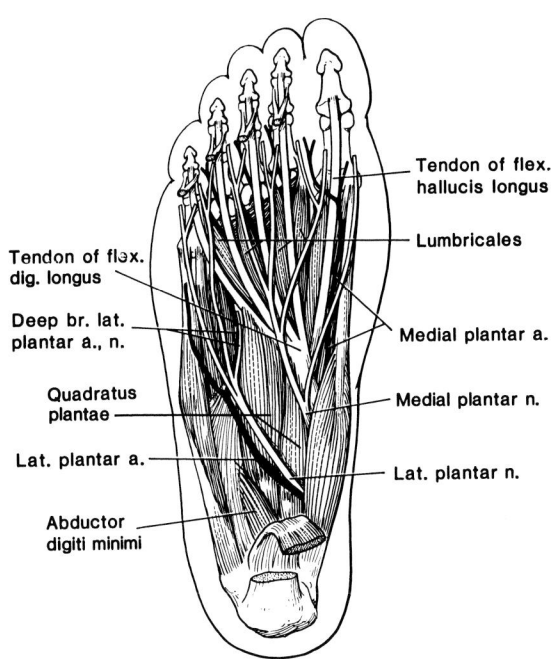

FIG. 9-11. The second layer and neurovascular structures (from 3, with permission.)

plantar nerve and artery passing deep to this muscle (8). It is not uncommon for the tendon to the fifth toe to be absent (38%) (5,8).

The abductor digiti minimi is the most lateral muscle in the superficial layer (Fig. 9-10). It arises from the lateral process of the calcaneal tubercle and the distal portion of the medial process. It inserts in the lateral aspect of the base of the proximal phalanx of the fifth toe and serves to flex and abduct the toe at the metatarsal phalangeal joint. It is supplied by the lateral plantar nerve and artery.

The second layer of the foot is composed of the tendons of the flexor hallucis longus and flexor digitorum longus plus the quadratus plantae and lumbrical muscles (Fig. 9-11) (15).

The quadratus plantae has two heads that arise from the medial and lateral plantar aspects of the calcaneal tuberosity. The muscle inserts in the lateral and posterior margin of the flexor digitorum longus just before it divides into its four tendon slips (Fig. 9-11) (5,8).

The muscle assists the flexor digitorum longus in flexing the lateral four toes. It is supplied by the lateral plantar nerve and artery. Occasionally the lateral head or, in certain cases, the entire muscle may be absent (5).

The four lumbrical muscles arise from the flexor digitorum longus tendon. They pass distally to insert on the medial side of the metatarsophalangeal joints of the four lateral toes (Fig. 9-11). They act as flexors of the metatarsophalangeal joints. The most medial muscle is innervated by the medial plantar nerve, while the lateral plantar nerves supply the lateral three muscles. Blood supply

is via the medial and lateral plantar arteries. Absence of one or more of the lumbricals has been reported. Occasionally two muscles insert on the fourth and fifth toes (5).

The third layer of plantar muscles includes the flexor hallucis brevis, adductor hallucis, and flexor digitis minimi brevis (Fig. 9-12).

The flexor hallucis brevis has two bellies arising from the plantar aspect of the cuboid and adjacent cuneiform. The tendons insert at the sides of the base of the great toe and the sesamoids. The muscle serves as a flexor of the great toe and is supplied by the medial plantar nerve and artery (1,5,8).

The adductor hallucis has oblique and transverse heads (Fig. 9-12). The oblique head arises from the long plantar ligament and the second through fourth metatarsals bases (5). The smaller transverse head arises from the capsules of the third through fifth metatarsophalangeal joints and the deep transverse ligaments. The two heads join lateral to the great toe to insert with the lateral head of the flexor hallucis brevis (5,8).

The adductor hallucis adducts and flexes the great toe. In addition, it assists in flexion of the proximal phalanx and maintains the transverse arch (5). It is supplied by the lateral plantar arteries and nerve.

The flexor digiti minimi brevis arises from the cuboid and base of the fifth metatarsal and inserts in the lateral base of the proximal phalanx of the fifth toe (Fig. 9-12). The muscle serves as a flexor of the small toe and is supplied by branches of the lateral plantar nerve and artery (5,8).

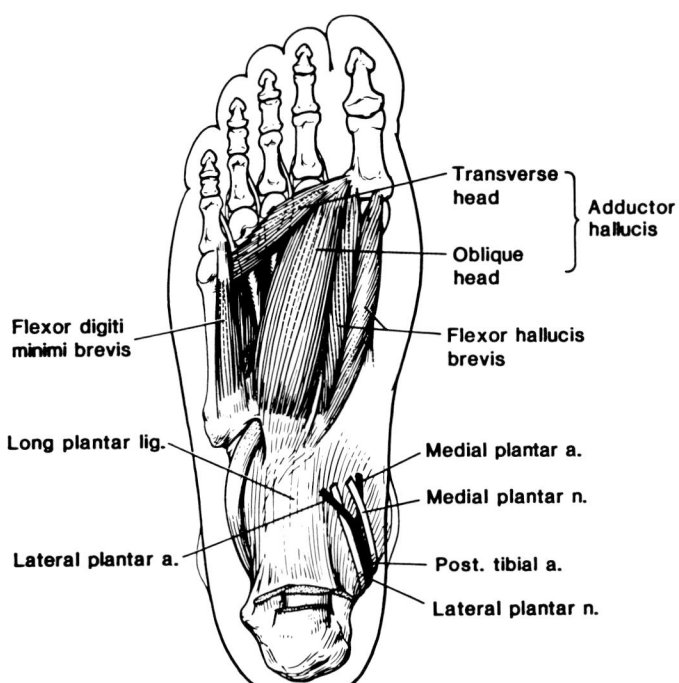

FIG. 9-12. The third layer of muscles in the foot (from 3, with permission.)

The fourth and deepest layer of plantar muscles consists of seven interosseous muscles: three plantar and four dorsal (Fig. 9-13). The four dorsal interossei arise with two heads from the adjacent aspects of the metatarsal bases. The tendons insert into the bases of the proximal phalanges with the two medial bellies inserting on

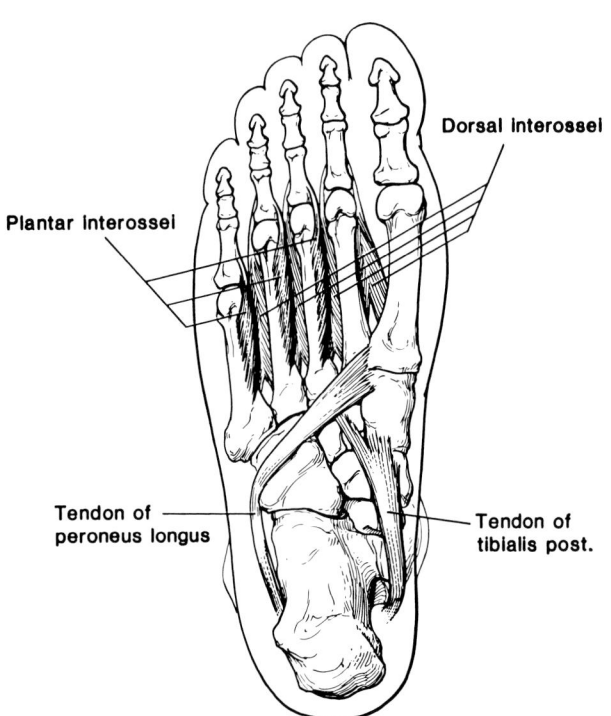

FIG. 9-13. The fourth layer of muscles in the foot (from 3, with permission.)

the medial and lateral side of the second and the third and fourth inserting on the lateral sides of the third and fourth proximal phalanges. The three plantar interosseous muscles arise from the bases of the third through fifth metatarsals and insert on the medial sides of the proximal phalanges of the third, fourth, and fifth toes. Thus the dorsal interossei are abductors and the plantar interossei adductors. All interossei muscles are supplied by branches of the lateral plantar artery and nerve (5).

The extensor digitorum brevis (Fig. 9-8) is the dorsal muscle of the foot. This broad, thin muscle arises from the superior calcaneus, lateral talocalcaneal ligament, and extensor retinaculum. It takes a medial oblique course ending in four tendons that insert in the lateral aspect of the proximal phalanx of the great toe and the lateral extensor digitorum longus tendons of the second to fourth toes (5,8).

The muscle extends the great toe and the second through fourth toes. It is supplied by the deep peroneal nerve and dorsalis pedis artery.

Neurovascular Supply of the Foot

The anterior tibial artery continues over the mid anterior aspect of the tibia passing deep to the extensor tendons and retinaculae of the ankle (Fig. 9-9). At the ankle, the anterior tibial artery anastomosis with the perforating branch of the peroneal artery, both supplying the periarticular structures of the ankle (5,8). As the anterior tibial artery emerges from the extensor retinaculum, it becomes the more superficial dorsalis pedis artery. After giving off the deep plantar artery, it becomes the first

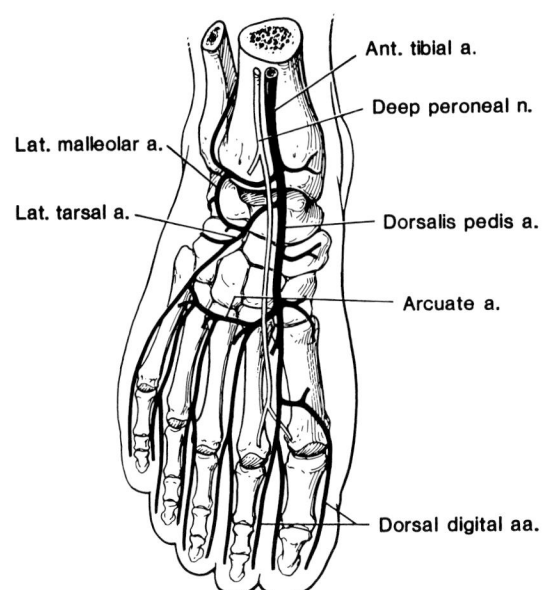

FIG. 9–14. The dorsal neurovascular supply to the foot (from 3, with permission.)

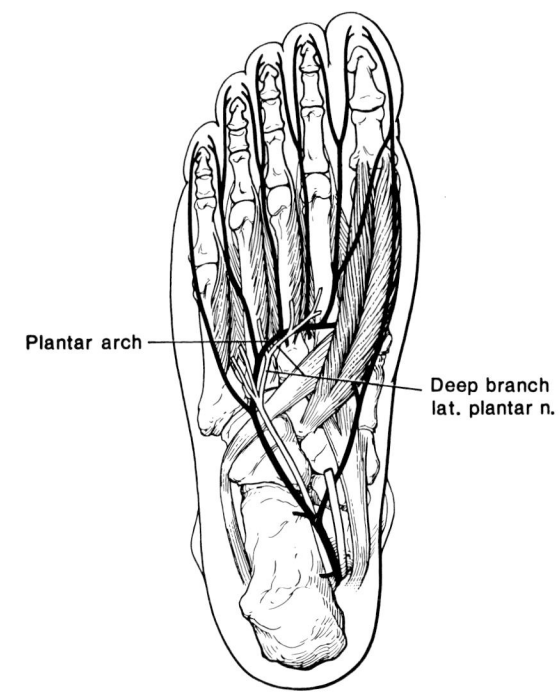

FIG. 9–15. The plantar neurovascular supply (from 3, with permission.)

dorsal metatarsal artery. This vessel courses distally ending in digital branches of the first and second toes (5). Dorsal branches of the foot include medial and lateral tarsal arteries and the arcuate artery with its dorsal metatarsal branches (Fig. 9-14).

The deep peroneal nerve accompanies the anterior tibial, dorsalis pedis, and first dorsal metatarsal arteries. It supplies the anterior muscles of the foot and leg. The superficial peroneal runs over the anterior aspect of the fibula supplying the peroneal muscles and the lateral aspect of the foot (1,5,8).

The posterior tibial artery divides into medial and lateral plantar branches deep to the flexor retinaculum (5). It is accompanied by similarly named nerves and veins. The neural branches (medial and lateral plantar nerves) are branches of the tibia nerve (Fig. 9-15) (5,8,9,11,14).

Osseous and Ligamentous Structures of the Ankle

The ankle is composed of three bones: the tibia, fibula, and talus (Fig. 9-16) (21,32). The tibia is the second longest bone in the skeleton. It is expanded proximally and distally. The body of the tibia (diaphysis) has three surfaces (anterior, medial, and posterior). The anterior surface ends in the medial malleolus. The medial margin is subcutaneous. The interosseous membrane attaches to the lateral margin (5).

Distally the tibia expands at the metaphysis forming the medial malleolus and the articular surface for the talus (Fig. 9-16). The inferior or articular surface is biconcave and articulates with the talar dome (17,19).

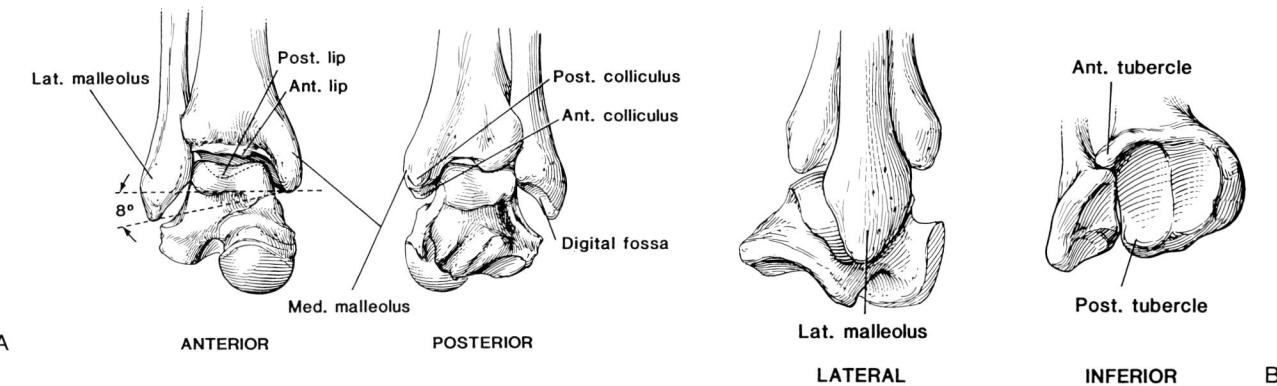

FIG. 9–16. The osseous anatomy of the ankle. **A:** Anterior and posterior. **B:** Lateral and inferior (from 3, with permission.)

Hyaline cartilage covers the articular surface of the tibia and extends medially to the articular portion of the medial malleolus. The articular cartilage does not completely cover the posterior tibia (posterior malleolus). This is significant because, if only small segments of the posterior malleolus are fractured, the articular portion may be excluded (5,8,19).

The anterior surface of the tibia is smooth except at the anterior inferior margin where it is more irregular at the site for attachment of the anterior ankle capsule. The posterior tibia has grooves for the flexor hallucis longus (lateral) and flexor digitorum longus and tibialis posterior tendons (medial) (5,16). The lateral surface articulates with the fibula. This articular surface is bounded anteriorly and posteriorly by ridges for insertion of the anterior and posterior distal tibiofibular ligaments (Fig. 9-16) (5,8,16,17,19). The strong medial extension (medial malleolus) articulates with the talus and forms the medial portion of the ankle mortise.

The fibula is thin and flat and does not have a direct weight-bearing surface (see Fig. 9-2). The lateral malleolus is the expanded distal portion of the fibula. The fibula is irregular along its medial margin at the point of attachment for the interosseous ligament. Hyaline cartilage covers the articular surface on the inferomedial aspect. There are irregular areas anteriorly and posteriorly for insertions of the tibiofibular ligament. The fibula (lateral malleolus) is more posterior than the medial malleolus and its distal extent is below the level of the medial malleolar tip. Thus an angle of about 8° is formed by a line drawn from the tips of the malleoli (Fig. 9-16A) (16,19). The posterior position of the lateral malleolus results in angle of 20° between the malleoli in the axial plane. For this reason, the mortise view of the ankle is taken with the foot internally rotated approximately 20° (8,9,19).

The hyaline cartilage trochlear surface of the talus is usually 2–3 mm wider anteriorly than posteriorly. It articulates with the weight-bearing surface of the tibia and medial and lateral malleoli. Thus the ankle mortise is formed by the tibial and fibular components of the ankle, which roofs the talus. The tibial portion of the mortise is termed the *plafond*. Forces on the talus that result in position changes of this structure in the mortise are responsible for many osseous and/or ligamentous ankle injuries (3,16,19).

The supporting structures of the ankle include the joint capsule, medial and lateral ligaments, and interosseous ligament (Fig. 9-17). In addition, thirteen tendons cross the ankle and there are four retinaculae (3,5,7,8). Four ligaments support the distal tibia and fibula (5). The interosseous ligament, with its oblique fibers, joins the tibia and fibula to a level just above the joint. The interosseous ligament is the thickened distal portion of the interosseous membrane. The tibial and fibular attachments of this ligament form a triangular configuration that is weakened at its base by the syndesmotic recess (Fig. 9-17). This recess is an extension of the joint into the tibiofibular space. The distal anterior and posterior tibiofibular ligaments join the tibia and fibula just proximal to the tibiotalar joint (Fig. 9-17). The anterior ligament is weaker than the posterior. This explains the increased incidence of avulsion fractures posteriorly, compared to ligament disruptions. The transverse ligament is the fourth ligament of the syndesmotic group. This ligament lies anterior to the posterior tibiofibular ligament and extends from the lateral malleolus to the posterior articular margin of the tibia just lateral to the medial malleolus (5). The ligament actually forms part of the posterior articulation with the talus (5,7-9,16).

The deltoid ligament provides medial stability (3,5,8,16). This ligament is a strong triangular-shaped group of fibers with its apex at the medial malleolus. The ligament fans out as it progresses inferiorly and divides into superficial and deep fibers (5). The superficial fibers insert in the navicular tuberosity. Progressing posteriorly, the remaining superficial fibers insert in the sustentaculum tali and talus. The deep fibers attach to the medial surface of the talus (Fig. 9-17) (5,8,16,19). The deltoid ligament prevents excessive abduction and eversion of the ankle and subtalar joints. In addition, eversion, pronation, and anterior displacement of the talus are restricted (5,12,13).

There are three ligaments laterally (Fig. 9-17A). The anterior talofibular ligament is the weakest and most frequently injured. It passes anteriorly from the fibula to insert anterior to the lateral talar articular facet. This ligament restrains the anterior talar motion. The posterior talofibular ligament is much stronger and courses transversely from the posterior aspect of the lateral malleolus to the posterior talar tubercle. The ligament prevents posterior talar motion. The calcaneofibular ligament is the longest of the three ligaments and takes a nearly vertical course from the lateral malleolus to the lateral surface of the calcaneus. The calcaneofibular ligament prevents excessive inversion. The peroneal tendons are just superficial to the calcaneofibular ligament (5,8,12,13).

The synovial lined capsule of the ankle is attached to the margins of the tibia, fibula, and talus. The anterior and posterior portions of the capsule are thin and provide much less support than the above ligaments (5,8,9,12,13).

Osseous and Ligamentous Structures of the Foot

For purposes of discussion, the foot can be divided into three segments; the hind foot (talus and calcaneus), mid foot (remaining five tarsal bones), and forefoot (metatarsals and phalanges) segments (5,16,23).

The Hind Foot

The hind foot includes the talus and calcaneus (16,20,23). The talus is the second largest of the tarsal bones and articulates with the tibia, medial and lateral malleoli, and calcaneus inferiorly (Fig. 9-16). The talar head articulates with the navicular (5,19).

Superiorly, the trochlear articulates with the tibia and malleoli (Fig. 9-16). It is covered with hyaline cartilage and makes up the upper portion of the body of the talus. There are three articular facets on the inferior surface of the talus (Fig. 9-16) (1,5,19). The anterior and posterior facets articulate with similarly named calcaneal facets. The middle facet is just posterior to the anterior calcaneal articular facet. The middle facet articulates with the sustentaculum tali (5). The talar sulcus lies between the middle and anterior facets. This structure with its calcaneal counterpart forms the tarsal sinus, which contains the interosseous talocalcaneal ligament. The head of the talus articulates with the navicular.

The calcaneus, the largest tarsal bone, contains three superior articular facets (1,3,5,8). The middle, most medial facet is on the sustentaculum tali. The calcaneal sulcus lies between the middle and anterior facets and forms the floor of the tarsal canal. This canal has an oblique course and measures 10–15 mm in height, 3–5 mm in width, and 15–20 mm in length (19). The distal or plantar surface of the calcaneus contains two grooves. The lateral groove is for the peroneus longus tendon. More medially the flexor hallucis longus runs in the groove beneath the sustentaculum tali (Fig. 9-13) (5,8,19).

The posterior aspect of the calcaneus forms the prominence of the heel (5,23). It contains irregular areas superiorly for insertion of the Achilles tendon (superior tuberosity), and medially for the plantar aponeurosi, flexor digitorum brevis and abductor hallucis, and lateral inferior processes (abductor digiti minimi) for muscle attachments. The calcaneus articulates with the cuboid anteriorly (5,16,19).

There are two ligaments that directly support the talocalcaneal joint. These are the interosseous talocalcaneal ligament, which is located in the sinus tarsi, and the smaller lateral talocalcaneal ligament. In addition, the

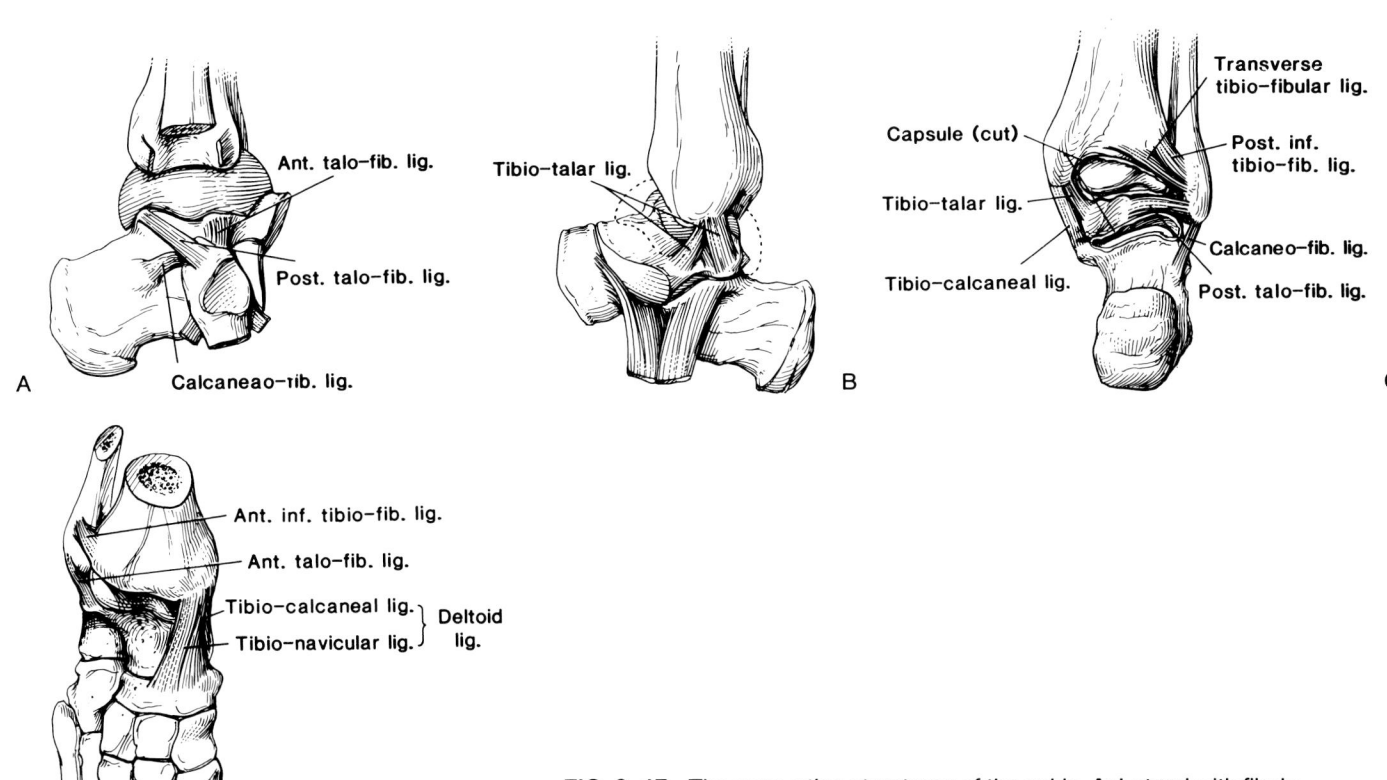

FIG. 9-17. The supporting structures of the ankle. A: Lateral with fibula retracted. B: Medial with superficial ligament reflected. C: Posterior; and D: dorsal.

ligaments of the ankle and the adjacent tendons provide stabilization. The latter include the peroneal tendons, flexor hallucis longus, flexor digitorum longus, and tibialis posterior tendons (5,8,16,19).

The Midfoot

The remaining tarsal bones make up the midfoot. These include the cuboid, navicular, and three cuneiforms (5,8,9,11,23).

The cuboid articulates with the calcaneus proximally and distally with the fourth and fifth metatarsals (Fig. 9-18). Dorsally the cuboid is roughened at the points of ligament attachment. On the plantar surface the cuboid contains a groove for the peroneus longus tendon (Fig. 9-13). The medial cuboid surface contains a facet for articulation with the lateral cuneiform (1,5,8).

The navicular is on the medial side of the foot anterior to the talus. It articulates proximally with the talus, anteriorly with the cuneiforms, and occasionally with the cuboid laterally (5,8).

The spring ligament is contiguous with the deltoid ligament of the ankle. (Fig. 9-17C) It extends from the calcaneus to the navicular tuberosity. The cubonavicular ligament runs dorsally from the cuboid to the navicular (5). Proximally, the bifurcate ligament originates on the anterior superior calcaneus and sends medial fibers to the

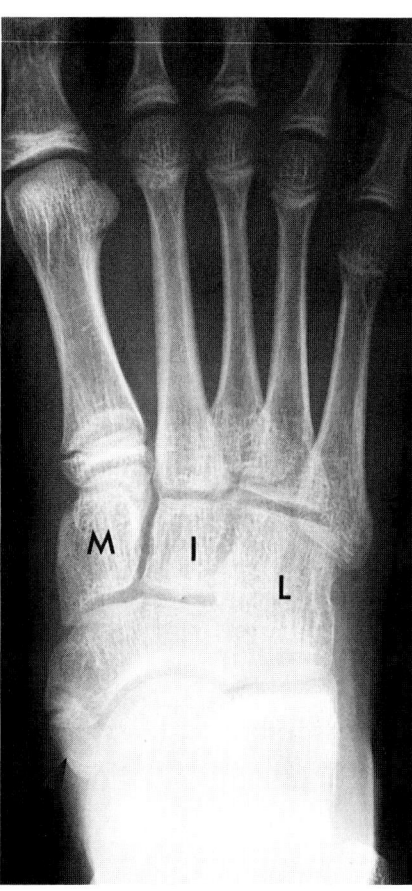

FIG. 9–19. AP view of the midfoot demonstrating the cunieforms and their articulations. M, medial; I, intermediate; L, lateral. Note the accessory navicular (*arrow*).

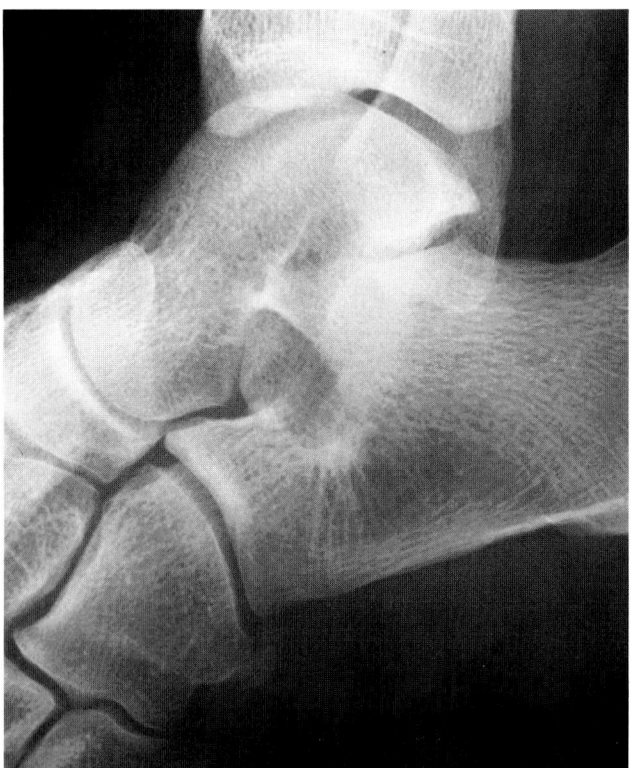

FIG. 9–18. Oblique radiograph demonstrating the cuboid and its articulations.

lateral navicular and lateral fibers to the cuboid (5,8). The cancaneonavicular ligament is on the plantar aspect of the capsule (1,5,8).

There are three cuneiform bones located distal to the navicular and medial to the cuboid (Fig. 9-19). The medial cuneiform is the largest and articulates with the navicular proximally, the intermediate cuneiform laterally, and the first and second metatarsals distally (Fig. 9-19) (5). The intermediate cuneiform is the smallest cuneiform and lies between the medial and lateral cuneiforms. It articulates with the latter bones, the navicular, and the second metatarsal (5,8,9,16). The lateral cuneiform lies between the intermediate cuneiform and the cuboid articulating with both. It also articulates with the navicular and second through fourth metatarsals (Fig. 9-19) (1,5,8,9).

The five metatarsals articulate proximally with the above tarsal bones (Fig. 9-19) and each, except the first (great toe) typically has three phalanges distally. The metatarsals have similar configuration except the first is broader from the proximal articular surface distally to its head. The fifth metatarsal has a broad base compared to the second through fourth metatarsals.

Dorsal, plantar, and interosseous ligaments support the tarsometatarsal joints and bases of the metatarsals. Distally, the transverse metatarsal ligament connects the heads of the metatarsals (5). Each of the metatarsophalangeal joints is supported by collateral and plantar ligaments. The extensor tendons replace the usual dorsal ligaments in these joints (5,8,9,23).

Normal Variants

There are many anatomic variants that can mimic more serious pathologic conditions. These changes are most common in the metaphyseal and epiphyseal areas adjacent to the growth plates. Occasionally small ossification centers are evident adjacent to the growth plates simulating fractures (Fig. 9-20) (3,8,18). Ossicles are also commonly noted near the medial and lateral malleoli. These frequently cause confusion in patients with recent injury (Fig. 9-21). They occur medially in 17–24% of females and up to 47% of males. Most are bilateral, and they are commonly seen in patients from 6–12 years of age (3,18).

Normal variants are also common in the tarsal bones (3,18). The secondary ossification center of the talus is located posteriorly. It appears at 8–11 years and normally fuses at 16–20 years of age. This somewhat controversial ossification center is the posterior part of the talar tubercle located lateral to the flexor hallucis longus tendon (3,16,18). If this center does not fuse to the talus, it is called the os trigonum tarsi and is frequently mistaken for a fracture (Fig. 9-22) (22,31). In forced plantar flexion the ossicle can separate or fracture can occur in the fused center.

Another common finding is the accessory-navicular or os tibiale externum (6,22,27). This lies in the posterior tibial tendon just proximal to the medial margin of the navicular. This ossicle may effect tendon function, especially during puberty when growth is accelerated (Fig. 9-19) (3,18). Resection may be required to relieve the painful symptoms. The os supranavicular (Fig. 9-23) is located at the proximal dorsal margin of the navicular distal to the joint space (3,18). This is more distal than the os supratalare, which would be proximal to the talonavicular joint.

The most frequently noted ossicles in the foot are summarized in Fig. 9-20.

Common Terms

Terms used to describe the movements in the foot and ankle are often misused. This results in some confusion when using descriptive terms such as *supination, eversion, pronation,* etc. Definitions of these commonly used terms are listed below as they apply during physiologic motion of the foot and ankle (9,11,21,22).

Plantar flexion The hinge motion at the tibiotalar joint allows the foot to plantar flex—sole of foot depressed. Several other motions and position changes occur with plantar flexion. During plantar flexion the gastrocnemius muscle pulls the calcaneus upward, which shifts the calcaneus into a slight varus (posterior heel rotated medially) position. The head of the talus turns in and downward during plantar flexion, which causes the foot to move inward (9,11).

Dorsiflexion The hinge motion of the ankle allows the foot to be elevated, or dorsiflexed—foot lifted toward the anterior leg. The gastrocnemius muscle is relaxed and the heel shifts into valgus (heel rotated laterally).

SUPERNUMERARY OSSICLES OF FEET

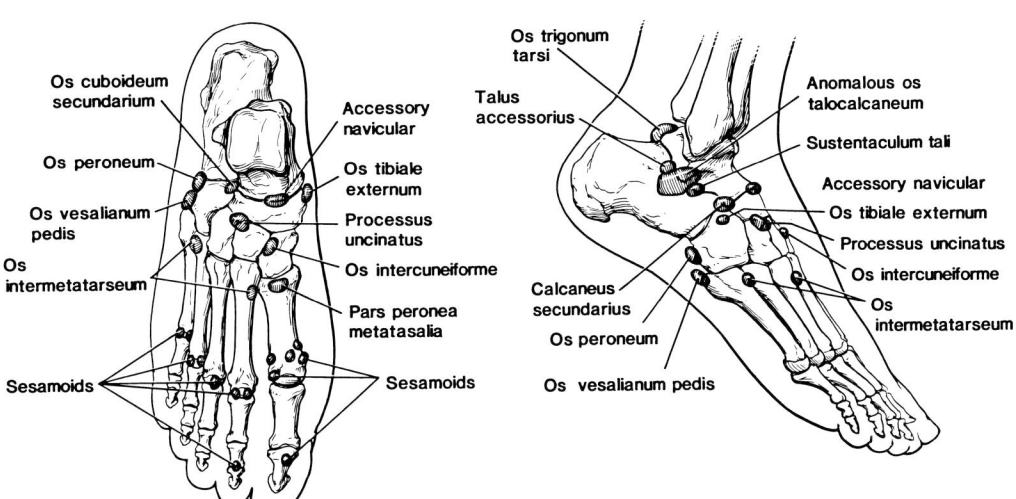

FIG. 9-20. The accessory ossification centers of the foot (from 3, with permission.)

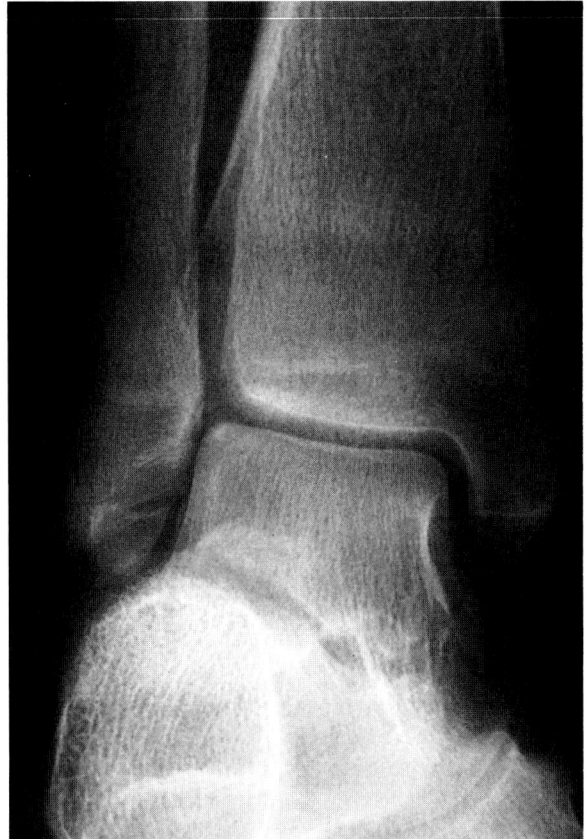

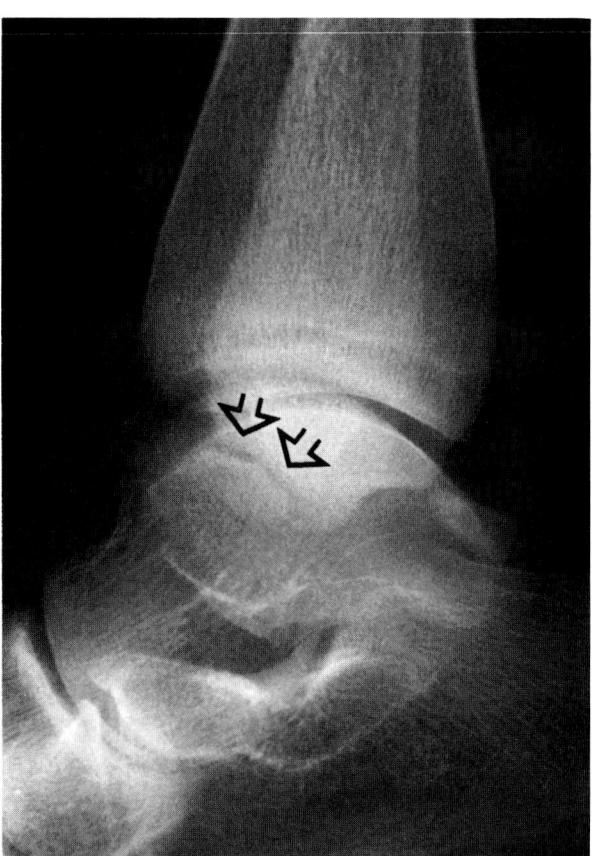

A

B

FIG. 9–21. AP (**A**) and lateral (**B**) views of the ankle demonstrate a normal ossicle at the tip of the lateral malleolus (*arrows*). Note the well-defined bony margins.

The talus turns upward and outward, and the foot, therefore, also turns outward during dorsiflexion (9,11,21,22).

Inversion During inversion the sole of the foot is turned inward. In the European literature, the terms *supination* and/or *adduction* (see below) are often used interchangeably. The foot tends to dorsiflex slightly during inversion.

Eversion During eversion the sole of the foot is turned outward. The terms *pronation* or *abduction* have been used interchangeably with eversion. The foot tends to plantar flex slightly during eversion (9,11,21,22).

Adduction By definition, *adduction* means movement of a part toward the axis or midline. The term is most frequently used to describe forces acting on the foot or ankle. *Inversion* has been used as a term equated to *adduction* in the literature. We prefer to use this term (*adduction*) when describing forces applied to the foot and ankle (9,11–13).

Abduction This term indicates motion of a given part away from the midline. Again, terms such as *eversion* have been used interchangeably. We believe it is best to use *abduction* when describing forces moving the foot or ankle outward (3,9,11–13).

Supination and pronation *Supination* and *pronation* are commonly used terms for describing the rotation that occurs at the wrist. Technically the foot is pronated when the sole is flat. Pronation can occur to a minimal degree with the forefoot abducted and dorsiflexed. Limited supination is possible. Typically the literature has used *pronation* and *eversion* and *supination* and *inversion* interchangeably (9,11–13). We prefer to reserve the terms *supination* and *pronation* for the upper extremity. *Eversion* and *inversion* are less confusing when describing foot and ankle position.

External rotation This term is typically used to define outward rotation of the foot in relation to the longitudinal axis of the leg. With many athletic injuries the leg actually rotates medially with the foot fixed. Therefore, the foot then is actually rotated in an outward (external) position compared to the leg (9,11–13).

Varus *Varus* indicates rotation, bending, or positioning inward or toward the midline axis. The term should be used to describe position, not motion.

Valgus *Valgus* is used to denote rotation, bending, or positioning away from the axis of the midline. Like *varus,* the term *valgus* denotes position.

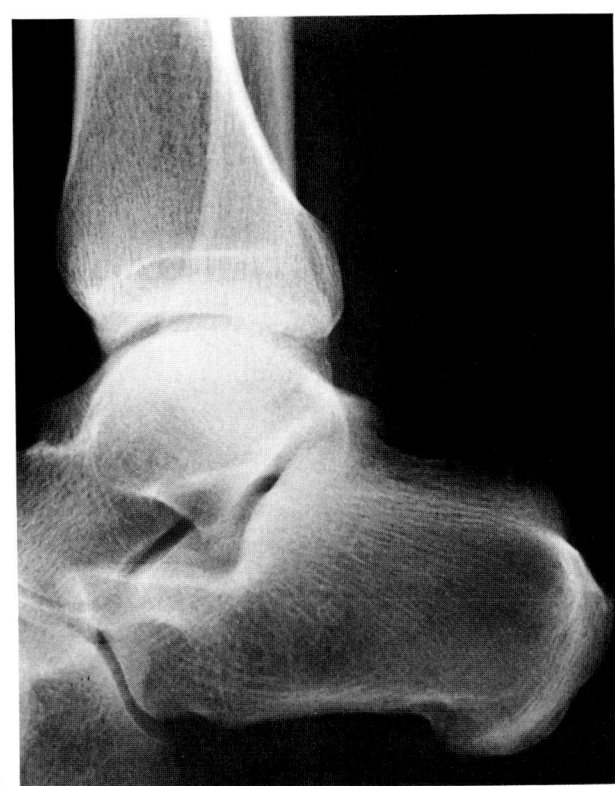

FIG. 9–22. A: Lateral view of the ankle showing a fused posterior talar ossification center. **B** and **C** demonstrate variation in the appearance of the os trigonum (*arrow*), which should not be mistaken for a fracture.

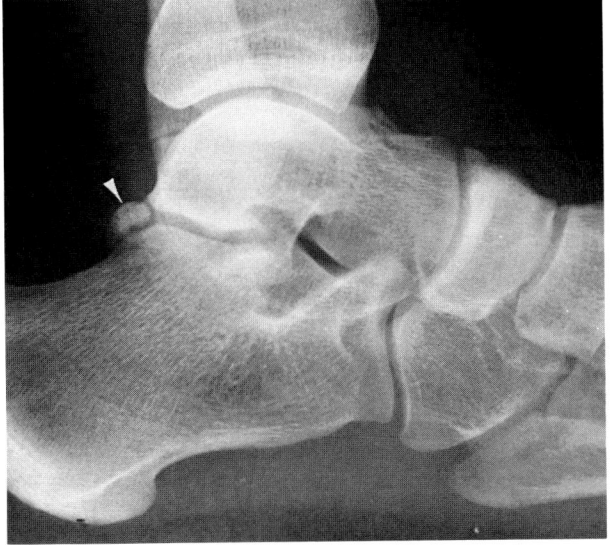

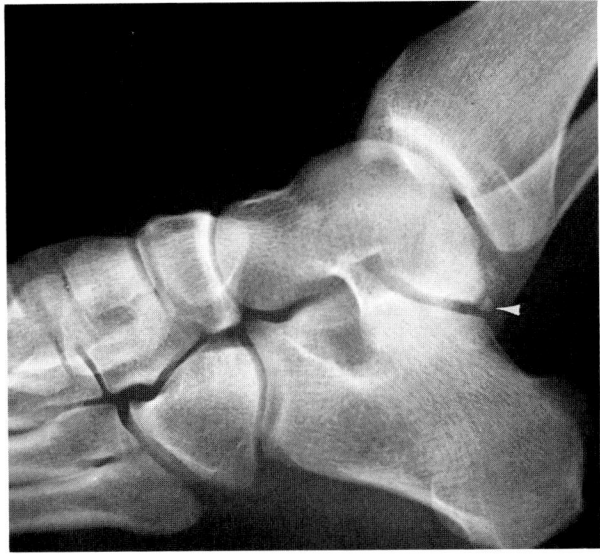

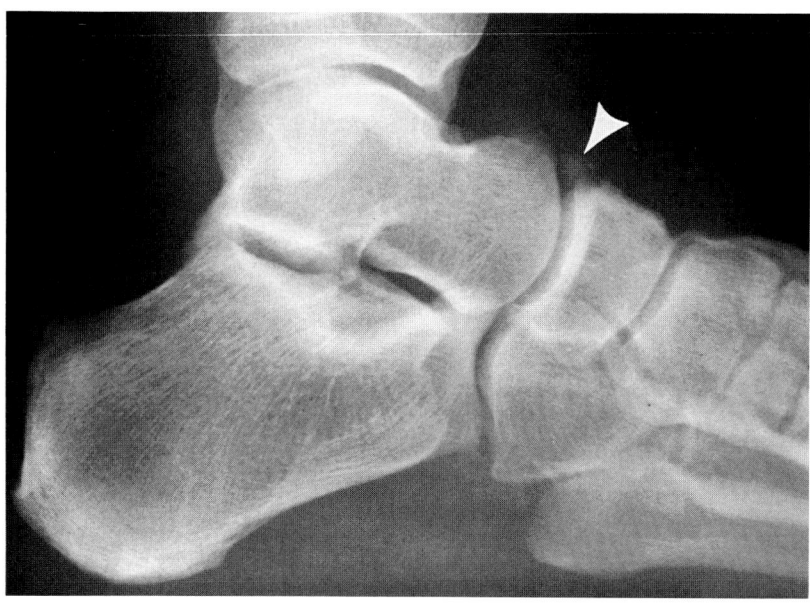

FIG. 9–23. Lateral view of the ankle demonstrating the os supranaviculare (*arrow*). The margins are distinct, differentiating this ossicle from an avulsion fracture.

IMAGING TECHNIQUES

Routine Radiographic Techniques

The Ankle

Evaluation of the ankle requires AP, lateral, and mortise views. Following trauma, an external oblique projection is also routinely obtained (25,27,28,29,47).

AP View

The patient is supine with the foot vertical and centered on an 8 × 10 cassette. The central beam is perpendicular to the cassette and centered on the ankle (tibiotalar) joint. The joint is 1–2 cm above the malleolar tips (Fig. 9-24A) (25,27,28). The radiograph demonstrates the normal tibiotalar joint and medial mortise. The lateral mortise is not clearly seen, as the fibula overlaps the tibia and talus (Fig. 9-24B).

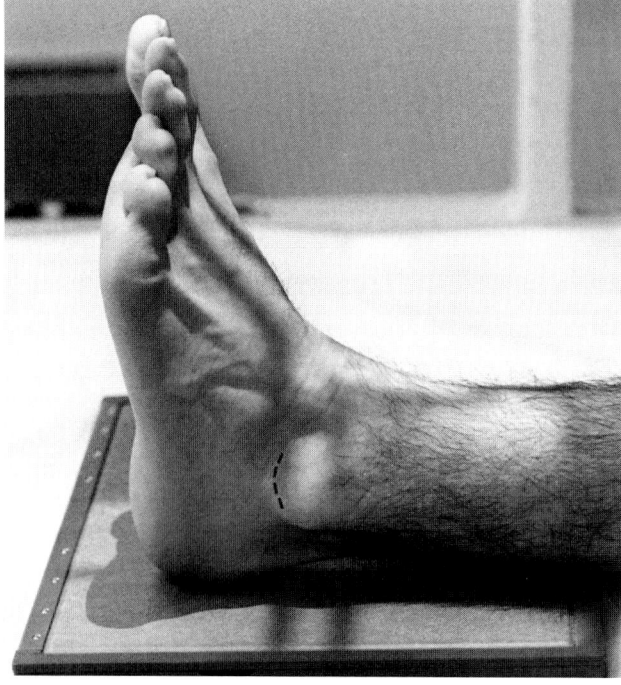

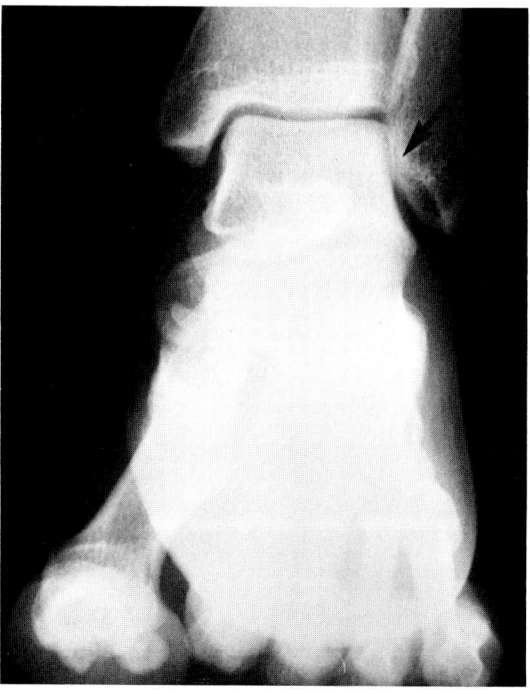

FIG. 9–24. **A:** Patient positioned for AP view of the ankle. The cross-lateral lines on the positioning light in correct centering. Curved line marks the lateral malleolus. **B:** AP radiograph. Note the fibula overlaps a portion of the talus.

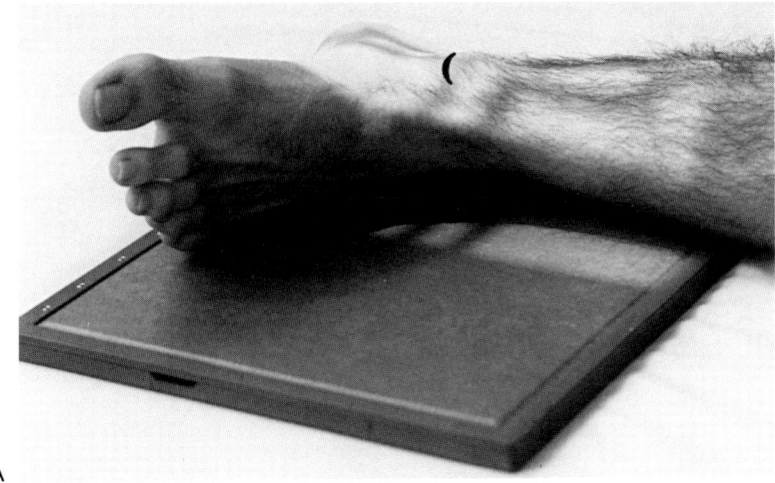

A

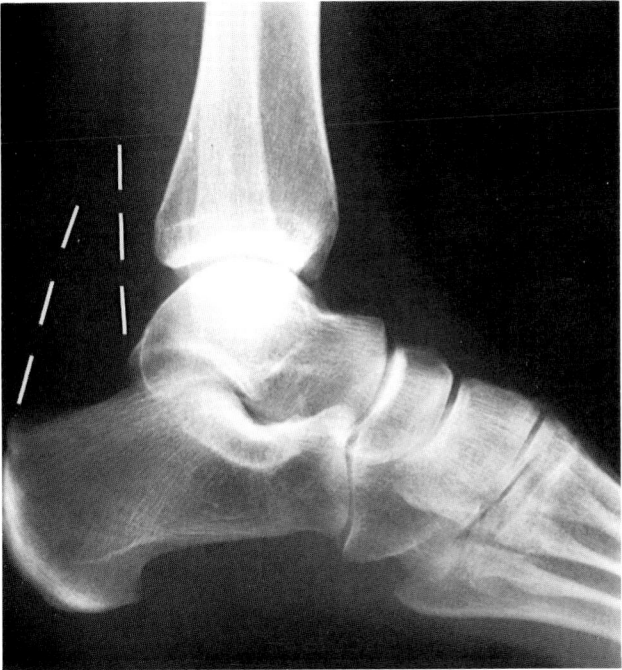

B

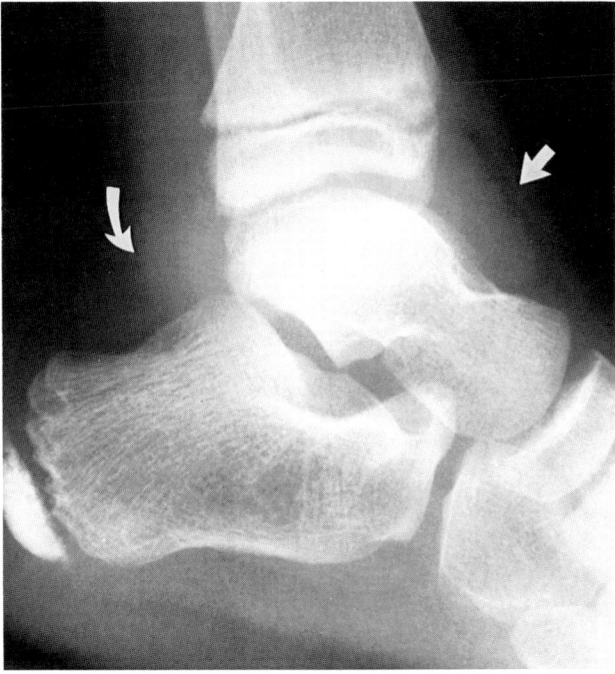

C

FIG. 9–25. **A:** Patient positioned for lateral ankle view (mediolateral) with slight dorsiflexion of ankle. Curved line (() marks the medial malleolar tip. **B:** Lateral radiograph includes base of fifth metatarsal. Normal pre-Achilles fat pad outlined with broken lines. **C:** Severe sprain with anterior "teardrop" (*arrow*) and posterior effusion (*curved arrow*).

Lateral View

The patient is on his or her side with the ankle adjacent to the 8 × 10 cassette. The central beam is perpendicular to the cassette and centered 1–2 cm above the tip of the medial malleolus (palpable unless swelling is extensive) (Fig. 9-25). Alternate positions include the cross-table lateral and reverse lateral (lateromedial) views, with the medial malleolus adjacent to the cassette (25,27,28,29).

The lateral view demonstrates the AP dimensions of the tibiotalar joint and the posterior subtalar joint. The base of the fifth metatarsal is also included on most films. This is useful when an inversion injury causes a fracture of the base of the fifth metatarsal, but the patient's clinical findings suggest an ankle injury. Soft tissue structures on the lateral view include the pre-Achilles

fat pad (Fig. 9-25B). This is a large, triangular fat collection anterior to the Achilles tendon. Hemorrhage in this region may be due to Achilles injury. Significant ankle or calcaneal fractures will also cause distortion of this fat pad (Fig. 9-25C) (28,29).

Detection of fluid in the ankle is important. Effusions present with a "teardrop-shaped" soft tissue mass anterior to the tibiotalar joint (Fig. 9-25B). This results in elevation of the pretalar fat pad (29,73). Less obvious changes may also be evident posteriorly. However, the anterior teardrop is the most consistent sign of effusion. An effusion may be the only sign of a subtle talar dome fracture. The presence of an effusion suggests an intact capsule and ligaments (Fig. 9-25C). In the immediate post-injury period, this may be useful. However, small tears may seal, reducing the reliability of this sign after 48 hours.

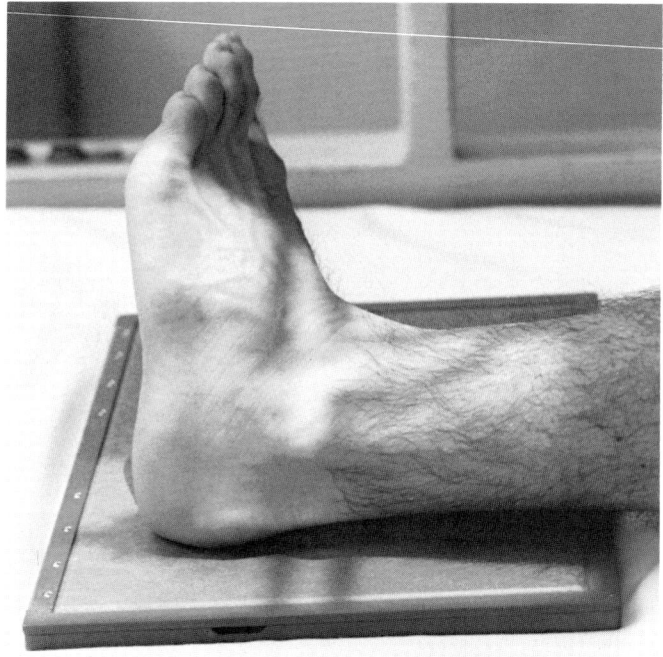
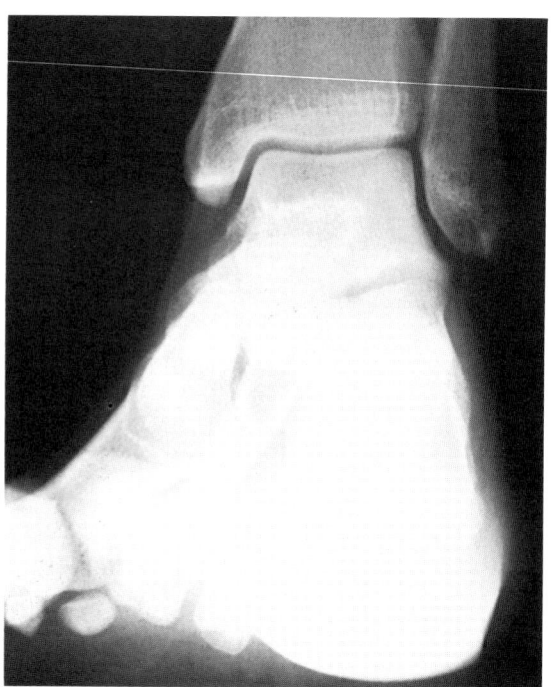

A

B

FIG. 9–26. A: Patient positioned for mortise view with 15°–20° internal rotation of ankle. **B:** Mortise radiograph defines the entire mortise as well as providing better visualization of the talar dome.

Mortise View

On the AP view, the entire ankle mortise is not seen. The fibula overlaps the lateral joint space (Fig. 9-24B). By internally rotating the ankle 15°–20°, however, the fibula is projected more laterally, allowing visualization of the entire ankle mortise (25,27). The central beam is still perpendicular to the ankle joint (Fig. 9-26A). The radiograph (Fig. 9-26B) allows assessment of the entire joint space and distal talofibular articulation. In this position, the posterior portion of the lateral talar facet is seen tangentially. The talar dome is better demonstrated.

Oblique Views

The oblique views of the ankle are obtained by rotating the foot 45° internally and 45° externally (Figs. 9-27A and 9-28A) (27). The beam remains perpendicular to the cassette and is centered on the ankle joint. The radiographs demonstrate the fibula (internal oblique) and medial malleolus (external oblique) more completely (Figs. 9-27B and 9-28B). The external oblique is normally obtained as a part of our department's trauma series. In most cases, the mortise view is used in place of the internal oblique. Additional information regarding the hindfoot relationships can also be obtained using the oblique views.

Stress Views

Stress views may be useful in evaluating ligament injury following ankle sprains (44,47,52,65,75,82). Often

the appearance of malleolar fractures will allow one to determine the degree of ligament injury (47). However, if no fracture is evident or if findings are not conclusive, stress views may be indicated (27–29,48).

In the immediate post-injury period, stress views may be difficult to perform owing to pain and swelling. For accurate results, injection of local anesthetic may be required. Positioning should be performed by an experienced physician. Stress views should be performed in the varus and valgus positions (Fig. 9-29), with the foot in the neutral and plantar flexed positions. Comparison with the uninjured side is essential. Olson (75) reported a normal talar tilt of up to 25° in the hypermobile asymptomatic ankle.

The distance from the lateral aspect of the talar dome to the lateral articular surface is measured during varus stress. The medial articular surfaces are measured with valgus stress. Several measuring techniques have been mentioned in the orthopedic literature (52,66,82). A difference of 3 mm between the injured and uninjured sides indicates ligament injury (Fig. 9-29C,D) (52,65,75). The angle of talar tilt can also be measured. If the angle of the injured ankle exceeds that of the normal ankle by 5°, injury is most likely present. If the difference is 10°, a ligament tear is almost certainly present (28,29,65).

Lateral stress views can be obtained by placing the patient's leg on a support, so that the ankle and knee are level. This removes stress from the ankle. The cassette is positioned perpendicularly to the table, and a cross-table technique is used (Fig. 9-30A). After taking the initial film, stress is applied to the tibia just above the ankle (Fig. 9-30B). A second exposure is made on the same

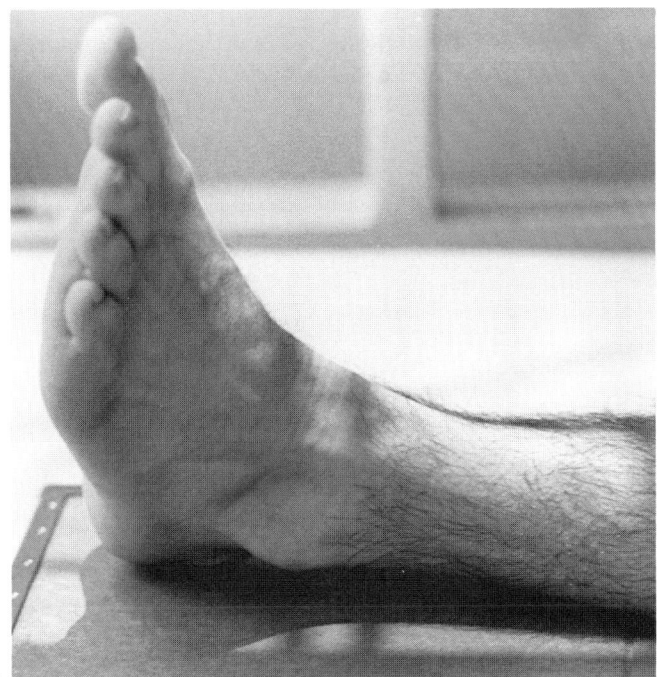
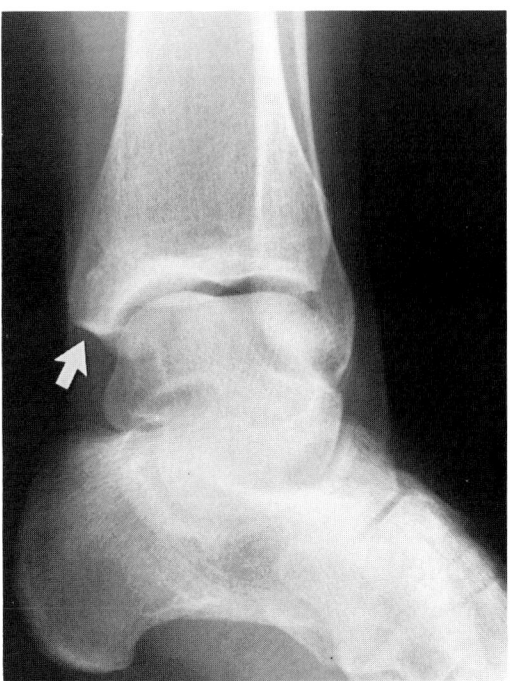

FIG. 9–27. A: Patient positioned for external oblique view (45°). X-ray beam centered on ankle joint. **B:** Radiograph gives best detail of the medial malleolus (*arrow*).

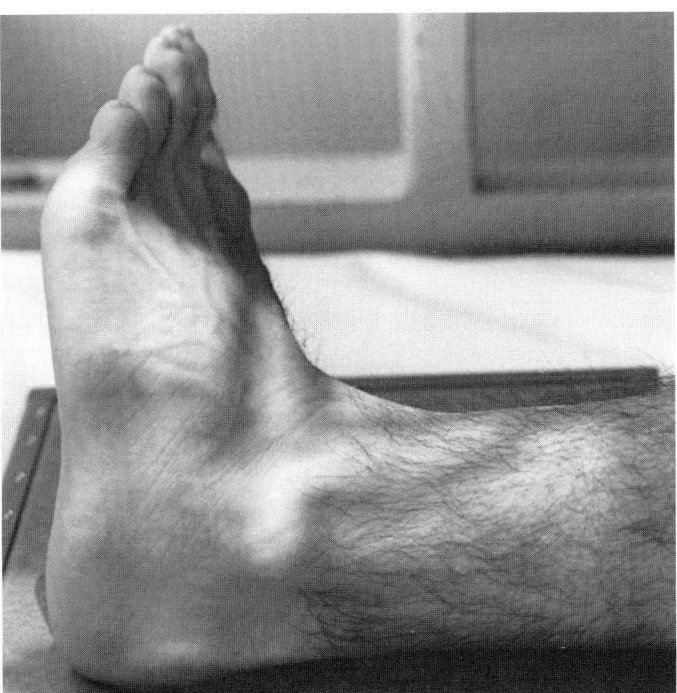
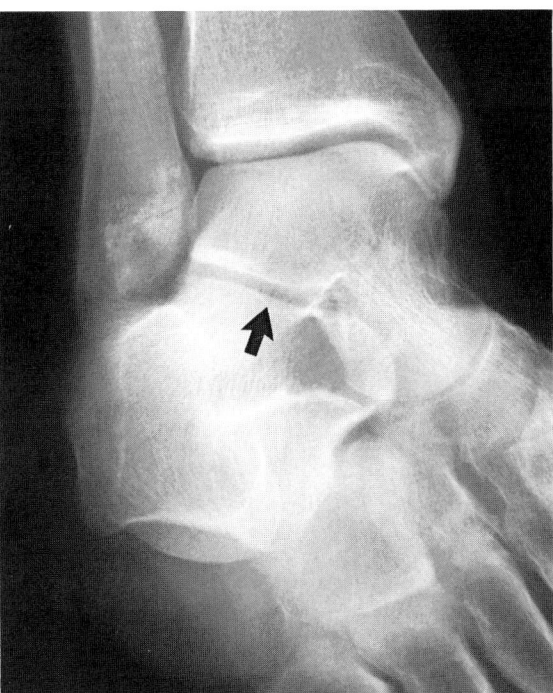

FIG. 9–28. A: Patient positioned for internal (45°) oblique radiograph. **B:** Radiograph gives additional information of lateral structures of ankle including subtalar area (*arrow*).

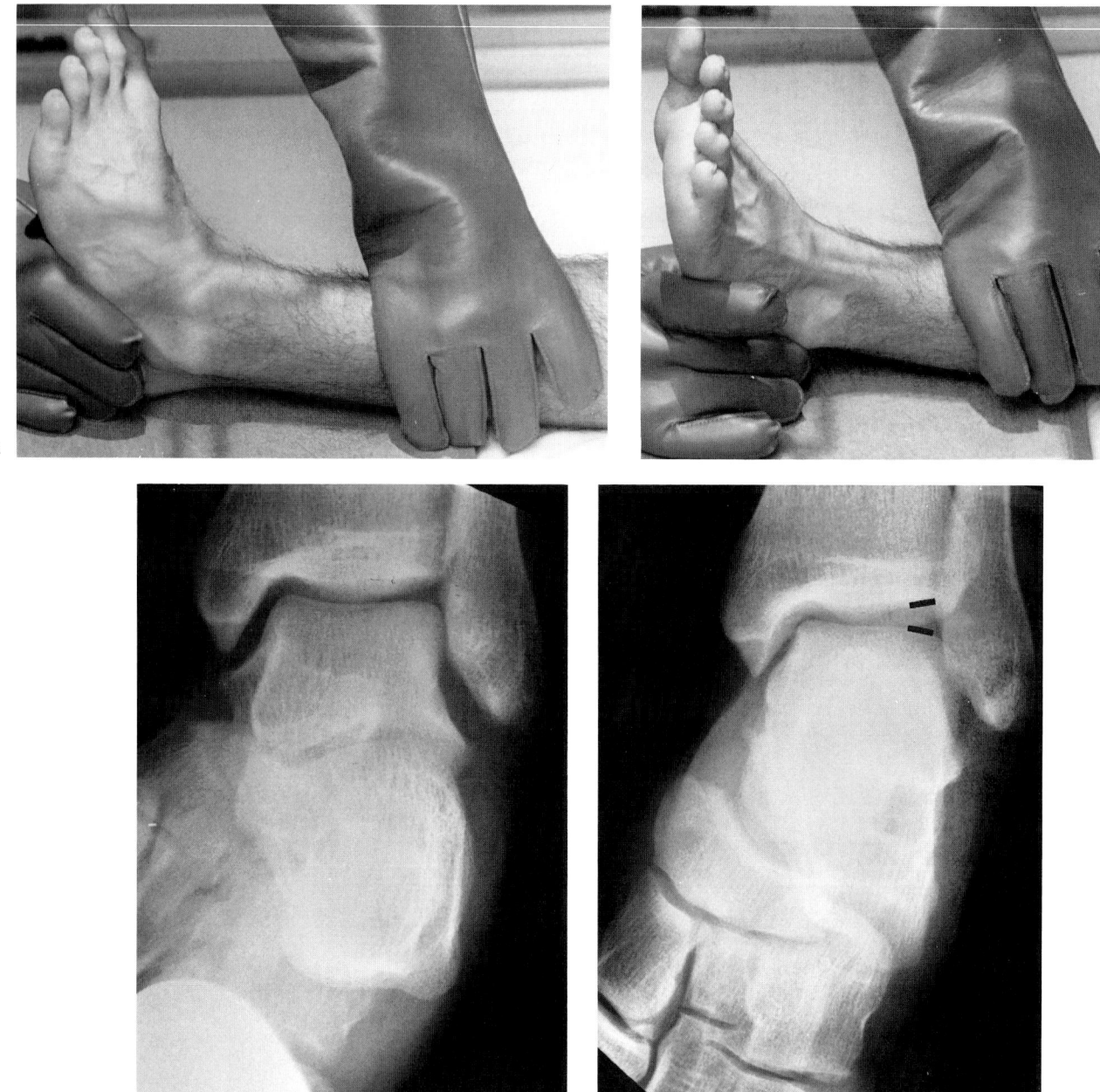

FIG. 9-29. A: Patient positioned for varus stress view with slight plantar flexion of foot. **B:** Patient positioned for valgus stress view. **C:** Varus stress radiograph with foot in neutral position (incorrect maneuver). Normal appearing tibiotalar joint. **D:** Varus stress radiograph with foot plantar flexed shows slight opening of the lateral mortise (*lines*) in normal ankle.

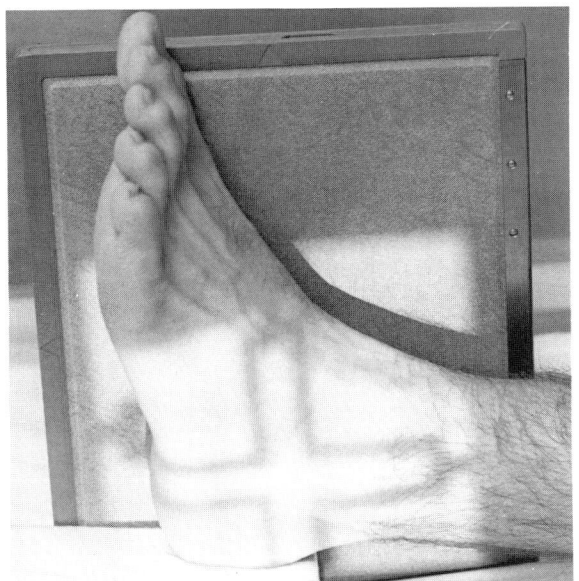
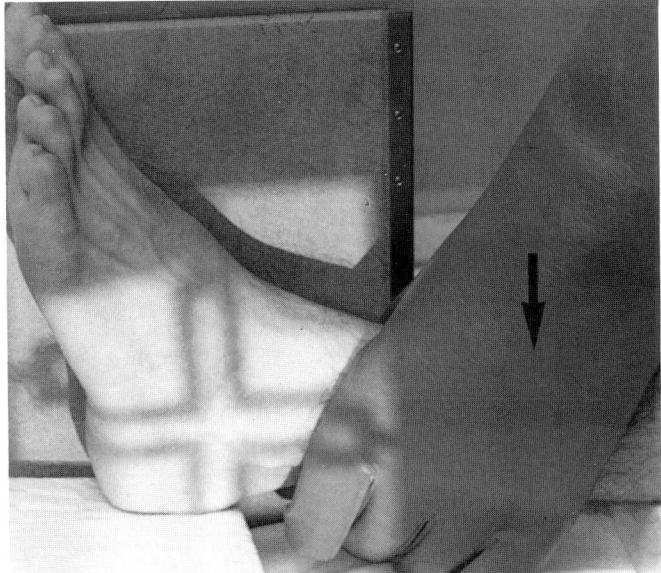

A

B

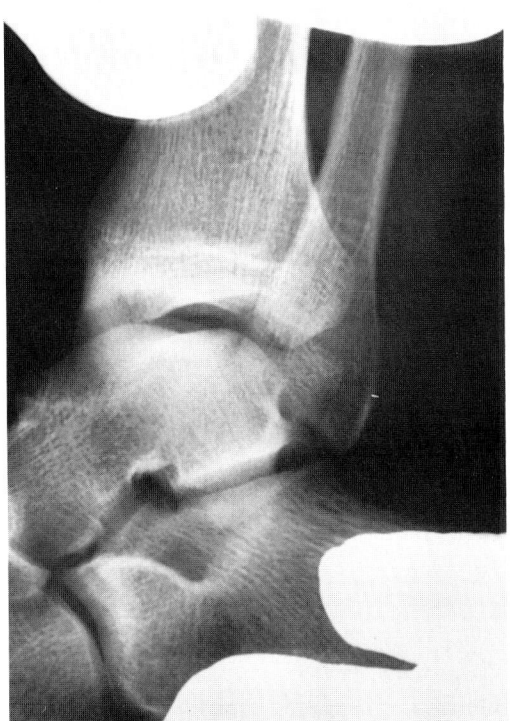
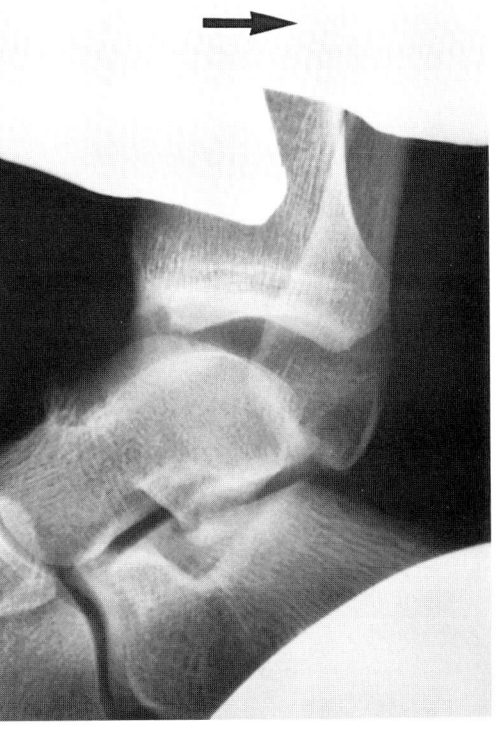

C

D

FIG. 9–30. A: Patient positioned for the AP stress view without manipulation. Note 2-inch support under the heel. **B:** Vertical force applied to distal lower leg between supports. **C:** Radiograph of lateral ankle made without stress. **D:** Repeat radiograph with shear-type stress applied shows positive anterior drawer sign. (Posterior tibial displacement > 2 mm.)

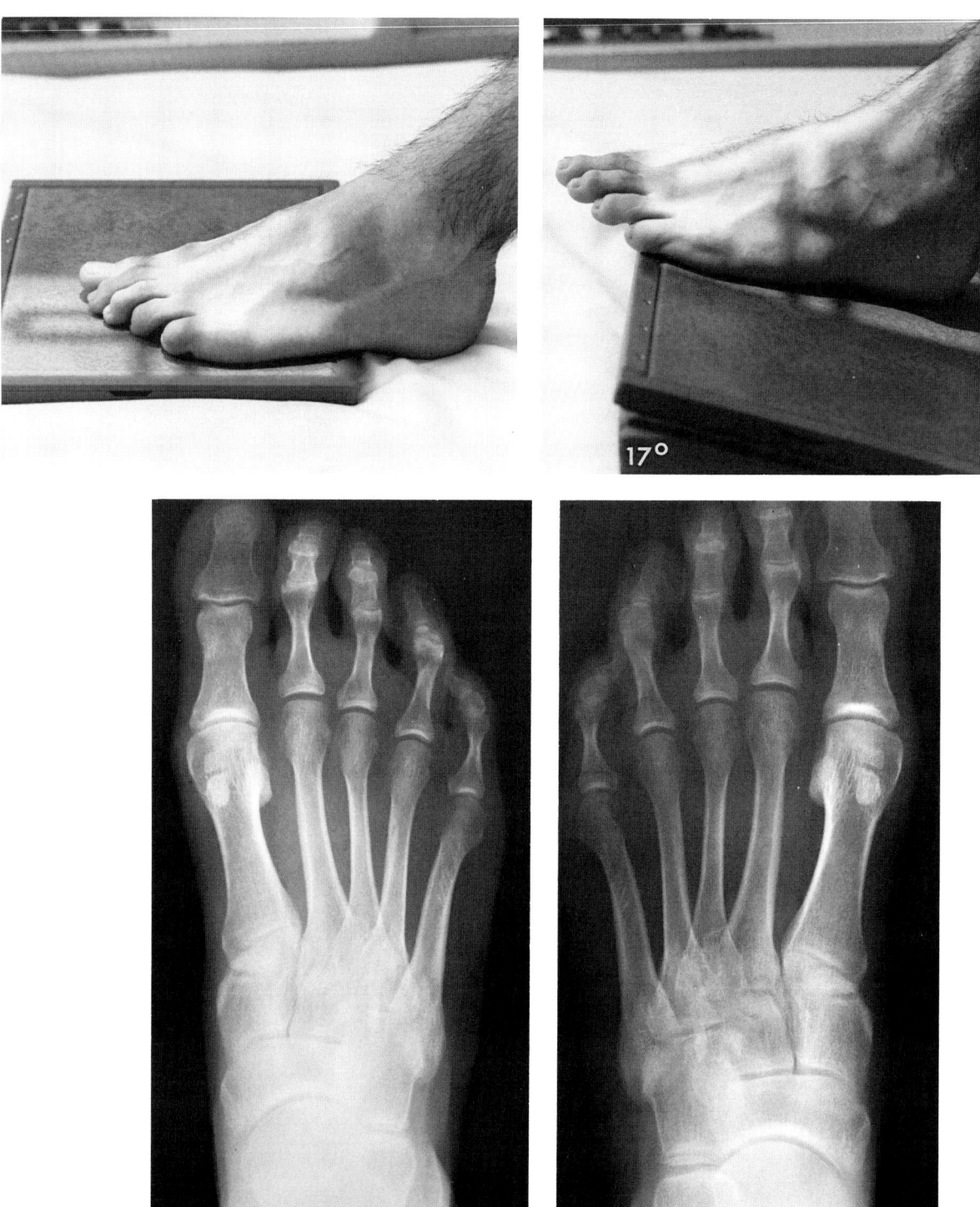

A

C

17°

B

D

FIG. 9–31. A: Patient positioned for AP view of forefoot. **B:** AP radiograph of the forefoot shows distal articular relationships. **C:** Patient positioned on a 17° angle board for AP midfoot view. **D:** The radiograph provides better detail of midfoot anatomy. Note there is still overlap of some of the tarsal joints. When indicated, fluoroscopic positioning can alleviate this problem.

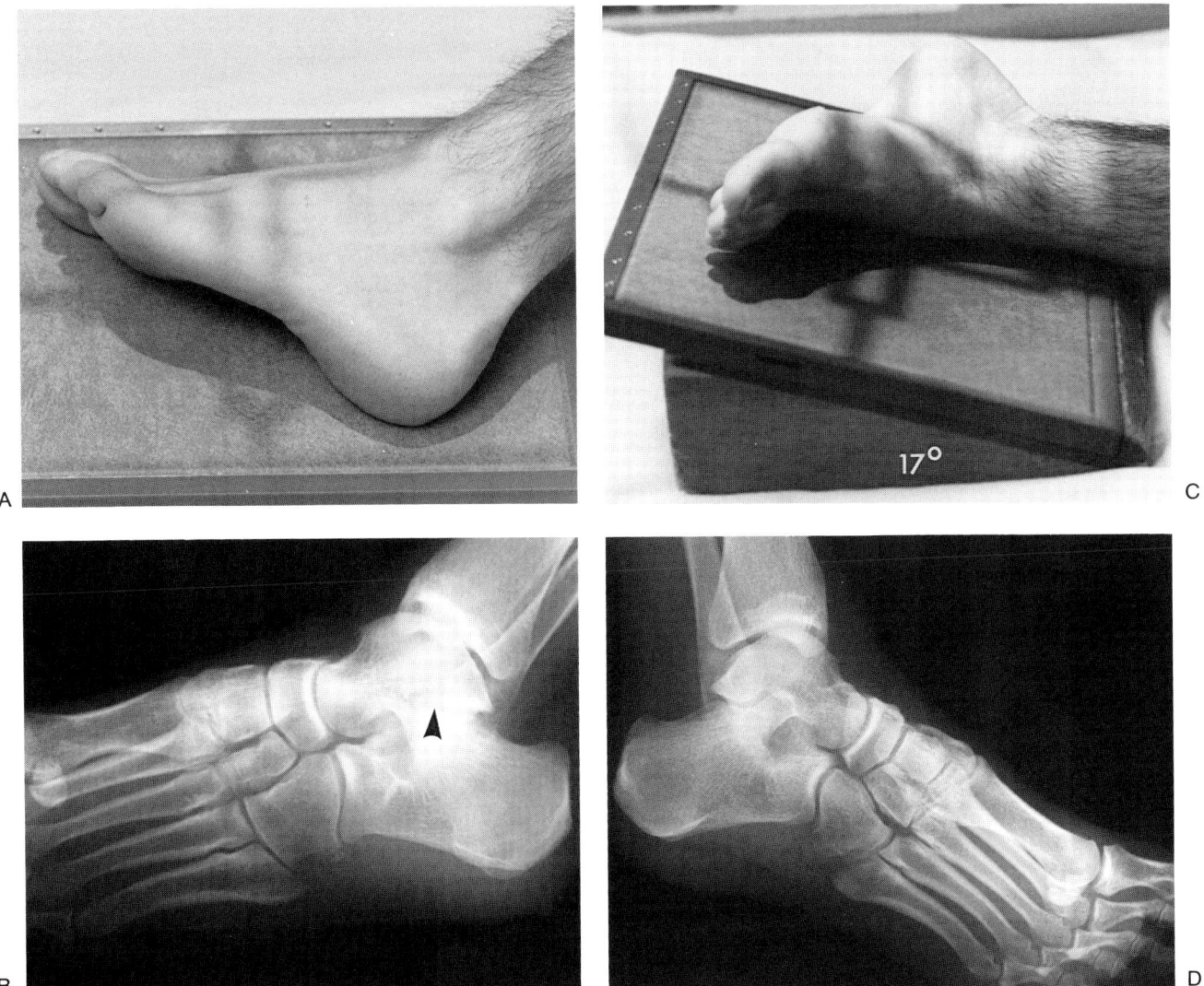

FIG. 9–32. A: Patient positioned for medial oblique view of foot. The lateral portion of the foot is elevated approximately 30° off the cassette. **B:** Radiograph of medial oblique foot demonstrates most articular relationships of the left foot. There is still overlap in the subtalar joint (*arrow*). **C:** Patient positioned for lateral oblique view with 17° angle board under the foot. **D:** Radiograph of lateral oblique view reduces the overlap of the medial portion of the foot in order to better detail the respective joints.

film (double exposure). This allows easy comparison and measurement (Fig. 9-30) (65). The difference between the nonstressed and stressed position is measured on both ankles. If the injured side moves 2 mm more than the uninjured side, the drawer sign is considered positive (65).

The Foot

AP, lateral, and oblique views are routinely obtained in patients with foot trauma. Special localized views or fluoroscopically positioned spot films may be required in certain situations.

AP View

Two AP views of the foot are routinely obtained. This allows visualization of the metatarsals (forefoot) and tarsals (midfoot). The patient sits on the table with the knee flexed. The plantar surface of the foot is placed on an 8 × 10 inch cassette with the heel resting on the table (Fig. 9-31A). The central beam is perpendicular to the cassette and is centered over the distal third metatarsal (25,27). The midfoot view is obtained with the entire foot on the cassette (Fig. 9-31C) and the central beam either perpendicular to the cassette or angled 17° toward the head. The latter technique allows better visualization of the tarsometatarsal joints (25). In either case the beam is centered on the base of the metatarsals (third, usually) (Fig. 9-31B).

The radiographs demonstrate the articular relationships of the tarsometatarsal and phalangeal joints. Care should be taken in evaluating the articular surfaces. They should be uniform and parallel, especially the tarsometatarsal joints. The space between the bases of the first and second metatarsals should also be studied. Widening of this space may be the only sign of subtle subluxation or dislocation (28,29).

Oblique View

Multiple techniques have been described for obtaining oblique views of the foot (25). We routinely use the medial oblique projection. This involves elevating the lateral aspect of the foot 30° off the cassette. The leg and knee are rotated internally (Fig. 9-32A). This view separates the third through fifth tarsometatarsal joints, which overlap on the AP view. The calcaneocuboid and talonavicular joints are also clearly seen (Fig. 9-32B).

Lateral View

The lateral view is most frequently taken with the patient lying on the side. The lateral aspect of the foot is placed against the cassette (8 × 10 or 10 × 12). The plantar surface of the foot should be parallel with the bottom of the cassette, if possible. The central beam is perpendicular to the cassette and is centered on the midfoot (Fig. 9-33A).

The radiograph shows overlapping of the metatarsal bases. The relationships of the mid- and hindfoot are well seen (Fig. 9-33B). Normally, a line drawn along the tuberosity and posterior facet forms a 20°–40° angle (Böhler's angle) with a line from the posterior facet to the

anterior superior calcaneus (28,29). This angle and calcaneal evaluation will be more accurate if the radiograph is centered over the calcaneus rather than over the midfoot.

The Phalanges

Although most phalangeal pathology can be detected on the AP view of the foot, oblique and lateral views can give additional information about the interphalangeal and metatarsophalangeal joints as well as the phalanges.

Oblique Phalangeal View

With the patient in the recumbent position on the unaffected side, a sandbag is placed under the ankle. The foot is plantarflexed and positioned at an angle of approximately 30° with the cassette. The central beam is vertical to the cassette and directed to the second metatarsophalangeal joint (Fig. 9-34A,B).

Lateral Phalangeal View

Each toe can be clearly evaluated on this view. The patient is placed in the lateral decubitus position on the unaffected side. To examine a particular toe, the remaining toes are flexed. Padding or tape may be used to separate or immobilize the unaffected toes. The toe being radiographed should be clearly marked on the film.

With collimated 8 × 10 inch cassette, industrial, or dental film placed under or between the toes, the central beam is directed perpendicularly to the field and centered on the corresponding proximal interphalangeal joint (Fig. 9-35A–D).

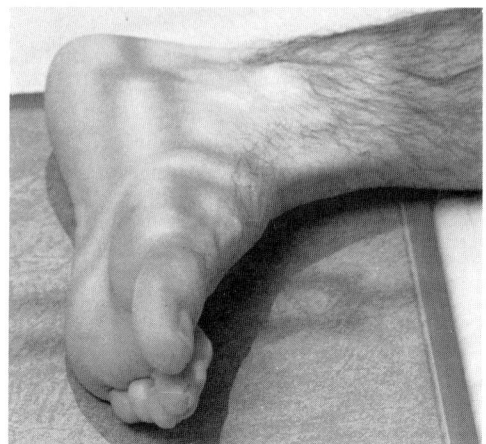 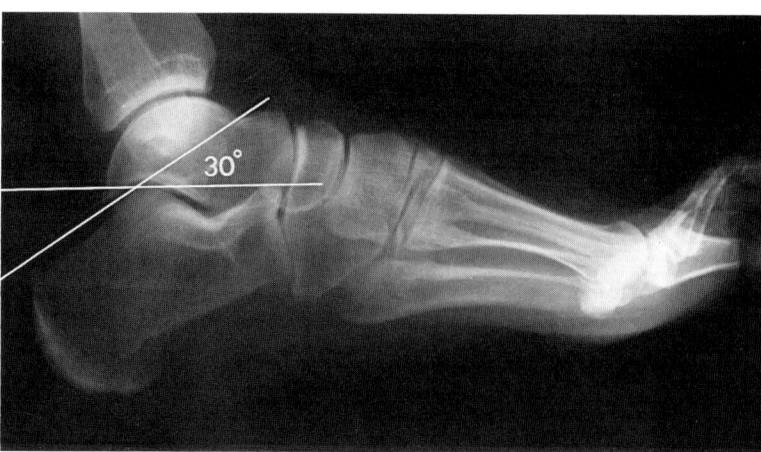

A

B

FIG. 9–33. A: Patient positioned for lateral foot view. **B:** Radiograph shows unique bony relationships between mid- and hindfoot. Bony overlap in the distal foot obscures articulations. Note the normal Böhler's angle.

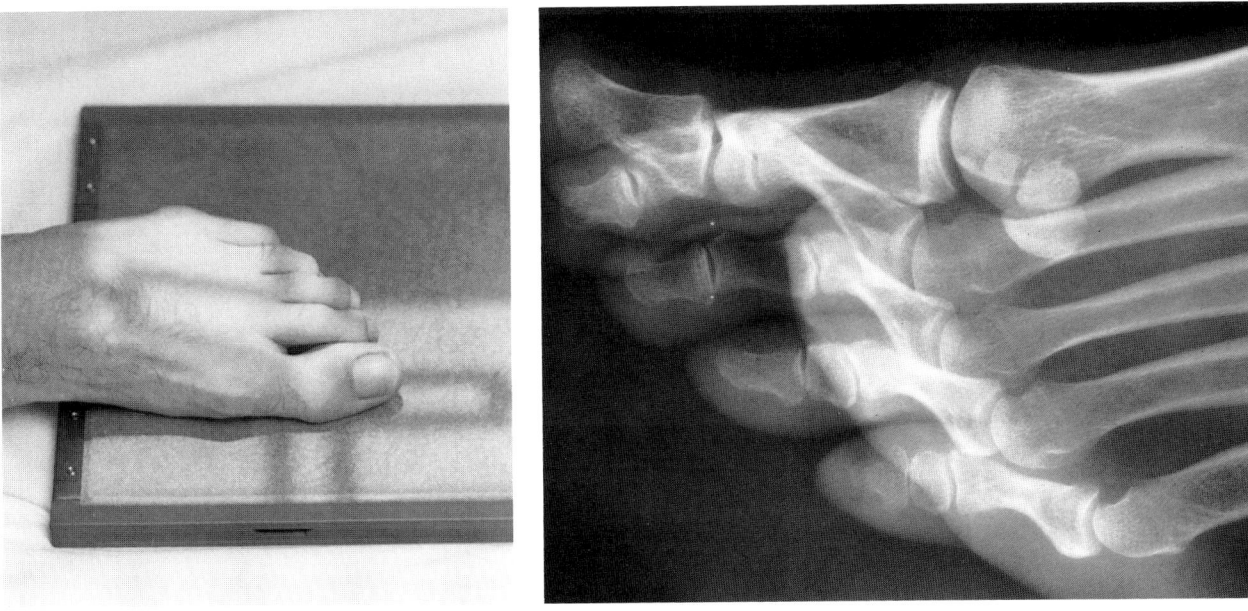

FIG. 9-34. A: Patient positioned for oblique view of toes. **B:** Radiograph shows bony and articular detail even with toe overlap.

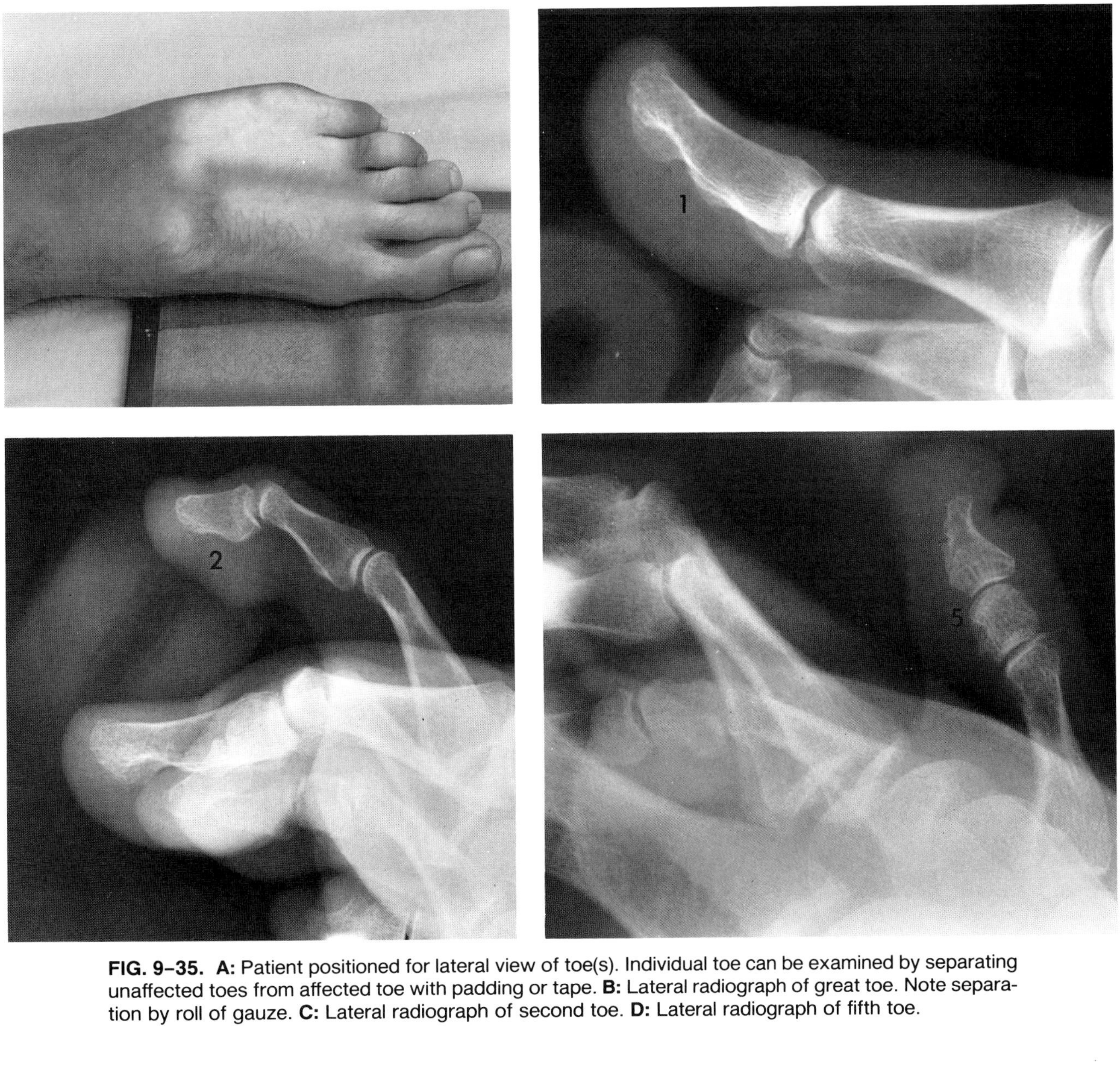

FIG. 9-35. A: Patient positioned for lateral view of toe(s). Individual toe can be examined by separating unaffected toes from affected toe with padding or tape. **B:** Lateral radiograph of great toe. Note separation by roll of gauze. **C:** Lateral radiograph of second toe. **D:** Lateral radiograph of fifth toe.

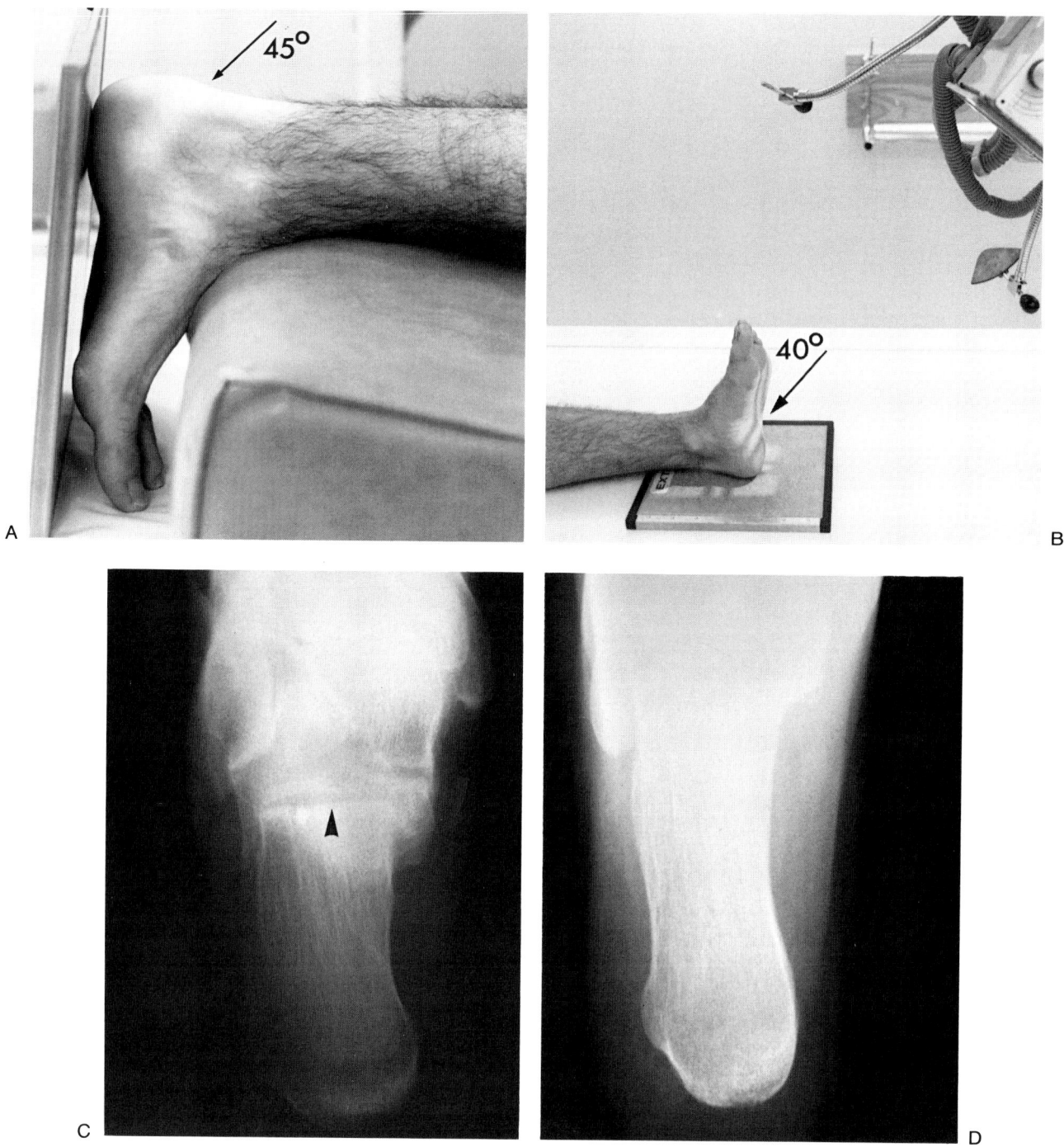

FIG. 9-36. A: Patient positioned for axial calcaneal view with the patient prone (nontrauma). X-ray tube is angled 45° caudally. **B:** Trauma axial calcaneal view with tube angled 40° in cephalad direction. **C:** Radiograph shows the trochlear process, sustentaculum tali (*curved arrow*), and calcaneocuboid articulation (*arrowhead*). **D:** Trauma radiograph (supine with tube angled 40° as in Fig. 9-36B) demonstrates distorted elongated view of tuberosity. Articulations are not demonstrated due to bony overlap.

Special Views

The complex anatomy of the hindfoot articulations may require further views for more complete evaluation (25,27,29,70).

Axial Calcaneal View. In addition to the lateral view described above, an axillary view of the calcaneus should be obtained in patients with suspected calcaneal fractures.

The patient is prone on the table. The ankle is supported with the 8 × 10 inch cassette flat against the foot. The cassette and holder (Fig. 9-36A) are perpendicular to the table. The central beam is angled at 45° and is centered on the calcaneotalar joint. This view can also be taken in the upright position (25).

The radiograph more clearly demonstrates the trochlear process, sustentaculum tali, and calcaneocuboid articulation (Fig. 9-36B).

Lateral Calcaneal View. Although the calcaneus is demonstrated on the routine lateral foot view, better definition is obtained when the x-ray beam is centered on the calcaneus (Fig. 9-37A,B).

Subtalar Views. Numerous techniques have been described for evaluation of the subtalar joint (25–29). The oblique views are easily accomplished. The patient's foot is rotated medially or laterally (Fig. 9-38). The hindfoot is centered on the cassette, with the beam centered on the malleolus (medial or lateral) and angled 10° to the head.

The radiographs (Fig. 9-38B,D) demonstrate the subtalar joint (lateral oblique) and sinus tarsi region (medial oblique). Variations in anatomy may cause difficulty in reproducing these views (25,28,29). Tomography or fluoroscopic positioning (Fig. 9-38E) may be needed in these situations.

Sesamoid Views. Fractures of the sesamoid bones are uncommon. However, these structures are often not clearly seen on routine views. Sesamoid views can easily be obtained (25,27,39). The patient is supine with the foot dorsiflexed (Fig. 9-39A). The beam is centered just plantar to the first metatarsal head and perpendicular to the cassette.

The radiograph projects the sesamoid bones away from the metatarsal, allowing fractures to be more readily identified (Fig. 9-39B).

Additional views including weight bearing, tangential views of the forefoot, and sesamoids may be obtained but are rarely required in the acute setting (29,40, 61,64,76).

Tomography

Most skeletal structures can be evaluated with routine radiographs or spot films obtained with fluoroscopic monitoring. Thin section (1–3 mm thick) tomography is a useful addition to conventional films when more detailed information is required. This is particularly true in the mid- and hindfoot where skeletal anatomy and joint alignment are more complex (29,37,74).

Generally tomograms are obtained in the AP and lateral planes. However, because of the position of the bones in the foot and off-axis angles of the joints, it is often necessary to fluoroscopically position the area of interest (29,73). In this situation, two different views are chosen, one in the best image plane and the second, if possible, at a 90° angle to that plane. In certain cases local pain or the patient's general condition may limit positioning.

In orthopedic practice, tomography is frequently used to evaluate subtle fractures (Fig. 9-40) (29,37,74). Fracture healing and other clinical problems such as tarsal coalition, are also effectively studied with tomography. In most orthopedic tomography, the detail is improved with trispiral or complex motion. Occasionally, especially in patients with metallic internal or external fixation devices, linear motion may be more useful (Fig. 9-41). Trispiral motion (Fig. 9-41A) can cause significant loss of bone detail adjacent to the metal. Linear motion perpendicular to the metal (Fig. 9-41B) and linear motion parallel to the metal (Fig. 9-41B) demonstrate that the metal artifact is reduced when the motion of the tube is parallel to the metal. Note that the adjacent bone and bone graft (Fig. 9-41C) are better defined with

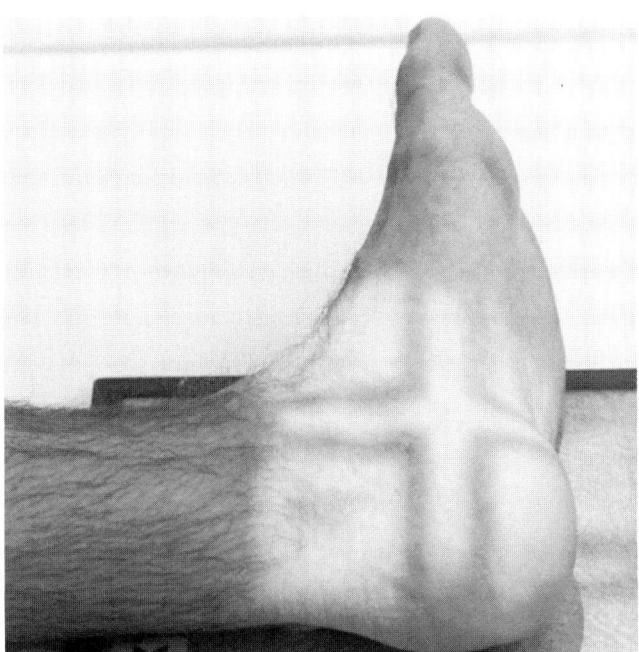
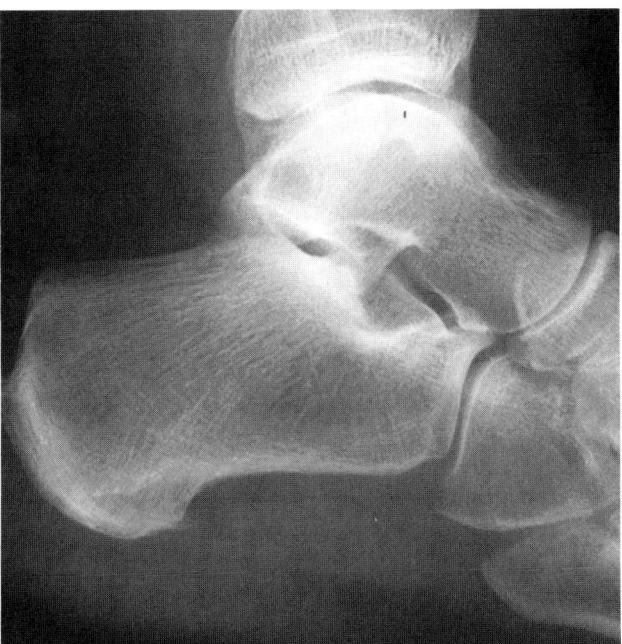

FIG. 9-37. A: Patient positioned for lateral calcaneous view. **B:** Radiograph outlines architecture of hindfoot.

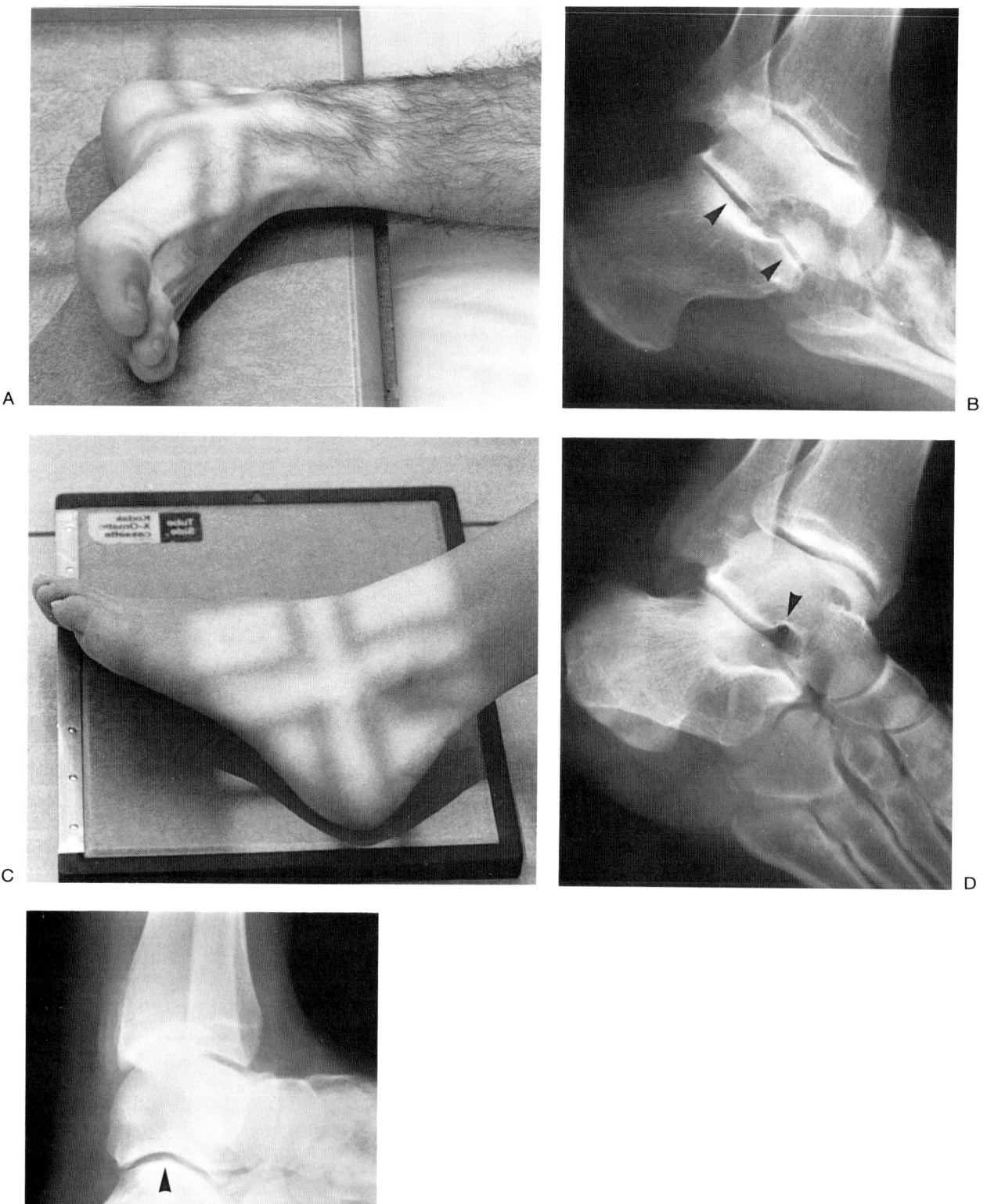

A

B

C

D

E

FIG. 9–38. A: Patient positioned for lateral oblique subtalar view on 17° angle board. **B:** Radiograph shows subtalar joint clearly (*arrowheads*). **C:** Patient positioned for medial oblique subtalar view. **D:** Radiograph of medial oblique subtalar view shows sinus tarsi (*arrowhead*). **E:** Fluoroscopically positioned subtalar view shows posterior aspect of talocalcaneal joint (*arrowhead*).

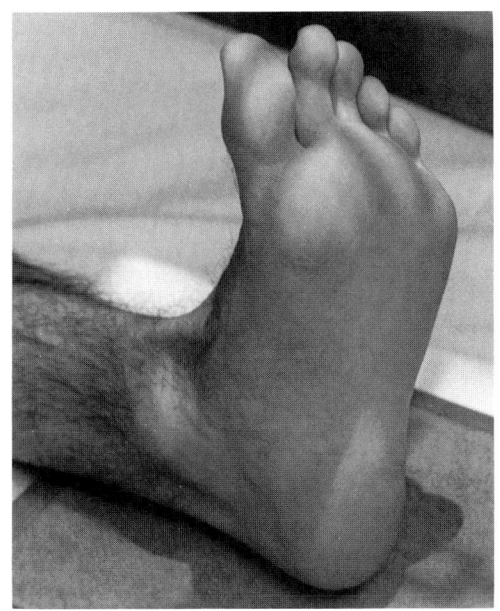
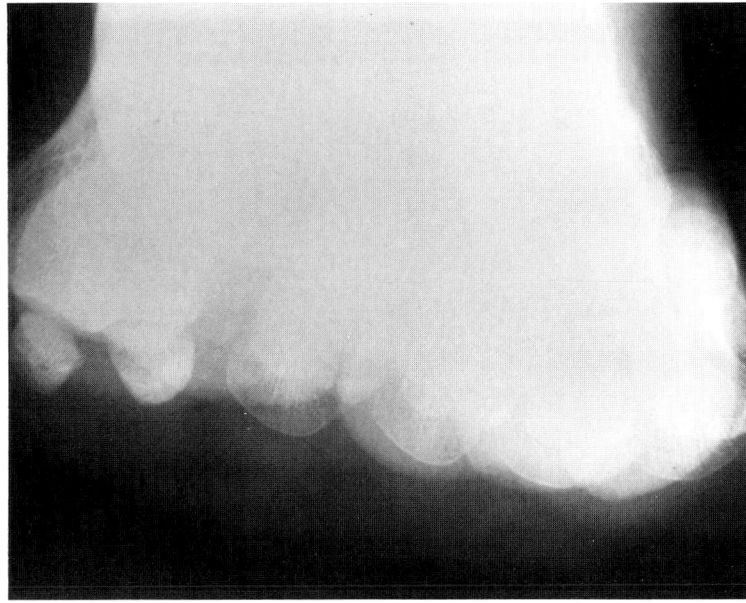

FIG. 9-39. A: Patient positioned for AP sesamoid view. Note slight dorsiflexion of toes to eliminate overlap on sesamoids. B: Radiograph of sesamoids.

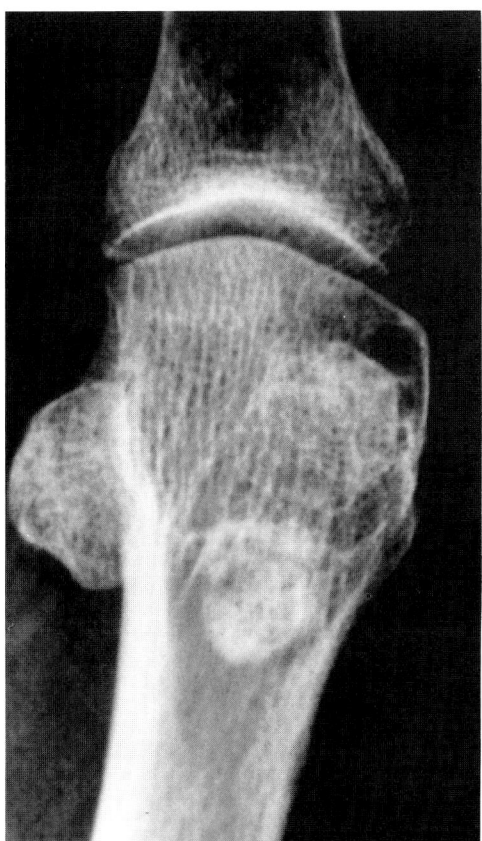
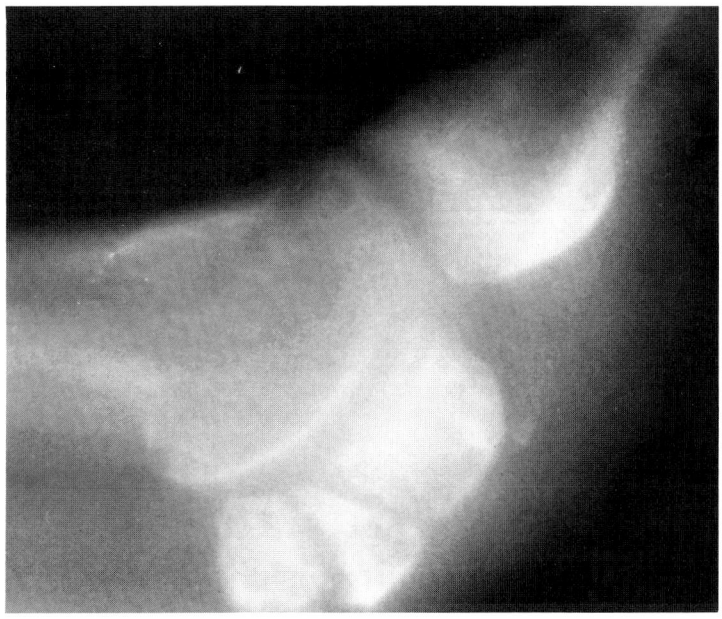

FIG. 9-40. Runner with pain under the first metatarsal head. Routine AP (A) view of the first metatarsal phalangeal joint is normal. Lateral tomogram (B) demonstrates a sesamoid fracture.

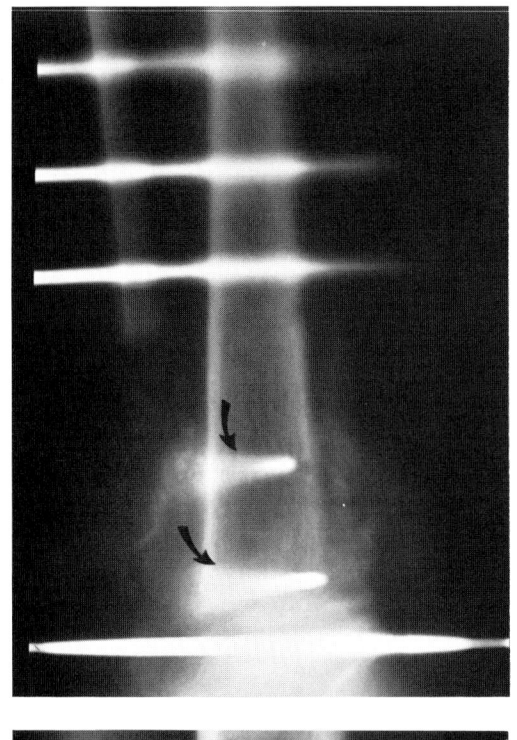

A

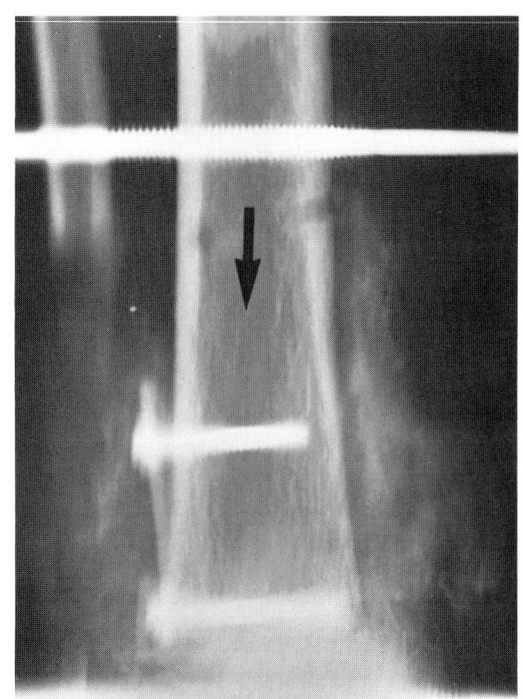

B

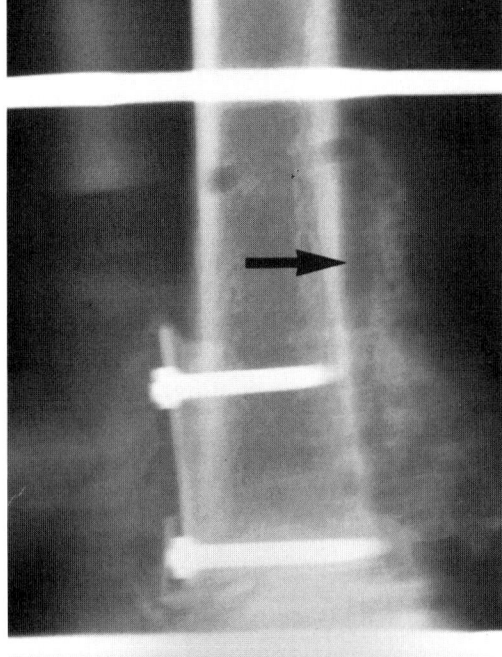

C

FIG. 9–41. Multiple types of tomographic motion in a patient with internal and external fixation of the distal tibia and fibula. **A:** Trispiral tomography blurrs the pin more severely causing loss of adjacent bone detail. **B:** Linear motion perpendicular to the screws causes less artifact and improved detail of the bone graft. **C:** Bone detail is optimal with the linear motion parallel to the screws.

linear motion parallel to the metal. In certain cases the configuration of the fixation device is such that examination choices are more difficult. Tomography is still often useful in providing increased detail in these situations.

Ultrasound

Perhaps the most severe limitation of diagnostic ultrasound imaging is due to the inability of sound waves to penetrate gas and bone. Because this fundamental physi-

cal principle prevents ultrasound from passing from soft tissue into bone, the applications of this modality to orthopedics are relatively limited. The lower extremity is an exception to the rule. The bones of the lower extremity are deep, except for the subcutaneous portions of the tibia, allowing easy examination of most soft tissue structures. Muscles, tendons, ligaments, and vessels are generally accessible (32,34,35,50,67). Thus, thrombophlebitis, tendon and muscle tears, hematomas, abscesses, and tumors can be evaluated. Most structures are within 5–6 cm of the skin surface so high frequency scans can be performed. Imaging should be performed in both transverse and longitudinal planes of section.

Real-time ultrasound has gained acceptance in evaluation of the Achilles tendon and other superficial soft tissue structures of the foot and ankle (67,72). Ultrasound is particularly suited for these structures because of its low cost and ability to study tendon motion (Fig. 9-42) (32,67,72).

Radionuclide Studies

Bone scanning can provide important information in patients with known or suspected trauma. Routine ra-

diographs easily demonstrate the site of fracture in most patients with a clinical history of trauma. In these uncomplicated cases, bone scintigraphy will not add significant additional information. However, when the initial x-rays are normal, as may occur with subtle fractures, the bone scan may play a role in directing the course of management (29,36,37,54). Fractures are demonstrated as focal areas of increased uptake, with 80% visible in 24 hours and 95% in 72 hours. However, in elderly patients more time is often required for the onset of activity to occur at the fracture site (29,36). Bone scanning is also very helpful in patients suspected of having stress fractures. Isotope scans will detect stress fractures earlier than radiography. Radiographs may not be positive for

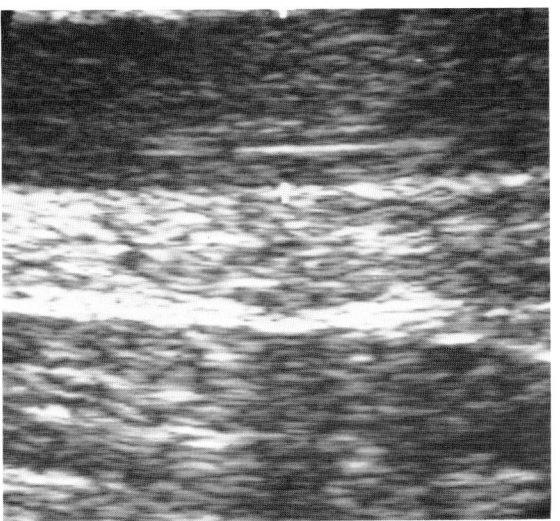
A

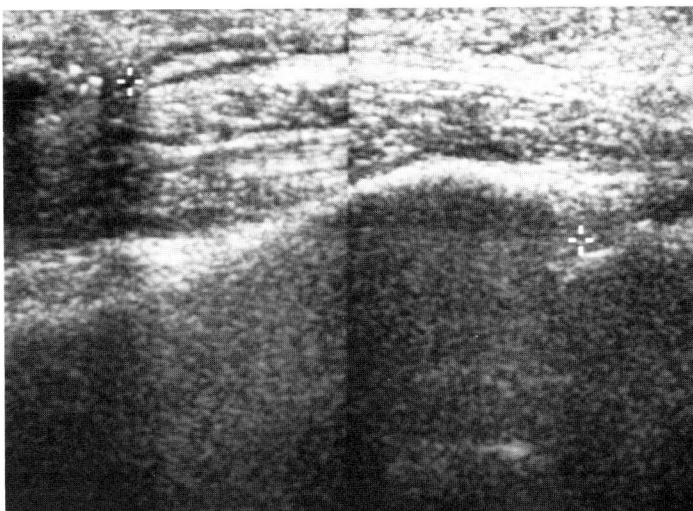
B

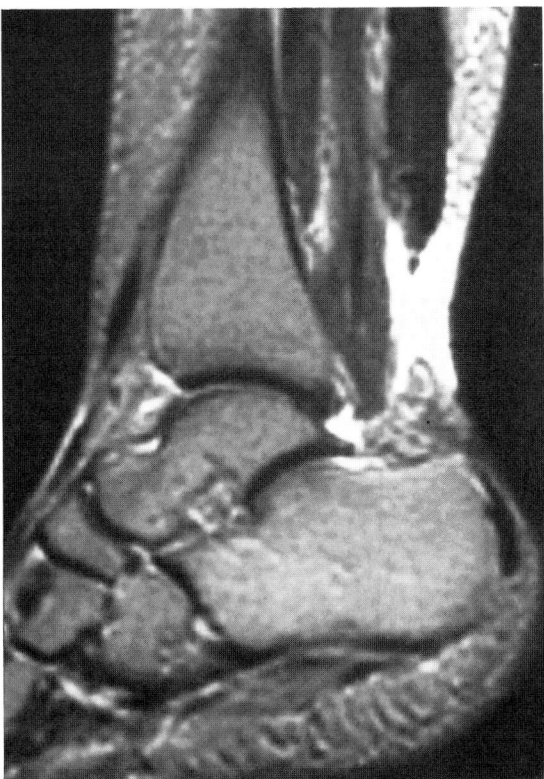
C

FIG. 9–42. A: Longitudinal ultrasonography study shows a normal Achilles tendon. Longitudinal ultrasonography (B) and sagittal SE 2000/60 MRI of a torn Achilles tendon (C).

several weeks and, if cessation of the stress is instituted, the radiograph may never become positive. A negative scan, with few exceptions, implies that the symptoms are not due to a stress fracture (29,54).

Infection

Radionuclide studies play a valuable role in early detection of bone and soft tissue infection (see Chapter 15, Infection). Three-phase technetium-99m pertechnetate studies are sensitive but less specific than newer isotope techniques. More recently, Gallium-67, and Indium-111-labeled white blood cells have provided improved specificity (112,114,123). The latter are particularly useful following trauma or surgery when detection of subtle infection can be very difficult (114).

Computed Tomography (CT)

CT examinations of the foot and ankle are particularly useful due to their complex anatomies. Examination of the hindfoot can be easily accomplished with CT and can demonstrate anatomic changes that may be difficult with special radiographic views or complex motion tomography (see Routine Radiography section). The mobility of the foot allows changes in position so that direct image data can be accomplished in several planes (29,49,53,71).

Proper examination of the foot and ankle requires adequate clinical information. Positioning, slice thickness (1.5 mm may be needed if three-dimensional, sagittal, or coronal reconstruction is contemplated), need for IV contrast medium, etc., must be considered prior to the examination. All pertinent radiographs and isotope studies should also be reviewed (29,87).

Ideally, positioning should be comfortable, easily maintained, provide the proper alignment for the area of interest, and be reproducible. This may be difficult following acute trauma. Reproducibility can be achieved to some degree with use of foot boards and angled wedges (Fig. 9-43) (29,49,53,71).

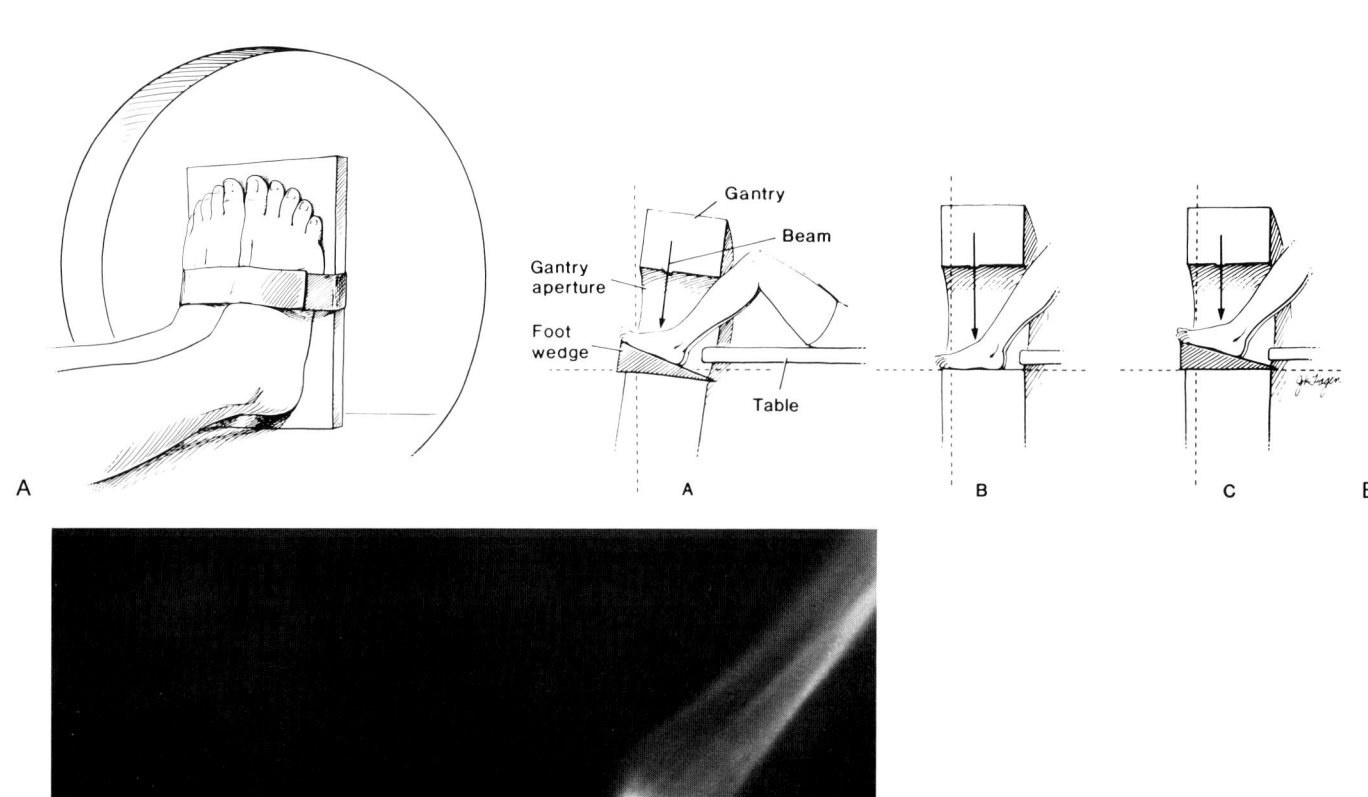

FIG. 9-43. A: Patient positioned for axial CT images. A foot board can be used to maintain proper positioning. **B:** Illustration of positioning for coronal images. The gantry can be angled (**A**) or the foot position changed (**A–C**). Selection of image planes is determined using a scout image (**C**) (from 29, with permission.)

Although positioning and technique vary with individual clinical problems, certain standard techniques can often be applied. Axial and coronal images are usually obtained. A scout view aids with proper positioning and slice selection.

Axial images of the foot and ankle are obtained with the feet perpendicular to the gantry table. The knees are extended and the great toes together. A foot board can be used to maintain this position and reduce motion (Fig. 9-43A) (29).

For coronal images the knees are flexed with the feet flat against the gantry table (Fig. 9-43B). Specific tarsal bones and joints may require use of either a foot wedge, angling the gantry, or both to obtain the alignment desired (29,53,59,60,81). These factors can be determined using the scout view. Positioning is particularly critical in the hindfoot.

Typically, examinations are performed using 5-mm-thick slices, 120 KV, 205 mAs, with 3–5-second scan time. Faster scan times reduce motion artifact, which can be a problem in patients with significant pain or when the position is difficult to maintain. Contiguous 1.5-mm slices provide superior reconstructed images if sagittal or three-dimensional reconstructions are needed. A 5-mm slice with 3-mm overlap can also be used (87). With 5-mm-thick slices, it generally takes 15–20 slices in both the coronal and axial plane to completely examine the hindfoot. If 1.5-mm slices are used over 40 slices may be needed (29,53).

CT provides excellent bone detail, and assessment of the complex articulations of the foot and ankle is readily accomplished. It may be the technique of choice for the subtalar joint (58–60). CT is capable of evaluating the bones and joints to establish diagnoses and assist in planning conservative or surgical therapy when appropriate.

When indicated, CT is a valuable addition to arthrography in evaluating patients with arthritis and other post-traumatic conditions. Soft tissue abnormalities can also be detected with CT (29,80). Specific indications and technical variations needed for the examinations will be discussed in later sections.

Magnetic Resonance Imaging (MRI)

MR imaging is a valuable technique for detection of musculoskeletal disorders in the foot and ankle. Soft tissue injuries are easily detected and classified. Evaluation of treatment response is also possible (26,29,45,68).

Patients should be positioned in the most comfortable and effective position to evaluate the specific clinical problem. Surface coils (Fig. 9-44) or the head coil (which allows comparison of both feet and ankles) are most commonly employed (29). Spin-echo sequences, specifically double-echo T2-weighted sequences (SE 2000/60–80, 20–30) are most effective for detection of pathology.

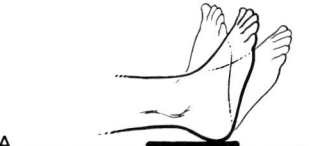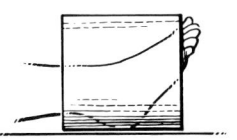

FIG. 9–44. Surface coils for foot and ankle imaging. The flat coil (**A**) and circumferential coil (**B**) can be used. Positioning is more flexible with the flat coil (from 29, with permission.)

New fast scan techniques (gradient echoes with reduced flip angles) are useful in providing T2*-weighted images, reducing examination time, and they allow cine loop motions studies (29,45,68).

MRI (see Chapter 1) is most commonly used to evaluate soft tissue injury (Fig. 9-45), complications of trauma, such as avascular necrosis, and other subtle injuries (29,42,46,84). Specific applications will be discussed in future sections, specifically, soft tissue injury.

Arthrography, Tenography, and Diagnostic-Therapeutic Injections

Interventional techniques in the foot and ankle are used for diagnostic and therapeutic purposes. Techniques include arthrography, tenography, and diagnostic and therapeutic injections. Proper use of these techniques requires a thorough knowledge of the anatomy and clinical problems. Routine films, fluoroscopy, CT, ultrasound, and rarely MRI may be used to monitor or record the procedures (29).

Ankle Arthrography

Arthrography is a safe, valuable method of studying the ligaments, capsule and articular anatomy (24,51,73). Ankle arthrograms are most frequently performed in patients with suspected soft tissue trauma. In Goergen and Resnick's series, 95% of arthrograms were performed in patients with suspected ligament injury (56). Arthrograms are less commonly performed to evaluate articular cartilage (talar dome fractures, osteochondritis dissecans) and loose bodies (29,51,63,73,84,85). Table 9-1 summarizes the indications and technical variations used in ankle arthrography.

Technique

Radiographs (routine and stress views) should be evaluated prior to obtaining the arthrogram. Pertinent clinical information concerning the type of trauma and other indications for the arthrogram are important. Arthrographic technique varies according to clinical indications (Table 9-1).

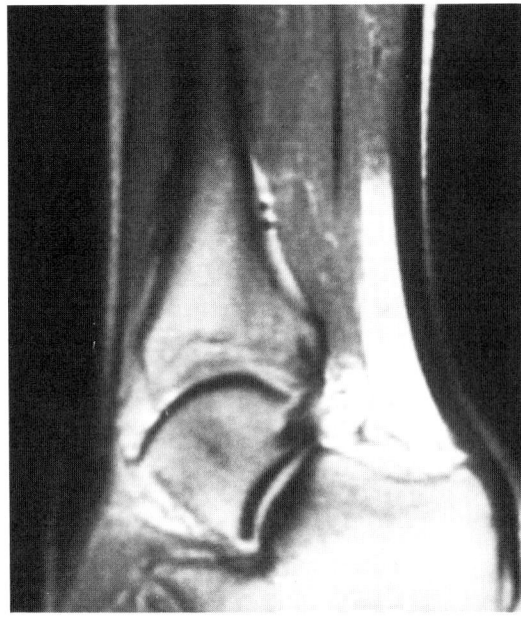

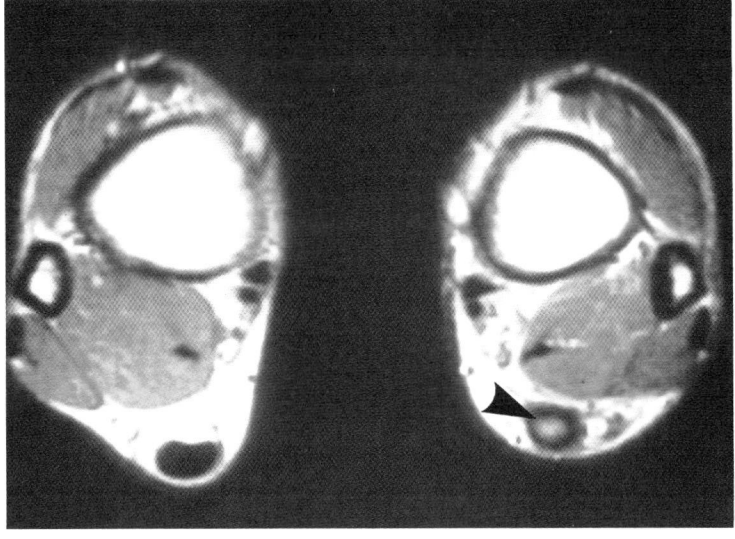

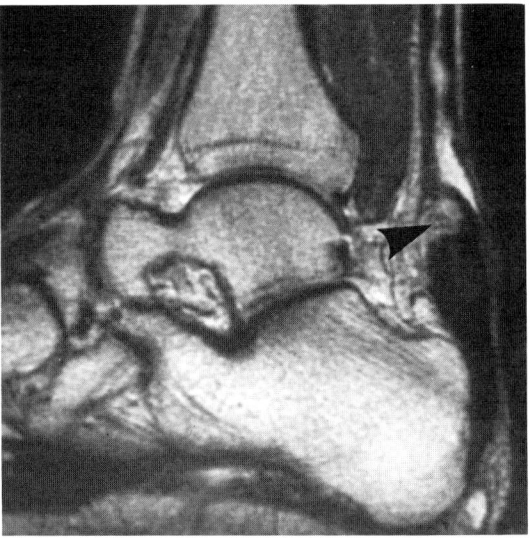

FIG. 9–45. A: Sagittal MR image showing the normal Achilles tendon. Axial (**B**) and sagittal (**C**) images of an Achilles tendon tear (*arrows*).

The patient is supine on the fluoroscopic table. The ankle should be examined fluoroscopically to determine whether there is any abnormality, i.e., instability, opaque foreign bodies, or osseous bodies, prior to injection (63). The anterior aspect of the ankle is prepared with sterile technique (5-minute povidone-iodine [Betadine] scrub). Prior to needle positioning, the dorsalis pedis pulse is palpated. The extensor tendons are usually easily located. In most situations, the joint is entered anteriorly and medial to the dorsalis pedis artery (Fig.

TABLE 9–1.[a] *Ankle arthrography: Indications and techniques*

Indication	Technique
Ligament injury	Single contrast, 6–8 ml
Articular evaluation	Double contrast
Talar dome fractures	(1 cc contrast + 8 cc air)
Osteochondritis dissecans	± Tomography
Loose bodies	Single contrast ± tomography or CT
Arthritis	Double contrast
Capsulitis	Single contrast + anesthetic

[a] (From 73.)

9-46) (29,51,56,75). The skin over the injection site is anesthetized with 1% lidocaine (Xylocaine) using a 25-gauge 1.5-inch needle. A 22-gauge 1.5-inch needle is used to perform the arthrogram. Once the needle has penetrated the skin, the ankle can be rotated into the lateral position. This allows one to judge the depth of the needle penetration. The joint is entered just inferior to the anterior tibial margin. The needle should be directed slightly inferior to avoid the tibial lip (Fig. 9-46).

When the needle is within the capsule, any fluid or blood should be aspirated. Appropriate laboratory studies should be obtained in patients with suspected infection or other arthritides. Contrast-material injection depends upon the clinical setting (Table 9-1). For patients with acute trauma, 6–8 ml of contrast material (meglumine diatrizoate or low osmolality non-ionic) is injected. Mixing 2–4 ml of lidocaine with the contrast material may facilitate stress views (38,73,82). If double-contrast technique is indicated, 1 ml of contrast medium combined with 6–8 ml of air is injected (63,73). Rarely, air alone may be used in patients with significant allergy to iodine. Occasionally 0.1–0.2 ml of 1:1000 epinephrine is injected with the contrast material. This is helpful if tomography or CT are to be used in conjunction with the arthrogram (29,63,73).

Excessive amounts of contrast medium should be avoided, for this can obscure the internal structures of the ankle, especially the articular cartilage. Also, contrast material may extravasate along the needle tract or actually leak out of the capsule. The latter is reported in older individuals (29,56,73). These changes should not be confused with ligament injuries.

Following the injection, the ankle is exercised and observed fluoroscopically. Films are obtained in the AP, lateral, and oblique projections. If a ligament injury is suspected, stress views are also taken (55). Vuust suggests the oblique axial view to improve detection of calcaneofibular ligament tears (85,86).

Normal Arthrographic Anatomy

The capsule of the anterior ankle extends from the neck of the talus to a point 5 mm superior to the distal tibial margin. This anterior recess is best seen on the lateral view (Fig. 9-46). Posteriorly, a second recess is also evident. This recess is more irregular and its size more variable compared with the anterior recess. Medially and laterally, the capsule extends to the tips of the malleoli. The margins should be smooth (43,44, 51,73,75). Superiorly, the capsule extends between the distal tibia and fibula (Fig. 9-46B), forming a syndesmotic recess. Normally this is smooth and does not extend more than 2.5 cm above the joint space (43,44, 51,73,75).

In about 10% of patients the tibiotalor joint communicates with the posterior subtalar joint. Communication with the flexor tendons (posterior tibial and flexor digitorum longus) along the medial aspect of the ankle is noted in about 20% of patients (29,43,44).

Clinical Applications

There is considerable controversy concerning the management of acute ankle injuries (24,38,51,73). Both open

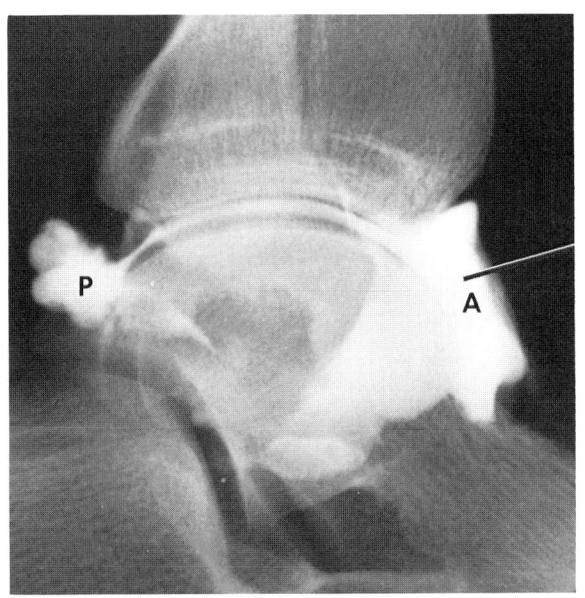
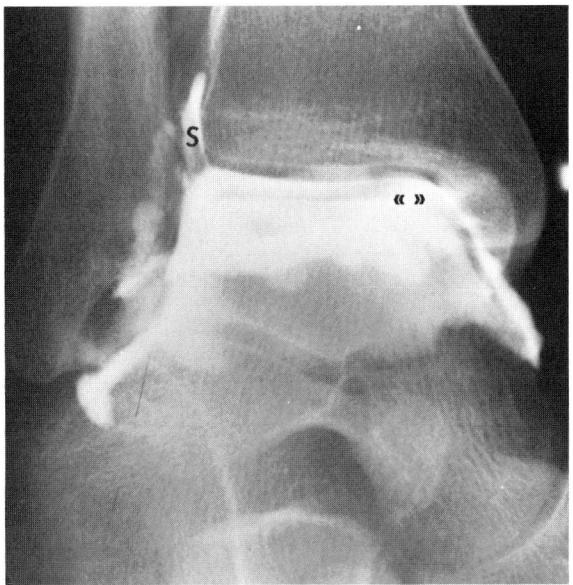

FIG. 9–46. Lateral (**A**) and AP (**B**) views of the ankle after injection demonstrating normal anatomy and needle entry point [*line* in **A**, (⟨ ⟩) in **B**]. P, posterior recess; A, anterior recess; S, syndesmotic recess. Note there is no filling of the peroneal tendons.

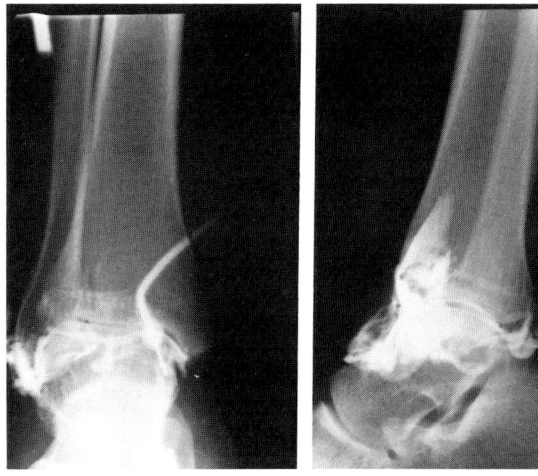
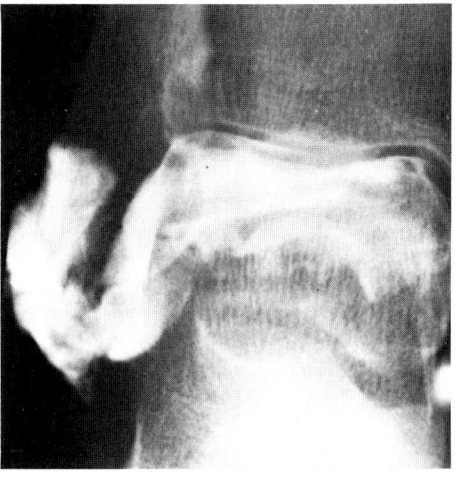

A,B   C

FIG. 9–47. Ankle arthrogram in a patient with an ankle sprain. AP (**A**) and lateral (**B**) views demonstrate extravasation of contrast medium laterally. The external oblique view (**C**) projects the contrast medium laterally, indicating that the extravasation is anterior to the fibula. This in turn indicates an anterior talofibular ligament tear.

and closed methods have been advocated. In young, active individuals, surgical reduction is more commonly performed when both the anterior talofibular and calcaneofibular ligaments are disrupted. Certainly, inadequate management can lead to recurrent injury and instability (38,43,73).

Arthrography can provide valuable information regarding the extent of ligament injury (29,51). In the acute, post-injury period, arthrography is easily performed and more accurate than stress views (73,82). Accuracy in assessing ligament injury decreases if the arthrogram is performed more than 72 hours following the injury. Ideally the test should be performed within 48 hours (51,63,73).

The ligaments of the ankle are not directly visible arthrographically. The medial complex (deltoid ligament) is broad and triangular. The fibers pass from the medial malleolus to insert into the talus and calcaneus (29,51,56). Laterally there are three major ligaments. The anterior talofibular ligament extends from the lateral malleolus to the talus and blends with the anterior capsule. The calcaneofibular ligament is not intimately associated with the capsule. The posterior talofibular ligament extends posteriorly from the fibula to the talus (29,51,73).

The anterior talofibular ligament is most frequently disrupted. This is usually the result of an inversion injury. The capsule is also torn, allowing contrast material to extravasate laterally and anterior to the distal fibula (56). The abnormality is best localized on the external oblique view. The contrast material will be projected lateral to the fibula if extravasation has occurred anteriorly. The lateral view is also useful (Fig. 9-47). Contrast medium may reach the tip of the lateral malleolus and ex-

tend superiorly. Anterior talofibular ligament tears may seal within 48 hours. Thus, arthrograms performed more than 2 days after injury may appear negative (51,73).

More significant ankle injuries may involve both the anterior talofibular and calcaneofibular ligaments. This injury classically results in filling of the peroneal tendon sheaths as well as capsular extravasation (Fig. 9-48) (29,31,51,73,75).

Diagnosis of calcaneofibular ligament tears may be difficult due to decompression of the capsule by the associated anterior talofibular ligament and capsular tear. The contrast material takes the path of least resistance (29,51,73,75). Olson suggests that lack of resistance in filling the joint with massive extravasation indicates disruption of both ligaments (75). Pre-arthrographic injection of the joint with lidocaine followed by exercise and stress or repeated exercise views following the arthrogram may be helpful in more accurate assessment of the calcaneofibular ligament.

Extravasation of contrast material posterior and lateral to the malleolus may also indicate a tear even though the peroneal tendon sheaths are not filled (29). This finding is best seen on the internal oblique or axial oblique view (86,87). Direct injection of the peroneal tendon sheath probably provides the most accurate method of diagnosing calcaneofibular ligament tears (29,65,73). Isolated tears of the calcaneofibular ligament are rare. If peroneal tendon sheath filling occurs without an associated anterior talofibular ligament tear, one can assume that the injury is not acute (29,51,75,82). Occasionally, incomplete, old, or partially healed tears are noted. These injuries present with subtle irregularity of the capsule or ulcerlike projections.

Tears of the posterior talofibular ligament are unusual

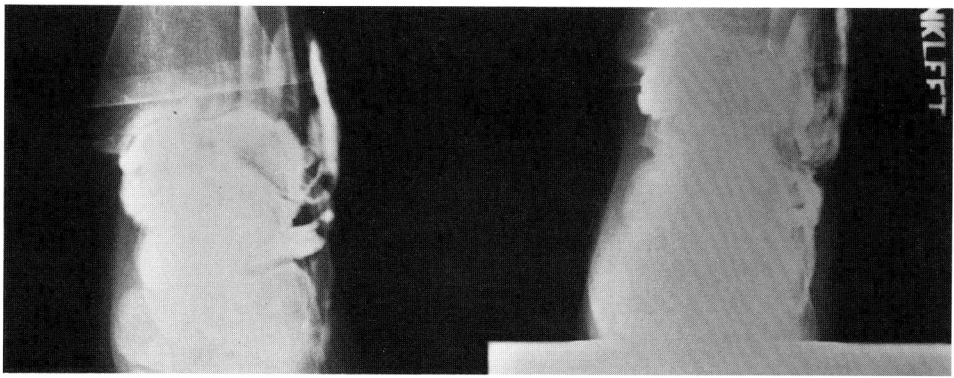

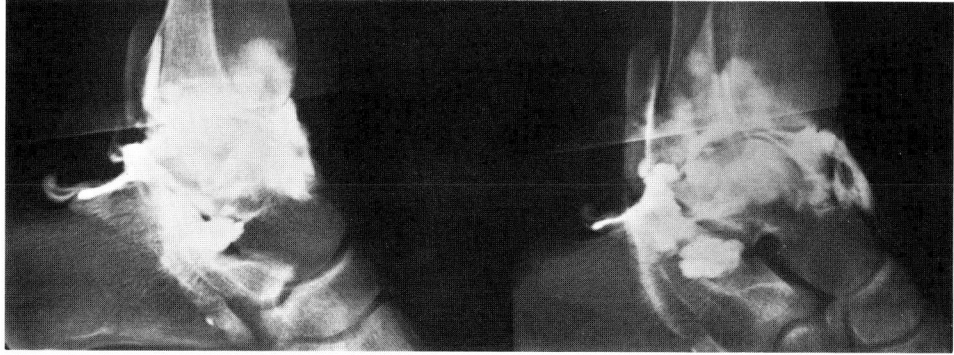

FIG. 9-48. Ankle tenogram (AP, lateral, and oblique views) shows filling of the ankle indicating a calcaneofibular ligament tear.

and do not occur as isolated injuries. In this setting, gross instability is usually evident clinically, obviating the need for arthrography (51,56,73,75).

Medial ligament injuries are less common and usually involve both the deltoid ligament and distal tibiofibular syndesmosis. The arthrogram will demonstrate extravasation around the tip of the medial malleolus and extension, disruption, or irregularity of the syndesmotic recess. Rupture of the anterior talofibular ligament may also be associated with syndesmotic tears (73,75). The lateral view will demonstrate loss of the normal lucent zone anterior to the distal tibia. (Isolated complete tears of the anterior tibiofibular ligament are uncommon.)

Following treatment of ankle injuries, arthrography with or without computed tomography may be useful in evaluating patients with persistent pain or instability. Persistent instability, adhesive capsulitis, and other complications will be clearly demonstrated (29,47).

Arthrography is less commonly performed to evaluate subtle articular or synovial changes. Articular cartilage is best studied using double-contrast technique (see Table 9-1). The combination of reduced contrast medium and air provides better detail of the articular surface. This is particularly useful in evaluating osteochondral defects such as talar dome fractures and osteochondritis dissecans (56,75). Additional information is provided by using tomography in conjunction with the double-

contrast technique. Tomography should be performed in the AP and lateral projections. Subtle synovial changes and loose bodies can also be evaluated with arthrotomography.

Following trauma, persistent pain and decreased range of motion may indicate adhesive capsulitis. In this clinical setting, single-contrast technique is most useful. Injection may be more difficult owing to the constricted capsule.

Goergen and Resnick (56) describe the use of ankle arthrography in patients with arthritis, ganglia, and total joint replacement; but these are uncommon indications. Subtraction arthrography is less effective for the evaluation of arthroplasty in the ankle than in the hip. The surface area of the components is smaller, and overlying contrast material may obscure the bone-cement interface (73).

Arthrography of the Subtalar and other Joints

Arthrograms of the tarsal joints, subtalar joints, and foot are infrequently performed. The subtalar joint can be easily entered medially or laterally depending on the anatomy and whether any joint or post-traumatic deformity exists (29,73). The patient should be on the side and the posterior talocalcaneal facet positioned fluoroscopically. The same sterile preparation and needles are used as in ankle arthrography. Fluoroscopic guidance will allow a straight vertical approach into the joint. Fluoroscopic spot films are useful, but tomography is often used to improve anatomic detail following the injection of 2–4 cc of contrast medium (Fig. 9-49).

The normal subtalar joint should be clearly outlined, with equal thickness of the articular surfaces and a smooth synovial lining (29,73). The examination is most often performed in patients with persistent posttraumatic pain or to ensure proper needle position for aspiration or therapeutic injections. If the articular cartilage is abnormal, there will be irregularity, hazy enhancement (degenerative changes), or thinning. Synovitis will cause irregularity of the synovial lining with small filling defects (29,73).

Injection of other tarsal joints and metatarsal phalangeal, and metaphalangeal joints can be accomplished easily with a fluoroscopically guided dorsal approach (Fig. 9-50). Usually the 25-gauge anesthetic needle has adequate length to penetrate the more superficial joints. When this is inadequate, as in the case of soft tissue swelling, a 22-gauge 1.5-inch needle can be used. Because the joint capacity is small, single contrast technique is almost always used. AP, lateral, and oblique spot films are taken. In certain situations, CT or conventional tomography may provide additional information.

Indications for these arthrograms are more limited. Assuring needle position for diagnostic or therapeutic aspiration or biopsy and injection, and determination of articular or capsular abnormalities are the primary indications (29,73).

Tenography

Injections of contrast medium into tendon sheaths is generally used to diagnose inflammatory or post-

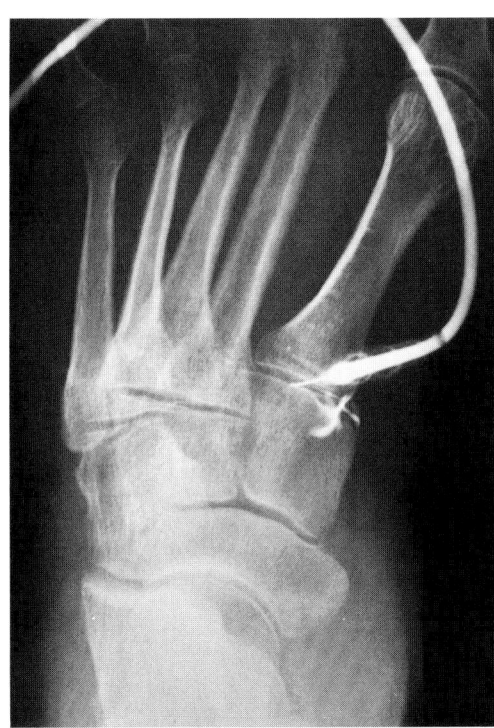

FIG. 9–50. Dorsal injection of the first tarsometatarsal joint prior to diagnostic injection.

traumatic conditions (31,55,78,83). The technique is slightly more difficult than arthrography, and experience is required to perform and interpret the studies. Studies may be performed on the lateral group (peroneus longus and brevis), medial tendons (tibialis posterior, flexor digitorum longus, and flexur hallucis longus), or the anterior tendons (tibialis anterior, extensor hallucis longus, extensor digitorum longus). The Achilles tendon does not have a tendon sheath.

Technique and Normal Anatomy

Clinical history and all pertinent imaging studies should be reviewed. Fluoroscopic examination of the foot and ankle should be performed prior to the injection. This allows palpation and localization of the tendons to be injected, evaluation of range of motion, snapping, and detection of osseous abnormalities. The skin is prepared using the same sterile technique described in the arthrogram section above. Prior to injection, the vascular structures should be localized and the foot dorsiflexed and plantar flexed to localize the tendon (Fig. 9-51).

Lateral Tendons

The peroneal tendon sheaths are injected by entering the sheaths posteriorly and just above the lateral malleo-

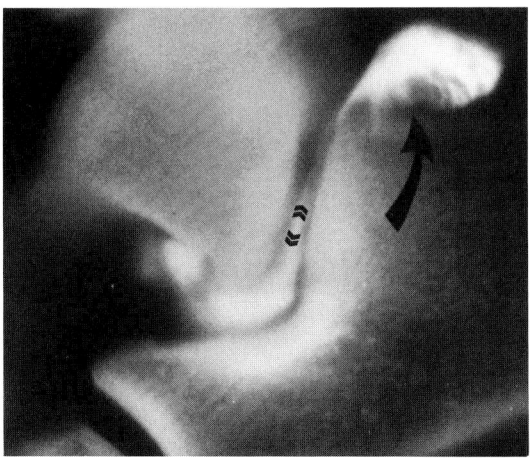

FIG. 9–49. Subtalar arthrogram showing the injection site (《 》) and synovial hypertrophy posteriorly (*curved arrows*).

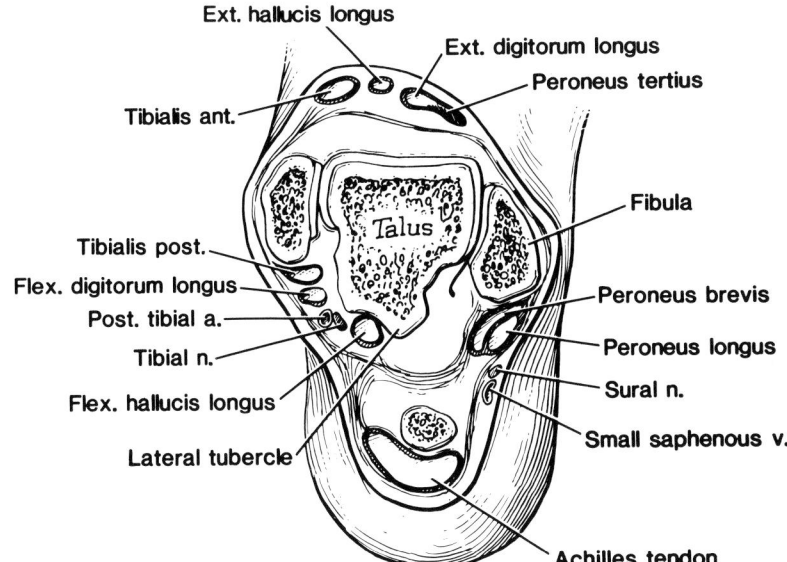

Ext. hallucis longus
Ext. digitorum longus
Peroneus tertius
Tibialis ant.
Fibula
Talus
Tibialis post.
Flex. digitorum longus
Post. tibial a.
Peroneus brevis
Tibial n.
Peroneus longus
Flex. hallucis longus
Sural n.
Lateral tubercle
Small saphenous v.
Achilles tendon

FIG. 9-51. Axial illustration of the tendons and neurovascular structures about the ankle.

lus (Fig. 9-52). The injection site may vary slightly depending on the site of suspected injury (i.e., slightly higher for suspected peroneal tendon subluxation). Following sterile preparation, the skin is anesthetized with 1% Xylocaine using a 25-gauge .75-inch needle. In certain cases, this needle is adequate for the study, but generally a 22-gauge 1.5-inch needle is required. This needle is directed from above and enters the tendon sheath obliquely so the bevel will be entirely within the sheath. When the needle enters the tendon, a slight resistance is felt. The needle is then withdrawn slightly, and a small

test injection is made using fluoroscopic observation. If the needle is properly positioned, the contrast will outline the tendon and flow away from the needle tip. The injection is monitored fluoroscopically to be certain the proper amount of contrast is used, to prevent overdistension and to detect sites of obstruction or extravasation. In general 10–20 ccs of contrast (Hypaque M-60) is required.

The peroneus longus and brevis tendons share a common tendon sheath to the distal third of the calcaneus (29,55,73). The sheath divides at this point, and the peroneus brevis inserts in the base of the fifth metatarsal. The peroneus longus takes an oblique course via the sole of the foot to insert in the inferior aspects of the medial cuneiform and first metatarsal base (29,30,73).

Following the injection, the foot is exercised during fluoroscopic monitoring to be certain that the sheaths are completely filled and to allow spot films of any abnormal findings.

Medial Tendons

The same preparation and examination technique described for the peroneal tendons is used for the medial tendons. The main difference is the injection sites. The tibialis posterior tendon is the most anterior and is entered just posterior to the metaphysis of the medial malleolus (Fig. 9-51). The flexor digitorum longus and flexor hallucis longus are more posterior (28,29,55). The posterior tibial tendon sheath begins 3–4 cm above the tibiotalar joint space and extends to the level of the navicular. Here the tendon spreads its expanded insertions on the navicular, cuneiforms, and metatarsal (2–4) bases (55).

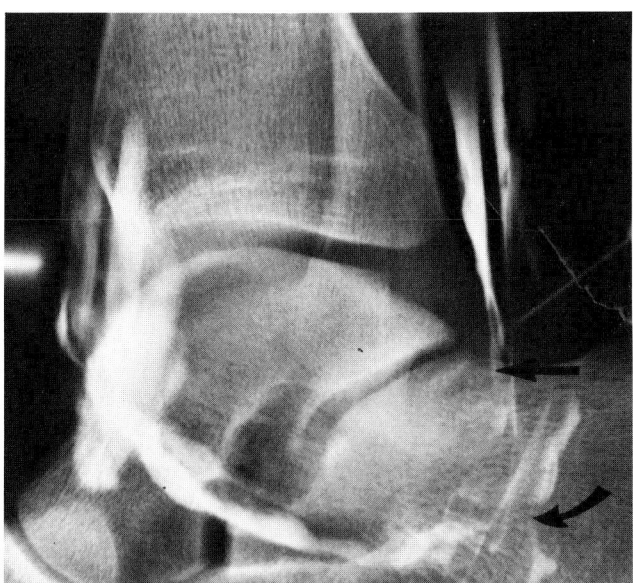

FIG. 9-52. Injection of the peroneal tendon sheath (*arrows*) with extravasation but no filling of the ankle joint. The former is normal.

The flexor digitorum longus and flexor hallucis longus lie posterior to the tibialis posterior (Fig. 9-51). In up to 25% of patients, these tendons share a common sheath (55). The flexor digitorum longus can be injected initially as it is more easily located. These tendon sheaths also begin 3–4 cm above the tibiotalar joint and extend distally crossing inferior to the talonavicular junction. The flexor digitorum longus divides and inserts in the bases of the distal phalanges of the lateral four toes. The flexor hallucis longus inserts in the base of the distal phalanx of the great toe (55).

Anterior Tendons

The anterior tendons (tibialis anterior, extensor hallucis longus, and extensor digitorum longus) are less often studied than the medial and lateral groups. These tendons can be entered 2–3 cm above the tibiotalar joint or can be injected inferiorly using the dorsalis pedis artery as a landmark. The injection is made in the proximal dorsal foot. The tibialis anterior is most medial, the extensor hallucis longus just medial to the dorsalis pedis artery and the extensor digitorum longus is lateral to the artery.

The tibialis anterior tendon sheath begins about 5 cm above the tibiotalar joint and extends to the level of the first cuneiform (55). The extensor hallucis longus is just lateral to the tibialis anterior and begins about the same level extending a variable distance, usually to the distal shaft of the first metatarsal. The combined tendon sheaths of the extensor digitorum longus begins just above the tibiotalar joint and ends at the level of the tarsometatarsal joints (55).

Clinical Indications

Tenography is most commonly used to evaluate trauma or post-traumatic conditions. The lateral tendons are most commonly studied. Black (31) found tenography more accurate than arthrography in detection of calcaneofibular ligament tears. If a ligament tear has occurred, injection of the tendon sheath will result in communication with the ankle joint. This does not occur normally (31,55). Extravasation can be normal and does not indicate a ligament tear (Fig. 9-52) (29). Other traumatic conditions such as subluxation, dislocation, or stenosis of the tendon sheath after calcaneal fractures can also be evaluated with tenography (73,78). Other chronic inflammatory changes can also be assessed tenographically. With the increased availability of MRI, we will, no doubt, see a decrease in the use of tenography. MRI provides a more direct look at the tendon, sheath, and bone and soft tissue anatomy (30).

Diagnostic Injection and Aspirations

Use of contrast to confirm position in joint spaces and tendon sheaths also provides accurate access to the joints and soft tissues for diagnostic aspirations (culture and other laboratory studies), biopsy, and instillation of anesthetic and/or steroids for therapeutic purposes. The latter is particularly valuable in patients with chronic pain. Injections can localize the site of abnormality so that surgery can be planned or allow steroid and anesthetic injection for therapeutic purposes.

These techniques are employed in the same manner and using the same sterile precautions described above. For injections, we generally use marcaine (buvivocaine 25%) because it is longer-acting than Xylocaine. This agent is used alone if surgery is comtemplated or if a total joint arthroplasty is in place. We also do not inject steroid if aspirated fluid is abnormal or infection is suspected. When steroid is used, we combine 1 cc of celestone with 2–3 ccs of marcaine or use this ratio depending on the volume of the joint or sheath to be injected.

SOFT TISSUE TRAUMA

Injuries affecting the soft tissues of the foot and ankle are common (88,89,99,107). Cass and Morrey (99) reported an incidence of about 500 ankle sprains per year. Many ankle injuries can be treated conservatively with satisfactory results. However, proper imaging evaluation is needed to determine the extent of injury so that chronic instability and function loss can be avoided (115).

Ligament Injuries

The ligaments and other supporting structures of the ankle have been discussed earlier in this chapter. However, certain aspects of ankle anatomy bear repeating in order to fully understand ligamentous trauma.

The distal tibia and fibula are supported in their anatomic relationship by the distal anterior and posterior tibiofibular ligaments and the interosseous membrane (95,119,125). Other ligament structures maintain the ankle joint. Medially, the deltoid ligament is triangular and broadens as it extends from the medial malleolus to its talar and calcaneal insertions. The deltoid ligament is composed of anterior and posterior superficial and an intermediate deep or tibiotalor ligament (125). The ligament is essentially a triangular thickening with medial capsule (See Fig. 9-17). There are three ligaments laterally. The anterior talofibular ligament extends from the anterior fibula to insert in the lateral talus just below the articular surface. With the ankle in a neutral position, this ligament is horizontally oriented and resists internal rotation. Recent studies also indicate that it is significant in resisting varus tilt particularly with the ankle in plantar flexion (118). The posterior tibiofibular ligament extends from the posterior fibula to the posterior talus. The calcaneofibular ligament originates at the lateral malleolar tip and inserts on the calcaneus, restricting inversion. The calcaneofibular ligament supports both the ankle and subtalar joints and is intimately associated with the peroneal tendon sheaths (see Fig. 9-17) (99,119,125).

Ankle Sprains

Ankle sprains are most commonly due to inversion with internal rotation of the foot. The injury commonly occurs during sporting events or from falls on uneven surfaces (98,99). Isolated rupture of the deltoid ligament (an eversion injury) is rare (98). Clinically, ankle sprains present with varying degrees of pain, swelling, and ecchymosis. In assessing ankle sprains, it is important to classify the degree of injury so that proper treatment can be instituted and chronic instability avoided. Typically, ankle sprains are divided into three grades (92,93,99). Patients with Grade 1 sprains present with mild stretching of the ligaments but no disruption or instability. These patients can still ambulate and generally have mild swelling with pain and tenderness over the anterior talofibular ligament (125). Grade 2 sprains are incomplete ligament tears. There is generally significant pain, marked swelling, and ecchymosis. Patients' injuries are difficult to evaluate on physical examination. Discomfort on palpation over the calcaneal fibular ligament is not uncommon (125). Grade 3 sprains are complete ligament tears. Both the anterior talofibular and calcaneofibular may be involved resulting in ankle instability (99). The degree of swelling is variable, but there is usually tenderness over both the anterior talofibular and calcaneofibular ligaments (125).

Diagnosis of ligament disruption usually requires special studies. Routine ankle views (AP, lateral, mortise view) are not effective in differentiating the types of ankle sprains. However, secondary signs are important in determining which additional techniques may be most useful (136). Patients with Grade 1 sprains generally present with mild, soft tissue swelling over the lateral malleolus. This can be identified on the AP and mortise views. A bright light is frequently needed to evaluate the soft tissues. No fracture or effusion is evident on the lateral view. Grades 2 and 3 sprains have more significant swelling that can be identified clinically and on both AP and lateral radiographs. However, this finding has little value. Attempts at correlating ligament injury with the degree of swelling seen radiographically have been unsuccessful. The presence of an effusion in the joint is

somewhat useful in that it generally indicates that the capsule is intact (see Fig. 9-25C). Effusions are best seen on the lateral view. Small avulsion fractures (Grade 4 sprain) can also be seen on plain films (Fig. 9-53). Measuring the tibiotalar joint to differentiate second- and third-degree sprains is not usually helpful (113,137). However, if the talus is shifted, resulting in asymmetry of the ankle mortise, a ligament injury is generally present.

Stress views of the ankle are useful in diagnosing ligament disruption (115,125). However, this technique requires adequate anesthesia of the involved joint and is highly dependent upon the experience of the examiner. Comparison with the normal ankle under stress is also necessary. The ankles should be stressed in varus and valgus positions with the foot in neutral and plantar flexed positions. AP stress views (drawer sign) should also be performed (125).

For best results, the examination should be fluoroscopically guided to assure proper positioning and monitoring. When performing varus and valgus stress tests, it is important to remember normal variations in ankle motion. Normal talar tilt ranges from 5°–23° (99,101,117,125). This problem is overcome by comparing the injured and uninjured sides. Measuring varus and valgus stress views can be accomplished using angles or distance measurements. When using the angle tech-

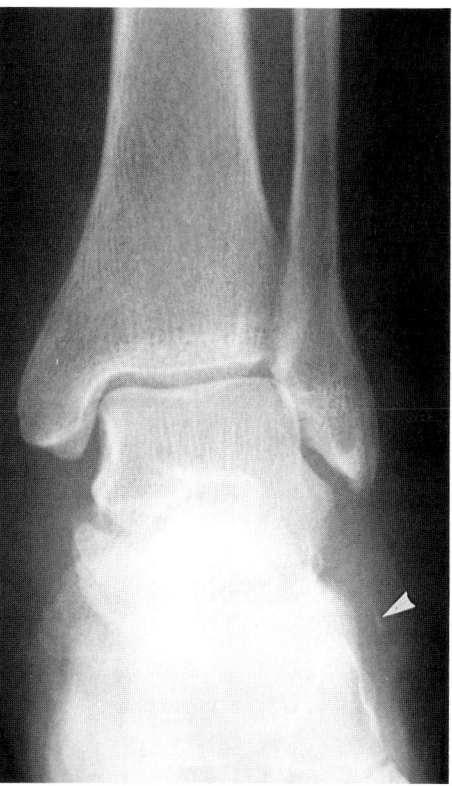

FIG. 9-53. AP view of the ankle demonstrating a "flake" fracture (*arrow*) due to calcaneofibular ligament avulsion.

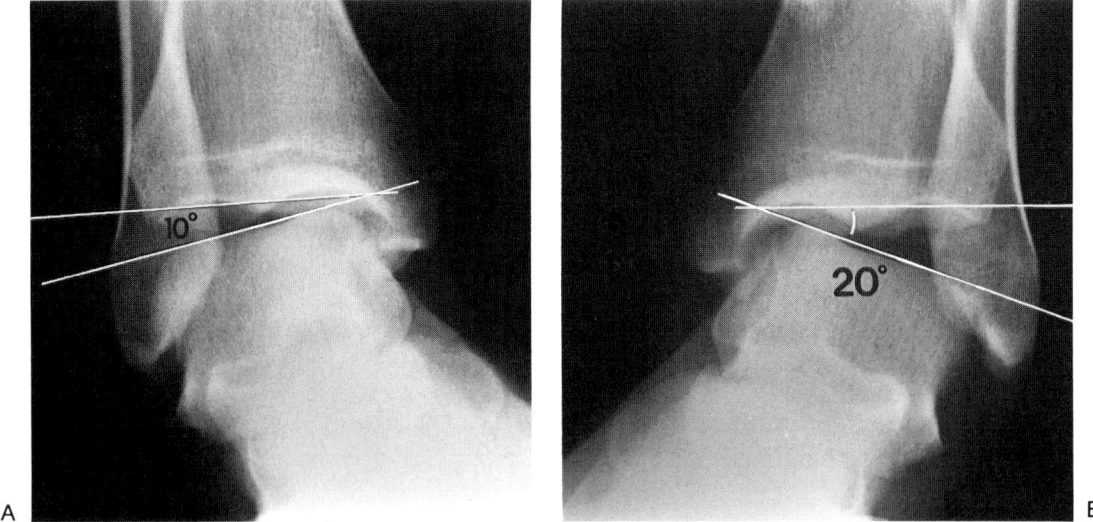

FIG. 9–54. Varus stress views of the normal (**A**) and injured (**B**) ankle. There is a 10° difference in talar tilt on the injured side.

nique, a line is drawn along the talar dome and tibial plafond. The change in the angle with stress is measured and both ankles compared (Fig. 9-54). If the angle (talar tilt) of the injured ankle is about 10° greater than the normal side, it generally indicates both the anterior talofibular and calcaneofibular ligaments are torn (99,113). These changes should be noted with the foot in both plantar flexed and neutral positions during stress. In neutral if the angle is 6° greater than the normal side, both ligaments are probably torn. If this occurs only in plantar flexed stress, it is likely that only the anterior talofibular ligament is torn (113). It has been demon-

strated experimentally that accuracy is best with 10° of plantar flexion and the leg internally rotated 25° (121). The change in height from the talar dome to the plafond can also be measured. A difference of 3 mm between the normal and injured ankle indicates ligament disruption (125). AP stress can be applied using several techniques. For consistancy, we prefer the double exposure technique with the foot plantar flexed 10° (Fig. 9-55). This allows the change in talar or tibial position to be easily measured on one film. A shift of greater than 2–3 mm of the injured over the uninjured side is considered significant (125).

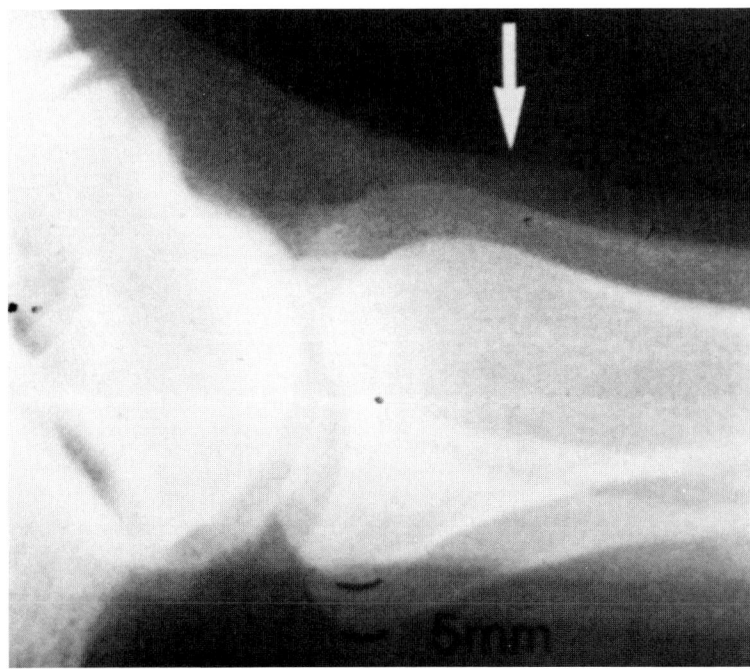

FIG. 9–55. AP stress test with double exposure showing a 5-mm shift (2 mm is normal) (from 125, with permission.)

Although stress views are useful, their accuracy is significantly lower than arthrography or tenography (89,125,135,136). Sauser et al. (134) studied 55 patients with stress views and arthrography within 72 hours of injury. This study noted stress views were accurate if talar tilt increased by 10° or more, but the test was only positive in 38% of patients with positive arthrograms.

Blanchard et al. (95), Black et al. (94), Schweigel et al. (135) report significantly improved accuracy, approaching 96%, using stress tenography to evaluate the calcaneofibular ligament. False negative studies using conventional arthrography approach 21% (94,131). The ankle tenogram is positive when contrast injected into the peroneal tendon sheath enters the joint space (Fig. 9-48). However, this decompresses the sheath and can make it more difficult to demonstrate anterior talofibular ligament tears. The latter and deltoid ligaments are intimately associated with the capsule and, therefore, ankle arthrography is more useful in demonstrating these ligament injuries. Since stress views are most accurate following anesthetic injection, it would seem wise to combine arthrograms or tenograms with stress views to allow the most accurate assessment of the injury. Therefore, we recommend using one of these combinations in assessing ankle injury. This decision should be based on clinical findings and whether surgery or treatment modifications will be made based on the degree of ligament injury. Surgical intervention is a more important consideration in professional athletes or young active individuals. Generally assessment of the calcaneofibular ligament is most critical as conservative treatment is most often used if only the anterior talofibular ligament is torn. Therefore, a stress tenogram is the technique of choice (94,95,108). CT and MRI are useful in evaluating the tendons around the ankle but less effective in evaluating the capsule and ligaments (93).

Treatment

Treatment of ligament injuries of the ankle is controversial (99,142). Accurate assessment of the degree of injury (anterior talofibular alone or with calcaneofibular ligament), the history of recurrent sprains, chronic instability, patients' ages and activities, the presence of systemic disease or steroid therapy all play a part in the decision to treat surgically or conservatively. Many authors believe conservative treatment is superior to early operative intervention. Brand and Collins (98) reported only 12% of ankle sprains were surgically repaired. Cass and Morrey (99) also recommend conservative therapy. Grades 1 and 2 sprains are treated with taping or casting if the patient is unable to ambulate with taping alone. Patients with Grade 3 sprains are treated with walking casts for 3–6 weeks. Patients are generally allowed to return to normal activity as symptoms dictate. This treatment approach is based on data that indicates that repair following acute injury will not provide any advantage to delayed repair if chronic instability occurs (99). Chronic instability can develop in 18–25% of patients following ligament injury (114). However, surgery is not required in all cases.

Patients treated conservatively or surgically may require radiographic follow-up when symptoms persist. Early degenerative changes and certain signs of chronic instability may be evident on standing AP and lateral views (Fig. 9-56) (114). Usually changes are more subtle, and arthrography or tenography with stress testing are required. These tests are generally believed to be most accurate within 72 hours of acute injury, however, chronic changes can be documented (106,135). Arthrography can demonstrate partially healed tears, chronic tears in the calcaneofibular ligament, adhesive capsulitis, and residual instability (Fig. 9-57) (95,106,135). When

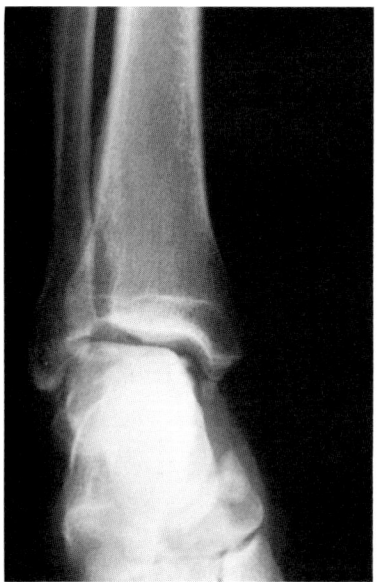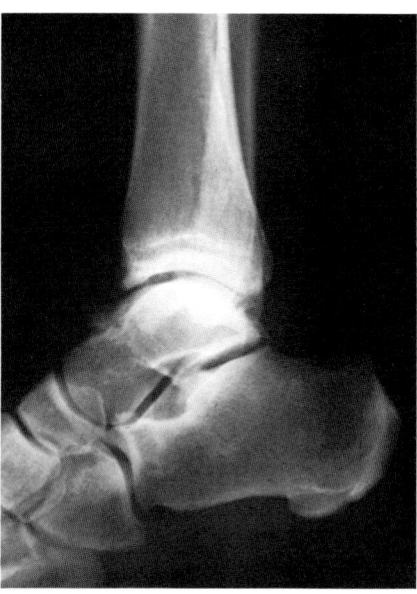

A,B

FIG. 9-56. Standing AP (A) and lateral (B) views of the ankle demonstrating talar shift and degenerative arthritis due to chronic instability.

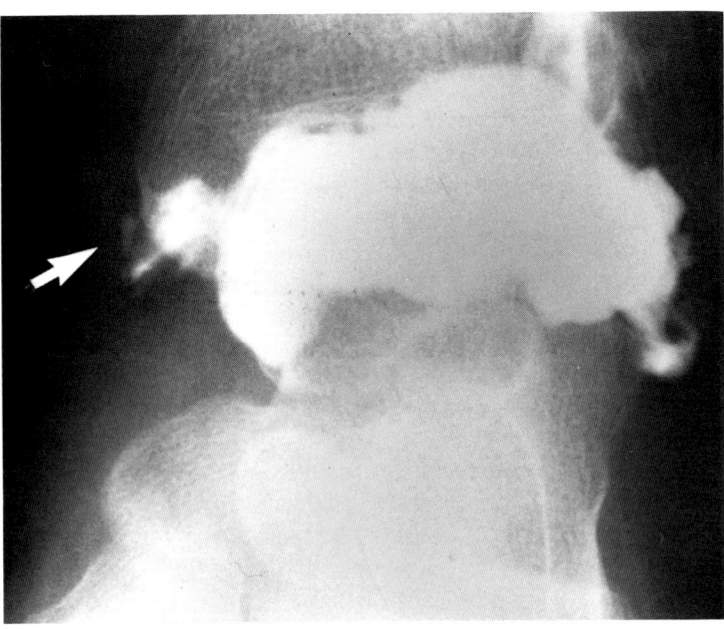

FIG. 9-57. Oblique view of an ankle arthrogram demonstrating an incomplete tear medially (*arrow*) (from 92, with permission.)

subtle changes are suspected, computed or conventional arthrotomography may be required. The axial images of computed tomography are particularly useful in evaluating the tibiofibular syndesmosis, and conventional tomography, the articular cartilage. MRI may have a similar role in evaluating residual articular and soft tissue pathology (93). Table 9-2 summarizes the late complications of ligament injuries.

Tendon Injuries

Thirteen tendons cross the ankle (119). These tendons include the peroneus brevis and longus laterally; the Achilles tendon posteriorly; the tibialis posterior, flexor digitorum longus, and flexor hallucis longus medially; and anteriorly, the tibialis anterior, extensor hallucis longus, tendons of the extensor digitorum longus and peroneus tertius. All tendons are enclosed in sheaths with the exception of the Achilles tendon. Tendon injury may occur as an isolated event, in association with a fracture, or may be due to previous fracture with degenerative joint disease. Tendons may also rupture in patients on steroid therapy (systemic or direct injection) or with chronic inflammatory diseases (112,122,124,132).

TABLE 9-2. *Sequelae of ankle ligament injuries*

Recurrent instability (follows Grade 3 sprains)
Sural nerve damage (usually follows surgical repair)
Recurrent sprains
Peroneal nerve palsy
Degenerative arthritis

(From 92.)

Peroneal Tendons

The peroneal muscles assist in pronation and eversion of the foot (119,132). The peroneus brevis tendon is anterior to the peroneus longus as they pass posterior to the lateral malleolus (Fig. 9-58). In about 80% of patients there is a notch (varies in size) in the fibula that accommodates a portion of the peroneus brevis. In 20% of patients, this notch is very shallow or absent, which may lead to recurrent subluxation (119,132). The tendons also pass through the superior and inferior peroneal retinacula (Fig. 9-58). It is between these two structures that they are immediately adjacent to the calcaneofibular ligament (119). The peroneal tendons share a common

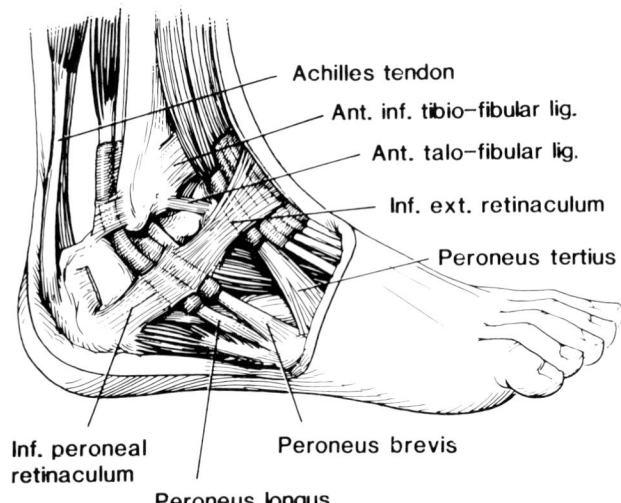

FIG. 9-58. Anterior and lateral tendons of the ankle.

sheath to the inferior margin of the superior peroneal retinaculum. At this point, the sheath of the peroneus longus separates from the peroneus brevis. The peroneus longus progresses inferior to the peroneal tubercle of the calcaneus to the plantar aspect of the foot where it inserts in the base of the first metatarsal and medial cuneiform. The peroneus brevis passes inferiorly inserting on the base of the fifth metatarsal (112). Evaluation of the tendons and normal osseous sulci is easily accomplished using MRI or CT (91,92,132,139).

Dislocation

Diagnosis of peroneal tendon injury first requires that the problem be considered. Patients frequently present with a "sprained ankle" and dislocation of the peroneal tendons is not considered (Table 9-3) (88,99,100,124). The mechanism of injury is not clear, but dislocation is most likely due to an inversion-dorsiflexion or abduction dorsiflexion injury. Patients present with pain and swelling over the posterior superior aspect of the lateral malleolus. Certain patients can voluntarily dislocate the peroneal tendons (124).

Swelling may make actual palpation of the tendon difficult and pain with motion can limit the detection of subluxation on physical examination. Routine radiographs will demonstrate soft tissue swelling laterally but the distribution is not characteristic or different from an inversion sprain. A characteristic longitudinal flake fracture along the distal fibular metaphysis is very useful when present (124). This is best seen on the internal oblique view (119). Murr (126) reported this finding in 15–50% of peroneal tendon dislocations (Fig. 9-59). Usually other imaging procedures are more useful. CT, MRI, or tenography should be considered to confirm the

diagnosis. CT provides excellent bone detail and is useful in assessing the peroneal notch in the fibula (132,133). The tendons are less well demonstrated with CT than with MRI (92,93). Subtle tears or complete disruptions are seen more easily on MR where the tendons are normally low signal intensity (black) compared to the high intensity seen in the tendon that has torn. These noninvasive techniques do have disadvantages. For example, if the tendons have returned to normal position or are only slightly displaced, fluoroscopic observation following tenography may be more useful in demonstrating subluxation. This may also be possible to demonstrate with new fast scan (gradient-echo techniques) MR techniques (112).

Rupture of the Peroneal Tendon

Rupture of the peroneal tendons is not common. However, the lesion may be overlooked as a cause of ankle instability and therefore the true incidence is not known (88). Patients may present acutely with an "ankle sprain" or have symptoms of chronic instability. The latter is more common in patients with chronic inflammatory arthritis or patients on systemic steroids. When the tendons are torn, the patient will be unable to effectively evert the foot (88,119).

Routine radiographs are usually not useful. However, displacement of the os peroneum may indicate peroneal rupture (141). Tenography may demonstrate the site of the tear, but since this technique outlines the tendon and does not provide direct assessment it is less useful than MRI. Both CT and MRI have been described as useful techniques for evaluating the peroneal tendons (92,93,

TABLE 9–3. *Ankle sprains: Differential diagnosis*[a]

Fractures
  Talus
    neck
    dome
    lateral process
    posterior process
  Calcaneus
    anterior process
  Cuboid
  Malleolar fractures or avulsions
  Fifth metatarsal base
Soft tissue injuries
  Peroneal tendon
    subluxation
    dislocation
  Subtalar subluxation or dislocation
  Deltoid ligament ruptures
  Talonavicular subluxation or dislocation

[a] (99,100,105,119).

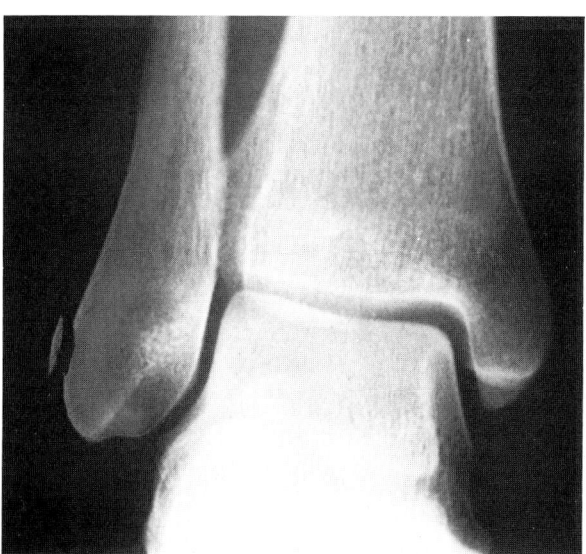
FIG. 9–59. Internal oblique view of the ankle demonstrating the appearance of a flake fracture associated with peroneal tendon dislocation.

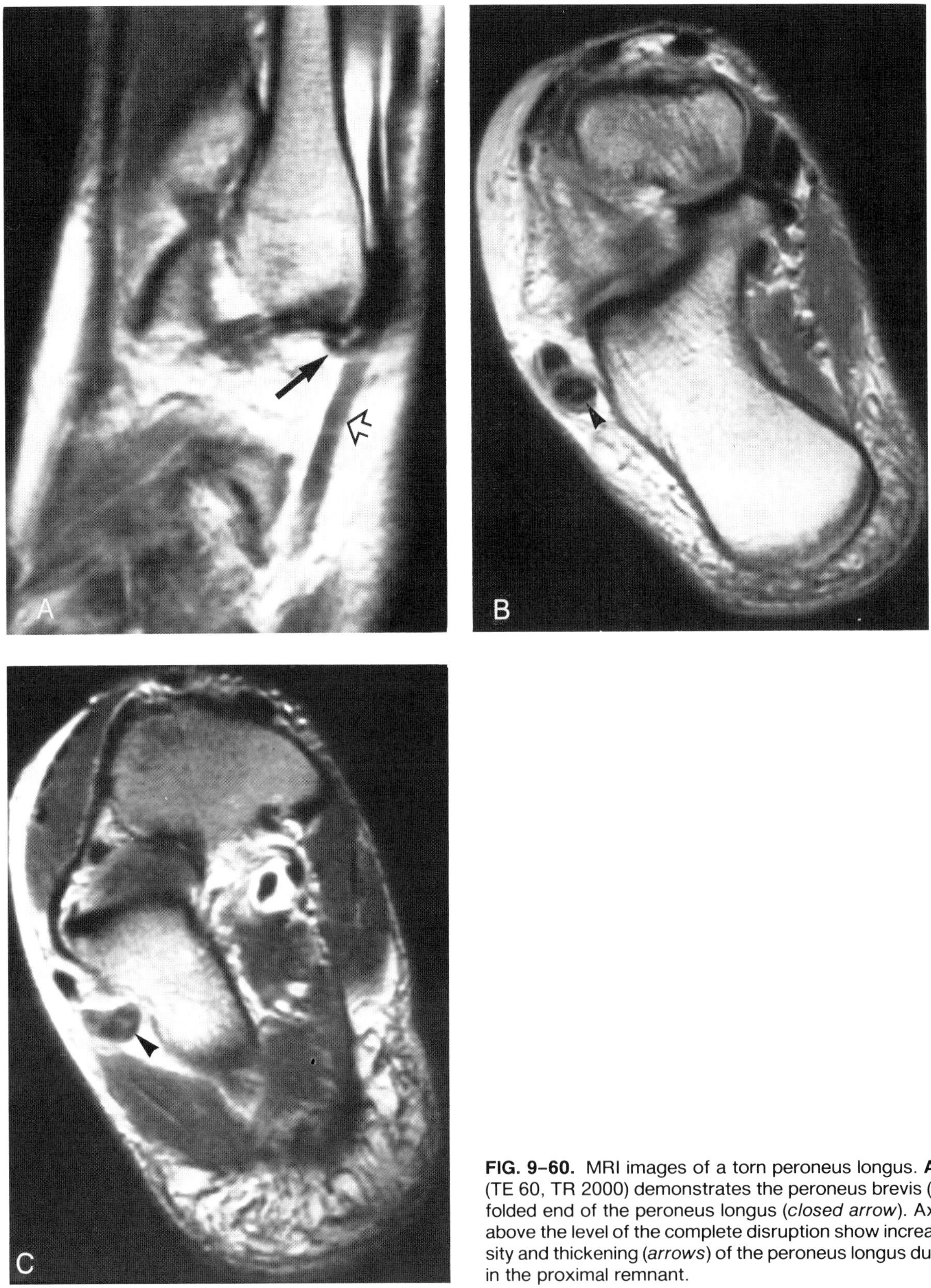

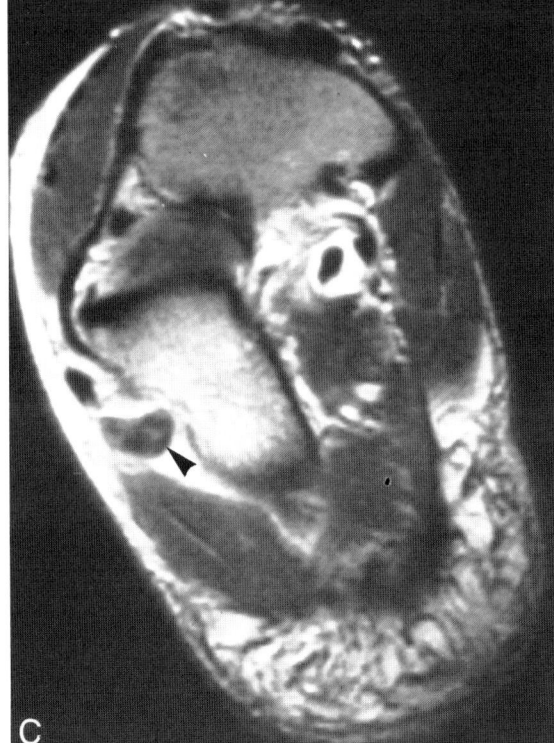

FIG. 9-60. MRI images of a torn peroneus longus. **A:** Sagittal image (TE 60, TR 2000) demonstrates the peroneus brevis (*open arrow*) and folded end of the peroneus longus (*closed arrow*). Axial images (**B,C**) above the level of the complete disruption show increased signal intensity and thickening (*arrows*) of the peroneus longus due to hemorrhage in the proximal remnant.

132,139). MRI has superior soft tissue contrast and can define incomplete, complete, and chronic inflammatory changes in both the tendon and the sheath (Fig. 9-60). If a complete tear is present, the tendon ends can be defined as well as absence of the tendon in its sheath in the torn region. If a partial tear has occurred, there will be increased signal intensity in the tendon due to blood and fluid. These findings are most easily demonstrated on T_2-weighted (TE60, TR2000) sequences. The contrast of the blood and fluid compared to the normally low intensity (black) tendon is most striking using this sequence. In patients with old tears, the tendon will look thickened, with areas of intermediate intensity (gray on MR image) and there is often fluid in the tendon sheath. The latter is not seen in normal patients.

Treatment

Treatment of peroneal tendon injury depends on the existing anatomy and degree of injury. In patients with dislocation, considerations include deepening the fibular groove and/or reinforcing the superior retinaculum. The latter can be accomplished using a pedical fascial flap, a strip of Achilles tendon, or a portion of the distal plantaris. The tendons can also be rerouted medial to the calcaneofibular ligament (119). Preoperative MRI or CT is useful in evaluating the bone and soft tissue anatomy prior to planning the procedure.

Incomplete tendon tears can be treated conservatively. In patients with complete disruption, operative intervention provides the best results. This can be accomplished by repairing the torn ends or using soft tissue grafts. Follow-up evaluation is most easily accomplished using MRI. MRI can determine whether the tendon is intact and provides valuable baseline data if postoperative infection or recurrent rupture should take place (92,93).

Achilles Tendon

The Achilles tendon is the largest and strongest tendon in the foot and ankle. The tendon originates as the gastrocnemius and soleus tendons join and inserts on the posterior calcaneus. In its axial presentation, the tendon thickens distally becoming elliptical with concave anterior and convex posterior surfaces (Fig. 9-61). Approximately 2–6 cm above its calcaneal insertion, the fibers in the tendon cross. The posterior fibers course medial to lateral and the anterior fibers course lateral to medial prior to inserting in the calcaneus. Most tendon tears occur just above this, perhaps partially due to the reduced blood supply in this region. The Achilles tendon does not have a true tendon sheath (119).

The Achilles tendon, although strong, is commonly torn. Ruptures are usually the result of indirect trauma.

The injury can occur during athletic activity at any age. The injury usually occurs in strenuous activities with frequent plantar flexion during raising up on the toes or with pushing off or jumping with the knee extended. Falling or landing on the forefoot, which leads to abrupt dorsiflexion of the foot, can also lead to Achilles rupture. In non-athletes the injury is most common from 30–50 years of age (119). Certain systemic and local conditions predispose to tendon disruption. Gout, systemic lupus erythematosis, rheumatoid arthritis, hyperpathathyroidism, chronic renal failure, steroids, and diabetes have all been implicated (127). Patients on systemic steroids or with other systemic diseases noted above may rupture both Achilles tendons simultaneously. Local steroid injections may also lead to partial or complete disruption (120).

Clinically, patients present with pain, local swelling, and an inability to raise up on their toes on the affected side (119). If completely torn, a defect may be palpable on physical examination. However, clinical examination is not always accurate. The exact nature of the injury can be misdiagnosed in over 25% of patients. This is because a gap in the tendon may not be palpable (especially in incomplete tears) and the patient may be able to plantar flex the foot with the toe flexors. Differentiation of Achilles tears from gastrocnemius or plantaris tears may also be difficult (129). The Thompson test may be useful. This test is performed by squeezing the gastrocnemius muscle belly. If the Achilles tendon is intact, the foot will plantar flex during the maneuver (positive response). If the tendon is torn, the foot will not respond (negative response) (143). O'Brien (128) described a similar test using a needle placed in the Achilles tendon 10 inches above the calcaneus. The motion of the needle hub is observed while the foot is into the dorsiflexed and plantar flexed positions. When the hub moves in opposite the direction of foot motion, the tendon is intact.

Imaging of Achilles tendon pathology can be accomplished using several modalities. Routine radiographs are usually nonspecific. However, Newmark, et al. (127) described fracture of a calcaneal osteophyte in association with Achilles tendon avulsion. Low kVp x-rays and Xerox techniques may demonstrate swelling, thickening of the tendon and irregularity of the pre-Achilles fat or Kager's triangle (92,93). These findings are best seen on the lateral view. Ultrasound can also be effective in looking at the architecture of the tendon (96,109). This requires experience on the part of the examiner and interpreter. Ultrasound images can be difficult to interpret by those who do not routinely use the technique (Fig. 9-61A,B).

CT and MRI, although more expensive than the above techniques, provide more information about the tendon and surrounding structures. MRI is particularly useful because of its superior soft tissue contrast and ability to obtain images in the axial, sagittal, coronal, and

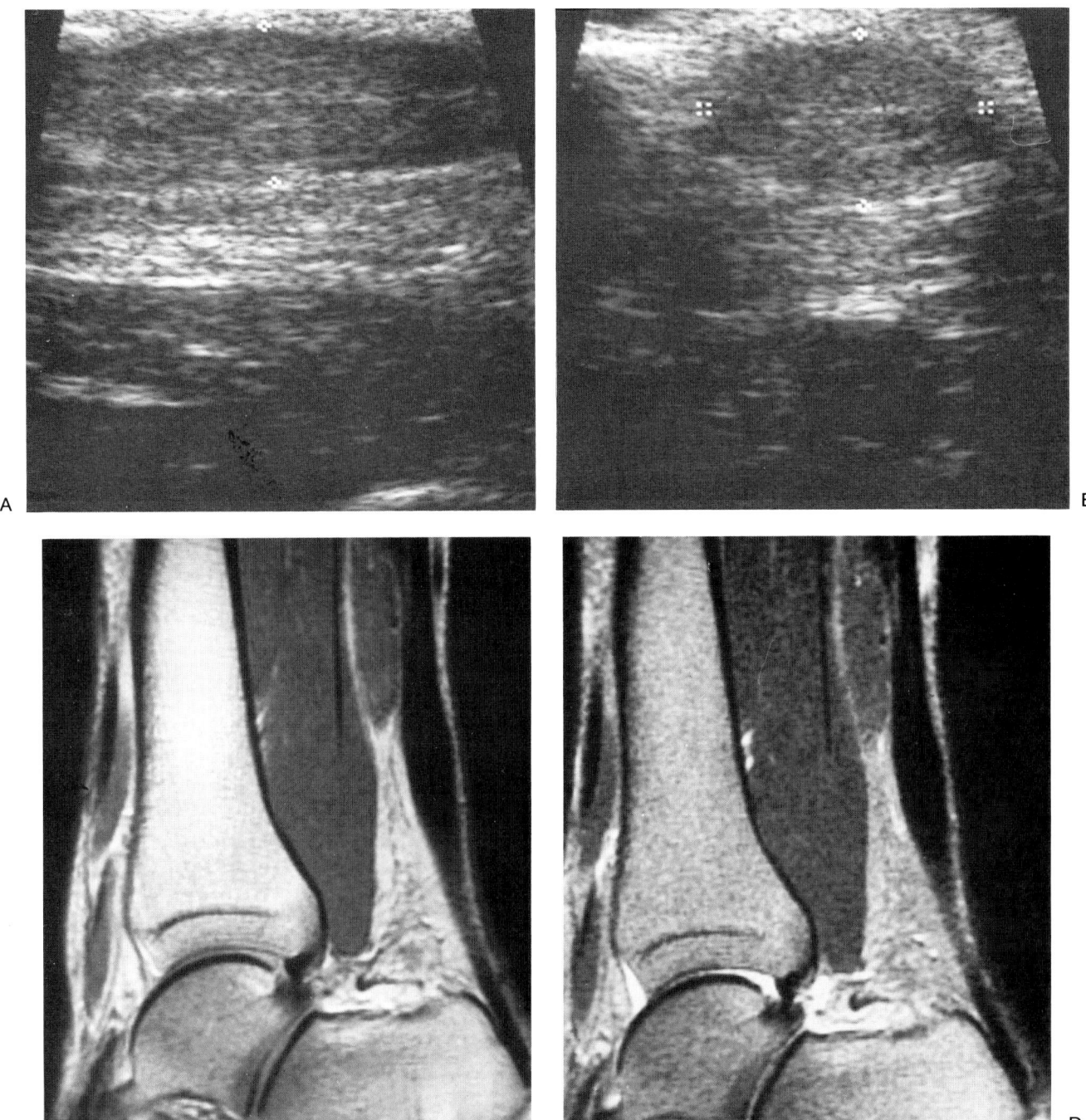

FIG. 9–61. Jogger with chronic Achilles tendon pain. Longitudinal (**A**) and transverse (**B**) ultrasound images show thickening and hyperechoic changes in the tendon suggesting an incomplete tear. Sagittal MR images using partial saturation (**C**) (T1-weighted, TE 20, TR 600) and spin-echo (**D**) (T2-weighted, TE 60, TR 2000) show thickening but no increased signal intensity in the tendon. Therefore, changes are due to an old tear with scar formation and thickening.

off-axis oblique plains (92,93,102). We find MR useful in detecting complete, incomplete, and old Achilles injuries as well as for evaluating bursitis and other causes of Achilles tendon pathology (Fig. 9-62) (93). The extent of involvement can be accurately assessed with MRI. In addition, patients can be followed to determine whether healing is progressing normally or whether operative intervention is necessary (93).

Decisions regarding treatment of Achilles tendon tears depend upon the age and activity status of the patient, the degree of tear (partial or complete) and whether there are any predisposing factors such as systemic disease or steroids. As with many soft tissue injuries, the treatment can be controversial.

Generally speaking minor tears (<50%, Grade 2) can be treated conservatively. This might be accomplished using a below-the-knee cast with the foot plantarflexed for eight weeks. After cast removal, the use of a shoe with an elevated heel (2.5 cm) for an additional four weeks is common. It is essential to follow the healing process to be certain that recurrent injury does not occur and that the incomplete tear has not become complete. This can be easily accomplished using MRI (Fig. 9-62).

Percy and Conochi (129) reported excellent surgical results in 64 patients with complete Achilles ruptures. In their series, four incomplete tears eventually ruptured after conservative management. Inglis (116) treated 48 patients surgically and 31 conservatively. The surgically treated patients were more satisfied with the result. Cybex testing demonstrated that patients treated conservatively achieved only 72% of normal strength. Therefore, it might be best to consider conservative therapy for older, inactive individuals or patients with underlying systemic disease. Surgical repair should be considered in more active patients (116,119). Surgical treatment consists of repairing the torn tendon ends and re-establishing continuity. Plantaris or other fascial or tendon grafts may be needed to approximate the torn ends of the tendon (119).

Medial Tendons

The posterior tibial, flexor digitorum longus, and flexor hallucis longus tendons make up the medial tendon group and are located anterior to posterior in the above order. The posterior tibial tendon (most anterior) with its tendon sheath passes just posterior to the medial malleolus, lateral to the flexor retinaculum, and broadens at its insertion in the navicular tuberosity and base of the medial cuneiform. The flexor digitorum longus takes a similar course proximally lying between the posterior tibial tendon and posterior tibial artery (Fig. 9-63). As it turns toward the plantar aspect of the foot, it passes superficially to the flexor hallucis longus before dividing into tendon slips that insert in the bases of the second to fifth distal phalanges. The flexor hallucis lon-

gus tendon is located more posteriorly and laterally. It passes through a fibro-osseous tunnel beneath the sustentaculum tali and along the medial plantar aspect of the foot to insert in the base of the distal phalanx of the great toe (111,112,119).

Acute rupture of the deltoid ligament is not common (98). Similarly, the posterior tibial, flexor digitorum longus, and flexor hallucis longus tendons are rarely torn following acute trauma (111,119,138). DeZwart and Davidson have reported posterior tibial tendon rupture in association with bimalleolar fracture (105). Injury is more common following repeated trauma or in patients who have either an associated systemic disease or are on predisone therapy (111,112).

The posterior tibial tendon is the most commonly injured of the three medial tendons. Patients present with pain, local tenderness, and swelling, and physical examination may reveal a non-palpable tendon (119). Rupture of the posterior tibial tendon can lead to progressive flatfoot deformity, inability to raise up on the toes, and weakness on inversion of the foot (110,122).

Routine radiography is usually of little value in patients with medial tendon injuries. Acute trauma rupture of the posterior tibial tendon has been described in association with medial malleolar fractures (105). The fracture is a mirror image of the flake fracture seen with peroneal tendon dislocation (see Fig. 9-59). It occurs longitudinally along the distal medial tibial metaphysis (138). Posterior tibial tendon rupture may present with an increased talocalcaneal angle on the AP and lateral view (110). These findings, along with soft tissue swelling are the only plain film findings that might suggest the diagnosis. In patients with chronic disease and inflammation, the stress tenogram may show changes in the posterior tibial or adjacent tendon sheaths. However, the structure of the tendon is better demonstrated with CT or MRI. In our experience, MRI has been most useful in assessing the nature and degree of posterior tibial tendon pathology (Figs. 9-64 and 9-65) (Table 9-4).

Rupture of the flexor digitorum and flexor hallucis longus tendons occurs less frequently but can present with similar clinical findings. Garth (111) reported rupture of the flexor hallucis longus in ballet dancers and soccer players. Patients presented with swelling, tenderness, and crepitation near the sustentaculum tali. Symptoms were increased with flexion and extension of the great toe.

Tenography of the flexor hallucis longus is tedious due to the difficulty in localizing the tendon with the needle tip. Therefore, MRI or CT are more useful (92,93).

Treatment

Most older patients or patients with systemic disease are treated conservatively. However, more active individ-

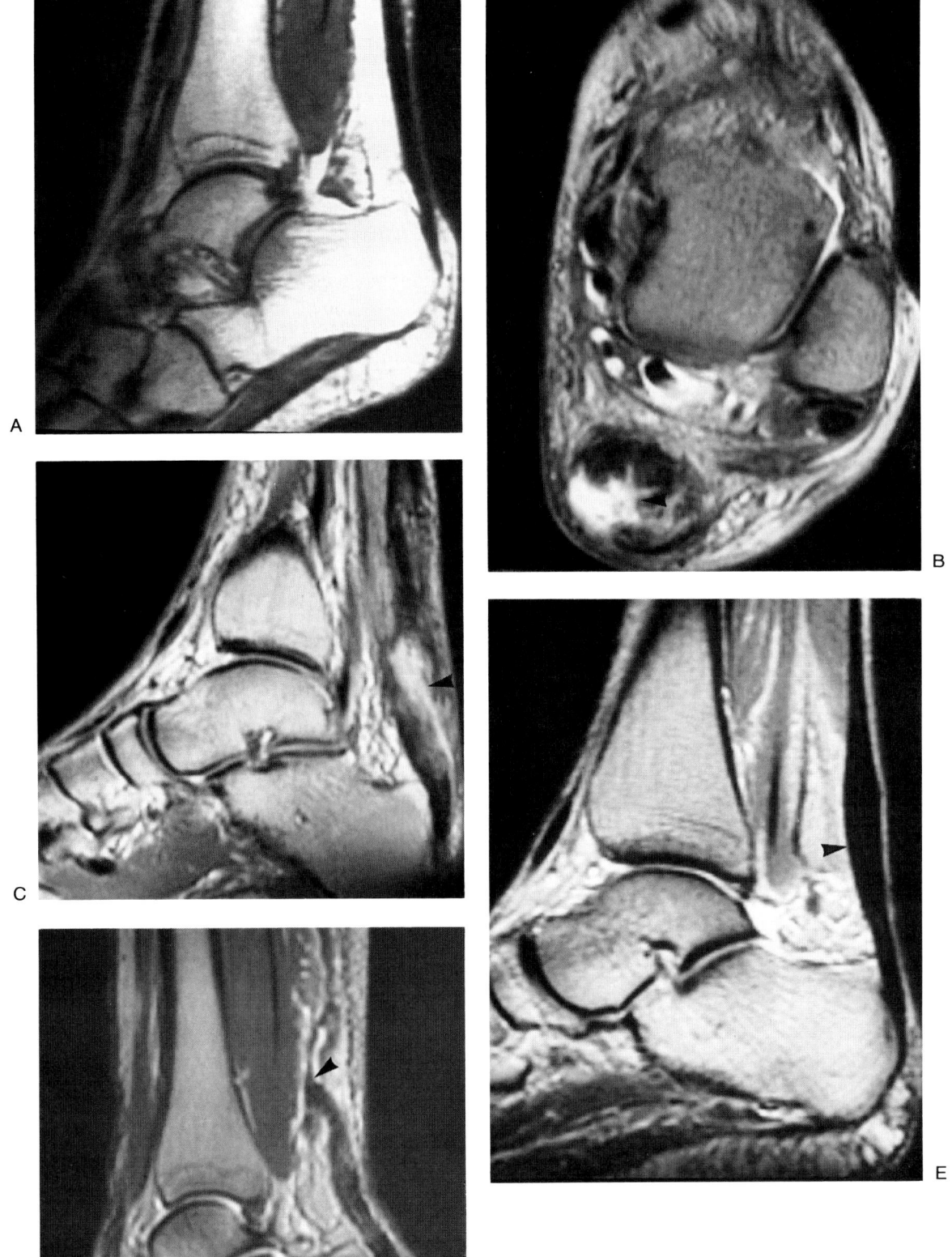

FIG. 9-62. Achilles tendon injuries: **A:** Normal sagittal SE 500/20 image of the Achilles tendon. **B,C:** Axial and sagittal SE 2000/60 images of a near complete tear (*arrows*). **D:** Sagittal SE 2000/60 image of a complete tear. **E:** Sagittal image of a thickened, healed tendon.

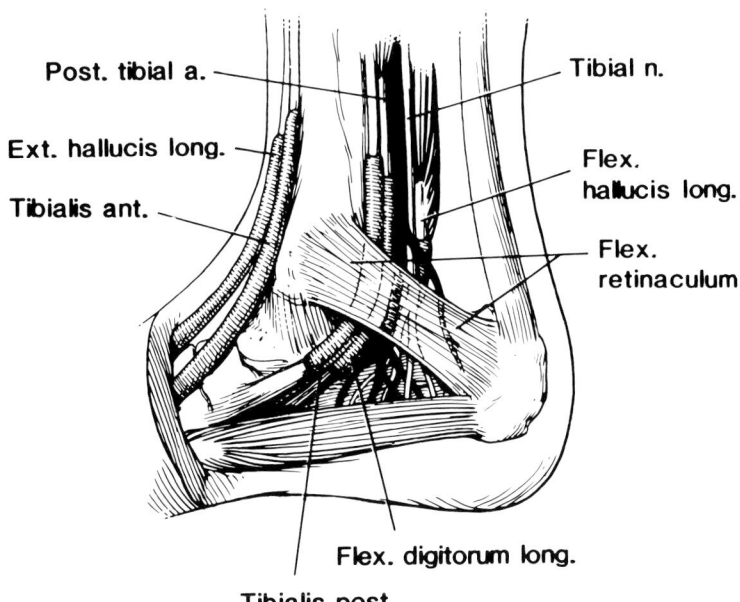

Post. tibial a.

Ext. hallucis long.

Tibialis ant.

Tibial n.

Flex. hallucis long.

Flex. retinaculum

Flex. digitorum long.

Tibialis post.

FIG. 9-63. Medial and anterior tendons and their relationships.

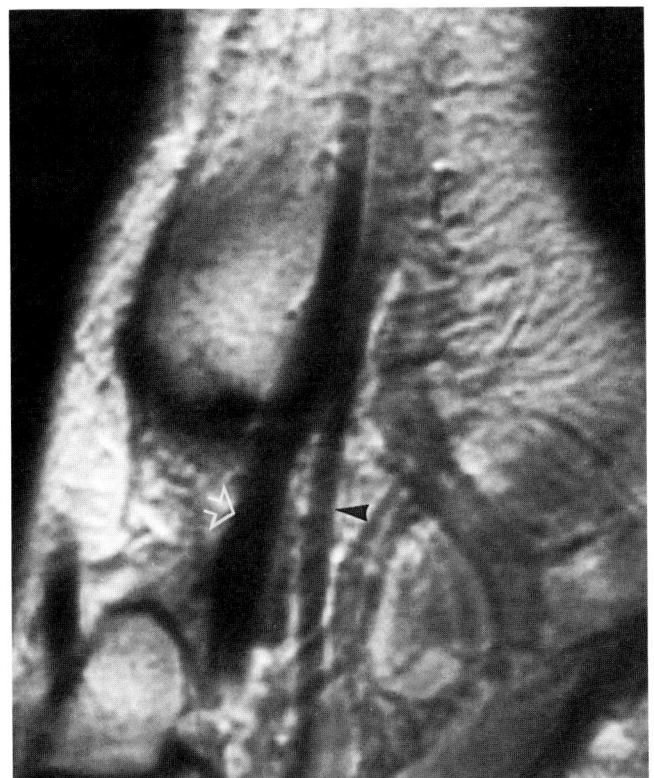

FIG. 9-64. Sagittal (TE 60, TR 2000) MR image showing normal low intensity signal in the posterior tibial (*open arrow*) and flexor digitorum longus tendons (*black arrow*).

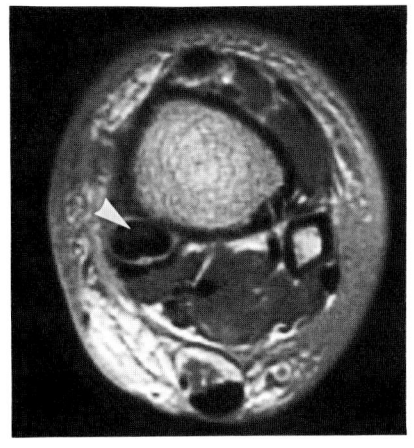 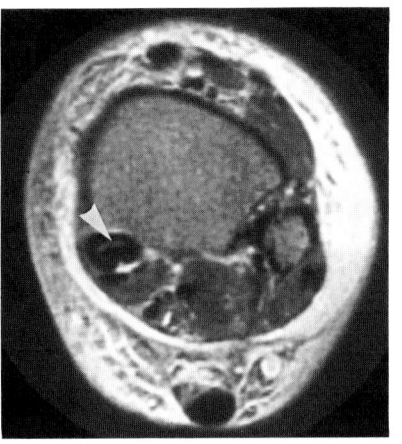 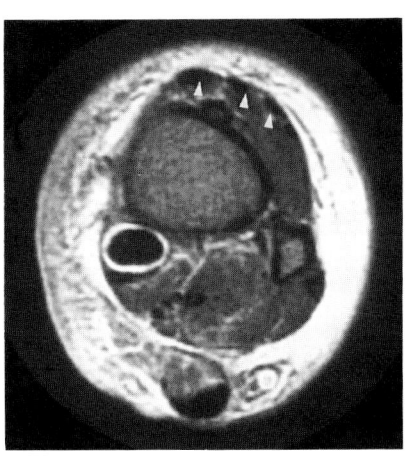

A   B   C

FIG. 9–65. Patient with medial ankle pain of indetermined etiology. Axial MR images (**A,B**) (TE 30, TR 2000) demonstrate a mid-substance tear, thickening of the tendon, and fluid on the tendon sheath (*arrow*). A more T2-weighted image (**C**) (TE 60, TR 2000) demonstrates the fluid more clearly. Note the absence of fluid around the other tendons (*small arrows*). Changes seen in the posterior tibial tendon would be compatable with Group III tear (11).

TABLE 9–4. *Ligament and tendon injuries*

	MRI features
Acute complete disruption	T_2 weighted (TE $\geq$ 60, TR2000) Tendon ends separated ↑ signal intensity between tendon ends and in sheaths Tendon ends may be thickened
Acute partial disruption	Tendon not separated ↑ signal for a portion of the width of the tendon ↑ signal in tendon sheath Tendon usually thickened in area of tear
Chronic disruption	Tendon thickened or separated and thickened Slightly increased intensity in area of tear ↑ signal in tendon sheath
Inflammation	↑ signal in tendon sheath Tendon may appear normal Thickened tendon or ligament with normal intensity (chronic)

(From 92.)

uals usually prefer surgical repair. Funk et al. (110) described the operative findings of posterior tibial tendon pathology. Group I tears were avulsions of the tendon insertion, Group II, mid-substance tears, Group III, partial tears with synovitis, and Group IV included patients with no tear but with synovitis. Mann and Thompson (122) reported results of posterior tibial tendon repair using the flexor digitorum longus tendon in 17 patients. Results were excellent in 13 of 17, fair in 3 of 17, and poor in one patient. In this patient an alternative procedure, arthrodesis was performed. Using their grading system, Funk et al. (110) found that surgical repair of Group I (avulsion at insertion) was not successful. Patients with mid-substance (Group II) tears had good results. Patients with incomplete tears had even better resolution of symptoms following surgery.

Anterior Tendons

Anteriorly, the anterior tibial, extensor hallucis longus, and extensor digitorum longus tendons are all enclosed in tendon sheaths. Acute tears are unusual but, in patients with previous fractures, degenerative arthritis or other predisposing factors, tendon rupture can occur (112,119). Injury to the anterior tibial tendon is not uncommon in runners. Rupture of the anterior tibial tendon usually occurs as it exits the superior retinaculum. The distal segment retracts and can be palpated between the superior and inferior retinaculum. Clinically there is pain and swelling over the ankle anteriorly. There may also be decreased dorsiflexion of the foot on physical examination.

Radiographically, patients will demonstrate minimal to prominent soft tissue swelling anteriorly. This is most easily identified on the lateral and oblique views. Tenography will demonstrate abnormalities in the tendon sheaths, but more specific information can be obtained with MRI. Examinations should be performed in the axial and sagittal planes. T2-weighted sequences are generally best because the high intensity of fluid and blood provides excellent contrast with the black tendon. Conservative treatment is adequate in older, less active patients. Surgical repair is indicated in active patients (119).

Miscellaneous Soft Tissue Injuries

Other soft tissue injuries have also been reported, especially in runners. These include plantar fascitis and compartment syndrome (90,97). Plantar fascitis occurs in up to 7% of runners. This is due to reaction at the plantar fascia insertion in the calcaneus.

Imaging of plantar fascitis can be accomplished early using three-phase technetium-99m scans or MRI performed in the sagittal plane. Later, spur formation may be evident on the lateral radiograph of the calcaneus.

Conservative treatment consists of anti-inflammatory medication, heel cord and plantar stretching exercises, and soft heel support. Rarely, surgical release or bone spur excision is required (90).

Foreign bodies in the soft tissues of the foot deserve brief mention. Opaque materials such as metal or leaded glass can be identified radiographically (130,140). In certain cases, soft tissue techniques and xerography can be used to localize non-opaque glass and wooden foreign bodies. When significant swelling is present and no foreign body is identified radiographically but there is strong clinical evidence, further studies may be needed. We have, on occasion, identified small (<5 mm) foreign bodies using MRI. MRI provides multiple image planes to clearly define the location. The foreign body is seen as a small area of no signal corresponding to the shape of the foreign body. Obviously ferromagnetic foreign bodies should not be sought with MRI. These materials are evident on routine radiographs.

FRACTURES

Management of foot and ankle fractures is a common problem for orthopedic surgeons, emergency room physicians, family practice physicians, and radiologists. Imaging plays an important role in assessing the degree of bone and soft tissue injury and in following the healing process.

The detection of most fractures is not difficult. However, detection of subtle fractures and evaluating the extent of soft tissue injury may be more difficult. Thus, it is essential for those interpreting images to be aware of the manner in which various fractures and soft tissue injuries present so the images can be correctly and thoroughly evaluated. Soft tissue changes may be the only clue to a subtle fracture or ligament rupture. Soft tissue swelling, obliteration of the fat planes or pre-Achilles fat triangle, and the presence of an effusion can be very useful in identifying the location of subtle fractures (see Fig. 9-25C) (158,161).

It is also important that one understand the clinical significance of certain fracture patterns. A systematic approach should be used when describing the imaging features of a fracture or fracture dislocation so that the injury is completely assessed (157,158). Eponyms are commonly used to describe fractures in the foot and ankle (Table 9-5). However, eponyms can be confusing and should not be used without describing the associated fractures and soft tissue injury. Articular involvement, including the degree of separation or articular irregularity and the percent of the articular surface involved should be described.

Discussion of specific foot and ankle fractures and fracture dislocations is most easily accomplished by us-

TABLE 9–5. *Fractures of the foot and ankle*

Eponym or descriptive term	Definition
Aviators astragalus	Fractures and fracture-dislocations of the talus (99) (Fig. 9-66).
Bosworth's fracture	Fracture of the distal fibula with locking of the proximal fibular fragment behind the tibia (144,151,156).
Chopart's fracture-dislocation	Injury involving the mid tarsal (talo-navicular and calcaneocuboid) joints (159) (Fig. 9-67).
Cotton's fracture	Tri-malleolar fracture with the posterior tibial fragment posteriorly and superiorly displaced. Medial malleolar fracture line continuing posteriorly and separating the posterior tibia. Usually fibular fracture above the joint level. Certain physicians refer to the posterior tibial fracture as Cotton's fracture (145–148,152,159) (Fig. 9-68).
Dupuytren's fracture 　High	Fracture of the fibular shaft above the ankle with rupture of the interosseous membrane and distal tibiofibular ligaments. Lateral talar shift with medial malleolar fracture or deltoid ligament tear (152,161) (Fig. 9-69A).
Low	Fracture of the fibula near the ankle joint with rupture of the anterior tibiofibular ligament or anterior tibial avulsion and medial malleolar fracture or deltoid ligament rupture (161). (Fig. 9-69B).
Gosselin's fracture	*V*-shaped fracture of the distal tibia that may enter the tibial plafond (159,161) (Fig. 9-70).
Greenstick fracture	Incomplete fracture involving one cortex with angulation and bowing (159).
Jone's fracture	Fracture of the fifth metatarsal about .75 inch distal to the tuberosity (148–150,152,159) (Fig. 9-71).
Le Fort's fracture	Vertical fracture of the anteromedial distal due to anterior tibiofibular ligament avulsion (159) (Fig. 9-72).
Lisfranc's fracture-dislocation	Any of a variety of fracture-dislocations of the tarso-metatarsal joints (159) (Fig. 9-73).
Maisonneuve's fracture	Fracture of the proximal fibula near the head with rupture of the interosseous membrane and distal tibiofibular syndesmosis. There is usually an associated deltoid ligament tear or medial malleolar fracture (152,159) (Fig. 9-74).
March fracture	Stress fracture of the metatarsal commonly seen in military recruits (159) (Fig. 9-75).
Pilon fracture	Comminuted fracture of the tibial plafond (147,153).
Pott's fracture	Fracture of the fibula 2–3 inches above the ankle with rupture of the deltoid ligament (or avulsion of the medial malleolus) and tibiofibular syndesmosis (150,160) (Fig. 9-76).
Shepherd's fracture	Fracture of the lateral tubercle of the posterior talar process. May be confused with os trigonum (150,159) (Fig. 9–77)
Tillaux's fracture	Fracture of the distal lateral tibial articular surface. May involve anterior or posterior tubercle. Usually triad of (1) deltoid rupture or medial malleolar avulsion; (2) fibular fracture 5–6 cm above the ankle joint, and (3) avulsion of tibial tubercles with diastasis of syndesmosis. (150,159) (Fig. 9-78).

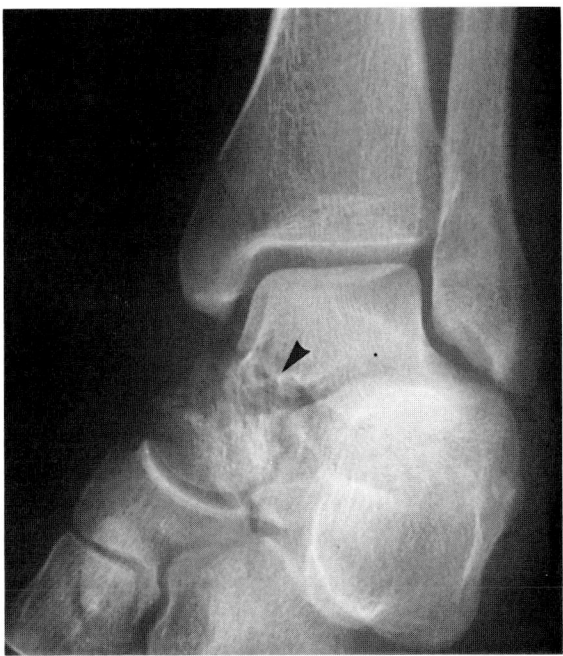

FIG. 9-66. Mortise view of the ankle demonstrating a comminuted talar fracture (*arrow*).

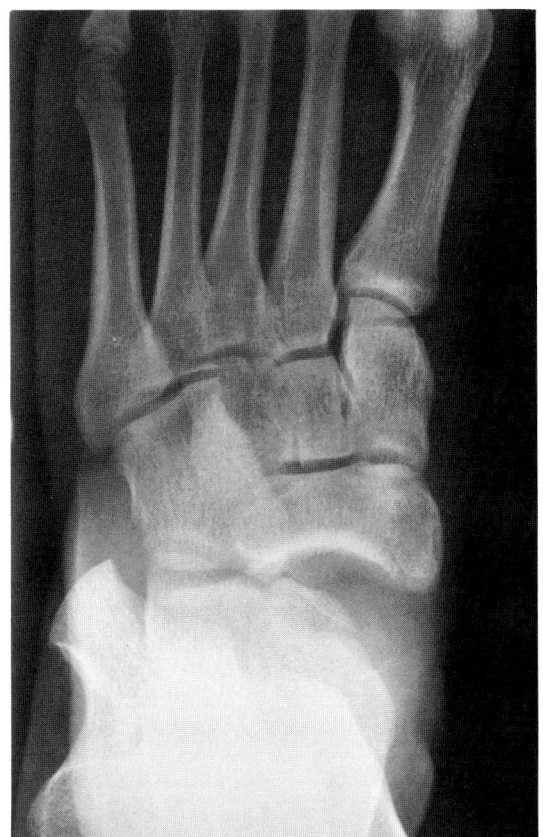

FIG. 9-67. AP view of the foot demonstrating a fracture-dislocation of the talonavicular joint.

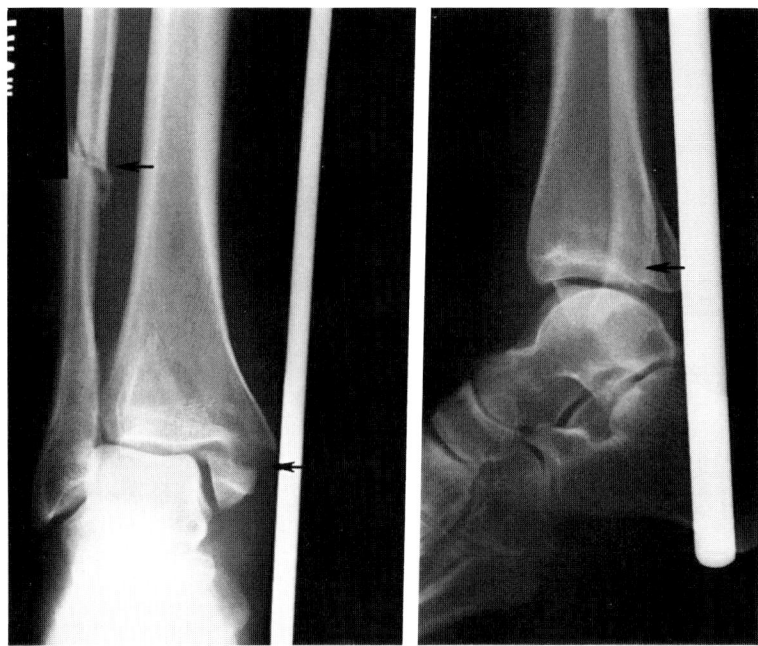

FIG. 9-68. Cotton's fracture. AP and lateral views demonstrate a medial malleolar fracture with posterior extension and displacement of the posterior tibial fragment (*lower arrows*). Note the high fibular fracture (*upper arrow*).

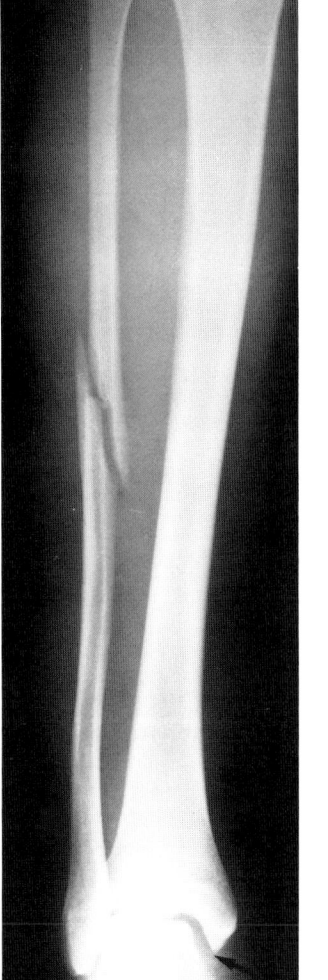

A

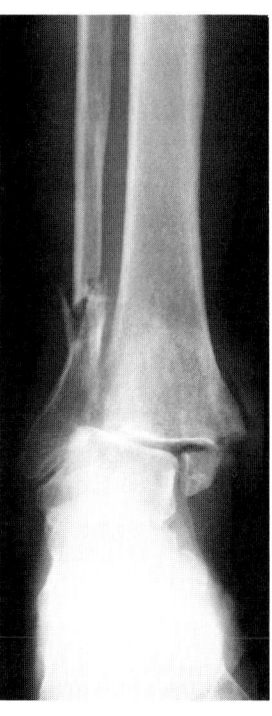

B

FIG. 9-69. A: High and (**B**) low Dupuytren's fractures. Note the higher fibular fracture and talar shift (*arrow*) due to deltoid ligament rupture in the high (**A**) Dupuytren's fracture.

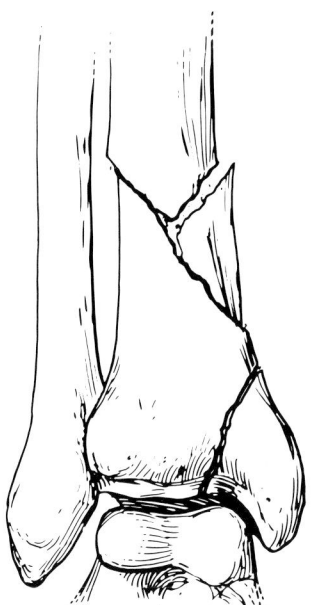

FIG. 9-70. Gosselin's fracture.

ing anatomic regions. Therefore, the ankle, hindfoot, midfoot and forefoot injuries will be discussed separately. Both adult and pediatric disorders will be discussed.

Ankle Fractures

Ankle fractures may be simple or complex with associated ligament rupture. The latter is more common in adults. Generally, fractures in patients over 15–16 years of age are classified and treated using adult criteria.

Complete evaluation of ankle fractures in adults in-

cludes assessment of the fracture fragments and accurate description of associated ligament injuries. Bone and soft tissue involvement is important in determining the mechanism of injury, which in turn has significant treatment implications (162,163,167,203,206).

When evaluating ankle fractures, one commonly considers the bones and ligaments as a "ring-like" structure in the coronal plane (Fig. 9-79). This concept has been popularized by Neer and other authors (168,189,192). The ring is made up of the medial malleolus, tibial plafond, distal tibiofibular ligaments and syndesmosis, lateral malleolus, lateral ligaments, talus and medial ligaments (168,189,192). Breaks in the ring commonly occur at five sites either alone or in combination. Shift of the talus indicates disruption of the ring at more than one site. The five common sites of injury include: (1) lateral malleolus, (2) lateral ligaments, (3) deltoid ligaments, (4) medial malleolus, and (5) syndesmosis (189). Fractures of the tibial plafond occur after axial loading with varying degrees of plantar flexion (167,187,189).

Clinical Features

Following ankle injury, patients generally present with varying degrees of pain, swelling, and ecchymosis depending to some degree on the significance of the injury. The incidence of swelling and the presence of ecchymosis is somewhat higher when fractures are present, but this is not a reliable clinical finding. With incomplete injuries and stable fractures (single break in the "ring") weight bearing is usually still possible. Weight bearing is more difficult or impossible with unstable fractures (167,187,189).

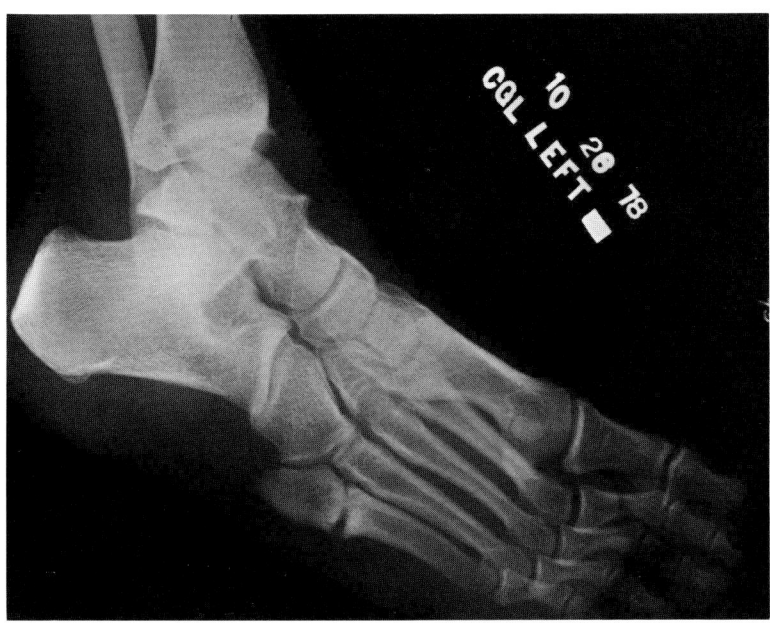

FIG. 9-71. Oblique view of the foot demonstrating a Jone's fracture.

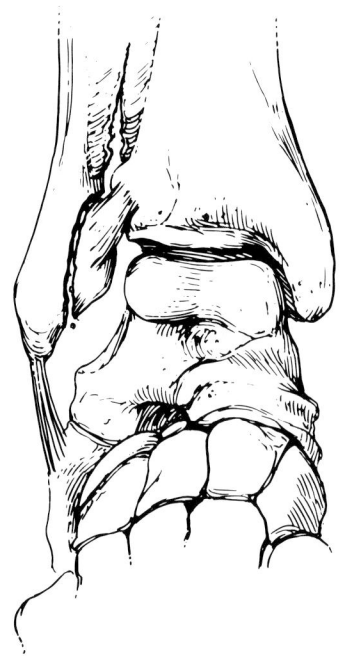

FIG. 9–72. LeFort's fracture.

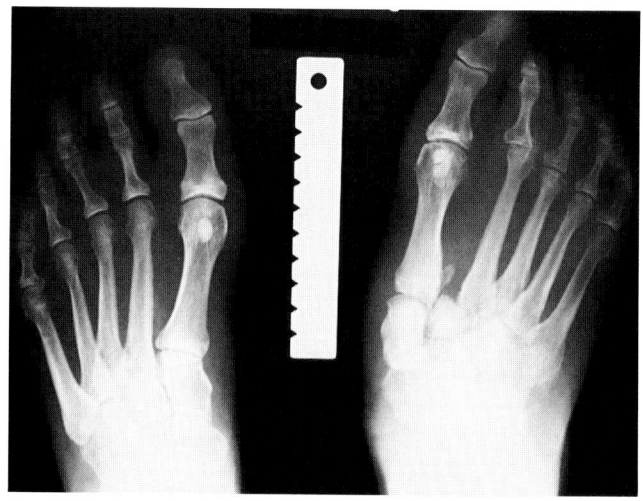

FIG. 9–73. AP views of the normal left foot and Lisfranc fracture-dislocation on the right. Note the wide space between the bases of the right first and second metatarsals. There are also fractures of the second and third metatarsal heads with dislocation of the second MTP joint.

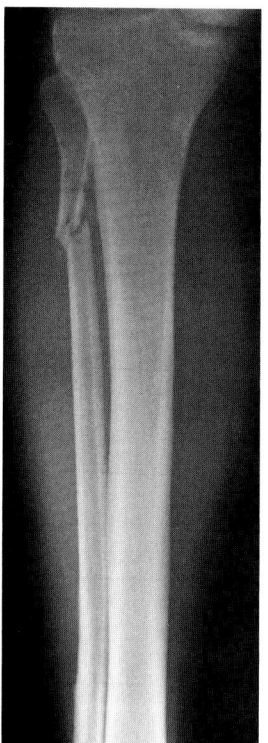
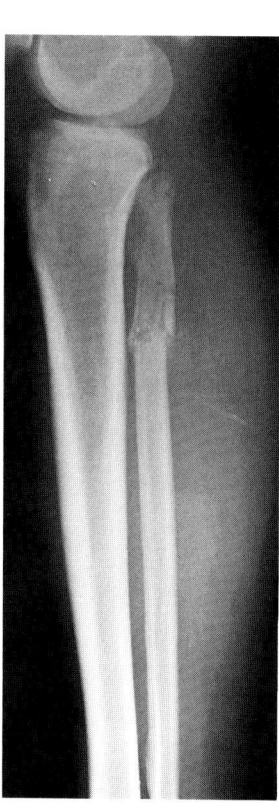
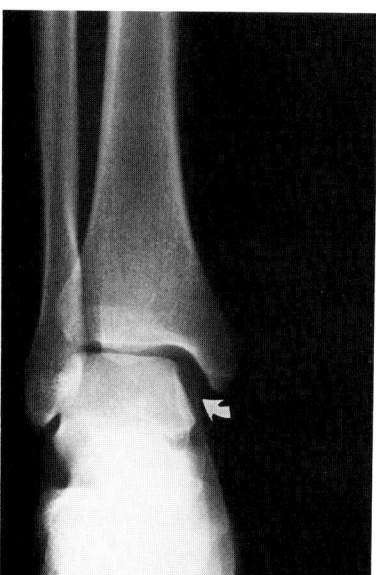
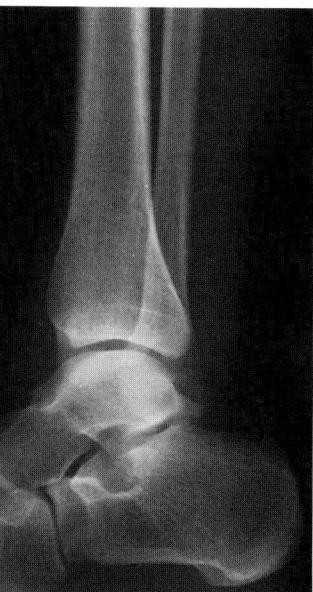

FIG. 9–74. Maisonneuve's type fracture with a fracture just below the fibular head (**A**) and rupture of the deltoid ligament (**B**) (*arrow*).

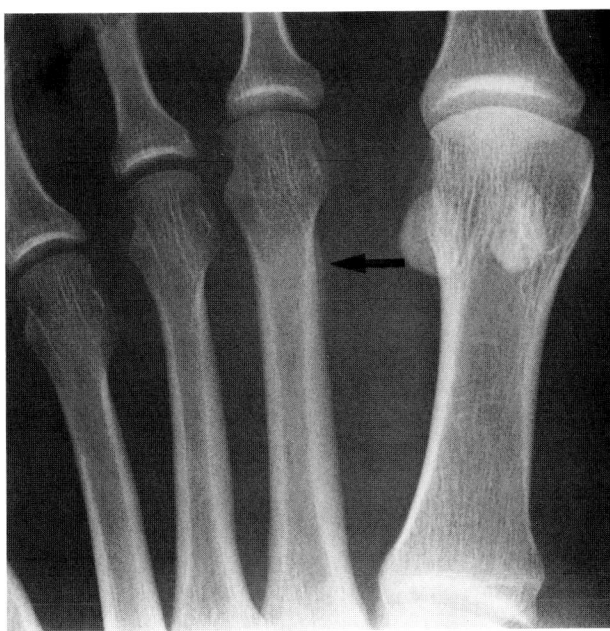

FIG. 9–75. Stress fracture (*arrow*) of the distal second metatarsal with callus formation.

Classification

Most ankle fractures occur as a result of inversion or eversion forces (165,171). However, the mechanism of injury is rarely pure. Most often abduction, adduction, lateral rotation, or axial loading occur in addition to eversion or inversion (164,165,167,171,175,176).

The value of classifications for ankle fractures is the

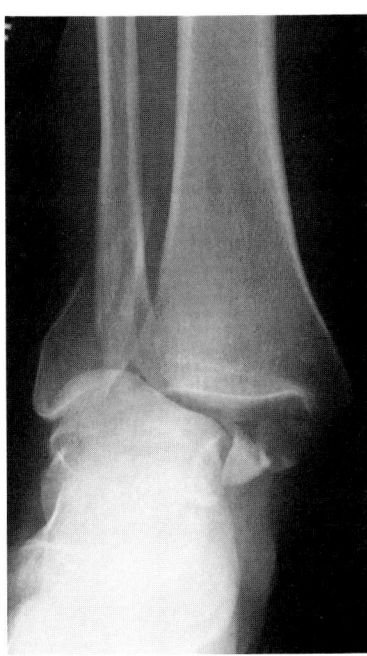

FIG. 9–76. Pott's fracture of the right ankle. Bimalleolar fracture with lateral talar displacement (pronation-abduction).

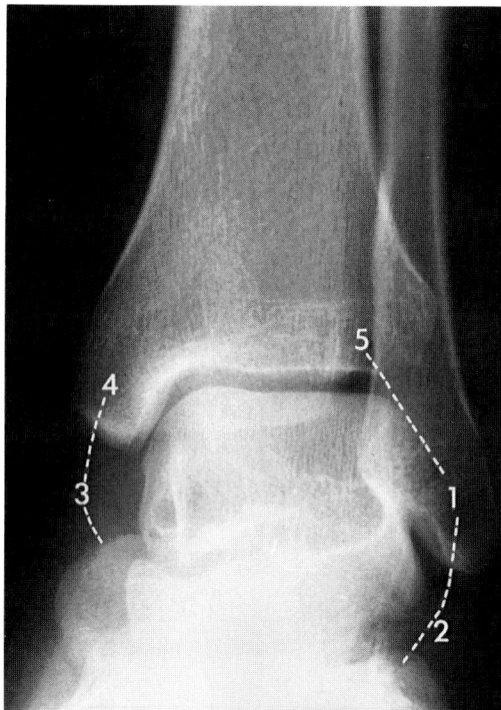

FIG. 9–79. AP radiograph demonstrating the ring concept created by bones and ligaments of the ankle. Common breaks in the ring are (1) lateral malleolus, (2) lateral ligaments, (3) medial ligaments, (4) medial malleolus, and (5) syndesmosis (from 165, with permission.)

cation did not include the ligament injuries associated with fractures and was limited to describing the fracture mechanism as due to a single force. The majority of fractures are due to force vectors from more than one direction (165,186,189).

The more commonly employed classifications are those proposed by Lauge-Hansen (186) and Weber (205). The former is very accurate in predicting the mech-

anism of injury and extent of ligament involvement. Therefore, it is recommended to radiologists so that the description of the injury can be most accurate. The Weber classification is not as complex but is frequently used because of its value in planning appropriate therapy (178,189).

Lauge-Hansen

The Lauge-Hansen classification was devised using cadaver specimens. It is based on the position of the foot at the time of injury (first word) and the direction of the injuring force (second word) (162,181). Using this system, four basic categories of injury are described. The classification considers different levels of injury in each category based upon the degree and length of time the force is applied (Table 9-6).

Supination-adduction injuries (inversion) (Fig. 9-80) cause traction on the lateral ligaments resulting in either a ligament tear or an avulsion fracture of the lateral malleolus (Stage I). The fracture is generally transverse and below the joint level (Fig. 9-81) (162,182,189). If the force is sufficient, the talus can impact against the medial malleolus (Stage II) (Table 9-6). If an oblique fracture of the medial malleolus is evident but no fracture is seen in the lateral malleolus, one can assume that the lateral ligaments are disrupted. This has to be the case if the talus is shifted (two breaks in the ring). Supination-adduction injuries account for 18–21% of ankle fractures fitting the Lauge-Hansen classification (214,215).

Supination-lateral rotation injuries cause medial tension with the talus causing posterior displacement of the lateral malleolus (162). This causes disruption of the anterior distal tibiofibular ligament (Stage I) (Figs. 9-82 and 9-83). As the force continues, a spiral fracture of the lateral malleolus occurs at or just above the tibiotalar joint.

TABLE 9-6. *Lauge-Hansen classification*[a]

Pronation-abduction
  Stage I. Ruptured deltoid ligament or transverse medial malleolar fracture.
  Stage II. Disruption of the distal tibiofibular ligaments (anterior and posterior).
  Stage III. [b]Oblique fibular fracture at the joint level (best seen on AP view).
Pronation-lateral rotation
  Stage I. Rupture of the deltoid ligament or transverse medial malleolar fracture.
  Stage II. Disruption of the anterior tibiofibular ligament and interosseous membrane.
  Stage III. [b]Fibular fracture above the joint space (usually 6 cm or more above the joint line).
  Stage IV. Posterior tibial chip fracture or rupture of posterior tibiofibular ligament.
Supination-adduction
  Stage I. Lateral ligament injury or [b]transverse lateral malleolar fracture below the ankle joint.
  Stage II. Steep oblique fracture of the medial malleolus.
Supination-lateral rotation
  Stage I. Disruption of the anterior tibiofibular ligament.
  Stage II. [b]Spiral fracture of the distal fibula near the joint (best seen on the lateral view).
  Stage III. Rupture of the posterior tibiofibular ligament.
  Stage IV. Transverse fracture of the medial malleolus.

[a] (162,181)
[b] Fibular fracture appearance is key to determining mechanism of injury.

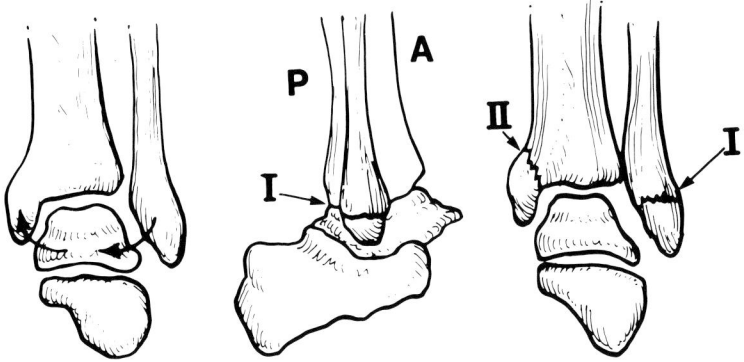

FIG. 9–80. Supination-adduction injury. Stage I fracture of the lateral malleolus or ligament injury. Stage II oblique medial malleolar fracture (from 28). (P, posterior; A, anterior.)

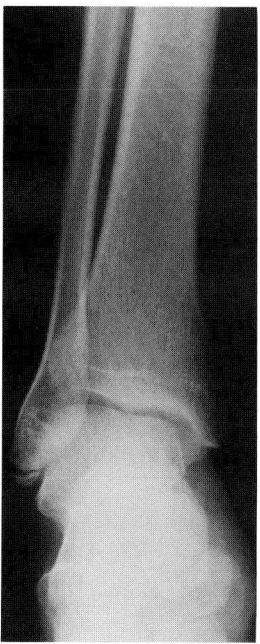
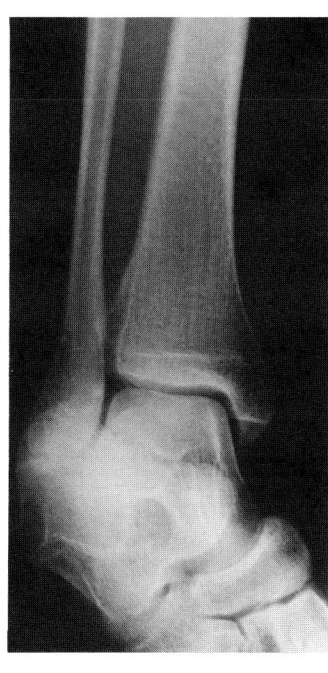

A   B

FIG. 9–81. AP (**A**) and mortise views (**B**) of the ankle demonstrating a Lauge-Hansen supination-adduction Stage I with a transverse avulsion fracture of the lateral malleolus. There is no medial malleolar fracture.

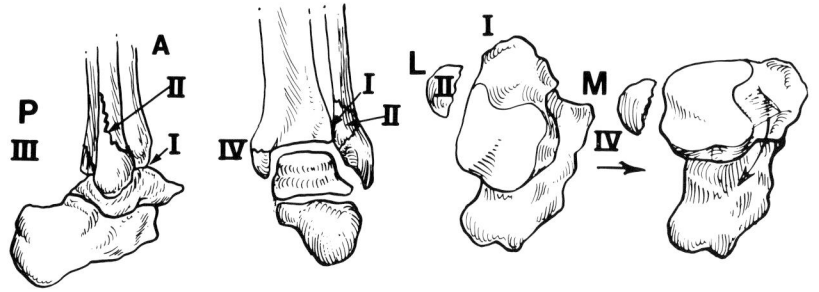

FIG. 9–82. Lauge-Hansen supination-lateral rotation injuries. Stage I, disruption of the distal tibiofibular ligaments. Stage II, an oblique fibular fracture seen best on the lateral view. Stage III posterior tibial fracture. Stage IV, a transverse medial malleolar fracture (from 28).

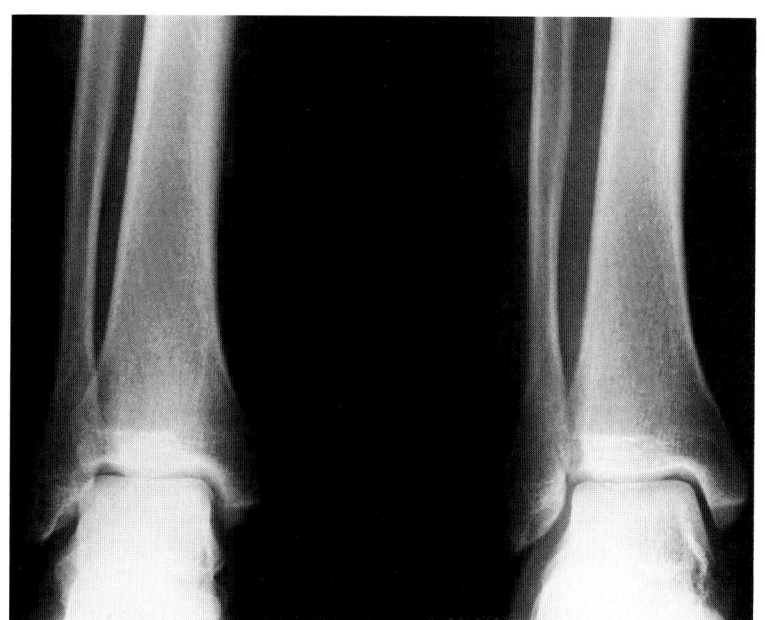

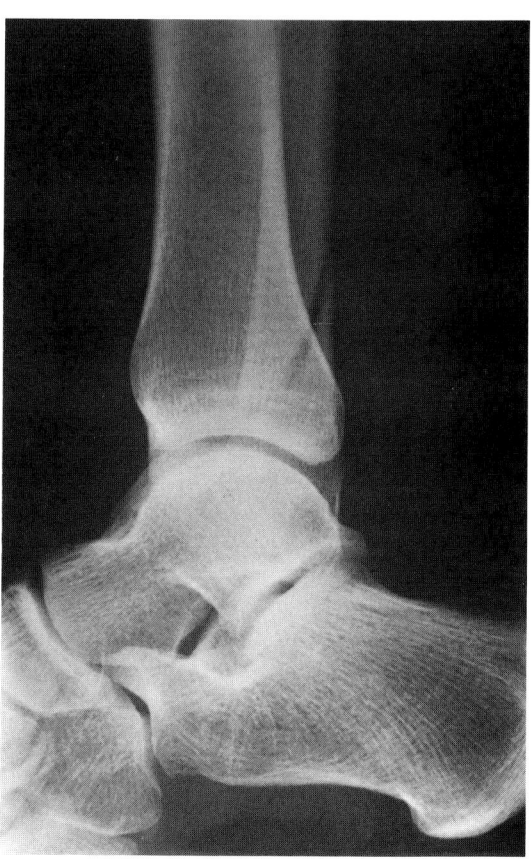

FIG. 9–83. AP and mortise views (**A**) are normal. The lateral view (**B**) clearly demonstrates an oblique fracture due to a supination-lateral rotation Stage II injury.

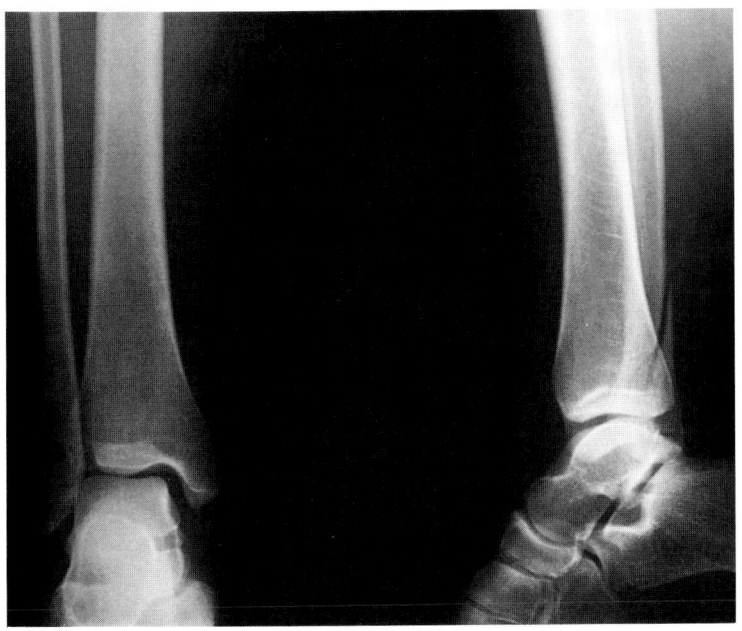

FIG. 9–84. Stage IV supination-lateral rotation injury. The fibular fracture is seen best on the lateral view. This is the key to the mechanism of injury. The medial joint space is increased due to deltoid ligament rupture.

This fracture is seen best on the lateral view (Fig. 9-82). This Stage II injury is the most common ankle fracture (162,214,215). When the force and talar rotation continue, a small posterior malleolar fracture will occur (Stage III) and, if the force continues, an avulsion fracture of the medial malleolus or rupture of the deltoid ligament occurs (Stage IV) (Fig. 9-84). Supination-lateral rotation injuries account for 55–58% of ankle fractures (215).

Pronation-abduction injuries (eversion) result in abduction of the talus in the ankle mortise placing tension on the medial structures. This leads to a transverse avulsion fracture of the medial malleolus or rupture of the deltoid ligament (Stage I) (Fig. 9-85). With continued force, the anterior and posterior distal tibiofibular ligaments are torn or avulsion fractures of the anterior and posterior tibial attachments occur (Stage II) (Fig. 9-86). With further force, an oblique fibular fracture develops at or just above the tibiotalar joint (162,176,181). This fracture is best seen on the AP view (Fig. 9-86), which

differentiates it from the spiral fracture seen with supination-lateral rotation injuries. The latter is seen best on the lateral view (100). When an oblique lateral malleolar fracture is noted on the AP view, one should assume the tibiofibular ligaments and deltoid ligaments are ruptured even though no obvious talar shift may be noted (162). Stress views may be needed to confirm this finding.

Pronation-lateral rotation injuries cause medial tension as the talus rotates laterally (Fig. 9-87). Initially, the medial ligaments rupture or an avulsion fracture of the medial malleolus occurs (Stage I). As the force continues, the injury progresses clockwise around the ankle in the axial plane. The anterior distal tibiofibular ligament and interosseous membrane rupture (Stage II), followed by a fibular fracture. This fracture (Stage III) is typical in that it occurs well above the joint space (≥5–6 cm), which allows differentiation of this injury from the others on the basis of the radiograph (Fig. 9-88). When the force continues, the posterior distal tibiofibular liga-

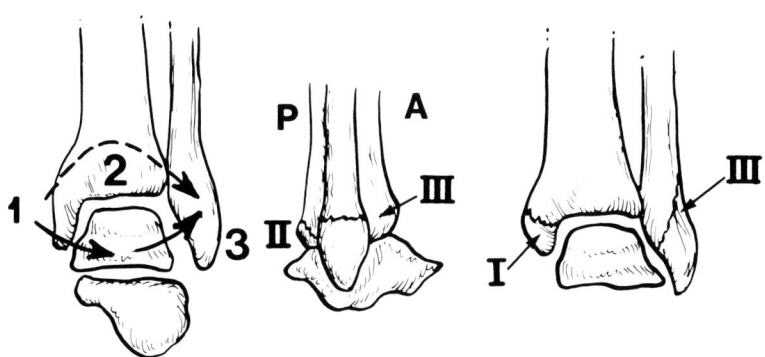

FIG. 9–85. Pronation-abduction injury. Stage I, transverse medial malleolar fracture below the joint level. Stage II, tibiofibular ligament rupture. Stage III, oblique lateral malleolar fracture best seen on the AP view (from 28).

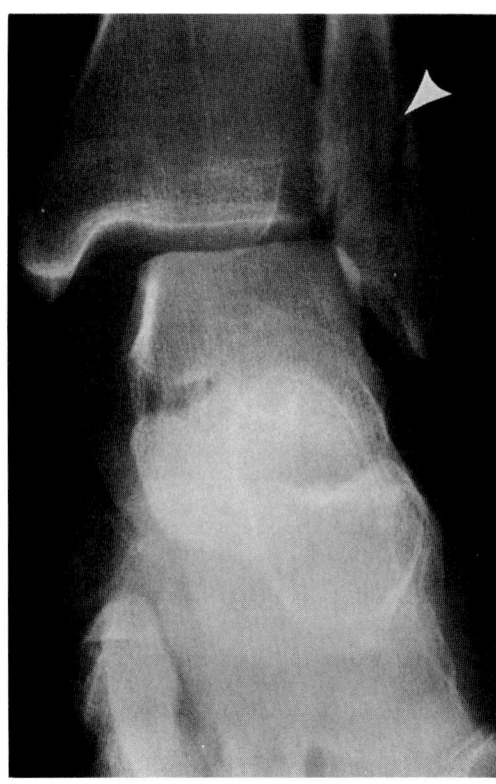

FIG. 9-86. AP view demonstrating a Stage III pronation abduction injury with widening of the medial ankle mortise due to ligament rupture and an oblique lateral malleolar fracture at the joint level (*arrow*).

ment ruptures or a posterior tibial avulsion fracture is noted (Stage IV) (Fig. 9-88). Pronation injuries (abduction lateral rotation) account for about 20% of ankle fractures (215).

In his original series, Lauge-Hansen found that 75% of injuries were either supination-adduction or supination-lateral rotation injuries (181). The classification is accurate in detection of fracture and ligament components of ankle injuries in 90–95% of cases (162). There are exceptions, most notably, fractures of the tibial plafond due to axial loading or plantar flexion injuries. However, the characteristic appearance of the fibular fracture and orderly progression of the injuries make this classification ideal for radiologists. Accurate reporting of ankle injuries is greatly facilitated (162,165,189,213).

The Weber classification is commonly used by orthopedic surgeons (162,165,189,213). This classification is much simpler using the level of fibular fracture in predicting the degree of syndesmosis injury and mortise displacement (178,189,196).

Type A injuries cause fractures below the tibiotalar joint and do not involve the syndesmosis (similar to Lauge-Hansen supination-adduction) (162,181). Type B fractures occur at the joint level producing an oblique fibular fracture (similar to Lauge-Hansen pronation-abduction), which is seen best on the AP view (Fig. 9-86) (178,189). Two categories of Type C fractures are described. Type C1 is an oblique fibular fracture above the level of the distal tibiofibular ligaments. Type C2 lesions present with higher fibular fractures and therefore more

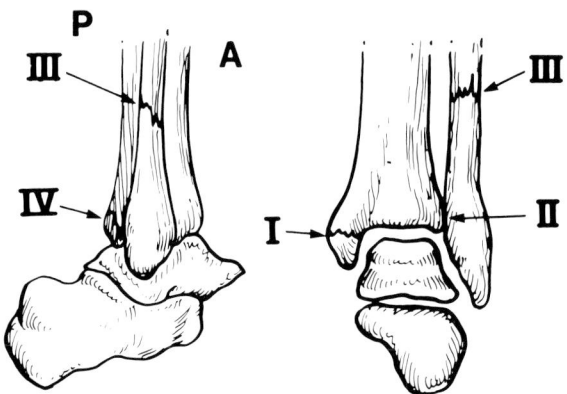

FIG. 9-87. Pronation-lateral rotation injuries. Stage I, transverse fracture of the medial malleolus. Stage II, rupture of the distal tibiofibular ligaments. Stage III, high fibular fracture. Stage IV, posterior tibial fracture (from 28).

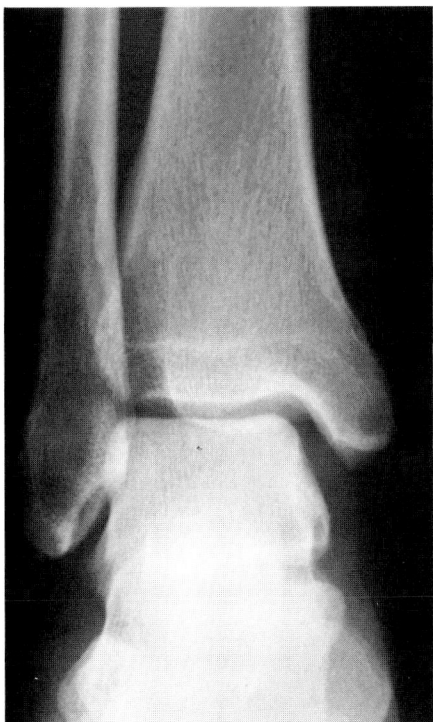
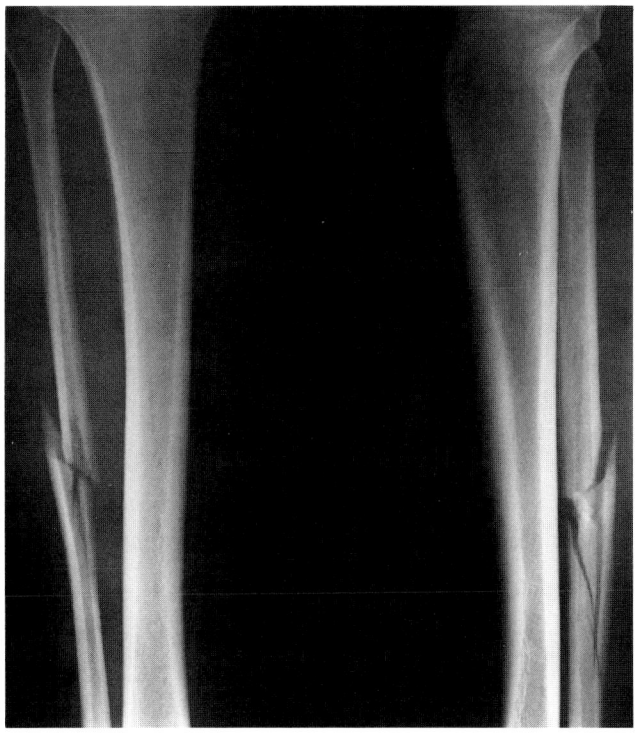

A   B

FIG. 9–88. Stage III pronation-lateral rotation injury. The AP (**A**) ankle view shows widening of the distal tibiofibular space and medial joint space. Fibular fractures may not be seen on routine ankle views. It is important to include the entire fibula (**B**) to properly identify the mechanism of injury. Note the high fibular fracture, the key to correctly identifying the mechanism of injury.

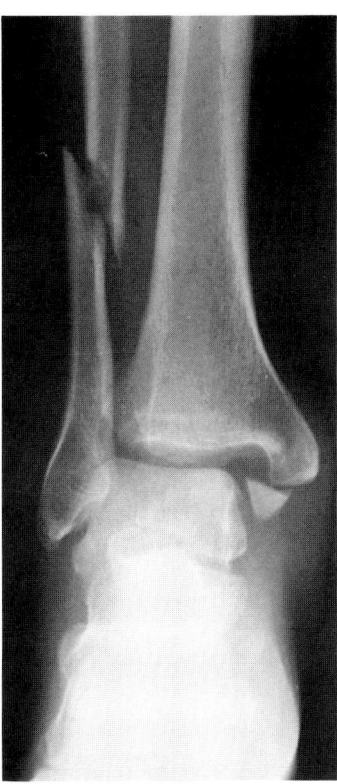

FIG. 9–89. Weber Type C2 fracture with a high fibular fracture and marked syndesmosis involvement (Lauge-Hansen pronation-lateral rotation, Stage III).

extensive rupture of the syndesmosis (Fig. 9-89). Treatment of Type A injuries can usually be accomplished closed, while Types B and C injuries usually require internal fixation. The Weber classification is useful for treatment purposes but is not as useful in understanding the mechanism of injury and ligament involvement as the Lauge-Hansen system (181,189).

Fractures of the tibial plafond do not fit neatly into either of the above classifications. Most occur in patients less than 50 years of age (77%) (186,194). These injuries, although uncommon, are very difficult to manage (182,183,189,198). Fractures are due to axial loading and generally occur in association with falling from a significant height or during motor vehicle accidents when the foot becomes trapped against the floor (165,183,189). Fractures usually extend up the tibial shaft in an oblique or spiral manner. Severe comminution with multiple articular fragments (pilon fracture) is common (194). Twenty percent of plafond fractures are open (194). Ovadia (194) classified plafond fractures based on radiographic evidence of displacement and metaphyseal and articular involvement (Fig. 9-90). Type I fractures are nondisplaced. Type II fractures showed minimal displacement. Type III fractures have articular surface displacement with several large bone fragments. Types IV and V fractures have comminuted articular components with displacement of the articular frag-

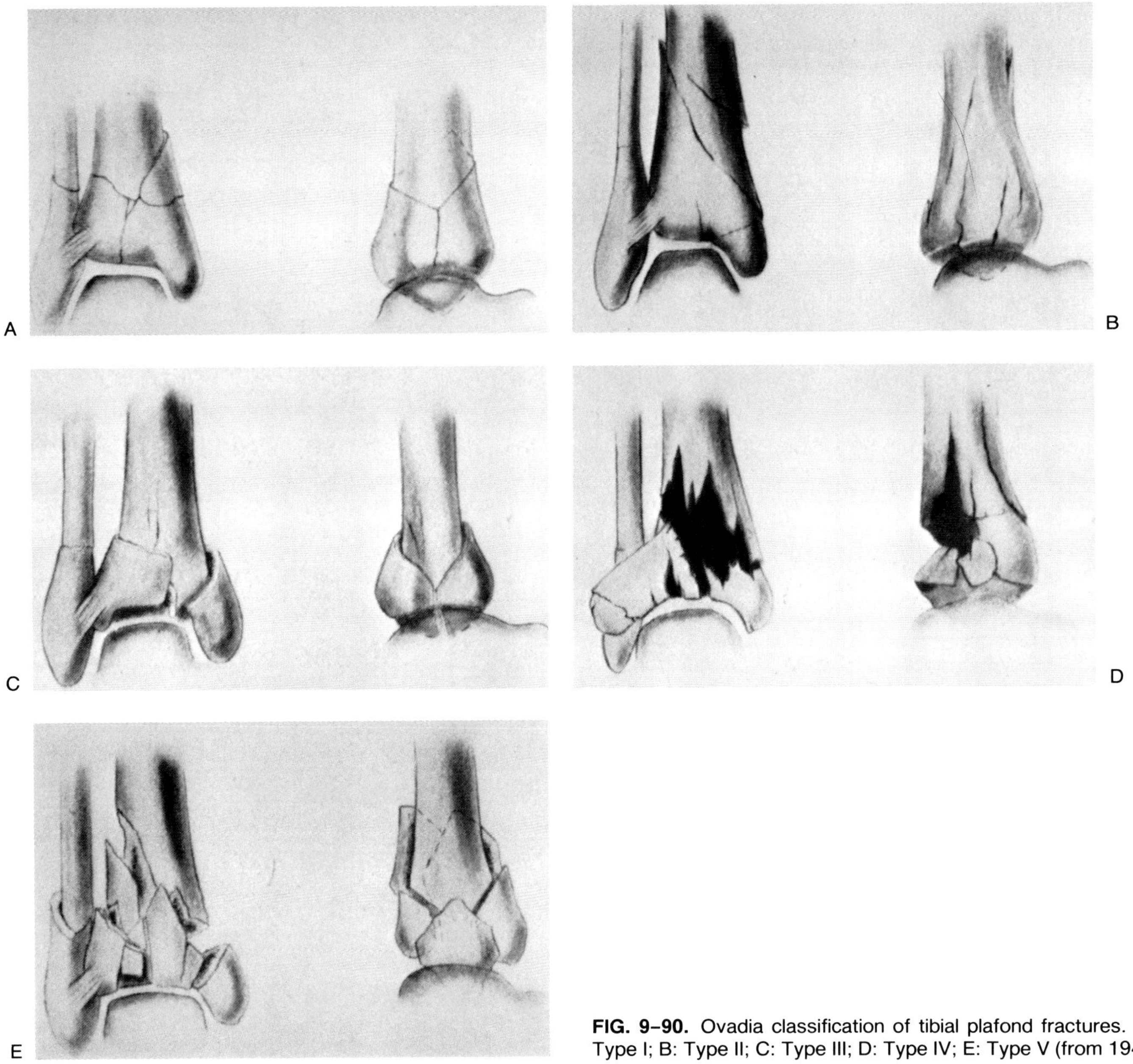

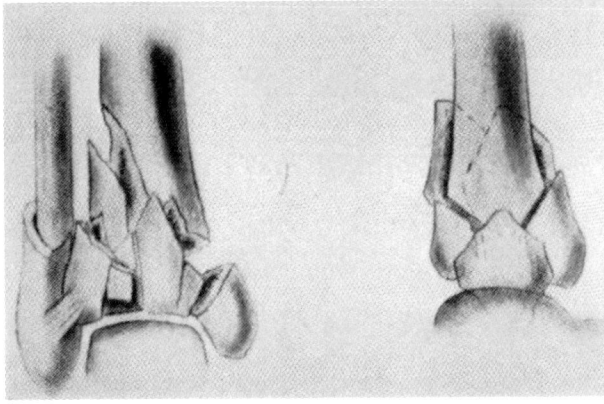

A

B

C

D

E

FIG. 9-90. Ovadia classification of tibial plafond fractures. A: Type I; B: Type II; C: Type III; D: Type IV; E: Type V (from 194).

ments. Fibular fractures were not considered in this classification. Types I and II fractures are usually due to less severe trauma. Internal fixation is required for Types III–V fractures (194).

Radiographic Evaluation

AP, lateral, and mortise views are performed in all patients with suspected ankle fractures. We also routinely obtain the external oblique view. In most cases, these views provide sufficient information regarding the degree of bone and soft tissue involvement (165,171,176,189). This is especially true in patients with fractures that fit the Lauge-Hansen classification

(>95%). It is also essential to include the entire tibia and fibula when studying patients with ankle fractures. The fibular fracture, which is key to classifying the injury, may be just below the fibular head (162,189). The AP view is useful in evaluating soft tissue swelling that may lead the interpreter to a subtle fracture. The oblique fracture of the fibula (pronation-abduction Stage III) is best seen on the AP view. Avulsion fractures of the tibia and fibula can also be seen on this view (171,176,183,189).

The mortise view (foot internally rotated 15°–20°) is critical for evaluating the position of the talus and the syndesmosis. The space between the talar margin and the medial malleolus, plafond, and lateral malleolus should be equal (189). The distance between the distal tibia and fibula should not exceed 4.5 mm (172,184). Talar asymmetry indicates the presence of two injuries: either two ligaments, two fractures, or a combination of fracture and ligament rupture (189,192,213–215).

The lateral view is most useful for detecting anterior and posterior tibial chip or avulsion fractures (Fig. 9-91). In addition, the fibular fracture seen with supination-lateral rotation Stage II injuries is best seen on the lateral view (162). The presence of an ankle effusion or Achilles tendon injury (obliteration of the pre-Achilles fat triangle) is also most easily noted on the lateral view.

We routinely obtain a 45° external oblique view in addition to the above views. This will provide added information, especially when subtle posterior tibial fractures are present. Because of the frequency of associated fractures in the foot and foot fractures that may mimic ankle injury, it may also be wise to obtain routine (AP, lateral, oblique) views of the foot in patients presenting with ankle injury.

Occasionally special studies are needed prior to planning conservative (closed) or operative therapy. Tomography (AP and lateral projections) is useful in evaluating the degree of articular involvement in complex plafond fractures and may also be necessary to exclude articular involvement. The position of fragments, especially articular fragments, can be better demonstrated using thin (1.5–3 mm)-slice CT. This technique offers the capability of three-dimensional reconstruction, which can be useful in planning surgical approaches for complex fractures (165,170,189).

Treatment

The goals of treatment should be accurate anatomic reduction and a parallel articular surface. Early motion is also essential to prevent range of motion loss (204). Decisions regarding open or closed reduction can be based upon the type of fracture (single vs. bi- or trimalleolar) and degree of displacement (173,189,200).

Fractures of the medial or lateral malleolus without a second fracture or ligament injury may be treated conservatively if displacement does not exceed 2 mm (168,189). Immobilization with a cast for six weeks is generally adequate. If the fracture is displaced more than 2 mm, internal fixation is indicated. The medial malleolus can usually be reduced with a single screw; fibular fractures may require multiple screws, plate and screw fixation, or a Rush rod (Figs. 9-92 through 9-94).

Most bimalleolar and trimalleolar fractures require internal fixation (165,189). These injuries are, by definition, unstable. Medial malleolar fractures are treated with screw fixation. The fibular fracture can also be reduced with multiple screws if it is spiral in nature. Short oblique or transverse fractures are reduced with plate and screw or Rush rod fixation. It is important that the

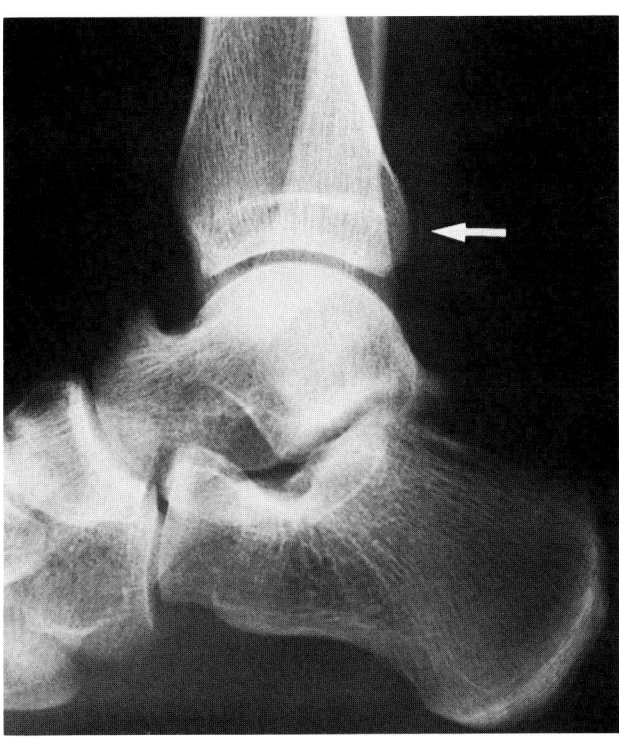

FIG. 9–91. Lateral view of the ankle demonstrating a posterior tibial avulsion fracture (*arrow*).

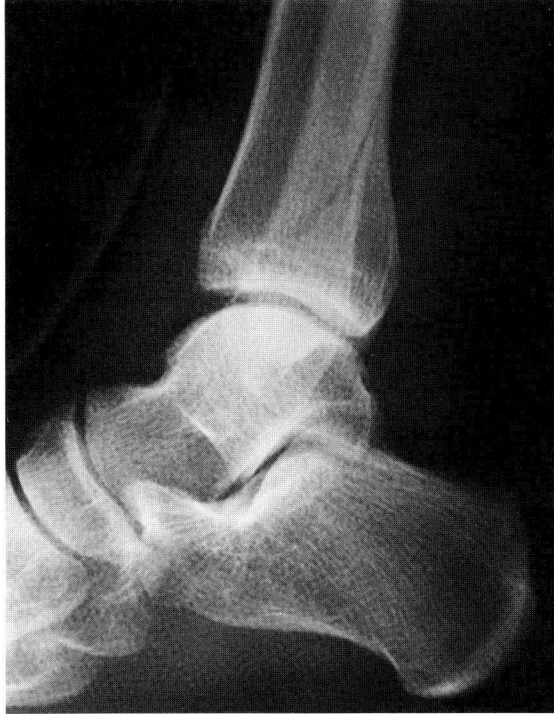

FIG. 9–92. Lateral view of the ankle showing an undisplaced supination-lateral rotation Stage II injury, which is appropriately treated using cast immobilization.

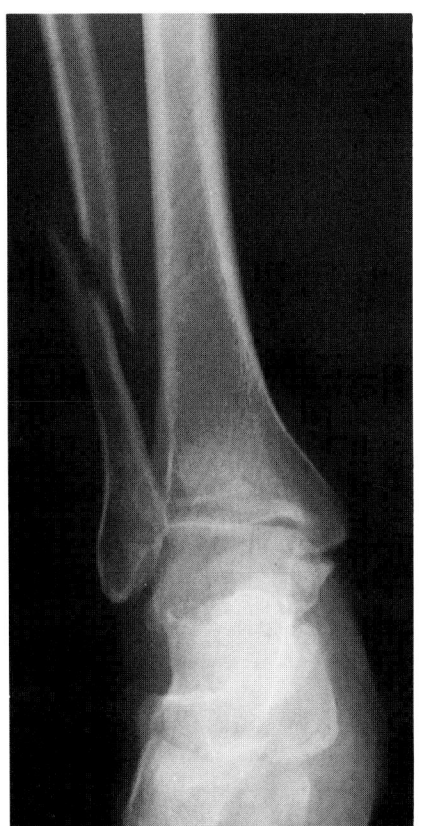
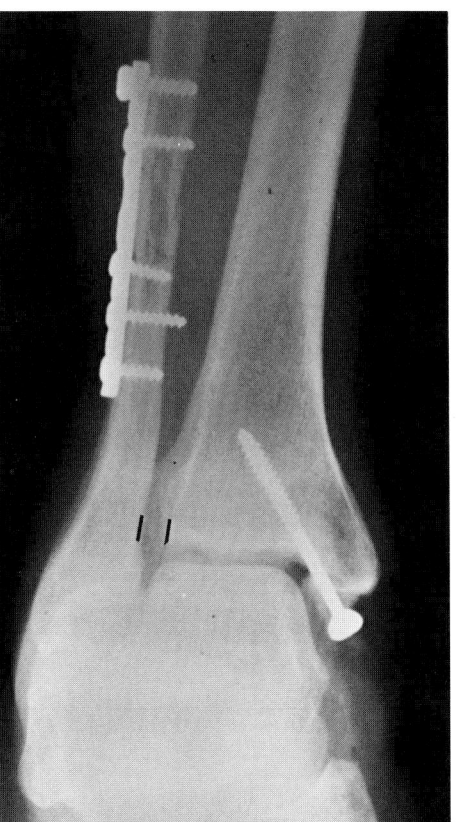
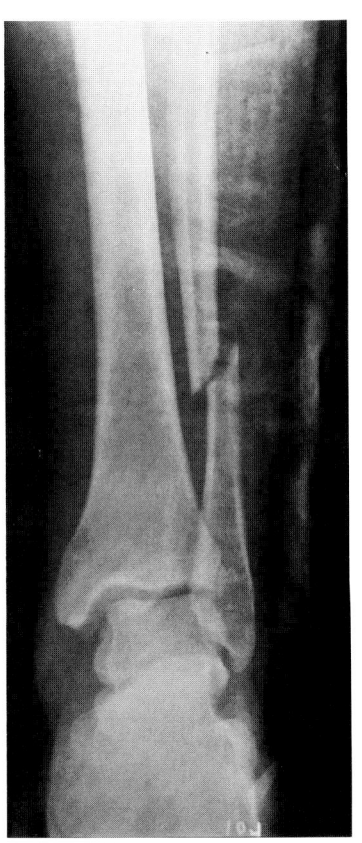

A

B

C

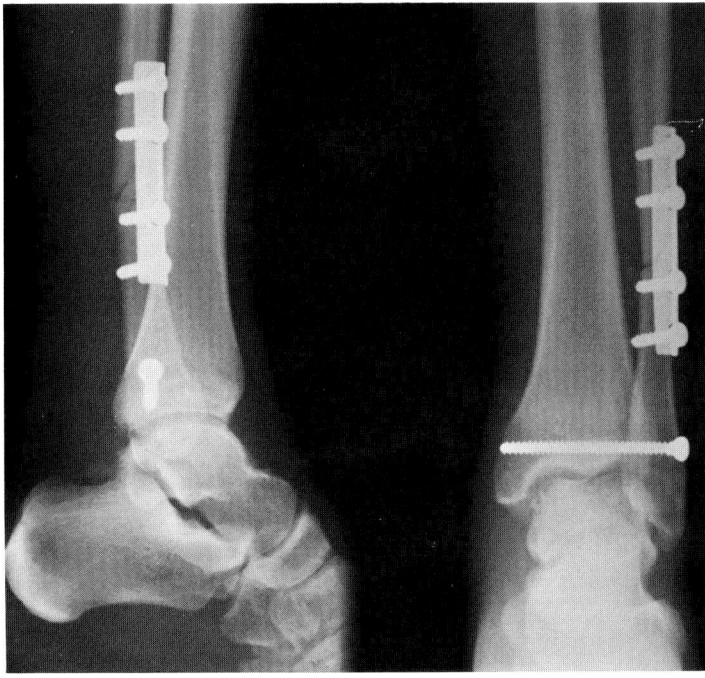

D

FIG. 9–93. AP view of a Lauge-Hansen Stage III prona-tion-lateral rotation injury (**A**). Following internal fixation (**B**) the distal tibiofibular space remains wide (>5 mm). A similar injury (**C,D**) is reduced by reducing the fibular fracture with a four-hole compression plate and a syn-desmosis screw. The deltoid ligament is torn but there is no medial malleolar fracture.

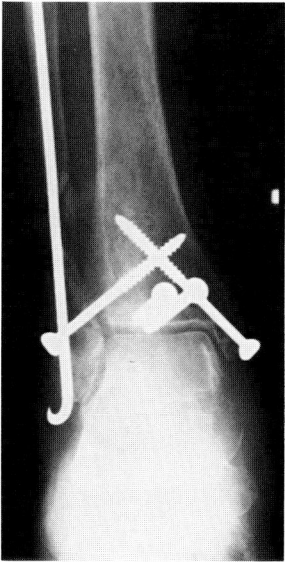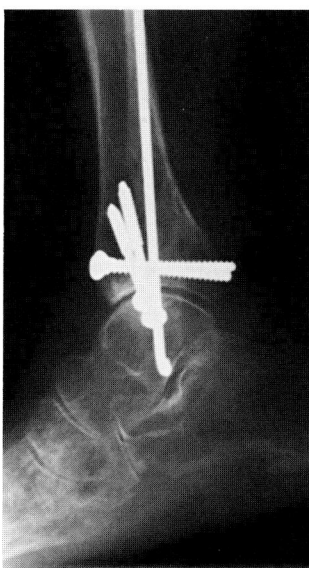

FIG. 9–94. Trimalleolar fracture reduced with tibial screws and a rush rod in the fibula.

fibular and syndesmosis be reduced in order to avoid chronic instability. This is especially true with supination lateral rotation and pronation lateral rotation injuries (184,200,205). In patients with extensive syndesmosis disruption, a syndesmosis screw may be needed to reduce the ankle mortise (189). The latter screw needs to be removed to avoid complications (see below) (Fig. 9-93). Internal fixation of the posterior tibial fragment is generally required if more than 25% of the articular surface is involved (214).

Fractures of the tibial plafond are particularly difficult to manage (194,198). Considerable separation of fragments and loss of articular cartilage may be present (Figs. 9-95 and 9-96). Three-dimensional CT may be particularly useful in planning reconstruction of these fractures. The fragments need to be repositioned and the articular surface restored as completely as possible. Severely comminuted fractures may require calcaneal traction for several weeks. This will help reduce the ankle mortise and perhaps allows fibrous ingrowth, which reduces post-traumatic arthritis. In certain cases, arthrodesis is necessary. Twenty-one of 145 patients with plafond fractures required arthrodesis in Ovadia's series (194). Regardless of the treatment, Type I fractures have excellent results. Only 22% of patients with Type V (Ovadia classification, see Fig. 9-90) had good results. Radiographs are necessary for a period of 4–8 weeks after reduction to be certain that fragments do not change position. In certain cases, more complex studies (tomography, CT, or MRI) are needed if the fracture pattern is unclear.

Complications

Complications may result from the initial injury or be related to treatment (Table 9-7). Loss of reduction gener-

ally occurs with closed reduction but can occur following internal fixation as well (189). Reduction may be difficult or impossible to maintain using closed manipulation in certain cases. For example, the fibula can become trapped behind the tibia. Also soft tissue underposition or tendon entrapment may make it impossible to reduce fractures (169,189). Usually routine radiographs are adequate to evaluate change in position of fragments (Fig. 9-97). Failure to maintain reduction due to soft tissue interposition can be easily diagnosed using CT or MRI. If these techniques are not available, tenography can be performed.

Arthritis is the most common long-term complication occurring in up to 30–40% of patients regardless of the treatment method used (208). The incidence is higher with displaced plafond fractures (Types III–V), when the syndesmosis is poorly reduced or with chronic instability and in older patients (194,196,208). Radiographic findings of arthritis may not become obvious for 3–8 years (Fig. 9-98). Pain symptoms may lead to operative intervention with ankle fusion or, in certain cases, ankle arthroplasty.

Malunion and non-union are uncommon when adequate reduction is obtained. Non-union occurs most commonly following avulsion of the medial malleolus. The incidence (10–15%) is much higher following closed than open (0.5%) reduction (165,208,212). Displaced fragments with well-defined sclerotic margins indicate obvious non-union radiographically. Subtle cases can be detected tomographically or more accurately with MRI. On T2-weighted (TE60, TR2000, 1.5T) sequences, there is increased signal in the fracture line with non-union. Fibrous union will be seen as a dark area in the fracture line on both T1- and T2-weighted sequences.

Patients with internal fixation are more prone to infection. Fortunately, the incidence is low, and infections are usually superficial (208).

Reflex sympathetic dystrophy is a syndrome of refractory pain, neurovascular changes of swelling, and vasomotor instability as well as trophic changes involving soft tissues and bone (174,197). The etiology is unclear, but the syndrome has been attributed to trauma, infec-

TABLE 9–7. *Complications of ankle fractures*[a]

Osteoarthritis
Chronic instability
Non-union
Malunion
Reflex sympathetic dystrophy
Infection
Adhesive capsulitis
Tendon rupture or dislocation
Synovial chondromatosis
Tarsal tunnel syndrome
Neurovascular injury
Pes cavovarus deformity

[a] (169,177,179,180,183,189,194,196)

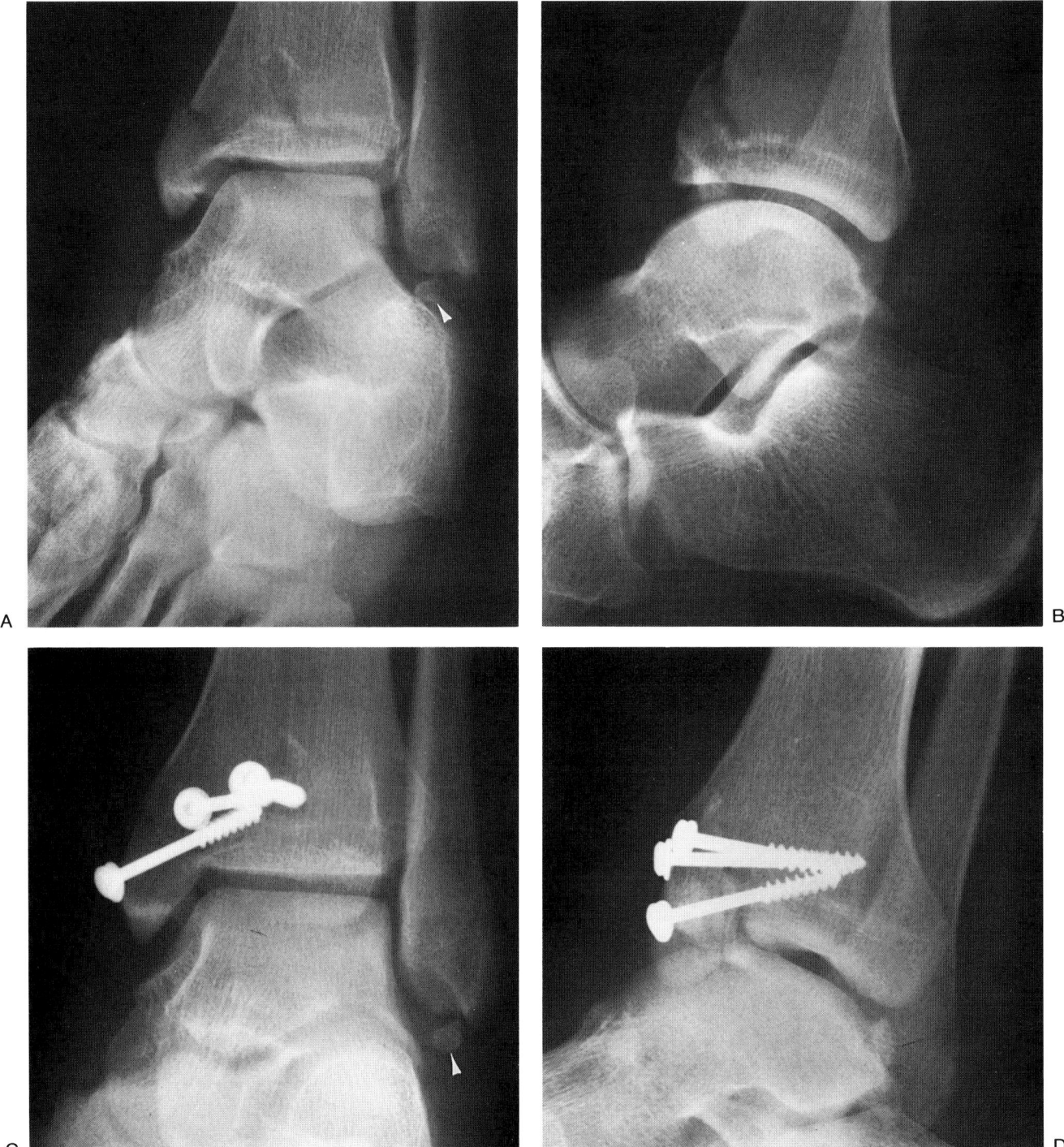

FIG. 9-95. Mortise (**A**) and lateral (**B**) views of a minimally displaced tibial plafond and malleolar fractures. Note the secondary ossification center below the fibula (**A,** *arrow*). Following screw fixation, the fragments appear to be in excellent position on the mortise view (**C**). The lateral view (**D**) demonstrates residual irregularity of the articular surface.

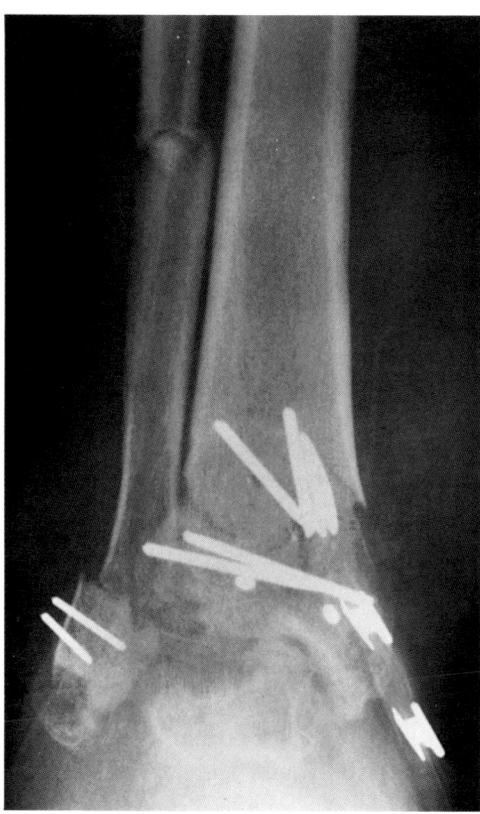

FIG. 9-96. Complex (Type V) plafond fracture with K-wire reduction. Note the avascular necrosis (sclerotic area) in the medial aspect of the talus.

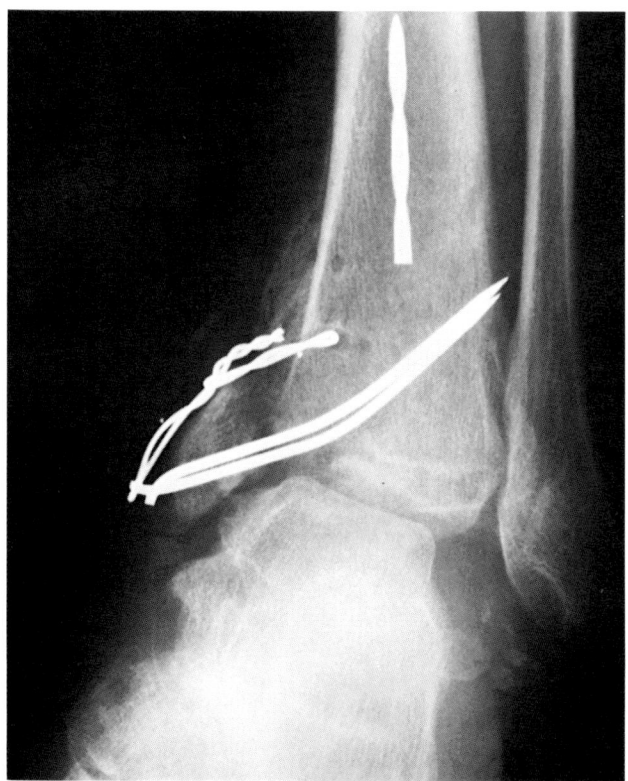

FIG. 9-97. AP view of the ankle following loss of reduction. The medial malleolus was inadequately reduced and progressive deformity has resulted with non-union of the fracture.

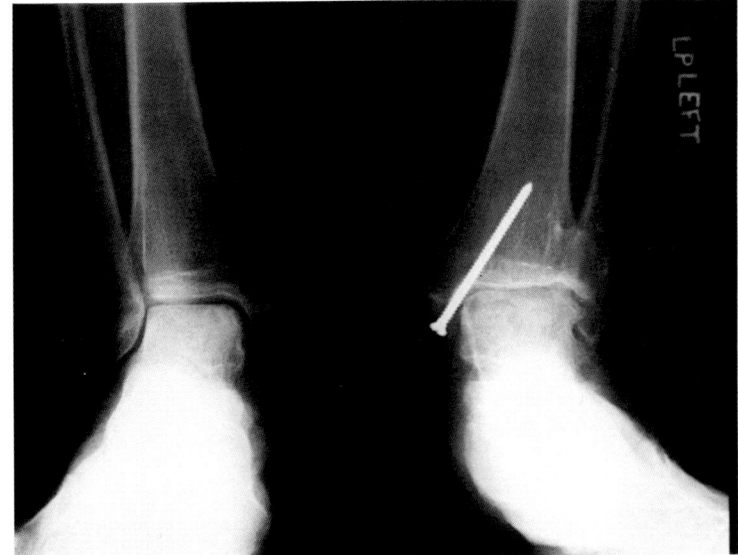

A

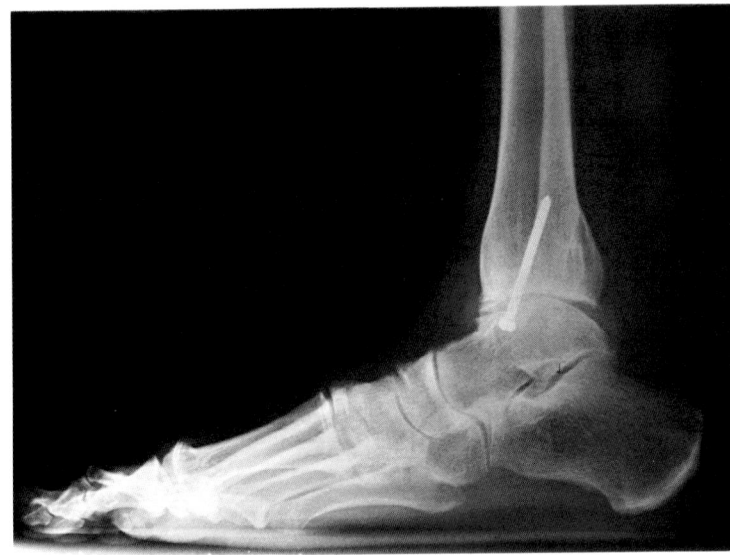

B

FIG. 9-98. AP (**A**) standing views of the ankle. Note the advanced osteoarthritis. The medial malleolar fracture has healed. The lateral view (**B**) shows joint space narrowing, hypertrophic lipping, and the old posterior tibial deformity.

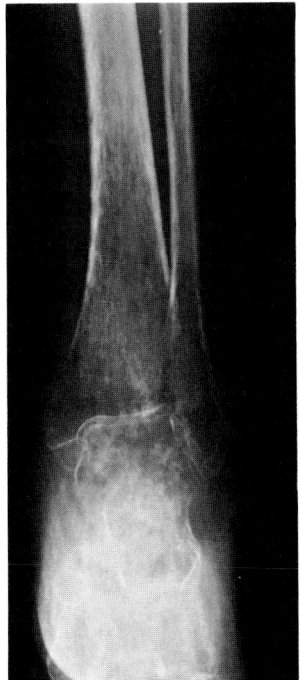

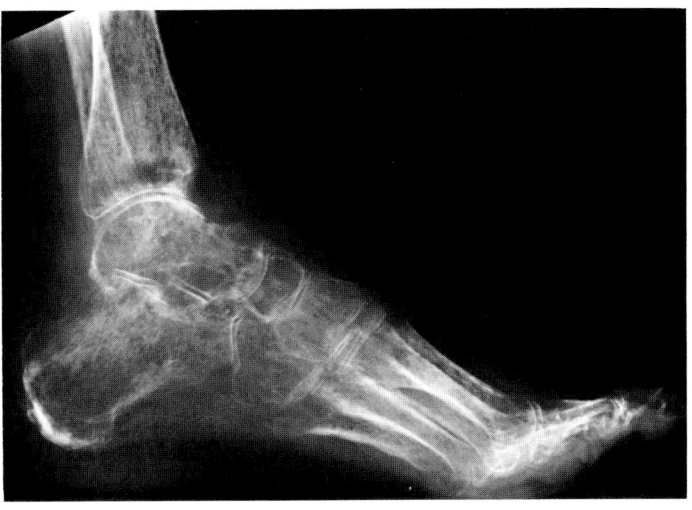

FIG. 9-99. Sudeck's atrophy. AP (A) and lateral (B) radiographs demonstrate aggressive osteoporosis due to reflex sympathetic dystrophy following ankle trauma. There was no fracture.

tion, cervical arthritis, etc. The severity of trauma does not correlate with the severity of the symptoms. Most authors feel that the syndrome is due to post-traumatic reflex spasm leading to loss of vascular tone and aggressive osteoporosis (197). Osteoporosis may have a diffuse or patchy appearance involving both medullary and cortical bone (Fig. 9-99). Prompt diagnosis can lead to more effective therapy. Isotope scans may demonstrate multiple articular changes earlier suggesting the diagnosis and permitting treatment to be instituted earlier.

Neurovascular injury can occur during the injury or because of inadequate treatment (Fig. 9-100). In the acute setting, angiography is most often employed to evaluate vascular occlusion. Doppler techniques can also be used to evaluate vascular patency.

Ossification of the syndesmosis can occur after ankle fracture (208). Most often it is incomplete. However, complete bony fusion can occur (Fig. 9-101), usually when a syndesmosis screw has been used. These changes are usually obvious on routine radiographs. However, scarring and stenosis may be purely fibrous in which case CT or MRI are more useful.

When treatment of initial injuries is unsuccessful or severe arthritis develops, further surgery may be required. Arthrodesis is an accepted technique for post-traumatic ankle problems (190,191). Multiple techniques have been described with good results reported in over 75% of patients (199). Imaging is helpful to confirm bony union and for detection of complications. Routine radiographs are usually sufficient to follow union of fusions. Tomography is very useful in detection of bony

fusion, and sequestra in cases of infection. MRI may prove to be most useful, depending on the type and amount of metal in place for fixation. Pseudarthrosis can develop in 10–25%, infection in up to 23%, and malunion in 12% of cases (188,190,199).

Talar Fractures and Dislocations

The talus is a unique and important functional unit of the hindfoot (223,233). It supports the body weight and distributes the forces to the foot. The talus ossifies from a single primary center with ossification beginning in the neck. The posterior aspect ossifies last with maturation completed 16–20 years after birth (247). Articular cartilage covers 60% of the talar surface, and there are no direct tendon or muscle attachments. Therefore, the blood supply is vulnerable (236,239,247,256).

Superiorly, the trochlear surface articulates with the tibia. This articular surface is wider anteriorly. Medially and laterally there are articular facets for the medial and lateral malleoli. There are bony processes posteriorly and laterally. The posterior process is divided into medial and lateral tubercles by a groove for the flexor hallucis longus tendon. This tendon in its fibrous tunnel is the closest anatomically to a tendinous attachment (236,239,260). In up to 50% of patients, the os trigonum is present as a secondary ossification center. This lies just posterior to the lateral tubercle of the posterior process.

Inferiorly, the talus articulates with the calcaneus via the larger posterior, and middle and anterior facets. The

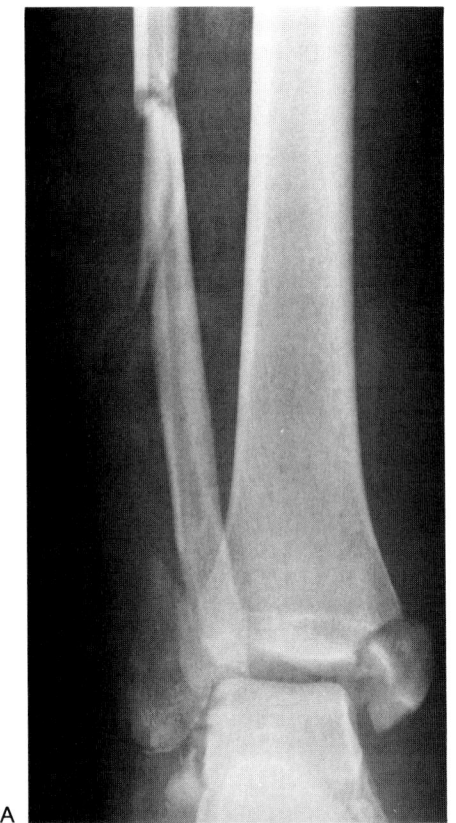

A

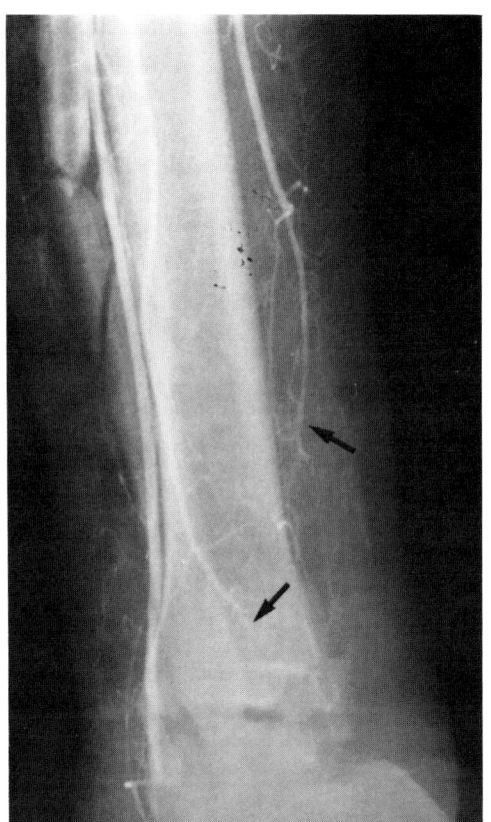

B

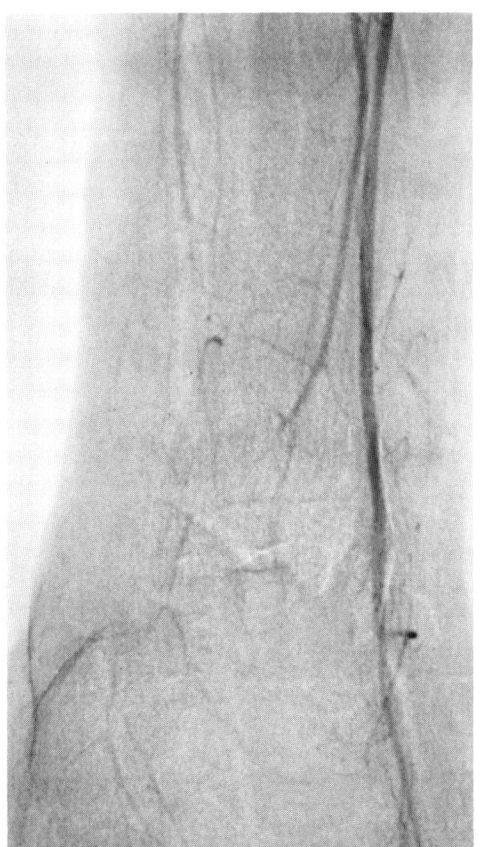

C

FIG. 9–100. AP (**A**) view demonstrating a complex ankle fracture with comminution of the mid-fibula. There was marked swelling and mottling of the skin on the foot. Routine (**B**) and subtracted (**C**) angiograms show occlusion of the peroneal and posterior tibial arteries (**B,** *arrows*). The dorsalis pedis artery is patent.

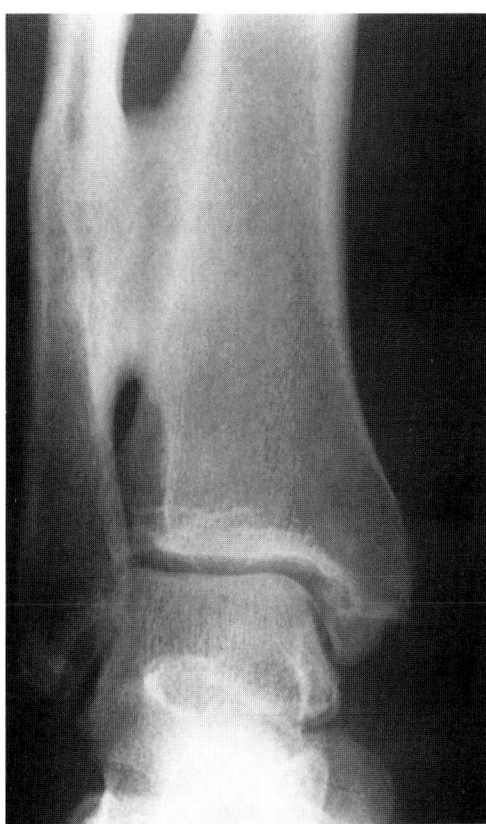

FIG. 9-101. Old ankle fracture with bony fusion of the distal tibia and fibula.

talus forms the roof of the tarsal tunnel between the middle and posterior facets. The talar head articulates with the navicular. Articular stability is maintained by articular capsules and ligaments (239,248,260). Movements in the subtalar joint include eversion (lateral rotation of the hindfoot), inversion (medial rotation of hindfoot), and slight flexion and extension.

The blood supply to the talus is limited by the significant articular surface area and lack of muscle and tendon insertions. The main blood supply enters the talus via the tarsal canal as a branch of the posterior tibial artery. This artery supplies the inferior neck and most of the body. Branches of the dorsalis pedis artery enter the superior aspect of the talar neck and supply the dorsal portion of the neck and the head of the talus. The peroneal artery supplies a portion of the lateral talus (Fig. 9-102) (239,249).

Talar Neck Fractures

Fractures of the talar neck are uncommon in adults and rare in children. Letts (241) identified 12 pediatric fractures over an 18-year period. The largest series of talar fractures was reported by Coltart (225). He noted 228 talar injuries in a total of 25,000 fractures and dislo-

cations (.9%). Talar injuries accounted for only 6% of all foot and ankle injuries. Fractures of the talar neck are the second most common talar injury (Table 9-8) (225,235,242). The injury usually occurs during abrupt dorsiflexion of the forefoot. This is most often associated with motor vehicle accidents or following a significant fall (238). Direct trauma from an object striking the top of the foot may also lead to fracture of the talar neck (242). As usual, the mechanism of injury is rarely pure. Adduction or external rotation forces are also implicated (235,238). Talar neck fractures have also been reported with other ankle injuries implicating supination, supination-lateral rotation, and, less commonly, pronation injuries (238).

Management of talar neck fractures and fracture/dislocation depends on accurate demonstration of the bone and soft tissue injury. The most commonly used classification of these injuries was devised by Hawkins (235) and modified by Canale and Kelly (223) to include four categories of injury. This classification is very useful in determining the prognosis of the injury, specifically in predicting the incidence of avascular necrosis (235,242). The types of fracture or fracture-dislocation are summarized in Table 9-9.

Talar neck fractures must be undisplaced to be considered Type I. These fractures enter the subtalar joint between the middle and posterior facets and may extend into the body. Type II fractures are displaced with subluxation or dislocation of the subtalar joint. The ankle joint is normal. In this setting, two and occasionally all three sources of blood supply are disrupted (223). Type III fractures are displaced with dislocation of the body from both the tibiotalar and subtalar joints; all three sources of blood supply are interrupted. Type IV fractures have associated talonavicular subluxation or dislocation (223). Twenty-four percent of Types II and III injuries were open fractures in Hawkins' series (235,262).

Radiographic Diagnosis

Routine AP, lateral, and mortise views of the ankle, and AP, lateral, and oblique views of the foot are obtained in patients with suspected talar fracture. Talar neck fractures, especially undisplaced (Hawkins Type I) can be subtle and easily overlooked on routine views. The presence of an ankle injury should alert one to search for a talar neck fracture. Too frequently the more obvious ankle injury provides too much interest for the unwary observer and a subtle talar fracture may be overlooked. Up to 20% of patients have associated medial malleolar fractures, which are often more obvious (235). Sixteen percent of patients have fractures in other bones of the ipsilateral foot. Tomography may be needed to confirm subtle fractures or to exclude a suspected injury (Fig. 9-103).

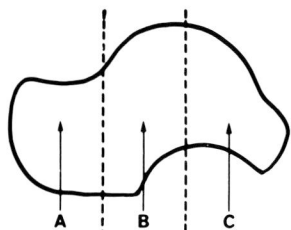

MEDIAL VIEW OF THE TALUS
SHOWING THE AREAS COVERED
BY THE FOLLOWING SECTIONS

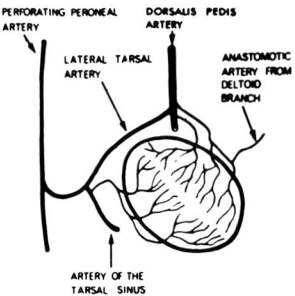

A BLOOD SUPPLY TO THE
HEAD OF THE TALUS

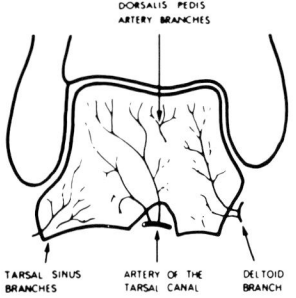

B BLOOD SUPPLY TO THE
MIDDLE ONE - THIRD
OF THE TALUS

A

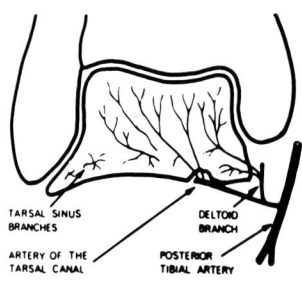

C BLOOD SUPPLY TO THE
POSTERIOR ONE - THIRD
OF THE TALUS

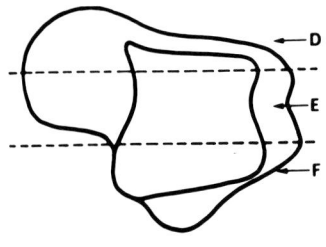

DORSAL VIEW OF THE TALUS
SHOWING THE AREAS COVERED
BY THE FOLLOWING SECTIONS

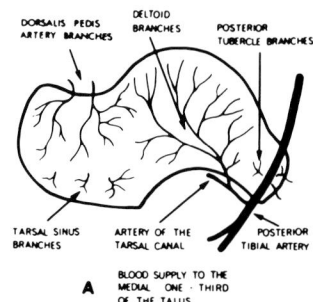

A BLOOD SUPPLY TO THE
MEDIAL ONE - THIRD
OF THE TALUS

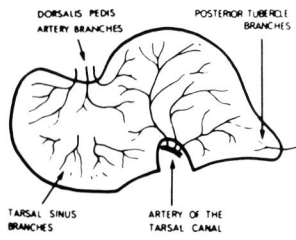

B BLOOD SUPPLY TO THE
MIDDLE ONE - THIRD
OF THE TALUS

B

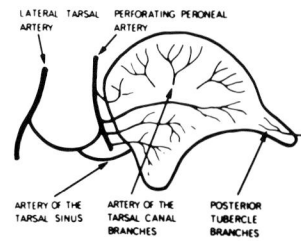

C BLOOD SUPPLY TO THE
LATERAL ONE - THIRD
OF THE TALUS

FIG. 9–102. Coronal (**A**) and sagittal (**B**) illustrations of talar blood supply (from 249).

TABLE 9-8. *Talar fractures*[a]

Fracture type	Incidence[b]
Chip or avulsion fracture	40–49%
Neck fracture	28–32%
Body fracture	11–14%
Compression fracture	5–10%
Fracture-dislocations	
Neck fracture with subtalar dislocation	45–50%
Neck fracture with posterior body dislocation	30–40%
Body fracture with subtalar dislocation	9–12%
Total dislocation	3–12%

[a] (218–221,229,233,237,249)
[b] Variable due to multiple series

TABLE 9-9. *Talar neck fractures and fracture-dislocations*[a]

Type	Definition	Incidence[b]
I	Undisplaced vertical neck fracture	11–21%
II	Displaced vertical neck fracture with subtalar subluxation or dislocation	40–24%
III	Displaced vertical neck fracture with subluxation or dislocation of both tibiotalar and subtalar joints	23–47%
IV	Displaced vertical fracture of the talus with subtalar or tibiotalar dislocation and subluxation or dislocation of the talonavicular joint	5%

[a] (223,224,234,242)
[b] Incidence > 100% due to multiple series.

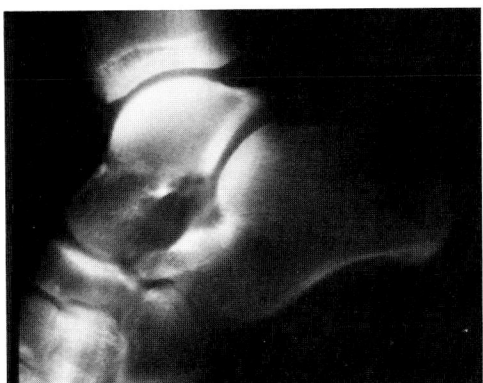
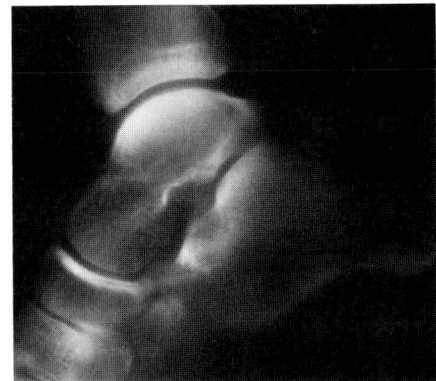
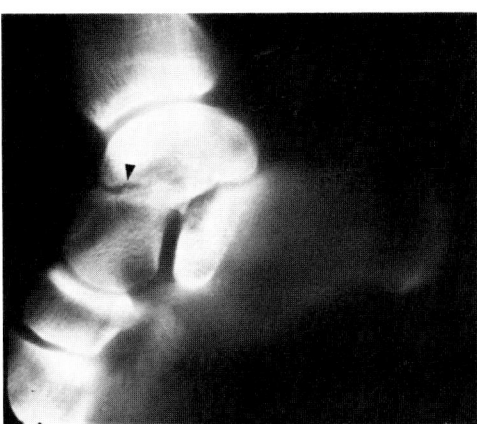
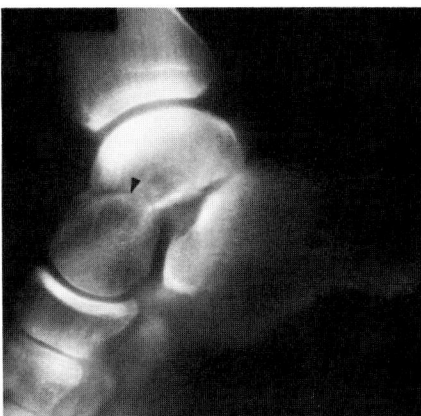

FIG. 9-103. Lateral tomograms of the talus showing a Hawkins Type I talar neck fracture (*arrows*). The fracture is not clearly seen on all slices and was not evident on routine views.

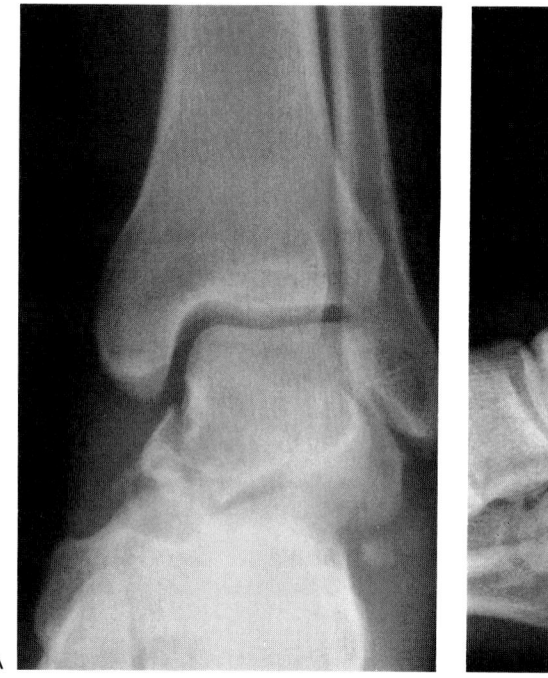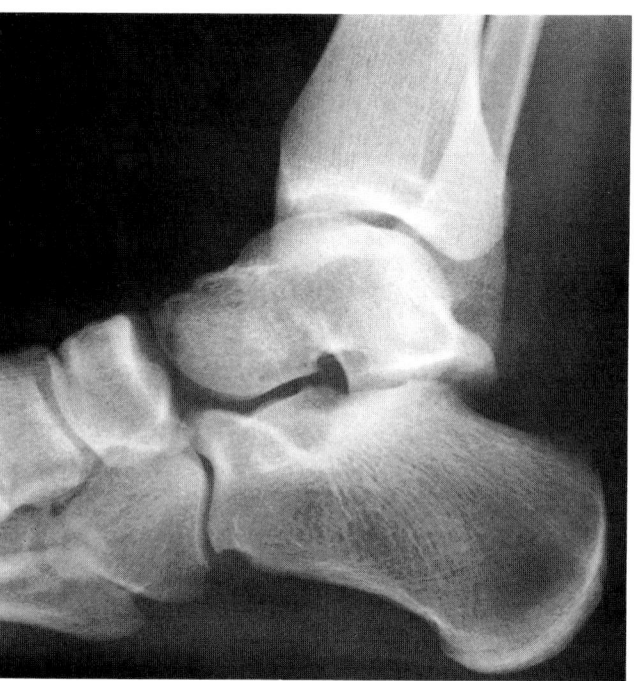

FIG. 9-104. AP (**A**) and lateral (**B**) views of the ankle showing a comminuted talar neck fracture with subluxation of the talonavicular and subtalar joints (Hawkins type IV).

Displaced talar neck fractures or fractures with dislocation are usually easily detected on routine views (Fig. 9-104). Detection of subluxation may require that joint spaces and articular relationships be more carefully assessed. Stress views may be helpful. However, the risk of displacing a talar fracture, when present, is significant and, therefore, stress views are not always safe in this setting. If the tarsal relationships are not clear, CT or conventional tomography should be obtained.

Treatment

Treatment should be instituted as soon as possible after radiographs have been assessed and the fracture properly classified (247). Undisplaced (Hawkins Type I) fractures can be treated with a below-the-knee cast for 8–12 weeks and non-weight bearing for up to 5 months (223).

Fractures that are minimally displaced may be reduced using closed techniques and cast immobilization. However, open reduction with lag or cancellous screws, or K-wires, is often needed to maintain reduction in Types II–IV injuries (Fig. 9-105) (223,235). Even slight displacement can lead to varus malunion (236). Prognosis is improved in Types II–IV if adequate open reduction can be obtained (238). Although most patients have some residual disability, good results can be achieved in 75% of Type I fractures. Good results are obtained in 42% of Types II and III fractures (255).

During reduction, routine radiographs can be used to be certain that adequate position of the fragments has been achieved (Fig. 9-105B,C) Canale and Kelly (223) recommend that more than 5-mm displacement and more than 5° malalignment on the AP view should not be accepted. In certain cases, tomography or CT may be needed to evaluate articular alignment and residual joint fragments (Fig. 9-106). CT is particularly useful in this regard. Follow-up radiographs should be obtained for up to 2 years after the injury to exclude avascular necrosis (AVN). In children, monthly radiographs should be obtained for 6 months as AVN will usually be evident by that time (233).

Complications

Complications are particularly common following displaced talar neck fractures (Hawkins Types II–IV) (224,235,242,245). Table 9-10 summarizes the common complications associated with talar neck fractures.

Avascular Necrosis. Avascular necrosis (AVN), if untreated, progresses through stages. Changes are based on radiographic features similar to those described in the hip. Stage I AVN shows slight increased density of the talar body with no deformity (Fig. 9-107). Stage II changes include increased sclerosis with moderate deformity of the trochlea. Stage III AVN presents with more severe deformity and sequestration. Fragmentation of the talus occurs in Stage IV (Fig. 9-108) (242). The inci-

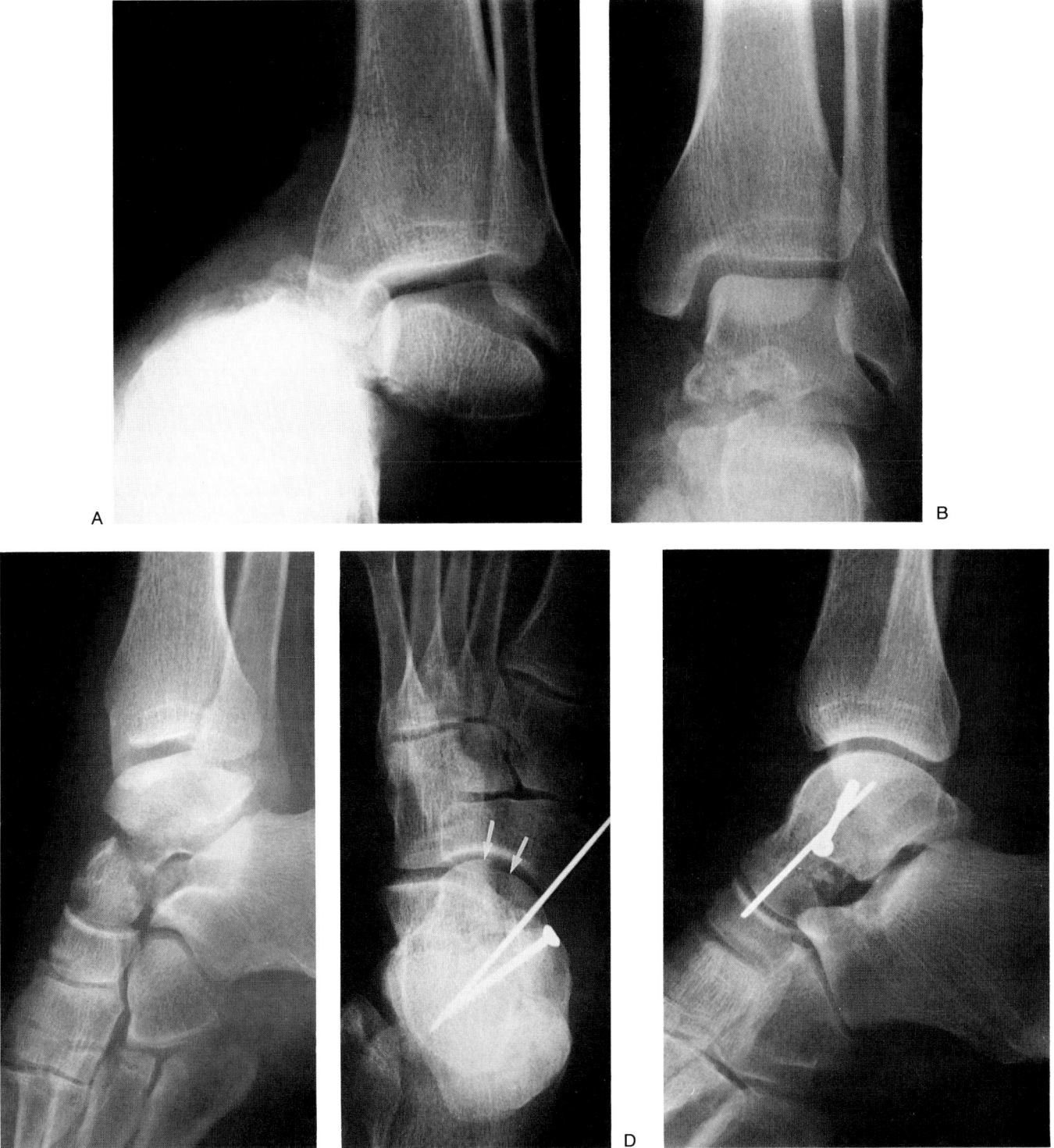

FIG. 9-105. AP (**A**) view of the ankle showing a displaced talar fracture with subtalar dislocation (Hawkins type II). The trochlea is in normal position in the ankle mortise. AP (**B**) and lateral (**C**) views taken following closed manipulation show comminution of the talar neck with residual displacement. AP (**D**) and lateral (**E**) views taken following screw and K-wire fixation show excellent reduction of the fracture. Note the fracture enters the talar head (**D,** *arrows*) with irregularity of the articular surface.

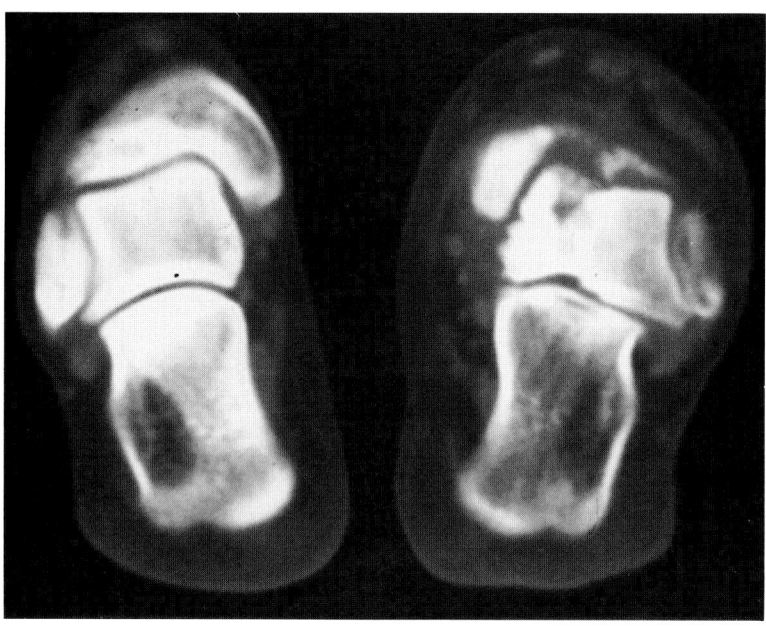

FIG. 9-106. CT images following talar fracture demonstrating irregularity of the subtalar joint and a large defect with fragmentation of the trochlea.

TABLE 9-10. *Complications of talar neck fractures*[a]

	Complications				
Type	AVN	Tibiotalar arthritis	Subtalar arthritis	Malunion	Non-union
I	0-4%	15%	25%	0	0
II	24-42%	36%	66%	28%	6%
III	75-100%	69%	63%	18%	12%

[a] (223,224,235,242)

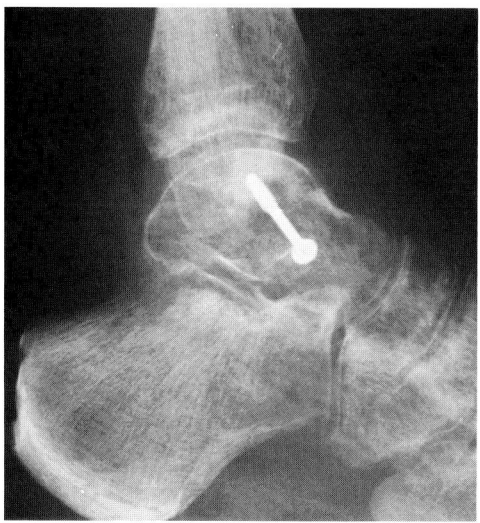
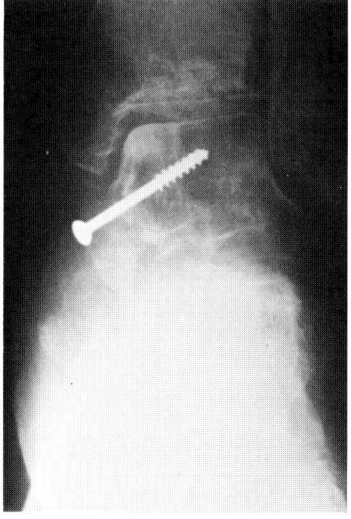

FIG. 9-107. Old talar neck fracture with screw fixation. There is sclerosis in the medial talar dome due to Stage I avascular necrosis. There is no articular deformity. The remainder of the talus and ankle appear osteoporotic.

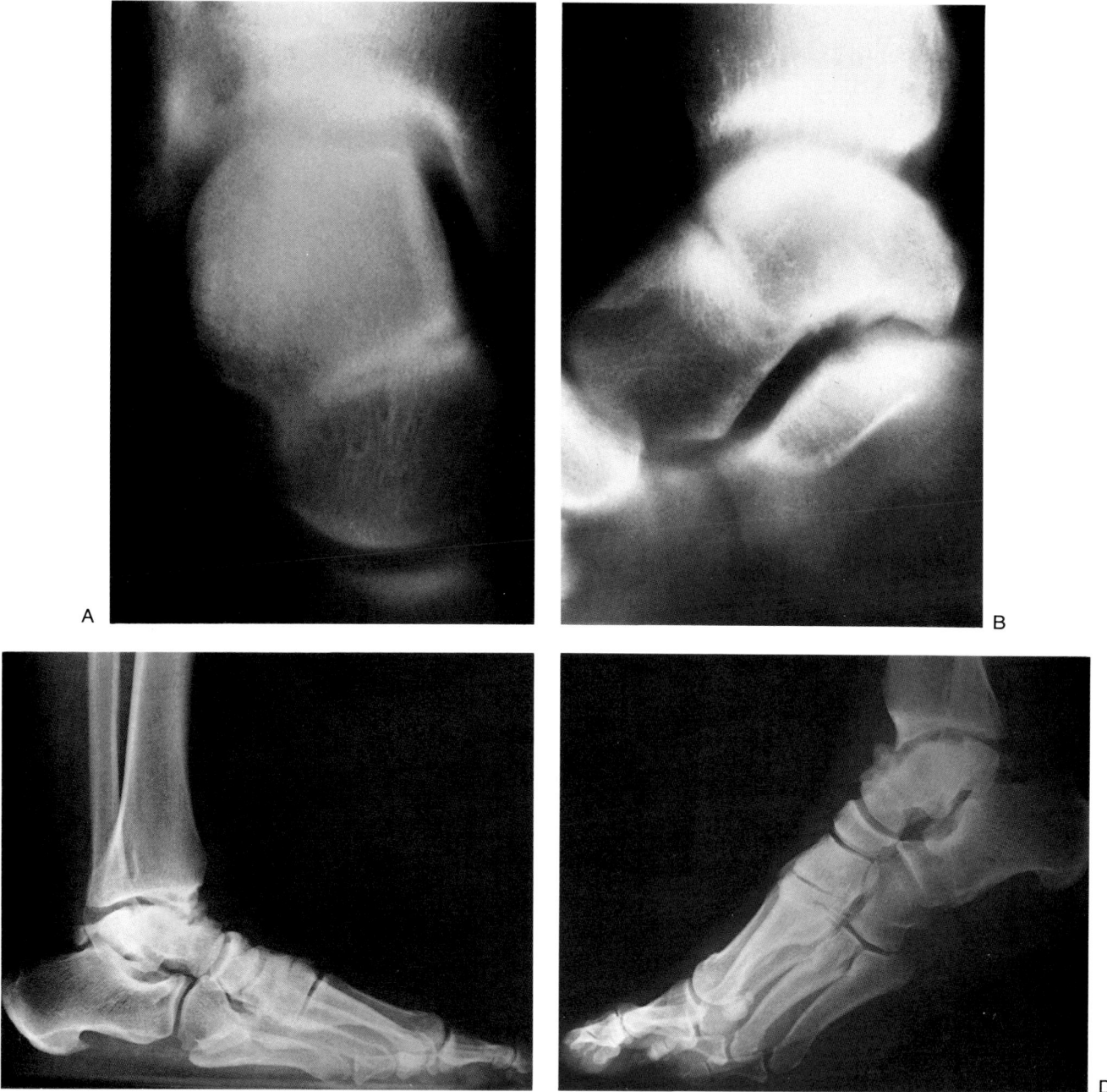

FIG. 9–108. AP (**A**) and lateral (**B**) tomograms of the talus showing a partially healed talar neck fracture with increased density in the posterior fragment and subtalar arthritis. Progressive avascular necrosis (Stage IV) resulted in marked deformity and talar collapse as demonstrated on the lateral and oblique views of the foot (**C,D**).

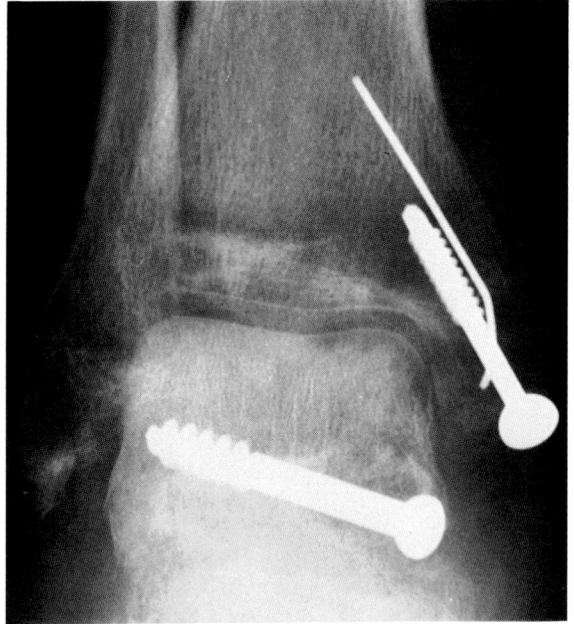

A

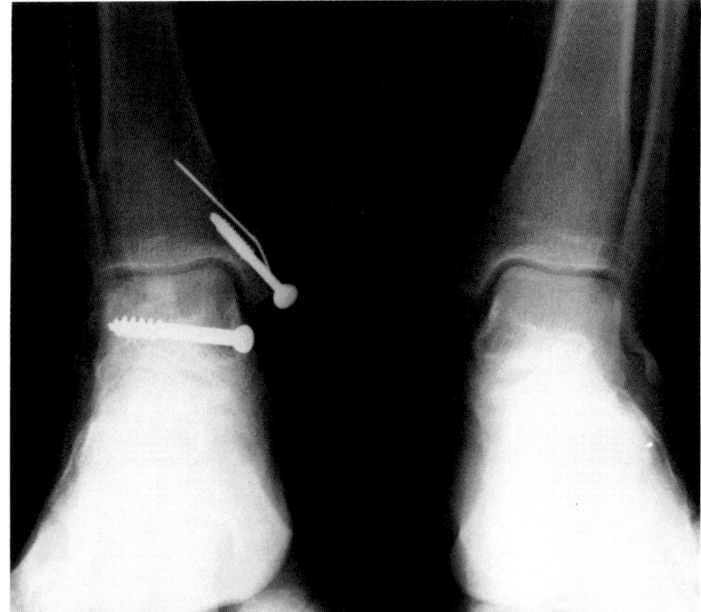

B

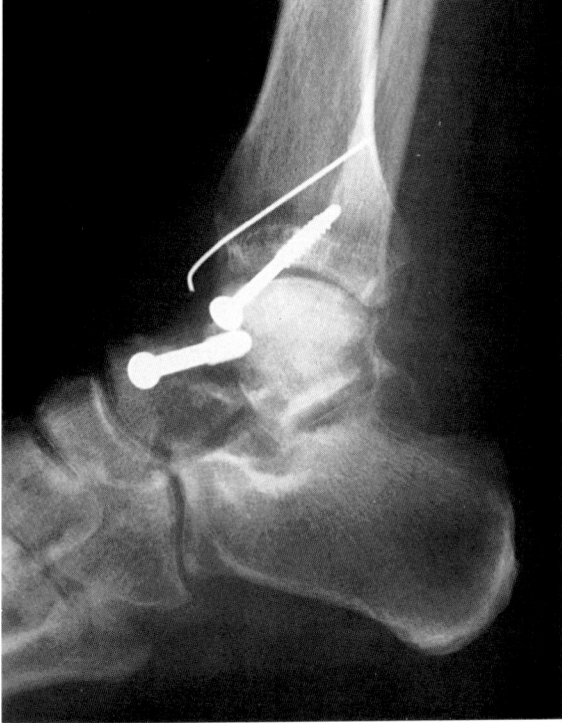

C

FIG. 9-109. Talar neck and associated medial malleolar fracture. AP view (**A**) taken 8 weeks following surgery shows screw fixation of the neck and medial malleolus. There is disuse osteoporosis in the distal tibia and medial talar dome. This segment should be viable. Delayed standing AP (**B**) and lateral (**C**) views taken one year later show obvious avascular necrosis with medial (area of previous Hawkins sign) sparing.

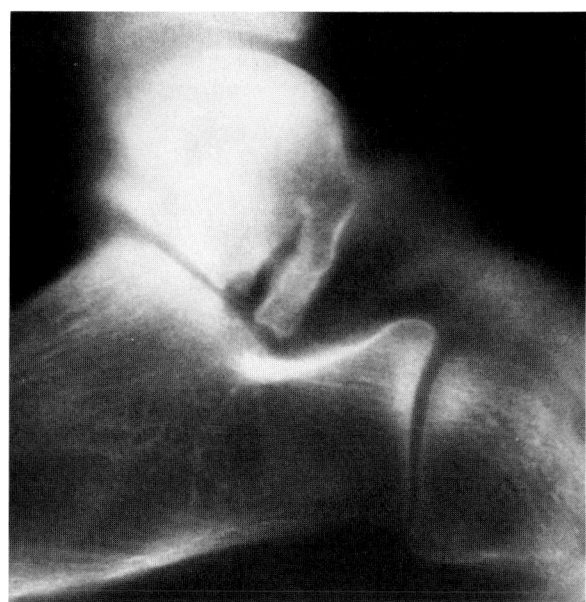

FIG. 9–110. Lateral tomogram demonstrating non-union in the subtalar portion of the talar neck with degenerative narrowing of the posterior facets.

dence of AVN increases significantly in Types II–IV fractures (Table 9-10) (223,235,242). An exception appears with pediatric injuries. Although rare, Type I fractures developed AVN in 7 of 22 patients reported by Canale (223) and Letts et al. (236).

Avascular necrosis usually becomes evident on routine radiographs in 6–8 weeks (Fig. 9-109). During this non-weight-bearing period, disuse osteoporosis develops, which leads to subchondral lucency in the talar dome. This finding (Hawkin's sign) was described by Hawkins and indicates intact vascular supply (235). The finding is most easily identified on AP or mortise views of the ankle. Canale noted this sign in 23 patients and only one developed AVN. Twenty of 26 with a negative Hawkin's sign developed AVN (223).

Although routine radiographic features are well described, changes are evident earlier with isotope scans and MRI. Interosseous phlebography is not commonly used for diagnosis at this time (253). Technetium-99m isotope studies have been advocated to assist in determining when weight bearing should be allowed (223). However, compared to MRI, bone detail is not as good with isotopes. MRI would appear to be the technique of choice in early detection of follow-up evaluation of patients with suspected AVN (218,265).

Arthritis. Post-traumatic arthritis is common following talar neck fractures. The incidence, as expected, increases with the severity of the injury (see Table 9-10). Peterson (255) reported that 97% of patients developed osteoarthritis. Most series show a lower incidence but indicate that degenerative changes developed in nearly two-thirds of Types II and III injuries (223,226,235,242).

The incidence of arthritis is also higher in the subtalar joint than in the tibiotalar joint (Fig. 9-108) (224,242).

Early radiographic changes may show only slight narrowing of the joint space. This may be too subtle to detect without comparison views or tomography. In certain cases, ankle or subtalar arthrography is useful for diagnosing early changes. This also allows injection of anesthetic for diagnostic purposes or a combination of steroid and anesthetic for treatment. MRI provides a new technique for assessing early changes in articular cartilage (218).

Malunion, Non-union. Delayed healing is not uncommon following talar neck fractures (15%) (255). Delayed union is considered in fractures that have not healed by 6 months. It is not unusual for fractures to take over a year to heal in adults. This is due partially to their intra-articular nature, lack of periosteum, and decreased blood supply (236). Non-union occurs in only about 4% of cases overall (236,241). However, the incidence is higher in Hawkins Types II and III fractures (242).

Malunion is also more common in complex injuries (Hawkins Types II–IV): Lorentzen (242) reported malunion in 15% of all cases, but none occurred in Hawkins Type I and 28% and 18% respectively in Hawkins Types II and III fractures. Canale and Kelly (223) noted varus deformity in 47% of Type II fractures. This resulted in increased stress in the lateral subtalar joint (223,236).

Radiographic diagnosis of malunion or non-union can be difficult. Serial radiographs may demonstrate widening, sclerosis, and irregularity of the fracture line if non-union has occurred.

Tomography and CT may be useful, but both have difficulty clearly defining union from fibrous union or early pseudarthrosis (Fig. 9-110). MRI is particularly useful in this situation. T2-weighted sequences (TE ≥ 60, TR 2000) will demonstrate high intensity (fluid) in the fracture line if nonunion is present and low signal (black) if a fibrous union is present (218).

Malunion is most easily demonstrated using AP and lateral radiographs that allow measurements to be obtained and compared with the uninjured side. CT may be particularly useful in evaluating the degree of malunion and resulting articular deformities of the complex subtalar joint (Fig. 9-107).

Other complications include associated fractures (Fig. 9-109), infection, skin necrosis, and neurovascular damage. Ipsilateral foot and ankle fractures have been reported in 16% of patients (226). Hawkins Type IV fractures have associated fractures of the medial malleolus in 15%, indicating that complex forces including pronation and rotation were also present (Fig. 9-109) (223). Fractures distant from the involved foot and ankle are noted in about 22% of patients (226).

Skin necrosis is particularly common following complex (Types II–IV) open fractures. This group of patients is also more prone to infection.

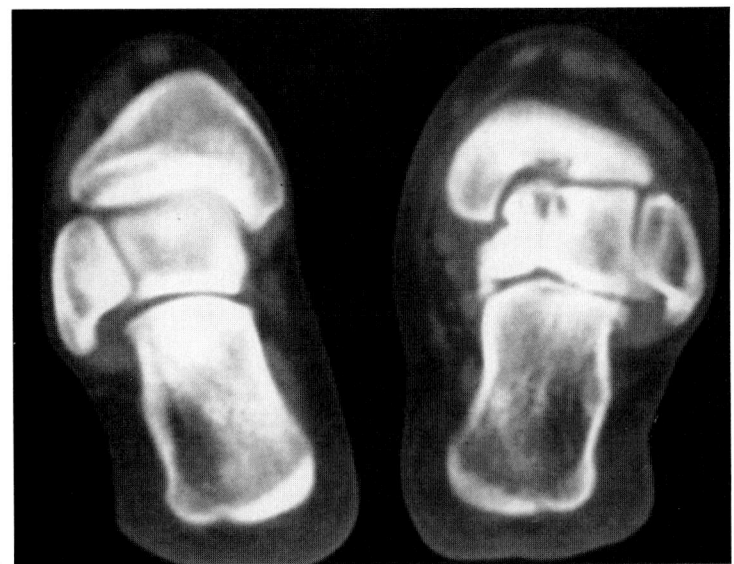

A

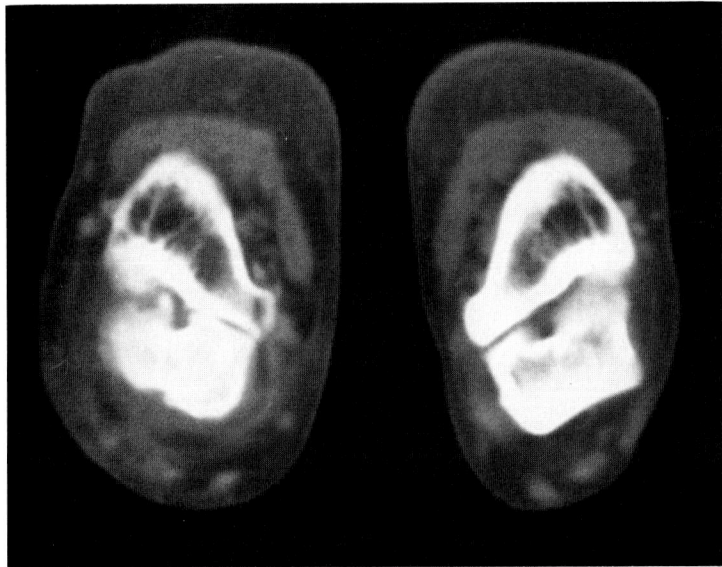

B

FIG. 9–111. Patient with persistent pain and disability following talar neck fracture. CT scans (**A,B**) show degenerative changes and fragmentation of both tibiotalar (**A**) and subtalar joints (**B**). Patient was treated with bone grafting and arthrodesis of both joints. AP (**C**) and lateral (**D**) radiographs show position of the joints and bone grafts (lateral view, **D**).

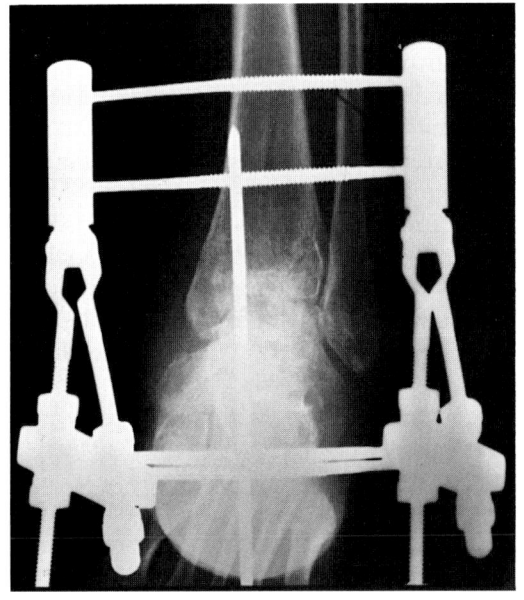

C

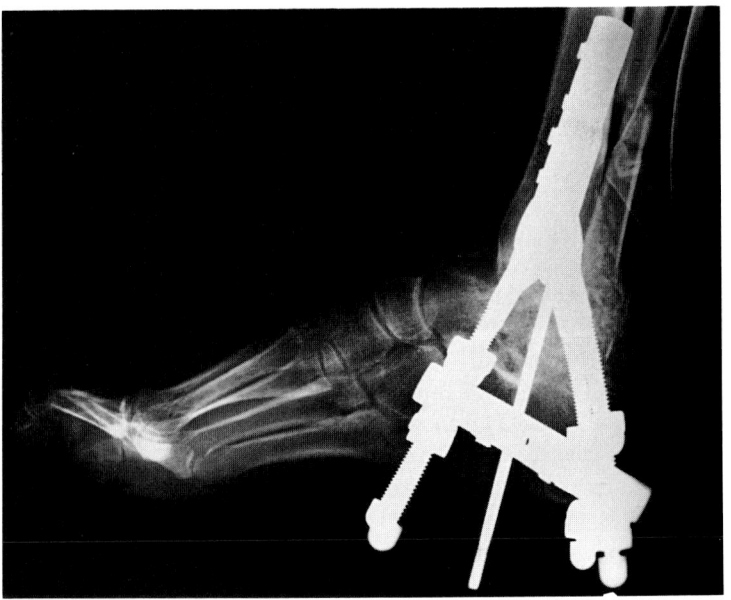

D

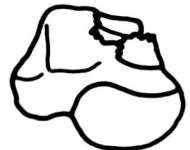 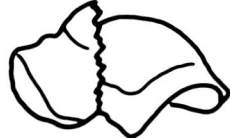 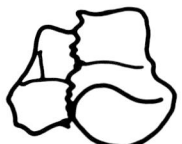

A. Compression fracture

B. Coronal shearing fracture

C. Sagittal shearing fracture

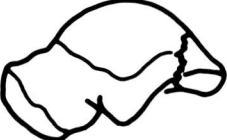 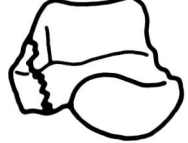 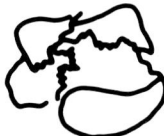

D. Fracture in the posterior tubercle

E. Fracture in the lateral tubercle

F. Crush fracture

FIG. 9–112. Types of talar body fractures (from 269).

Treatment of complications depends upon the patient's age, activity level, and the severity of symptoms. Even patients with avascular necrosis may have satisfactory results with conservative treatment. Alternatives to treatment of AVN, malunion, non-union, infection, and talar break formation include triple arthrodesis, tibiocalcaneal fusion, and resection of dorsal talar breaks (223,228). Talectomy alone has not proved to be a successful treatment method in most authors' experiences (223,228). Talectomy with an interposed bone graft has been more successful.

Imaging techniques also play an important role in evaluating surgical procedures. Follow-up studies are needed to be certain that fusion occurs properly without loss of position. Complications such as infection and pseudarthrosis also require careful diagnostic evaluation. To date, routine AP, lateral, and oblique views have been used to evaluate the various fusion procedures (Fig. 9-111). Tomography is frequently needed to evaluate the complex anatomy. External and internal fixation devices do not interfere with tomography to the degree that images are degraded by them with CT. MRI may be useful in certain cases if non-ferromagnetic materials are used (218).

Early infection may be identified with gallium-67 or Indium-111-labeled white blood cells (WBCs). Also, the extent of infection can be easily demonstrated using sonography or MRI.

Diagnostic anesthetic injection of suspected pseudarthrosis can be accomplished fluoroscopically. This technique may be helpful in localizing the patient's symptoms. This information is particularly useful if further surgery is considered.

Talar Body, Head, and Process Fractures

Fractures of the talar body and posterior and lateral processes are uncommon in adults and rare in children (236,250,258). Although the incidence is lower than for talar neck fractures, complications are similar for body and neck fractures.

Most talar body fractures are due to significant falls or motor vehicle accidents that lead to axial compression of the talus between the tibial plafond and calcaneus. Fractures of the lateral process usually occur with the foot dorsiflexed and inverted (234,244). The calcaneus causes shearing of the lateral process. Snepper et al. (268) described six basic fracture patterns (Fig. 9-112). These included simple compression fractures (Fig. 9-113), vertical fractures in the coronal and sagittal planes, posterior tubercle fractures (Fig. 9-114), lateral tubercle fractures, and comminuted crush fractures. In addition, chip or

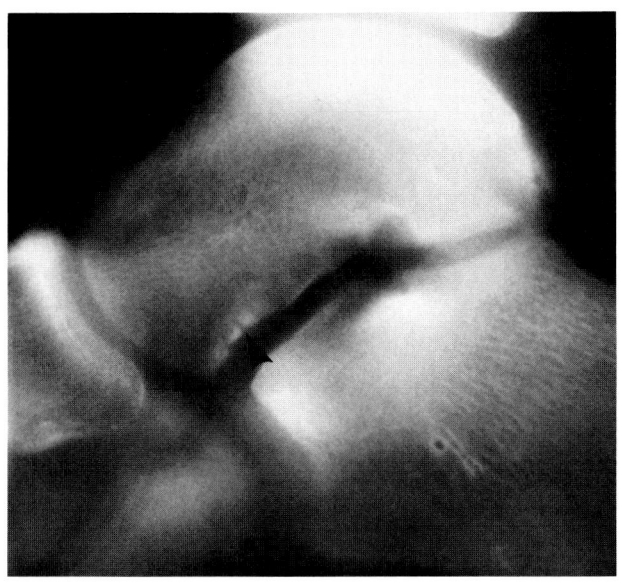

FIG. 9–113. Lateral tomogram of a comminuted osteochondral compression fracture (*arrow*).

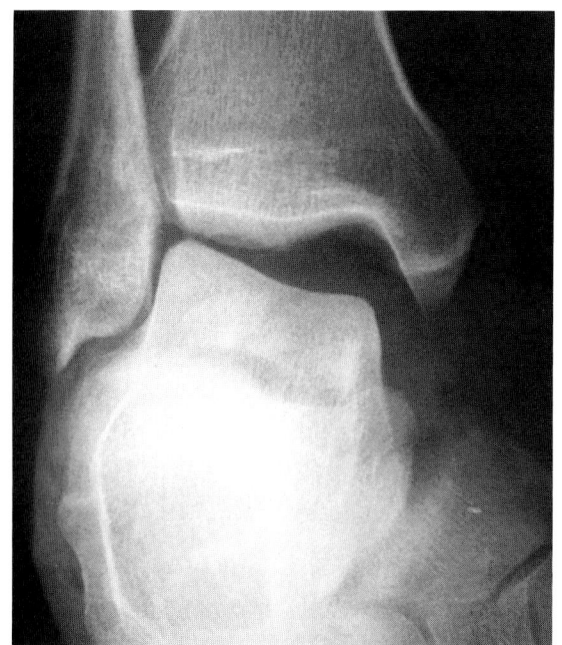
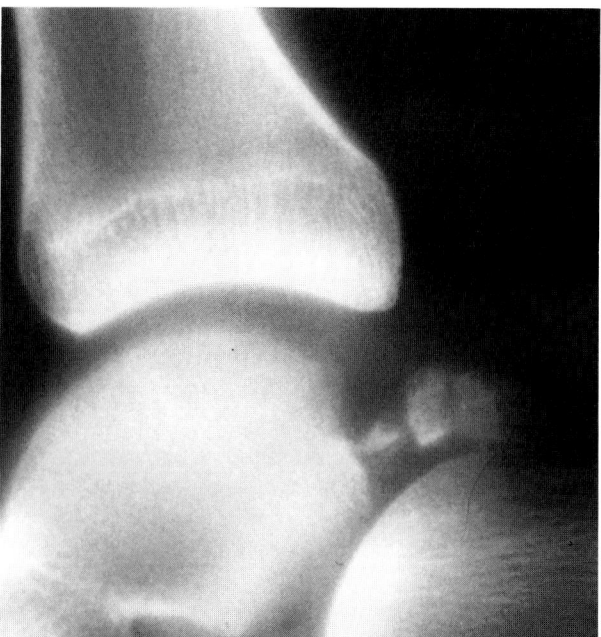

A

B

FIG. 9–114. Pronation injury with disruption of the medial ligaments (**A**). Lateral tomogram (**B**) demonstrates a posterior talar fracture.

avulsion fractures may also occur. Fractures of the head generally involve the talonavicular joint. Many body fractures, especially due to shearing forces, are displaced and associated with subluxation (236).

Radiographic Diagnosis

AP, lateral and mortise views of the ankle are usually adequate for diagnosis of displaced fractures. More subtle fractures (chip avulsion, or undisplaced body fractures) require conventional or computed tomography for detection (Fig. 9-115). Views of the foot should also be obtained as multiple injuries are common (268). Treatment planning is facilitated by CT or conventional tomography in many cases.

Avulsion fractures dorsal and distal to the neck are not common (Fig. 9-116). Bone fragments are avulsed by the articular capsule and talonavicular ligament. These fractures are best seen on the lateral view of the ankle and should not be confused with the normal talar ridge (259).

Treatment

Treatment principles are similar to those applied to talar neck fractures. Anatomic reduction is necessary and is accomplished using operative techniques for displaced fractures. Although process fractures are rare (.86% of 1500 patients presenting with ankle sprains), there is often significant cartilage loss leading to osteoarthritis (244). Posterior (Fig. 9-114) and lateral pro-

cess fractures can be treated with cast immobilization if not displaced (248,268). In patients with displaced process fractures, either early internal fixation or late removal of the fragment is preferred (247).

Complications are similar to talar neck fractures with almost all patients eventually developing arthrosis. The incidence is somewhat lower with posterior and lateral process fractures. Snepper et al. (268) reported malunion in one-third of patients and avascular necrosis in 16% of cases. When complications developed, a second procedure such as tibiocalcaneal fusion or tibiotalar (Blair) fusion may be indicated (219,247).

Talar Dome Fractures

Osteochondral fractures of the talar dome differ from other chip or avulsion fractures in that they are more difficult to detect and prognosis is potentially worse than a nonarticular chip fracture (219,247). Talar dome fractures are the most common talar fracture. This injury is much more common in adults. Only 8% (16 of 201) of patients in Berndt and Harty's series were less than 16 years of age (217,221,247).

The etiology of the lesion is somewhat controversial. Suggested mechanisms include ischemic necrosis, abnormal vascular anatomy, congenital disorders, spontaneous necrosis, and trauma (221,247,251). Most agree that trauma is responsible for most fractures, especially those occurring laterally. Eighty-four to 90% of patients have a definite traumatic event that precipitated their

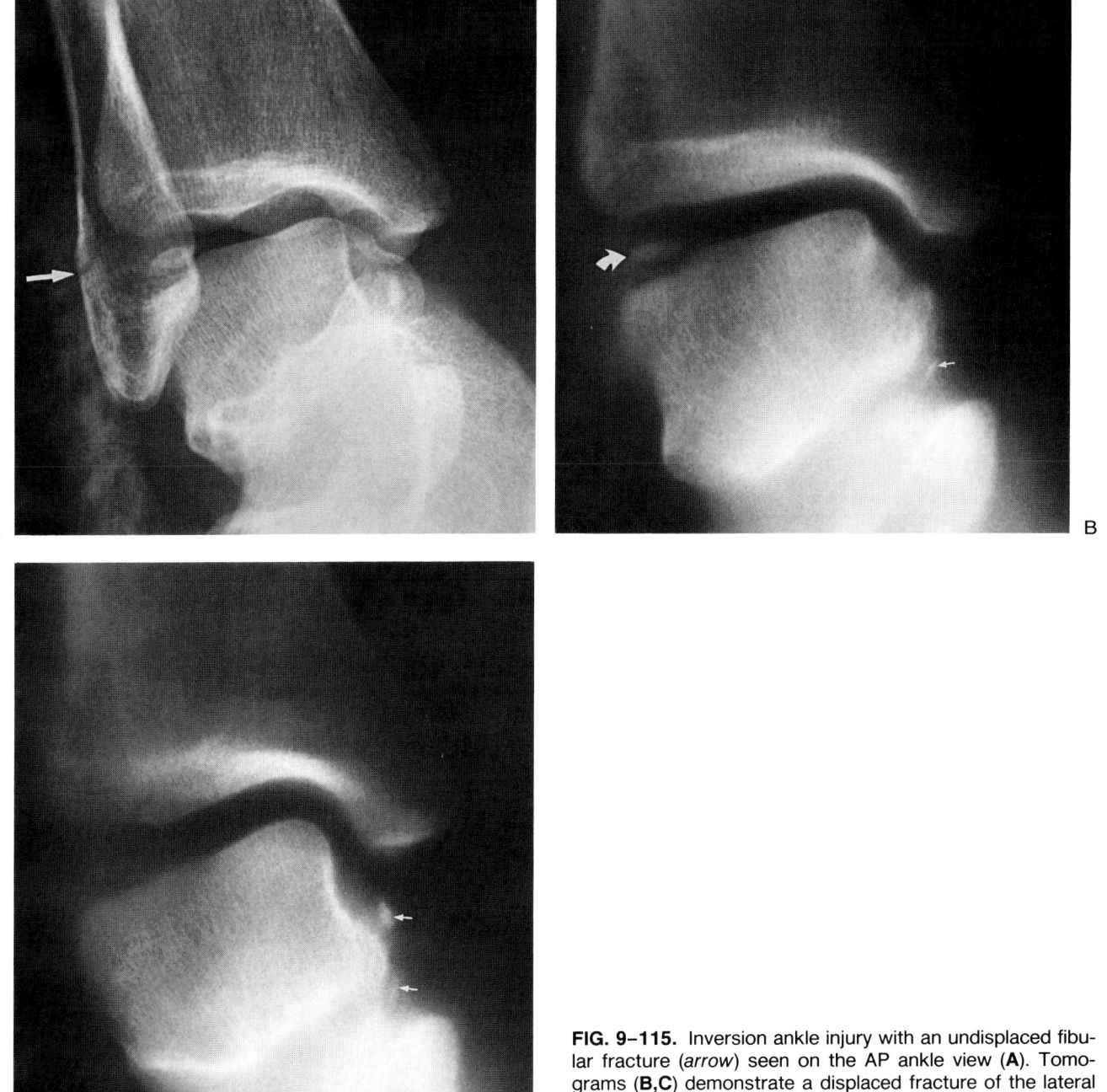

FIG. 9–115. Inversion ankle injury with an undisplaced fibular fracture (*arrow*) seen on the AP ankle view (**A**). Tomograms (**B,C**) demonstrate a displaced fracture of the lateral articular surface of the talus (*curved arrow*) and two small avulsion fractures medially (*small arrows*).

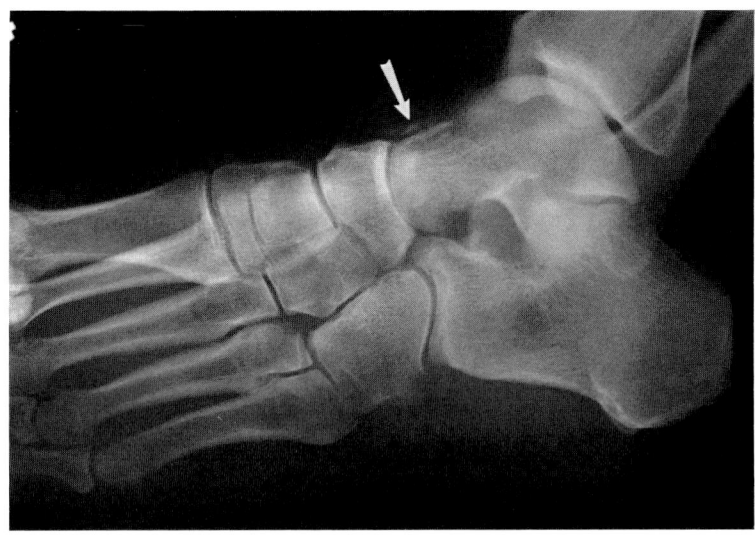

FIG. 9–116. Oblique view of the foot demonstrating a dorsal talar avulsion fracture.

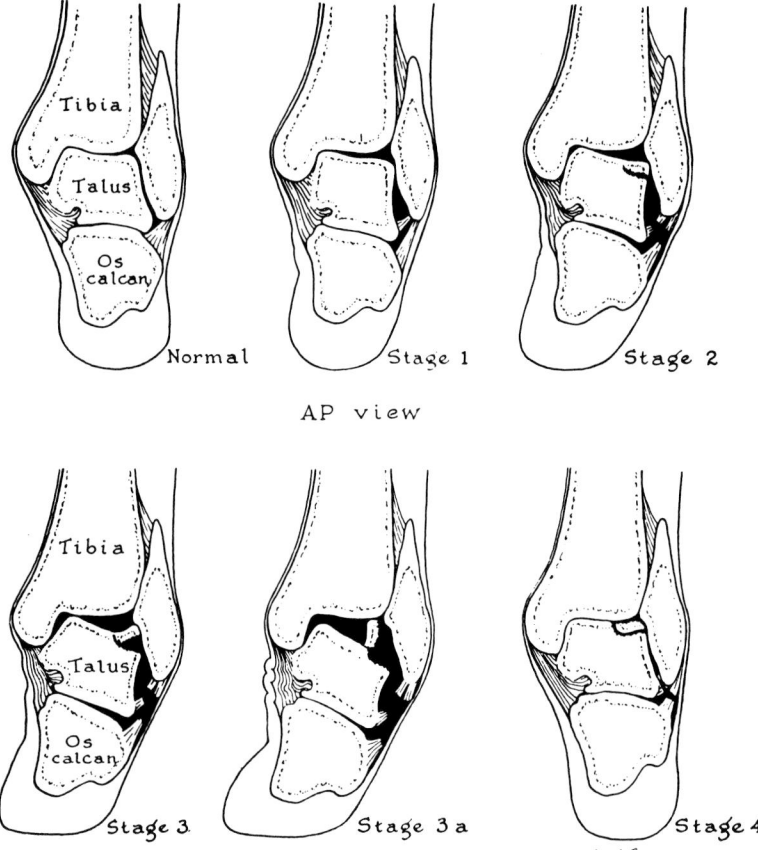

FIG. 9–117. Mechanism of injury in lateral talar dome fractures. During inversion of the foot, the lateral talar dome impacts on the fibula (Stage 1). If the force continues, the lateral ligaments rupture and the dome elevates (Stage 2). This fragment may remain in place (Stage 3) or become displaced (Stage 4) (from 221).

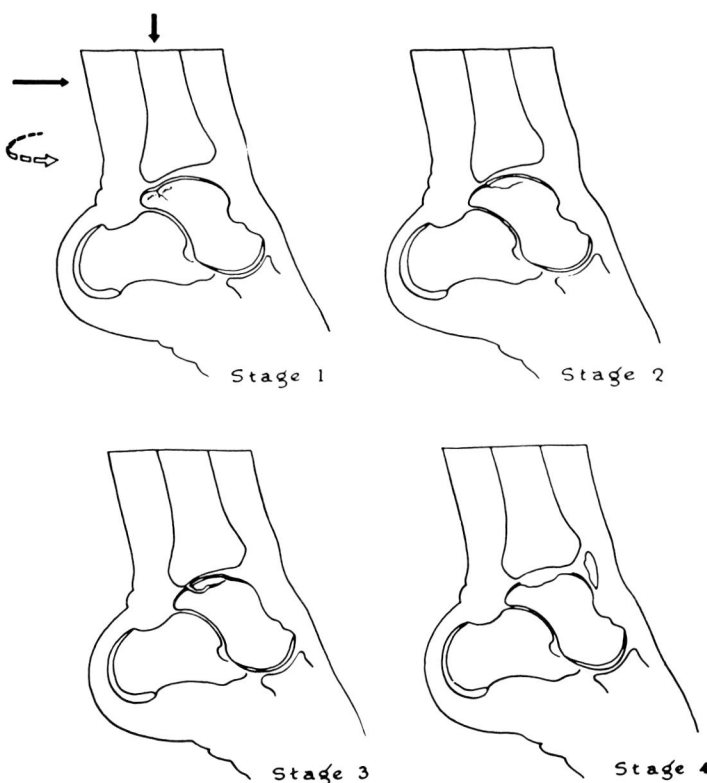

FIG. 9–118. Mechanism of injury of the medial talar dome. The foot is plantar flexed with inversion lateral rotation force applied during the injury. This can produce impaction of the dome (Stage 1). As the force continues the tibial lip elevates the fragment partially (Stages 2, 3) or displaces the fragment anteriorly (Stage 4) (from 221).

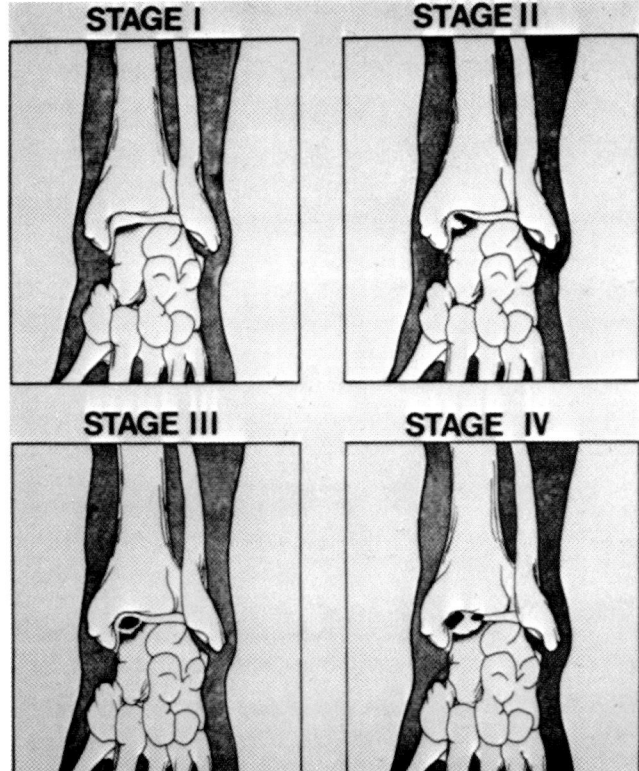

FIG. 9–119. Classification of talar dome fractures after Berndt and Harty (221). Stage 1, compression fracture. Stage 2, incomplete fracture with elevation. Stage 3, complete but undisplaced fracture. Stage 4, complete fracture with fragment loose in the joint (from 224).

symptoms. Males outnumbered females nearly 2:1 (216,247).

The mechanism of injury and radiographic appearance of medial and lateral talar dome fractures differs significantly. Lateral fractures are due to inversion or inversion dorsiflexion injuries (Fig. 9-117). The fracture is shallow with a "flake-like" fragment (217,224). Medial lesions are deeper, not always clearly associated with trauma, and often less symptomatic (224). Traumatic lesions are due to lateral rotation of the plantar-flexed ankle (Fig. 9-118) (217).

The most commonly used classification for talar dome fractures was devised by Berndt and Harty (Fig. 9-119) (217). Stage I lesions are compressions of the talar dome with no associated ligament ruptures and intact cartilage. These lesions are the most subtle and rarely symptomatic. Stage II lesions are incomplete fractures with the fragment remaining partially attached. Stage III lesions are complete fractures but not displaced. Stage IV lesions are detached (217). Stages II–IV lesions can be overlooked due to the significant ligament injuries that accompany them (Figs. 9-117 through 9-119).

Diagnosis

Routine AP, lateral, and mortise views of the ankle are taken in patients with suspected fracture or ligament injury. Talar dome fractures are most easily detected on mortise, or occasionally on the AP, view (Fig. 9-120).

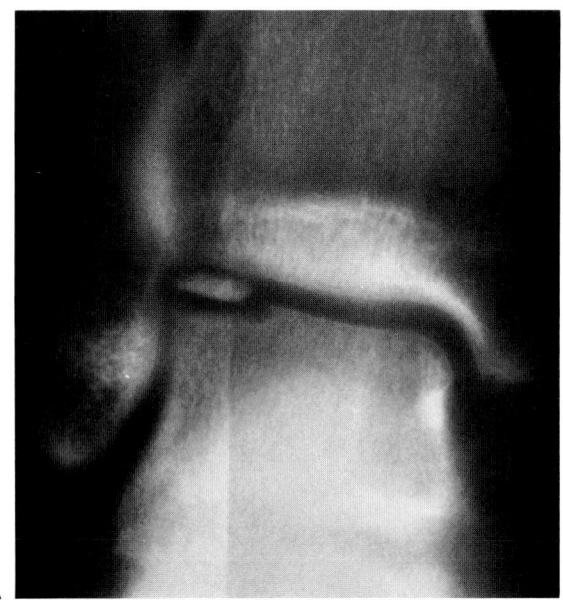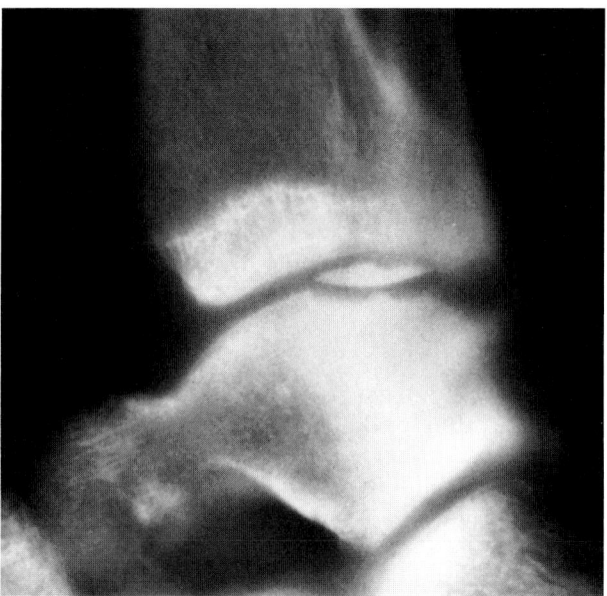

A   B

FIG. 9-120. AP (**A**) and lateral (**B**) tomograms demonstrate a Stage IV talar dome fracture. The fragment is completely rotated so the articular surface faces the talus instead of the tibial plafond.

The lateral view is rarely useful for identification of this fracture. However, the lateral view should be carefully evaluated for the presence of an effusion. The presence of an effusion should lead one to search more carefully for a talar dome fracture. Stage I lesions can be especially subtle. The only finding on routine views may be a subtle change in bone density at the margin (usually lateral) of the talar dome. If an effusion is present or clinical suspicion is high, tomography should be performed in both the AP and lateral projections (Fig. 9-120).

It is not uncommon to overlook this lesion on the initial examination (Fig. 9-121). Patients are commonly treated for an ankle sprain. It is imperative to keep this lesion in mind in all patients with ankle sprains. When a history of inversion injury, exercise-related ankle pain, clicking, or catching, and persistent swelling is present, one should definitely pursue the possibility of an osteochondral fracture (254,270). If the injury is more than 48 hours old, isotope scans can be used to identify the site of injury. This is important because other fractures (see Table 9-3) can also mimic ankle sprains. Following isotope studies, tomography should be performed to clarify the type and significance of the lesion (Fig. 9-120) (222). Over 20% of lesions are missed if tomography is not performed (247,254).

Once the lesion is detected, it is important to determine its exact site and size. This can be determined tomographically (Fig. 9-120) (266). The cartilage over the lesion may be intact or interrupted. This can be determined using double contrast arthrotomography or MRI (Fig. 9-122) (218,247,266).

Treatment

Opinions vary on the optimal treatment for talar dome lesions (221,231,257). Berndt and Harty (221) reviewed 201 cases, 43.7% lateral and 56.3% medial. The lateral lesions most often involved the middle third of the dome and the medial fractures, the posterior portion of the articular surface. Fifteen percent were Stage I, 36% Stage II, 28% Stage III, and 21% Stage IV lesions (221). One-hundred-forty-nine of the patients were treated conservatively and 73.9% had poor results. Patients treated surgically had good results in 78.6% of cases. Alexander and Lichtman (216) found better results with drilling and curettage, followed by non-weight bearing and early range of motion exercises. Their results were also excellent in chronic lesions. Canale and Belding (224) recommended conservative treatment for Stages I and II lesions reserving surgery for patients if this is unsuccessful. Surgery was recommended for all Stages III and IV lesions. More recently, arthroscopy has been used to evaluate the articular cartilage and determine whether arthroscopic or conventional surgery is required (257).

Complications

Symptoms are often more prolonged and displacement of lateral lesions, more common. The most common complication is osteoarthritis (224,243). This is evident in 50% of patients regardless of the treatment employed (224). Displaced fragments lose their blood

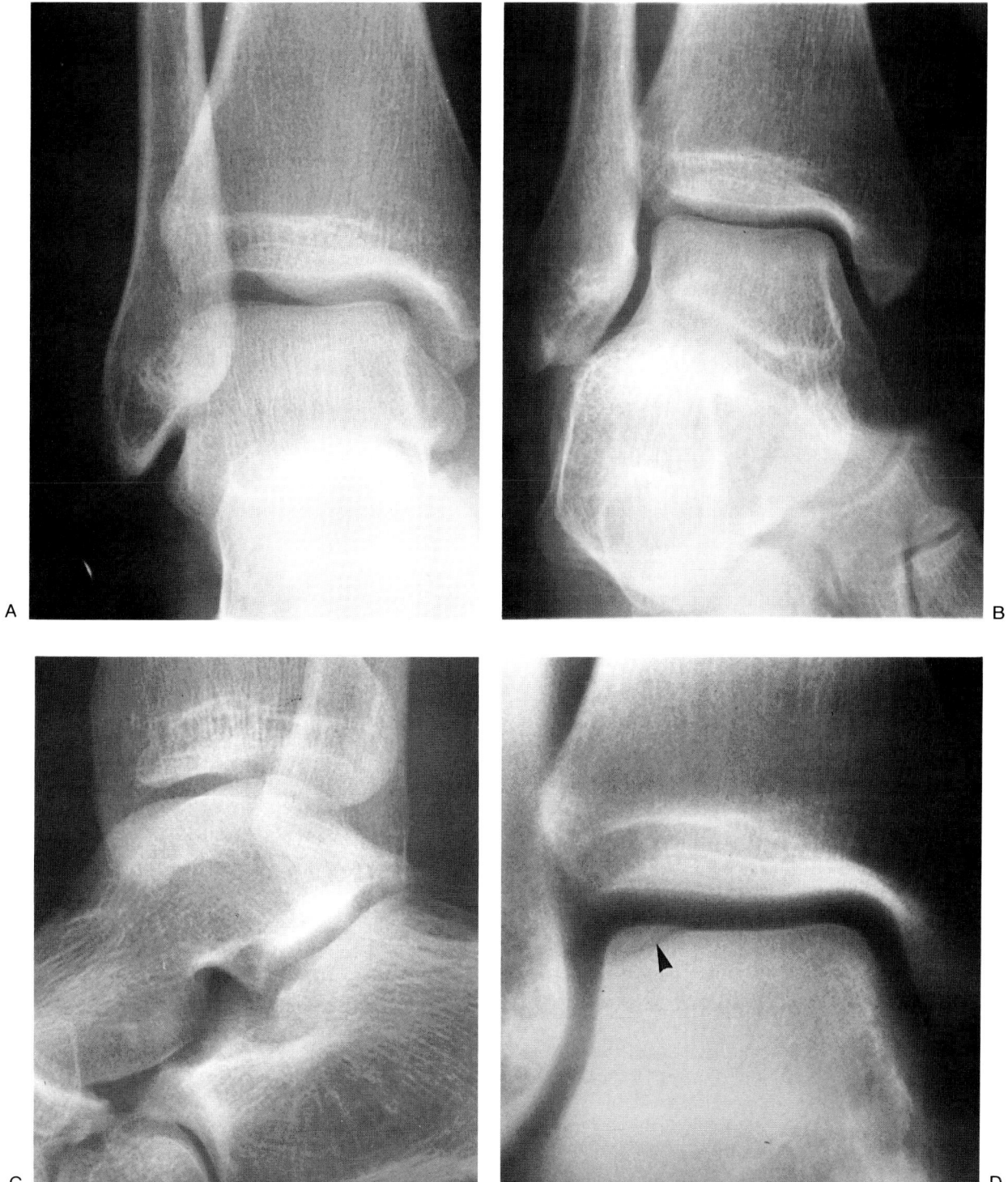

FIG. 9–121. AP (**A**), mortise (**B**), and lateral (**C**) views of the ankle in a patient presenting with symptoms of an ankle sprain. Tomograms (**D**) clearly demonstrate an undisplaced lateral talar dome fracture (*arrow*).

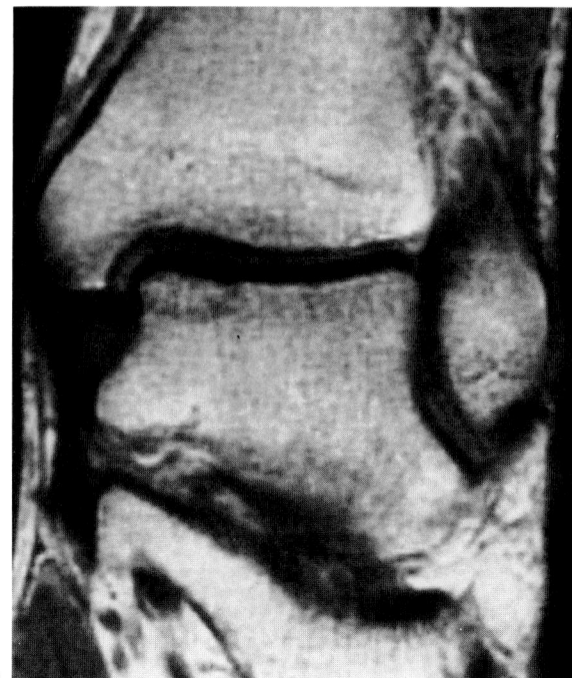 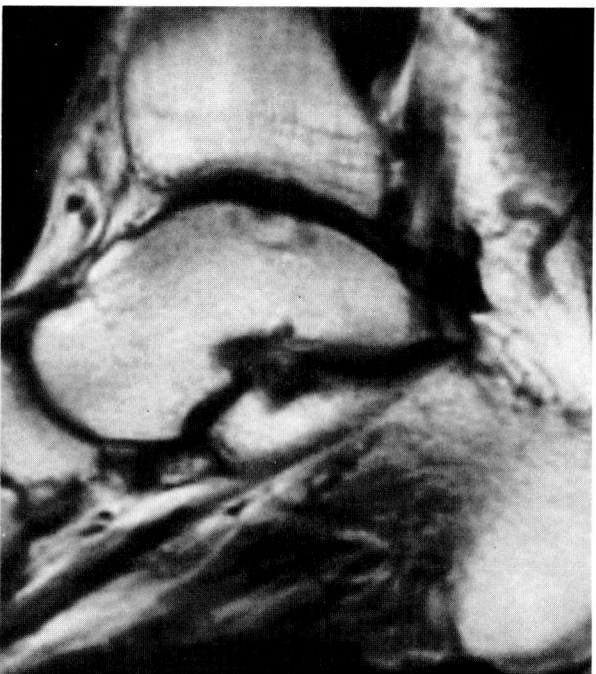

A

B

FIG. 9-122. Coronal (**A**) and sagittal (**B**) MR images (TE 20, TR 600) of a medial talar dome fracture. The cartilage is intact.

supply and are susceptible to avascular necrosis. Subchondral cyst formation has also been reported, presumably due to intrusion of synovial fluid through defects in the articular cartilage and subchondral bone (271).

Talar and Subtalar Dislocations

The majority of eversion and inversion motion occurs at the subtalar joint. Inversion is limited by the interosseous ligament, peroneal tendons, and lateral ankle ligaments. Eversion is limited by the deltoid ligament, posterior tibial tendon, and anterior tibial tendon (218,246,247).

The talus and calcaneus are connected by joint capsules and the lateral, medial, interosseous, and cervical ligaments. The talonavicular ligament provides less support than the talocalcaneal group (230,236).

Pure subtalar dislocations occur with simultaneous dislocation of the talocalcaneal and talonavicular joints. Total talar dislocation occurs when the talus is dislocated from the ankle mortise in addition to the above joints (229,236,246).

Subtalar dislocations are uncommon (1.3–2% of all dislocations) (227,237,263). Fifteen percent of all talar injuries are due to dislocation (254). Most injuries occur during significant falls with inversion forces, motor vehicle accidents, or landing on the inverted ankle in sporting events (227,263,267). Bilateral dislocations have been reported with Ehlers-Danlos syndrome (238). The injury is rare in children. DeLee and Curtis (227) re-

ported the average age to be 33.6 years. The incidence of subtalar dislocations in males is 6–10 times higher than in females (230).

Subtalar dislocations may be medial (56%), lateral (34%), posterior (6%), or anterior (4%) (267). With medial dislocations, the talus remains in the ankle mortise and the calcaneus and navicular are dislocated medially (inversion force). Lateral dislocations occur with eversion injuries (227). DeLee and Curtis (227) reported a higher incidence of associated fractures with lateral dislocations. Articular fractures of the talus, navicular, or calcaneus occurred in 75% of patients with lateral dislocation compared to 45% with medial dislocations. Lateral dislocations are also more commonly open injuries (227,236). Associated malleolar fractures or fractures of the fifth metatarsal base can occur with any subtalar dislocation.

Total dislocation is uncommon but potentially one of the worst hindfoot injuries (263). Detenbeck and Kelly (229) noted only 9 cases of total talar dislocations from 1959–1967. Seven of nine cases were open injuries and required open reduction. Despite aggressive reduction and adequate position 7 of 9 eventually required talectomy due to infection (Fig. 9-123). Most infections were severe enough to require open drainage and/or irrigation.

Diagnosis

Routine radiographs of the foot and ankle are usually sufficient to diagnose subtalar or total talar dislocation

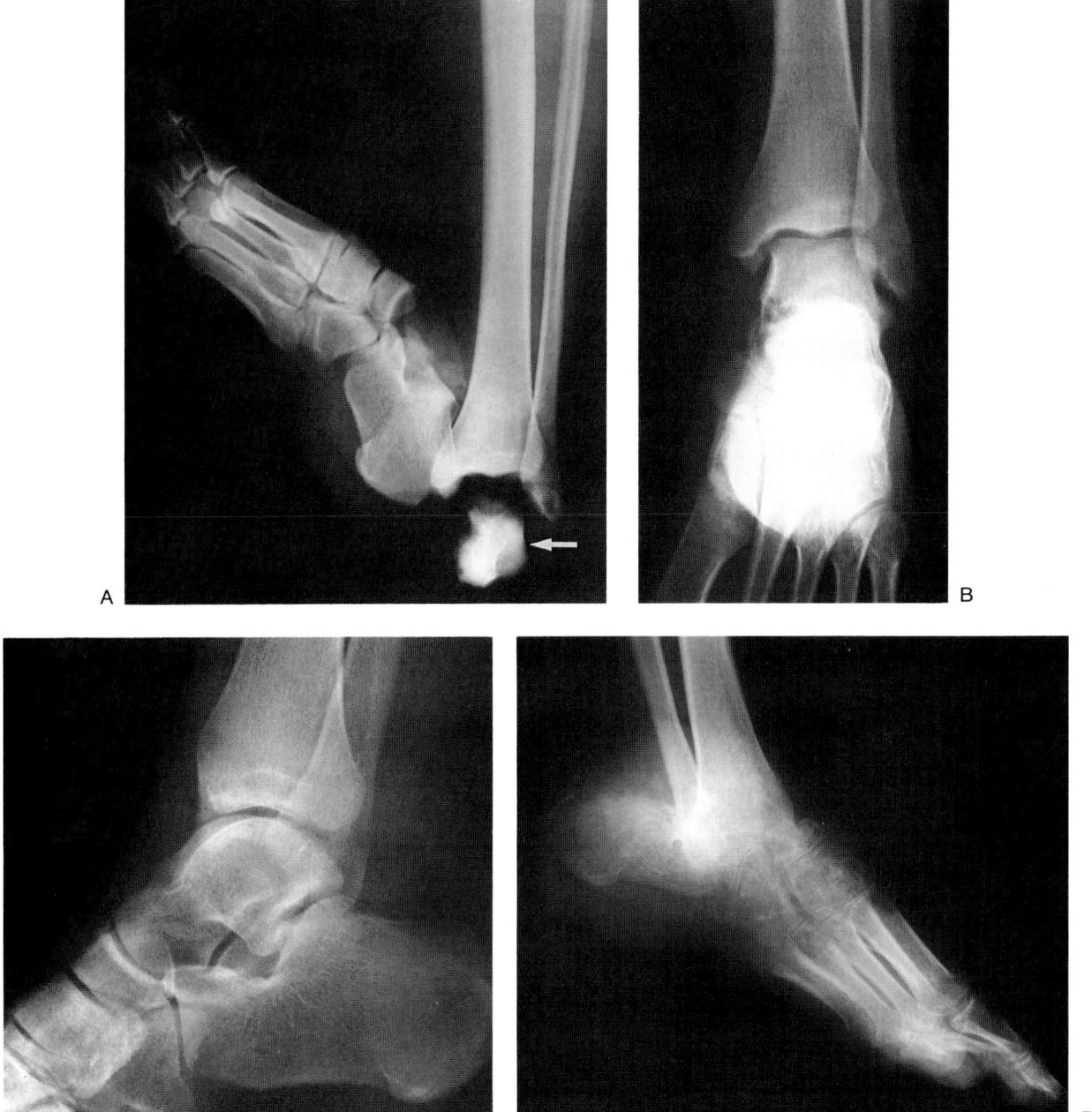

FIG. 9-123. AP (**A**) radiograph of the foot and ankle following total talar dislocation. The talar dome is directed laterally (*arrow*). Following reduction, the talus is in normal position on the AP (**B**) and lateral (**C**) views. Because of chronic infection and persistent drainage, a talectomy (**D**) was performed nearly one year later (from 229).

(Fig. 9-123). In certain cases, stress views may be useful. Associated fractures should be looked for carefully following reduction (263). Tomography or occasionally CT are best for this purpose (232,247,264,269).

Treatment

Prompt reduction and early motion (3 weeks after injury) should be the goals of treatment. The latter is particularly important to maintain subtalar motion. Medial dislocations can more often be reduced using closed techniques than can lateral subtalar dislocations. When there are associated fractures, immobilization in casts is longer, leading to poorer results (229,236). Inability to reduce dislocations has been reported. The posterior tibial tendon becomes entrapped making it impossible to reduce lateral dislocations (227,240,242).

Because of the high incidence of infection and the need for eventual talectomy, Detenbeck and Kelly (229) suggest early talectomy. The morbidity and problems with infection and AVN are reduced. Avascular necrosis almost always accompanies total talar dislocation.

Calcaneal Fractures

The calcaneus is the largest tarsal bone, and, because of its complex anatomy, it can be difficult to image with routine radiographic techniques. It is composed of a thin cortical shell with sparse trabecular bone, especially in adults (281,291). The superior surface has three facets that articulate with the anterior, mid-, and posterior talar facets. The middle facet is located on the sustentaculum tali and lies anterior to the sinus tarsi. There is a groove on the inferior surface of the sustentaculum for the flexor hallucis longus. The posterior facet (largest of the three) forms the posterior border of the sinus tarsi (279,287,297).

The calcaneus is the most commonly fractured bone in the adult foot accounting for 60% of foot fractures and 2% of all skeletal fractures (274,279,287). Fractures occur most commonly in males. Calcaneal fractures in children are much less common (5% of all calcaneus fractures), and the patterns differ from adult calcaneal fractures (278,294,298). Most calcaneal fractures in children are less extensive, and compression is less likely to occur due to the cancellous bone (294,298). Also, unlike

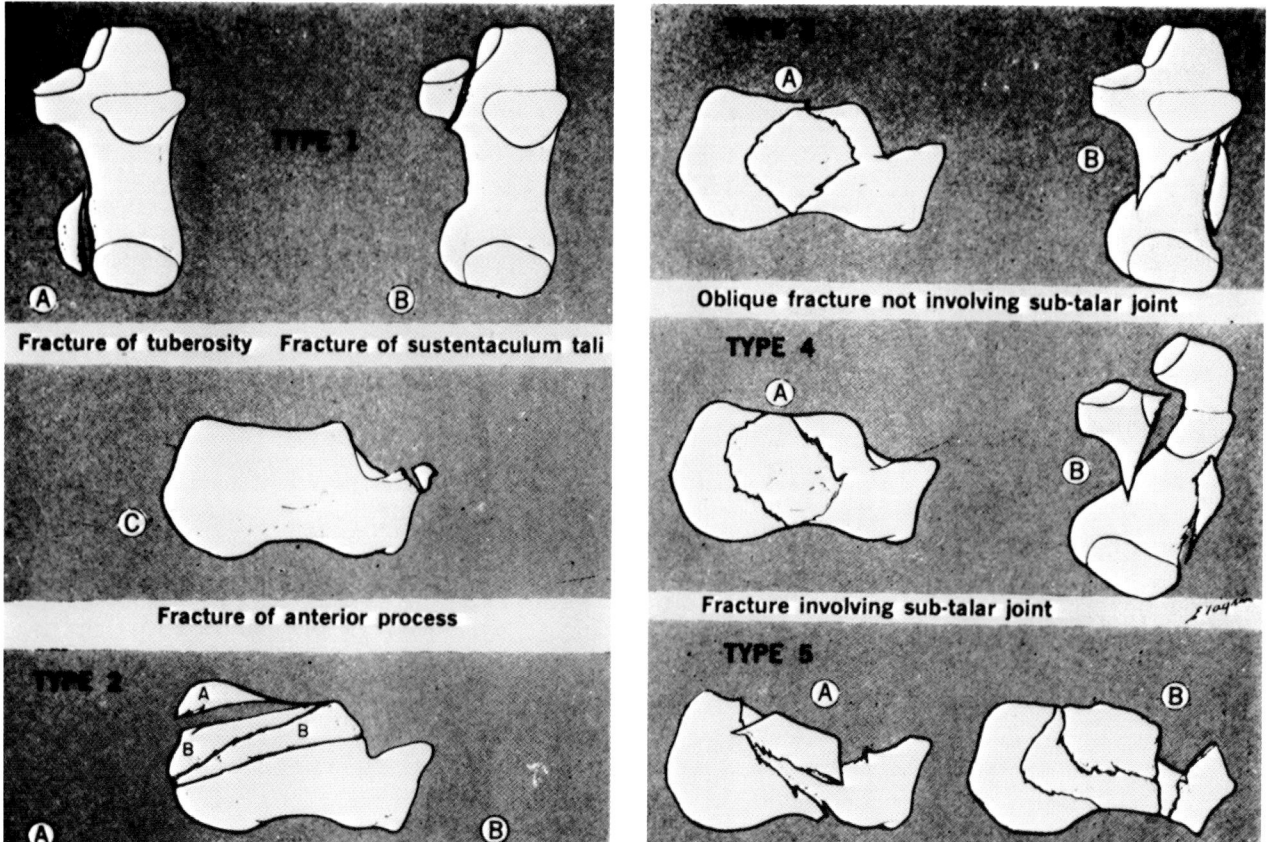

FIG. 9–124. Rowe classification of calcaneal fractures (from 293).

TABLE 9–11. *Essex-Loprestic classification of calcaneal fractures*[a]

I. No subtalar joint involvement
  A. Tuberosity fractures
    1. Beak type
    2. Medial avulsion
    3. Vertical
    4. Horizontal
  B. Calcaneocuboid joint involvement
II. Involving subtalar joint
  A. Undisplaced
  B. Displaced
  C. Gross comminution

[a] 275,287

the adult, calcaneal fractures in children are generally extra-articular. In adults, 70–75% of calcaneal fractures are intra-articular and 25–30% extra-articular. The adult calcaneus is more susceptible to axial loading resulting in frequent compression and displacement of the fractured fragments (287,291).

Mechanism of Injury and Classification

Most severe adult calcaneal fractures are due to falls or motor vehicle accidents resulting in axial loading of the calcaneus. Less severe avulsion and extra-articular fractures occur with twisting injuries or muscle pulls (277,287).

Classification of calcaneal injuries has been proposed by Rowe et al. (293) and Essex-Loprestie (275). The Rowe classification (Fig. 9-124) is less commonly used. Using this classification, Types I and II fractures are due to avulsion injuries. These may be subtle radiographically, especially anterior process fractures, and, if there is articular involvement, management is more difficult. Types III–V fractures are more extensive with more complex treatment considerations (287,293). Essex-Loprestie classification is more popular than the Rowe classification. This classification divides fractures into two major categories, intra-articular (involving the subtalar joint) and those not involving the subtalar joint (Table 9-11) (270,287). Types IIB and IIC are the most common intra-articular fractures (270). Schmidt and Weiner (294) combined the above classifications to provide a more general classification that could be used for adults and children (Fig. 9-125). The incidence of fractures in this classification is summarized in Table 9-12.

Type I fractures generally have a benign course and are due to avulsion or twisting injuries (270,287,293). However, Types IB, IC and ID do involve articular surfaces resulting in different treatment considerations. Apophyseal fractures (Type IA) occur only in children. Anterior process fractures (15% of calcaneal fractures)

(Type IC) can be particularly subtle (281,290). Patients often present with symptoms of an ankle sprain (see Table 9-3) (290). The most common mechanism of injury is inversion with internal rotation of the foot with the anterior process avulsed by the bifurcate ligament (287,290). A less common mechanism is a compression fracture ("nut cracker injury") with the foot dorsiflexed during varus stress leading to compression of the anterior process (Fig. 9-126). Other inversion fractures effecting the dorsal lateral calcaneus can be confused with sprain, anterior process fracture, or the os peroneum (a normal variant). Norfay et al. (288) noted this small, flake-like fracture in 10% of patients with suspected ankle fracture.

Type II fractures are due to direct trauma (IIA), usually with abruption contraction of the Achilles (IIB) when the ankle is in a fixed position (285,287). These fractures account for only about 4% of calcaneal injuries (285,293).

Types III–V injuries are usually due to axial loading. This may be a direct vertical force or posterior force directed toward the base of the posterior facet (Fig. 9-127). Generally, the fracture also involves the sustentaculum tali, which is commonly involved due to associated sharing forces (Fig. 9-128) (277). Type III fractures account for about 19% of calcaneal fractures and Types IV–V (intra-articular), 70–75% of calcaneal fractures (278, 287,293).

Type VI fractures involve the posterior calcaneus, tuberosity, and Achilles tendon. There is extensive posterior soft tissue injury. This injury commonly occurs with lawnmower accidents in children.

Radiographic Diagnosis

Routine radiographs in patients with suspected calcaneal fractures should include lateral, oblique, and axial views. Routine views are generally adequate for diagnosis of displaced fractures (Figs. 9-129 and 9-130). Care should be taken to measure Böhler's angle (see Fig. 9-33) and assess the degree of articular involvement. The latter problem and the need to detect more subtle injury may require further studies.

Special oblique views for the subtalar joint and anterior process have been described earlier in this chapter (276). In the acute setting, fluoroscopically positioned spot views are more easily obtained. Conventional or computed tomography are the techniques of choice in defining more complex fractures and foot anatomy. These techniques are not only important for diagnoses but also to assist in determining the type of therapy (277,279,287,289). Undisplaced Type I fractures are frequently missed. Schmidt and Weiner (294) noted that 81% of fractures overlooked radiographically fell into the

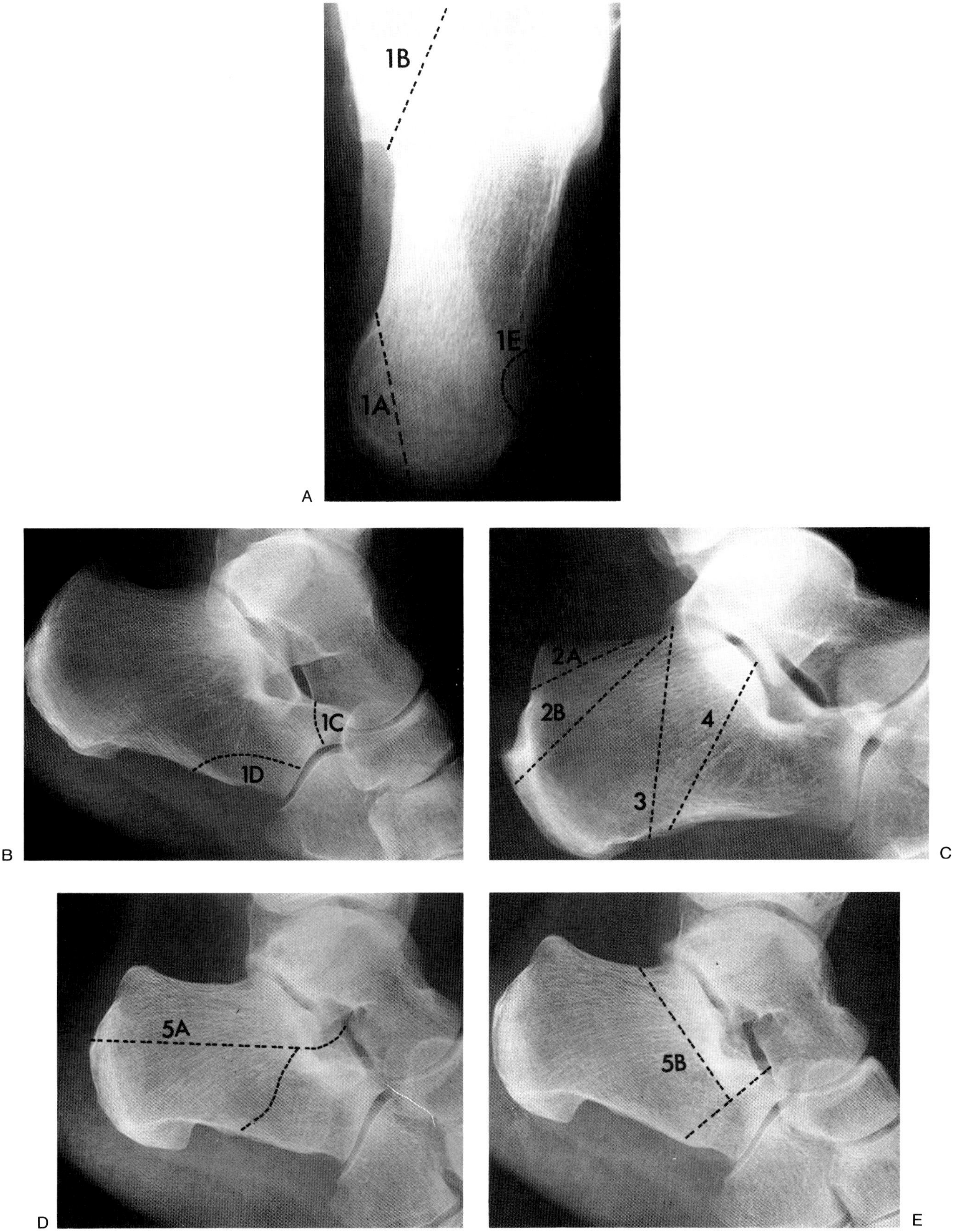

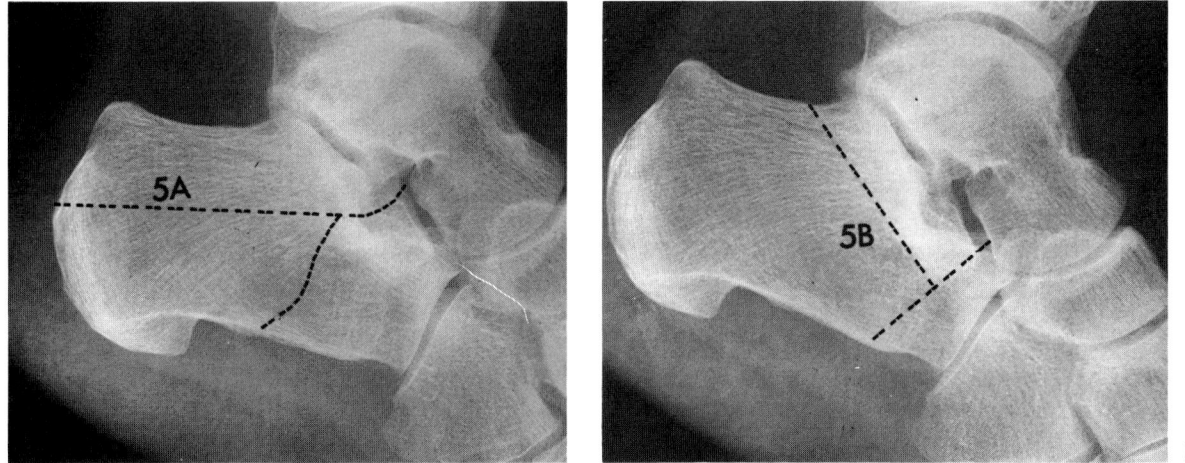

FIG. 9–125. Schmidt and Weiner modification of Rowe and Essex-Loprestie classifications for calcaneal fractures. **A:** Axial views of the calcaneus demonstrating Type 1A (tuberosity or apophysis fracture), Type 1B (fracture of sustentaculum), and Type 1E (avulsion fractures). **B:** Lateral view of the calcaneus demonstrating Type 1C (anterior process fracture) and 1D (inferolateral fracture). **C:** Lateral view of the calcaneus demonstrating 2A (beak fracture), 2B (Achilles avulsion fracture), Type 3 (undisplaced fracture without subtalar joint involvement), and Type 4 (linear fracture involving the subtalar joint). **D:** Lateral view demonstrating tongue-type compression fracture of subtalar joint (5A). **E:** Lateral view demonstrating joint depression-type fracture (5B) (from ref. 165, with permission).

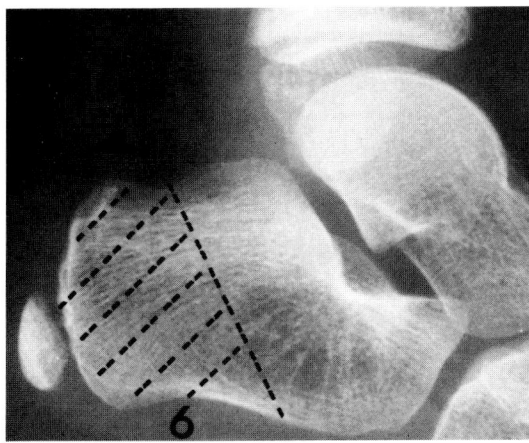

FIG. 9-125. *Continued.* **F:** Lateral view of the calcaneus in a child demonstrating extent of Type 6 fracture with loss of Achilles insertion (*arrow*).

TABLE 9–12. *Calcaneal fractures: Classification and incidence*[a]

Type (Schmidt and Weiner modification of Rowe and Essex-Loprestie)	Incidence
IC (anterior process)	15%
IA (tuberosity)	6%
IB (sustentaculum tali)	3%
ID, IE	1%
II (A, beak or B, Achilles avulsion)	3–4%
III (linear extra-articular)	19%
IV (intra-articular, linear)	10–24%
VA(tongue-type)	5%
VB (joint depression or comminution)	43–60%

[a] 275,294

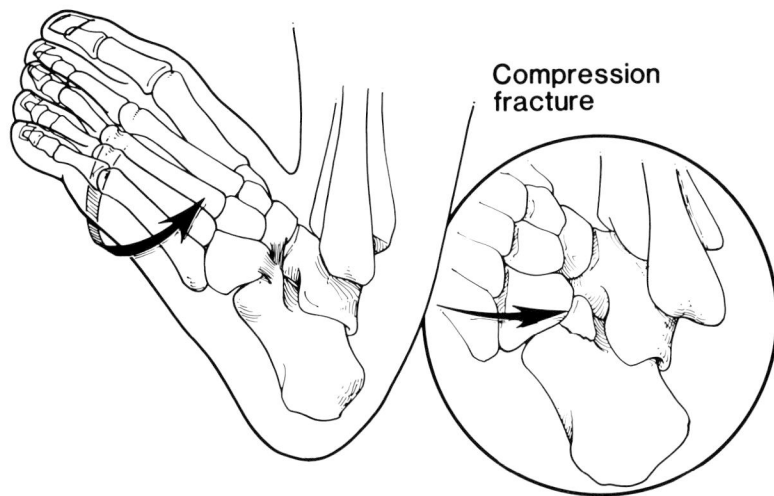

Compression fracture

FIG. 9-126. Compression injury of the anterior process (from 247).

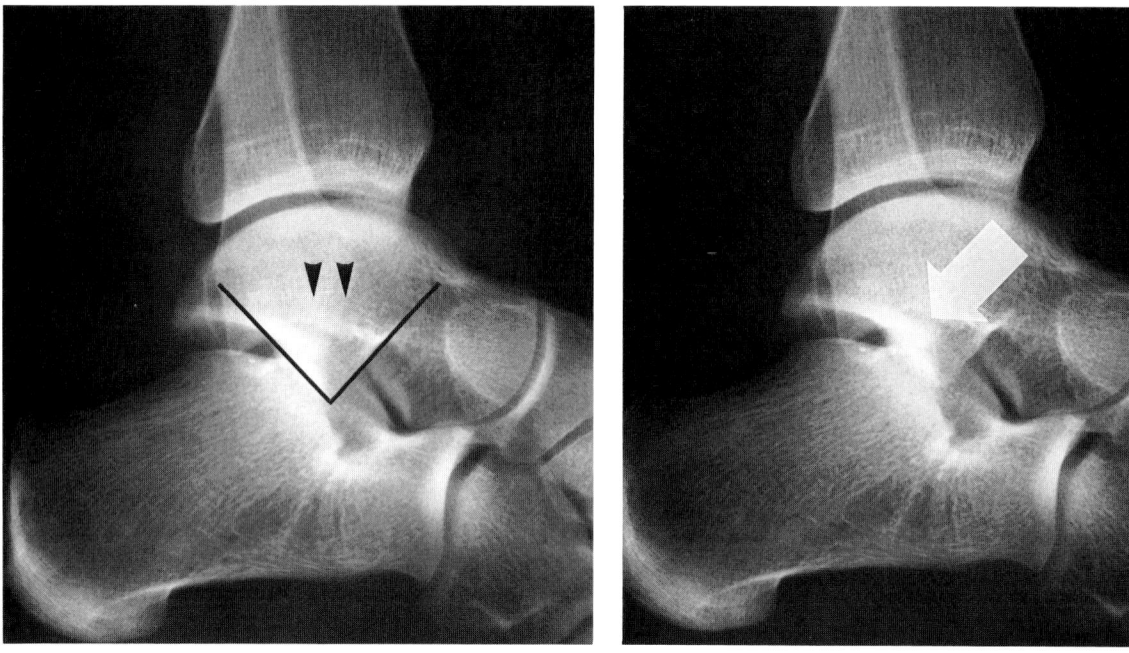

FIG. 9–127. Lateral radiographs (**A,B**) demonstrating the forces leading to intra-articular tongue and compression fractures of the calcaneus.

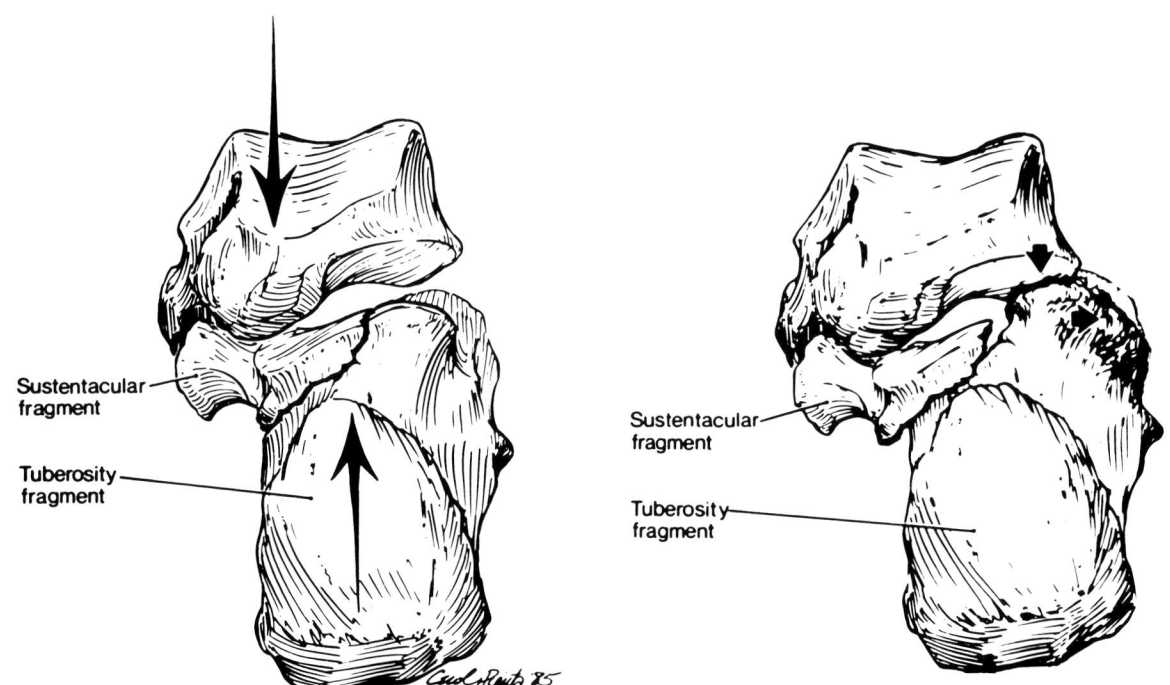

FIG. 9–128. Illustration of vertical forces leading to calcaneal fracture and sustentaculum involvement (from 277).

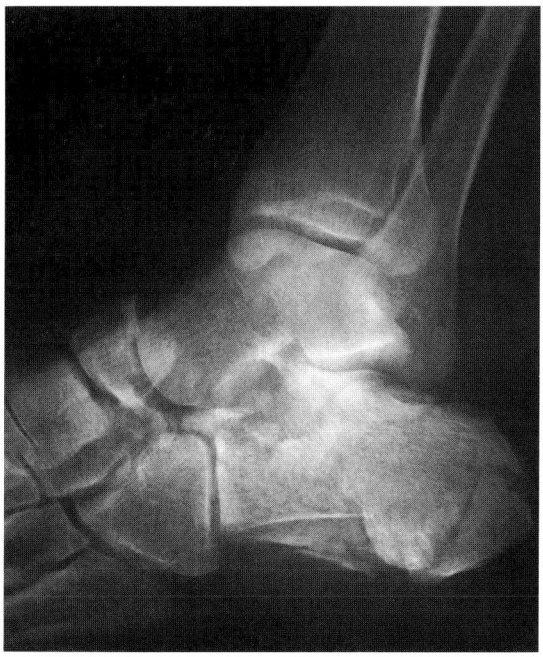

FIG. 9–129. Oblique view of the foot demonstrating a complex intra-articular calcaneal fracture (Type V). The navicular is also compressed.

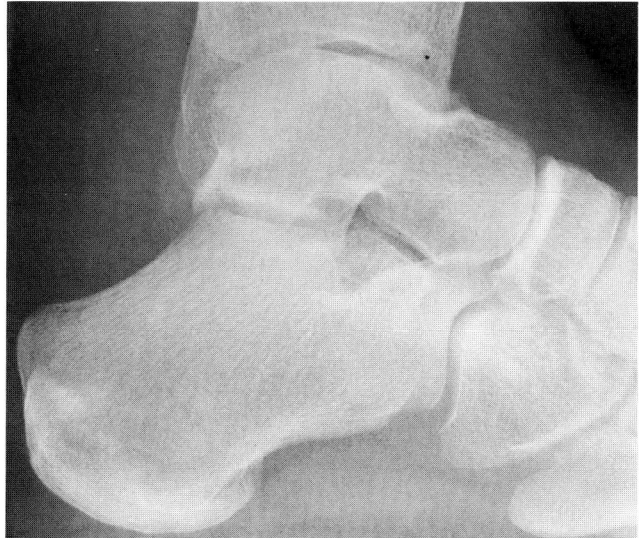

A

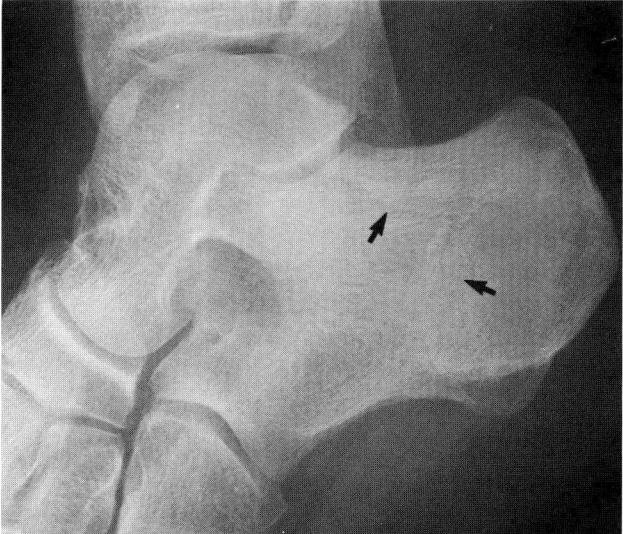

B

FIG. 9–130. Lateral (**A**) and oblique (**B**) views of the calcaneus. The undisplaced stellate fracture (*arrows*) is barely visible on the oblique view (**B**). One can assume the upper fracture line enters the joint space, but this cannot be confirmed without tomography or CT (Type IV).

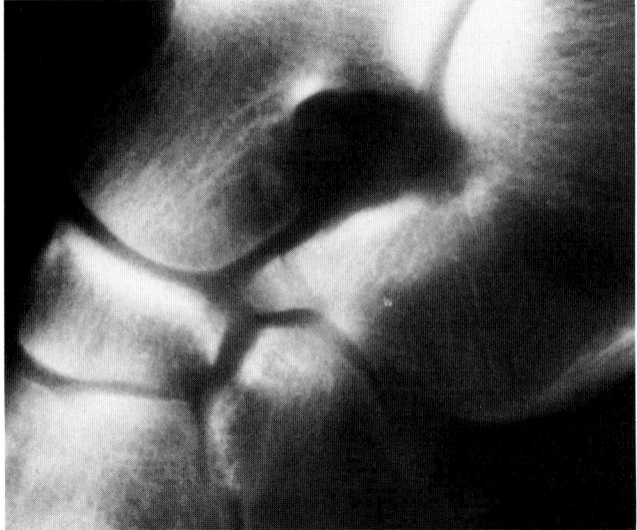

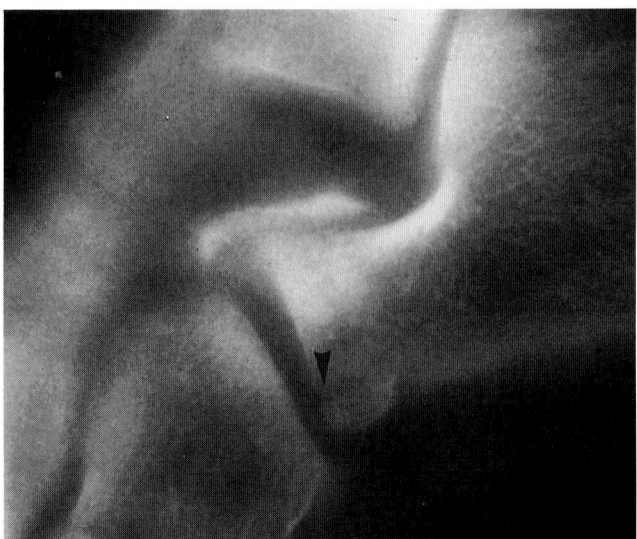

FIG. 9–131. Lateral tomogram demonstrating an undisplaced Type IC (anterior process) fracture. Up to 50% of these injuries can be overlooked without tomography.

FIG. 9–132. Lateral tomogram demonstrating both Type IC (anterior process) and Type ID (*arrow*) fractures.

Type I category. These fractures can be easily detected using conventional tomography (Figs. 9-131 and 9-132). Conventional tomograms can also be used in patients with intra-articular fractures (Fig. 9-133). However, generally CT is preferred. CT provides advantages in defining joint alignment, detecting intra-articular fragments, and the integrity of the sustentacular portion of the calcaneus. These are key factors in therapy planning (282,289,295). Soft tissue injury can also be assessed using CT (277,289,295). However, when tendon and ligament complications are suspected, MRI may provide

better information (Fig. 9-134). CT images are more easily reformated into three-dimensional display than are MRI. This needs to be decided prior to performing the examination so that 1.5-mm slices can be obtained in the axial and 30° coronal planes (295).

Treatment

Treatment of simple or extra-articular calcaneal fractures is much less controversial than is management of

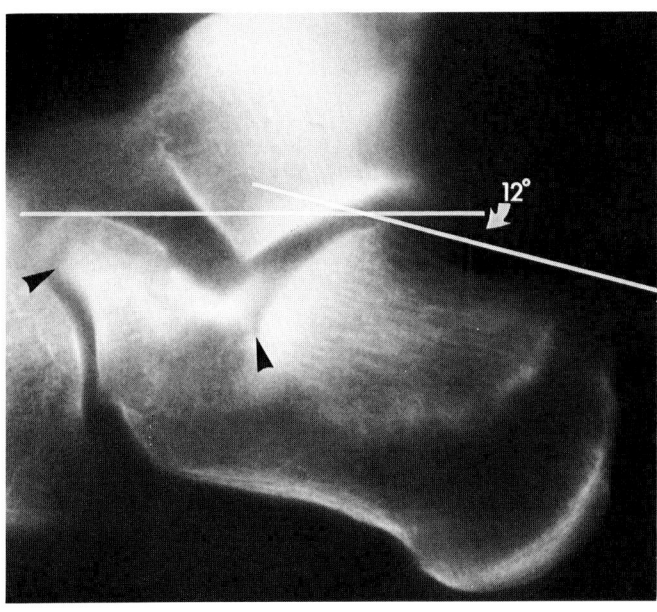

A

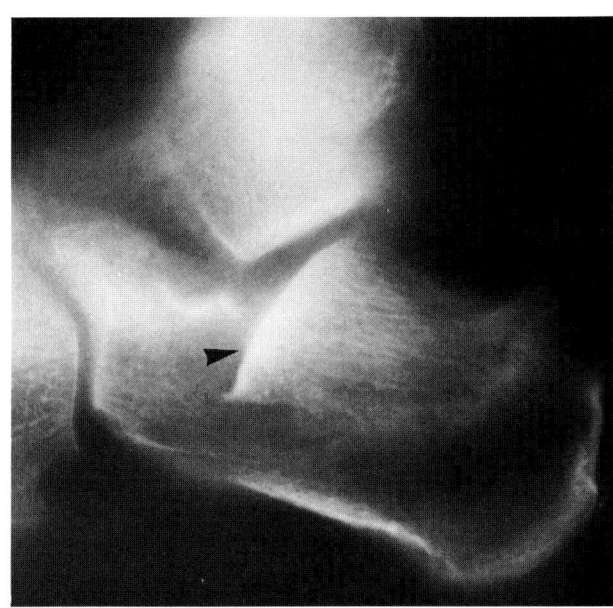

B

FIG. 9–133. Complex Type V calcaneal fracture with involvement of the subtalar and calcaneocuboid joints (*arrow*) on lateral tomograms (**A,B**). The joint involvement and decrease in Böhler's angle (12°) are clearly demonstrated.

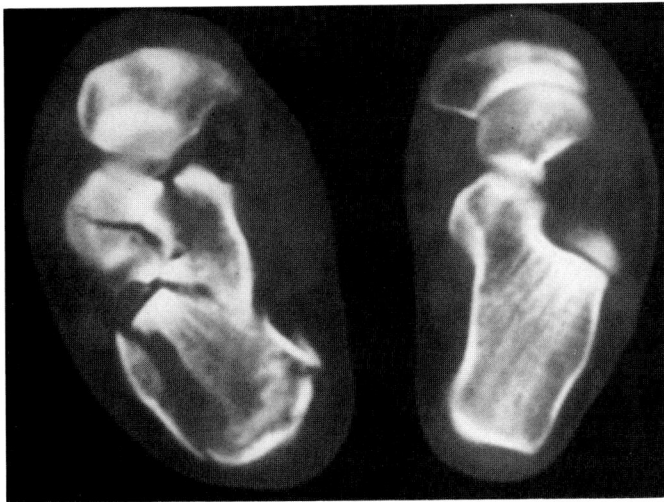

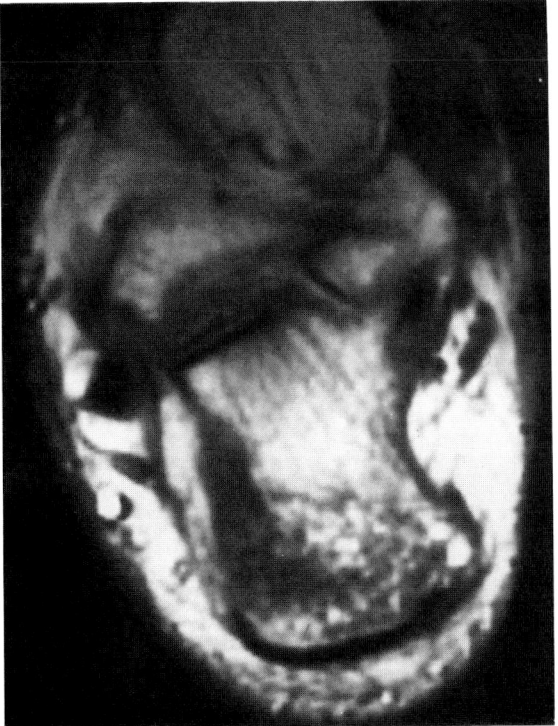

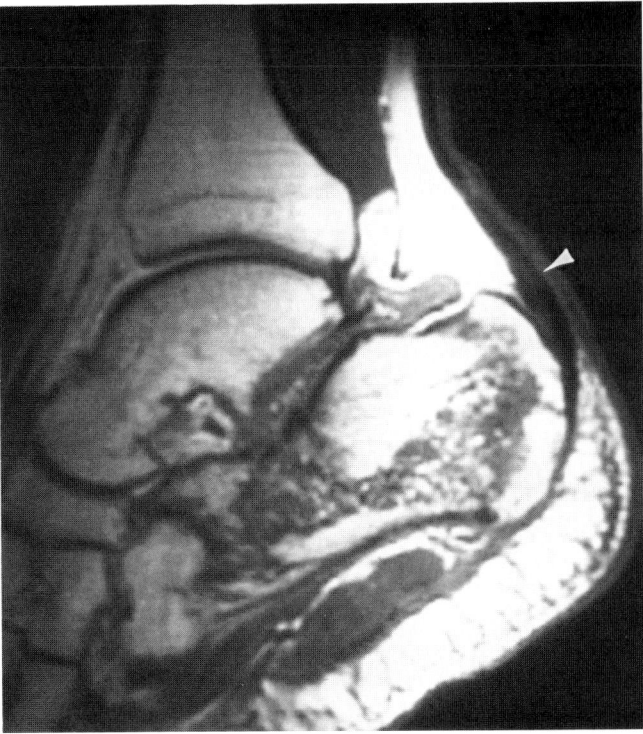

FIG. 9-134. Complex Type V calcaneal fracture. CT scan (**A**) shows the fracture, including slight displacement of the sustentaculum with involvement of the medial portion of the facet and widening of the calcaneus. Axial MR image (**B**) shows the fracture less clearly than the sagittal (**C**) image (TE 25, TR 500). However, the tear in the Achilles tendon (*arrow*) is more easily seen (from ref. 165, with permission).

complex intra-articular fractures (273,286,287,293). The goals of treatment are to reestablish the articular alignment (particularly the posterior facet (Böhler's angle) (272) and maintain normal calcaneal width (292,293,296). Early motion is also important to maintain normal function (292). Fulfilling these criteria is more difficult with complex fractures. The importance of pre-therapy imaging to clearly define the extent of injury cannot be overstated.

Type I fractures (Figs. 9-124 and 9-125) are generally not difficult to treat if recognized. Diagnoses, as mentioned above, can be a problem (294,298). Most extra-articular (Type IA and IE) fractures can be treated with cast immobilization for approximately six weeks (287).

Fractures of the sustentaculum tali (Type IB) and those involving the calcaneocuboid joint (Types IC and ID, see Fig. 9-125) may require more aggressive therapy (270,286,287,293). Undisplaced fractures can still be treated with cast immobilization, although up to 12 weeks may be required for fractures with larger fragments. Displaced fragments may require internal fixation or excision depending upon their size and position. Computed tomography is very useful if the latter treatment decision is being entertained.

Type II and III fractures (Figs. 9-124 and 9-125) can also be treated conservatively. Occasionally, the Achilles avulsion fractures are significantly displaced, in which case internal fixation may be necessary (287,293).

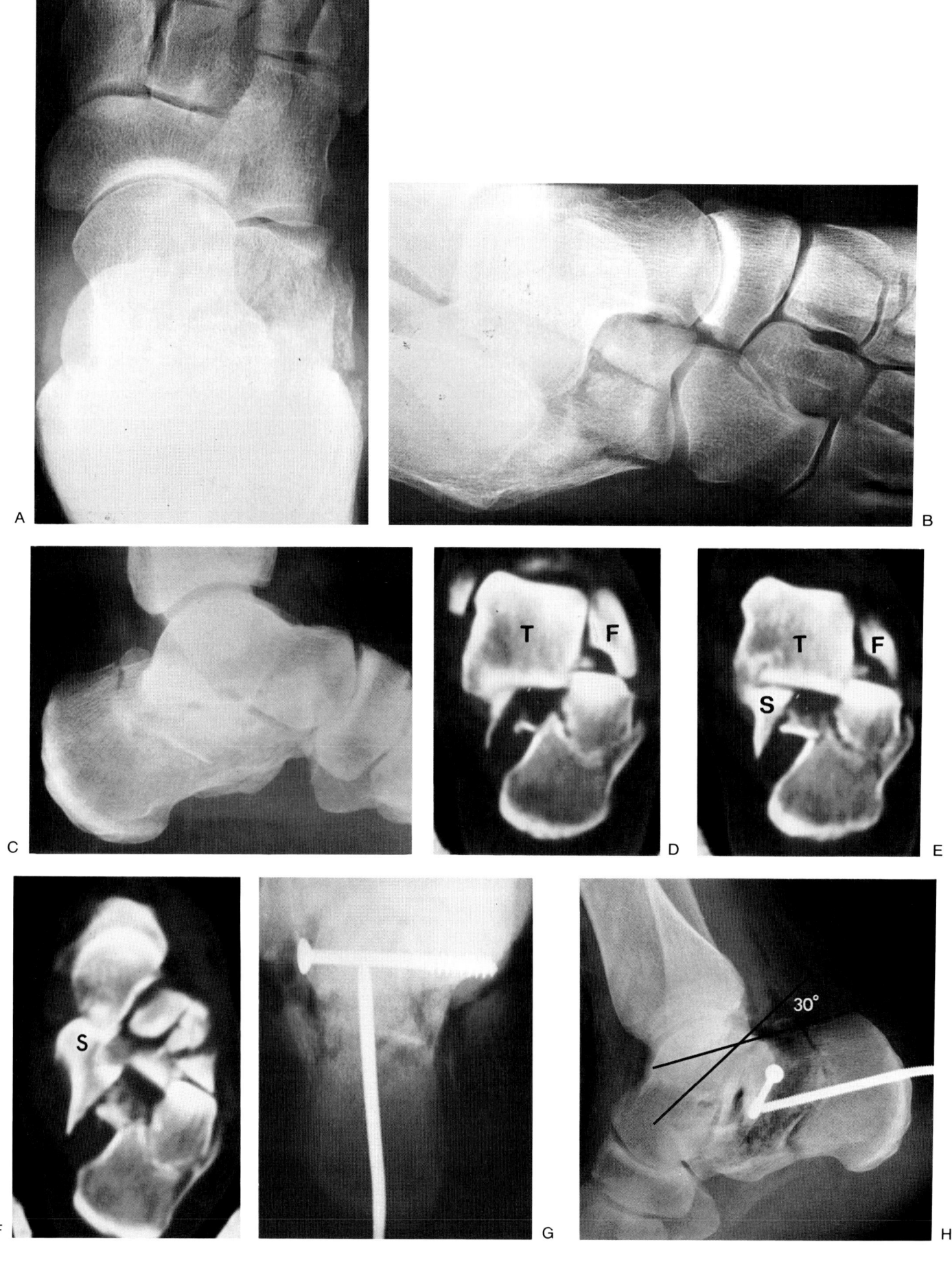

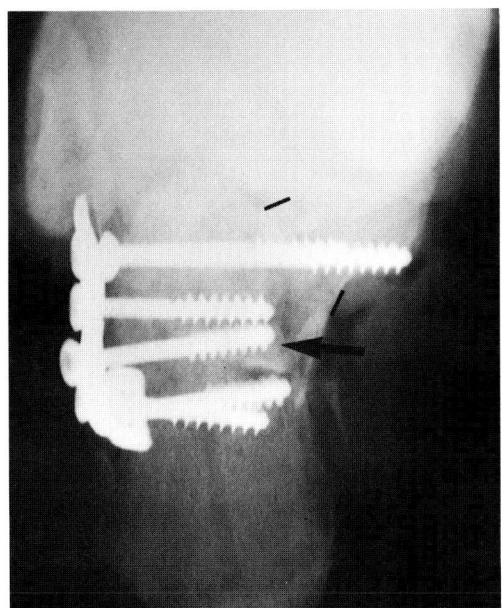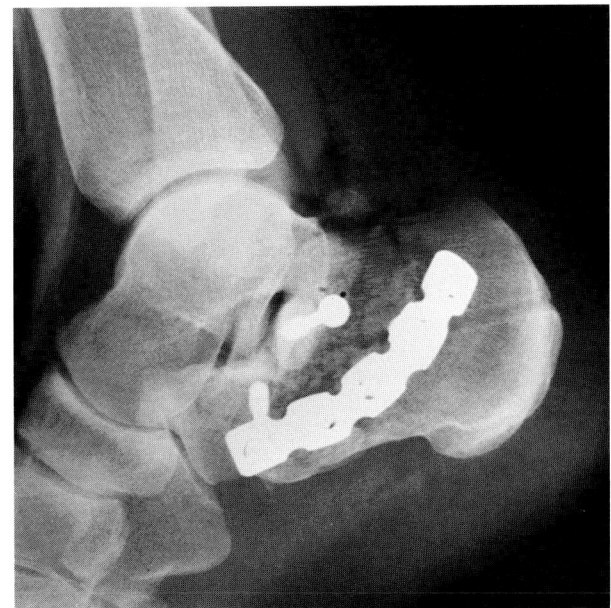

I   J

FIG. 9–135. *Continued.*

Treatment of patients with Type IV and V fractures is more controversial. Vertical forces applied to the talus via the tibial lead to an initial fracture in the coronal plane, which is located just anterior to the posterior calcaneal facet (Figs. 9-126 and 9-127). If the force continues, the calcaneus becomes divided into three major fragments. The first fragment consists of the tuberosity and lateral portion of the posterior facet, the second portion includes the sustentaculum and anteromedial calcaneus, and the third portion consists of the anterolateral calcaneus with the calcaneocuboid articulation. With tongue-type fractures (Type VA), the fracture line may extend medial to the posterior facet, through it, or lateral to the facet (292). The exact location of this is critical in planning the operative approach. This further points out the need for CT in preoperative evaluation of intra-articular fractures (Fig. 9-135). The talocalcaneal joints are best seen on coronal scans and the talonavicular and calcaneocuboid articulations are most clearly demonstrated on axial scans (209,222). Lateral radiographs are also important in demonstrating the degree of displacement of the posterior facet and reduction in Böhler's angle (217) (Fig. 3-115).

Multiple approaches to treatment of these fractures have been proposed. Subtalar arthrodesis and triple arthrodesis were considered appropriate for comminuted

fractures at one time. Open reduction with accurate reduction and fixation has become more popular recently (Fig. 3-117). If comminution is too severe and adequate reduction cannot be achieved, closed treatment with early motion may be the only option (217,222,223).

The results achieved by the various treatment methods are more closely related to the fracture pattern than to the treatment method. Although somewhat controversial, subtalar arthrodesis has been very successful in certain series. Hall and Pennal (280) and Johansson et al. (284) both reported 90% of patients treated with subtalar arthrodesis had satisfactory results with a return to work or normal activity in 6–7 months.

Immediate motion without specific reduction is no longer advocated, although up to 50% satisfactory results were reported at one time (217). Open reduction and internal fixation result in good to satisfactory results in 68–100% of patients (217).

CT is particularly useful in defining articular and certain soft tissue changes. However, because of its unparalleled soft tissue contrast and multiplanar imaging, MRI is better suited to evaluate soft tissue (nerve and tendon) injury and compartment syndromes.

The most common problem following calcaneal fracture is prolonged pain and disability (287). This occurs most commonly after Type V fractures. The average pe-

FIG. 9–135. AP (**A**), oblique (**B**), and lateral (**C**) radiographs of a complex intra-articular calcaneal fracture. CT images (**D–F**) demonstrate marked comminution with separation of the sustentacular fragment(s). There is a fragment between this and the body of the calcaneus that would prevent reduction. The lateral aspect of the subtalar joint is displaced between the talus (T) and fibula (F). Reduction was accomplished using open reduction with plate and screw fixation. Axial (**G**) and lateral (**H**) views taken during repositioning show of the fragments with re-establishment of Böhler's angle and width reduction. The reduction of the sustentacular fragment (*arrow*) is confirmed after all screws are in place (**I,J**).

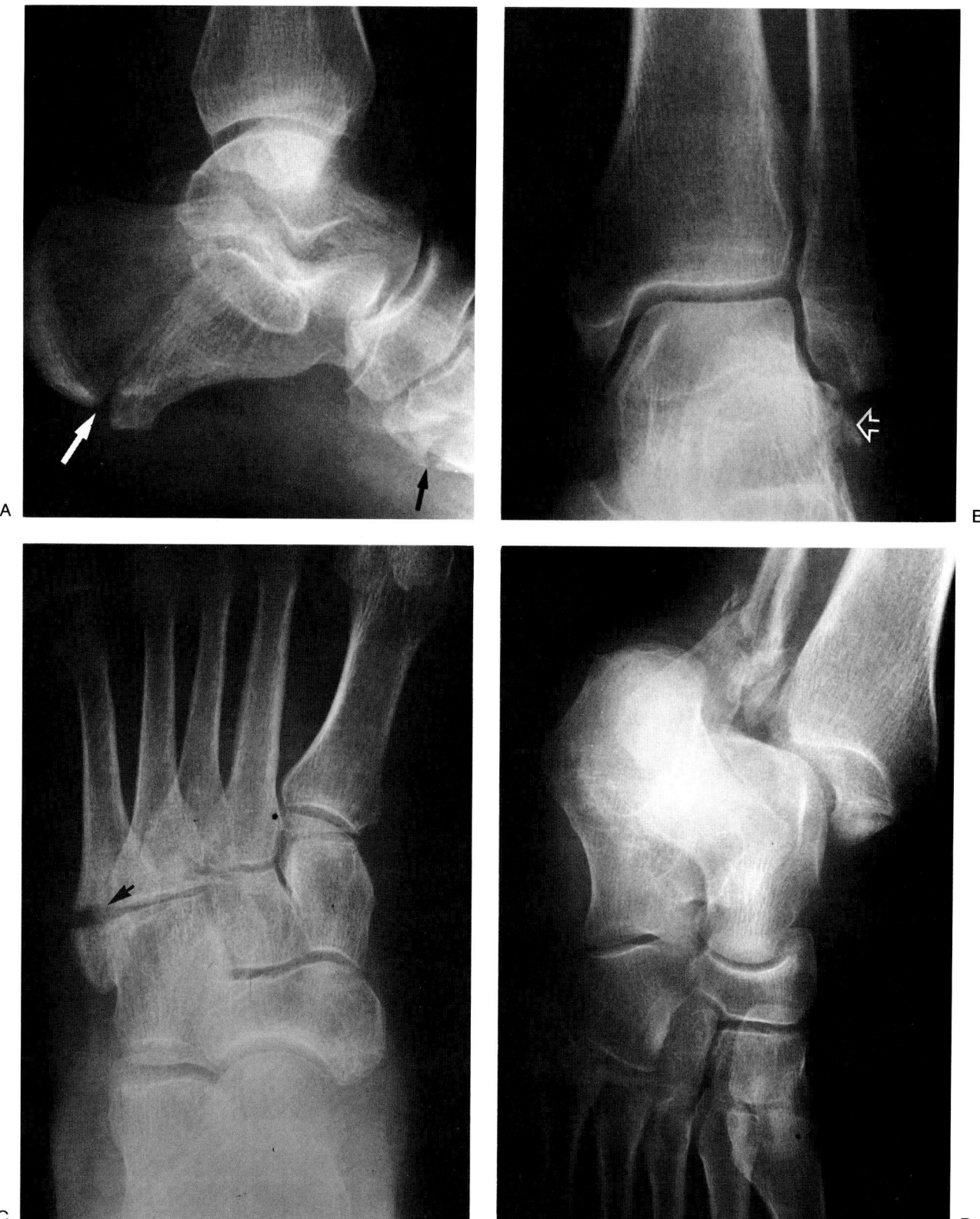

FIG. 9-136. Elderly patient with bilateral foot and ankle injuries after a fall. Lateral (**A**), mortise (**B**) views of the ankle and AP (**C**) view of the left foot show an intra-articular calcaneal fracture (*white arrow*), a fracture of the base of the fifth metatarsal (*black arrow*), and a lateral calcaneal avulsion (*open arrow*). Oblique (**D**) view of the right foot and ankle demonstrates comminuted fractures of the lateral malleolus and posterior tibia.

riod of disability is several months, but pain may persist for 2 years or more. Slatis et al. (296) reported that 2–6 years after fracture, only 28 of 86 patients (32.5%) were pain free. The etiology of the pain varies. Loss of motion was noted in 74–89% of patients. Early in the post-fracture period, pain may be related to altered hindfoot anatomy. Pain may also occur due to peroneal tendinitis or incomplete disruption of these tendons, plantar nerve entrapment, and, in the later stages, due to degenerative arthritis (286,287,289). Fibulocalcaneal abutment syndrome may develop due to widening of the calcaneus with fracture (Fig. 9-135). Compartment syndrome and tarsal tunnel syndrome can also result in persistent hindfoot pain (283,287).

Associated fractures are common with calcaneal injury (Fig. 9-136). Bilateral calcaneal fractures occur in 10% of patients due to the mechanism of injury—fall, landing on both feet (273).

Lower extremity fractures in the ipsilateral extremity have been reported in 20–46% of patients (Fig. 9-136) (273,296). Spine injuries, usually lumbar compression fractures, are associated with calcaneal fractures in 10–30% of adults (286,287,296).

Surgically related complications include skin infection, osteomyelitis, loss of reduction, and parasthesias, which may develop in up to 10% of patients (287). Infection, after surgical reduction with metal fixation devices, causes problems in imaging patients with suspected osteomyelitis. Metal artifact can cause problems with CT, conventional tomography, and, to a lesser degree, MRI (nonferromagnetic metal). Indium-111 labeled WBCs may be particularly useful in detecting subtle postoperative infection. (See Chapter 15, Infection).

MID- AND FOREFOOT INJURIES

Midfoot Fractures and Fracture-Dislocations

The midfoot is made up of the lesser tarsal bones (navicular, cuboid, and three cuneiforms). There is minimal motion in the articulations of these bones, and stability is greater laterally than medially. Additional plantar support is due to stronger ligaments and tendon reinforcement. The major joint (Choport's joint) is formed by the combination of the talonavicular and calcaneocuboid articulations.

Mechanism of Injury and Classifications of Midfoot Fracture-Dislocations

Injuries to the bones and midtarsal joints have been classified by Main and Jowett (323). Their classification is based on the deforming force and resulting displacement. Five categories of injury were established: (1) medial (30% of injuries), (2) longitudinal (41% of injuries), (3) lateral (17% of injuries), (4) plantar (7% of injuries),

and (5) crush injury (5% of injuries) (323). When forces are applied medially, the following injuries can occur: (1) inversion resulting in dorsal avulsion fractures of the talus or navicular and lateral margins of the calcaneous or cuboid (Fig. 9-137), (2) medial subluxation of the forefoot, and (3) rotational dislocation of the talonavicular joint, leaving the calcaneocuboid articulation intact (Fig. 9-138). This is less common than subtalar dislocation (323).

Longitudinal forces cause compression of the metatarsals with forces transmitted to the cuneiforms, compressing the navicular between the cuneiform and talar head. This causes lines of force and fractures to occur parallel to the articular margins of the cuneiforms (323).

Lateral forces are usually due to falls causing medial distraction that may lead to avulsion fractures of the navicular or talus and lateral impaction that causes compression of the calcaneous and/or cuboid. Lateral subluxation of the talonavicular joint may also occur (Fig. 9-139) (316,323).

Plantar forces result in talonavicular or calcaneocuboid subluxation or dislocation, with associated periarticular avulsion fractures (Fig. 9-140). With crush injuries, there is no consistent pattern of injury (316,323).

Isolated Tarsal Fractures

Isolated fractures of the tarsal bones without associated joint involvement are uncommon (314,316). The navicular articulates with the talar head proximally, and there are three facets on the distal surface that articulate with the cuboid and cuneiforms. There are ligament and tendon attachments on both the dorsal and plantar surfaces. The posterior tibial tendon attaches, in part, to the tuberosity of the navicular (301,308,314,316). Eichenholtz and Levene (308) described several categories of navicular fracture. In their study, 47% of navicular fractures were avulsions, 29% involved the body, and 24% were tuberosity fractures. (Stress fractures will be discussed in Chapter 16.) Avulsion fractures are caused by twisting or eversion forces with fragments avulsing due to the pull of the talonavicular capsule, or anterior fibers of the deltoid. These fractures should not be confused with the well-marginated cortex, which is seen on secondary ossification centers. Tuberosity fractures are also, in a sense, avulsion fractures (Fig. 9-140) as, again, either the posterior tibial tendon or anterior deltoid fibers is implicated during eversion of the foot (316). Most body fractures are associated with fracture dislocations of the midfoot (316,327).

Isolated fractures of the cuneiforms and cuboid are uncommon (Fig. 9-141) (314,316).

Radiographic Diagnosis of Midfoot Injuries

Imaging of the midfoot begins with routine AP, lateral, and oblique views of the foot. In many cases, subtle

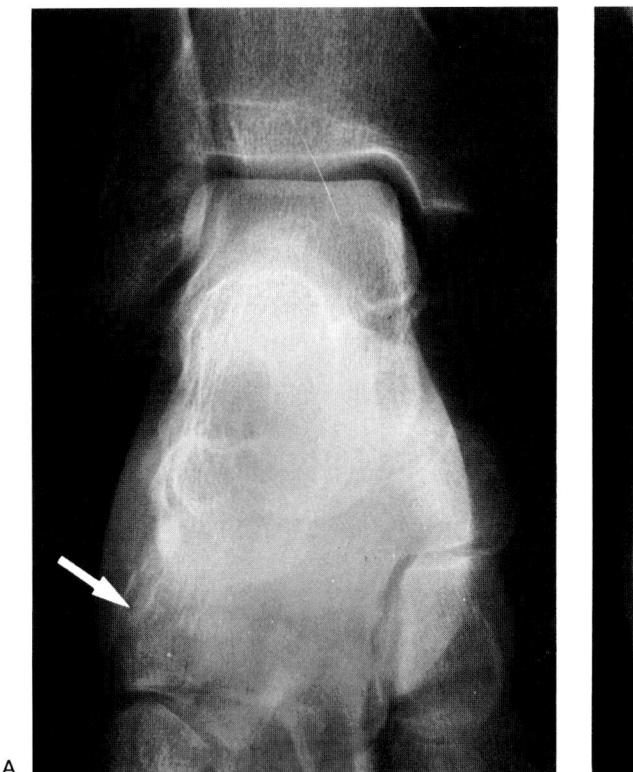 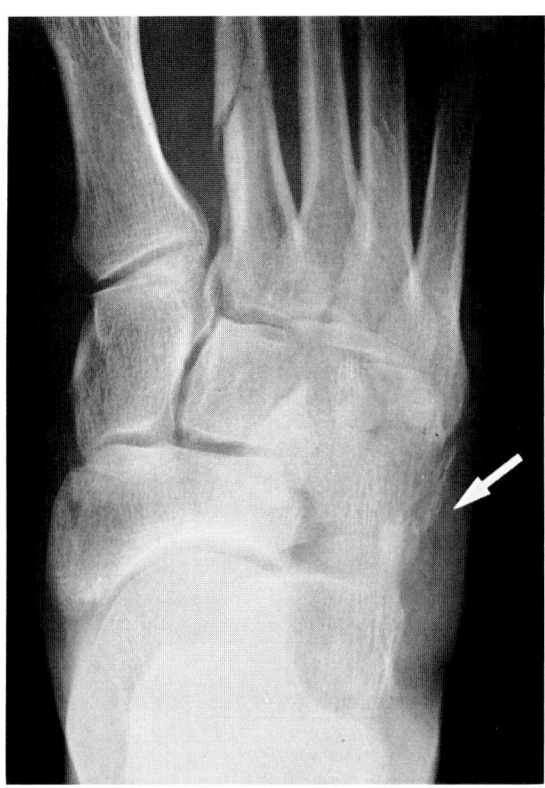

FIG. 9-137. AP (**A**) view of the ankle showing a cuboid avulsion fracture (*arrow*) due to a medial force inversion injury. The AP (**B**) view of the midfoot also shows this injury (*arrow*). There is also a fracture of the second metatarsal. Alignment of the tarsal bones is difficult to evaluate on this view.

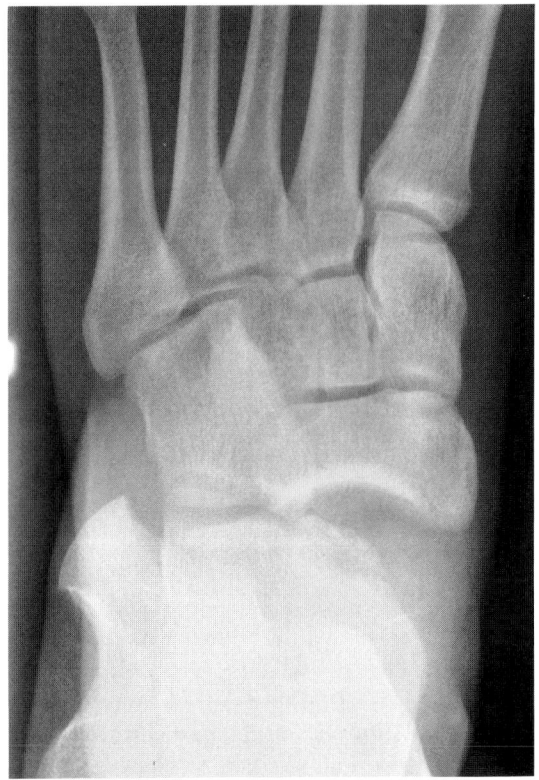

FIG. 9-138. AP view of the foot demonstrating swivel injury leading to fracture-dislocation of the talonavicular joint. The talus is displaced laterally and no longer articulates with the navicular.

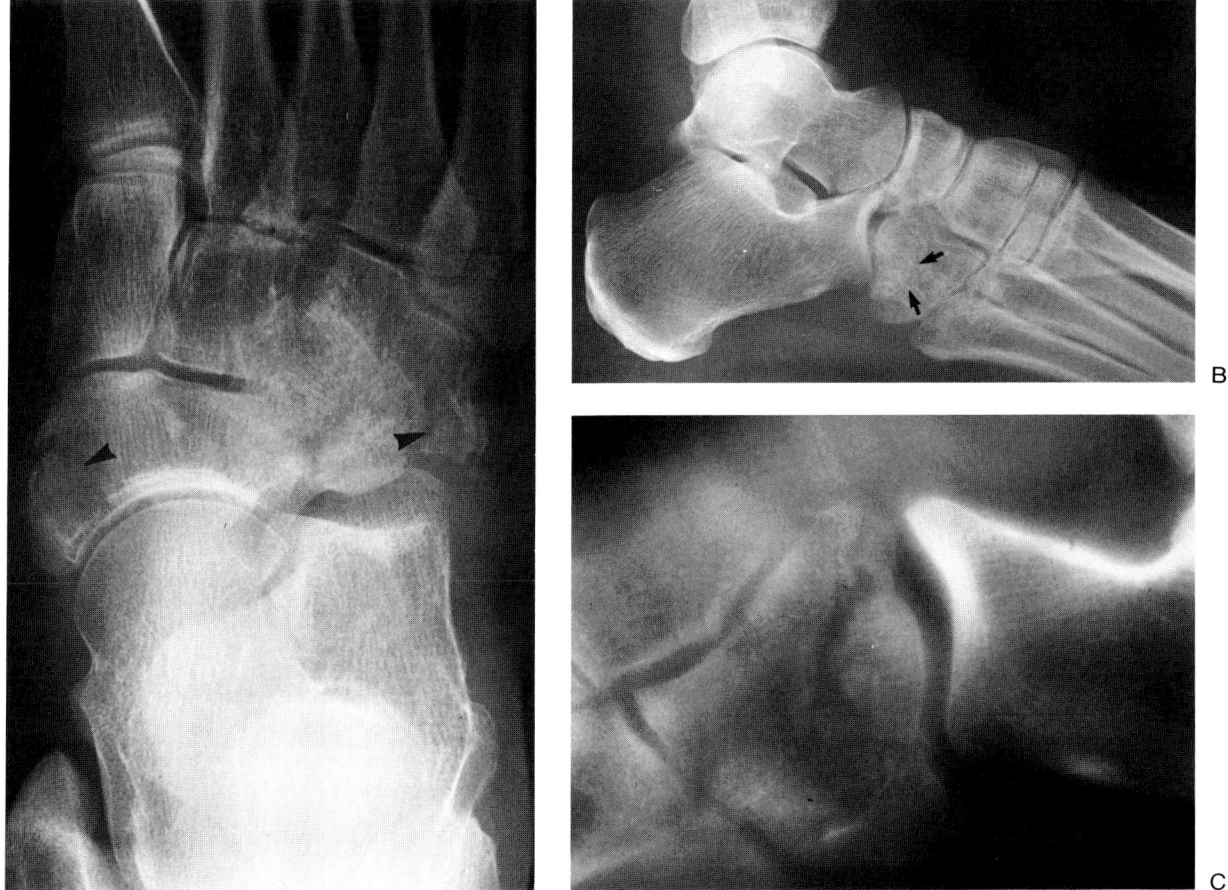

FIG. 9–139. Lateral injury of the midfoot. **A:** AP view of the midfoot showing a medial navicular fracture (*arrow*) and compression fracture of the cuboid (*arrow*). **B:** Lateral view shows only increased density (*arrows*) due to the overlying bony trabeculae. **C:** Tomogram more clearly demonstrates the complexity of the cuboid fracture.

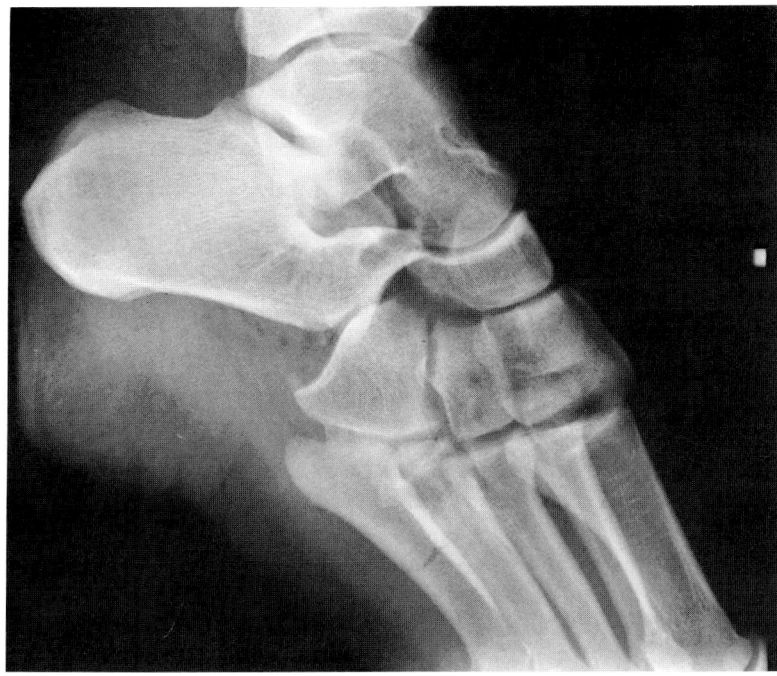

FIG. 9–140. Injury due to plantar force with plantar dislocation of the cuboid and associated avulsion fractures.

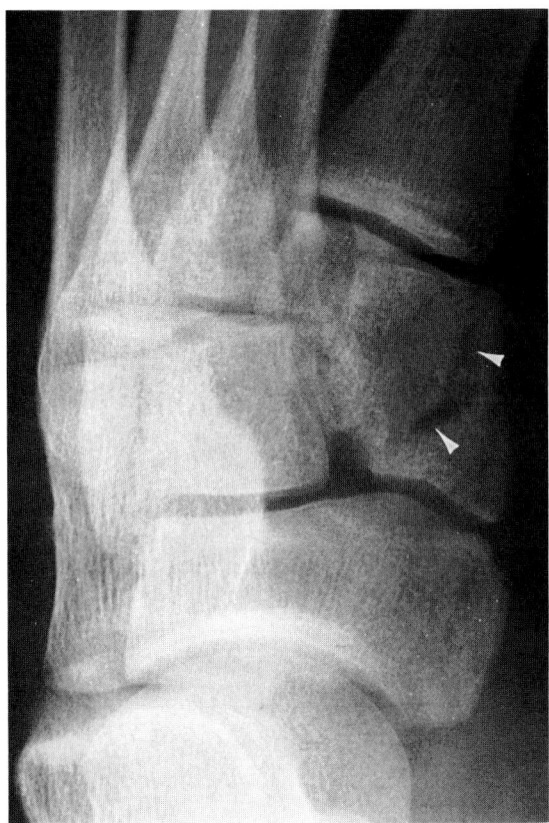

FIG. 9-141. Fluoroscopically positioned view of the midfoot. The foot is externally rotated or inverted to demonstrate the oblique undisplaced fracture of the medial cuneiform (*arrows*) (from ref. 165, with permission).

subluxations, avulsion fractures, or undisplaced fractures are difficult to identify. Main and Jowett (323) reported delay in diagnosis in over 41% of patients using routine views. One should carefully study the soft tissues. Swelling or hemorrhage, which causes distortion of the fat planes, may provide a valuable clue to the location of a fracture or subtle subluxation. The articular surfaces of all bones should be parallel (Fig. 9-141).

If routine views are normal or a questionable area is identified, further studies should be performed. Fluoroscopically positioned spot films (Fig. 9-141) may be useful in the acute setting and can be performed quickly. Trispiral tomography is especially useful in detection of subtle fractures. CT may also be used to evaluate articular changes (313).

Treatment

Most subluxations and minimally displaced fractures (≤2 mm) are treated conservatively with closed reduction and casting. The prognosis of lateral injuries is more guarded than medial injury and may require calcaneocuboid arthrodesis. Triple arthrodesis is an excellent procedure in complex injury or when conservative treatment is unsuccessful (323).

Isolated tarsal fractures, if nondisplaced, can be treated with elastic support or cast immobilization for 4–6 weeks (308,316). Treatment of displaced fractures is more controversial, but open reduction with either triple arthrodesis or talonavicular cuneiform arthrodesis is advocated by most authors (307,308,316,323).

Tarso-metatarsal Fracture-Dislocations

Tarso-metatarsal fracture-dislocations are commonly referred to as Lisfranc injuries (301,315). This injury is based on the description of amputation through these joints by a surgeon of the same name during the Napoleonic wars (300). There is uncertainty as to whether Lisfranc ever described the dislocation, but the joint has become known as Lisfranc's joint based on his surgical description (306). The injury is uncommon, accounting for fewer than 1% of fracture dislocations (299,309).

The four lateral metatarsals (second to fifth) are connected at the bases by transverse metatarsal ligaments. This is not the case at the base of the first and second metatarsal. Here the transverse ligament is absent. The second metatarsal is situated in a mortise formed by the medial and lateral cuneiform and its ligamentous support is via the transverse ligament laterally and the medial and second cuneiform proximally (Fig. 9-142) (299,300,329). The oblique ligament from the medial cuneiform to the base of the second metatarsal is implicated in avulsion fractures of the second metatarsal base. The plantar ligaments and tendons provide more support than the dorsal soft tissues, which explains why most dislocations occur dorsally (300). The dorsalis pedis artery passes between the proximal first and second metatarsals as it enters the plantar aspect of the foot to form the plantar arch. Therefore, it is susceptible to injuries of fracture-dislocations in this region (316).

Typically, the injury occurs with forced plantar flexion of the forefoot with or without associated rotation (329). This can occur during a fall, or landing on the toes, which forces the forefoot into plantar flexion. Other mechanisms include falls with the forefoot fixed or compression of the foot due to a heavy object striking the heel when the patient is kneeling. In adults, motor vehicle and motorcycle accidents are more commonly implicated, but the forces producing the injury are similar (300,316). The injury that occurs takes several different patterns (299,300,316). The homolateral pattern (total incongruity) occurs when all five metatarsals are displaced. The displacement is almost always in the lateral direction (Figs. 9-143 and 9-144). The alignment of both the first and second metatarsal bases is abnormal (Fig. 9-144). Fractures of the second metatarsal are common in this pattern due to its position in the mortise formed by the cuneiforms (Fig. 9-145) (299,300,301,310,315). Partial incongruity (Fig. 9-143) occurs when the first

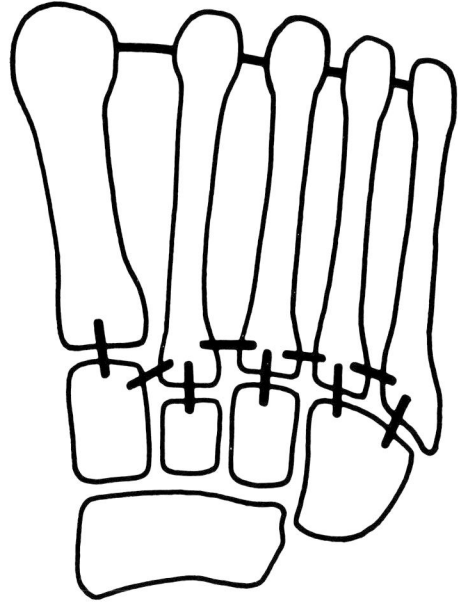

FIG. 9–142. Bony and ligamentous anatomy of the tarsometatarsal joints. There is no transverse ligament between the first and second metatarsal bones. The base of the second metatarsal is situated in a mortise formed by the cuneiforms (from 329).

TYPE A
TOTAL INCONGRUITY

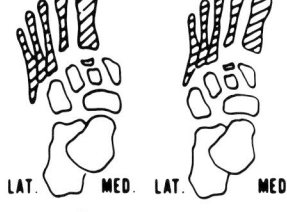

TYPE B
PARTIAL INCONGRUITY

Medial dislocation

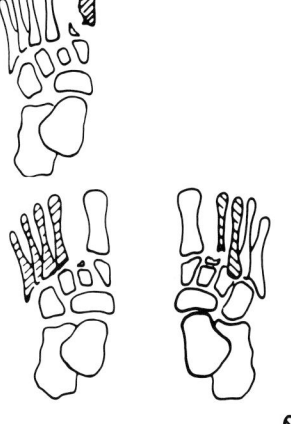

Lateral dislocation

TYPE C
DIVERGENT

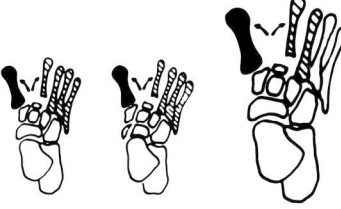

Total
displacement

Partial
displacement

FIG. 9–143. The patterns of Lisfranc fracture dislocation. (from 315).

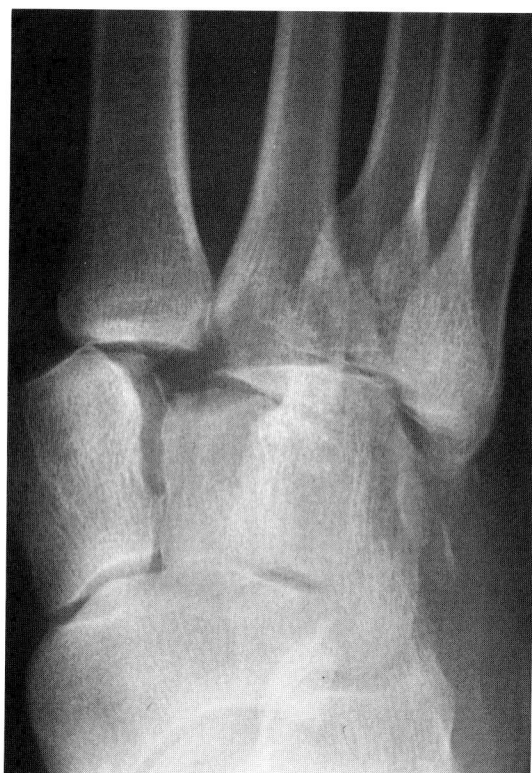

FIG. 9-144. AP view of the midfoot demonstrating lateral displacement of the first and second metatarsals.

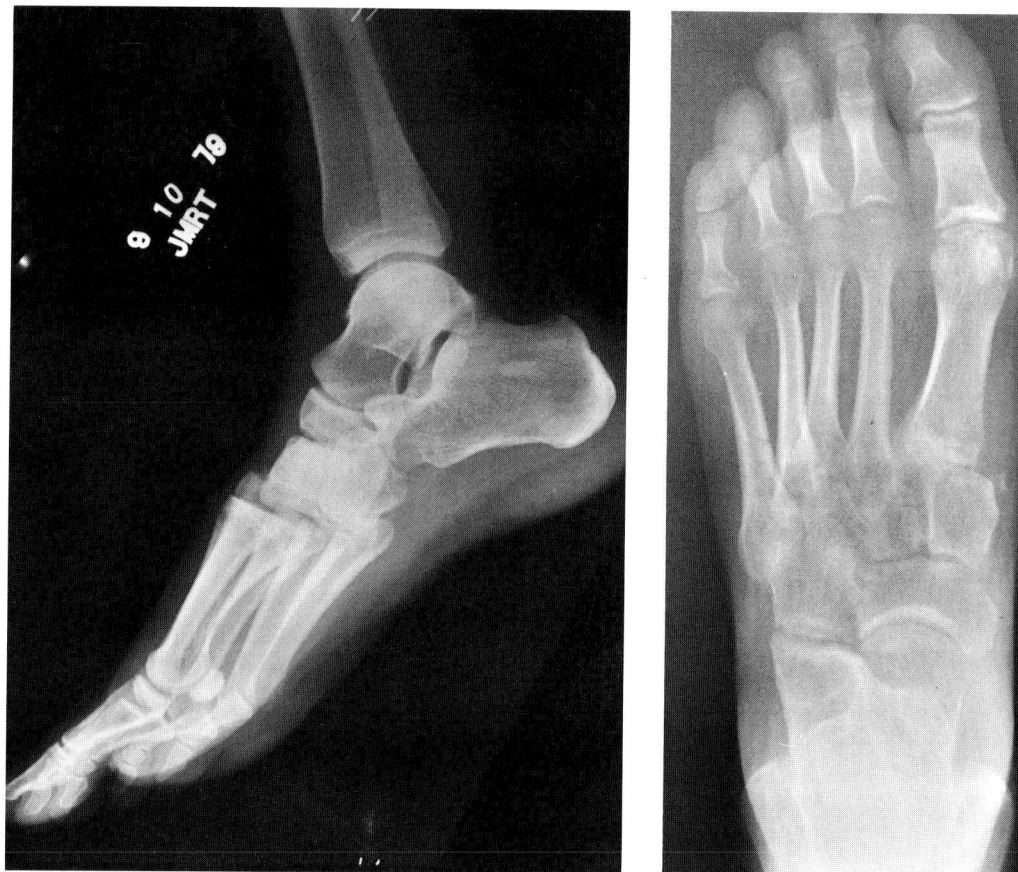

FIG. 9-145. Obvious Lisfranc injuries. **A:** Lateral view demonstrating dorsal dislocation of the tarso-metatarsal joints. **B:** AP view demonstrating total incongruity with shift laterally. The first metatarsal shift is most obvious. Note the avulsion fracture medially.

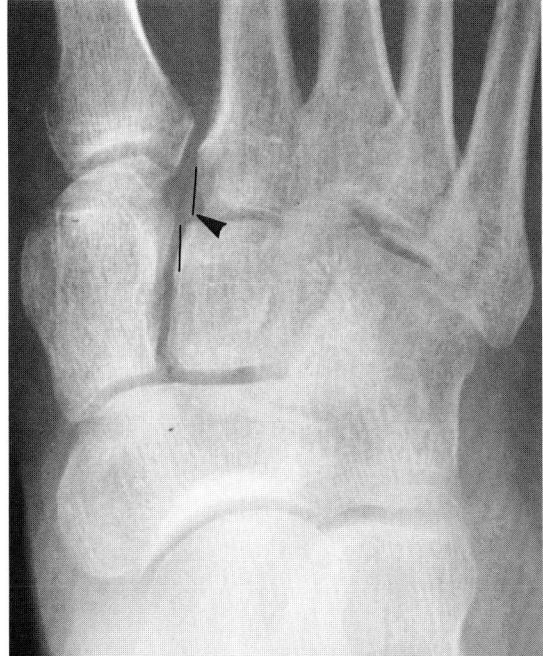
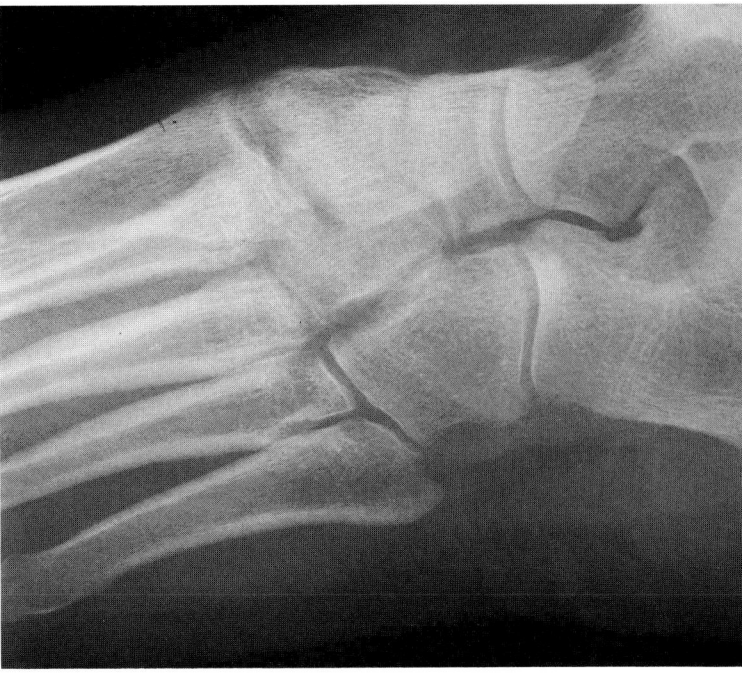

A

B

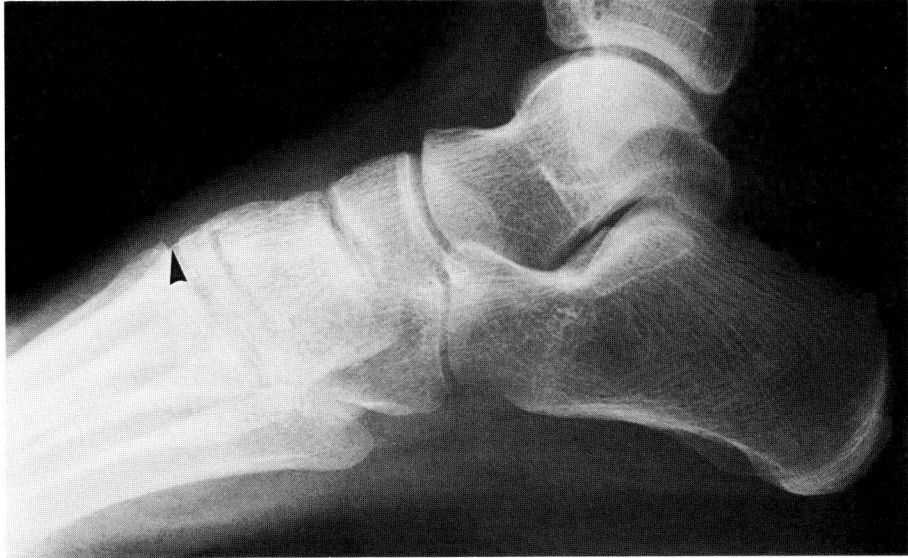

C

FIG. 9–146. Lisfranc injury with partial incongruity laterally. **A:** AP view shows that the medial aspect of the second metatarsal base and cuneiform are not aligned. There is a small avulsion fracture (*arrow*). **B:** Oblique view shows normal alignment of the fourth and fifth metatarsals. **C:** Lateral view shows a slight dorsal "step-off" at the second tarsometatarsal joint (*arrow*).

metatarsal fractures at the base and the shaft displaces medially, accompanied with lateral displacement of the second to fifth metatarsals (315). A third pattern of injury (divergent) occurs when the base of the first metatarsal subluxes or dislocates medially and the second metatarsal or a combination of the second to fifth metatarsals displaces laterally (299,300,315). The significance of this injury is the associated cuneiform and navicular fractures. Rarely, an isolated tarso-metatarsal dislocation can occur (322).

Radiographic Evaluation

Radiographic evaluation must start with careful evaluation of the tarso-metatarsal relationships. Routine views of the foot are usually sufficient for diagnosis of obvious fracture-dislocations of the tarso-metatarsal joint (Fig. 9-145). However, subtle ligament injuries may be easily overlooked (Fig. 9-146) (310). These injuries may spontaneously reduce so that nonstress radiographs appear normal. On the AP view, the medial margin of

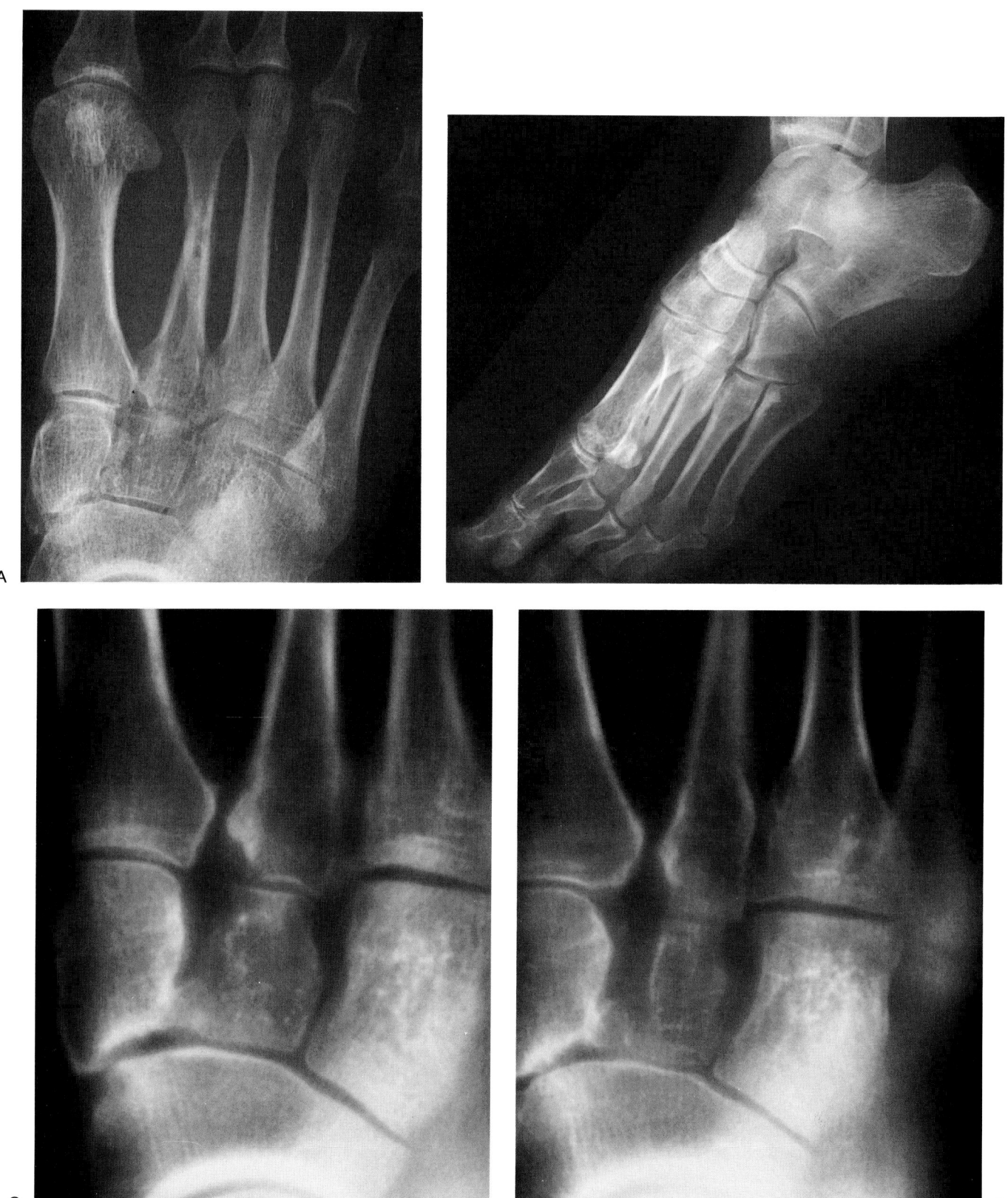

FIG. 9-147. Patient with foot pain due to previous foot fracture. AP (**A**) and oblique (**B**) views show a healed fracture of the second metatarsal. AP tomograms (**C,D**) show degenerative changes between the first and second metatarsal bases and fragments between the cuneiforms with partial ankylosis proximally due to a missed Lisfranc injury.

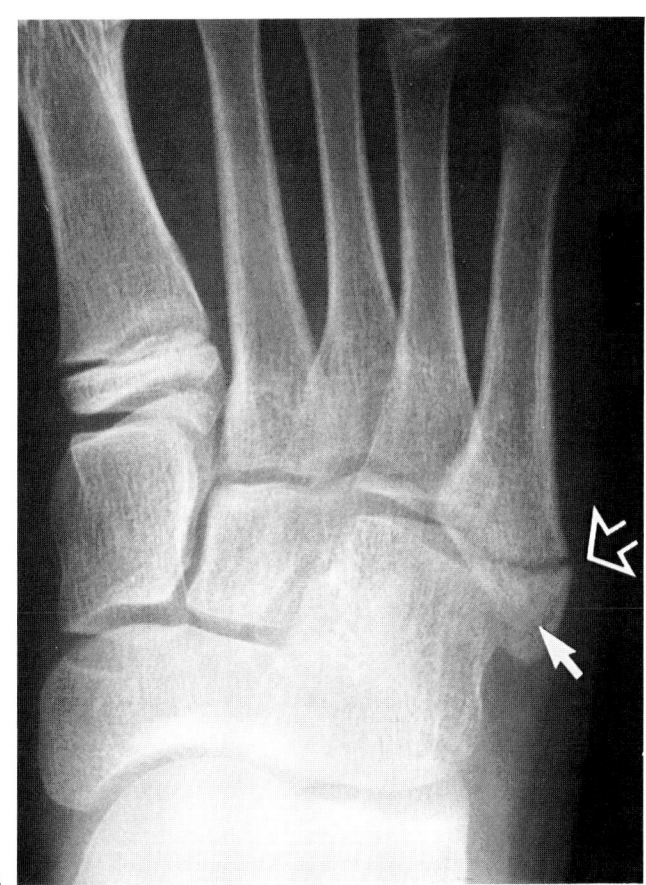

A

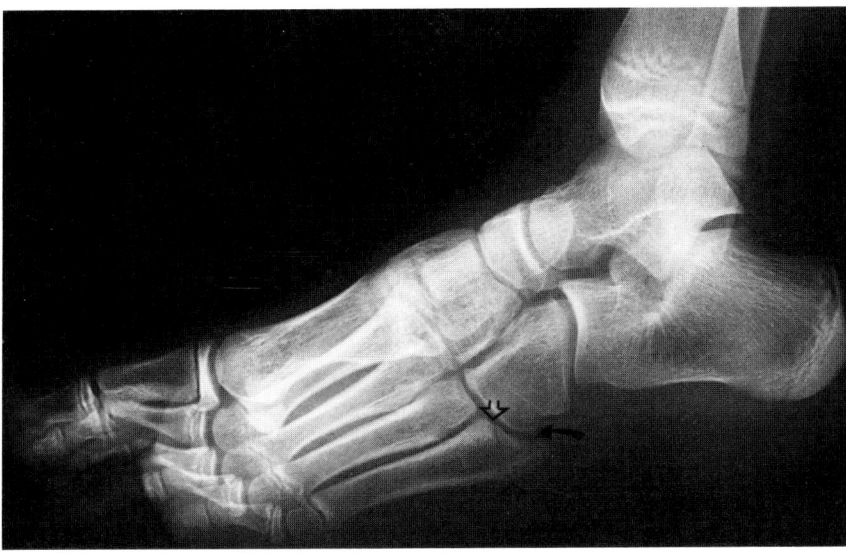

B

FIG. 9-148. Normal tuberosity and fracture of the fifth meta-tarsal base. AP (**A**) view of the foot shows a transverse fracture (*open arrow*) and normal physis (*closed arrow*). Oblique view (**B**) also demonstrates the transverse line characteristic of fracture (*open arrows*) and the normal epiphysis (*curved arrow*).

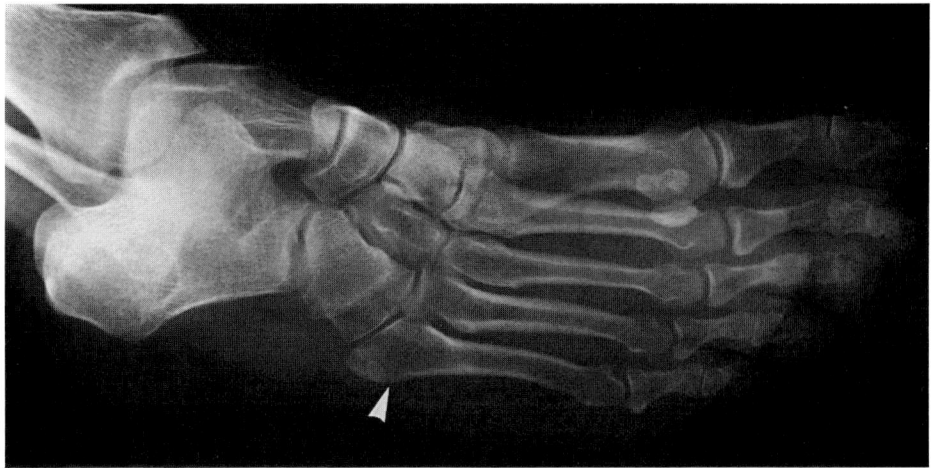

FIG. 9-149. Oblique view of the foot demonstrating an acute linear fracture of the fifth metatarsal metaphysis (*arrow*).

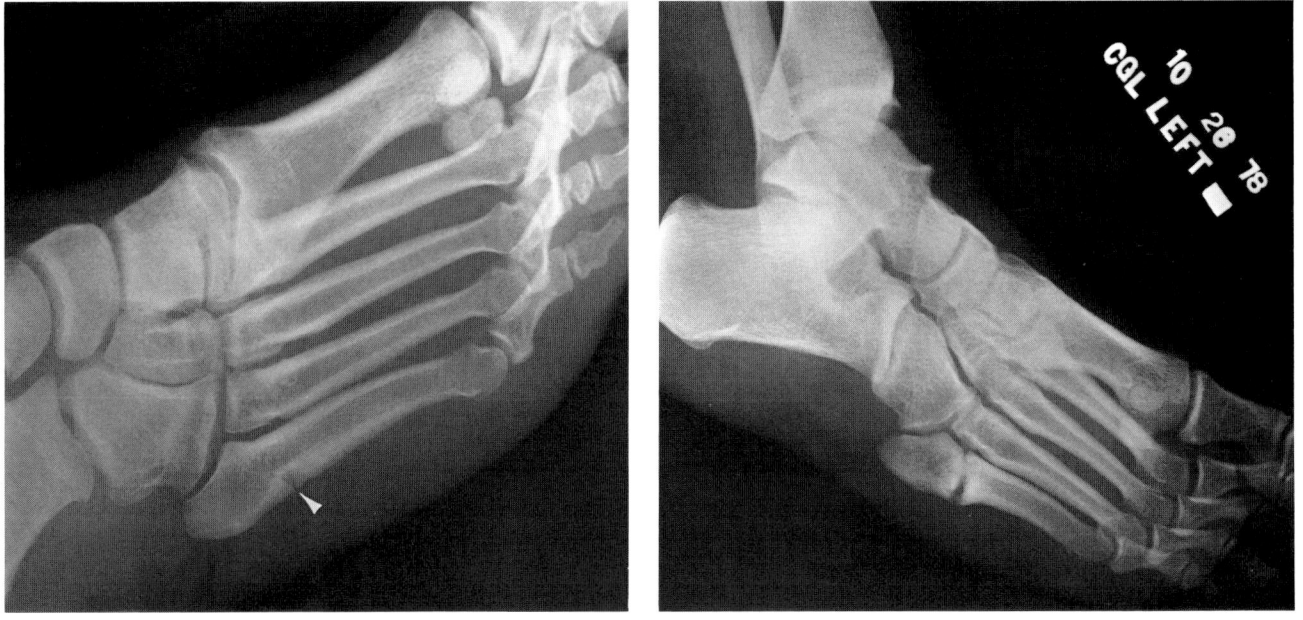

A   B

FIG. 9-150. Jone's fractures. **A:** Acute undisplaced fracture of the proximal fifth metatarsal (*arrow*). **B:** Ununited Jone's fracture with sclerotic margins (from ref. 301, with permission).

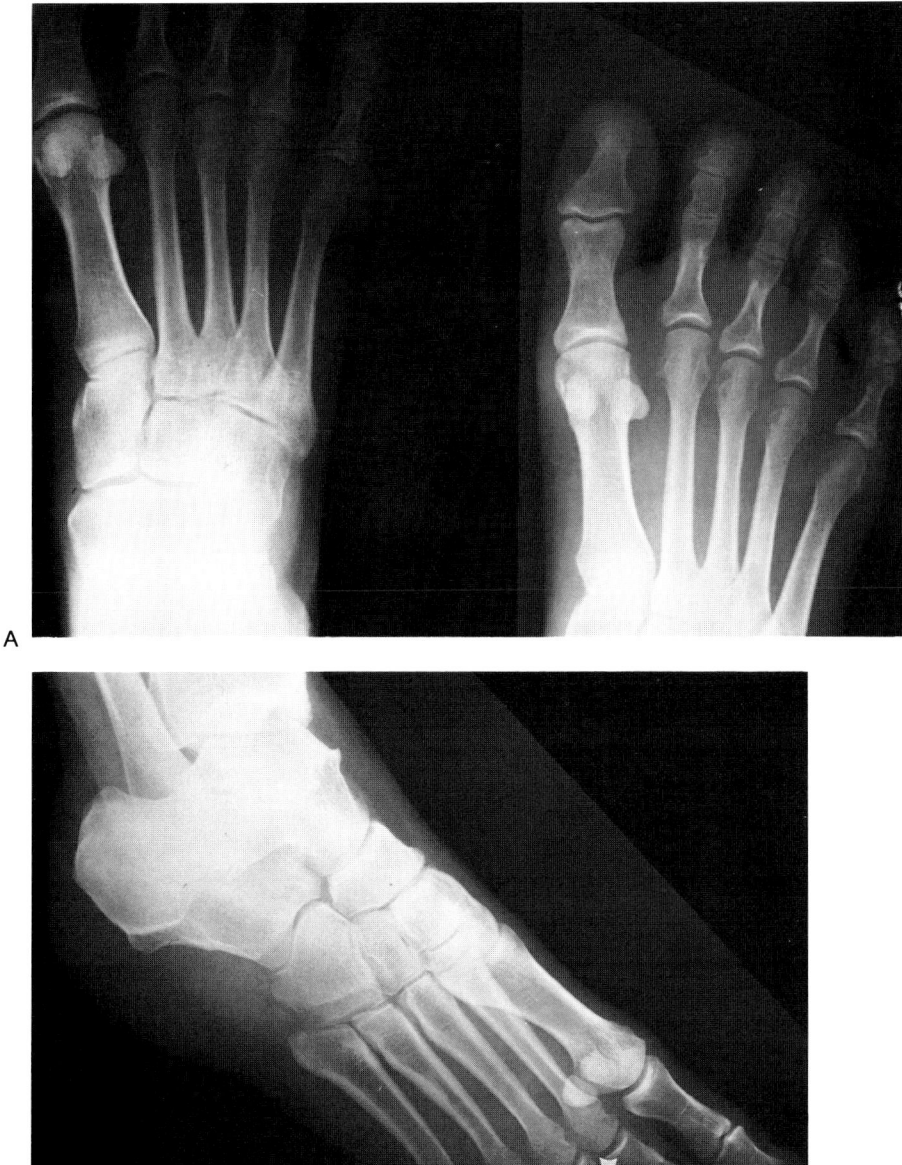

FIG. 9-151. AP (**A**) and oblique (**B**) views of the foot. The undisplaced oblique fracture of the third proximal phalanx is well seen only on the oblique view (B, *arrow*). The soft tissue crease from the foot pad (*arrows*) should not be confused with a fracture. This line extends beyond the cortex of the bones distinguishing it from fracture.

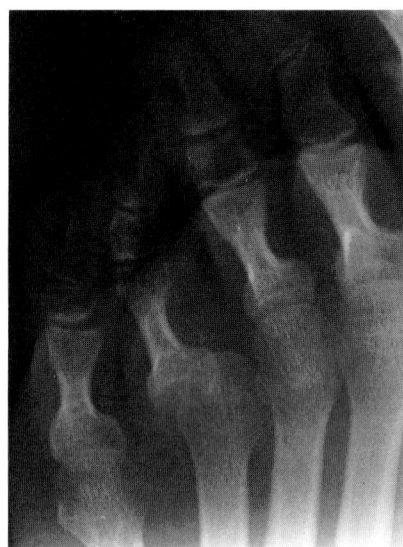

FIG. 9–152. Localized view of the toes demonstrating a lateral dislocation of the fourth metatarsal phalangeal joint.

the second metatarsal base should align with the margin of the second cuneiform. The space between the first and second metatarsal bases should be assessed, but is less useful than the foregoing relationship (311). However, the lateral margins of the first metatarsal and cuneiform should align. The medial base of the fourth metatarsal should align with the medial margin of the cuboid. The bases of the remaining metatarsals are more difficult to evaluate due to bony overlap and the overlapping tuberosity of the fifth metatarsal. However, the metatarsal bases should be parallel to the tarsal articular surfaces (311,324,325). On the lateral view, the second metatarsal and cuneiform should be aligned such that an uninterrupted line can be drawn along their dorsal surfaces.

On occasion, fluoroscopically positioned spot views, or stress views, may be indicated to detect subtle ligament injury. Conventional or computed tomography can also be useful to more fully evaluate the bony relationships and to exlude cuneiform and navicular fractures (301,310,313).

Treatment

Closed reduction can be used for patients with subtle injury or displacement less than 2–3 mm (314). With more significant fracture dislocation, reduction can be more difficult. The anterior tibial and peroneal tendons may interfere with reduction (306,314). If reduction is difficult, MRI may be useful to determine whether tendons (specifically tibialis anterior) have become entrapped between fragments (301,316). Open reduction with accurate re-alignment and internal fixation should be used in these patients (303,330). During surgery, AP

views of the foot should be obtained to determine whether satisfactory re-alignment of the second metatarsal base has been achieved (303). Follow-up routine films should be obtained to be certain that the reduction is maintained. In problem cases, CT or conventional tomography are useful to better define the complex bony relationships (Fig. 9-147).

Complications

The most common problems include degenerative arthritis and persistent pain. These may occur in 20–30% of patients (301). Vascular injury has been reported, but it is generally uncommon. Gissane reported gangrene of the foot in 3 patients, which lead to below the knee amputations (312). Avascular necrosis of the second metatarsal head has also been reported (306,330). This was believed to be due to the relationship of the dorsalis pedis artery and interosseous branch to the bases of the first and second metatarsals (322). Suspected vascular injury can be quickly assessed using Doppler ultrasound (304,326).

Metatarsal and Phalangeal Fractures

Metatarsal fractures are common. Injuries are usually the result of direct trauma due to a heavy object striking the foot. However, twisting or shearing injuries may also lead to fracture (300,301,314,316). The neck of the metatarsal is weaker than the shaft, which explains the higher incidence at this location (304). Patients generally present with pain, swelling, and ecchymosis over the injured metatarsals (300,314).

Fractures of the fifth metatarsal base are common in children and adults. Two basic fracture patterns with differing prognosis can be distinguished. Avulsion of the proximal tuberosity is most common. This is due to abrupt pull of the peroneus brevis. The adductor digiti minimi and lateral cord of the plantar fascia also insert on the fifth metatarsal base (314). This fracture must be distinguished from the normal tuberosity in younger patients (Fig. 9-148). The growth plate runs parallel to the shaft while fractures will be perpendicular to the shaft (Fig. 9-149). Avulsion of the epiphyses is uncommon, but, if suspected, comparison with the normal extremity should be obtained. Differentiation of this fracture from the os peroneum or os vesalianum is usually not difficult due to their smooth cortical margins.

The second type of fifth metatarsal base fracture is often referred to as the *Jones fracture* (318,319). This fracture involves the proximal diaphyses or metaphysis (Fig. 9-150). Treatment of this fracture can be more difficult and may require internal fixation (305).

Phalangeal fractures occur when the bare toe strikes a hard object or when a heavy object lands on the toe.

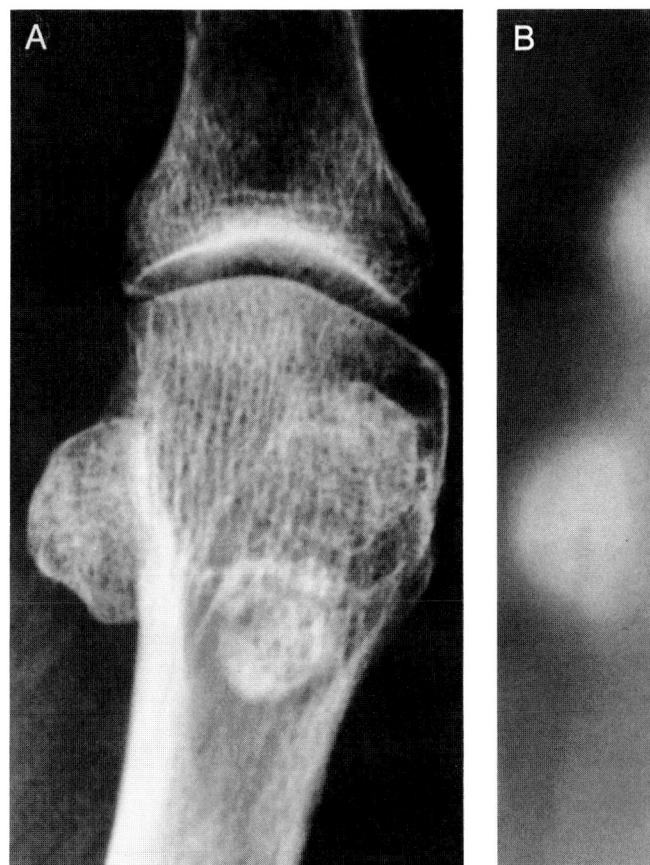

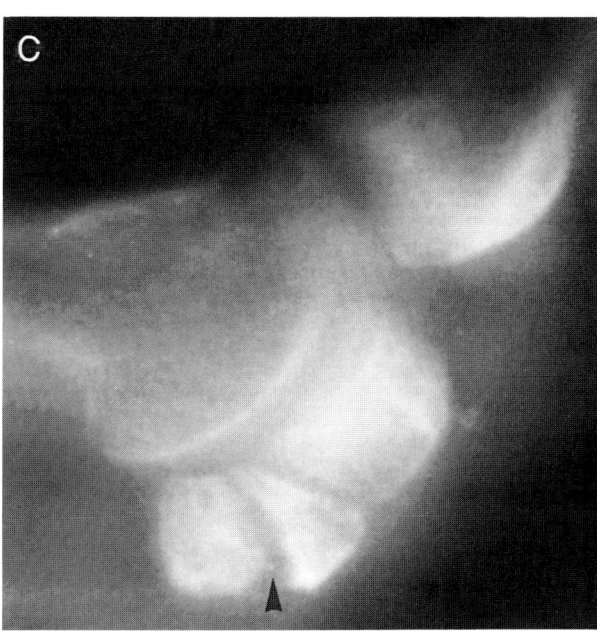

FIG. 9–153. Patient with pain under the first metatarsal head due to long distance running. Magnified AP view (**A**) is normal. AP (**B**) and lateral (**C**) tomograms clearly demonstrate the sesamoid fracture (*arrow*) (from ref. 301, with permission).

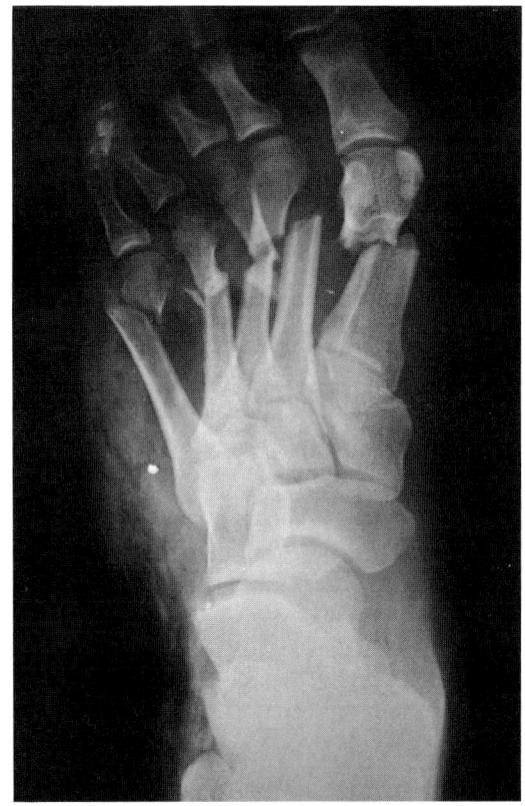

A

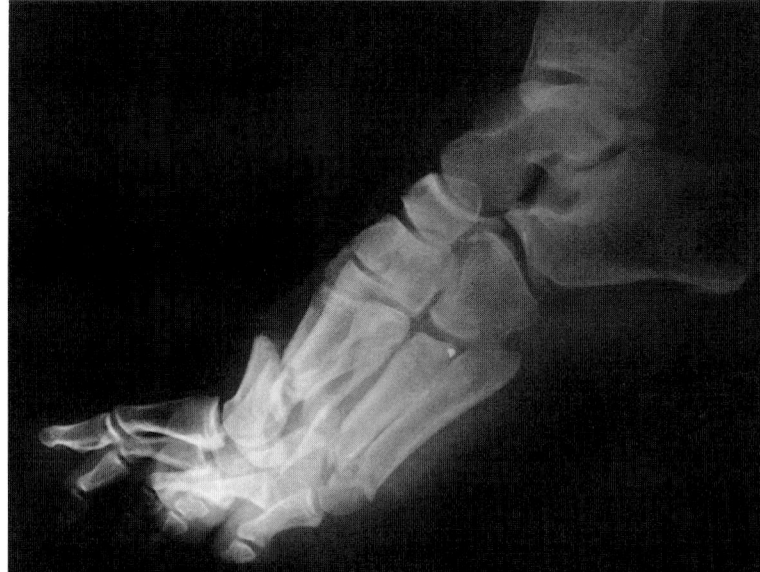

B

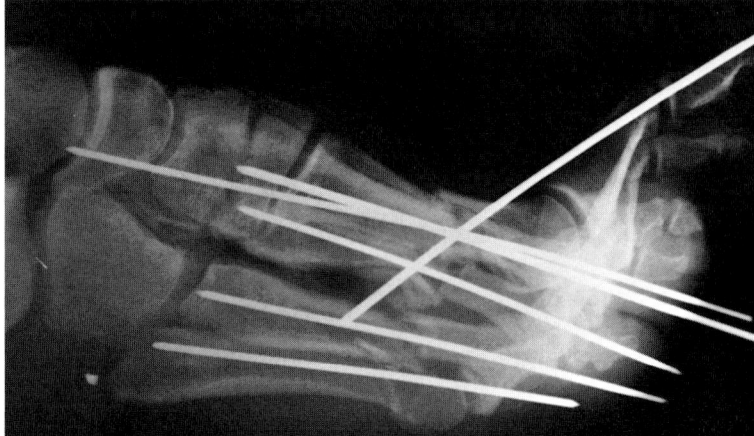

D

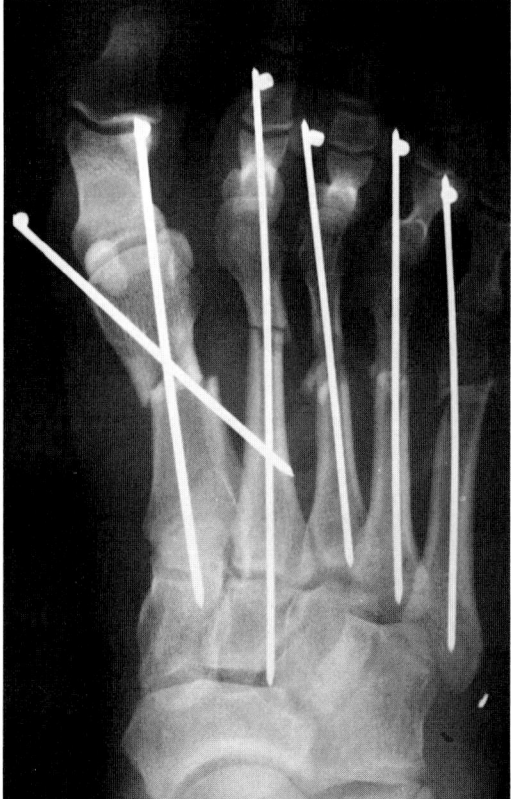

C

FIG. 9-154. AP (**A**) and oblique (**B**) views of the foot following a lawn mower injury show an open wound with comminuted fractures of all 5 distal metatarsals. Fractures were reduced with K-wire fixation (**C**) and (**D**). Note that the angulation has been reduced.

Most fractures are minimally displaced. Care must be taken to carefully evaluate all radiographs or these fractures can be overlooked. It is important to determine whether fractures are intra-articular (Fig. 9-151).

Dislocations of the metatarsophalangeal and interphalangeal joints may be isolated or associated with fracture. Metatarsophalangeal dislocations are usually due to hyperextension with proximal phalanx forced dorsally over the metatarsal tearing the plantar capsule (300). The great toe is most commonly involved. Medial and lateral dislocations are less common (Fig. 9-152). Similar forces lead to dislocations of the interphalangeal joints.

Radiographic Evaluation

AP, oblique, and lateral radiographs of the foot are routinely obtained. The AP and oblique views are most useful as bony overlap makes evaluation more difficult on the lateral view. The lateral view is useful in determining fracture angulation and the direction of dislocations. Following reduction of dislocations it is important to obtain the same views to be certain that there is no associated fracture or soft tissue interposition (wide joint space). Tomography is useful on occasion, especially for sesamoid fractures (Fig. 9-153) (301,331).

Treatment

Treatment of most closed fractures and dislocations is conservative. Undisplaced metatarsal fractures are treated with walking casts for 4–6 weeks (300,301,316). Displaced fractures (Fig. 9-154) or open fractures are better managed with internal fixation. This reduces the problem of malposition, which can result in uneven weight bearing on the metatarsal heads. Debridement and parenteral antibiotics are needed following reduction of open wounds (300,314). Differentiation of tuberosity and Jones fractures is important. Jones fractures can be more difficult to manage. Torg et al. (328) classified these fractures according to their radiographic appearance; (1) acute fractures with a narrow fracture line (Fig. 9-150), (2) fractures with medullary sclerosis and widening of the fracture line, and (3) non-union with sclerosis of the fracture line and obliteration of the medullary canal (Fig. 9-150B). Acute fractures healed with a nonweight-bearing knee-to-toe cast. If the fracture line is widened with sclerosis, curettage and bone grafting is most successful (328).

Most dislocations and phalangeal fractures can also be reduced and treated conservatively. "Buddy taping" of the injured phalanx to the adjacent toe may be all that is required. Articular involvement may require K-wire reduction.

REFERENCES

Anatomy

1. Anderson JE. *Grant's atlas of anatomy,* 8th ed. Baltimore: Williams and Wilkins, 1983.
2. Berquist TH. *MRI of the musculoskeletal system.* New York: Raven Press, 1990.
3. Berquist TH. *Radiology of the foot and ankle.* New York: Raven Press, 1989.
4. Burman MS, Lapidus DW. The functional disturbances caused by unconstant bones and sesamoids of the foot. *Arch Surg* 1931;22:936–975.
5. Clemente CD. *Gray's anatomy of the human body,* 13th ed. Philadelphia: Lea & Febiger, 1985.
6. Dunn AW. Anomalous muscles simulating soft tissue tumors of the lower extremities. *J Bone Joint Surg* 1965;47A:1397–1400.
7. Goergen TG, Danzig LA, Resnick D, Owen CA. Roentgen evaluation of the tibiotalar joint. *J Bone Joint Surg* 1977;59A:874–877.
8. Hollinshead WH. *Anatomy for surgeons,* vol. 3, 3rd ed. New York: Harper and Row, 1982.
9. Jahss MH. *Disorders of the foot.* Philadelphia: W. B. Saunders, Co., 1982.
10. Jonsson K, Fredin HL, Cederlund CG, Bauer M. Width of the normal ankle joint. *Acta Radiol* 1984;25:147–149.
11. Kelikian H, Kelikian AS. *Disorders of the ankle.* Philadelphia: W. B. Saunders, Co., 1985.
12. Lauge-Hansen N. Fractures of the ankle. Analytical historical survey as basis of a new experimental roentgenologic and clinical investigation. *Arch Surg* 1948;56:259–317.
13. Lauge-Hansen N. Fractures of the ankle II: Combined experimental surgical and experimental roentgenological investigation. *Arch Surg* 1950;60:959–985.
14. Leung RC, Wong WL. The vessels of the first metatarsal web space. An operative and radiographic study. *J Bone Joint Surg* 1983;65A:235–238.
15. McDougall A. The os trigonum. *J Bone Joint Surg* 1955;37B:256–265.
16. Morrey BF, Cass JR, Johnson KA, Berquist TH. The foot and ankle. In: Berquist TH. *Imaging of orthopedic trauma and surgery.* Philadelphia: W. B. Saunders, 1986;407–498.
17. Mukherjee SK, Pringle RM, Baxter AD. Fracture of the lateral process of the talus. *J Bone Joint Surg* 1974;56B:263–273.
18. O'Rahilly R. A survey of tarsal and carpal anomalies. *J Bone Joint Surg* 1953;35A:626–641.
19. Resnick D. Radiology of the talocalcaneal articulations. *Radiology* 1974;111:581–586.
20. Steel M, Johnson KA, Dewitz MA. Radiographic measurements of the normal adult foot. *Foot and Ankle* 1980;1:151–158.
21. Sutherland DH, Cooper L, Daniel D. The role of plantar flexors in normal walking. *J Bone Joint Surg* 1980;62A:354–363.
22. Venning P. Radiologic studies of variation in ossification of the foot III. Cone shaped epiphysis of the proximal phalanges. *Am J Phys Anthropol* 1961;19:131–136.
23. Weissman SD. *Radiology of the foot.* Baltimore: Williams and Wilkins, 1983.

Imaging Techniques

24. Ala-Ketola L, Puronen J, Koivisto E, Purepera M. Arthrography in the diagnosis of ligament injuries and classification of ankle injuries. *Radiology* 1977;125:63–68.
25. Ballinger WR. *Merrill's atlas of roentgenographic positions and standard radiographic procedures,* 5th Ed. St. Louis: C. V. Mosby, 1982.
26. Beltran J, Nato AM, Mosure JC, Shuman OM, Weiss KL, Zuelger WA. Ankle: Surface coil MR imaging at 1.5 T. *Radiology* 1986;161:203–209.

27. Bernau A, Berquist TH. *Orthopedic positioning in diagnostic radiology.* Baltimore: Urban and Schwarzenberg, 1983.

28. Berquist TH. *Imaging of orthopedic trauma and surgery.* Philadelphia: W. B. Saunders, 1986.

29. Berquist TH. *Radiology of the foot and ankle.* New York: Raven Press, 1989.

30. Berquist TH. *MRI of the musculoskeletal system,* 2nd ed. New York: Raven Press, 1990.

31. Black HM, Brand RL, Eichelberger MR. An improved technique for the evaluation of ligamentous injury in severe ankle sprains. *Am J Sports Med* 1978;6:276–282.

32. Blei CL, Nirschl RP, Grant EG. Achilles tendon: US diagnosis of pathologic conditions. *Radiology* 1986;159:765–767.

33. Bleikrodt RP, Kingma LM, Binnendijk B, Klein JP. Injuries of the lateral ankle ligaments. Classification with tenography and arthrography. *Radiology* 1989;173:347–349.

34. Bluth EI, Merritt CR, Sullivan MA. Grey scale ultrasound evaluation of the lower extremities. *JAMA* 1982;247:3127–3129.

35. Braumstein EM, Silver TM, Martel W, Jaffe M. Ultrasonographic diagnosis of extremity masses. *Skel Radiol* 1981;6:157–163.

36. Brown ML, Swee RG, Johnson KA. Bone scintigraphy of the calcaneus. *Clin Nucl Med* 1986;11:530–536.

37. Burkus JK, Sella EJ, Southwick WO. Occult injuries of the talus diagnosed by bone scan and tomography. *Foot and Ankle* 1984;4:316–324.

38. Cass JR, Morrey BF. Ankle instability: Current concepts, diagnosis and treatment. *Mayo Clin Proc* 1984;59:165–170.

39. Causton J. Projection of the sesamoid bones in the region of the first metatarsophalangeal joints. *Radiology* 1943;9:39–40.

40. Chang JW, Griffiths H, Chan DPK. A new radiological technique for the forefoot. *Foot and Ankle* 1984;5:77–83.

41. Cone RO III, Nguyen V, Flourroy JG, Guerra J. Triplane fracture of the distal tibial epiphysis: Radiographic and CT studies. *Radiology* 1984;153:763–767.

42. Daffner RH, Reimer BL, Lupetin AR, Dash N. Magnetic resonance imaging of acute tendon ruptures. *Skel Radiol* 1986;15:619–621.

43. Dory MA. Arthrography of the ankle joint in chronic instability. *Skel Radiol* 1986;15:291–294.

44. Edeiken J, Colter JM. Ankle injury. The need for stress views. *JAMA* 1978;240:1183–1184.

45. Erickson SJ, Quinn SF, Kneeland JB, et al. MR imaging of the tarsal tunnel and related spaces. *AJR* 1990;155:323–328.

46. Erickson SJ, Smith JW, Ruiz ME, et al. MR imaging of the collateral ligament of the ankle. *AJR* 1991;156:131–136.

47. Evans GA, Frenyo SD. The stress-tenogram in the diagnosis of ruptures of the lateral ligament of the ankle. *J Bone Joint Surg* 1979;61B:347–351.

48. Feist JH, Mankin HJ. The tarsus: Basic relationships and motions in the adult and definition of optimal recumbent oblique projection. *Radiology* 1962;79:250–263.

49. Floyd EJ, Ransom RA, Dailey JM. Computed tomography scanning of the subtalar joint. *J Am Podiatry Assoc* 1984;74:533–537.

50. Fornage BD. Achilles tendon: US examination. *Radiology* 1986;159:759–764.

51. Freiberger RH, Kaye J. *Arthrography.* New York: Appleton-Century-Crofts, 1979.

52. Frolich H, Gotzen L, Adam D. Evaluation of stress roentgenogram of the upper ankle joint. *Unfallheikurde* 1980;83:457–461.

53. Genant HK, Helms CA. Computed tomography of the appendicular musculoskeletal system. In: Moss AA, Gainser G, Genant HK. *Computed tomography of the body.* Philadelphia: W. B. Saunders, 1983;525–533.

54. Geslian JE, Thrall JH, Espenosa JL, Older RA. Early detection of stress fractures using Tc-99m polyphosphate. *Radiology* 1976;121:683–687.

55. Gilula LA, Oloff L, Caputi R, Destouet JM, Jacobs A, Solomon MA. Ankle tenography: A key to unexplained symptomatology. *Radiology* 1984;151:581–587.

56. Goergen TG, Resnick D. Arthrography of the ankle. In: Dalinka M. *Arthrography.* New York: Springer-Verlag, 1981.

57. Goiney RC, Connell DG, Nichols DM. CT evaluation of tarsometatarsal fracture dislocation injuries. *AJR* 1985;144:985–990.

58. Guyer BH, Levinsohn EM, Fredrickson BE, Bailey GL, Formi-

kell M. Computed tomography of calcaneal fractures: Anatomy, pathology, dosimetry and clinical relevance. *AJR* 1985;145:911–919.

59. Heger L, Wulff K. Computed tomography of the calcaneus: Normal anatomy. *AJR* 1985;75:123–129.

60. Heger L, Wulff K, Seddigi MSA. Computed tomography of calcaneal fractures. *AJR* 1985;145:131–137.

61. Holley EW. Radiography of the tarsal sesamoid bones. *Med Radiogr Photogr* 1955;31:73–80.

62. Horsfield D, Murphy G. Stress views of the ankle joint in lateral ligament injury. *Radiography* 1985;51:7–11.

63. Hudson TM. Fluoroscopy before arthrography. Detection and evaluation of loose bodies. *Skel Radiol* 1984;12:199–203.

64. Isherwood I. A radiologic approach to the subtalar joint. *J Bone Joint Surg* 1961;43B:566–574.

65. Johannsen A. Radiologic diagnosis of lateral ligament lesion of the ankle. A comparison between talar tilt and anterior drawer sign. *Acta Orthop Scand* 1978;49:259–301.

66. Jonsson K, Fredin HO, Cederlund CG. Width of the normal ankle joint. *Acta Radiologic Diag* 1984;25:147–149.

67. Kainberger FM, Engel A, Barton P, Huebsch P, Newbold A, Salomonowitz E. Injury to the Achilles tendon: Diagnosis with sonography. *AJR* 1990;155:1031–1036.

68. Kneeland JB, Macrandor S, Middleton WD, Cates CD, Jesmanowicz A, Hyde JS. MR imaging of the normal ankle: Correlation with anatomic sections. *AJR* 1988;151:117–123.

69. Leopold GR. Ultrasonography of superficially located structures. *Radiol Clin North Am* 1980;18:161–173.

70. Lewis RW. Non-routine views in roentgen examination of the extremities. *Surg Gynecol Obstet* 1938;69:38–45.

71. Martinez S, Herzenberg JE, Apple JS. Computed tomography of the hindfoot. *Orthop Clin North Am* 1985;16:481–496.

72. Mathieson JR, Connell DG, Cooperberg PL, Lloyd-Smith DR. Sonography of the Achilles tendon and adjacent bursae. *AJR* 1988;151:127–131.

73. Morrey BF, Cass JF, Johnson KA, Berquist TH. The foot and ankle. In: Berquist TH. *Imaging of orthopedic trauma and surgery.* Philadelphia: W. B. Saunders, 1986;407–498.

74. Norman A. The value of tomography in the diagnosis of skeletal disorders. *Radiol Clin North Am* 1970;8:251.

75. Olson RW. Ankle arthrography. *Radiol Clin North Am* 1981;19:255–268.

76. Pritsch M, Heim M, Horoszowski H, Farine I. The significance of the axial foot projection in diagnosis of metatarsal pathology. *Arch Orthop Trauma Surg* 1981;98:139–141.

77. Quinn SF, Murray WT, Clark RA, Cochran CF. Achilles tendon: MR imaging at 1.5 T. *Radiology* 1987;164:767–770.

78. Resnick D, Goergen TG. Peroneal tenography in patients with previous calcaneal fractures. *Radiology* 1975;115:211–213.

80. Rosenberg ZS, Johss MH, Noto AM, et al. Rupture of the posterior tibial tendon: CT and surgical findings. *Radiology* 1988;176:489–493.

81. Rosenberg ZS, Feldman F, Singson RD. Intra-articular calcaneal fractures: Computed tomographic analysis. *Skel Radiol* 1987;16:105–113.

82. Sauser DD, Nelson RC, Lavine MH, Wa CW. Acute injuries of the lateral ligaments of the ankle: Comparison of stress radiography and arthrography. *Radiology* 1983;148:643–657.

83. Schweigel JF, Knickerbocher WJ, Cooperberg P. A study of ankle instability utilizing ankle arthrography. *J Trauma* 1977;17:878–881.

84. Sierra A, Potchen EJ, Moore J, Smith HG. High-field magnetic resonance imaging of aseptic necrosis of the talus. *J Bone Joint Surg* 1986;68A:927–928.

85. Vuust M. Arthrographic diagnosis of ruptured calcaneofibular ligament: A new projection tested on experimental post mortem. *Acta Radiol Diag* 1980;21:123–128.

86. Vuust M, Niedermann B. Arthrographic diagnosis of ruptured calcaneofibular ligament. II. Clinical evaluation of a new method. *Acta Radiol Diag* 1980;21:231–234.

87. Woolson ST, Porvati D, Fillingham LL, Vassiliodis A. Three-dimensional imaging of the ankle joint from computed tomography. *Foot and Ankle* 1985;6:2–6.

Soft Tissue Trauma

88. Abraham E, Sternaman JE. Neglected rupture of the peroneal tendon causing recurrent sprains of the ankle. *J Bone Joint Surg* 1979;61A:1247–1248.

89. Ala-Ketola L, Peranen J, Kovivisto E, Puupera M. Arthrography in the diagnosis of ligament injuries and classification of ankle injuries. *Radiology* 1977;125:63–68.

90. Andrews JR. Overuse syndromes of the lower extremity. *Clin Sports Med* 1983;2:137–148.

91. Beltran J, Nato AM, Mosure JC, Shamam OM, Weiss KL, Zuelzer WA. Ankle: Surface coil MR imaging at 1.5 T. *Radiology* 1986;161:203–209.

92. Berquist TH. *Radiology of the foot and ankle.* New York: Raven Press, 1989.

93. Berquist TH. *MRI of the musculoskeletal system,* 2nd ed. New York: Raven Press, 1990.

94. Black HM, Brand RL, Eichelberger MR. An improved technique for the evaluation of ligamentous injury in severe ankle sprains. *Am J Sports Med* 1978;6(5):276–282.

95. Blanchard KS, Finlay DBL, Scott DJA, Ley CC, Siggins D, Allen MJ. A radiological analysis of lateral ligament injuries of the ankle. *Clin Radiol* 1986;37:247–251.

96. Blei CL, Nirschl RP, Grant EG. Achilles tendon: US diagnosis of pathologic conditions. *Radiology* 1986;159:765–767.

97. Bonutti PM, Bell GR. Compartment syndrome of the foot. *J Bone Joint Surg* 1986;68A:1449–1450.

98. Brand RL, Collins MDF. Operative management of ligamentous injuries to the ankle. *Clin Sports Med* 1982;1(1):117–130.

99. Cass JR, Morrey BF. Ankle instability: Current concepts, diagnosis, and treatment. *Mayo Clin Proc* 1984;59:165–170.

100. Church CC. Radiographic diagnosis of acute peroneal tendon dislocation. *AJR* 1977;129:1065–1068.

101. Cox JS, Hewes TF. Normal talar tilt angle. *Clin Orthop* 1979;140:37–41.

102. Daffner RH, Riemer BL, Lupetin AR, Dash N. Magnetic resonance imaging in acute tendon ruptures. *Skel Radiol* 1980;15(8):619–621.

103. Davies JAK. Peroneal compartment syndrome secondary to rupture of the peroneus longus. *J Bone Joint Surg* 1979;61A:783–784.

104. DeLuca PA, Bauta JV. Pes cavovarus as a late consequence of peroneus longus tendon rupture. *J Ped Orthop* 1985;5:582–583.

105. Dezwart DF, Davidson JSA. Rupture of the posterior tibial tendon associated with ankle fractures. *J Bone Joint Surg* 1983;65A:260–261.

106. Dory MA. Arthrography of the ankle joint in chronic instability. *Skel Radiol* 1986;15(9):291–294.

107. Edwards GS, DeLee JC. Ankle diastasis without fracture. *Foot and Ankle* 1984;4(6):305–312.

108. Evans GA, Frenyo SD. The stress-tenogram in diagnosis of ruptures of the lateral ligament of the ankle. *J Bone Joint Surg* 1979;61B:347–351.

109. Fornage BD. Achilles tendon: US examination. *Radiology* 1986;159:759–764.

110. Funk DA, Cass JA, Johnson KA. Acquired adult flatfoot secondary to posterior tibial-tendon pathology. *J Bone Joint Surg* 1986;68A:95–102.

111. Garth WP. Flexor hallucis tendonitis in a ballet dancer. *J Bone Joint Surg* 1981;63A:1489.

112. Gilula LA, Oloff L, Caputi R, Destouet JM, Jacobs A, Solomon MA. Ankle tenography: A key to unexplained symptomatology. Part II: Diagnosis of chronic tendon disabilities. *Radiology* 1984;151:581–587.

113. Goergen TG, Resnick D. Arthrography of the ankle and hindfoot In: Dalinka MK. *Arthrography.* New York: Springer-Verlag, 1980;137–153.

114. Harrington KD. Degenerative arthritis of the ankle secondary to long-standing ligament instability. *J Bone Joint Surg* 1979;61A:354–361.

115. Horsfield D, Murphy G. Stress views of the ankle joint in lateral ligament injury. *Radiography* 1985;51:7–11.

116. Inglis AE, Scott N, Sculo TP, Patterson AH. Rupture of the tendo

117. Johannsen A. Radiologic diagnosis of lateral ligament lesion of the ankle. *Acta Orthop Scand* 1978;49:295–301.

118. Johnson EE, Morkolf KL. The contribution of the anterior talofibular ligament to ankle laxity. *J Bone Joint Surg* 1983;65A:81–88.

119. Kelikian H, Kelikian AS. *Disorders of the ankle.* Philadelphia: W. B. Saunders, 1985.

120. Kleinman M, Gross AE. Achilles tendon rupture following steroid injection. *J Bone Joint Surg* 1983;65A(9):1345–1347.

121. Larson E. Experimental instability of the ankle: A radiographic investigation. *Clin Orthop* 1986;204:193–200.

122. Mann RA, Thompson FM. Rupture of the posterior tibial tendon causing flat foot. *J Bone Joint Surg* 1985;67A:556–561.

123. Montague AP, McQuillan RF. Clinical assessment of the apparently sprained ankle and detection of fracture. *Injury* 1985;16:545–546.

124. Morti R. Dislocation of the peroneal tendon. *Am J Sports Med* 1977;5(1):19–22.

125. Morrey BF, Cass TR, Johnson KA, Berquist TH. Foot and ankle. In: Berquist TH. ed. *Imaging of orthopedic trauma and surgery.* Philadelphia: W. B. Saunders, 1986;407–493.

126. Murr S. Dislocation of the peroneal tendon with marginal fracture of the lateral malleolus. *J Bone Joint Surg* 1965;43B:563–565.

127. Newmark H, Olken SM, Mellon WS, Malhotra AK, Halls J. A new finding in radiographic diagnosis of Achilles tendon rupture. *Skel Radiol* 1982;8:223–224.

128. O'Brien T. The needle test for complete rupture of the Achilles tendon. *J Bone Joint Surg* 1984;66A:1099–1101.

129. Percy EC, Conochie LB. Surgical treatment of ruptured tendo Achilles. *J Bone Joint Surg* 1975;57B:535.

130. Puhl RA, Altman MI, Seto JE, Nelson GA. The use of fluoroscopy in detection—an excision of foreign bodies in the foot. *J Am Podiatr Med Assoc* 1983;73:514–517.

131. Romanus B, Lundahl S, Stener B. Accessory soleus muscle: A clinical and radiographic presentation of 11 cases. *J Bone Joint Surg* 1986;68A:731–734.

132. Rosenberg ZS, Feldman F, Singson RD. Peroneal tendon injuries: CT analysis. *Radiology* 1986;161:743–748.

133. Rosenberg ZS, Feldman F, Singson RD, Price GJ. Peroneal tendon injury associated with calcaneal fractures. CT findings. *AJR* 1987;149:125–129.

134. Sauser DD, Nelson RC, Lavine MH, Wu CW. Acute injuries of the lateral ligaments of the ankle: Comparison of stress radiography and arthrography. *Radiology* 1983;148:653–657.

135. Schweigel JF, Knickerbocher WJ, Cooperberg P. A study of ankle instability utilizing ankle arthrography. *J Trauma* 1977;17(11):878–881.

136. Simon RR, Hoffman JR, Smith M. Radiographic comparison of plain films on second and third-degree ankle sprains. *Am J Emerg Med* 1986;4(5):387–389.

137. Spiegel PK, Staples OS. Arthrography of the ankle joint: Problems in diagnosis of acute lateral leg injuries. *Radiology* 1975;114:587–590.

138. Stein RE. Rupture of the posterior tibial tendon in closed ankle fractures. *J Bone Joint Surg* 1985;67A:493–494.

139. Szczukowski M, St Pierre RK, Fleming LL, Somogyi J. Computerized tomography in the evaluation of peroneal tendon dislocation. A report of two cases. *Am J Sports Med* 1983;11(6):444–447.

140. Tandberg D. Glass in the hand and foot. Will x-ray film show it? *JAMA* 1982;248:1872–1874.

141. Tehranzadeh J, Stoll DA, Gabriele OM. Case report 271: Posterior migration of the os peroneum of the left foot, indicating a tear of the peroneal tendon. *Skel Radiol* 1984;12:44–47.

142. Termansen NB, Hansen H, Damvolt V. Radiologic and muscular status following injury to the lateral ligaments of the ankle. *Acta Orthop Scand* 1979;50:705–708.

143. Thompson TC. A test for rupture of the tendo Achilles. *Acta Ortho Scand* 1962;32:461–465.

Achilles: An objective assessment of surgical and non-surgical treatment. *J Bone Joint Surg* 1976;58A:990–993.

Fractures

144. Bosworth DM. Fracture-dislocation of the ankle with fixed displacement of the fibula behind the tibia. *J Bone Joint Surg* 1947;29:130–135.
145. Cotton FJ. A new type of ankle fracture. *JAMA* 1915;64:318–321.
146. Cotton FJ. Ankle fractures. A new classification and a new class. *N Engl J Med* 1929;201:753–760.
147. Destot E. Traumatis mes dupied et rayons v malleoles, as tragale, calcaneum, avant-pied. Paris: Masson, 1911.
148. Jones R. Fracture of the fifth metatarsal bone. *Med Chir J* 1902;22:103–107.
149. Kavanagh JH, Brower TD, Mann RV. The Jones fracture revisited. *J Bone Joint Surg* 1978;60A:776–782.
150. Kelikian H, Kelikian AS. *Disorders of the ankle.* Philadelphia: W. B. Saunders, 1985.
151. Marmor L. An unusual fracture of the tibial epiphysis. *Clin Orthop* 1970;73:132–135.
152. Morrey BF, Cass JR, Johnson KA, Berquist TH. The foot and ankle. In: Berquist TH, ed. *Imaging of orthopedic trauma and surgery.* Philadelphia: W. B. Saunders, 1976.
153. Ovadia DN, Beals RK. Fractures of the tibial plafond. *J Bone Joint Surg* 1986;68A:543–551.
154. Peiro A, Araal J, Martos F, Mat T. Triplane distal tibial epiphyseal fracture. *Clin Orthop* 1981;160:196–200.
155. Penetcost RL, Murry RA, Brindley HH. Fatigue, insufficiency and pathologic fractures. *JAMA* 1964;187:1001–1004.
156. Perry CR, Rice S, Aswath R, Burdge R. Posterior fracture-dislocation of the distal part of the fibula. *J Bone Joint Surg* 1983;65A:1149–1157.
157. Pitt MJ, Speer DP. Radiologic reporting of orthopedic trauma. *Med Radiogr Photo* 1982;58:14–18.
158. Rand JA, Berquist TH. Fracture healing. In: Berquist TH, ed. *Imaging of orthopedic trauma and surgery.* Philadelphia: W. B. Saunders, 1986;51–90.
159. Schultz RJ. *The language of fractures.* Baltimore: Williams and Wilkins, 1972.
160. Torg JS, Baldini FC, Zelko RR, Pavlov H, Peff TC, Dos M. Fractures of the base of the fifth metatarsal distal to the tuberosity. *J Bone Joint Surg* 1984;66A:209–214.
161. Towbin R, Dimbar JS, Towbin J. Teardrop sign: Plain film recognition of ankle effusion. *AJR* 1980;134:985–990.

Adult Ankle Fracture

162. Arimoto HR, Forrester DM. Classification of ankle fractures: An algorithm. *AJR* 1980;135:1057–1063.
163. Ashhurst APC, Bromer RS. Classification and mechanism of fractures of the leg bones involving the ankle. *Arch Surg* 1922;4:51–129.
164. Baird RA, Jackson ST. Fractures of the distal part of the fibula associated with disruption of the deltoid ligament. *J Bone Joint Surg* 1987;69A:1346–1352.
165. Berquist TH. *Radiology of the foot and ankle.* New York: Raven Press, 1989.
166. Boden SD, Labropoulus PA, McCowin P, Lestine WF, Hurwitz SR. Mechanical considerations for the syndesmosis screw. *J Bone Joint Surg* 1989;71A:1548–1555.
167. Charnley J. *The closed treatment of common fractures.* Baltimore: Williams and Wilkins, 1963.
168. Coonrad RW. Fracture dislocation of the ankle joint with impaction injury of the lateral weight bearing surface of the tibia. *J Bone Joint Surg* 1970;52A:1337–1344.
169. DeZwart DF, Davidson JSA. Rupture of the posterior tibial tendon associated with fractures of the ankle. *J Bone Joint Surg* 1983;65A:260–262.
170. Dihlman W. Computed tomography of the ankle joint. *Chirurg* 1982;53:123–126.
171. Edeiken J, Cotler JM. Ankle trauma. *Sem Roent* 1978;13(2):145–155.
172. Edwards GS, DeLee JC. Ankle diastasis without fracture. *Foot and Ankle* 1984;4(6):305–312.
173. Eventon I, Salama R, Goodwin DRA, Weissman SL. An evaluation of surgical and conservative treatment of fractures of the ankle in 200 patients. *J Trauma* 1978;18(4):271–274.
174. Genant HK, Kozin F, Bekerman C, McCarty DJ, Sims J. The reflex sympathetic dystrophy syndrome. *Radiology* 1975;117:21–32.
175. Giachino AA, Hammond DI. The relationship between oblique fracture of the medial malleolus and concomitant fractures of the anterolateral aspect of the tibial plafond. *J Bone Joint Surg* 1987;69A:381–384.
176. Griffiths HJ. Trauma to the ankle and foot. *Crit Rev Diagn Imaging* 1979;26(1):45–105.
177. Griffiths HJ, Utz R, Burke J, Bonfiglio T. Adhesive capsulitis of the hip and ankle. *AJR* 1985;144:101–105.
178. Hall H. A simplified workable classification of ankle fractures. *Foot and Ankle* 1980;1:5–10.
179. Horne G. Pes cavovarus following ankle fracture. *Clin Orthop* 1984;184:249–251.
180. Jenkins D, Campbell LG. Synovial chondromatosis of the ankle. *J Am Podiatr Assoc* 1981;71(12):666–670.
181. Lauge-Hansen N. Fractures of the ankle II: Combined experimental-surgical once experimental roentgenologic investigations. *Arch Surg* 1950;60:957–985.
182. Leach RE. Fractures of the tibial plafond. *AAOS Instructional Course Lectures* 1979;28:88–93.
183. Leach RE. Fractures of the tibia and fibula. In: Rockwood CA, Green DP, ed. *Fractures in adults,* vol. II, Philadelphia: J.B. Lippincott, 1984.
184. Leeds HC, Erlich MG. Instability of the distal tibiofibular syndesmosis after bimalleolar and trimalleolar fractures. *J Bone Joint Surg* 1984;66A:490–503.
185. Limbird RS, Aaron RK. Laterally comminuted fracture dislocation of the ankle. *J Bone Joint Surg* 1987;69A:881–885.
186. Mainwaring BL, Daffner RH, Riemer BL. Pylon fractures of the ankle: A distinct clinical and radiologic entity. *Radiology* 1988;168:215–218.
187. Montague AP, McQuillan RF. Clinical assessment of apparently sprained ankle and detection of fracture. *Injury* 1985;16:545–546.
188. Morgan CD, Henke JA, Bailey RW, Kaufer H. Long-term results of tibiotalar arthrodesis. *J Bone Joint Surg* 1985;67A:546–550.
189. Morrey BF, Cass JR, Johnson KA, Berquist TH. In: Berquist TH ed. *Imaging of orthopedic trauma and surgery.* Philadelphia: W. B. Saunders, 1986;407–498.
190. Morrey BF, Weedeman GP. Complications and long-term results of ankle arthrodesis following trauma. *J Bone Joint Surg* 1980;62A:777–784.
191. Müller ME, Allgower M, Willenegger H. *Manual of internal fixation.* New York: Springer-Verlag, 1970.
192. Neer CS II. Injuries of the ankle joint: Evaluation. *Conn St Med J* 1953;17:580–583.
193. Olerud C. Supination-eversion ankle fractures sustained during downhill skiing. *Acta Orthop Traum Surg* 1985;104:129–131.
194. Ovadia DN, Beals RK. Fractures of the tibial plafond. *J Bone Joint Surg* 1986;68A:543–551.
195. Perry CR, Rice S, Rao A, Burdge R. Posterior fracture-dislocation of the distal part of the fibula. *J Bone Joint Surg* 1983;65A:1149–1157.
196. Pettrone FA, Gail M, Pee D, Fitzpatrick T, Van Herpe LB. Quantitative criteria for prediction of the results after displaced fracture of the ankle. *J Bone Joint Surg* 1983;65A:667–677.
197. Poplawski ZJ, Wiley AM, Murry JF. Post-traumatic dystrophy of the extremities. *J Bone Joint Surg* 1983;66A:642–654.
198. Ruedi T. Fractures of the lower end of the tibia into the ankle joint: Results of 9 years after open reduction and internal fixation. *Injury* 1973;5:130–134.
199. Said F, Hunka L, Siller TN. Where ankle fusions stand today. *J Bone Joint Surg* 1978;60B:211–214.
200. Sarkisian JS, Cody GW. Closed treatment of ankle fractures: A new criteria for evaluation—a review of 250 cases. *J Trauma* 1976;16(4):323–326.
201. Schaffer JJ, Manoli A. The antiglide plate for distal fibular fixa-

tion. A biomechanical comparison with fixation with a lateral plate. *J Bone Joint Surg* 1987;69A:596–605.

202. Schutzer SF, Gosslurg HR. The treatment of reflex sympathetic dystrophy syndrome. *J Bone Joint Surg* 1984;66A:625–629.

203. Sclafani SJA. Ligamentous injury of the lower tibiofibular syndesmosis: Radiographic evidence. *Radiology* 1985;156:21–27.

204. Segal D, Wiss DA, Whitelaw GP. Functional bracing and rehabilitation of ankle fractures. *Clin Orthop* 1985;199:39–45.

205. Weber BG, Simpson LA. Corrective lengthening osteotomy of the fibula. *Clin Orthop* 1985;199:61–67.

206. Whitelaw GP, Sawka MW, Wetzler M, Segal D, Miller J. Unrecognized injuries of the lateral ligaments associated with lateral malleolar fractures of the ankle. *J Bone Joint Surg* 1989;71A:1396–1399.

207. Wilson FC. Fractures and dislocations of the ankle. In: Rockwood CA, Green DP eds. *Fractures in adults,* vol. II. Philadelphia: J.B. Lippincott, 1984;1665–1702.

208. Wilson FC, Skibred LA. Long-term results in the treatment of displaced bimalleolar fractures. *J Bone Joint Surg* 1966; 48A:1065–1078.

209. Woersdoefer O, Weber BG. Diaphyseal fracture of both bones of the lower leg with associated injury of the ankle mortise. *Arch Orthop Traumat Surg* 1981;98:293–296.

210. Yablon IG, Heller FG, Shouse L. The key role of the lateral malleolus in displaced fractures of the ankle. *J Bone Joint Surg* 1977;59A:169–173.

211. Yablon IG, Wasilewski S. Management of unstable ankle fractures. *Foot and Ankle* 1980;1:11–19.

212. Yablon IG, Leach RE. Reconstruction of malunited fractures of the lateral malleolus. *J Bone Joint Surg* 1989;71A:521–527.

213. Yde J. The Lauge-Hansen classification of malleolar fractures. *Acta Orthop Scand* 1980;51:181–192.

214. Yde J, Kristensen KD. Ankle fractures: Supination eversion fractures of stage IV. *Acta Orthop Scand* 1980;51:981–990.

215. Yde J, Kristensen KD. Ankle fractures: Supination eversion fractures stage II. Primary and late operative and non-operative treatment. *Acta Orthop Scand* 1980;51:695–702.

Talar Fractures and Dislocations

216. Alexander AH, Lichtman DM. Surgical treatment of transchondral talar dome fractures. *J Bone Joint Surg* 1980;62A:646–652.

217. Anderson IF, Crichton KJ, Grattan-Smith T, Cooper RA, Brazier DI. Osteochondral fractures of the talar dome. *J Bone Joint Surg* 1989;71A:1143–1152.

218. Berquist TH. *MRI of the musculoskeletal system,* 2nd ed. New York: Raven Press, 1990.

219. Blair HC. Comminuted fractures and fracture dislocations of the body of the talus. *Am J Surg* 1943;59:37–43.

220. Bonnin JG. *Injuries of the ankle.* New York: Grune and Stratton, 1950.

221. Berndt AL, Harty M. Transchondral fractures (osteochondritis dissecans) of the talus. *J Bone Joint Surg* 1959;41A:988–1020.

222. Burkus JK, Sella FJ, Southwick WO. Occult injuries of the talus diagnosed by bone scan and tomography. *Foot and Ankle* 1984;4(6):316–324.

223. Canale ST, Kelly FB. Fractures of the neck and the talus. *J Bone Joint Surg* 1978;60A:143–156.

224. Canale ST, Belding RH. Osteochondral lesions of the talus. *J Bone Joint Surg* 1980;62A:97–102.

225. Coltart WD. Aviators astragalus. *J Bone Joint Surg* 1952;34B:545–566.

226. Cooper RR, Capillo W. Talectomy. *Clin Orthop* 1985;201:32–35.

227. DeLee J, Curtis R. Subtalar dislocation of the foot. *J Bone Joint Surg* 1982;64A:433–437.

228. Dennis DM, Tullas HS. Blair tibiotalar arthrodesis for injuries of the talus. *J Bone Joint Surg* 1980;62A:103–107.

229. Detenbeck LC, Kelly PJ. Total dislocation of the talus. *J Bone Joint Surg* 1969;51A:283–288.

230. El-Khary GY, Yousefzadek DH, Mulligan GM, Moore TE. Subtalar dislocation. *Skel Radiol* 1982;8:99–103.

231. Flick AB, Gould N. Osteochondritis dissecans of the talus: Review of the literature and a new surgical approach for medial dome lesions. *Foot and Ankle* 1985;5(4):165–185.

232. Floyd FJ, Ransom RA, Dailey JM. Computed tomography scanning of the subtalar joint. *J Am Podiatr Assoc* 1984;14(11):533–537.

233. Gross RH. Fractures and dislocations of the foot. In: Rockwood CA, Wilkins KE, Kuig RE. *Fractures in children,* vol. 3. Philadelphia: J.P. Lippincott, 1984.

234. Hawkins LG. Fractures of the lateral process of the talus. *J Bone Joint Surg* 1965;47A:1170–1175.

235. Hawkins LG. Fractures of the neck of the talus. *J Bone Joint Surg* 1970;52A:991–1002.

236. Heckman JD. Fractures and dislocations of the foot. In: Rockwood DA, Green DP. *Fractures in children,* 2nd ed. Philadelphia: J.B. Lippincott, 1984;1703–1832.

237. Janssen T, Kopta J. Bilateral recurrent subtalar dislocation. *J Bone Joint Surg* 1985;67A:1432–1433.

238. Kenwright J, Taylor RG. Major injuries of the talus. *J Bone Joint Surg* 1970;52B:36–48.

239. Kleiger B, Ahmed M. Injuries of the talus and its joints. *Clin Orthop* 1976;121:243–262.

240. Leitner B. Obstacles to reduction of subtalar dislocation. *J Bone Joint Surg* 1954;39A:299–306.

241. Letts RM, Gibeault D. Fractures of the neck of the talus in children. *Foot and Ankle* 1980;1(2):74–77.

242. Lorentzen JE, Christensen SB, Krogsoe O, Snepper. Fractures of the neck of the talus. *Acta Orthop Scand* 1977;48:115–120.

243. Mankin HJ. The response of articular cartilage to mechanical injury. *J Bone Joint Surg* 1982;64A:460–466.

244. McDougall A. The os trigonum. *J Bone Joint Surg* 1955; 37B:257–265.

245. Mindell EB, Cisek EE, Kartalian G, Dziob JM. Late results of injuries of the talus. *J Bone Joint Surg* 1963;45A:221–245.

246. Monson ST, Ryan JR. Subtalar dislocation. *J Bone Joint Surg* 1981;63A:1156–1158.

247. Morrey BF, Cass JR, Johnson KA, Berquist TH. Foot and ankle. In: Berquist TH. ed. *Imaging of orthopedic trauma and surgery.* Philadelphia: W.B. Saunders, 1986.

248. Mukherjee SK, Pringle RM, Baxter RM. Fracture of the lateral process of the talus. *J Bone Joint Surg* 1974;56B:263–273.

249. Mulfinger GL, Trueta JC. The blood supply of the talus. *J Bone Joint Surg* 1970;52B:160–167.

250. Mulligan ME. Horizontal fracture of the talar head. *Am J Sports Med* 1986;14(2):176–177.

251. Naumetz VA, Schweigel JF. Osteocartilagenous lesions of the talar dome. *J Trauma* 1980;20(11):924–927.

252. Newberg AH. Osteochondral fractures of the dome of the talus. *Brit J Radiol* 1979;52:105–109.

253. Nyari T, Kazar G, Frenyo S, Balla I. The role of interosseous phlebography in the prognosis of injuries of the talus. *Injury* 1982;13:317–323.

254. Pennal GF. Fractures of the talus. *Clin Orthop* 1963;30:53–63.

255. Peterson L, Goldie IF, Irstam L. Fracture of the neck of the talus. *Acta Orthop Scand* 1977;48:696–707.

256. Peterson L, Goldie I, Lindell D. The arterial supply of the talus. *Acta Orthop Scand* 1974;45:260–270.

257. Pritsch M, Horoshovski H, Farine I, Tel-hanomer. Arthroscopic treatment of osteochondral lesions of the talus. *J Bone Joint Surg* 1986;68A:862–864.

258. Quirk R. Talar compression syndrome in dancers. *Foot and Ankle* 1982;3(2):65–68.

259. Resnick D. Talar ridges, osteophytes and beaks: A radiologic commentary. *Radiology* 1984;151:329–332.

260. Resnick D. Radiology of the talocalcaneal articulations. *Radiology* 1984;111:581–586.

261. Rijsbosch JKC. Fractures of the talus. *Arch Chir Nierlandicum* 1956;8:163–173.

262. Scott JE. Dislocations of the ankle without fracture. *J Bone Joint Surg* 1974;39A:299–306.

263. Segal D, Waselewski S. Total dislocation of the talus. *J Bone Joint Surg* 1980;62A:1370–1372.

264. Seltzer SE, Weissman BN, Braunstein EM, Adams DF, Thomas

WH. Computed tomography of the hind foot. *J Comp Assist Tomogr* 1984;8(3):488–497.
265. Sierra A, Potchen EJ, Moore J, Smith GH. High-field magnetic resonance imaging of aseptic necrosis of the talus. *J Bone Joint Surg* 1986;68A:927–928.
266. Smith GR, Winquist RA, Allan NK, Northrop CH. Subtle transchondral fractures of the talar dome: A radiological perspective. *Radiology* 1977;124:667–673.
267. Smith H. Subastragalar dislocation. *J Bone Joint Surg* 1937;19:373–380.
268. Snepper O, Christensen SB, Krogsoe O, Lorentzen J. Fracture of the body of the talus. *Acta Orthop Scand* 1977;48:317–324.
269. Solomon MA, Gilula LA, Oloff LM, Oloff J, Compton J. CT scanning of the foot and ankle: Normal anatomy. *AJR* 1986;146:1192–1203.
270. Thompson JP, Loomer RL. Osteochondral lesions of the talus in a sports medicine clinic. *Am J Sports Med* 1984;12(6):460–463.
271. Yuan HA, Cody RB, DeRosa C. Osteochondritis dissecans of the talus associated with subchondral apts. *J Bone Joint Surg* 1979;61A:1249–1251.

Calcaneal Fractures

272. Bohler L. Diagnosis, pathology, and treatment of fractures of the os calcis. *J Bone Joint Surg* 1931;13:75–89.
273. Cave EF. Fracture of the os calcis—the problem in general. *Clin Orthop* 1963;30:64–66.
274. DuVries HL. *Surgery of the foot*, 4th ed. St. Louis: C.V. Mosby, 1978.
275. Essex-Loprestie P. The mechanism, reduction technique, and results in fractures of the os calcis. *Br J Surg* 1952;39:395–419.
276. Gellman M. Fractures of the anterior process of the calcaneus. *J Bone Joint Surg* 1931;13:877–879.
277. Gilmer PW, Herzenberg J, Frank JL, Silverman P, Morteney S, Goldner JL. Computerized tomographic analysis of acute calcaneal fractures. *Foot and Ankle* 1986;6:184–193.
278. Gross RH. Fractures and dislocations of the foot. In: Rockwood CA, Wilkins KE, King RE, *Fractures in children*, vol. 3. Philadelphia: J.B. Lippincott, 1984;1043–1103.
279. Guyer BH, Levinsuhn EM, Fredrickson BE, Bailey GL, Formikell M. Computed tomography of calcaneal fractures: Anatomy, pathology, dosimetry, and clinical relevance. *AJR* 1985;145:911–919.
280. Hall MC, Pennal GF. Primary subtalar arthrodesis in treatment of severe fractures of the calcaneus. *J Bone Joint Surg* 1960;42B:336–343.
281. Heckman JD. Fractures and dislocations of the foot. In: Rockwood CA, Green DP. *Fractures in adults*, vol. 2. Philadelphia: J.B. Lippincott, 1984;1703–1832.
282. Heger L, Wolff K. Computed tomography of the calcaneus: Normal anatomy. *AJR* 1985;145:123–129.
283. Isbister JF. Calcaneofibular abutment following crush fracture of the calcaneus. *J Bone Joint Surg* 1974;56B:274–278.
284. Johannson J, Harrison J, Greenwood FAH. Subtalar arthrodesis for adult arthritis. *Foot and Ankle* 1982;2:294–298.
285. Korn R. Der Bruch durch Lintere obere Drittel des Fersenbeines. *Arch Orthop* 1942;47:189.
286. Lance EM, Corey EJ, Wade PA. Fractures of the os calcis. *J Trauma* 1964;4:15–56.
287. Morrey BF, Cass JF, Johnson KA, Berquist TH. Foot and Ankle. In: Berquist TH. *Imaging of orthopedic trauma and surgery*. Philadelphia: W. B. Saunders, 1986;407–498.
288. Norfay JF, Rogers LF, Adams GP, Graves HC, Herser WJ. Common calcaneal avulsion fracture. *AJR* 1980;134:119–123.
289. Pablot SM, Daneman A, Strurger DA, Carroll N. The value of computed tomography or early assessment of comminuted calcaneal fractures. *J Ped Orthop* 1985;5:435–438.
290. Renfrew DL, El-Khoury GY. Anterior process fractures of the calcaneus. *Skel Radiol* 1985;14:121–125.
291. Rosenberg ZS, Feldman F, Surgson RD. Intra-articular calcaneal

fractures: Computed tomographic analysis. *Skeletal Radiol* 1987;16:105–113.
292. Ross SDK, Sowerby RR. The operative treatment of fractures of the os calcis. *Clin Orthop* 1985;199:132–143.
293. Rowe CR, Sakillarides HT, Freeman PA. Fractures of the os calcis. A long-term follow-up study in 146 patients. *JAMA* 1963;184:920–924.
294. Schmidt TL, Weiner DS. Calcaneal fractures in children. An evaluation of the nature of injury in 56 children. *Clin Orthop* 1982;171:150–155.
295. Segal D, Marsh JL, Leiter B. Clinical application of computerized axial tomography scanning of calcaneal fractures. *Clin Orthop* 1985;199:114–123.
296. Slatis P, Kroduoto O, Santavista S, Laasonen EM. Fractures of the calcaneus. *J Trauma* 1979;19(12):939–943.
297. Stephenson JR. Displaced fractures of the os calcis involving the subtalar joint: The key role of the superomedial fragment. *Foot and Ankle* 1983;4:91–101.
298. Trott AW. Fractures of the foot in children. *Orthop Clin North Am* 1976;7:677–686.

Midfoot and Forefoot Fractures

299. Aitken AP, Paulsen D. Dislocation of the tarso-metatarsal joints. *J Bone Joint Surg* 1963;45A:246–260.
300. Anderson LD. Injuries of the forefoot. *Clin Orthop* 1977;122:18–27.
301. Berquist TH. *Radiology of the foot and ankle.* New York: Raven Press, 1989.
302. Bonutti PM, Bell GR. Compartment syndrome of the foot. *J Bone Joint Surg* 1986;68A:1449–1450.
303. Cain PR, Seligson D. Lisfranc's fracture-dislocation with intercuneiform dislocation. *Foot and Ankle* 1981;2(3):156–160.
304. Campbell WB, Fletcher EL, Hands LD. Assessment of the distal lower limb arteries: A comparison of arteriography and Doppler ultrasound. *Am Royal Coll Surgeons* 1986;68:37–39.
305. Carp L. Fracture of the fifth metatarsal bone with special reference to delayed union. *Am Surg* 1927;86:308–320.
306. Cassebaum WH. LisFranc fracture dislocations. *Clin Orthop* 1963;30:116–129.
307. Dick IL. Impacted fracture of the tarsal navicular. *Proc Royal Soc Med* 1941;35:760.
308. Eichenholtz SN, Levene DB. Fracture of the tarsal navicular bone. *Clin Orthop* 1964;34:142–157.
309. English TA. Dislocation of the metatarsal bone and adjacent toe. *J Bone Joint Surg* 1964;46B:700–704.
310. Faciszewoki T, Burks RT, Manaster BJ. Subtle injuries of the Lisfranc joint. *J Bone Joint Surg* 1990;72A:1519–1522.
311. Foster SC, Foster RR. Lisfranc's tarsometatarsal fracture dislocation. *Radiology* 1976;120:79–83.
312. Gissane W. A dangerous type of fracture of the foot. *J Bone Joint Surg* 1951;33B:535–538.
313. Goiney RC, Connell DG, Nichols DM. CT evaluation of tarsometatarsal fracture-dislocation injuries. *AJR* 1985;144:985–990.
314. Gross RH. Fractures and dislocation of the foot. In: Rockwood CA, Wilkins KE, King RE. *Fractures in children*, vol. 3. Philadelphia: J.B. Lippincott, 1984;1043–1103.
315. Hardcastle PH, Reschauer R, Kutscha-Lissberg E, Schoffman W. Injuries of the tarsometatarsal joint: Incidence, classification, and treatment. *J Bone Joint Surg* 1982;64B:349–356.
316. Heckman JD. Fractures of the foot and ankle. In: Rockwood CA, Green DP. *Fractures.* Philadelphia: J.B. Lippencott, 1984;1703–1832.
317. Johnson GF. Pediatric Lisfranc injury: "Bunkbed" fracture. *AJR* 1981;137:1041–1044.
318. Jones R. Fracture of the base of the fifth metatarsal bone by indirect violence. *Am J Surg* 1902;35:697–700.
319. Kavanaugh JH, Borower TD, Mann RV. The Jones' fracture revisited. *J Bone Joint Surg* 1978;60A:776–782.

320. Lawson JP. Symptomatic radiographic variants in the extremities. *Radiology* 1985;157:625–631.
321. Lewis AG, DeLee JC. Type I complex dislocation of the 1st metatarsophalangeal joint—open reduction through a dorsal approach. *J Bone Joint Surg* 1984;66A:1120–1123.
322. Macy NJ, DeVoer P. Mid-tarsal dislocation of the first ray. *J Bone Joint Surg* 1983;65A:265–266.
323. Main BJ, Jowett RL. Injuries of the mid-tarsal joint. *J Bone Joint Surg* 1975;57B:89–97.
324. Nielsen S, Agnholt J, Christensen H. Radiologic findings in lesions of the ligamentum bifurcatum of the mid foot. *Shel Radiol* 1987;16:114–116.
325. Norfray JF, Feline RA, Steinberg RI, Galinski AW, Gilula LA. Subtleties of Lisfranc fractures-dislocation. *AJR* 1981;137:1151–1156.

326. Roedersheimer LR, Feins R, Green RM. Doppler evaluation of the pedal arch. *Am J Surg* 1981;142:601–604.
327. Sangeorzan BJ, Benirschke SK, Mayo KA, Hansen ST. Displaced intra-articular fractures of the tarsal navicular. *J Bone Joint Surg* 1989;71A:1504–1510.
328. Torg JS, Balduini FC, Zelko RR, Povlov LT, Peff TC, Das M. Fractures of the base of the fifth metatarsal distal to the tuberosity. *J Bone Joint Surg* 1984;66A:209–214.
329. Wiley JJ. The mechanism of tarsometatarsal joint injuries. *J Bone Joint Surg* 1971;53B:474–482.
330. Wilppula E. Tarsometatarsal fracture-dislocation. *Acta Orthop Scand* 1973;44:335–345.
331. Zinman H, Keret Q, Reis ND. Fracture of the medial sesamoid bone of the Hallux. *J Trauma* 1981;21(7):581–582.

Imaging of Orthopedic Trauma, Second Edition, edited by T.H. Berquist, Mayo Clinic © 1992. Published by Raven Press, Ltd., New York.

CHAPTER 10

The Shoulder

Robert H. Cofield and Thomas H. Berquist

Anatomy, 579
Osteology, 579
Articular Anatomy, 582
Neurovascular Anatomy, 584
Biomechanics, 584
Imaging Techniques, 586
Routine Radiography, 586
Radiography of the Scapula, 590
Radiography of the Acromioclavicular Joint, 592
Radiography of the Clavicle, 592
Radiography of the Sternoclavicular Joints, 595
Special Views, 597
Tomography, 605
Special Diagnostic Techniques, 605
Ultrasonography, 605
Computed Tomography, 606

Shoulder Arthrography, 607
Bursography, 624
Acromioclavicular Arthrography, 625
Other Procedures, 626
Magnetic Resonance Imaging (MRI), 626
Applications, 628
Shoulder Arthroscopy, 633
Trauma, 635
Fractures of the Proximal Humerus, 635
Glenohumeral Dislocations, 639
Acromioclavicular Dislocations, 643
Sternoclavicular Dislocations, 644
Clavicle Fractures, 646
Scapular Fracture, 650
References, 653

ANATOMY

The shoulder is anatomically complex, and a review of certain anatomic features is helpful in understanding how to perform imaging procedures and interpret radiographic findings properly.

Osteology

Clavicle

The clavicle is a slight curved (S-shaped) bone that lies ventral to the shoulder girdle (Fig. 10-1). It is one of the first bones to ossify (1,4,6). The medial epiphysis does not unite until the end of the second decade. This should

not be mistaken for a fracture. There are no secondary ossification centers distally. The clavicle articulates with the acromion distally and rarely with the corocoid (5,10). Medially, the pestle-shaped portion of the clavicle articulates with the sternum and first rib. The midportion of the clavicle is tubular, and the distal portion is relatively flat (1,4,10). The dorsal surface of the clavicle is roughened proximally and distally. The trapezius and deltoid muscles insert distally, and the sternocleidomastoid and pectoralis major insert proximally (Fig. 10-1). Inferiorly, the conoid and trapezoid bands of the coracoclavicular ligament attach as the clavicle bows dorsally. They insert in the conoid tubercle and trapezoid ridge, respectively.

Scapula

The scapula is dorsal to the chest wall. The wing (body) of the scapula is a large, flat triangular bone that is almost entirely covered with muscles dorsally and ventrally (Fig. 10-2). The subscapularis covers the ventral

R. H. Cofield: Department of Orthopedic Surgery, Mayo Medical School, Mayo Clinic, Rochester, Minnesota 55905.

T. H. Berquist: Department of Diagnostic Radiology, Mayo Medical School, Mayo Clinic Jacksonville, Jacksonville, Florida 32224.

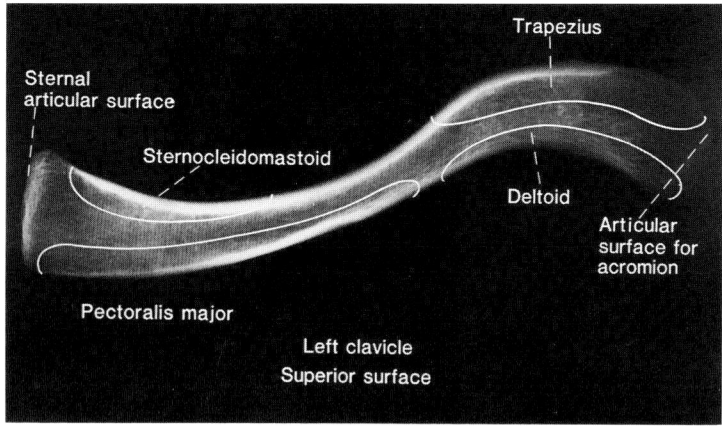

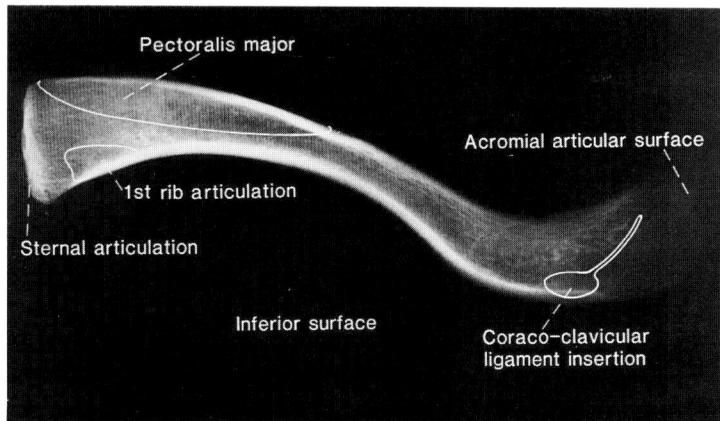

FIG. 10–1. Radiographs of the clavicle with location of major muscle attachments. **A:** Superior surface. **B:** Inferior surface.

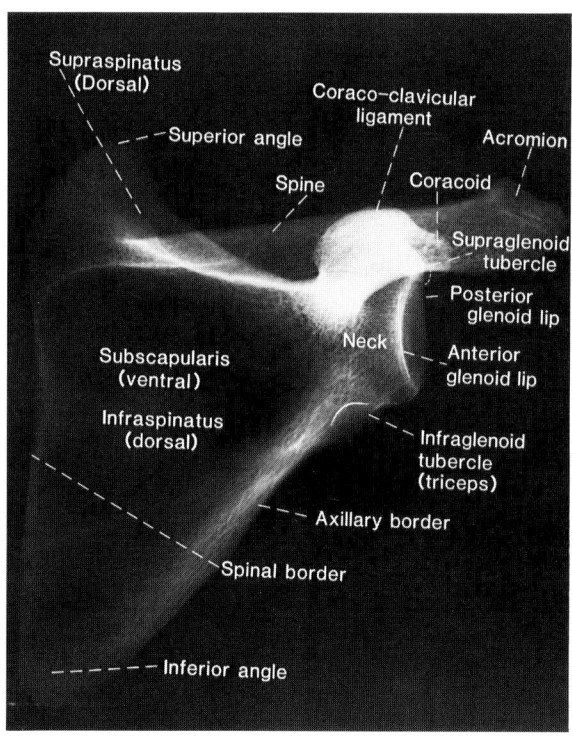

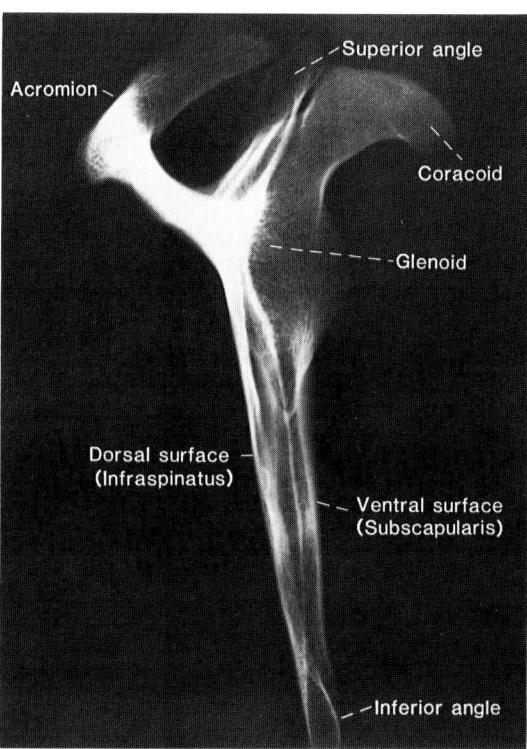

FIG. 10–2. Radiographs of the scapula. **A:** AP view. Note that the anterior glenoid lip is medial to the posterior glenoid rim. **B:** Lateral scapula.

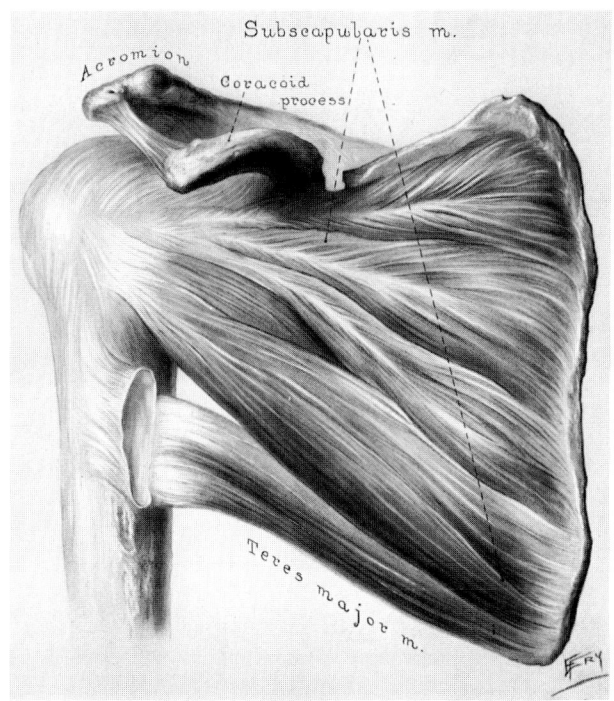

A

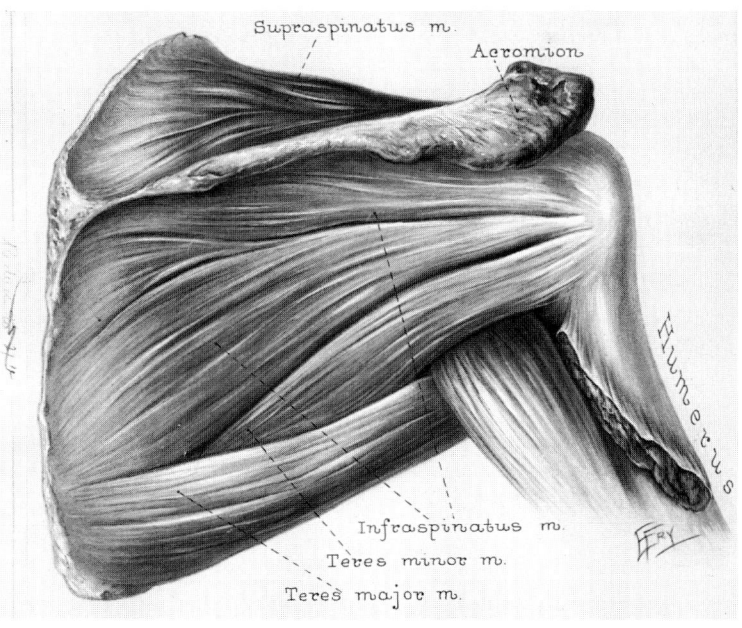

B

FIG. 10-3. **A:** Ventral musculature of the scapula. **B:** Dorsal musculature arising from the scapula.

surface. Dorsally, the supraspinatus takes its origin above the spine of the scapula and the infraspinatus below (Fig. 10-3). The teres major and minor arise from the inferior scapula. The triceps originates from a tubercle just below the glenoid (Fig. 10-2). This tubercle is usually easily visible radiographically. The supraglenoid tubercle is located just superior to the glenoid and serves as the origin of the long head of the biceps brachii. When seen en face, the glenoid lies at the junction of the scapular body, the scapular spine posteriorly, and coracoid anteriorly (Fig. 10-2). This forms a Y with the glenoid at the junction of the limbs.

With the patient positioned for the AP view, the scapula appears oblique. Therefore, the anterior lip of the glenoid is projected medially to the posterior lip (Fig. 10-2). Approximately 40° of posterior rotation is required to obtain a true tangential view of the glenoid (Fig. 10-2). The broad dorsal convex surface of the coracoid serves as the origin of the coracoclavicular ligaments.

There are several secondary ossification centers that should not be confused with fractures. These include the superior glenoid, inferior glenoid, acromial, coracoid, and infrascapular. These ossification centers usually fuse in the second decade (11,17). The glenoid ossification centers may be a source of confusion in patients with shoulder instability.

Proximal Humerus

The humeral head is nearly hemispheric and has four times the surface area of the glenoid (10,16,18,19). The anatomic neck is located at the margin of the articular surface and lies in an oblique plane running superiorly from medial to lateral zones (Fig. 10-4). The surgical neck lies more inferiorly below the tuberosities.

The greater tuberosity is located laterally below the anatomic neck. This structure is seen in profile with the shoulder externally rotated (Fig. 10-4A). There are three facets on the greater tuberosity for insertion of three of the muscles of the rotator cuff (9,10). The insertion for the supraspinatus is most anterior, lying near the intertu-

bercular sulcus. The infraspinatus and teres minor insert just posteriorly to the supraspinatus (Fig. 10-4). The intertubercular sulcus lies between the greater and lesser tuberosities. Radiographically, this groove normally measures about 11 mm in width and 4.6 mm in depth (6). The tendon of the long head of the biceps brachii runs through this groove (4,6,13). The lesser tuberosity lies medially to the intertubercular sulcus and serves as the insertion for the subscapularis (Fig. 10-4C).

The osteology for the remainder of the humerus is discussed in Chapter 11, The Humerus and Arm.

Articular Anatomy

Glenohumeral Joint

The glenohumeral joint is a ball and socket (spheroidea) joint (1,7,10). The normally shallow glenoid cavity

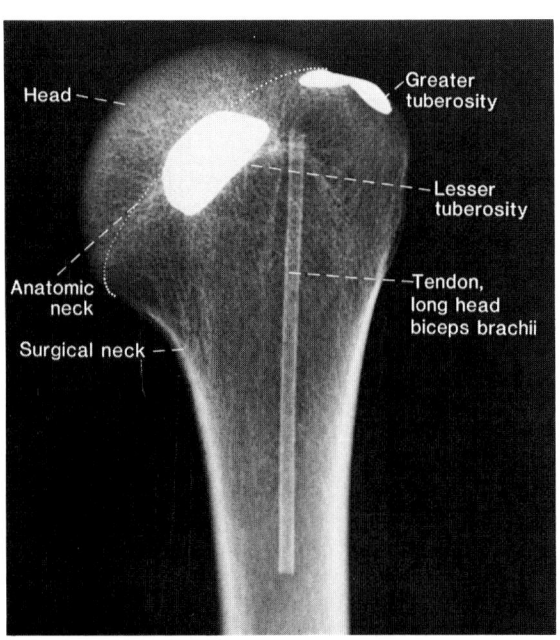

A

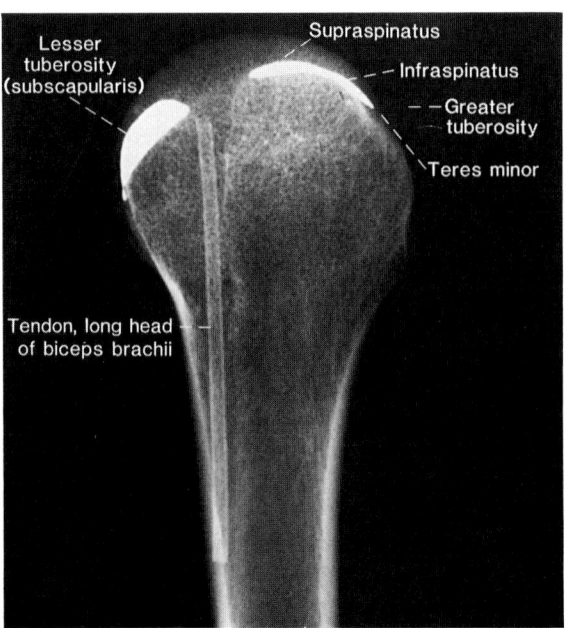

B

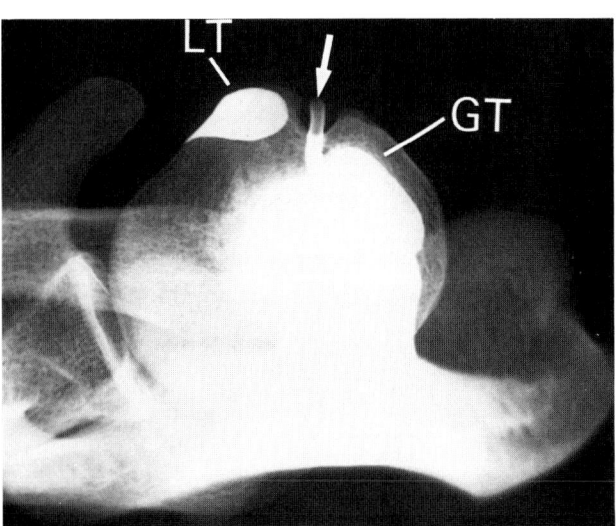

C

FIG. 10-4. Radiographs of the proximal humerus (metal markers on the tuberosities). **A:** External rotation. **B:** Internal rotation. **C:** Tangential view of bicipital groove.

is much smaller than the humeral head (4,15,16). The cavity is deepened by a fibrocartilaginous labrum that extends around the entire peripheral margin of the glenoid cavity (Fig. 10-5).

The synovial-lined capsule attaches proximally to the glenoid labrum and extends peripherally to the anatomic neck of the humerus (1,4,7,14). The total capsular volume is nearly twice that of the humeral head (15). The capsule is stronger anteriorly and inferiorly and is reinforced by surrounding muscles, tendons, and ligaments. Superiorly, reinforcement is achieved by the rotator cuff muscles, specifically by the supraspinatus (Fig. 10-6). Inferiorly, there is support of the glenoid attachment by the triceps brachii, which originates from the infraglenoid tubercle. Anterior reinforcement is provided by the subscapularis tendon. Posteriorly, the teres minor and infraspinatus are adjacent to the capsule (Fig. 10-5) (1,4,10). Superiorly, the tendon of the long head of the biceps brachii arises from the supraglenoid tubercle and labrum (16). The tendon crosses the superior joint and exits through the intertubercular sulcus (Fig. 10-7) (6). This sulcus is formed by the greater and lesser tuberosities. The roof of the groove is covered by the transverse humeral ligament. The biceps tendon is covered by a synovial sheath that extends several centimeters beyond the normal capsule to about the level of the surgical neck (1,4,10,16). Additional support is provided by four ligament complexes: (1) the coracohumeral ligament, which arises from the coracoid to insert in the greater and lesser tuberosities; (2) the superior glenohumeral ligament, which originates just below the coracohumeral ligament

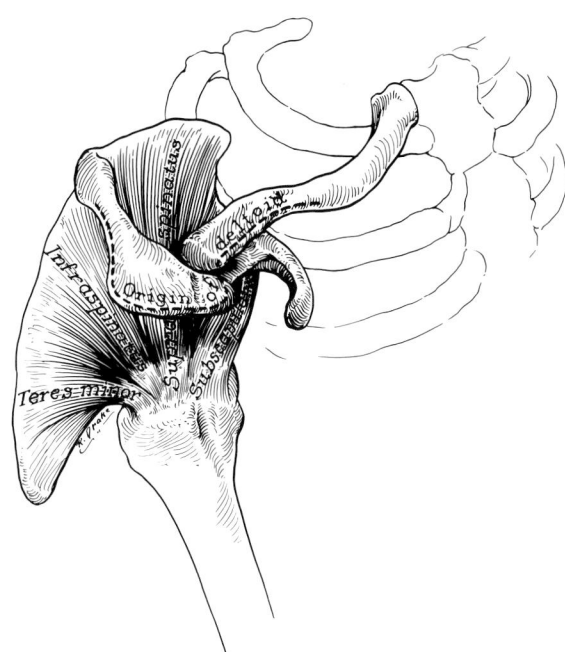

FIG. 10-6. The muscles of the rotator cuff. (Courtesy of Mark B. Coventry, Mayo Clinic, Rochester, Minnesota.)

and blends with the capsule as it inserts in the lesser tuberosity; (3) the middle glenohumeral ligament, which arises from the anterior glenoid and crosses inferiorly to the superior glenohumeral ligament to insert in the lower portion of the lesser tuberosity; and (4) the inferior gle-

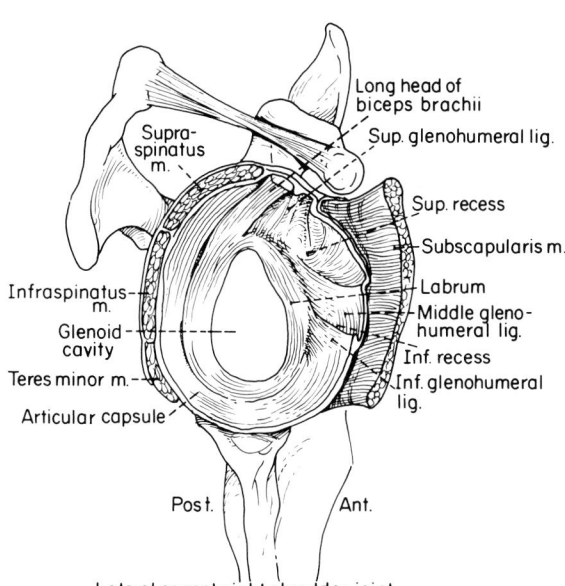

FIG. 10-5. Glenoid cavity enface with humeral head removed. (from Morrey BF, Chao EY. A case history approach—Recurrent anterior dislocation of the shoulder. In *Clinical biomechanics, A case history approach,* Black J, Dampleton JH, eds. New York: Churchill Livingstone, 1981).

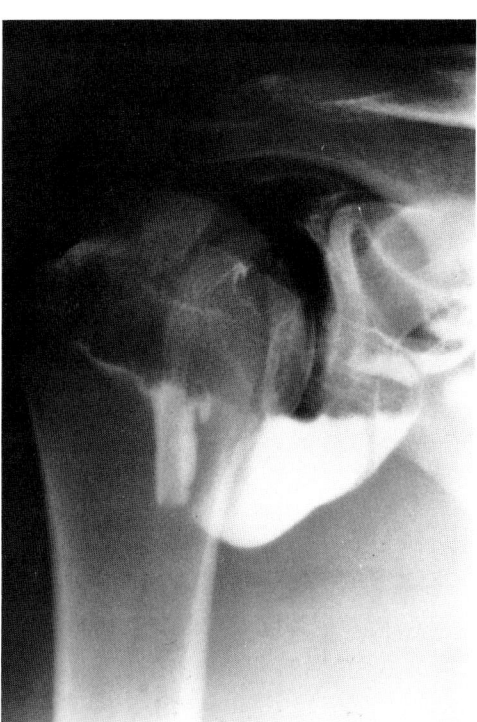

FIG. 10-7. AP view of double contrast arthrogram demonstrating the course of the tendon of the long head of the biceps brachii and its sheath.

nohumeral ligament, which arises from the anterior glenoid and inserts in the region of the surgical neck below the middle glenohumeral ligament (Fig. 10-5) (1,4,5,16,20). Stability supplied by the capsule and ligaments is augmented considerably by the rotator cuff (16).

There may be numerous bursae about the shoulder, but most do not communicate with the joint, and they are not always constant (Table 10-1). The most important are the subscapularis, subdeltoid, subcoracoid, and subacromial. The subscapularis bursa is situated anteriorly beneath the coracoid process and lies dorsal to the subscapularis tendon. The infraspinatus bursa communicates with the posterior joint and lies between the capsule and the infraspinatus tendon. This is not always present (1,4,10). Communication with the tendon sheath of the long head of the biceps is almost always present in the normal shoulder (1,4,16). A large bursa lies between the rotator cuff and acromion. It is composed of subdeltoid, subacromial, and subcoracoid portions (4,10). This does not communicate with the capsule if the rotator cuff is intact (10,15,18,19).

Acromioclavicular Joint

The acromioclavicular joint is a synovial joint that joins the distal clavicle and medial portion of the acromion. An intra-articular disk is occasionally present (4). Both gliding and rotary motion (scapula) are possible (4,12,15). The capsule of the joint is supported by the superior and inferior acromioclavicular ligaments; however, major support is derived from the coracoclavicular ligament (trapezoid and coracoid ligaments). Rarely, a joint is present between the coracoid and clavicle (5,10).

Sternoclavicular Joint

The medial articular portion of the clavicle forms a gliding synovial joint with the manubrium and cartilaginous portion of the first rib. The clavicular surface is larger than the articular surface of either the manubrium or the first rib (4,16). Ligamentous support includes the interclavicular ligament superiorly, the costoclavicular ligament inferiorly, and the anterior and posterior sternoclavicular ligaments. An articular disk extends from the upper clavicle to the cartilage of the first rib, dividing the joint into medial and lateral compartments.

Neurovascular Anatomy

The relationships of the neurovascular structures to the clavicle and sternoclavicular joint deserve mention.

The subclavian artery and vein pass posteriorly to the sternoclavicular joint. The second portion of the artery passes posteriorly to the scalenus anterior, which inserts into the upper portion of the first rib (Fig. 10-8). The brachial plexus (C5-T1 ventral roots) descends to join the vessels at this point (Fig. 10-9). The axillary artery, a continuation of the subclavian artery, begins at the lateral margin of the first rib and extends to the distal border of the teres major. The neurovascular structures pass between the midclavicle and first rib through the axilla and along the medial aspect of the upper humerus. The major blood supply to the humerus and surrounding musculature is derived from branches of the axillary artery. These include the anterior and posterior humeral circumflex, clavicular, acromial, and deltoid branches from the thoracoacromial axis (3,4,10).

Fracture-dislocations of the sternoclavicular joint and glenohumeral joint may result in neurovascular complications. These will be discussed in more detail later in this chapter.

Biomechanics

The glenohumeral configuration and supporting structures of the shoulder allow uniquely complex motion (5,9,12,15,16,19). The muscles involved in glenohumeral motion are the rotator cuff, deltoid, pectoralis major, latissimus dorsi, and teres major (19). Motion

TABLE 10-1. *Shoulder bursae*

Bursa	Location	Normal joint communication
Subscapular	Between subscapulosus tendon and capsule	yes
Infraspinatous	Between capsule and infraspinatous tendon	inconstant
Subdeltoid	Between deltoid and rotator cuff	no
Subacromial	Between acromion and rotator cuff (usually continguous with subdeltoid)	no
Subcoracoid	Between coracoid and subscapularis (may be contiguous with subacromial)	no
Coracobrachialis	Between coracobrachialis and subscapularis	no
Latissimus dorsi	Between the latissimus and teres major	no
Teres major	Between the teres and humeral insertion	no
Pectoarlis major	Between the pectoralis and humeral insertion	no

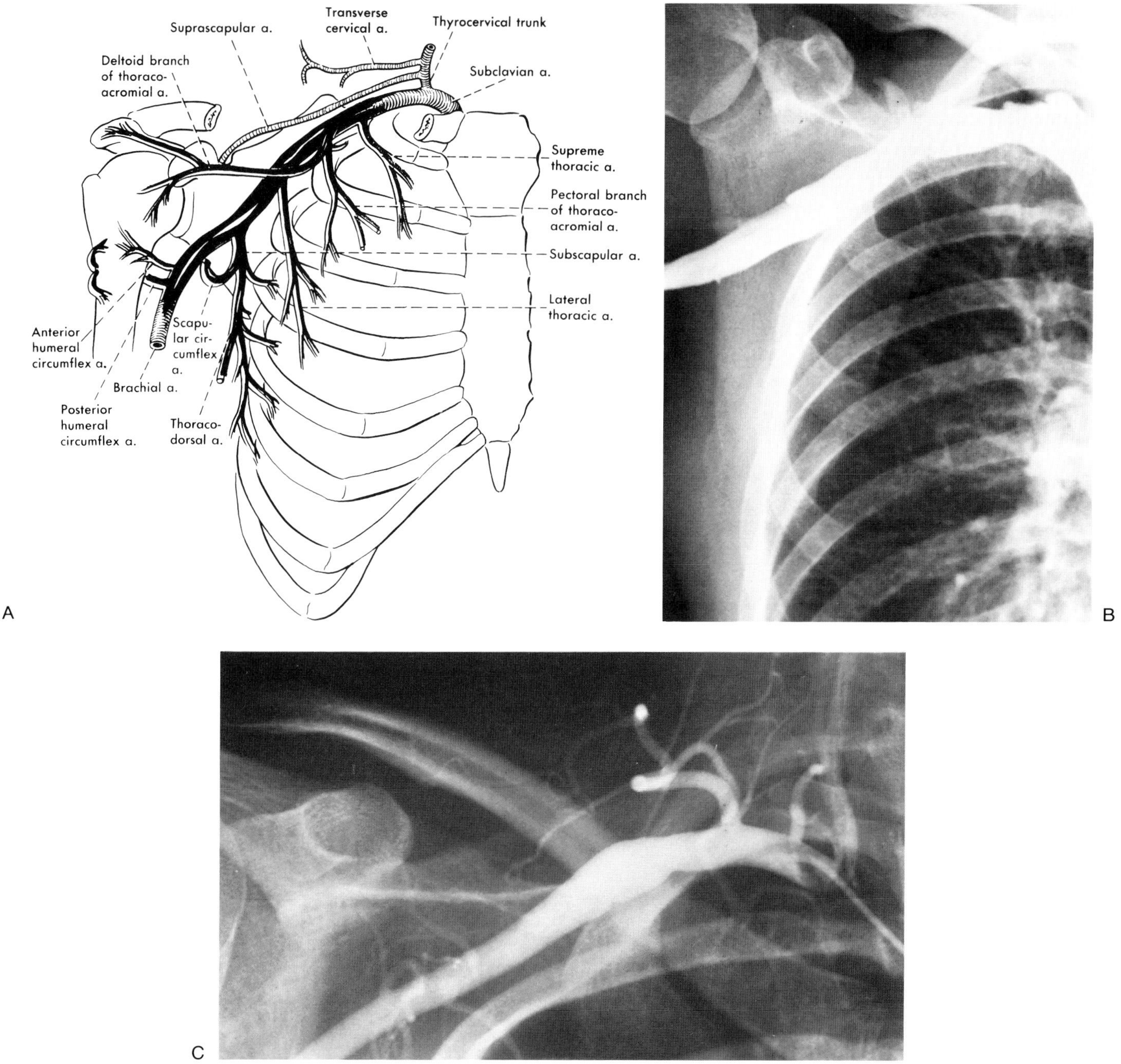

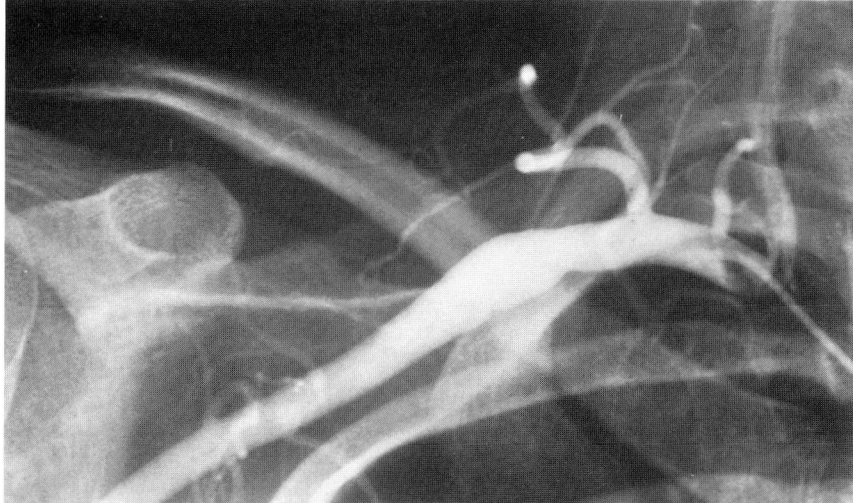

FIG. 10–8. A: The vascular anatomy of the shoulder (from 10). **B:** Venogram with humerus abducted. Note relationship of the vessels to the sternoclavicular joint, first rib, and clavicle and glenohumeral joints. **C:** Arteriogram demonstrating subclavian branches and their relationship to clavicle and first rib.

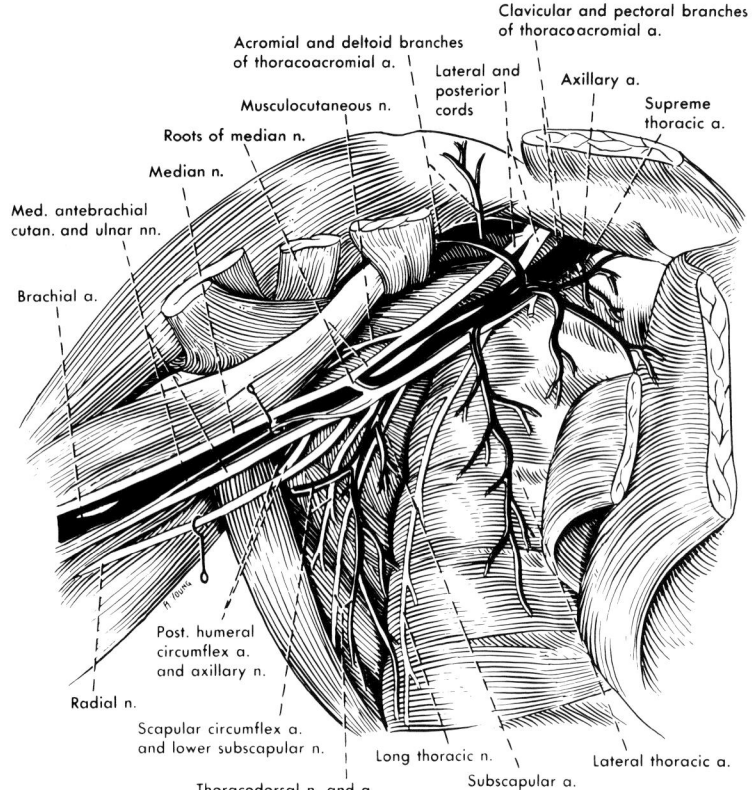

Clavicular and pectoral branches
of thoracoacromial a.

Acromial and deltoid branches
of thoracoacromial a.

Lateral and
posterior
cords

Axillary a.

Musculocutaneous n.

Supreme
thoracic a.

Roots of median n.

Median n.

Med. antebrachial
cutan. and ulnar nn.

Brachial a.

Post. humeral
circumflex a.
and axillary n.

Radial n.

Scapular circumflex a.
and lower subscapular n.

Long thoracic n.

Lateral thoracic a.

Subscapular a.

Thoracodorsal n. and a.

FIG. 10–9. The neurovascular relationships in the shoulder (from 10).

occurs primarily at the glenohumeral joint. However, motion also occurs in the acromioclavicular and sterno-clavicular joints (15). Glenohumeral motion is responsible for 120° of the 180° abduction arc. More than 120° of abduction requires scapular and clavicular motion. If the humerus cannot externally rotate, motion is restricted owing to impingement of the greater tuberosity on the acromion. With full abduction (180°) the scapula is capable of rotating 60°. The major muscles producing full abduction are the deltoid, supraspinatus, trapezius, and serratus anterior (2,4,12).

The biomechanics of abduction have been stressed owing to common clinical problems involving the rotator cuff (tears and impingement) (5,12,13). This movement can be studied fluoroscopically as a part of shoulder arthrography. The shoulder is also capable of flexion, extension, adduction, and rotation (4). The main flexors are the pectoralis major and anterior deltoid fibers, with some contribution from the biceps brachii (2,4). Extension is accomplished with fibers from the posterior deltoid, teres major, and latissimus dorsi. Adduction is achieved by contraction of the subscapularis, infraspinatus, teres minor, pectoralis major, latissimus dorsi, and teres major (4). External rotation is powered by the infraspinatus and teres minor; and internal rotation is powered by the pectoralis major, latissimus dorsi, teres major, and subscapularis.

IMAGING TECHNIQUES

Routine Radiography

Radiographic analysis of the shoulder has proved to be more difficult and less fruitful than x-rays of other anatomic regions of the musculoskeletal system. Golding has most succinctly stated this problem and has offered one—and a major—solution: "The commissioner who sends a patient to the x-ray department for an examination of his shoulder is frequently disappointed in the disparity between the lack of radiologic evidence and the marked clinical signs which are present. . . . A fundamental principle established in the early days of radiography was to obtain an anterior-posterior and a lateral film of every bone or joint. It is not a fact, therefore, that an axial film of the shoulder joint is a routine procedure in every x-ray department." (38) This failure to include a "lateral" view of the shoulder has been one major problem. Another has been a lack of analysis of the various views and lack of uniformity in the radiographic techniques that apply to the investigation of an individual with shoulder injury or disease.

This section presents the plain film alternatives for evaluation of the shoulder problems and suggests groupings of these films. Special techniques are then discussed as an augmentation of the basic x-ray examination.

These include tomography, nuclear scanning, the contrast studies of bursography and arthrography, computed tomography (CT), ultrasound, and magnetic resonance imaging (MRI).

AP Views

Standard Shoulder Projections

The standard shoulder projections have been AP views of the humerus in external and internal rotation. These views should be obtained in the upright position when possible. However, following trauma, the supine position is most often used. The external rotation view is obtained with the arm rotated externally so that the hand is palm up. The central beam is centered on the coracoid and is perpendicular to the 8 × 10-inch cassette. The internal rotation view requires the arm to be internally rotated. This can be best accomplished with the elbow flexed and the hand on the abdomen or side (21,22) (Fig. 10-10).

These films have advantages and limitations. Their major advantage is familiarity. They offer a useful survey for the presence or absence or severe or advanced shoulder diseases: metastatic or primary cancer, arthritis, calcific tendinitis (Fig. 10-11), chronic rotator cuff tears, or old trauma (22,26). However, these views alone are usually not satisfactory, as implied by Golding, for a careful analysis of acute trauma or for an evaluation of musculoskeletal pathology in the shoulder being considered for reconstructive surgery. The standard shoulder projections essentially represent AP views of the chest centered over the shoulder girdle. They are oblique to the glenohumeral joint because of the position of the scapula on the chest wall and do not depict the joint line free of bony overlap.

Posterior Oblique View

The basic shoulder projections, being oblique to the glenohumeral joint, may not clearly show joint space narrowing. A 40° posterior oblique view will visualize the joint space and offers the advantage of an angle nearly 90° to the anterior oblique view. The patient is rotated 40° to the affected side. In the supine position, a wedge should be used for support (Figs. 10-12A and 10-13). The central beam is centered on the shoulder joint and is perpendicular to the cassette.

Scapular Y-View

The scapular Y-view (54), the 60° anterior oblique view, or the lateral scapular view represents an alternative for obtaining a lateral x-ray of the shoulder. In the upright position, the patient is rotated 60° toward the wall-mounted cassette. Following trauma it is often necessary to elevate the involved shoulder 60° and to support the patient with a foam wedge (Fig. 10-14A). In the latter situation, the central beam is centered on the medial edge of the shoulder and is perpendicular to the cassette (21). The Y (Fig. 10-14B and 10-2B) is formed by the junction of the coracoid process, the body of the scapula, and the spine of the scapula. These limbs meet at the glenoid, and in this projection the humeral head should be centered over the glenoid. The x-ray technique is simple, and the bony anatomy is clearly delineated. In one study evaluating 19 shoulder fractures, 4 fractures were not seen on any other views of the shoulder (30).

Transthoracic Lateral View

A number of additional or alternative views have been described and suggested. Their goal is to visualize the

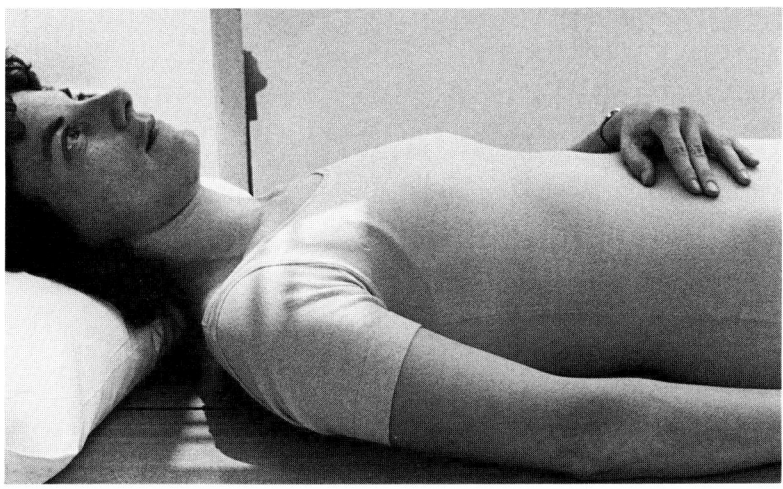

FIG. 10–10. Standard AP views of the shoulder. Patient positioned for internal rotation view. The hand is palm down.

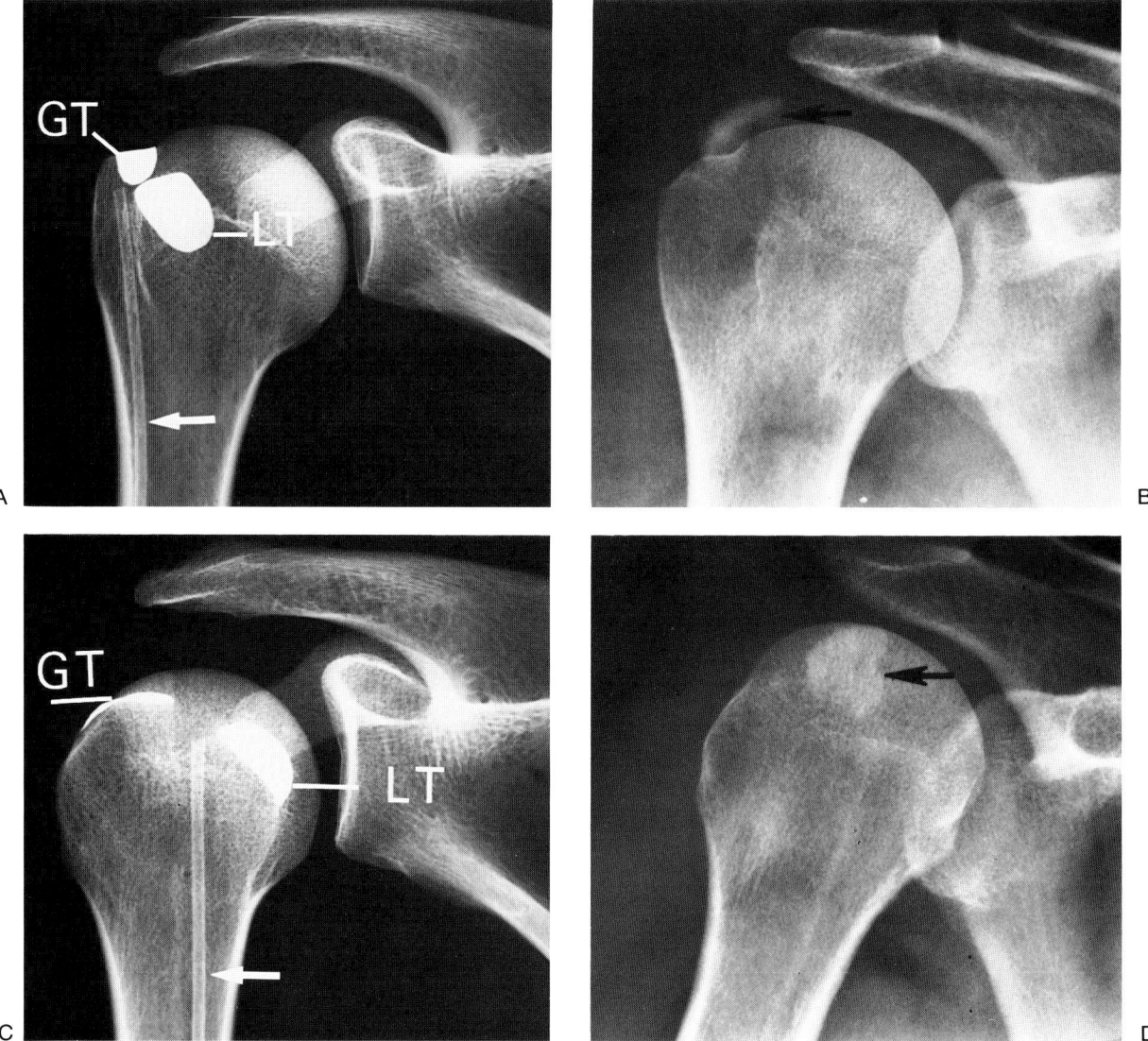

FIG. 10–11. A: Dried skeletal specimen demonstrating the position of the tuberosities and bicipital groove with the external rotation. (GT, greater tuberosity; LT, lesser tuberosity; *arrow,* position of tendon of long head of the biceps). **B:** External rotation view in a patient with calcific tendonitis (*arrow*). Note the overlap of the humeral head and glenoid. **C:** Dried skeletal specimen. The lesser tuberosity is rotated medially demonstrating the relationship of the tendon (*arrow*) to the tuberosities. Note the glenoid is tangential indicating a true AP position. **D:** Internal rotation view on the same patient shown in **B.** The calcific deposit is indicated by the arrow.

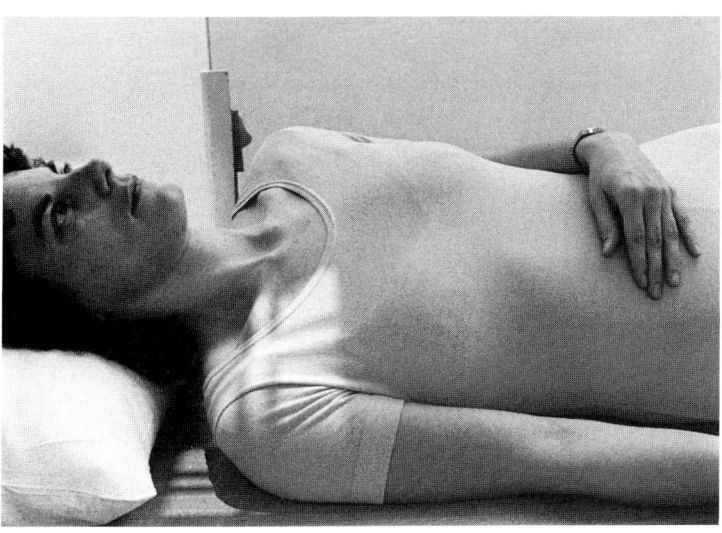

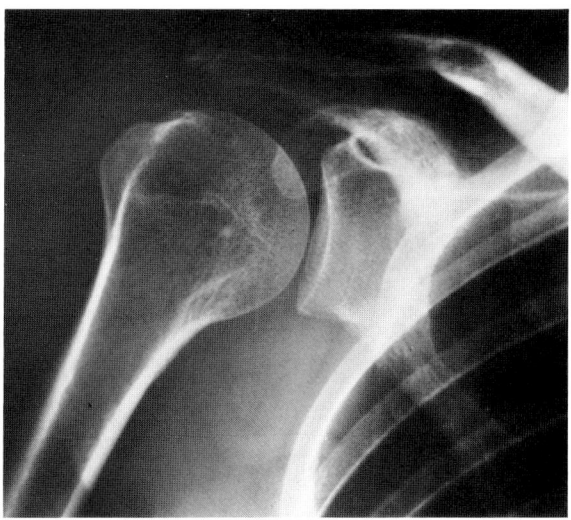

FIG. 10-12. A: Patient positioned for 40° posterior oblique view with wedge for support under opposite shoulder. **B:** Radiograph clearly demonstrates the glenohumeral joint. The coracoid is projected over the upper joint space.

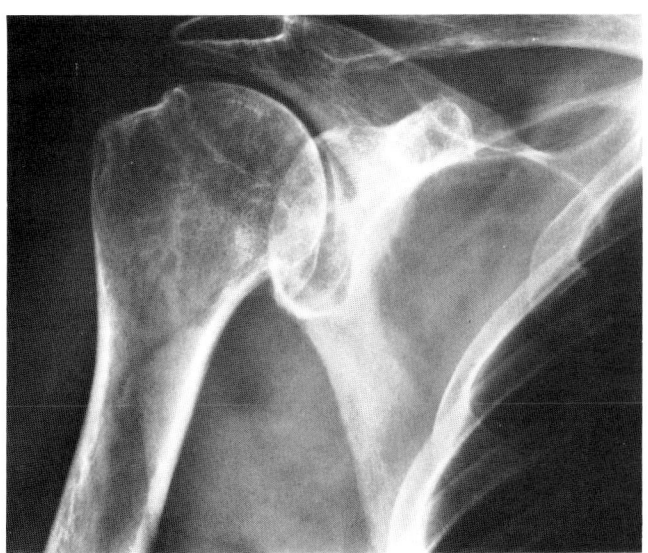

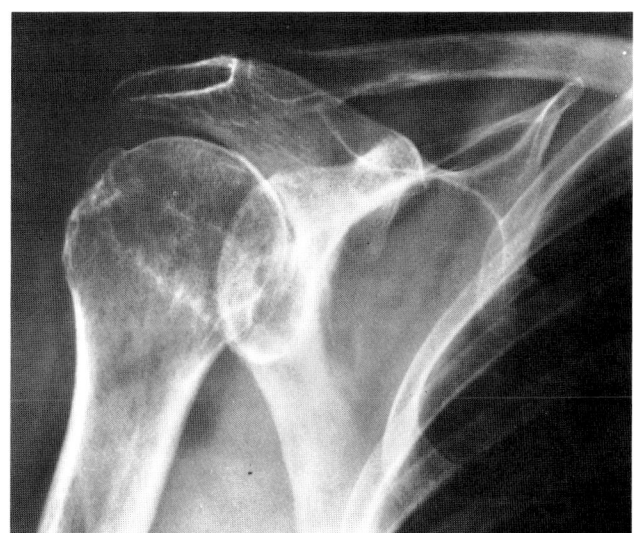

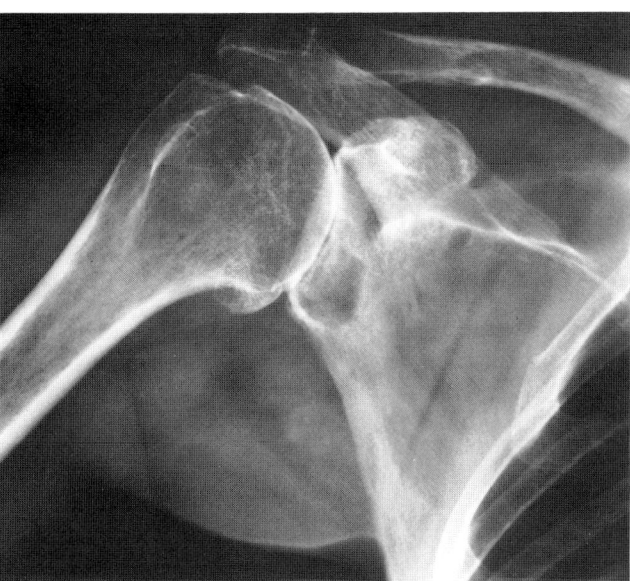

FIG. 10-13. Radiographs in an 82-year-old woman with osteoarthritis. Standard external (**A**) and internal (**B**) rotation views. The 40° posterior oblique view (**C**) (true AP of the glenohumeral joint) shows complete loss of the articular cartilage. This was not demonstrated on the standard views (from Cofield, R.H.: Unconstrained shoulder prosthesis. *Clin. Orthop.* 173:97, 1983).

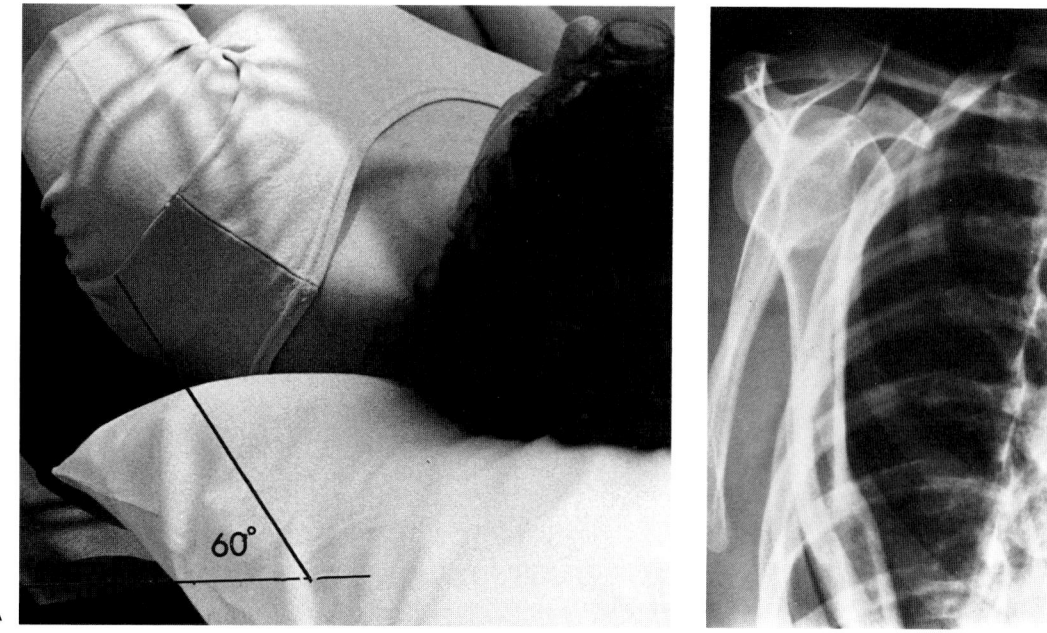

FIG. 10–14. A: Patient positioned for *Y*-view of the shoulder (patient shoulder elevated 60°). **B:** Radiograph clearly demonstrates the relationship of the humeral head to the glenoid and coracoacromial arch. The acromion and coracoid are well seen.

glenohumeral joint at or near 90° to the standard projection. The transthoracic lateral view is a projection at 90° to the standard views, but the superimposed chest structures render interpretation difficult at best and typically uncertain. As in the case of the standard projections, another disadvantage of this view is that it is oblique to the glenohumeral joint surface. This technique will be the auxiliary view discussed in Chapter 11.

Axillary View

The axillary shoulder projection has largely replaced the transthoracic lateral view. The patient is supine with the arm abducted 90°, and the cassette on the table top is cranial to the shoulder (Fig. 10-15A). The central beam is centered on the axilla and is perpendicular to the cassette. Alternate positions have also been described by Bernau (22) and Ballinger (21). In the absence of acute trauma, the arm is widely abducted, and excellent visualization of the bony architecture is easily accomplished. In the presence of an acute injury, this view can still be obtained without the use of special equipment by abducting the arm only the width of the x-ray tube (Fig. 10-15B). An alternative method has been described by Wallace and Hellier (55). Several authors have proclaimed the value of this view (Fig. 10-15C). In a series of patients without acute trauma, 15 abnormalities (25,32,38) in 130 abnormal x-rays would not have been identified without using this view (29).

It is apparent that several options are available to de-

pict the shoulder joint radiographically. An incomplete examination need no longer be accepted. In the absence of acute trauma, the largest amount of information is obtained from a combination of several views. These include a 40° posterior oblique x-ray in internal and external rotation and an axillary view. With further experience, it may prove possible to eliminate the internal rotation view. This grouping of three x-rays might be called an elective shoulder series. When acute trauma is being evaluated, arm rotation is often not desirable, and arm movement is kept to a minimum. In this situation, a shoulder trauma series is more effective, including a 40° posterior oblique, a 60° anterior oblique, and an emergency axillary view (35,49).

Radiography of the Scapula

AP View

The AP view of the scapula can be obtained with the patient supine or upright. The arm should be fully abducted, if possible (Fig. 10-16A) (21). The hand may be placed on the hip with the elbow slightly flexed, if abduction is limited. The beam is centered on the midscapula and is perpendicular to the cassette. Breathing during the procedure will diminish the shadows caused by the overlying ribs (21).

The radiograph demonstrates the lateral portions of the scapula, but the medial scapula is partially obscured by thoracic structures (Fig. 10-16B).

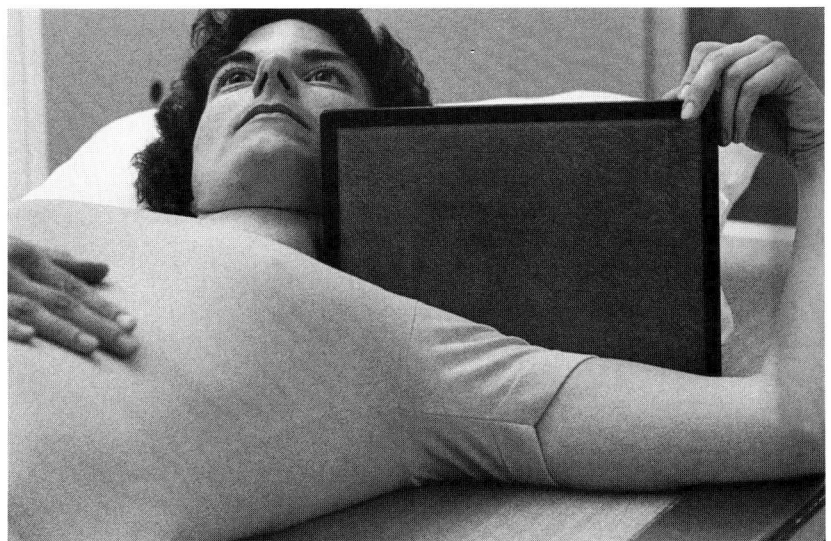

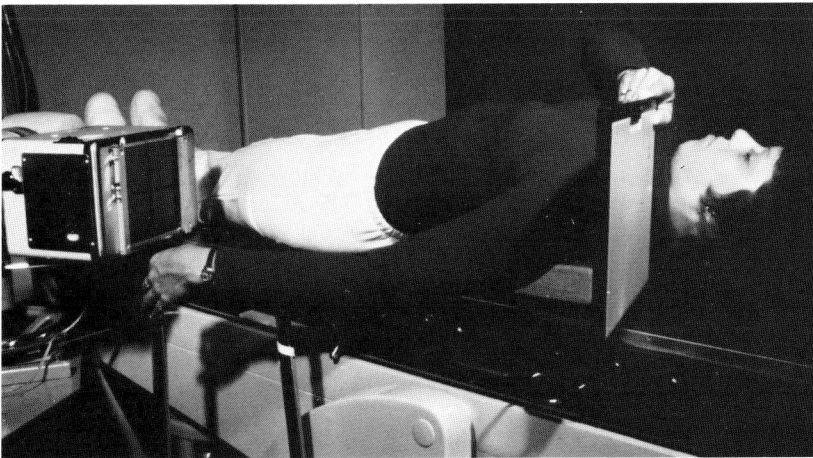

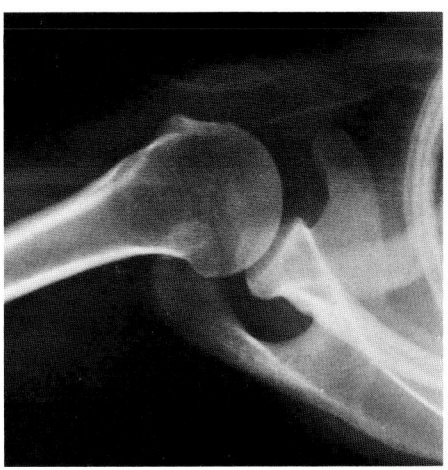

FIG. 10-15. A: Patient positioned for routine axillary view of the shoulder. B: Patient positioned for "emergency" axillary view of the shoulder. C: Radiograph demonstrating axillary view.

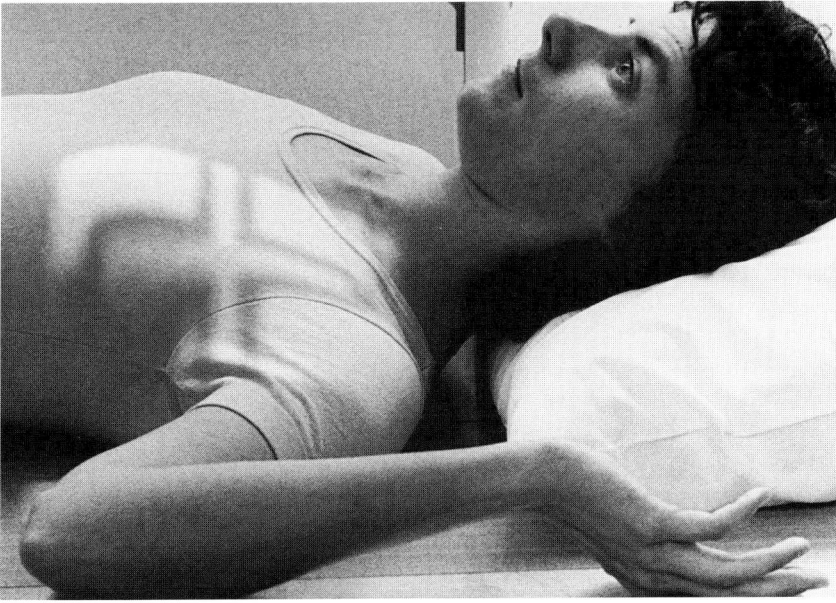

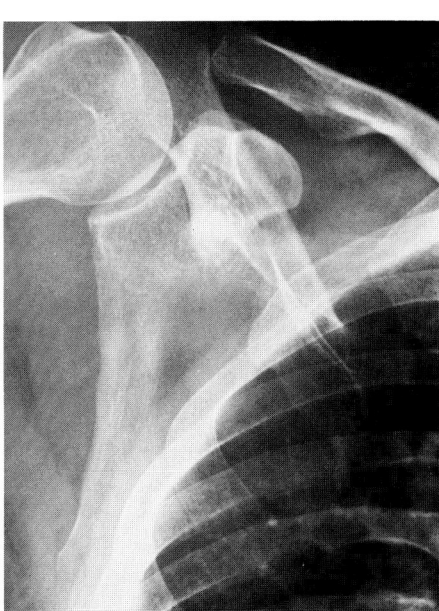

FIG. 10-16. A: Patient positioned for the AP scapular view. The beam is centered on the mid-scapula and perpendicular to the table. B: AP view of the scapula. The medial margin is partially obscured by ribs.

Lateral View

The lateral view of the scapula may be difficult to obtain in the acutely injured patient. The patient can be rotated from the supine position to an almost lateral position, with the affected shoulder adjacent to the table. The elbow should be flexed, with the forearm anterior to the chest (47). This will prevent the humerus from overlapping the scapula (Fig. 10-17B). The central beam is centered parallel to the scapular border (palpable) and is perpendicular to the cassette (Fig. 10-17A). When possible, this view should be obtained in the upright position.

The radiograph (Fig. 10-17B) demonstrates the scapular body and spine, the coracoid, and the acromion. Excellent rib detail is also obtained in the area adjacent to the clavicle.

Radiography of the Acromioclavicular Joint

X-rays of the clavicle and its articulations can be difficult to obtain and may require special projections. The acromioclavicular joint is seen on AP or posterior oblique views of the shoulder and on the axillary view. The typical x-ray exposure for the shoulder joint may, however, be too great, overpenetrating the acromioclavicular joint and rendering this portion of the film too dark for interpretation (Fig. 10-18A). The technician may have to decrease the intensity of the beam to obtain better detail. Best results are obtained with localized views.

The injured patient is most easily examined in a supine position. The beam is coned down over the acromioclavicular joint and angled 15° to the head (Fig. 10-18B) (21,22). The resulting image provides better detail and projects the joint free of overlying structures (Fig. 10-18C).

With injuries of the acromioclavicular joint, stress x-rays may be helpful to diagnose the degree of ligamentous damage. This is done by hanging 8 to 10 lbs of weight from both wrists, using a device such as the one illustrated in Fig. 10-19. If the patient is asked to hold the weights, contraction of the extremity muscles may create false negative results. Fig. 10-20 illustrates an acromioclavicular dislocation as demonstrated on stress views. On this x-ray, the distance between the undersurface of the clavicle and the upper surface of the coracoid is almost twice as great on the left as on the right. If the difference on the injured side is more than 5 mm greater than the noninjured side, a complete coracoclavicular ligament disruption is likely to have occurred. The coracoclavicular distance normally measures about 1.3 cm (23).

Radiography of the Clavicle

AP Views

The PA view of the clavicle (AP may also be used) places the clavicle against the cassette; this increases image quality. In severely injured patients, the AP view

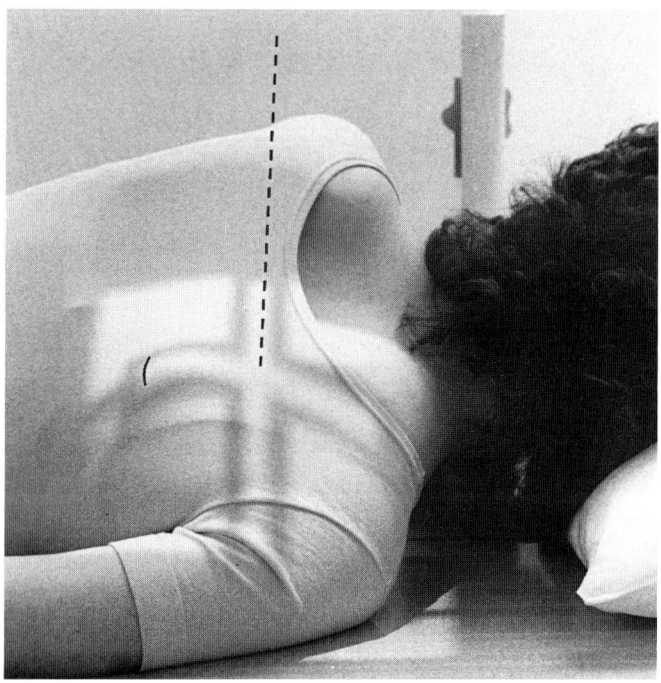
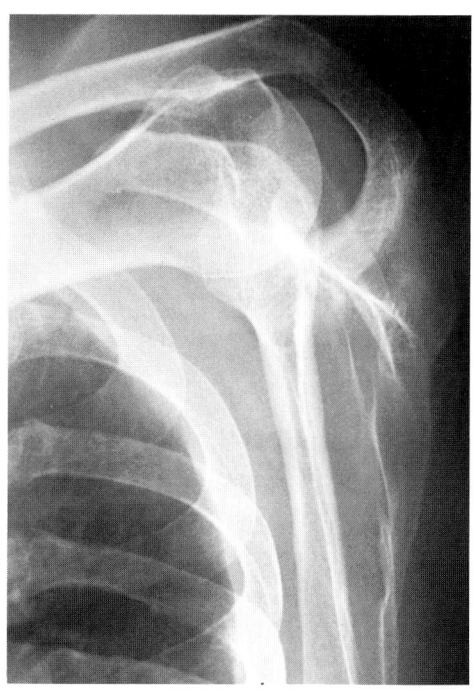

FIG. 10-17. A: Patient positioned for lateral view of the scapula. Inferior scapular angle (( ), central beam (*broken line*). B: Lateral view of the scapula. Note the humerus is not overlying the scapula.

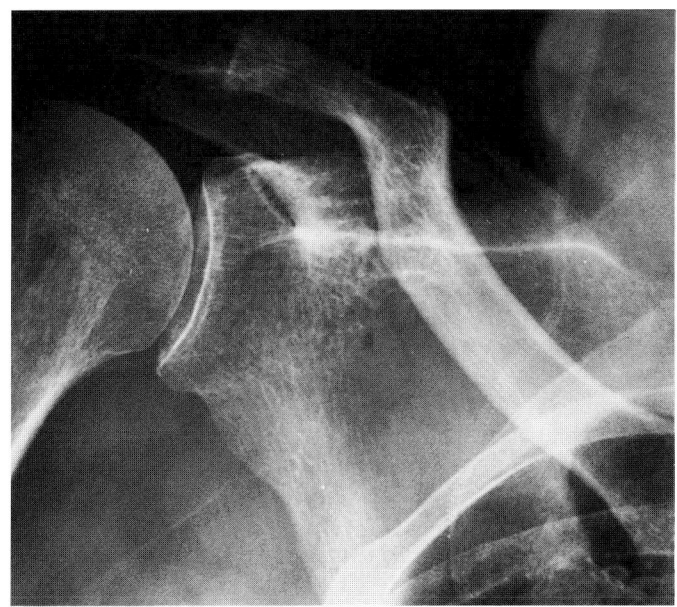

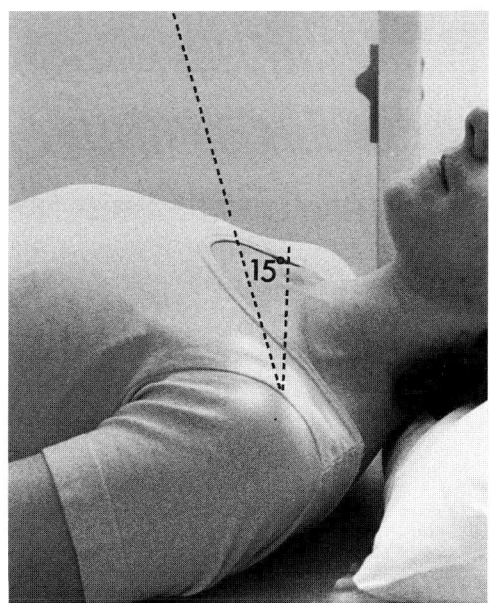

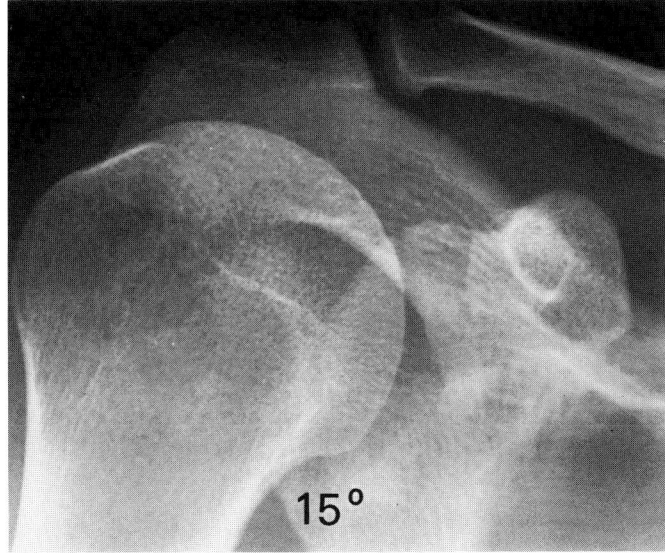

FIG. 10–18. A: AP view of the clavicle. The acromioclavicular joint is overpenetrated and now well demonstrated. **B:** Patient positioned for AP view of the AC joint. The tube is angled 15° and the beam coned down over the joint. **C:** Radiograph of acromioclavicular joint.

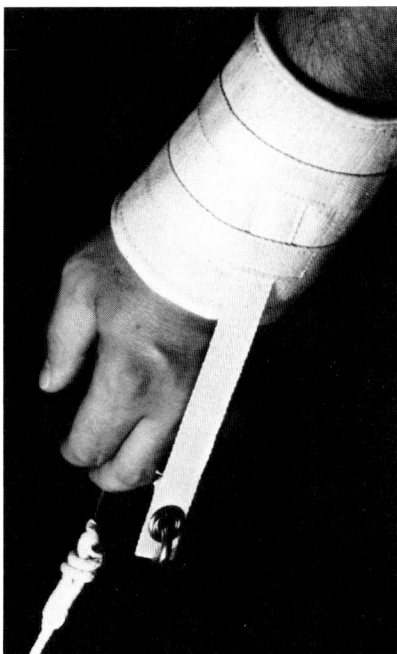

FIG. 10–19. Ankle traction cuff adapted as a wrist cuff for stress views of the acromioclavicular joint.

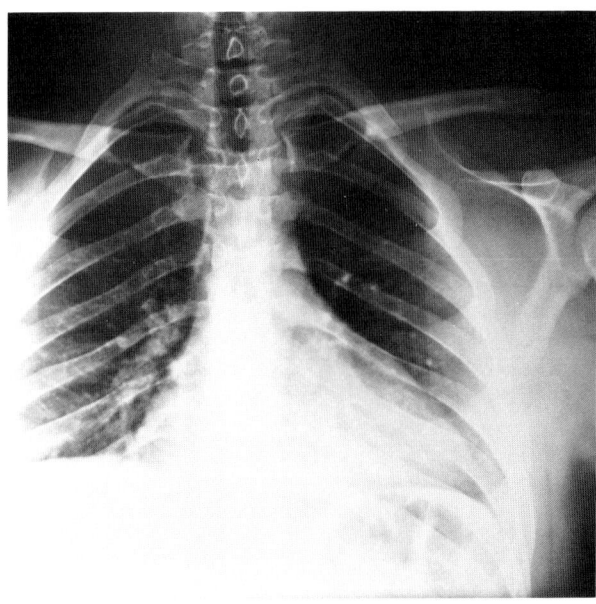

FIG. 10–20. Stress views of the acromioclavicular joint. Note the marked increase in coracoclavicular distance on the left compared to the right.

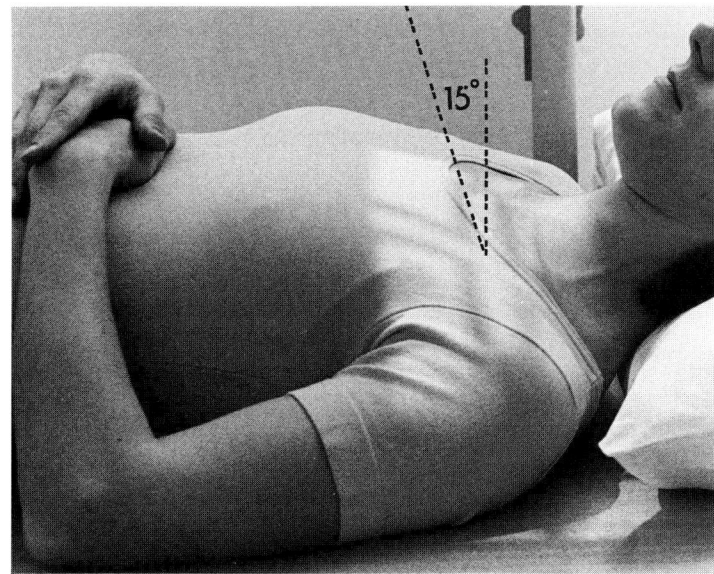

A

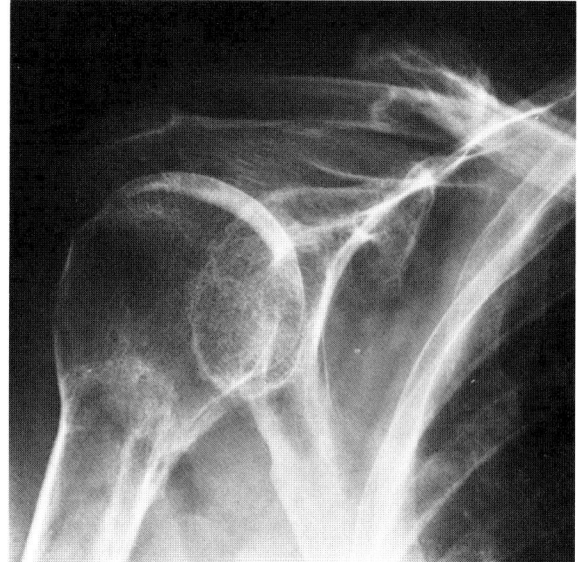

B

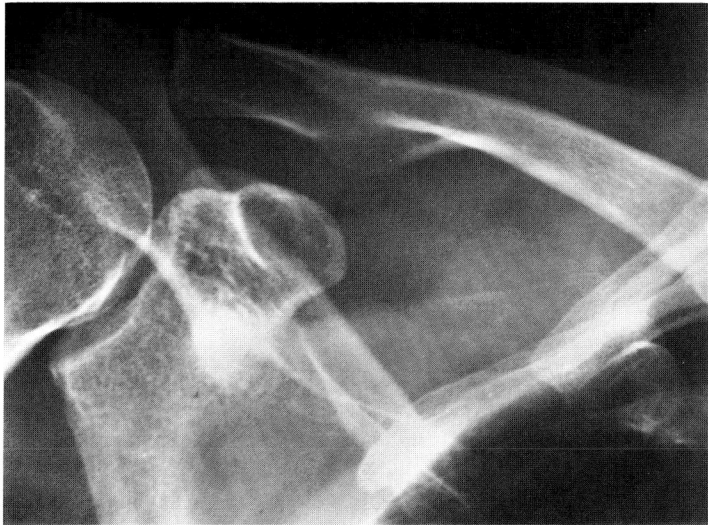

C

FIG. 10-21. **A:** Patient positioned for AP view of the clavicle. The tube is angled 15° to the head. (Note cone light size compared to AC joint view in Fig. 10-18B.) **B:** AP view of the clavicle, acromion, and scapula. Note the displaced midshaft fracture. **C:** Angled (15°) view of the clavicle more clearly demonstrates the distal clavicle as it projected above the spine of the scapula.

(supine) is most often used (Fig. 10-21A). With the AP projection, the acromioclavicular joint is superimposed on the posterior acromion and spine of the scapula. Angling the central beam 15° cephalad will eliminate this difficulty (21,22,61).

Oblique View

The oblique view (tangential view) provides better visualization of the midclavicle. The patient's affected side is elevated, and the cassette (angled 45° to the table) is placed above the shoulder (Fig. 10-22A). The central beam is also angled 45° to be perpendicular to the cassette. The resulting radiograph projects the clavicle above the ribs (Fig. 10-22B). This allows better evaluation of the midclavicle (21). The alternate method (Fig. 10-22C) is performed with the patient supine. With this

technique the acromioclavicular joint is more often obscured.

Radiography of the Sternoclavicular Joints

With lesions in the middle third of the clavicle or involving the sternoclavicular joint, views other than an AP or slightly oblique projection will be difficult to obtain. Bernau and Berquist (22) describe a prone technique with the cassette angled 15° to place it next to the sternoclavicular joints. The tube is centered on T2 and angled perpendicularly to the cassette (15° to the head) (Fig. 10-23A). This view is useful in most situations. Quesada has suggested placing the patient prone and obtaining two views, one with the central ray angled cephalad 45° and one with the central ray angled caudad 45° (51). A 40° cephalic tilt view (serendipity technique)

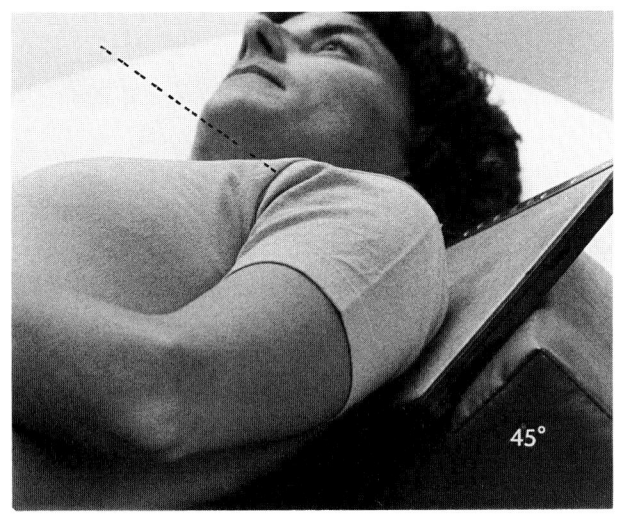

A

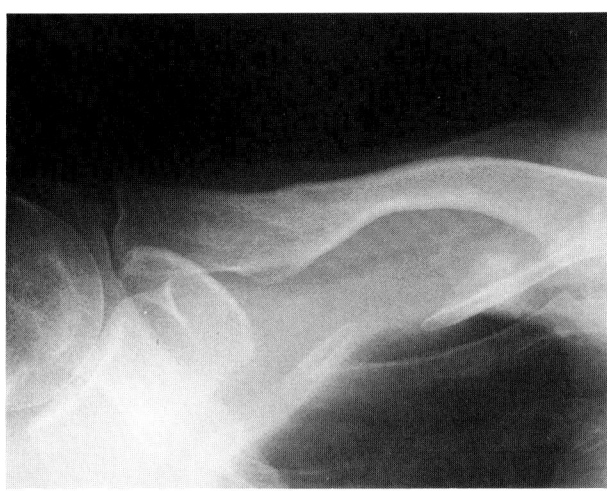

B

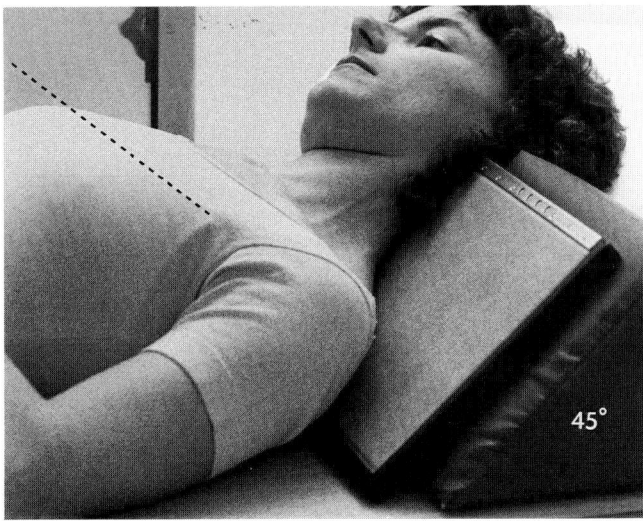

C

FIG. 10–22. **A:** Patient positioned for the oblique tangential view. The cassette is angled about 45°. The central beam is perpendicular to the cassette. **B:** Radiograph demonstrates the midclavicle and acromioclavicular joint. Fractures will be projected free from overlying bone shadows. **C:** Patient positioned for supine tangential view.

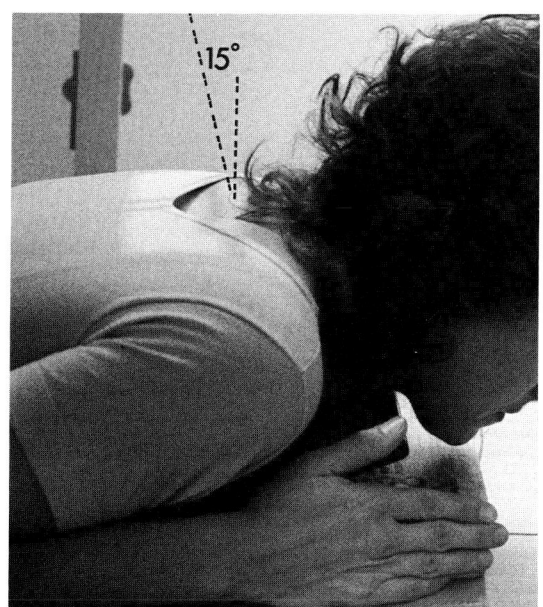

A

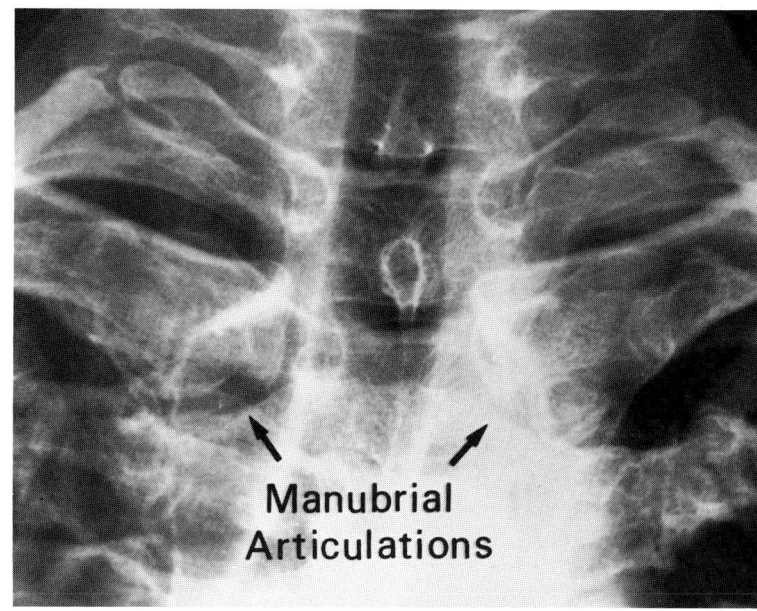

B

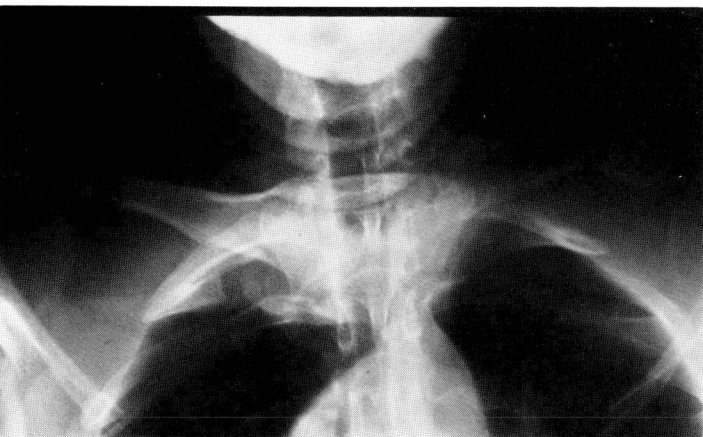

C

FIG. 10–23. A: Patient positioned for routine PA view of the sternoclavicular joint. Normally the tube is angled 15°. B: Normal sternoclavicular joints. Even with excellent technique, this view is difficult to interpret due to overlying structures. C: Forty-degree angled view showing asymmetrical clavicles due to posterior dislocation on the right.

with the patient supine has proved to be more practical. The patient is positioned as for the AP clavicle view, but the tube is angled 40° to the head and centered on the manubrium. With this technique, an anteriorly displaced structure will appear to be upwardly displaced, and a posteriorly displaced structure will appear inferior to its normal position (Fig. 10-23C). Heinig has suggested a technique for obtaining a lateral view of the medial end of the clavicle and the sternoclavicular joint (Fig. 10-24). This may prove helpful in difficult situations, but interpretation is still difficult because of the superimposition of chest structures (40). Computed tomography may provide the best evaluation of the sternoclavicular joint (Fig. 10-25).

Special Views

The views already discussed represent the general x-ray alternatives for investigation of the shoulder girdle.

There are additional views that can be obtained to visualize specific structures or to search for discrete pathologic changes (21,22,28).

On occasion, it may be desirable to obtain x-rays of the bicipital groove. With the extremity in the anatomic position, the groove is positioned approximately 15° lateral to the midportion of the anterior aspect of the humeral head. Fisk (34) suggested one method of visualizing this groove (Fig. 10-26A). We have as an alternative positioned the patient as illustrated in Figure 10-26B (22). The involved side is elevated slightly with cushion support. The cassette is positioned above the shoulder, with the hand in an anatomic position. The central beam is centered on the upper aspect of the humeral head (22). This view offers a projection of the length of the groove. The upper angle of the groove is better shown in the Fisk projection (Fig. 10-26C).

A number of views have been developed to augment the evaluation of the unstable or recurrently dislocating shoulder. These views are designed to visualize a bony or

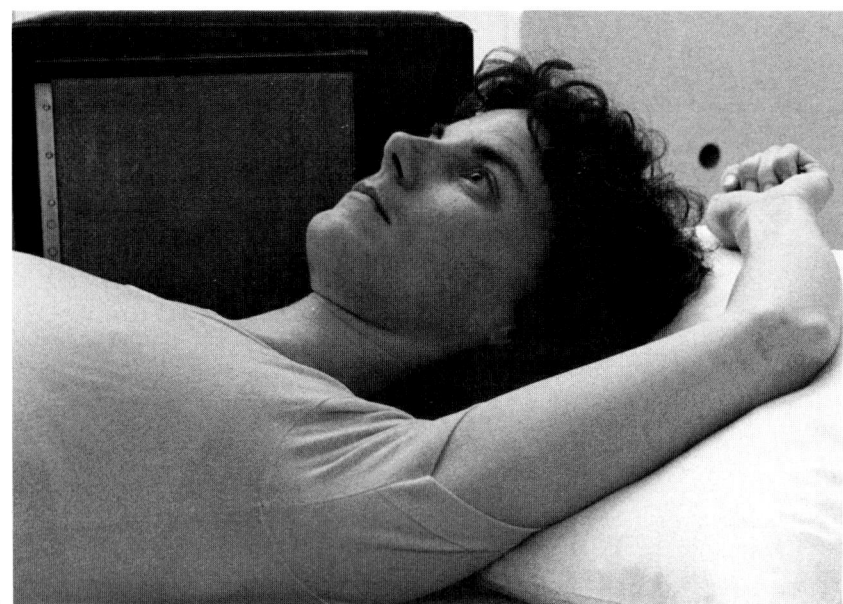
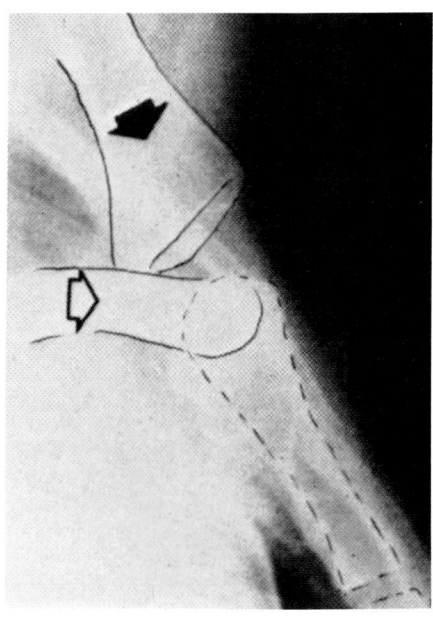

FIG. 10-24. A: Patient positioned for Heinig view (36,40). The arm closest to the tube is elevated with the tube angled through the joint at about 45°. The cassette is above the opposite shoulder and perpendicular to the beam. B: Retouched radiograph of Heinig projection (from 46).

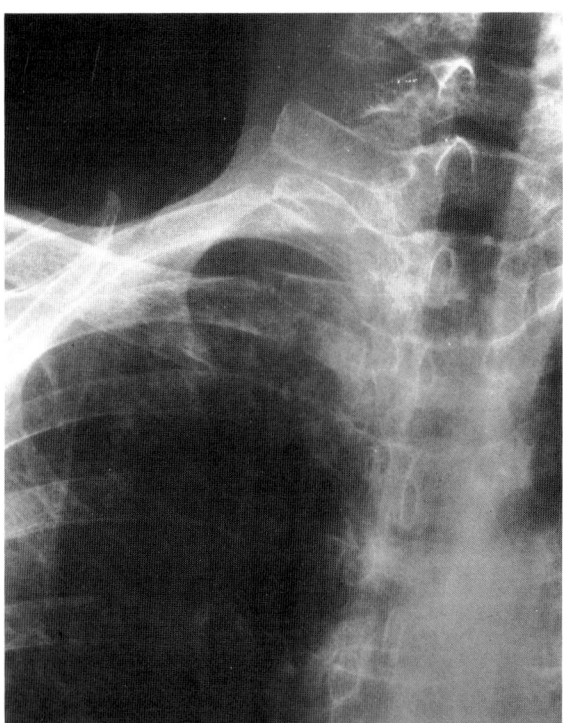

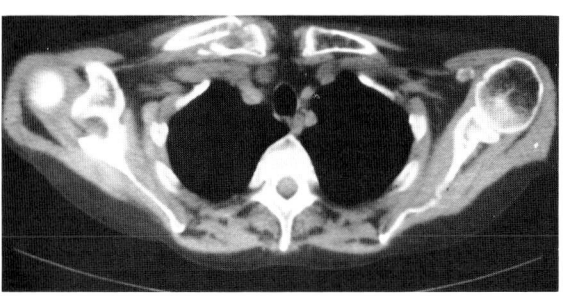

FIG. 10-25. Trauma to the medial clavicle. A: Radiograph shows a fracture of the median end of the clavicle. CT scan (B) clearly demonstrates this overriding fracture of the proximal clavicle.

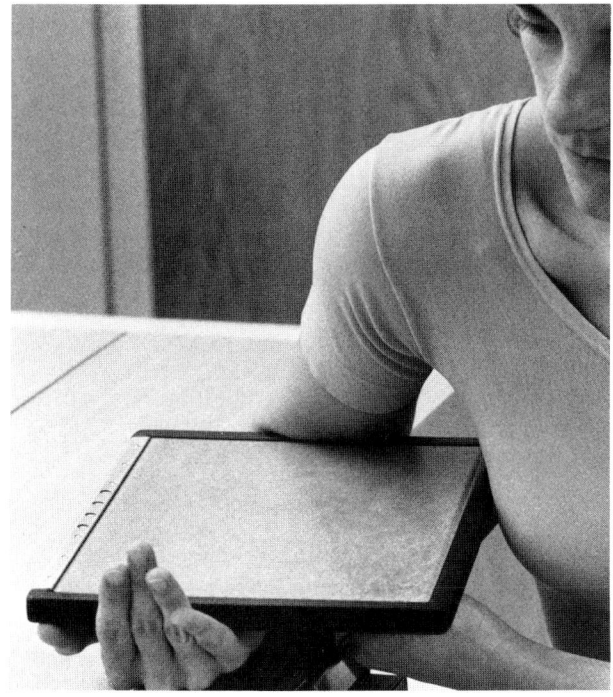

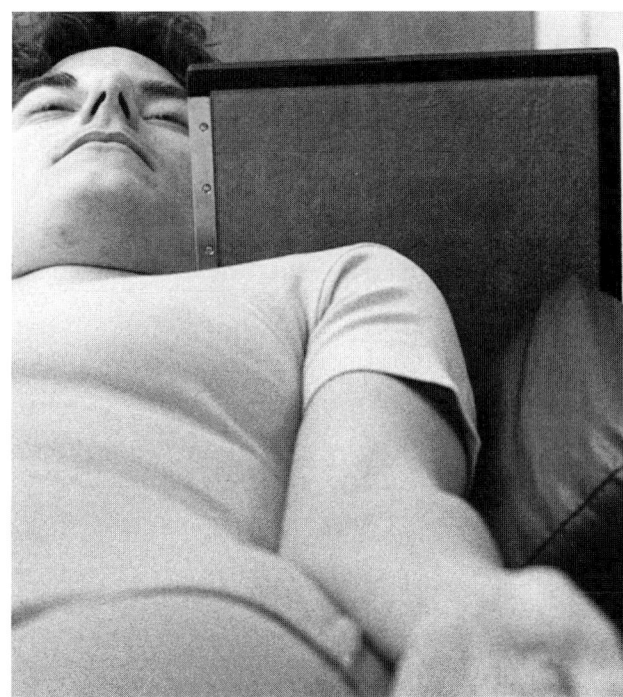

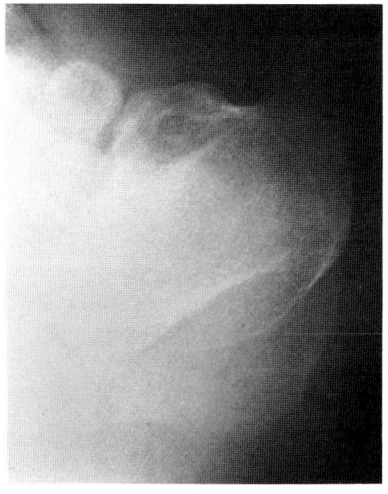

FIG. 10–26. **A:** Patient positioned for bicipital groove view described by Fisk. **B:** Alternate method for bicipital groove view. **C:** AP radiograph demonstrating the bicipital groove.

calcific reaction, a fracture of the anterior glenoid rim, or a compression fracture of the posterior aspect of the humeral head—the Hill-Sachs lesion (42). In the acute anterior dislocation, the Hill-Sachs deformity is seen on an AP view and is usually characteristic (Fig. 10-27). On occasion the humeral head can be seen to be indented posteriorly and impacted on the anterior glenoid rim— the genesis of the humeral head defect. The anterior nature of this dislocation can be confirmed with an emergency axillary or anterior oblique shoulder x-ray (Fig. 10-27B).

In the nonacute setting, the diagnosis of continuing shoulder instability may be difficult, and x-ray confirmation of the presence of lesions associated with shoulder instability is sought. Hill and Sachs suggested using an AP x-ray with the arm in marked internal rotation to visualize the humeral impaction-fracture. Rokous and colleagues (52) suggested a modified axillary

view (the West Point axillary) to accomplish these ends (Fig. 10-28A-C). The patient is prone, and the shoulder is elevated 3 inches from the tabletop. The arm is abducted 90° and rotated so that the forearm hangs off the x-ray table and is pointed directly at the floor. The x-ray tube is positioned with the central ray projecting 25° from the horizontal and 25° medially. This projects the anterior inferior glenoid rim better than the standard axillary x-ray, which projects the anterior glenoid rim. The fixed arm position and rotation usually demonstrates the Hill-Sachs lesion when it is present. In their 63 patients with chronic subluxation of the shoulder, 53 (84%) demonstrated abnormalities of the glenoid rim. No cases of acute anterior dislocation demonstrated this abnormality, but 6 of 19 cases (32%) with recurrent anterior dislocation did have this lesion (52).

Hall and colleagues described a view developed by William S. Stryker: the Stryker notch view (Fig. 10-29A,

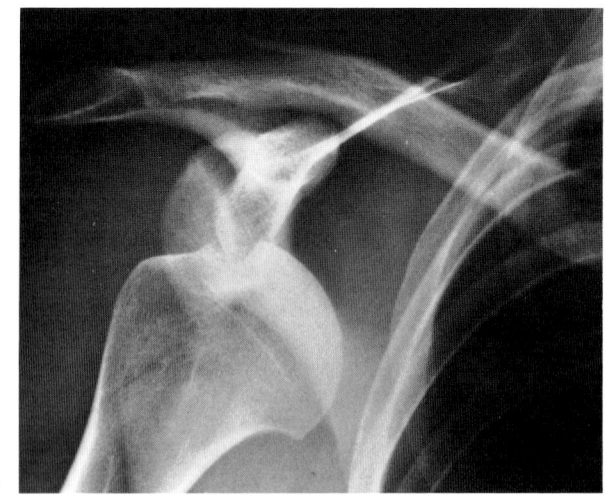
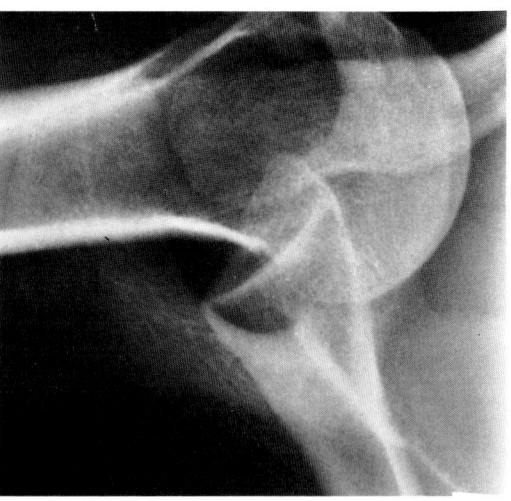

FIG. 10–27. A: Anterior dislocation with typical Hill-Sachs impression fracture as the head rests on the glenoid rim. **B:** Axillary view of the anteriorly dislocated shoulder.

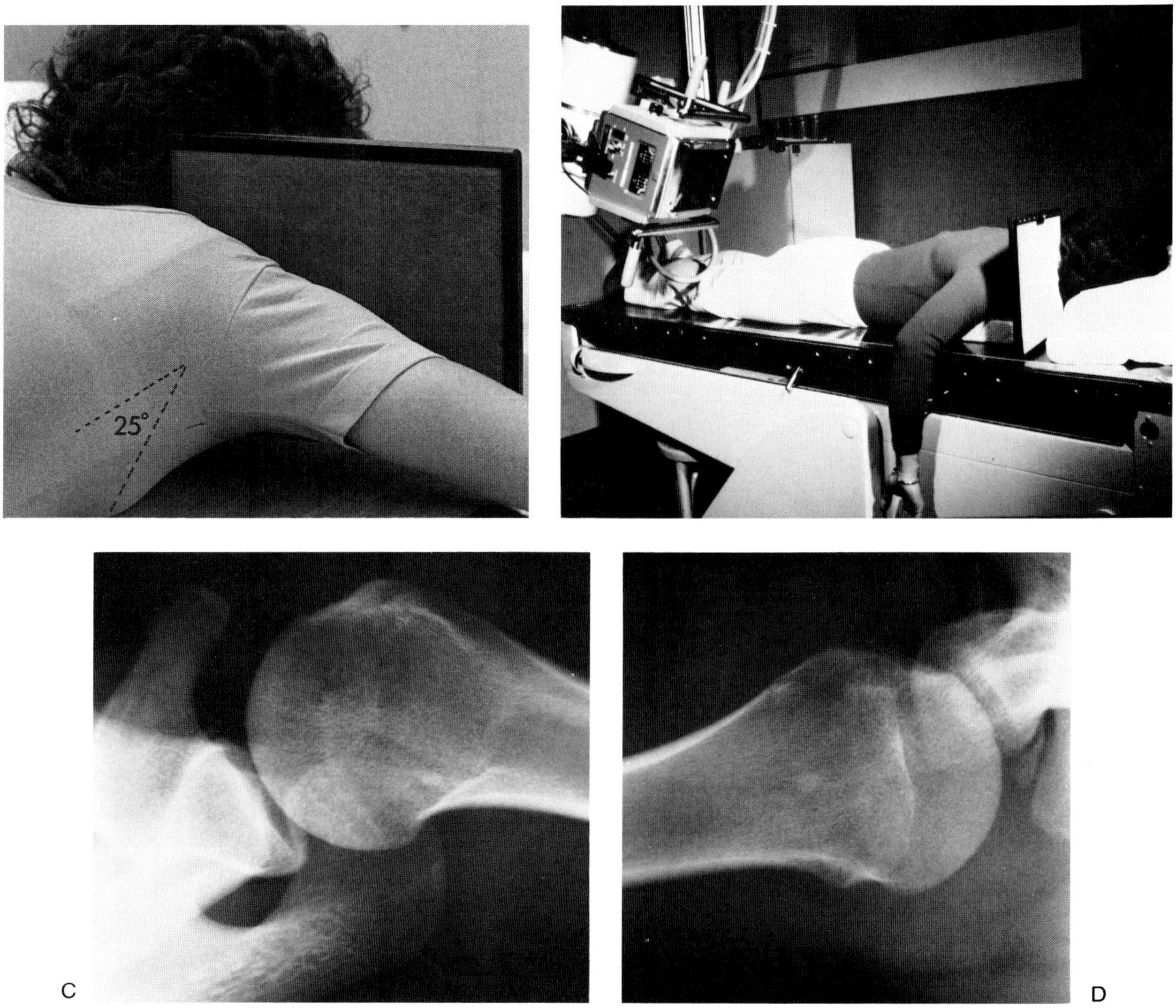

25°

A

B

C

D

FIG. 10–28. Patient positioned for West Point view. The tube is angled 25° medially (**A**) and 25° off horizontal (**B**). Normal axillary view (**C**) and West Point view (**D**) in a patient with a small Hill-Sachs fracture and reactive bone along the anterior-inferior glenoid rim.

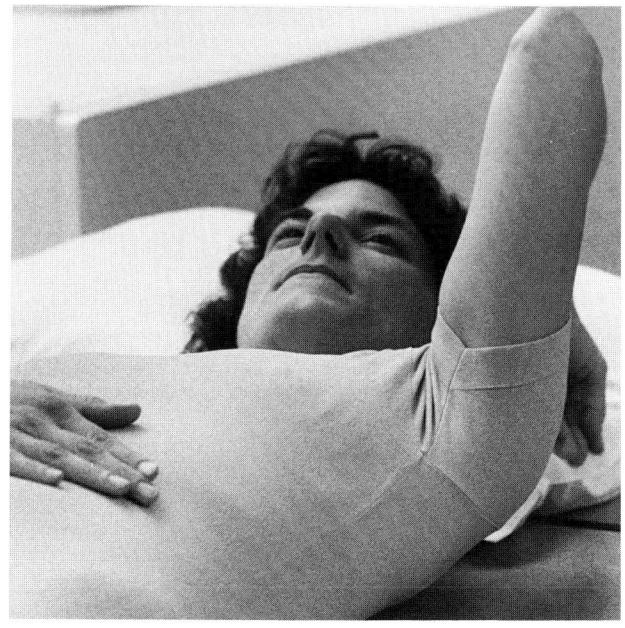

A

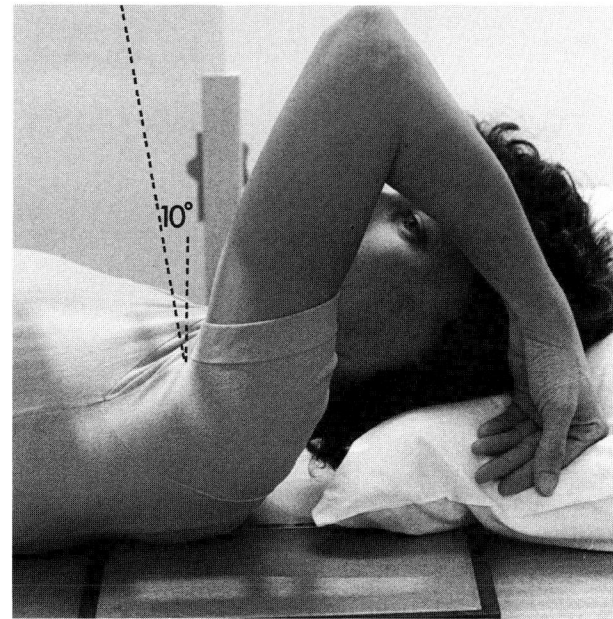

B

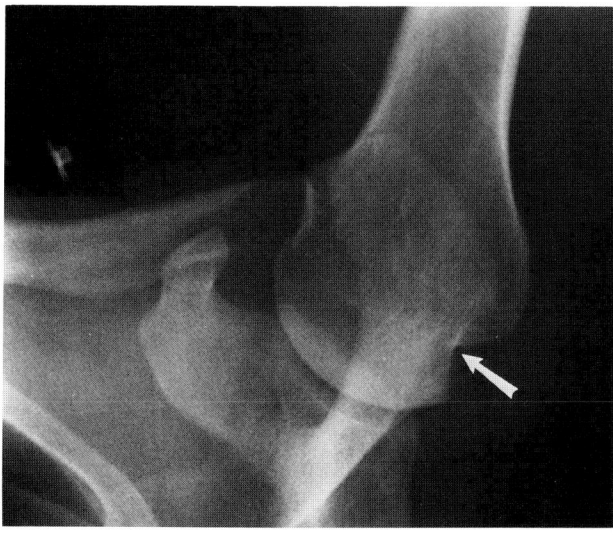

C

FIG. 10–29. A, B: Patient positioned for the Stryker Notch View (35). C: Radiograph demonstrating a large Hill-Sachs defect (*arrow*).

B) (39). The patient is supine, with the hand adjacent to or on top of the head and the elbow directed vertically. The central beam is angled 10° cephalad and centered on the coracoid (palpable). In patients with recurrent anterior dislocation, Hall and colleagues could identify the humeral head lesion in 18 of 20 shoulders (90%). Additional x-ray views also designed to depict the humeral head lesion and recurrent anterior instability are modifications of the Hermodsson (41) or the Didiee (31) views.

More recently, additional views have been described to identify shoulder subluxation, instability, Hill-Sachs, and glenoid lesions (36,43,45). The apical oblique view is obtained with the patient seated or supine with the injured shoulder against the cassette and the opposite shoulder rotated 45° anteriorly (Fig. 10-30A) (36,50). The central beam is directed 45° caudally through the

shoulder with the scapula parallel to the beam due to the adducted position of the extremity (36). This view provides a coronal profile of the glenohumeral joint that is ideal for detection of intra-articular fractures, dislocations, instability, Hill-Sachs deformities, and glenoid injuries (36).

Detection of acromial abnormalities is useful in diagnosis of impingement (44,61). Routine radiographs may demonstrate chronic changes such as sclerosis, irregularity of the greater tuberosity, acromioclavicular joint changes, and superior subluxation of the humeral head (Fig. 9-31) (44). Acromial changes can be obtained by angling the beam 30° caudally on the AP view or by angling the tube 5° with the same position used for the scapular lateral view (Fig. 9-32) (44,45).

In patients who are being evaluated for recurrent anterior shoulder instability, multiple views are necessary to

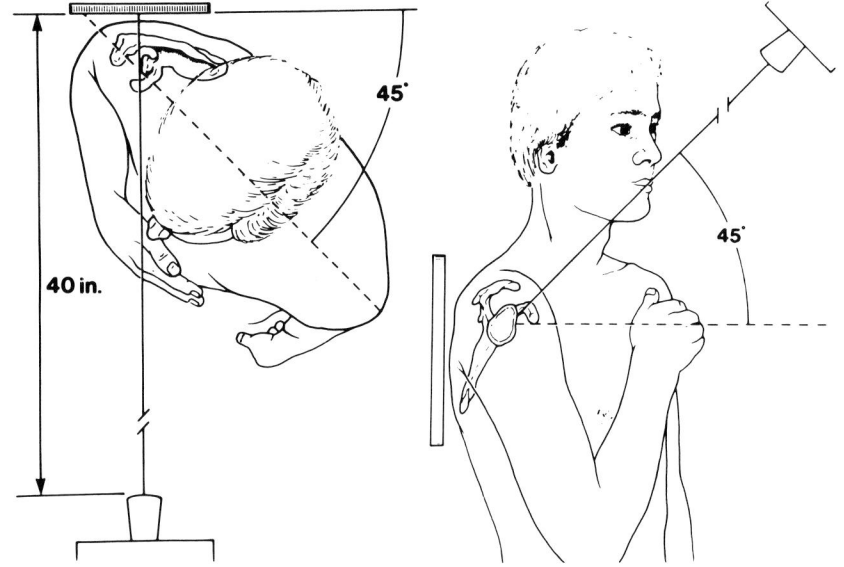

A

FIG. 10–30. A: Technique for apical oblique view (from 36, with permission.) Note: Hand on injured side should be placed on patient's lap instead of as shown. **B:** Normal shoulder and **C:** posterior dislocation as seen on the apical oblique view (from 45, with permission). C, coracoid; Cl, clavicle.

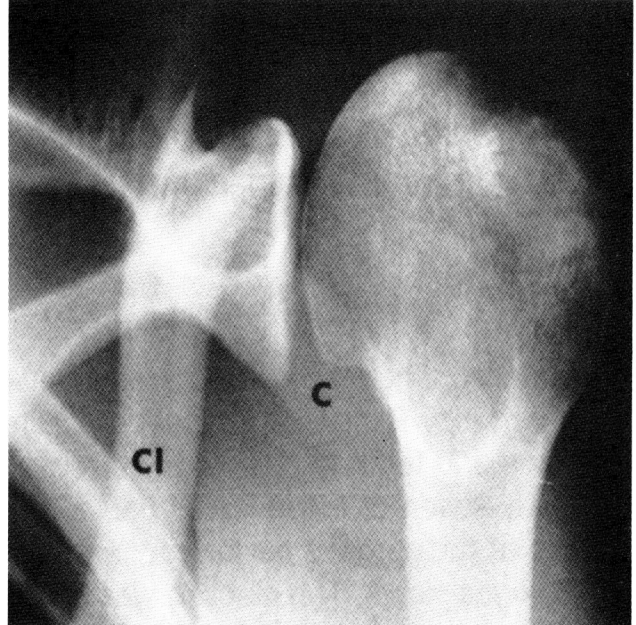

B

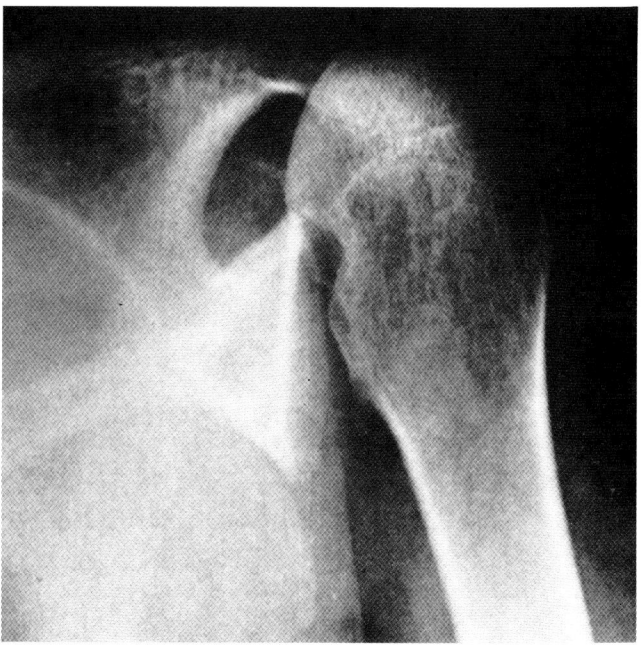

C

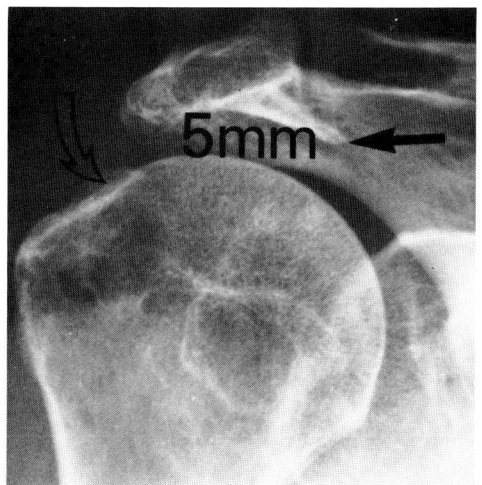

FIG. 10–31. AP view of the shoulder demonstrating a large subacromial spur (*arrow*), sclerosis in the tuberosity (*open arrow*) and reduction of the humeroacromial space to 5 mm.

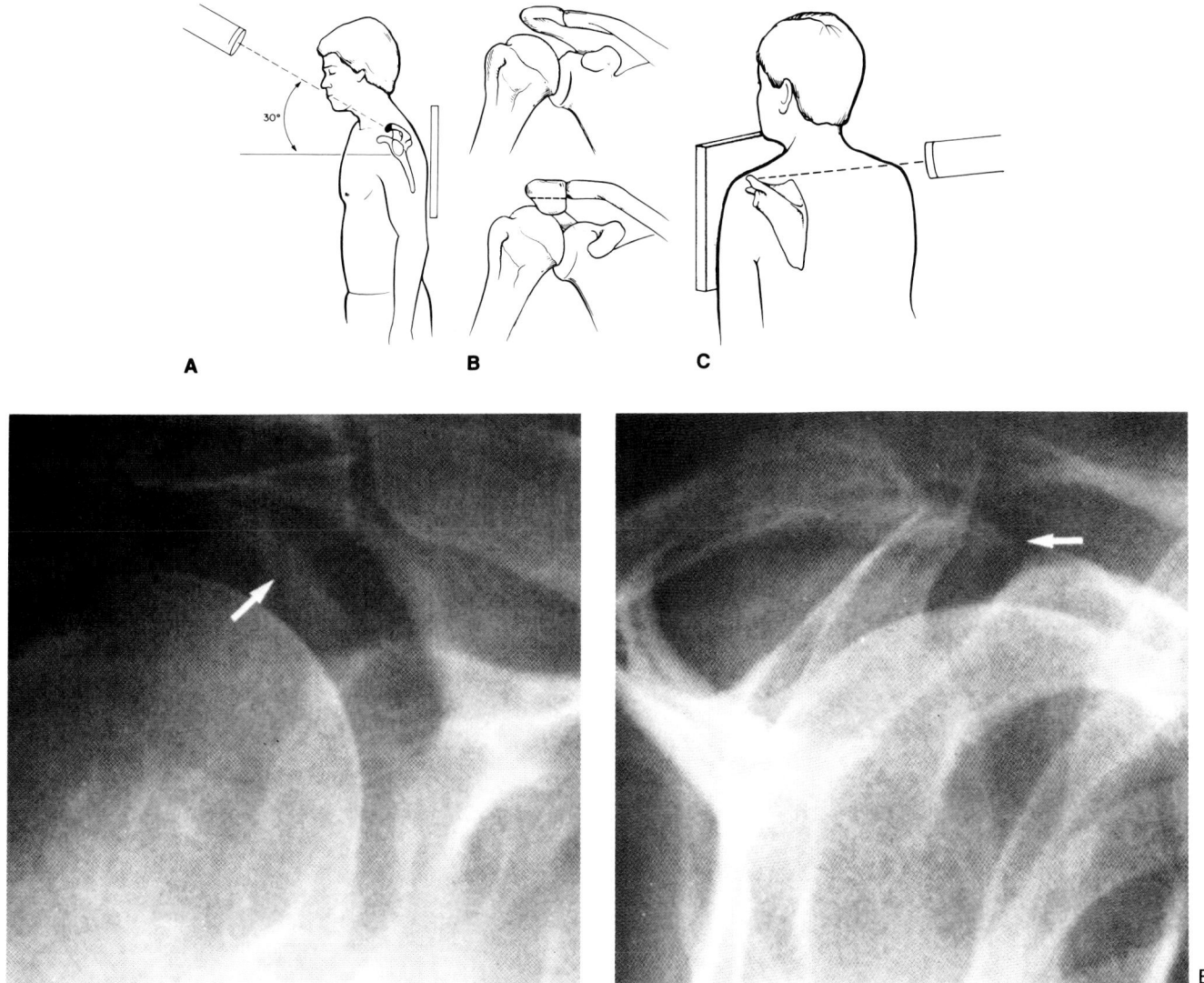

FIG. 10–32. A: Illustration of positioning for 30° angled AP view. **B:** Normal (*top*) and angled (*bottom*) views. The abnormal area (*below dotted line*) is not seen on the routine view (*top*). **C:** Positioning for supraspinatous outlet view. **D:** Radiograph obtained with 30° caudally angled AP view demonstrating subacromial spurring. **E:** Supraspinatus outlet view in the same patient (from 44, with permission).

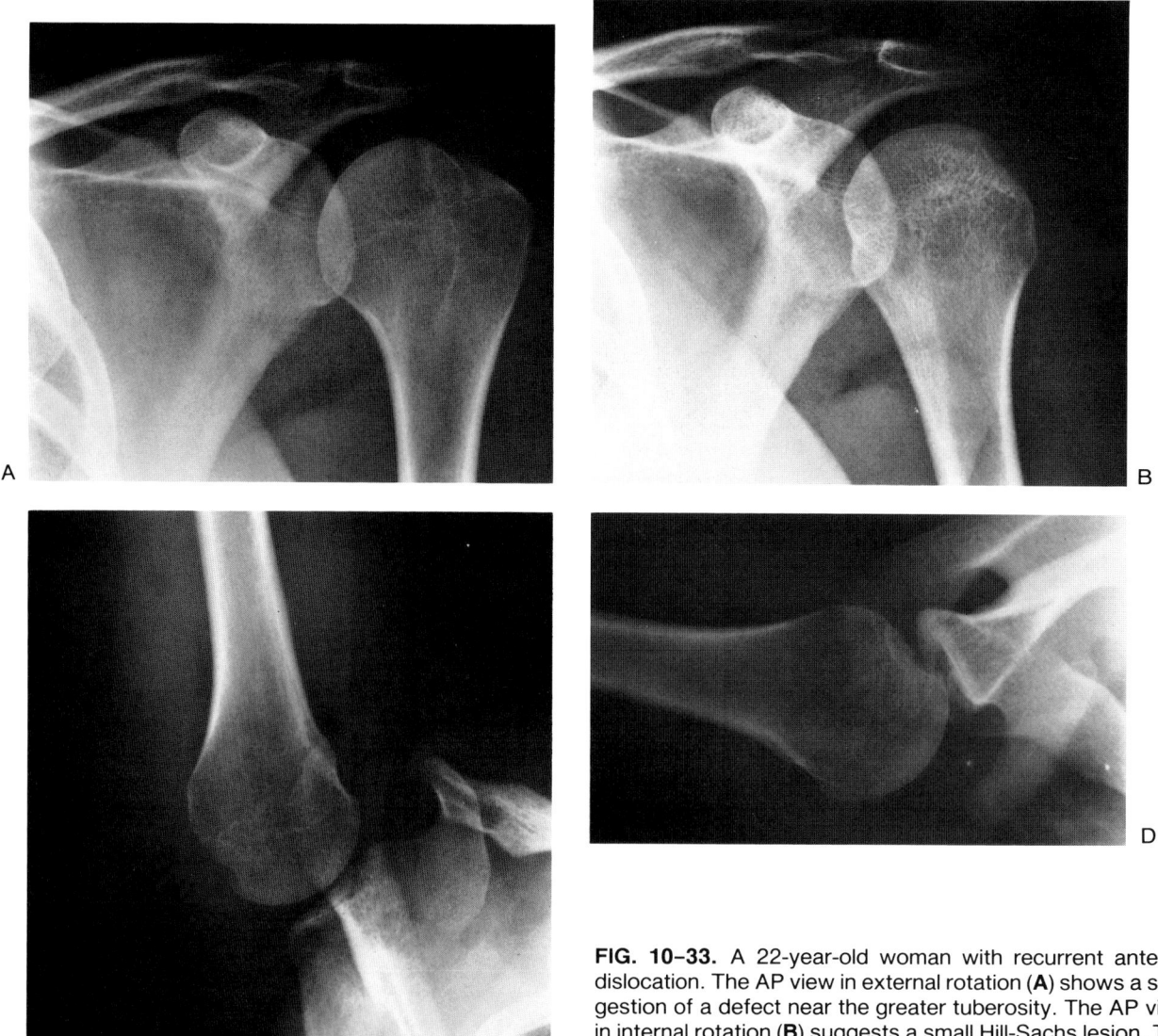

A

B

C

D

FIG. 10–33. A 22-year-old woman with recurrent anterior dislocation. The AP view in external rotation (**A**) shows a suggestion of a defect near the greater tuberosity. The AP view in internal rotation (**B**) suggests a small Hill-Sachs lesion. The Stryker Notch view (**C**) also suggests this lesion. However, the Hill-Sachs lesion is only well seen on the West Point view (**D**).

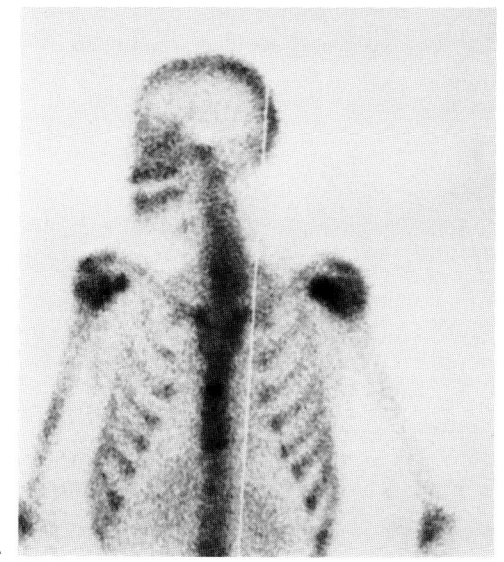

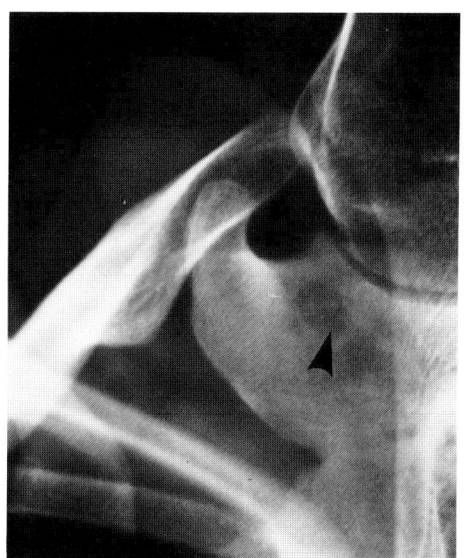

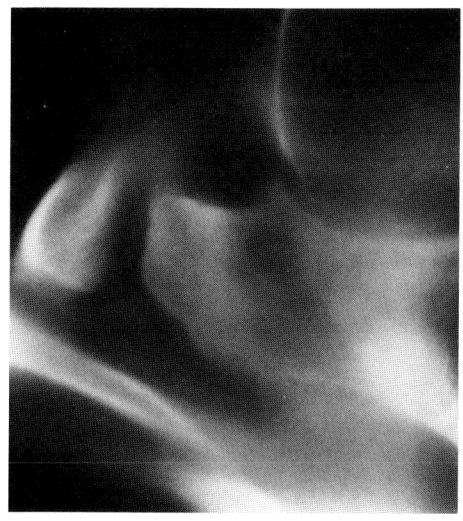

FIG. 10–34. A 24-year-old man with pain in the shoulder, worse at night, and relieved by aspirin. **A:** ^{99m}Tc scan demonstrates increased uptake in the left glenoid. **B:** A Stryker Notch view demonstrates a lucent area in the glenoid (*arrow*). **C:** Tomograms further define the osteoid osteoma.

outline all of the bone pathology, as one single view does not always depict these two lesions. In these situations, the basic AP views in internal and external rotation are supplemented by a West Point axillary and a Stryker notch view. With these two additional x-rays, it is unlikely that important findings will be missed (Fig. 10-33). Fluoroscopy is also useful for obtaining optimal positioning in selected cases (50).

Tomography

In the shoulder, tomography is seldom necessary. However, it may be a useful adjunct to routine x-ray evaluation or coned-down views. This is especially true of the medial third of the clavicle and the sternoclavicular joint, as thoracic contents may obscure alterations in bone structure or joint relationships. Shoulder pain is often traumatic or degenerative in origin, but small neo-

plasms such as an osteoid osteoma may cause difficulty in diagnosis. Plain x-rays may not localize the problem. A radioisotope scan can localize the lesion, allowing selection of a tomographic projection to define the lesion (Fig. 10-34).

Recently, several authors have combined arthrography and tomography to yield a better definition of structures outlined by the contrast material (44). Arthrotomography will be discussed later with arthrography. Other imaging techniques are discussed below (22,24,27,30).

SPECIAL DIAGNOSTIC TECHNIQUES

Ultrasonography

The role of ultrasonography for evaluating shoulder disorders continues to evolve. In early studies, features

consistently associated with tendon tears included abnormal motion patterns of the supraspinatus with arm
rotation and persistently disrupted echoes within the
tendon substance. Cuff tears typically follow four
patterns. These include focal cuff thinning, non-
visualization, discontinuity in echo patterns, and a central echogenic band in the substance of the rotator cuff
(88,100). Very large tears were imaged as regions of diminished echo density (60,85).

As experience with sonography of the shoulder has
expanded, its role for evaluation of both the biceps tendon and rotator cuff have gained acceptance. Using axial
and longitudinal scans to evaluate these structures is
quite successful in experienced hands. Middleton et al.
(100) reported both sensitivity and specificity to be 91%
for detection of rotator cuff tears. Errors related to ultrasound are usually due to technique or lack of familiarity
with normal anatomy (100). This is documented by vari-

ation in accuracy reports that range from 63–94%
(61,68,100).

Computed Tomography

Some of the difficulties involved in obtaining an alternative to the AP views for sternoclavicular and medial
clavicular lesions have been mentioned earlier. Computed tomographic scanning is very useful for overcom-
ing these difficulties (Fig. 10-25B). Scapular spine or
body lesions may also be further defined using this technique (86).

Computed tomography (CT) has proved to be especially useful for better definition of glenoid fractures and
more complex fractures, because often the shoulder
views are not adequate to make a decision about the
need for surgery (Fig. 10-35). Combined with arthrogra-

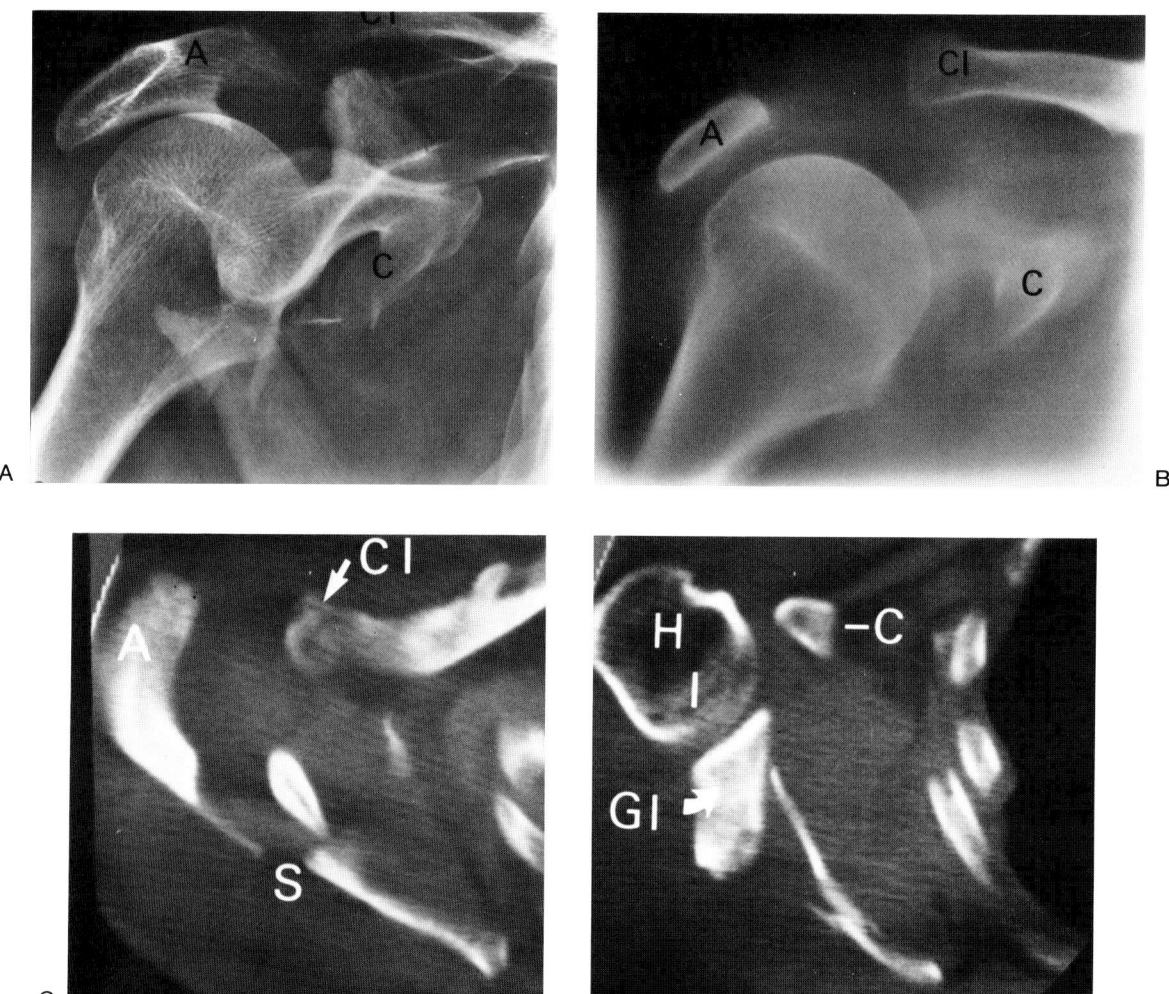

FIG. 10–35. Complex scapular fracture. **A:** AP view demonstrates multiple fragments. **B:** Tomography is not of great value in demonstrating the position of the fragments. **C:** CT scan at the acromial level shows communication of the spine of the scapula and AC separation. The mid-clavicle is fractured. **D:** Image taken just below this level shows an intact glenoid articular surface and the anterior-most portion of the coracoid. Gl, glenoid; A, acromion; Cl, clavicle; C, coracoid; S, scapula.

TABLE 10-2. Indications and techniques for shoulder arthrography in 552 arthrograms

Suspected clinical problem	% Cases	Technique
Rotator cuff tear (partial and/or complete)	57	Double contrast/single contrast
Adhesive capsulitis: diagnosis and treatment	15	Single contrast ± dilatation
Impingement syndrome	8	Double contrast ± bursography
Evaluation of the PO (postoperative) shoulder	6	Double contrast subtraction technique
1. Previous cuff tears		
2. TSA (total shoulder arthroplasty)		
Instability or chronic subluxation	5	Double contrast with conventional or computed tomography (CT)
Biceps tendon tear	4	Double contrast
Post-traumatic deformities	3	Double contrast ± conventional or computed tomography
Tendinitis	2	Double contrast

phy, CT is especially useful for evaluation of instability and glenoid labral lesions (63,71). CT arthrography will be discussed more completely in the following section.

Shoulder Arthrography

Proper choice of arthrographic technique requires an awareness of the patient's clinical problem, such as a rotator cuff tear or impingement syndrome, as well as an understanding of the plain-film findings. Shoulder arthrography is most often utilized in the evaluation of the rotator cuff (73–78,98,109,110,115,120,122). However, more subtle changes in the shoulder may also be detected, especially with double-contrast techniques, and combined arthrographic techniques with conventional or computed tomography.

In our series of 552 shoulder arthrograms, 38% of patients were referred with pain and diminished range of motion. The majority of these patients were suspected to have rotator cuff lesions. An additional 19% were referred with definite clinical evidence of cuff tears. Thus, 57% of the arthrograms were performed with cuff disease specifically in mind. Table 10-2 summarizes the other common indications in our practice. The techniques most often used are also included in Table 10-2. Arthrography is less commonly performed to exclude synovitis, loose bodies, and arthritis (69,80).

Knowledge of the patient's suspected problem and careful evaluation of routine radiographs can assist one

in proper performance of the arthrogram and choice of filming sequence to best define the patient's problem.

Review of plain-film findings on 552 patients undergoing shoulder arthrography has provided extensive data regarding these findings. Previous reports of plain-film findings in patients with rotator cuff tears describe superior subluxation of the humeral head (distance from humeral head to acromion ≤7 mm), reversal of the normal acromial convexity, sclerosis or cystic changes in the greater tuberosity, and bony eburnation of the glenoid or humeral head inferomedially (70,82,94,130). The latter finding (hypertrophic spurring involving the humeral head inferomedially) is not a reliable indicator of rotator cuff tearing and can be seen with many chronic shoulder problems (94,130). DeSmet reported plain-film abnormalities in 90.4% of 42 patients with rotator cuff tears (70). Our review of 552 arthrograms revealed 145 complete and 38 partial tears of the rotator cuff. As would be expected, changes on plain radiographs were much more common with complete chronic cuff tears (Table 10-3). Patients with acute cuff tears (no associated fractures) less frequently demonstrate bony abnormalities on plain films.

Superior subluxation of the humeral head causes a reduction of the distance between the acromion, which is normally convex inferiorly, and the humeral head. Consistency in measurement is essential if one is to utilize this measurement properly. We measure all cases in external rotation. This measurement is virtually always greater than 1 cm in normal individuals (Fig. 10-36).

TABLE 10-3. Plain film findings in rotator cuff tears

	Location of abnormal finding						
	Humeroacromial distance (Superior subluxation)			Greater tuberosity	AC[a] joint	Inferior glenoid spurring	Humeral spurring
	>1 cm	<1 cm	<7 cm				
Complete thickness cuff tears, 145 cases	5%	30%	65%	90%	75%	25%	25%
Partial thickness cuff tears, 38 cases	44%	40%	16%	11%	None	None	10%

[a] AC, acromioclavicular.

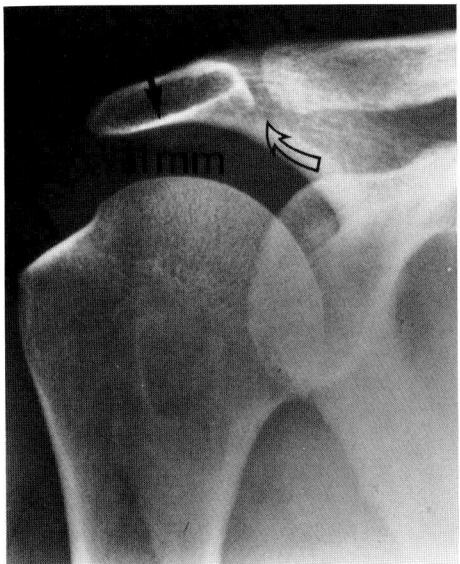

FIG. 10-36. Normal humeroacromial distance with convex acromion (*black arrows*) and a well-defined smooth greater tuberosity. Normal AC joint (*open arrow*).

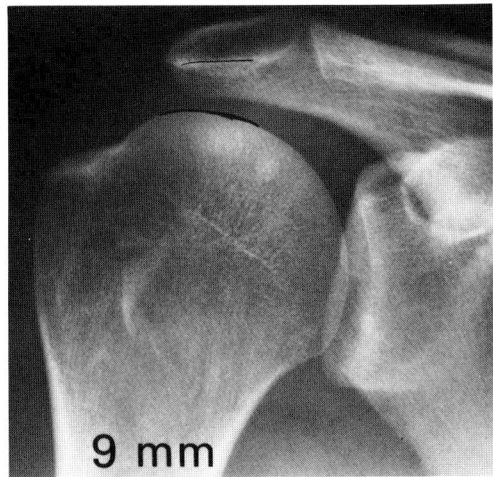

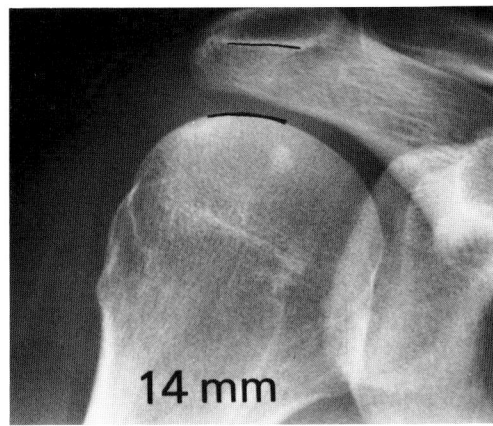

FIG. 10-37. The acromiohumeral distance in the external rotation (**A**) measures 9 mm. In internal rotation (**B**) the measurement is 14 mm, a difference of 5 mm with position change.

Measurements on the same shoulder may vary up to 5 mm between external and internal rotations (Fig. 10-37). Also, one must consider target-film distance and tube centering. We measured the acromiohumeral distance in external rotation with a 48-inch target-film distance. The patient was placed in a straight AP position and then positioned obliquely for a true AP view of the glenohumeral joint. We also centered the tube over the coracoid and directly over the acromiohumeral joint. There was less than 1 mm difference in the measurements. Thus, consistency in obtaining the measurements is all that is necessary for constitutional accuracy. In patients with rotator cuff tears, the acromiohumeral distance was less than 1 cm in 95% of cases, with 65% measuring less than 0.7 cm (Fig. 10-38). The small percentage of patients with 1 cm in distance and rotator cuff tears were younger patients with small cuff tears. In fewer than 5% of cases, measurements of less than 0.7 cm were noted, and no cuff tears were detected arthrographically. We must strongly question whether proper arthrographic technique and exercise were accomplished during the procedures in this group of patients.

Changes in the greater tuberosity were evident in 90% of patients with complete cuff tears. These findings included cystic changes (Fig. 10-39), sclerosis, small erosions, and in 6 patients a "double tuberosity" (Fig. 10-40). This latter finding is of interest in that 2 cuff tears were missed arthrographically. These patients also demonstrated some degree of superior subluxation. At surgery, large cuff tears were found as well as extensive capsular scarring. We suspect that the area of ossification adjacent to the tuberosity may represent an ossified or calcified supraspinatus remnant. This finding should

alert one to look harder for a cuff tear if the initial films are normal.

Subtle changes on the inferior surface of the acromion or distal clavicle were present in 75% of patients with complete cuff tears (Fig. 10-41). These findings were also noted in a high percentage of patients with impingement syndrome. Therefore, such changes are less specific for a rotator cuff tear than changes in the greater tuberosity or superior subluxation of the humeral head.

Eburnation along the glenoid rim and spurring of the inferior medial aspect of the humeral head were present in 25% of patients (Fig. 10-41A, B), but this finding can also be seen with degenerative arthritis and in adhesive capsulitis. Other routine radiographic findings not usually associated with cuff tears included chondrocalcinosis, soft tissue calcification (Fig. 10-42), loose bodies, and calcified phleboliths (from hemangioma or arteriovenous malformation). These changes suggest other etiologies as the cause of the patient's pain.

Other views should also be reviewed for findings suggesting instability or previous dislocation (Hill-Sachs lesions, Bankart deformity). Older films may indicate sub-

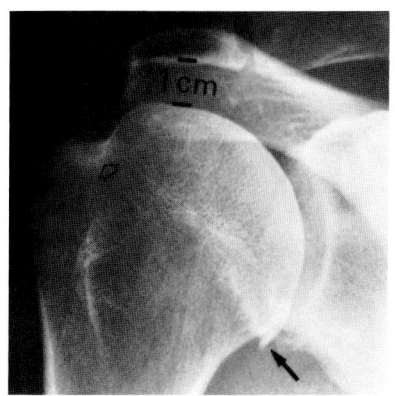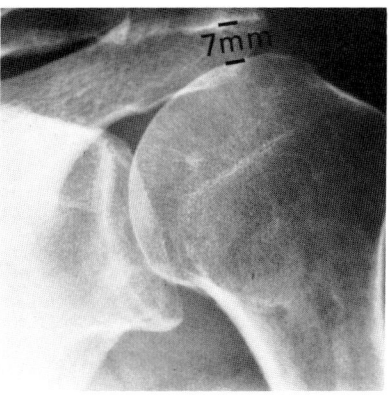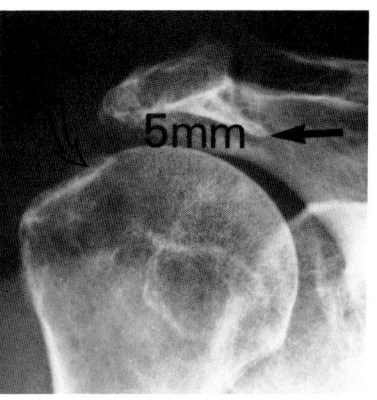

A　B　C

FIG. 10–38. Plain film changes in patients with chronic rotator cuff tears. **A:** Acromiohumeral distance 1 cm. Note cystic changes in the greater tuberosity (*open arrow*) and spurring of the head and glenoid (*black arrow*). **B:** Superior subluxation with acromiohumeral distance of 7 mm. Relatively normal glenoid and greater tuberosity. **C:** Superior subluxation with acromiohumeral distance of 5 mm. Note large acromial spur (*black arrow*) that was impinging on the cuff and bursa. New bone formation at the cuff insertion into the greater tuberosity (*open arrow*).

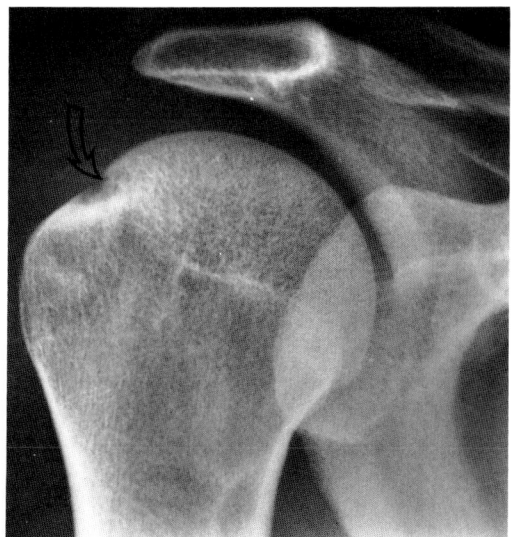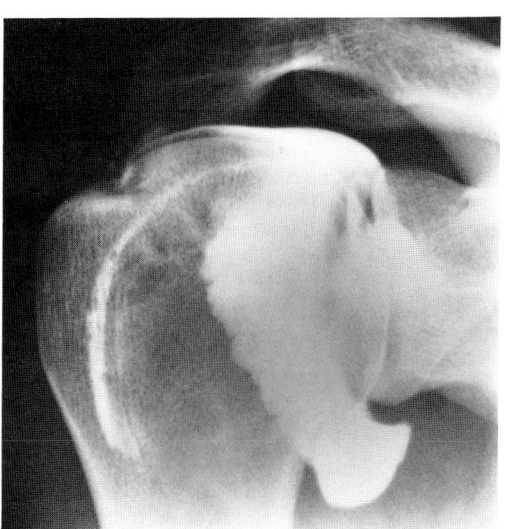

A　B

FIG. 10–39. A: Normal external rotation view except for cystic erosion (*open arrow*) in the greater tuberosity. **B:** Arthrogram demonstrates a corresponding incomplete thickness tear in the rotator cuff (*arrow*).

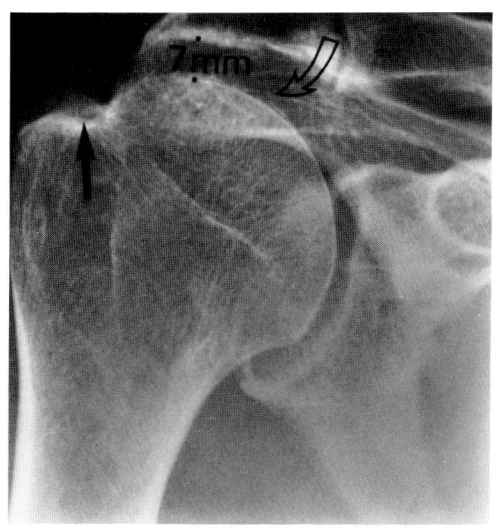

FIG. 10–40. Chronic rotator cuff tear with "double tuberosity" (*black arrow*). Also subluxation with acromiohumeral measurement of 7 mm and cartilagenous calcification (*open arrow*).

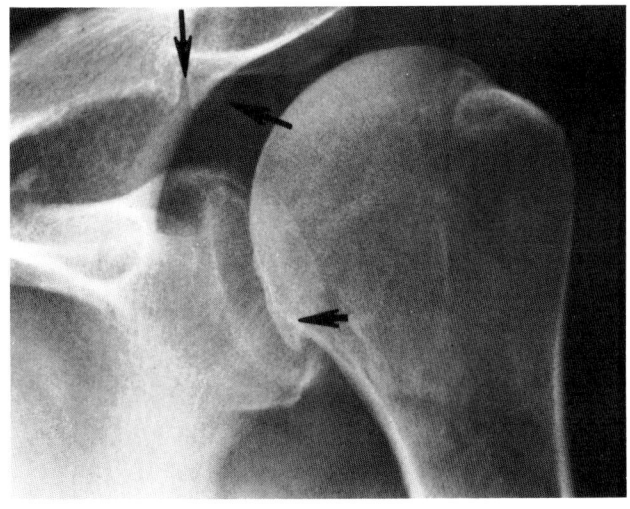

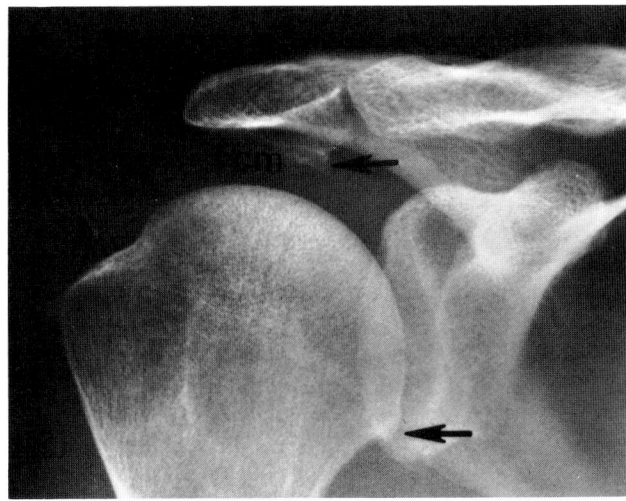

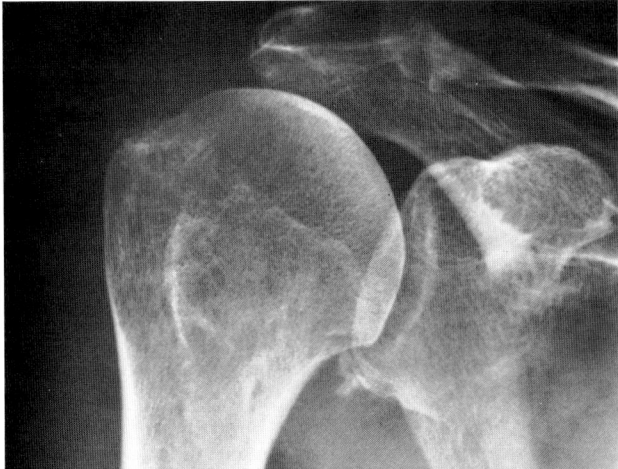

FIG. 10–41. A: Spurring of the inferior margins of the AC joint (*upper black arrows*) in a patient with symptoms of impingement and a proved rotator cuff tear. Inferior humeral head spurring (*lower black arrow*). B: Normal acromiohumeral distance. Large acromial spur (*upper black arrow*). Small spur in lower humeral head (*lower arrow*). C: Almost all secondary changes described with chronic cuff tears are present, i.e., superior subluxation of the humeral head, eburnation on the greater tuberosity, spurring of the AC joint margin, and osteophytic changes of the acromion.

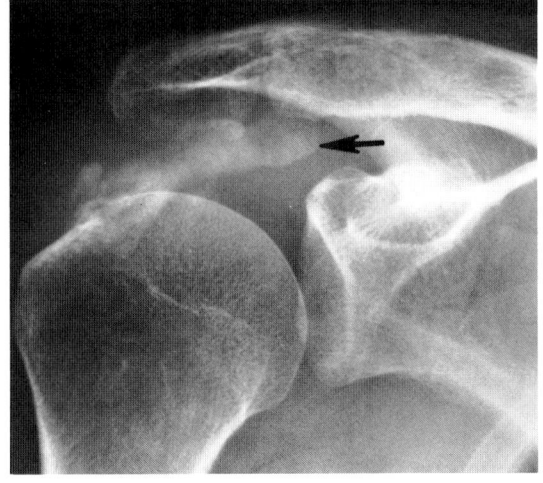

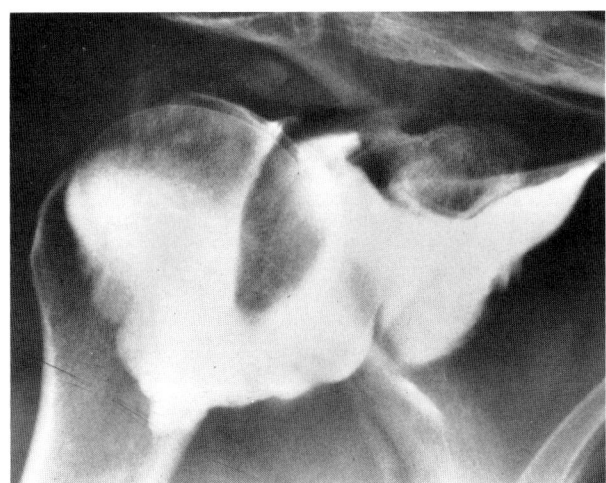

FIG. 10–42. A: Extensive calcification in the rotator cuff. Note increased acromiohumeral space due to inflammed fluid-filled bursa. B: Arthrogram demonstrates an intact rotator cuff.

tle loss of articular cartilage in patients with arthritis or joint space infection (see Radiographic Technique section). Once one has conferred with the clinician and examined the routine radiographs, the proper approach for the arthrogram will become evident.

Technique

Shoulder arthrography is performed on a fluoroscopic table with an overhead tube and small (≤6 mm) focal spot. This has the advantage of better geometry than conventional fluoroscopic equipment, resulting in better film quality. It also allows greater patient access for the physician performing the examination (see Introduction to Arthrography in Chapter 1).

With the patient in the supine position, the arm to be examined is externally rotated. A scout film is obtained to be certain that the radiographic technique is optimum. The technical quality of the films taken following injection is critical, and pre-injection scout films minimize the problem of inadequate technique and repeat injections. Scout films are especially important if the radiographic technician does not perform arthrography on a regular basis.

Following establishment of optimum radiographic technique, the patient is prepared for the procedure with a 5-minute surgical scrub followed by application of povidone-iodine (Betadine) to the skin in the area to be injected. A 5-ml syringe with 1% lidocaine (Xylocaine) and a 25-gauge needle is used to mark the site of injection. The site is chosen over the glenohumeral joint below the coracoid and approximately at the junction of the mid- and distal thirds of the glenoid articular surface (Fig. 10-43). A wheal is made in the skin over the joint-entrance point. The soft tissues are also infiltrated with lidocaine. We err toward the medial margin of the humeral head. This insures an intra-articular positioning of the needle. The needle enters the joint or strikes the humeral head. With this technique the glenoid labrum is avoided.

The injection is made after fluoroscopic control to be certain that the needle is properly positioned. If the needle is not in the joint, a small collection of contrast material will accumulate at the needle tip with the initial injection. If properly positioned, the contrast material flows away from the needle around the humeral head (Fig. 10-44). An extensive literature is available concerning variations in this technique (74,98,120,123).

If single-contrast technique is utilized, 6–10 ml of diatrizoate meglumine (Hypaque-M-60) is injected. Low osmolality, non-ionic agents are now available that may be more easily tolerated than ionic agents. Too much contrast material obscures detail, and the arthrogram is less informative (Fig. 10-45). With experience, one can judge capsular volume early and avoid excessive amounts of contrast material. In double-contrast examinations, 4 ml of contrast material is injected followed by 10–15 ml of air, depending upon the capsule size. Again, too much contrast material defeats the purpose of a double-contrast examination. The injection must be observed fluoroscopically. If contrast is seen to leak into the subacromial bursa during the injection, the exact site of a rotator cuff tear can be visualized.

Following the injection, the patient is exercised under fluoroscopic control, and any symptoms and radiographic changes are carefully noted. The relationship of the head and tuberosities to the acromion and coracoid can be examined, if impingement is suspected clinically. The patient is then fluoroscopically positioned for tangential AP views of the glenohumeral joint. Films are taken in external and internal rotation. The tangential

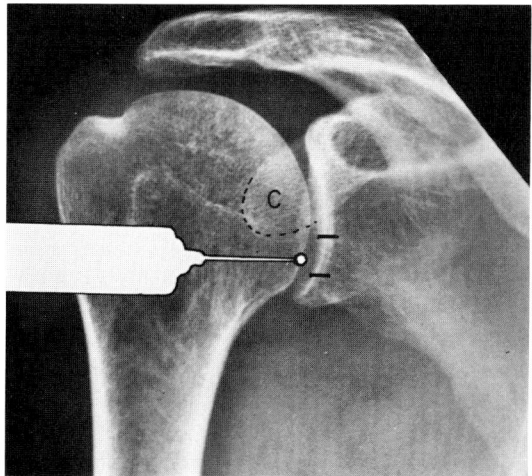
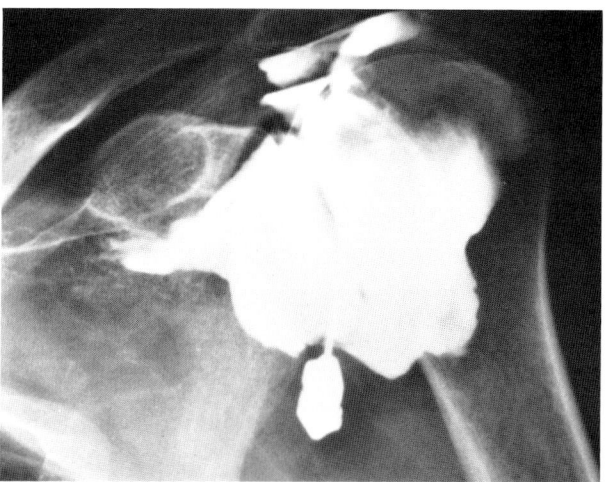

FIG. 10–43. A: Needle tip marking entry site. **B:** Improper needle placement. The tip of the needle is too far lateral and superior. This resulted in filling of both the joint and subdeltoid subacromial bursa. No cuff tear was identified at surgery.

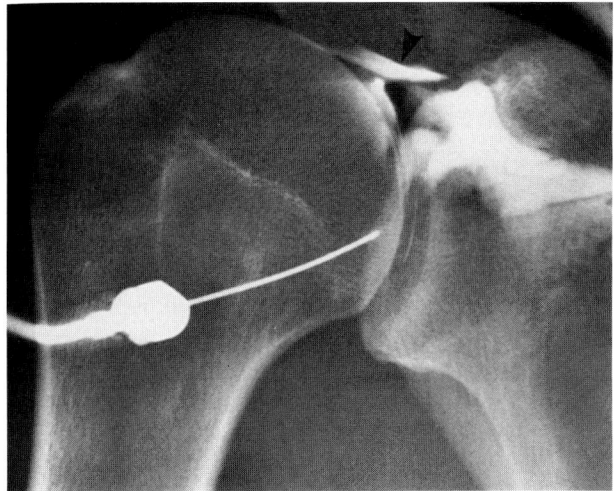

FIG. 10-44. With needle properly positioned contrast flows around the humeral head. Note the contrast (*arrow*) above the origin of the biceps tendon. This should not be confused with a tear.

projection allows better evaluation of the articular cartilage (Fig. 10-46). Goldman and colleagues recommend overpenetrated views for evaluation of the articular cartilage and underpenetrated views for evaluation of soft tissue anatomy (80).

The patient is then moved to a different radiographic suite, and the remainder of the films are performed. With a routine single-contrast examination, axillary, upright weight bearing (77) and scapular lateral *Y*-views are obtained in addition to the internal and external rotation views. Bicipital groove views are obtained if symptoms dictate. If routine film findings lead one to suspect a rotator cuff tear but none is found on the initial arthro-

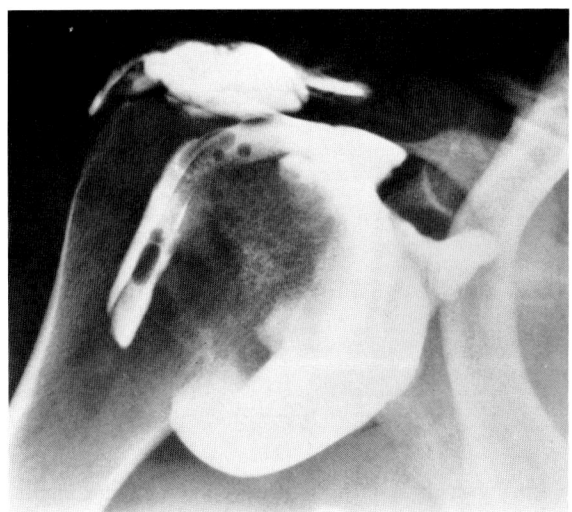

FIG. 10-45. Single contrast arthrogram with too much contrast material. A complete rotator cuff tear is noted. Other detail is obscured by the contrast material.

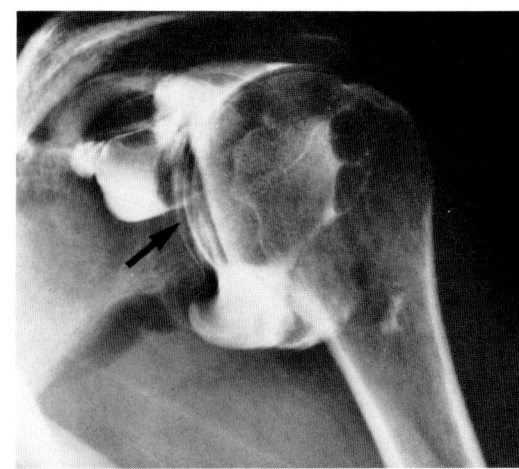

FIG. 10-46. Normal double contrast arthrogram. External rotation view with patient positioned for tangential view of the articular surface (*arrow*).

grams, further exercise and occasionally reinjection are performed to prevent false-negative studies.

If a double-contrast examination is performed, the same views are obtained. However, axillary views are taken in the prone and supine position to demonstrate the glenoid labrum to better advantage. Conventional or computed tomography is occasionally necessary to evaluate the labrum and other subtle changes, especially in patients with previous dislocations or chronic shoulder instability (63,72,87,91,93,97,124).

When conventional or computed tomography is anticipated, we often injection 0.3 ml of 1:1000 epinephrine with the contrast material. This allows more time to obtain the adequate films, as dilution and absorption of the contrast material are decreased. Double contrast technique is best if computed tomography or tomography are used. Lesions are less frequently obscured and air allows more time for imaging (63,71).

Normal Arthrogram

Review of the normal film series utilized with single- and double-contrast arthrography will emphasize the usefulness of each exam (Figs. 10-47 and 10-48). It is obvious that the double-contrast examination provides better detail of certain structures. The synovium and articular cartilages are seen to better advantage, as is the undersurface of the cuff, which is coated with contrast material and outlined by air (Figs. 10-49 and 10-50). The intercapsular portion of the biceps tendon is also more clearly demonstrated, especially with the upright weight-bearing view. Advantages in the visualization of various pathologic conditions will be discussed later in this section.

Single-contrast examinations are effective for demonstrating cuff tears and are perhaps the study of choice for

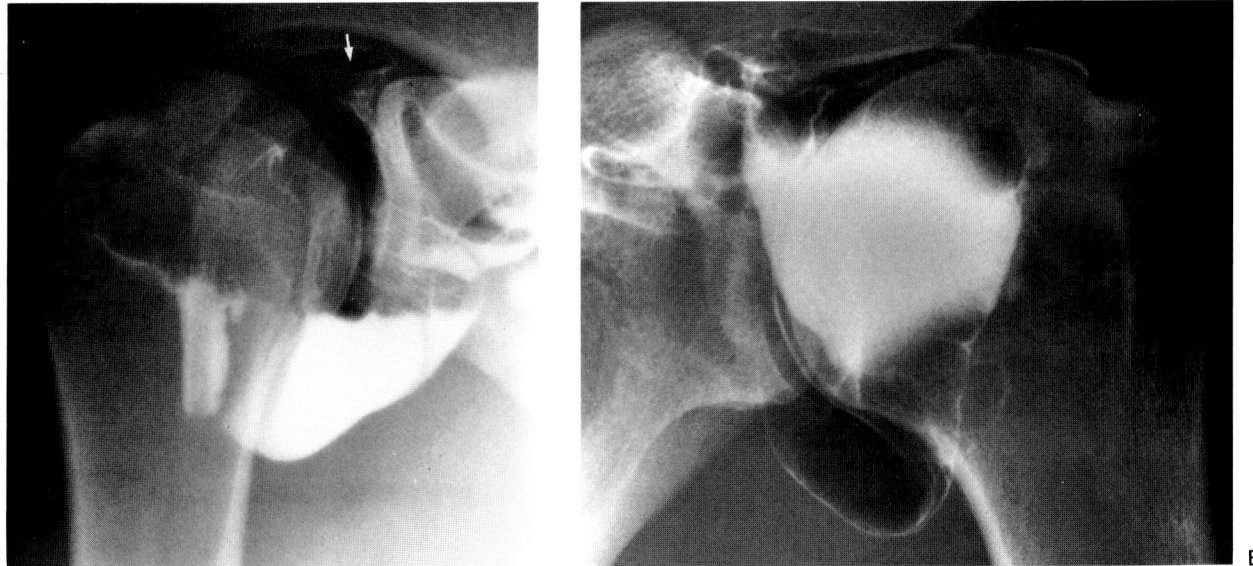

FIG. 10-47. External rotation with upright weight bearing (**A**) using double contrast technique. Note that the biceps tendon can be seen from its origin to the point at which it leaves the tendon sheath (*arrow*). The under surface of the cuff is well demonstrated. The subscapularis recess is small and compressed by the subscapularis during external rotation. **B:** Non-weight-bearing view. Note superior glenoid labrum.

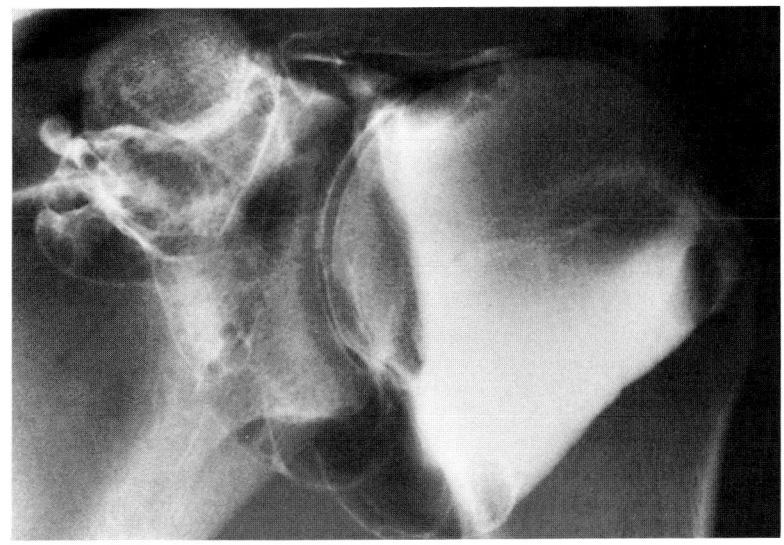

FIG. 10-48. Internal rotation view. The subscapularis bursa is larger. Biceps tendon is obscured by contrast material and the medial humeral cortex.

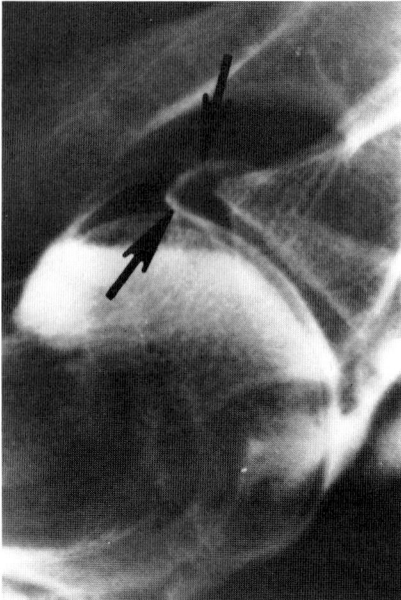

FIG. 10–49. Prone axillary view with double contrast technique. Note the glenoid labrum (*arrows*) and articular cartilage. Contrast medium pools in the anterior capsule.

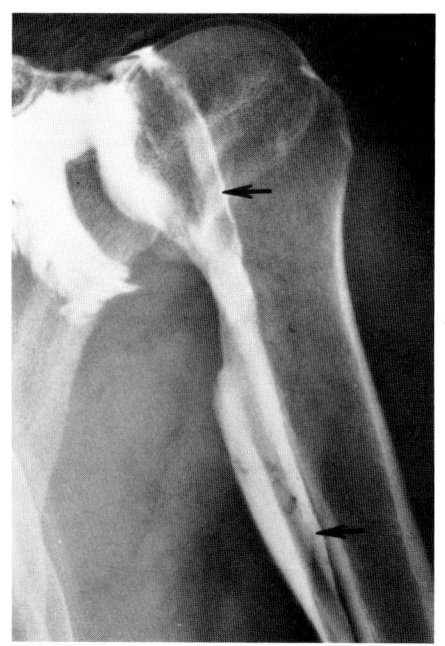

FIG. 10–51. Contrast medium may leak from the biceps tendon sheath (*arrows*) in normal individuals.

adhesive capsulitis. However, the synovium, articular cartilages, and labrum are often obscured using single-contrast technique. The biceps tendon is also more difficult to evaluate. Extravasation may be noted from the biceps tendon sheath and subscapularis bursa in normal individuals (Fig. 10-51).

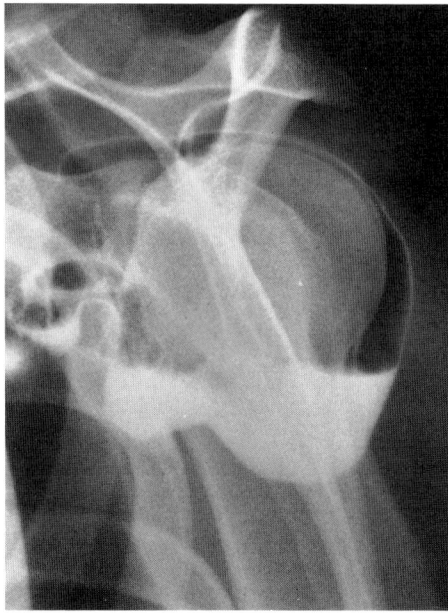

FIG. 10–50. The scapular lateral view allows one to assess the capsular volume and entire circumferential synovial surface. Note also the normal relationship of the humeral head to the acromion.

Abnormal Arthrograms

Rotator Cuff Tears

The most common indication for shoulder arthrography is evaluation of patients with suspected tears in the rotator cuff. Many patients with rotator cuff tear have a history of trauma. The incidence is higher in patients over 50 years of age (109,110,115,133). In our experience (552 cases), 91% were over 40 years of age.

The patient presentation as described by Neviaser (109) may include any of the following:

1. Trauma without fracture dislocation
2. Anterior dislocation
3. Dislocation with avulsion of the greater tuberosity
4. Chronic pain without history of trauma
5. Avulsion of the greater tuberosity

In our study, all but 9% were chronic tears, with a history of trauma within 2 years in over 60% of patients. Of the 552 arthrograms reviewed, 145 patients were found to have complete tears of the cuff, as demonstrated by communication of the glenohumeral joint with the subacromial bursa (Fig. 10-52).

The most important views are the AP views with internal and external rotation. Almost all rotator cuff tears start in or are confined to the supraspinatus tendon. With external rotation of the shoulder, this tendon is the most lateral when compared with the other tendons of the rotator cuff. In rotator cuff tears, upward subluxation is most severe on this view, as the amount of tendon

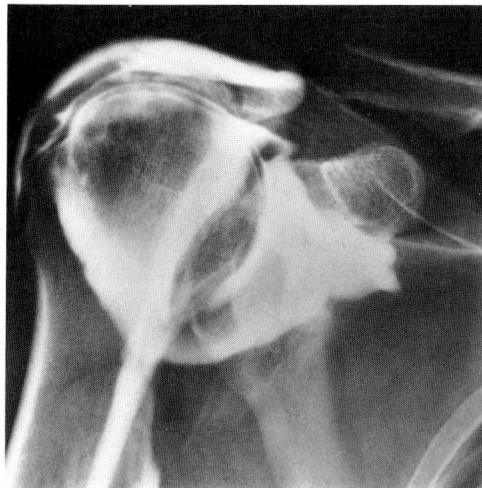

FIG. 10–52. Single contrast arthrogram demonstrating a complete rotator cuff tear. Contrast medium fills the subacromial and subdeltoid bursa. The articular cartilage and nature of the tear are difficult to evaluate.

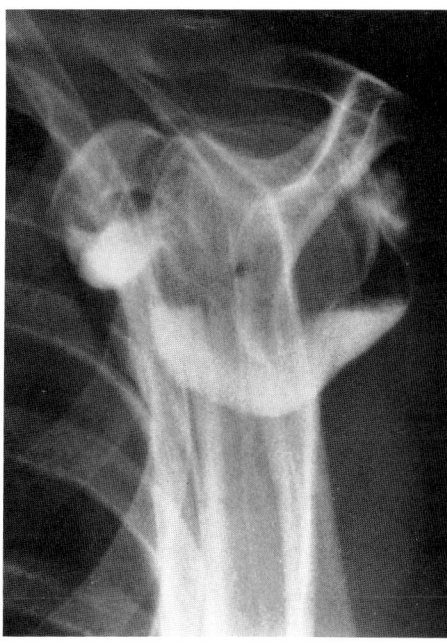

FIG. 10–53. Partial thickness cuff tear posteriorly that could be identified only on the scapular lateral view.

between the humeral head and the acromion is least. In the external rotation view, the distance from the edge of the humeral head cartilage to the tendon edge as defined by the dye is significant. This will depict the medial-to-lateral length of the tear. The extent of the tear in a posterior direction or the width of the tear, on the other hand, is assessed on the internal rotation view. When the shoulder is internally rotated, the infraspinatus becomes more lateral and lies under the acromion, as seen on the AP view. If the upper surface and undersurface of the tendon are well outlined and complete to the tendon insertion, the tear has not extended to any degree into the infraspinatus, and it is a small or medium-sized tear. If the tendon is not well outlined on both surfaces but another tendon gap is seen, the tear has extended into the infraspinatus and is at least large in size. If the axillary view shows a normal posterior capsule pouch, the tear is large; but if the posterior pouch is also obliterated, as mentioned previously, the tear likely extends to include the posterior aspect of the infraspinatus also and is global or massive in size. Finally, an anterior oblique view should be obtained to confirm observations of the extent of the tendon tearing.

In our series, 38 patients had partial tears in which the arthrogram revealed extravasation of contrast material into the partial thickness of the rotator cuff (Fig. 10-53; also see Fig. 10-39B). Partial thickness tearing of the rotator cuff usually occurs in the supraspinatus. This can be seen as an extension of dye into the tendon substance but not into the bursa. If the contrast material extends past the end of the cartilage surface laterally, a portion of the tendon attachment is torn or has degenerated. These findings may be clarified by using a traction view in the upright position. Such findings also suggest that a careful

evaluation is necessary, as a component of the impingement syndrome related to anterior acromial osteophyte information may well be present. Figure 10-54 points out the importance of multiple views in assessing the rotator cuff. The AP views were normal in this case.

Surgery or arthroscopy was performed in 140 of 183 patients and confirmed the arthrographic findings in 99% of the cases. False-negative arthrograms are usually due to improper technique. Technical failures included improper injections, failure to exercise the patient suffi-

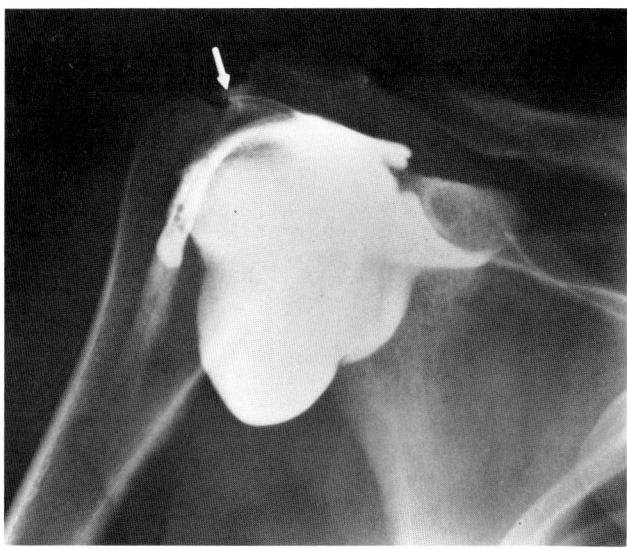

FIG. 10–54. Partial thickness cuff tear (*arrow*) in the distal supraspinatous portion of the cuff seen on external rotation.

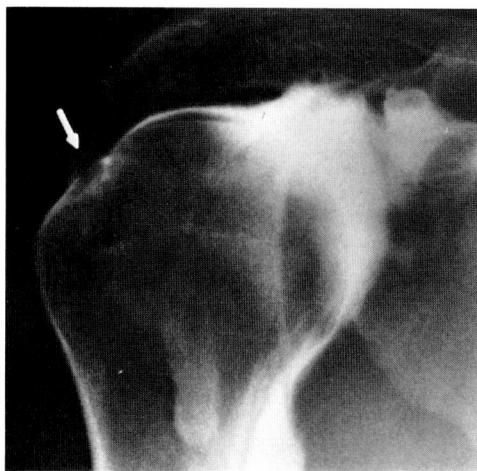

FIG. 10–55. External rotation view with no evidence of a cuff tear. Note the bony projection from the greater tuberosity (*arrow*). At surgery, a large tear was present with fibrous scarring.

ciently (Fig. 10-55), and a lack of awareness of the radiographic appearance of partial cuff tears. There were no false positives. Eighty-five percent of complete tears involved the supraspinatus near its insertion into the greater tuberosity; the adjacent infraspinatus was also involved in 39% of the cases. Tears in the subscapularis and teres minor were much less common, occurring in only 12% of the patients.

The accuracy rate did not differ significantly when comparing single- versus double-contrast techniques. However, partial tears were more readily detected by utilizing double-contrast techniques. This technique allows one to evaluate the size of the tear and the appearance of tendon ends (Fig. 10-56). These findings may aid the surgeon in determining the best treatment (78,91,119).

We find that in tears of 1–2 cm in length, evaluation of tendon ends is of value, but, in larger chronic tears with extensive plain-film findings, the tendon ends are more difficult to visualize owing to scarring (Fig. 10-56). In patients with superior subluxation and an acromiohumeral distance of 5 mm or less, we have found double-contrast technique to add little to the diagnosis. Also, in this setting, unless surgery is contemplated, we see little need to perform the arthrogram in the first place. Double-contrast arthrography is not utilized prior to arthroscopy, as the air hinders the arthroscopist.

Adhesive Capsulitis

The term *adhesive capsulitis* was coined by Neviaser in 1953 (107,108). Patients present with pain and varying degrees of reduction in the range of motion of the involved shoulder. The etiology is unclear, but it has been stated that the condition may be due to capsular thickening or adhesions involving the capsule, biceps, and subacromial bursa (120). Simmonds and DePalma postulated that inflammation may be secondary to degeneration of the supraspinatus tendon and biceps tendon, respectively (69,125). To add to the confusion, a recent report in which arthroscopy was performed on patients with adhesive capsulitis noted no adhesions or intra-articular abnormalities. It stated that the etiology was more likely extra-articular (83). The final common result is cuff and capsular stiffness secondary to scarring (134). Regardless of the etiology, however, arthrography is an effective diagnostic tool.

Suspected adhesive capsulitis was the third most common indication for arthrography in our series. Fifty-eight of 82 patients with decreased capsular volume had associated rotator cuff tears. Only 25% of patients with

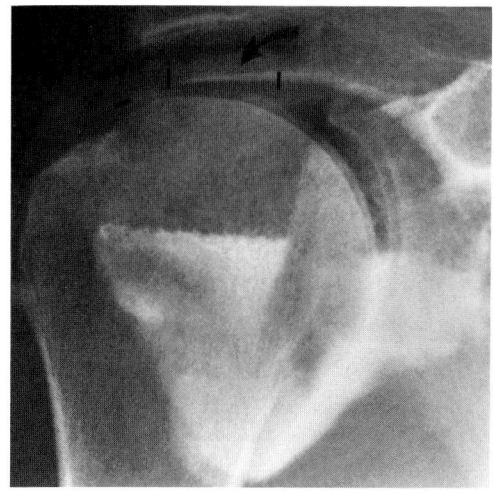
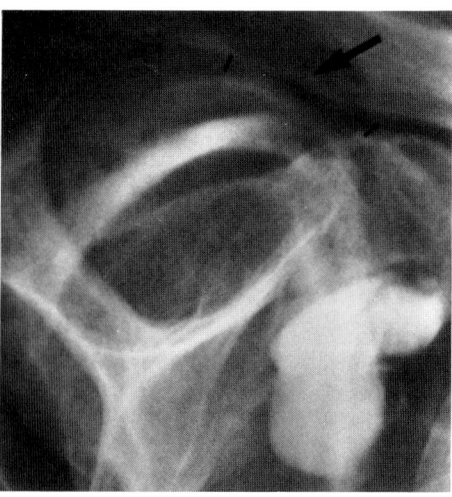

FIG. 10–56. Double contrast technique demonstrating a complete thickness tear superior to the head (*arrow*) on external rotation (**A**). Thickness is easily assessed. The scapular lateral view (**B**) demonstrates the AP dimensions.

TABLE 10-4. *Arthrographic finding in adhesive capsulitis*

1. Diminished capsular volume (usually <10 cc)
2. Small axillary recess and subscapularis bursa
3. Lymphatic filling
4. Synovitis
5. Irregularity at the capsular insertions

adhesive capsulitis alone demonstrated changes on the routine radiographs, and, when present, these were non-specific, such as spurring of the glenoid or humeral head.

Arthrograms revealed a group of characteristic findings that are presented in Table 10-4 (Fig. 10-57). The most common feature is decreased capsular volume, with reduced size of the axillary recess and subscapular bursa (Fig. 10-57). Patients may complain of shoulder discomfort after only several ml of contrast material has been injected (Fig. 10-58) (74,108,109,119). If double-contrast technique is used, the air will not be retained in the small capsule, and the joint will often decompress via the needle. After injecting 2–4 ml of contrast material, it may become apparent that the capsule volume is only minimally reduced. Double-contrast technique adds little to the diagnosis.

In our series, the biceps tendon sheath was not filled or only incompletely filled in 20% of patients with adhesive capsulitis. The significance of this finding is uncertain, but biceps adhesions have been described by several authors (78,112,115,122).

Once the diagnosis is established, the arthrogram may then become a therapeutic tool to distend the contracted capsule and relieve, at least temporarily, the patient's symptoms (78,112). This can be accomplished by gradually distending the capsule with a mixture of contrast material and 1% lidocaine (Xylocaine) or marcaine and celestone (74,79,107,115,120). The injection volume is gradually increased until the capsule ruptures, and at this point further injection is unnecessary. The extravasation usually occurs along the subscapularis. This is followed by a set of assisted exercises with a gradually increasing range of motion (Fig. 10-59). To use this technique, other precipitating or continuing sources of pain must be excluded. Unless a formal manipulation accompanies the procedure, the amount of success one will have in gaining more movement is uncertain. Our experience has shown that most success occurs in patients with mild to moderate reduction in capsular volume. In patients with a rotator cuff tear, dilatation is of little value, as the capsule will decompress into the subacromial bursa.

Biceps Tendon Abnormalities

Arthrography, if properly utilized, may aid in diagnosis of biceps tendon abnormalities. Again, plain film evaluation is important. A bicipital groove view should be obtained in cases of clinically suspected biceps tendon lesions. The bony appearance of the groove may provide some clue to the diagnosis. Cone and colleagues noted an average medial wall angle of 48° (66). The average width was 11 mm and the depth, 4.6 mm. Medial wall bone spurs and spurs in the groove were noted in 33% and 8%, respectively (Fig. 10-60). If the angle approaches 90°, constriction and tenosynovitis is said to be a diagnostic consideration. Angles less than 30° may be associated with subluxation of the biceps tendon (66,112).

The main difficulty in detecting biceps tendon abnormalities arthrographically is the lack of consistent filling of this tendon sheath. Preston (115) and Nelson (106) have reported nonfilling as abnormal; however, other au-

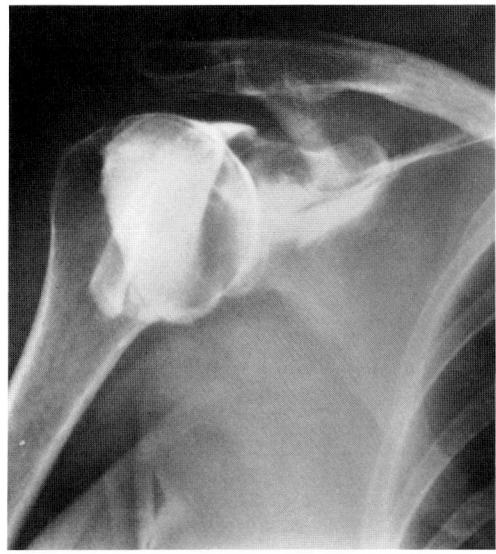 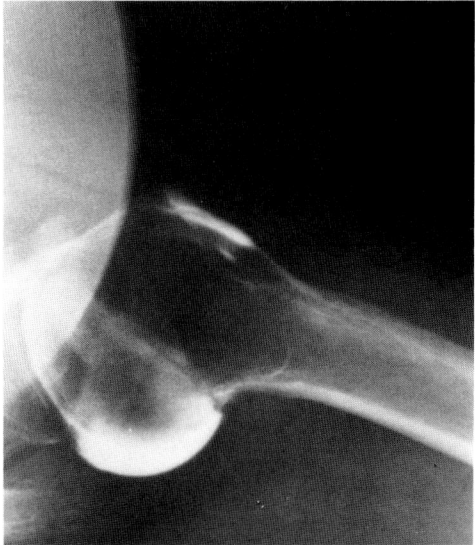

FIG. 10–57. Adhesive capsulitis. AP (**A**) and axillary (**B**) views showing small axillary and subscapularis recesses. Biceps tendon is normal.

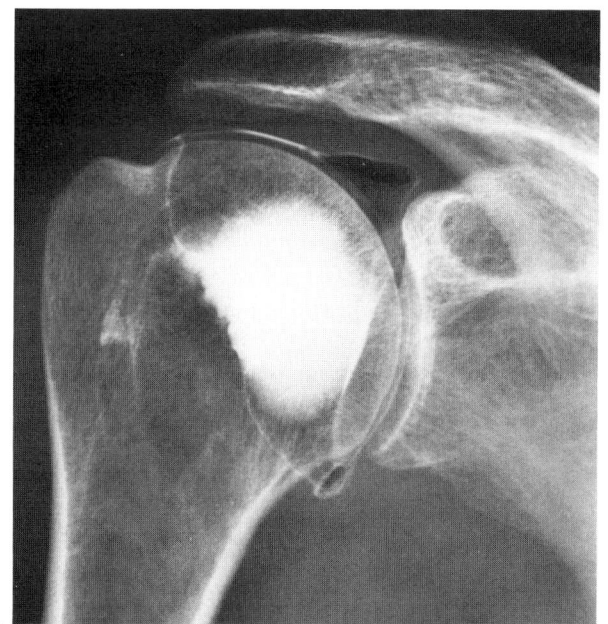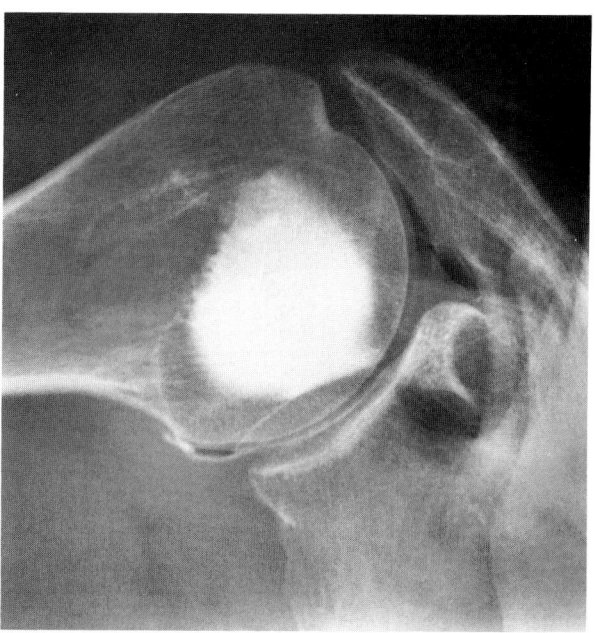

FIG. 10–58. AP (**A**) and abduction (**B**) views of a double contrast arthrogram in a patient with a frozen shoulder. Note that most of the motion with abduction is scapular.

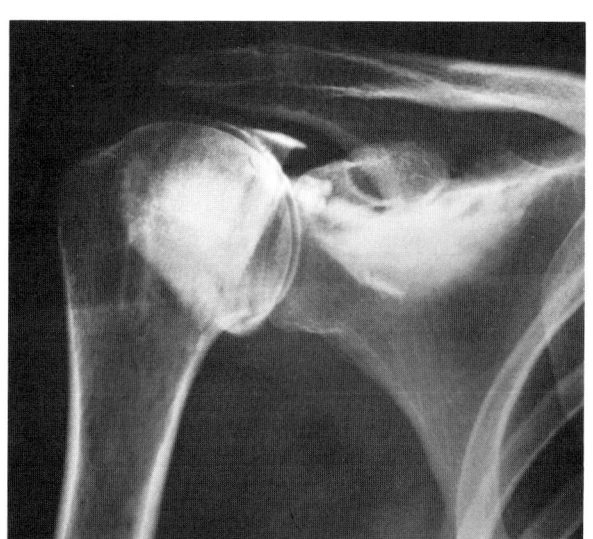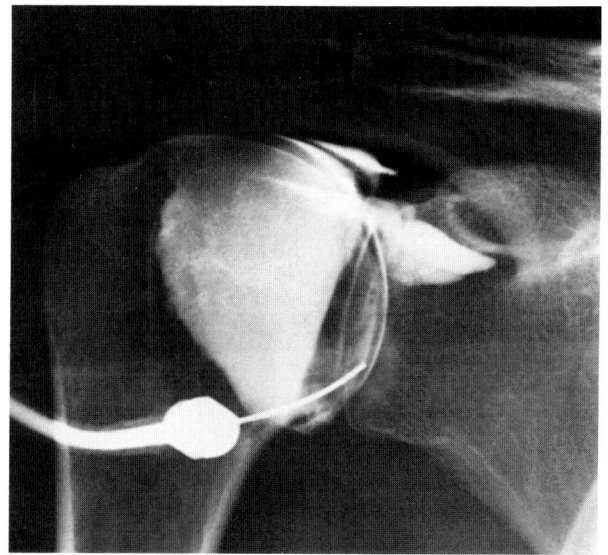

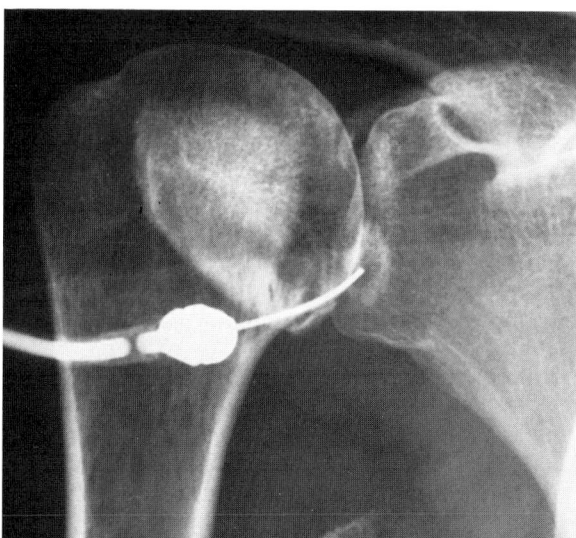

FIG. 10–59. A: Adhesive capsulitis with reduced volume and no axillary or subscapularis recesses. The biceps tendon sheath is not filled. **B:** Following dilatation with contrast material and Marcaine and celestone, the volume begins to increase (**B**). The tendon and sheath are identified later (**C**) as is extravasation. The patient noted dramatic improvement following the study.

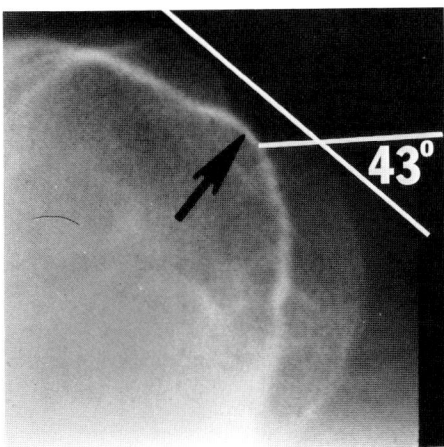

FIG. 10–60. Bicipital groove (*arrow*) with angle of (43°) measured by a line across the top of the tuberosities and a line along the medial wall.

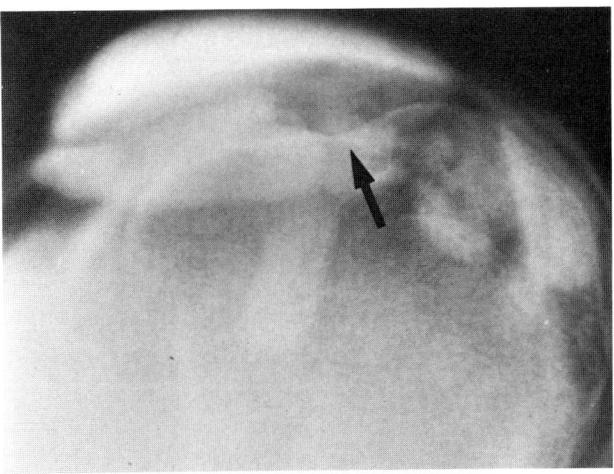

FIG. 10–61. The biceps tendon is totally absent (*arrow*). It was detached from its point of origin.

thors (74,120), including our group, cannot concur with this statement. Killoran reports that 11% of tendon sheaths failed to fill in otherwise normal arthrograms (92). Normal tendon sheaths with nonfilling of the sheath were noted surgically in a significant number of patients during the preoperative arthrograms. Only when the tendon sheath is filled can evaluation of the tendon be accomplished. This is most accurate with double-contrast technique and bicipital groove views combined with weight-bearing internal and external rotation views (77,78,80). The number of tendon sheaths filled does not differ significantly with single- or double-contrast technique, but the detail, especially in the intracapsular portion, is much improved with the double-contrast technique (Fig. 10-47A). Goldman (81) described 9 biceps tendon abnormalities in 158 patients with double-contrast technique. Single-contrast exams in 198 patients failed to detect any abnormalities and missed 2 complete tears (81). In our experience, biceps tendon involvement (nonfilling or synovitis of the sheath on the arthrogram) occurred in 20% of patients with complete rotator cuff tears and in 20% of patients with adhesive capsulitis. However, nonfilling and extravasation of the tendon sheaths are not necessarily significant findings (74,81,120). Positive findings (Table 10-5) include complete or partial tears noted by absence of the tendon in the sheath, irregularity of the tendon, or distortion of the sheath (Fig. 10-61). Subluxation of the tendon is best seen on the bicipital groove view, but it can

also be detected by failure of the tendon to change position properly on internal and external rotation views (Fig. 10-62) (74,81,120). Additional findings in our series included synovitis, loose bodies in the tendon sheath (Fig. 10-63), surgically absent or transplanted tendons, and tendon entrapment by greater tuberosity fractures (Fig. 10-64). In the total series of 552 arthrograms, excluding associated cuff tears, only 16 biceps abnormalities were detected (3%).

Although routine arthrography can be used to study the biceps tendon, there are now more suitable alternatives. Ultrasonography has already been mentioned above (100). Arthro-computed tomography and MRI are excellent techniques. Axial images are easily ob-

TABLE 10-5. *Arthrographic biceps tendon abnormalities*

Tears—complete or partial
Subluxation
Tendinitis and entrapment
Loose bodies

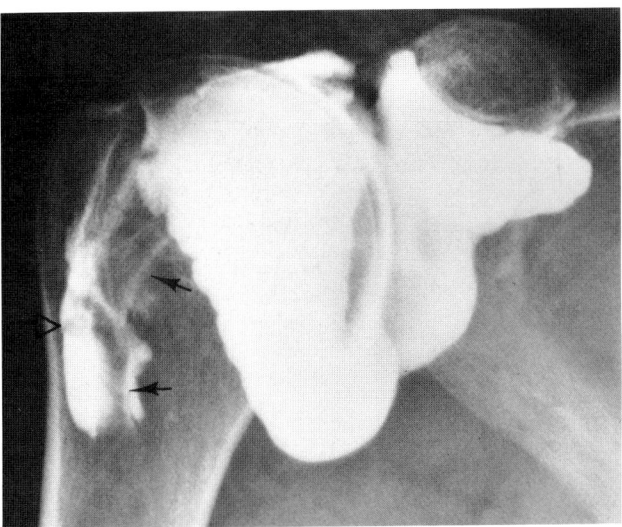

FIG. 10–62. External rotation view. Note medial subluxation and irregularity of the biceps tendon (*black arrows*). There is a partial tear and synovitis with a small loose body lateral to the tendon (*open arrow*).

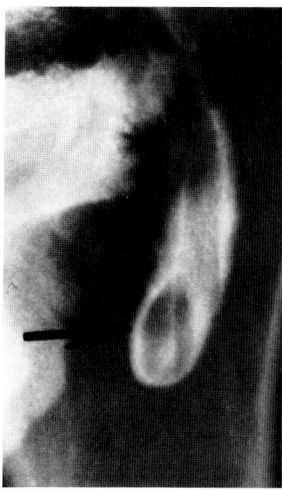

FIG. 10-63. Localized view of biceps tendon with loose body (*arrow*). Note also the irregular synovial pattern in the upper capsule and sheath.

tained and the anatomy of the tendon is more clearly displayed (59).

Articular Cartilage and Other Abnormalities

Arthrography is also valuable in evaluating the articular cartilage, glenoid labrum, and synovium. Cartilaginous lesions can be detected before they are obvious on plain films in rheumatoid arthritis, ankylosing spondylitis, and infection. More commonly, the arthrogram is utilized in patients with shoulder instability. Evaluation

of the glenoid labrum for Bankart lesions and the humeral head for Hill-Sachs deformities may indicate dislocations (76,81,95,106,111). The capsule may be generous as well, indicating an additional factor contributing to the instability.

In evaluating the glenoid labrum and articular cartilage, double-contrast arthrography provides much greater detail. Care must be taken not to utilize more than 4 ml of positive contrast or large portions of the articular cartilage may be obscured. This is true in single-contrast arthrography as well (Fig. 10-65).

We prefer both supine and prone axillary views as well as fluoroscopically positioned internal and external rotation views for the best evaluation of the labrum and articular cartilage. In patients with shoulder instability, better detail is offered by arthrotomography. Despite the introduction of MRI, many still prefer double-contrast computed tomography (Fig. 10-66) (71,72,87,97,124).

CT images are obtained following conventional images. Axial scans at 3–5-mm intervals are obtained with the patient supine and the arm in neutral position (87). Using this technique, the accuracy for evaluating the labrum and capsule approaches 100% (87). Deutsch et al. (71) reported a sensitivity of 96% and an accuracy of 86%. Callaghan et al. (63) reported a specificity of 100% for labral injuries and Hill-Sachs lesions (Fig. 10-67). The ability to evaluate the biceps tendon is obvious.

Double-contrast examination with a scapular lateral view or CT is also critical to evaluate capsule size and to detect any changes in the configuration of the anterior, posterior, and inferior recesses of the capsule (Fig. 10-

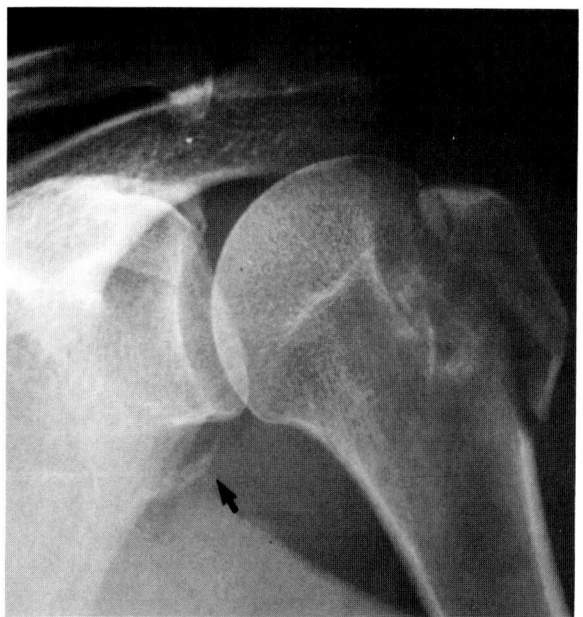

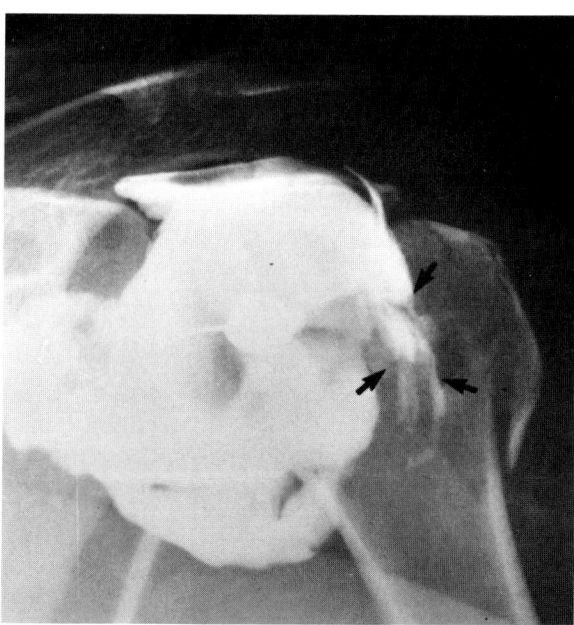

A

B

FIG. 10-64. A: Recent dislocation of the left shoulder with a Bankhart lesion (*arrow*) and displaced greater tuberosity fracture. **B:** Arthrogram demonstrates the capsular tear and entrapment of the biceps tendon (*arrows*).

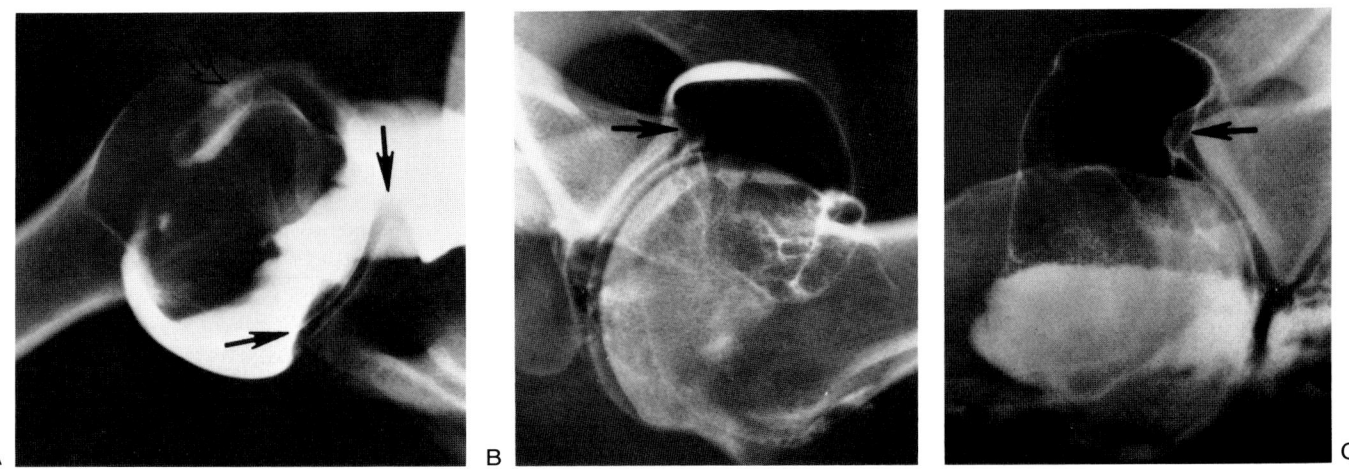

FIG. 10-65. A: Single contrast arthrogram, axillary view. The glenoid labrum are partially obscured (*black arrows*). Biceps tendon is well seen (*open arrow*). **B:** Double contrast arthrogram prone axillary view revealing normal rounded appearance of the posterior labrum (*arrow*). Articular cartilage is well demonstrated. Posterior capsule normal. **C:** Previous posterior dislocation with slightly irregular posterior labrum (*arrow*) and generous capsule posteriorly. Compare capsule to **A.**

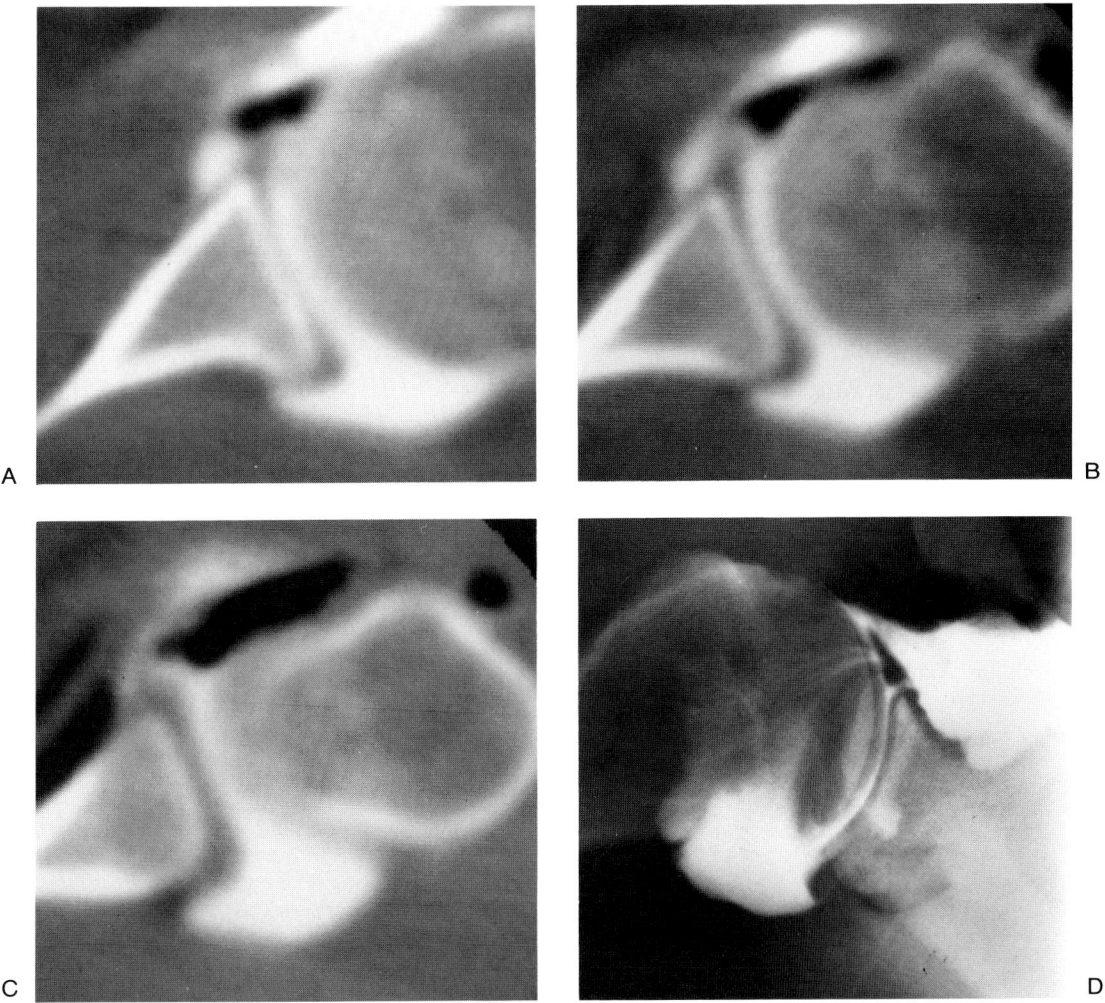

FIG. 10-66. Normal axial images of the glenoid labrum (**A-C**) following double contrast arthrogram and anterior lateral tear (**D**).

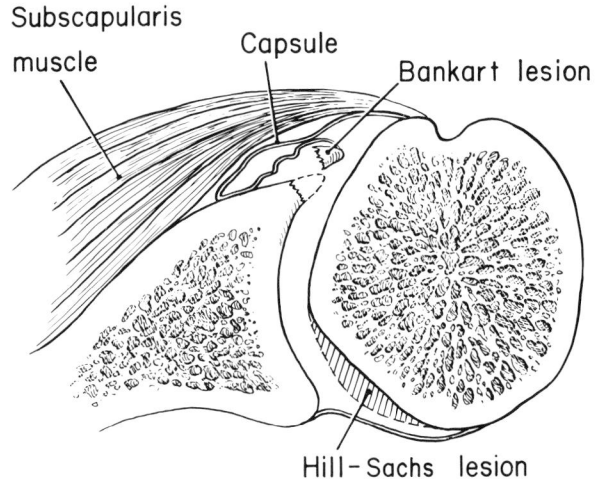

Subscapularis muscle

Capsule

Bankart lesion

Hill-Sachs lesion

FIG. 10–67. The value of CT for detection of Bankhart and Hill-Sachs lesions.

68). With anterior dislocations, the capsule may be stripped from the glenoid, resulting in a generous anterior capsule and loss of the separation between the axillary recess and subscapularis bursa (76). To attach any significance to this, the arm must be in external rotation, as it is common for this confluence to occur without instability when the arm is internally rotated. Partial or complete rotator cuff tears may also be detected in association with chronic instability. Evaluation of patients with previous trauma or surgery may be aided by an upright weight-bearing view, which assists in determining the degree of laxity (Fig. 10-69).

Loose bodies may be sufficiently ossified to be detected on routine radiographs. However, CT arthrography can be helpful, especially when the loose bodies are in such unusual locations as the biceps tendon sheath (63). Care must be taken not to mistake air bubbles for loose bodies. If the arthrogram is specifically requested

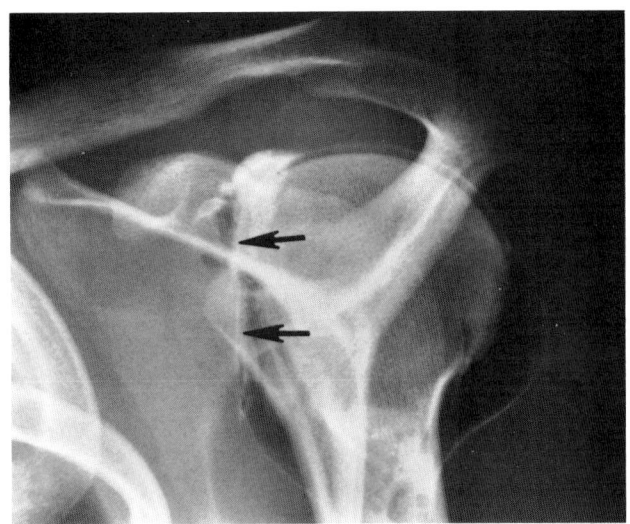

A

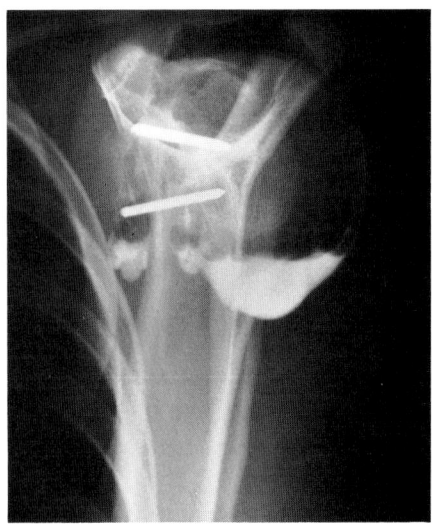

B

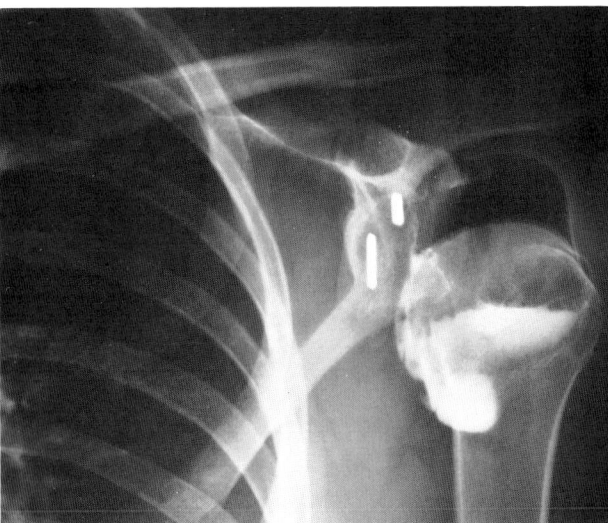

C

FIG. 10–68. Postoperative changes. **A:** Previous anterior repair with straightening and reduction of the anterior recess (*arrows*). The posterior capsule is now generous (*arrow*). **B:** Upright weight-bearing view demonstrates marked inferior instability. **C:** Scapular lateral view in patient with previous anterior repair and continued instability. Absent biceps tendon with inferior subluxation and slight reduction in capsular volume. (Compare with Fig. 10–63).

THE SHOULDER / 623

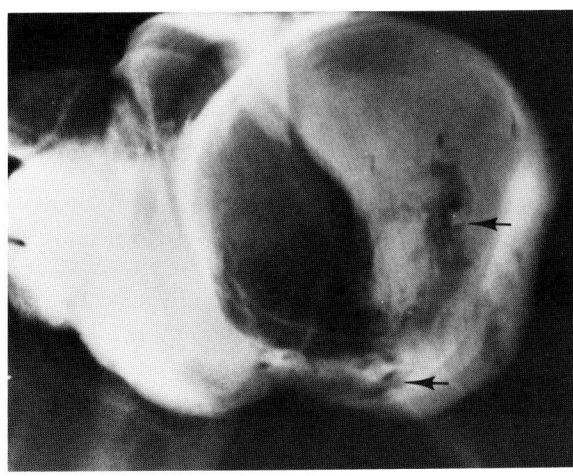

FIG. 10–69. Irregular synovial filling defects (*arrows*) due to synovitis in a patient with degenerative arthritis. No evidence of a rotator cuff tear.

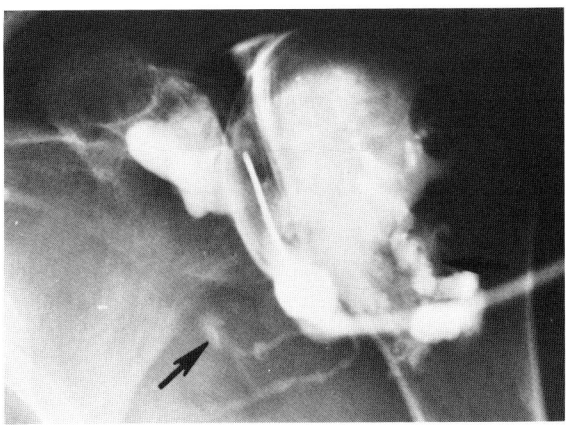

FIG. 10–70. Reduced capsular volume with small axillary and subscapularis recesses. Note dissecting synovial cysts and lymphatic filling in the axillary region (*arrow*).

for the detection of osteocartilaginous fragments, single-contrast examinations may be more useful.

Synovitis, although nonspecific, indicates inflammation and, along with other findings, may aid in determining the patient's clinical problem. We detected synovial changes in 56 patients (10%) of 552 cases (Fig. 10-69). Most patients with synovitis also had advanced degenerative arthritis and chronic rotator cuff tears. Dissecting synovitis was noted in 4 patients. The etiology of this condition is not clear, but synovitis has been associated with chronic cuff tears and rheumatoid arthritis, and it is also noted following local steroid injections (104). We have also demonstrated this condition with adhesive capsulitis (Fig. 10-70). Steroids may result in connective tissue weakness, leading to synovial dissection. Subtle synovial changes are best detected with double-contrast technique, although gross changes are usually obvious with single-contrast technique.

Chondromalacia is best detected arthroscopically, but it can also be seen with double-contrast arthrography. Findings include irregular thinning and subchondral sclerosis (Fig. 10-71).

Pitfalls in Shoulder Arthrography

Inaccuracy in shoulder arthrography should not occur if proper attention is given to clinical data, plain film findings, and choice of technique. Proper needle position is essential. Improper position can result in extravasation, which if not detected fluoroscopically results in an indeterminate examination. Also, if the needle is inadvertently placed in the subacromial bursa (see Fig. 10-43B), a false diagnosis of rotator cuff tear may result. A most important and often overlooked factor is the neces-

sity of quality films, in which proper projections are obtained by an experienced arthrographic technician. If such a person is not available, preliminary films in the prechosen postinjection positions should be obtained to avoid poor-quality films and repeat injections.

One must also take care not to use too much contrast material, which may obscure subtle changes. Injection of 20 ml of positive contrast material to exclude a complete cuff tear will totally obliterate any additional findings. This, then, dictates individualization of cases depending on the size of the capsule, which can be observed during the initial portion of the injection. Marked adhesive capsulitis will be obvious. In a normal capsule, no more than 4 ml of contrast material and 10–15 ml of air is necessary for high-quality, double-contrast examinations.

Proper evaluation of routine films can also aid in proper technique and diagnosis. A good example is the "double tuberosity" sign that was noted in 6 patients—

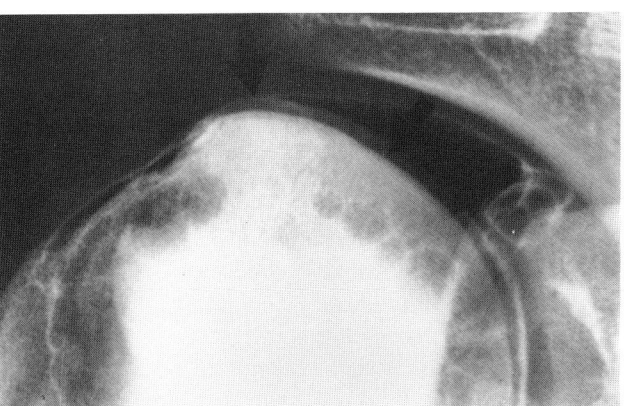

FIG. 10–71. Double contrast arthrogram with sclerosis of the humeral head and thinning and increased density of the articular cartilage (*arrows*).

624 / CHAPTER 10

all with complete rotator cuff tears. Because of the chronic nature of their clinical status, a bursal membrane or scarring partially seals the tear and makes arthrographic evaluation difficult. When this situation arises, further exercise or, in some cases, reinjection will identify the surprisingly large tears. Assuming proper technique has been employed, there are certain findings that may be confused with rotator cuff tears. Freiberger and Kaye report that contrast medium in the biceps tendon sheath may project laterally to the humeral head on the external rotation view and mimic a complete cuff tear (74). Also, occasionally a small streak of contrast may be present above the origin of the biceps tendon near the superior glenoid labrum. This should not be confused with a rotator cuff tear (see Fig. 10-44).

Healed partial or complete tears with fibrous nodules, deep central tears, and incomplete tears on the bursal side of the cuff may go undetected arthrographically (115).

Complications in Shoulder Arthrography

Shoulder arthrography is a simple, relatively benign procedure with few potential complications. No infections occurred in our 552 cases. Freiberger reports an incidence of infection of 1 in 25,000 cases (74).

However, allergic reactions to contrast medium may occur and proper emergency medications (see Introduction to Arthrography in Chapter 1) should be available. Urticaria has been reported (74,75). Four percent of our patients developed urticaria following the procedure. In only one instance (1 of 552) were symptoms sufficient to warrant treatment with antihistamines.

Pain may occur following the arthrogram. Hall (84) and Pastershank (114) report increased pain in 74% of patients 24–48 hours following arthrography. Mixtures of contrast material with small amounts of lidocaine may result in less discomfort, but especially with double-contrast technique this causes significant dilution of the contrast material and thus poor quality films. Increased pain typically occurs 4–6 hours following the procedure in Hall's experience, and the pain may persist for up to 2 days (84). This pain does not correlate with the arthrographic findings. Double-contrast technique results in less post-procedural pain than single-contrast examinations, perhaps owing to smaller volumes of contrast material (84). New low osmolality non-ionic contrast materials may be better tolerated. However, to date, no large studies have documented this theory.

Sterile effusions, perhaps owing to contrast medium irritation of the synovium, have been reported in the knee, and aspiration is indicated for relief of pain. To date we have not experienced this problem with shoulder arthrography.

Bursography

Contrast studies of the subacromial bursa (Fig. 10-72) are rarely performed but have been suggested as a means of evaluating partial tears in the superior surface of the rotator cuff, adhesive capsulitis (119), and impingement syndrome (67,75,96,129). The bursa may also be enlarged and inflamed in rheumatoid arthritis or any chronic inflammatory process (120,125,130). Subacromial bursography, rather than arthrography, has been used in Japan to diagnose rotator cuff tears (75,101).

We have utilized bursography infrequently, and to date the indications are still somewhat unclear. However, this technique may become more efficacious in the future, and certainly radiologists or orthopedists should be familiar with injection or aspiration of this bursa.

The subacromial bursa is a caplike structure between the rotator cuff and acromion with subdeltoid, subacromial, and subcoracoid portions. The normal bursa may be difficult to inject accurately (95,125).

The patient is placed on the fluoroscopic table in the supine position. The anterior shoulder is prepared with povidone-iodine (Betadine) solution as in arthrographic technique. The bursography set is the same as the tray used for arthrography. A 5-ml syringe with a 25-gauge needle is used to mark the subacromial region, and a wheal is made in the skin with 1% lidocaine (Xylocaine). The soft tissues are also anesthetized. Following injection of the local anesthetic, a 1.5-inch 22-gauge needle is advanced vertically and slightly superiorly under the acromion. When the undersurface of the acromion is reached, the needle can be withdrawn 1–2 mm, and the tip should be in the subacromial bursa. Any fluid should be aspirated at this time and sent for the appropriate laboratory studies. Three ml of Hypaque-M-60 and 5 or more ml of room air are used to distend the bursa. This promotes better elevation of the synovium and upper surface of the cuff, allowing these, as well as any extrinsic

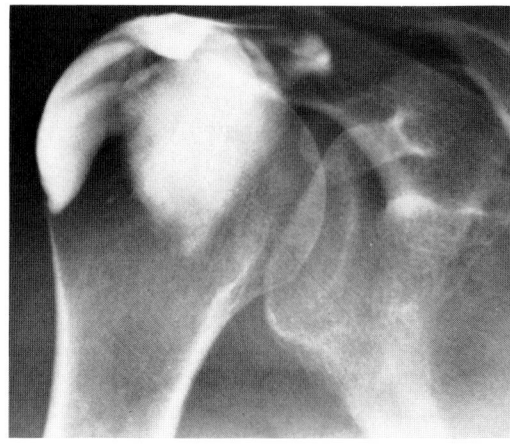

FIG. 10-72. Normal single contrast bursogram.

ligamentous or bony deformity of the bursa, to be evaluated (Fig. 10-73). Radiographs are obtained in internal and external rotation, axillary, and scapular positions. The scapular lateral view allows the most advantageous study of the acromial and coracoid relationships to the bursa.

Following the radiographic study, diagnostic or therapeutic injection with bupivacaine or lidocaine and beta-methasone (Celestone) may be performed, thus adding to the versatility of the study.

Acromioclavicular Arthrography

Radiographic approach to the acromioclavicular joint, although not commonly employed compared with

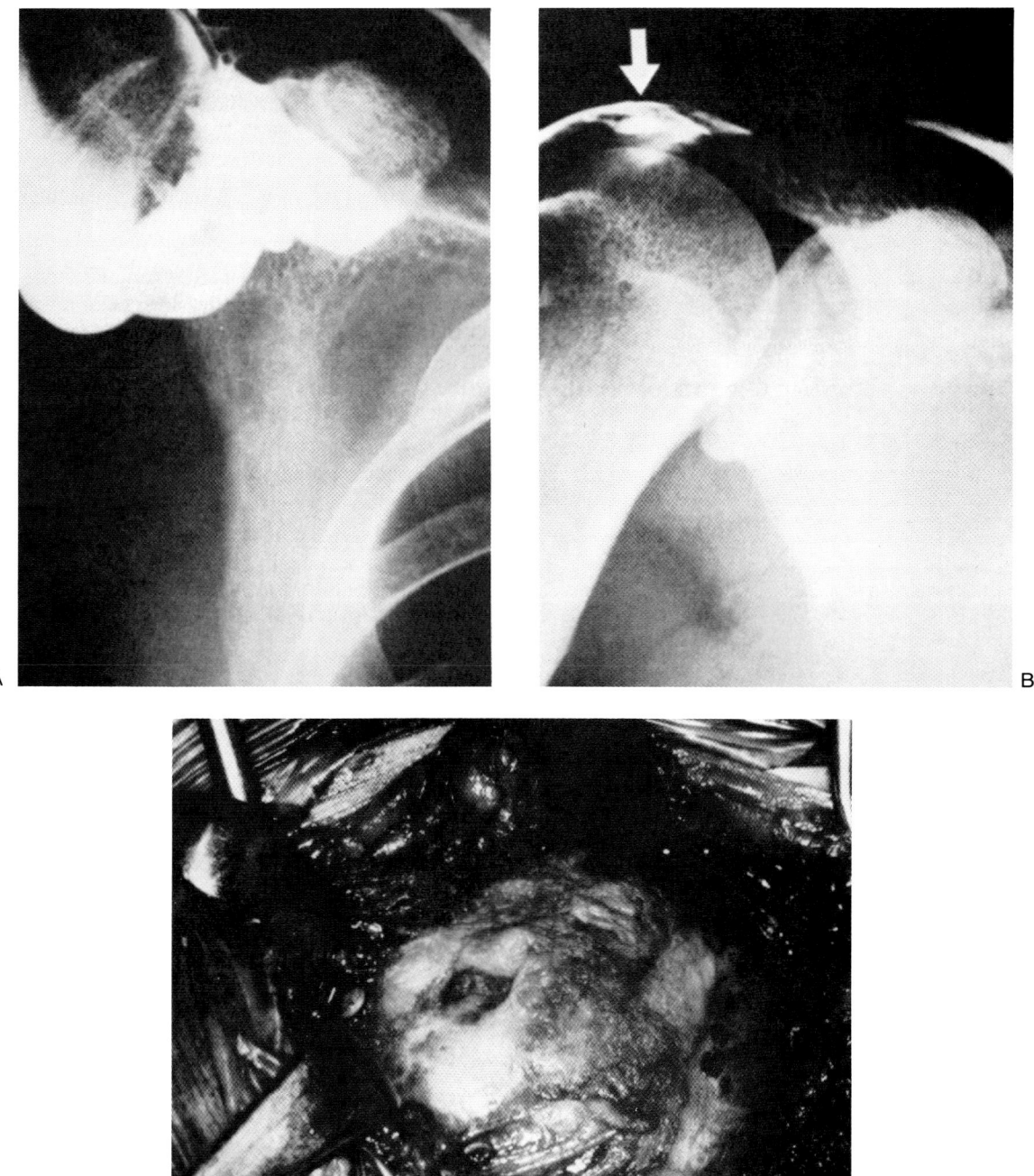

FIG. 10–73. A: Normal shoulder arthrogram. **B:** Bursogram shows a superior partial thickness cuff tear (*arrow*). **C:** Tear observed at surgery. (From Fukuda H, Mikasa M, Yamanaka K. Incomplete thickness rotator cuff tears diagnosed by subacromial bursography. *Clin Orthop* 1987;223:51–58.)

glenohumeral arthrography, may be of diagnostic and therapeutic value.

Arthrography has been reported to be useful in determining the extent of ligamentous injury following acromioclavicular separations (135). Resnick (119) described potential utilization of this technique in rheumatoid arthritis to diagnose cystic formation and synovitis, but it is likely that acromioclavicular arthrography will be restricted to therapeutic injections or diagnostic aspirations and will remain an infrequently performed procedure.

The anatomy of the acromioclavicular joint results in an *L*-shaped cavity, with the leg of the *L* projecting under the distal clavicle (131). The capsule is lined with synovium and is reinforced by the superior and inferior acromioclavicular ligaments. The normal joint capacity is 1–2 ml (119,131).

Patients to be studied are prepared in the usual manner with sterile technique. The joint can be entered superiorly or anteriorly (Fig. 10-74). Fluoroscopic guidance assures proper positioning. One to 2 ml of Hypaque-M-60 can be injected. This normally should not extend beyond the capsule. Extension of contrast material medially toward the coracoid indicates coracoclavicular ligament injury (114).

Other Procedures

Diagnostic injections of local anesthetic may be useful. Also, areas of tendon calcification may be helped through irrigation of the calcium with sterile saline via injection. This results in a breakup of the calcium, and some fragments may actually be aspirated. The procedure is followed by injection of the involved area with a 1:1 mixture of bupivacaine (0.5%) and betamethasone. This procedure may result in significant symptomatic relief of calcific tendonitis.

Magnetic Resonance Imaging (MRI)

Techniques for MR examination of the shoulder region will vary depending upon the clinical symptoms. New software and coil techniques have greatly enhanced the ability of MRI examinations to properly evaluate patients with shoulder symptoms. A particularly important development is the ability to perform off-axis small field-of-view images in the shoulder region. This allows the patient to be examined in a more comfortable position with the arm at the side (Fig. 10-75). Larger patients may need to be rotated slightly with the uninvolved arm above the head in order to properly position the patient in the gantry. Off-axis small field-of-view with the surface coil is still the most optimal technique in these patients. In some cases, the body coil with a smaller field of view can be utilized but image quality is usually suboptimal (59,89,136,137).

In most situations, the patient is placed supine in the magnet with a single or dual circular five-inch surface coil placed over the shoulder to be examined (Fig. 10-75). When using dual coils, one coil is above and the other below the shoulder with a connector between the two coils. An advantage of this configuration is the additive signal created by the two coils. New shoulder coils are being configured to improve image quality in the shoulder (59,94,136,137).

Generally, the patient is being examined for suspected tear of the rotator cuff, the glenoid labrum, or other soft tissue abnormalities involving the periarticular soft tissues of the shoulder (59,89). Our routine examination consists of three image planes using T1- and T2-weighted spin-echo sequences (Fig. 10-76). A coronal scout film is obtained initially using 128 × 256 matrix, a 30–48 cm field of view, and three 1-cm-thick sections. This sequence takes approximately 26 seconds. The scout image is used to select the image locations for the axial T2-weighted (SE 2000/60,20) sequence (Fig. 10-76A). A 16–20 cm field of view is usually optimal, depending upon patient size, and 3-mm-thick slices with 1.5-mm interslice gaps are used to study the area from

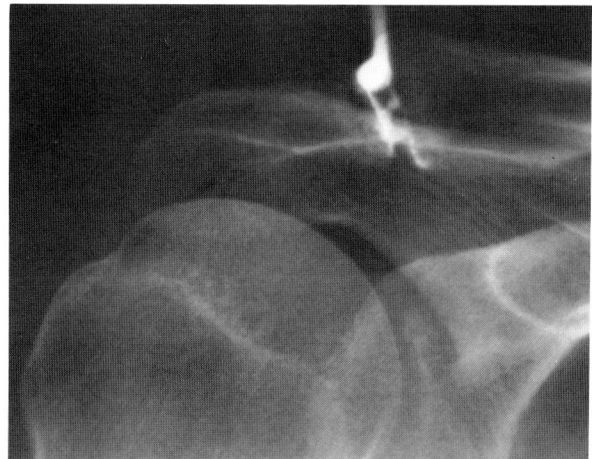

FIG. 10–74. Acromioclavicular joint injection. Contrast medium confirms needle position.

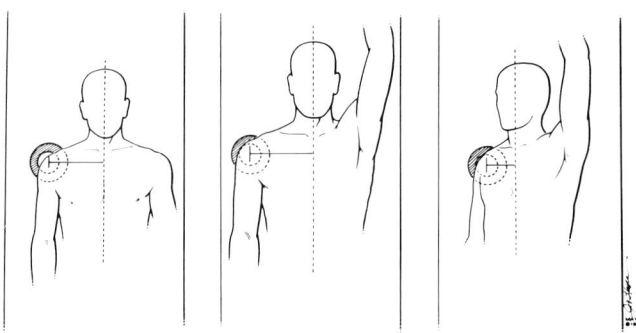

FIG. 10–75. Patient positions for shoulder MRI (from 59, with permission).

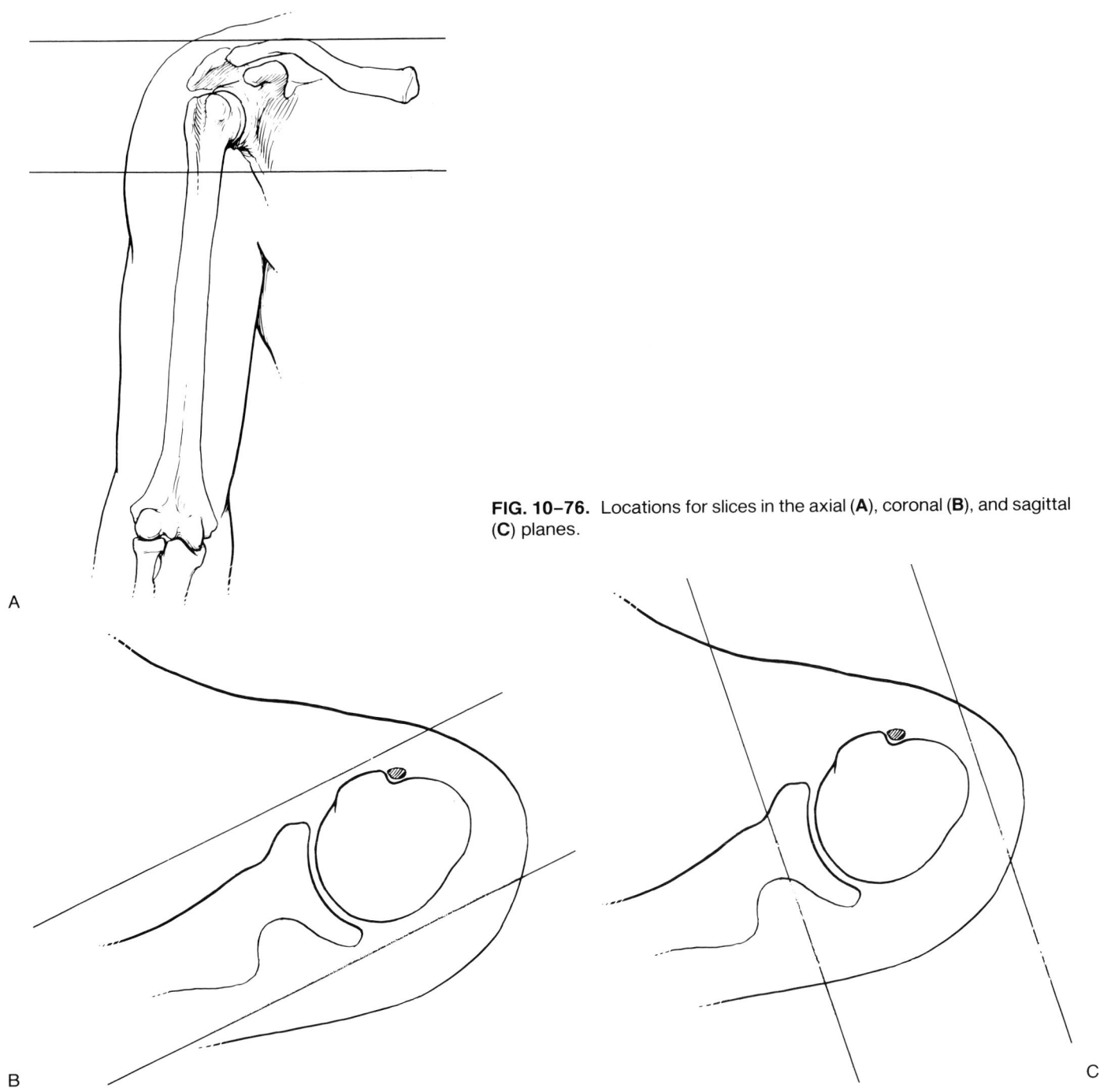

FIG. 10–76. Locations for slices in the axial (**A**), coronal (**B**), and sagittal (**C**) planes.

the axillary region through the superior aspect of the acromioclavicular joint. Following this portion of the examination, coronal sections are obtained in the same plane as the scapula or perpendicular to the glenohumeral articulation (Fig. 10-76B). These images are obtained using the same field of view with either 256 × 256 or 192 × 256 matrix and 3-mm slices with a 1.5-mm skip between slices. The same pulse sequence is used in the coronal plane. This provides optimal anatomic detail and also demonstrates synovial fluid as high signal inten-

sity allowing subtle changes in the rotator cuff and glenoid labrum to be more easily appreciated. These two sequences are usually adequate to evaluate rotator cuff tears and glenolabrum pathology. However, we generally also perform sagittal images (Fig. 10-76C) parallel to the glenohumeral joint. This is useful for evaluating the under surface of the AC joint and supraspinatus muscle for impingement (Fig. 10-77). This sequence is performed using the same field of view with a spin-echo sequence (500/20) and 5-mm-thick contiguous slices. In

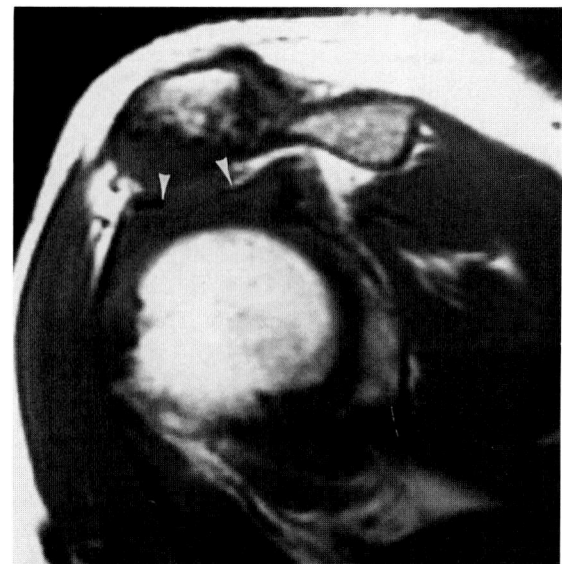

FIG. 10–77. Sagittal SE 500/20 image demonstrating marked hypertrophy of the acromioclavicular joint with compression (*arrows*) of the supraspinatus.

patients with significant discomfort or claustrophobia, gradient-echo sequences (MPGR) can be used to reduce image time.

In some situations, additional sequences or image planes may be indicated, but the above technique is generally appropriate for most shoulder or glenohumeral joint pathology. In certain cases, subtle marrow abnormalities may be more easily detected using short T1 inversion recovery sequences (STIR) or when the glenolabrum is not optimally noted with the routine examination, radial GRIL images may be used to further define this anatomy (59).

Applications

Routine radiography is an important initial examination for screening patients with shoulder disorders. Other techniques including radionuclide studies, CT, and arthrography also have an important role in evaluating these patients (59,65,74,126–128).

The majority of patients who are referred for MRI of the shoulder present with pain or restricted range of motion in the shoulder. The most common clinical indications for MRI are patients referred with suspected rotator cuff tears or impingement, defects in the glenoid-labrum, osteonecrosis, suspected soft tissue or bony neoplasms, and infectious or inflammatory disorders (59,89).

Trauma

The most common application for MRI is evaluation of patients with suspected rotator cuff tear or impinge-

ment syndrome (59,94,116). The majority (95%) of rotator cuff lesions are the result of chronic impingement of the supraspinatus tendon against the acromial arch (65,136,137). Neer (105) divided rotator cuff disease into three stages. The initial stage (Stage I) consists of edema or hemorrhage in the rotator cuff, specifically the supraspinatus tendon. During stage II there is progression of the inflammatory stage to a more fibrotic process. The final stage, Stage III, results in a tear of the rotator cuff. The most susceptible area in the cuff is approximately 1 cm from the insertion of the supraspinatus tendon into the greater tuberosity. This critical zone is where the majority of tendon ruptures occur. Chronic impingement of this avascular area leads to tendinitis or inflammation during the first stage of the degeneration period (59,105,136,137). This abnormality is identifiable on MR images, which is important since inflammatory changes may be reversible. As the degenerative process continues to Stage II and Stage III, progressive change in the supraspinatus tendon and AC joint region occur. Therefore, in evaluating MRI of the shoulder, it is important to compare the routine radiographs to get some predictive value in the secondary osseous changes, especially in the AC joint as well as the position of the humeral head in relation to the AC joint. On the normal AP radiograph in external rotation, the distance between the under surface of the acromion and humeral head should measure 1 cm. When this space is reduced to 7 mm or less, the presence of a rotator cuff tear is almost certain (59).

MRI is particularly suited for evaluation of the shoulder for it is capable of detecting lesions in the rotator cuff as well as other abnormalities in the glenohumeral joint, acromioclavicular joint, and the associated periarticular soft tissues (59,94,116).

The technique described in this chapter consisting of axial, coronal, and sagittal T2- and T1-weighted sequences is well suited for evaluating patients with suspected rotator cuff tears. Patients with Stage I disease (Fig. 10-78) or tendinitis have an intact rotator cuff. However, there is increased signal intensity within the supraspinatus tendon. This is generally most obvious on T2-weighted sequences but can be seen as an area of intermediate signal intensity (gray) on T1-weighted sequences. This increased signal intensity is most likely due to edema, inflammation, and hemorrhage in the tendon. During this stage of rotator cuff disease, the subacromial bursa is generally not fluid distended and the normal fat plane between the rotator cuff and deltoid is clearly demonstrated. In contrast to MRI, arthrograms would be normal during this stage of rotator cuff disease. Histologic changes during this phase of rotator cuff disease show inflammation and mucoid degenerative changes within the tendon (116,136,137).

Additional osseous and articular changes in the AC joint may also be evident in patients at this time. These

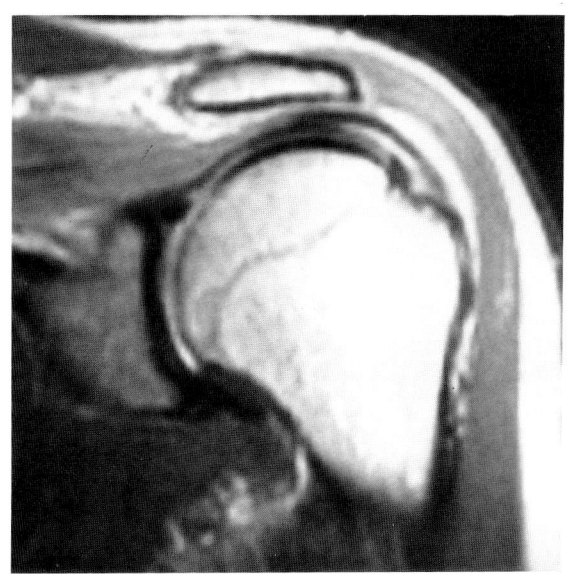

FIG. 10–78. Coronal SE 2000/60 image demonstrates increased signal in the cuff with normal subdeltoid fat.

are easily demonstrated on the coronal and sagittal images that usually demonstrate expansion, either fibrocartilaginous or osseous, of the subacromial joint with deformity of the adjacent supraspinatus muscle (Fig. 10-77) (59,136,137).

The ability to demonstrate early changes in the rotator cuff is important in treatment planning, specifically for developing surgical criteria for management of patients with impingement syndrome. Patients who fail to respond to conservative therapy in this setting may require acromioplasty and excision of the coracoacromial ligament to prevent Stages II and III disease (65,105).

In patients with complete rotatory cuff tears, it is important to identify the ends of the tendons and calculate as closely as possible the size of the tear. Coronal and sagittal images are usually sufficient in this regard and, again, T2-weighted sequences provide the best contrast distinction between the dark tendon and the high intensity signal of the fluid between the ends of the torn tendon (Fig. 10-79). In addition to demonstrating the tear,

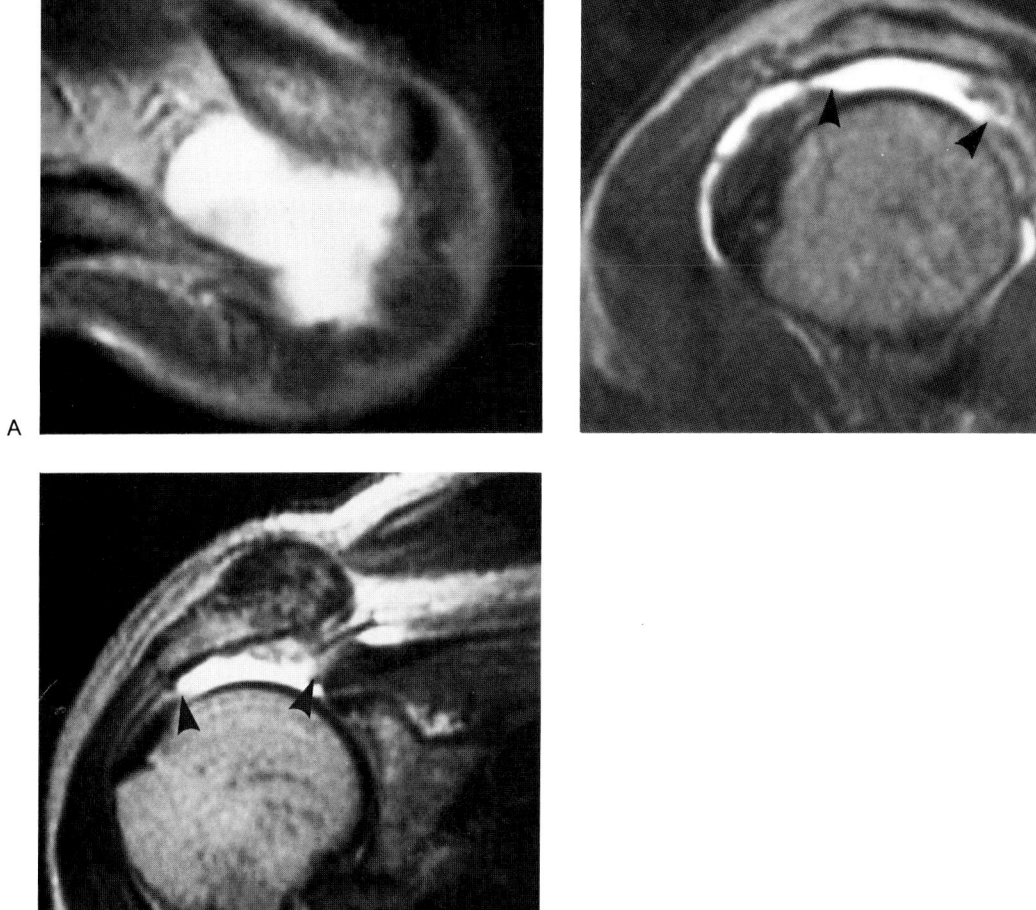

FIG. 10–79. Axial (**A**), sagittal (**B**), and coronal (**C**) SE 2000/60 images demonstrating a large, full thickness cuff tear (*arrows*). The tear is most easily measured (*arrows*) on the coronal and sagittal images.

the tendon thickness is also important. In chronic disease, the tendon is often significantly thinned. Additional findings include fluid in the subacromial and subdeltoid bursae and disruption of the normal subdeltoid fat stripe. It is not unusual in advanced disease to see communication from the glenohumeral joint through a tear into the subacromial bursa with continued extension into the acromioclavicular joint. In addition, cystic or ganglion-like lesions may appear on the dorsal aspect of the AC joint in patients with advanced chronic rotator cuff tears. These patients may also demonstrate atrophy and retraction of the supraspinatus muscle along with the secondary osseous changes previously described (59,65,105,116,136,137).

MR experience is more limited with incomplete rotator cuff tears (116,137). Incomplete tears may occur superiorly or inferiorly and are demonstrated as areas of increased signal intensity involving only a partial thickness of the tendon, usually in a linear fashion perpendicular to the course of the tendon (Fig. 10-80). These findings may be difficult to differentiate from tendinitis. In this setting, double-contrast arthrography with weight-bearing views may still be the most effective in identifying subtle tears of the inferior surface of the tendon. However, superior defects would require bursography, which is a more difficult technique to perform (75). Therefore, it is apparent that, at some point, MRI will also be the technique of choice in this regard.

Based on the work of Kneeland (94), Zlatkin (136,137), and others (116), diagnostic criteria for MRI have been developed. Criteria are based on changes involving the rotator cuff, as well as secondary signs involving the subacromial and subdeltoid fat planes and bursae. The grading system is as follows: A normal tendon with normal signal intensity and morphology is considered Grade 0. Grade 1 tendons have increased signal but normal width and morphology. A Grade 2 tendon shows increased signal intensity with change in morphology such as tendon thinning or irregularity (Fig. 10-78). Grade 3 tendons have discontinuity, with increased signal in the region of tendinous disruption best appreciated on T2-weighted images (Fig. 10-79) (136,137).

Zlatkin (136,137) reported the accuracy of shoulder MRI using these criteria. Sensitivity, specificity, and accuracies of 91%, 88%, and 89% respectively for all tears, partial and complete, was demonstrated. MRI was also noted to be more sensitive than arthrography in the diagnosis of small anterior supraspinatus tendon tears.

It is important to compare the results of MRI with other accepted imaging techniques, specifically arthrography, bursography, and ultrasonography. Both single- and double-contrast arthrography have been accurate in detection of rotator cuff tears. However, unless combined with bursography, partial superior tears and impingement are difficult to diagnose. Bursography is invasive and difficult to perform unless the procedure is performed by an experienced examiner (59,75,136,137).

Burk et al. (61) compare the results of arthrography, MRI, and ultrasound in a group of 38 patients referred for suspected rotator cuff tears. Both MRI and double-contrast arthrography demonstrated sensitivities of 92% and specificities of 100% for normal cuffs. Diagnosis of cuff tears was equal with both techniques. Ultrasound was 63% sensitive for diagnosis of cuff tears and demonstrated a specificity of only 50% for intact rotator cuffs. Others report ultrasound to have an accuracy of 87–94% for diagnosis of rotator cuff tears (100). Importantly, the negative predictive value of ultrasonography was 95%. However, in the operated group, the specificity of ultrasound was only 73% compared to 100% for arthrography.

Arthrography is an accurate (98%) but invasive technique for diagnosis of rotator cuff tears but is of little value in evaluating impingement (59,61,65). Ultrasound is accurate in some physicians' hands but has not achieved the wide acceptance of MRI or arthrography due to the experience required by examiners and the difficulty in achieving acceptance in the orthopedic community. Physicians not involved in performing and interpreting ultrasound find the image difficult to evaluate. MRI is non-invasive and provides a method of screening for many osseous and soft tissue abnormalities. Although refinements are still in progress, it appears to be the non-invasive technique of choice for evaluating impingement and rotator cuff pathology (Table 10-6).

Capsular Abnormalities

The capsular structures of the shoulder consist of the synovial membrane, the capsule, the associated glenohu-

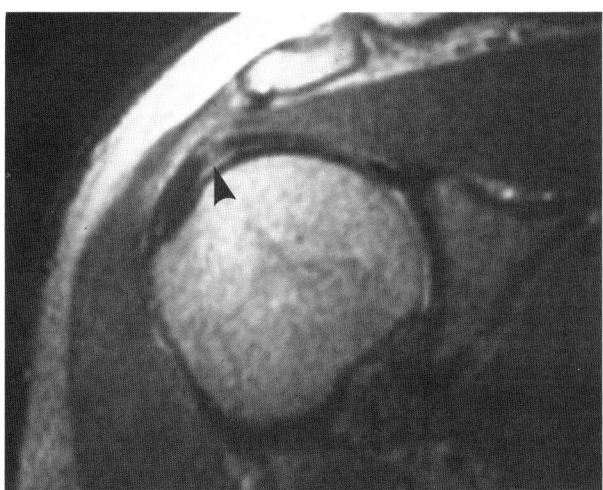

FIG. 10–80. Coronal SE 2000/60 image demonstrating a small cuff tear (*arrow*) that appears to be nearly complete thickness.

TABLE 10-6. *Special imaging techniques: Value in shoulder disorders*

Lesions	Arthrography conventional	CT	MRI	Ultrasound
Rotator cuff	++	++	+++	++
Impingement	+	+	+++	++
Hill-Sachs	+	+++	+++	0
Bankhart	+	+++	+++	0
Articular cartilage	+	++	+++	0
Labrum	+	+++	++	0
Loose bodies	+	+++	+	0
Capsule				
1. Size	++	+++	+	+
2. Tears	++	+++	++	0
3. Adhesive capsulitis	+++	++	0-+	0-+
4. Synovitis	++	++	+++	0-+
Biceps tendon	+	+++	+++	++
Periarticular soft tissues	0-+	+	+++	+

+, adequate; ++, excellent; +++, superior; 0, questionable value.

meral ligaments, glenoid labrum, and associated bursa and recesses (59,65). Subscapularis muscle and tendon are also closely applied to the anterior capsule. Imaging of the shoulder capsule has conventionally been accomplished using either conventional tomography or CT or arthrotomography (63,126,127). Contrast arthrography provides valuable information regarding the size and integrity of the capsule and also allows intra-articular injections of anesthetic and/or a combination of anesthetic and steroidal compounds to treat and diagnose certain shoulder disorders.

Capsular volume is difficult to evaluate with MRI since the degree of distention of the capsule cannot be evaluated unless contrast material of some type is injected. Recently, gadolinium diethylenetriamine penta-acetic acid (DTPA) has been advocated as an MR arthrography contrast agent. However, to date there has not been significant experience to clearly understand its implications in MRI of the shoulder. Certainly fluoroscopically monitored injections of contrast material are much more efficacious than MR arthrography at this point. Therefore, patients who are being evaluated for subtle changes in the synovial lining or for changes in capsular volume such as adhesive capsulitis are still studied to better advantage with conventional arthrography or arthrography combined with CT or tomography (Table 10-6).

Disruption of the shoulder capsule can be detectable by arthrography or MRI. Loss of integrity of the capsule or its adjacent or associated ligaments can be identified on MRI as poorly defined areas of increased signal intensity adjacent to the capsule on T2-weighted sequences. Capsular lesions are most easily evaluated in the axial and coronal planes.

Recurrent shoulder dislocations are a common problem in orthopedic practice (65,69). Originally, it was felt that the Bankhart lesion (glenoid labral tear or osteo-chondral fracture of the inferior labrum) was the main lesion resulting in recurrent anterior dislocation. More recently, the entire anterior capsule mechanism has been implicated (65,69). Type II and Type III capsular insertions are more often associated with instability (Fig. 10-81).

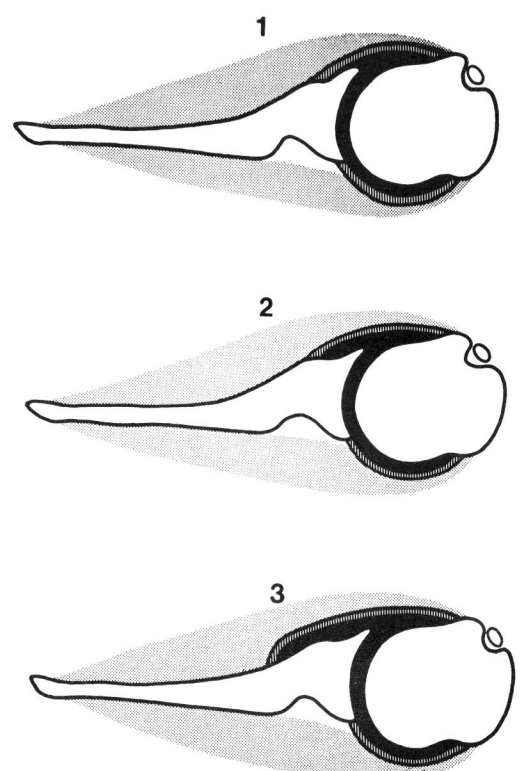

FIG. 10-81. Variations in the anterior capsular attachments. Type 1, in or near anterior glenoid labrum, 2 along the scapular neck, and 3 medial to the neck. (From Zlatskin MB, Dalinka MK, Kressel HY. Magnetic resonance imaging of the shoulder. *Magn Reson Q* 1989;5:3–22.)

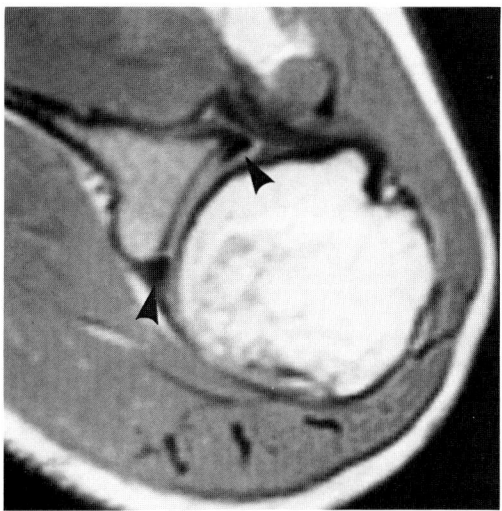

FIG. 10–82. Axial SE 2000/20 image demonstrating the normal glenoid labrum (*arrows*).

ally sharper anteriorly and slightly more rounded posteriorly (Fig. 10-82) (59,94,136,137). Disruptions of the labrum are seen as linear areas of high signal intensity on MR images. Complete avulsion or total absence of the labrum is easily identified (Fig. 10-83). Degenerative changes within the meniscus that do not communicate with the articular surface (Fig. 10-84), similar to those changes described in the knee, may also be evident. The clinical significance of these is probably similar to changes in the knee meniscus and, therefore, a glenoid labrum tear should not be suggested unless there is a clear linear defect that articulates with the articular surface of the labrum or a labral detachment. Tears are most commonly identified anteriorly and, therefore, if GRIL techniques are not available, the axial plane is usually best suited to identify these lesions (59,136,137).

Until recently, arthrography with CT has been the technique of choice for evaluating the glenoid labrum (71,126). T2-weighted or gradient-echo sequences can be used to evaluate the glenoid labrum as well. Conventional axial and coronal images (Fig. 10-82) will demonstrate the entire labrum, however, it might be optimal to use radial GRIL sequences, similar to those described in the knee, to optimally look at the labrum tangentially. Currently, most software does not provide the capability to select multiple off-axis radial GRIL images (59).

Normally the glenoid labrum has a triangular shape and appears black, or low intensity, on spin-echo and gradient-echo sequences (Fig. 10-82). There are some variations in the appearance of the labrum as it is gener-

Inflammatory Disorders

The shoulder, specifically the glenohumeral joint, is frequently involved in osteoarthritis and other types of inflammatory arthropathies. Soft tissue changes as well as early changes in the articular and osseous structures of the shoulder are more easily defined using MRI than by using conventional radiography. Chronic synovial changes such as proliferative synovitis can also be demonstrated without the use of contrast material. These changes are, however, not specific and do not preclude the need for aspiration to obtain fluid for more specific analysis, especially infection (59,89).

Osteomyelitis and infectious arthritis involving the shoulder can also be detected early (59). The extent of bone and soft tissue involvement can be more clearly defined using MRI than conventional radiographs or ra-

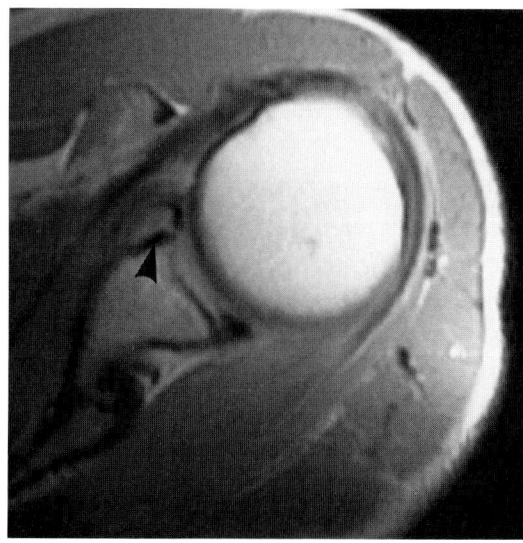

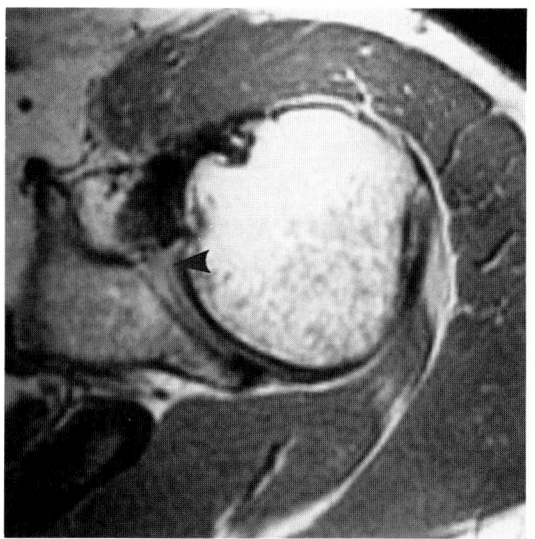

FIG. 10–83. A: Axial SE 500/20 image demonstrating an osteochondral fracture of the anterior labrum (*arrow*). **B:** Axial SE 2000/20 image demonstrating an anterior tear (*arrow*).

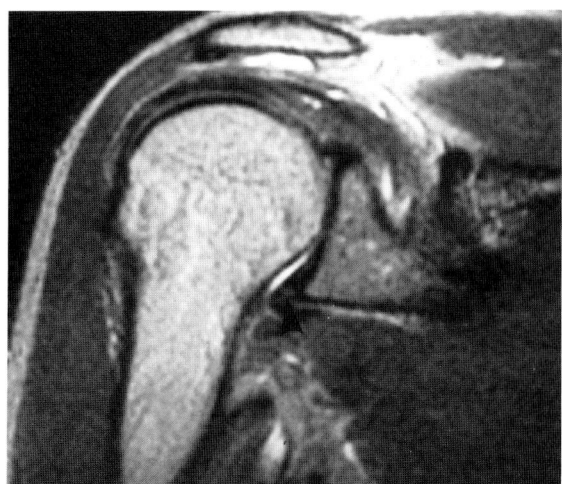

FIG. 10-84. Coronal SE 2000/60 image demonstrating internal increase in signal intensity in the inferior labrum (*arrow*). This is not a labral tear.

dionuclide scans. Certain other inflammatory diseases such as pigmented villonodular synovitis and giant cell tumors of the tendon sheath can be somewhat more specifically identified due to hemosiderin deposition in the proliferative synovium. The paramagnetic effects of hemosiderin result in shortening of the T2 relaxation time, which causes areas of low signal intensity in the normally high intensity synovial fluid (59).

Osseous Disorders

Detection of early avascular necrosis or osteonecrosis of the humeral head can be difficult with routine radiographs and radionuclide studies. Later, once these changes have become obvious, the radiographic appearance is typical, and MRI is not usually indicated.

The appearance of osteonecrosis in the humeral head does not differ significantly from osteonecrosis in the hip (59).

Screening for avascular necrosis in the shoulder can be accomplished with coronal SE 500/20 images using a large field of view (include both shoulders), the body coil, 256 × 256 matrix and 1 NEX (Fig. 10-85). This examination can be performed in less than 5 minutes. Early or subtle changes may require surface coils to more clearly delineate the changes in one or both shoulders. In this setting, coronal and sagittal images are useful to evaluate the articular cartilage and the area of involvement.

Subtle fractures may also be detected with MRI (Fig. 10-86) making this technique an ideal screening tool for shoulder disorders (Table 10-6). Although MRI is an excellent technique for evaluating many shoulder disorders, there are still good indications for arthrography and ultrasonography. The best technique for a given clinical problem depends on the equipment available, experience of examiners, and the type of disorder suspected (Table 10-6). For example, conventional arthrography would still appear to be the best technique for evaluation and potential treatment of frozen shoulder.

Shoulder Arthroscopy

Arthroscopy has become a valuable tool for the investigation and treatment of knee pathology. Burman, a pioneer in arthroscopy, recognized that shoulder arthroscopy was possible and not too difficult (62). More recently, suggestions have been offered concerning the usefulness of arthroscopy in evaluating shoulder lesions. These include investigation of rotator cuff tears, biceps tendon lesions, periarthritis, shoulder instability, glenoid labral tears, degenerative joint disease, rheumatoid arthritis, congenital abnormalities, and postoperative pain (58,90). Certainly arthroscopy has a role in the evalua-

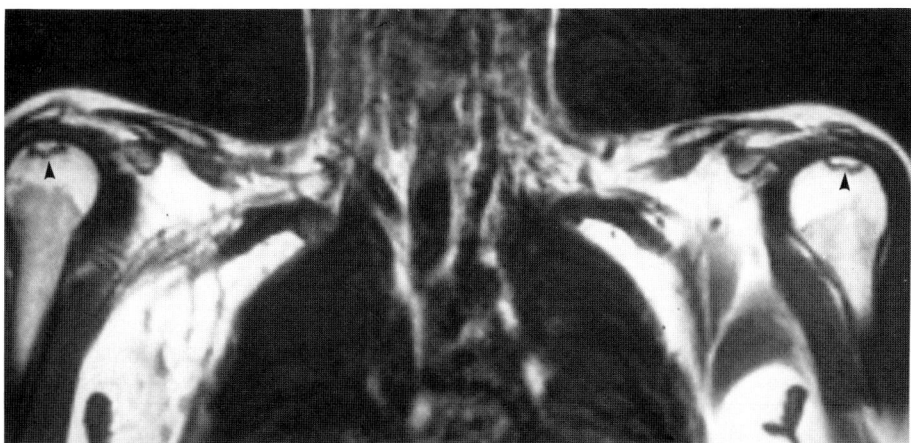

FIG. 10-85. Coronal SE 500/20 image of the shoulders demonstrating bilateral avascular necrosis (*arrow*). Radiographs were normal.

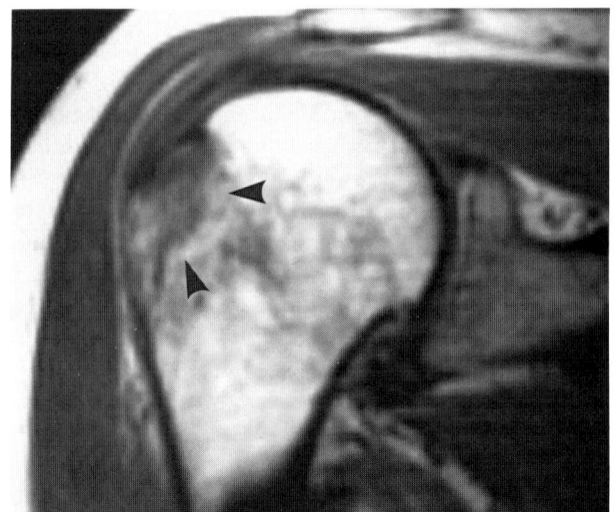

FIG. 10-86. Coronal SE 500/20 image demonstrating a greater tuberosity fracture (*arrows*). Radiographs were normal.

tion or treatment of shoulder diseases (Fig. 10-87), but it is probably not as extensive as has been suggested.

The authors reviewed their recent experience with shoulder arthroscopy, and a number of points emerged (64). For rotator cuff tears, arthrography is a highly useful diagnostic tool, and arthroscopy offers little or nothing in addition to this test. Bicipital tendon problems occur within the groove on the upper humerus and only rarely occur within the shoulder joint. Periarthritis is diagnosed by physical examination, and, if necessary, by arthrography. It is best treated by physiotherapy with or without manipulation. In difficult cases with shoulder instability, arthroscopy was occasionally of value, but examination under anesthesia was more often helpful.

On the other hand, when x-rays are not compatible with the degree of joint-related symptomatology, arthroscopy can stage arthritic diseases. It can also diagnose the disease with certainty when an atypical clinical picture is present (Fig. 10-88). Arthroscopy is valuable in the diag-

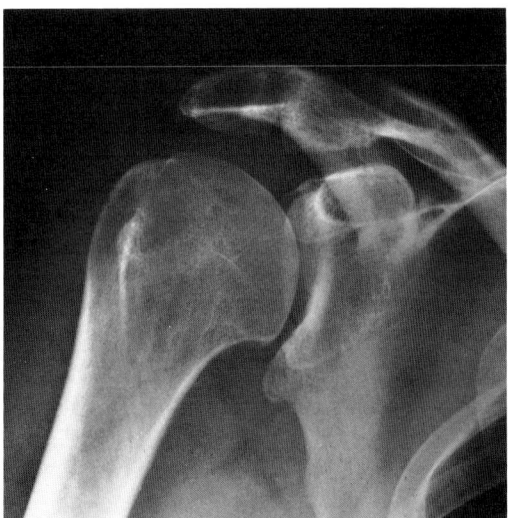

A

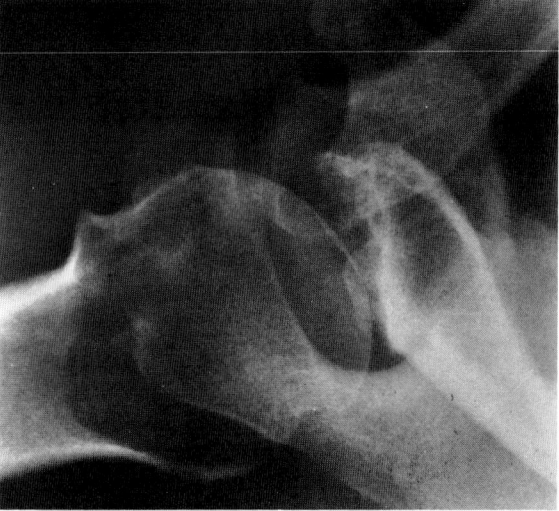

B

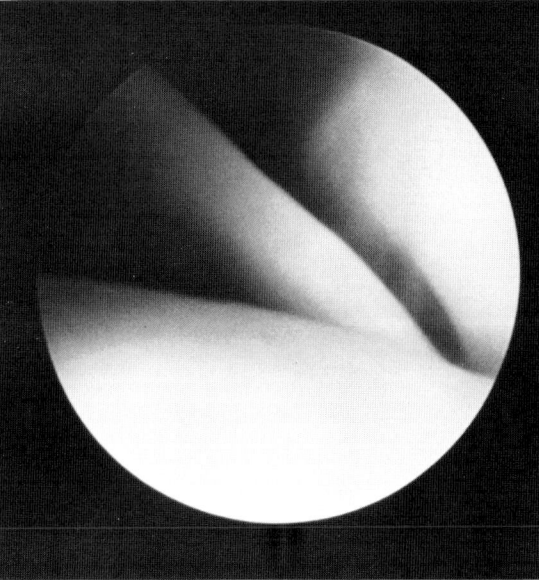

C

FIG. 10-87. A 53-year-old construction worker with severe shoulder pain and inability to work. The anteroposterior view (**A**) and the axillary view (**B**) show glenoid dysplasia with posterior humeral subluxation. Some secondary arthritic changes are present but seem to be mild, much milder than for the degree of symptoms expressed by the patient. **C:** One arthroscopic view of the joint showing normal cartilage of the humeral head. The biceps tendon without inflammation or fraying and a normal appearance of the anterior aspect of the supraspinatous tendon.

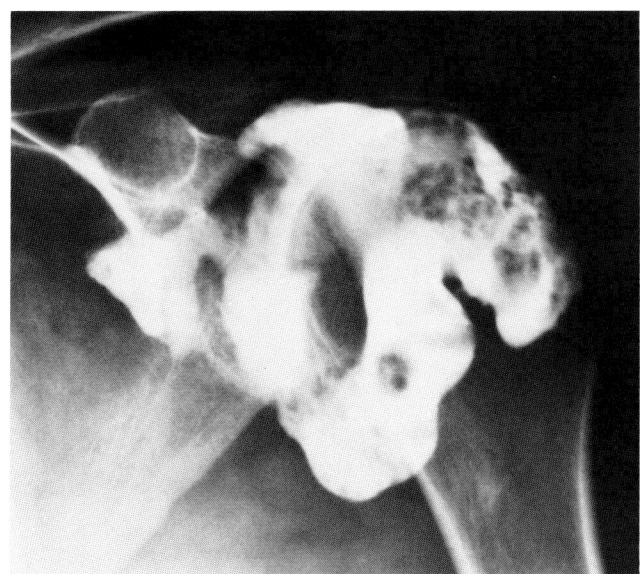 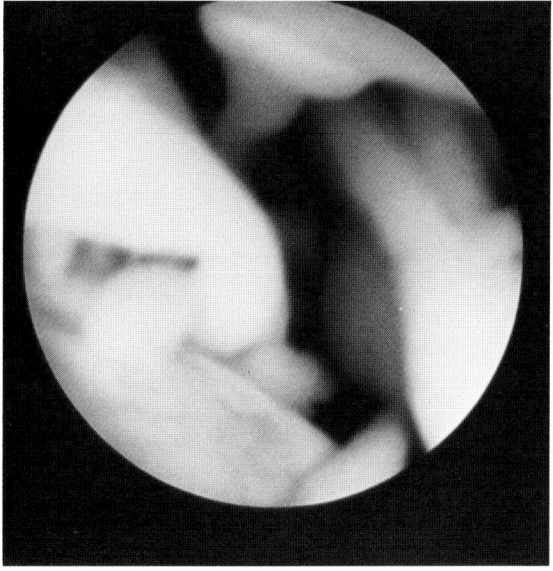

A   B

FIG. 10–88. A: An arthrogram of the shoulder of a 22-year-old man with rheumatoid arthritis. The joint abnormalities in this patient were limited to the shoulder, and before arthrography and arthroscopy with synovial biopsy, the diagnosis was uncertain. **B:** The arthroscopic view shows the drumstick-shape of the hypertrophic synovial fronds often seen in rheumatoid arthritis.

nosis and treatment of acute septic arthritis, although in chronic sepsis operative treatment is probably better. Computed tomographic scanning will now define glenoid fractures quite well, eliminating the need for arthroscopic evaluation. As one can see, the potential for arthroscopy, as for many other powerful diagnostic tools, is evolving and is not fully established.

TRAUMA

Fractures of the Proximal Humerus

Fractures of the proximal humerus usually occur in older patients. If one considers all fractures, about 5% involve the proximal humerus (153,189). In older patients, the fracture most often occurs after minor trauma, such as a fall. In younger individuals, the skeletal strength is greater than provided by ligaments, so that dislocations usually occur instead of fractures (166,189). When fractures occur in this age group, they usually result from significant trauma (motor vehicle or motorcycle accidents).

Codman (150) demonstrated that fractures of the proximal humerus tend to follow the physeal lines that divide the humerus into four parts: the humeral head, lesser tuberosity, greater tuberosity, and shaft (Fig. 10-89). Neer (185) proposed the most widely accepted classification of fractures of the proximal humerus. This classification is based on the number of fragments and the degree of displacement or angular deformity. If there is 1 cm of displacement between the fragments or greater

than 45° of angular malposition, the fragment is considered to be displaced (Fig. 10-90) (170,171,185).

The majority of proximal humeral fractures (80–85%) are undisplaced (170). Fractures most commonly involve the surgical neck (164,201). The rotator cuff, capsule, and periosteum assist in maintaining position of the fragments (Table 10-7) (189). A two-part fracture indicates that one fragment is displaced more than 1 cm

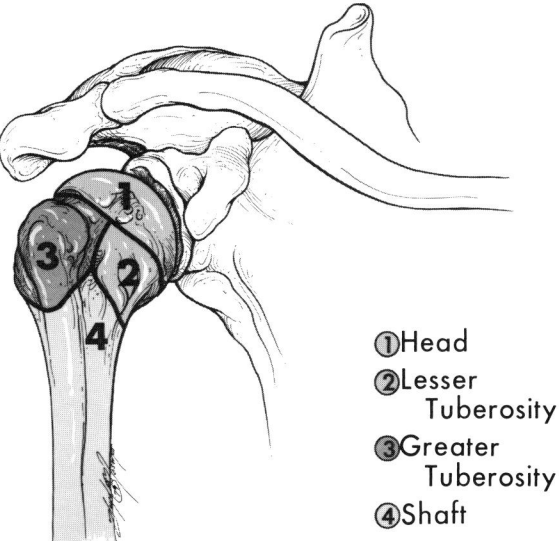

①Head
②Lesser
  Tuberosity
③Greater
  Tuberosity
④Shaft

FIG. 10–89. The four major anatomic fragments used to describe proximal humeral fractures in the displacement system of Neer (8).

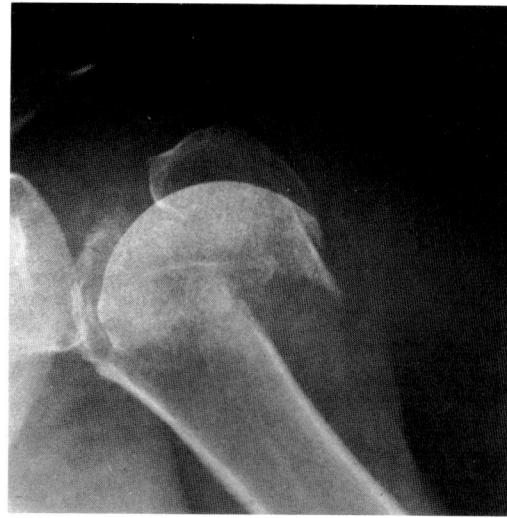
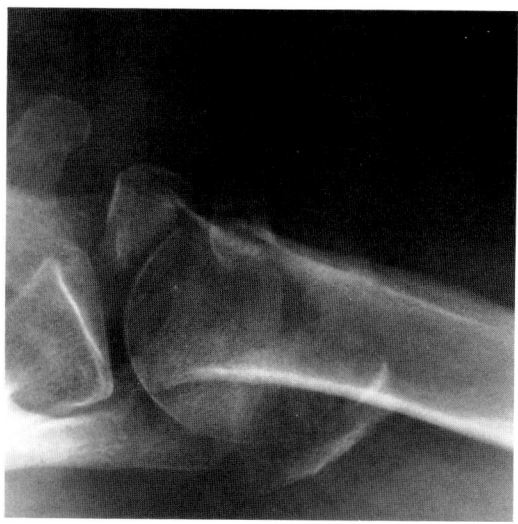

FIG. 10–90. AP view (**A**) and axillary view (**B**) of a four-part proximal humeral fracture. Both the lesser and greater tuberosities are fractured from the humeral head and displaced from their normal positions in relation to the humeral head. The humeral head is also displaced relative to the humeral shaft and angled upward 45°.

or angulated more than 45°. Three-part fractures have two displaced or angulated fragments (Fig. 10-91). With four-part fractures (Fig. 10-90), all fragments are displaced. Isolated fractures of the tuberosities are rare unless there is an associated dislocation (156,178).

As a general rule, with two-part displacement closed manipulation restores acceptable position. Immobilization with a sling or Velpeau immobilizer is followed with early exercise to avoid adhesive capsulitis (162,189). Open reduction is occasionally attempted to restore position. The pectoral muscles may cause medial displacement of the shaft (Fig. 10-92). Open reduction is generally required with three-part fractures. When all four fragments are displaced, a proximal humeral prosthesis is considered because of the relatively high frequency of late avascular necrosis of the separated head fragment. If there is an associated shoulder dislocation, the displacement classification is still useful to classify the injury and to predict the type of treatment that will be needed (Figs. 10-91 and 10-93).

TABLE 10–7. *Proximal humerus fractures: Classification and incidence*[a]

Type	Incidence
1 Part (no segment displaced)	80%
2 Part (1 segment displaced in relation to other 3)	13%
3 Part (2 segments displaced in relation to other 2)	3%
4 Part (all segments displaced)	4%

[a] (158,185)

Other classifications of surgical or anatomic neck fractures do not adequately describe the variety of injuries seen. The classification of humeral fractures as abduction or adduction fractures is usually spurious, as the direction of arm rotation will affect the x-ray appearance. In most of these fractures, the apex of the head-shaft angulation is actually anterior (Fig. 10-92). Accurate radiographic evaluation can be obtained with the shoulder trauma series (40° posterior oblique in external rotation, axillary view, scapular view). Proper classification requires experience. Since the majority of fractures are undisplaced (Table 10-7), it is not surprising that interobserver errors are higher with three- and four-part fractures (171). Computed tomography is very useful to assure proper classification and to accurately assess fragment position prior to surgery (148,170,171).

Significant complications in undisplaced proximal humeral fractures are uncommon (173). Adhesions may cause a reduced range of motion and pain. This can be reduced by including early mobilization as a part of the treatment plan (185,189,201).

Injury to the axillary artery and vein or brachial plexus may occur with significant displacement of the surgical neck. These structures lie just anterior and inferior to the capsule (189,201).

Non-union or malunion may occasionally occur (Fig. 10-92B). Neer reported non-union more commonly in patients treated with hanging casts (186). Malunion (Fig. 10-93) due to fracture of the greater tuberosity or significant angulation of the neck fractures can result in decreased range of motion. Joint reconstruction may be necessary in the most severe cases (Fig. 10-94).

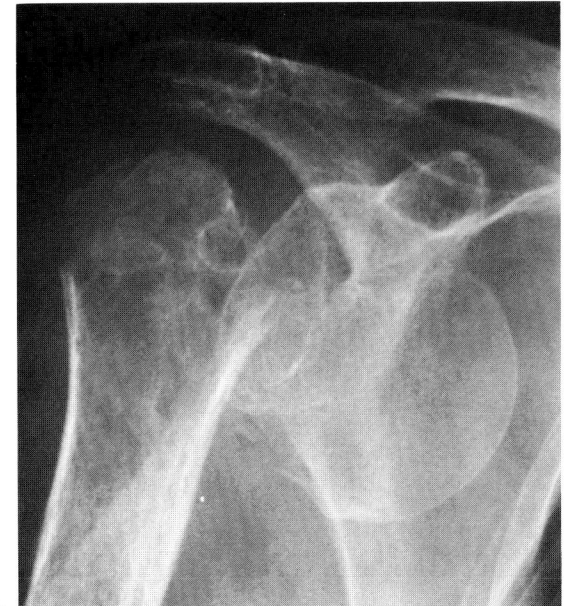
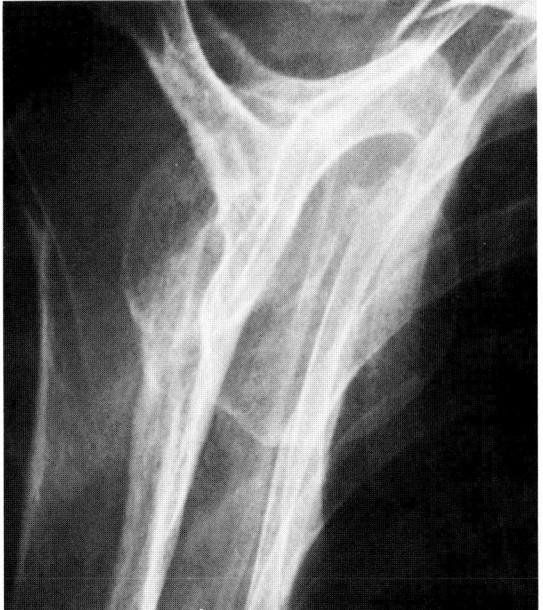

A

B

FIG. 10-91. Fracture-dislocations are similarly classified. Three part anterior dislocation. AP view (**A**) and scapular *Y*-view (**B**) demonstrate anterior dislocation of the humeral head with superior positioning of the shaft. The greater tuberosity remains in the joint space.

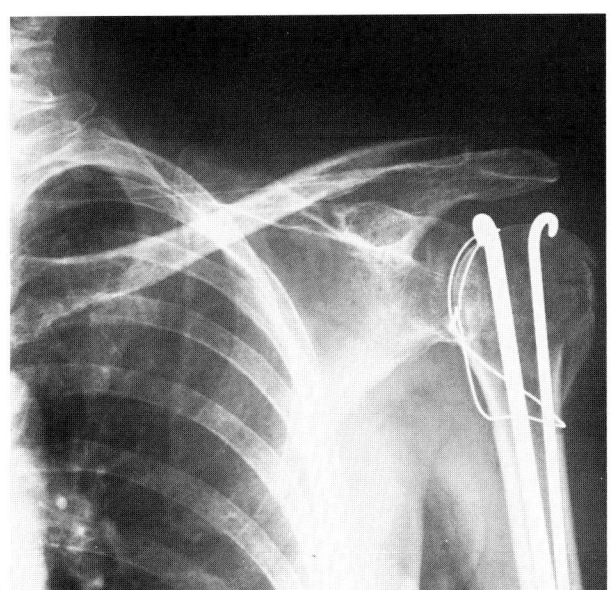
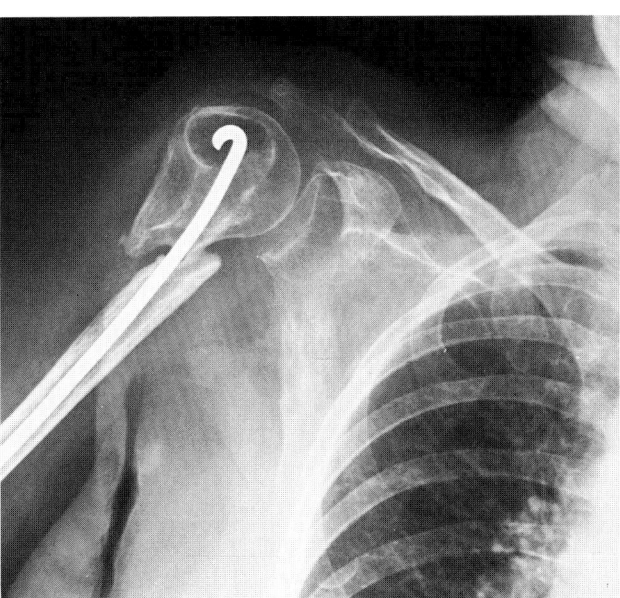

A

B

FIG. 10-92. A: Internal fixation of a three-part fracture with two Rush rods and wire. There is good anatomic reduction. **B:** Ununited fracture with loose Rush rod. Note the sclerotic fracture ends and lucency around the rod due to motion.

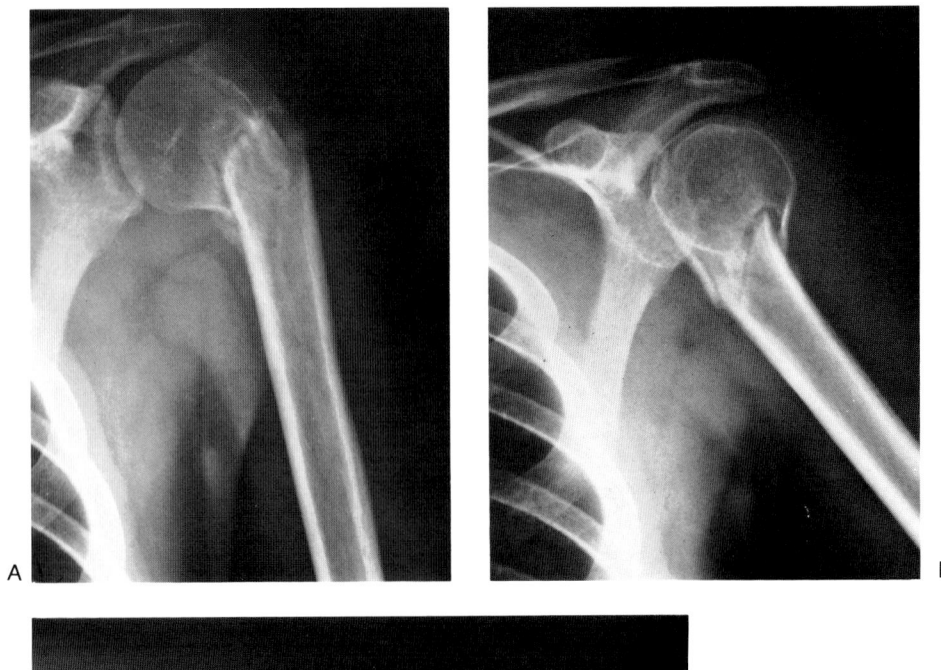

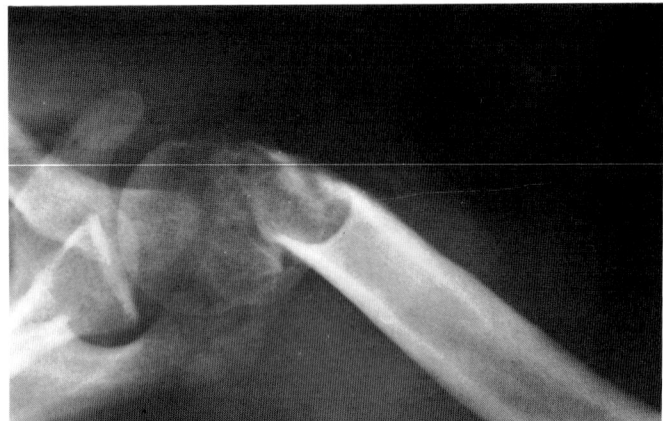

FIG. 10-93. An 8-week-old fracture of the proximal humerus showing the difficulties of using the abduction-adduction classification system for proximal humeral fractures. AP view (**A**) in external rotation of the arm shows that the fracture appears to be of the abduction type. AP view in internal rotation (**B**) shows the fracture to be of the abduction type. The axillary view (**C**) shows the actual angulation is anterior. This is the usual direction of displacement seen with this type of fracture.

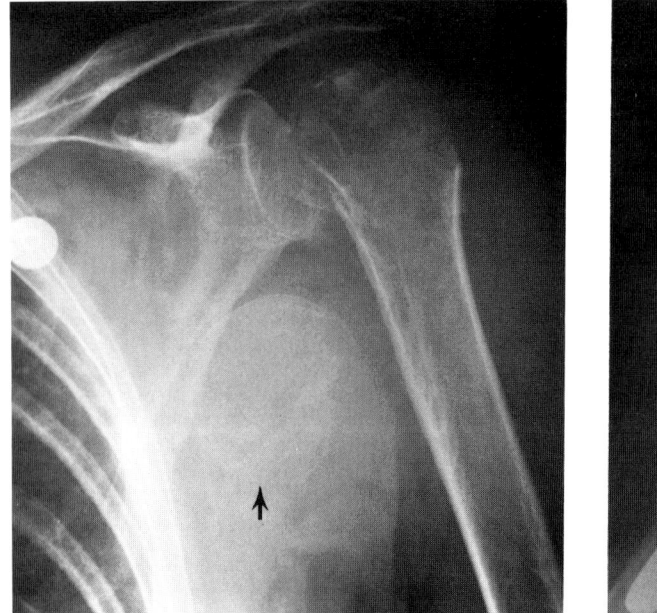
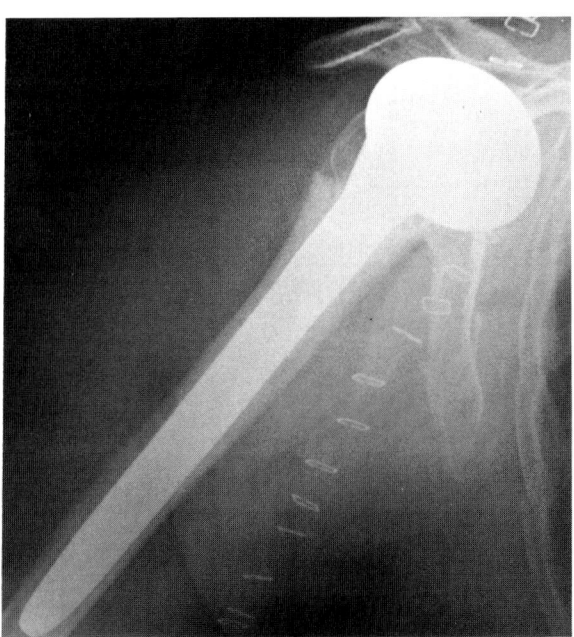

FIG. 10-94. **A:** Fracture dislocation with humeral head (*arrow*) in the axillary region. **B:** Treated with a Neer prosthesis and tuberosity fixation.

Avascular necrosis is common following four-part fractures or displaced fractures of the anatomic neck. The blood supply to the head is disrupted in these cases (189).

Glenohumeral Dislocations

Dislocations of the glenohumeral joint occur more frequently than dislocations at any other articulation. They account for 50% of all dislocations (189,201). Most dislocations are anterior (97%). Posterior dislocations occur in 2–4.3% of patients, and superior and inferior dislocations are rare (155,189,195,200,201).

Anterior Dislocations

Most anterior dislocations (96%) are due to trauma, although certain individuals can voluntarily dislocate their shoulders (204). Traumatic dislocations usually result from a fall with the arm in abduction and external rotation. Rarely, the dislocation is due to direct posterolateral trauma. In adolescence, dislocations in males outnumber those in females 5:1 (189,197). As the humeral head dislocates, it is forced anteriorly and inferiorly against the capsule, glenohumeral ligaments, and subscapularis (Fig. 10-95). These structures provide the majority of the shoulder's anterior stability (154,215). The posterolateral aspect of the humeral head comes in contact with the glenoid rim, which may result in an associated impaction fracture. This was described by Hill and Sachs and bears their name, the Hill-Sachs deformity (165). This lesion occurs in 67–76% of cases (184,195,207). Associated lesions of the anterior inferior glenoid rim reportedly occur less frequently, appearing in approximately 50% of cases (189,197,201). However, Rowe determined that the Bankart lesion was the most common finding in patients with recurrent dislocations (180,182,207).

Most anterior dislocations are obvious on the conventional AP radiograph. However, a routine trauma series is most accurate (40° posterior oblique, axillary, Y-view) for complete assessment of the dislocation and associated fractures. Dislocations are described according to their location. In order of decreasing frequency, dislocation may be subcoracoid (Fig. 10-95), subglenoid, subclavicular, or intrathoracic. Intrathoracic dislocations are rare but are associated with more significant complications (189).

Following closed reduction, the radiographic trauma series, except for the axillary view, should be repeated. The radiographs must be carefully studied to assure adequate reduction and to exclude associated fractures (greater tuberosity, Hill-Sachs, or glenoid rim) (Fig. 10-96). For example, if the anterior dislocation results in the humeral head lying medial to the coracoid, reduction may be more difficult. Interposition of the tendon of the long head of the biceps may occur with this type of dislocation, making reduction difficult or impossible. Displacement of the biceps tendon should also be considered in dislocations with large greater tuberosity fractures, for the bicipital groove may be involved (168). Fractures of the greater tuberosity occur in up to 15% of anterior dislocations (Fig. 10-97).

Additional views (described in the earlier section on radiographic techniques) are useful in detecting subtle

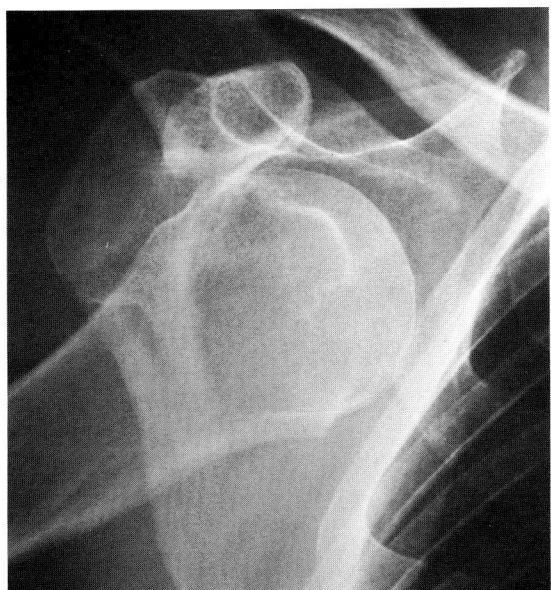
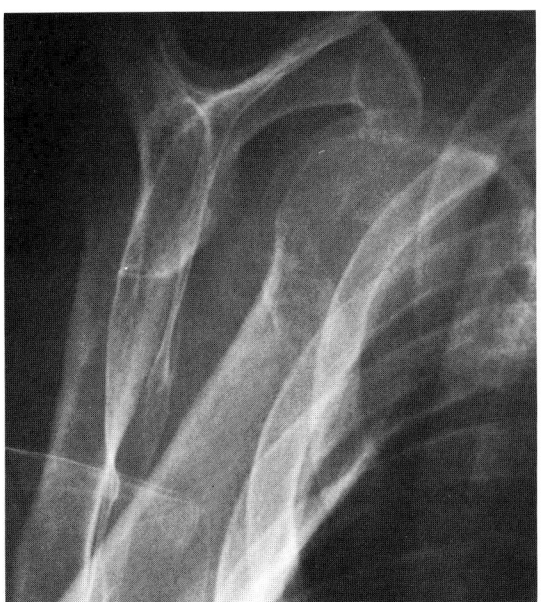

FIG. 10-95. Subcoracoid anterior dislocation. AP view (**A**) and scapular Y-view (**B**). The Y-view most clearly demonstrates the humeral head relationship to the glenoid.

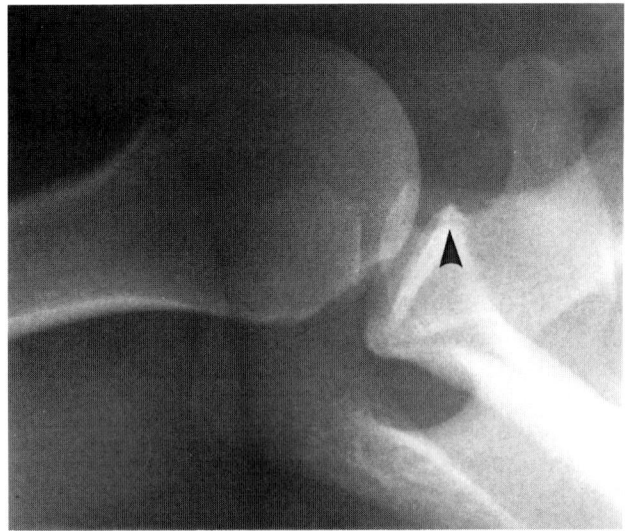

FIG. 10–96. Axillary radiograph shows persistent anterior subluxation with a glenoid rim fracture (*arrow*).

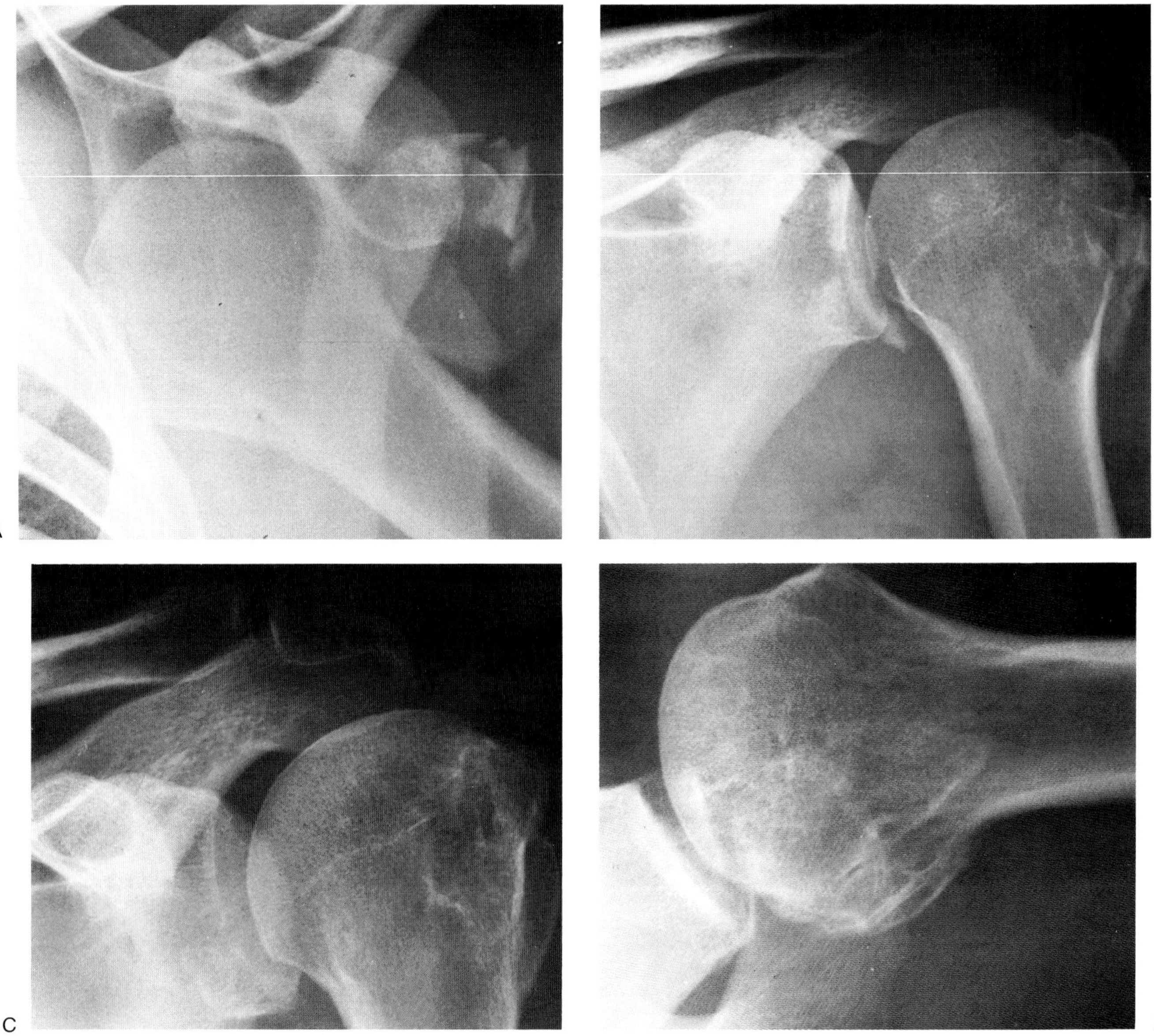

A

B

C

D

FIG. 10–97. A: AP view of the shoulder demonstrating an anterior dislocation with fracture of the greater tuberosity and glenoid. **B:** Following closed reduction, the greater tuberosity is near anatomic position. There is a fragment below the glenoid. This should have been localized with axillary views or CT. AP (**C**) and axillary views (**D**) after healing.

THE SHOULDER / 641

Hill-Sachs deformities and glenoid rim fractures. The Stryker notch view is easy to duplicate and can identify Hill-Sachs deformities in 90% of patients with recurrent dislocation (159). AP internal rotation views will detect Hill-Sachs deformity in 50% of patients with recurrent dislocation (185). Glenoid rim fractures may be obvious on the routine axillary or West Point views (142,202). However, labral injuries may be present with no obvious bony changes. Therefore, double-contrast arthrography, with or without CT, or arthrotomography may be indicated in patients with recurrent dislocations. MRI is also useful in this setting.

Treatment of anterior dislocation can usually be accomplished with closed reduction (Fig. 10-97). Exceptions include patients with soft tissue interposition, subacromial greater tuberosity displacements, and large (>5 mm) glenoid rim fractures. Glenoid fractures can lead to recurrent dislocation or traumatic arthritis (142,172, 189,216). Internal fixation is considered in these patients.

Posterior Dislocations

Only about 2–4.3% of shoulder dislocations are posterior (150,179,189,193,195,201,217). The injury may follow electric shock therapy, seizures, or falls with the arm adducted and internally rotated. Direct trauma to the anterior shoulder may also cause dislocation, but this is not common (197,217).

Clinically, the patient's arm may be held in slight abduction with internal rotation. External rotation is blocked. Unfortunately, the diagnosis is missed clinically in many patients (161,189,201).

The injury may be easily overlooked on the conventional AP view. There are, however, several signs present:

1. The humeral head is fixed in internal rotation (100%).
2. The joint may appear abnormally widened or narrowed.
3. The usual "half moon" overlap of the humeral head and glenoid may be absent or distorted (55%).
4. A "trough line" may appear in the humeral head, representing a compression-fracture of the anterior aspect of the humeral head (75%).
5. There may be an associated fracture of the lesser tuberosity (25%) (149).

Routine use of the 40° posterior oblique AP, scapular Y-view, and axillary view (trauma series) should prevent missed diagnoses of posterior dislocation. The Y-view is particularly useful, as the relationship of the humeral head to the glenoid is easy to access. Also, the view can be obtained without moving the arm (Fig. 10-98). Rather than memorize the various signs on the conventional AP view, we suggest use of these alternative views for more accurate diagnoses.

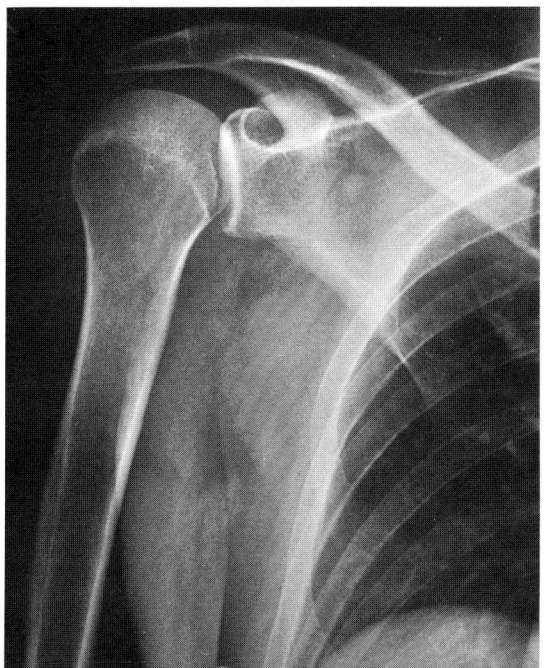
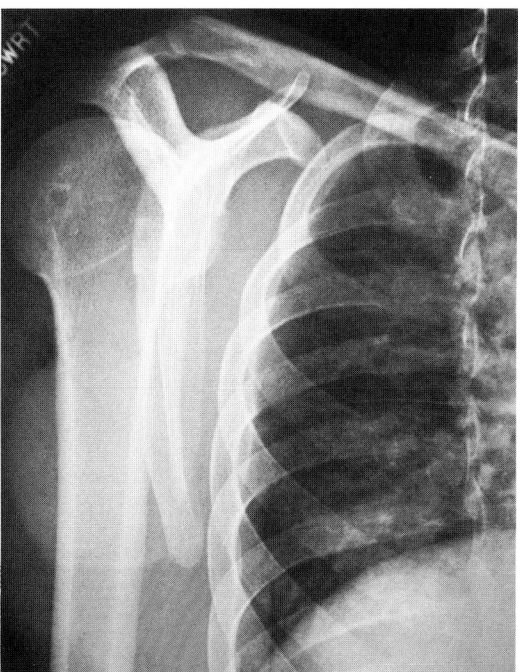

FIG. 10–98. Posterior dislocation of the right shoulder. **A:** Conventional AP view. The humeral head is internally rotated, the glenoid projected over the humeral head with a through line in the humeral head. **B:** The scapular Y-view clearly demonstrates the posterior dislocation. (So why memorize all of the signs on the conventional AP view—take the correct views instead.)

Normally, the distance from the medial margin of the humeral head to the anterior glenoid rim is no more than 6 mm (139). Posterior dislocation results in an increase in this distance, the rim sign (Fig. 10-99) (139,201). The normal overlap between the head and posterior rim of glenoid will be absent.

Posterior dislocations are also described by location. The majority (98%) are subacromial, but subglenoid and subspinal (scapular spine) dislocations also occur (193,197). On the AP view, posterior subglenoid and subspinal dislocations may mimic an anterior dislocation (189). The problem is easily solved with the scapular Y-view. Fractures of the lesser tuberosity and less commonly of the glenoid and posterior capsule tears with rim fractures are associated with posterior dislocations (Fig. 10-99) (149,189,201).

Posterior dislocations can usually be treated with closed reduction (157). The incidence of recurrence is much lower than that with anterior dislocations (163,189).

Superior and Inferior Dislocations

Superior and inferior (luxatio erecta) dislocations are rare (155,189,197). Superior dislocations overlie the acromion or clavicle on the AP view (Fig. 10-100). This dislocation is usually due to a severe upward force on the adducted arm (155). With luxatio erecta, the humerus becomes parallel to the spine of the scapula, and the arm is abducted (Fig. 10-101). Downey reported this type of dislocation in 0.5% of all dislocations (155). This injury is due to force on the flexed arm (above the head). As a result, the humeral head is forced downward. Inferior subluxation may be associated with humeral fractures, glenoid fractures, capsular tears, or brachial plexus injury (221). These types of dislocations can usually be managed initially with closed reduction, but more injuries and rotation cuff tears may be present.

Complications of Glenohumeral Dislocations

Complications of glenohumeral dislocations and fracture-dislocations are more common than complications of proximal humeral fractures. Associated fractures and recurrent dislocations are the most common problem (189,201). Rowe (207) reviewed 39 patients with recurrent anterior dislocation. He noted Bankart fractures in 84%, Hill-Sachs deformities in 76%, and capsular laxity in 83% of operated shoulders. Other associated fractures include the greater tuberosity (15%), and, less frequently, the coracoid and lesser trochanteric or subscapularis avulsions (156,178).

Recurrence is a common problem after anterior dislocations. It is most common in young patients (55% less than 22 years old) compared to older patients (12% in patients over 30 years of age) (167). Delayed arthrosis is also common following dislocations. The incidence is increased following posterior dislocation (210).

Radiographic assessment of these complications has been discussed earlier in this chapter. Rupture of the capsule and tears on the rotator cuff may occur either acutely or with recurrent dislocations (179,199). CT, ar-

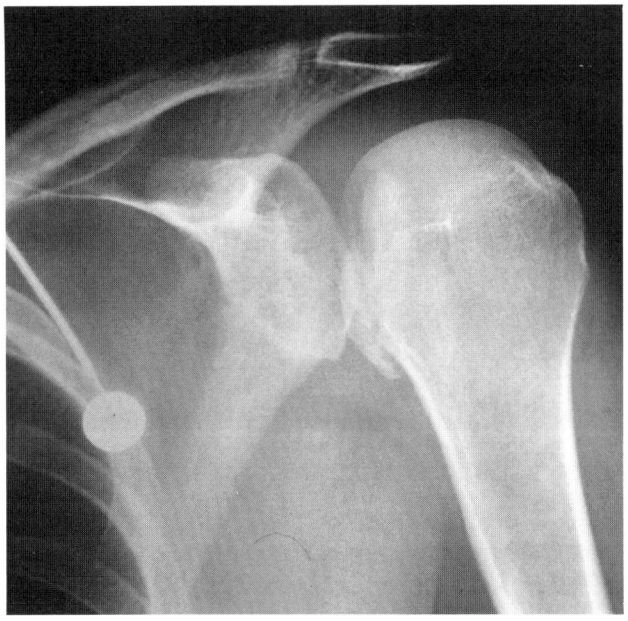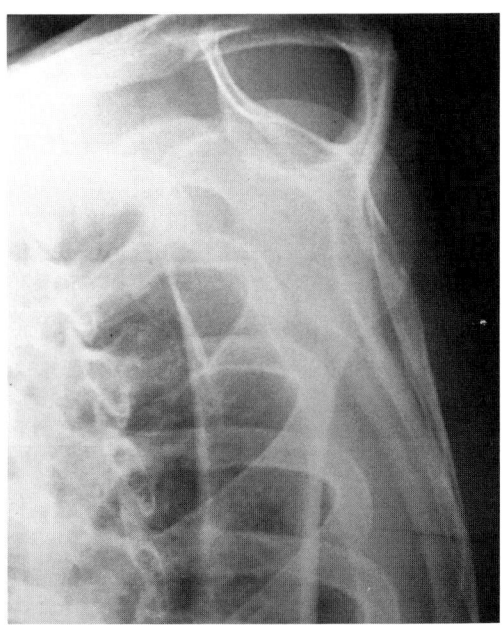

FIG. 10–99. AP view (**A**) demonstrates a vacant glenoid fossa with a tuberosity fracture medially. The posterior position of the humeral head is clearly seen on the scapular Y-view (**B**).

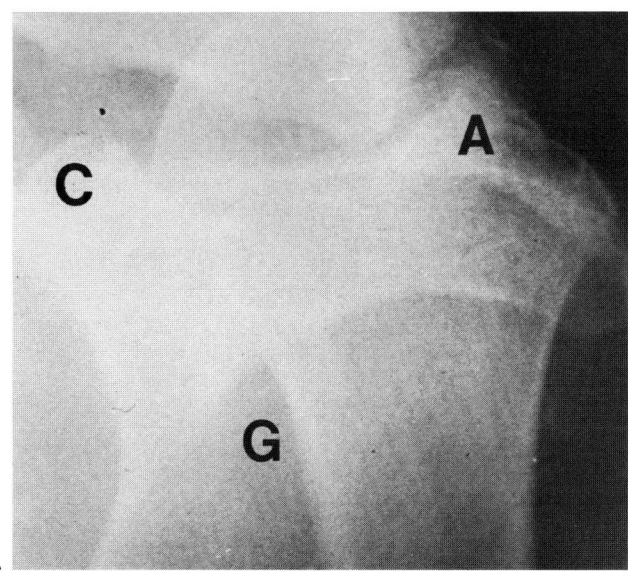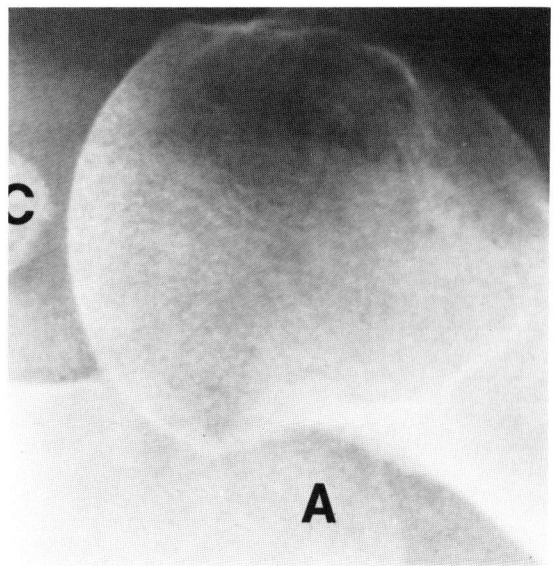

FIG. 10-100. Superior dislocation of the shoulder. AP view (**A**) with acromion (A) and glenoid (G) labeled. The humeral head overlies the AC joint. The axillary view (**B**) shows the relationship to the coracoid (C) and acromion (A) (from 155).

thrography, or MRI are important in the evaluation of patients with suspected soft tissue or cartilaginous injury following dislocation.

Neurovascular injury may occur in the axillary region following dislocations. Vascular injuries include laceration, thrombosis, intimal laceration, and false aneurysms of the axillary artery (164,173,189,197,218). Axil-

lary artery injuries may be overlooked initially owing to collateral circulation. Peripheral pulses may be present even with significant axillary artery injury (164,173). Early diagnosis with selective angiographic techniques is essential to determine the extent of injury. Amputation rates following axillary artery occlusion have been reported to be as high as 43% (164).

The axillary nerve crosses the subscapularis anteriorly (189). Stretching or compression can occur, especially with anterior dislocations. Fortunately, complete disruption is uncommon, and loss of function is rare (189,214). Simeone recommends exploration only if neural deficit persists beyond 3 months after reduction (214).

Acromioclavicular Dislocations

Dislocations of the acromioclavicular joint (12%) occur less commonly than glenohumeral dislocations (85%). Rowe and Marble reported only 52 cases in 1,603 patients with shoulder trauma (205). The mechanism of injury is usually a fall in which force is directed to the point of the shoulder. Dislocations due to indirect forces directed superiorly through the humeral head have also been reported (183,189,197). Nielsen found that the majority of injuries were due to direct trauma and that only 5% were due to falls on the outstretched hand (192).

Allman (138) classified acromioclavicular joint injuries based on the degree of ligament injury. Table 10-8 describes the categories of injury, the radiographic findings, and the prognosis used in Allman's classification. Radiographic changes in Type I and Type II injuries may be subtle. The radiographs are normal in Type I (Fig.

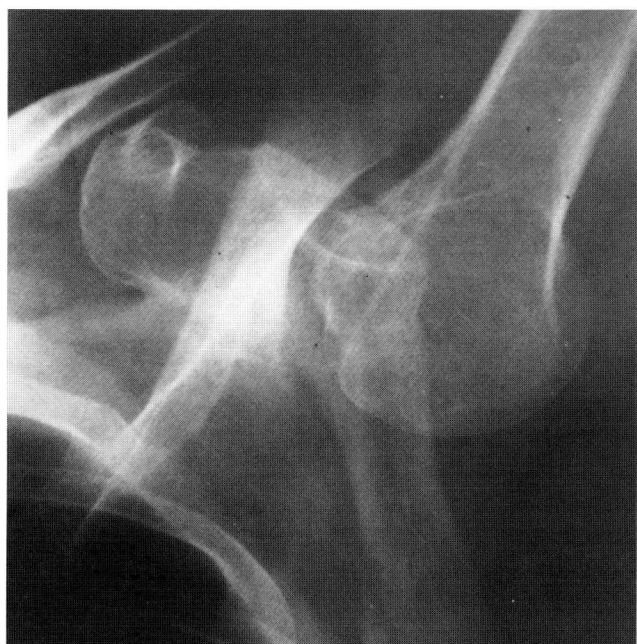

FIG. 10-101. Erect (luxatio erecta) dislocation. The humerus is parallel to the scapular spine, with the humeral head inferior to the glenoid (from 155).

TABLE 10–8. *Acromio-clavicular dislocation: Classification and Prognosis*

Classification	x-ray	Prognosis

Type I
  Ligament strain, a few ligament
    fibers torn
	Normal	No instability; Excellent[a]

Type II
  Rupture of the capsule and
    acromio-clavicular ligaments
	Joint wide: clavicle may be slightly
	  elevated
		May require arthroplasty if symptoms
		  persist; 90% recover, 10% may
		  require surgery[a]

Type III
  Rupture of capsule, AC ligaments
    and coraco-clavicular ligaments
	Elevated clavicle: increased clavicle-
	  coracoid distance
		Internal fixation: 80% good, 20%
		  reoperation[a]

[a] (185)

10-102). Generally, radiographs of the shoulder will overpenetrate the acromioclavicular joint. Therefore, it is best to obtain well-coned views centered on the joint, with the tube angled 15° to the head. This will reduce the amount of bony overlap. Weight-bearing views are essential to diagnose Type II lesions and to differentiate Type II from Type III injuries (Fig. 10-103) (143, 189,197). In Type III injuries, the coracoclavicular ligaments are torn if the distance between the upper aspect of the coracoid and the undersurface of the clavicle is greater than 50% or increased >5 mm compared with the normal shoulder (143,169,189).

Treatment of most Type I and II injuries is successful with closed methods. Occasionally, closed reduction fails with Type II lesions, and late distal clavicle excision is necessary. Internal fixation is more often necessary with Type III injuries (189,197).

Adjacent fractures can accompany acromioclavicular dislocation (Fig. 10-104). In our experience the coracoid and clavicle are fractured most frequently. Intraarticular acromial fractures may also occur.

Heterotopic ossification in the coracoclavicular and acromioclavicular region has been reported (Fig. 10-105) (140,189). The incidence reported varies from 57–82%.

Migration of pins has also been reported following internal fixation (175).

Sternoclavicular Dislocations

Dislocations of the sternoclavicular joint are uncommon (151,178,205). Rowe reported that this injury occurred in 3% of all shoulder dislocations (205). Dislocation usually results from indirect trauma to the shoulder. Posterolateral forces transmitted medially cause anterior dislocation. Direct anterior trauma can occur in sports such as football. This causes posterior dislocation (189,196,197,205). Anterior dislocations occur much more frequently than posterior dislocations (185,190). Nettles and Linscheid reported that 3 of 60 sternoclavicular dislocations were posterior (163).

Anterior dislocations may be easily palpable. Posterior dislocations can be more difficult to diagnose clinically

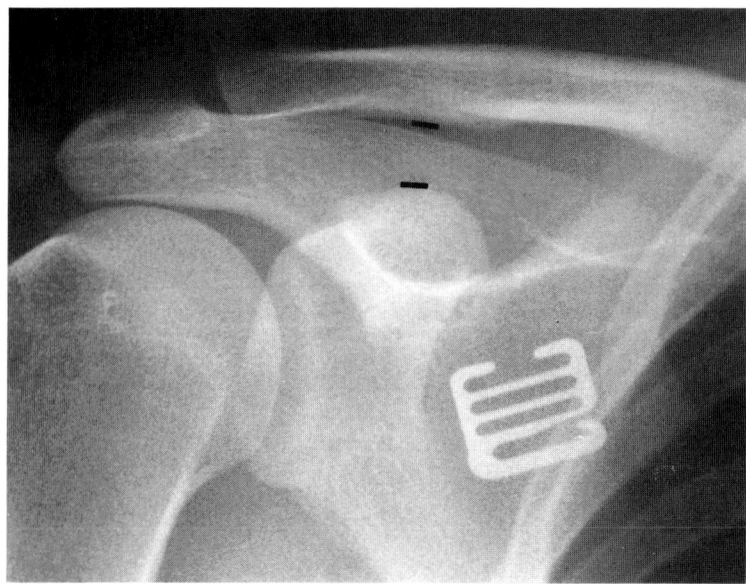

FIG. 10–102. Mild strain of the acromioclavicular ligaments. The joint space and coracoclavicular distance (*lines*) are normal even with weight bearing.

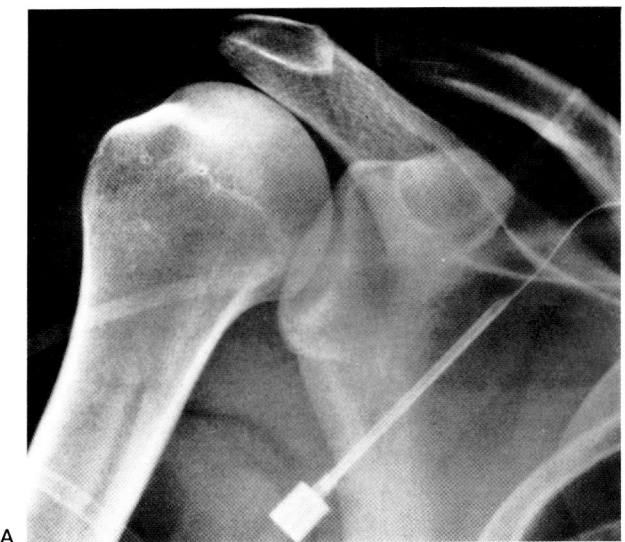

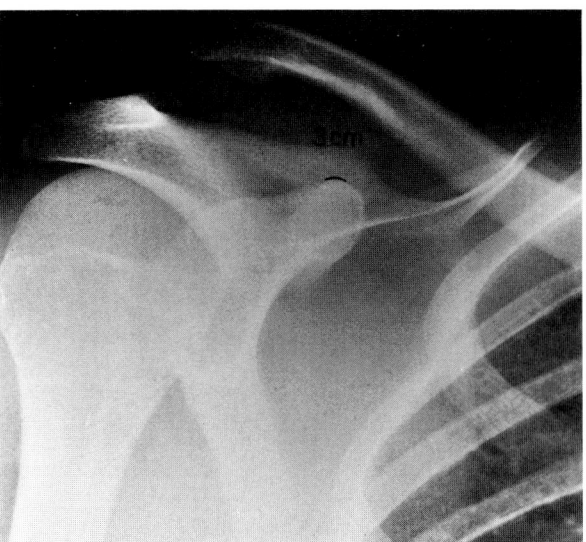

A

B

FIG. 10–103. A: Widening of the right AC joint with apparently normal coracoclavicular distance. Non weight bearing (Type II vs. Type III). **B:** Weight-bearing views clearly demonstrate the complete dislocation and coracoclavicular ligament disruption (Type III).

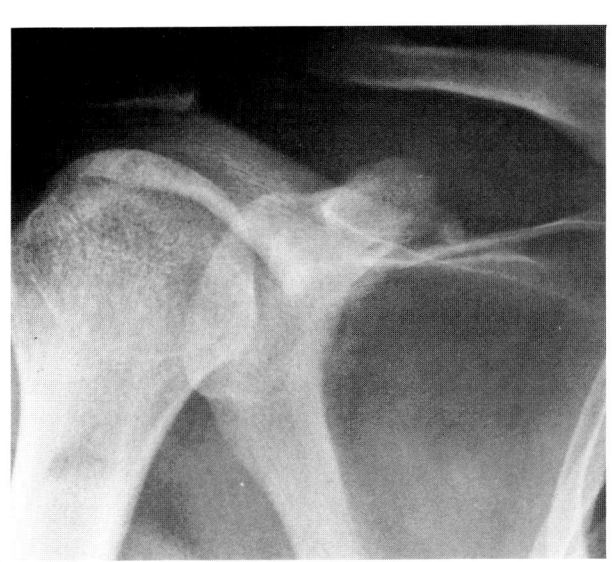

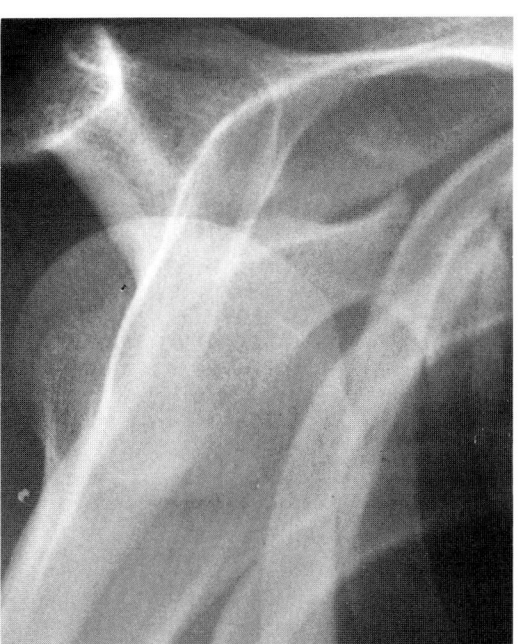

A

B

FIG. 10–104. A: Acromioclavicular separation and undisplaced clavicle fracture seen on the AP view. **B:** The scapular Y-view more clearly demonstrates the coracoid fracture.

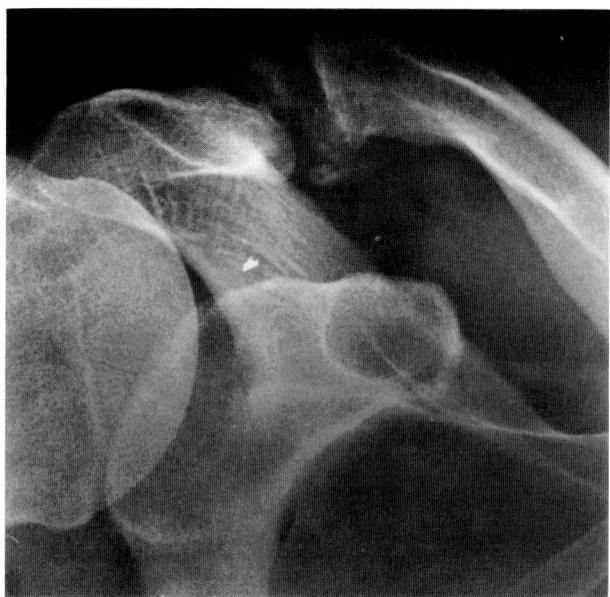

FIG. 10–105. Ossification following unsuccessful closed reduction of the acromioclavicular joint.

due to swelling. Unfortunately, early diagnosis is necessary, as reduction after 48 hours is difficult (147,213). In addition, posterior dislocations may be potentially fatal injuries owing to involvement of the trachea and great vessels.

Allman (138) classified sternoclavicular dislocations in the same manner as acromioclavicular dislocations. Type I injuries cause only slight tearing of the sternoclavicular ligament. In Type II lesions, the sternoclavicular ligament is torn, and Type III injury results in tears of both the sternoclavicular and costoclavicular ligaments. In the latter situation, either anterior or posterior dislocation occurs.

Radiographic evaluation of this injury is difficult. Overlying structures often cause confusion (see routine radiography section in this chapter). Since the lesion is uncommon, radiographic technicians are often unfamiliar with appropriate techniques. However, a simple technique described by Hobbs is usually sufficient for complete dislocations (see section on Radiography). Angling the tube 40° to the head projects the sternoclavicular joints superiorly. If the anterior dislocation is present, the involved clavicle will be higher than the normal side. With posterior dislocations, the involved clavicle is lower. Conventional and computed tomography may be helpful in more difficult cases (174,213). Actually, CT provides sufficient images for accurately evaluating subluxations as well as complete dislocations (see Fig. 10-109C). Subtle changes in the joint are much more obvious with CT than with routine films or tomography. The direction of displacement is also more obvious. An additional advantage of CT is the ability to assess the trachea, great vessels, and adjacent soft tissues. Magnetic reso-

nance imaging may prove to be equally effective in this regard.

Treatment of sternoclavicular dislocation is usually successful with closed techniques (147,189,194,197, 211). Problems can occur with internal fixation. Migration or fracture of pins and screws may result in injury to the retrosternal vessels or airway (189,223).

Most significant complications are associated with posterior dislocation. Fortunately, this injury is not common. Injuries to the arch vessels, trachea and esophagus have been reported (189,197,209,220). Nerve injury may also occur. Injuries to the great vessels and trachea may be life threatening, indicating the urgency of early diagnosis of posterior dislocation (209). The incidence of complications is 25% (189,209,220).

Surgical complications may occur as well, and closed reduction is attempted in most cases (147). A major problem is migration of Steinmann pins or Kirschner wires into the anterior superior mediastinum. Omer (194) reported operative complications in 5 patients who had metal fixation of a sternoclavicular dislocation. Complications included infection, pin fracture, and pin migration.

Clavicle Fractures

Clavicle fractures are common, especially in children (189,197,201). The injury usually is caused by a fall on the outstretched hand. The lateral force directed through the shoulder results in fracture of the midclavicle (Fig. 10-106). Less frequently direct trauma to the clavicle or shoulder results in fracture.

Fractures of the middle third of the clavicle are most common (80%) (138,188,201). Allman (138) classified clavicle fractures anatomically. Group I fractures involve the middle third of the clavicle. Displacement of these fractures is common (Fig. 10-107). The sternoclei-

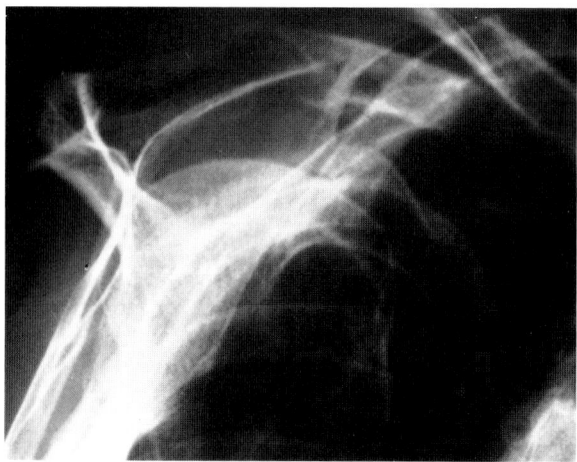

FIG. 10–106. Scapular Y-view demonstrating overriding of a midclavicle fracture.

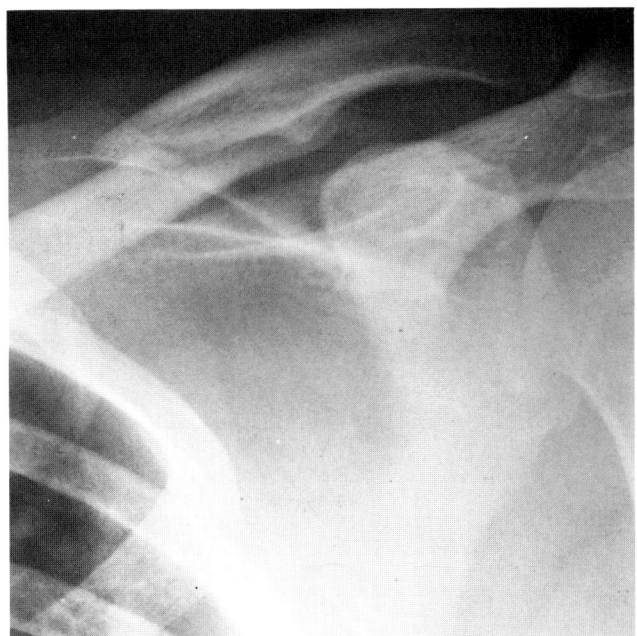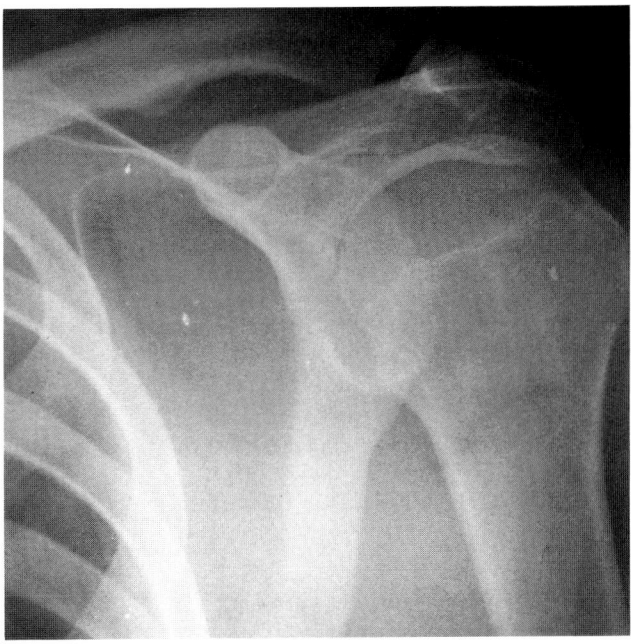

FIG. 10–107. Fracture of the midclavicle. The fracture is barely visible on the AP view (**A**). The 15° cephalic angle (**B**) makes the diagnosis obvious.

domastoid elevates the proximal fragment, and the weight of the arm tends to lower the distal fragment. This results in a superior tented radiographic appearance. Group II fractures involve the distal clavicle (lateral to the coracoclavicular ligament) (Fig. 10-108). These fractures make up 15% of clavicle fractures (138,201). Group III fractures (5%) involve the medial clavicle.

Radiographic evaluation of the mid- and distal clavicle is not difficult. AP or oblique views of the clavicle (see section on Radiography), with the tube angled 15° to the head, will allow good visualization of the mid- and distal clavicle (Fig. 10-107). The angulation projects the clavicle above the chest. A coned-down 15° angled view is best to overcome the problem of overpenetrating the acromioclavicular joint. Subtle midclavicle fractures may be overlooked. If symptoms dictate, a 40° cephalic angle may make detection less difficult (Fig. 10-107). Evaluation of the proximal clavicle is more difficult. Forty-degree angled views and oblique views are usually adequate if the fracture is displaced. In selected cases, especially undisplaced fractures, tomograms or computed tomography may be necessary (Fig. 10-109).

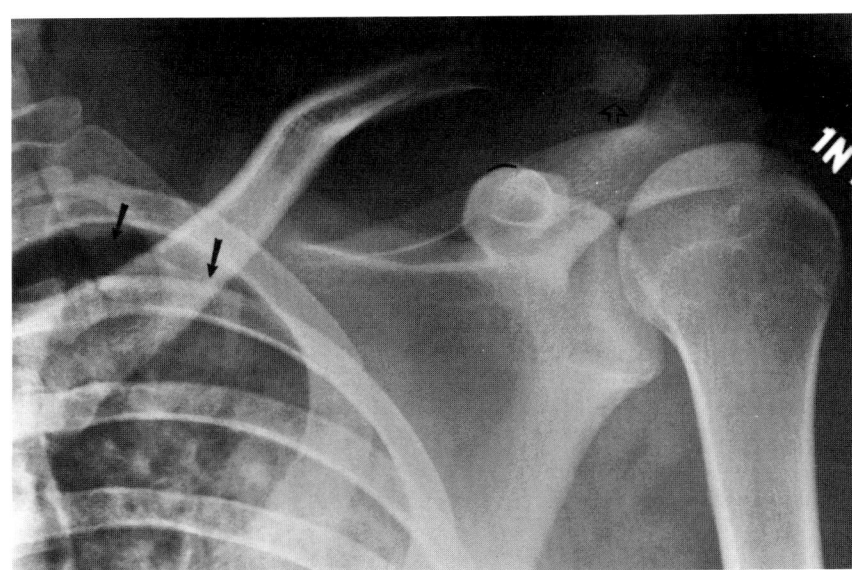

FIG. 10–108. Fracture of the distal left clavicle (*open arrow*) with rupture of the coracoclavicular ligament (Neer Group II). Note the pneumothorax (*closed arrows*) and upper lobe pulmonary contusion.

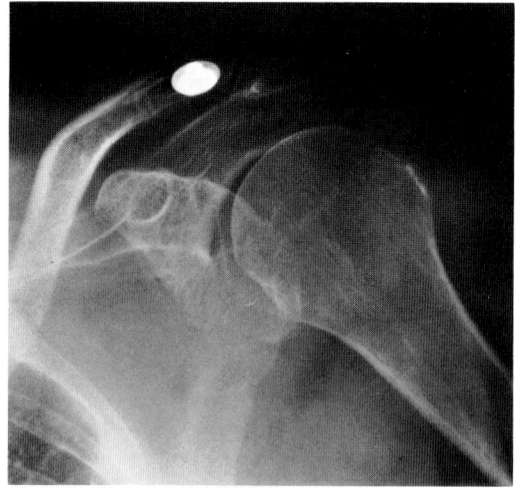
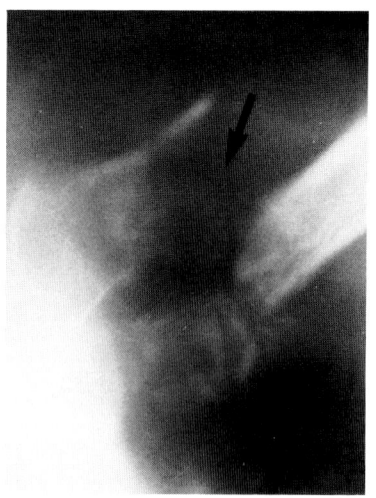
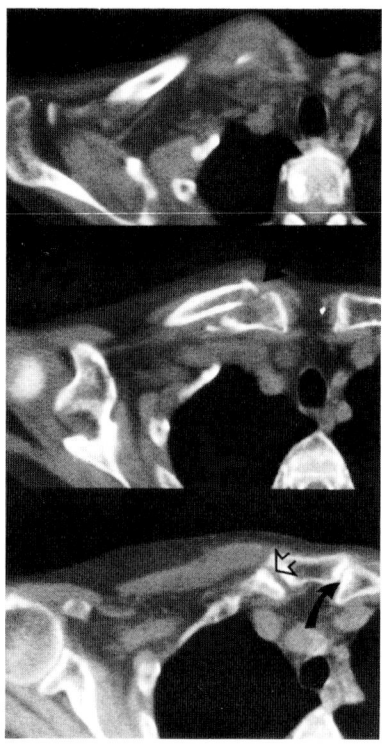

FIG. 10-109. Injury to the sternoclavicular region. **A:** AP view of the clavicle is difficult to evaluate. **B:** Tomogram clearly demonstrates a displaced fracture of the proximal clavicle. **C:** CT images demonstrate the relationship of the fracture fragments, soft tissue involvement, and subluxation of the sternoclavicular joint (*open arrow*). The left sternoclavicular joint (*curved arrow*) is normal. The great vessels and trachea are normal.

Most clavicle fractures can be treated with closed reduction using shoulder support (sling, "figure of 8", etc.) (189,197).

Open reduction is generally reserved for the following conditions (176,222):

1. Neurovascular compromise or entrapment.
2. Distal clavicle fractures with coracoclavicular ligament disruption (Fig. 10-110).
3. Fractures with severe augulation or comminution.
4. Patients who cannot tolerate closed treatment methods.
5. Symptomatic non-union which was previously treated with closed reduction.

Group II fractures of the distal clavicle may require internal fixation. Resection of the distal clavicle may be required in patients with persistent symptoms (Fig. 10-110).

Significant complications are less common with clavicle fractures than with glenohumeral fracture-dislocations. Malunion of midclavicle fractures or excessive callus formation does occur. This may result in compression of the adjacent neurovascular structures between the clavicle and first rib.

Non-union occurs in only 1–2% of cases (Figs. 10-111 and 10-112) (219). Osteoarthritis may occur following intra-articular fracture. This is more common at the acromioclavicular joint. Post-traumatic osteolysis may

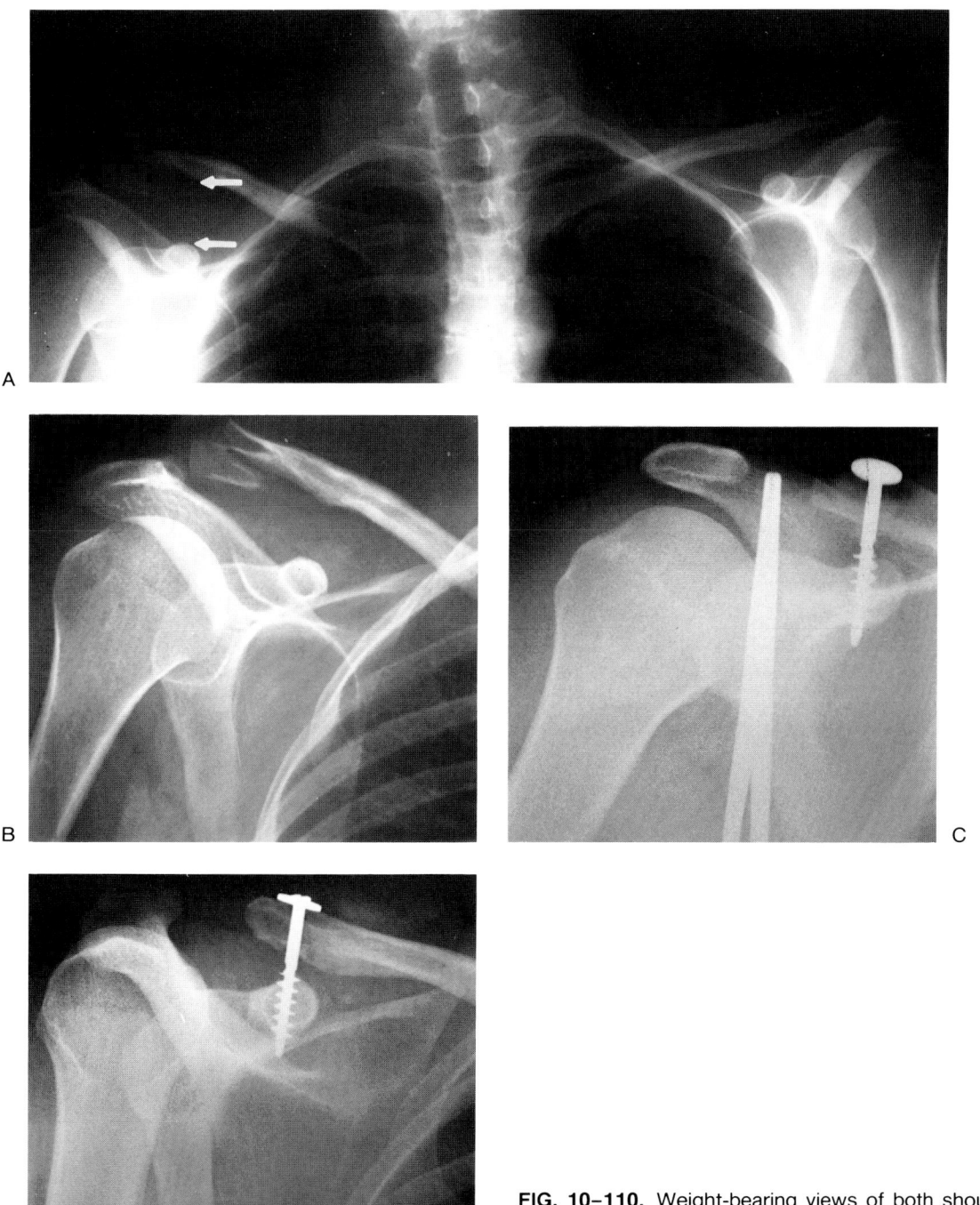

FIG. 10–110. Weight-bearing views of both shoulders (**A**) and localized view (**B**) of the right shoulder demonstrating a distal clavicle fracture with disruption of the coracoclavicular ligament (*arrows*) and acromioclavicular joint. The distal clavicle was resected (**C**) and the coracoclavicular ligament reduced with screw fixation (**D**).

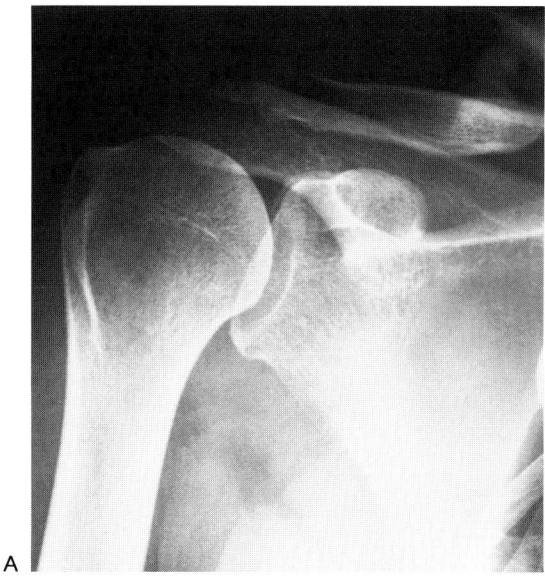
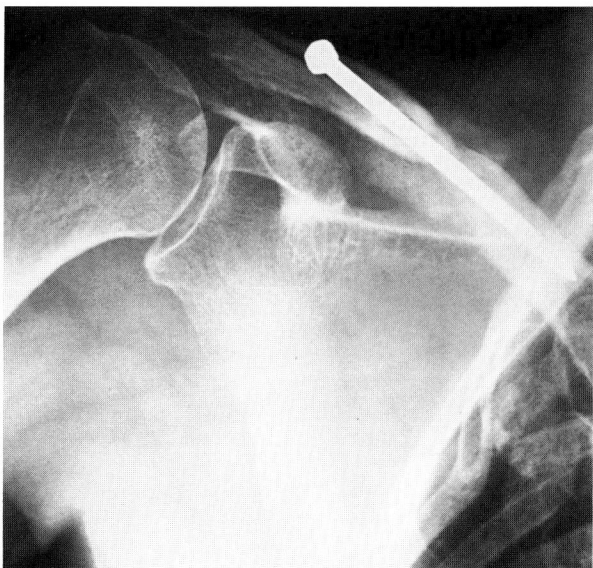

FIG. 10–111. A: Old, ununited comminuted fracture of the midclavicle. **B:** The fracture was reduced with bone graft and pin fixation.

be seen in the distal clavicle. Patients present with continued pain and weakness after trauma. Erosive changes develop on the distal clavicle, which are visible on the radiograph (Fig. 10-113). Involvement may progress to the level of the coracoclavicular ligaments (198). Changes may be due to synovial hyperplasia, but this is uncertain. Following treatment with immobilization some degree of bone healing occurs, although the joint often remains widened (198).

Scapular Fractures

Fractures of the scapula are uncommon (1% of all fractures) (161). Injury to the body of the scapula is

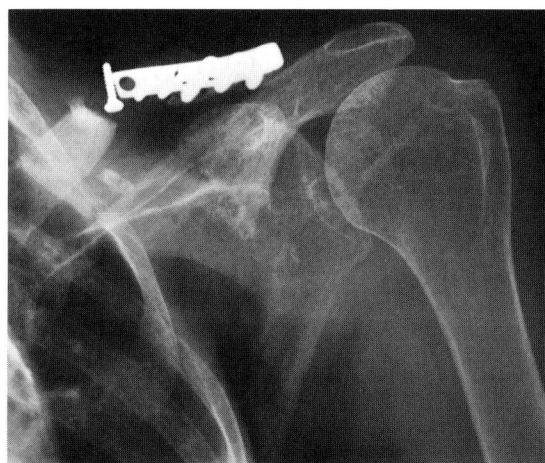

FIG. 10–112. Old fracture of the distal clavicle with plate and screw fixation. The proximal fragment has undergone osteolysis with resulting non-union and angulation.

caused by direct force. The scapula is well protected by an envelope of muscles. Therefore, considerable force is required to cause the fracture, and displacement of body fractures is usually not significant. Associated fractures of the ribs, clavicle, and spine, however, are not unusual. Injury to the lungs and bronchi may also occur. Evaluation of the body of the scapula is usually successful with AP and lateral views. Frequently, the initial opportunity to evaluate the scapula is on the chest film that is obtained to evaluate the multiple trauma patient. Despite this, many obvious fractures are overlooked. Up to 43% of scapular fractures are not detected on initial chest films. Associated fractures of the ipsilateral ribs or clavicle occur in 88% of patients. Therefore, when these injuries are noted the scapula should be studied more carefully or scapular views obtained (160,208). Another unusual but potentially lethal injury can also be detected on chest films. Scapulothoracic dissociation presents with lateral displacement of the scapula. There are frequently associated fractures of the clavicle or acromioclavicular joint separations. This injury is basically a closed forequarter amputation and significant neurovascular injury is common. Early angiography and surgery are required to treat this injury (208).

Fractures of the body may extend to the glenoid articular surface (Fig. 10-114, see also Fig. 10-35). Most commonly, glenoid fractures are associated with dislocations. However, Varriale and Adler (216) have described glenoid fractures that are not associated with dislocation. Fractures may be undisplaced, displaced, or bursting. Detection of glenoid fractures is critical because, if displaced, they lead to traumatic arthritis. Scapular *Y*, West Point, and axillary views are most useful in demonstrating these fractures (Fig. 10-115) (141,216). CT images

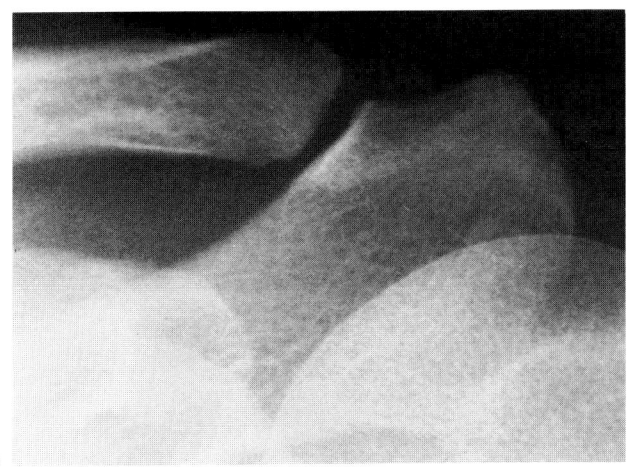

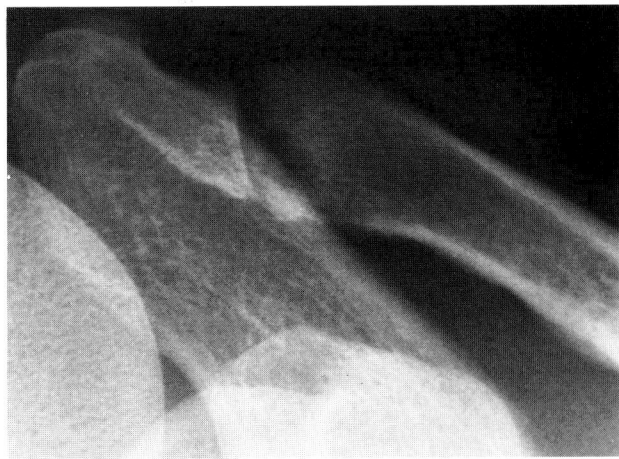

A

B

FIG. 10–113. Post-traumatic osteolysis, partially treated. **A:** Normal clavicle. **B:** Erosions in the involved clavicle.

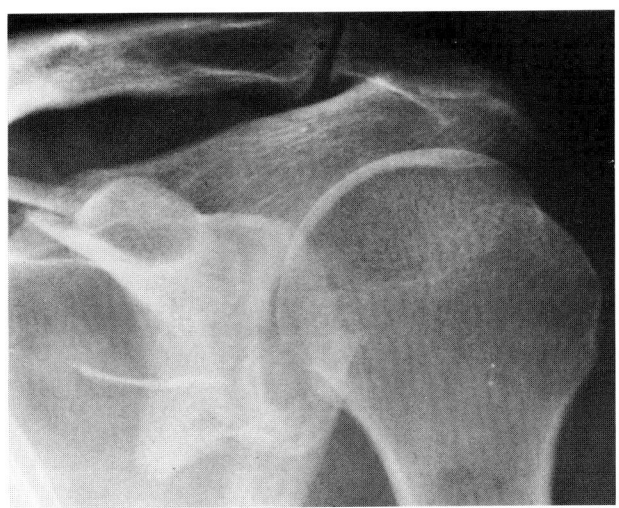

FIG. 10–114. Fracture of the body and neck of the scapula involving the lower glenoid.

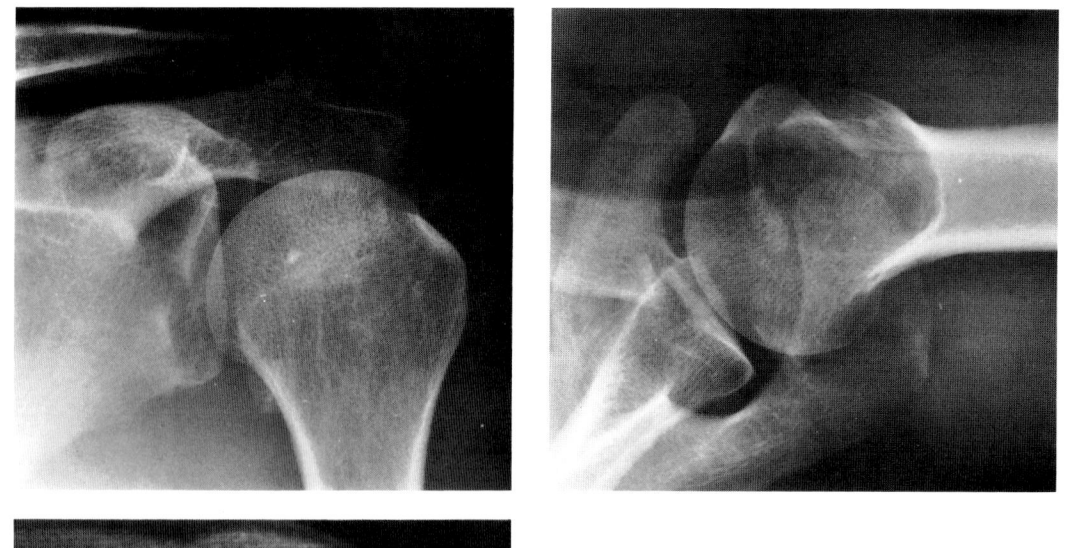

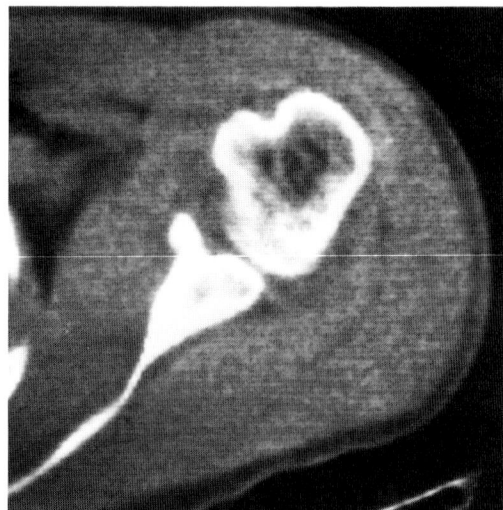

FIG. 10–115. Glenoid fracture demonstrated on AP view (**A**). The axillary view (**B**) shows the fracture anteriorly. CT scan (**C**) demonstrates the position of the fragment most accurately.

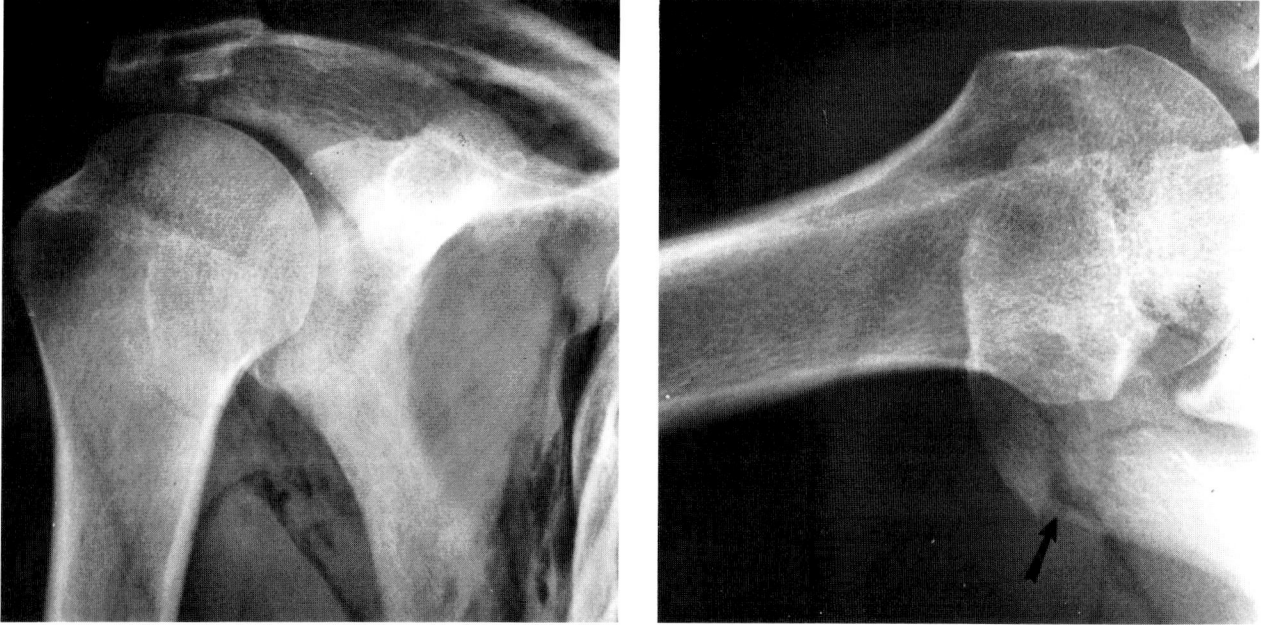

FIG. 10–116. Undisplaced comminuted acromial fracture. The AP view (**A**) demonstrates extensive subcutaneous emphysema. Air overlying the bone makes fracture detection difficult. **B:** Axillary view demonstrates the acromial fracture (*arrow*).

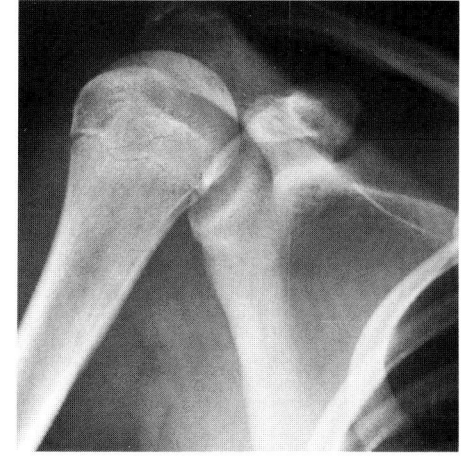

A

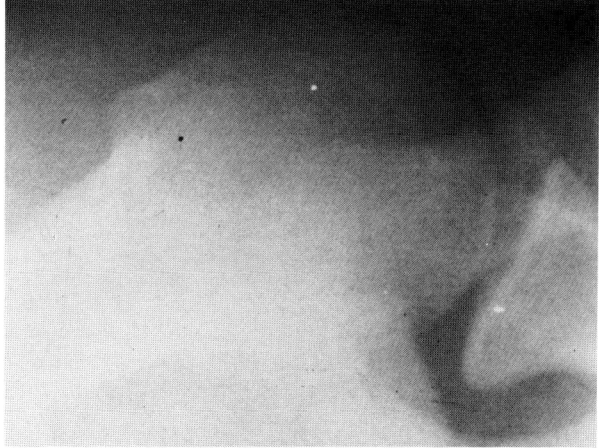

B

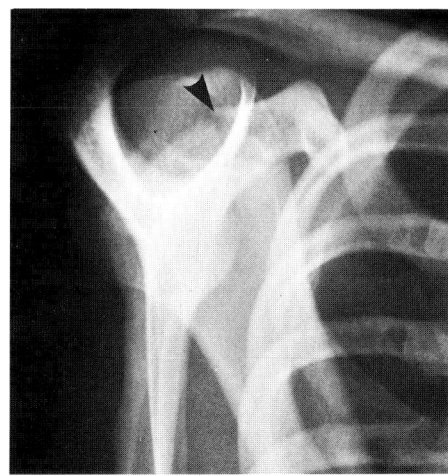

C

FIG. 10–117. Shoulder pain after anterior trauma. The AP (A) and axillary (B) views are negative. Scapular Y-view (C) clearly demonstrates the coracoid fracture (arrow).

are very useful, especially if open reduction is considered. Avulsion fractures of the infraglenoid tubercle are due to forceful triceps contraction. This fracture may also lead to recurrent dislocation, especially if a portion of the rim is involved (189). Subtle avulsions of the infraglenoid tubercle may require a Bennett view for detection. This view is taken with the arm abducted 90° and the elbow flexed. The tube is angled 5° to the head and centered on the shoulder (147).

Fractures of the acromion usually are due to a direct blow from above. However, stress fractures may also occur in association with dislocations and rotator cuff tears (152). Radiographic diagnosis is not difficult in most cases. The axillary and Y-view are particularly useful in the diagnosis of subtle acromial fractures (Fig. 10-116).

Fractures of the coracoid process may be due to direct trauma or avulsion. Most fractures occur at the base. Displacement is usually prevented by ligament attachment.

Muscular origins of the scapula include the coracobrachialis, short head of the biceps, and pectoralis minor (203). Repeated trauma in trapshooters may result in a coracoid stress fracture (146,212). Radiographic evaluation of coracoid fractures should include the scapular

Y-view and axillary views (Fig. 10-117) (212). In addition, weight-bearing views should be considered. Fractures of the coracoid are associated with acromioclavicular dislocation (177). Subtle injury may also be identified with the oblique angled view described by Goldberg and Vicks (158). The patient is rotated 20° posteriorly, and the tube is angled 20° toward the head. This view projects the coracoid above the adjacent skeletal structures.

Most scapular fractures are managed conservatively. Internal fixation may be necessary if significant displacement has occurred (Fig. 10-35).

REFERENCES

Anatomy

1. Anderson JE. Grant's atlas of anatomy, 8th ed. Baltimore: Williams & Wilkins, 1983.
2. Basmajian JV. The surgical anatomy and function of the arm-trunk-mechanism. Surg Clin North Am 1963;43:1471.
3. Blair DN, Rapoport S, Sostman HD, Blair OC. Normal brachial plexus: MR imaging. Radiology 1987;165:763–767.
4. Clemente CD. Gray's anatomy of the human body, 13th ed. Philadelphia: Lea & Febiger, 1985.
5. Cockshott P. The coracoclavicular joint. Radiology 1979; 131:313.

6. Cone RO, Danzig L, Resnick D, et al. The bicipital groove: Radiographic, anatomic, and pathologic study. *AJR* 1983;141:781–788.
7. DePalma AF. *Surgery of the shoulder.* Philadelphia: J.B. Lippincott, 1973.
8. Gardner E, Gray DJ. The prenatal development of the human shoulder and acromioclavicular joint. *J Anat* 1953;92:219–276.
9. Hitchcock HH, Bechtol CO. Painful shoulder. *J Bone Joint Surg* 1948;30A:263–273.
10. Hollinshead WH. *Anatomy for surgeons,* vol. 3, 3rd ed. New York: Harper & Row, 1982.
11. Keats TE. *Atlas of normal roentgen variants which may simulate disease,* 3rd ed. Chicago: Year Book Medical Publishers, 1984.
12. Lucas DB. Biomechanics of the shoulder joint. *Arch Surg* 1973;107:425–432.
13. Meyer AW. Spontaneous dislocation and disruption of the tendon of the long head of the biceps brachii: 59 instances. *Arch Surg* 1928;17:493–506.
14. Mitchell MJ, Causey G, Berthoty DP, Sartoris DJ, Resnick D. Peribursal fat plane of the shoulder: Anatomic study and clinical experience. *Radiology* 1988;168:699–704.
15. Neer CS, Rockwood CA. Fractures and dislocations of the shoulder. In Rockwood CA Jr, Green DP. *Fractures in adults.* vol. 1. Philadelphia: J.B. Lippincott, 1984;675–985.
16. Post M. *The shoulder: surgical and nonsurgical management.* Philadelphia: Lea & Febiger, 1978.
17. Prodromos CC, Ferry JA, Schiller AC, Zarins B. Histologic studies of the glenoid labrum from fetal life to old age. *J Bone Joint Surg* 1990;72A:1344–1348.
18. Saha AK. Dynamic stability of the glenohumeral joint. *Acta Orthop Scand* 1973;44:668–678.
19. Saha AK. *Theory of shoulder mechanism.* Springfield, Ill: Charles C. Thomas, 1961.
20. Turkel SJ, Pono MW, Marshall JL, Girgis FG. Stabilizing mechanisms preventing anterior dislocation of the glenohumeral joint. *J Bone Joint Surg* 1981;63A:1208–1217.

Imaging Techniques

21. Ballinger PW. *Merrill's atlas of roentgenographic positions and standard radiologic procedures,* 5th ed. St. Louis: C.V. Mosby, 1982.
22. Bernau A, Berquist TH. *Orthopedic positioning in diagnostic radiology.* Baltimore: Urban and Schwarzenberg, 1983.
23. Bosworth BM. Complete acromioclavicular dislocation. *N Engl J Med* 1949;241:221–225.
24. Cahill BR. Osteolysis of the distal part of the clavicle in male athletes. *J Bone Joint Surg* 1982;64A:1053–1058.
25. Clements RW. Adaptation of the technique for radiography of the glenohumeral joint in the lateral position. *Radiol Technol* 1979;51:305.
26. Cone RO III, Resnick D, Danzig L. Shoulder impingement syndrome: Radiographic evaluation. *Radiology* 1984;150:29–33.
27. Danzig L, Resnick D, Greenway G. Evaluation of unstable shoulders by computed tomography. *Am J Sports Med* 1982;10:138–141.
28. Deichgraber E, Olsson B. Soft tissue radiography in painful shoulder. *Acta Radiol (Diagn)* 1975;16:393.
29. DeSmet AA. Axillary projection in radiography of the nontraumatized shoulder. *AJR* 1980;143:511–518.
30. DeSmet AA. Anterior oblique projection in radiography of the traumatized shoulder. *AJR* 1980;134:515–518.
31. Didiee J. Le radiodiagnostic dans la luxation recidivante de l'épaule. *J Radiol Electrol* 1930;14:209–218.
32. Fagerlund M, Ahlgren O. Axial projection of the humeroscapular joint. *Acta Radiol (Diagn)* 1981;22:203–205.
33. Farrar E, Matsen F, Rogers J, et al. Dynamic sonographic study of lesions of the rotator cuff. Presented at the Annual Meeting of the AAOS, Anaheim, CA, 1983.
34. Fisk C. Adaption of the technique for radiography of the biceptal groove. *Radiol Technol* 1965;37:47–50.
35. Flinn RM, MacMillan CL, Campbell DR, et al. Optimal radiography of the acutely injured shoulder. *J Can Assoc Radiol* 1983;34:128.
36. Garth WP, Slappey CE, Ochs CW. Roentgen demonstration of instability of the shoulder: The apical oblique projection. *J Bone Joint Surg* 1984;66A:1450–1453.
37. Genoe GA, Moeller JA. Normal shoulder variations in the technetium-99m polyphosphate bone scan. *South Med J* 1974;67:659.
38. Golding FC. The shoulder: The forgotten joint. *Br J Radiol* 1962;35:149–158.
39. Hall RH, Isaac F, Booth CR. Dislocation of the shoulder with special reference to accompanying small fractures. *J Bone Joint Surg* 1959;41A:489–491.
40. Heinig CF. Retrosternal dislocation of the clavicle: Early recognition, x-ray diagnosis, and management. *J Bone Joint Surg* 1968;50A:830.
41. Hermodsson I. Roentgenologische Studien über die traumatischen und habituellen Schultergelenkverrenkungen nach vorn und nach unten. *Acta Radiol (Suppl)* 1934;20:1.
42. Hill NH, Sachs MD. The grooved defect of the humeral head. A frequently unrecognized complication of dislocations of the shoulder joint. *Radiology* 1940;35:690–701.
43. Howell SM, Galinat BJ, Renzi AJ, Marone PJ. Normal and abnormal mechanics of the glenohumeral joint in the horizontal plane. *J Bone Joint Surg* 1988;70A:227–232.
44. Kilcoyne RF, Reddy PK, Lyons F, Rockwood CA. Optimal plain film imaging of the shoulder impingement syndrome. *AJR* 1989;153:795–797.
45. Korngerth PJ, Salazar AM. The apical oblique view of the shoulder: Its usefulness in acute trauma. *AJR* 1987;149:113–116.
46. Lee FA, Gwinn JL. Retrosternal dislocation of the clavicle. *Radiology* 1974;110:631–634.
47. Mazuijian M. Lateral profile view of the scapula. *X-Ray Tech* 1953;25:24.
48. McGlynn FJ, El-Khoury G, Albright JP. Arthrotomography of the glenoid labrum in shoulder instability. *J Bone Joint Surg* 1982;64A:506–518.
49. Neer CS II. Displaced proximal humeral fractures. Part I. Classification and evaluation. *J Bone Joint Surg* 1970;52A:1077–1089.
50. Newhouse KE, El-Khoury GY, Nepala JV, Montgomery WJ. The shoulder impingement view: A fluoroscopic technique for detection of subacromial spurs. *AJR* 1988;151:539–541.
51. Quesada F. Technique for the roentgen diagnosis of fractures of the clavicle. *Surg Gynecol Obstet* 1926;42:4261–4281.
52. Rokous JR, Feagin JA, Abbott HG. Modified axillary roentgenogram. A useful adjunct in the diagnosis of recurrent instability of the shoulder. *Clin Orthop* 1972;82:84–86.
53. Rubin SA, Gray RL, Green WR. The scapular "Y": A diagnostic aid in shoulder trauma. *Radiology* 1974;110:725–726.
54. Slivka J, Resnick D. An improved radiographic view of the glenohumeral joint. *J Can Assoc Radiol* 1979;30:83–85.
55. Wallace WA, Hellier M. Improving radiographics of the injured shoulder. *Radiography* 1983;49:229.
56. Zanca P. Shoulder pain: Involvement of the acromioclavicular joint. Analysis of 1000 cases. *Am J Roentgenol* 1971;112:493–506.

Special Diagnostic Techniques

57. Andren L, Lundberg BJ. Treatment of rigid shoulders by joint distension arthrography. *Acta Orthop Scand* 1965;36:45–53.
58. Bateman JE. *The shoulder and neck,* 2nd ed. Philadelphia: W.B. Saunders and Co., 1978.
59. Berquist TH. *MRI of the musculoskeletal system.* New York: Raven Press, 1990.
60. Brandt TD, Cardone BW, Grant TH, Post M, Weiss CA. Rotator cuff sonography: A reassessment. *Radiology* 1989;173:323–327.
61. Burk LD, Karasick D, Kurtz AB. Rotator cuff tears: Prospective comparison of MR imaging with arthrography, sonography, and surgery. *AJR* 1989;153:87–92.
62. Burman MS. Arthroscopy of the direct visualization of joints: An experimental cadaver study. *J Bone Joint Surg* 1931;13:669.
63. Callaghan JJ, McNiesh LM, Dehaven JP, Savory CG, Polly DW. A prospective comparison of double contrast computed tomography, arthrography and arthroscopy of the shoulder. *Am J Sports Med* 1988;16:13–20.

64. Cofield RH. Arthroscopy of the shoulder. *Mayo Clin Proc* 1983;58:501–508.
65. Cofield RH. Rotator cuff disease of the shoulder. *J Bone Joint Surg* 1985;67:974–979.
66. Cone RO, Danzig L, Resnick D, Goldman AB. The bicipital groove. Radiographic, anatomic, and pathologic study. *AJR* 1983;141:781–788.
67. Cone RO, Resnick D, Danzig L. Shoulder impingement syndrome: Radiographic evaluation. *Radiology* 1984;150:29–33.
68. Crass JR, Craig EV, Feinberg SB. Sonography of postoperative rotator cuff. *AJR* 1986;146:561–564.
69. DePalma AF. Loss of scapulohumeral motion. *Ann Surg* 1952;135:193–204.
70. DeSmet AA, Ting YM. Diagnosis of rotator cuff tear on routine radiographs. *J Can Assoc Radiol* 1977;28:54–57.
71. Deutsch AL, Resnick D, Mink JH, et al. Computed and conventional arthrotomography of the glenohumeral joint: Normal anatomy and clinical experience. *Radiology* 1984;153:603–609.
72. El-Koury GY, Albright JB, Yousef MA, Montgomery WJ, Tuck SL. Arthrotomography of the glenoid labrum. *Radiology* 1979;131:333–337.
73. Ellis VH. The diagnosis of shoulder lesions due to injuries to the rotator cuff. *J Bone Joint Surg* 1953;35B:72–74.
74. Freiberger RH, Kaye JJ. *Arthrography.* New York: Appleton-Century-Crofts, 1979.
75. Fulenda H, Mikasa M, Yamanaka K. Incomplete thickness rotator cuff tears diagnosed by subacromial bursography. *Clin Orthop* 1987;223:51–58.
76. Garcia JF. Arthrography. *Curr Probl Diagn Radiol* 1980;9:1.
77. Garcia, JF. Arthrographic visualization of rotator cuff tears. Optimal application of stress to the shoulder. *Radiology* 1984;150:595.
78. Ghelman B, Goldman AB. Double-contrast shoulder arthrogram: Evaluation of rotator cuff tears. *Radiology* 1977;124:251–254.
79. Gilula LA, Schoenecker PL, Murphy WA. Shoulder arthrography as a treatment modality. *AJR* 1978;131:1047–1048.
80. Goldman AB, Dines DM, Warren RF. *Shoulder arthrography: Technique, diagnosis, and clinical correlation.* Boston: Little, Brown and Co., 1982.
81. Goldman AB, Ghelman B. The double-contrast shoulder arthrogram. A review of 158 studies. *Radiology* 1978;127:655–663.
82. Ha'eri GB. Ruptures of the rotator cuff. *Can Med Assoc J* 1980;123:620–627.
83. Ha'eri GB, Maitland A. Arthroscopic findings in the frozen shoulder. *J Rheumatol* 1981;8:149–152.
84. Hall FM. Morbidity from shoulder arthrography. Etiology, evidence, and prevention. *AJR* 1981;136:56–62.
85. Harke AT, Grissom LE, Finkelstein MS. Evaluation of the musculoskeletal system with sonography. *AJR* 1988;150:1253–1261.
86. Hatfield MK, Gross BH, Glazer GM, Martel W. Computed tomography of the sternum at its articulation. *Skel Radiol* 1984;11:197–203.
87. Haynor DR, Shuman WP. Double contrast CT arthrography of the glenoid labrum and shoulder girdle. *Radiographics* 1984;4:411–421.
88. Holder J, Fretz CJ, Terrier F, Gerber C. Rotator cuff tears: Correlation of sonographic and surgical findings. *Radiology* 1988;169:791–794.
89. Holt RG, Helms CA, Steinbach L, Neumann C, Mink PL, Genant HK. Magnetic resonance imaging of the shoulder: Rationale and current applications. *Skel Radiol* 1990;19:5–14.
90. Johnson LL. *Arthroscopic surgery: Principles and practice,* 3rd ed. St. Louis: C.V. Mosby Co., 1986.
91. Kilcoyne RF, Matsen FA II. Rotator cuff tear measurement by arthropneumotomography. *AJR* 1983;140:315–318.
92. Killoran PJ, Marcove RC, Breiberger RH. Shoulder arthrography. *AJR* 1968;103:658–668.
93. Kleinman PK, Kanzaria PK, Goss TP, Pappas AM. Axillary arthrotomography of the glenoid labrum. *AJR* 1984;141:993–999.
94. Kotzen LM. Roentgen diagnosis of rotator cuff tears. *AJR* 1971;112:507–511.
95. Kummel BM. Arthrography in anterior capsular derangements of the shoulder. *Clin Orthop* 1972;83:170–176.
96. Lie S, Mast WA. Subacromial bursography. *Radiology* 1982;144:626–630.
97. McGlynn FJ, El-Koury G, Albright JP. Arthrotomography of the glenoid labrum in shoulder instability. *J Bone Joint Surg* 1982;64A:506–518.
98. McLaughlin HL. Rupture of the rotator cuff. *J Bone Joint Surg* 1963;44A:979–983.
99. McNiesh LM, Callaghan JJ. CT arthrotomography of the shoulder: Variations of the glenoid labrum. *AJR* 1987;149:963–966.
100. Middleton WD, Reinus WR, Totty WG, Madson CL, Murphy WA. Ultrasonographic evaluation of the rotator cuff and biceps tendon. *J Bone Joint Surg* 1986;68A:440–450.
101. Mikasa M. Subacromial bursography. *J Jap Orthop Assoc* 1979;53:225.
102. Mink JH, Richardson H, Grant TT. Evaluation of the glenoid labrum by double-contrast arthrography. *AJR* 1979;133:883–887.
103. Mosely HF, Goldie I. Arterial pattern of the rotator cuff. *J Bone Joint Surg* 1963;48B:780–789.
104. Nance PF, Jones TR, Kaye JJ. Dissecting synovial cysts of the shoulder. A complication of chronic rotator cuff tars. *AJR* 1982;138:739.
105. Neer CS II. Anterior acromioplasty for the chronic impingement syndrome in the shoulder. *J Bone Joint Surg* 1972;54A:41.
106. Nelson CL, Burton RI. Upper extremity arthrography. *Clin Orthop* 1975;107:72.
107. Neviaser JS. Adhesive capsulitis of the shoulder. *J Bone Joint Surg* 1953;27:211–222.
108. Neviaser JS. Arthrography of the shoulder joint. Study of the findings in adhesive capsulitis. *J Bone Joint Surg* 1962;44A:1321–1330.
109. Neviaser RJ. Tears of the rotator cuff. *Orthop Clin North Am* 1980;11:295–303.
110. Nixon JE, DiStefano VS. Rupture of the rotator cuff. *Orthop Clin North Am* 1975;6:423–449.
111. Nixon JR, Young WS. Arthrography of the shoulder in anterior dislocations: A study of African and Asian patients. *Injury* 1978;9:287.
112. O'Donoghue DH. Subluxing biceps tendon in the athlete. *Clin Orthop* 1982;164:26.
113. Older MWJ, McIntyre JL, Lloyd GJ. Distension arthrography of the shoulder joint. *Can J Surg* 1976;19:203.
114. Pastershank SP. The effect of water-soluble contrast medium on the synovial membrane. *Radiology* 1982;143:331–334.
115. Preston BJ, Jackson JP. Investigation of shoulder disability by arthrography. *Clin Radiol* 1977;28:259–266.
116. Rafii M, Finoznia H, Sherman O, et al. Rotator cuff lesions: Signal patterns at MR imaging. *Radiology* 1990;177:817–823.
117. Rathburn JB, McNab I. Microvascular pattern of the rotator cuff. *J Bone Joint Surg* 1970;52B:540–553.
118. Reeves B. The natural history of frozen shoulder syndrome. *Scand J Rheum* 1975;4:193–196.
119. Resnick D. Arthrography, tenography, and bursography. In: Resnick D, Niwayama G, eds. *Diagnosis of bone and joint disorders.* Philadelphia: W.B. Saunders, 1988.
120. Resnick D. Shoulder arthrography. *Radiol Clin North Am* 1981;19:243–255.
121. Rothman RH, Park WW. Vascular anatomy of the rotator cuff. *Clin Orthop* 1965;41:176.
122. Samolson RC, Binder WF. Symptomatic full thickness tears of the rotator cuff. *Orthop Clin North Am* 1975;6:449–466.
123. Schneider R, Ghelman B, Kaye JJ. A simplified technique for shoulder arthrography. *Radiology* 1975;114:738–739.
124. Shuman WB, Kilcoyne RF, Matsen FA, Rogers JV, Mack LA. Double-contrast computed tomography of the glenoid labrum. *AJR* 1983;141:581–584.
125. Simmonds FA. Shoulder pain with particular reference of "frozen" shoulder. *J Bone Joint Surg* 1949;31B:834–838.
126. Singson RD, Feldman F, Bigliani L. CT arthrographic patterns in recurrent glenohumeral instability. *AJR* 1987;149:749–753.
127. Singson RD, Feldman F, Bigliani LU, Rosenberg ZS. Recurrent shoulder dislocation after surgical repair: Double-contrast CT arthrography. *Radiology* 1987;164:425–428.
128. Stiles RG, Resnick D, Sartoris DJ, Andre MP. Rotator cuff

disruption: Diagnosis with digital arthrography. *Radiology* 1988;168:705–707.

129. Strizak AM, Torrance LD, Jackson W, et al. Subacromial bursography. An anatomical and clinical study. *J Bone Joint Surg* 1982;64A:196–201.

130. Weiner DS, MacNab I. Superior migration of the humeral head: A radiographic aid to diagnosis of rotator cuff tear. *J Bone Joint Surg* 1970;52B:524–527.

131. Weston WJ. Arthrography of the acromioclavicular joint. *Australas Radiol* 1974;18:213–214.

132. Weston WJ. The subdeltoid bursa. *Australas Radiol* 1973;17:214.

133. Wolfgang GL. Rupture of the musculotendinous cuff of the shoulder. *Clin Orthop* 1978;134:230–243.

134. Wright V, Haj AM. Periarthritis of the shoulder. *Assoc Rheum Dis* 1975;35:220–226.

135. Zachrisson BE, Ejeskar A. Arthrography in dislocation of the acromioclavicular joint. *Acta Radiol (Diagn)* 1979;20:81–87.

136. Zlatkin MB, Iannotti JP, Roberts MC, et al. Rotator cuff disease: Diagnostic performance of MR imaging. *Radiology* 1989; 172:223–229.

137. Zlatkin MB, Dalinka MK. The glenohumeral joint. *Top Magn Reson Imag* 1989;1(3):1–13.

Trauma

138. Allman FL. Fractures and ligamentous injuries of the clavicle and its articulations. *J Bone Joint Surg* 1967;49A:774–784.

139. Arndt JH, Sears AD. Posterior dislocation of the shoulder. *AJR* 1965;94:639–645.

140. Arner O, Sandahl U, Ohrling H. Dislocation of the acromioclavicular joint: A review of the literature and report of 56 cases. *Acta Chir Scand* 1957;113:140–152.

141. Aston JW Jr, Gregory CF. Dislocation of the shoulder with significant fracture of the glenoid. *J Bone Joint Surg* 1973;55A:1531–1533.

142. Bankart ASB. Recurrent or habitual dislocation of the shoulder joint. *Br Med J* 1923;2:1132–1133.

143. Bearden JM, Hughston JC, Whatley GS. Acromioclavicular dislocation: Method of treatment. *J Sports Med* 1973;1:5–17.

144. Benchetrit E, Friedman B. Fracture of the coracoid process associated with subglenoid dislocation of the shoulder. *J Bone Joint Surg* 1979;61A:295–298.

145. Bosworth BM. Complete acromioclavicular dislocation. *N Engl J Med* 1949;241:221–225.

146. Boyer DW Jr. Trapshooter's shoulder: Stress fracture of the coracoid process. *J Bone Joint Surg* 1975;57A:862.

147. Buckerfield CT, Castle ME. Acute traumatic retrosternal dislocation of the clavicle. *J Bone Joint Surg* 1984;66A:379–384.

148. Castagno AA, Shuman AA, Kilcoyne RF, Haynor DR, Morris ME, Matson FA. Complex fractures of the proximal humerus: Role of CT in treatment. *Radiology* 1987;165:759–762.

149. Cisternino SJ, Rogers LF, Stuffleban BC, Kruglik GD. The trough line: A radiographic sign of posterior dislocation. *AJR* 1978;130:951–954.

150. Codman EA. *The shoulder: Rupture of the supraspinatus tendon and other lesions in or about the subacromial bursa.* Boston: Thomas Todd, 1934.

151. Cope R, Riddervold HO. Posterior dislocation of the sternoclavicular joint: Report of two cases with emphasis on the radiologic management and early diagnosis. *Skel Radiol* 1988;17:247–258.

152. Dennis DA, Ferlic DC, Clayton ML. Acromial stress fractures associated with cuff-tear arthropathy. *J Bone Joint Surg* 1986;68A:937–940.

153. DePalma AF, Cantilli RA. Fractures of the upper end of the humerus. *Clin Orthop* 1961;20:73–93.

154. DePalma AF, Cooke AJ, Prabhakar M. The role of the subscapularis in recurrent anterior dislocation of the shoulder. *Clin Orthop* 1967;54:35–49.

155. Downey EF Jr, Cartes DJ, Bower AC. Unusual dislocations of the shoulder. *AJR* 1983;140:1207–1210.

156. Earwaker J. Isolated avulsion fracture of the lesser tuberosity of the humerus. *Skel Radiol* 1990;19:121–125.

157. Fronek J, Warren RF, Bowin M. Posterior subluxation of the glenohumeral joint. *J Bone Joint Surg* 1989;71A:205–216.

158. Goldberg RP, Vicks B. Oblique angled view for coracoid fractures. *Skeletal Radiol* 1983;9:195–197.

159. Hall RH, Isaac E, Booth CR. Dislocation of the shoulder with special reference to accompanying small fractures. *J Bone Joint Surg* 1959;41A:489–494.

160. Harris RD, Harris JH. The prevalence and significance of missed scapular fractures in blunt chest trauma. *AJR* 1988;151:747–750.

161. Hawkins RJ, Neer CS II, Mendoza FX. Locked posterior dislocation of the shoulder. *J Bone Joint Surg* 1987;69A:9–18.

162. Hawkins RJ, Bell RH, Gurr K. The three-part fracture of the proximal part of the humerus. *J Bone Joint Surg* 1986;68A:1410–1414.

163. Hawkins RJ, Koppert G, Johnston G. Recurrent posterior instability (subluxation) of the shoulder. *J Bone Joint Surg* 1984;66A:169–174.

164. Hayes JM, Van Winkle GN. Axillary artery injury with minimally displaced fracture of the neck of the humerus. *J Trauma* 1983;23:431–433.

165. Hill AA, Sachs MD. The grooved defect of the humeral head—a frequently unrecognized complication of dislocations of the shoulder joint. *Radiology* 1940;35:690–701.

166. Horak J, Nilsson BE. Epidemiology of fractures of the upper end of the humerus. *Clin Orthop* 1975;112:250–253.

167. Hovelius L. Anterior dislocation of the shoulder in teenagers and young adults. *J Bone Joint Surg* 1987;69A:393–399.

168. Janecki CJ, Barnett DC. Fracture-dislocation of the shoulder with biceps tendon interposition. *J Bone Joint Surg* 1979; 61A:141–143.

169. Keats TE, Pope TL. The acromioclavicular joint: Normal variation and diagnosis of dislocation. *Skel Radiol* 1988;17:159–162.

170. Kilcoyne RF, Shuman WP, Matsen FA III, Rockwood CA. The Neer classification of displaced proximal humeral fracture: Spectrum of findings on plain radiographs and CT scans. *AJR* 1990;154:1029–1033.

171. Kristiansen B, Andersen ULS, Olsen CV, Vanmarken J. The Neer classification of fractures of the proximal humerus. An assessment of interobserver variation. *Skel Radiol* 1988;17:420–422.

172. Kummel BM. Fracture of the glenoid causing chronic dislocation of the shoulder. *Clin Orthop* 1970;69:189–191.

173. Linson MA. Axillary artery thrombosis after fracture of the humerus. *J Bone Joint Surg* 1980;62A:1214–1215.

174. Lourie JA. Tomography in diagnosis of posterior dislocation of the sterno-clavicular joint. *Acta Orthop Scand* 1980;51:579–580.

175. Lyons FA, Rockwood CA. Migration of pins used in operations on the shoulder. *J Bone Joint Surg* 1990;72A:1262–1267.

176. Manske DJ, Szabo RM. The operative treatment of mid-shaft clavicular non-unions. *JBJS* 1985;67A:1367–1371.

177. Mariani PP. Isolated fracture of the coracoid process in an athlete. *Am J Sports Med* 1980;8:129–130.

178. McKenzie JJM. Retrosternal dislocation of the clavicle. *J Bone Joint Surg* 1963;45B:138–141.

179. McLaughlin HL. Posterior dislocations of the shoulder. *J Bone Joint Surg* 1952;34A:584–590.

180. McLaughlin HL, MacLellan DI. Recurrent anterior dislocation of the shoulder. II. A comparative study. *J Trauma* 1967;7:191–201.

181. Miller DS, Boswick JA. Lesions of the brachial plexus associated with fractures of the clavicle. *Clin Orthop* 1969;64:144–149.

182. Moseley HF. The basic lesions of recurrent anterior dislocation. *Surg Clin North Am* 1963;43:1631–1634.

183. Natter PD. Coracoclavicular articulation. *J Bone Joint Surg* 1941;23:177.

184. Nedecker A, Cooke GM. Hill-Sachs deformity with an unusually large defect. *J Can Assoc Radiol* 1979;30:116.

185. Neer CS II. Anterior acromioplasty for the chronic impingement syndrome in the shoulder: A preliminary report. *J Bone Joint Surg* 1972;54A:41–50.

186. Neer CS II. Displaced proximal humeral fractures. Part I. Classification and evaluation. *J Bone Joint Surg* 1970;52A:1077–1089.

187. Neer CS II. Fractures of the distal clavicle with detachment of the coracoclavicular ligament in adults. *J Trauma* 1963;3:99–110.

188. Neer CS II. Fractures of the distal third of the clavicle. *Clin Orthop* 1968;58:43–50.
189. Neer CS II, Rockwood CA. Fractures and dislocations of the shoulder. In: Rockwood CA, Green DP, eds. *Fractures in adults,* vol. 1, 2nd ed. Philadelphia: J.B. Lippincott, 1975;675–985.
190. Nettles JL, Linscheid R. Sternoclavicular dislocations. *J Trauma* 1968;8:158–164.
191. Neviaser JS. The treatment of fractures of the clavicle. *Surg Clin North Am* 1963;43:1555–1563.
192. Nielsen WB. Injury to the acromioclavicular joint. *J Bone Joint Surg* 1963;45B:207.
193. Nobel W. Posterior traumatic dislocation of the shoulder. *J Bone Joint Surg* 1962;44A:523–528.
194. Omer GE. Osteotomy of the clavicle in surgical reduction of anterior sternoclavicular dislocation. *J Trauma* 1967;7:584–590.
195. Pavlov H, Freiberger RH. Fractures and dislocations about the shoulder. *Semin Roentgenol* 1978;13:85.
196. Paterson DC. Retrosternal dislocation of the clavicle. *J Bone Joint Surg* 1961;43B:90–92.
197. Post M. *The shoulder: Surgical and non-surgical management.* Philadelphia: Lea and Febiger, 1978.
198. Quinn SF, Glass TA. Post-traumatic osteolysis of the clavicle. *South Med J* 1983;76:307.
199. Reeves B. Arthrography of the shoulder. *J Bone Joint Surg* 1966;48B:424–435.
200. Resnick D. Shoulder pain. *Orthop Clin North Am* 1983;14:81.
201. Rogers LF. *Radiology of skeletal trauma.* New York: Churchill Livingstone, 1982.
202. Rokous JR, Feegin JA, Abbott HG. Modified axillary roentgenogram. A useful adjunct in diagnosis of recurrent instability of the shoulder. *Clin Orthop* 1972;82:84–86.
203. Rowe CR. Fractures of the scapula. *Surg Clin North Am* 1963;43:1565–1571.
204. Rowe CR. Prognosis in dislocation of the shoulder. *J Bone Joint Surg* 1956;38A:957–977.
205. Rowe CR. Shoulder girdle injuries. In: Cave EF. *Trauma management.* Chicago: Year Book Publishers, 1974.
206. Rowe CR, Sakellarides HT. Factors related to recurrence of anterior dislocation of the shoulder. *Clin Orthop* 1961;20:40–47.
207. Rowe CR, Zarins B, Ciullo JV. Recurrent anterior dislocation of the shoulder after surgical repair. Apparent causes of treatment failure. *J Bone Joint Surg* 1984;66A:159–168.
208. Ruberstein JD, Ebraheim NA, Kellam JF. Traumatic scapulothoracic dissociation. *Radiology* 1985;157:297–298.
209. Salvatore J. Sternoclavicular joint dislocation. *Clin Orthop* 1968;58:51–55.
210. Samilson RL, Prieto V. Dislocation arthropathy of the shoulder. *J Bone Joint Surg* 1983;65A:456–460.
211. Sanders JO, Lyons FA, Rockwood CA. Management of dislocations of both ends of the clavicle. *J Bone Joint Surg* 1990;72A:399–402.
212. Sandrock AR. Another sports fatigue fracture: Stress fracture of the coracoid process of the scapula. *Radiology* 1975;117:274.
213. Selesnick FH, Jablow M, Frank C, Post M. Retrosternal dislocation of the clavicle. Report of 4 cases. *J Bone Joint Surg* 1984;66A:287–291.
214. Simeone FA. Neurological complications of closed shoulder injuries. *Orthop Clin North Am* 1975;6:499.
215. Turkel SJ, Pinto MW, Marshall JL, Girgis FG. Stabilizing mechanisms preventing anterior dislocation of the glenohumeral joint. *J Bone Joint Surg* 1981;63A:1208–1217.
216. Varriale PL, Adler ML. Occult fracture of the glenoid without dislocation. *J Bone Joint Surg* 1983;65A:688.
217. Vastamaki M, Solonen KA. Posterior dislocations and fracture-dislocations of the shoulder. *Acta Orthop Scand* 1980;51:479–484.
218. White EM, Kattapuram SV, Jupiter JB. Case report 241. Post-traumatic pseudoaneurysm. *Skeletal Radiol* 1983;10:178.
219. Wilkins RM, Johnson RM. Ununited fractures of the clavicle. *J Bone Joint Surg* 1983;65A:773–778.
220. Worman LW, Leagus C. Intrathoracic injury following retrosternal dislocation of the clavicle. *J Trauma* 1967;7:416–423.
221. Yosipovitch Z, Tikva P, Goldberg I. Inferior subluxation of the humeral head after shoulder injury. *J Bone Joint Surg* 1989;71A:751–753.
222. Zenni EJ, Krieg JK, Rosen MJ. Open reduction and internal fixation of clavicular fractures. *JBJS* 1981;63A:147–151.
223. Zuckerman JD, Matsen FA. Complications about the glenohumeral joint related to the use of screws and staples. *J Bone Joint Surg* 1984;66A:175–180.

Imaging of Orthopedic Trauma, Second Edition, edited by T.H. Berquist, Mayo Clinic © 1992. Published by Raven Press, Ltd., New York.

CHAPTER 11

The Humerus and Arm

Claire E. Bender, Donald C. Campbell II, and Thomas H. Berquist

Anatomy, 659
Humeral Shaft Fractures, 663
  Mechanism of Injury and Classification, 663
  Radiologic Evaluation, 666
Management of Humeral Fractures, 666

Initial Management, 666
Delayed Management, 667
Complications, 670
Soft Tissue Injuries, 673
References, 673

Humeral shaft fractures comprise 1% of all fractures (16). Most of these fractures heal with closed reduction. Radial nerve and vascular complications occur occasionally. Other soft tissue injuries, primarily muscular injuries, can occur in association with fractures or as isolated injuries (1,9).

ANATOMY

The humeral shaft extends proximally from the upper border of the insertion of the pectoralis major muscle on the greater tubercle to the supracondylar ridges distally (Figs. 11-1A and 11-2A) (4,12). On a cross-sectional view, the proximal half of the shaft is circular; the distal half flattens in the AP dimension. The humeral shaft is described as having three surfaces and three borders. The anterior border, between the anterolateral and anteromedial surfaces, begins with the crest of the greater tubercle, includes the medial edge of the deltoid tuberosity, becomes indistinct on the more flattened lower part of the body, and ends at the sharp lateral edge of the coronoid fossa. The medial border begins with the crest of the lesser tubercle (which often fades out in the midshaft) and ends as the medial supracondylar ridge. The lateral border, although poorly defined superiorly, ends as the lateral supracondylar ridge (Figs. 11-1 and 11-2).

The anterolateral surface contains the deltoid tuberos-

ity above; below, where the anterior border becomes poorly defined, the anterolateral and anteromedial surfaces tend to blend, as they both give rise to the brachialis muscle. There are no distinguishing landmarks on the anteromedial surface. The posterior surface is crossed obliquely by a shallow groove, the radial or spiral groove, which runs downward and laterally from behind the deltoid tuberosity (Fig. 11-2A) (5,12).

Anterior and posterior compartments are formed by medial and lateral intermuscular septa (Fig. 11-3). The biceps brachii, brachialis, and coracobrachialis are muscles included in the anterior compartment; the posterior compartment includes the triceps (12,13).

A relatively common variation in the distal humerus is the supracondylar process (Fig. 11-4). It represents an anomalous beaklike projection of variable size along the anteromedial surface of the humerus about 5 cm above the medial epicondyle. A well-developed supracondylar process is often connected to the medial epicondyle by a fibrous band, the ligament of Struthers. Fracture of the supracondylar process is clinically important, as it may result in damage to the median nerve and brachial artery, which pass beneath it (12).

The muscles of the arm are the biceps brachii, coracobrachialis, brachialis muscles anteriorly and the triceps and anconeus posteriorly. Of these muscles, the brachialis and medial and lateral heads of triceps arise from the humeral shaft. Only the coracobrachialis inserts on the shaft of the humerus (see Figs. 11-1B and 11-2B).

The musculocutaneous nerve supplies the anterior compartment arm muscles. Posteriorly the radial nerve supplies the triceps. In the upper arm, the radial nerve lies behind the axillary artery and on the front of the long

C. E. Bender, D. C. Campbell II: Departments of Diagnostic Radiology and Orthopedic Surgery, Mayo Medical School, Mayo Clinic, Rochester, Minnesota 55905.
T. H. Berquist: Department of Diagnostic Radiology, Mayo Medical School, Mayo Clinic Jacksonville, Jacksonville, Florida 32224.

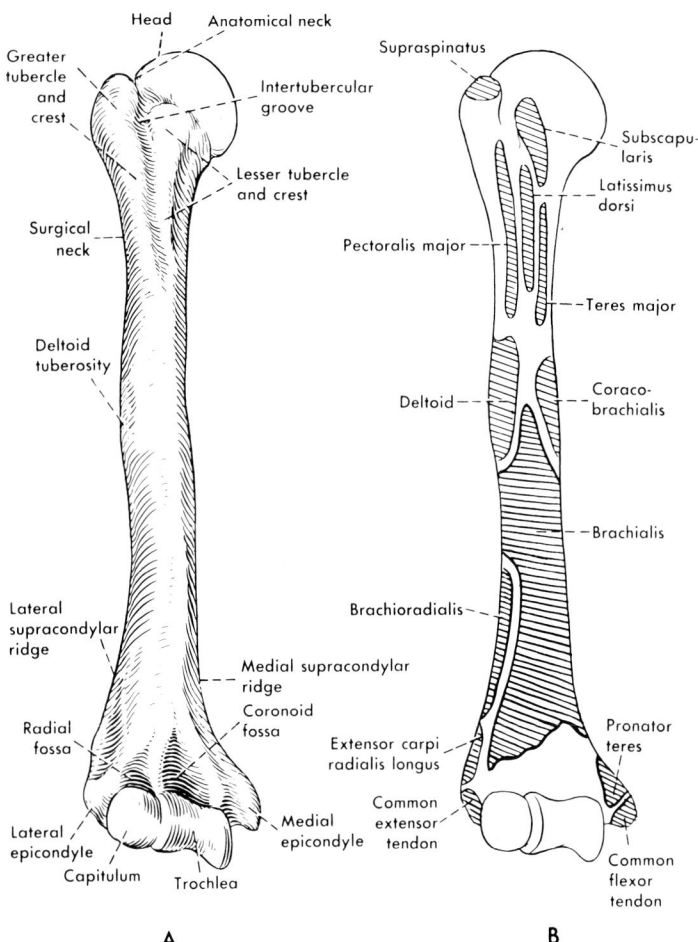

FIG. 11–1. Anterior humerus and muscle insertions. **A:** Bony landmarks of the humerus. **B:** Muscle insertions (from 12).

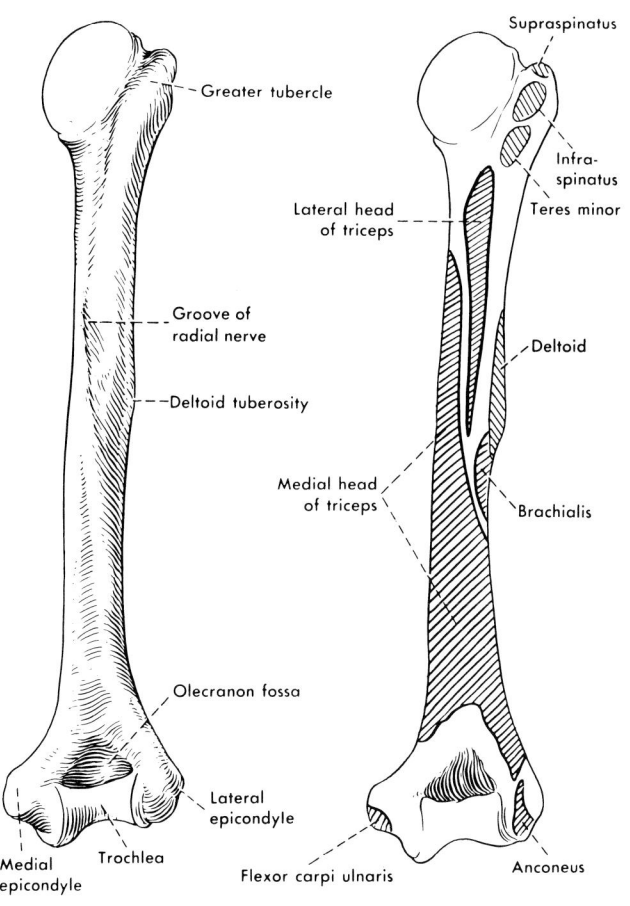

FIG. 11-2. Posterior humerus and muscle insertions. **A:** Bony landmarks. **B:** Muscle insertions (from 12).

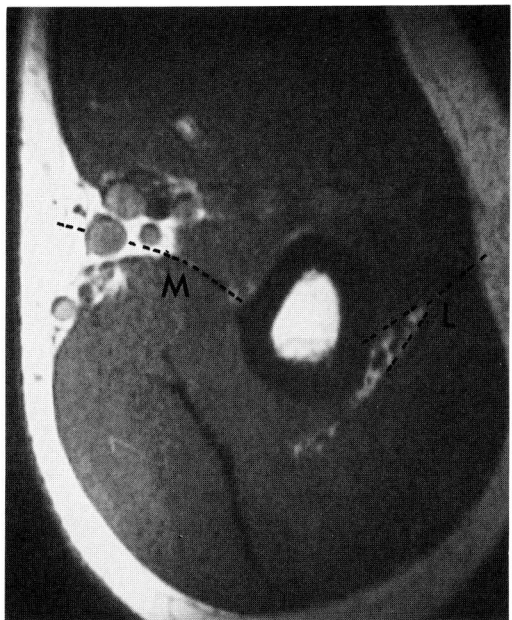

FIG. 11-3. Axial MR image demonstrating the medial and lateral intermuscular septae (*dotted lines*). M, medial; L, lateral.

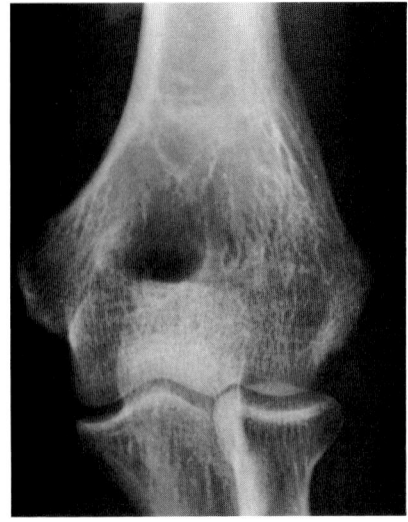
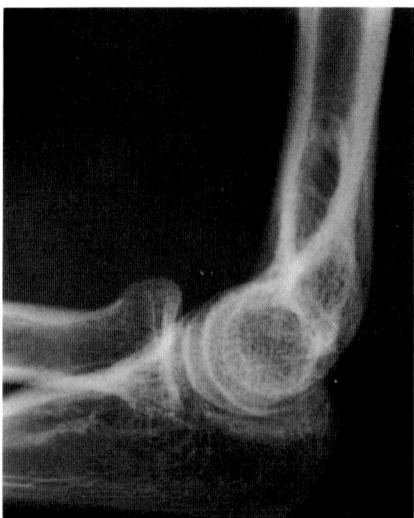

FIG. 11-4. Supracondylar process seen on AP (**A**) and lateral (**B**) views.

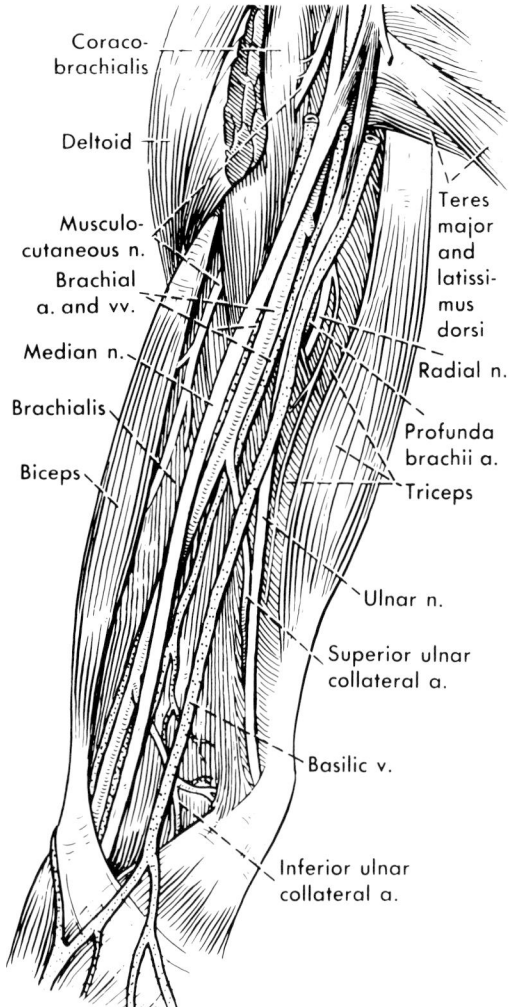

Coraco-
brachialis

Deltoid

Musculo-
cutaneous n.

Brachial
a. and vv.

Median n.

Brachialis

Biceps

Teres
major
and
latissi-
mus
dorsi

Radial n.

Profunda
brachii a.

Triceps

Ulnar n.

Superior ulnar
collateral a.

Basilic v.

Inferior ulnar
collateral a.

FIG. 11-5. Major vessels and nerves of the arm (from 12).

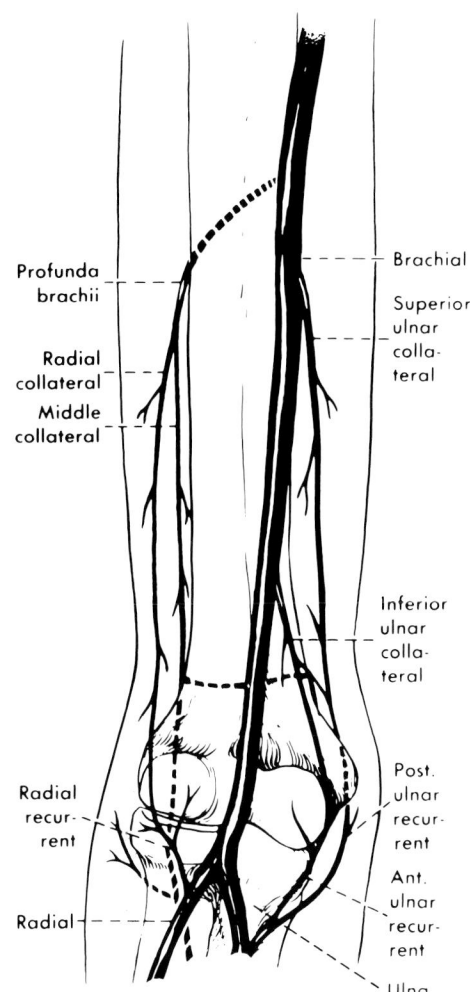

FIG. 11-6. Brachial artery and its branches (from 12).

The brachial artery roughly parallels the shaft of the humerus. At the lower border of the teres major, the axillary artery becomes the brachial artery. Proximally, the artery lies first on the medial side of the arm in front of the long head of the triceps and then on the medial head of the triceps (Fig. 11-6). As it continues distally, it slopes forward along the medial border of the biceps to lie on the anterior surface of the brachialis muscle. It then passes into the cubital fossa, where it divides into the radial and ulnar arteries. The brachial artery is usually accompanied by two brachial veins, one lying medial and one lateral to it, but with numerous anastomoses between them.

Branches of the brachial artery in the arm include the profunda brachii, the nutrient artery of the humerus, and the superior and ulnar collateral arteries (Fig. 11-6).

Blood is supplied to the humerus from branches of the brachial artery, including one or more nutrient arteries, and from the vessels intimately associated with the ends of the bone. The chief nutrient artery of the humerus is a slender branch that arises from the brachial artery (or sometimes from the superior ulnar collateral) about the middle of the arm, which enters the anteromedial surface of the humerus. The nutrient artery foramen travels inferiorly and obliquely. Its external end is usually located in the middle third of the bone, but it may vary considerably, appearing anywhere from a position at the inferior level of deltoid tuberosity to the junction of the mid- and lower third of the humerus (5,12).

The profunda brachii artery is the largest branch vessel in the arm. Usually it originates on the posteromedial side of the brachial artery in the upper arm and runs downward and laterally behind the brachial artery to parallel the radial nerve in a spiral around the humerus. It passes deep to the long head of the triceps, then deep to the lateral head, and then between it in the medial head of the triceps. At the level of the lateral intermuscular septum, the profunda divides into the radial and middle collateral arteries. The profunda brachii artery usually gives off a nutrient branch to the body of the humerus as it starts its course around the bone. Usually this nutrient branch enters the bone above and medial to the radial groove. It may be the largest nutrient artery of the humerus (5,12).

HUMERAL SHAFT FRACTURES

Mechanism of Injury and Classification

There are several unique features of the humerus that present special problems in fracture treatment. First, the humerus is the most freely movable long bone. Scapulohumeral motion can amplify its motions. Second, the humerus functions as a lever; therefore, nearly all stress to the bone is in tension from or is at an angle to the long

head of the triceps. It then passes laterally and posteriorly with the profunda brachii artery, deep to the long head of the triceps. As it passes along the posterior aspect of the humerus, it moves between the lateral and medial heads of the triceps. The radial nerve is positioned close to, but not actually in, the spiral groove. The nerve then pierces the lateral intermuscular septum (along with the radial collateral branch of the brachial artery) to pass forward and distally in close association with the brachialis (12).

Usually the median and ulnar nerves do not supply any muscles of the arm. The median nerve is formed anterior or anterolateral to the brachial artery. It then descends lateral or anterolateral to the artery to the midshaft level. Thereafter, it usually crosses in front of the artery to lie on the medial side and passes down to the cubital fossa. The ulnar nerve lies medial or posterior to the brachial artery in the upper arm. At the midarm level, it pierces the medial intermuscular septum to lie in front of the medial head of the triceps. It courses inferiorly with the superior ulnar collateral artery (Fig. 11-5) (5,12).

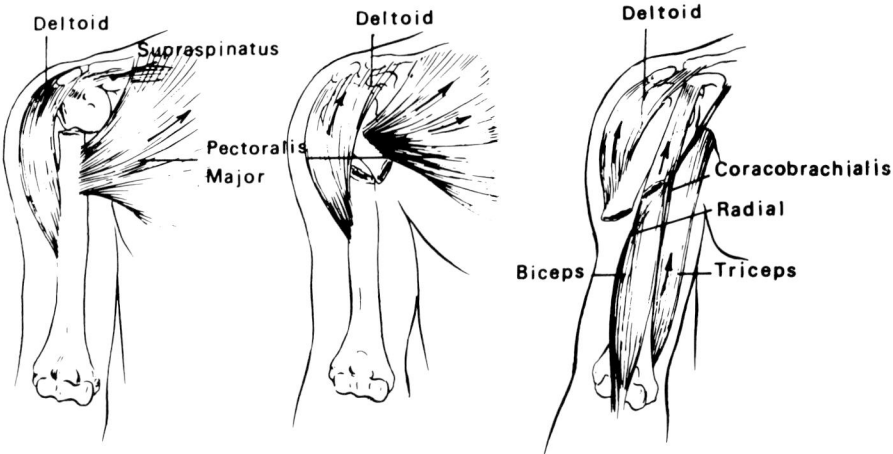

FIG. 11-7. Muscle forces on humeral shaft fractures (from 5).

axis of the bone. Thus, weight-bearing or compression forces are not problems in fracture management. Finally, when the patient is upright, the bone hangs vertically and thus is influenced by gravity alone, allowing realignment of fracture fragments (3,13).

The location of the fracture and its relationship to muscle attachments will affect the direction of displacement of bone fragments. Fractures of the proximal third (between the pectoralis major and deltoid insertions) result in medial displacement of the proximal fragment owing to the pull of the pectoralis major muscle. Fractures distal to the deltoid tuberosity result in abduction of the proximal fragment from pull by the deltoid and proximal displacement of the distal fragment from pull by the brachialis and biceps (Fig. 11-7).

Direct force, from either blunt or penetrating injury, is the most frequent cause of fracture of the humeral shaft. A transverse fracture is the result of a bending force; a spiral fracture results from a combination of bending and torsion forces (5). Compression forces acting on the humerus tend to affect either end but not the shaft (5). Indirect forces, such as falling directly on the elbow or on an outstretched hand, vigorous throwing of objects, or even violent muscle contraction can also result in fracture of the humeral shaft (5,8,22).

Depending on the age of the patient and the type of injury, the fracture can be open or closed, complete or incomplete, simple or comminuted (5).

The level of the fracture is described as being in the upper, middle, or lower third of the shaft (Fig. 11-8). In

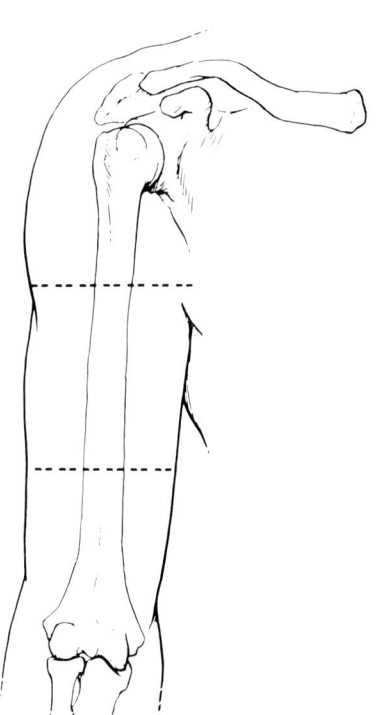

FIG. 11-8. Levels of humeral fractures. For purposes of description, the shaft is divided into upper, middle, and distal thirds.

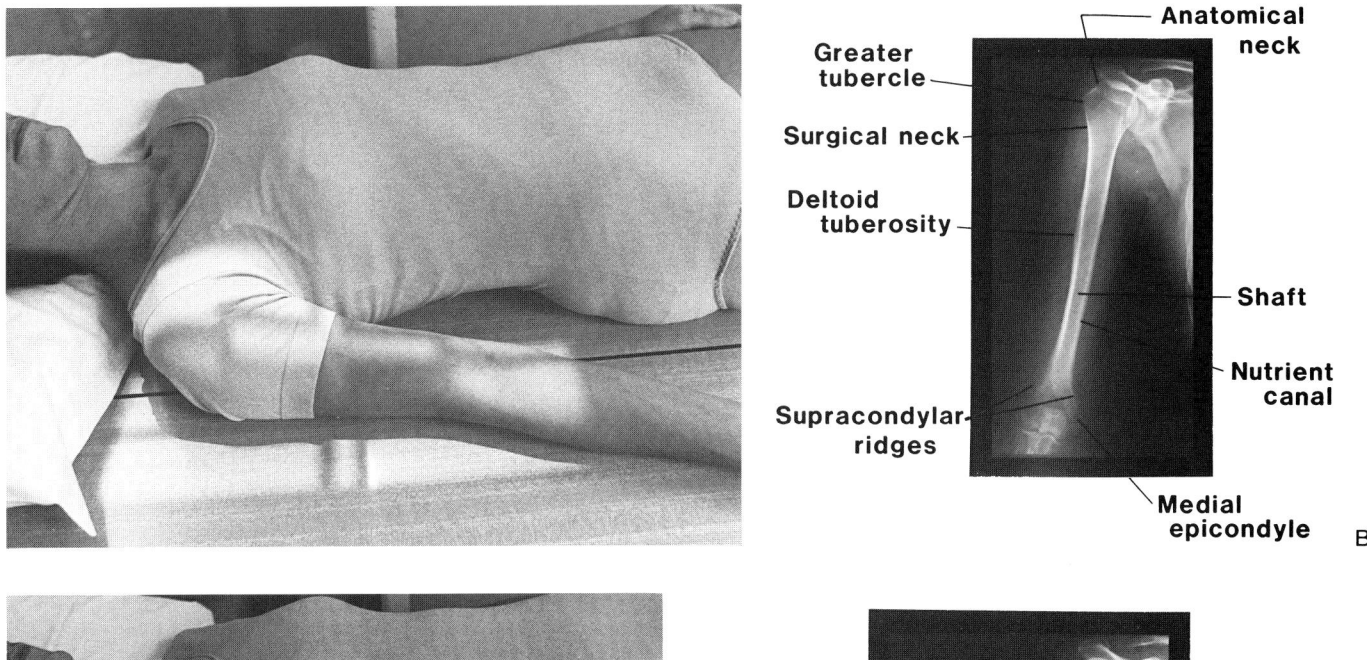

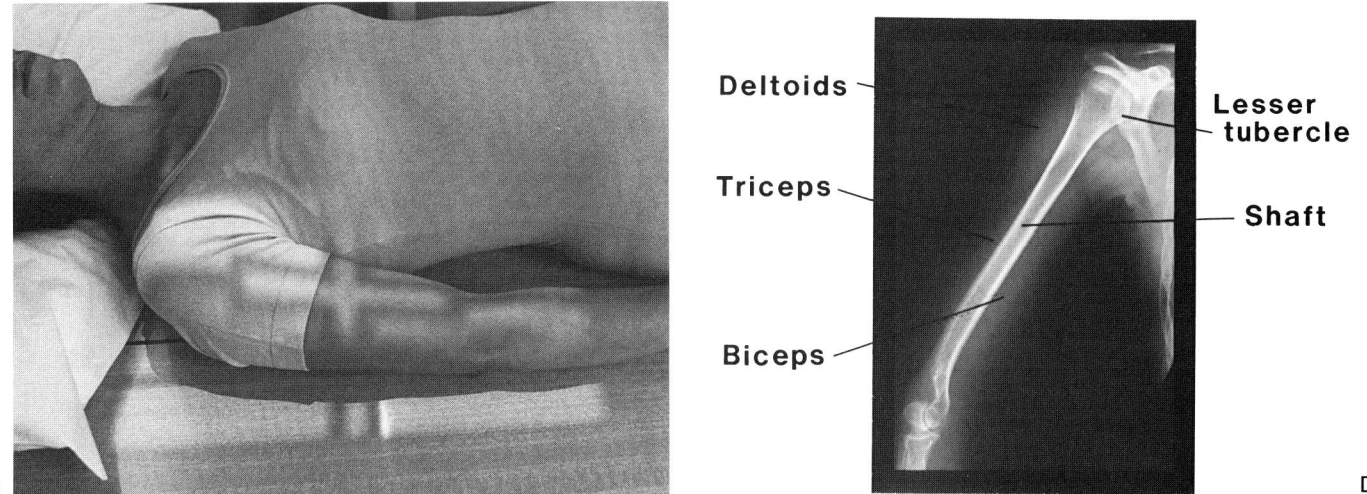

FIG. 11-9. Standard radiographs of the humerus. **A:** Patient positioned for AP radiograph of the humerus. The film is centered on the mid-shaft with both the elbow and shoulder included on the film. **B:** AP radiograph of the humerus. **C:** Patient positioned for lateral view of the humerus. The forearm is pronated. **D:** Radiograph of the humerus.

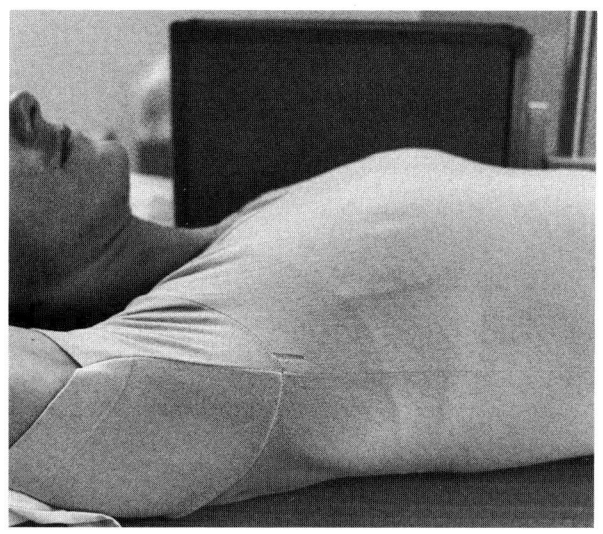

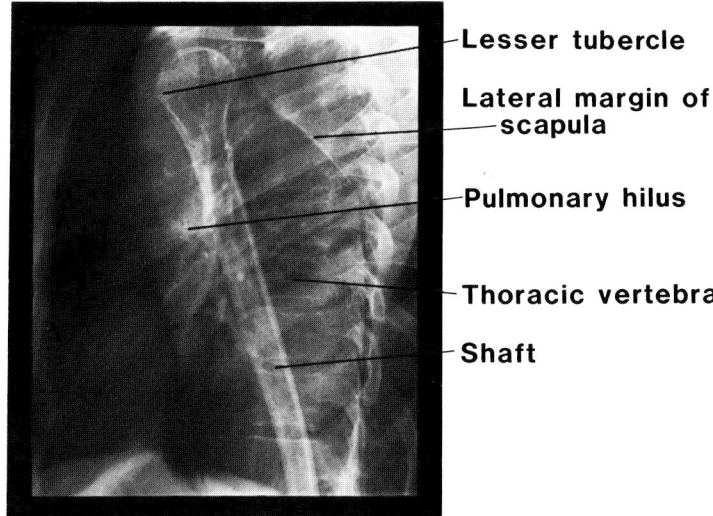

Lesser tubercle

Lateral margin of scapula

Pulmonary hilus

Thoracic vertebra

Shaft

A

B

FIG. 11–10. A: Patient positioned for transthoracic view. The unaffected arm is elevated. **B:** Radiograph taken with transthoracic technique.

Mast's series of 240 patients, 69% of the fractures occurred at midshaft level (17). Of the total fractures, 61% were transverse, 18% were oblique, 17% were spiral, and 4% were segmental. Severe comminution occurred in 12% (17).

Fractures at the junction of the middle and distal thirds of the humeral shaft may be particularly troublesome. Injury to the main nutrient artery may contribute to delayed union or non-union. Holstein and Lewis have emphasized that the radial nerve is at great risk of entrapment in the fracture because it passes close to the bone near the lateral supracondylar ridge (14). The mobility of the nerve is reduced as it passes through the lateral intermuscular septum. Closed reduction may damage the nerve. For this reason, open reduction and internal fixation of these fractures is recommended, especially if there is any evidence of radial nerve paresis (5,7,11).

Radiologic Evaluation

Standard recumbent views include the AP and lateral projections (Fig. 11-9). The selected film must be long enough to include both the shoulder and elbow joints. This is necessary in order to exclude associated injuries as well as to assist in determining the position in which the film was obtained. All films are obtained using the Potter-Bucky technique. For the AP projection, the arm is placed at the patient's side with the elbow extended and hand supinated (Fig. 11-9A). This places the epicondyles parallel to the plane of the film.

The lateral projection is obtained with the elbow extended and hand pronated (Fig. 11-9C). If the patient is

in a hanging cast or splint, the arm is abducted slightly and internally rotated. The hand will then be over the abdomen.

The central ray of the x-ray beam is directed perpendicularly to the midshaft of the humerus in the standard projections.

The transthoracic lateral projection should be obtained when additional injuries or immobilization precludes the standard lateral view. With the patient in the recumbent position, the affected extremity is placed next to the cassette. The uninjured arm is raised, resting the forearm on the head (Fig. 11-10A). This elevates the normal shoulder and depresses the injured extremity. Superimposition of the shoulders is therefore minimized. The cassette is centered at the area of interest of the humerus. The unaffected shoulder should be turned slightly posterior to visualize the injured humerus properly. The central ray is directed perpendicularly to the midpoint of the film. Film exposure is made at full inspiration in order to improve the anatomic contrast as well as to minimize the exposure factors (Fig. 11-10B). A lead apron is used for gonadal shielding.

With severe trauma, additional injury to the radius and ulna may occur. Pierce (18) described 21 cases of combined injury, with 6 cases in which the fractures were of the midshafts of all three bones. He also noted that 11 of 21 patients had acute neural injuries (18).

MANAGEMENT OF HUMERAL FRACTURES

Initial Management

Humeral shaft fractures usually heal without problems. Nevertheless, treatment must be individualized

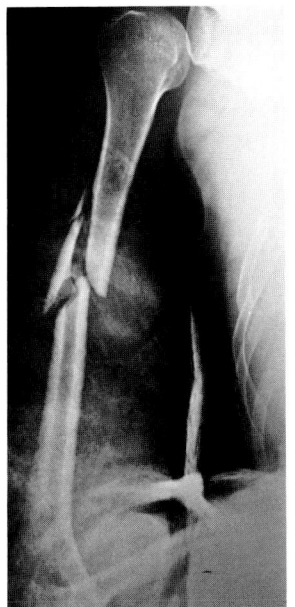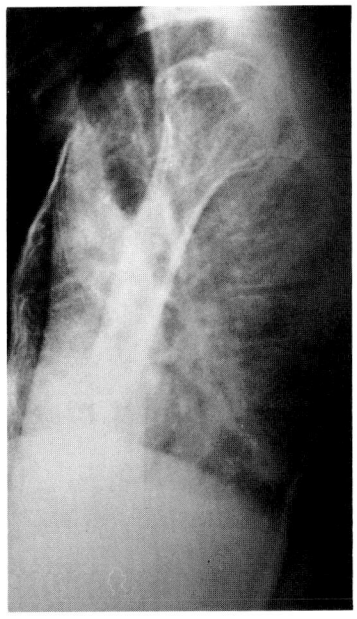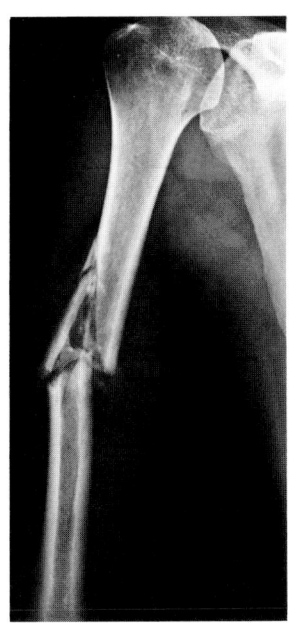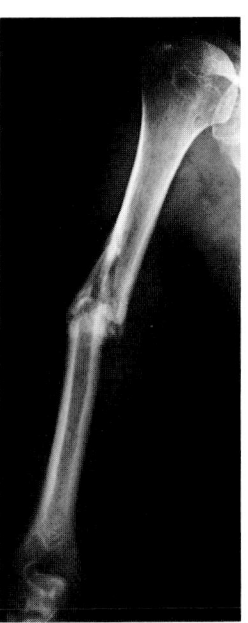

A   B   C   D

FIG. 11–11. A: AP view of comminuted fracture of the mid-shaft of the humerus in hanging cast. **B:** Transthoracic views reveal slight anterior angulation. **C:** Follow-up film in 5 weeks demonstrates healing of callus formation. **D:** Film taken 4 months after injury with healed fracture.

because of several factors. Treatment depends upon (1) the patient's age, (2) the type and level of fracture, (3) the degree of fracture displacement, (4) muscular development, and (5) associated injuries (5,13). Closed primary treatment may include (1) dependency traction (e.g., long-arm hanging cast) and (2) thoracobrachial immobilization (e.g., open Velpeau-type cast) (13). Abduction splints or casts and various forms of functional bracing may also be used in closed primary treatment (5,13,15,17,21,22).

Perfect alignment and apposition of fracture components are not essential. Anterior angulation of up to 20° and varus angulation of up to 30° can usually be accepted without compromising function or appearance (15). However, the closer the fracture is to the elbow joint, the more important alignment becomes.

Immediately after initial closed reduction and immobilization, repeat radiographs are obtained in the AP and lateral (or transthoracic) views (Figs. 11-11 and 11-12). Follow-up radiographs are obtained at appropriate intervals until evidence of healing is seen.

Indications for primary operative treatment include (1) displaced transverse fractures and short oblique fractures, (2) long spiral fractures with displacement suggestive of soft tissue interposition (Fig. 11-13) (15), and (3) compound wounds and vascular complications. Mast reports vascular injury at a frequency of 3% (17).

Radial nerve paralysis secondary to injury from humeral shaft fractures does not imply the need for early operative management. Although the frequency of radial nerve injury varies from 3–16% (16), most cases of radial nerve injury resolve spontaneously (6). Exploration of the fracture and nerve may itself result in nerve injury. Since the results of late nerve repair are equal to those following early repair, it is wise to wait at least 2 weeks to evaluate nerve status further. Electromyography may become useful at this point. The incidence of median and ulnar nerve palsy is less than 3% (5,11,21).

Methods of internal fixation include plating with the option of bone grafting, which is the most common technique (Figs. 11-14 and 11-15), and use of intramedullary rods and nails. The latter help to preserve alignment and maintain length. The level of the fracture may influence the choice of internal fixation. Midshaft fractures may be treated with plates and screws or intramedullary rods. Fractures at the ends of the humeral shaft must be carefully evaluated in order to choose the best method of fixation (2,5,7,11).

Delayed Management

Delayed union (defined as clinical absence of union at 8 weeks) or nonunion may be associated with (1) poor apposition or distraction of fracture fragments, (2) initial internal fixation, (3) interference of blood supply to the humeral shaft, (4) open injury and infection, and (5) soft tissue interposition (10). Treatment of delayed union

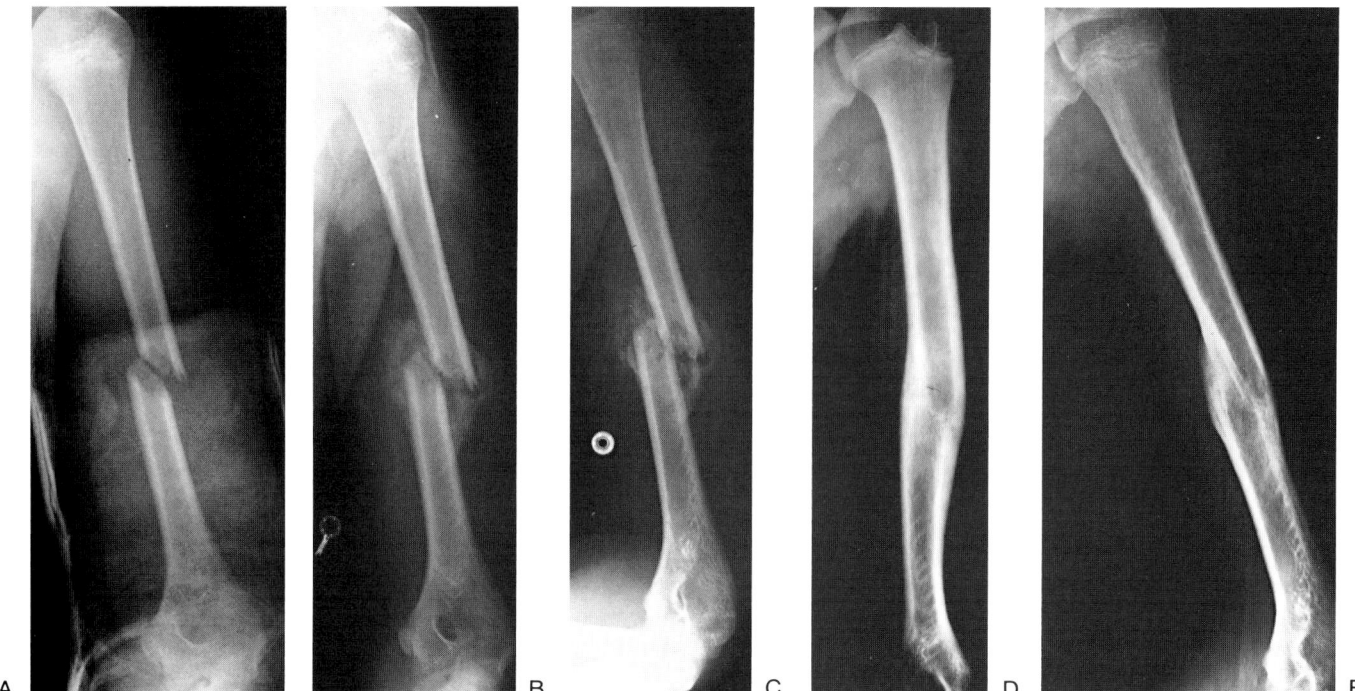

FIG. 11-12. Simple fracture of the mid-shaft of the humerus. AP view (**A**) at time of injury. AP (**B**) and lateral (**C**) views 3 weeks after injury show abundant callus. Healing is evident on the AP (**D**) and lateral (**E**) views 3 months after the fracture.

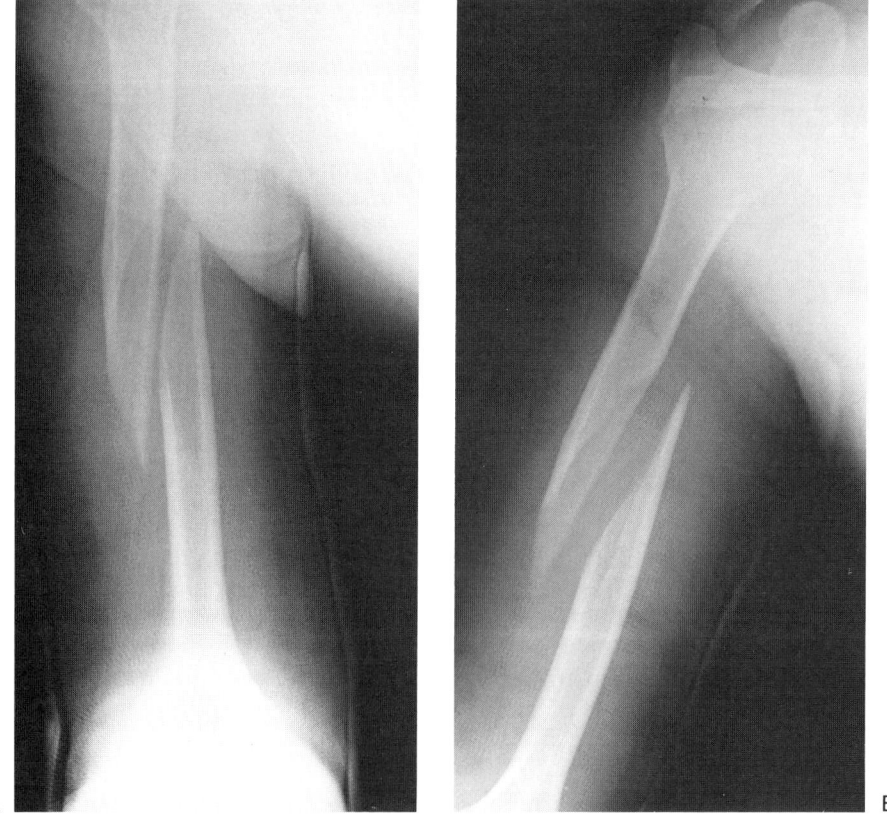

FIG. 11-13. A: AP view of the humerus demonstrating an overriding spiral midshaft fracture. Hanging cast does not reduce the fracture. Fragments were separated by soft tissue interposition.

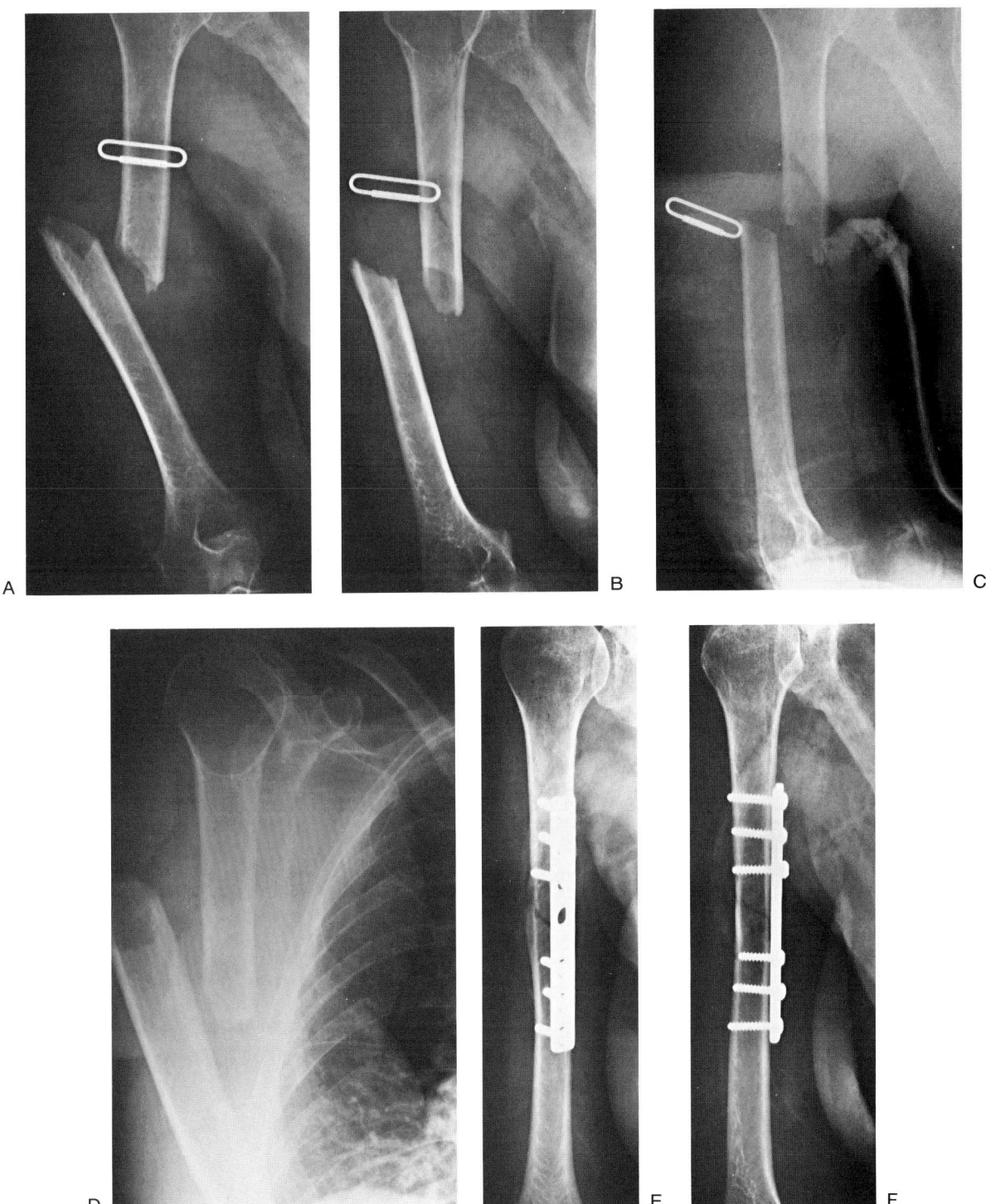

FIG. 11-14. AP (**A**) and lateral (**B**) radiographs demonstrating a short, oblique fracture of the mid humerus with significant displacement. Immediate post-reduction view (**C**) in hang cast. Three week follow-up film (**D**) shows progressive displacement and overriding of the fragments. AP (**E**) and lateral (**F**) views show good reduction with plate and screw fixation.

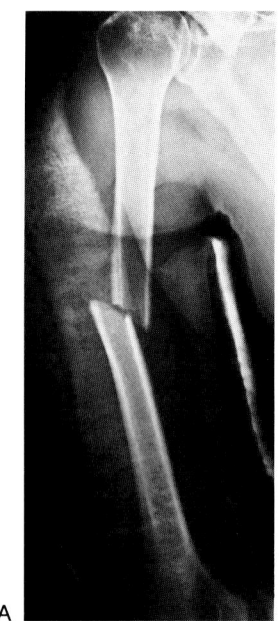 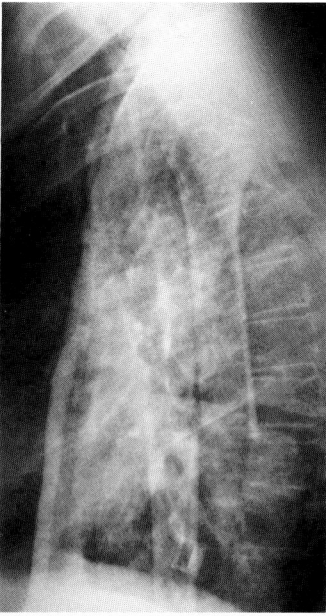 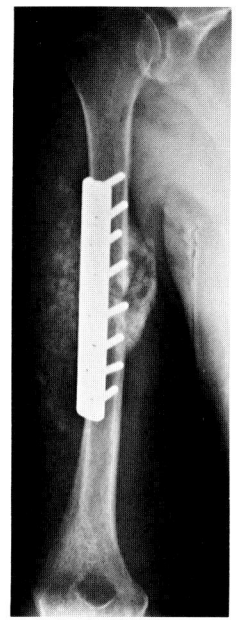 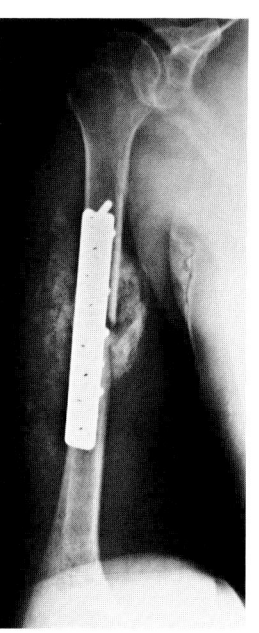

A   B   C   D

FIG. 11–15. AP (**A**) and transthoracic views (**B**) demonstrate a fracture of the mid humerus with anterior displacement of the distal fragment. The fracture was treated with bone graft and plate and screw fixation (**C, D**).

consists of further conservative measures or internal fixation. Non-union of the humerus may be treated with plating, nailing, intramedullary rod fixation, or, more rarely, external fixation devices (Fig. 11-16) (20). Delayed unions and non-unions may be complicated by osteoporosis. In such cases, it may be useful to utilize methyl methacrylate to enhance fixation of the screws and plate (Fig. 11-17).

Unstable fractures in osteoporotic bone can defeat efforts at stabilization by internal fixation as a result of loosening and migration of fixation devices (Fig. 11-18) (14).

Body-section tomography is performed for evaluation of delayed fracture healing (Fig. 11-16D). Linear or complex motion tomography is used, depending upon the presence of metallic fixation devices (see in Chapter 1, Conventional Tomography). AP and lateral views are obtained at 0.5-cm slices, depending on the thickness of the body part. A persistent fracture line is usually readily identified by this technique. Gupta and colleagues have performed osteomedullograms in cases of delayed union and non-union of diaphyseal fractures (10). While visualizing the proliferating venous endothelium across the fracture site, conservative treatment was continued, which led to complete healing in all 12 cases (10).

Complications

Delayed union, non-union, and malunion have been described above (5,11,19). Delayed union is evident with no evidence of clinical healing at eight weeks. Transverse fractures most frequently go on to non-union due to reduced bone contact and soft tissue interposition (Fig. 11-13) (5,7).

Soft tissue complications include neurovascular injury and myositis ossificans (2,5). The latter is far more common with elbow fracture/dislocation (5). Radial nerve injury occurs with 5–10% of humeral fractures. Injury may be the result of direct injury (bruising), stretching, or entrapment between fracture fragments. Radial nerve bruising or stretching usually resolves in several days. More severe injuries can result in wrist drop and require operative intervention.

Associated brachial plexus injuries can also occur with humeral fractures. These injuries can result in loss of muscle tone and sensation—flail arm (2).

Imaging evaluation of neurovascular complications may require angiography or MRI. The latter can evaluate both neural and vascular injury (1).

Bone and soft tissue infections may also develop. Open fractures are most commonly involved. Infection is discussed completely in Chapter 15.

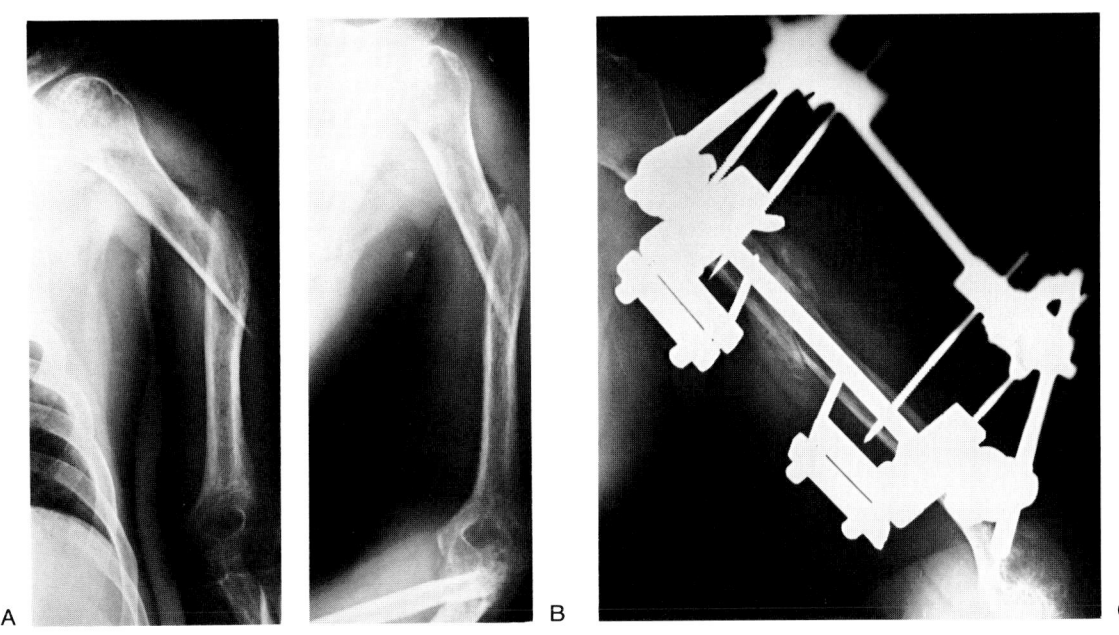

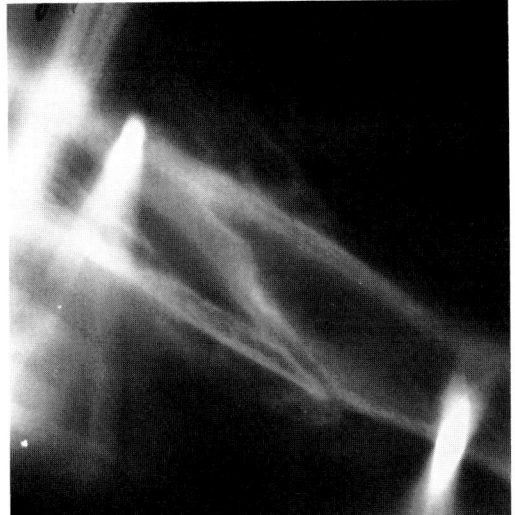

FIG. 11–16. AP (**A**) and lateral (**B**) views of an overriding ununited humeral fracture. Reduction was maintained with a Hoffman apparatus (**C**). Tomograms (**D**) demonstrate healing with early callus formation.

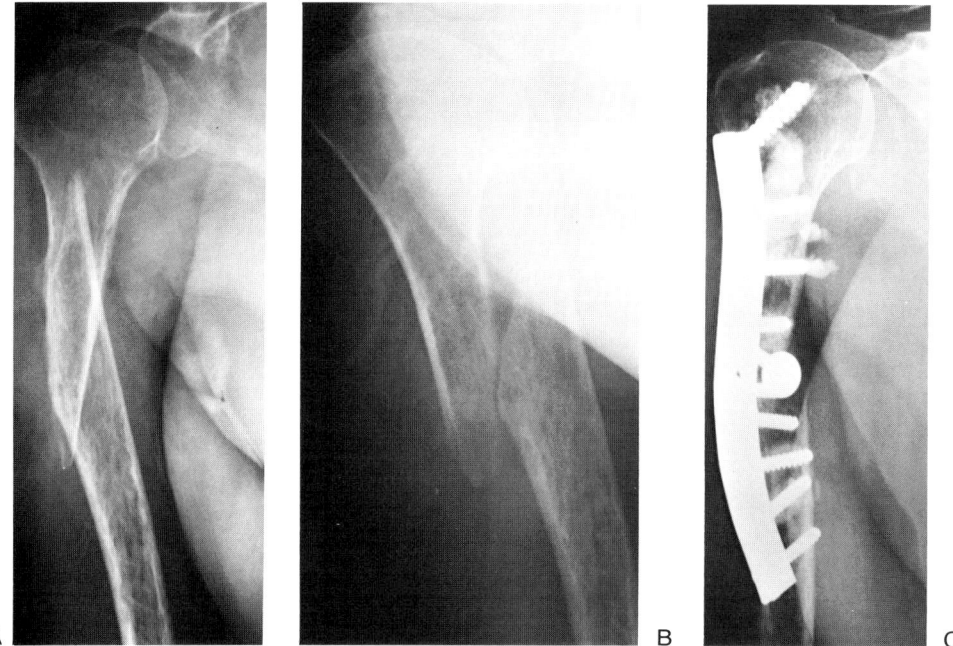

FIG. 11–17. AP (**A**) and oblique (**B**) views with an ununited fracture of the humeral shaft and osteoporosis. Stabilization with plate and screws. Methyl-methacrylate used to improve fixation of screws (**C**).

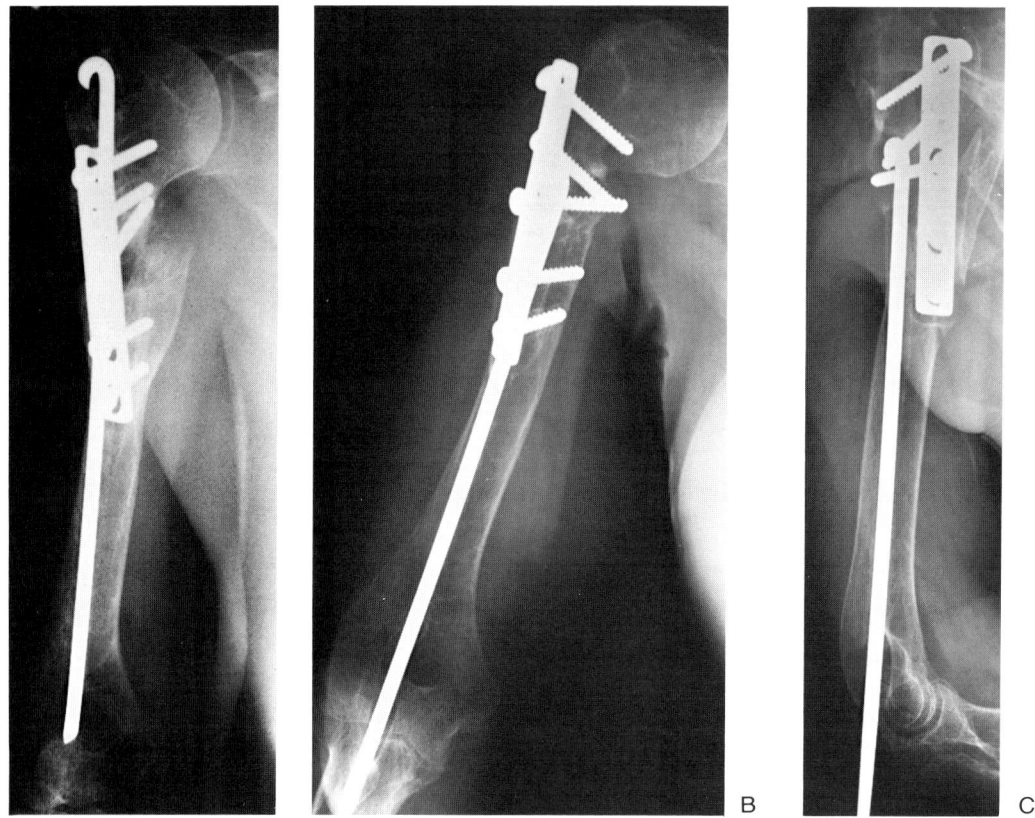

FIG. 11–18. A: Osteoporotic humerus with rush rod and plate and screw fixation of a proximal humeral fracture. Follow-up AP (**B**) and lateral (**C**) views demonstrate migration of the rod through the distal humerus and loosening of the plate and screws. The fracture is ununited.

SOFT TISSUE INJURIES

Isolated soft tissue injuries can occur with direct blows or abrupt muscle contractions. Contusions, hemorrhage, and partial or complete disruptions in muscles, ligaments, and tendons may result. These injuries are infrequent in the upper extremity compared to the lower extremities.

Choices of therapy are aided by imaging techniques. MRI is particularly useful in this regard. Axial and sagittal or coronal images can define and stage these injuries. T2-weighted sequences are most useful due to the contrast provided by signal intensity of blood and/or edema to normal muscle, ligaments, and tendons (1).

REFERENCES

1. Berquist TH. *MRI of the musculoskeletal system.* New York: Raven Press, 1990.
2. Brien WW, Gellman H, Becker V, Garland DE, Waters RL, Wiss DA. Management of fractures of the humerus in patients who have ipsilateral brachial plexus injury. *J Bone Joint Surg* 1990;72A:1208–1210.
3. Caldwell JA. Treatment of fractures of the shaft by hanging cast. *Surg Gynecol Obstet* 1940;70:421–425.
4. Christensen NO. Küntscher intramedullary reaming and nail fixation for nonunion of the humerus. *Clin Orthop* 1976;116:222–226.
5. Epps CH Jr. Fractures of the shaft of the humerus. In: Rockwood CA, Green DP eds. *Fractures in adults,* 2nd ed. Philadelphia: J.B. Lippincott, 1984;655–674.
6. Fenyo G. On fractures of the shaft of the humerus. *Acta Chir Scand* 1971;137:221–226.
7. Foster RJ, Dixon GL, Bach AW, Appleyard RW, Green TM. Internal fixation of fractures and non-unions of the humeral shaft. *J Bone Joint Surg* 1985;67A:857–864.
8. Garth WP, Leberte MA, Cool TA. Recurrent fractures of the humerus in a baseball pitcher. *J Bone Joint Surg* 1988;70A:305–306.
9. Greene TL, Louis DS. Compartment syndrome of the arm: A complication of the pneumatic tourniquet. *J Bone Joint Surg* 1983;65A:270–272.
10. Gupta RC, Kumar S, Gupta KK. A clinical evaluation of osteomedullography in diaphyseal fractures. *J Trauma* 1980;20:507–512.
11. Hall RF, Pankovick AM. Ender nailing of acute fractures of the humerus. *J Bone Joint Surg* 1987;69A:558–567.
12. Hollinshead WH. *Anatomy for surgeons,* vol. 3. *The back and limbs,* 3rd ed. New York: Harper and Row, 1982.
13. Holm CL. Management of humeral shaft fractures. *Clin Orthop* 1970;71:132–139.
14. Holstein A, Lewis GB. Fractures of the humerus with radial-nerve paralysis. *J Bone Joint Surg* 1963;45A:1382–1388.
15. Klemerman L. Fractures of the shaft of the humerus. *J Bone Joint Surg* 1966;48B:105–111.
16. Mann RJ, Neal FG. Fractures of the shaft of the humerus in adults. *South Med J* 1964;58:264–268.
17. Mast JW, Spiegel PG, Harvey JPJ, et al. Fractures of the humeral shaft. *Clin Orthop* 1975;112:254–262.
18. Pierce RO, Hodurski F. Fractures of the humerus, radius and ulna in the same extremity. *J Trauma* 1979;19:182.
19. Rooney PJ, Cockshott WP. Pseudarthrosis following proximal humeral fractures: A possible mechanism. *Skel Radiol* 1986;15:21–24.
20. Shaw JL, Sakellarides H. Radial nerve paralysis associated with fractures of the humerus. *J Bone Joint Surg* 1967;49A:889.
21. Stern PJ, Maltughy DA, Pomeroy DL, Zenni EJ, Krieg JK. Intramedullary fixation of humeral shaft fractures. *J Bone Joint Surg* 1984;66A:639–646.
22. Zagorski JB, Latta LL, Zych GA, Finnieston AR. Diaphyseal fractures of the humerus. Treatment with prefabricated braces. *J Bone Joint Surg* 1988;70A:607–610.

*Imaging of Orthopedic Trauma,
Second Edition,* edited by T.H. Berquist,
Mayo Clinic © 1992. Published
by Raven Press, Ltd., New York.

CHAPTER 12

The Elbow

Bernard F. Morrey and Thomas H. Berquist

Anatomy, 675
Imaging Techniques, 680
   Routine Radiographic Techniques, 680
   Assessment of Standard Radiographic Views, 685
   Arthrography, 687
   Magnetic Resonance Imaging (MRI), 693
Trauma, 696
   Soft Tissue Injury, 696

Fractures, 701
   Humeral Fractures, 701
   Fractures of the Proximal Radius, 712
   Fractures of the Ulna, 717
   Treatment of Displaced Fractures, 721
   Coronoid Fractures, 723
   The Monteggia Lesion, 725
References, 728

ANATOMY

Understanding the basic anatomy of the elbow is essential for the proper interpretation of the various manifestations of trauma that can affect this joint.

The distal humerus flares just above its articulation to form the medial and lateral supracondylar bony columns. These stabilize the articular surface, which is composed of the capitellum and trochlea (Fig. 12-1). The distal half of the elbow is composed of the proximal radius and ulna. These in turn articulate with the capitellum and trochlea in a very tightly constrained configuration. The lateral aspect of the distal humerus demonstrates a normal anterior articulatory rotation of approximately 30° with respect to the long axes of the humeral shaft (Fig. 12-2). The proximal radius is composed of a disk-shaped radial head with an indentation in the center that articulates with the capitellum. The neck of the radius makes a 15° angle with the shaft (Fig. 12-3) (5). The proximal ulna consists of the sigmoid notch with an arc of approximately 180°. This notch is rotated posteriorly to articulate with the trochlea (Fig. 12-4). On the AP view, the distal humerus makes a valgus angle of

approximately 6°. The proximal humerus makes a 4° valgus angle, thus explaining the normal 10°–13° carrying angle (Fig. 12-5) (2,3). The carrying angle changes with flexion (11). Thus, flexion-contractures make radiographic estimates of carrying angle meaningless (12).

The elbow articulation is one of the most congruent in the body (11,12). As such, the cartilage thickness varies inversely with the congruence (4,13). Thus, the anticipated radiographic appearance of the joint space would be less at the elbow than at other joints. The distribution of the articular cartilage about the greater sigmoid notch is also of interest, since in most individuals the hyaline cartilage is not continuous (Fig. 12-6) (15). This finding is significant in that comminuted intra-articular fractures of the olecranon usually occur through this area, just as some surgical approaches to the joint are undertaken here. The highly congruent articulation, coupled with its lateral ligaments, provides the stability of the elbow joint.

The medial aspect of the elbow and the medial collateral ligaments are dominated by the anterior ulnar collateral ligament (Fig. 12-7) (7). The posterior ulnar collateral ligament is taut only in flexion, and a transverse component is of relatively little clinical significance. It is the medial complex that tends to render the elbow stable. On the lateral aspect, the lateral collateral ligament attaches to the annular ligament and then onto the ulnar ligament with accessory fibers (Fig. 12-8) (12).

The supracondylar bone that supports the articulation

B. F. Morrey: Department of Orthopedic Surgery, Mayo Medical School, Mayo Clinic, Rochester, Minnesota 55905.

T. H. Berquist: Department of Diagnostic Radiology, Mayo Medical School, Mayo Clinic Jacksonville, Jacksonville, Florida 32224.

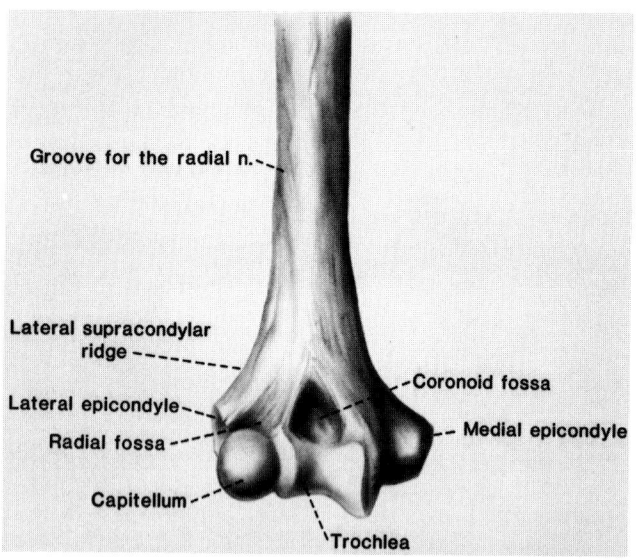

FIG. 12-1. Osseous anatomy of the distal humerus. Note the supracondylar bone that supports the articular trochlea and capitellum. The bone laterally is more substantial than that medially (from 12, with permission).

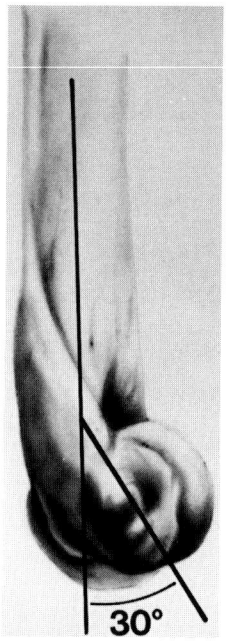

FIG. 12-2. Lateral projection of the humerus demonstrates the anterior angulation of the distal condyles that is important in order to assess the adequacy of reduction (from 12, with permission).

is vulnerable to fracture and comminution. The medial bone is much thinner and less substantial than the lateral supracondylar column. Fractures of the distal humerus, then, are difficult to reduce and treat, whether by open or closed techniques.

The medial epicondyle is much more prominent than the lateral. The medial collateral ligament attaches to the undersurface of the medial epicondyle. Thus, any disruption of the epicondyle is indicative of disruption of the medial collateral ligament complex (9). The radial collateral ligament attaches to the lateral epicondyle, which is much less prominent and thus less vulnerable to injury.

Four major muscle groups are distributed about the elbow (Fig. 12-9) (1,8). The first, or flexor group, consists of the brachialis and biceps muscles. The biceps brachii

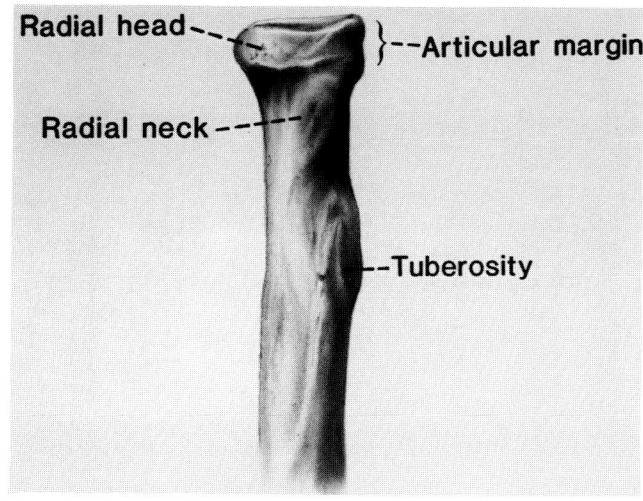

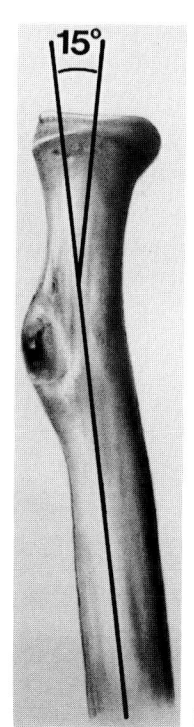

FIG. 12–3. Proximal radius (**A, B**) reveals approximately 15° angulation of the neck with respect to the shaft (from 12, with permission).

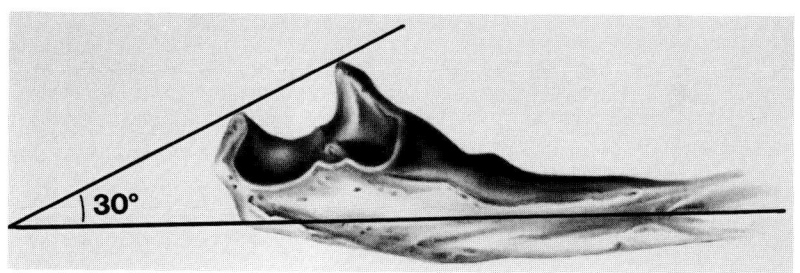

FIG. 12–4. The lateral aspect of the proximal ulna reveals the greater sigmoid notch that is approximately 180° of arc and accounts for the stability of this joint. The midportion of the olecranon reveals no articular cartilage in most individuals (from 12, with permission).

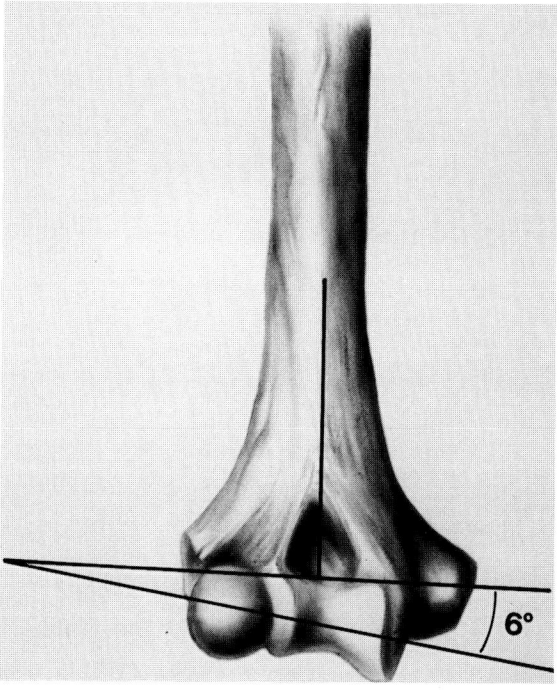

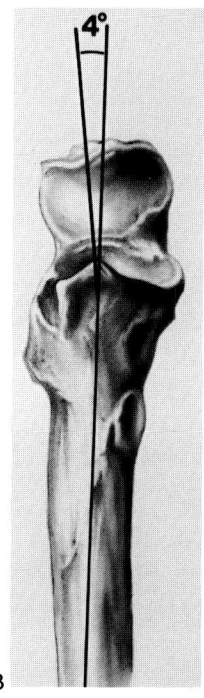

FIG. 12–5. The carrying angle is formed by the valgus tilt of both the humeral (**A**) and ulnar articulations (**B**).

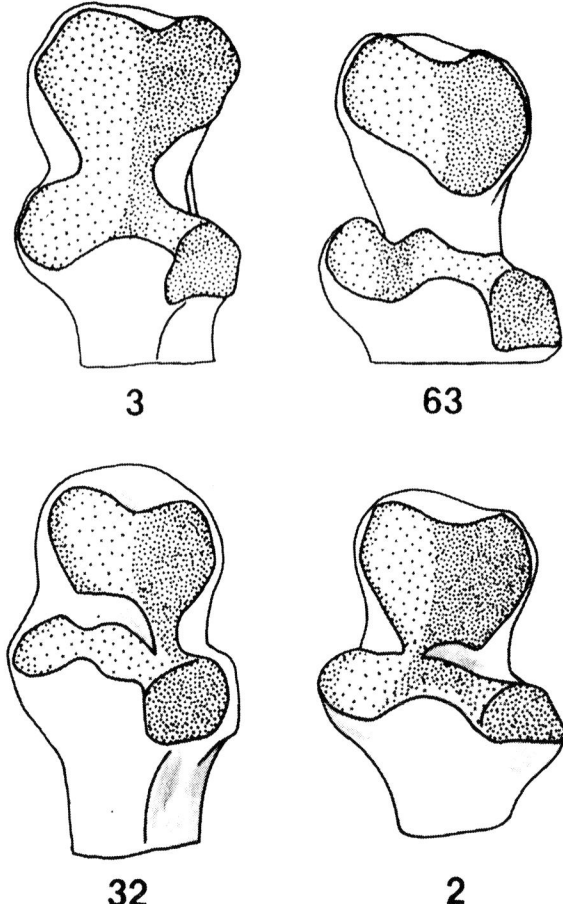

3   63

32   2

FIG. 12-6. In approximately 95% of patients, virtually no articular cartilage is present at the midportion of the olecranon (from 15).

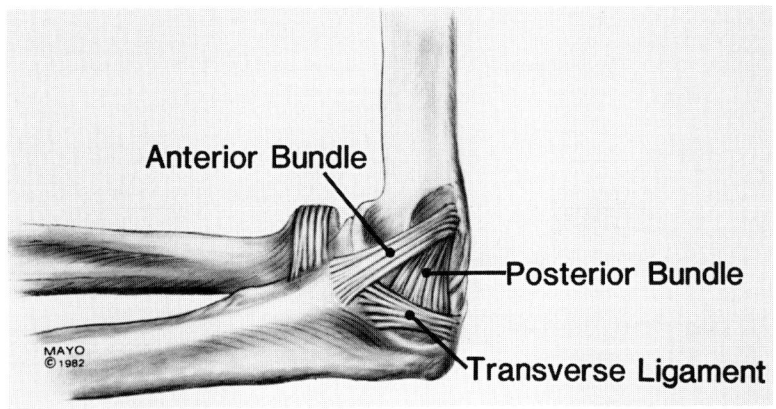

Anterior Bundle

Posterior Bundle

Transverse Ligament

MAYO
© 1982

FIG. 12-7. Classical demonstration of the medial collateral ligaments. Notice the anterior bundle of the medial collateral ligament inserts onto the coronoid. This accounts for the stability of the joint even when the proximal ulna has been removed (from 12, with permission).

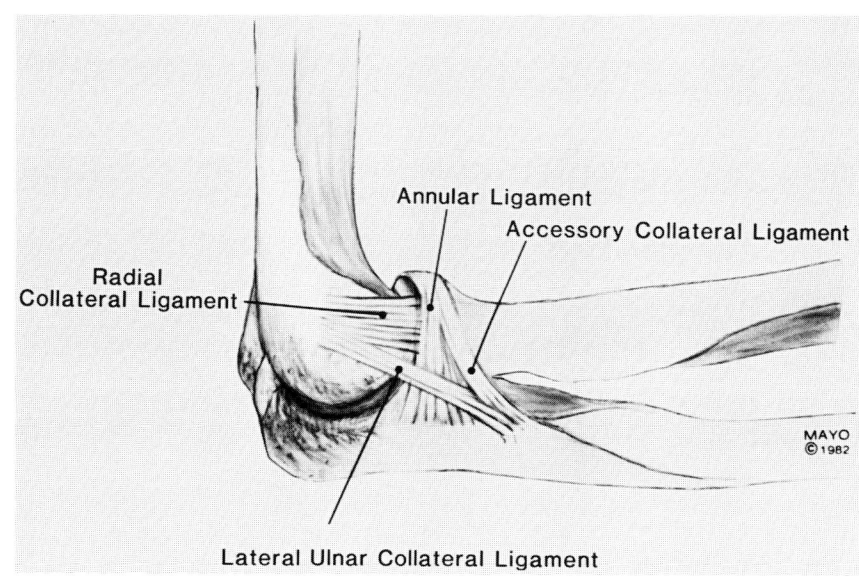

FIG. 12–8. Lateral collateral ligament complex. The radial collateral ligament inserts into the annular ligament but accessory components provide additional stability to this joint (from 12, with permission).

Radial Collateral Ligament

Annular Ligament

Accessory Collateral Ligament

Lateral Ulnar Collateral Ligament

crosses the elbow anteriorly to insert on the radial tubercle. The brachialis crosses the joint closely applied to the capsule, thus making it vulnerable to injury during elbow dislocations and in trauma (10). The brachialis inserts on the proximal ulna near the coronoid process.

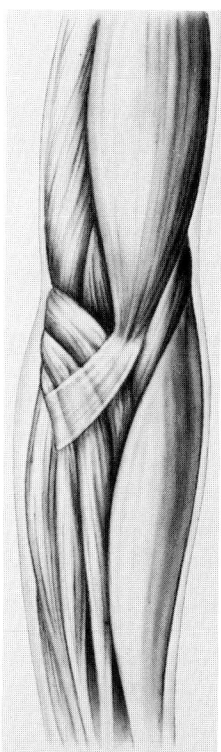

FIG. 12–9. The muscular envelope of the elbow joint accounts for the deforming forces seen in supracondylar type fractures as well as ectopic calcification seen after injury.

Myositis ossificans may be distributed along the course of this muscle (14). The extension of the elbow is provided almost exclusively by the second muscle group, the triceps mechanism along with the anconeus (8). The triceps inserts onto the tip of the olecranon and is rarely involved with traumatic conditions or diseased prostheses. The insertion, however, is protected from the skin by the olecranon bursa, which is a common source of inflammation in occupational and recreational injuries. On the lateral aspect of the joint, the third muscle group, the so-called *extensor-supinator* group, is intimately associated with the lateral epicondyle. The undersurface of the supinator muscle is associated with the collateral ligament structures. These are rarely the source of direct trauma, and calcification is unusual. The medial aspect attaching to the region of the medial epicondyle gives rise to the origin of the fourth muscle group, the flexor-pronator group. Both of these common tendinous regions are subject to tennis elbow. In youth, these regions are vulnerable to avulsion fractures, particularly along the medial aspect (8,12).

The neurovascular structures across the elbow are well recognized (Fig. 12-10). The brachial artery closely accompanies the median nerve; both cross the medial aspect of the biceps as each structure enters the antecubital fossa (8). In this position, these structures are vulnerable to injury after supracondylar fractures and elbow dislocation. Entrapment in the fracture or in the joint has been occasionally reported. The ulnar nerve is particularly susceptible to direct trauma to the joint. In addition, non-union of condylar fractures commonly result in a "tardy ulnar nerve palsy" (6). The radial nerve emerges from the lateral aspect of the biceps and under the brachioradialis. This nerve is particularly vulnerable

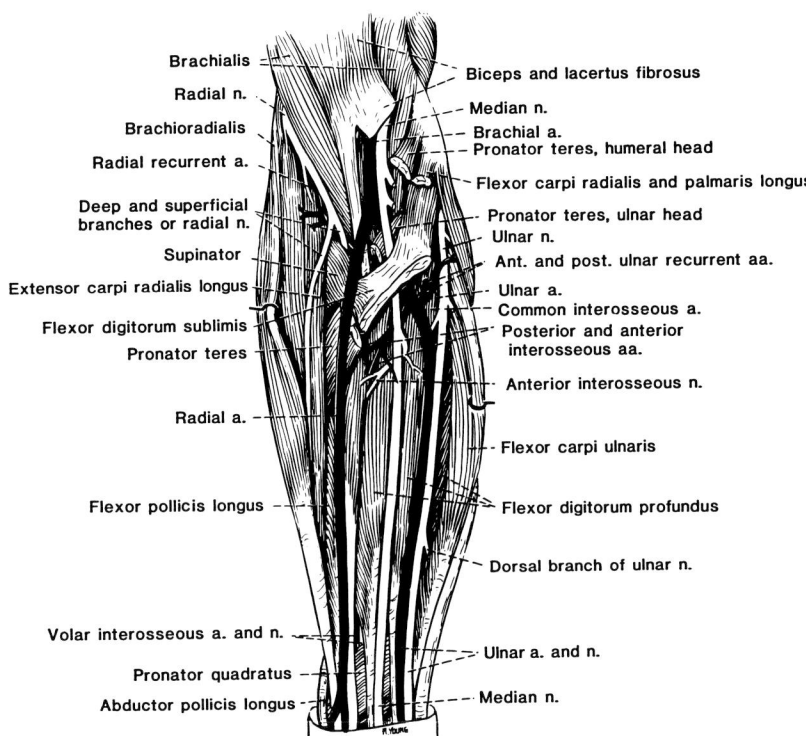

Brachialis

Radial n.

Brachioradialis

Radial recurrent a.

Deep and superficial
branches or radial n.

Supinator

Extensor carpi radialis longus

Flexor digitorum sublimis

Pronator teres

Radial a.

Flexor pollicis longus

Volar interosseous a. and n.

Pronator quadratus

Abductor pollicis longus

Biceps and lacertus fibrosus

Median n.

Brachial a.

Pronator teres, humeral head

Flexor carpi radialis and palmaris longus

Pronator teres, ulnar head

Ulnar n.

Ant. and post. ulnar recurrent aa.

Ulnar a.

Common interosseous a.

Posterior and anterior
interosseous aa.

Anterior interosseous n.

Flexor carpi ulnaris

Flexor digitorum profundus

Dorsal branch of ulnar n.

Ulnar a. and n.

Median n.

FIG. 12–10. The neurovascular relationship with the muscles as they have crossed the antecubital fossa is a complex anatomic relationship that accounts for the rather frequent incidence of compromise of these structures with elbow trauma (from 8, with permission).

to injury with midshaft humeral fractures, but it is not uniquely vulnerable to trauma at the elbow joint.

The supracondylar bone that supports the articulation of the joint is vulnerable to fracture-comminution. As mentioned earlier, the medial bone is much thinner and less substantial than the lateral supracondylar column, making fractures of the distal humerus difficult to reduce and treat. Finally, the fat pads of the elbow joint, present both anteriorly and posteriorly, are extrasynovial but intracapsular. Hence, any effusion or hemathrosis tends to displace them. This displacement makes the fat pads visible on the local roentgenogram. The anterior fat pad may occasionally be seen in a routine radiograph. Demonstration of the posterior fat pad, on the other hand, is generally considered pathognomonic of an intra-articular effusion.

IMAGING TECHNIQUES

Routine Radiographic Techniques

A minimum of two projections is necessary to evaluate the elbow (46). The AP and lateral views of the elbow provide two views taken at 90° angles and fulfill this criterion. In trauma patients, we also routinely obtain oblique views.

AP View

The AP view is obtained with the patient sitting adjacent to the x-ray table (the supine position may be used in the injured patient). The patient should be positioned so that the extended elbow is at the same level as the shoulder; thus, the extremity is in contact with the full length of the cassette (17,19). The extended elbow with the hand supinated is positioned with the central beam perpendicular to the joint, as shown in Fig. 12-11A. The AP view is of value in studying the medial and lateral epicondyles as well as the radial capitellar articular surface. With this view, the invariant relationship of the radial head centered on the capitellum is observed (Fig. 12-11B). Assessment of the ulnotrochlear fossa is also possible. The normal carrying angle (5°–20°, average 15°) can be measured on this view (3,20,21).

Lateral View

The lateral view is obtained by flexing the elbow 90° and placing it directly upon the cassette. Again, the beam is perpendicular to the joint, as shown in Fig. 12-12A. The hand must also be carefully placed in the lateral

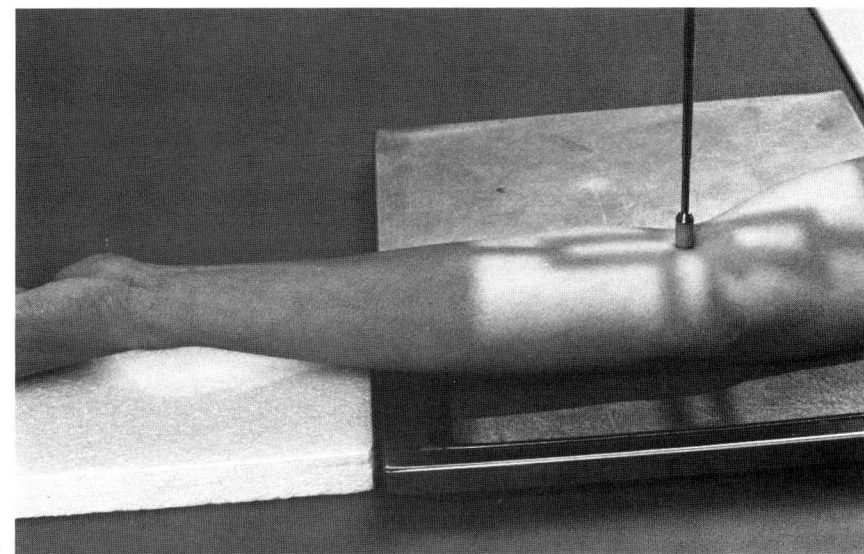

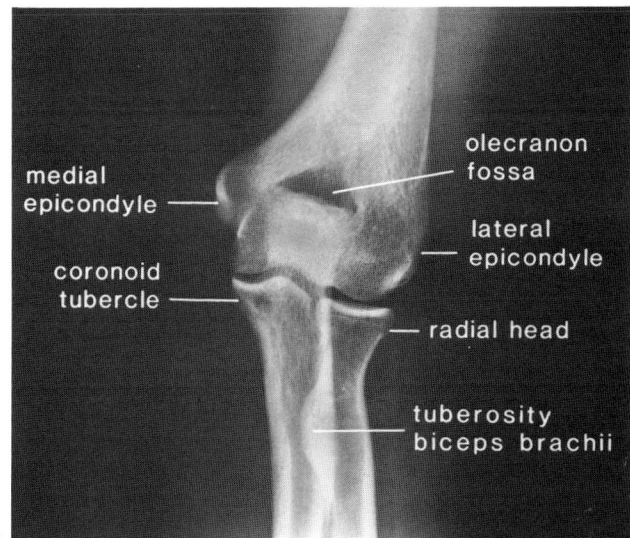

medial
epicondyle

olecranon
fossa

lateral
epicondyle

coronoid
tubercle

radial head

tuberosity
biceps brachii

FIG. 12–11. A: Patient positioned for AP view of the elbow. Arm is level with cassette with the hand palm up. The central beam (*pointer*) is perpendicular to the elbow. **B:** Radiograph demonstrating bony relationships and anatomy.

position (17,19). This view provides good detail of the distal humerus, elbow joint, and proximal forearm. The coronoid of the ulna, which cannot be readily visualized on the AP view, and the olecranon are well visualized in the lateral projection (Fig. 12-12B, C). With a true lateral projection, the presence of three concentric arcs can be identified (Fig. 12-13) (37). The smaller arc is the trochlear sulcus, the intermediate arc represents the capitellum, and the larger arc is the medial aspect of the trochlea. If the arcs are interrupted, one has not obtained a true lateral projection.

Unfortunately, in patients with elbow injury, the true AP and lateral views are difficult to obtain. Patients will frequently be unable to extend the elbow fully or flex the elbow to 90°. In these situations, the cassette should be placed under or adjacent to the extremity, and the tube should be angled to approximate these views as closely as possible.

Oblique Views

Oblique views are obtained by initially positioning the arm as one would for the usual AP film. For the medial oblique view (Fig. 12-14), the patient's arm is positioned with the forearm and arm internally rotated approxi-

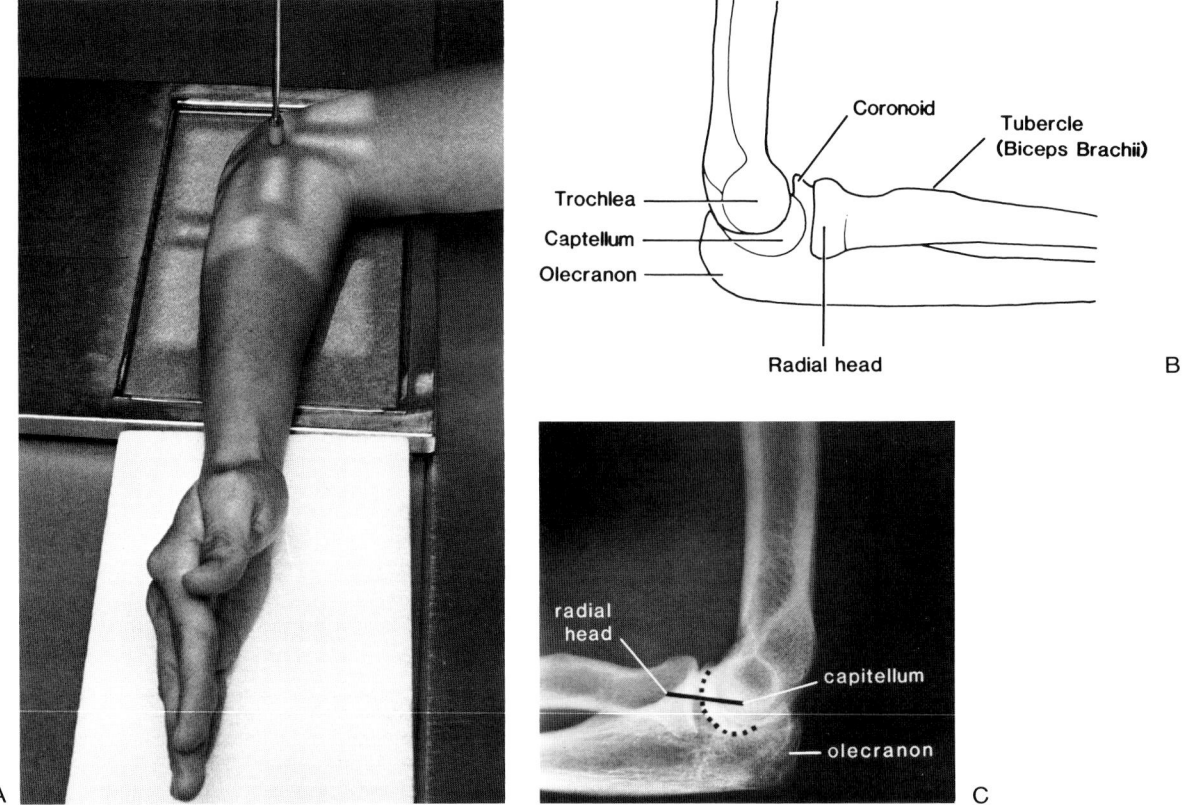

FIG. 12–12. A: Patient positioned for lateral view of the elbow flexed 90° and the beam (*pointer*) perpendicular to the joint. The shoulder is at the same level as the cassette. This is required to obtain a true lateral view. **B:** Illustration and radiograph (**C**) demonstrating lateral view of the elbow (from Berquist TH. *Imaging techniques in the elbow*; 12).

mately 45° (17). This view allows improved visualization of the trochlea, olecranon, and coronoid. The radial head is obscured by the proximal ulna. The lateral oblique view (Fig. 12-15) is taken with the forearm, arm, and hand externally rotated (Fig. 12-15A) (17). This projection provides excellent visualization of the radiocapitellar articulation, medial epicondyle, radioulnar articulation, and coronoid tubercle (Fig. 12-15B).

Radial Head View

Radial head fractures are a common clinical problem and are often difficult to visualize. Several other techniques may be utilized when such a lesion is suspected (28–32,42,46,48). The radial head view (Fig. 12-16) is easily performed by positioning the patient as one would for a routine lateral examination. The tube is then angled 45° toward the joint (28). This view projects the radius away from the remaining bony structures, allowing some subtle changes to be more readily detected (Fig. 12-16B).

This view may also allow the fat pads to be more easily visualized.

Axial Views

Occasionally, suspected pathology of the olecranon or epicondyles prompts further evaluation using axial projections. Figure 12-17 demonstrates the axial projection utilized to evaluate the medial and lateral epicondyles as well as the olecranon fossa and ulnar sulcus. The patient's elbow is flexed approximately 110° with the forearm on the cassette, the beam directed perpendicularly to the cassette, and the cassette centered on the olecranon fossa (17). This projection is also helpful in detecting subtle tendon calcifications in athletes with tendinitis and is often used to evaluate the reduction of unstable supracondylar fractures. The olecranon process itself is best demonstrated on the axial projection taken with the elbow completely flexed, as shown in Fig. 12-18 (17).

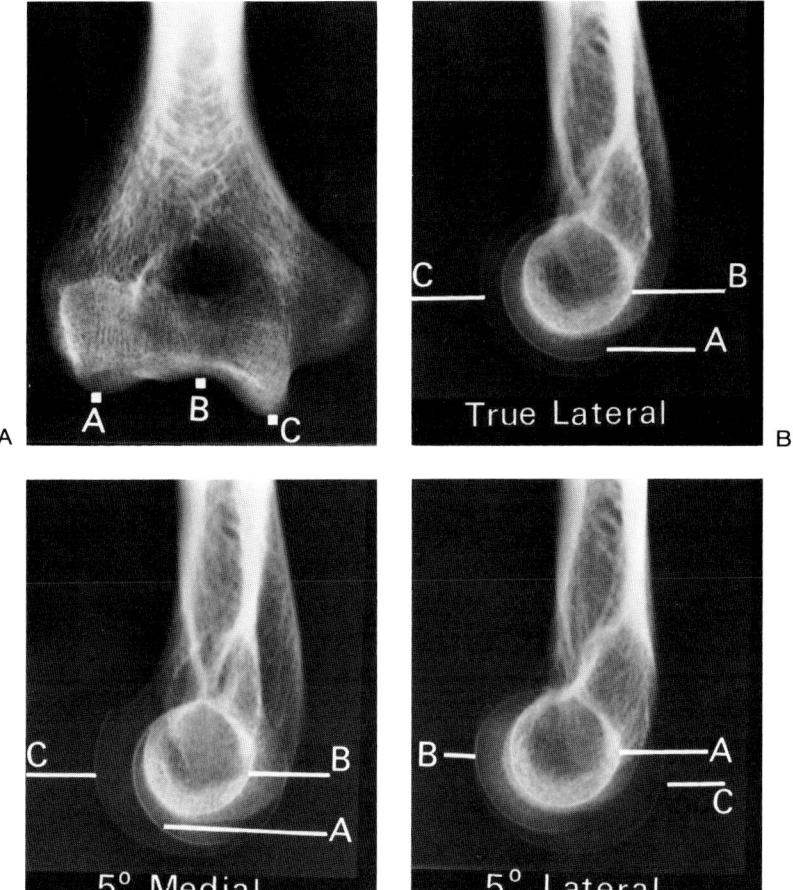

FIG. 12–13. A–D: Dried bone specimen demonstrating the points of the three concentric arcs of the AP view. A: Medial aspect of the trochlea, B: trochlear sulcus, C: capitellum. On true lateral (B), these arcs are perfectly aligned. With slight angulation (C, 5° lateral, and D, 5° medial) the arcs are no longer aligned indicating the view is not a true lateral (from Berquist TH. *Imaging techniques in the elbow;* 12).

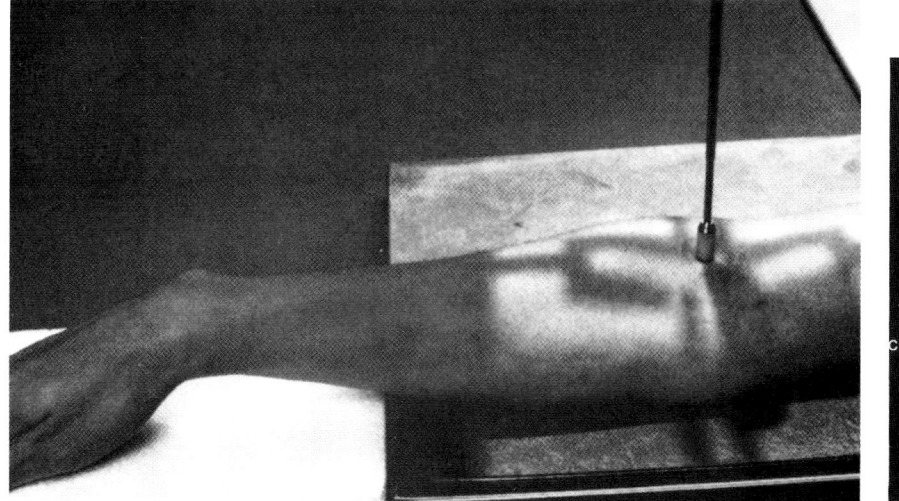

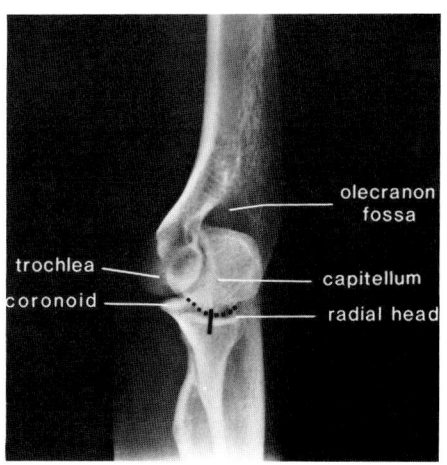

FIG. 12–14. A: The patient's arm and forearm are internally rotated and the hand pronated. The central beam is perpendicular to the elbow joint. B: Radiograph of medial view. The radial head is obscured by the ulna. Note the constant radiocapitellar alignment (*dotted line,* capitellum) (from Berquist TH. *Imaging techniques in the elbow;* 12).

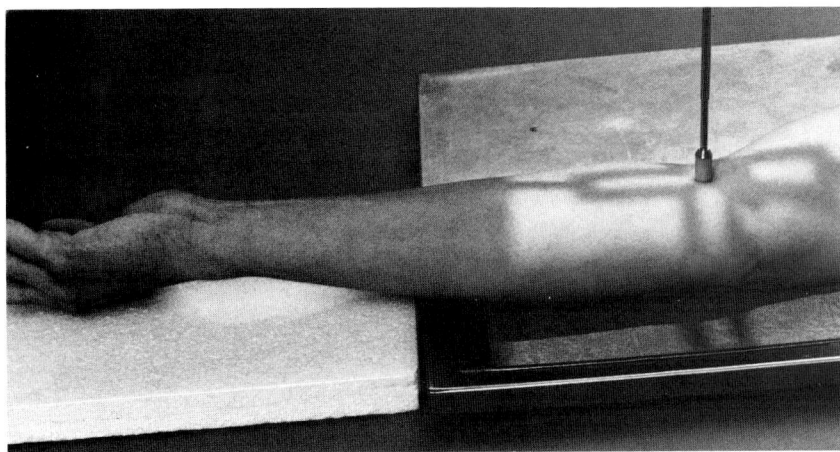
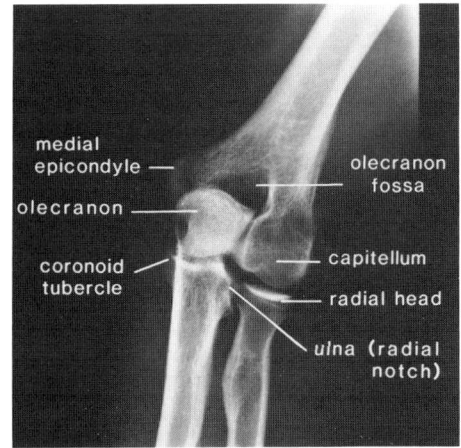

A   B

FIG. 12–15. A: The patient is positioned for the lateral oblique view with the arm and forearm externally rotated and the central beam perpendicular to the elbow joint. **B:** Radiograph of lateral oblique view. Note good visualization of radial head and capitellum, medial epicondyle, and radioulnar articulation (from Berquist TH. *Imaging techniques in the elbow;* 12).

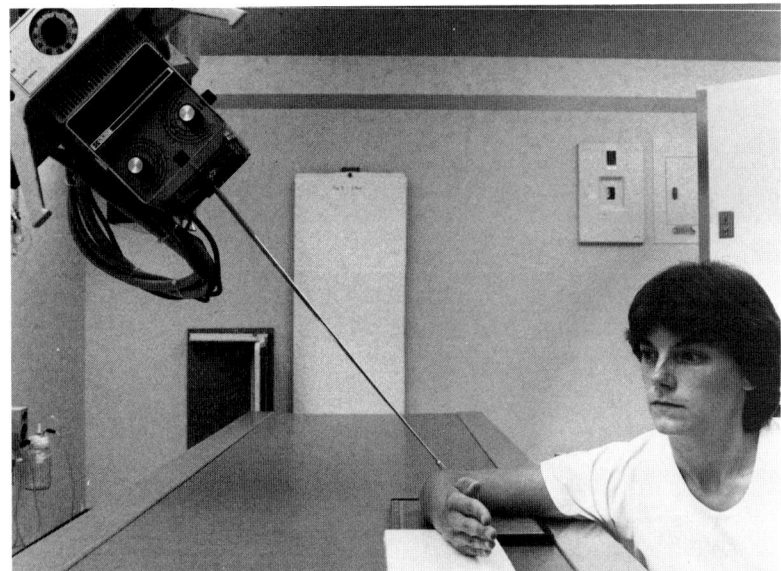
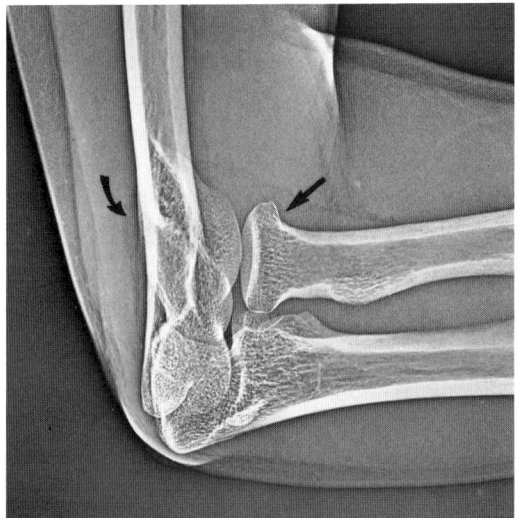

A   B

FIG. 12–16. Radial head view. **A:** The patient is positioned as if a routine lateral view (Fig. 12–12A) is to be obtained. The tube is angled 45° toward the joint rather than perpendicularly. **B:** Radial head view with xerographic technique (see Xeroradiography in Chapter 1). Note excellent visualization of the radial head with an unpacked fracture (*arrow*). Posterior fat pad (*curved arrow*) is definitely seen (from Berquist TH. *Imaging techniques in the elbow;* 12).

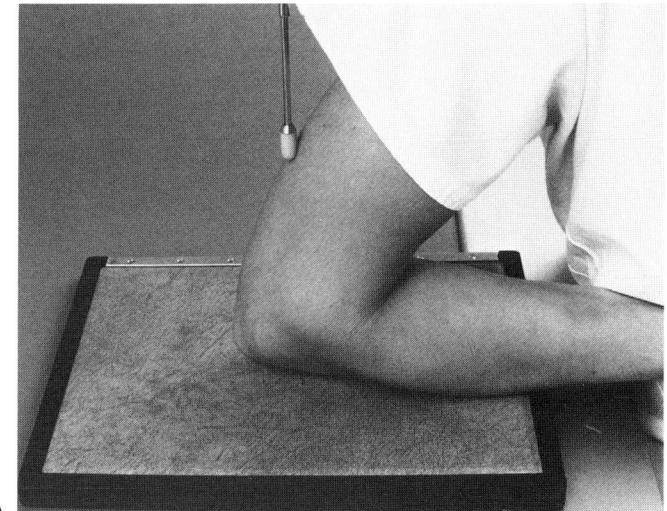
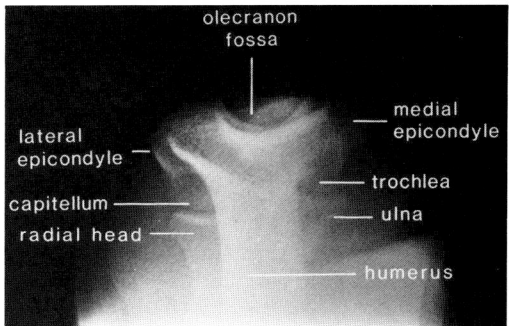

FIG. 12-17. A: Patient positioned for axial view of the distal humerus. The elbow is flexed approximately 110° with the forearm and elbow on the cassette. The central beam is perpendicular to the cassette and centered in the region of the olecranon fossa. B: Radiograph provides excellent visualization of the epicondyles, ulnar sulcus, and radiocapitellar and ulnar trochlea articulations (from Berquist TH. *Imaging techniques in the elbow;* 12).

Assessment of Standard Radiographic Views

Other views of the elbow can be performed in different clinical situations, but the studies discussed are the most commonly utilized views. Assessment of these views should be complete and systematic. Certain features should be checked consistently and, when necessary, further views or modalities should be employed.

The relationship of the radial head to the articular surface of the capitellum is constant regardless of the view obtained (Fig. 12-19). The radius is normally bowed at the level of the tubercle. Therefore, while a line through the midpoint of the head and neck provides consistency, the line should not be extended to include this portion of the shaft.

Careful evaluation of the fat pads is essential. These structures are intracapsular but extrasynovial (23,36, 39,41,46). The anterior fat pad is normally seen on the lateral view. The posterior fat pad is obscured due to its position in the olecranon fossa (Fig. 12-20). Displace-

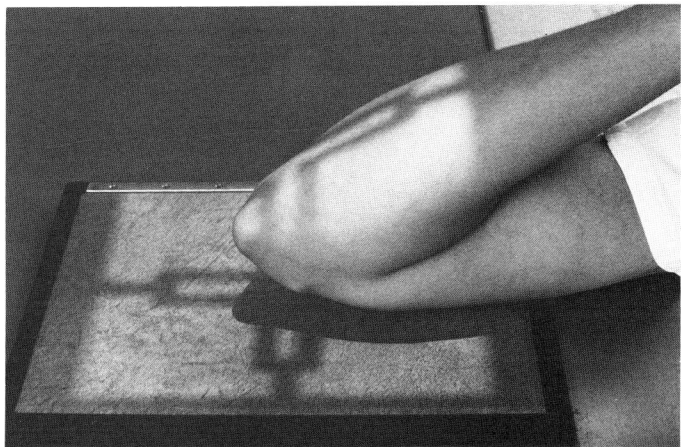
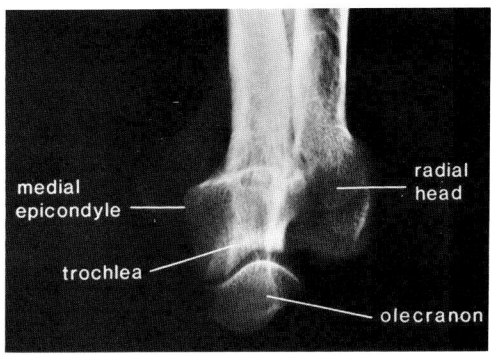

FIG. 12-18. A: The patient's arm is placed on the cassette with the elbow completely flexed. The central beam is perpendicular to the cassette. B: Radiograph demonstrates the olecranon, trochlea, and medial epicondyle (from Berquist TH. *Imaging techniques in the elbow;* 12).

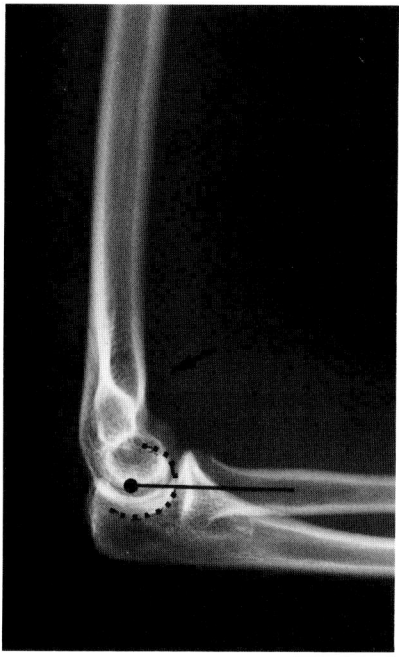
A

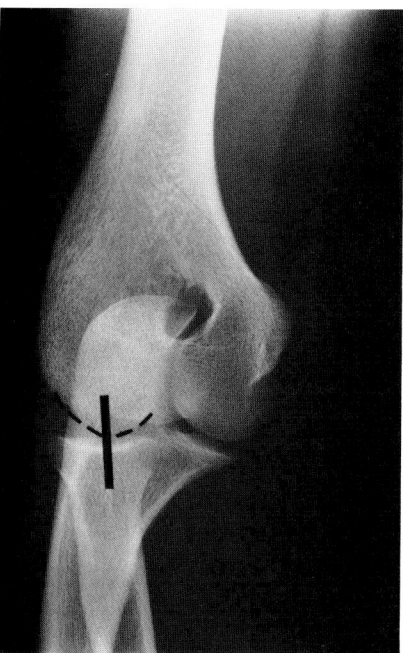
B

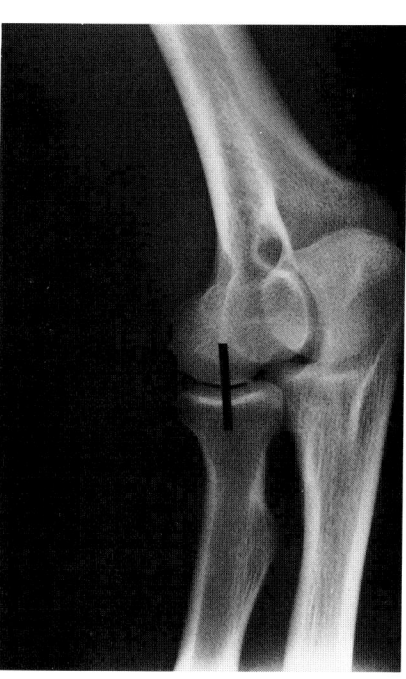
C

FIG. 12-19. Radiocapitellar relationship. **A:** Lateral (note fat pads, *arrows*). **B:** Medial oblique; **C:** Lateral oblique (from Berquist TH. *Imaging techniques in the elbow;* 12).

ment of the fat pads, particularly the posterior, is indicative of an intra-articular fracture with hemarthrosis (22,23,40,46). Norell (40) reported that 90% of children with posterior fat pad signs had elbow fractures. This finding is somewhat less common in the adult, but, if it is present, a fracture is likely. Cross-table lateral views may be more specific. A lipohemarthrosis may be evident, which is more specific for an intra-articular fracture (16,41,52).

The supinator fat stripe lies ventral to the radial head and neck on the surface of the supinator muscle (Fig. 12-21). Fractures about the elbow will frequently dis-

place or obliterate this structure, providing a clue to the underlying injury. Rogers and MacEwan (46) reported changes in this fat stripe in 100% of fractures of the radial head and neck and in 82% of other elbow fractures.

The anterior humeral line is helpful in detecting subtle supracondylar fractures in children, but it is not frequently used in adults (45). This line, drawn along the anterior humeral cortex, should pass through the middle third of the capitellum.

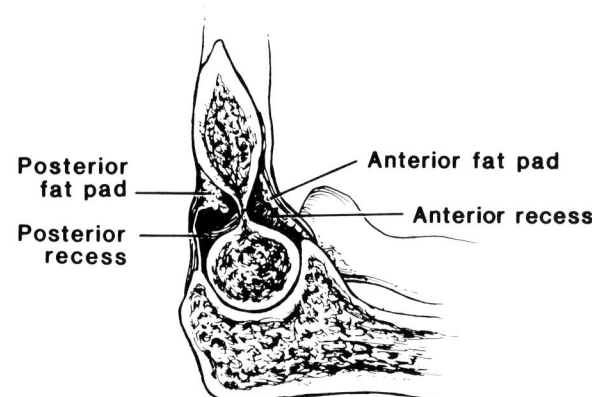

FIG. 12-20. Lateral illustration of elbow demonstrating the anterior and posterior fat pads (from Berquist TH. *Imaging techniques in the elbow;* 12).

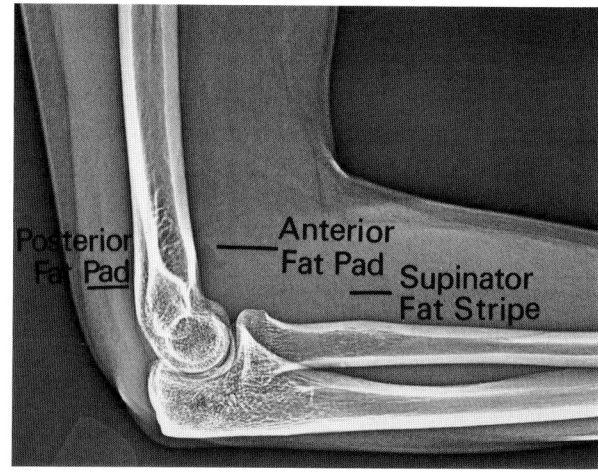

FIG. 12-21. Xerogram of elbow demonstrating fat pads and supinator fat stripe (from Berquist TH. *Imaging techniques in the elbow;* 12).

Stress Views

Fluoroscopy may be required to achieve proper positioning in order to define certain aspects of elbow anatomy. Specifically, positioning of stress views is optimized using fluoroscopy. Varus and valgus stress views should be performed on the involved elbow and on the normal side to allow comparison. Exact positioning is required to achieve optimal accuracy. An increase in the joint space of 2 mm compared to the normal side is abnormal (Fig. 12-22).

Arthrography

Elbow arthrography is a simple and valuable technique in selected patients with elbow disorders. The procedure, when properly performed, can provide valuable information regarding the synovial lining, articular surfaces, and configuration of the elbow joint. Elbow arthrography is most commonly indicated for evaluation of loose bodies or subtle synovial or articular changes (Table 12-1) (26,43,50,51). Such osteocartilaginous bodies may result from osteochondromatosis, osteochondritis dissecans, or osteochondral fragments from acute trauma. The articular cartilage in patients with osteochondritis dissecans and the various arthritides is also effectively studied with elbow arthrography (25). Less commonly, arthrograms are performed to evaluate ligament tears or the articular capsule. In our experience as well as that of several other authors, patients with chronic elbow instability frequently demonstrate an enlarged, irregular capsule (26,38,50). Elbow arthrography may reveal diminished capsular volume in patients with

TABLE 12-1. *Elbow arthrography:
Indications and techniques*

Indication	Technique

Loose bodies
  Osteochondromatosis
  Osteochondritis dissecans
	Double contrast ± CT or
	  tomography

Fracture fragments	Double contrast with CT or tomography
Ligament and capsule tears	Single contrast
Synovial disease	Double contrast with CT or tomography
Cartilage disorders	Double contrast with tomography or CT
Capsule size	Single contrast

Needle position for
  aspiration or diagnostic
  injection
	Single contrast

a decreased range of motion and pain, changes similar to those described for adhesive capsulitis involving the shoulder (38). Arthrograms are occasionally performed to evaluate patients with pain thought to be due to loosening or infection of a prosthesis following total joint replacement. Arthrograms may also be indicated in certain instances following other surgical procedures on the elbow in which unexplained chronic pain or disability persists (38,50).

Technique

To obtain maximum information, arthrography should be performed by an experienced physician with a

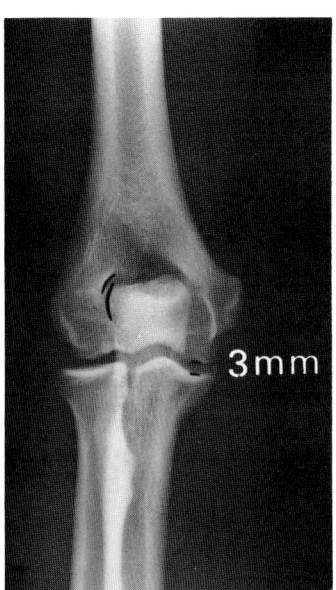
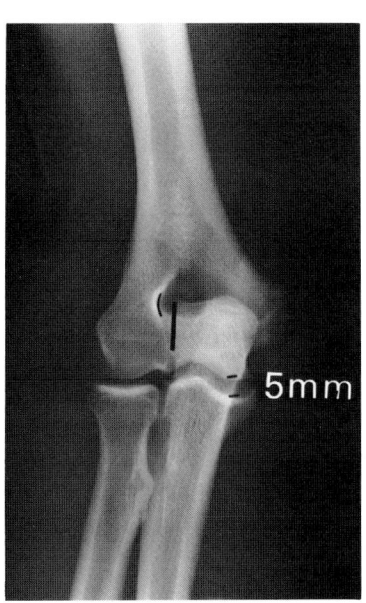

A   B

FIG. 12-22. Neutral (**A**) and varus (**B**) stress view of the elbow. The space opens 2 mm. Note the ulnar rotation (*lines*).

thorough understanding of the patient's clinical situation. Review of routine radiographs is essential, as these films may provide clues that dictate subtle changes in film technique. The choice of contrast material and indications for tomography or computed tomography (CT) are also highly dependent upon the patient's clinical situation (see Table 12-1). Simply stated, arthrography should be tailored to the individual patient.

The radiographic equipment utilized in arthrography requires excellent detail and must also allow adequate work space to simplify patient positioning and needle placement. An overhead tube provides better geometry, resulting in improved film quality compared with the conventional fluoroscopic unit (see Introduction to Arthrography in Chapter 1).

The contrast agent for arthrography can be air, a positive contrast material, or a combination of the two. Several contrast media are available that can be utilized effectively in single- or double-contrast arthrography. We most commonly use Hypaque-M-60. Renografin 60 and Reno-M-60 are also commonly used. Because of increased osmolality and rapid absorption, the contrast medium rapidly becomes diluted in the joint, resulting in loss of detail with filming. This may occur as early as 5–10 minutes following injection. If an effusion is present, dilution may occur even more rapidly. This dilution and loss of detail can be prevented to some degree by combining 0.3 ml of 1:1,000 epinephrine with the contrast material (26). The latter step is especially indicated if tomography is used. New low osmolality contrast may alleviate these problems. However, because of the significant increase in cost, they are not currently used routinely for arthrography.

Multiple techniques for performing elbow arthrography have been described by other authors (26,38,43, 44,50,51). In most cases, we utilize double-contrast technique. This provides better detail in the visualization of the articular surfaces and synovial lining of the capsule. Subtle changes can be obscured if single-contrast technique is utilized (Fig. 12-23) (26,34). We frequently employ trispiral tomography to define the articular and intracapsular detail most effectively. Computed tomography is also useful (47).

The patient is positioned either sitting next to the table or lying prone (Fig. 12-24). In either position, the elbow is flexed 90° with the lateral aspect of the elbow toward the examiner. The determination of which position is best depends somewhat upon the equipment available and the patient's condition. Prior to the procedure, fluoroscopic evaluation of the range of motion, examination for stability, and observations for possible loose bodies should be performed (26,34). The elbow is then prepared using sterile technique, and one of two needle sites may be chosen for entering the joint. In most instances, a lateral approach into the radiocapitellar joint is chosen (Fig. 12-25). However, following resection of the radial head or other operative techniques, or, if a lateral injury is suspected, a posterior approach may occasionally be required. With the posterior approach, the elbow is again flexed 90°, and the medial and lateral epicondyles and olecranon are palpated. The needle is then placed at an equal distance between these landmarks (Figs. 12-24B and 12-25) (34). The needle is positioned with fluoroscopic guidance in both situations.

When the needle enters the joint space, a small amount of contrast material is introduced to check nee-

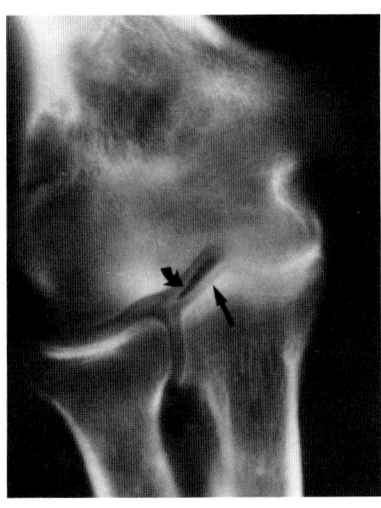 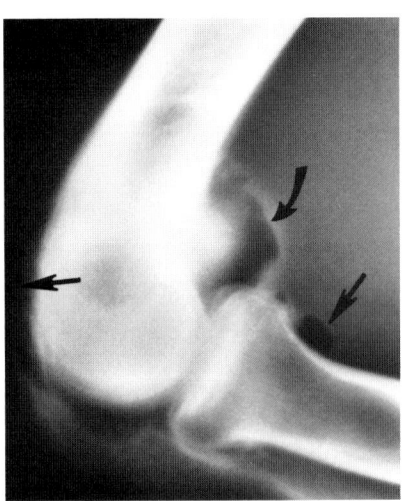 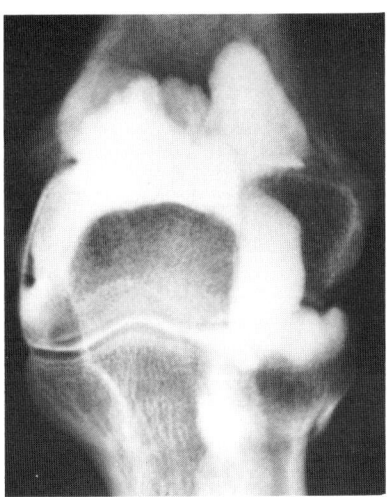

A   B   C

FIG. 12–23. Double contrast arthrogram with tomography. The AP (**A**) and lateral (**B**) views demonstrate excellent articular and synovial detail (*arrows*). Single contrast arthrogram (**C**) with too much contrast medium obscures anatomic detail.

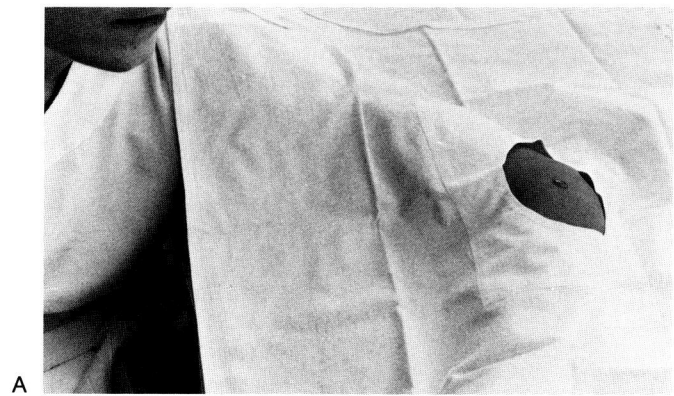

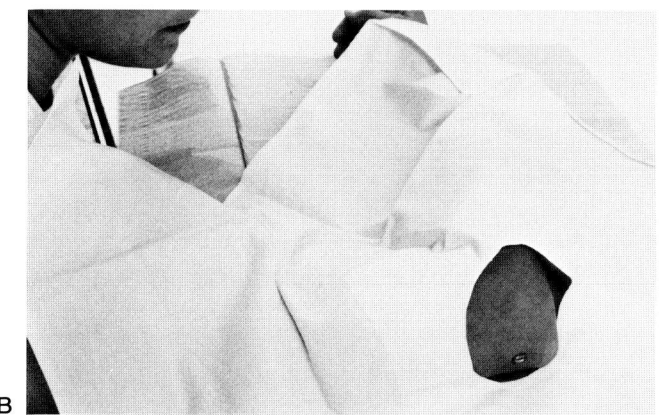

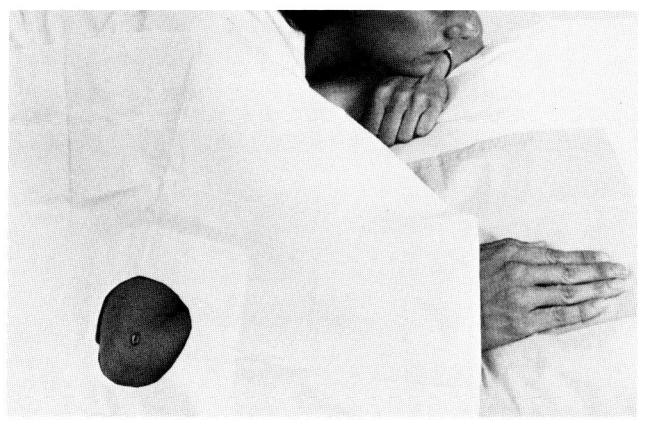

FIG. 12-24. Patient positioning for elbow arthrography. **A:** Sitting with elbow flexed and marker over radiocapitellar joint (lateral approach). **B:** Sitting with elbow flexed and marker set for posterior approach. **C:** Supine with marker positioned for lateral approach (from Berquist TH. *Imaging techniques in the elbow;* 12).

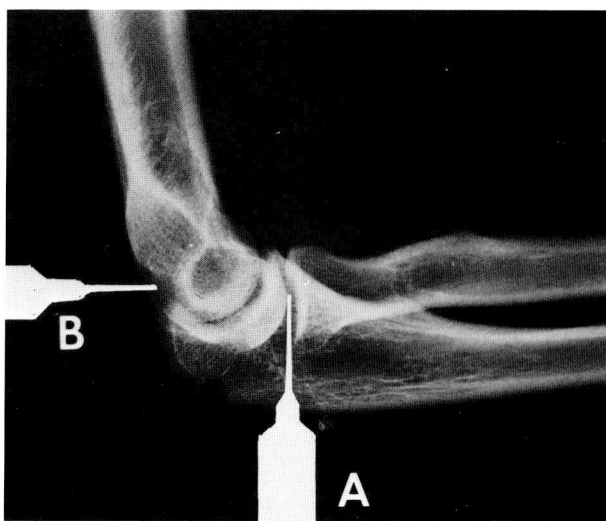

FIG. 12-25. Lateral and posterior approaches for elbow arthrography or joint aspiration.

the balance of the contrast medium. If fluid is present, laboratory studies can be obtained (culture, crystals, etc.) Large amounts of fluid will result in dilution of the contrast medium and a suboptimal arthrogram.

Depending on the clinical setting, the injection may consist of three different techniques (see Table 12-1). As mentioned previously, we most frequently use the double-contrast technique, which requires approximately 0.5–1 ml of positive contrast material and 6–12 ml of air. This mixture varies depending upon the size of the joint capsule and the patient being studied. If a significant allergy to contrast material is elicited in the patient's history, air alone may be utilized; however, with air alone the detail is not ideal, and even with tomography the examination may be suboptimal. In this setting, magnetic resonance imaging (MRI) may be the technique of choice (20,21). Single-contrast injections of 5–6 ml may be adequate in certain situations (examination of capsule size and disruptions) (26,51), however, we rarely use single-contrast technique (see Table 12-1).

Following the injection, the needle is removed, and the elbow is slowly exercised to avoid rupturing the capsule. This also avoids the formation of excessive air bubbles. While being exercised, the elbow is studied fluoroscopically. This assists in evaluating the joint's range of motion as well as the presence of loose bodies. In addition, stress can be applied to the elbow in patients with suspected elbow instability. Routine filming includes AP, lateral, and both oblique views. Medial and lateral cross-table views (with double-contrast technique) enhance the air-contrast component in the superior portion of the capsule. Routine films are followed by tomography or CT, when indicated.

dle position. If the needle is properly located within the joint space, the contrast material will flow away from the needle tip. Contrast material will collect at the needle tip if the needle is not properly positioned. Significant resistance is also noted if the needle is not within the joint space. The joint should be aspirated prior to injection of

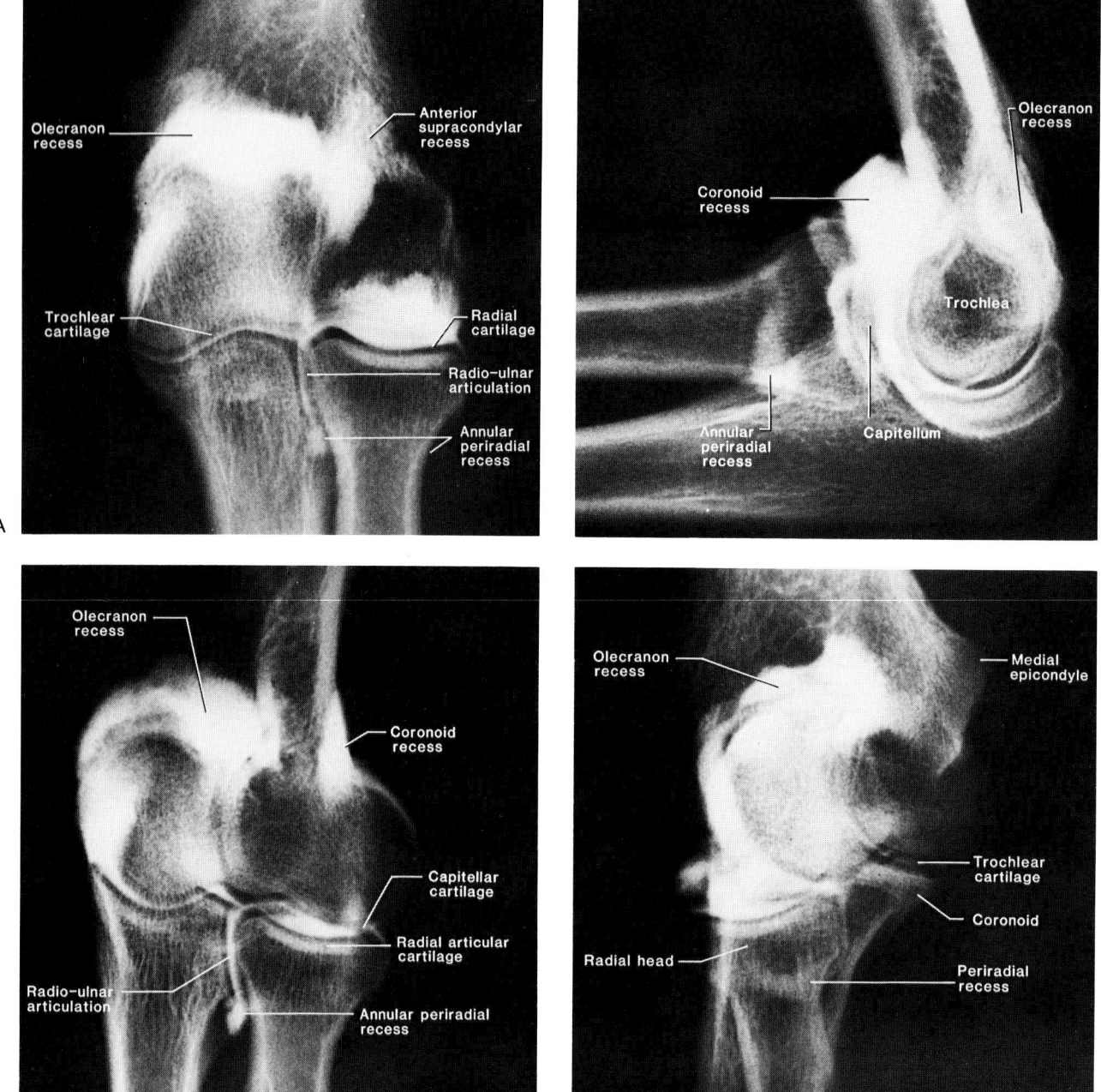

FIG. 12–26. Normal single contrast arthrogram: AP (**A**), lateral (**B**) and oblique (**C, D**) views (from Berquist TH. *Imaging techniques in the elbow;* 12).

Normal Arthrogram

In the normal arthrogram (Fig. 12-26), the three articular compartments of the joint are readily identified (radiocapitellar, ulnotrochlear, radioulnar). There are three recesses: anterior (coronoid), posterior (olecranon), and annular (27,50,51). The posterior recess is particularly difficult to visualize. Tomograms taken in the lateral projection with the elbow flexed 90° are the most helpful in evaluating this region.

The normal joint capacity is 10–12 ml. This capacity may decrease in cases of capsulitis or increase to 18–22 ml in patients with chronic instability or recurrent dislocations (34).

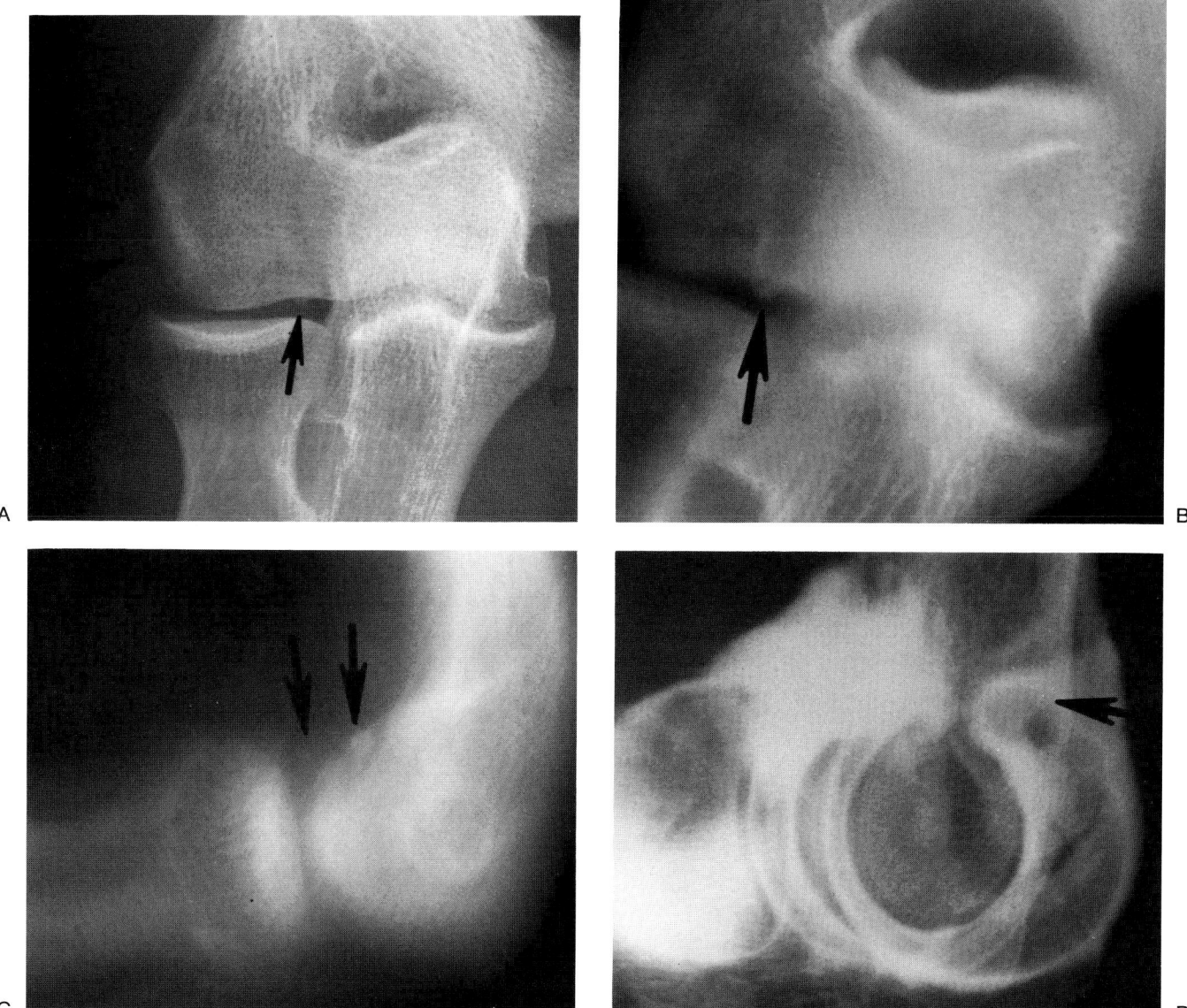

FIG. 12–27. Patient with chronic elbow pain and clicking. **A:** AP view of the elbow with irregularity or loose body near the capitellum (*single arrow*) and subtle densities laterally (*double arrows*). AP (**B**) and lateral (**C**) tomograms reveal that the fragment is attached to the capitellum. The densities seen laterally should be extra-articular. Lateral arthrogram (**D**) demonstrates several lucent loose bodies (*arrow*).

Abnormal Arthrogram

Abnormalities encountered during arthrography are frequently related to loose bodies. These so-called *loose bodies* may actually be free or attached. If contrast material completely surrounds the object, it may properly be considered a loose body. In most cases, arthrography combined with tomography or CT is used to detect loose bodies and evaluate articular defects (Fig. 12-27) (25).

Intra-articular bodies in the olecranon fossa may be due to trauma associated with enlarging osteochondral

fragments. Fragments are nourished by synovial fluid (18). An ossicle, the os supratrochleare dorsale, has also been described by Obermann (Fig. 12-28) (41). This may be symptomatic owing to repeated olecranon trauma. In patients with symptoms, the ossicles are sclerotic and irregular (Fig. 12-28B, C). This feature allows the ossicles to be radiographically differentiated from asymptomatic densities. The majority of symptomatic ossicles (87%) are on the right (41).

Occasionally arthrography is performed for suspected capsular tears or ligament injury. Extravasation of con-

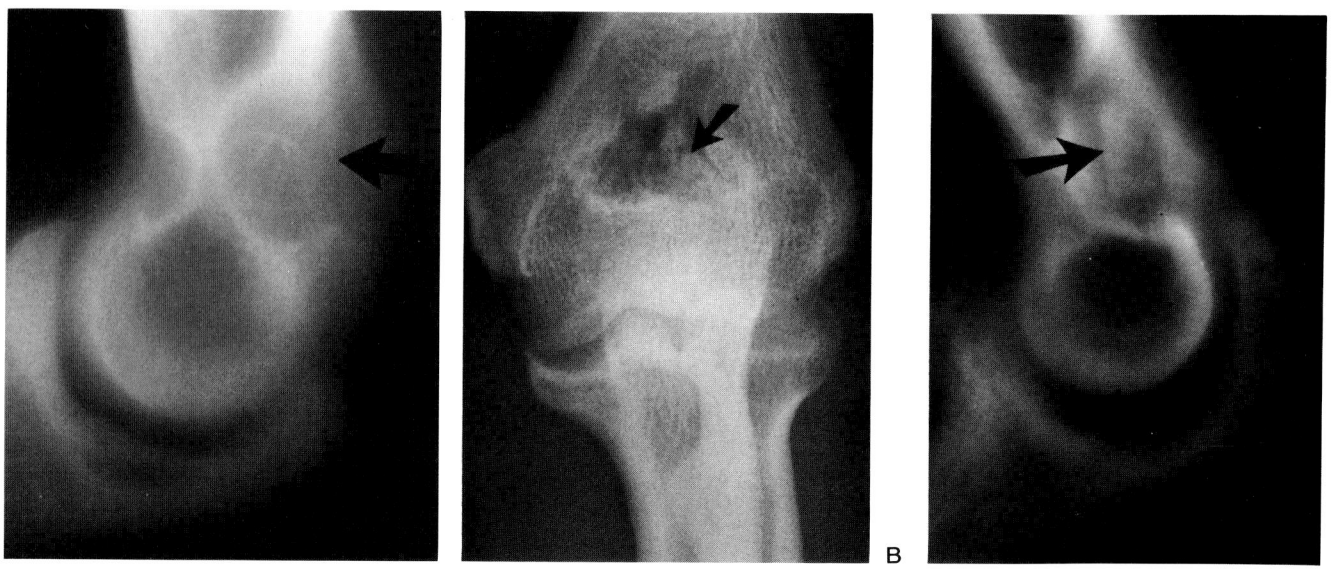

FIG. 12-28. Lateral tomogram (**A**) of the elbow in patient with os supratrochlear dorsale. Note the thin cortical margin and lack of trabecular pattern. AP film (**B**) and lateral tomogram (**C**) demonstrating marked thickening and trabeculation in a symptomatic patient.

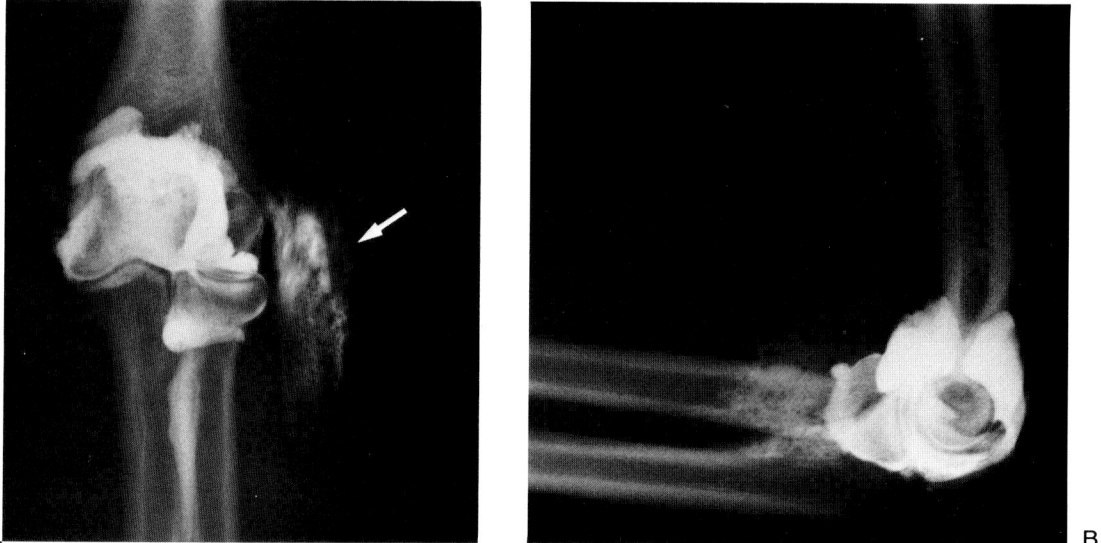

FIG. 12-29. Patient with suspected lateral capsule tear. Posterior injection was used. AP (**A**) and lateral (**B**) views of a single contrast arthrogram demonstrates lateral extravasation from a capsular tear (*arrows*) (from Berquist TH. *Imaging techniques in the elbow;* 12).

trast material indicates a tear (Fig. 12-29). Care must be taken not to mistake this extravasation with extravasation at the needle site. This latter extravasation is frequent with capsulitis but can usually be avoided with good technique. If a lateral ligament tear is suspected, a posterior approach should be utilized. Ideally, the injec-

tion should be placed on the side opposite that of the suspected tear.

Persistent pain and limited range of motion following surgery may also require arthrographic evaluation (Fig. 12-30). The integrity of the capsule, ligaments, and articular surface can be accurately assessed.

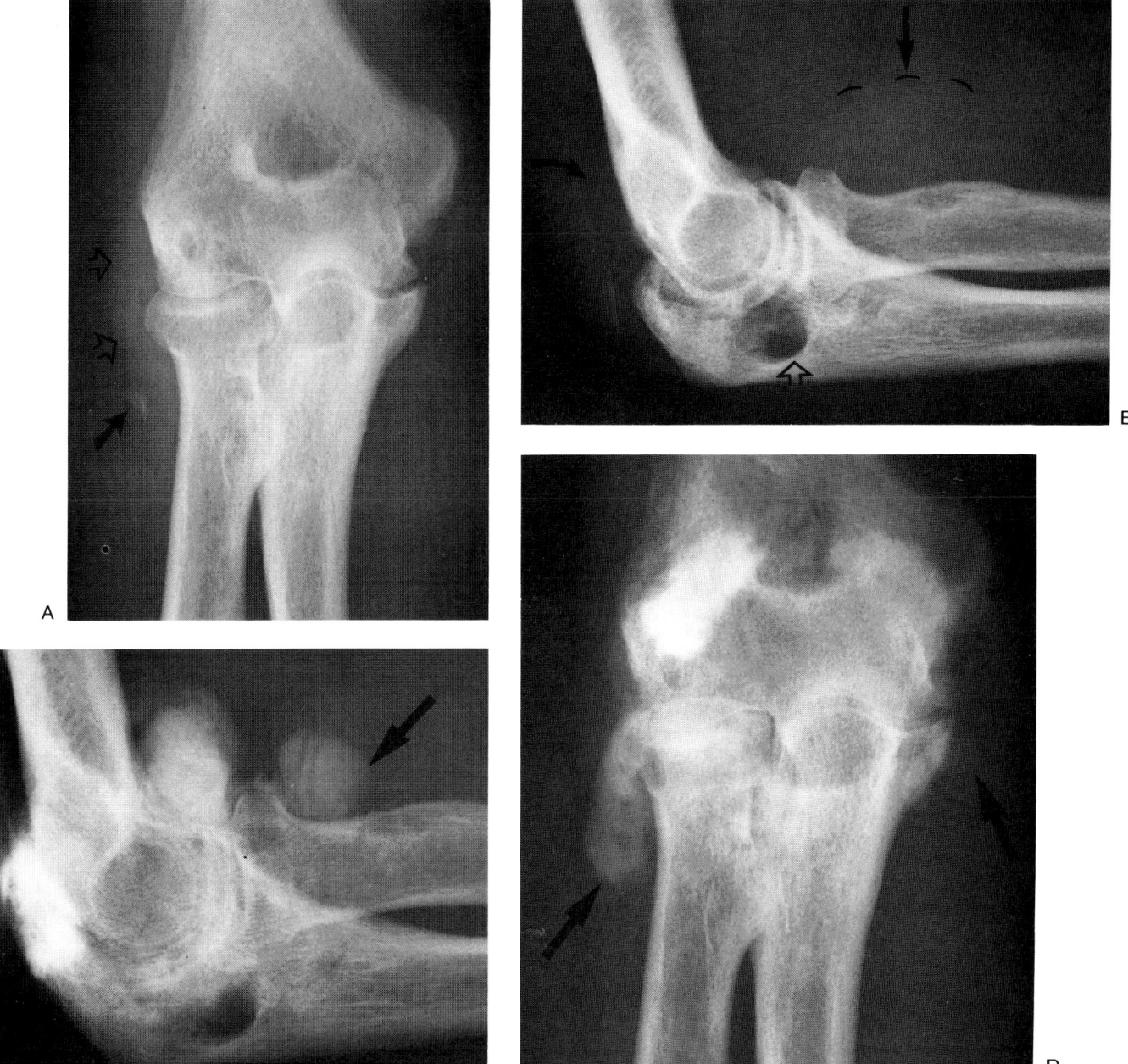

FIG. 12–30. Patient with previous surgery for ligament repair and degenerative cyst in the ulna. The AP (**A**) view demonstrates lateral soft tissue swelling (*open arrows*) with a bony density (*black arrow*) in the soft tissues. The joint space is narrowed with degenerative changes. The lateral view (**B**) is narrowed with degenerative changes and demonstrates the cyst with postop changes (*open arrow*), displacement of the posterior fat pad (*curved arrow*), and supinator fat stripe (*upper straight arrow and broken lines*). The single contrast arthrogram (**C**) demonstrates a walled-off leak in the annular recess (*black arrow*) and a second area laterally that contains the bony density seen in **A** (*arrow* in **D**). Note also the walled off capsular extension medially (*arrow*) in **D**.

Magnetic Resonance Imaging (MRI)

Computed tomography (CT) is most frequently used in conjunction with elbow arthrography. Ultrasound is less frequently applied to elbow injuries. Recently, MRI has become a valuable technique for evaluating elbow disorders (20,21). MR imaging of the elbow and forearm can clearly define normal bone and soft tissue anatomy and pathology. Clinical information (symptomatic region, the relationship of symptoms to flexion, extension, pronation, and supination) and the type of pathology suspected are important in planning the MRI examination. In order to solve a given clinical problem the patient must be comfortable, properly positioned, and the best image planes and pulse sequences selected to optimize lesion identification and characterization.

Patient Positioning and Coil Selection

Patient positioning is as important with MR imaging as with other radiographic techniques. The types of coils available, gantry limitations, patient size and clinical status may lead to suboptimal examinations, particularly in the upper extremity. The confining nature of the MR gantry reduces positioning options, especially for larger patients. Patients are usually most comfortable when supine with the elbow extended and the arm at the side (Fig. 12-31). The circular or license-plate-shaped flat coils can be used in this position. The circular coil is optimal for localized evaluation of the elbow and the larger license-plate coil is preferred for examination of larger areas such as the forearm or elbow and forearm (Fig. 12-31). Partial volume and circumferential coils for the upper extremity are also available. Positioning the patient with the arm at the side can only be accomplished when software allows the use of off-axis small field of view (20,21).

Different positions and coils may be required when software does not permit off-center placement of surface coils (off-axis small field of view) or when patients are too large. The elbow can be moved closer to the center of the magnet by rotating the patient and/or placing the elbow above the head (Fig. 12-31A). In the latter position, a volume (circumferential) coil can be used. A volume or circumferential coil provides more uniform signal intensity, avoiding the problem of signal drop off seen with flat surface coils. Unfortunately, patient discomfort can be significant when the arm is above the head. As a result, images may be degraded by motion artifact. In our initial review of 200 upper extremity cases, we found image degradation due to motion in 25%. Motion artifact is usually not a problem when the patient is supine with the arm at the side (20,21).

In certain situations, such as biceps insertion pathology, positioning the patient with the elbow flexed displays anatomy to better advantage (Fig. 12-32). This may be impossible with large patients. Smaller patients can be rotated into the oblique position with the elbow flexed at the side. Axial examinations during pronation and supination are also useful for evaluating the biceps tendon and subtle abnormalities in the radioulnar joint. Both axial and sagittal images should be obtained. When motion studies are required, it is usually best to use gradient-echo sequences (see below) and cine studies. Video tapes of the examination can be easily produced. This technique provides more information than static images in areas where motion is important in order to analyze the extent of the lesion.

Comparison of both extremities is useful in patients with subtle pathology. This doubles the examination time with conventional coils and software. Dual coils are being developed that allow simultaneous examinations of both upper extremities. This will reduce image time significantly without reduction in image quality (20,21).

Pulse Sequences and Image Planes

Many examinations of the elbow can be performed in the axial plane using T1- (SE 500/20) and T2- (SE 2000/20–30, 60–80) weighted sequences. This will generally provide sufficient information to screen for most suspected abnormalities (21).

In most situations, a coronal scout is obtained (Fig. 12-33). Three 1-cm-thick slices are obtained using a spin-echo sequence (200/20), large field of view (FOV) (32–40 cm), 256 × 128 matrix, and one excitation or average. This can be accomplished in approximately 26 seconds with a 128 × 256 matrix or 52 seconds with a 256 × 256 matrix and one excitation. The first axial images are usually performed using a T2 (SE 2000/30, 60 or 2000/20, 80) sequence. Soft tissue contrast is superior with this pulse sequence so the likelihood of over-

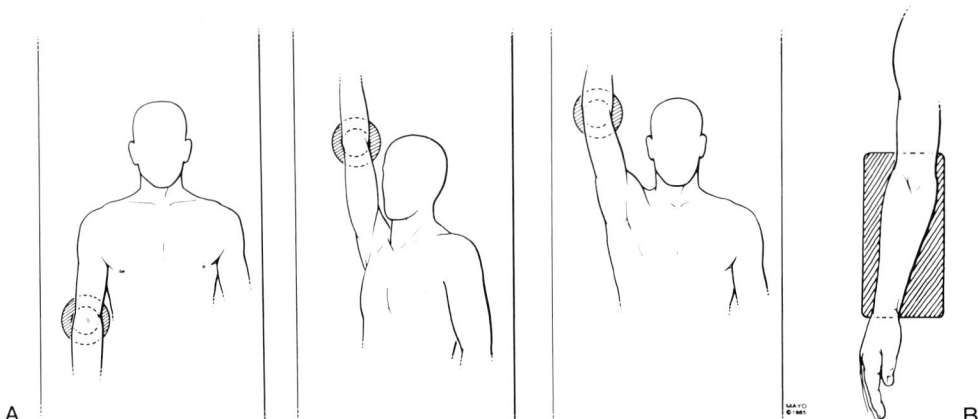

FIG. 12-31. Patient positions for circular (**A**) and license plate (**B**) extremity coils (from 20).

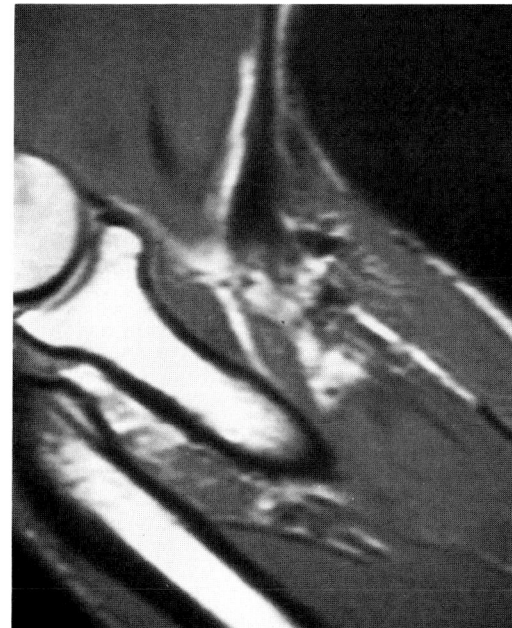
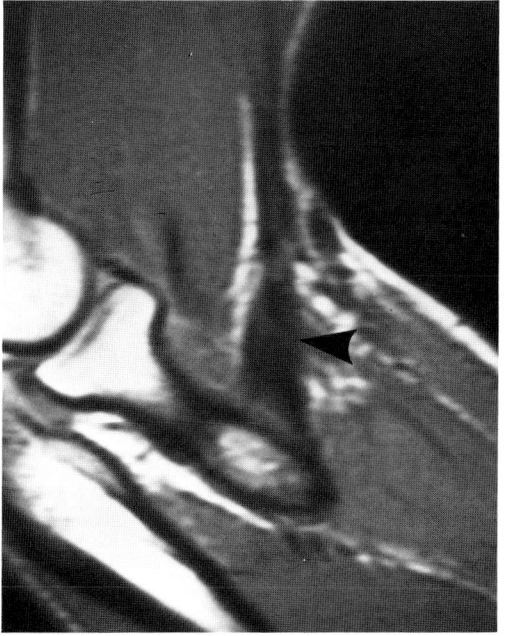

FIG. 12–32. Sagittal SE 500/20 images of the elbow with varying degrees of pronation and supination (**A, B**). The biceps tendon (*arrow*) is more easily evaluated in **B**.

looking an abnormality is remote. Initial axial slice thicknesses vary depending upon the region of interest and size of the suspected or palpable lesion. Larger, palpable lesions can be evaluated with 1-cm-thick slices and .25–.5-cm interslice gaps. Thinner (3 mm–5 mm/skip 1.5–2.5 mm) slices are used when more subtle pathology is suspected. We typically use a 16–24 cm FOV, 192 × 256 matrix, and two excitations that provide excellent image quality. The axial T2-weighted sequence takes 12.8 minutes using these parameters. The second sequence is a T1-weighted scan using SE 500/20 sequence in either the axial, coronal, or sagittal plane depending on the clinical symptoms and findings on the axial images. The FOV, matrix size, and excitations are the same as described with the T2-weighted sequence. This sequence takes 2.13–4.26 minutes. No further studies

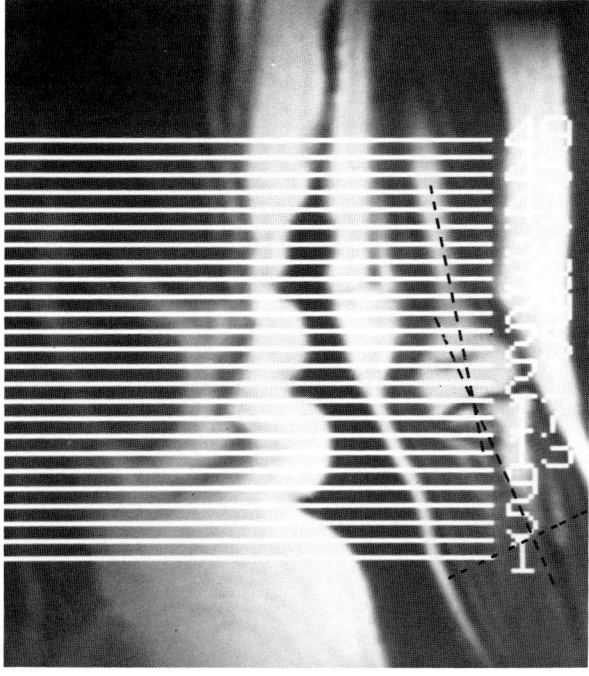
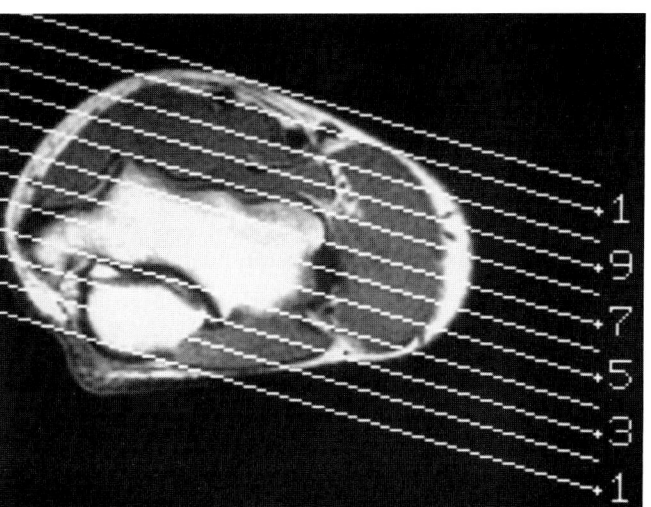

FIG. 12–33. Technique for axial (**A**) and coronal (**B**) imaging of the elbow. The carrying angle (**A**) must be considered (*dotted lines*) if true axial images must be obtained. The relationship of the humerus and radius and ulna are important in obtaining true coronal (**B**) or sagittal images.

may be needed if the examination is normal or if the lesion is clearly identified and characterized. If the nature or extent of the lesion is unclear, further image planes and sequences may be needed.

Inversion recovery, short TI inversion recovery (STIR), gradient echo sequences (GRASS, GRIL, FLASH, etc.), and chemical shift sequences may be indicated in certain situations. Inversion recovery sequences provide more purely T1-weighted images than spin-echo sequences with short TR/TE (500/20). These sequences are not commonly used in musculoskeletal imaging. However, short T1 inversion recovery sequences can be very useful for evaluating subtle lesions, specifically in bone marrow. This pulse sequence (TE 30, TR 1500, TI 100–150) can be performed in 75% of the time required for a typical T2-weighted spin-echo sequence (SE 2000/60–80). In addition, STIR sequences provide superior contrast by adding the effects of prolonged T1 and T2 and by suppressing fat signal.

Gradient-echo sequences with reduced flip angles and short TRs provide excellent flexibility for rapid imaging in different positions. These techniques are especially useful when evaluating articular problems that require evaluating anatomic changes during flexion, extension, supination, and pronation (minimum TE/TR, flip angle 30°–70°, 2–4 Nex). Static GRASS images are particularly useful for evaluating vascular anatomy and pathology (20,21).

TRAUMA

Soft Tissue Injury

Soft tissue injury about the elbow is most often secondary to hyperextension or valgus stress commonly due to a fall on the outstretched hand. An associated blow directed to the posterior aspect of the elbow coincident with the fall is occasionally reported. While the radiographs will not show an injury to bone, tearing of the anterior capsule, stretching of the medial collateral ligament, or possibly tearing of the synovium can all result in a painful hemarthrosis. The fat pad sign will be positive, physical examination may reveal a local tenderness, and the joint will not fully extend. It should be recognized that a significant injury to this joint is possible even without roentgenographic evidence of fracture. Recovery may be slow, and some loss of extension may occasionally be seen even without fracture.

Ligament Injury

The most extreme example of ligamentous disruption is posterior dislocation of the elbow (Fig. 12-34). Some have classified elbow dislocation according to the position of the displaced ulna with respect to the humerus. This criterion gives rise to the following types of dislocations: posterior, posterolateral, (Fig. 12-35) lateral, posteromedial, pure lateral, or anterior. The posterolateral type of dislocation (Fig. 12-35) is most common (80–90%) (57). Anterior dislocation is extremely rare. This classification implies little about the prognosis of such injuries, and it probably has relatively little value to the clinician. However, it does serve to describe the radiographic appearance of the displacement accurately (57,65,73).

While the degree of dislocation will vary, injury to the anterior portion of the medial collateral ligament is considered present in all such events (73). Associated injuries are common, and fractures of the coronoid, epicondyles (72), or radial head occur in approximately 28% of patients with the dislocation (65). Of these fractures, involvement of the radial head (Fig. 12-36) or coronoid is most common. The mechanism of injury is a fall on the

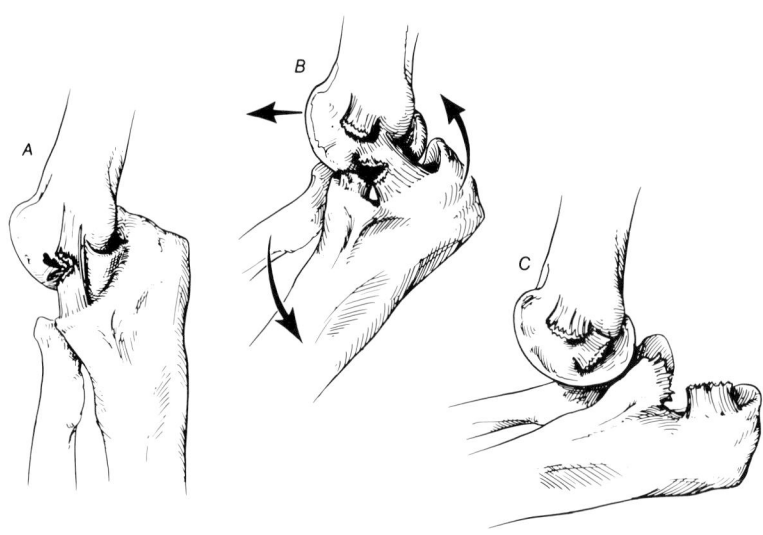

FIG. 12-34. Dislocation of the elbow caused by hyperextension injury. Results in progressive (A → C) disruption of the medial and lateral collateral ligament complex (from 73 with permission).

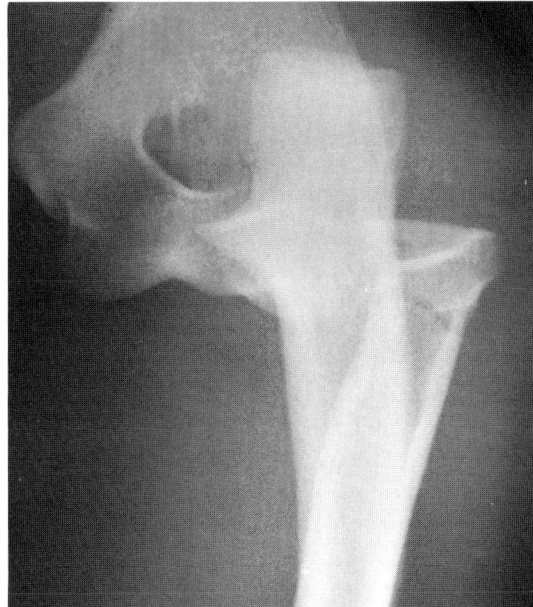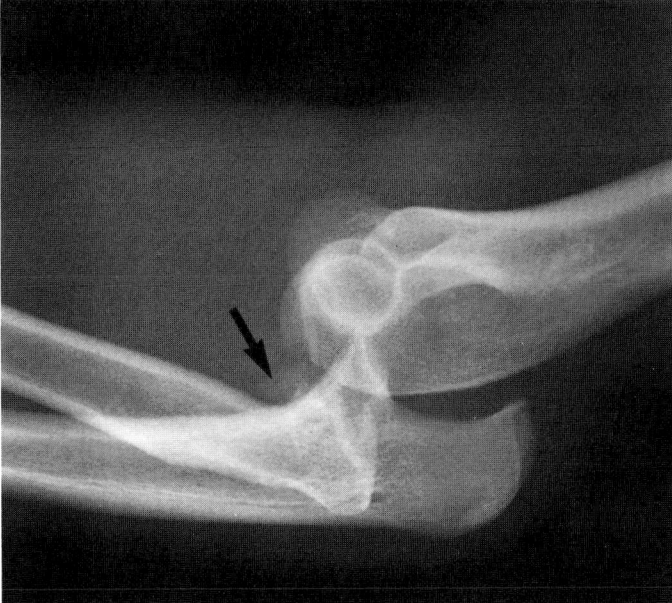

FIG. 12–35. AP (**A**) and lateral (**B**) views after posterolateral dislocation with radial head fracture (*arrow*).

outstretched hand possibly combined with a hyperextension injury or a significant axial load (74).

Physical examination clearly reveals an elbow that is markedly painful to examination and is usually held in a position of approximately 60°–70° of flexion. The prominent proximal ulna is palpable posteriorly. If the injury has gone without attention for more than 3–4 hours, a significant amount of swelling may be present. Treatment consists of immediate reduction of the dislocation

regardless of the presence of a fracture. If the dislocation is complete, this is performed under a general anesthetic or an axillary block. If the coronoid is perched on the trochlea, reduction may be performed using intravenous sedation. Following the reduction, AP, lateral, and occasionally oblique radiographs are necessary to ensure that no fracture is present, or, if one is present, that the fracture fragment will not interfere with motion. Tomography and occasionally arthrography with CT or tomogra-

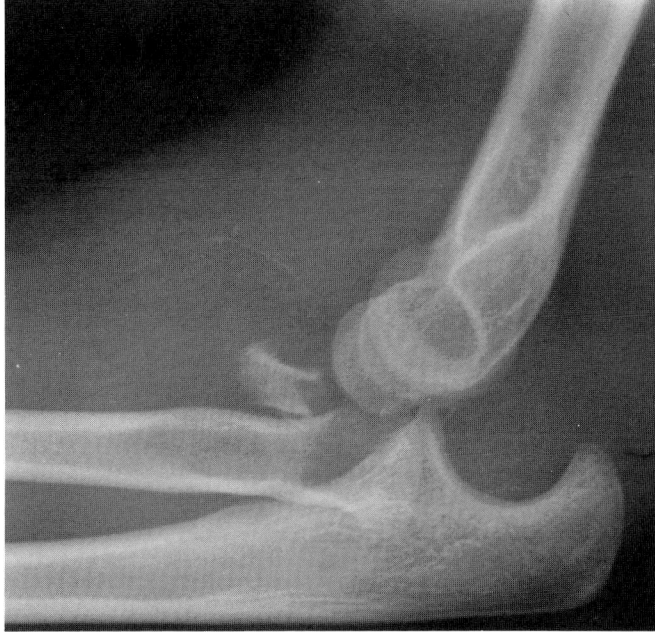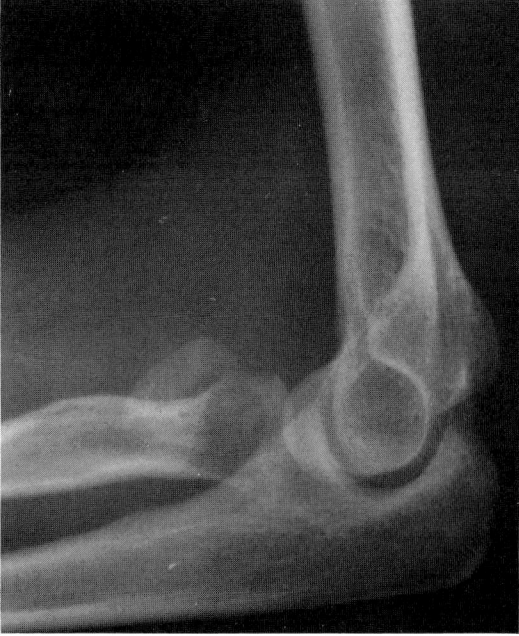

FIG. 12–36. Type IV fracture-dislocation of the elbow with displacement of the radial head fragment (**A**). With reduction, the radial head aligns to the capitellum but the fragment remains displaced (**B**).

phy may be required to evaluate the joint space completely. Calcification of the ligaments has been variously described in 10–15% of these individuals (72). The calcification can occur either medially or laterally but is most common in the medial ligament complex.

Isolated ligamentous injury is occasionally diagnosed after a fall on the outstretched hand when a valgus stress imparted to the joint results in disruption of the medial collateral ligament (67). This is an injury that is not commonly recognized, and radiographically there are virtually no clues to its presence except a possible fat pad sign or calcification at the medial epicondyle (Fig. 12-37) (65).

Additional mechanisms of ligamentous injury include the stress at the medial epicondyle that is seen with ballplayers, particularly in the case of adolescents (55,59). Frank avulsions of the medial epicondyle can also occur that might be considered a variant of ligamentous disruption (75).

Confirmation of ligamentous disruption can be obtained with stress views, MRI, or arthrography (54). The valgus stress view as recommended by Schwab and colleagues is demonstrated in Fig. 12-38 (73). This view cannot be obtained in the acute instance unless the joint has been anesthetized. Stress views of the elbow are difficult to interpret, since a significant valgus angulation can occur without a concurrent amount of widening of the ulnohumeral joint (Fig. 12-38). On the AP roentgenogram, the tip of the olecranon is not symmetrically aligned in the olecranon fossa (Fig. 12-39). This finding should alert the radiologist to the instability even if the joint line does not appear tilted. Ideally, stress views

should be performed with fluoroscopic guidance. This allows proper positioning and facilitates detection of subtle changes during the stressing maneuver. Comparison with the normal elbow is essential. A widening of the joint space greater than 1 mm above the neutral measurement may be arbitrarily considered abnormal (see Fig. 12-22). Magnetic resonance imaging may provide a new method of examining elbow ligament injury. The anatomic detail provided allows one to visualize the tendons and ligaments. This should allow detection of significant ligament tears. Arthrography may also be of value in detecting ligament disruption and in evaluating capsule size (65).

Complications of ligamentous disruption can include recurrent dislocations of the elbow (68). The brachial artery may be entrapped in the joint upon reduction (63), or the median nerve may likewise become incarcerated (70). The most commonly recognized radiographic complication of elbow dislocation is probably the entrapment of the medial epicondyle in the joint (Fig. 12-40). This occurs in adolescents who have sustained avulsion of this structure at the time of the traumatic event (75).

Treatment of most soft tissue injuries about the elbow consists simply of rest and immobilization for variable periods of time. Usually less than 2- or, at most, 3-weeks' immobilization is required after dislocation because late instability occurs in only about 1 or 2%, and because a flexion-contracture can result with prolonged immobilization (62,68). Most clinicians recommend early motion at least through a safe or protected arc, for example, from 30°–100° (65).

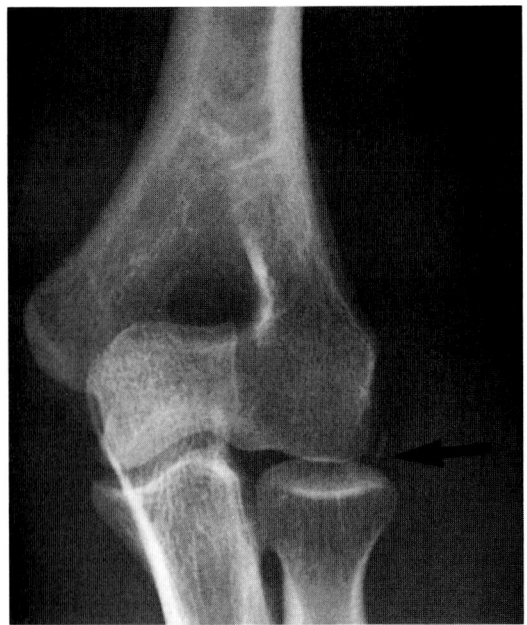
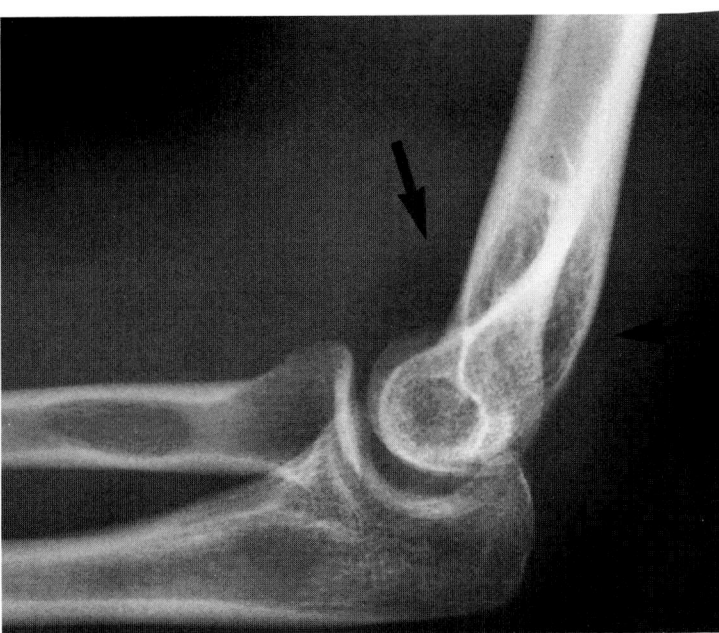

FIG. 12-37. AP (**A**) and lateral (**B**) views of the elbow demonstrate displacement of both anterior and posterior fat pads (*arrows* in **B**) and a capitellar avulsion fracture (*arrow* in **A**).

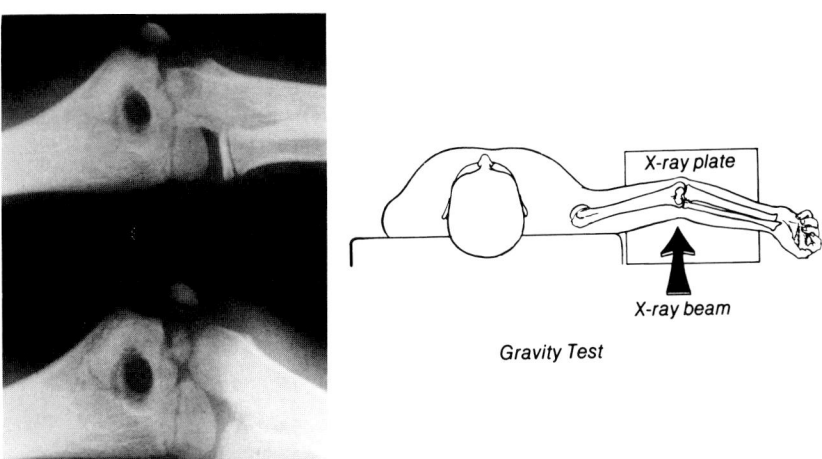

FIG. 12-38. The valgus stress view of the elbow is demonstrated with the gravity test in which the arm is allowed to fall into "valgus" (from 73 with permission).

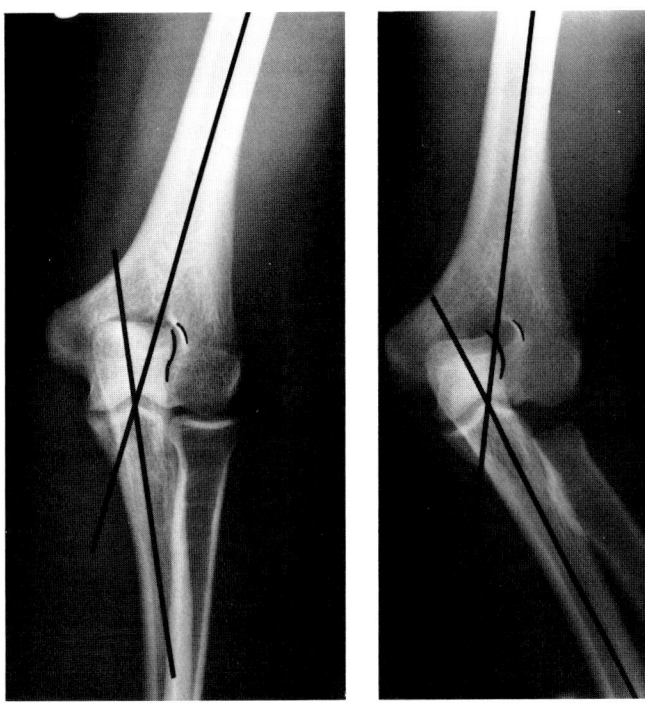

FIG. 12-39. Normal valgus carrying angle of the uninjured extremity (**A**) with an increased valgus carrying angle after radial head has been excised. Once again, notice the surprisingly normal ulnohumeral joint but the tip of the proximal ulna moves out of the olecranon fossa (**B**).

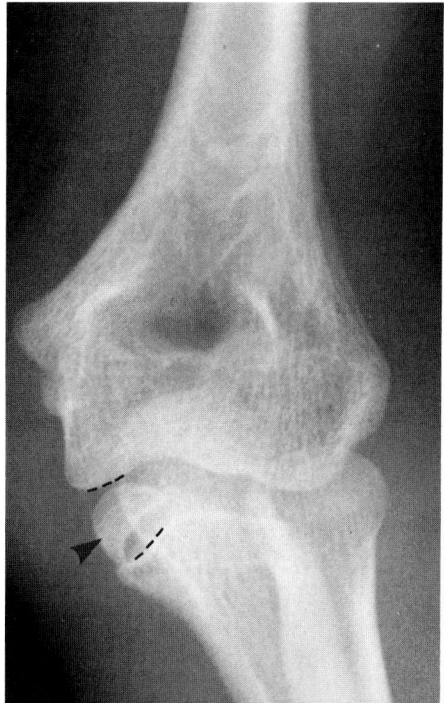
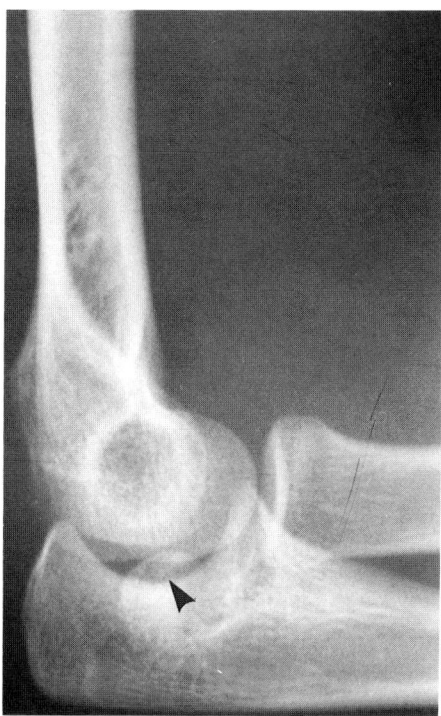

A

B

FIG. 12–40. AP (**A**) and lateral (**B**) views of the elbow demonstrating a medial epicondyle fracture with the fragment (*arrow*) trapped in the joint space. Note the widening of the humeroulnar articulation (*lines*).

Tendon Injury

Traumatic tendon avulsions about the elbow are distinctly uncommon (57,59,65). Some authors have implicated systemic disease processes, such as hyperparathyroidism (55) or osteogenesis imperfecta (64), for these avulsions. Associated injuries may also occur with tendon injury, such as fracture of the radial head. Levy demonstrated that these fractures occur with avulsion injuries of the triceps (61).

It is of special interest that characteristic radiographic features have been described for both the biceps (56) and triceps avulsion (58). The most commonly recognized tendon injury about the elbow is avulsion of the biceps tendon from the radial tuberosity (57,59). Radiographically, the radial tuberosity will often reveal hypertrophic changes or irregularity. This is best demonstrated on the lateral radiograph with the forearm in neutral rotation (Fig. 12-41) (56). Davis has found that this finding implicates a degenerative process as the etiology of the disruption. MRI is now more frequently used to detect ruptures of the biceps tendon (Fig. 12-42) (54). The diagnosis is suspected when the patient complains of a ripping or tearing pain in the antecubital space during a lifting episode. Examination reveals tenderness in the antecubital fossa, and flexion causes a proximal retraction of the muscle as opposed to the distal retraction that is seen in rupture of the long head of the biceps. The

injury is treated with primary reattachment of the biceps tendon to the tuberosity (65) within the first several days.

Avulsion of the triceps from the tip of the olecranon is even less common. The mechanism of injury is unexpected resistance to extension of the elbow. The clinical features include local tenderness and loss of extension function. On the routine lateral roentgenogram, an osseous density is regularly observed about the olecranon fossa (58). This finding is pathognomonic for triceps

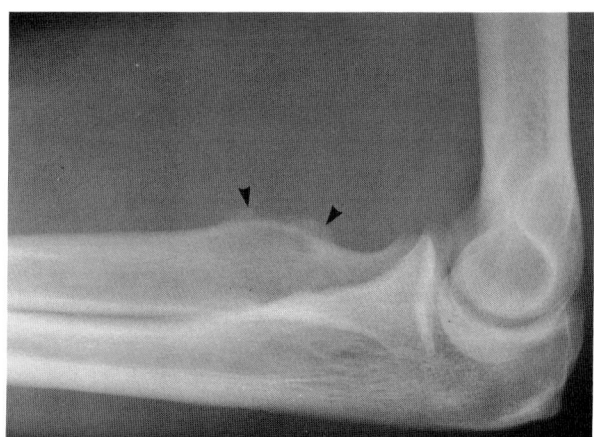

FIG. 12–41. Rupture of the biceps tendon is often associated with degenerative changes in the radial tuberosity. Note the prominence (*arrows*) of the radial tuberosity due to new bone formation.

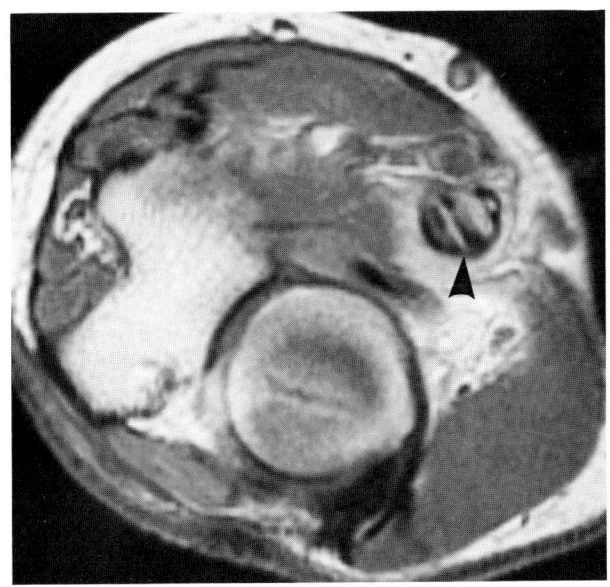

FIG. 12–42. Axial MR image of the elbow demonstrating increased signal in the biceps tendon (*arrow*) due to an incomplete tear.

avulsion. MRI is the most useful imaging procedure when radiographs are normal (54). As with biceps rupture, the treatment is an immediate reattachment to the tip of the olecranon.

FRACTURES

Humeral Fractures

Supracondylar and Transcondylar Fractures of the Distal Humerus

Mechanism of Injury

Approximately 80% of distal humeral fractures occur in children (101). The usual mechanism of injury for the most common type of fracture is a fall on the outstretched hand causing extension at the elbow joint (Fig. 12-43) and a shearing fracture of the distal humerus. The flexion fracture occurs from a direct blow to the posterior aspect of the flexed elbow and is much less common.

Classification

Fractures of the distal humerus have been classified as flexion and extension injuries. The extension injury occurs approximately ten times more often than the flexion injury. In the extension injury the fracture line is usually oblique, and displacement occurs posteriorly and proximally. The flexion injury occurs in the older age group. It entails a more transverse fracture line. Dis-

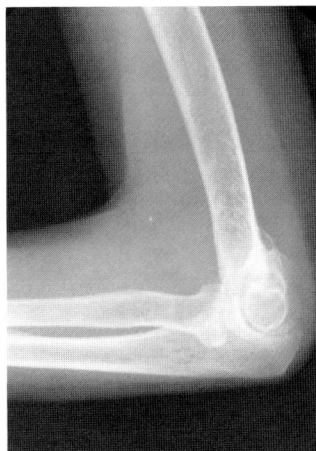
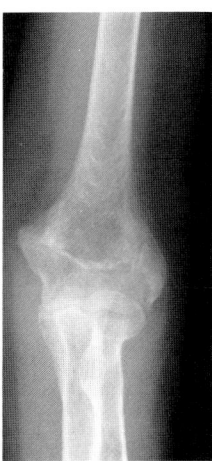

FIG. 12–43. Extension type of supracondylar fractures with relatively little deformity on the AP projections but the loss of the anterior angulation, the condyles are noted in the lateral view.

placement occurs anteriorly and proximally (Fig. 12-44) (83,101).

Physical Examination

Physical examination usually demonstrates variable amounts of swelling in the distal humeral region. The important bony landmarks retain their nominal relationships. With the elbow flexed, the medial and lateral epicondyle form the base of a triangle with the olecranon at the tip (Fig. 12-45). The deforming force from the muscle causes displacement but does not alter the relationship. A careful neurologic and vascular examination is of paramount importance in the patient with a supra-

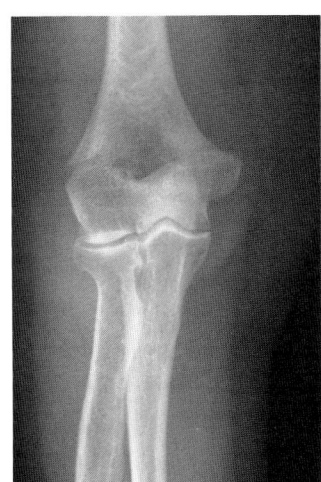
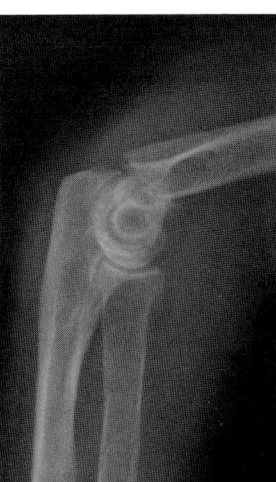

FIG. 12–44. Flexion-type of supracondylar fracture. Again, the anterior posterior view looks essentially normal but the important anterior angulation of the articular surface clearly demonstrates the fracture (from 101, with permission).

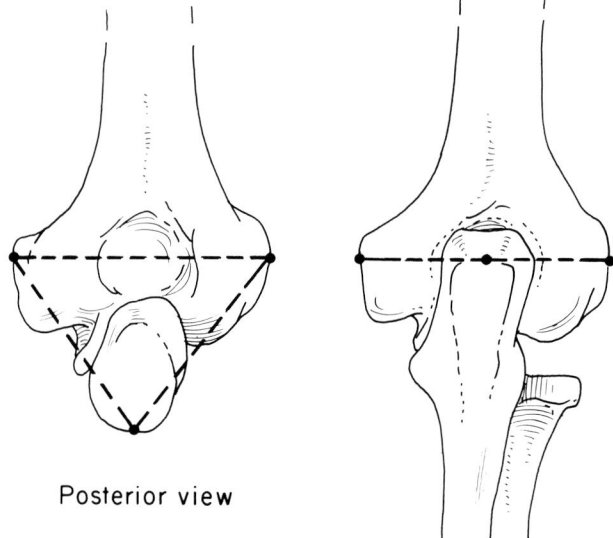

FIG. 12–45. The posterior bony landmarks of the medial and lateral epicondyle and the tip of the olecranon form a triangle in the flexed position and a straight line in the extended position (from 101, with permission).

condylar fracture, since the brachial artery as well as the median and ulnar nerve can be injured by the distal humeral fracture fragment (Fig. 12-46) (94). Injury to the brachial artery can result in muscle and nerve ischemia of the extremity in the severe form known as *Volkmann's ischemic contracture* (96).

The lateral radiograph reveals variable amounts of displacement caused by the triceps mechanism, which pulls the condylar fragment proximally and posteriorly in the

extension injury. The flexion fracture usually has less deformity, with anterior and proximal displacement as seen in the lateral radiograph. The transcondylar fracture occurs more commonly in older patients and usually shows less displacement (77). The diagnosis is readily made by routine AP and lateral radiographs (83,101).

Treatment

Treatment of these fractures consists of closed reduction or reduction by skeletal traction (84,90,102,105). In either instance, an AP image is important to ensure the proper varus-valgus orientation of the articulation, thus avoiding a varus or "gun stock" malunion deformity. Since the elbow is stable in flexion, routine views do not show this relationship. Hence, special flexion axial views of the distal humerus are required in order to appreciate fully the quality of the reduction (Fig. 12-17). The normal anterior orientation of the articular surface (see Fig. 12-2) should be considered in assessing the reduction. This is readily accomplished with a routine lateral radiograph (Fig. 12-47).

Epicondylar Fractures

Mechanisms of Injury

Avulsion fractures of the epicondyle are distinctly unusual in the adult, since the physis has closed. Varus or valgus stresses that ordinarily cause an avulsion fracture of the epicondyle in the child result in a complex injury or fracture in the adult (77). The mechanism of the medial epicondyle fracture is an avulsion force that is trans-

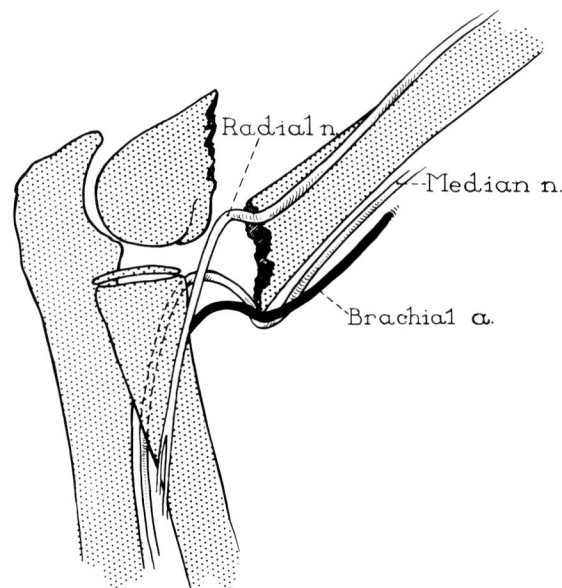

FIG. 12–46. The displaced extension supracondylar injury of the elbow can result in neurovascular compromise (from 94, with permission).

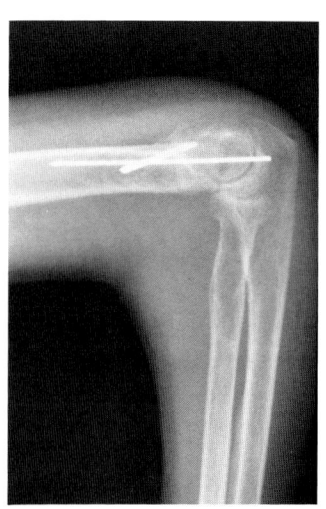
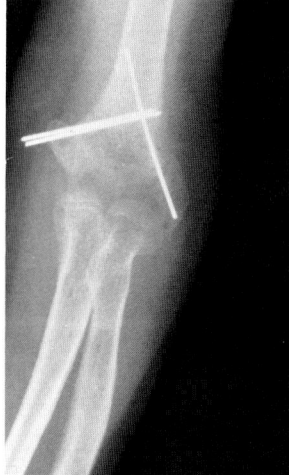

FIG. 12–47. Supracondylar fracture fixed with crossed K-wires. Notice that, in the lateral projection, an anatomic reduction has not been obtained (from 101, with permission).

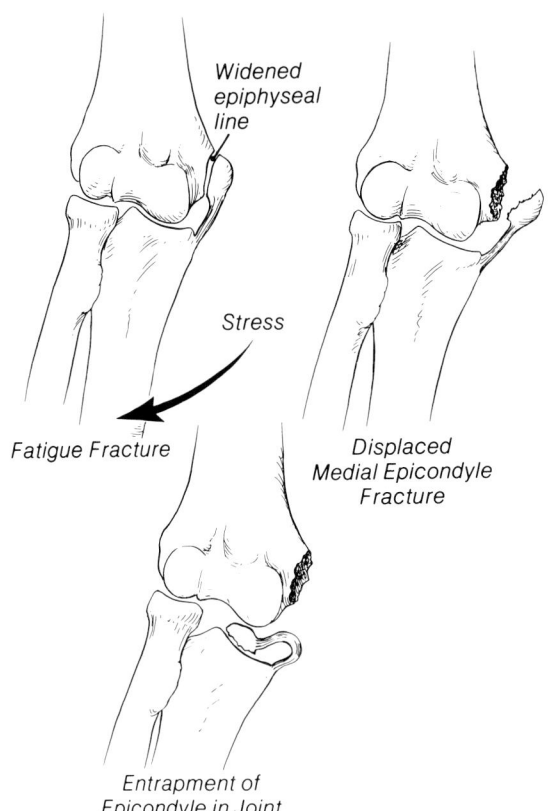

Widened epiphyseal line

Stress

Fatigue Fracture

Displaced Medial Epicondyle Fracture

Entrapment of Epicondyle in Joint

FIG. 12–48. Valgus stress to the elbow can result in avulsion of the medial epicondyle that can occasionally result in entrapment in the joint (from 73, with permission).

mitted across the medial collateral ligament from a valgus stress imparted to the extended elbow (Fig. 12-48). The lateral epicondylar fracture is extremely rare (Fig. 12-48C) (101,109). It probably occurs with a mechanism of injury similar but opposite in direction to that involved in fractures of the medial epicondyle. The lateral epicondyle may be treated in a closed fashion if the displacement is less than 2–3 mm (105). An accurate reduction of the medial epicondyle, however, is more critical, since the ligamentous integrity of the joint depends upon the position of the medial epicondyle (77). Thus, we recommend anatomic replacement of this fracture if more than 2–3 mm of displacement has occurred (Fig. 12-49) (101).

Complications

Occasionally, a severe displacement of the medial epicondyle associated with elbow dislocation can result in entrapment of this fracture fragment in the joint after reduction (see Fig. 12-40). This entrapment is often difficult to diagnose on the lateral x-ray but is suggested by medial joint widening or visualization of the loose body on the radiograph. When this occurs, closed reductions are unsuccessful, and the fracture should be opened and anatomically pinned. Usually two smooth K-wires or a small compression screw is adequate for fixation. If closed treatment is used, immobilization for approximately 2 weeks is followed by gentle, progressive, active

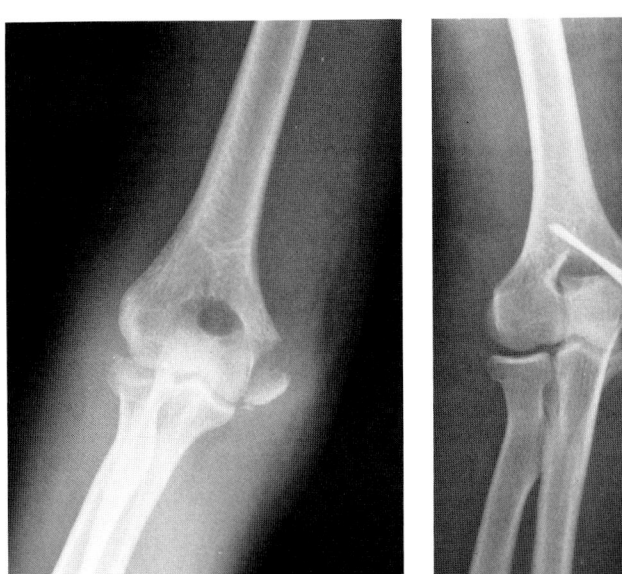
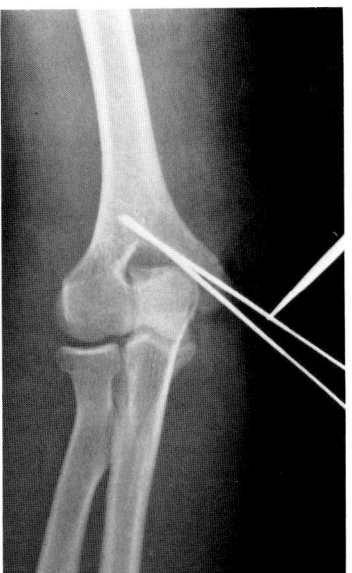
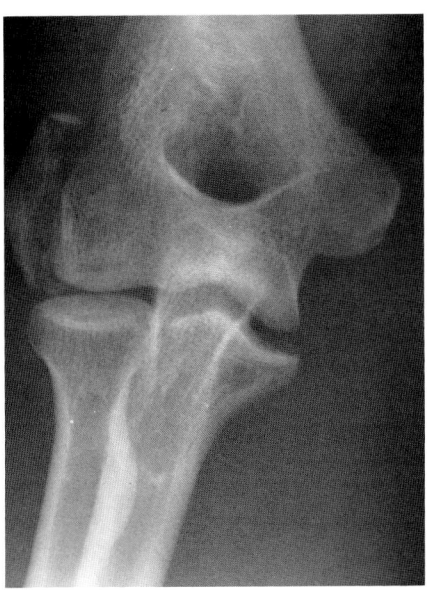

A   B   C

FIG. 12–49. Avulsed medial epicondyle (**A**). Because this was displaced more than 3 mm, open reduction internal fixation was carried out (**B**). A rare avulsion injury of the lateral epicondyle (**C**) (from 101, with permission).

motion in an arc of 30°–90°. Gradual increase in activity, as tolerated, is allowed after this period of time. Residual deformity, weakness, or instability following the fracture is considered very unusual (105).

T and Y Condylar Fractures

Mechanism of Injury

These fractures occur from a direct blow to the proximal ulna usually, but not always, with the elbow in flexion. The fracture line is initiated in the central groove of the trochlea, propagates across the olecranon and coronoid fossa, and emerges across the medial and lateral supracondylar bony columns.

Classification

The most useful classification of this fracture is that proposed by Riseborough and Radin in 1969 (104). This classification aids in clarifying the mechanism and severity of the injury as well as the appropriate treatment program (Fig. 12-50). Riseborough and Radin distinguished four types of fracture. Type I fractures consist of undis-

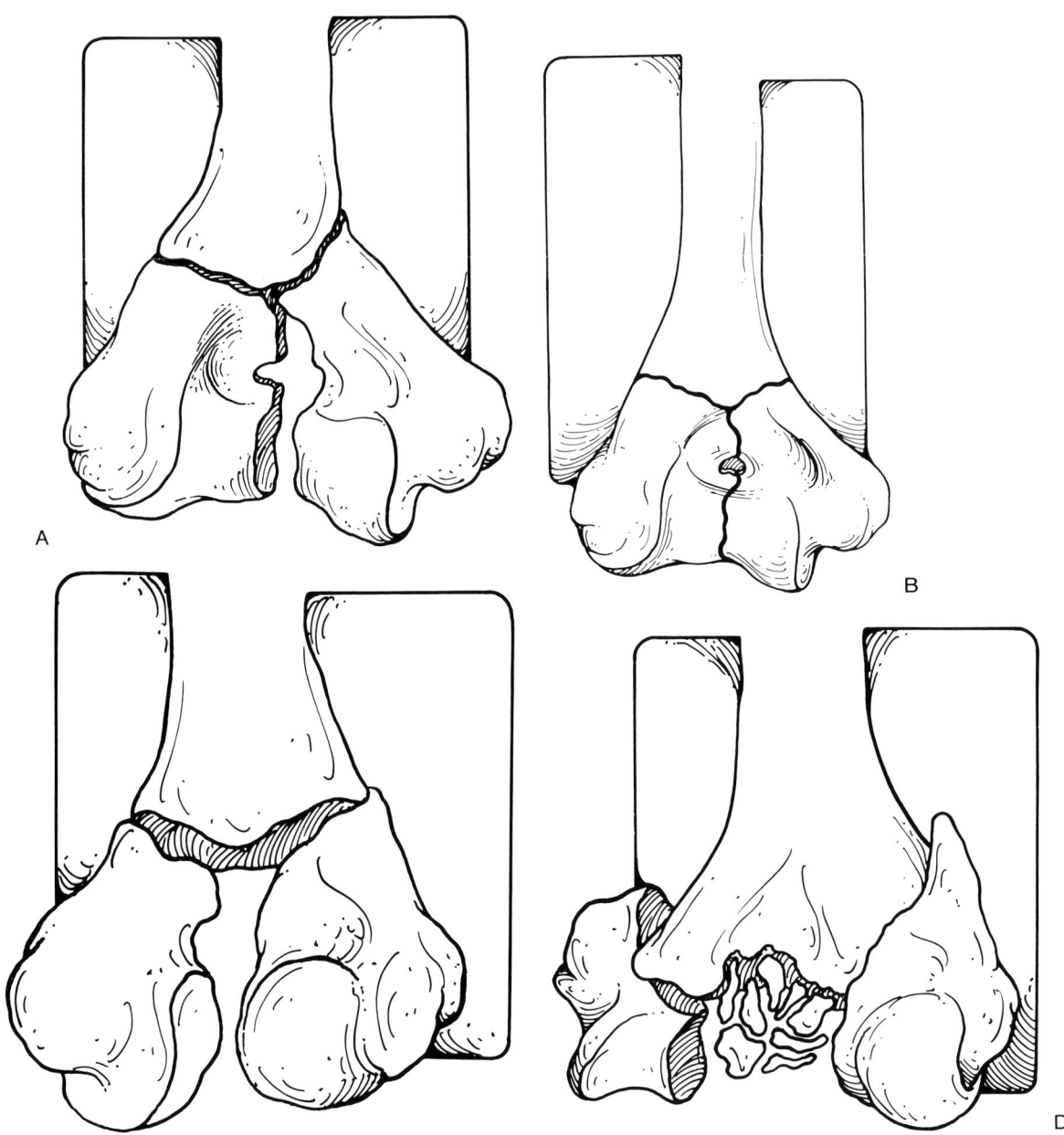

FIG. 12–50. Classification of T and Y condylar fractures. Type I, undisplaced fracture (**A**); Type II, displacement without significant rotation (**B**); Type III, displacement with rotation of the condyle (**C**); and Type IV, displacement and comminution (**D**) (from 101, with permission).

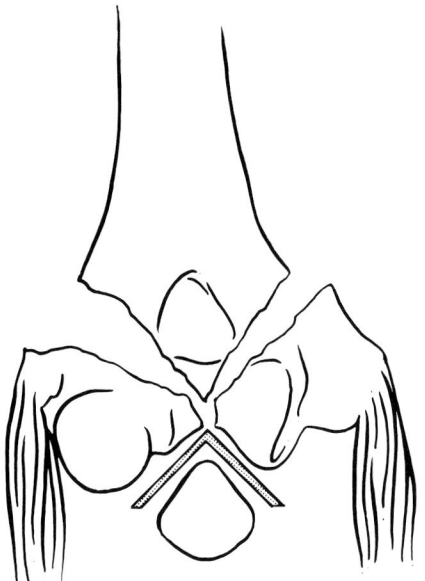

FIG. 12–51. The medial and lateral musculature results in the deforming rotation of the articular condyles. The ulna serves as a wedge that initiates the fracture (from 101, with permission).

placed T or Y condylar fractures. The Type II injury is one in which the condyles are displaced but not rotated. Type III fractures are those in which the medial and lateral condylar compartments are rotated. This rotation is caused by the action in the flexor and extensor muscle masses and results in the so-called *inverted V* sign (Fig. 12-51). The Type IV fracture is one with marked comminution.

Clinical and Radiographic Evaluation

In the T and Y supracondylar fracture, the epicondyles are displaced, so that the posterior triangle relationship is altered. There is usually massive swelling, and flexion-extension of the elbow is not possible. The radiographs clearly demonstrate the fracture (Fig. 12-52). No special techniques or views are required for the diagnosis. However, the severity and degree of comminution is often more extensive than can be appreciated on the simple AP and lateral views. Oblique views are sometimes helpful to appreciate fully the precise nature of the fracture. Conventional or computed tomography may also

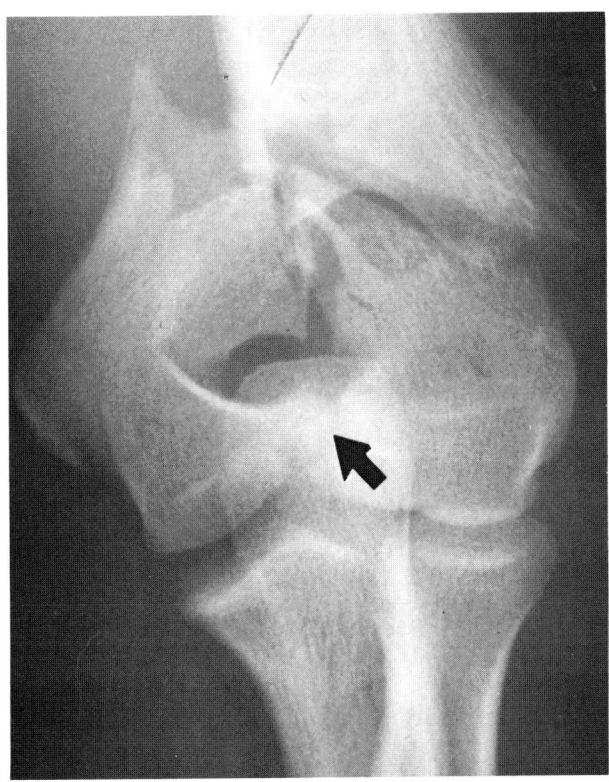
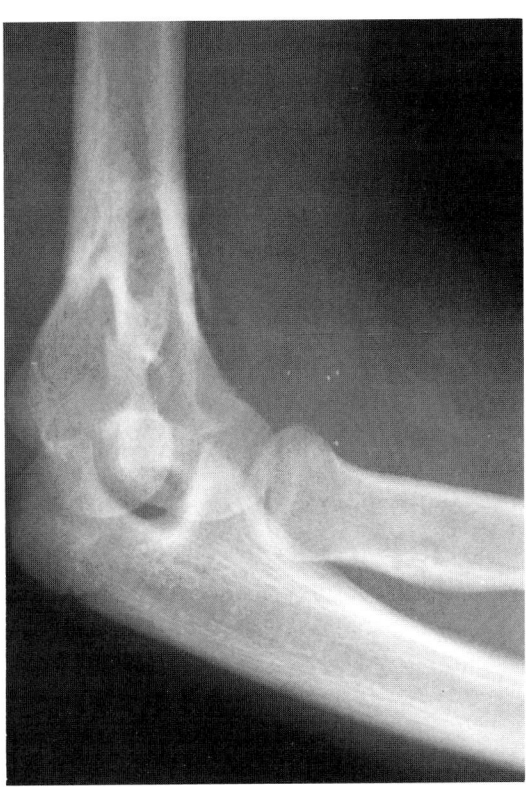

FIG. 12–52. AP (**A**) and lateral (**B**) views of an overriding Y type fracture (*arrow*) with displacement but no rotation (Type II) of the condyles.

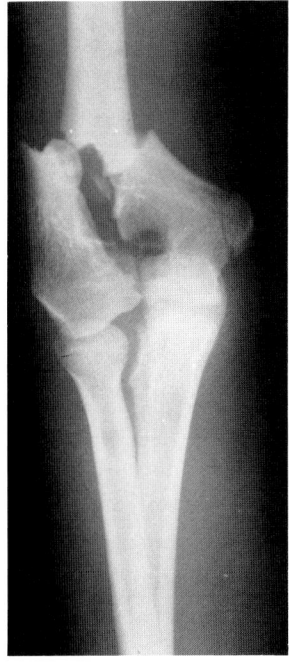

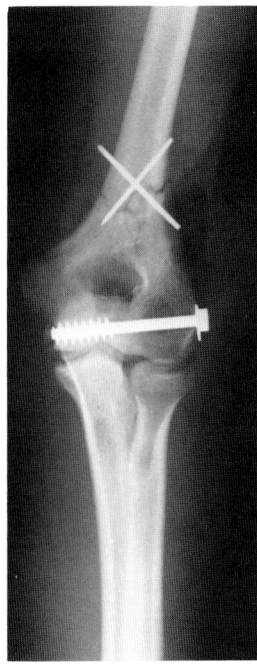

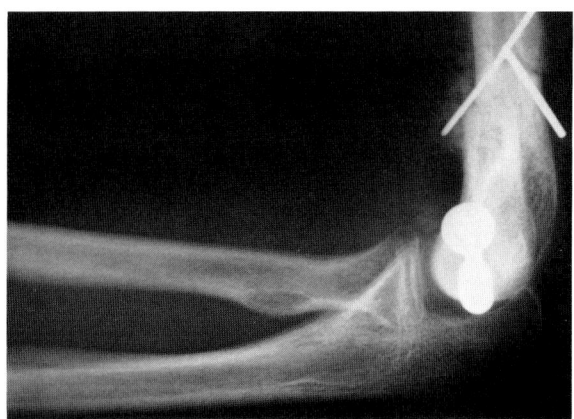

A

B

FIG. 12–53. A: Type III T-condylar fracture in which the fracture fragments are rotated but gross comminution has not occurred. This is readily fixed by restoring the articular integrity with a lag screw. The supracondylar component is then initially sutured with K-wires **(B, C)** (from 101, with permission).

Treatment

Treatment is controversial. In the Type I and Type II injuries (Figs. 12-50 and 12-52), closed reduction is often employed and is usually adequate, particularly if there is not a great deal of displacement (89,93,107). With the Type III fracture, many recommend open reduction and internal fixation (Fig. 12-53) (78,80,91,108). This is the treatment of choice in our experience, but we would emphasize that significant experience and expertise with open techniques is mandatory. Skeletal traction is a safe and frequently employed technique for the fractures (102,107).

An accurate evaluation of the reduction during traction or after closed reduction is, in any case, of paramount importance. The quality of reduction can be readily followed with serial AP and lateral roentgenograms. The flexed axial view is frequently employed in this setting. Posterior angulation is not uncommon and must be avoided in the adult. Rigid fixation should be obtained with these fractures if an open technique is employed. Cortical cancellous lag screws, medial and lateral plates, Y-plates (Fig. 12-54), and multiple K-wires have been used for this purpose. The radiograph not only helps assess the adequacy of the reduction; it also ensures that the fixation device has not impinged on the olecranon fossa.

be useful in complex cases. Three dimensional CT evaluation may be needed for surgical planning.

Complications

Complications of this fracture include improper reduction (Fig. 12-55) and the development of exuberant callus that can fill the olecranon fossa and thus limit motion. Internal fixation devices can likewise limit motion if the fossae are crossed by screws or pins (Fig. 12-56). These features of treatment can be detected radiographically with routine views, but occasionally tomography or flexion-extension views will be helpful. Non-union occurs in about 2–5% and is usually associated with inadequate surgical procedure (76,83, 99,101). Most non-unions occur with Types III and IV

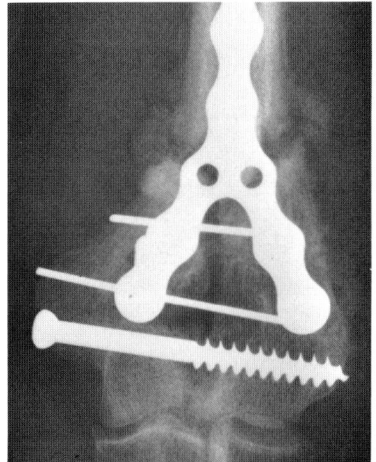

FIG. 12–54. The Y plate is often used for Type III fractures.

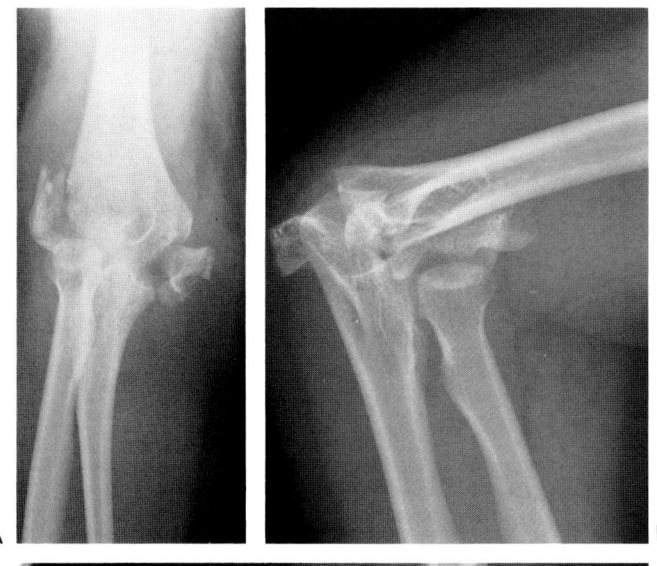

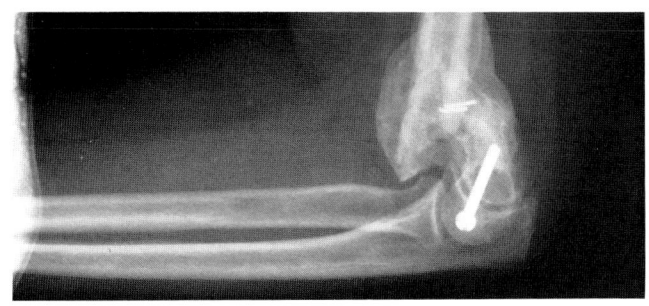

FIG. 12–55. A severely comminuted fracture involving primarily the condyles (**A**) with further extent of damage being demonstrated by the lateral (**B**). These fractures are usually very difficult and this one has healed in a malunited position as demonstrated on the lateral (**C**).

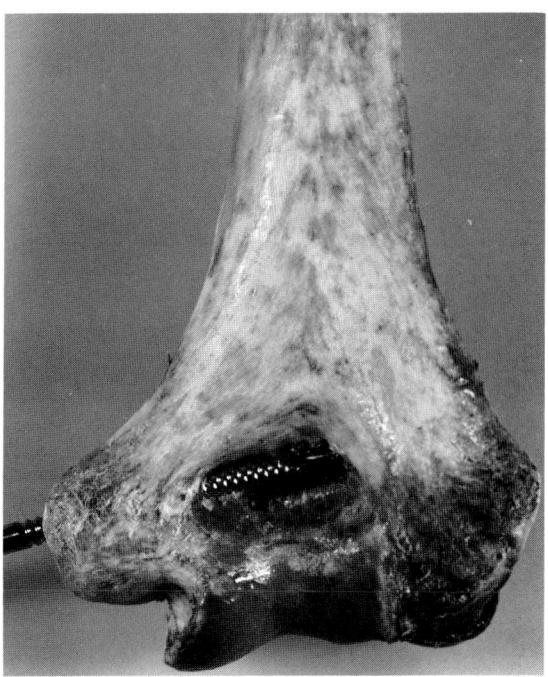

FIG. 12–56. Limitation of motion can result from fixation devices being present in the olecranon fossa (from 101, with permission).

(see Fig. 12-50) injuries. Total elbow arthroplasty should be considered when non-union occurs in patients treated with previous open reduction (85).

Capitellar Fractures

This fracture is one of the most difficult to diagnose accurately by the radiograph. The incidence is reported to be only 1% of all elbow injuries (83). The mechanism of injury is either a direct blow or a fall on the outstretched hand.

Classification

Three types of capitellar fractures have been described (Fig. 12-57) (101). The Type I fracture involves the entire capitellum or a major portion of it, often with a small portion of the trochlea. This fracture is virtually never seen on the AP radiograph but is readily seen on the lateral view (Fig. 12-58). Type II injury consists of a

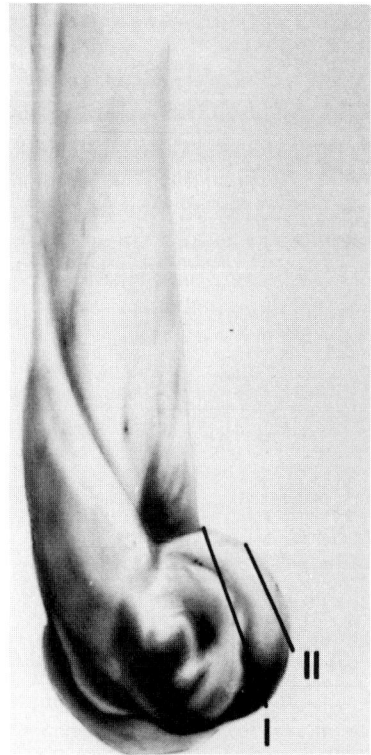

FIG. 12–57. Capitellar fractures may be classified as Type I in which a large fragment is sheared from the capitellum. Type II in which a very thin cartilaginous fragment is fractured. The Type III, not shown, is an impaction type fracture that cannot usually be diagnosed by the radiograph.

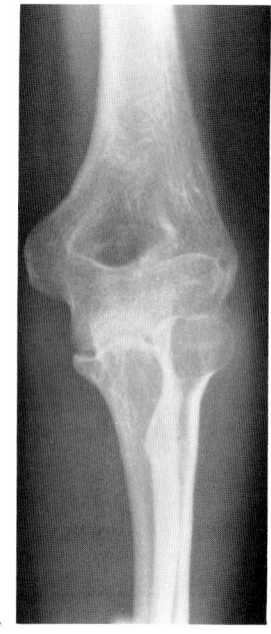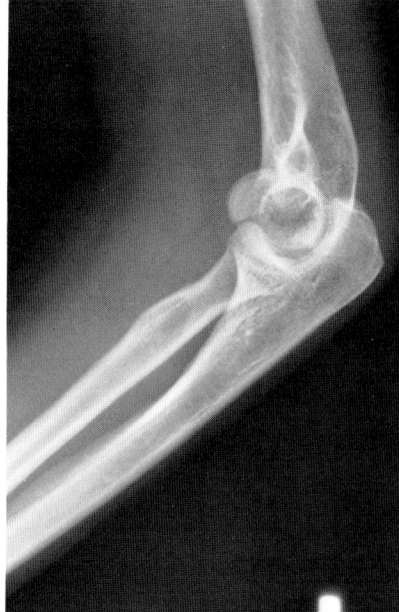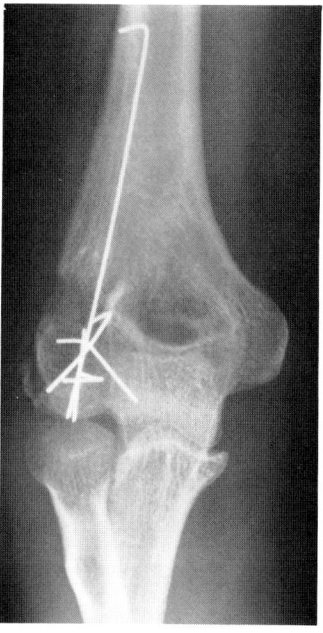

A   B   C

FIG. 12–58. Type I fracture of the capitellum but the anterior posterior roentgenogram of the elbow is essentially normal (**A**). However, on the lateral view, the fractured capitellum is easily visualized (**B**). In this instance, the fracture was stabilized with multiple K-wires (**C**) (from 101, with permission).

shearing fracture. Often there is little or no cancellous bone on the cartilage; as a result, this fracture is notoriously misdiagnosed. The fat pad sign is helpful in detecting an injury, and aspiration showing fat globules and a hemarthrosis should also raise one's suspicion of the likelihood of this fracture (82). The Type III injury is a comminuted fracture of the capitellum, often associated with fracture of the radial head (103). Associated rupture of the ulnar collateral ligament may occur in up to 13% of cases (83,92). The mechanism of injury is a fall on the outstretched hand, causing a compression injury.

Roentgenographic Assessment

The AP view is usually unrewarding for all three types of fractures. The lateral view is sufficient for Type I, but oblique views of the elbow joint may be needed for detection of Type II fractures. Occasionally, a lateral tomogram may be needed for Types II and III fractures (Fig. 12-59). The differential diagnosis for Type II fracture includes fracture of the radial head. An important point of distinction is that the displacement of the capitellar fracture fragment is commonly superior to the capitellum (Fig. 12-58B), while the displacement of the radial head fracture fragments is not (see Fig. 12-36B). For Type II fractures, the sheared cartilage may have little or no osseous compartment. In this instance, evidence of a lipohemarthrosis from radiography or arthrocentesis will be helpful.

Physical Examination

While the physical examination is not very helpful in most other fractures, it is helpful in the diagnosis of capitellar fractures. Hemarthrosis with crepitus and pain over the radiohumeral articulation, which is aggravated by pronation and supination but not by flexion-extension, are specific and characteristic physical features (101).

Treatment

The treatment of Type I fractures is somewhat controversial (81,87,88). Closed reduction is possible, and the fracture may appear to be anatomically reduced on the lateral roentgenogram. However, limitation of motion may persist. Internal fixation may be effected by K-wires if the fracture is not too large (Fig. 12-58C). If the fragment is large, screw fixation lagged from posterior to anterior is our preferred treatment. The small Type I fragment and the Type II fragment may simply be excised (86). Loose fragments are removed for Type III fractures if motion is limited. If the radial head requires removal, the capitellar fracture is ignored, but loose fragments are removed.

Fracture of the Condyles

Fracture of a humeral condyle is uncommon but may be seen to involve either the medial or the lateral structure.

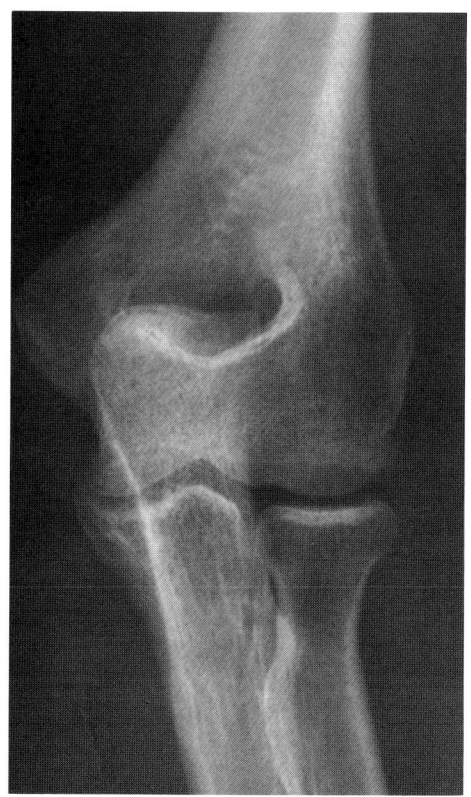

A

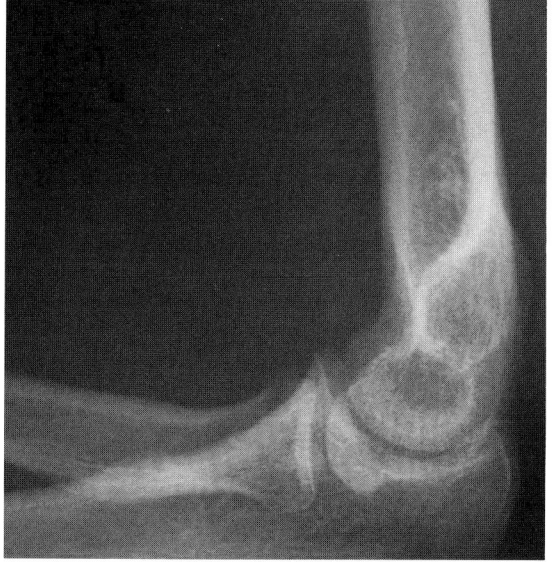

B

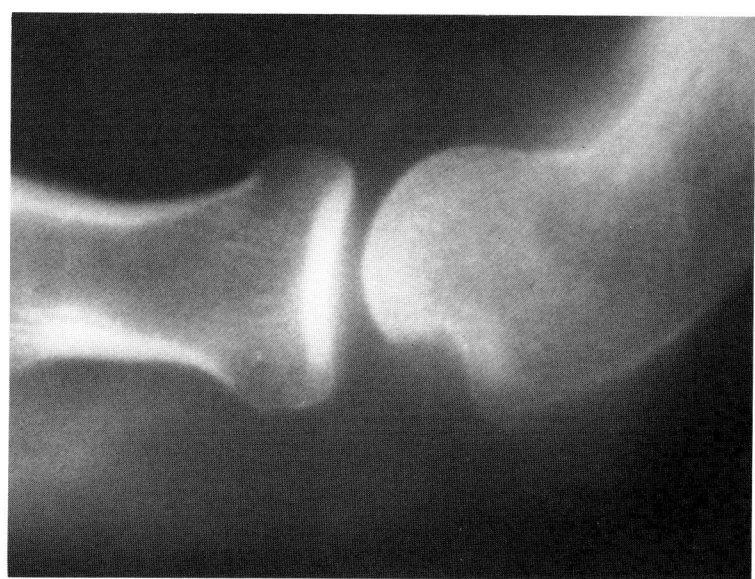

C

FIG. 12–59. Impacted capitellar fracture. AP (**A**) and lateral (**B**) views of the elbow do not demonstrate any definite abnormality. Lateral tomogram (**C**) clearly demonstrates the capitellar impaction.

Mechanism of Injury

An isolated fracture of the condyle can occur from one of two mechanisms. Both essentially involve an avulsion or a shearing type of fracture. A fall on the outstretched hand with the forearm in valgus can produce an axial load that, depending upon the distribution of the forces, may result in a shearing type of lateral condylar fracture or an avulsion type of medial condylar fracture. Conversely, a fall on the outstretched hand with axial load

and a varus angular component may produce a shearing type of medial condylar fracture and an avulsion type of lateral condylar fracture. Thus, four possible mechanisms obtain: shearing or avulsion of the medial condyle and shearing or avulsion of the lateral condyle.

Classification

This fracture has been classified into two types by Milch (97,98). The Type I lateral fracture involves only

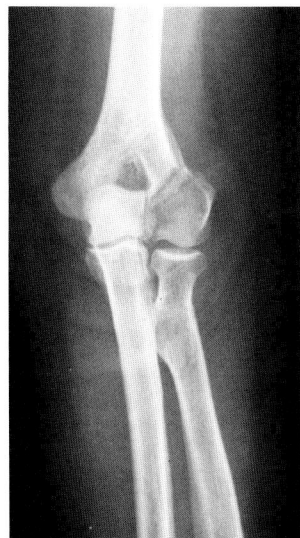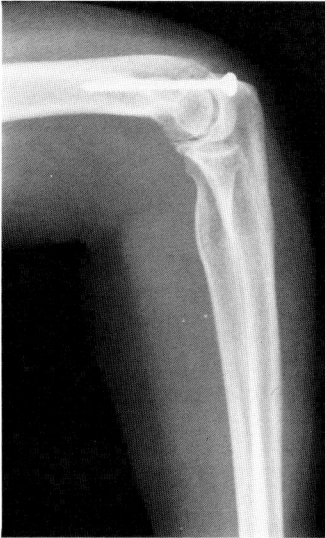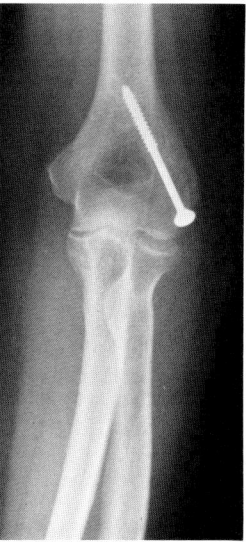

A   B

FIG. 12–60. An example of an undisplaced lateral condylar fracture. Notice that this fracture involves the supracondylar and bony column (**A**). Although undisplaced in order to allow early motion, this fracture was stabilized with a single screw (**B, C**) (from 129, with permission.)

the capitellum and lateral epicondyle; the Type I medial fracture includes the medial lip of the trochlea and the medial epicondyle. The Type I lateral fracture includes no part or only a small part of the lateral trochlea (Fig. 12-60). The Type II lateral fracture involves the lateral half of the trochlea; the Type II medial fracture involves the entire trochlea. This classification is of major significance, because the Type II fracture, usually lateral, is associated with marked elbow instability (Fig. 12-61). If this fracture is not appropriately treated with surgery, permanent and significant residual impairment can result.

Diagnosis

The diagnosis of an articular fracture of some type is suspected as a result of a physical examination that demonstrates that the posterior triangular relationship has been altered. In the adult, routine radiography readily demonstrates the nature of the injury. However, because the distal humerus is primarily cartilaginous in the young child, this fracture, representing a Salter-Harris Type IV, can be very difficult to diagnose correctly.

Treatment

The Type I injury is frequently an undisplaced fracture and can be treated by closed reduction and immobilization for 3–6 weeks, depending upon the age and severity of the injury. Any displaced Type I fracture should be

treated with open reduction and internal fixation (Fig. 12-60B). Surgical correction of all Type II fractures is recommended (97). Usually a lateral Kocher incision or a medial triceps reflecting approach, as described by Bryan and Morrey, is used (79). In most instances, the condyles are readily fixed with interfragmentary compression by lag screws. Early motion is begun at 1–2 weeks. In the child, the fracture must be followed carefully for 1–2 years because of potential disturbance of growth.

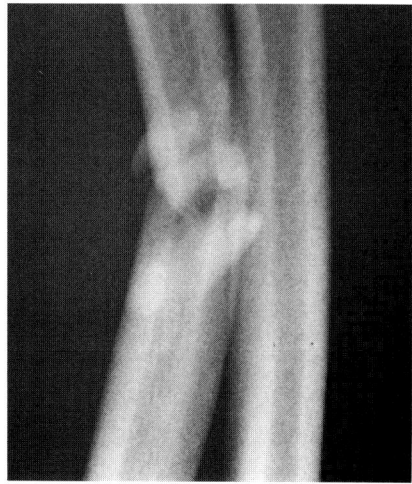

FIG. 12–61. AP view of the elbow demonstrates a comminuted Type II lateral condyle fracture involving the lateral trochlea.

Complications

Untoward events with this fracture include neurovascular compromise, as the proximal fragment may impinge on or impale the neurovascular bundle (94). The development of ischemic contracture of the forearm, the so-called *Volkmann's ischemic contracture,* is notorious following supracondylar types of fractures (96). The more common types of complications, however, involve inadequate reduction and the subsequent loss of proper position, motion, and stability owing to an incongruous joint. Even internal fixation can contribute to this complication if the fixation device impinges on the olecranon fossa and thereby limits motion (see Fig. 12-56). Lack of proper reduction can cause malorientation of the articular surface, which further limits motion or function (Fig. 12-62) (100). Soft tissue calcification and scarring about this joint are common even with minimal trauma, but they are particularly significant and disastrous after the more severe intra-articular injuries. They require prompt treatment (95). Hypertrophic callus can sometimes develop either posteriorly or anteriorly. Often the olecranon fossa will be obliterated. Once again, motion is lost.

To conclude, the current philosophy of treatment for distal humeral fractures emphasizes early motion and relies upon open reduction and internal fixation with rigid devices as the treatment of choice. If the injury has resulted in hopeless comminution, then traction and motion is recommended. With single large fragments that are not badly displaced, early motion is likewise suggested. In any event, prolonged casting is to be discouraged.

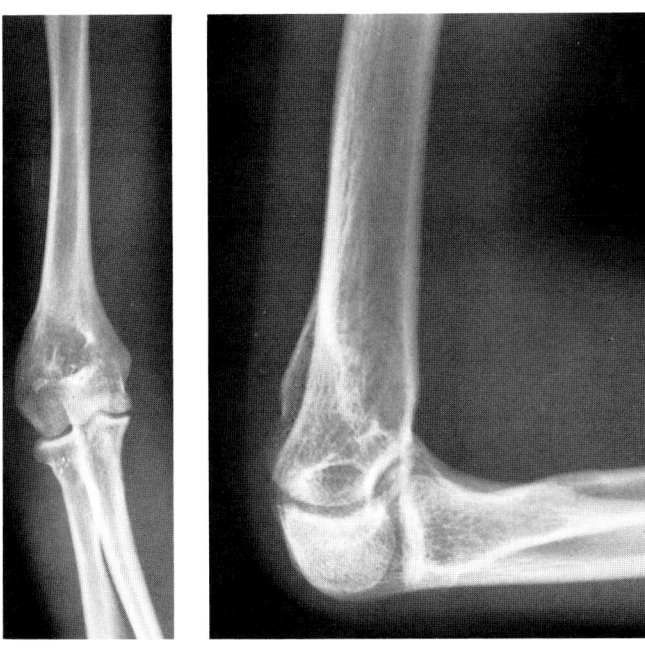

A

B

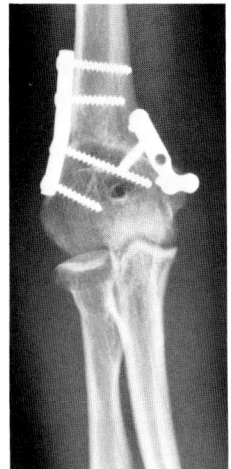

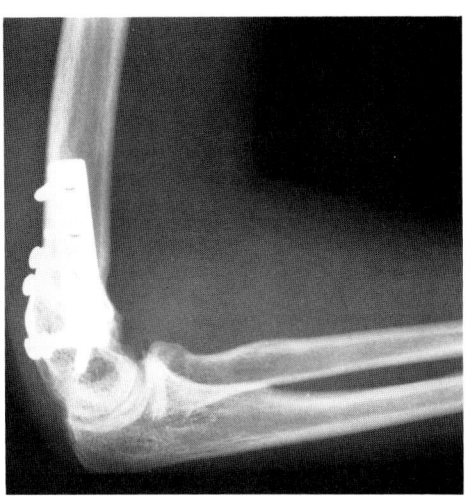

C

D

FIG. 12–62. Healed fracture of the humeral condyles demonstrates approximately 5° of varus angulation (**A**) and also limitation of flexion due to the posterior displacement of the condyles (**B**). A corrective osteotomy was performed in both the anterioposterior plane (**C**) and the lateral projection (**D**). Note the restoration of the normal anterior rotation of the articular surface. This resulted in resumption of normal motion of this joint (from 129, with permission).

Fractures of the Proximal Radius

Fractures of the head and neck of the radius are a common injury, accounting for approximately one-third of all elbow fractures and 1–2% of all fractures seen by physicians. The mechanism of injury has been carefully described by Thomas. These fractures occur from a fall on the outstretched hand with the elbow partially flexed and pronated (Fig. 12-63) (74). Because the neck of the radius makes an angle of about 15° with the shaft of the bone (Fig. 12-63), in the pronated position the anterolateral margin comes into contact with the capitellum. Thus, the proximal radius is vulnerable to a shearing type of fracture. Increasing amounts of force with this orientation result in a more extensive injury.

Classification

We feel that the most useful classification is one modified from Mason (126). It consists of four types (Fig. 12-64). The type I fracture is an undisplaced or minimally displaced (<2 mm) fracture of the head or neck (Figs. 12-65 and 12-66). The Type II fracture involves approximately one-third of the radial head, with greater than 2 mm of displacement or 20°–30° of angulation (Fig. 12-67 and 12-68). The Type III fracture involves comminution of the radial head (Fig. 12-69). The Type IV fracture is any fracture of the radial head with dislocation of the ulnohumeral joint (Fig. 12-70) (122). In the pediatric age group, most of these injuries occur as fractures of the radial neck, with varying degrees of angulation and displacement. If the fracture is of the radial neck, angulation of less than 20°–30° is considered a Type I fracture; angulation of greater than 20°–30° is considered a Type II fracture; and angulation of greater

than 60° or dislocation is considered a Type III radial neck fracture (126,129).

The diagnosis is suspected by a history of injury. Marked local tenderness of the radiohumeral joint with extreme pain on pronation-supination is demonstrated on the physical examination.

Radiographic Findings

Routine AP and lateral radiographs are usually sufficient to demonstrate this fracture (Figs. 12-65–12-70). However, a single view often will not reveal the fracture line, and oblique or radial head views (Fig. 12-66) are sometimes required before the true extent of the fracture is appreciated. A fat pad sign with the features of the physical examination discussed earlier may be the only indication, but these should allow diagnosis even of minimally displaced Type I fractures. Distinction between a Type II capitellar and a Type I radial head fracture may be difficult. Additional views should be taken when there is doubt. Occasionally a tomogram may be necessary to resolve the issue (129).

Treatment

The appropriate treatment of this fracture is one of the most controversial areas in orthopedic surgery. The Type I fracture is treated nonoperatively with early motion after the joint has been aspirated (110,125,130). Surgical excision of Types II and III fractures has been the standard treatment (116,117,126,132,133,135). In our opinion, Types II or III uncomplicated fractures should be surgically excised only if displacement limits motion in the anesthetized joint (110,111,113,118,129).

We begin motion on the day of the injury, if possible.

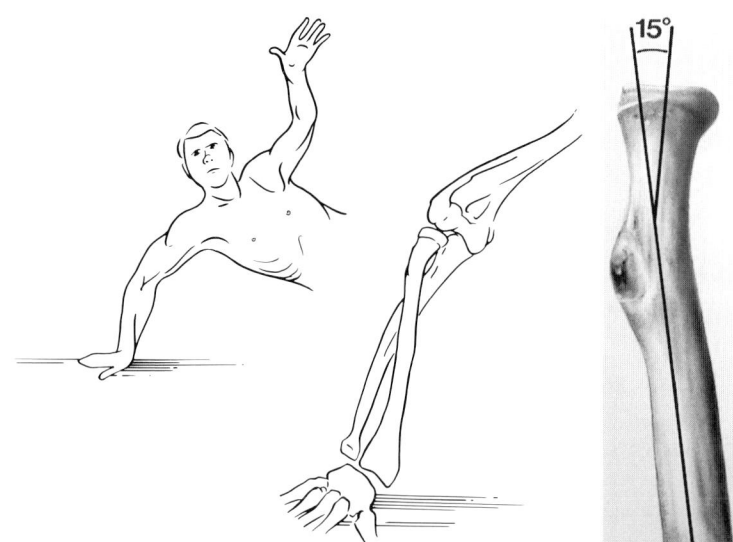

FIG. 12–63. Mechanism of radial head fracture or fall on the slightly flexed pronated upper extremity (**A**). Normal neck-shaft angles of the proximal radius (**B**) (from 129, with permission).

A

B

TYPE I

TYPE II

TYPE III

TYPE IV

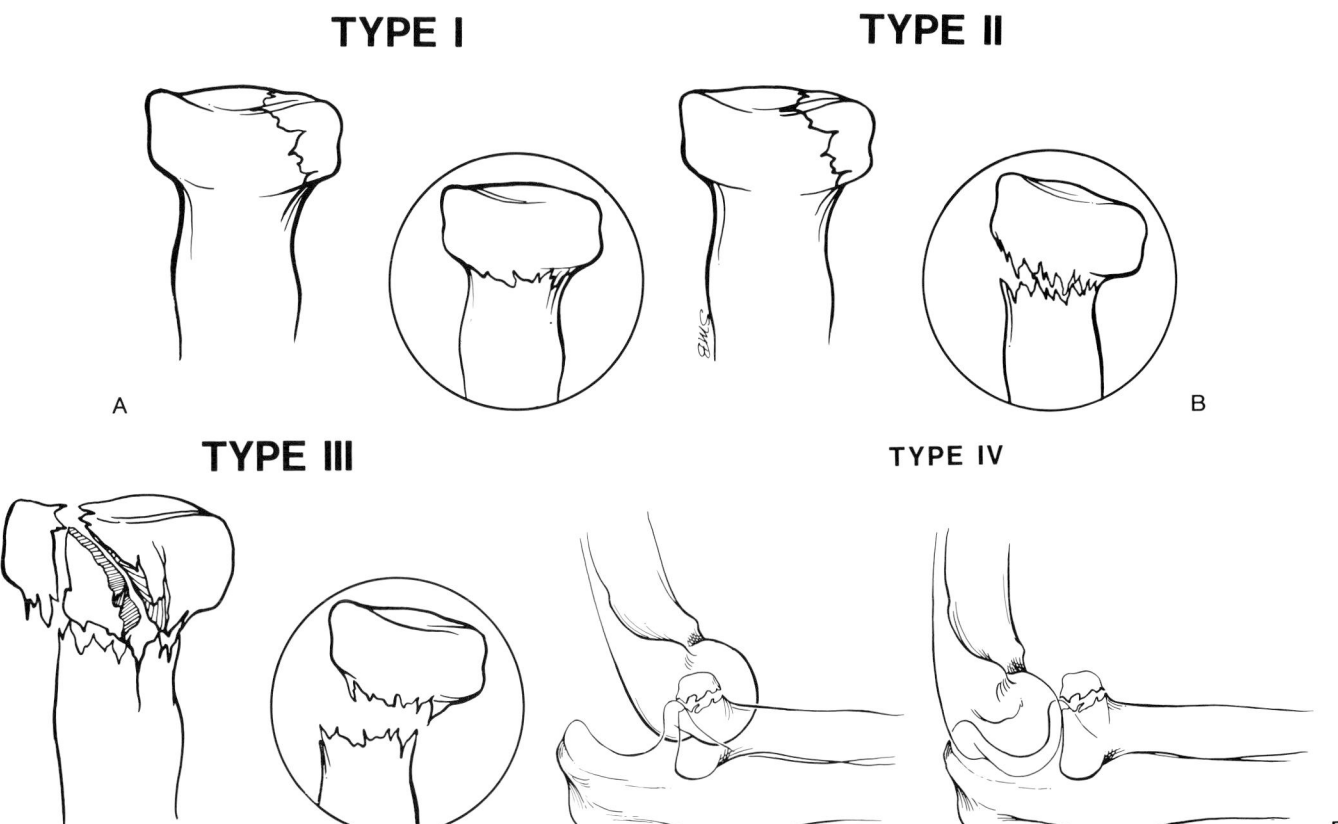

FIG. 12–64. Type I radial head fractures undisplaced (**A**). Type II demonstrates less than a 2–3 mm displacement and less than 30% involvement and/or less than 30° angulation. Type III is a comminuted fracture of the radial head or displaced radial neck fracture. Type IV is represented as a fracture-dislocation of the radial head and ulnohumeral joint (from 129, with permission).

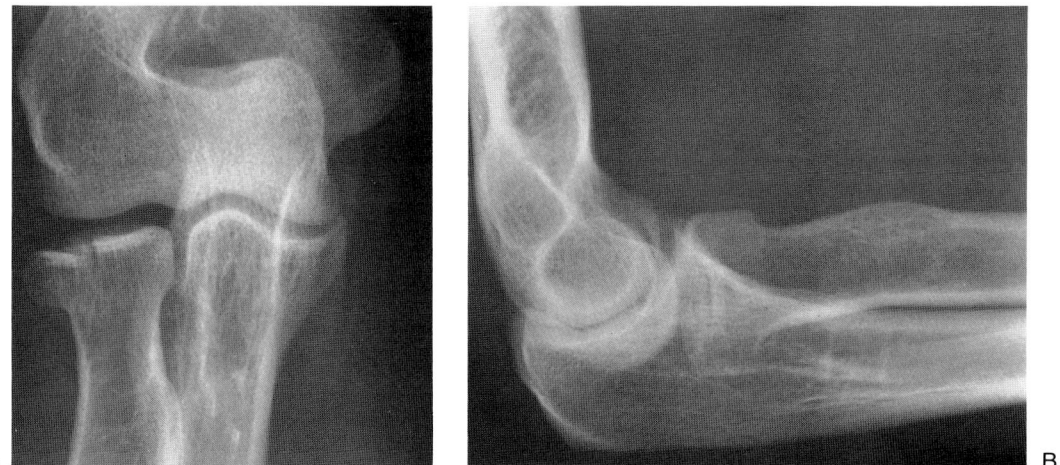

FIG. 12–65. An example of a Type I radial head fracture on the AP projection (**A**). Notice that the fracture line cannot be visualized in the lateral projection (**B**). Thus the importance of the two plane radiographic assessment (from 129, with permission).

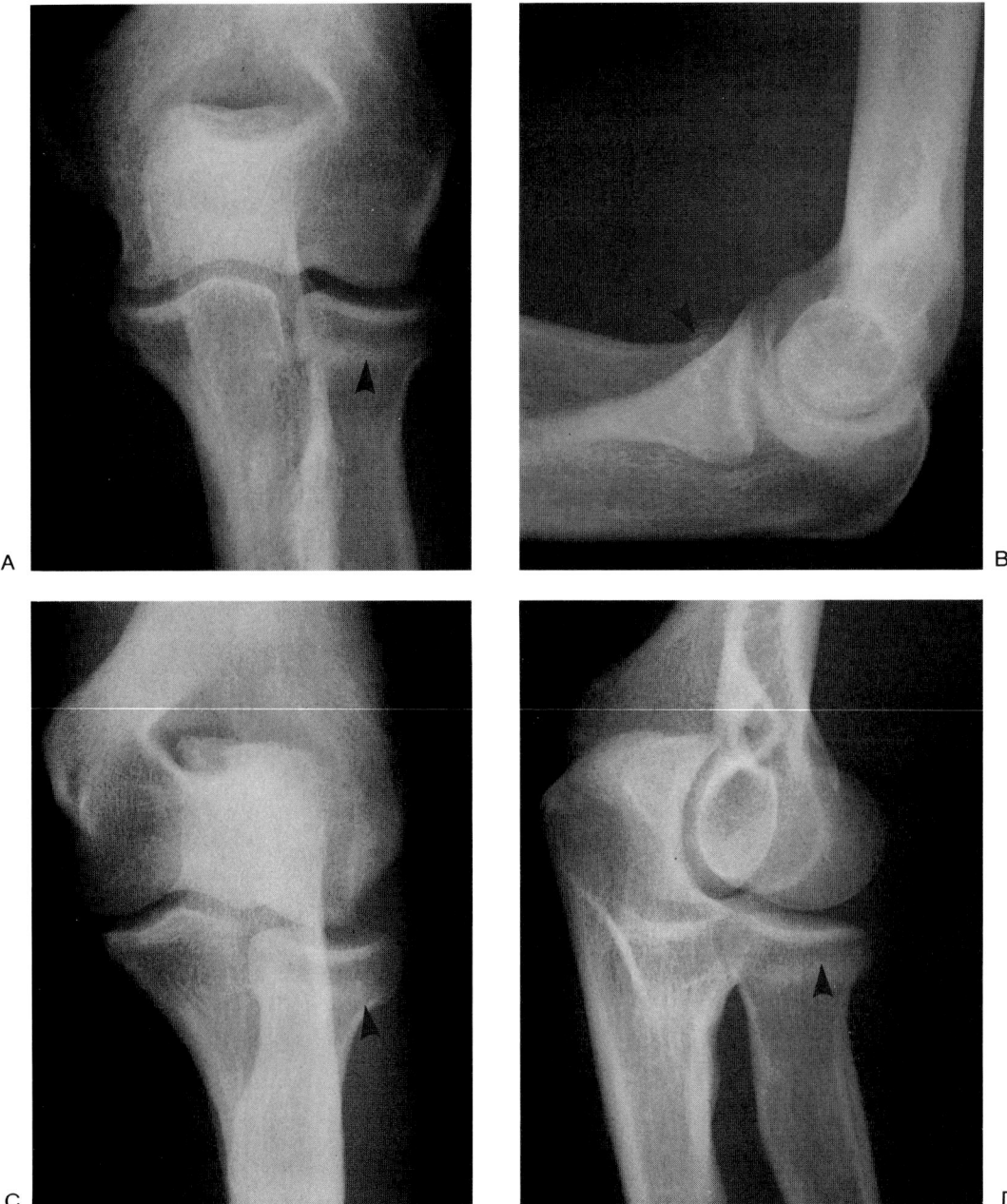

FIG. 12-66. AP (**A**), lateral (**B**), and oblique (**C, D**) views of an impacted radial neck fracture (*arrows*), Type I. There is an area of bony condensation (*arrows*) due to trabecular compression.

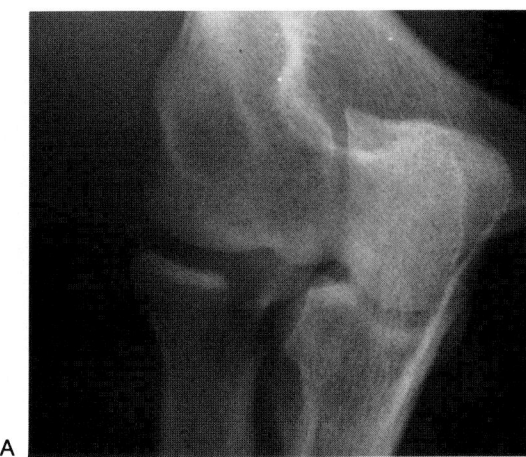
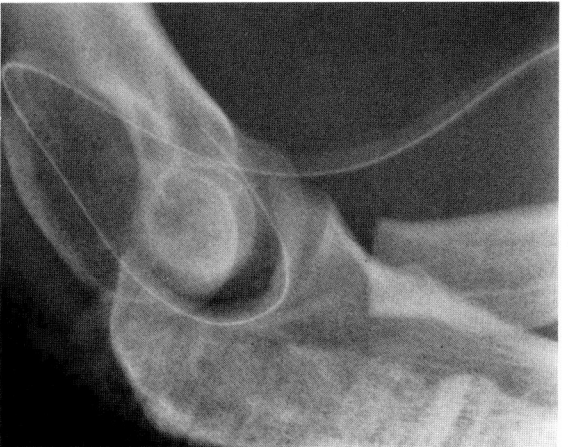

A

B

FIG. 12-67. Type II radial head fracture with greater than 2 mm displacement of 30% of the radial head (**A**). This is treated by radial head excision (**B**) (from 129, with permission).

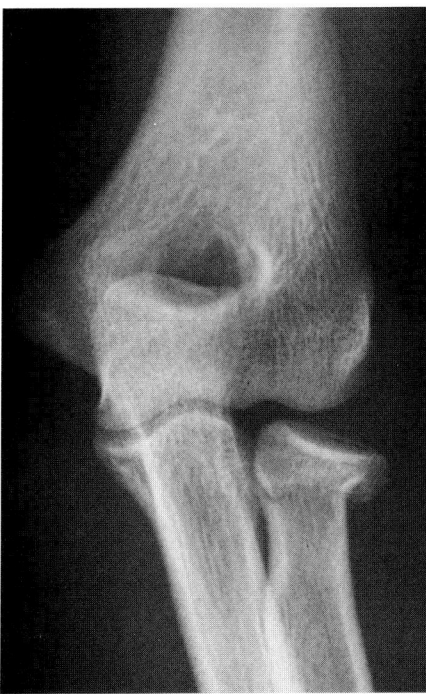

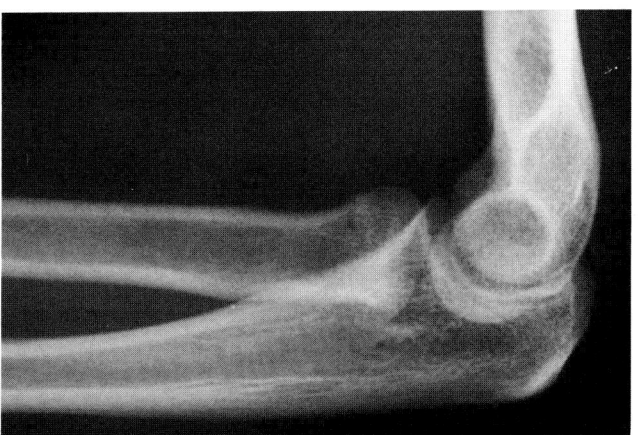

B

FIG. 12-68. AP (**A**) and lateral (**B**) views of a displaced Type II neck fracture. The finding is most obvious on the AP view (**A**).

A

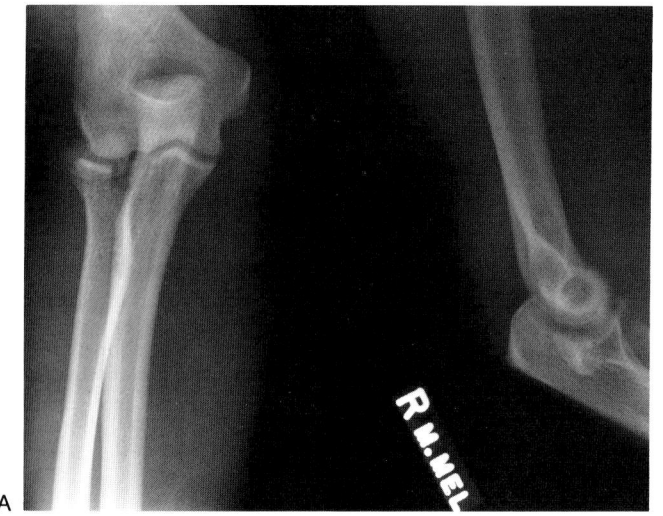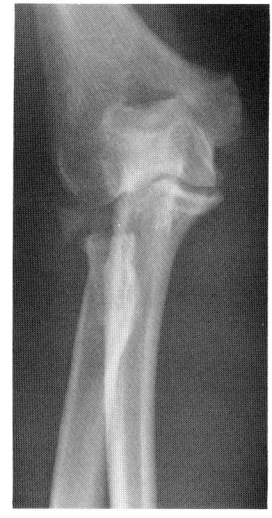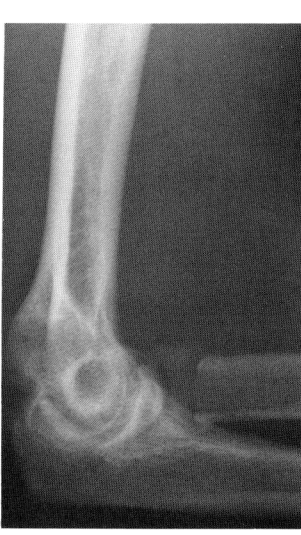

A

B

C

FIG. 12–69. Comminuted fracture of the radial head demonstrated in both the AP and lateral projections (**A**). This particular fracture was treated at 8 years in both the anterior and posterior (**B**) and lateral (**C**) projections. As is often the case, this radiographic finding did not correlate with any clinical symptomatology (from 129, with permission).

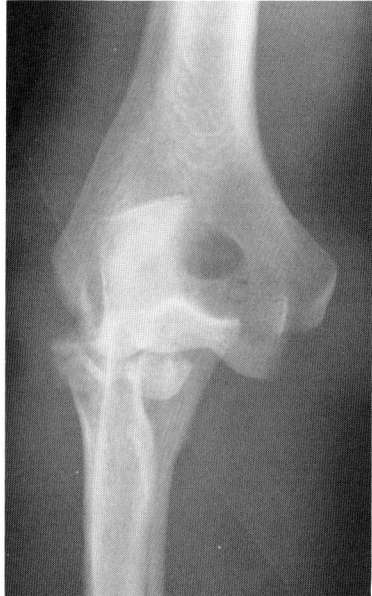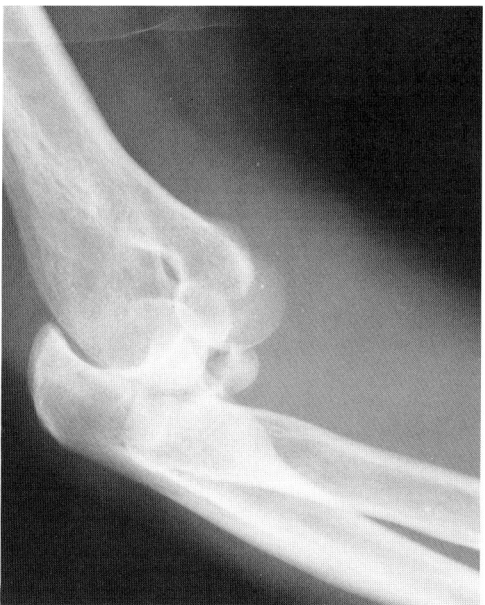

A

B

FIG. 12–70. Fracture-dislocations of the radial head and ulnohumeral joint (**A**). These are best demonstrated on the lateral projection (**B**) (from 129, with permission).

If there have been associated injuries of the distal radioulnar stabilizers (120) or of the medial collateral ligament (112,115), a radial head prosthesis should be considered (121,124). A cleavage fracture of a single fragment involving approximately one-third of the radial head with associated ligament injury is amenable to open reduction and internal fixation. This treatment should be considered (Fig. 12-71) in a patient under 40–50 years of age (131). If elbow ligaments have been torn, the joint can be unacceptably unstable after radial head excision (121,129). In this case, a radial head prosthesis may also be used to improve stability and to allow early rehabilitation (128). Although acrylic and metal prostheses have been used in the past, the Silastic prosthesis designed by Swanson is most commonly used in this country (124,129,137). However, this material is subject to fracture and the implant can dislocate. To assess these radiographic features properly, routine and oblique views may be necessary. Since Silastic is radiolucent, xeroradiography has been recommended to evaluate this implant (114,129). While not necessary routinely, it is of value in the symptomatic joint.

Results

The results of treatment of the Type I fracture tend to be very good, although a surprisingly high number of patients will have some complaints (133). In general, Types II and III fractures are associated with about 80–90% satisfactory results (110,111,113,116,126) with both operative and closed treatment. Patient selection remains controversial, although early motion is generally becoming accepted regardless of the nature of initial treatment (129).

Complications

Multiple complications are seen both as associated injuries and following treatment of radial head fractures, particularly after radial head excision. Associated fractures of the ulna (134) are not uncommon and represent a variant of the Monteggia lesion described later. Ectopic ossification (Fig. 12-72) or overgrowth of the resected stump of the radius can be so prominent that it gives rise to a radiographic appearance of an apparent regrowth of the radial head, particularly in the younger individual (136). Ligamentous instability is so common that it may be termed a Type IV fracture. Our experience with this injury indicates that immobilization for more than 4 weeks will result in a poor prognosis (129), and thus a Silastic implant might be considered a source of stability in this setting (121,128,137). If radial head excision has occurred, shortening of the radius can cause some symptoms at the wrist (129,137). This injury can result in a decrease in forearm rotation due to shortening of the interosseous membrane (138). For this reason, some people recommend that the radial head be left alone and excised only if it becomes symptomatic later. Interestingly, very few data have been gathered to demonstrate whether this is an effective means of treatment. We have recently analyzed our experience with delayed excision of the radial head. Our review demonstrated that, in fact, improved motion and relief of pain can be rather predictably observed in about 75% of the patients treated this way (129).

Fractures of the Ulna

Because of its subcutaneous position, the olecranon is particularly susceptible to trauma. Most fractures are

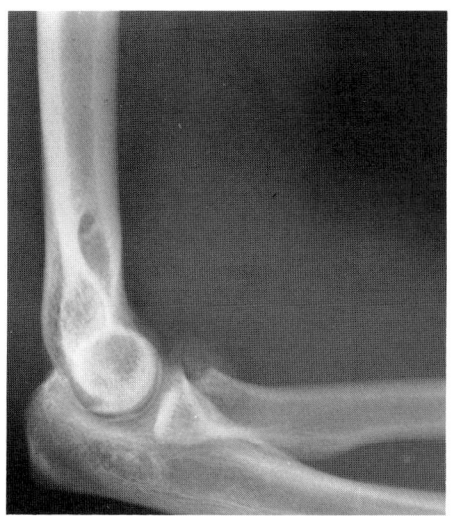
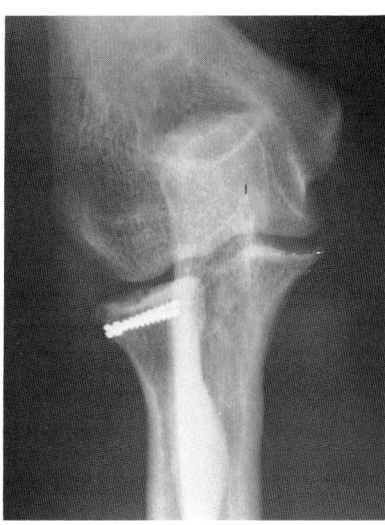

A B

FIG. 12–71. Fracture of the radial head demonstrated the lateral projection (**A**). In this instance treated with internal fixation (**B**). Two views are helpful to assure containment of the screws (from 129, with permission).

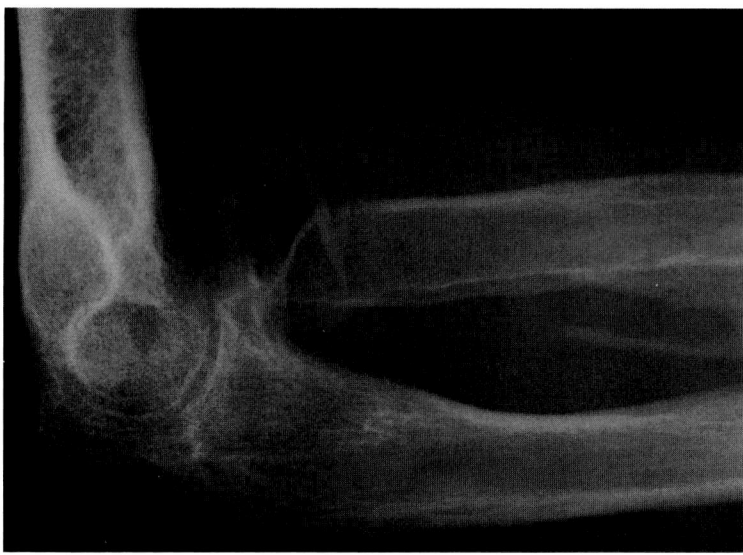

FIG. 12–72. Lateral view of the elbow after resection of the radial head. There is heterotopic bone near the radial neck and in the interosseous membrane.

intra-articular and thus can compromise both the stability and function of the joint. If the triceps with its fascial expansions has been disrupted, the fracture becomes even more displaced. Without this feature, the displacement is usually minimal. Persistent fascial lines, usually bilateral, have been reported and are usually differentiated from fractures (159).

Mechanism

Fractures of the olecranon occur from a direct blow, usually from a fall on the flexed elbow or, less commonly, as a result of a hyperextension injury. The hyperextension injury is usually associated with other injury, for example, elbow dislocation or radial head fracture. Greater comminution is observed in the older and younger age groups. A clean transverse line is often observed.

Classification

The most common classification of olecranon fractures is that described by Colton (144) and consists, with minor modifications, of the following types (Fig. 12-73):

Type I. Undisplaced fracture. This fracture usually results from a direct blow, with the fragment separated less than 2 mm.

Type II. Displaced fracture involving avulsion and a transverse or oblique fracture line. This fracture probably occurs from a direct pull of the triceps during a forced elbow flexion or from a fall on the tip of the olecranon (Fig. 12-73A,B).

Type III. Transverse or oblique olecranon fracture (Fig. 12-73C,D). This fracture usually occurs by way of a more indirect mechanism of injury. The elbow is flexed

against resistance and receives a direct blow, with the trochlea serving as a wedge that fractures the midportion of the olecranon. With more severe violence, comminution is again usually found in the midportion of the olecranon, which is the nonarticular part of the elbow.

Type IV. Comminuted fracture. A direct blow, severe in a younger individual, less severe in the older patient, may cause significant comminution involving not only the midportion but also the proximal portion of the olecranon (Fig. 12-73E).

Type V. Fracture-dislocation. As a fracture is more distal about the area of the coronoid, associated disruption of the collateral ligament occurs, which results in a more unstable type of fracture (Fig. 12-74). Often the forearm is dislocated or subluxated anteriorly (Fig. 12-73F). This may also be considered a Monteggia variant.

Radiographic Evaluation

The AP radiograph of the elbow is not particularly helpful in defining the severity of the injury unless there is either medial or lateral displacement. Even rather severe fractures may demonstrate a reasonably normal AP view (Fig. 12-75A). The lateral view, on the other hand, not only demonstrates the precise orientation, displacement, and comminution of the fracture but also is most helpful in revealing any associated fracture of the radial head or displacement of the distal fragment (Fig. 12-75B). Failure to obtain a true lateral view before treatment is probably the most common error in the initial radiographic assessment of this type of injury.

Treatment

The specific goals of treatment of this fracture include maintenance or restoration of congruity, attainment of

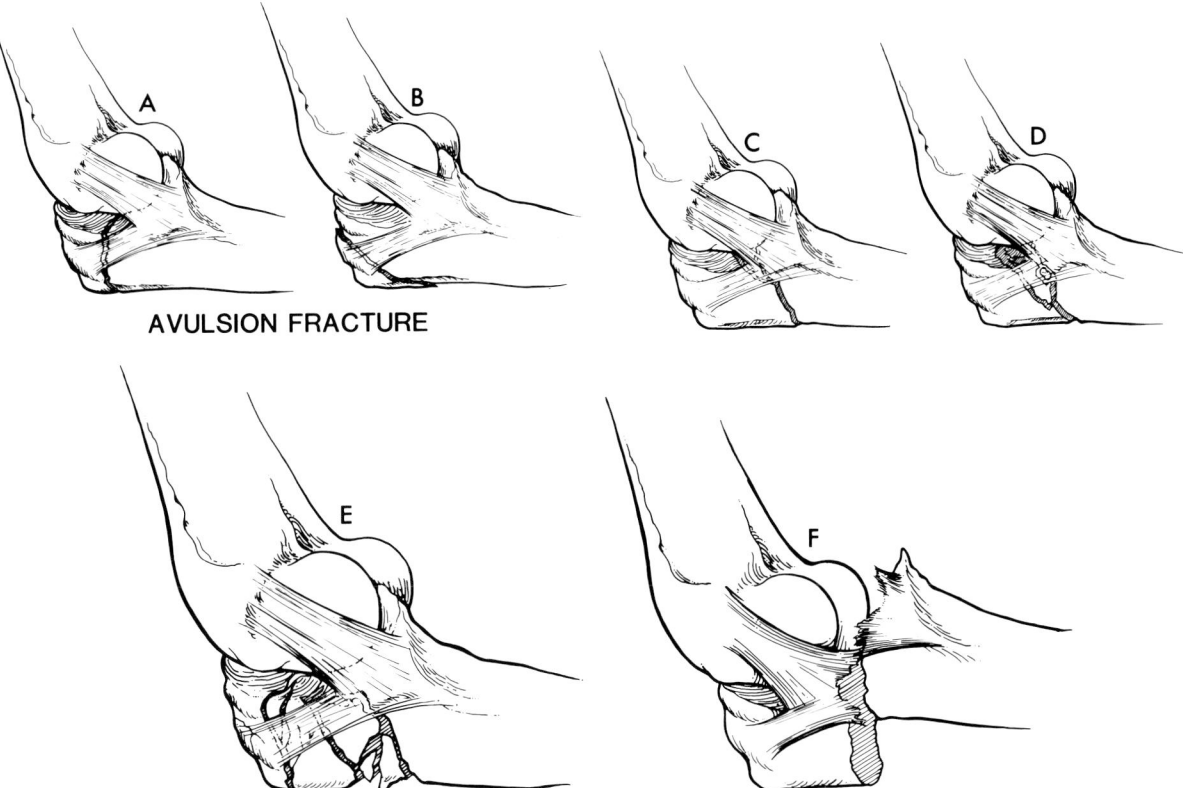

FIG. 12–73. Classification of olecranon fractures. The avulsion type fracture (**A, B**) may or may not involve the articular joint. The oblique or transverse fracture usually involves the mid-portion of the olecranon (**C**). An oblique fracture with comminution, usually in the non-articular portion of the olecranon (**C, D**). Comminuted fracture involving the majority of the olecranon process (**E**). Fracture-dislocation in which the fracture occurs more distally with the associated injury of the medial collateral ligament thus resulting in stability (**F**) (from 157, with permission).

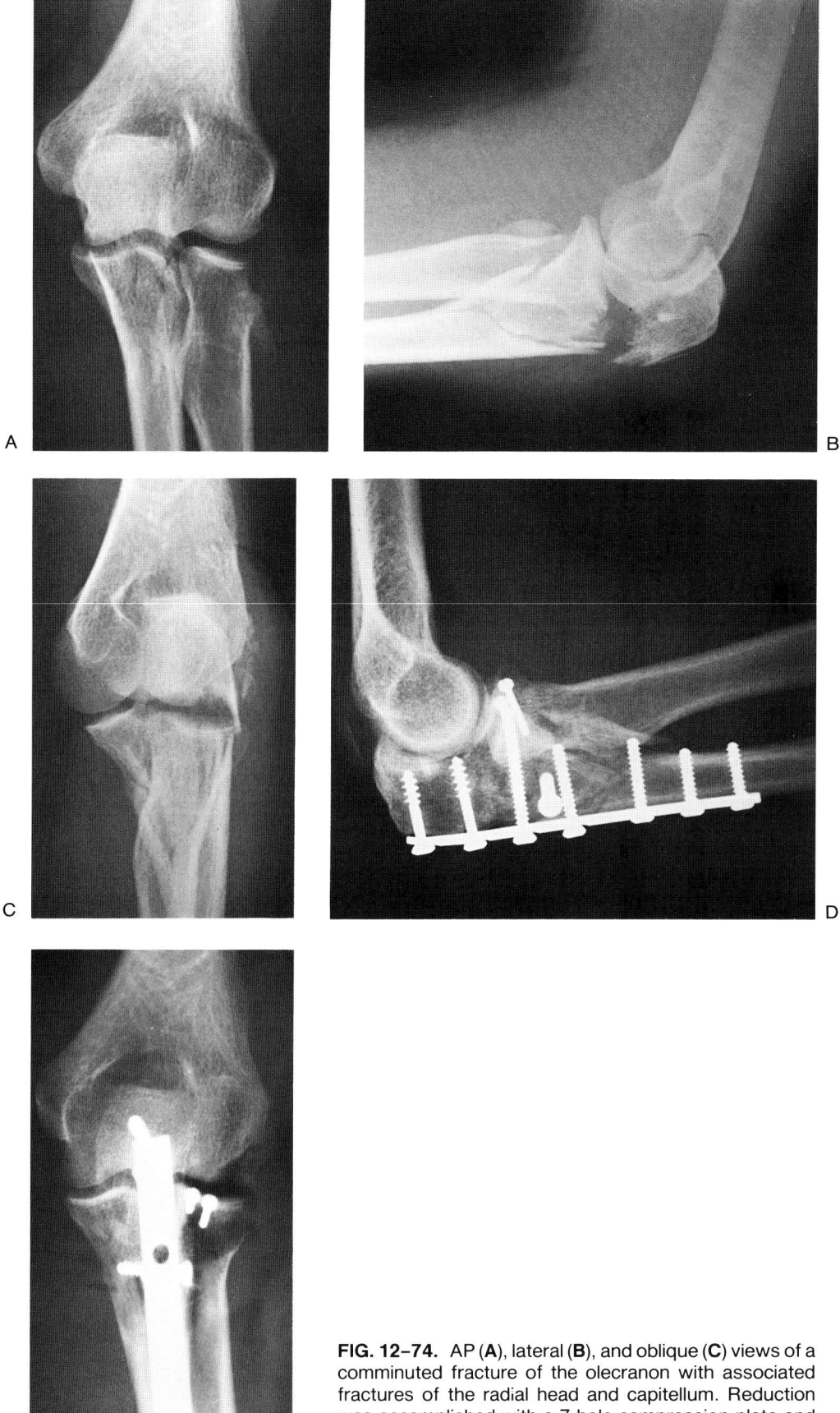

FIG. 12–74. AP (**A**), lateral (**B**), and oblique (**C**) views of a comminuted fracture of the olecranon with associated fractures of the radial head and capitellum. Reduction was accomplished with a 7-hole compression plate and screw fixation of the radial head (**D, E**).

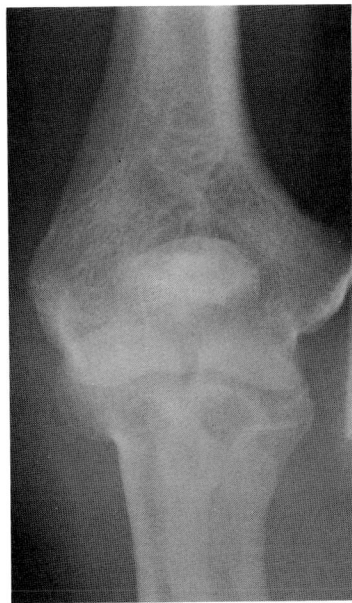 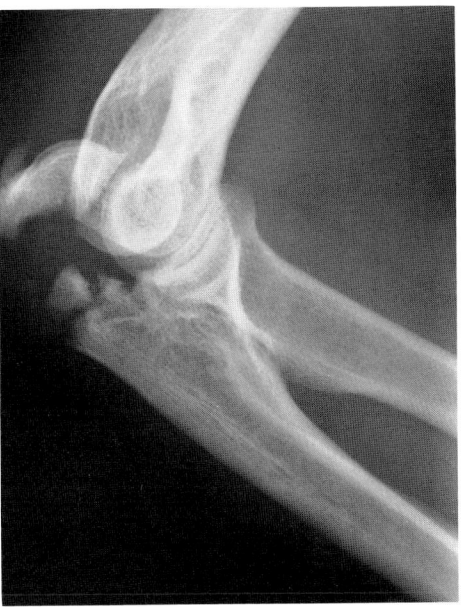

FIG. 12–75. AP roentgenogram of an olecranon fracture demonstrating relatively little pathology (**A**). Lateral projection showing a marked comminution and displacement of the olecranon fracture (**B**) (from 157, with permission).

stability, and preservation of function, particularly avoiding limitation of motion. Thus, surgical intervention is indicated in most displaced fractures unless rather significant extenuating circumstances obtain (147,154,165).

If the fracture is undisplaced, a relatively brief period of immobilization (2 or 3 weeks) followed by gentle controlled motion and careful recheck evaluation is indicated. Follow-up roentgenograms should be obtained 6–10 days after the initial injury and then on a weekly basis for approximately 1 month. Flexion at greater than 90° is usually avoided until union is complete. Union often occurs in the second and almost always by the third month.

Treatment of Displaced Fractures

Treatment of displaced fractures of the olecranon depends upon the degree of comminution and displacement and the age of the patient. As long ago as 1876, surgical fixation was reported by Shelton (168). Various devices were used in the early 1900s, including wires, nails, bone pegs, kangaroo tendon, and fascia lata (146). Simple wiring of the fracture was the most common method of treatment until the last decade (139,148, 152,169). Because of the inadequate stability, the reduction was often lost.

The most common means of fixation now is that recommended by the AO Group, termed *tension band wiring* (Fig. 12-76). This technique converts the distraction forces of the fracture into compression forces during elbow flexion (147,154). The two Kirschner wires directed down the shaft of the olecranon allow reduction of the fracture, which is converted to a stable configuration by

the addition of the figure-of-8 wire loop. This wire is placed through a transverse hole in the distal portion of the fracture and across the pins as they protrude from the olecranon more proximally (Fig. 12-76).

Intramedullary fixation with Rush rods and Leinbach screws or a flexible device (145) has been recommended, but, in general, these modalities are unable to stabilize the fracture adequately. Because of this inadequate stabilization, fatigue failure of such devices is not uncommon.

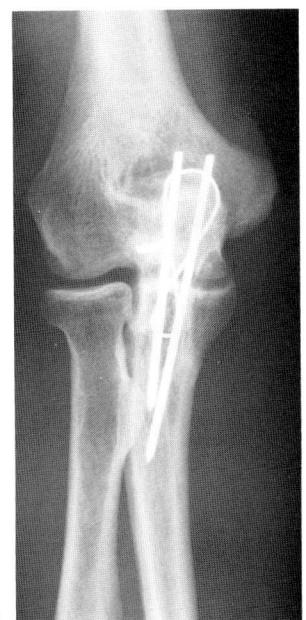 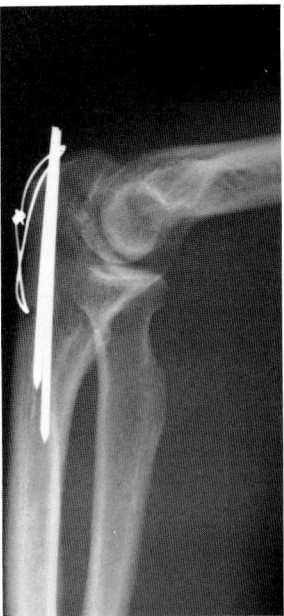

FIG. 12–76. AP (**A**) and lateral (**B**) radiographs of the most common type of fixation that is the AO recommended tension band wiring (from 157, with permission).

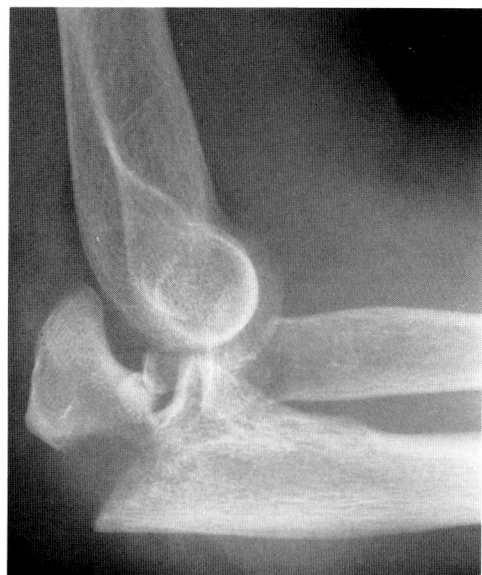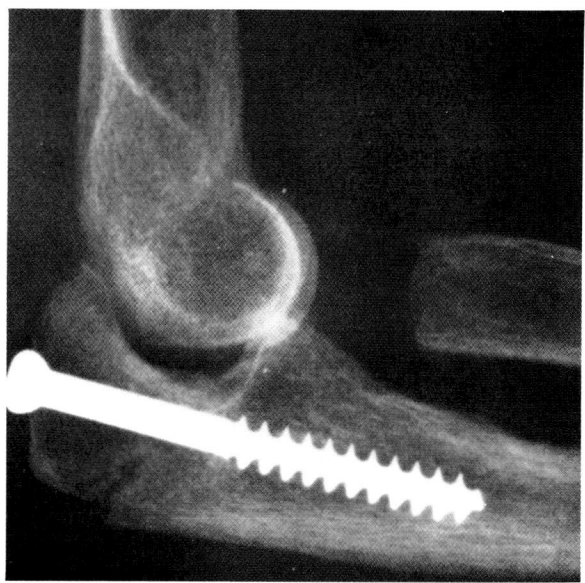

FIG. 12–77. An oblique relatively noncomminuted fracture of the proximal ulna but with a fracture of the medial head (**A**) treated with a compression screw (**B**).

The use of a single screw across the oblique fracture is sometimes used, and this fixation is effective in stabilizing uncomminuted fractures owing to compression of the fracture surface (Fig. 12-77).

The use of plates is less commonly used for this frac-

ture because of the subcutaneous nature of the bone and the difficulty in obtaining soft tissue cover. For badly displaced fractures or in uncertain circumstances, one of the special plates may be used (Fig. 12-78), but generally in this instance one of the other modalities is preferred.

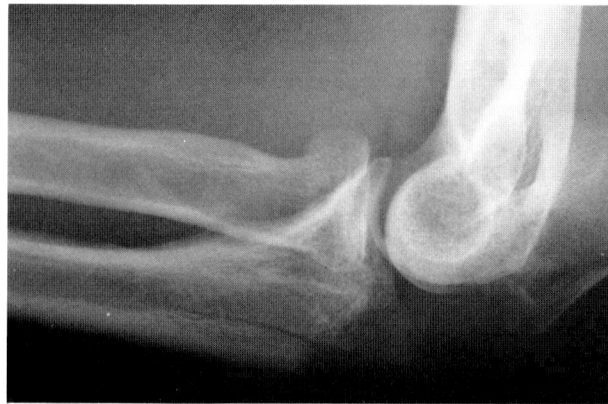
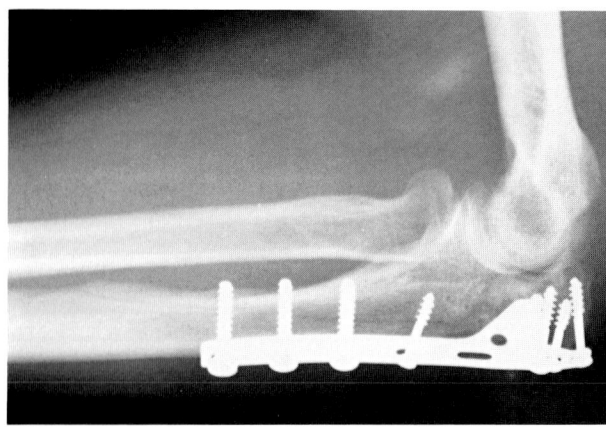
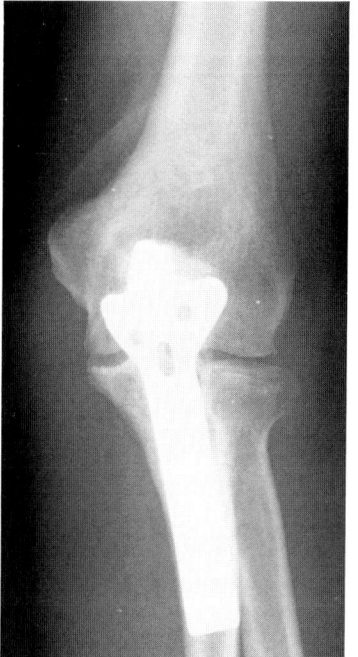

FIG. 12–78. Badly displaced but minimally comminuted fracture but with a linear component down the shaft of the ulna (**A**). This was treated with a special AO type plate demonstrated on the anterior-posterior (**B**) and lateral (**C**) projections (from 157, with permission).

A third treatment option other than casting or splinting and open reduction with internal fixation is excision of fracture fragments. The principle for this approach has been well defined by MacAusland (154). If at least 20% of the olecranon is present and intact, the procedure maintains stability for badly comminuted fractures in older individuals. The major attractions of this particular procedure are its relative ease and freedom from complications (150).

Results

The results of prolonged splinting have been universally bad; thus, as mentioned earlier, this is not commonly performed unless the fracture is stable and relatively undisplaced, and unless reasonable early motion can be begun. Surprisingly, relatively little information is available with respect to the long-term follow-up of many of these techniques. Weseley has reported the results of a specialized hooked plate for fixation of this fracture. He reported excellent to good results in all 25 patients so treated (170). A careful assessment of the long-term follow-up of excision compared with one of the other modalities of fixation has been recently reported by Gartsman and colleagues (150). They found no significant difference between these two groups and, in general, quite gratifying results in both. However, there were more complications in the group treated by reduction and fixation. These were usually related to removal of the fixation devices.

Complications

In general, complications from this fracture involve loss of motion, sometimes ulnar neuropathy, post-traumatic arthritis, and rarely instability or non-union (Fig. 12-79). Loss of 30° of extension is not uncommon, and some loss of motion is reported in about half of the cases (150,164). Ulnar neuropathy has been reported in 2% (164) to 10% (148) of patients. Obviously, this nerve must be carefully inspected and protected during any surgical procedure. Instability of the forearm after resection of the olecranon is very uncommon but has been reported.

Non-union of the olecranon is uncommon. When it occurs, it is almost always a result of inadequate surgical intervention (Fig. 12-80). Olecranon non-union less commonly occurs as a result of a transolecranon approach to distal humeral fractures. This occurs in only about 5% of such exposures (157).

Coronoid Fractures

Isolated coronoid fractures are uncommon. When present, they are most often associated with posterior dislocations of the elbow (157,163). In this setting, the incidence is 2–10%. Recurrent dislocation is associated with this injury.

Classification

Based on a review of 35 cases, Regan and Morrey (163) classified coronoid fractures into three types (Fig. 12-81). Type I fractures are avulsion injuries of the coronoid tip. Type II fractures involve 50% or less of the coronoid, and Type III fractures involve greater than 50% of the coronoid. Fractures without elbow dislocation were further classified as Type A, and Type B fractures were associated with elbow dislocations.

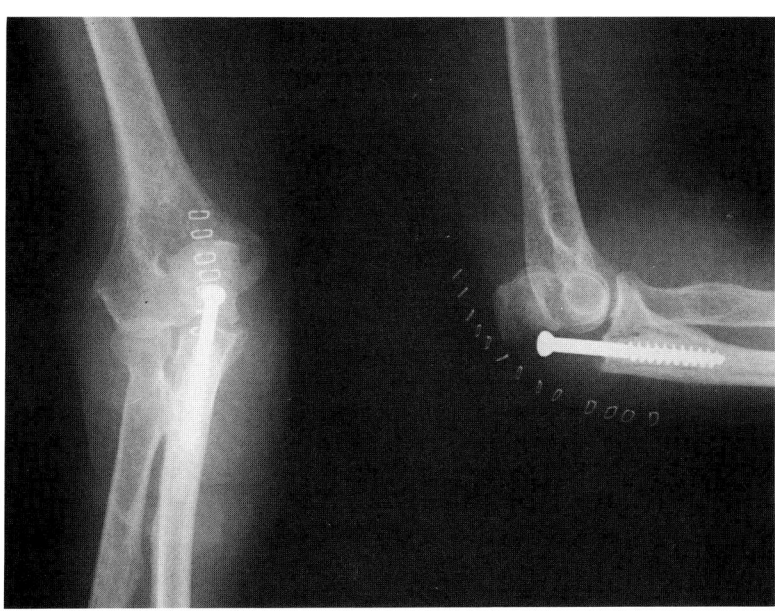

FIG. 12-79. AP and lateral views of the elbow with loss of reduction after screw fixation.

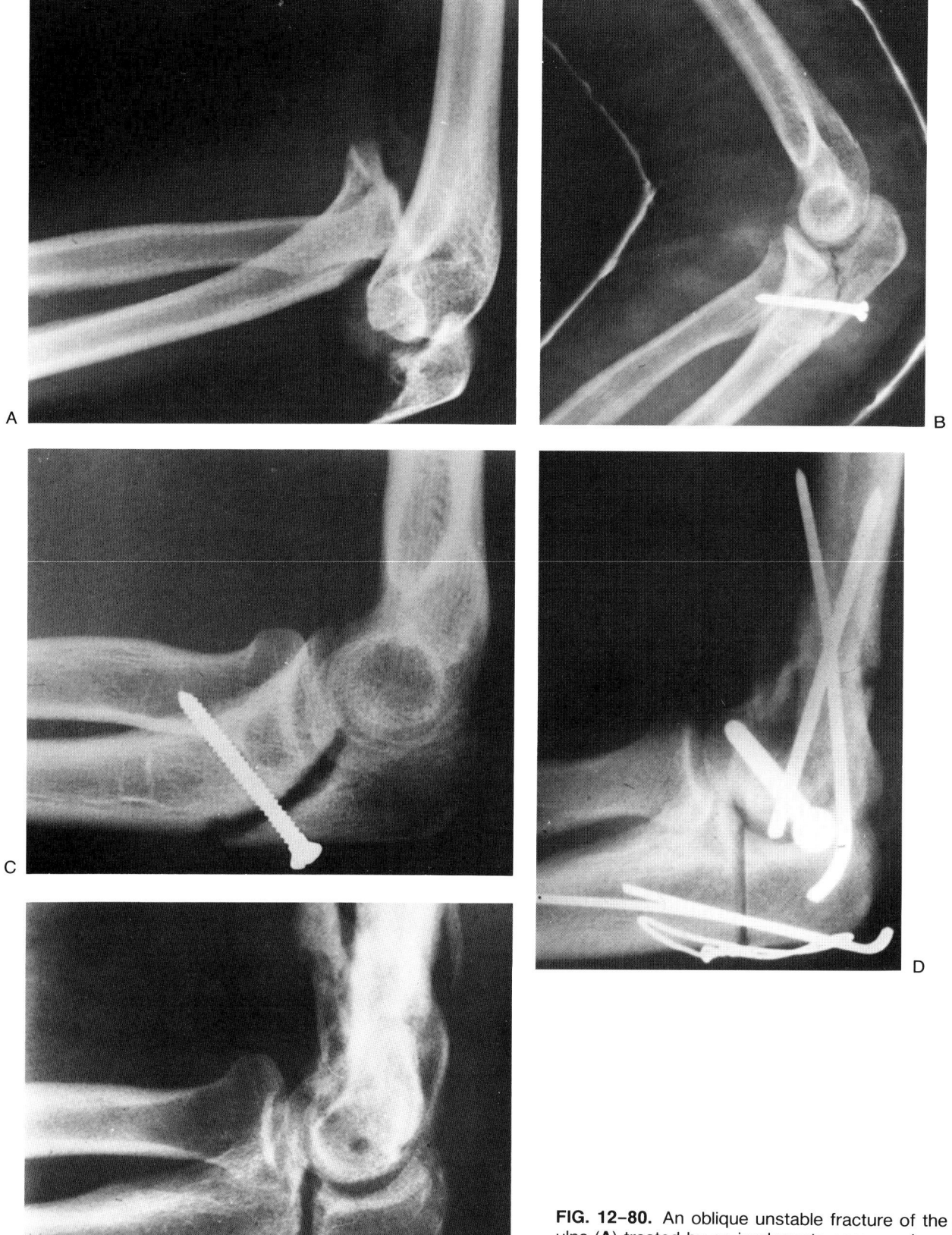

FIG. 12–80. An oblique unstable fracture of the proximal ulna (**A**) treated by an inadequate compression screw (**B**). This fracture went on to a nonunion (**C**). Olecranon osteotomy was performed to fix the supracondylar fracture (**D**) and this went on to a nonunion (**E**) (from 157, with permission).

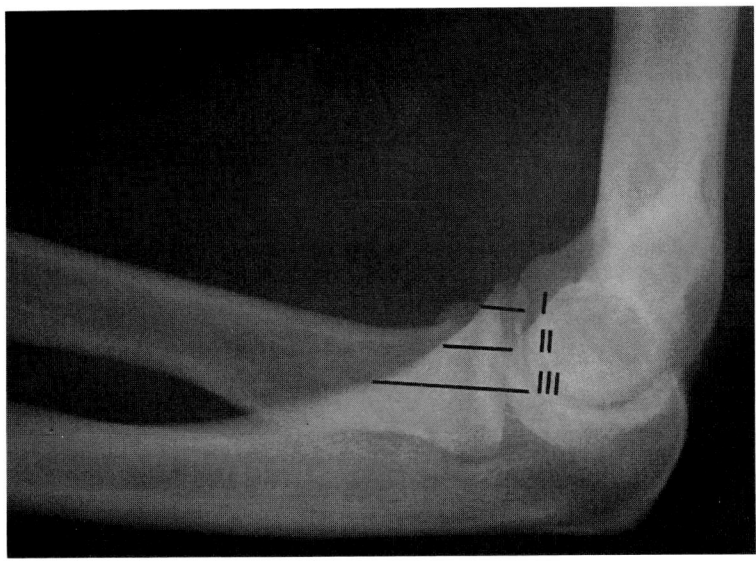

FIG. 12–81. Lateral radiograph of the elbow demonstrating the three types of coronoid fracture.

Radiographic Evaluation

Most displaced coronoid fractures can be detected with routine radiography. However, tomography or in some cases CT may be required to fully evaluate the injury. The coronoid is frequently partially obscured on routine radiographs.

Treatment

Patients with Types I and II fractures can be immobilized with a cast or sling for less than 3 weeks. Patients with Type III fractures were immobilized for 4 weeks (163). Satisfactory outcome was achieved in 72% of patients using this approach. The results were superior (91%) in patients with Type I fractures. Most patients with poor results had associated dislocation and other elbow fractures (163).

The Monteggia Lesion

A very specialized type of fracture that occurs about the elbow involves fracture of the proximal ulna with dislocation of the radial head. Described in 1814 by Monteggia of Milan (156), this fracture has been termed the *Monteggia lesion* by Bado (140). These fractures are not common and compose about 7% of all ulnar fractures and thus about 0.7% of elbow injuries (141).

Classification

The relatively simple classification of this fracture has been proposed by Bado (140) and consists of the following types:

Type I. Fracture of the ulna with anterior dislocation of the radial head. This is the most common fracture, occurring in 50–75% of instances. It is a common type of fracture in children (Fig. 12-82).

Type II. Fracture of the proximal ulna with a posterior or posterolateral dislocation of the radial head and a posterior angulation of the ulnar fracture (Fig. 12-82B). This is usually a more proximal fracture. It occurs most often in adults and represents about 10–15% of the Monteggia lesions.

Type III. Fracture of the ulna with a lateral and anterolateral dislocation of the radial head. This is a common type of fracture in children, representing 6–20% of Monteggia type lesions (Fig. 12-82C).

Type IV. Anterior dislocation of the radial head with fracture of the proximal third of the radius and ulna. This is the rarest of the Monteggia lesions and represents about 5% of cases (Fig. 12-82D) (161,162).

In addition to these types, many variants of the fracture were described by Bado as well (140). Variations of Type I fractures consist of (1) isolated anterior dislocation of the radial head in children; (2) fracture of the ulnar diaphysis with fracture of the neck and the radius; (3) isolated fractures of the neck of the radius; (4) fracture of the ulnar diaphysis and a more proximal fracture of the radial diaphysis; (5) fracture of the ulnar diaphysis and olecranon with anterior dislocation of the radial head; and (6) fracture-dislocation of the elbow, including fracture of the ulnar diaphysis with or without variations of the fracture of the proximal radius. Variations of Type II fractures consist of epiphyseal fractures of the dislocated radial head or fractures of the neck of the radius. Usually these occur in children.

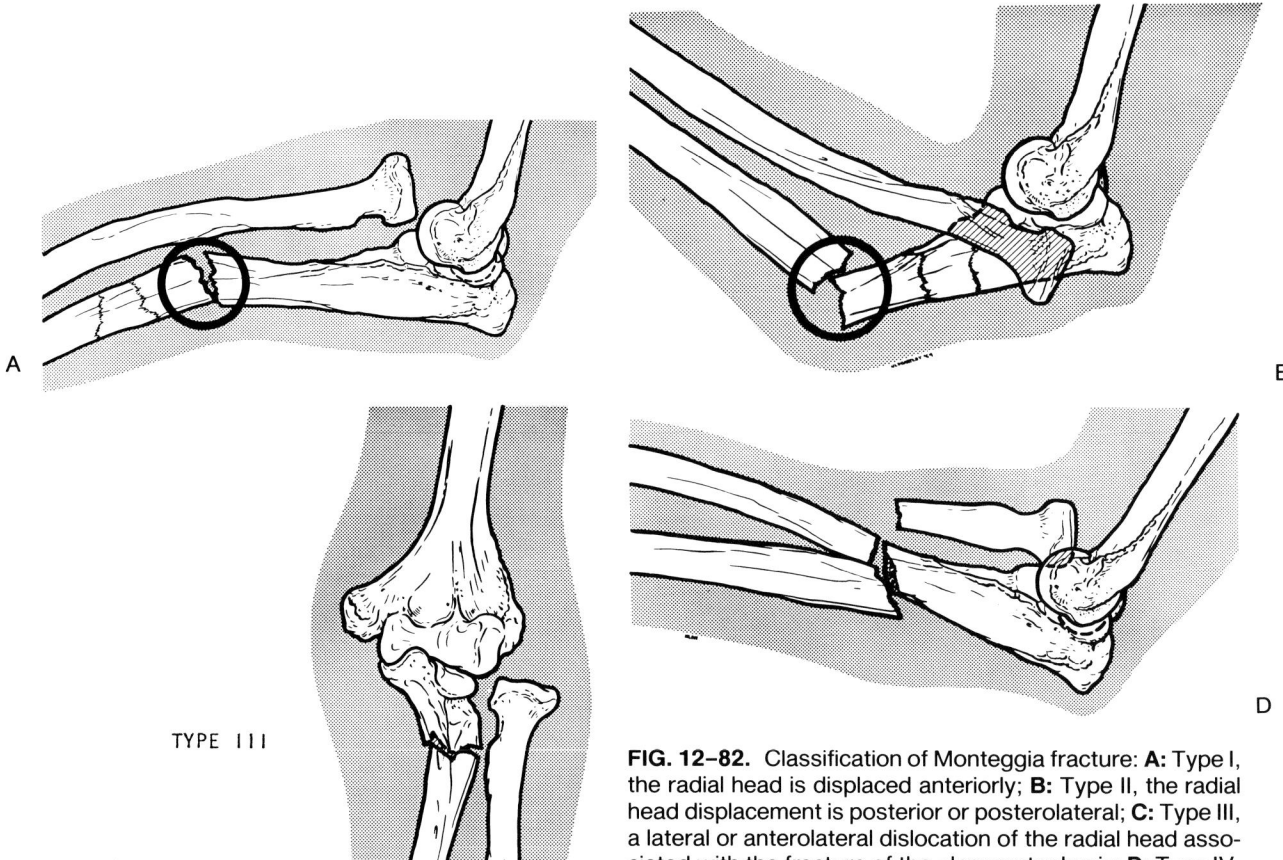

TYPE III

FIG. 12–82. Classification of Monteggia fracture: **A:** Type I, the radial head is displaced anteriorly; **B:** Type II, the radial head displacement is posterior or posterolateral; **C:** Type III, a lateral or anterolateral dislocation of the radial head associated with the fracture of the ulnar metaphysis; **D:** Type IV, which is the unusual anterior dislocation of the radial head of the fracture of the proximal third of the radius and ulna at the same level (from 162, with permission).

Mechanism of Injury

There have been three mechanisms proposed for this injury, and probably all three can give rise to one or the other of the types. These include:

1. A direct blow to the posterior aspect of the ulna.
2. A fall on the outstretched hand with the elbow flexed by impact. This occurs with the forearm in pronation, causing a levering of the radius and fracture of the ulna (149).
3. A hyperextension mechanism. This has been proposed by Tompkins (167), as mentioned previously.

Probably all three mechanisms—direct blow, hyper-pronation, and hyperextension—are implicated in this type of fracture.

Roentgenographic Findings

Adequate roentgenograms in two or more planes are particularly important in this injury since the dislocation of the radial head may be missed in a single view (Fig. 12-83). Certainly in the severe cases, the diagnosis is not

difficult (Fig. 12-84). If the dislocation becomes inadvertently reduced at the time of positioning for the x-ray, the full severity of the injury may be missed. This occurred in 50% of the early cases (166). In 1940, this incidence was reduced to 33% in a series reported in 1955 from the Mayo Clinic by Mobley and Janes (155). It is currently approximately 16%, according to the most recent report by Reckling and Cordell (162).

Treatment

In the child, the fracture is usually able to be reduced and hence treated by nonoperative modalities. However, for the adult, surgical intervention is the treatment of choice. Since the early recommendations for this treatment in 1940, improved techniques of osteosynthesis have resulted in a more aggressive approach to the fracture with a concurrent decrease in the complication rate. In fact, a specific surgical approach to the region has been proposed by Boyd (142) for this specific injury. The most recent studies recommend such operative management (Fig. 12-85) (140,143,160,162).

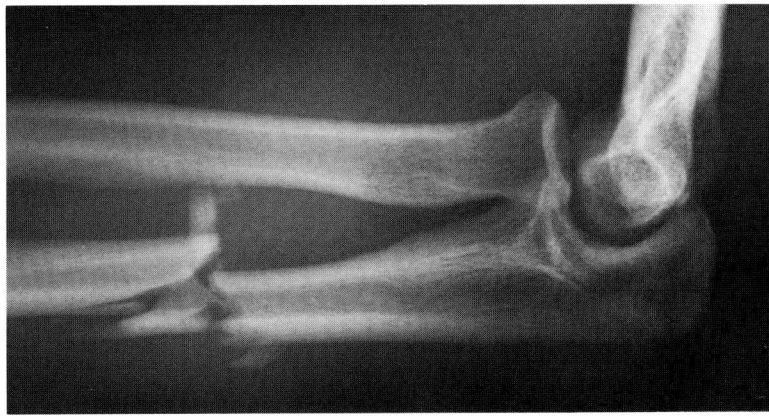

FIG. 12-83. Lateral view of the elbow demonstrating a comminuted fracture of the proximal ulna. Does the radial head articulate with the capitellum?

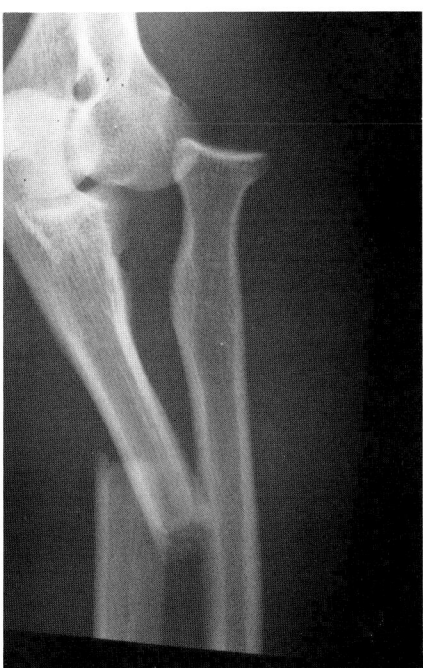 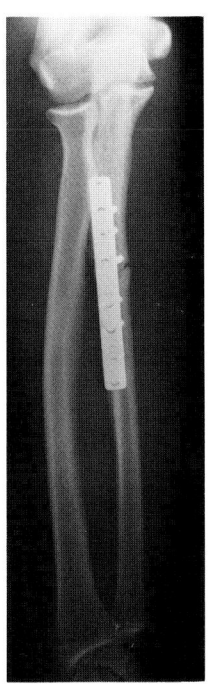

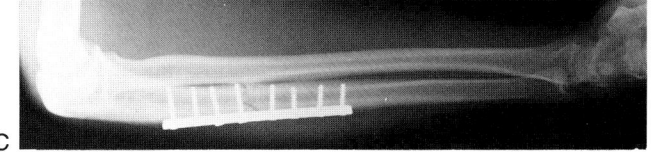

FIG. 12-84. A: Classic Monteggia fracture Type I in an 18-year-old boy. AP (B) and lateral (C) fixation with plate. Notice the reduction of the radial head (from 159, with permission).

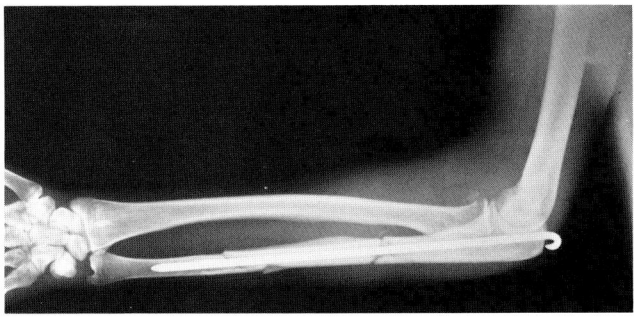 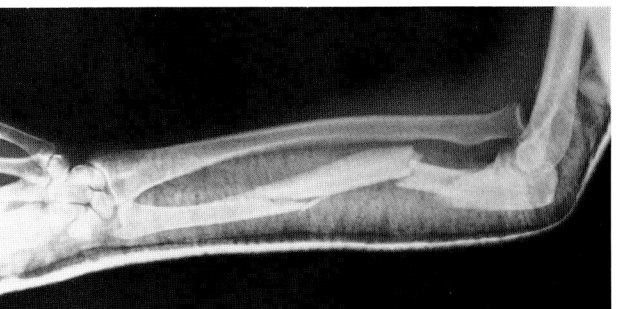

FIG. 12-85. A: Segmental fracture of the ulna with anterior dislocation of the radial head. The fracture was reduced with a Rush rod (B) (from 157, with permission).

Results

Boyd (142) reported 77% satisfactory results in the surgical management of these fractures. Reckling (161,162) in 1968 and again in 1982 demonstrated that the results of treatment in the adult were in those that underwent an anatomic reduction. However, only 9 of 40 of their patients obtained an excellent result. To some extent, the results depend on the type of fracture, which reflects the severity of the injury.

Complications

Radial palsy has been reported rather commonly as a sequela of this fracture (143,151,155). It is most common with the Type III fracture. Median (151) and ulnar (143) palsies have also been reported. Malunion is uncommon today with the better fixation techniques available, but cross-union has been observed following this fracture.

REFERENCES

Anatomy

1. An KN, Hui FC, Morrey BF, Linscheid RL, Chao EY. Muscles across the elbow joint: A biomechanical analysis. *J Biomech* 1981;14:659–669.
2. Atkinson WB, Elftman H. The carrying angle of the human arm as a secondary sex characteristic. *Anat Rec* 1945;91:49.
3. Beals RK. The normal carrying angle of the elbow. *Clin Orthop* 1976;119:194–196.
4. Ekholm R, Ingelmark BE. Functional thickness variations of human articular cartilage. *Acta Soc Med Upsal* 1952;57:39–59.
5. Evans EM. Rotational deformity in the treatment of fractures of both bones of the forearm. *J Bone Joint Surg* 1945;27:373–379.
6. Gay JR, Love JG. Diagnosis and treatment of tardy paralysis of the ulnar nerve. *J Bone Joint Surg* 1947;29:1087–1097.
7. Guttierez LF. A contribution to the study of the limiting factors of elbow fixation. *Acta Anat* 1964;56:146–156.
8. Hollinshead WH. *Anatomy for surgeons*, vol. 3. The back and limbs. 3rd ed. New York: Harper and Row, 1982.
9. Johansson O. Capsular and ligament injuries of the elbow joint. *Acta Chir Scand* (Suppl.) 1962;287:50–65.
10. Loomis LK. Reduction and after-treatment of posterior dislocation of the elbow: With special attention to the brachialis muscle and myositis ossificans. *Am J Surg* 1944;63:56–60.
11. Morrey BF, Chao EY. Passive motion of the elbow joint. A biomechanical analysis. *J Bone Joint Surg* 1976;58A:501–508.
12. Morrey BF. *The elbow and its disorders.* Philadelphia: W.B. Saunders, 1985.
13. Simon WH, Friedenberg S. Joint congruence. *J Bone Joint Surg* 1973;55A:1614–1620.
14. Thompson HC III, Garcia A. Myositis ossificans: Aftermath of elbow injuries. *Clin Orthop* 1967;50:129–136.
15. Tillman B. *A contribution to the functional morphology of articular surfaces.* In: Bargmann W, Doerr W, eds. Konorz G, trans. Littleton, Mass.: P.S.G. Pub. Co., 1978.

Imaging Techniques

16. Arger PH, Oberkircher PE, Miller WT. Lipohemarthrosis. *AJR* 1974;121:97–100.
17. Ballinger PW. *Merrill's atlas of roentgenographic positions and standard radiologic procedures,* 5th ed. St. Louis: C.V. Mosby, 1982.
18. Bassett LW, Mirra JM, Forrester DM, Gold RH, Berstein ML, Rollins JS. Post-traumatic osteochondral "loose body" of the olecranon fossa. *Radiology* 1981;141:635–638.
19. Bernau A, Berquist TH. *Positioning techniques in orthopedic radiology.* Baltimore: Urban & Schwarzenberg, 1983.
20. Berquist TH. *MRI of the musculoskeletal system.* New York: Raven Press, 1990.
21. Berquist TH. The elbow and wrist. *Topics Mag Res Imag* 1989;1(3):15–27.
22. Bledsoe RC, Izenstark JL. Displacement of fat pads in disease and injury of the elbow. A new radiographic sign. *Radiology* 1959;73:717–724.
23. Bohrer SP. The fat pad sign following elbow trauma. *Clin Radiol* 1970;21:90–94.
24. Brown R, Blazina ME, Kerlan RK. Osteochondritis of the capitellum. *J Sports Med* 1974;2:27.
25. Eto RT, Anderson PW, Harley JD. Elbow arthrography with the application of tomography. *Radiology* 1975;115:283–288.
26. Freiberger RH, Kaye JJ. *Arthrography.* New York: Appleton-Century-Crofts, 1979.
27. Godfroy D, Pallardy G, Chevrot A, Zenny JC. Arthrography of the elbow: Anatomical and radiological consideration and technical considerations. *J de Radiol* 1981;62:441–447, (Fre.).
28. Greenspan A, Norman A. Radial-head-capitellar view: An expanded imaging approach to elbow injury. *Radiology* 1987;164:272–274.
29. Greenspan A, Norman A, Rosen H. Radial head-capitellum view in elbow trauma: Clinical application and radiographic anatomic correlation. *AJR* 1984;143:355–359.
30. Greenspan A, Norman A. The radial head, capitellar view. Useful technique in elbow trauma. *AJR* 1982;138:1186–1188.
31. Greenspan A, Norman A. The radial head, capitellar view. Another example of its usefulness. *AJR* 1982;139:193.
32. Hall-Craggs MA, Shorvon PJ, Chapman M. Assessment of the radial head capitellum view and the dorsal fat pad sign in acute elbow trauma. *AJR* 1985;145:607–609.
33. Hindman BW, Schreiber RR, Wiss DA, Ghilarducci MJ, Avolio RE. Supracondylar fractures of the humerus: Prediction of the cubitus varus deformity with CT. *Radiology* 1988;168:513–515.
34. Hudson TM. Elbow arthrography. *Radiol Clin North Am* 1981;19:227.
35. Jasefsson PO, Andren L, Gentz CF, Johnell O. Arthrography of the distal elbow joint. *Acta Radiol Diag* 1984;25:143–145.
36. Kohn AM. Soft tissue alterations in elbow trauma. *AJR* 1959;82:867–874.
37. London JT. Kinematics of the elbow. *J Bone Joint Surg* 1981;63A:529–535.
38. Mink JH, Eckhardt JJ, Grant TT. Arthrography in recurrent dislocation of the elbow. *AJR* 1981;136:1242–1244.
39. Murry WA, Siegel MJ. Elbow fat pads with new signs and extended differential diagnosis. *Radiology* 1977;124:659–665.
40. Norell HG. Roentgenologic visualization of the extracapsular fat. Its importance in the diagnosis of traumatic injuries to the elbow. *Acta Radiol* 1954;42:205–210.
41. Obermann WR, Loose HWC. The os supratrochleare dorsale: A normal variant that may cause symptoms. *AJR* 1983;141:123–127.
42. Page AC. Critical evaluation of the radial head capitellum view in elbow trauma. *AJR* 1986;146:81–82.
43. Pavlov H, Ghelman B, Warren RF. Double-contrast arthrography of the elbow. *Radiology* 1979;130:87–95.
44. Roback DL. Elbow arthrography: Brief technical considerations. *Clin Radiol* 1979;30:311–312.
45. Rogers LF. *Radiology of skeletal trauma.* New York: Churchill Livingstone, 1982.
46. Rogers SL, MacEwan DW. Changes due to trauma in the fat plane overlying the supinator muscle: A radiographic sign. *Radiology* 1969;92:954.
47. Surgson RD, Feldman F, Rosenberg ZS. Elbow joint: Assessment with double-contrast CT arthrography. *Radiology* 1986;160:167–173.
48. Smith DN, Lee JR. The radiological diagnosis of post-traumatic effusion of the elbow joint and its clinical significance: The displaced fat pad sign. *Injury* 1978;10:115–119.

49. Teng MM, Murphy WA, Gilula LD, et al., Elbow arthrography: A reassessment of technique. *Radiology* 1984;153:611–613.
50. Weisman J, Reimate A. Contrast arthrography in diagnosis of soft tissue injuries of the elbow joint. *RoFo* 1982;136:313.
51. Weston WJ. *Arthrography.* New York: Springer-Verlag, 1980.
52. Yousefzadeh DK, Jackson JH. Lipohemarthrosis of the elbow joint. *Radiology* 1978;128:643–645.

Soft Tissue Injuries

53. Barnes DA, Tullos HS. An analysis of 100 symptomatic baseball players. *Am J Sports Med* 1978;6:62–67.
54. Berquist TH. *MRI of the musculoskeletal system.* New York: Raven Press, 1990.
55. Cirincione RJ, Baker BE. Tendon ruptures with secondary hyperparathyroidism. A case report. *J Bone Joint Surg* 1975;57A:852–853.
56. Davis WM, Jassine Z. An etiologic factor in the tear of the distal tendon of the biceps brachii. *J Bone Joint Surg* 1956;38A:1365–1368.
57. DeLee JC, Green DP, Wilkins KE. Fractures and dislocations of the elbow. In: Rockwood CA, Green DP, 2nd ed., vol. 1. *Fractures in adults.* Philadelphia: J. P. Lippincott Co., 1984;559–652.
58. Farrar EL III, Lippert FG III. Avulsion of the triceps tendon. *Clin Orthop* 1981;161:242–246.
59. Jorgensen U, Hinge K, Rye B. Rupture of the distal biceps brachii tendon. *J Trauma* 1986;26:1061–1062.
60. King JW, Brelsford HJ, Tullos HS. Analysis of the pitching arm of the professional baseball player. *Clin Orthop* 1969;67:116–123.
61. Levy M, Fischel RE, Stern GM. Triceps tendon avulsion with or without fracture of the radial head—a rare injury? *J Trauma* 1978;18:677–670.
62. Linscheid RL, Wheeler DK. Elbow dislocations, *JAMA* 1965;194:1171–1176.
63. Mains DB, Freeark RJ. Report of compound dislocation of the elbow with entrapment of brachial artery. *Clin Orthop* 1975;106:180–185.
64. Match RM, Corrylos EV. Bilateral avulsion fracture of the triceps tendon insertion from skiing with osteogenesis imperfecta tarda. *Am J Sports Med* 1983;11:99–102.
65. Morrey BF. *The elbow and its disorders.* Philadelphia: W. B. Saunders, 1985.
66. Morrey BF, Askew LJ, An KN, Dobyns JH. Rupture of the distal biceps tendon: Biomechanical assessment of different treatment options. *J Bone Joint Surg* 1985;67A:418–421.
67. Norwood LA, Shook JA, Andrews JR. Acute medial elbow ruptures. *Am J Sports Med* 1981;9:16–19.
68. Osborne G, Cotterill P. Recurrent dislocation of the elbow. *J Bone Joint Surg* 1966;48B:340–346.
69. Patrick J. Fracture of the medial epicondyle with displacement into the elbow joint. *J Bone Joint Surg* 1946;28:143–147.
70. Pritchard DJ, Linscheid RL, Svien HJ. Intra-articular medial nerve entrapment with dislocation of the elbow. *Clin Orthop* 1973;90:100–103.
71. Roberts AW. Displacement of the elbow. *Br J Surg* 1969;56:806–815.
72. Roberts AW. Displacement of the internal epicondyle into the elbow joint. *Lancet* 1934;2:78–79.
73. Schwab GH, Bennett JB, Woods GW, Tullos HS. Biomechanics of elbow instability: The role of the medial collateral ligament. *Clin Orthop* 1980;146:42–52.
74. Thomas TT. Fractures of the head of the radius. *U Penn M Bull* 1905;18:184–197 and 221–234.
75. Woods GW, Tullos HS. Elbow instability and medial epicondyle fractures. *Am J Sports Med* 1977;5:23–30.

Humeral Fractures

76. Ackerman G, Jupiter JB. Non-union of the distal end of the humerus. *J Bone Joint Surg* 1988;70A:75–83.
77. Bryan RS. Fractures about the elbow in adults. *AAOS Instr Course Lect* 1981;30:200–223.
78. Bryan RS, Bickel WH. T-condylar fractures of the distal humerus. *J Trauma* 1971;11:830–835.
79. Bryan RS, Morrey BF. Extensive posterior exposure of the elbow. A triceps sparing approach. *Clin Orthop* 1982;166:188–192.
80. Cassebaum WH. Open reduction of T- and Y-fractures of the lower end of the humerus. *J Trauma* 1969;9:915–925.
81. Collert S. Surgical management of fractures of the capitellum humeri. *Acta Orthop Scand* 1977;48:603–606.
82. Corbett RH. Displaced fat pads in trauma to the elbow. *Injury* 1978;9:297–298.
83. DeLee JC, Green DP, Wilkins KE. Fractures and dislocations of the elbow. In: Rockwood CA, Green DP, 2nd ed., vol. 1. *Fractures in adults.* Philadelphia: J. P. Lippincott Co., 1984;559–652.
84. Edman P, Lohr G. Supracondylar fractures of the humerus treated with olecranon traction. *Acta Chir Scand* 1963;126:505–516.
85. Figgie MP, Ingles AE, Mow CS, Figgie HE. Salvage of non-union of the supracondylar fracture of the humerus by total elbow arthroplasty. *J Bone Joint Surg* 1989;71A:1058–1065.
86. Fowles JV, Kassab MT. Fracture of the capitellum humeri. Treatment by excision. *J Bone Joint Surg* 1974;56A:794–798.
87. Gejrot W. An intra-articular fracture of the capitellum and trochlea of the humerus with special reference to treatment. *Acta Chir Scand* 1932;71:253–270.
88. Grantham SA, Norris TR, Bush DC. Isolated fracture of the humeral capitellum. *Clin Orthop* 1981;161:262–269.
89. Horne G. Supracondular fracture of the humerus in adults. *J Trauma* 1980;20:71–74.
90. Hoyer A. Treatment of supracondylar fracture of the humerus by skeletal traction in an abduction splint. *J Bone Joint Surg* 1952;34A:623–637.
91. Johansson H, Olerud S. Operative treatment of intercondylar fractures of the humerus. *J Trauma* 1971;11:836–843.
92. Johansson O. Capsular and ligament injuries of the elbow joint. *Acta Chir Scand* (Suppl.) 1962;287:50–65.
93. Lansinger O, Mare K. Intercondylar T-fractures of the humerus in adults. *Arch Orthop Trauma Surg* 1982;100:37–42.
94. Lipscomb PR, Burleson RJ. Vascular and neural complications in supracondylar fractures of the humerus in children. *J Bone Joint Surg* 1955;37A:487–492.
95. McLaughlin HL. Some fractures with a time limit. *Surg Clin North Am* 1955;35:553.
96. Meyerding HW. Volkmann's ischemic contracture associated with supracondylar fracture of the humerus. *JAMA* 1936;106:1138.
97. Milch H. Fracture of the external humeral condyle. *JAMA* 1956;106:641.
98. Milch H. Unusual fracture of the capitulum humeri and capitulum radii. *J Bone Joint Surg* 1931;13:882–886.
99. Mitsunaga MM, Bryan RS, Linscheid RL. Condylar non-unions of the elbow. *J Trauma* 1982;22:787–791.
100. Mohan K. Myositis ossificans traumatica of the elbow. *Int Surg* 1972;57:475–478.
101. Morrey BF. *The elbow and its disorders.* Philadelphia: W. B. Saunders, 1985.
102. Reich RS. Treatment of intracondylar fractures of the elbow by means of traction. *J Bone Joint Surg* 1936;18:997–1004.
103. Rieth PL. Fractures of the radial head—associated with chip fracture of the capitellum in adults: Surgical considerations. *Sough Surg* 1948;14:154–159.
104. Riseborough EJ, Radin EL. Intracondylar T-fractures of the humerus in the adult. A comparison of operative and non-operative treatment in 29 cases. *J Bone Joint Surg* 1969;51A:130–141.
105. Smith FM. *Surgery of the elbow*, 2nd ed. Philadelphia: W. B. Saunders, 1972.
106. Smith FM. Traction and suspension in the treatment of fractures. *Surg Clin North Am* 1951;31:545.
107. Suman RK, Miller JH. Intercondylar fractures of the distal humerus. *J R Coll Surg Edinb* 1982;27:276.
108. Van Gorder GW. Surgical approach in supracondylar T-fracture of the humerus requiring open reduction. *J Bone Joint Surg* 1940;22:278–292.
109. Wilson PD. Fracture and dislocations in the region of the elbow. *Surg Gynecol Obstet* 1933;56:335–359.

Fractures of the Proximal Radius

110. Adler JB, Shaftan GW. Radial head fractures. Is excision necessary? *J Trauma* 1964;4:115–136.
111. Arner O, Ekengren K, VonSchreeb T. Fractures of the head and neck of the radius. A clinical and roentgenographic study of 310 cases. *Acta Chir Scand* 1957;112:115–134.
112. Arvidsson H, Johansson O. Arthrography of the elbow-joint. *Acta Radiol* (Stockh.) 1955;43:445–452.
113. Bakalim G. Fractures of radial head and their treatment. *Acta Orthop Scand* 1970;41:320–331.
114. Bohl WR, Brightman E. Fracture of a Silastic radial-head prosthesis: Diagnosis and localization of fragments by xerography. *J Bone Joint Surg* 1981;63A:1482–1483.
115. Buxton St, JD. Ossification in the ligaments of the elbow joint. *J Bone Joint Surg* 1938;20:709–714.
116. Carstam N. Operative treatment of fractures of the upper end of the radius. *Acta Orthop Scand* 1950;19:502–526.
117. Castberg T, Thing E. Treatment of fractures of the upper end of the radius. *Acta Chir Scand* 1953;105:62–69.
118. Coleman DA, Blair WF, Shurr D. Resection of the radial head for fracture of the radial head. *J Bone Joint Surg* 1987;69A:385–392.
119. Conn J, Wade P. Injuries of the elbow: A ten-year review. *J Trauma* 1961;1:248–268.
120. Essex-Lopresti P. Fractures of the radial head with distal radio-ulnar dislocation. *J Bone Joint Surg* 1951;33B:244–247.
121. Harrington IJ, Tountas AA. Replacement of the radial head in the treatment of unstable elbow fractures. *Injury* 1981;12:405–412.
122. Johnston G. A follow-up of one hundred cases of fracture of the head of the radius with a review of the literature. *Ulster Med J* 1962;31:51–56.
123. Keon-Cohen BT. Fractures at the elbow. *J Bone Joint Surg* 1966;48A:1623–1639.
124. Mackay I, Fitzgerald B, Miller JH. Silastic replacement of the head of the radius in trauma. *J Bone Joint Surg* 1979;61B:494–497.
125. Mason JA, Shutkin NM. Immediate active motion in the treatment of fractures of the head and neck of the radius. *Surg Gynecol Obstet* 1943;76:731–737.
126. Mason MB. Some observations on the fractures of the head of the radius with a review of one hundred cases. *Brit J Surg* 1954;42:123–132.
127. Morrey BF, Chao EY, Hui FC. Biomechanical study of the elbow following excision of the head of the radius in adults. *J Bone Joint Surg* 1979;61B:63–68.
128. Morrey BF, Askew RPT, Chao EY. Silastic prosthetic replacement for the radial head. *J Bone Joint Surg* 1981;63A:454–458.
129. Morrey BF. *The elbow and its disorders.* Philadelphia: W. B. Saunders, 1985.
130. Neuwirth AA. Nonsplinting treatment of fractures of elbow joint. *JAMA* 1942;118:971–972.
131. Odenheimer K, Harvey JP Jr. Internal fixation of fracture of the head of the radius. *J Bone Joint Surg* 1979;61A:785–787.
132. Poulsen JO, Tophoj K. Fracture of the head and neck of the radius. *Acta Orthop Scand* 1974;45:66–75.
133. Radin EL, Riseborough EJ. Fractures of the radial head. *J Bone Joint Surg* 1966;48A:1055–1061.
134. Scharplatz D, Allgower M. Fracture-dislocations of the elbow. *Injury* 1976;7:143–159.
135. Stephen IBM. Excision of the radial head for closed fracture. *Acta Orthop Scand* 1981;52:409–412.
136. Sutro CJ. Regrowth of bone at the proximal end of the radius following resection in this region. *J Bone Joint Surg* 1935;17:867–878.
137. Swanson AB, Jaegar SH, La Rochelle D. Comminuted fractures of the radial head. The role of silicone-implant replacement arthroplasty. *J Bone Joint Surg* 1981;63A:1039–1049.
138. Taylor TKF, O'Connor BT. The effect upon the inferior radio-ulnar joint of excision of the head of the radius in adults. *J Bone Joint Surg* 1964;46B:83–88.

Fractures of the Ulna

139. Aldredge GH Jr, Gregory CF. Triceps advancement in olecranon fractures. *J Bone Joint Surg* 1969;51A:816.
140. Bado JL. The Monteggia lesion. *Clin Orthop* 1967;50:71–86.
141. Beck C, Dabezies EJ. Monteggia fracture-dislocation. *Orthopedics* 1984;7:329–331.
142. Boyd HB. Surgical exposure of the ulna and proximal third of the radius through one incision. *Surg Gynecol Obstet* 1940;71:86–88.
143. Bryan RS. Monteggia fracture of the forearm. *J Trauma* 1971;11:992–998.
144. Colton CL. Fractures of the olecranon in adults: Classification and management. *Injury* 1973;5:121–127.
145. Coughling NJ, Slabaugh PB, Smith TK. Experience with the McAtee olecranon device in olecranon fractures. *J Bone Joint Surg* 1979;61A:385–389.
146. Daland EN. Fractures of the olecranon. *J Bone Joint Surg* 1933;16:601–607.
147. DeLee JC, Green DP, Wilkins KE. Fractures and dislocations of the elbow. In: Rockwood CA, Green DP, 2nd ed., vol. 1. *Fractures in adults.* Philadelphia: J. P. Lippincott Co., 1984;559–662.
148. Eriksson E, Sahlen O, Sandohl U. Late results of conservative and surgical treatment of fractures of the olecranon. *Acta Chir Scand* 1957;113:153–166.
149. Evans EM. Pronation injuries of the forearm with special reference to the anterior Monteggia fracture. *J Bone Joint Surg* 1949;31B:578–595.
150. Gartsman GM, Sculco TP, Otis JC. Operative treatment of olecranon fractures. *J Bone Joint Surg* 1981;63A:718–721.
151. Jessing P. Monteggia lesions and their complicating nerve damage. *Acta Orthop Scand* 1975;46:601–609.
152. Lou I. Olecranon fractures treated in the orthopedic hospital. Copenhagen, 1936–1947. A follow-up examination. *Acta Orthop Scand* 1949–1950;19:166–179.
153. MacAusland WR Jr, Wyman ET. Fractures of the olecranon by longitudinal screw or nail fixation. *Ann Surg* 1942;116:293–296.
154. Macko D, Szabo RM. Fractures and dislocations of the elbow. In: Rockwood CA, Green DP, 2nd ed., vol. 1. *Fractures in adults.* Philadelphia: J. P. Lippincott Co., 1984;559–662.
155. Mobley JE, Janes JM. Monteggia fractures. *Proc Staff Meet Mayo Clin* 1955;30:497–504.
156. Monteggia GB. *Instituzioni Chirurgiche*, vol. 5. Milan: Maspero, 1814.
157. Morrey BF. *The elbow and its disorders.* Philadelphia: W. B. Saunders, 1985.
158. Muller ME, Allgower M, Schneider R, Willeniegger H. *Manual of internal fixation. Techniques recommended by the AO group,* 2nd ed. New York: Springer-Verlag, 1979.
159. O'Donoghue DH, Sell LS. Persistent olecranon epiphysis in adults. *J Bone Joint Surg* 1942;24:677–680.
160. Penrose JH. The Monteggia fracture with posterior dislocation of the radial head. *J Bone Joint Surg* 1951;33B:65–73.
161. Reckling FW. Unstable fracture-dislocation of the forearm (Monteggia and Galeazzi lesions). *J Bone Joint Surg* 1982;64A:857–863.
162. Reckling FW, Cordell LB. Unstable fracture-dislocations of the forearm. The Monteggia and Galeazzi lesions. *Arch Surg* 1968;96:999–1007.
163. Regan W, Morrey BF. Fractures of the coronoid process of the ulna. *J Bone Joint Surg* 1989;71A:1348–1354.
164. Rettig AC, Waugh TR, Evanski PM. Fracture of the olecranon: A problem of management. *J Trauma* 1979;19:23–28.
165. Rowe CR. The management of fractures in elderly patients is different. *J Bone Joint Surg* 1965;47A:1043–1059.
166. Speed JS, Boyd HB. Treatment of fractures of the ulna with dislocation of head of radius (Monteggia fracture). *JAMA* 1940;115:1699–1704.
167. Tompkins DG. The anterior Monteggia fracture. Observations on etiology and treatment. *J Bone Joint Surg* 1971;53A:1109–1114.
168. Van der Kloot JFVR. Results of treatment of fractures of the olecranon. *Arch Chir Neerlandicum* 1964;16:237–249.
169. Wainwright D. Fractures of the olecranon process. *Brit J Surg* 1942;29:403–406.
170. Weseley MS, Barenfeld PA, Eisenstein AL. The use of the Zuelzer hook plate in fiation of olecranon fractures. *J Bone Joint Surg* 1976;58A:859–863.

Imaging of Orthopedic Trauma,
Second Edition, edited by T.H. Berquist,
Mayo Clinic © 1992. Published
by Raven Press, Ltd., New York.

CHAPTER 13

The Radius, Ulna, and Forearm

Claire E. Bender, Donald C. Campbell II, and Thomas H. Berquist

Anatomy, 731
  Roentgenographic Evaluation, 734
Forearm Fractures, 736
  Mechanism of Injury, 736
  Classification, 736

Management, 737
Complications, 743
Soft Tissue Injuries, 747
References, 747

Fractures may involve the shafts of both the radius and the ulna, the radius alone, or the ulna. Isolated soft tissue injuries or soft tissue trauma associated with fractures can now be more easily imaged and will be included in this chapter.

ANATOMY

The anatomy of the forearm is very complex (Fig. 13-1). Fractures of the forearm, therefore, create difficult treatment situations not seen in other diaphyseal long bones (7,8,24).

The ulna is a relatively straight bone. Its shaft or body has three borders: the interosseous (or lateral), anterior, and posterior, and three surfaces: the anterior, medial, and posterior. The radius is more complex, as it is composed of several angles and curves. There are three main curves in the normal radius. These can be quite variable. The largest curve is convex laterally in the middle three-fifths of the bone. The second curve is convex dorsally in the distal fifth. The third is convex ventrally in the proximal fifth (15). The body or shaft of the radius is somewhat triangular in shape, so that it presents three borders and three surfaces. Of the borders, the medial or interosseous is the best defined. The anterior border begins proximally at the tuberosity, runs obliquely across the front of the bone to its lateral side, and ends at the base of the styloid process. The posterior border is defined only in the middle third of the bone. The lateral, posterior, and anterior surfaces need no particular comment (3,14).

The radius and ulna are relatively parallel but approximate at both ends. Proximally, the elbow joint capsule envelops both bones, and the annular ligament, which surrounds the radial head, attaches on the ulna. Distally, the wrist joint capsule, the anterior and posterior radioulnar ligaments, and the fibrocartilaginous articular disk provide continuity. There are five complex joints associated with the forearm bones: (1) proximal radioulnar, (2) distal radioulnar, (3) ulnahumeral, (4) radiohumeral, and (5) radiocarpal (1,14).

The intraosseous ligament is located between the shafts of the radius and ulna. The strong oblique fibers of the fibrous tissue originate proximally on the radius and insert distally on the ulna. Proximal to the interosseous membrane there is a small band of fibrous tissue, the oblique cord. The interosseous membrane tends to resist independent upward movement on the radius (Fig. 13-2) (1,14).

Complex muscle groups act across the forearm (Figs. 13-3 and 13-4). Fractures of the forearm thus result in complex deforming forces. The supinator, pronator teres, and pronator quadratus insert or originate solely on the radius or ulna. With fracture, these muscles tend to approximate the radius and ulna, with subsequent decrease in the interosseous space (14).

Other muscles cross the elbow or wrist joint, tending to produce pronation or supination. Pronators include the flexor carpi radialis, abductor pollicis longus and brevis, and extensor pollicis longus. Supinators include the biceps brachii (14).

C. E. Bender, D. C. Campbell II: Departments of Diagnostic Radiology and Orthopedic Surgery, Mayo Medical School, Mayo Clinic, Rochester, Minnesota 55905.
T. H. Berquist: Department of Diagnostic Radiology, Mayo Clinic Jacksonville, Jacksonville, Florida 32224.

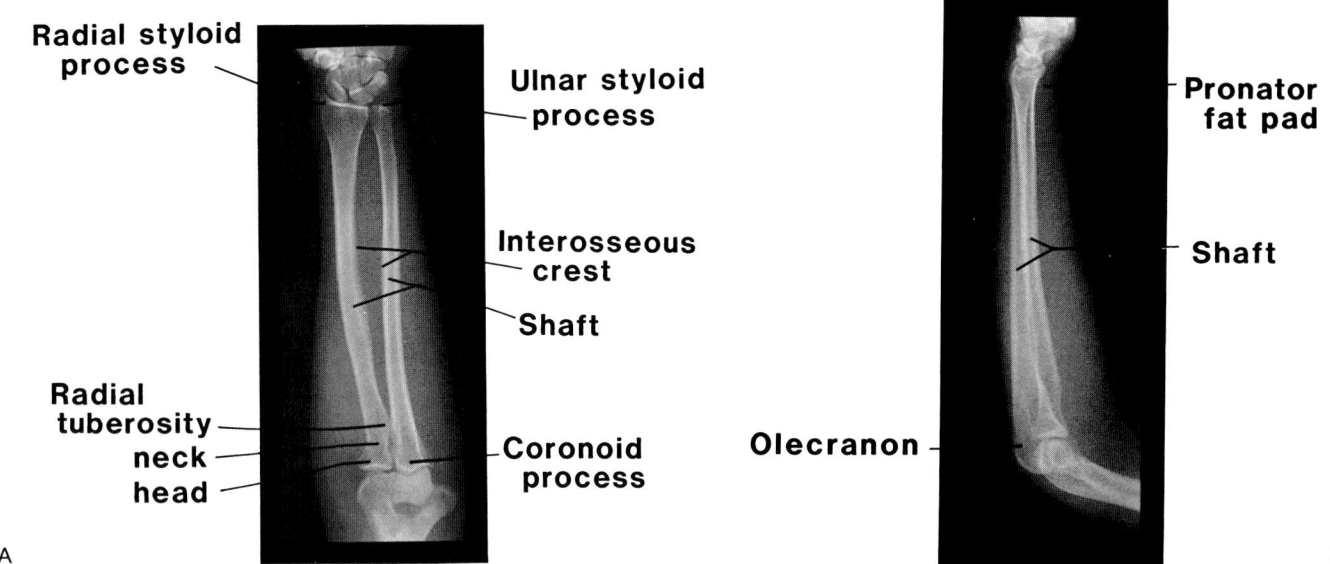

Radial styloid process

Ulnar styloid process

Interosseous crest

Shaft

Radial tuberosity

neck

head

Coronoid process

Pronator fat pad

Shaft

Olecranon

A

B

FIG. 13–1. A, B: Anteroposterior and lateral radiographs of radius and ulna.

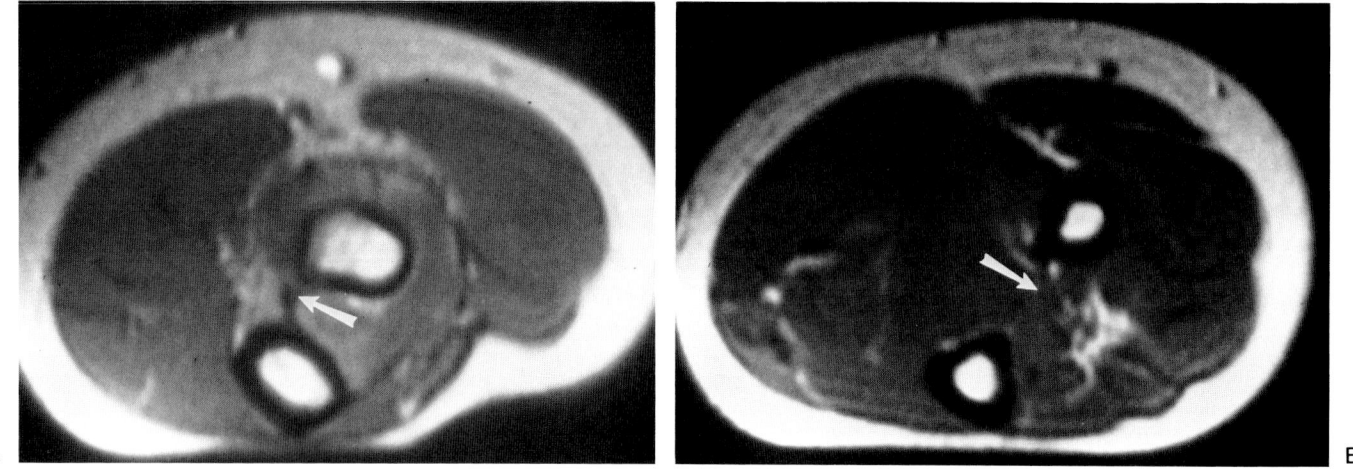

A

B

FIG. 13–2. Axial MR images of the proximal (**A**) and mid (**B**) forearm demonstrating the muscle groups and variation in thickness of the interosseous membrane (*arrow*).

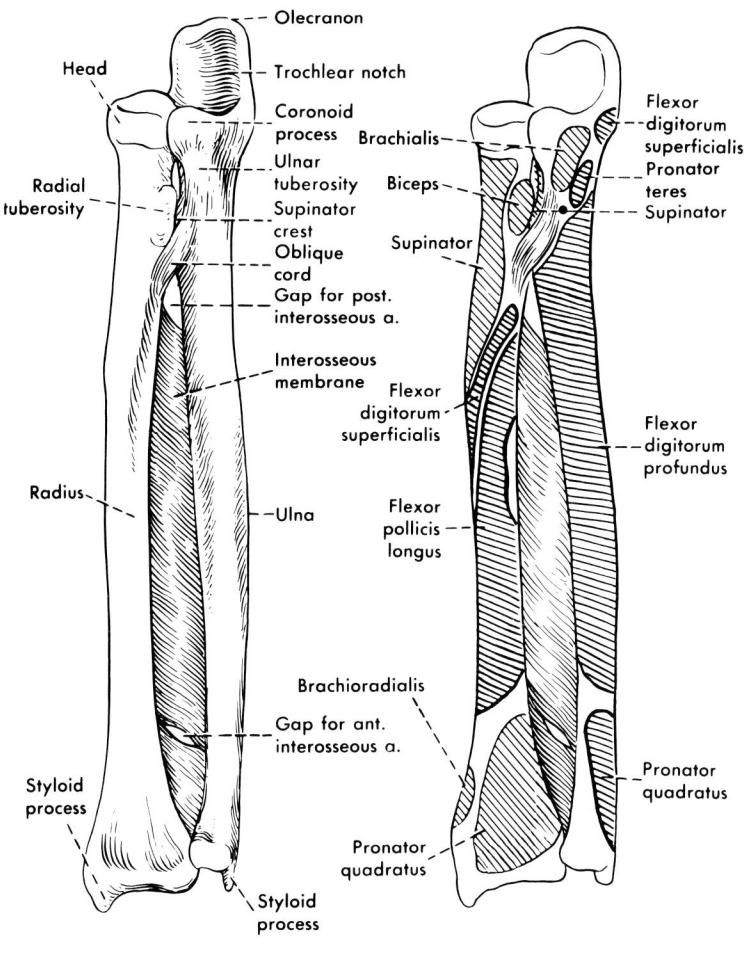

Olecranon

Head

Trochlear notch

Coronoid process

Radial tuberosity

Ulnar tuberosity

Supinator crest

Oblique cord

Gap for post. interosseous a.

Interosseous membrane

Radius

Ulna

Styloid process

Styloid process

A

Brachialis

Biceps

Supinator

Flexor digitorum superficialis

Flexor digitorum superficialis

Pronator teres

Supinator

Flexor digitorum profundus

Flexor pollicis longus

Brachioradialis

Gap for ant. interosseous a.

Pronator quadratus

Pronator quadratus

B

FIG. 13-3. A, B: Anterior muscle attachments of the forearm (from 14, with permission).

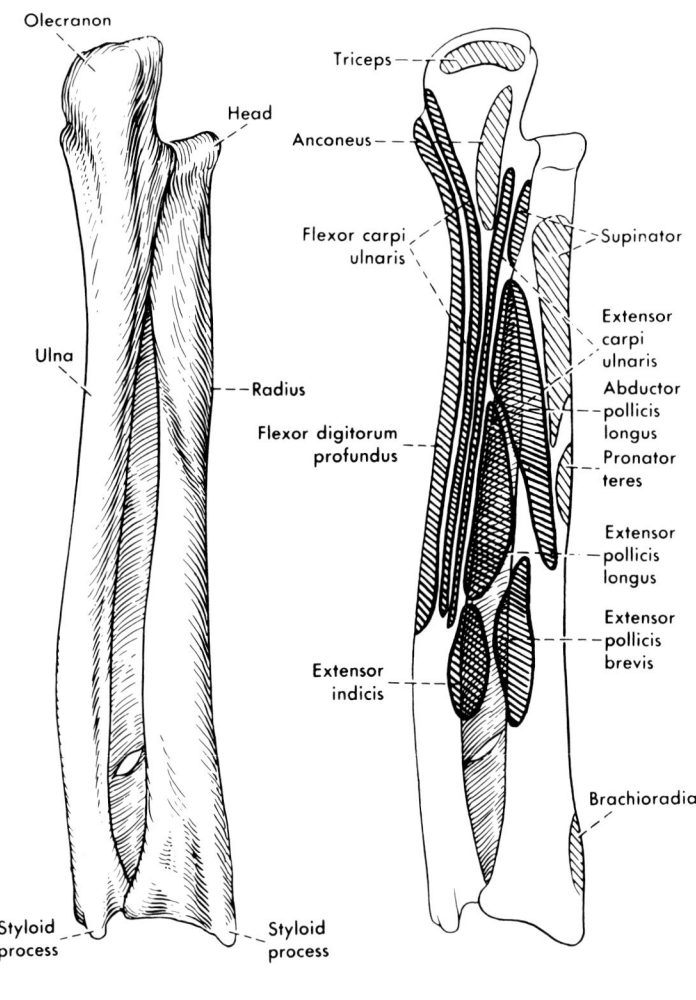

Olecranon

Head

Ulna

Radius

Flexor digitorum
profundus

Extensor
indicis

Styloid
process

Styloid
process

Triceps

Anconeus

Flexor carpi
ulnaris

Supinator

Extensor
carpi
ulnaris

Abductor
pollicis
longus

Pronator
teres

Extensor
pollicis
longus

Extensor
pollicis
brevis

Brachioradia

A

B

FIG. 13–4. A, B: Posterior muscle attachments of the forearm (from 14, with permission).

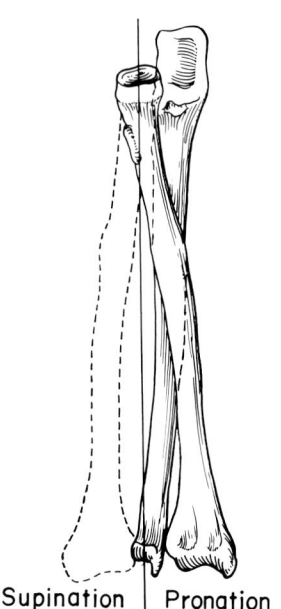

Supination | Pronation

FIG. 13–5. Relationships of the radius and ulna with pronation and supination.

Pronation and supination are the forearm motions (Fig. 13-5). The movement of the radius around the ulna has been compared with the handle of a bucket. The radial head pivots in the annular ligament, while the distal end sweeps around the ulnar head (attached by the fibrocartilaginous articular disk) (1,4,14,16).

The radial, median, and ulnar nerves course through the soft tissues of the forearm. The nutrient arteries of the radius and ulna are branches of the anterior interosseous artery (Fig. 13-6). The better defined chief nutrient canal of the radius is at the junction of the upper and middle thirds of the anterior surface and courses obliquely through the medial cortex.

Roentgenographic Evaluation

Although the clinical presentation of fracture of the forearm bones is usually quite obvious, thorough radiologic examination of the radius and ulna and adjacent wrist and elbow joints is mandatory. Standard views of the forearm of the patient include the AP and lateral

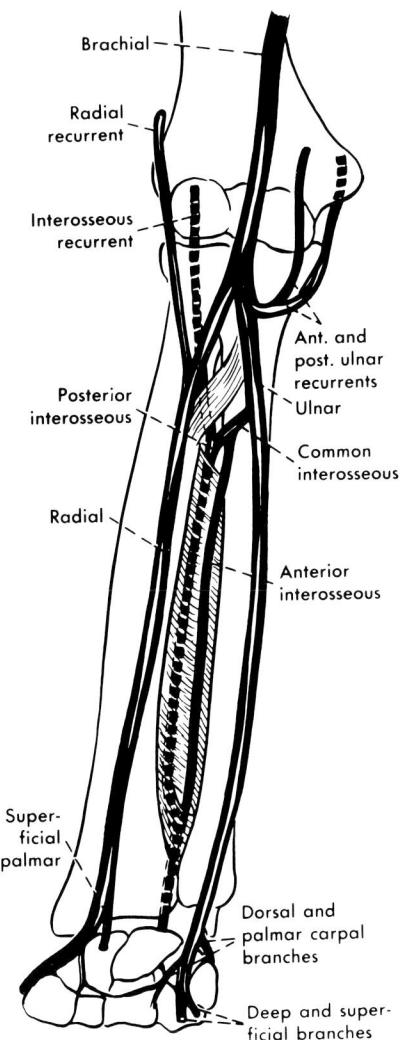

Brachial

Radial recurrent

Interosseous recurrent

Ant. and post. ulnar recurrents

Ulnar

Posterior interosseous

Common interosseous

Radial

Anterior interosseous

Super-ficial palmar

Dorsal and palmar carpal branches

Deep and super-ficial branches

FIG. 13-6. Arteries of the forearm (from 14, with permission).

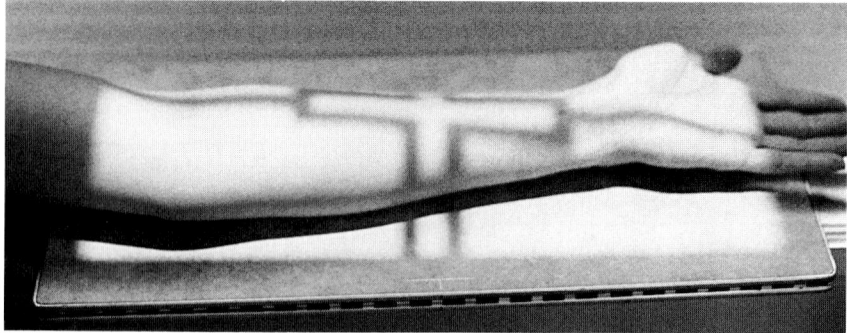

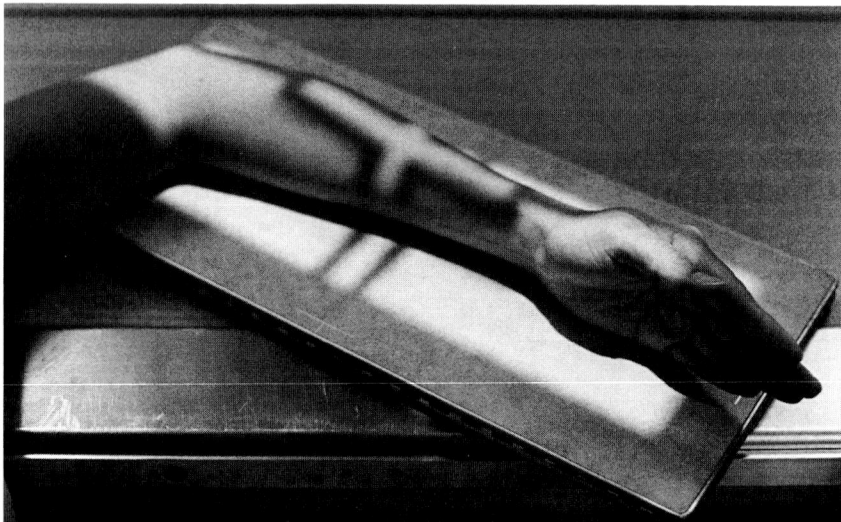

FIG. 13–7. Patient positioned for AP (**A**) and lateral (**B**) projections of forearm.

projections (Fig. 13-7). The degree of shortening, angulation, rotation, and comminution should be noted (1). The selected films must be long enough to include the adjacent elbow and wrist joints. The two views can be obtained either on one large film by alternately covering half the cassette with a lead mask or by using two separate 7 × 17 extremity cassettes (5,6). This is necessary to be certain of the position of the forearm and to detect associated wrist and elbow pathology. If there is a clinical indication, separate views of the elbow and wrist, with proper centering, must be obtained.

The AP projection (Fig. 13-7A) is obtained with the patient seated close to the extended elbow. The hand must be supinated to prevent superimposition of the distal radius and ulna. Immobilization may be necessary by placing a sandbag over the palm of the hand.

For the lateral projection, the patient is seated with the elbow and shoulder joints in the same plane and parallel to the table top. This permits the necessary superimposition of the proximal and distal radius and ulna. By flexing the elbow to 90°, the forearm is placed on the unmasked half of the cassette. In order to obtain a true lateral film, the thumb side of the hand must be up.

In immobilized patients with multiple severe injuries, films are obtained with the forearm at the patient's side. With severe forearm injuries or associated upper extremity injuries, accurate positioning of the forearm is impossible. In addition to the AP view, a cross-table lateral view can be taken. The central beam is centered perpendicularly to the cassette. Lead aprons are used for gonadal shielding.

FOREARM FRACTURES

Mechanism of Injury

A direct blow to the forearm, usually as a result of some form of motor vehicle accident, is the most common mechanism of injury. A severe fall on the outstretched hand may also result in fractures to the shafts of the radius and ulna.

Classification

Fractures of either or both forearm bones are classified according to the level of fracture, degree of displacement and angulation, degree of comminution, and open versus closed wound. Each factor is of considerable importance in the treatment and prognosis. Figure 13-8 illustrates the Orthopedic Trauma Association system for

Shaft Fractures

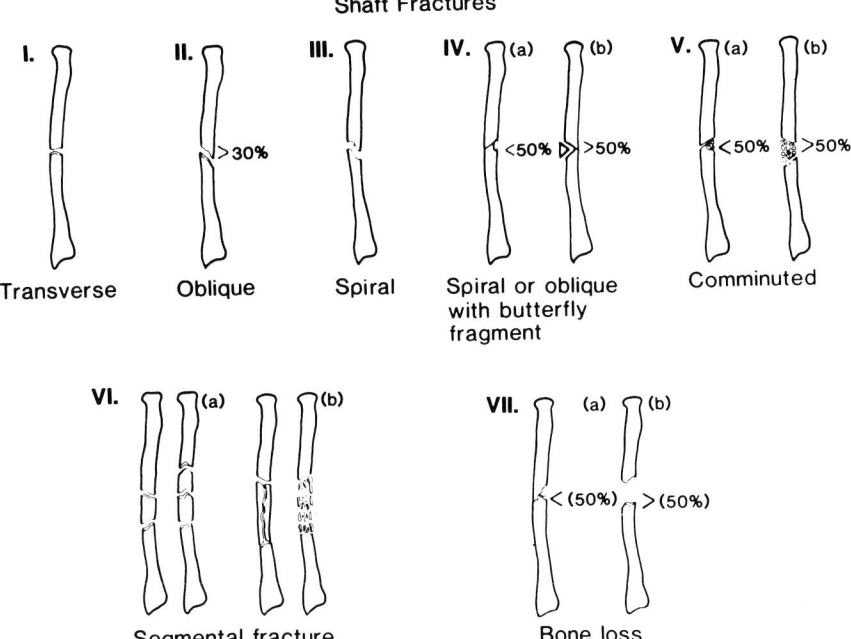

FIG. 13-8. Forearm fracture classification of the Orthopedic Trauma Association. (From Chapman MW, Gordon JE, Zissimos AG. Compression plate fixation of acute fractures of the diaphysis of the radius and ulna. *J Bone Joint Surg* 1989;71A:159–169, with permission.)

classification of forearm fractures (7). Comminuted fractures (groups IV–VII) are more frequently open injuries (7).

In Smith and Sage's series of 555 forearm fractures in 338 adult patients, approximately 75% involved both bones, 15% involved the ulna alone, and 10% involved the radius alone (22). About three-fifths of the fractures involved the adjacent proximal and distal third of the shafts equally. Figure 13-9 illustrates the incidence and locations of forearm fractures (7).

Management

Undisplaced fractures of the shafts of both the radius and ulna (Type I) are rare (1). Treatment usually consists of immobilization in a well-molded long-arm cast, with the elbow flexed 90° and the hand in neutral position (Fig. 13-10).

The undisplaced fracture of the ulna alone, also called the nightstick fracture because the mechanism of injury is usually a direct blow, is fairly common. Treatment is by long-arm immobilization. Loss of position tends to be more common in the proximal half of the bone, where the forearm muscles attach.

Undisplaced fractures of the proximal radius alone are rare. The forearm muscles pad the area. Therefore, severe injuries to this area are likely to injure the ulna, too. Also, the anatomic position of the radius makes it less likely to receive a direct blow (1,15).

Because the fracture can become displaced even while immobilized, weekly AP and lateral roentgenograms must be obtained for the first several weeks. Each new set of films must be compared with the original films in order to exclude even the slightest displacement or rotation (Fig. 13-11).

Displaced fractures of the shafts of the radius and ulna are difficult and challenging to treat. The fractures are often rotated. If satisfactory results are obtained, longitudinal and rotational alignment must be maintained.

Good rotational alignment is necessary for a functional extremity. Generally, fractures proximal to the pronator teres insertion on the radius result in supination of the proximal radial fragment of the supinators. In fractures distal to the insertion of the pronator teres, the major forces of the biceps and supinator muscles are neutralized, and therefore fragments are minimally displaced. Because the proximal ulnar fragment remains stable, the position for immobilization must be governed by the position of this fragment. Thus, for satisfactory reduction, the distal radial fragment must be rotated to align with the proximal fragment (2,14).

Evans has described a method by which one can determine the correct rotational position in which to immobilize fractures of both the forearm bones (9). He emphasizes standardized technique by obtaining AP views of both the involved elbow and the normal side. The elbow joint is flexed to 90°, and the tube is angled 20° toward the joint space. By locating the position of the radial tuberosity on the radiograph, the rotational position of

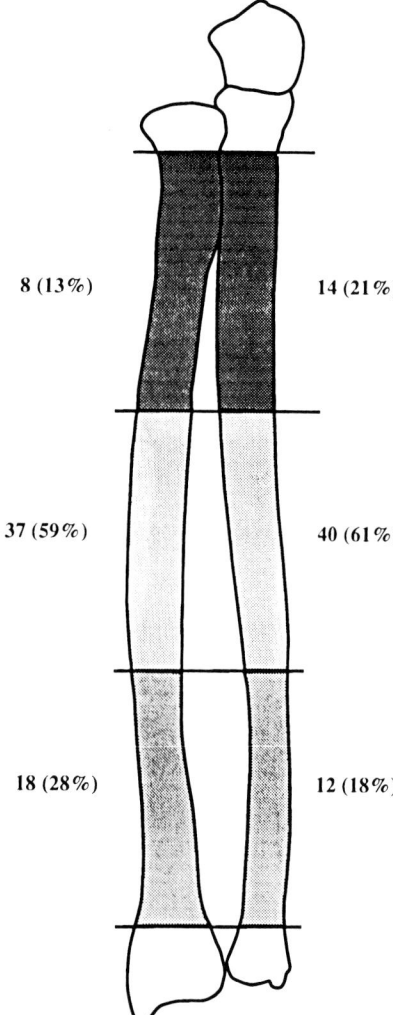

8 (13%) 14 (21%)

37 (59%) 40 (61%)

18 (28%) 12 (18%)

FIG. 13-9. Incidence and location of forearm fractures. (From Chapman MW, Gordon JE, Zissimos AG. Compression plate fixation of acute fractures of the diaphysis of the radius and ulna. *J Bone Joint Surg* 1989;71A:159–169, with permission.)

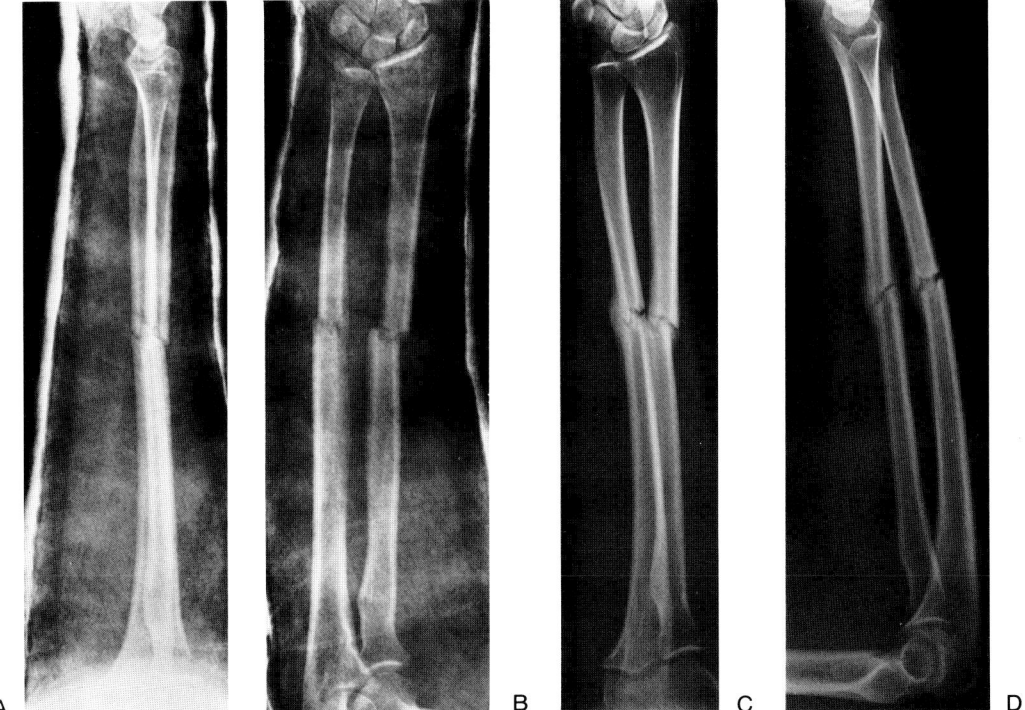

FIG. 13-10. A: AP view of undisplaced fracture of midshafts of radius and ulna in long arm cast. **B:** Lateral view. **C:** Three-month follow-up. AP view shows healing fractures. **D:** Lateral view.

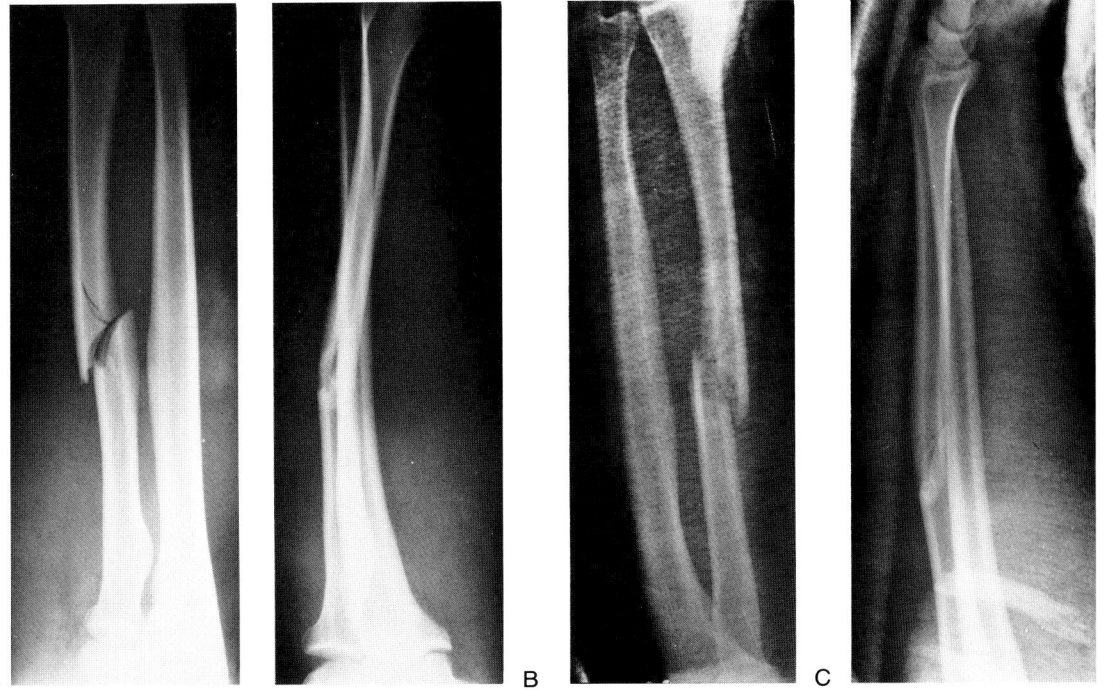

FIG. 13-11. A: AP view shows minimally displaced fracture of radial shaft. **B:** Lateral view. **C:** Slight shift and rotation of fragments have occurred after cast application. AP view. **D:** Lateral view.

the proximal radial fragment can be determined (Fig. 13-12, see also Fig. 13-5), and thus the radial fragment can be appropriately reduced.

Closed treatment consists of a long-arm cast with the forearm in mild or full supination, depending upon whether the fracture is proximal or distal to the pronator teres. Closed reduction and treatment of displaced radial and ulnar shaft fractures has been disappointing, although Sarmiento has been a strong advocate of early functional bracing of forearm fractures and has reported satisfactory results in spite of imperfect reductions (21).

Open reduction with some form of internal fixation offers the best chance for successful alignment and functional result. Various internal fixation devices include medullary nails (Rush pins, Kirschner wires, Steinmann pins, Lottes nails, Sage triangular nails), plate and screw fixation, and compression plating, with or without bone grafting (Fig. 13-13).

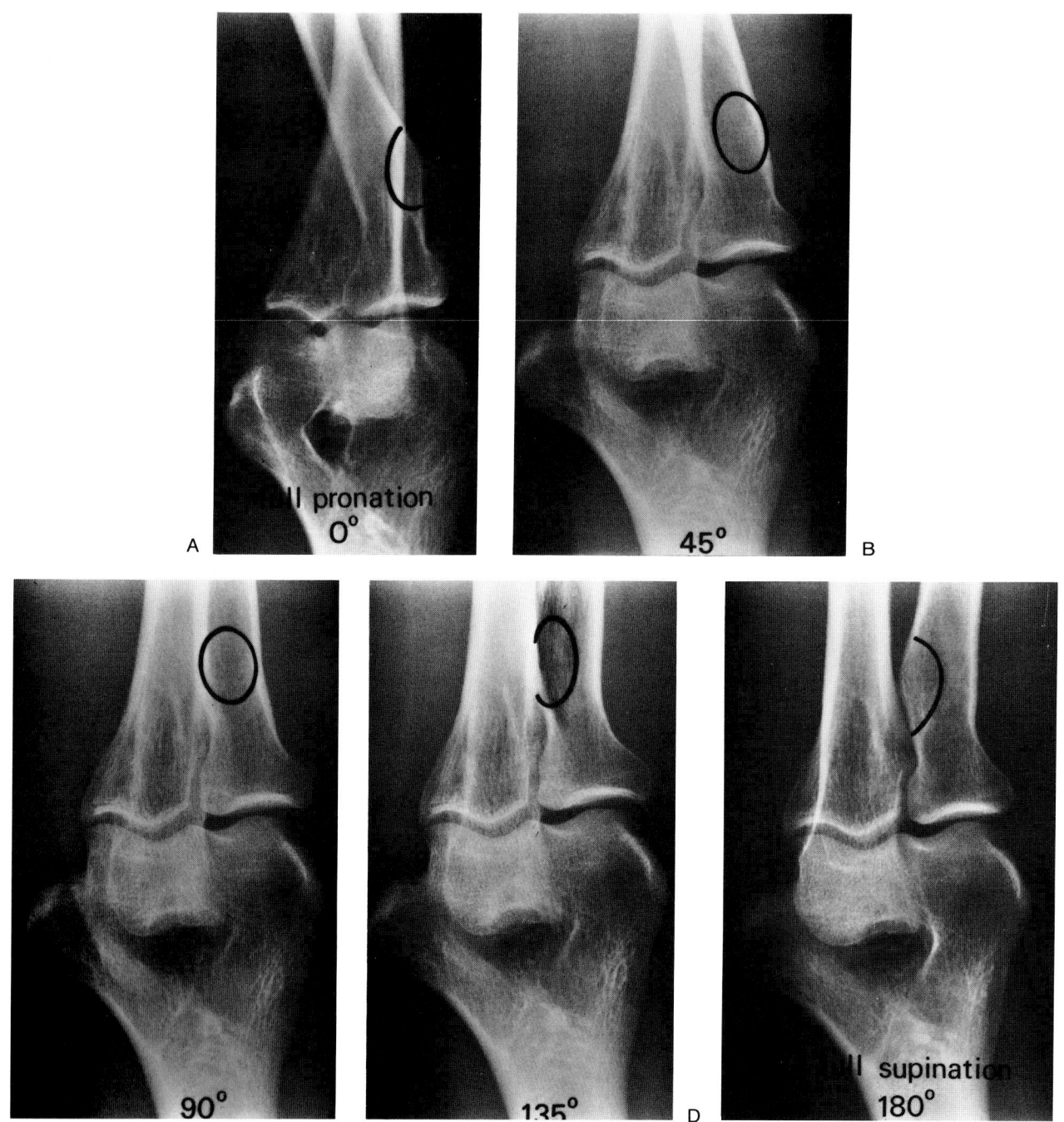

FIG. 13–12. A–E: Location of radial tuberosity (*outlined in black*) determines rotational position of proximal radial fragment allowing for proper reduction of distal radial fragment.

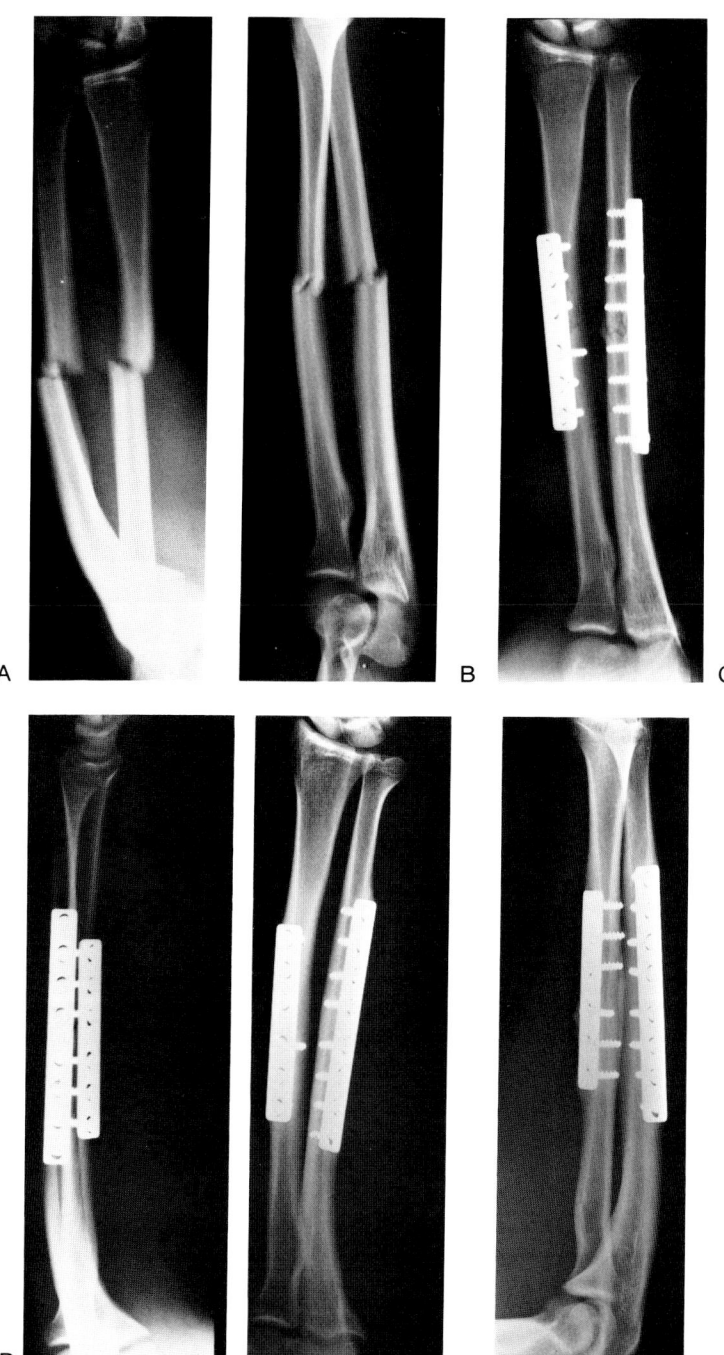

FIG. 13-13. A, B: Moderately displaced fractures of mid-shafts of radius and ulna with pronation of distal fragments. **C, D:** Six-week films (AP and lateral) of plate and screw fixation. **E, F:** Two-year follow-up (AP and lateral views). Fractures are healed.

The most popular method of treatment of displaced fractures of the radius and ulna is compression plate fixation. Autogenous bone grafts are used if a significant degree of comminution is present (Types V–VII, Fig. 13-8). Anderson and colleagues reported satisfactory results with compression plate fixation in 240 patients with acute diaphyseal fractures of the radius and ulna (2). Union occurred in 97.9% of radius fractures and 96.3% of ulna fractures. Satisfactory or excellent results were obtained in over 90% of the patients.

Follow-up roentgenographic evaluation for open reduction treatment is similar to that following closed reduction. With open reduction and internal fixation, however, early loss of reduction is unlikely; therefore, roentgenograms can be obtained at less frequent intervals. Because of the rigid fixation achieved, healing callus is reduced and radiographic evidence of healing is not as apparent. Long-arm cast immobilization may be used following open reduction and internal fixation if fixation is suboptimal or if the patient is unreliable. In those patients who are treated with casts, it has been observed that allowing a few days of gentle motion prior to casting will reduce stiffness following final cast removal.

Displaced fractures of the ulna alone rarely occur without fracture of the radius or radial head dislocation. The likelihood of associated injury is greater as displacement increases.

The Monteggia fracture is a classic example of fracture of the ulna accompanied by other injury. This was originally described by Monteggia in 1814 as a "traumatic lesion distinguished by a fracture of the proximal third of the ulna and an anterior dislocation of the proximal epiphysis of the radius."(4) Type I includes anterior dislocation of the radial head and fracture of the ulnar diaphysis at any level with anterior angulation (60% of the cases) (Fig. 13-14). Type II includes posterior or posterolateral dislocation of the radial head and fracture of the ulnar diaphysis with posterior angulation (15% of the cases). Type III (Fig. 13-15) includes lateral or anterolateral dislocation of the radial head and fracture of the ulnar metaphysis (20% of cases). Type IV includes anterior dislocation of the radial head, fracture of the proximal third of the radius, and fracture of the ulna at the same level. There are also several equivalent lesions that possess similar characteristics (1,12).

Detailed histories and careful examination of the lateral elbow roentgenogram are very important in the eval-

uation of these injuries. Unrecognized and untreated fractures may result in malunion with subsequent loss of function. Radiographically, the ulnar fractures are usually quite easy to detect. The dislocation radial head can easily be missed, however. Reasons for this include (1) failure to include the elbow on the film, which occurs especially when the fracture involves the mid- or distal ulnar shaft; (2) failure to center the x-ray beam on the elbow joint, thereby producing image distortion; and (3) a low index of suspicion for this lesion.

Use of the radiocapitellar line is helpful in evaluation of the radial head. In any elbow film, a line bisecting the radial head must always pass through the capitellum (11) (See Chapter 12, The Elbow).

In 1929, Valande described the solitary, unstable fracture of the radius at the junction of the middle and distal thirds, known as the *reverse Monteggia fracture* (23). In 1934, Galeazzi described the subluxation or dislocation of the distal radioulnar joint associated with this fracture. He further stressed that subluxation of the joint may be present initially or may occur during treatment (18).

Other factors also contribute to the instability of this fracture. Shortening of the radius tends to occur because of the brachioradialis insertion on the radial styloid process. The pronator quadratus muscle action rotates the distal radius in a volar direction, and the action of the

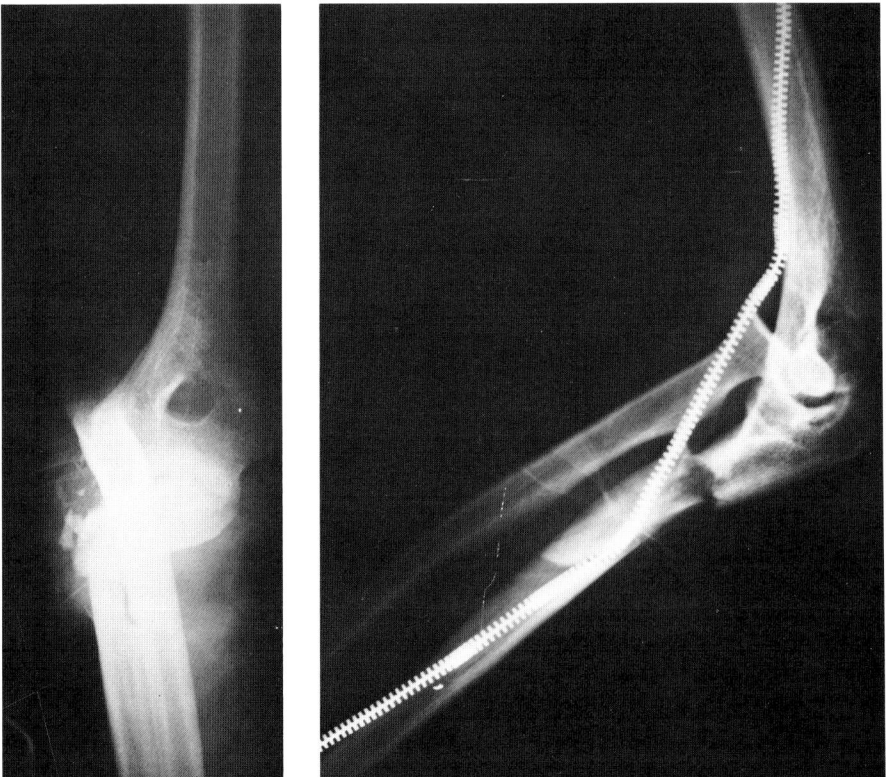

A   B

FIG. 13–14. A, B: AP and lateral films of Monteggia fracture, Type I with anterior dislocation of radial head.

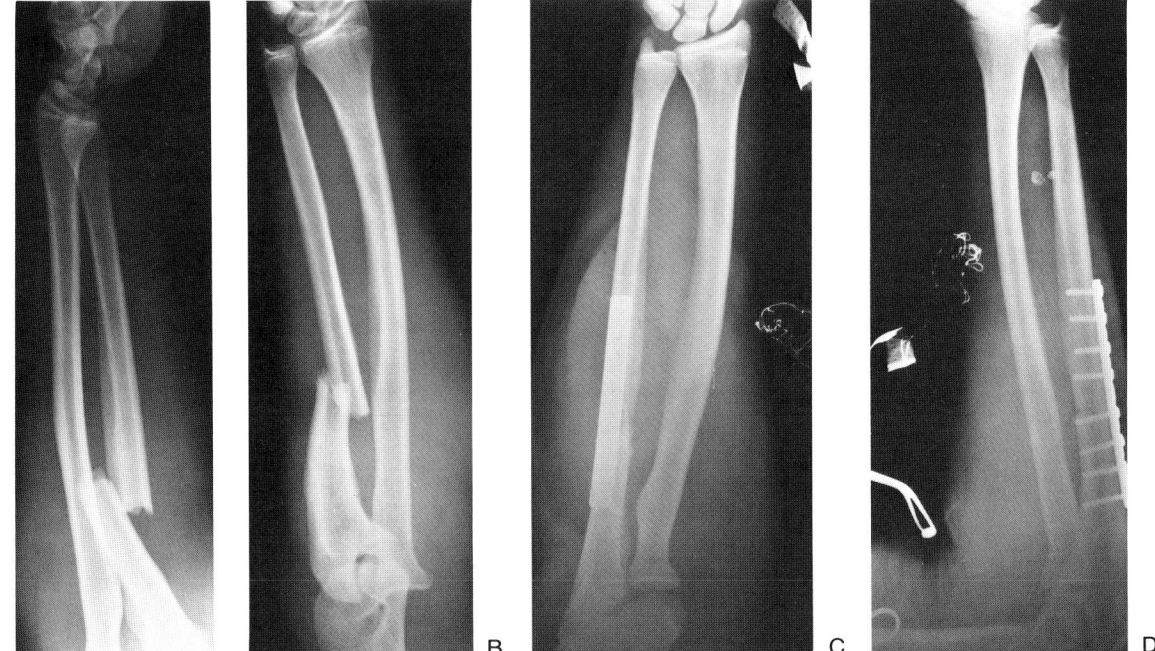

FIG. 13–15. A, B: Variant of Type III Monteggia fracture anterolateral dislocation of radial head and ulnar shaft fracture. **C, D:** Intraoperative AP and lateral films show excellent reduction.

thumb abductors and extensors tends to deviate the wrist radially (19). According to Galeazzi, this lesion is at least three times as common as the Monteggia fracture (1,18).

Radiologically, the fracture usually has a transverse or short oblique configuration and is angulated (Fig. 13-16). Generally there is not significant comminution. If much fracture displacement has occurred, there will be dislocation of the distal radioulnar joint. The distal ends of the radius and ulna are normally parallel. On the AP film, there may be increased distance between the articulation of the distal radius and ulna, or there may be overlap owing to ligamentous injury. There may also be an avulsion fracture of the ulnar styloid.

On the lateral view, the radius fracture is angulated dorsally, and the head of the ulna is prominent dorsally. Normally the projection of the distal ulna will overlie the posterior cortex of the distal radius. Although rare, damage to the ulnar nerve has been reported in this injury (17).

Displaced fractures of the proximal two-thirds of the radius are usually treated with compression plating or medullary nailing (Fig. 13-17). Detection is important because untreated fractures may result in loss of pronation and supination (1,7,12).

Closed treatment has led to poor results. Muscles acting across the distal forearm tend to displace the distal fragment. In order to maintain good pronation and supination, anatomic reduction must be obtained and held. The preferred method of treatment of these fractures, therefore, is open reduction and internal fixation with compression plating of the radial fracture. Tempo-

rary pin fixation of the radioulnar joint may be necessary. However, the pin must be removed before motion is instituted.

Open forearm fractures present special problems. When bone loss is minimal, treatment can proceed in the same way closed fractures are treated, once the soft tissue wounds are treated. For more serious injuries with soft tissue and bone loss, treatment is much more involved. Following initial debridement of the wounds, stabilization of the fractures must be carried out. The use of external fixation devices, plates, or occasionally, medullary devices may be useful. Treatment must then focus upon the soft tissue injuries. Muscle flaps, skin grafts, and free flap transfers of muscle—in some cases along with bone or skin—may be needed. When the soft tissue environment is satisfactory, definitive fixation of the fracture with bone grafting as necessary can be carried out.

Complications

Complications of fractures or treatment include nonunion, malunion (including radioulnar synostosis) (Fig. 13-17), infection, nerve or vascular injury, or compartment injury. Cross-union may also occur (10,12,24). This results in complete loss of pronation and supination (24). Vince and Miller classified cross-unions based on anatomic location (Fig. 13-18). Type I occur in the distal intra-articular region, Type II (Fig. 13-19) in the diaphyseal region, and Type III in the proximal radius and ulna.

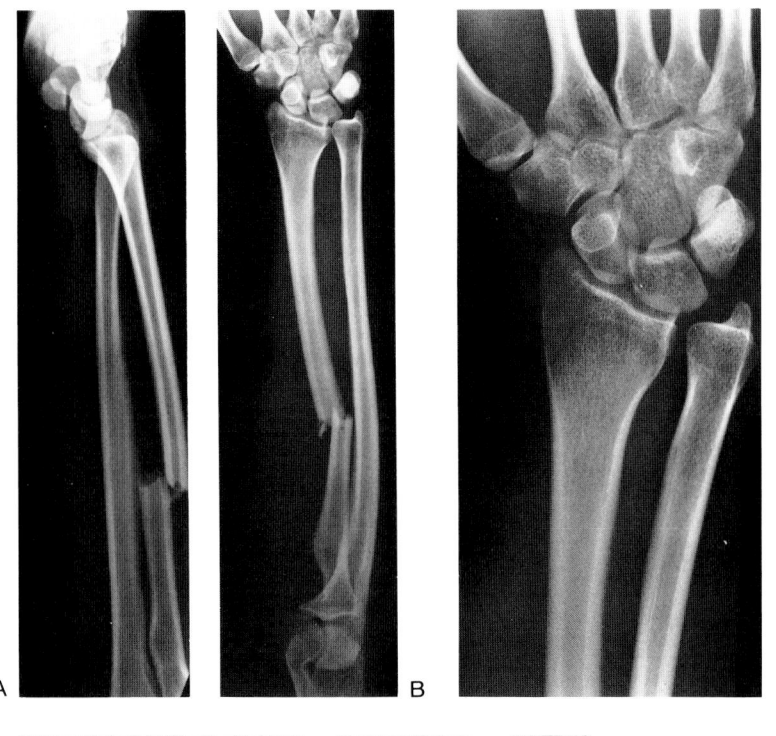

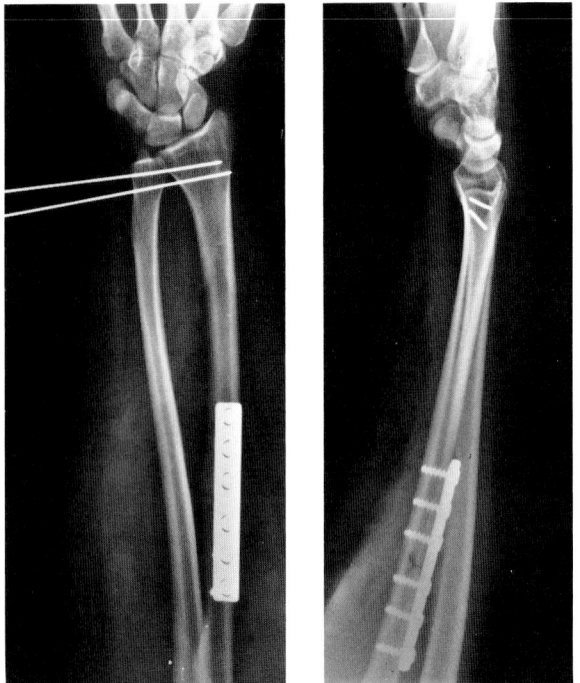

FIG. 13–16. **A, B:** Galeazzi fracture (AP and lateral views) show radial shaft fracture with radial deviation of wrist. **C:** AP wrist view shows increased distance between ulna and radius indicating ligamentous injury. **D, E:** Post-reduction films (AP and lateral).

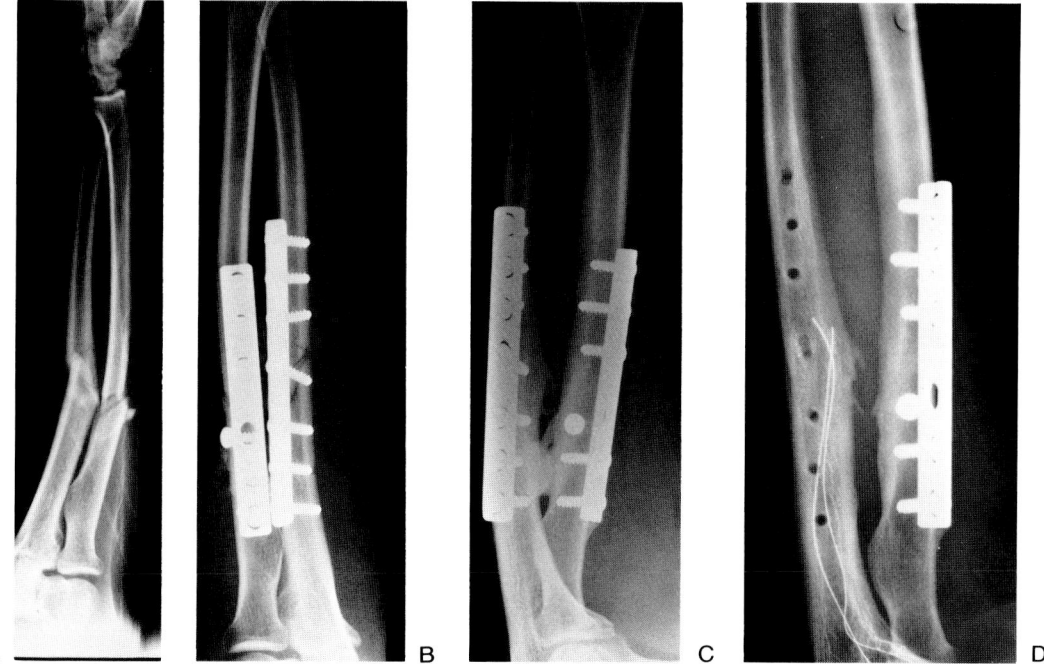

FIG. 13–17. A: Fractures of proximal shafts of radius and ulna (AP view). **B:** Plate and screw fixation, callus found on two-month follow-up (AP film). **C:** Oblique film shows synostosis, patient had no pronation or supination. **D:** Post-operative film shows removal of bony bridge and ulnar plate and screws. Good functional result.

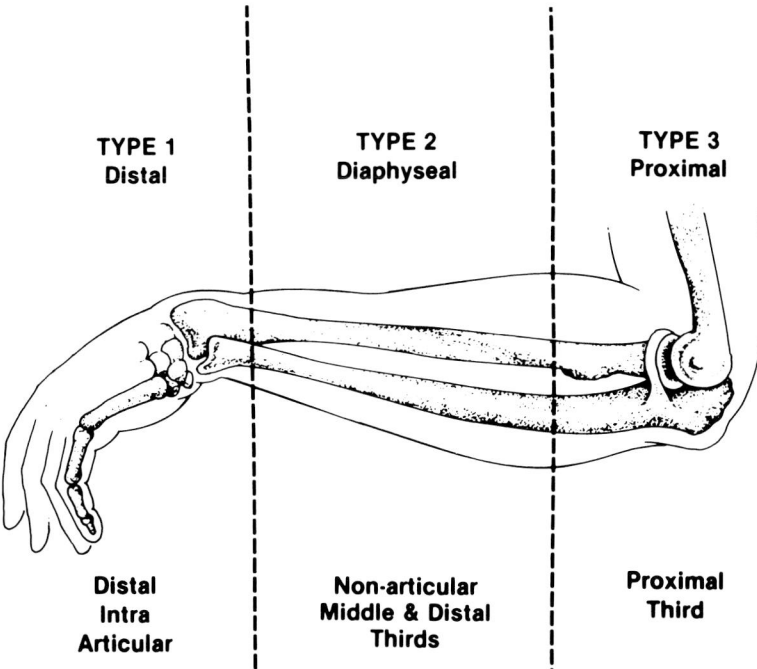

TYPE 1
Distal

TYPE 2
Diaphyseal

TYPE 3
Proximal

Distal
Intra
Articular

Non-articular
Middle & Distal
Thirds

Proximal
Third

FIG. 13–18. Three anatomic locations of cross-union (from 24, with permission).

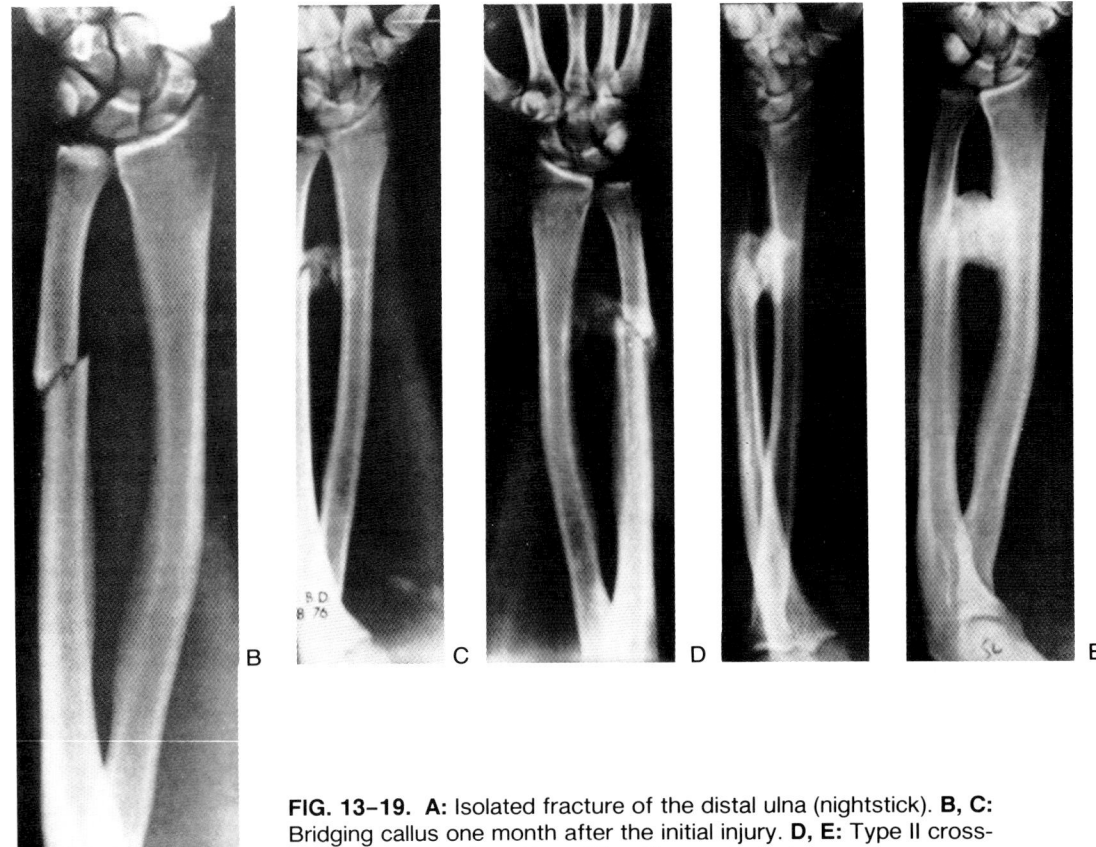

FIG. 13-19. A: Isolated fracture of the distal ulna (nightstick). **B, C:** Bridging callus one month after the initial injury. **D, E:** Type II cross-union 14 months later (from 24, with permission).

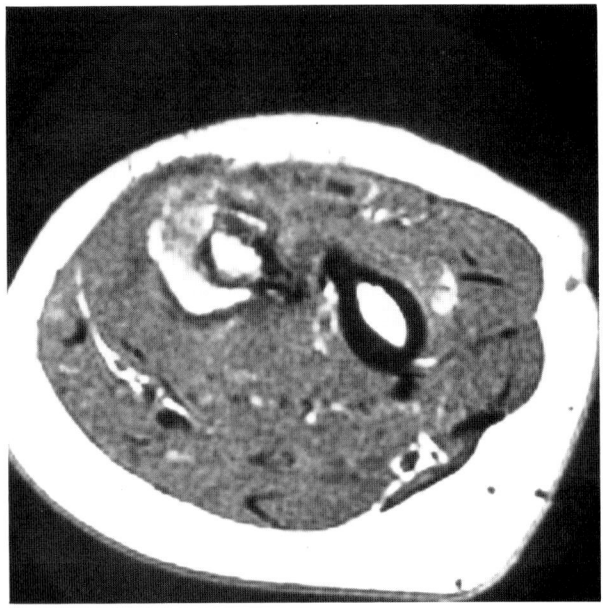

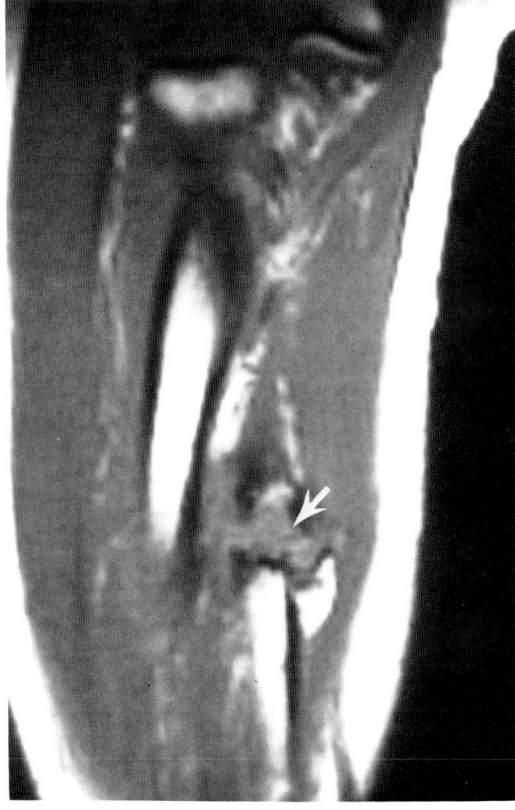

FIG. 13-20. Axial SE 2000/30 (**A**) and coronal SE 500/20 (**B**) image demonstrating an ulnar non-union with fluid (*arrow*) in the fracture site.

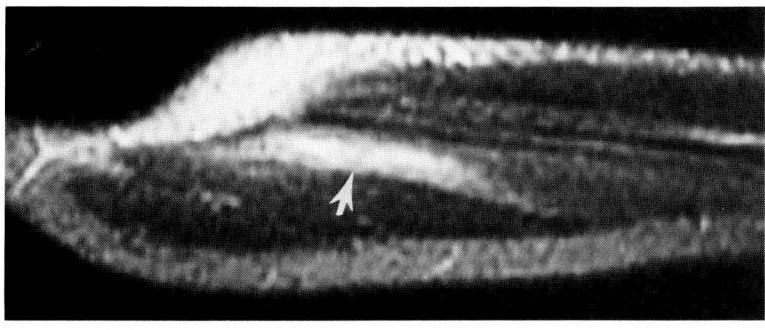

FIG. 13-21. Sagittal SE 2000/60 image demonstrates a larger area of increased signal intensity (*arrow*) in the extensor region due to a muscle tear.

Cross-unions may be more common in patients with fractures of both bones at the same level. Certainly, patients with complex fractures with extensive soft tissue injury more frequently develop this complication. Cross-unions can be excised within the second year after fracture. Radionuclide scans are useful in evaluating callus activity prior to planning surgical intervention (24).

Nerve injuries have been reported in one-sixth of forearm fractures (22). The radial nerve is involved in three-fifths of the injuries, with the remainder involving ulnar and medial nerves.

Refracture after plate removal is an additional complication of forearm fractures (7,8,13). This may occur in up to 11% of cases (8). Refracture typically occurs within the first 121 days after plate removal. If plates require removal, one should carefully evaluate radiographs or consider tomography. Fracture sites with residual lucent areas are more prone to fracture after plate removal (8). This complication can be reduced by keeping plates in place for 12–18 months and then protecting the forearm for 4–6 weeks (8).

SOFT TISSUE INJURIES

Isolated soft tissue injury or injury associated with fracture can occur in the forearm. Evaluation of soft tissue structures after fracture is not commonly required unless angiography is needed to assess vascular injury. Detection and classification of isolated soft tissue injury may be more difficult. Physical examination may provide the answer. However, imaging may be necessary to define the extent and nature of the injury.

Soft tissue injuries (neural, muscle, ligament, tendon ruptures; compartment syndromes, etc.) can be effectively evaluated using magnetic resonance imaging (MRI) and in some cases ultrasonography and computerized tomography (CT). The latter is particularly useful for detection of early myositis ossificans (3). MRI can define all anatomic regions (Fig. 13-20) and is useful for detecting muscle and ligament tears (Fig. 13-21) as well as neural injury. Axial T1 (SE 500/20) and T2 (SE 2000/60–80, 20–30) or T2* gradient-echo sequences are most useful. Additional image planes (oblique, coronal, sagittal) are useful for determining the extent of injury. Gra-

dient echo sequences are employed for motion studies or vascular lesions (3).

REFERENCES

1. Anderson LD. Fractures of the shafts of the radius and ulna. In: Rockwood CA, Green DP, eds. *Fractures in Adults,* vol. 1 Philadelphia: J. B. Lippincott Co., 1984;511–558.
2. Anderson LD, Sisk TD, Tooms RE, Park WI III. Compression plate fixation in acute diaphyseal fractures of the radius and ulna. *J Bone Joint Surg* 1975;57A:287–297.
3. Berquist TH. *MRI of the musculoskeletal system.* New York: Raven Press, 1990.
4. Bado JL. The Monteggia lesion. *Clin Orthop* 1967;50:71–86.
5. Ballinger PW. *Merrill's atlas of roentgenographic positioning and standard radiologic procedures,* 5th ed. St. Louis: C. V. Mosby Co., 1982.
6. Bernau A, Berquist TH. *Orthopedic positioning in diagnostic radiology.* Baltimore: Urban and Schwarzenberg, 1983.
7. Chapman MW, Gordon JE, Zissimos AG. Compression plate fixation of acute fractures of the diaphysis of the radius and ulna. *J Bone Joint Surg* 1989;71A:159–169.
8. DeLuca PA, Lindsey RW, Rowe PA. Refracture of bones in the forearm after removal of compression plates. *J Bone Joint Surg* 1988;70A:1372–1376.
9. Evans EM. Rotational deformity in the treatment of fractures of both bones of the forearm. *J Bone Joint Surg* 1945;27A:373–379.
10. Failla JM, Amadio PC, Morrey BF. Post traumatic proximal radio-ulnar synostosis. *J Bone Joint Surg* 1989;71A:1208–1213.
11. Giustra PE, Killoran PJ, Fierman RS, Root JA. The missed Monteggia fracture. *Radiology* 1974;110:45–47.
12. Grace TG, Eversmann WW. Forearm fractures. *J Bone Joint Surg* 1980;62A:433–438.
13. Hidaka S, Gustilo RB. Refracture of the bones of the forearm after plate removal. *J Bone Joint Surg* 1984;66A:1241–1243.
14. Hollinshead WH. *Anatomy for surgeons,* vol. 3: *The back and the limbs,* 3rd ed. New York: Harper and Row, 1982.
15. Jinkins WJ, Lockhart LD, Eggers GWN. Fractures of the forearm in adults. *South Med J* 1960;53:669–679.
16. Patrick J. Study of supination and pronation with especial reference to the treatment of forearm fractures. *J Bone Joint Surg* 1946;28A:737–748.
17. Poppi M. Fracture of the distal radius with ulnar nerve palsy. *J Trauma* 1978;18:278–279.
18. Rang M. *Anatomy of orthopaedics.* Baltimore: Williams and Wilkins, 1966.
19. Reckling FW, Cordell LD. Unstable fracture-dislocation of the forearm (Monteggia and Galeazzi lesions). *J Bone Joint Surg* 1982;64A:999–1007.
20. Rogers LF. *Radiology of skeletal trauma.* New York: Churchill Livingstone, 1982.
21. Sarmiento A, Cooper JS, Sinclair WF. Forearm fractures. Early functional bracing—a preliminary report. *J Bone Joint Surg* 1975;57A:297–304.
22. Smith H, Sage FP. Medullary fixation of forearm fractures. *J Bone Joint Surg* 1957;39A:91–98.
23. Valande M. Luxation en arriere du aibitus avec fracture de la diaphyse radiale. *Bull Mem Soc Nat Chir* 1929;55:435–437.
24. Vince KG, Miller JE. Cross-union complicating fracture of the forearm. Part I: Adults. *J Bone Joint Surg* 1987;69A:640–660.

Imaging of Orthopedic Trauma,
Second Edition, edited by T.H. Berquist,
Mayo Clinic © 1992. Published
by Raven Press, Ltd., New York.

CHAPTER 14

The Hand and Wrist

Michael B. Wood and Thomas H. Berquist

Anatomy, 749
  Osteology, 749
  Ligament and Joint Capsules, 755
  Muscular Anatomy, 758
  Neurovascular Anatomy, 761
Imaging Techniques, 763
  Routine Radiography, 763
  Tomography, 777
  Computed Tomography, 778
  Radionuclide Imaging, 779
  Magnetic Resonance Imaging, 782
Arthrography of the Hand and Wrist, 789
  Wrist Arthrography, 789
  Arthrography of the Hand, 794
Fractures and Dislocations, 796
  Distal Radius Fractures, 796

Dislocations about the Distal Radius, 810
Radiocarpal Dislocation, 811
Carpal Fractures, 811
Carpal Dislocations, 827
Metacarpal Fractures, 830
Metacarpophalangeal Joint Dislocations, 840
Phalangeal Fractures, 843
Dislocations of the Interphalangeal Joints, 852
Chronic Post-traumatic Conditions, 852
Post-traumatic Reconstruction, 861
  Osteotomy, 861
  Arthrodesis, 861
  Soft Tissue Stabilization, 863
  Arthroplasty, 863
Summary, 866
References, 866

This chapter, devoted to the hand and wrist, will summarize the pertinent normal and abnormal anatomic features related to traumatic conditions in the distal upper extremity. No attempt will be made to address those conditions of the hand and wrist that are of little radiographic significance in terms of diagnosis or assessment.

ANATOMY

Osteology

The wrist begins proximally at the distal metaphysis of the radius and ulna and extends distally to include the entire carpus. The term *wrist/joint* is a misnomer, as the wrist includes a number of articulations. However, from the functional aspect, these fall into three main articular groups: the distal radioulnar joint, the radiocarpal articulation, and the so-called *midcarpal articulation.*

The distal radial metaphysis and epiphysis is composed largely of cancellous bone with a relatively thin cortex. This structural arrangement, coupled with its liability to injury with falls on the outstretched hand, likely accounts for the frequency of fractures seen in this area. Its extreme radial aspect is elongated distally as a styloid process. The distal articular surface of the radius has two fossae for the scaphoid and lunate, respectively. These are separated by a variably defined vertical ridge. This surface of the radius is inclined 14° toward the ulna in the frontal plane and 12° toward the palmar surface in the lateral plane (2). On the ulnar aspect of the distal radius is a separate concave joint surface called the *sigmoid notch* for articulation with the distal ulna (Fig. 14-1). The dorsal surface of the distal radius is characterized by a series of sulci and ridges that define the floor of the first through fourth dorsal tendinous compartments of the wrist. The most readily palpable protuberance of this surface is Lister's tubercle, which lies between the compartment of the radial wrist extensor tendons (second) and that of the extensor pollicis longus tendon (third).

M. B. Wood: Department of Orthopedic Surgery, Mayo Medical School, Mayo Clinic, Rochester, Minnesota 55905.
T. H. Berquist: Department of Diagnostic Radiology, Mayo Medical School, Mayo Clinic Jacksonville, Jacksonville, Florida 32224.

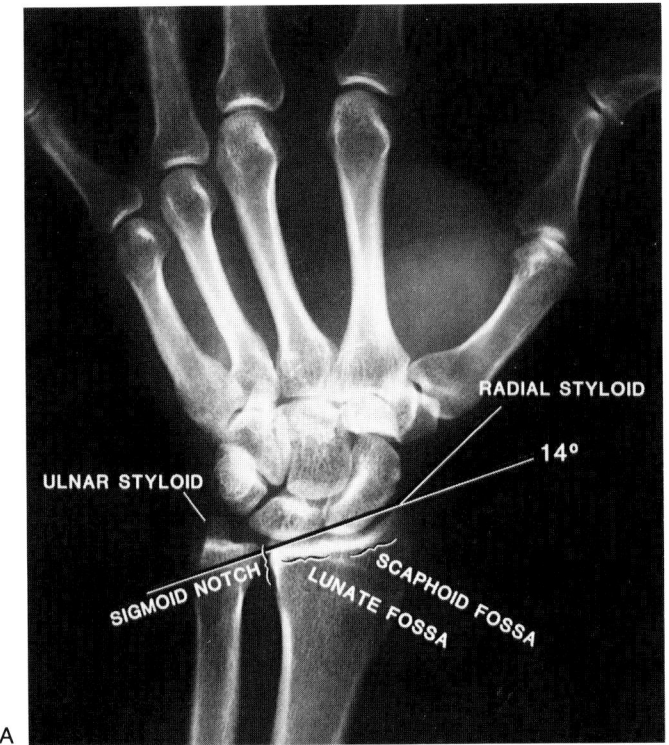
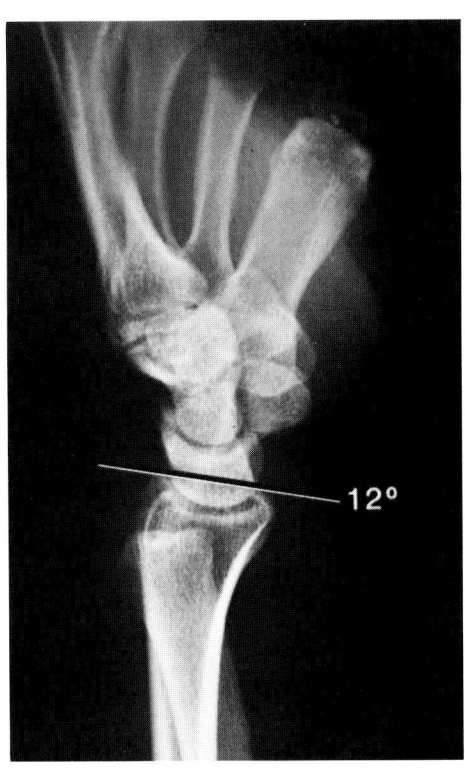

FIG. 14-1. AP (A) and lateral (B) radiographs of the hand and wrist. The distal radius normally demonstrates a 14° ulnar tilt on the AP (A) and 12° volar tilt on the lateral view (B).

The first (most radial) dorsal compartment contains the tendons of the abductor pollicis longus and extensor pollicis brevis tendons, while the fourth compartment contains the extensor digitorum communis tendons to all fingers and the proprius tendons of the index digit (Fig. 14-2).

The distal ulna is also predominantly composed of cancellous bone but with a reasonably thick cortex. It has a spikelike, well-defined styloid process. Fracture of

this process not infrequently accompanies a fracture of the distal radius. The ulnar head articulates with the distal radius, lunate, and triquetrum. It is usually separated from the latter two bones by an articular disk that represents a portion of the triangular fibrocartilage complex. The dorsal surface of the ulna has sulci for the fifth and sixth dorsal compartments of the wrist, which house the extensor digiti quinti and extensor carpi ulnaris tendons, respectively (Fig. 14-2). The position of the distal articular surface of the ulna relative to that of the radius may have significance in certain clinical situations and is defined by the term *ulnar variance* (4,5). In most patients it is either equal (neutral) or 1 mm shorter than the radius. Ulnar variance is positive if the ulnar articular surface is more distal than that of the radius. Conversely, it is negative if it lies more proximally (Fig. 14-3). The distal radioulnar joint in conjunction with the proximal radioulnar joint at the elbow permits rotation of the radius about the ulna in the process of forearm pronation

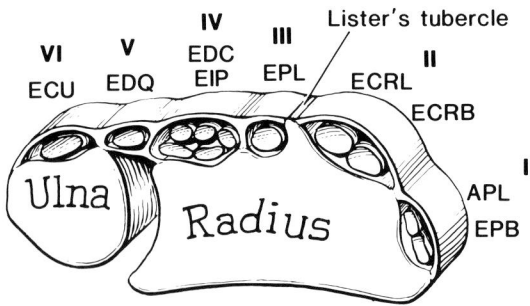

FIG. 14-2. Distal radius and ulnar enface demonstrating the first through sixth dorsal compartments. First compartment, abductor pollicus longus (APL) and extensor pollicus brevis (EPB); Second compartment, extensor carpi radialis longus (ECRL) and extensor carpi radialis brevis (ECRB); Third compartment, extensor pollicus longus (EPL); Fourth compartment, extensor indicis proprius (EIP) and extensor digitorum communis (EDC); Fifth compartment, extensor digiti quinti (EDQ); Sixth compartment, extensor carpi ulnaris (ECU).

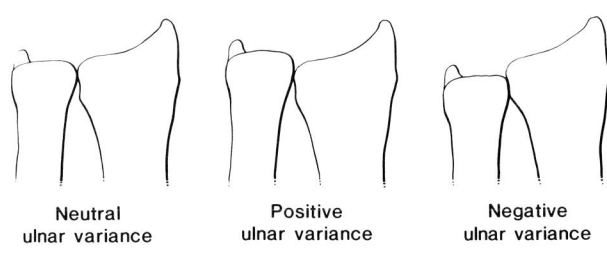

FIG. 14-3. Neutral, positive, and negative ulnar variance.

and supination. Normally an arc of 160°–180° of rotation is possible (2).

The carpus functionally is composed of three anatomic groups (Fig. 14-4). The first, the proximal row, consists of the scaphoid, lunate, triquetrum, and overlapping pisiform. The scaphoid and triquetrum are firmly bound to the lunate by strong interosseous ligaments. The stability of these articulations is essential for normal wrist mechanics (21). The proximal articular surfaces of these three bones should define a smooth unbroken arc in the frontal plane (Fig. 14-5). In this same projection, the scaphoid tubercle will present a ringlike appearance in the distal half of the bone, and the lunate should appear "trapezoidal." The distance between the scaphoid and lunate or lunate and triquetrum should be relatively constant in all positions of the wrist. Normally this distance should not exceed 2 mm (3). The position of the scaphoid and lunate should be congruous with the scaphoid and lunate fossae of the distal radius. Ulnar translation of the carpus relative to the radius may be seen in conditions of chronic wrist synovitis and in disruption of the radiocarpal ligament complex, particularly if accompanied by dorsal subluxation of the distal

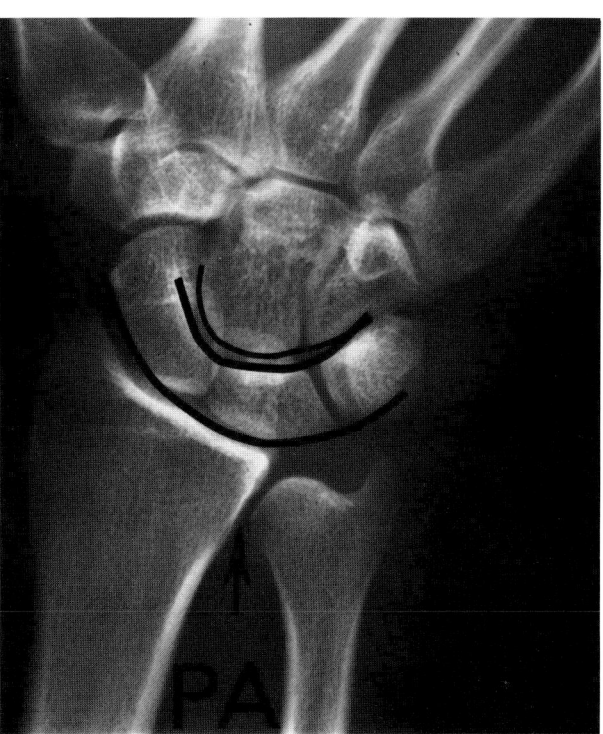

FIG. 14–5. True PA of the wrist. The proximal and distal carpal rows form concentric arcs. The normal distal radial-ulnar joint (*large arrows*) is 2–3 mm. The hook of the hamate is seen on end (*upper arrow*).

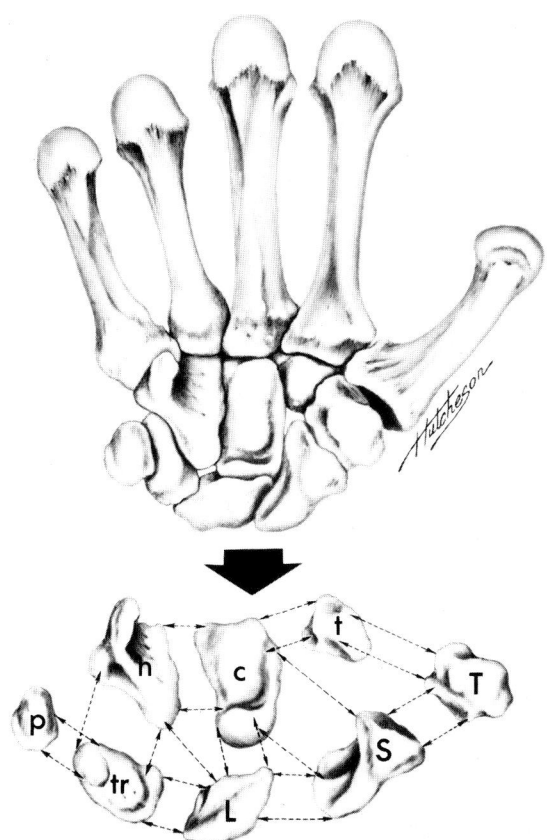

FIG. 14–4. Skeletal anatomy of the wrist with bones detached below. The proximal carpal row: scaphoid (S), lunate (L), triquetrum (tr), and overlapping pisiform (p). The distal carpal row: trapezoid (t), capitate (c) and hamate (h). The trapezium (T) provides independent motion of the thumb (from 2).

ulna. This instability pattern is characterized by the presence of an apparent widened joint space between the lateral radial articular surface and the scaphoid as well as a decrease in the carpal ulnar distance (22,23). This latter term refers to the perpendicular distance between the midpoint of the head of the capitate and a line drawn through the midpoint of the ulna along its longitudinal axis on a PA radiograph. Normally, the carpal ulnar distance should form a ratio of 0.30 (±0.03) with the length of the third metacarpal (Fig. 14-6). In the lateral plane with the wrist neutral, the lunate should generally be collinear with the radius and should appear symmetric within the lunate fossa. The scaphoid outline may be difficult to visualize due to bony overlap. With the wrist in a neutral position, however, it should point obliquely in a palmar direction. A line drawn through its long axis should form an angle of 30°–60° (mean, 47°) with a line drawn through the axis of the lunate (Fig. 14-7) (2,3). This angle is called the *scapholunate angle* and may be abnormal in certain collapse deformities of the wrist. The position of the scaphoid relative to the lunate, however, will vary with ulnar or radial deviation of the wrist (11,19). This should be borne in mind when assessing the scapholunate angle. As the wrist moves from complete ulnar deviation to complete radial deviation, the scaphoid will subtend an arc of 40° (Fig. 14-8). The pisiform is a true sesamoid bone lying within the flexor carpi ulnaris tendon. It forms a synovial articulation with the trique-

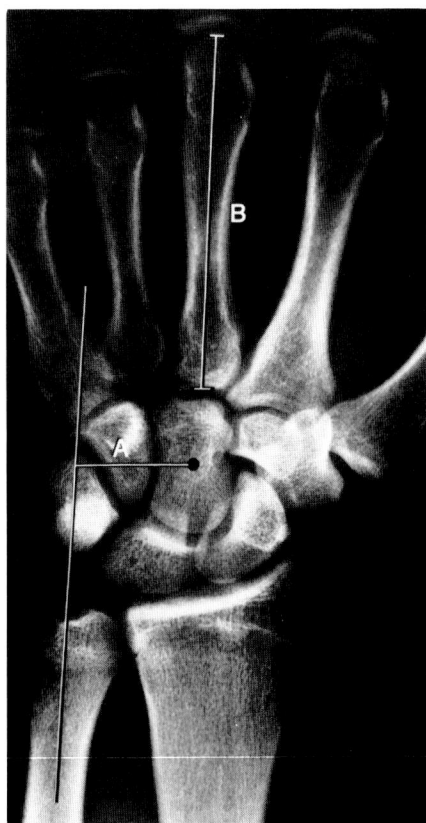

FIG. 14–6. AP radiograph of the wrist demonstrating the carpal ulnar distance. Normally the ratio of the distance from a line parallel to the ulnar shaft to the midpoint of the capitate (A) over the length of the third metacarpal (B) is 0.30 [A/B = 0.30 (±.03)].

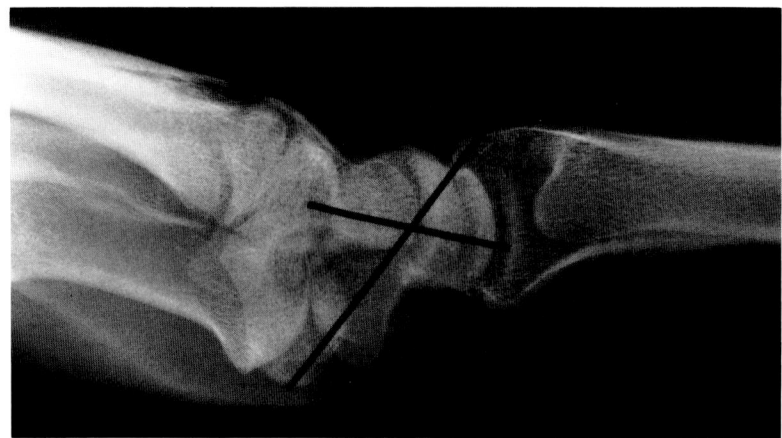

FIG. 14–7. Normal lateral view of the wrist demonstrating the normal scapholunate axis (lines through the long axis of the scaphoid and midlunate). This angle normally is 30°–60° with a mean of 47°.

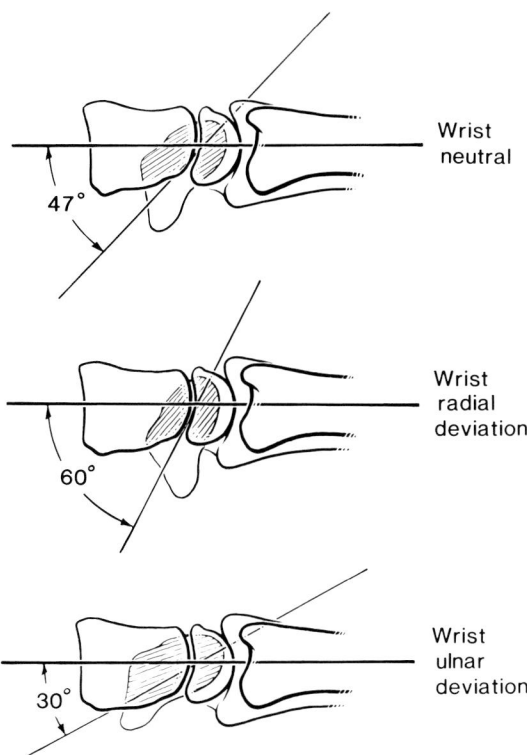

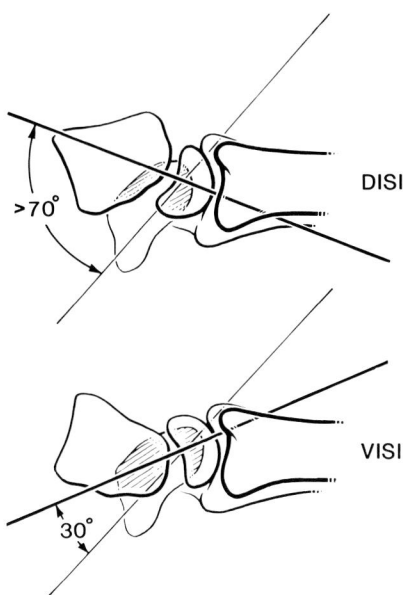

FIG. 14-9. Collapse deformities: DISI (dorsal intercalated segment instability), VISI (volar intercalated segment instability).

FIG. 14-8. Scapholunate angle changes with radial and ulnar deviation. The scaphoid subtends a 40° arc.

trum. Motion between the proximal carpal row and the forearm long bones is primarily associated with dorsiflexion (extension) and also contributes to radial and ulnar deviation (8).

The second anatomic group, the distal carpal row, consists of the trapezoid, capitate, and hamate. These too are tightly bound to each other by strong interosseous ligaments. The hook (hamulus) of the hamate will present an overlying ringlike appearance in the frontal projection (see Fig. 14-5). On the lateral view, the capitate should articulate congruently with the lunate; with the wrist in a neutral position, these two bones along with the radius should be collinear (11) (see Fig. 14-7). This collinear relationship may be lost in certain collapse deformities of the wrist.

Two basic patterns of collapse deformity are recognized and are defined by the direction of the lunate relative to the capitate (14). The first and most common is a dorsal intercalated segment instability (DISI) pattern. This is characterized on the lateral projection by the lunate appearing to be dorsiflexed on the radius and the capitate palmar flexed on the lunate (Figs. 14-9 and 14-10). DISI is most commonly associated with injuries that result in destabilization of the lunate to the scaphoid, for example, fractures of the scaphoid (6) and complete disruption of the scapholunate interosseous ligament. In such cases, therefore, an additional radiographic finding will be an exaggeration of the scapholunate angle.

The second major category of collapse deformity is in the opposite direction and is referred to as a volar intercalated segment instability (VISI) pattern. This type is characterized by the lunate assuming a palmar flexed position relative to the radius, with the capitate dorsiflexed relative to the lunate (12) (Figs. 14-9 and 14-11). It is most commonly associated with destabilization of the lunate and triquetrum (lunotriquetral interosseous ligament disruption), midcarpal sprains, rheumatoid arthritis, and exaggerated congenital ligamentous laxity in certain individuals. With this pattern, a reduction of the scapholunate angle is frequently seen. It is important to emphasize that the diagnosis of either of these two collapse patterns can be made only on the basis of a true lateral x-ray with the wrist in a neutral position. The diagnosis is further supported by the apparent persistence of the collapse pattern on true lateral radiographs obtained with the wrist in a fully extended and fully flexed position.

In the absence of a collapse pattern of the carpus, a fracture, or a loss of bone mass, the carpal height should be constant (22,23). This term refers to the distance between the base of the third metacarpal and the distal articular surface of the radius along the axis of the third metacarpal as determined on a PA x-ray. Normally the carpal height should be a ratio of 0.54 (±0.03) when compared with the length of the third metacarpal (Fig. 14-12). Motion between the proximal and distal carpal rows is primarily associated with palmar flexion and also contributes to radial and ulnar deviation.

Distal to the carpus are the five metacarpals. The first (thumb) metacarpal lies outside the plane of the others in

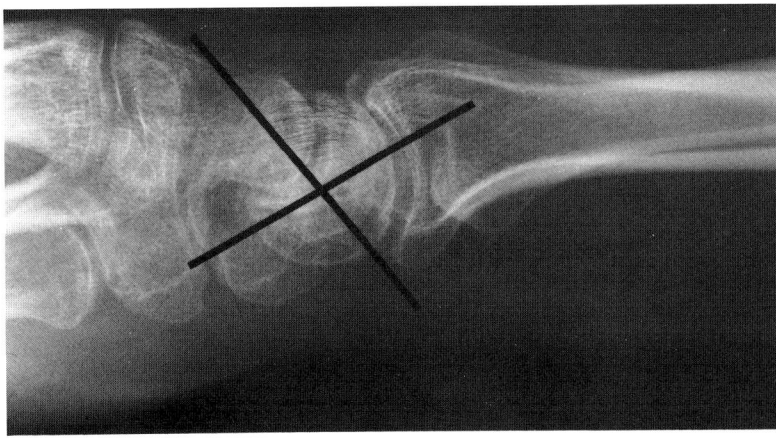

FIG. 14–10. Lateral radiograph with DISI. The distal articular surface of the lunate is directed dorsally.

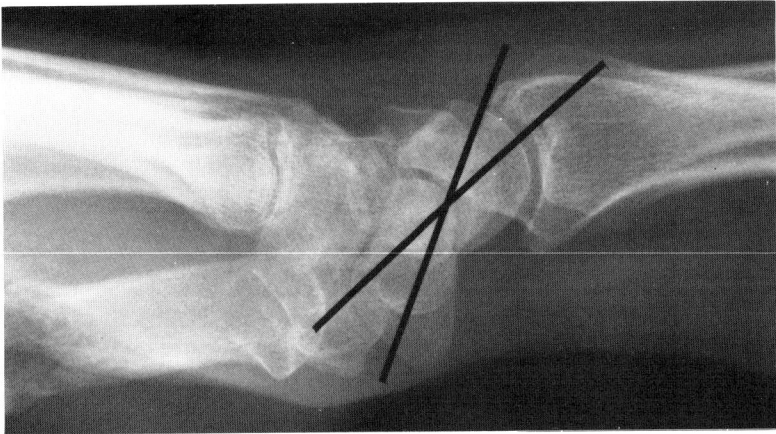

FIG. 14–11. Lateral radiograph with VISI. The distal articular surface of the lunate is in a palmar direction and the scapholunate angle reduced.

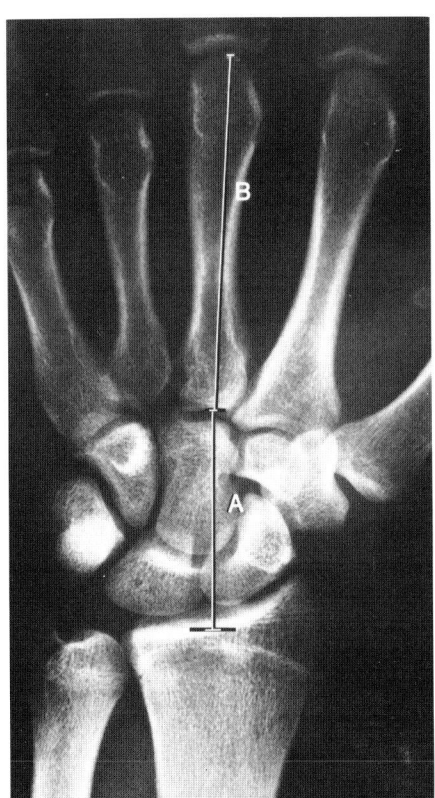

FIG. 14–12. PA radiograph demonstrating carpal height measurement. The ratio of the distance from the distal radial articular surface to the base of the third metacarpal (A) over the length of the third metacarpal (B) is 0.54. (A/B = 0.54 ± 0.03).

an obliquely palmar direction. The structure of each is similar, with flared metaphyses proximally and distally composed chiefly of cancellous bone and a narrow diaphysis of cortical bone (see Fig. 14-4). This joint space of the second and third carpometacarpal articulations is usually poorly visualized on routine radiographs because of the amount of bony overlap. Moreover, these joints have essentially negligible motion (9). The fourth and fifth carpometacarpal joints, however, usually do have a well-defined joint space, which is best visualized on AP and oblique projections, and they also have a range of motion between 15° and 40° (7). Adjacent metacarpals are stabilized with respect to each other by strong proximal interosseous ligaments and by the transverse metacarpal ligaments distally. The metacarpal heads are roughly spherical. A lateral depression just proximal to the articular surface at the site of origin of the collateral ligaments may be seen on the Brewerton view (see section on Routine Radiographic Techniques and Fig. 14-26). This depression may be particularly obvious in rheumatoid arthritis and represents one of the x-ray diagnostic signs of this condition. The metacarpal head is eccentric in shape, with its palmar aspect broader than its dorsum. This configuration allows relaxation of the collateral ligaments with lateral motion for abduction of the fingers with the metacarpophalangeal joint in a position of extension. Conversely, flexion of the joint tightens the collateral ligaments and allows for little lateral motion. In all positions of the metacarpophalangeal joint, however, the respective articular surfaces should appear congruent.

The proximal and middle phalanges of the fingers are similar in structure, with flared proximal and distal ends composed chiefly of cancellous bone (see Fig. 14-1). The diaphysis consists predominantly of cortical bone and is cylindrical. The distal articular surface of the phalanges is bicondular and is intimately congruent with its articular fellow on both frontal and lateral planes. The thumb lacks a middle phalanx and thus has only a single interphalangeal joint. The distal phalanx is foreshortened, with its distal end flared in the shape of a blunt arrowhead on the frontal projection.

Small spherical sesamoid bones, although varying in position and number, are frequently seen in pairs volar to the metacarpophalangeal joints or in the interphalangeal joint of the thumb (Fig. 14-13). Moreover, occasionally accessory ossicles can be visualized about the hand and wrist. At least sixteen accessory ossification centers have been reported (16). The most significant of this group is probably the os centrali. If this ossification center fails to unite to the scaphoid, confusion with a so-called *bipartite scaphoid* may be possible. Another accessory ossicle described by some is the so-called *styloid bone* lying in the region of the second and third carpometacarpal joint. Whether this represents a true accessory ossicle or a reactive process is debatable, but it may

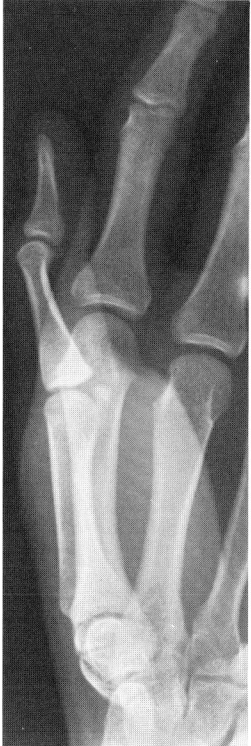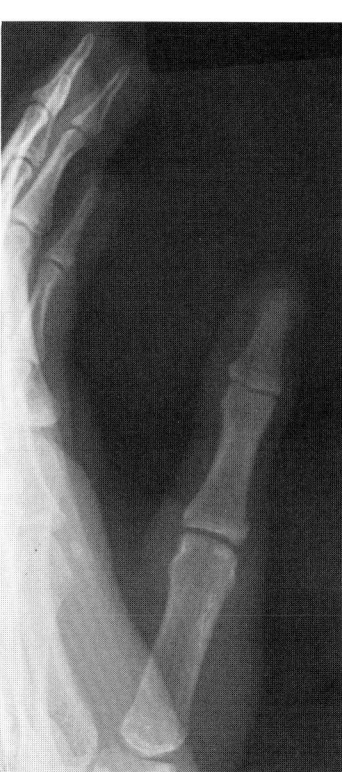

FIG. 14-13. Two views of the thumb demonstrating paired sesamoid bones at the first MCP joint and a single sesamoid at the second MCP joint.

present as a symptomatic carpe bosseau. Other well known accessory ossification centers are the lunula (lying between the triquetrum and ulnar styloid) and the os radiali externum at the distal end of the scaphoid. The order of ossification of the normal carpal bones is somewhat variable. However, in general the center of ossification appears for the capitate at 6 months, for the hamate at 6–18 months, for the triquetrum at 2 years, for the lunate at 4 years, for the trapezium at 5 years, for the trapezoid at 6 years, for the scaphoid at 5–6 years, and for the pisiform at 10 years.

Ligament and Joint Capsules

A detailed description of all the various ligaments about the wrist and hand is beyond the scope of this chapter. However, a review of those ligaments most frequently associated with pathologic conditions or of particular radiographic significance will be emphasized. Because the wrist comprises at least ten bones and allows a variety of degrees of motion, it naturally depends on a complex array of strong ligaments and soft tissue supports for its mechanical characteristics (8).

The stability of the distal radioulnar joint and a major component of the ulnocarpal articulation depend on the integrity of the triangular fibrocartilage complex (11,18).

This so-called *ligamentous complex* consists of multiple components that blend imperceptibly into one another and include the triangular fibrocartilage proper, the ulnocarpal meniscus, the ulnar collateral ligament, and the volar and dorsal distal radioulnar ligaments (Fig. 14-14). The apex of the triangular fibrocartilage proper (or articular disk) originates from the base of the ulnar styloid process and fans out to insert broadly along the ulnar margin of the distal radius. Perforations may be seen in the center portion of the disk that may or may not be of clinical significance (16,18). The dorsal and volar margins of the fibrocartilage are thickened, blending with the respective radioulnar ligaments, capsular ligaments of the wrist, and lunotriquetral interosseous ligaments. The ulnocarpal meniscus component arises near the insertion of the articular disk on the radius and courses distally, inserting into the triquetrum and hamate. Its extreme ulnar aspect blends with the ulnar collateral ligament fibers. Other factors contributing to the stability of the distal radioulnar joint include the interosseous membrane of the radius and ulna, the extensor carpi ulnaris tendon and its retaining fibro-osseous sheath, and finally the degree of concavity of the sigmoid notch of the radius.

Both volar and dorsal extrinsic capsular ligaments contribute to the stability of the radiocarpal aspect of the wrist, but the former are of greater clinical significance. Descriptions of the precise components and nomenclature of the capsular ligaments vary from author to author (10,15,20). Hence, considerable confusion exists in the literature regarding this topic. However, most agree on a general anatomic arrangement. The palmar capsular ligaments are most obvious when viewed intracapsularly. Basically, they consist of two concentric arches originating from the volar radial lip of the radius and inserting into the triquetrum and triangular fibrocartilage complex (Fig. 14-15). The first arch is composed of the radiolunotriquetral ligament, which courses from the radius across the volar surface of the lunate, inserts into the volar surface of the lunate, and then inserts firmly on the triquetrum. The ulnotriquetral ligament then completes the arch. The second arch is made up of the radiocapitate ligament, which originates more laterally on the radius, passes across the waist of the scaphoid, and inserts into

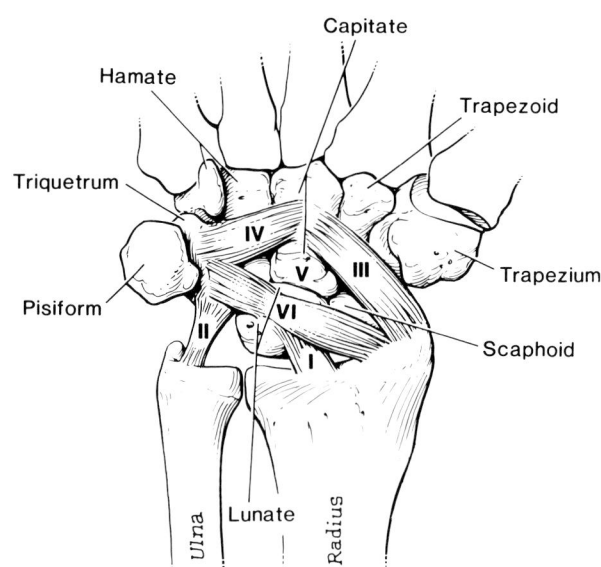

FIG. 14-15. Palmar ligaments of the wrist. I. Radio-lunotriquetral ligament; II. ulnotriquetral ligament; III. radiocapitate ligament; IV. capitotriquetral ligament; V. space of Poirier; VI. ligament of Testut or radioscapholunate ligament.

the capitate. This arch is completed by the capitotriquetral ligament and the ulnotriquetral ligament. Between these two arches is a rather thinned area of the volar wrist capsule known as the *space of Poirier*. In addition to the double ligamentous arch of the palmar capsule, there is a short but stout radioscapholunate ligament (ligament of Testut). This structure arises from the volar lip of the radius and courses obliquely distally and dorsally to insert on the volar and middle aspect of the scapholunate interosseous ligaments. The dorsal capsular ligaments of the wrist are relatively thin and of lesser significance than their palmar counterparts. The most important components are the radiolunotriquetral and ulnotriquetral ligaments (Fig. 14-16). Both dorsal and volar complexes are reinforced by a radial and ulnar collateral ligament complex.

In addition to the extrinsic capsular ligaments, intrinsic intercarpal ligaments contribute to the stability of the radiocarpal and intercarpal articulations. These include the scapholunate and lunotriquetral interosseous ligaments in the proximal carpal row and both dorsal and volar interosseous ligaments connecting the hamate, capitate, trapezoid, and trapezium. The preserved integrity of the extrinsic capsular and intrinsic intercarpal ligaments is essential for normal wrist stability and mechanisms.

Ligamentous support of the carpometacarpal articulations is provided by longitudinally oriented dorsal and volar carpometacarpal ligaments. These vary in location, number, and strength according to the joint involved (8). The first carpometacarpal joint is relatively lax, allowing considerable motion in several degrees of

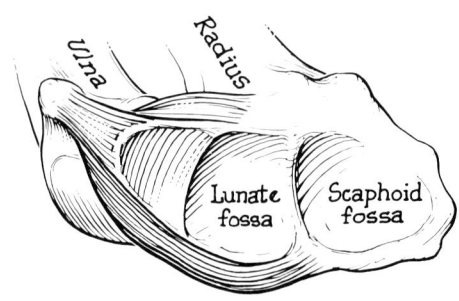

FIG. 14-14. Triangular fibrocartilage complex.

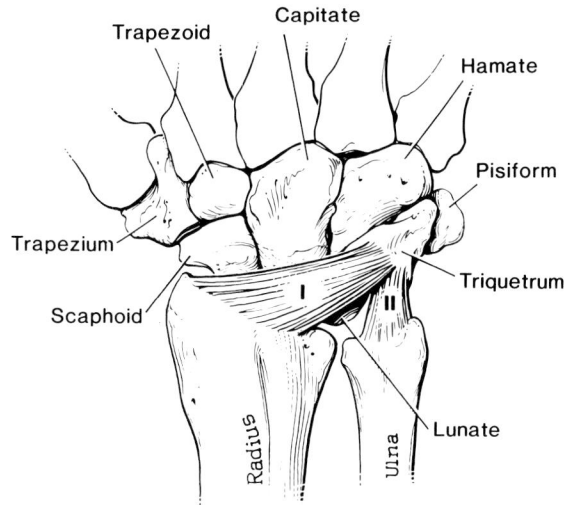

FIG. 14–16. Dorsal ligaments of the wrist. I. Radiolunotri-quetral; II. ulnotriquetral.

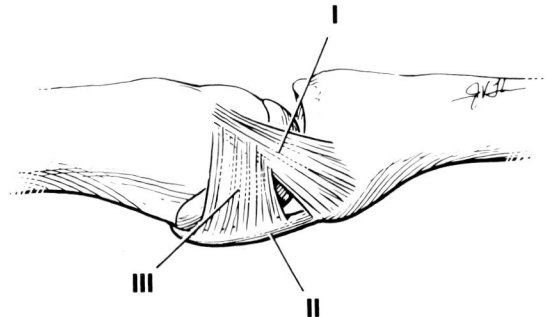

FIG. 14–17. Metacarpophalangeal ligaments seen from the lateral view. I. Collateral ligaments; II. volar plate; III. accessory collateral ligaments.

freedom. Often its inherent instability is a source of clinical concern. The chief ligamentous support is provided by the palmar and dorsal oblique capsular ligaments. The former is strongest and most important. By contrast, the second and third carpometacarpal joints are extremely stable, with negligible motion. Strong, short capsular ligaments pass from the trapezoid to both radial and ulnar condyles of the second metacarpal on both the volar and dorsal aspects of the joint. The third metacarpal base is stabilized by obliquely disposed dorsal ligaments passing from the trapezoid and capitate as well as by a volar ligament from the capitate and hamate. The fourth and fifth carpometacarpal joints have a moderate range of motion in the plane of flexion and extension and, therefore, are stabilized by less stout capsular ligaments. These arise on both dorsal and volar aspects from the capitate and hamate to the base of the fourth metacarpal and from the hamate along to the base of the fifth metacarpal. The carpometacarpal articulations are further stabilized by strong transverse intermetacarpal ligaments between the bases of the second through fifth metacarpals (3). Moreover, these same metacarpals are weakly stabilized distally by distal transverse intermetacarpal ligaments.

Ligamentous support of the metacarpophalangeal joints is similar in all digits and depends primarily upon the collateral ligaments, the accessory collateral ligaments, and the fibrocartilaginous volar plate (10) (Fig. 14-17). The collateral ligaments are well-defined capsular structures that arise from a dorsal position on either side of the metacarpal just proximal to its articular head. These structures then pass in a palmar and distal direction to insert onto the volar lateral aspect of the base of the proximal phalanx. The fibrocartilaginous volar plate arises from the base of the proximal phalanx and inserts into the volar aspect of the metacarpal just proximal to

the articular surface. It is a thick, unyielding structure distally but becomes thin and compliant more proximally. It is intimately associated with the distal intermetacarpal ligaments and proximal flexor-tendon-sheath pulley system. Between the collateral ligaments and the volar plate are the interconnecting fibers of the accessory collateral ligaments. Dorsal to the collateral ligaments, the joint capsule is filmy and closely associated with the extensor apparatus. As such, the dorsal capsule contributes relatively little stability to the joint. The metacarpophalangeal articulation allows considerable lateral motion, particularly in a position of extension, owing to the eccentricity and relative spherical shape of the metacarpal head. Of particular clinical significance for collateral ligament injury is the metacarpophalangeal joint of the thumb. This joint is shrouded by a well-defined extensor aponeurosis, or hood, which may become interposed with complete ruptures of the ulnar collateral ligament.

The ligamentous support of the interphalangeal joints is basically identical in all digits and is quite similar to the arrangement described earlier for the metacarpophalangeal joints (12). The volar fibrocartilaginous plate of this joint, however, is thickened on its lateral extreme where it is most firmly attached to the base of the middle (or distal) phalanges (1). Proximally, the laterally thickened portions are inserted into the proximal phalanx in close association with the flexor-tendon-sheath pulley system and form the so-called *check-rein ligaments*. In contrast to the metacarpophalangeal joints, the interphalangeal joints are not eccentric and have little lateral motion. The collateral ligaments in the interphalangeal joint, therefore, are shorter and more rectangular in appearance. The dorsal capsule, although filmy, is reinforced at the base of the middle phalanx. In addition to the ligamentous structures discussed above and the inherent stability conferred by bony architecture, stability to all joints of the upper extremity is further augmented by musculotendinous structures crossing or inserting near the articulation. A detailed description of these structures, however, is of relatively little significance for radiographic evaluations. There are, however, certain specific clinical situations in which the musculotendinous anatomy is relevant, and these will be discussed later in this chapter.

Muscular Anatomy

Many of the muscles and tendons that cross the wrist originate at the elbow or proximal forearm. These muscles of the forearm are largely responsible for flexion and extension of the wrist (7,8,19). This section will deal primarily with those muscles directly related to the bones of the hand and wrist with regard to their origins and insertions.

Flexor Muscles

The chief flexors of the wrist are the flexor carpi radialis and flexor carpi ulnaris. The palmaris longus is a minor flexor of the wrist (Fig. 14-18) (8). Extension of the wrist is largely due to the extensor carpi radialis longus and brevis and the extensor carpi ulnaris (Fig. 14-19). During radial deviation of the wrist, primary muscles involved are the abductor pollicis longus and extensor pollicis brevis. Ulnar deviation of the wrist is accomplished primarily by the extensor carpi ulnaris (7,8,10,11).

There are typically four lumbrical muscles that arise from the flexor digitorum profundus tendons and extend along the radial aspects of the second through fifth metacarpals to insert in the extensor aponeurosis of the proximal phalanx on the radial side. The flexor pollicis longus originates from the anterior aspect of the middle third of the radius. The tendon passes through the radial side of the carpal tunnel (Fig. 14-20) radial to the superficial and deep flexor tendons. A synovial sheath of the flexor pollicis longus tendon begins just proximal to the flexor retinaculum and extends distally to near the insertion of the tendon on the distal phalanx of the thumb (8).

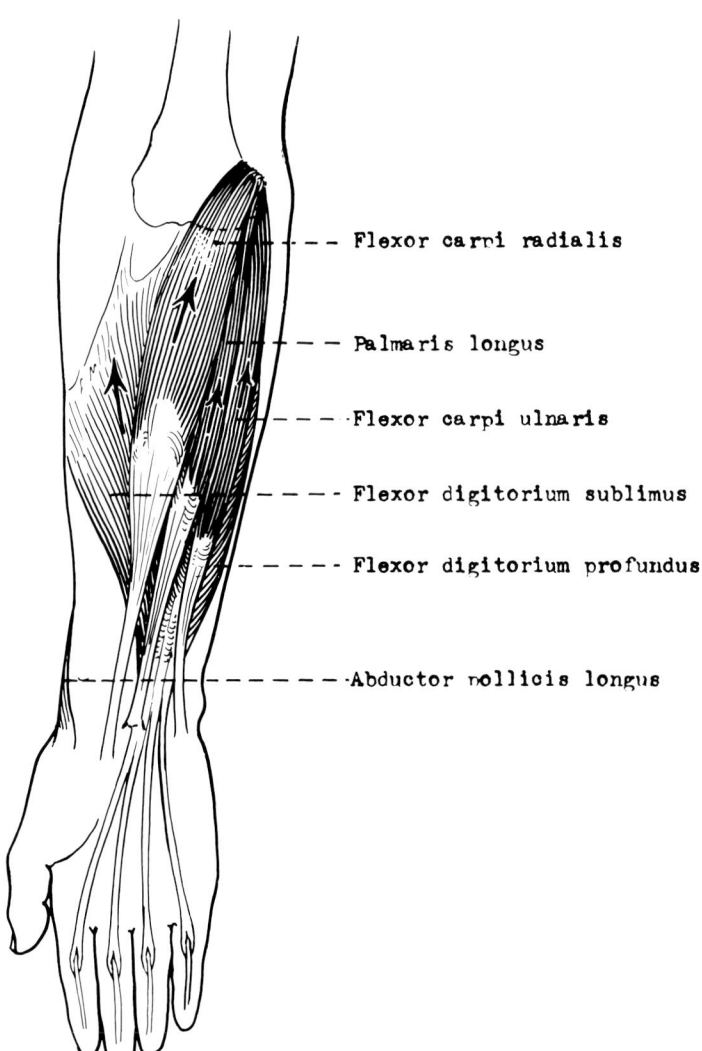

Flexor carpi radialis

Palmaris longus

Flexor carpi ulnaris

Flexor digitorium sublimus

Flexor digitorium profundus

Abductor pollicis longus

FIG. 14–18. Flexors of the wrist (from 8, with permission).

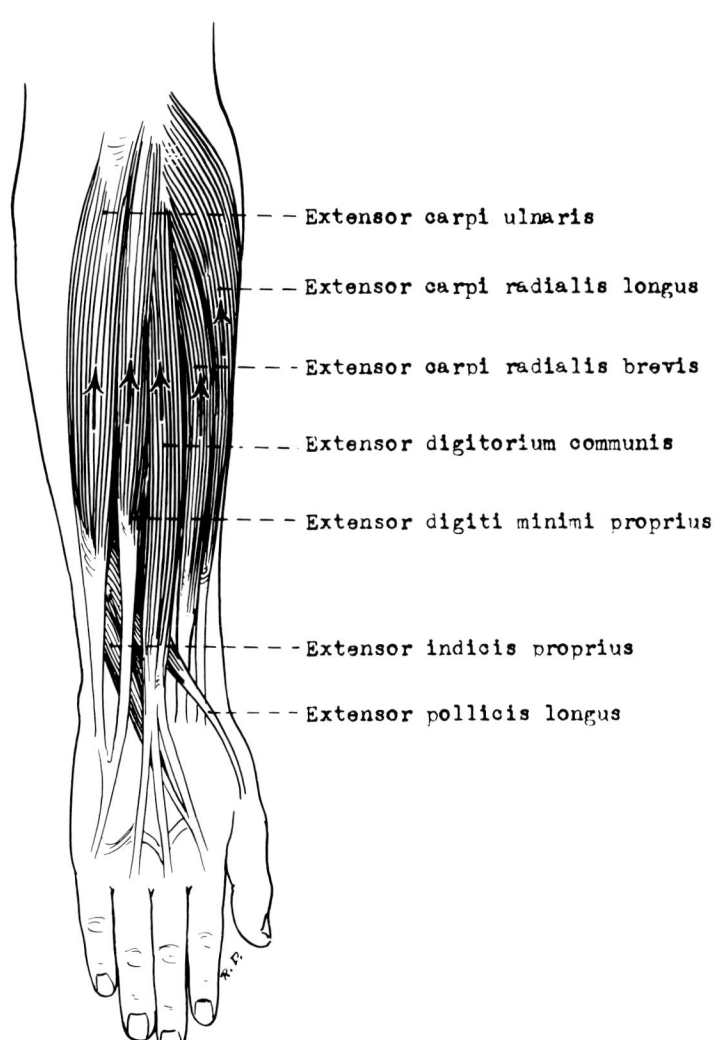

Extensor carpi ulnaris

Extensor carpi radialis longus

Extensor carpi radialis brevis

Extensor digitorium communis

Extensor digiti minimi proprius

Extensor indicis proprius

Extensor pollicis longus

FIG. 14-19. Extensors of the wrist (from 8, with permission).

Interosseous Muscles

The interosseous muscles form the deepest layer of the muscles in the hand and are divided into palmar and dorsal groups. The palmar group consists of three muscles that take their origin on the radial aspect of the fifth and fourth metacarpals and the ulnar aspect of the second metacarpal. The muscles pass distally between the metacarpophalangeal joints to insert on the extensor aponeurosis. The dorsal interossei originate from adjacent metacarpals, the first from the first and second metacarpal, the second from the second and third metacarpal, the third from the third and fourth metacarpal, and the fourth from the fourth and fifth metacarpal diaphyses. The muscles pass dorsally and distally to insert with a palmar and dorsal slip into the bases of the proximal phalanges. The interosseous muscles, both palmar and dorsal, are innervated by the deep branch of the ulnar nerve and function in abduction and adduction of the fingers of the hand (8).

Thenar Eminence

The thenar eminence or muscle group is comprised of the abductor pollicis brevis and superficial head of the flexor pollicis brevis that overlie the opponens pollicis (Fig. 14-21). The abductor pollicis brevis arises from the flexor retinaculum and has deeper origins from the trapezium and trapezoid. This somewhat triangular muscle extends distally to insert in the radial aspect of the proximal phalanx of the thumb. It serves as the primary abductor of the thumb. The flexor pollicis brevis has two

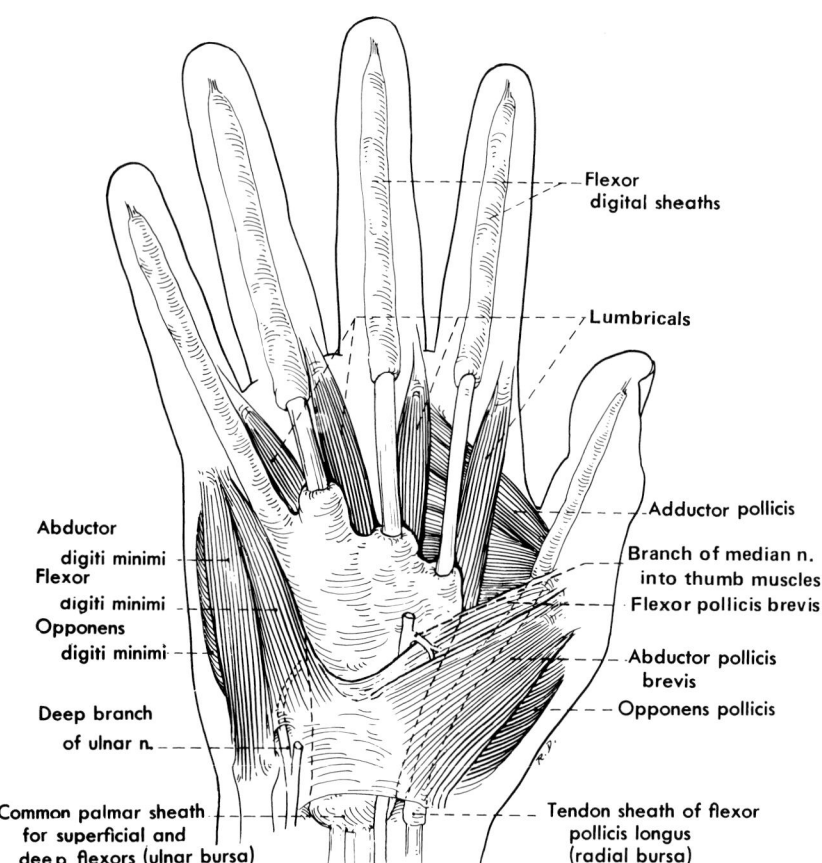

Flexor
digital sheaths

Lumbricals

Adductor pollicis

Branch of median n.
into thumb muscles

Flexor pollicis brevis

Abductor pollicis
brevis

Opponens pollicis

Abductor
digiti minimi
Flexor
digiti minimi
Opponens
digiti minimi

Deep branch
of ulnar n.

Common palmar sheath
for superficial and
deep flexors (ulnar bursa)

Tendon sheath of flexor
pollicis longus
(radial bursa)

FIG. 14-20. Tendons and tendon sheaths of the hand and wrist (from 8, with permission).

heads, one superficial and the other deep. The superficial head arises from the trapezium and flexor retinaculum and the deep head, from the trapezoid. The muscle extends distally to form a tendon that inserts on the radial flexor side of the base of the proximal phalanx of the thumb. The primary function is flexion and rotation of the thumb. The opponens pollicis is partially covered by the abductors and flexors of the thumb and arises from the flexor retinaculum and trapezium to insert on the radial surface of the diaphysis of the first metacarpal. The adductor pollicis arises with both oblique and transverse heads. The transverse head arises from the ulnar surface of the third metacarpal diaphysis and the oblique head from the base of the third metacarpal and flexor aspects of the trapezium, trapezoid, and capitate. The triangular muscle extends to insert at the base of the proximal phalanx of the thumb. This muscle serves to adduct the metacarpal and flex the metacarpophalangeal joint of the thumb (7,8).

Hypothena Muscle Group

The hypothenar muscle group consists of one superficial and three deep muscles. The superficial muscle is the palmaris brevis that arises from the ulnar side of the palmar aponeurosis and extends medially to attach into the skin along the medial border of the palm. This muscle is superficial to the ulnar nerve and artery (8). The deep muscles include the abductor digiti minimi, flexor digiti minimi brevis, and opponens digiti minimi (Fig. 14-21). The abductor digiti minimi is the most superficial of the three deep muscles. It arises from the distal surface of the pisiform and passes distally along the medial aspect of the hand to insert along the ulnar side of the base of the fifth proximal phalanx. This muscle abducts the little finger at the metacarpophalangeal joint. It acts along with the dorsal interosseous muscle in assisting in abduction or spreading of the fingers. The flexor digiti minimi brevis arises more distally than the abductor digiti minimi and takes its origin from the hook of the hamate and flexor retinaculum. This muscle passes more obliquely and medially and inserts in the same position as the abductor. The main function of this muscle is a flexor of the fifth metacarpophalangeal joint. The third and final muscle of the deep hypothenar group is the opponens digiti minimi. This muscle is the deepest and arises deep to the abductor and flexor from the flexor retinaculum and distal hook of the hamate, taking an oblique course

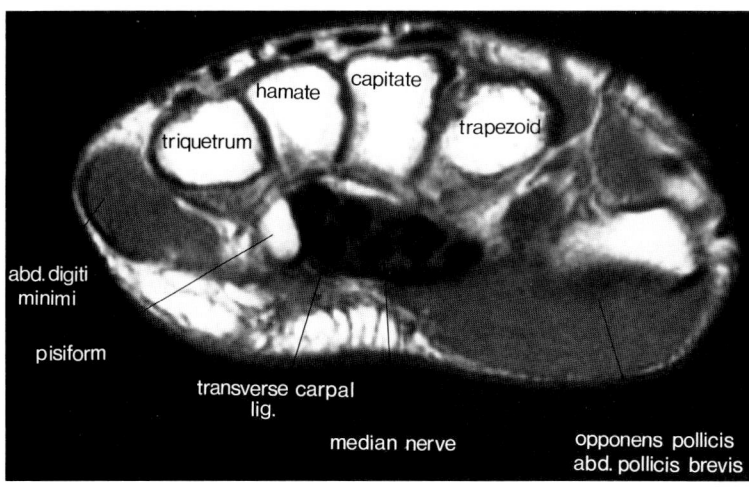

FIG. 14–21. Axial MR image through the thenar region demonstrating the thenar muscles and carpal tunnel.

to insert along the ulnar aspect of the fifth metacarpal diaphysis. This muscle draws the fifth metacarpal anteriorly. All muscles of the hypothenar group are supplied by the deep branch of the ulnar nerve (7,8).

Neurovascular Anatomy

The neurovascular anatomy of the hand and wrist is complex. Since there are numerous causes of nerve compression in this region, it is especially essential to understand the anatomy and the relationship of these structures in the hand and wrist (1,7,8,11). Evaluation of neurovascular anatomy is most easily accomplished by following the major nerve branches proximal to distal on axial magnetic resonance (MR) images (Fig. 14-21). On the ulnar side of the distal forearm proximal to the carpal tunnel, the ulnar artery, nerve, and their accompanying veins lie deep within the flexor carpi ulnaris. The nerve is generally medial to the artery at this level. At the level of the pisiform (Fig. 14-22), these structures pass along the lateral or radial side of the pisiform passing deep to the volar carpal ligament and then distally into the palm of the hand anterior to the flexor retinaculum but deep to the palmaris brevis muscle (7,8). At the level of the pisiform, the ulnar nerve typically divides into superficial and deep branches. Also at the pisiform level, the nerve and accompanying vascular structures lie between the volar carpal ligament and flexor retinaculum in a space commonly known as *Guyon's canal*. Lesions proximal to or within the canal can produce both sensory and motor abnormalities in the ulnar nerve distribution (8,10).

The two flexor digitorum muscles (superficial and profundus) are lateral to the ulnar nerve and vessels at the level of the wrist (Fig. 14-18). The tendon of the

palmaris longus lies superficially. The midline volar structures of the wrist, as they enter the carpal tunnel, tend to form three layers. The most superficial or anterior layer is formed by the flexor digitorum superficialis. The middle layer is formed by the superficial flexor of the index and middle fingers, and the most posterior or deepest layer is formed by the flexor digitorum profundus tendons. All tendons have a common sheath just before they pass under the flexor retinaculum. The palmaris longus tendon is the most superficial and midline structure at the wrist level (Fig. 14-20, and 14-21) (7,10).

The median nerve lies deep to the flexor digitorum superficialis through much of the forearm. Just proximal

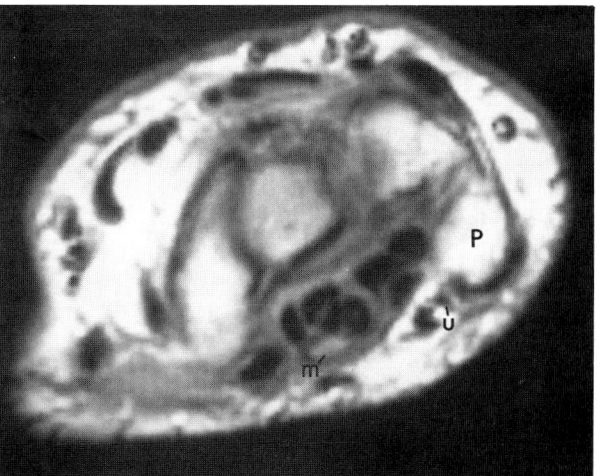

FIG. 14–22. Axial MR image at the level of the pisiform (P) demonstrating the median nerve (m) and ulnar nerve (u).

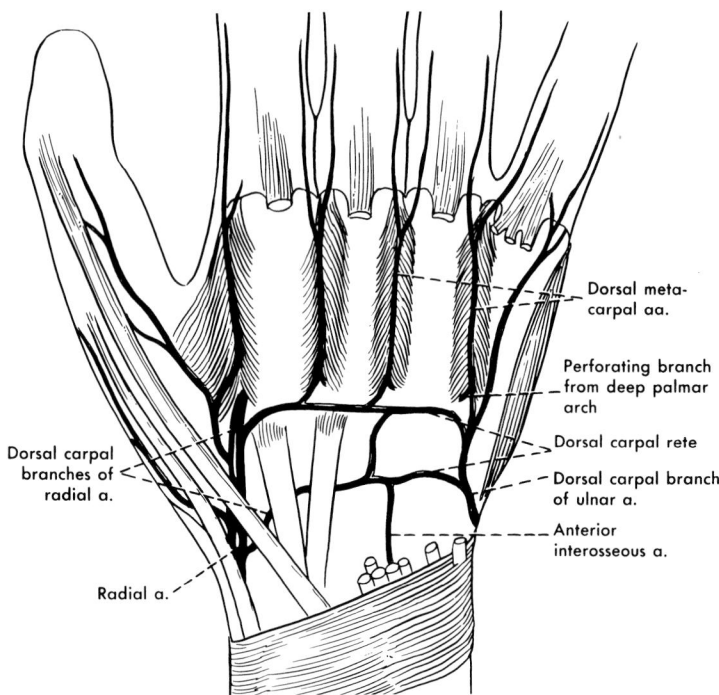

A

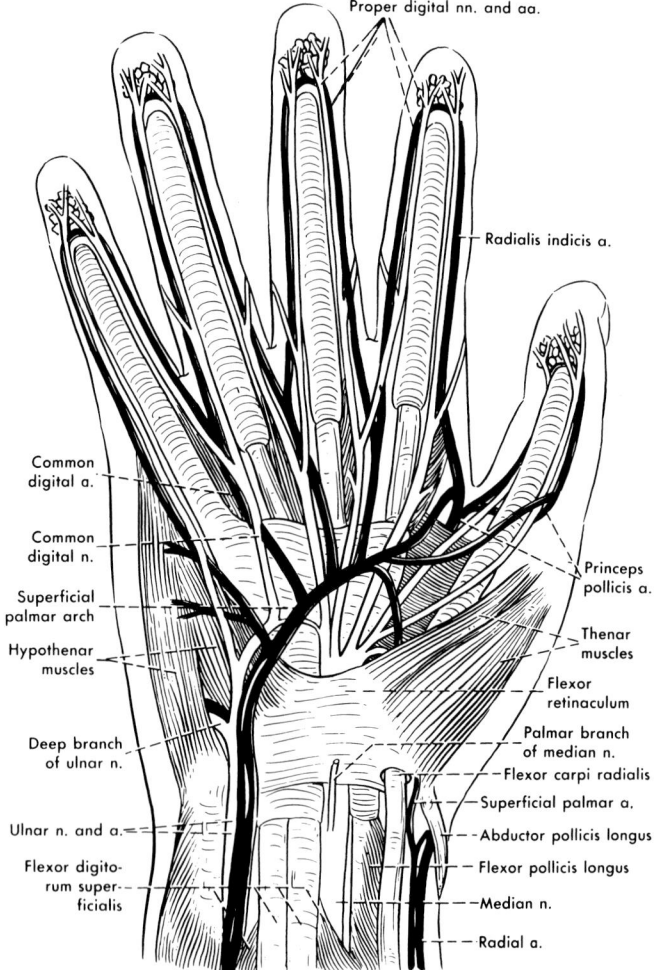

B

FIG. 14–23. Dorsal (**A**) and volar (**B**) vascular anatomy of the hand and wrist (from 8, with permission).

to the wrist, it emerges on the radial side of the superficial flexor and passes forward and medially to lie in front of the flexor tendons in the carpal tunnel (Fig. 14-21 and 14-22). At the distal margin of the flexor retinaculum, the median nerve divides into five or six branches (8,10).

The muscle planes and fascial compartments of the palm basically divide the palm into three compartments, the thenar, hypothenar, and central compartments (Fig. 14-21). These compartments, along with the tendon sheaths of the flexor tendons, are anatomically important in the spread of inflammatory and infectious diseases (8).

The complex vascular anatomy of the hand and wrist is demonstrated in Fig. 14-23.

IMAGING TECHNIQUES

Routine Radiography

There are numerous positioning techniques for evaluating the hand and wrist. Complex anatomy and subtle fractures often require multiple views for complete evaluation (24,25,28).

Hand

Routine evaluation of the hand requires PA, lateral, and oblique views (25,54).

PA Views

The PA view is obtained with the patient sitting and the hand positioned on one-half of an 8 × 10-inch cassette. The remainder of the cassette is shielded, allowing a second view to be obtained. The fingers should be slightly spread and the palm laid flat against the cassette. The beam is perpendicular to the cassette and centered on the third metacarpophalangeal joint (Fig. 14-24A) (25,28,54). The hand, carpal bones, and distal radius and ulna are included on the film (Fig. 14-24B). Careful ra-

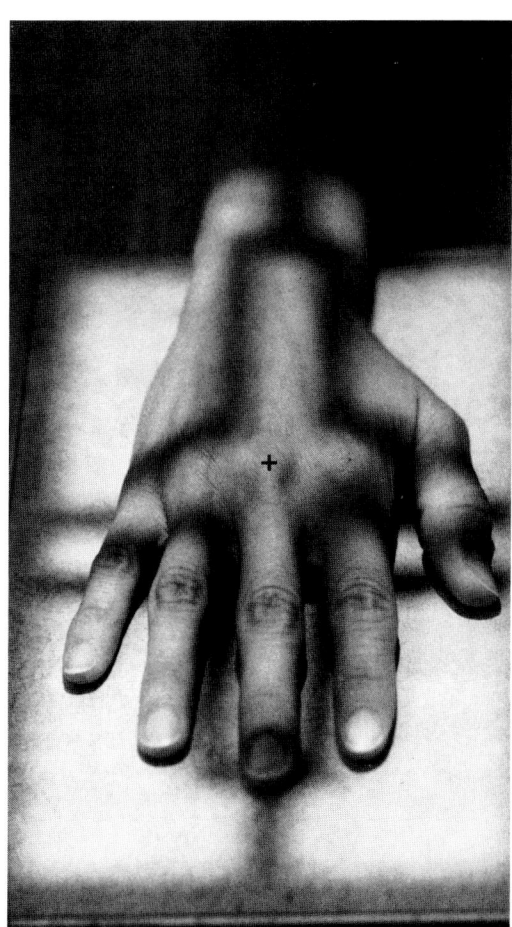
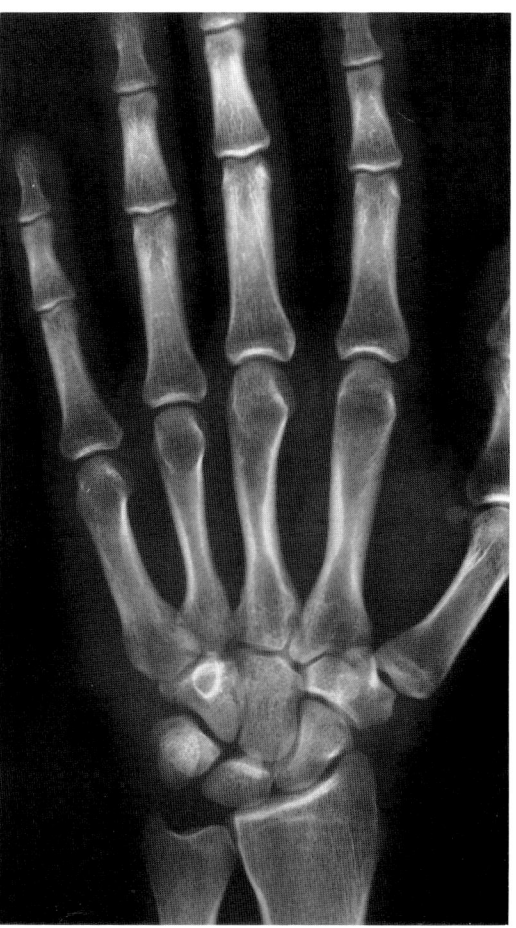

FIG. 14-24. A: Patient positioned for PA view of the hand. The beam is centered perpendicularly to the third MCP joint (+). **B:** Normal radiograph of the hand. Note the thumb is not entirely included on the film due to "over coning" from side to side.

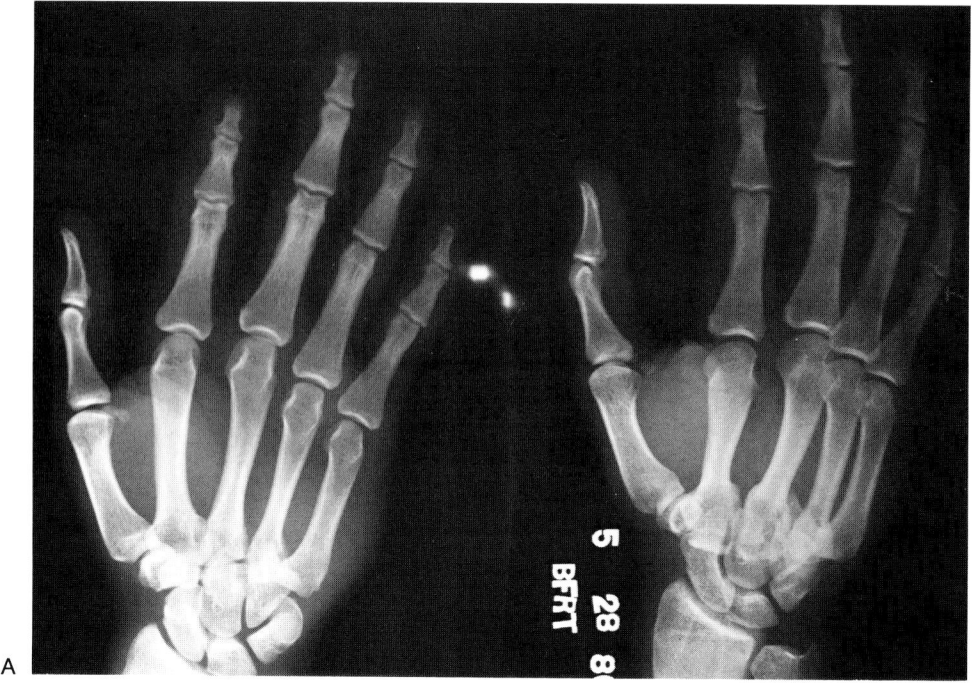

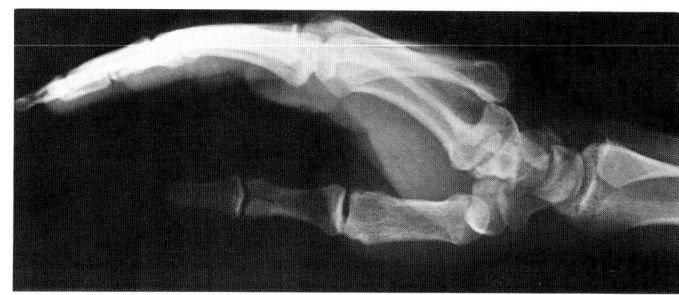

FIG. 14–25. Radiographs of the right wrist following trauma. The PA and oblique views (**A**) demonstrate loss of the parallel configuration of the second to fifth carpometacarpal joints due to dislocation. The lateral view (**B**) is essential in demonstrating the relationship of the articular surfaces.

diographic analysis will demonstrate uniform cortical margins along the diaphysis of the phalanges and metacarpals. The proximal metaphysis expands just distal to the cortex of the joint space. Asymmetry in the metaphysis is common with torus fractures. The carpometacarpal joints should be parallel and uniform in width (44,48,92). Fisher and colleagues describe an *M* configuration formed by the second through fifth carpometacarpal joints (44). Any disruption of this configuration suggests subluxation or dislocation (Figs. 14-25 and 14-26).

Oblique View

The hand is rotated superiorly about 45° (thumb up) with the fingers slightly spread. A sponge can be used to maintain the proper position (Fig. 14-27A). The central beam is perpendicular to the cassette and centered on the metacarpophalangeal joints. The oblique view more clearly demonstrates the metacarpal heads (Fig. 14-27B) and the first and second carpometacarpal joints.

Lateral View

The lateral view is obtained with the ulnar side of the hand adjacent to the cassette and the thumb and fingers extended (Fig. 14-28). The central beam is perpendicular to the cassette and centered on the metacarpophalangeal joints. This view is useful in evaluating dislocations (Fig. 14-25B) and fracture-angulation (25,54).

Fingers

Overlapping of the metacarpals and phalanges is common on the lateral and oblique views. Obtaining views of

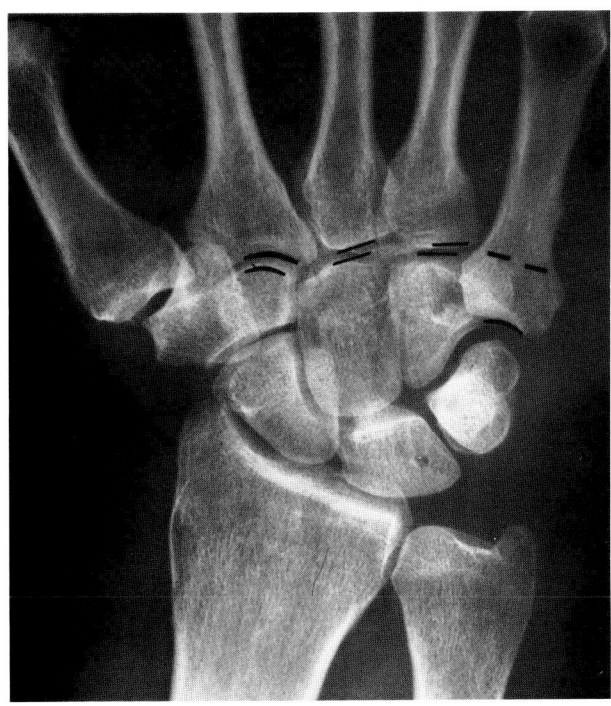

FIG. 14-26. PA view of the hand. The carpometacarpal joints are parallel except the fifth. There is a dislocation of the fifth metacarpal.

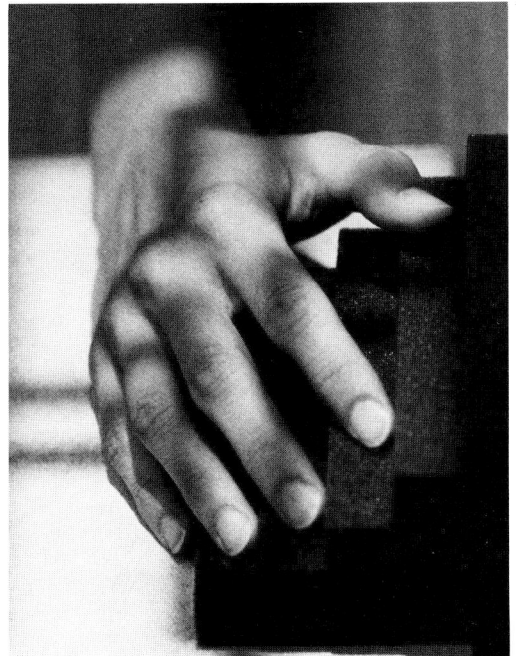

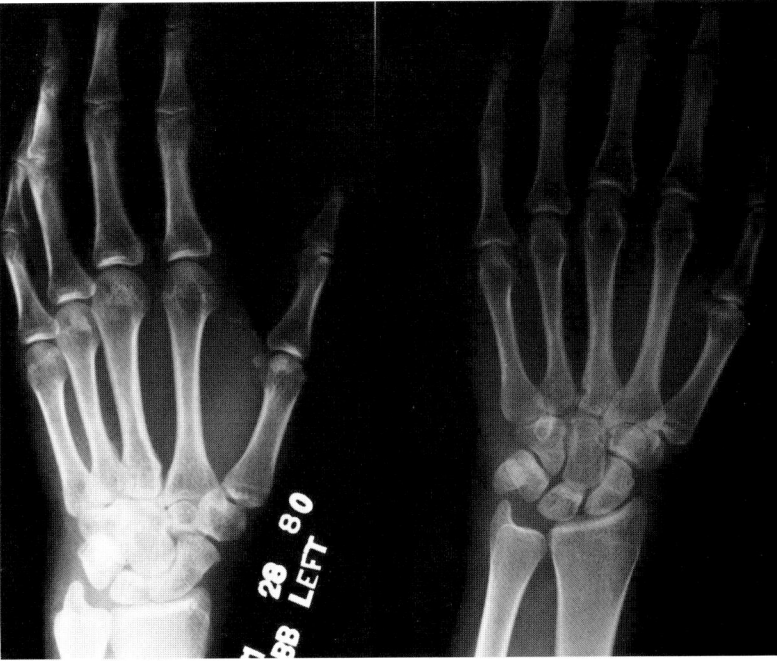

A

B C

FIG. 14-27. A: Hand positioned in the oblique view. Oblique radiograph (B) with PA for comparison (C). Note the overlap of the third to fifth metacarpals and phalanges on the oblique view.

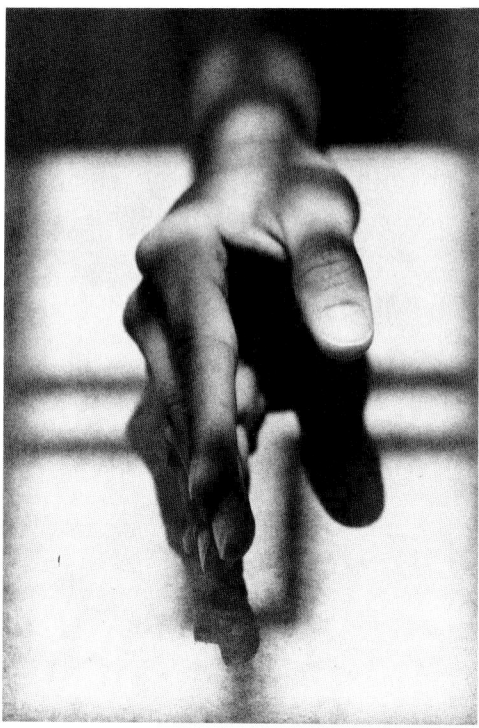

FIG. 14–28. Hand positioned for the lateral view. The central beam is perpendicular to the cassette and centered on the metacarpophalangeal joints.

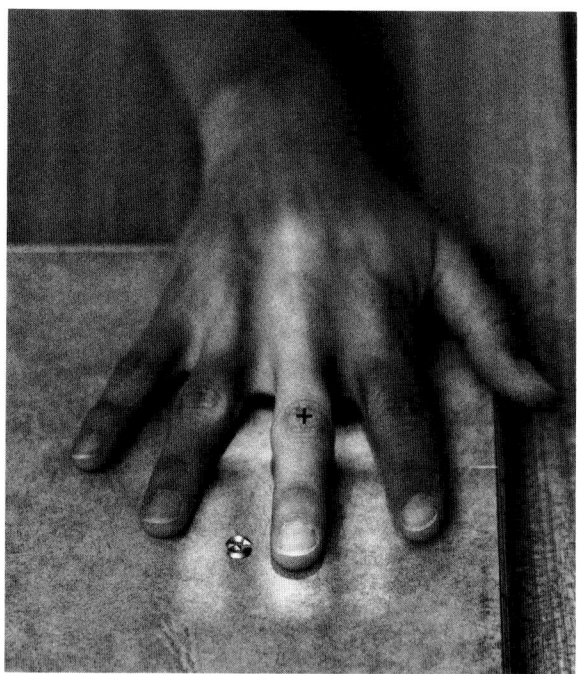

A

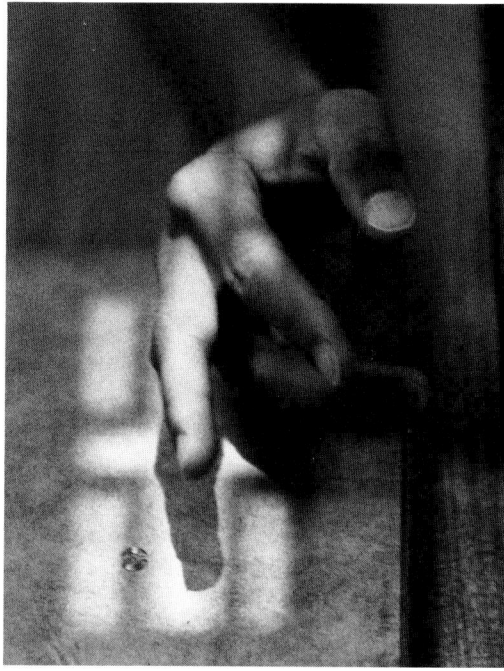

B

FIG. 14–29. A: Hand positioned for PA radiograph of the middle finger. The beam is centered on the PIP joint (+). The finger being examined is marked on the film with a lead number. **B:** Third finger positioned for lateral radiograph.

the digit in question provides better detail. In this way subtle injuries are more easily detected.

Views of the individual fingers can be obtained with extremity cassettes or dental film (see Chapter 1, Routine Radiography). The finger being radiographed should be clearly marked on the film. The PA view is obtained with the finger flat on the cassette and the beam centered perpendicularly to the proximal interphalangeal joint (Fig. 14-29). The lateral view is essential in evaluating articular fractures (hyperextension volar plate fractures of the middle phalanx) and for determining the position and angulation of fractures (28). This view is obtained with the ulnar side of the hand adjacent to the cassette and the finger separated by flexing the remaining digits (Figs. 14-29B and 14-30). This may require taping or props to assist in positioning. Centering is the same as in the PA view. The oblique view is obtained by rotating the hand as one would for the oblique view of the hand. The finger in question is isolated by flexing the remaining digits.

Thumb

The PA view of the thumb is obtained with the thumb elevated from the film and the ulnar side of the hand adjacent to the cassette (Fig. 14-31A). This results in some magnification. However, this position is much more easily maintained than the AP position, which requires that the hand be inverted with the dorsum of the thumb against the cassette (25,28). The central beam is perpendicular to the cassette and centered on the metacarpophalangeal joint.

The lateral view is obtained with the radial side of the thumb adjacent to the cassette and the fingers deviated to the ulnar side (Fig. 14-31B). The beam is centered on the metacarpophalangeal joint.

Figures 14-31C and 14-31D demonstrate the normal radiographic appearance of the thumb in the PA and lateral projections.

Special Views

Numerous additional views have been described (25,28,54). In our practice, the Brewerton (34,62), Burman (36), and stress views are commonly used (34,42,48).

The Brewerton view is obtained by placing the dorsal aspect of the hand flat against the cassette (palm up) with the fingers flexed about 65° (Fig. 14-32A) (34). The beam is centered on the metacarpal heads, and the tube is angled 15° to the ulnar side of the wrist (Fig. 14-32B). The Brewerton view (34,62) is useful in evaluating subtle arthritic abnormalities or fractures of the metacarpal heads (34). The bases of the fourth and fifth metacarpals

and hook of the hamate are also clearly demonstrated (Fig. 14-32C).

The Burman view improves visualization of the first carpometacarpal joint (25,36). The hand is hyperextended and rotated radially. The thumb is laid against the 8 × 10-inch cassette. The beam is angled 45° and centered on the base of the first metacarpal (Fig. 14-33 A and B).

Stress views, especially of the first metacarpophalangeal joint, are frequently used to exclude ligament injury (28,33,41,42). This study is more accurately performed fluoroscopically. Both thumbs should be in the PA position for comparison. Spot films are obtained in the neutral position and during radial and ulnar stress. Increase in the joint space on the stressed side (Fig. 14-34) or subluxation indicates ligament injury. Swelling and pain may reduce the accuracy in the acute setting. Intra-articular injection of 1% lidocaine (Xylocaine) allows more accurate assessment. However, if this is needed, an arthrogram should be performed. The latter is more definitive (Fig. 14-34C). The use of local anesthetic results in an invasive procedure. Contrast material can be injected through the anesthetic needle. (See Arthrography of the Hand and Wrist).

Wrist

PA, lateral, and oblique views are obtained following trauma.

PA View

Position for the PA view of the wrist is similar to that used for the PA view of the hand (Fig. 14-35; see Fig. 14-5) except that the beam is centered on the wrist instead of the metacarpophalangeal joints.

Careful examination of the PA view reveals significant bony and soft tissue anatomy. If approached systemically, information regarding pathology and appropriate further views can easily be obtained (28,44,46,52,56). Subtle fractures on the radial side of the wrist, especially the scaphoid, are easily overlooked. The navicular fat stripe is a useful structure in this regard. This fat plane lies between the radial collateral ligament and the tendon sheaths of the abductor pollicis longus and extensor pollicis brevis (Fig. 14-35). Although the fat plane is inconsistently seen in children, it is present in 96% of normal adults (86). Terry and Ramin (86) noted absence or displacement of the fat stripe in 88% of fractures on the radial side of the wrist. These changes were noted in 87% of scaphoid fractures. Changes in the navicular fat stripe may be the only clue to a wrist fracture on the radial side (Fig. 14-35B).

The articular surfaces of the carpal bones should be

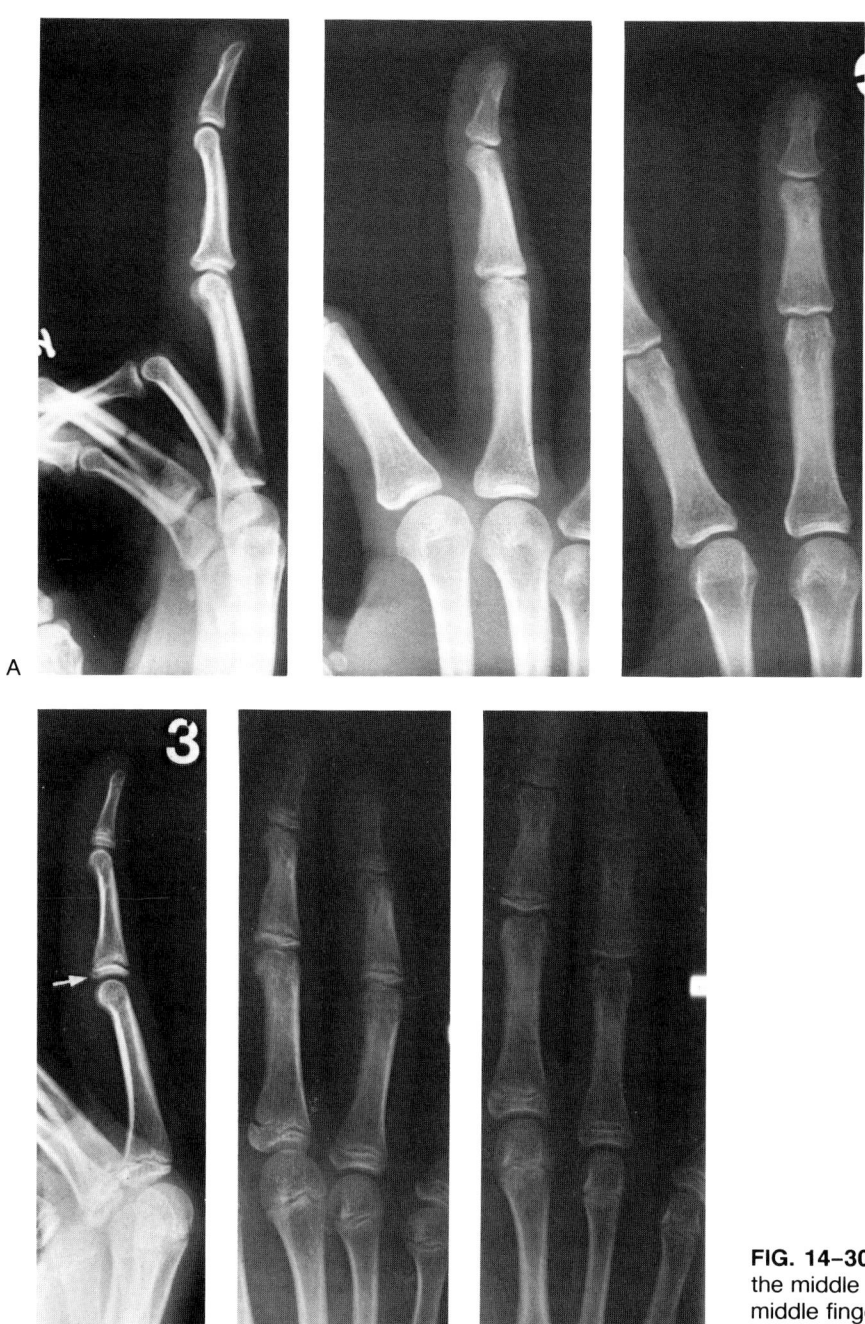

FIG. 14-30. A: Normal PA, oblique, and lateral views of the middle finger. **B:** PA, lateral, and oblique views of the middle finger with a subtle volar plate fracture of the middle phalanx (*arrow*). The lateral view is most useful in evaluating hyperextension injuries.

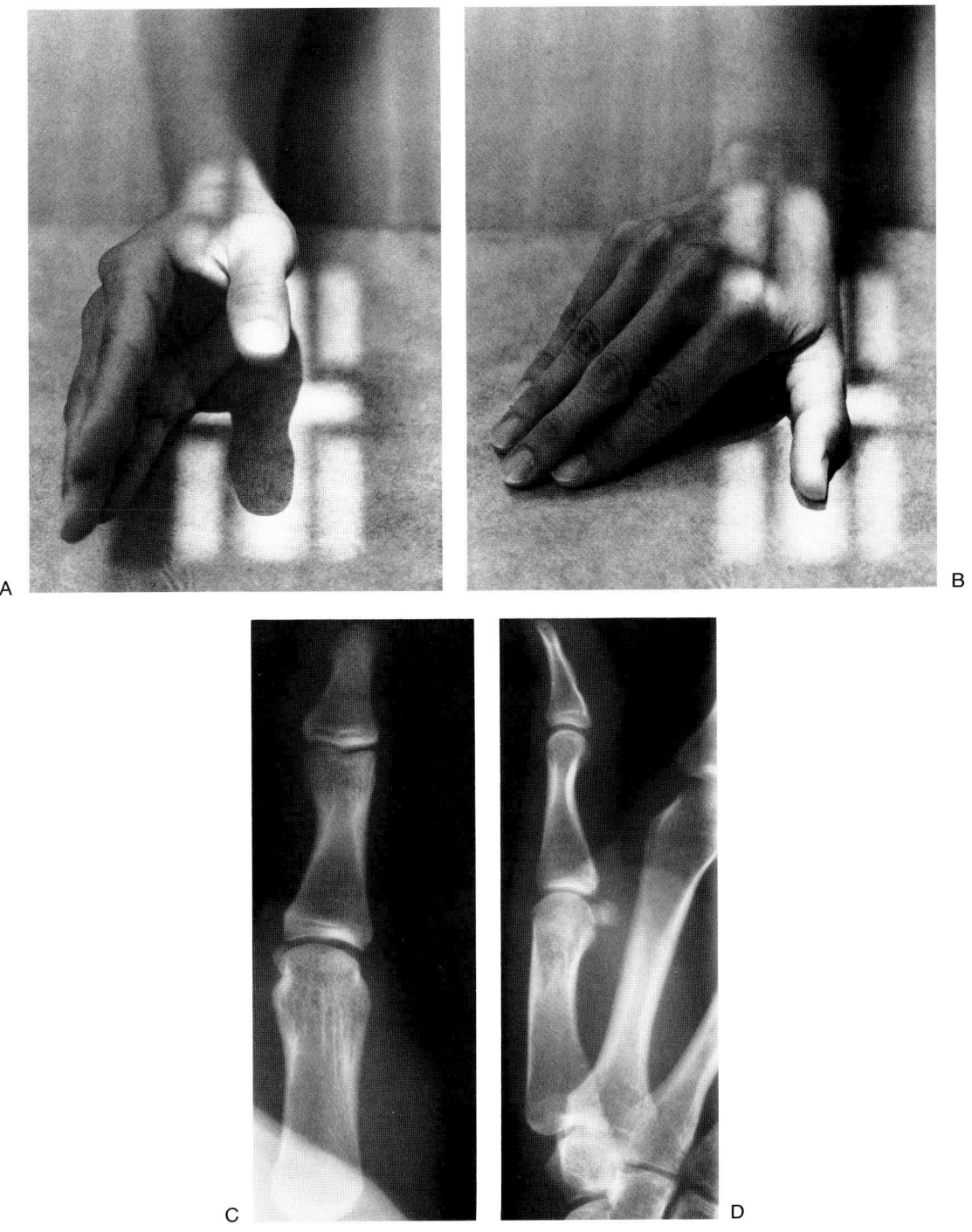

FIG. 14–31. Hand positioned for PA (**A**) and lateral (**B**) views of the thumb. **C:** PA and (**D**) lateral radiographs of the thumb.

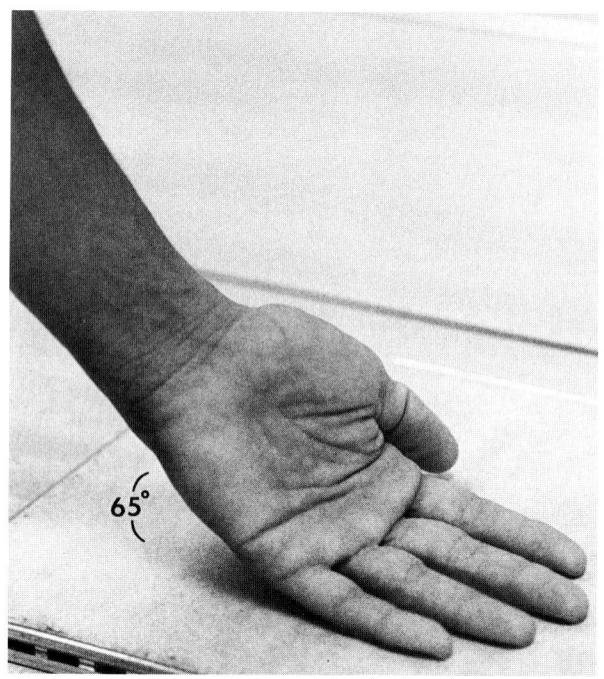

A

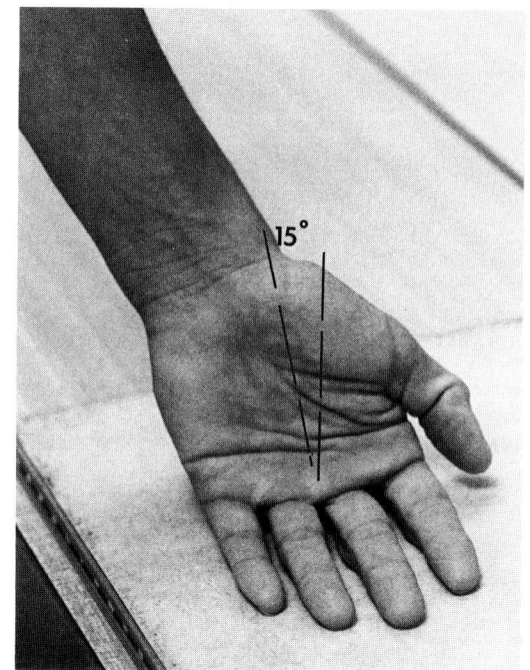

B

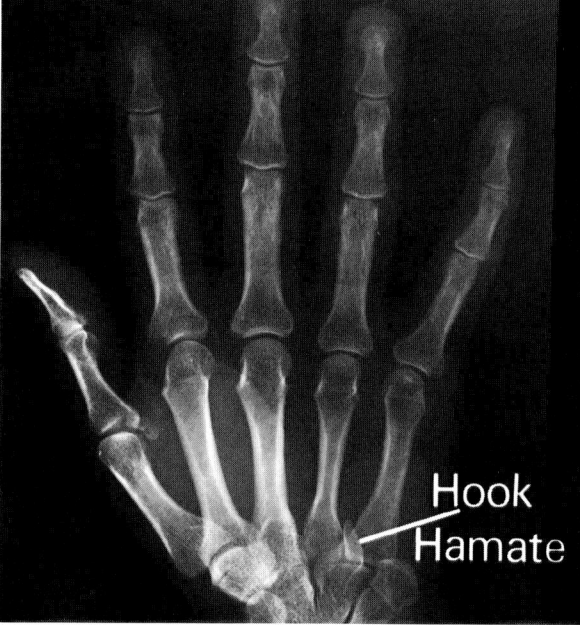

C

FIG. 14–32. Brewerton view of the hand. **A:** The dorsum of the hand is against the cassette with the MCP joints flexed about 65°. **B:** The central beam is angled 15° to the ulnar side of the hand. **C:** Radiograph of the Brewerton view demonstrating the metacarpal heads, hook of the hamate and fourth and fifth carpometacarpal joints.

parallel with 1–2 mm joint spaces (28,48,51,59,61). Angling the tube 10° to the ulnar side of the wrist may optimize measurement of the scapholunate space (61). Any change in the joint space or shape of the carpal bones may indicate subluxation or dislocation. Three arcs can be drawn on the normal PA view (see Fig. 14-5). The first arc is formed by the proximal articular surfaces of the scaphoid, lunate, and triquetrum. The second arc is formed by the distal articular surfaces of these carpal bones. The third arc is formed by the proximal (convex) articular surfaces of the capitate and hamate. Any significant interruption of these arcs, other than where the trapezium, trapezoid, and pisiform are seen as overlapping structures on the PA view, suggests abnormality at the involved joint (Figs. 14-36 and 14-37). Flexion, extension, and radial and ulnar deviation result in significant changes in position and configuration (see treatment of motion views later in this chapter).

The distal radioulnar joint should also be clearly demonstrated on the PA view (see Fig. 14-5). This joint space normally measures about 2 mm. Ulnar variance should also be assessed on the PA view. The relationship of the distal radiocarpal and ulnocarpal joints is effected significantly by changes in wrist position. Supination increases and pronation decreases negative ulnar variance. Subtle positioning changes may also effect ulnar variance (43).

Lateral View

Positioning for the lateral view is similar to that involved in the lateral view of the hand (see Fig. 14-28) except that the beam is centered on the wrist.

On the lateral view, the normal pronator fat stripe (Fig. 14-38) can be seen passing proximally from the ventral surface of the radius. This normally lies within 1 cm of the cortical surface of the distal radius. Subtle radial fractures will cause displacement or obliteration of the fat plane (Fig. 14-39). This may be the only indication of fracture. Dorsal swelling is also best seen on the lateral view.

The relationship of the radius, lunate, capitate, and metacarpals is clearly demonstrated on the lateral view (see Figs. 14-7 and 14-38). The capitate is firmly attached to the third metacarpal. The convex proximal surface of the capitate articulates with the lunate, and the lunate articulates with the radius. A straight line can be drawn along the axis of the radius, lunate, capitate, and third metacarpal in the neutral position. However, slight flexion or extension will normally interrupt this line. The angle formed by the radius and scaphoid is normally about 136° (range 121°–153°) (40). The scapholunate angle is normally about 45° (52).

Oblique Views

For the external oblique view, the position of the wrist should be similar to that used for the oblique view of the hand (see Fig. 14-27). The wrist is pronated approximately 45° from the PA position, and the beam is centered on the wrist. The radiograph (Fig. 14-40) demonstrates the scaphoid, trapezium, and first carpometacarpal articulation (25,28).

The internal oblique view is obtained by internally rotating the wrist 45° (25,28,38). This view demonstrates the triquetropisiform articulation (Fig. 14-40). Normally this joint measures about 2 mm. If the wrist is flexed, the joint space may actually widen.

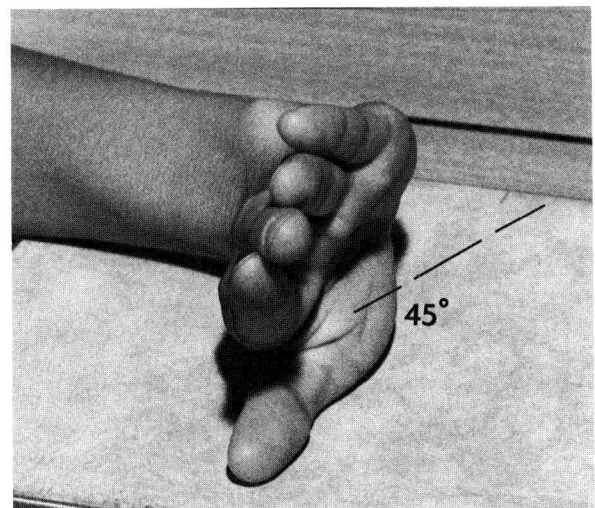
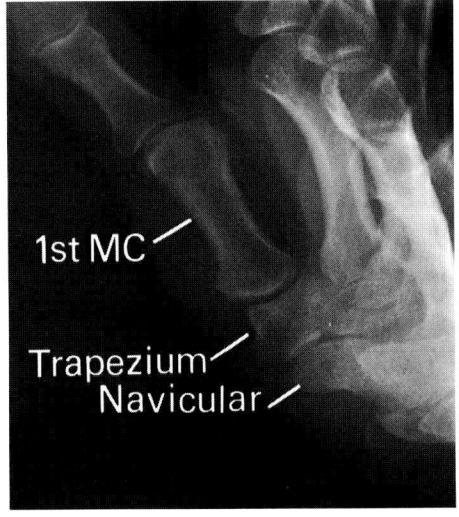

A B

FIG. 14–33. Burman views. **A:** The radial side of the thumb is on the cassette with the hand hyperextended. The beam is angled 45° and centered on the thenar eminence. **B:** The radiograph clearly demonstrates the articulations of the scaphoid (navicular), trapezium, and first metacarpal.

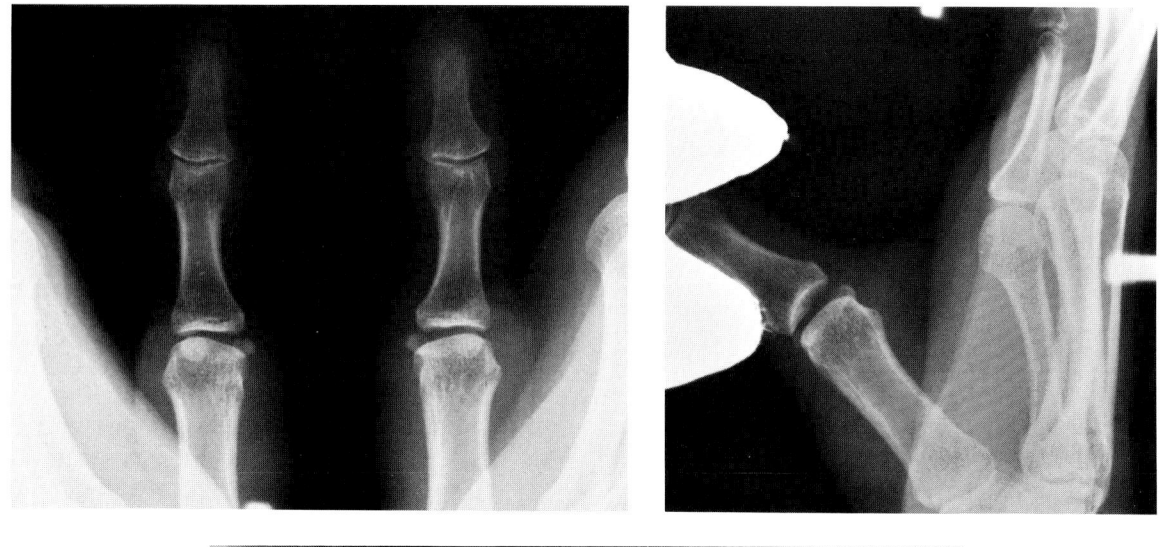

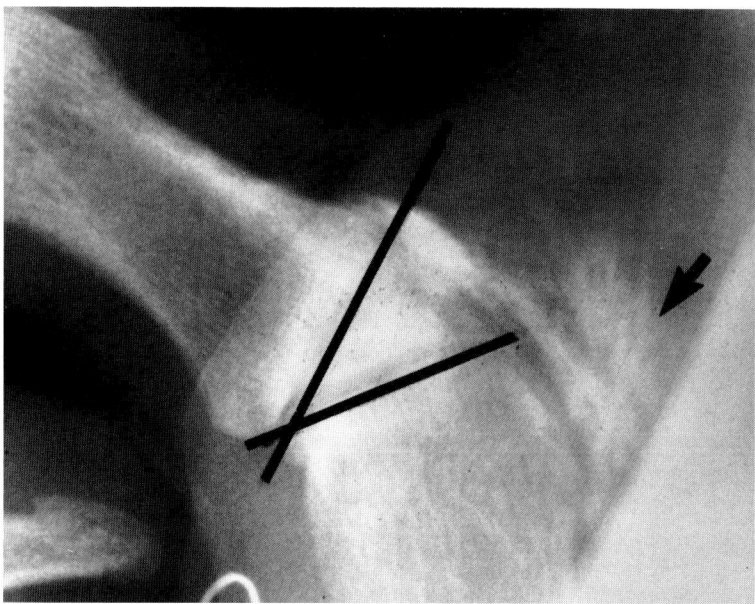

FIG. 14–34. Stress views of the first MCP joint. **A:** PA view of both thumbs in neutral position. **B:** Radial stress demonstrates slight opening of the ulnar side of the joint. **C:** Arthrogram with anesthetic more clearly demonstrates the ulnar collateral ligament injury. Contrast material has extravasated through the ulnar ligament and capsular defect (*arrow*).

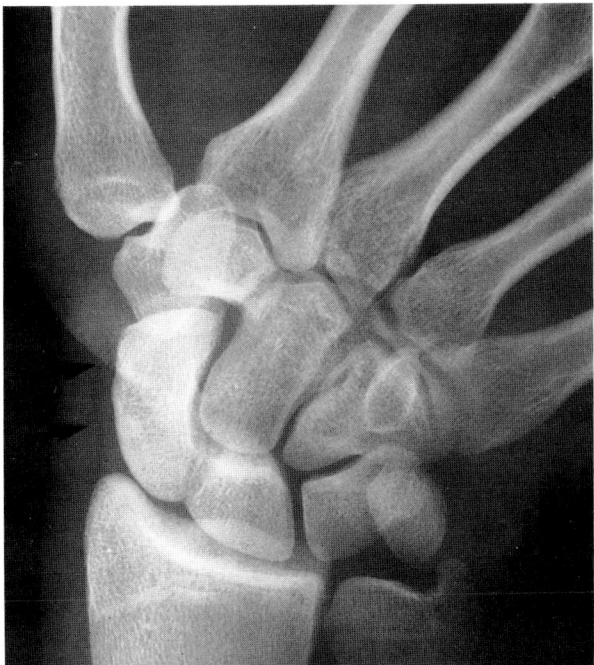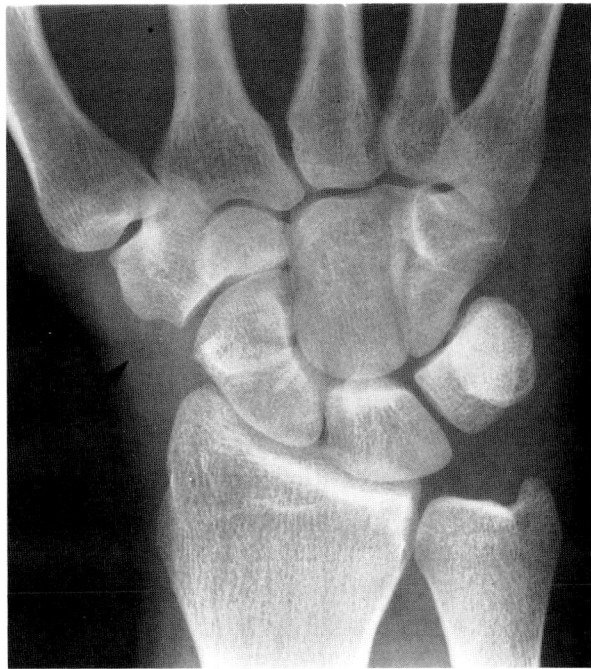

A   B

FIG. 14–35. A: PA view of the wrist demonstrating the normal navicular fat stripes (*arrows*). The hand is in slight ulnar deviation. Radial deviation may obliterate the fat stripe. **B:** Subtle scaphoid fracture with partial obliteration of the fat stripe (*arrow*).

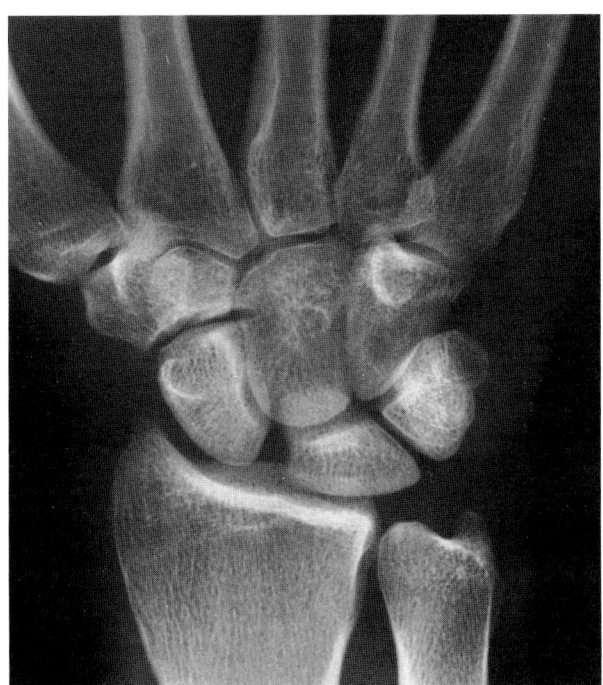

FIG. 14–36. Widened scapholunate space due to ligament injury.

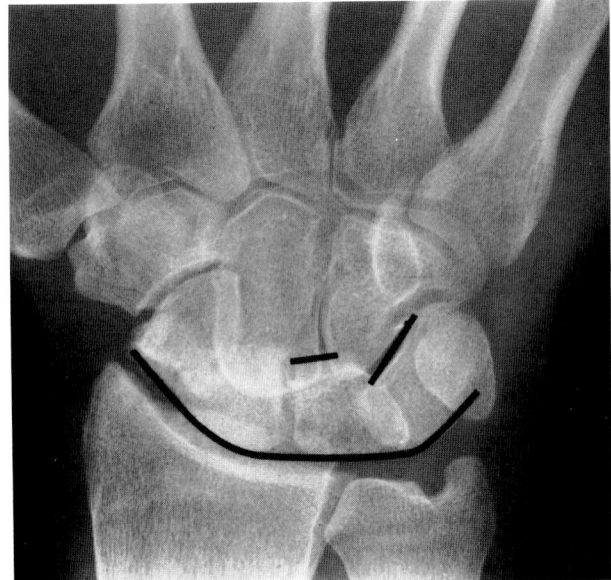

A

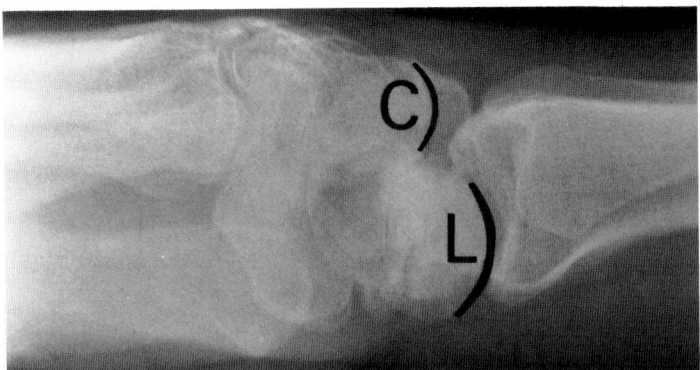

B

FIG. 14-37. A: PA view of the wrist. Normally unin-terrupted arcs can be drawn along the radial articular surface of the proximal carpal row and the articular sur-faces of the midcarpal joints. On the true PA, the radioulnar joint is well seen. Interruption of these arcs (A) indicates abnormality at the level of the break in the arc. B: There is dorsal dislocation at the midcarpal joint with the capitate (C) overriding the lunate (L).

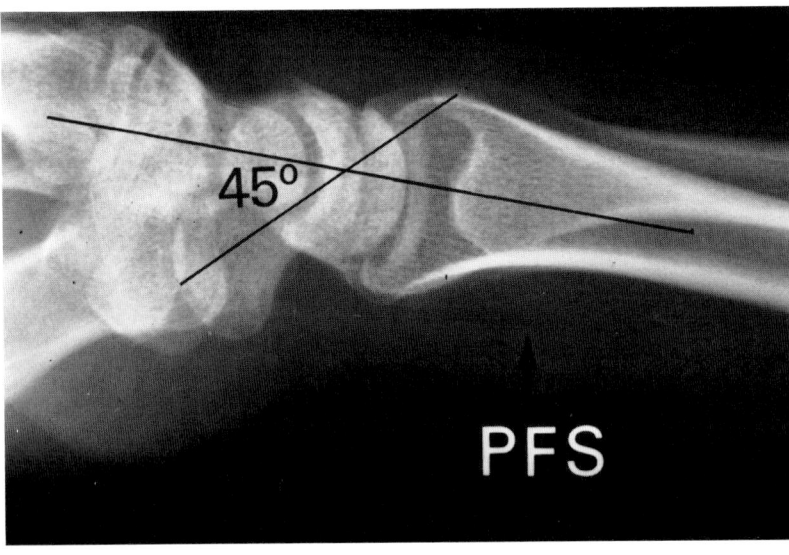

FIG. 14-38. Lateral view of the wrist. The normal scapholunate angle (about 45°). The pronator fat stripe (PFS) is a useful indicator of distal radial fractures.

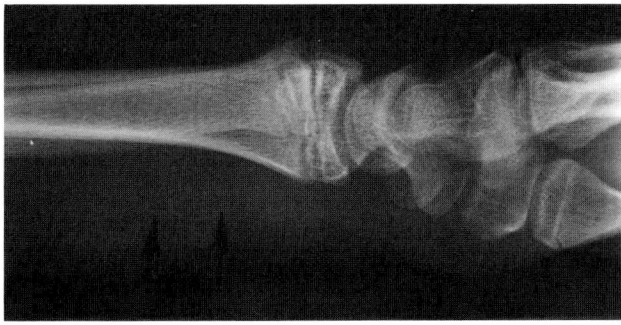

FIG. 14–39. Teenager with subtle fracture of the distal radius. The displaced pronator fat stripe (*arrows*) was the only clue to the fracture.

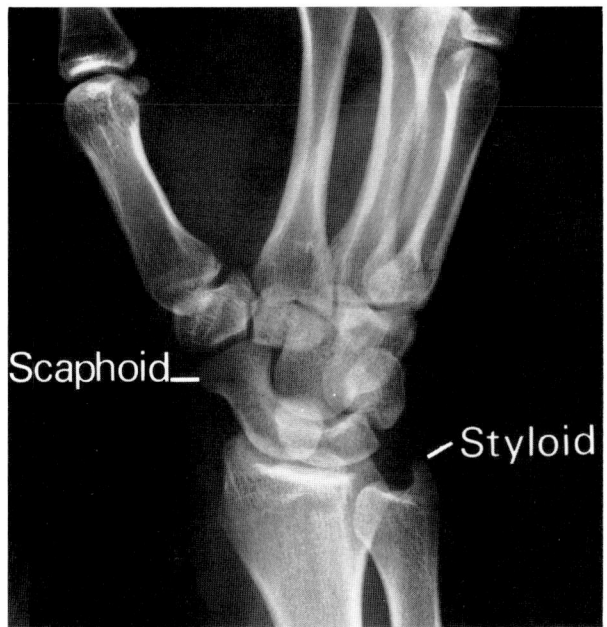
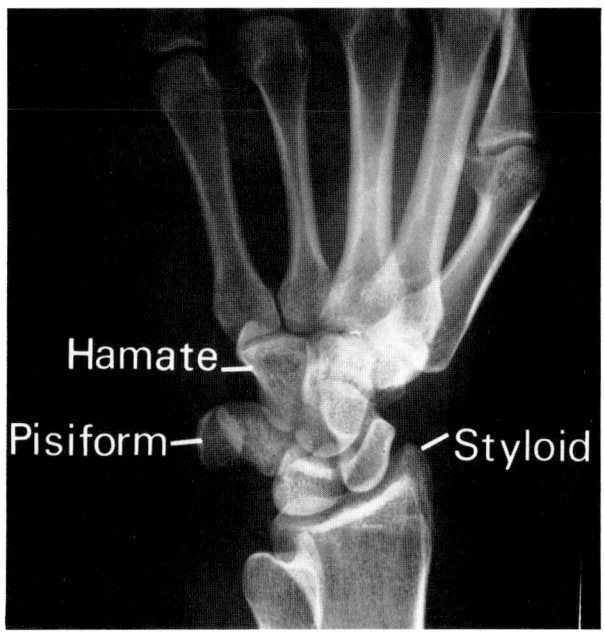

A   B

FIG. 14–40. Oblique radiographs of the wrist. **A:** External oblique with the wrist externally rotated (pronated) 45°. The scaphoid, scaphotrapezial, and traezio first metacarpal articulations are well demonstrated. The first and second carpometacarpal joints are also better demonstrated than on the PA view. **B:** The internal oblique (wrist rotated internally 45°) demonstrates the pisiform-triquetral articulation and the fourth and fifth carpometacarpal joints.

Subtle fractures of the radial and ulnar styloids are often demonstrated only on the oblique views.

Scaphoid View

The scaphoid is the most frequently fractured carpal bone. These fractures are often subtle. Therefore, a scaphoid view should be obtained initially if a fracture is suspected.

We routinely position the hand palm down on the cassette with the hand in ulnar deviation (Fig. 14-41). The thumb is extended and in line with the radius. The beam is centered on the scaphoid and is perpendicular to the cassette (28). This clearly demonstrates the elongated scaphoid (Figs. 14-41B and C).

Variations of this technique have been described by Bridgman (35) and Stecher (84).

Pisiform View

The pisiform view clearly demonstrates the pisiform and triquetropisiform articulation (Fig. 14-42). This technique is a variation of the external oblique view. The hand and wrist are rotated 30° externally from the lateral position (28). The beam is centered on the ulnar side of the wrist and is perpendicular to the cassette.

Carpal Tunnel View

Several methods have been described for obtaining this view. A simple technique involves hyperextending the hand with the base of the wrist against the cassette. The hand can be positioned using the opposite hand for support or by using a strap to maintain the hyperextended position. The tube is angled toward the wrist at 40° from the horizontal (tabletop) (Figs. 14-43A and B) (24,28,57).

The radiograph (Fig. 14-43C) demonstrates the carpal tunnel and surrounding carpal structures. This is particularly useful in evaluating the hook of the hamate and soft tissue in the region of the carpal tunnel (45,46).

Dorsal Tangential View

This projection was described by Lentino (63). The dorsum of the hand is placed on the cassette, with the wrist maximally flexed (Fig. 14-44A). The central beam is angled 45° with the tabletop and centered 3–4 cm above the radiocarpal joint.

The radiograph (Fig. 14-44B) demonstrates the dorsal aspect of the proximal carpal row (scaphoid, lunate, and triquetrum). Definition of dorsal chip fractures, foreign bodies, and soft tissue calcifications is accomplished with this technique (25).

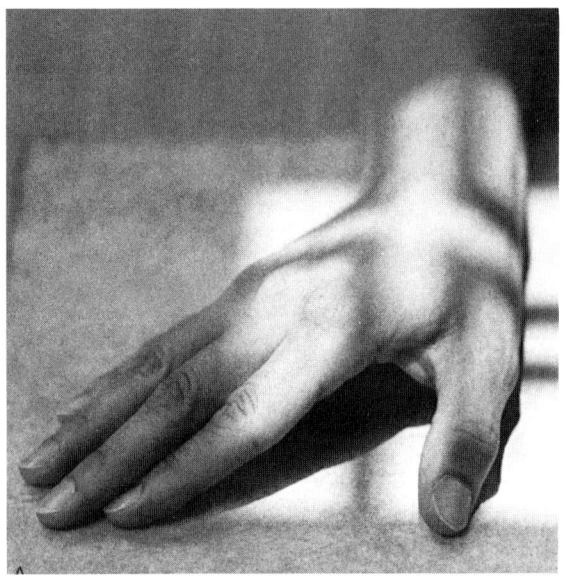 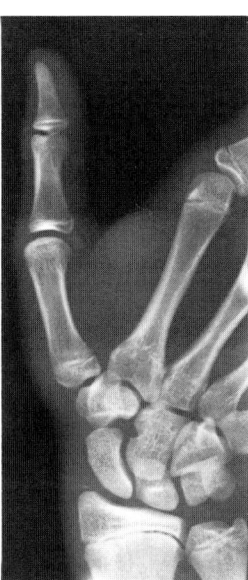 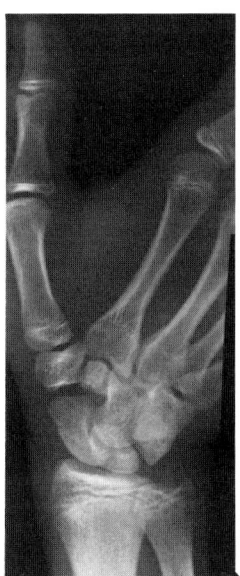

A   B   C

FIG. 14–41. Scaphoid view. **A:** Hand positioned for scaphoid view of the wrist. Radiographs of the scaphoid in the PA (**B**) and slightly oblique (**C**) position. The scaphoid is clearly demonstrated and normal. There is a small chip fracture of the radial styloid with soft tissue swelling.

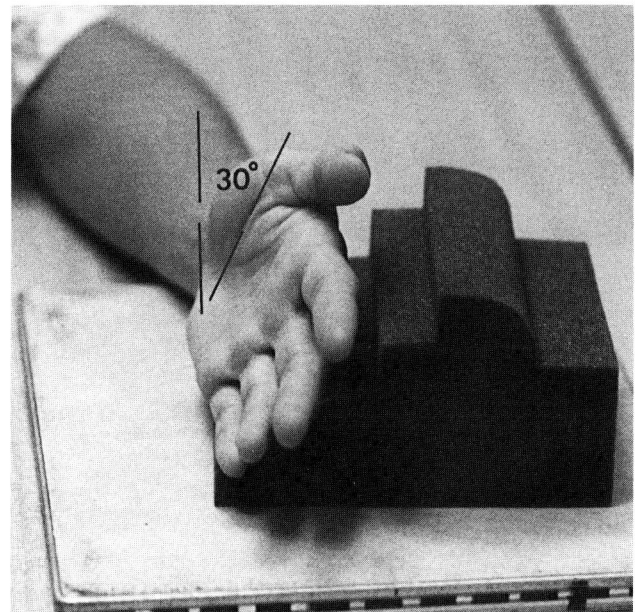

A

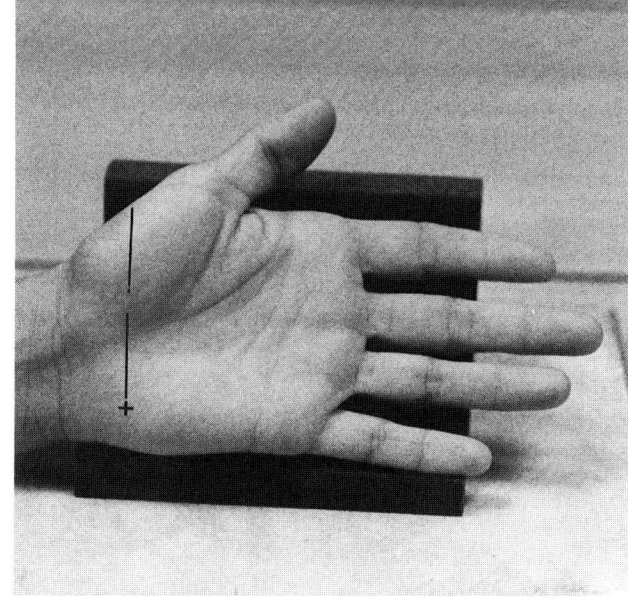

B

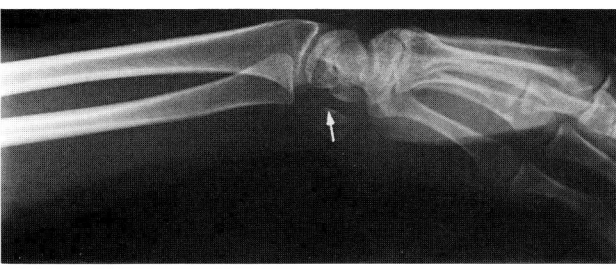

C

FIG. 14–42. Pisiform view. **A:** The hand is externally rotated 30° (lines) from the lateral position. **B:** The beam is perpendicular and centered on the pisiform. **C:** Radiograph demonstrating an undisplaced fracture of the pisiform. The joint space is widened due to hemorrhage and the slight flexion of the wrist.

Motion Studies

Bending views of the wrist are often obtained to evaluate subtle bony or ligamentous injuries in patients with persistent pain. This series of radiographs includes the PA and lateral views. In addition, lateral views are obtained with maximal flexion and extension (Fig. 14-45), and PA views are obtained with radial and ulnar deviation (Fig. 14-46). Certain institutions also obtain lateral and AP clenched-fist and oblique views (51). In certain cases, fluoroscopy with videotape or cineradiography may be helpful. These techniques allow review of the motion series for detection of more subtle abnormalities (32,77,91).

The lateral dynamic views are obtained in the same manner as the views of the lateral wrist except that the wrist is flexed and extended. Dorsiflexion (hyperextension) and palmar flexion average 70° and 75°, respectively.

With ulnar deviation (Fig. 14-46B), the scaphoid is elongated, and the lunate is more trapezoid in shape and articulates completely with the radius. During radial deviation (Fig. 14-46D), the lunate translates and only partially articulates with the radius. The scaphoid is foreshortened owing to palmar flexion. This provides a "ringlike" shadow distally that is similar to the ring sign seen with rotary subluxation. The scapholunate space (<2 mm) does not change with radial and ulnar deviation unless ligament injury is present.

The implications of this radiographic series will be discussed more fully under carpal instability. The use of tomography and isotope studies in the hand and wrist will also be discussed.

Fluoroscopically positioned spot films are also useful for clarifying suspected injuries. Alignment of the osseous structures is easily accomplished (51,52,92).

Tomography

Complex motion, thin-section tomography (1–3 mm thick) is preferred for evaluating the hand and wrist (Fig. 14-47) (52,83). Typically, tomograms are performed in the PA and lateral projections. However, fluoroscopic positioning may be necessary, and flexion and extension tomograms may also be useful in certain situations (85).

Tomography following localizing radionuclide scans

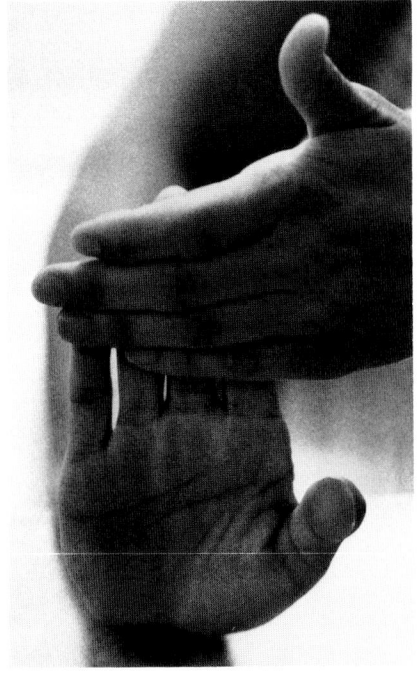

A

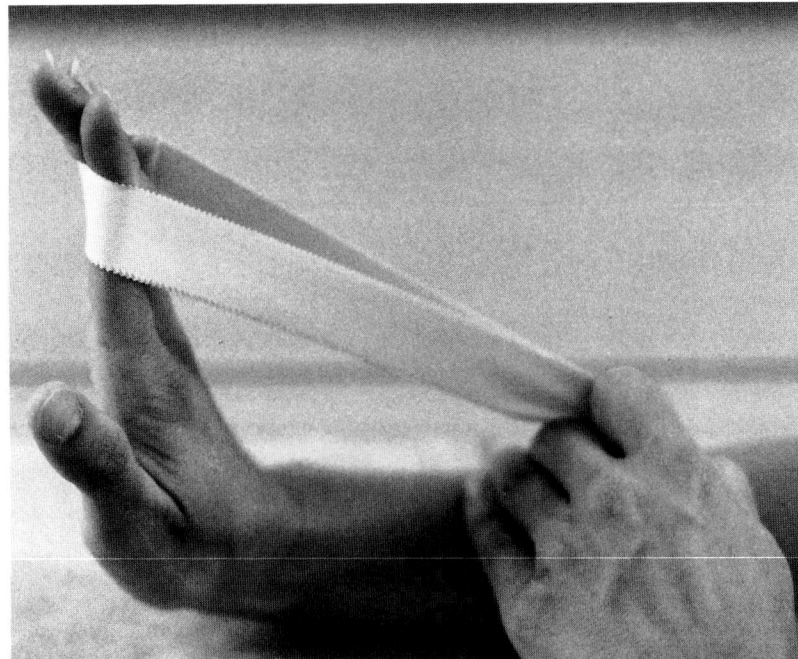

B

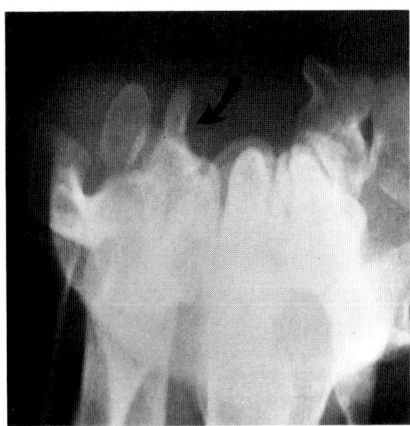

C

FIG. 14–43. Carpal tunnel view. The hand is hyperextended and supported by the opposite hand (**A**) or a strap (**B**). The tube is angled 40° off the horizontal table. **C:** The radiograph demonstrates the carpal tunnel, hook of the hamate (*arrow*), trapezium, pisiform, and first metacarpal base.

or in conjunction with arthrography is also useful in patients with chronic wrist pain or complex symptoms (27,31).

Computed Tomography

In certain situations, computed tomography (CT) may provide additional information with regard to bone and soft tissue injuries (37,38,52). In our practice, magnetic resonance imaging (MRI) has largely replaced CT for evaluating soft tissue injury and avascular necrosis (29,30).

Technique is critical. Routinely, 2–3-mm axial and direct coronal or sagittal images are obtained. The latter are accomplished with the arm above the head with the elbow flexed and the wrist in neutral (coronal) or pronated (sagittal) positions (52,68). Unfortunately, acutely injured patients may not be able to tolerate the necessary positions for direct coronal and sagittal imaging. Reconstructed coronal and sagittal images can be obtained if the patient cannot tolerate positioning for direct coronal and sagittal images (78,79).

Computed tomography is most frequently used to evaluate the distal radioulnar joint and subtle fractures or fracture healing (73,79,89). Recently, post-arthrographic CT has also been effective in evaluating subtle triangular fibrocartilage complex injuries (78).

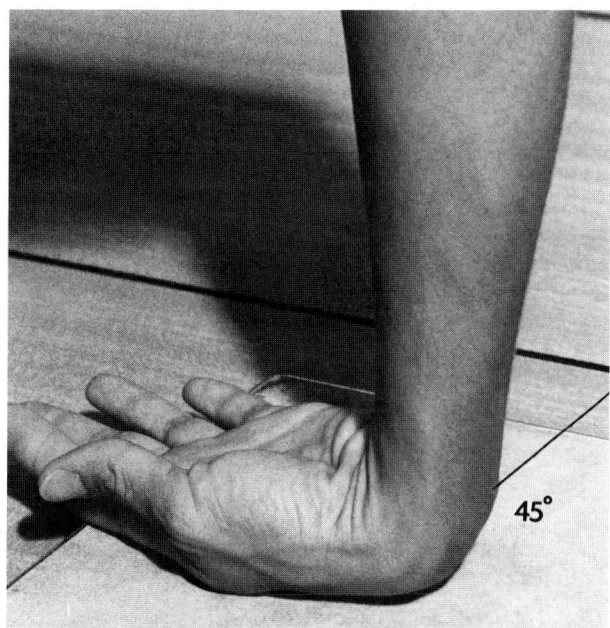

A

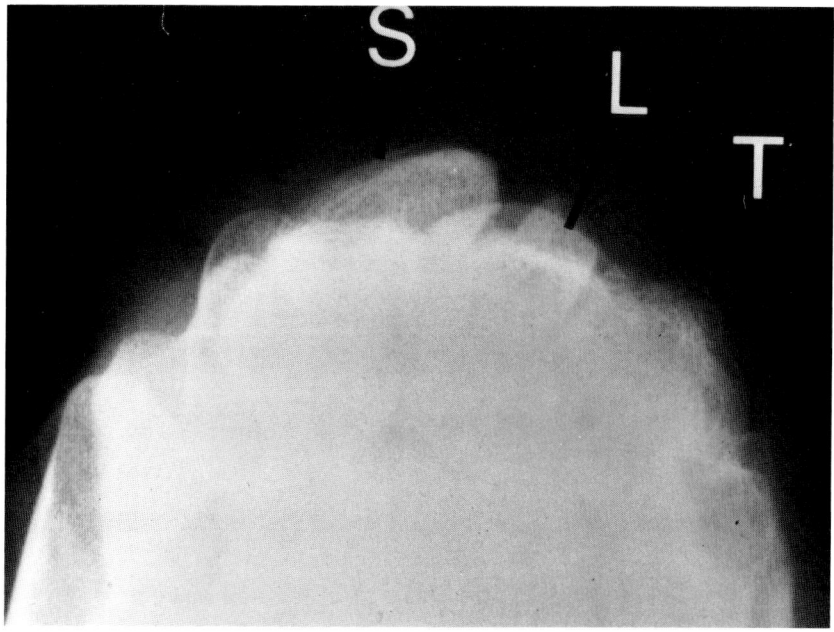

B

FIG. 14-44. Dorsal tangential view. A: Hand positioned for dorsal tangential view. B: Radiograph demonstrating the dorsal soft tissues and dorsal portions of the scaphoid (S), lunate (L), and triquetrum (T).

We use CT most frequently for evaluating subluxation and/or dislocation of the distal radioulnar joint. Axial images in the symptomatic position may be diagnostic. In some cases, neutral, pronation, and supination images are required to detect subtle subluxation. The normal wrist is generally examined for comparison (89). This can be done simultaneously, but positioning must be symmetrical. This may be difficult to achieve in symptomatic patients (Fig. 14-48). Figure 14-49 demonstrates the normal relationships of the distal radius and ulna (89).

Complex injuries can also be evaluated with three-dimensional reconstruction. However, this is not commonly required in routine trauma cases (90).

Radionuclide Imaging

Three-phase radionuclide imaging of the wrist is a useful technique for evaluating acute and chronic trauma-related disorders of the hand and wrist. In this setting, ^{99m}TC coupled to phosphate compounds such as methylene diphosphonate (MDP) is most often used. Three-phase imaging provides additional advantages compared to the usual delay (2–3 hour) bone images (Phase III)

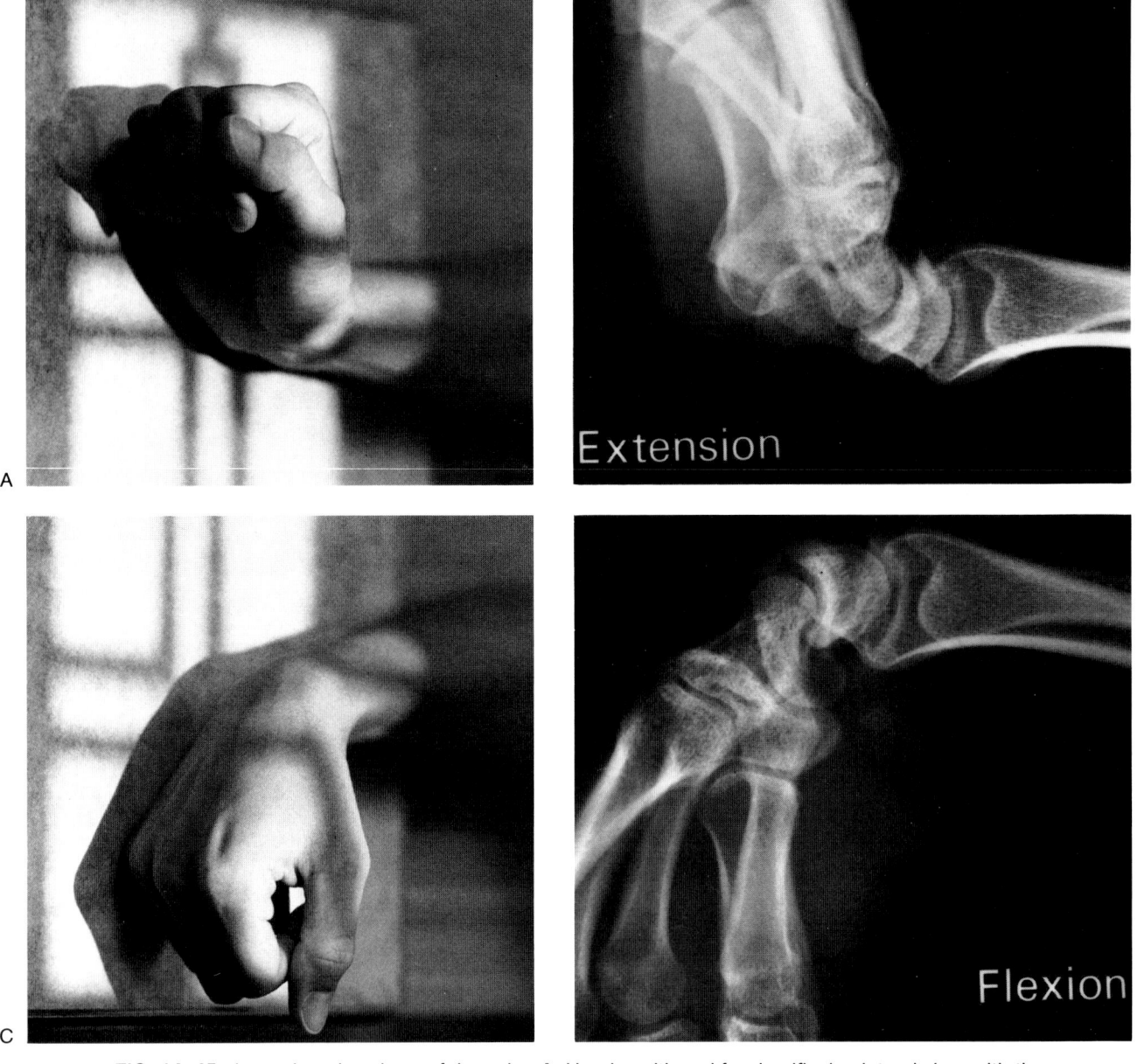

FIG. 14–45. Lateral motion views of the wrist. **A:** Hand positioned for dorsiflexion lateral view with the beam centered on the wrist. **B:** Radiograph demonstrates the elongated scaphoid with slight dorsal rotation of the lunate. The degree of extension is normal (approximately 70°). **C:** Hand positioned for the palmar flexion lateral. **D:** Radiograph on palmar flexion demonstrates normal flexion (approximately 75°). The scaphoid assumes a nearly vertical position.

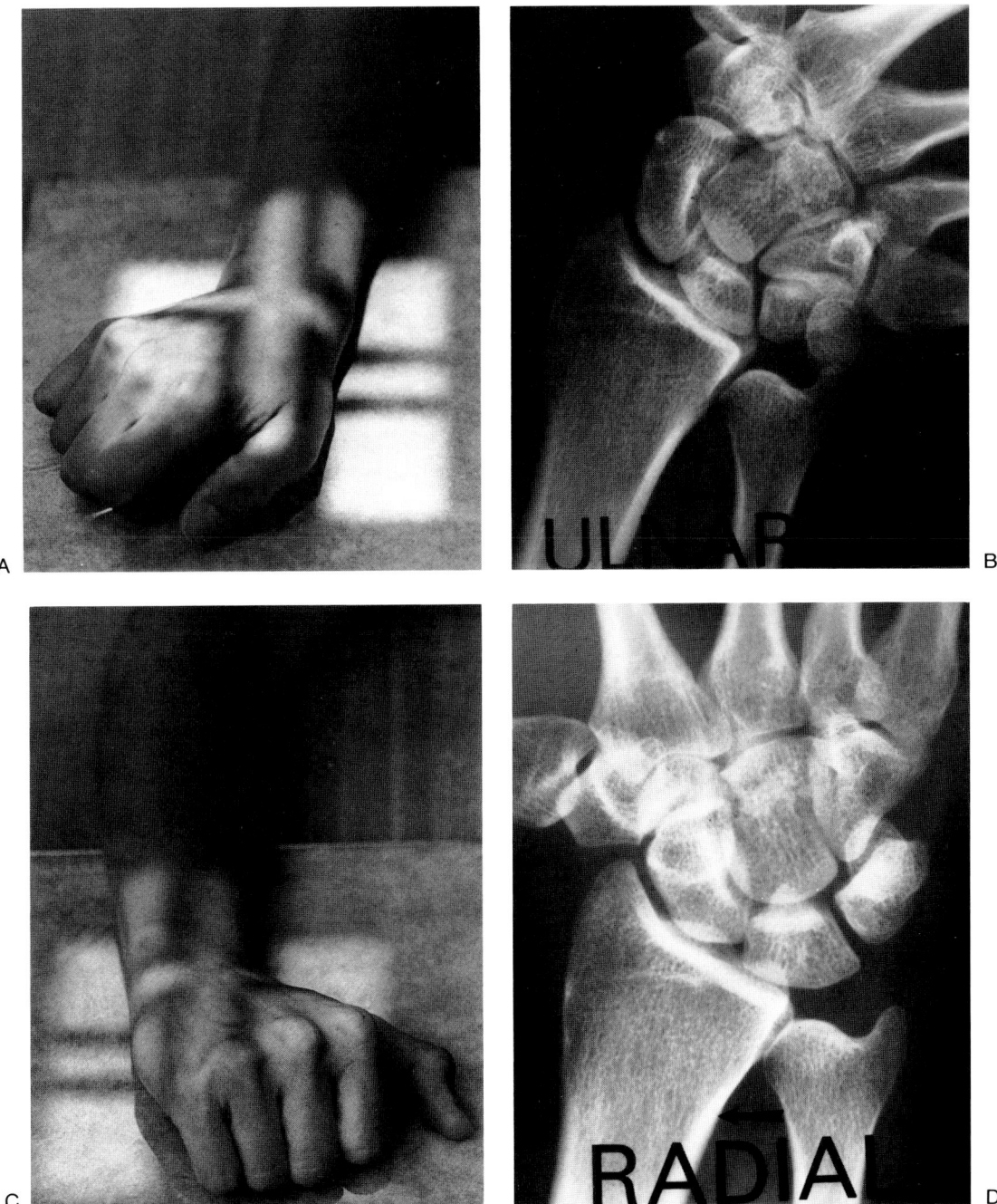

FIG. 14–46. PA wrist with radial and ulnar deviation. **A:** Hand with clenched fist and ulnar deviation. **B:** Radiograph in ulnar deviation. The scaphoid is elongated. There is no increase in the joint space. **C:** Hand in radial deviation with clenched fist. Normally the joint spaces do not increase. The lunate slides to the ulnar side of the radiocarpal joint and the scaphoid is rotated vertically resulting in a foreshortened appearance (D).

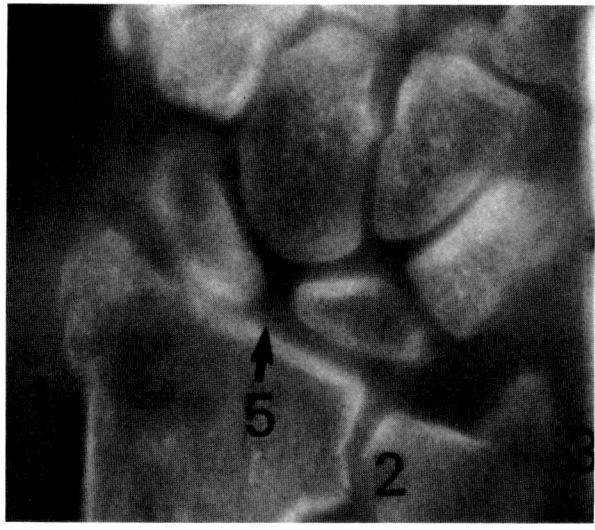
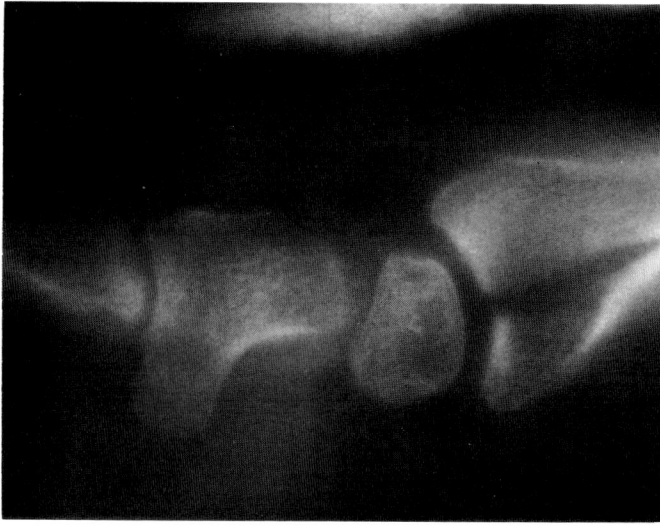

FIG. 14–47. Wrist fracture. AP (**A**) and lateral (**B**) tomograms define the injuries more clearly. 1, Radial styloid fracture; 2, fracture involving the distal radioulnar joint; 3, ulnar styloid fracture; 4, trapezial fracture; 5, scapholunate ligament tear.

(52,72). The first phase (Phase I) provides valuable flow information. This phase is obtained using rapid sequential imaging during the first 1–2 minutes after injection while the isotope is intravascular (72). Soft tissue distribution is evaluated during phase II (5–10 minutes after injection) when the radiopharmaceutical is in the extracellular fluid space (52,72). Abnormal uptake in diffuse regions is not unusual during the early phases (Phase I and II) in soft tissue injuries. The lack of focal uptake on delayed images is useful in excluding osseous involvement (Fig. 14-50) (52).

The most common indication for three-phase radionuclide imaging in the hand and wrist include the following: (1) to exclude subtle osseous injury, (2) reflex sympathetic dystrophy, (3) bone ischemia, and (4) early inflammation or infection (47,53,58,72,88).

Magnetic Resonance Imaging

MRI has become increasingly useful in defining soft tissue abnormalities, subtle bone lesions, and ischemic changes in the hand and wrist. When properly performed, MRI may replace more conventional techniques in diagnosing certain disorders of the hand and wrist (29,30,93).

Technique

MRI examinations of the hand and wrist can be difficult to perform due to limitations in positioning and coil selection. Patient comfort is an essential part of the examination. If the position is difficult to tolerate, one can expect significant problems with motion artifact. In our initial review of upper extremity MRI studies we noted motion artifacts or incomplete studies due to patient discomfort in 25% of cases (30).

Positioning depends upon patient size, information required (i.e., motion studies), software, and coil availability. Uniform signal intensity is most easily obtained using a wrap-around, partial volume, or helmholtz coil system. The small flat coils (3 inches and 5 inches) are also adequate for hand and wrist imaging (Fig. 14-51). Flat coils allow more flexibility for positioning and motion studies. When patient size allows, it is best to position the arm at the side. Dual coils are now available that allow simultaneous evaluation of both hands and wrists. The wrist can also be positioned over the abdomen with the elbow flexed. However, the coil must be supported and separated from the abdominal wall or motion artifact becomes a problem. Larger patients may need to be rotated with the arm above the head. This position is difficult to tolerate due to shoulder discomfort (Fig. 14-51) (29,30).

Optimal image quality in hand and wrist imaging requires a small field of view (FOV). We typically use an 8–12 cm FOV for examinations with both flat and volume coils. Off axis, small field of view is needed if the coil is positioned away from the central axis of the magnet. Therefore, if this software is not available one must position the arm above the head to achieve the proper FOV (Fig. 14-51).

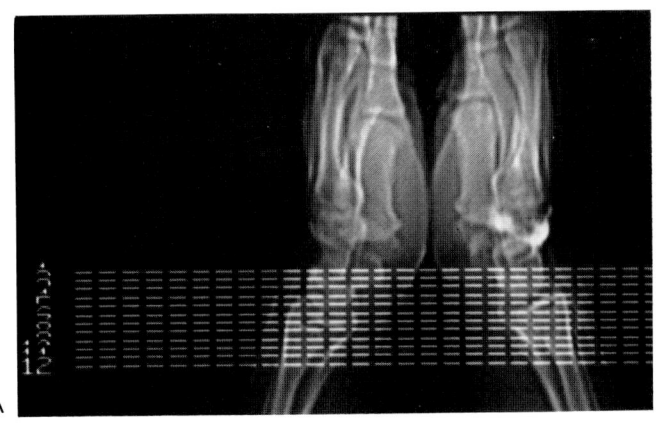

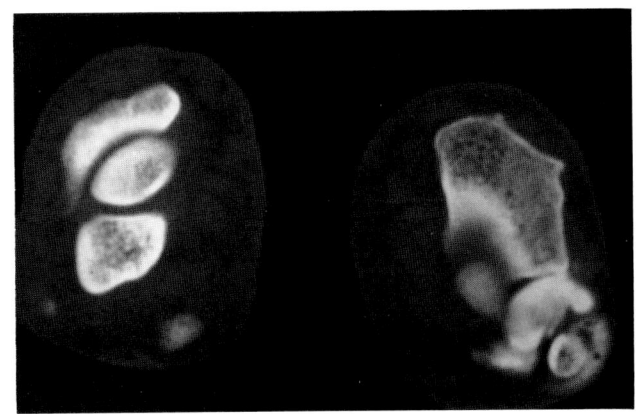

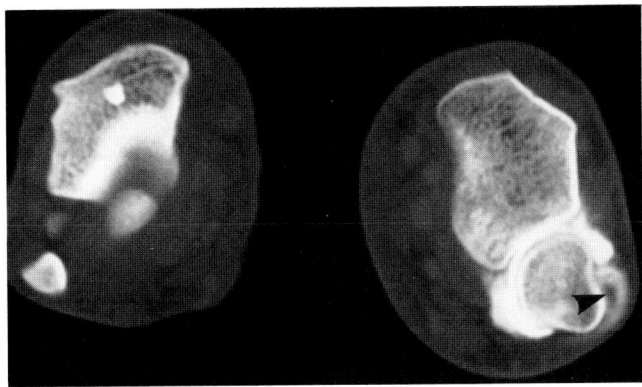

FIG. 14-48. CT images of the wrist. **A:** Scout image. Note slight positioning asymmetry that is evident on the axial images **B** and **C**. Contrast was placed in the left distal radioulnar joint. The distal radioulnar joint is normal. Note the filling of the extensor carpi ulnaris tendon sheath (*arrow*). This should not communicate with the tendon sheath.

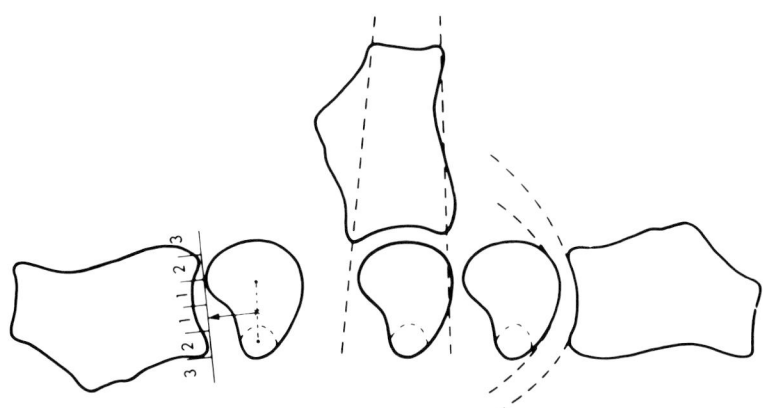

A

A. Supination   **B.** Neutral   **C.** Pronation

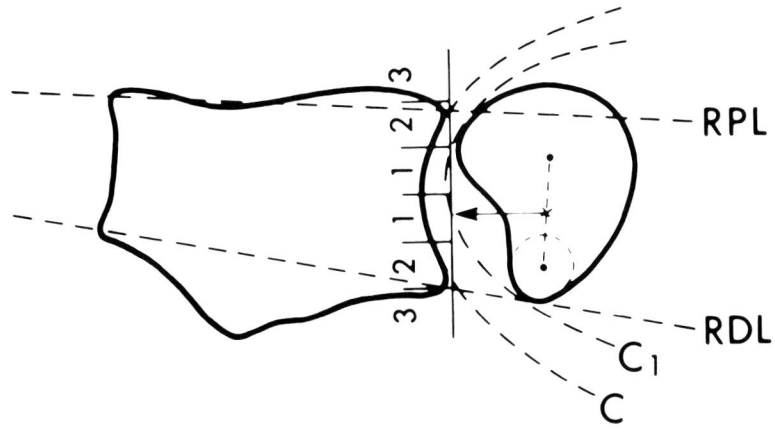

B

FIG. 14-49. Criteria for evaluating the distal radioulnar joint. **A:** Wrist in supination, neutral, and pronation. A, epicenter method. A perpendicular is drawn from the center of a line between the ulnar styloid and mid ulna. This should intersect the middle of the radial notch. B, radioulnar line method. The ulna should line within the marginal lines of the radius. C, congruency method. The arcs of the ulna and radius should be congruent. **B:** Summary of all three techniques in a supinated wrist (from 89, with permission).

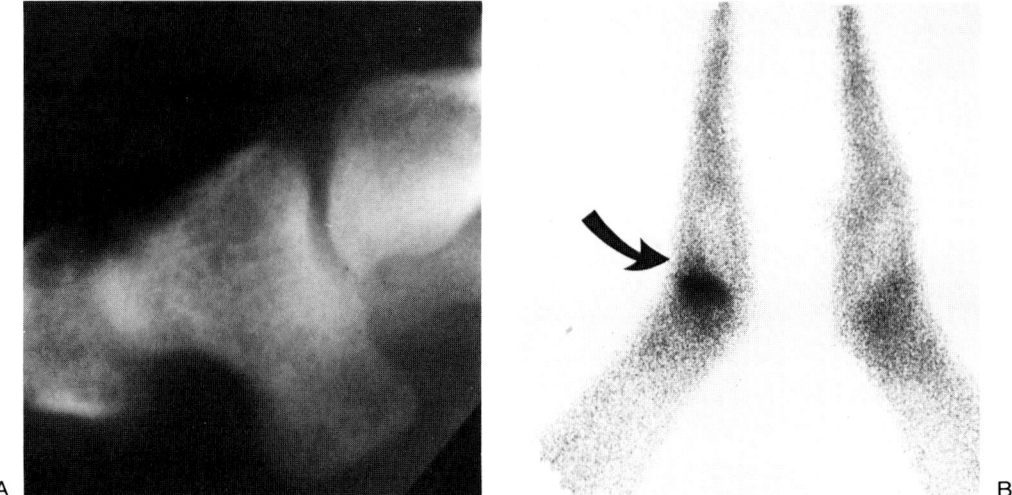

FIG. 14–50. Racket injury to the hand. **A:** Lateral tomogram in the acute phase is normal. **B:** Bone scan several days later demonstrates focal increased tracer (*arrow*) in the hamate region. A repeat tomogram 10 days after injury confirmed the fracture.

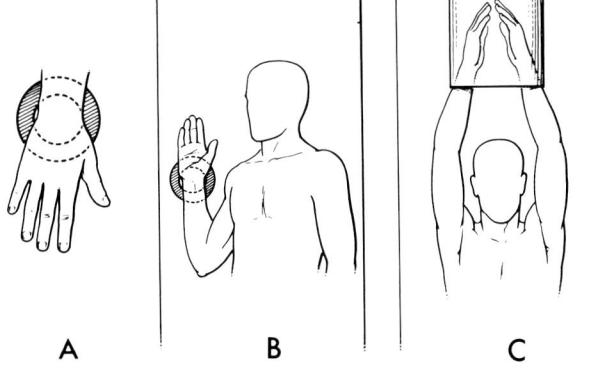

FIG. 14–51. Patient positioned with the hand at the side (**A**), rotated with the elbow flexed (**B**), and arms above the head with both hands in a circumferential coil (**C**). The latter is least comfortable (from 102, with permission).

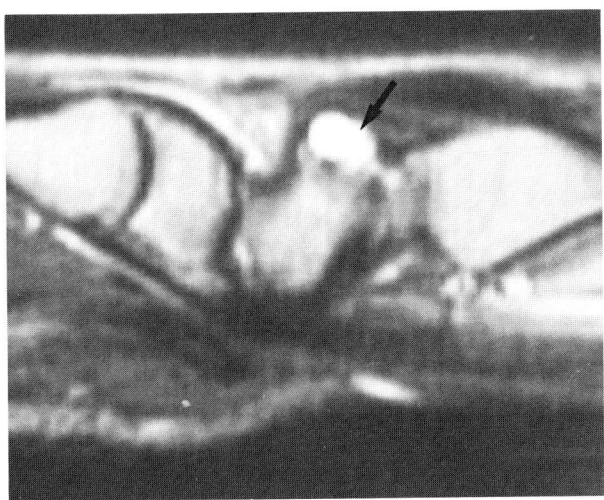

FIG. 14–52. Patient with chronic wrist pain after trauma. Sagittal SE 2000/60 image demonstrating a dorsal ganglion (*arrow*).

Once the patient has been positioned, the proper pulse sequences and image planes must be selected to demonstrate the anatomy and pathology. An effective screening examination can be accomplished by beginning with either a coronal or sagittal scout (SE 150–400/20). This should include the full area of the hand and wrist to be examined. We typically follow this sequence with an axial T2-weighted sequence (SE 2000/20–30, 60–80) using 5-mm thick slices, minimal interslice gap, 256 × 256 matrix with one excitation (8 min 56 sec) or 256 × 192 matrix with 2 excitations (13 min). A small field of view (8–12 cm), no phase, no frequency wrap, and presatura-

tion techniques are used to reduce flow artifacts and maximize image quality. The second sequence chosen varies depending on the findings of the first sequence or clinical indication for the examination. A coronal T1-weighted sequence (SE 500/20) with 3–5 mm slice thicknesses, no skip and other setup data above is usually adequate as a second sequence to provide a good screening technique for bone and soft tissue pathology (Figs. 14-52 and 14-53) (29,30,93).

Additional sequences may be indicated in specific clinical situations or when abnormalities are evident on the initial sequences that dictate the need for further sequences to characterize the lesion. For example, if an abnormality is suspected in a specific phalangeal segment, sagittal T2 (SE 2000/30,60) or gradient-echo sequences (TE 13, TR 100–400, flip angle 30°–70°) will define the structures, including vasculature, to better advantage. The sagittal sequence should be performed with thin slices (3 mm) and aligned with the tendon or osseous structure (Fig. 14-54) (29).

Specific anatomic areas can be examined with the 3-inch coil, an 8-cm field of view, and sequences that may differ from the screening examination described above. Specifically, the scaphoid is demonstrated most completely using the coronal and sagittal planes (Figs. 14-55 and 14-56). T1- and T2-weighted sequences should be performed to fully evaluate the bone and articular anatomy. Evaluation of the distal radioulnar joint often requires pronation, supination, and neutral T2-weighted axial images. This allows functional anatomic information and evaluation of subtle soft tissue abnormalities. Cine motion studies can be performed quickly using GRASS or GRIL sequences. Soft tissue abnormalities in

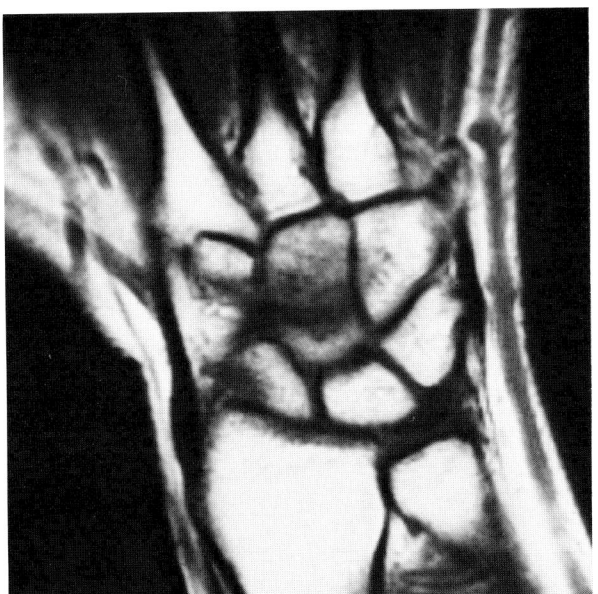
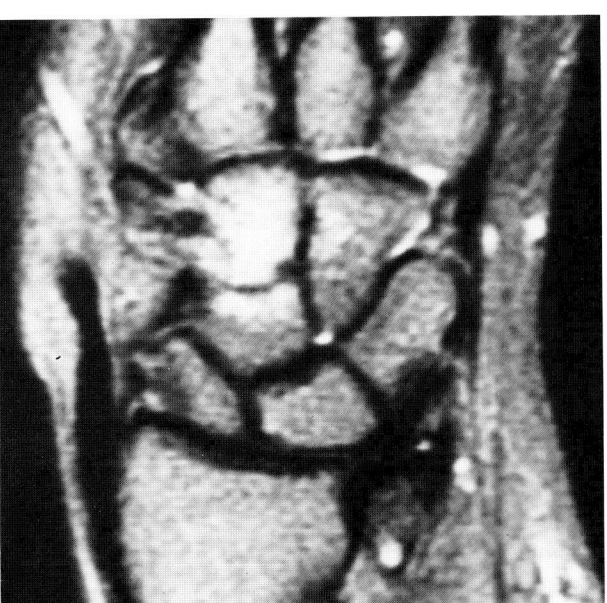

FIG. 14–53. Coronal SE 500/20 (**A**) and SE 2000/60 (**B**) images demonstrating an unsuspected capitate fracture.

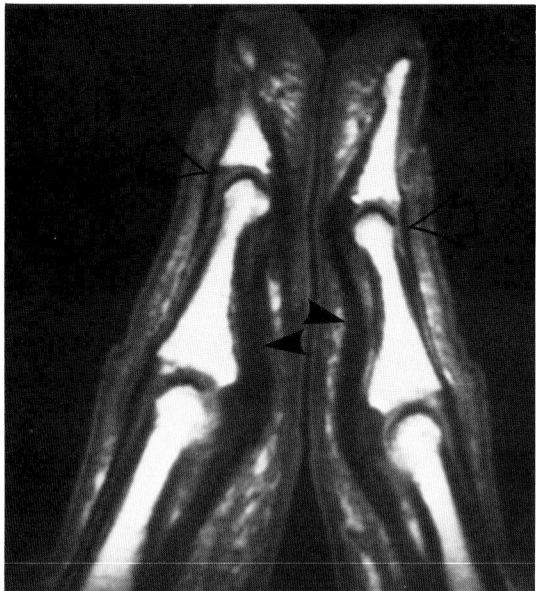

FIG. 14-54. Sagittal SE 500/20 images of the index fingers demonstrating the extensor (*open arrows*) and flexor (*black arrows*) tendons (from 102, with permission).

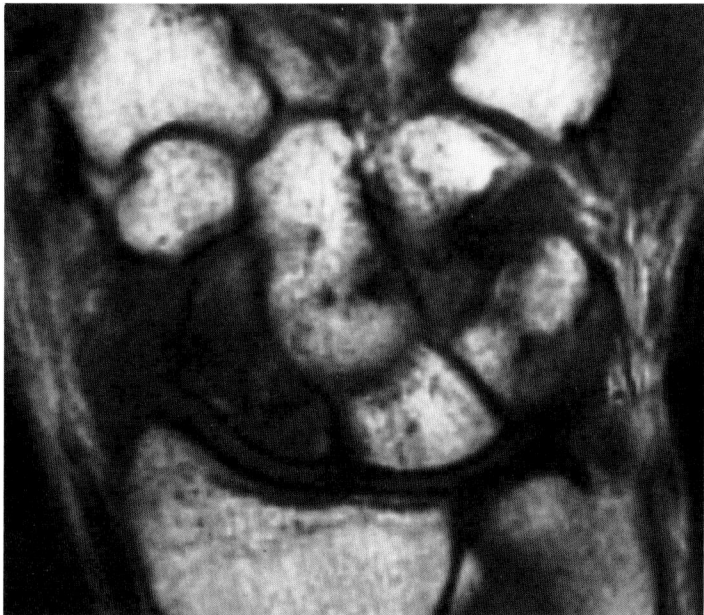

FIG. 14-55. Coronal SE 500/20 image after a subtle scaphoid fracture demonstrating edema and hyperemia, which causes low signal intensity in the entire scaphoid.

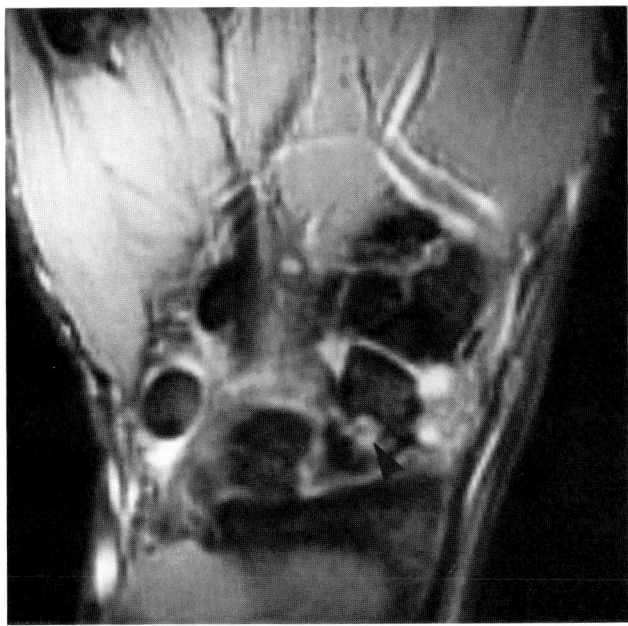

FIG. 14–56. Coronal gradient-echo image demonstrating high signal intensity in the scaphoid (*arrow*) due to cystic non-union.

the carpal tunnel can be studied using axial SE 2000/30, 60 and SE 500/20 sequences. These images provide more than adequate evaluation of the median nerve and surrounding structures (Fig. 14-57). Vascular anatomy is demonstrated most completely using GRASS or volume reconstruction techniques.

Magnetic resonance imaging techniques can be useful in acute and chronic musculoskeletal injuries to the hand and wrist (Table 14-1). Most acute skeletal injuries are adequately diagnosed with routine radiography. Conventional tomography or isotope studies are valuable supplemental radiographic techniques (29,30).

MRI is not frequently used for diagnosis of skeletal injuries in the hand and wrist. However, it is not unusual to detect subtle injuries that may not be evident with

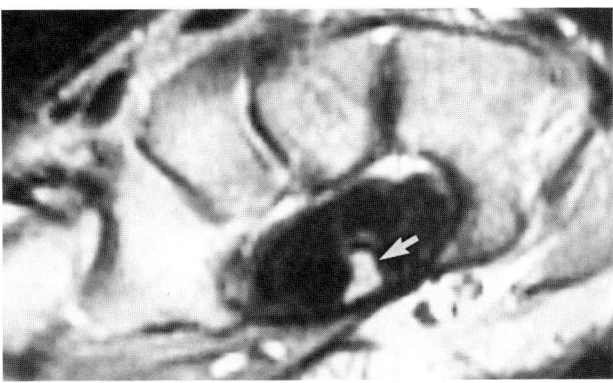

FIG. 14–57. Axial SE 2000/60 image of the wrist demonstrating increased signal intensity and compression of the median nerve (*arrow*).

TABLE 14–1. *Hand and wrist trauma*

Anatomic region/indication	Imaging work-up
Osseous Trauma	
Distal radius and ulna	Routine radiographs, tomography if needed
Carpal bones	Routine radiographs, radionuclide scans plus tomography if indicated
Metacarpals and phalanges	Routine radiographs
? Avascular necrosis	Routine radiograph, MRI if negative
Distal radioulnar joint (DRUJ) (subluxation-dislocation)	CT ± arthrography or MRI: gradient-echo technique with cine (neutral, pronation, supination)
Ligament injuries	Arthrography
Capsules and ligaments MCP and IP joints	Arthrography
Muscle and tendon	MRI
Neural injury	MRI

routine radiographs or tomography (Fig. 14-53). Detection of stress fractures and osteochondral fractures with MRI has also been reported. Cortical bone appears black on MR images. Therefore, cortical fractures are most easily appreciated on T2-weighted images (SE 2000/60–80). Edema and hemorrhage in marrow will also have higher signal intensity than normal marrow using these parameters. Fracture lines and adjacent reactive change have low signal intensity compared to normal marrow on T1-weighted (SE 500/20) sequences (Fig. 14-55). Compression injuries with trabecular condensation are seen as areas of low intensity on both T1- and T2-weighted sequences (29,30).

MRI is also useful for evaluating fracture healing, non-union (Fig. 14-56), and early osteonecrosis. Fibrous union has low signal intensity on both T1- and T2-weighted sequences. Increased signal intensity along the fracture line (due to fluid) is noted with T2-weighted sequences when non-union occurs. Osteonecrosis following scaphoid fractures is easily detected with coronal MR images. Initially, the signal intensity is diminished on T1-weighted images. As osteonecrosis progresses to sclerotic bone commonly seen on routine radiographs, the signal intensity is low on both T1- and T2-weighted sequences (29,30).

Articular or joint-related injuries of the hand and wrist are usually evaluated with arthrography, motion studies, stress views, and, in certain cases, post-injection CT or tomography (Table 14-1). Arthrography is still valuable for confirming suspected ligament injuries. In addition, diagnostic and therapeutic injections can be performed in conjunction with arthrography and tenography (29,55).

MRI is most useful for evaluating soft tissue trauma, specifically muscle and tendon injuries, neural compression syndromes, and capsule disruptions (10,28) (Table 14-1). Tears in the triangular fibrocartilage (TFC) can be detected, especially if they occur near the thicker ulnar margin (Fig. 14-58). Zlatkin (93) reported accuracies of 95% for MR detection of TFC tears and a sensitivity of 100% and specificity of 92% with MRI compared to 89% and 90% for arthrography (93). However, near the apex (radial edge) the radiocarpal and distal radioulnar joint are separated by a thin segment. Therefore, injection of gadolinium-diethylenetriamine pinta-acetic acid (Gd-DTPA) may be required to enhance detection accuracy in this region. Evaluation of the intercarpal ligaments and distal radioulnar joint is usually accomplished with arthrography and CT (89). However, MRI has also demonstrated significant potential in these areas. Although experience is early, Zlatkin et al. (93) reported accuracy of 90% for the scapholunate ligament and slightly less accurate results (80%) for the lunotriquetral ligament.

Technique is very important. Dual-coupled flat coils, a small field of view (8–12 cm) and T2-weighted sequences (SE 2000/20, 60) or gradient-echo sequences (TR 200–700; TE 12,31; flip angle 25°–30°) with T2* weighting are most useful. The coronal plane and thin (1–3 mm) slices are also best suited to evaluate the TFC and ligaments (29,93). At this time, arthrography is still very useful for detection of interosseous ligament and TFC injuries (29,55).

Muscle and tendon tears are also most easily demonstrated with T2-weighted sequences. To accurately define the extent of injury, we usually use axial and either coronal or sagittal image planes. Subtle tendon abnormalities may be better demonstrated using gradient-echo motion studies. Axial images in neutral, pronation, and supination are also best for evaluating the distal radioulnar joint.

MRI is a proved technique for detection of avascular necrosis (29,30). In the wrist, these changes are seen most commonly in the lunate and following scaphoid fractures (Fig. 14-59). Carpal bones are smaller and, therefore, the MRI features of osteonecrosis may be more difficult to interpret. Uniform loss of signal intensity on short TE/TR sequences is the most reliable sign of avascular necrosis (Fig. 14-59A), specifically in the lunate. Similar changes can occur also in the other carpal bones but are less common. Patchy or focal signal intensity changes have also been noted. When small focal areas of reduced signal intensity are noted in the carpal bones on a T1-weighted sequence, the diagnosis may be more difficult (29,30). Comparison with T2-weighted images is somewhat useful. In the early stages, the signal intensity will be increased. Later, when bone sclerosis occurs, the signal intensity will be reduced on both T1- and T2-weighted sequences. In either setting, comparison with routine radiographs is important. Well-marginated lucent areas are usually degenerative and should not be confused with osteonecrosis. This appearance can also be seen with conditions such as ulnolunate abutment syndrome (29,30).

MRI has been useful in detection and monitoring of the response of avascular necrosis to conservative therapy (Fig. 14-59B). In several cases, the signal intensity in an otherwise low signal intensity lunate has returned to normal with conservative therapy. This finding was correlated with improvement in the patient's symptoms. Although isotope studies can also be used for identification of avascular necrosis (72,88), the MR findings are

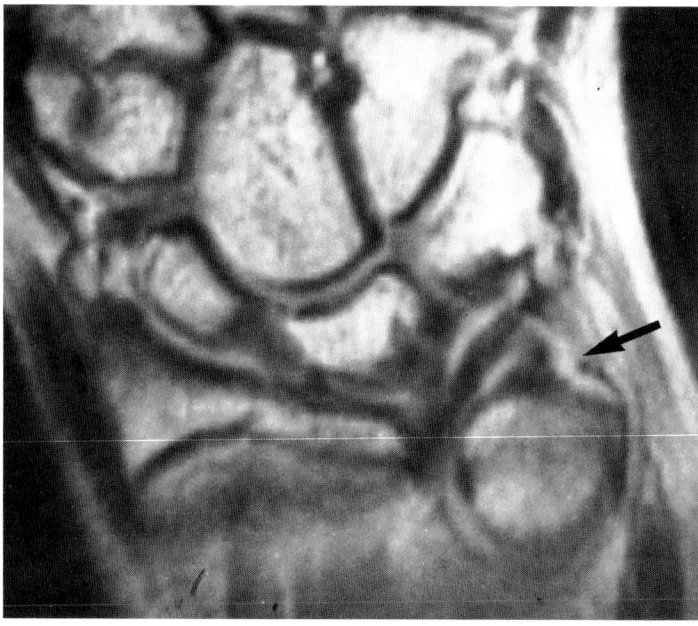

FIG. 14-58. Coronal SE 2000/30 image demonstrating a tear (*arrow*) in the TFC (triangular fibrocartilage complex).

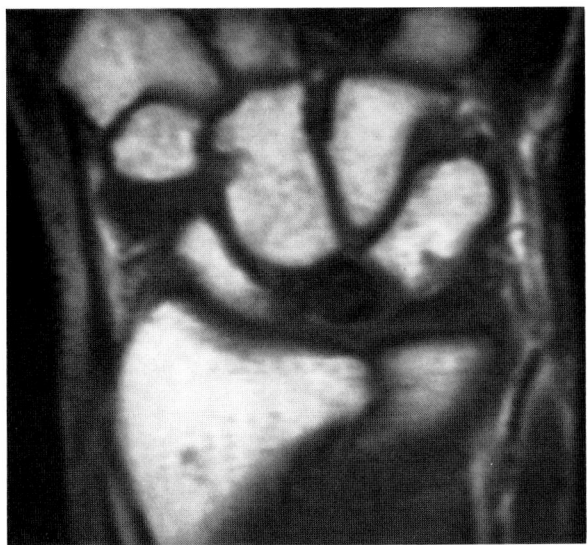 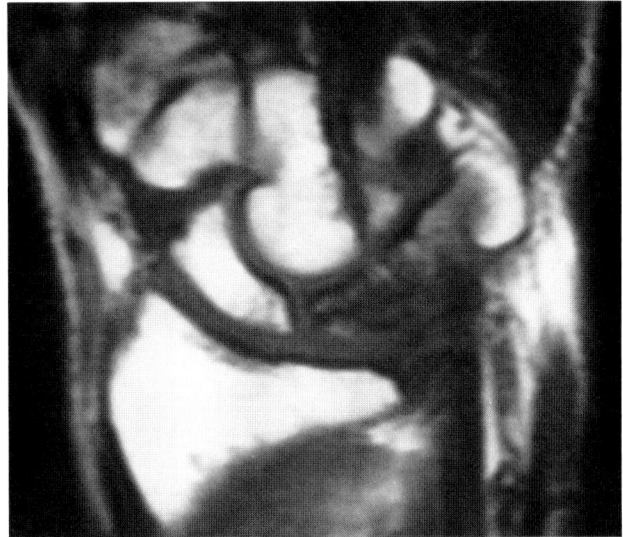

A   B

FIG. 14–59. SE 500/20 images of the wrist demonstrating decreased signal in the lunate due to avascular necrosis (**A**). After several months of conservative therapy (**B**) the signal intensity is beginning to return to normal.

more informative and the anatomy more clearly demonstrated (29,30).

ARTHROGRAPHY OF THE HAND AND WRIST

Wrist Arthrography

Wrist arthrography allows evaluation of the articular cartilage and synovium. The integrity of the ligaments, triangular fibrocartilage complex (TFC), and joint compartments can also be assessed.

Arthrography is most commonly used to evaluate patients with post-traumatic wrist pain. The number of injections and initial injection site depends upon the clinical indication and suspected pathology. All routine radiographs should be reviewed. We also routinely examine the wrist with video fluoroscopy prior to injection to search for additional clues to the underlying injury.

Technique

The examination may be performed with the patient seated next to the fluoroscopic table or supine with the arm extended and the hand resting palm down. The latter method allows easier access to the patient and decreases the concern for syncopal attacks.

The dorsum of the wrist is prepared with a povidone-iodine (Betadine) preparation and sterile towels.

The radiocarpal joint is entered with the wrist flexed over a cushion to open the dorsal radiocarpal joint (Fig. 14-60). The injection site is checked by positioning the needle tip just distal to the radius and on the radial side

of the scapholunate joint (Fig. 14-60). Care should also be taken not to inject the extensor tendon (81). To assist in needle placement, the dorsal joint space and distal radial tubercle are often easily palpated. An .5-inch 25-gauge needle is used to inject a small amount of 1% lidocaine (Xylocaine) in the skin. In most patients, the same needle will easily reach the joint space and can be used to perform the procedure. If cultures are required or if the soft tissues are thicker, a 1.5-inch 22-gauge needle may be required. Needle position and depth can be confirmed by gently rotating the wrist into the lateral position. The joint should be aspirated prior to the injection of contrast material. Cultures and synovial fluid analysis may be indicated. If infection is suspected and no fluid can be obtained, the joint should be flushed with nonbacteriostatic sterile saline and the aspirate sent for culture. Injection of a small test dose of contrast material (meglumine diatrizoate) should demonstrate free flow away from the needle tip. When the proper position has been obtained, 1.5–3 ml of contrast material is injected. This should be performed slowly and observed fluoroscopically to confirm the site of any intercompartmental communication (50).

Following the injection, the needle is removed, and the wrist is gently exercised under video fluoroscopic guidance. In addition, films are obtained in the PA, lateral, oblique, and bending (flexion, extension, radial and ulnar deviation) positions. In certain situations, repeat films may be required after the initial films have been studied.

Injection of the distal radioulnar joint or mid carpal joint (Fig. 14-60A) is performed with the hand palm down. When a previous injection has already been per-

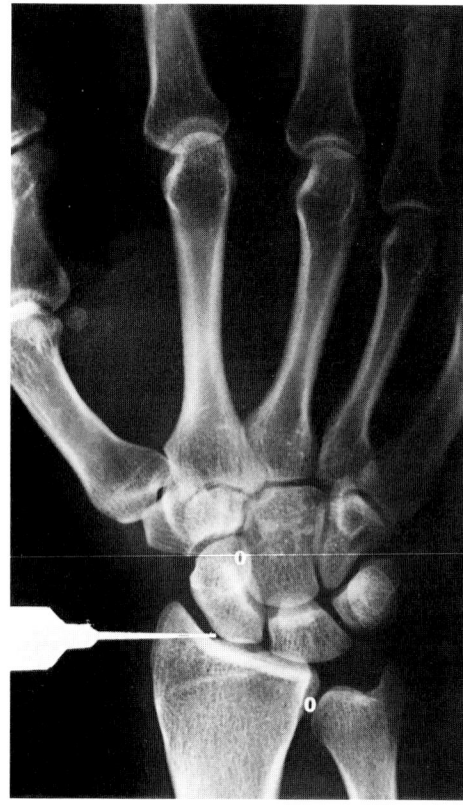

A

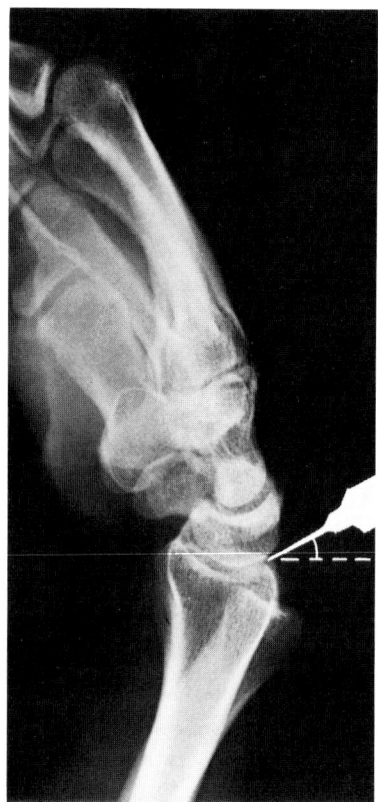

B

FIG. 14-60. Radiograph simulating fluoroscopic appearance of needle positioning. **A:** The AP position demonstrates the proper needle position over the radiocarpal joint. The scapholunate space should be avoided. White *o* shows injection sites for the distal radioulnar joint and mid carpal joints. **B:** Lateral view with the wrist flexed. The needle tip should be angled proximally to assure proper positioning in the radiocarpal joint.

formed, 2–3 hours are required to allow the initial contrast medium to dissipate (65,66,74).

There is some controversy as to how many compartments should be injected. Levinsohn et al. (65,66) state three injections (radiocarpal, mid carpal, and distal radioulnar joint) are required. Manaster (71) suggests that this may not be necessary in all cases using her technique. We also frequently use fewer than three injections (Fig. 14-61). Digital techniques may be useful for detection of subtle abnormalities (70). This technique is useful if used routinely and when equipment is readily available. However, we typically use videotape fluoroscopy, arthrography, and occasionally tenography. Diagnostic injection with xylocaine or marcaine may also be indicated. MRI may also be required when these techniques fail to isolate the abnormality.

Double-contrast technique is rarely used in wrist arthrography. Occasionally, trispiral tomography or CT is used in conjunction with arthrography (27,31,78). In these cases epinephrine may be required (see Introduction to Arthrography in Chapter 1).

Normal Arthrographic Anatomy

The anatomy of the hand and wrist has been discussed earlier in this chapter. The compartments of the wrist should be re-emphasized for proper arthrographic evaluation. These include the radiocarpal joint, distal radioulnar joint, intercarpal joint, carpometacarpal joints, first

carpometacarpal joint, and pisotriquetral joint (Fig. 14-62) (67,74).

Communications between the compartments of the wrist have been noted by numerous authors in normal patients (Fig. 14-63). The most common problem is differentiating communication of the radiocarpal and intercarpal compartments from a ligament tear in asymptomatic patients.

Injection of the radiocarpal joint will normally demonstrate no communication with the midcarpal or distal radioulnar joint (see Figs. 14-61, 14-65 and 14-67). Communication with the pisotriquetral joint is commonly noted. Lewis (67) and Mrose and Rosenthal (74) reported radiocarpal-pisotriquetral communication in 34% and 75% of cases respectively. Intracompartmental communications must be correlated with the clinical findings in each patient. Normal recesses are present in the prestyloid region and are volar to the distal radius (Fig. 14-64). The synovial lining is smooth. There is no communication with the tendon sheaths in the normal wrist. The triangular fibrocartilage is attached to the distal radius and ulnar styloid (67).

Abnormal Arthrogram

Trauma

Arthrography is most commonly performed to evaluate patients with post-traumatic wrist pain or instability.

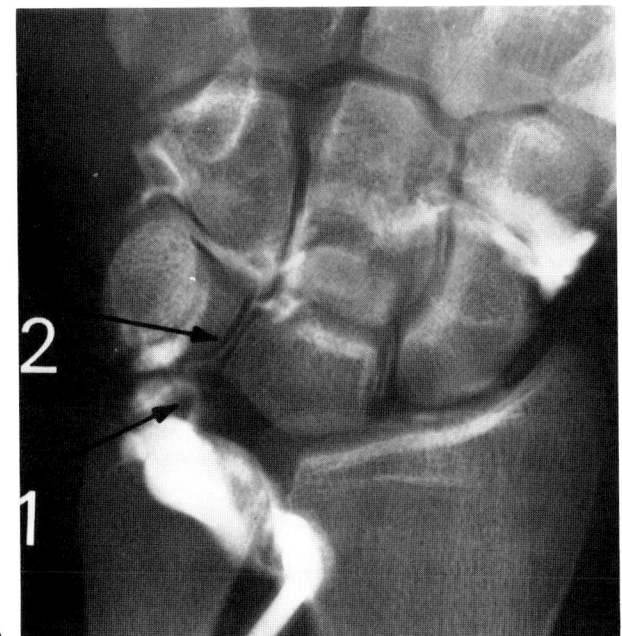 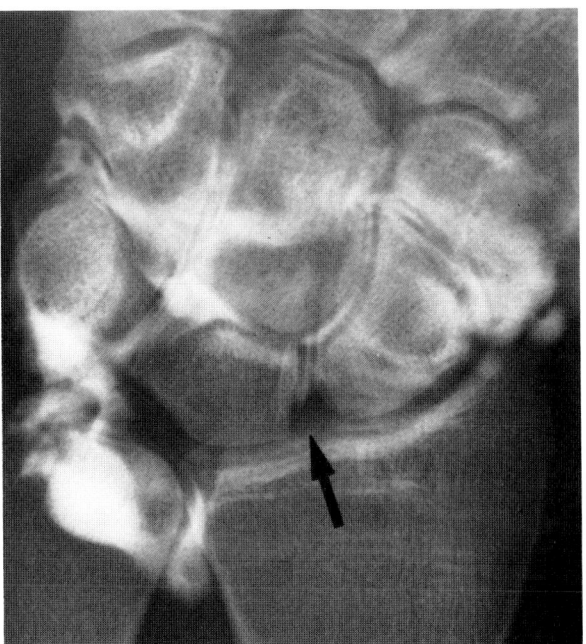

FIG. 14-61. Patient with post-traumatic wrist pain and suspected abnormality of the radioulnar joint. **A:** Fluoroscopically, the distal radioulnar joint was injected. Contrast medium entered the radioulnar joint via a triangular cartilage tear (1) and entered the intercarpal joint via a defect in the lunotriquetral ligament (2). **B:** Scapholunate dissociation was also present (note widened joint, *arrow*). The complexity of the injury would not be appreciated if the injection were not observed fluoroscopically.

In the assessment of ligament injuries, the arthrogram must be correlated with clinical findings, including the age of the patient. Patients with ligamentous disruption will demonstrate communication between the compartments of the wrist. The scapholunate ligament is commonly involved. This results in communication between the radiocarpal and midcarpal joints. To be significant, joint tenderness or other local symptoms should correlate with the area of abnormality on the arthrogram. The bones may also be malaligned. This may present with widening or loss of the parallelism of the joint space (Fig. 14-65). In addition, a decrease in the radioscaphoid angle or the ring sign may be present (Fig. 14-66). The latter is due to the vertical position of the scaphoid. In longstanding cases secondary degenerative changes are common, but these may require tomography for identification.

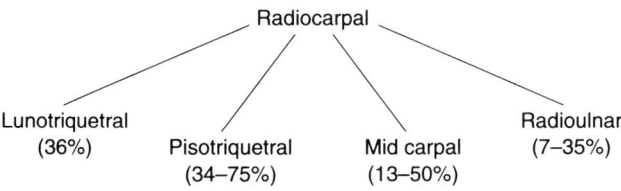

FIG. 14-62. Intercompartmental communications of the wrist.

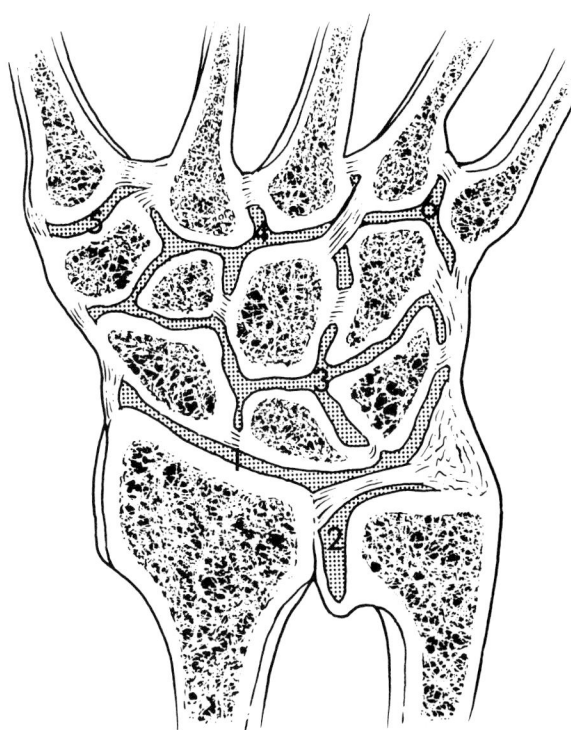

FIG. 14-63. Dorsal compartments of the wrist. 1, radiocarpal; 2, distal radioulnar; 3, intercarpal; 4, common carpometacarpal; 5, first carpometacarpal; and 6, outer carpometacarpal. The pisotriquetral articulation is located on the volar aspect of the wrist.

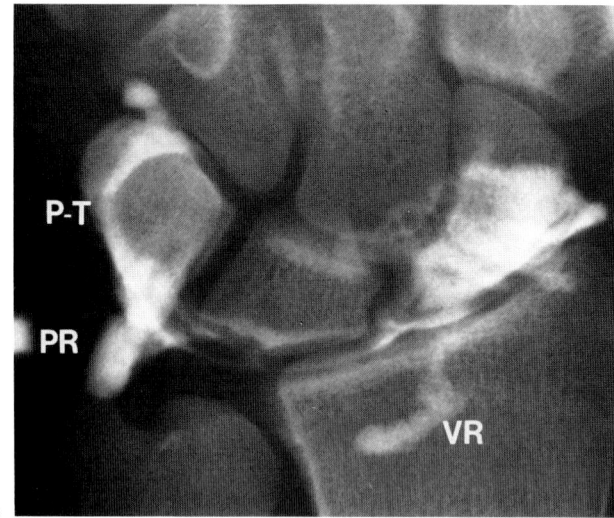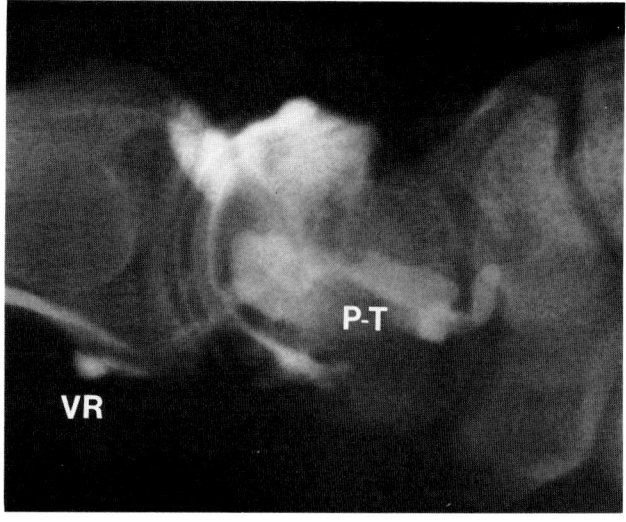

A

B

FIG. 14–64. Normal wrist arthrogram. PA (**A**) and lateral (**B**) views demonstrating contrast in the radio-carpal joint. The pisotriquetral joint communication (P-T) is of no clinical significance. Normal recesses include the pre-styloid (PR) and volar radial recesses (VR).

Lunotriquestral perforations are also common. This lesion was reported in 52% of the Levinsohn et al. (65) series. This lesion is frequently associated with TFC abnormalities (26,65). Up to 80% of these patients will also have ulnar positive variance (Fig. 14-61A) (26). Both midcarpal and radiocarpal injections may be necessary to clarify isolated lunotriquetral injuries.

In patients with tears in the triangular cartilage, communication between the radiocarpal and distal radioulnar joints will be observed (Figs. 14-61A and 14-67).

Tears in the triquetrolunate ligament may be associated with triangular cartilage tears (Fig. 14-61A).

Occasionally, local synovial irregularity or tendon communication may be evident (81). Levinsohn and Palmer (64) noted capsular lesions in 31%, lymphatic filling in 12%, and tendon sheath communication in 10% (Fig. 14-68) of patients with chronic post-traumatic pain.

Arthrography is also necessary to detect adhesive capsulitis. The volume is reduced and recesses obliterated

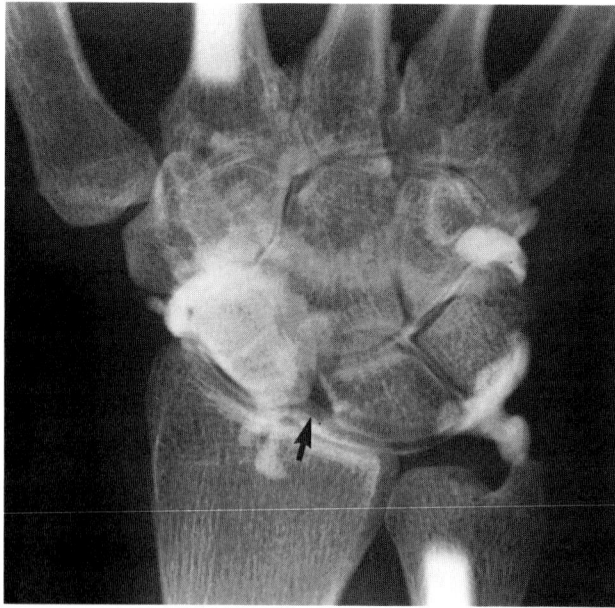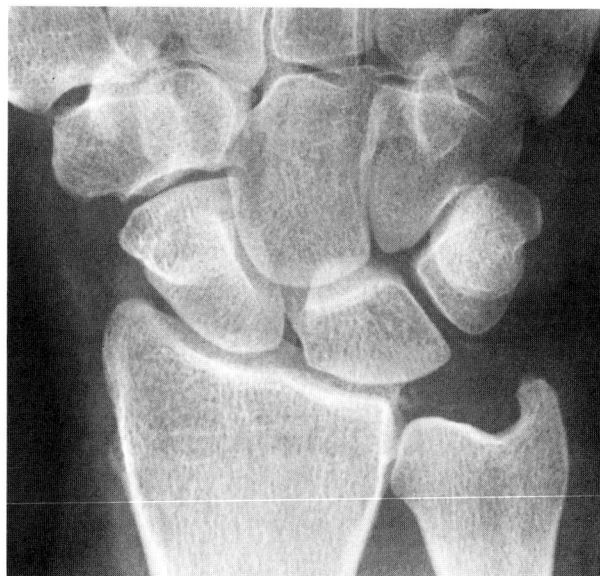

FIG. 14–65. Patient with scapholunate ligament disruption. There is communication between the radiocarpal and intercarpal compartments. Note the triangular configuration of the scapholunate space (*arrow*).

FIG. 14–66. Patient with chronic scapholunate ligament instability. PA view of the wrist demonstrating slight widening and a triangular configuration to the scapholunate joint. (The scaphoid is foreshortened with the ring sign.) Note that chondrocalcinosis is also present.

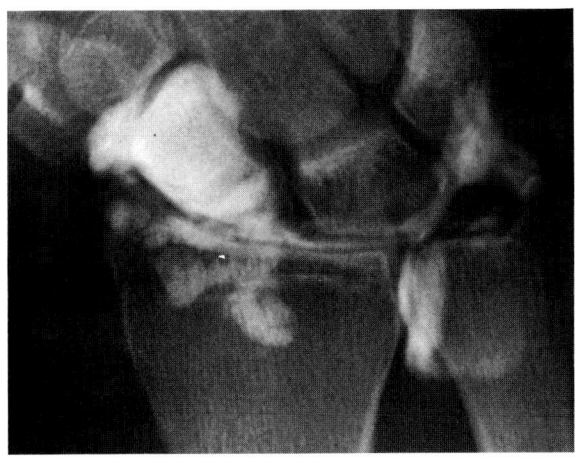

FIG. 14-67. Young male with chronic ulnar wrist pain. Arthrogram (PA view) with injection of the radiocarpal joint demonstrates communication with the distal radioulnar joint indicating a triangular cartilage tear.

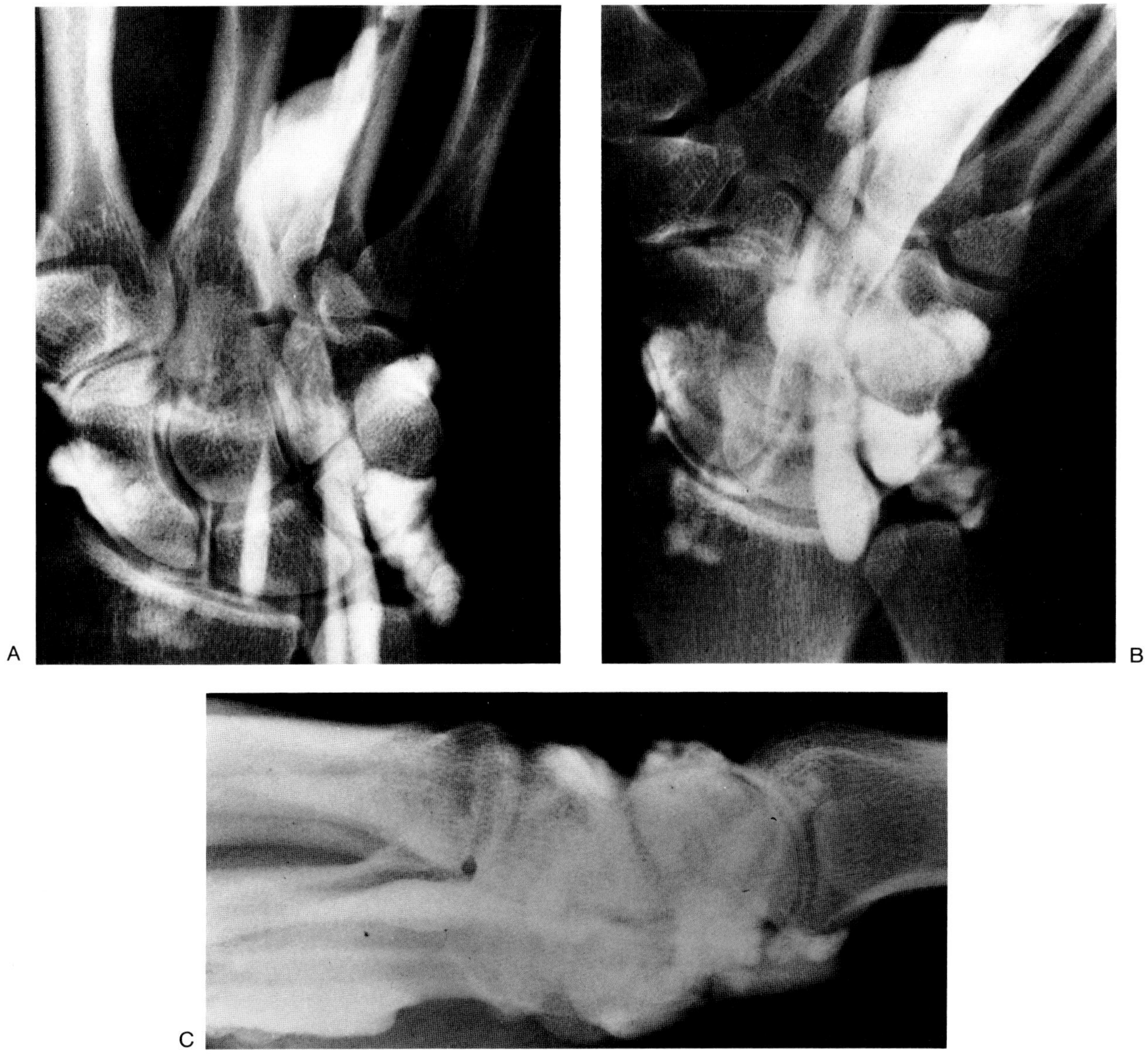

A

B

C

FIG. 14-68. AP (**A**), oblique (**B**), and lateral (**C**) views following radiocarpal injection. There is communication with the flexor tendon sheaths and mid carpal joint. The latter was due to a scapholunate tear.

(69). Radiocarpal injection is most effective in this setting (49).

Ganglia

Identification of periarticular ganglia may be difficult arthrographically. Frequently, more contrast material (5+ ml) and repeat exercise are necessary. Communication is more frequent with the midcarpal joint than with the radiocarpal joint. Therefore, the midcarpal joint should be injected when a ganglion is suspected. If injection of the wrist fails to demonstrate the mass, a direct injection of the ganglion may be useful. Currently, MRI is more frequently used to identify ganglia.

Arthritis

Arthrography may be useful in evaluation of early arthritic conditions, especially rheumatoid arthritis (50,81). Arthritic changes are nonspecific. The most common findings is intercompartmental communication. Resnick (81) noted this finding in 92% of patients with a similar incidence of synovitis. Lymphatic filling may be evident in 32–42% of cases. Communication with tendon sheaths may occur in up to 25% of patients.

Although the arthrographic findings may not be completely successful in differentiating the type of arthritis, synovial fluid analysis may be useful. This is especially true if infection is present.

Careful correlation of arthrographic findings with the clinical symptoms, proper injection technique, and fluo-roscopic control of injection and exercise result in highly accurate, informative wrist arthrograms.

Arthrography of the Hand

Arthrograms of the hand are most commonly performed to evaluate ligament injury, instability, and cartilage abnormalities (74,82). The technique is most often used to evaluate the first metacarpophalangeal joint of the thumb. Injury to the capsule and ulnar collateral ligament is common. This injury, formerly associated with gamekeepers, is commonly caused by skiing or other sporting injuries. The patient falls with the arm extended and the thumb forced into radial deviation. Subluxation or dislocation, resulting in weakness and decreased pinch strength, may occur (33,74). Bowers and Hurst (33) described associated chip fractures of the distal metacarpal in 55 of 109 cases.

Examination of the second through fifth metacarpophalangeal joints and the proximal interphalangeal joints may also be required. Arthrography is equally effective, although less commonly requested, in evaluation of these articulations.

Technique

The examination is performed with the patient prone to avoid syncopal attack (82). The joint is prepared using sterile technique. A .5-inch 25-gauge needle is used for

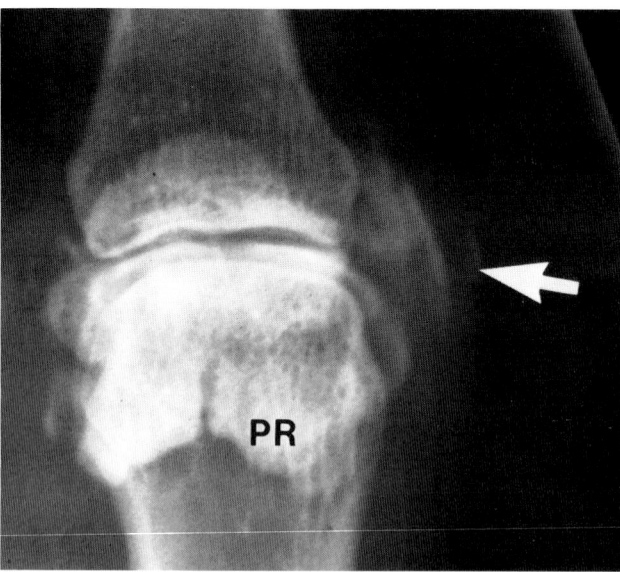

FIG. 14–69. Normal anatomy of the first metacarpophalangeal joint. PA view: There is no extracapsular contrast on the ulnar side of the joint. The palmar recess (PR) extends more proximal. The distal aspect of the capsule is small. Slight extravasation at the injection site (*arrow*) should not be confused with a capsular tear.

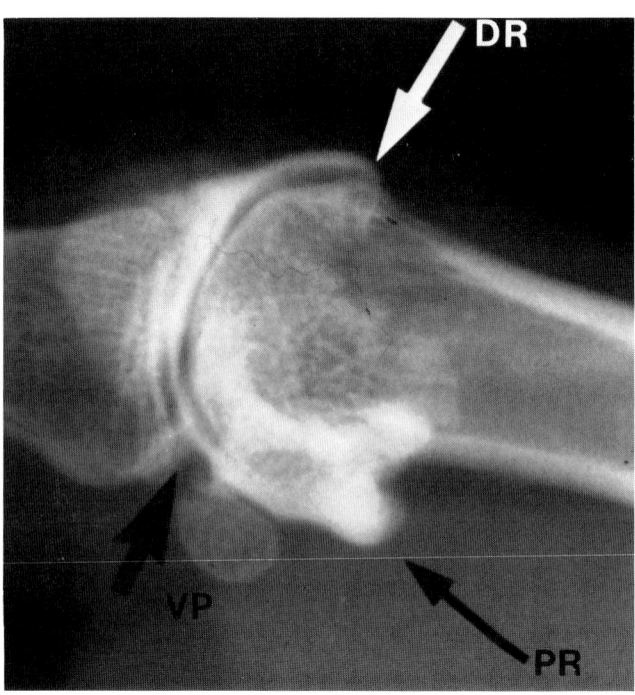

FIG. 14–70. Lateral view: The palmar (PR) and dorsal recesses (DR) extend to the metaphysis. The volar plate (VP) projects into the margin of the palmar articular surface.

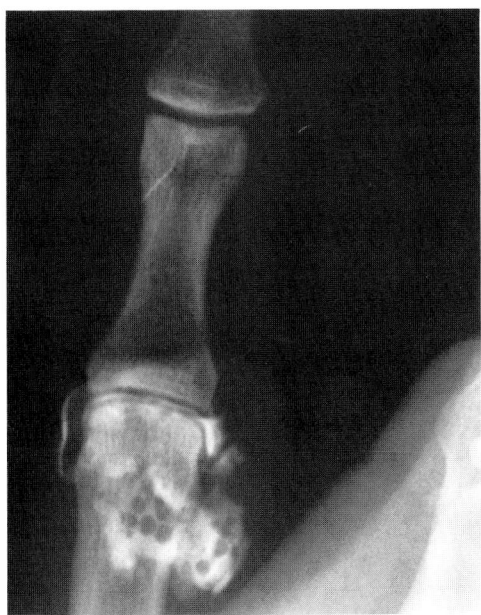

FIG. 14-71. Patient with ulnar capsular tear, right thumb. There is extravasation of contrast medium from the ulnar side of the capsule.

the injection of local anesthetic and the contrast material. The injection site should be dorsal and contralateral to the side of suspected injury. Most commonly, single-contrast technique is used. One to 1.5 ml of meglumine diatrizoate is injected. If ligament injury is not the primary concern, different techniques may be required. Study of the articular cartilage may be facilitated by double-contrast technique (0.1–0.3 ml of contrast material with 1 ml of air). Occasionally, trispiral tomography or magnification technique may be useful (82). Epinephrine is not used in the small joints because of the risk of vasospasm (82).

The injection and post-injection filming should be fluoroscopically monitored. Films are taken in AP and lateral projections and with ulnar and radial stress. Hyperextended lateral views are obtained if hyperextension injury is suspected.

Normal Arthrographic Anatomy

The capsule of the metacarpophalangeal joint is straight to slightly concave laterally owing to the radial and ulnar collateral ligaments (Fig. 14-69). Proximally, the capsule extends to a position near the metacarpal metaphysis, resulting in dorsal and palmar recesses (Fig. 14-70). A triangular plate extends into the palmar aspect of the joint (Fig. 14-71) (33,74,82).

Abnormal Arthrograms

Arthrograms are most accurate in the acute post-traumatic period. Extravasation of contrast material from the ulnar aspect of the capsule indicates capsular disruption with or without associated involvement of the ulnar collateral ligament (Fig. 14-71). If contrast material extends along the plane of the adductor pollicis muscle, a tear of the ulnar collateral ligament with involvement of the volar plate is more likely (Fig. 14-72) (33,82).

In patients with chronic instability or old capsular tears, the arthrogram will demonstrate irregularity, but extravasation may not occur. Chronic tears may fill in with fibrous tissue.

Examination of the interphalangeal joints is performed as easily and as accurately as in the case of the metacarpophalangeal joints. Ligament and capsule tears result in extravasation of contrast material. Associated periarticular fractures may occur.

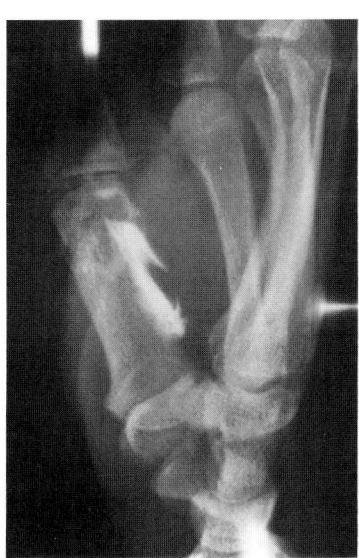
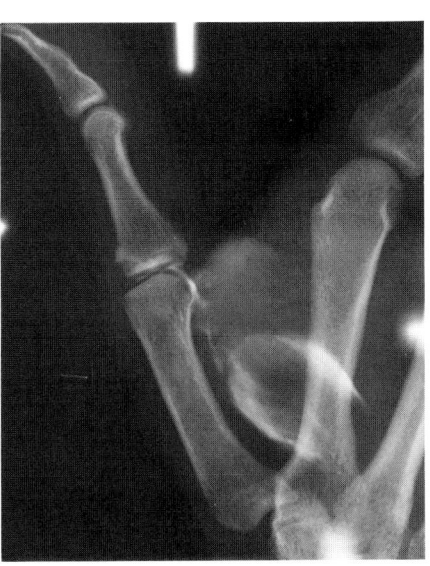

A   B

FIG. 14-72. Ulnar collateral ligament tear involving the volar aspect of the capsule. PA (**A**) and lateral (**B**) views demonstrate extravasation with extension along the muscle planes of the thenar eminence.

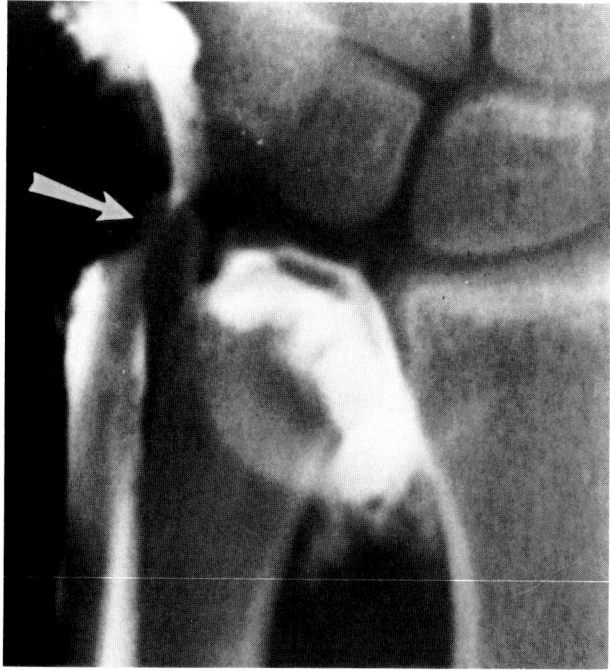

FIG. 14–73. Patient with ulnar pain. MRI and DRUJ injection were normal. Extensor carpi ulnaris tenogram showed stenosis of the tendon sheath (*arrow*) near the ulnar styloid. Anesthetic injection of the tendon sheath relieved the symptoms. Patient did well after tendon release.

Tenography of the hand and wrist is rarely indicated following trauma. Resnick (80,81) has described this technique in evaluation of patients with rheumatoid arthritis. When arthrograms are negative, diagnostic tenograms (Fig. 14-73) are useful when combined with diagnostic injection to localize symptoms and assist in selecting proper therapy.

FRACTURES AND DISLOCATIONS

Distal Radius Fractures

Fractures of the distal radius likely account for the lion's share of significant trauma about the wrist. They account for 17% of all emergency room fractures (160). It is also the wrist bone that most frequently requires manipulative reduction and hence careful sequential radiographic monitoring. Most fractures of the distal radius fall into one of five eponymic categories.

Colles' Fracture

The Colles' fracture, first described by Abraham Colles in 1813 prior to the discovery of the x-ray, is undoubtedly the most common fracture of the distal radius (159). This term is so well known that frequently, but

incorrectly, it is applied to all bony injuries of the radius. The term *Colles' fracture,* however, should be restricted to those fractures of the distal radial metaphysis or epiphysis, with or without intra-articular involvement, that are either displaced and angulated or have the tendency to displace or angulate in the dorsal direction (Fig. 14-74) (2,3,159). Most commonly, there is dorsal cortical comminution, but this is not a necessary feature of the fracture. There may or may not be an associated fracture of the ulnar styloid. There should be no demonstrable radiocarpal subluxation.

Radiographic evaluation can usually be adequately completed for this fracture with simple PA and lateral planar films. Interpretation, both pre- and post-reduction, should note the following characteristics of the fracture: (1) direction of displacement or angulation, if present (which, by definition, should be dorsal); (2) degree of comminution; (3) presence or absence of intra-articular involvement of the radiocarpal or distal radioulnar joint; (4) degree of apparent loss of radial length (or apparent positive ulnar variance); and (5) degree of loss of the ulnar inclination of the radial articular surface (normally 14°) on the PA projection and loss of the volar tilt of the articular surface (normally 12°) (2) on the lateral projection (see Fig. 14-1) (159).

Classification

A classification of Colles' fractures may be quite adequately accomplished by a comprehensive description of its characteristics. This should include details, for example, regarding displacement, angulation, comminution, and presence or absence of intra-articular involvement. Numerous classification systems have been proposed including the number of fragments and the extent of articular involvement (159). The AO Classification is most complex. This system is based on three major and three minor or subcategories. Type A fractures are extra-articular. Type B fractures are partially articular, and Type C fractures are completely articular. These categories are further divided into subcategories, i.e., C1, which is a simple articular and simple metaphyseal fracture; Type C2 is a simple articular fracture but a complex metaphyseal fracture; and Type C3 fractures have complex metaphyseal and articular involvement (159). However, a numerical classification described by Frykman (136) has gained acceptance and is useful in discussion of prognosis. This schema is based on the presence of intra-articular involvement of either the radiocarpal or distal radioulnar joint and the presence or absence of an associated ulnar fracture (Table 14-2) (Figs. 14-75 through 14-79). In addition to an anatomic classification as determined by radiographs, Colles' fractures may also be clinically classified as stable or unstable (116). This grouping may be made by the surgeon at the time of

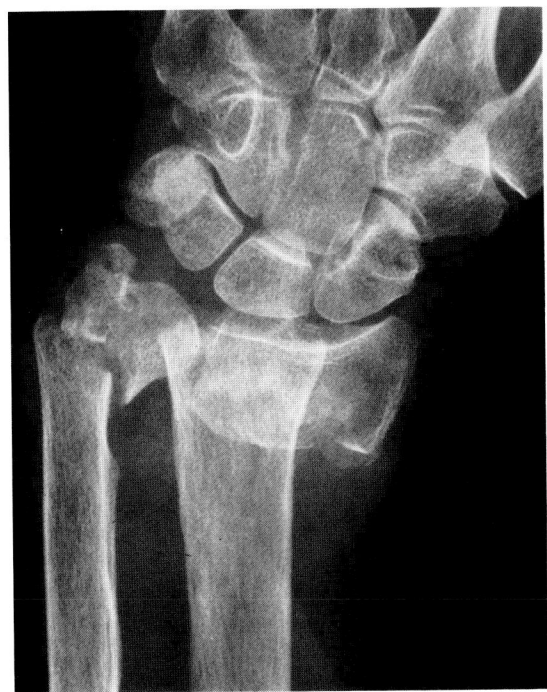

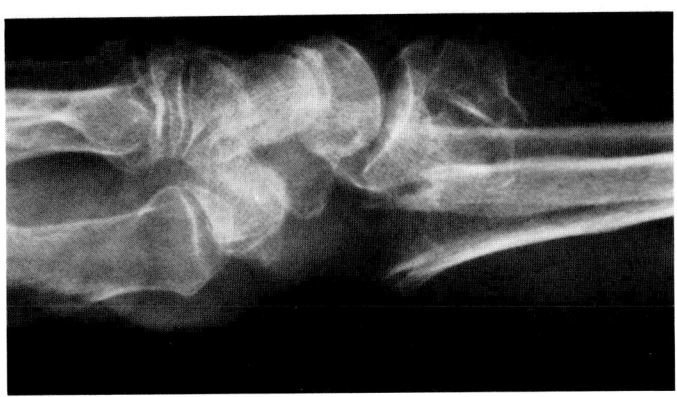

FIG. 14-74. PA (**A**) and lateral view (**B**) of the fractures of the distal radial and ulnar metaphysis with dorsal and radial displacement of the distal fragments.

A

B

reduction by the "feel" of the fracture or by demonstrated loss of position in the post-reduction period. Whether the fracture is stable will dictate the type of treatment and the degree of vigilance in monitoring the progress of healing. In general, those fractures with marked displacement, comminution, and intra-articular fracture lines will tend to be more unstable.

Mechanism of Injury

The mechanism of injury of the Colles' fracture is most usually a fall onto the outstretched hand. In an elderly patient with considerable osteoporosis, this may represent a relatively trivial trauma. However, in a younger patient a moderately violent force may be necessary to produce this fracture. In the latter instance, therefore, considerably more accompanying soft tissue injury can be anticipated, which may have implications in terms of the treatment options.

Treatment

The goal of treatment with the Colles'-type fracture is bony union in as close to an anatomic position as is possible and reasonable. Therefore, the minimally acceptable position will vary with the patient's age, other injuries, and other factors. In general, maintenance of radial length (neutral ulnar variance) (Fig. 14-79), 0°–10° of palmar tilt of the articular surface (lateral projection) (Fig. 14-80), 14° of ulnar inclination of the articular surface (PA projection), and articular congruity are the criteria for evaluating adequacy of reduction. The stable fracture (nondisplaced, minimally displaced, or reduced with maintenance of position) is managed by cast immobilization in 75–80% of patients (159). We generally prefer a position of forearm pronation and slight palmar flexion with ulnar deviation of the wrist for the first 3 weeks. Thereafter, a short-arm cast with the wrist in neutral position is used for an additional 3 weeks. Reduction, when necessary, is most easily achieved by longitudinal traction for approximately 10 minutes using finger traps and 8–10 pounds of counterweight (Fig. 14-81). A gentle attempt at manipulation involving a maneuver that extends the wrist, palmarly translates the

TABLE 14-2. *Frykman classification of Colles' fractures[a]*

Type	Fracture location	Distal ulnar fracture
I	Extra-articular	Absent
II	Extra-articular	Present
III	Intra-articular involving radiocarpal joint	Absent
IV	Intra-articular involving radiocarpal joint	Present
V	Intra-articular involving distal radioulnar joint	Absent
VI	Intra-artericular involving distal radioulnar joint	Present
VII	Intra-articular involving both radiocarpal and distal radioulnar joints	Absent
VIII	Intra-articular involving both radiocarpal and distal radioulnar joints	Present

[a] (136)

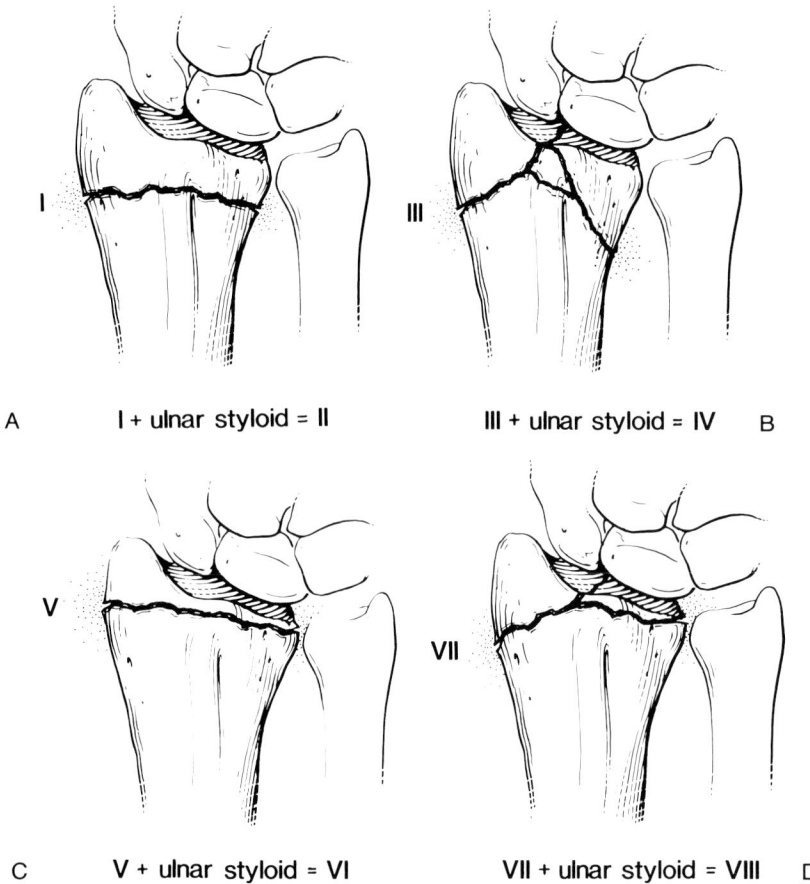

A   I + ulnar styloid = II   III + ulnar styloid = IV   B

C   V + ulnar styloid = VI   VII + ulnar styloid = VIII   D

FIG. 14–75. Fryckman classification (**A**). I, fracture of the distal radius without articular involvement. II, if the ulnar styloid is also fractured. **B:** III, fracture involves the radial carpal joint and IV, ulnar styloid. **C:** V, fracture involves the distal radioulnar joint; VI, if the ulnar styloid is fractured. **D:** VII, fractures involving both the radiocarpal and distal radioulnar joint; VIII, if the ulnar styloid is fractured.

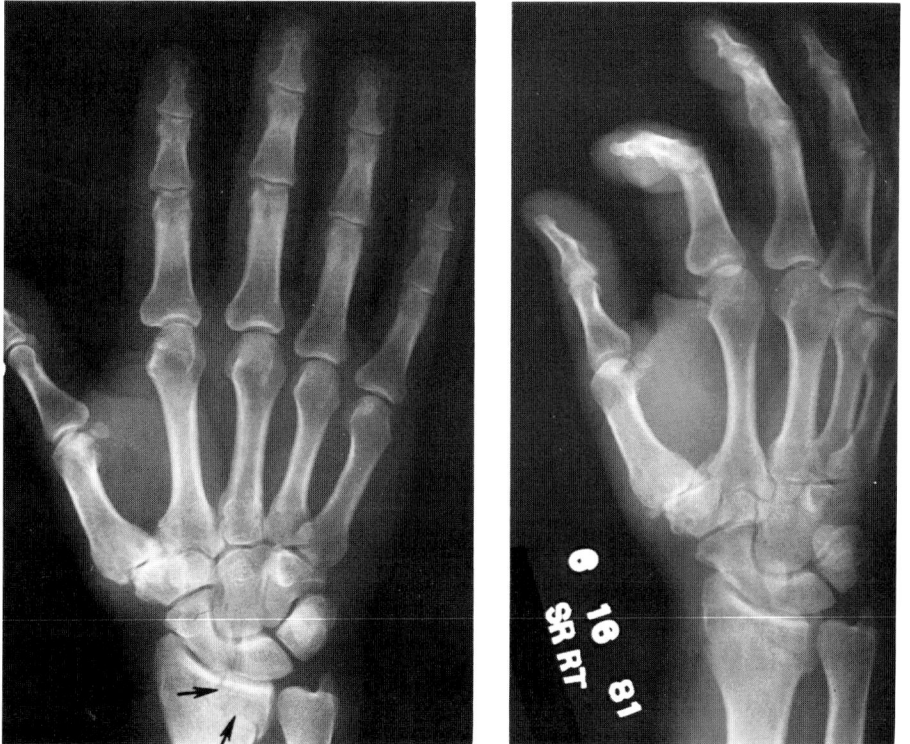

FIG. 14–76. Fryckman III fracture of the right wrist. AP (**A**) and oblique (**B**) views demonstrate a radial fracture (*arrow*) entering the radiocarpal joint. The ulnar styloid is not involved.

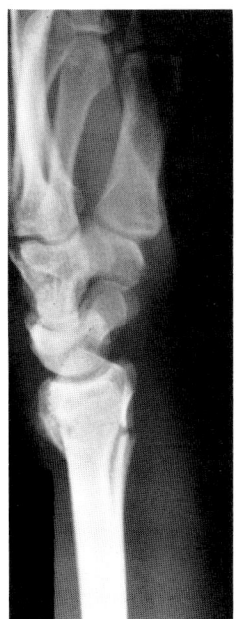
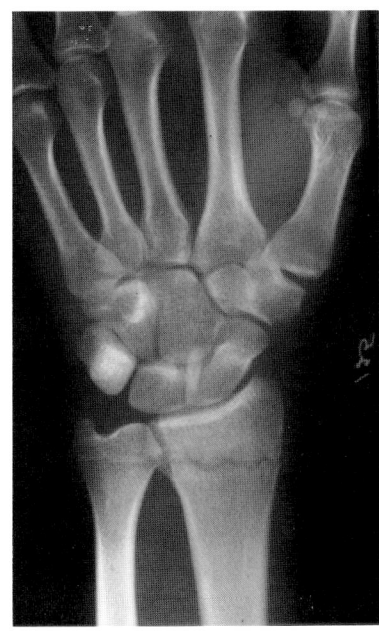

A   B

FIG. 14–77. Fryckman V fracture. Lateral (**A**) and PA (**B**) views of a distal radial fracture that enters the distal radioulnar joint. The ulnar styloid is not fractured.

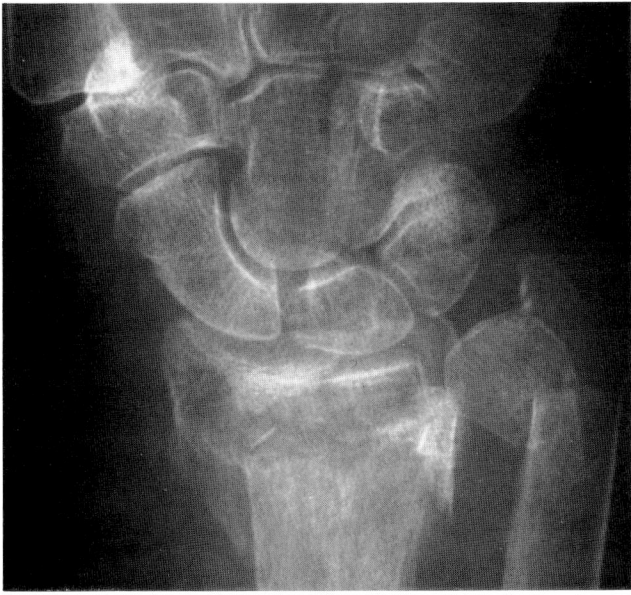

FIG. 14–78. Fryckman VIII fracture. PA view of the wrist with a comminuted fracture of the distal radius involving the radiocarpal and distal radioulnar joints with an associated ulnar fracture.

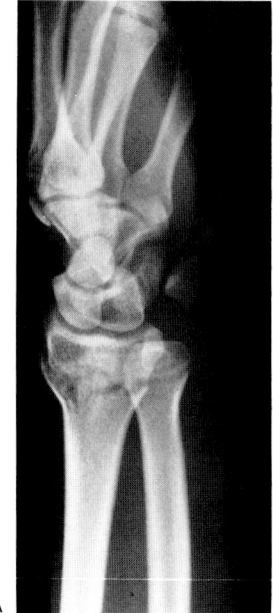
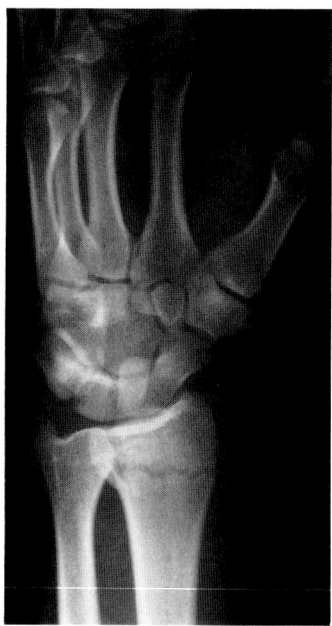

A

B

FIG. 14–79. Reduction views (oblique **A, B**) following a fracture of the distal radius (Fryckman V) with no loss of radial length and neutral ulnar variance.

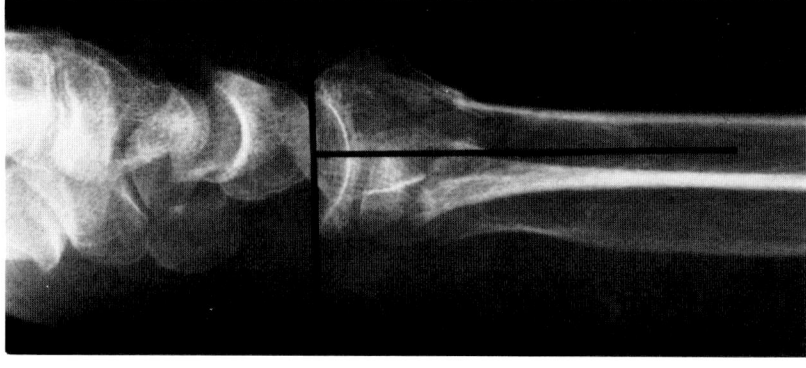

FIG. 14–80. Lateral view of the wrist following reduction of a Colles' fracture. The distal radial articular surface is vertical (0°).

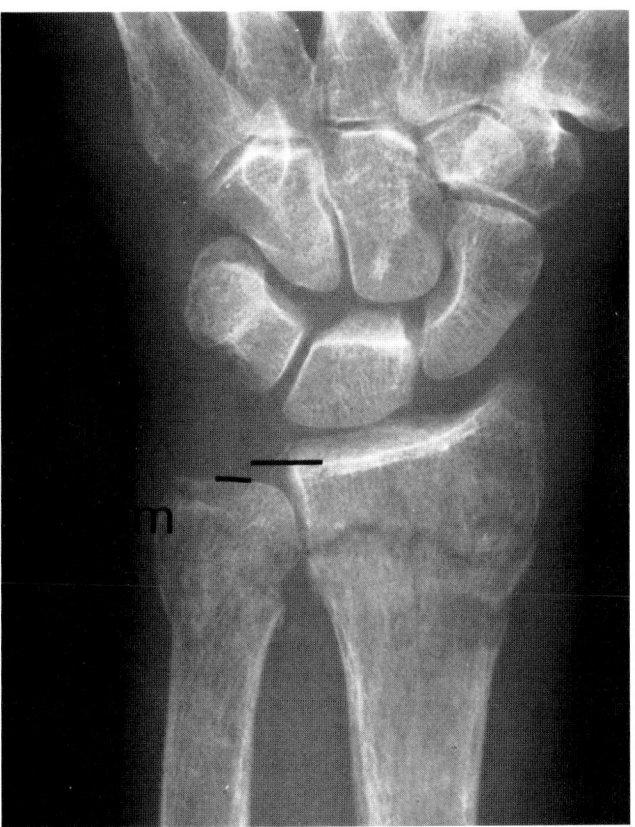

FIG. 14–81. Reduced Colles' fracture in traction. Note 2-mm negative ulnar variance. The widened carpal joint spaces are due to traction.

distal fracture fragment, and palmarly flexes the wrist may be necessary. Close post-reduction monitoring by weekly serial PA and lateral x-rays for the first 3 weeks is advisable unless the fracture is initially nondisplaced and stable. The unstable fracture can be managed by reduction and cast immobilization but only with some uncertainty owing to the possibility of a loss of reduction in the first 2 weeks following the injury (130,159,161,164).

For this reason, we generally favor a more aggressive approach to management with this injury. Reduction is generally not difficult to achieve by the same method described above. Once reduced, the unstable Colles' variant may be secured by either percutaneous Kirschner wires across the fracture site or by exoskeletal fixation (Fig. 14-82). The latter may be carried out using a variety of available appliances. Four-pin fixation (two proximally in the radius and two distally in the base of the second metacarpal, or one each in the base of the second and third metacarpals) is recommended (114,116). If exoskeletal means are used, the device should be maintained for at least 8 weeks before removal. Occasionally, soft tissue interposition, volar cortical comminution, or a depressed articular surface bone fragment may prevent closed reduction. In such cases, open reduction may be necessary. As the fracture heals, bone union or the presence of callus formation may be difficult to assess. Often the most reliable indicator of bony union will be maintenance of fracture position and absence of pain and tenderness.

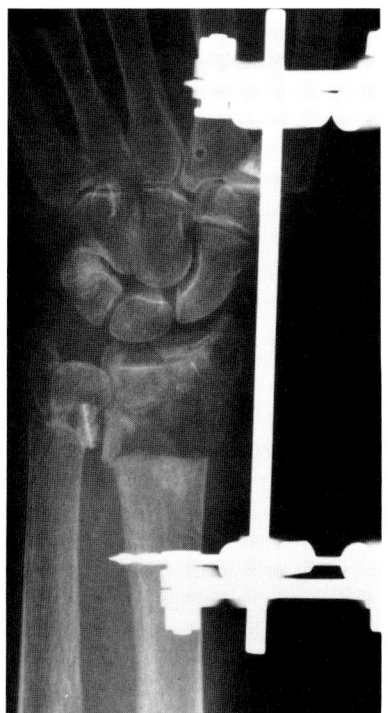

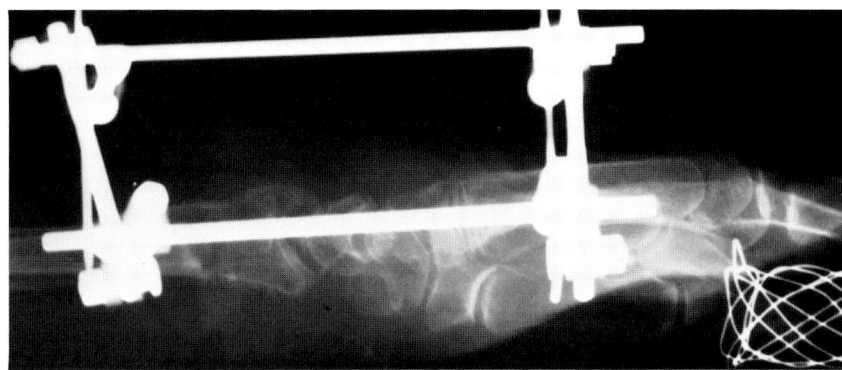

FIG. 14–82. Post reduction views of a Fryckman VIII fracture with finger traction and external fixation. (Same patient as Fig. 14-78.) **A:** AP view shows no radial shortening with slight ulnar minus variance. **B:** Lateral view shows 0° distal radial angle.

A

B

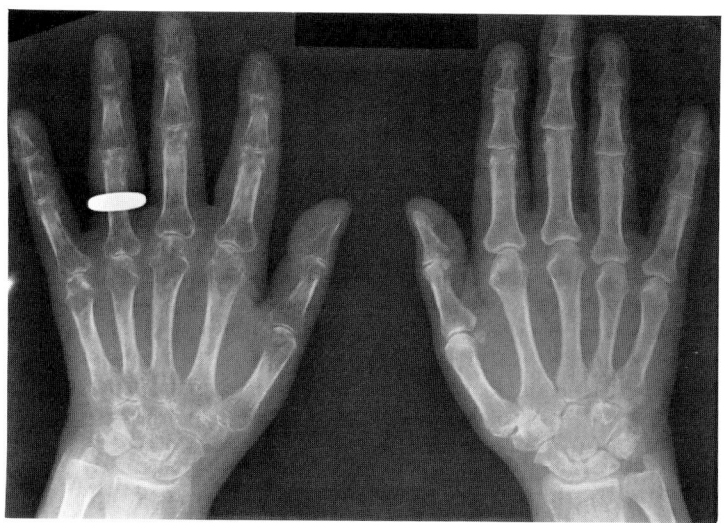

FIG. 14–83. PA views of both hands and wrist. Classic Sudeck's atrophy on the left with marked osteoporosis.

Complications

Complications following Colles' fracture are relatively frequent, with a reported rate of 31% (113). Eight major complications were described by Cooney et al. (113). These included (1) compressive neuropathy (7–9%), (2) arthrosis, (3) malunion, (4) tendon rupture, (5) unrecognized associated injuries, (6) fixation complications, (7) Volkman's ischemic contracture, and (8) shoulder hand syndrome. Median nerve injury is most easily identified using MRI (see Fig. 14-57). Similarly, injury to the tendons of the extensor pollicis longus or less frequently the flexor digitorum profunda or flexor pollicis longus may be evaluated with MRI. Tenography is less useful and more difficult to perform following acute injury (102).

Unrecognized injuries include scaphoid fractures, ligament injury, and radial head fracture (113).

The major problems with function may occur with post-traumatic autonomic dysfunction syndrome (sympathetic dystrophy), median nerve compression, residual wrist pain and deformity, and wrist or forearm limitations in range of motion (2). The first condition is often radiographically apparent by extreme bony rarefaction distal to the wrist (Fig. 14-83). The latter complications correlate fairly well with the adequacy of reduction (Figs. 14-84 and 14-85). Non-union of the Colles' fracture is extremely rare (113).

Smith Fracture Type

The Smith fracture was described by Robert Smith, a Dublin contemporary of Colles, in 1847 (188). This injury was described without the aid of x-rays as "a fracture of the lower end of the radius with displacement of the lower fragment along with the carpus forewards and the head of the ulna backwards. . . ." Most authors agree that this description refers essentially to a "reverse Colles' fracture." Therefore, the term *Smith fracture* should be restricted to those fractures of the distal radial metaphysis or epiphysis, with or without articular involvement, that are displaced or angulated in the palmar direction (Fig. 14-86). There may or may not be an associated fracture of the ulnar styloid. There should be no radiocarpal subluxation. In the orthopedic literature there is, however, some confusion regarding the Smith

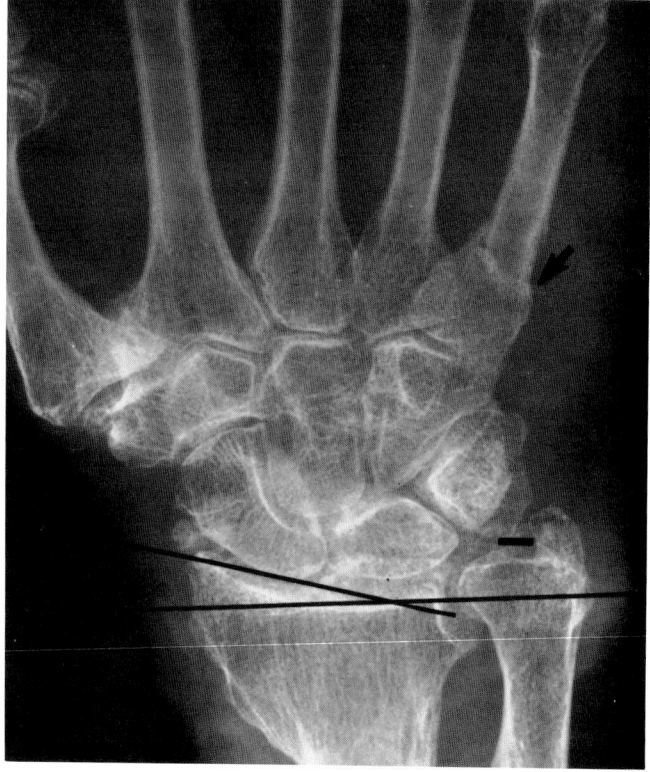

FIG. 14–84. Old Colles' fracture of the right wrist with loss of radial length and reduced ulnar tilt. Note the fracture of the fifth metacarpal (*arrow*).

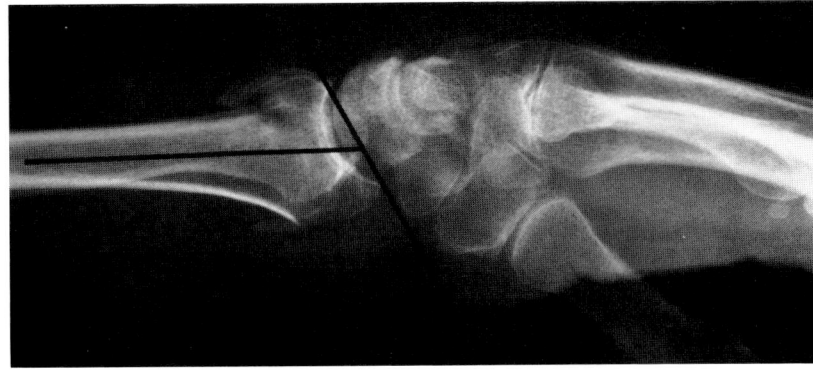

FIG. 14–85. Lateral view of Colles' fracture deformity with dorsal tilt of the distal radius. This position results in a poor prognosis.

fracture. Thomas has somewhat popularized a categorization of all palmarly displaced or angulated fractures of the distal radius, including the volar Barton-type fracture (to be discussed), as Smith-fracture variants (214). We believe, however, that this classification groups together heterogeneous injuries. We recommend limiting usage of the term *Smith fracture* to the fracture described earlier. Adequate radiographic evaluation generally requires only PA and lateral planar films. Interpretation of the x-rays should note the same general characteristics as described for the Colles' fracture.

Classification

In general, the Smith fracture can be adequately classified as extra-, juxta-, or intra-articular, with or without displacement or comminution. The Thomas classification of the Smith fracture is perhaps too inclusive but is in moderately widespread use (214). In this classification, Type I is the classic Smith fracture through the distal radial metaphysis and is wholly extra-articular. Type II is a typical volar Barton-type fracture (to be discussed), and Type III is an oblique juxta-articular fracture with a greater degree of instability than that of Type I (Fig. 14-87).

Mechanism of Injury

The mechanism of injury as originally suggested by Smith was hyperflexion from a fall on the palmar flexed wrist. Others suggest that a blow to the dorsum of the wrist and hand or a hypersupination-type injury with a

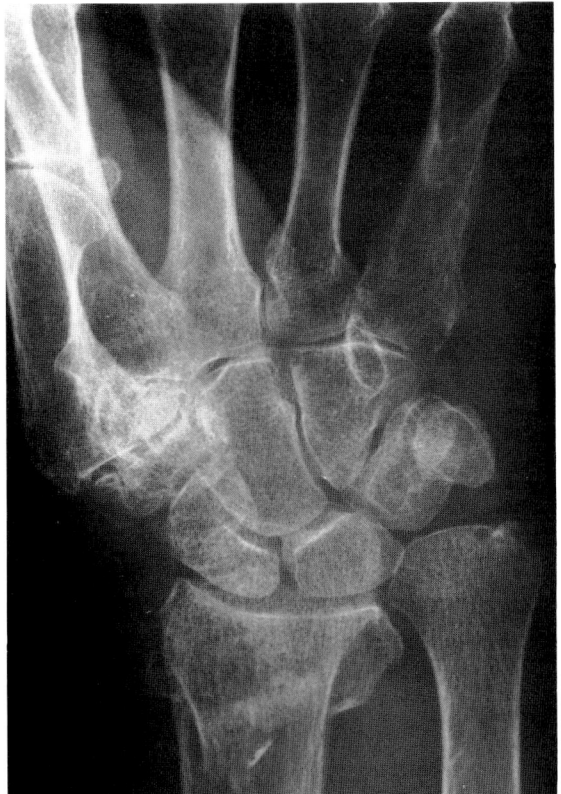

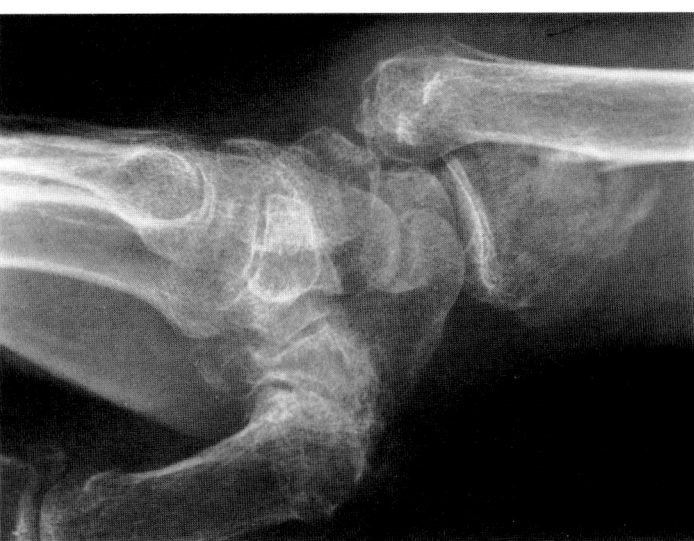

FIG. 14–86. Juxta-articular (Thomas Type III). Smith's fracture. PA (**A**) and lateral (**B**) radiographs demonstrate marked volar displacement of the distal radial fragment with considerable radial shortening and almost no ulnar tilt.

A

B

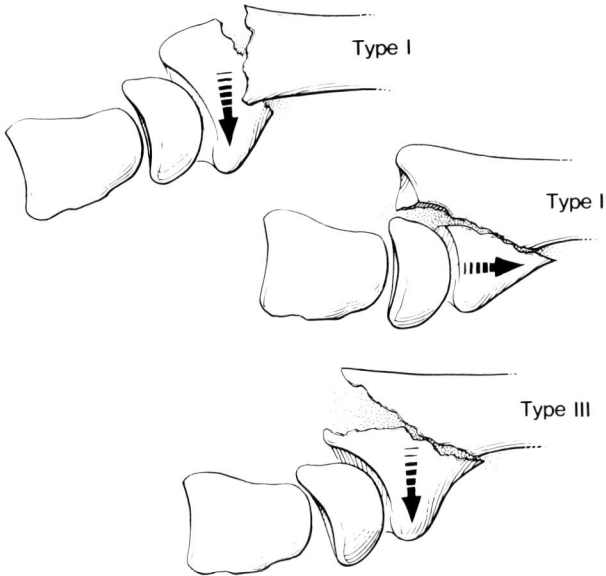

FIG. 14–87. Thomas classification of Smith fractures. Type I, extra-articular; Type II, volar intra-articular fracture; Type III, oblique juxta-articular fracture.

fall onto the extended wrist may reproduce this fracture type (2).

Treatment

The goals of treatment and the criteria for an acceptable reduction are basically identical to those outlined for the Colles' fracture. Reduction is usually achieved by simple longitudinal traction, as discussed in the previous section. If a gentle, manipulative reduction is also required, it is generally accomplished in a manner opposite to that of the Colles' fracture, i.e., hyperflexion followed by extension and dorsal translation of the wrist. Most often the typical extra-articular variety (Type I in Thomas's classification) (Fig. 14-87) is stable following reduction and can be maintained in a long-arm cast that immobilizes the forearm in a position of supination with the wrist neutral. This position should be maintained for a period of 3–4 weeks followed by a short-arm cast with the wrist neutral for an additional 3 weeks. As with the Colles' fracture, serial x-rays to ensure maintenance of reduction in the cast for the first 3 weeks following injury are advised. Smith fractures with greater degrees of comminution or with obliquely directed juxta-articular fracture lines (Thomas Type III) may be unstable (Fig. 14-87). Such fractures may be candidates for percutaneous fixation or exoskeletal fixation, as previously described. Rarely is open reduction and internal fixation indicated.

Complications

The complications of the Smith fracture are virtually identical to those of the Colles' fracture. Residual sub-luxation of the distal radioulnar joint with pain or impaired grip strength is not uncommon.

Barton's Fracture Type

The Barton fracture is credited to John Rhea Barton, a Philadelphia surgeon who described this injury in 1838 (187). This term implies, in Barton's own words, "a subluxation of the wrist, consequent to a fracture through the articular surface of the carpal extremity of the radius." Therefore, by definition, this injury represents a marginal rim fracture of the radius that displaces along with the carpus, in this way producing a fracture-subluxation (Fig. 14-88) (124). The latter feature, therefore, distinguishes this fracture from an intra-articular Colles' or Smith fracture. In his original description, Barton described the injury involving the dorsal or palmar lip of the radius. He believed the former to be more common. However, the palmar variety of this fracture is, in fact, more commonly seen. Furthermore, this variety is indeed the injury described by Thomas as a Type II Smith fracture (see Fig. 14-87). Considerable confusion is present in the literature regarding the terminology of Barton and reverse Barton fractures. The terms have been applied depending on whether the dorsal or palmar lip of the radius is fractured (187,215). We suggest that a distinction in terminology between palmar and dorsal Barton-type fractures will obviate any confusion in this regard.

Adequate radiographic evaluation generally requires only PA and lateral radiographs. It may be particularly important to obtain a high-quality, true-lateral projection to appreciate the degree of carpal subluxation accompanying the fracture fragment. At times, particularly in assessing the adequacy of reduction, lateral trispiral tomograms or CT in the coronal and sagittal planes may be helpful to evaluate the articular congruity of the distal radius.

Classification

Adequate classification of the Barton fracture simply notes the location of the marginal fracture as palmar or dorsal, with or without comminution. By definition, the fracture is always intra-articular, exhibits some displacement, and is accompanied by a subluxation of the carpus.

Mechanism of Injury

The palmar Barton-type fracture (Fig. 14-89) probably occurs by a mechanism similar to that described for Smith-type injuries with perhaps an exaggerated degree of loading in compression across the wrist. The dorsal variety most often results from a fall that produces wrist

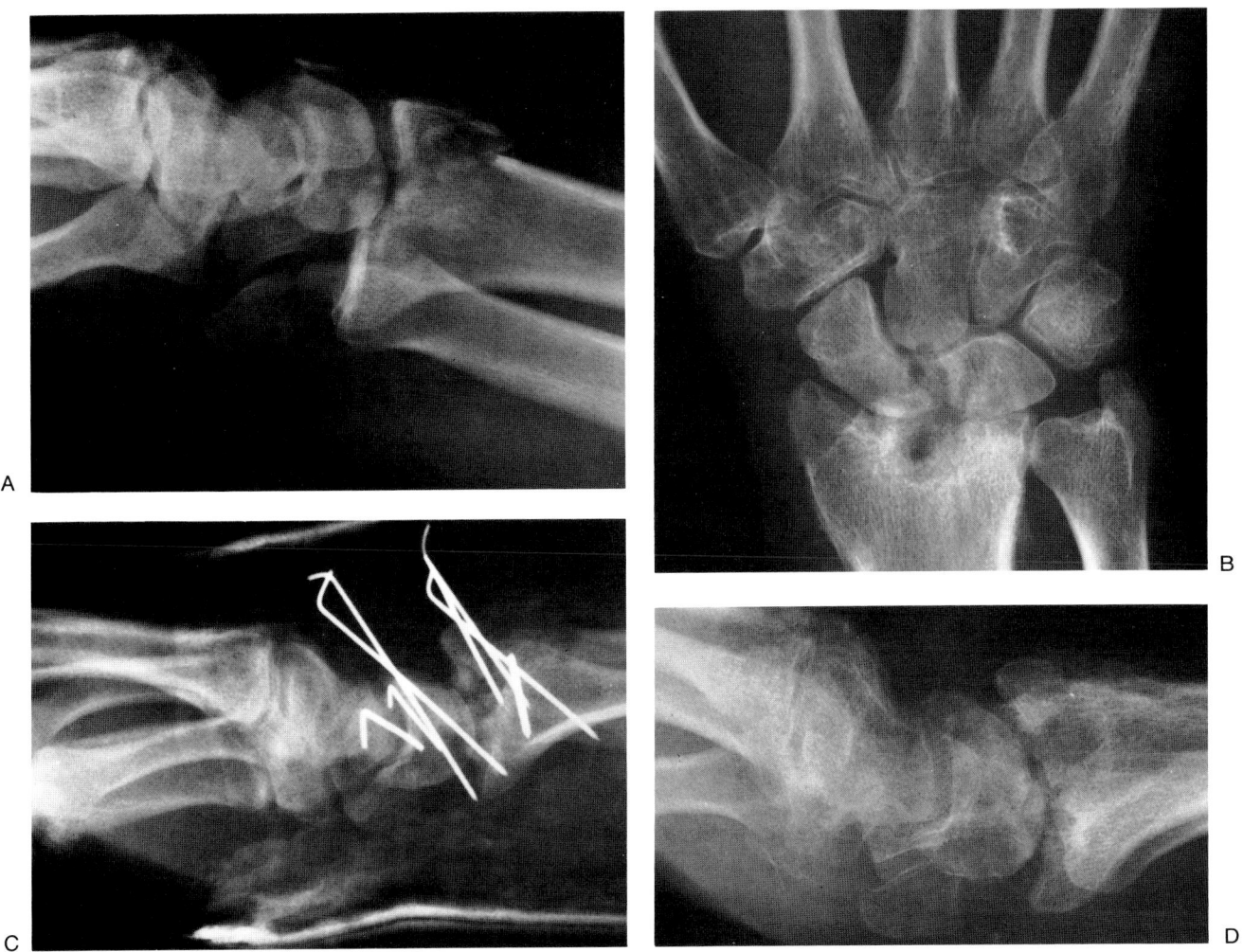

FIG. 14–88. A: Dorsal Barton's fracture of the distal radius with a chip fracture of the triquetrum. **B:** The fracture was reduced with K wires. The PA (**C**) and lateral (**D**) views demonstrate advanced degenerative changes in the radiocarpal joint after healing.

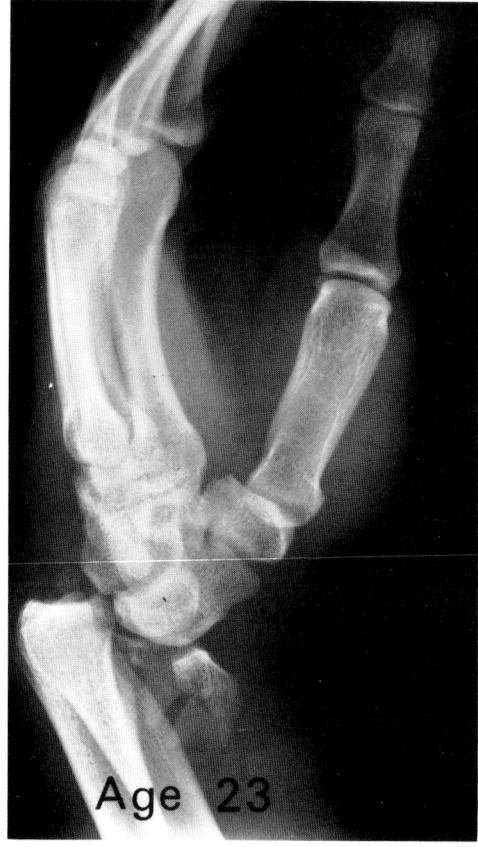
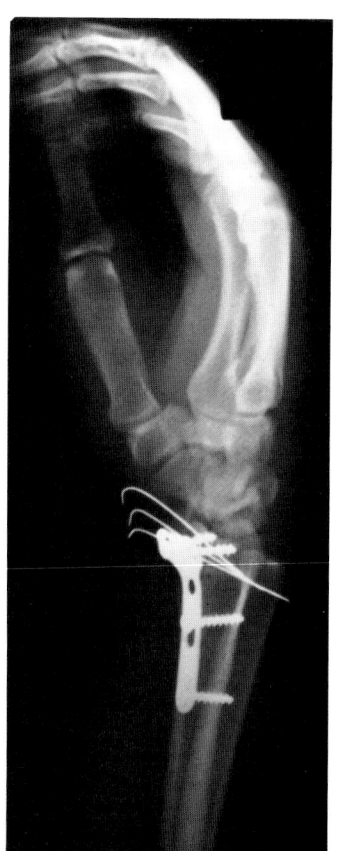

A

B

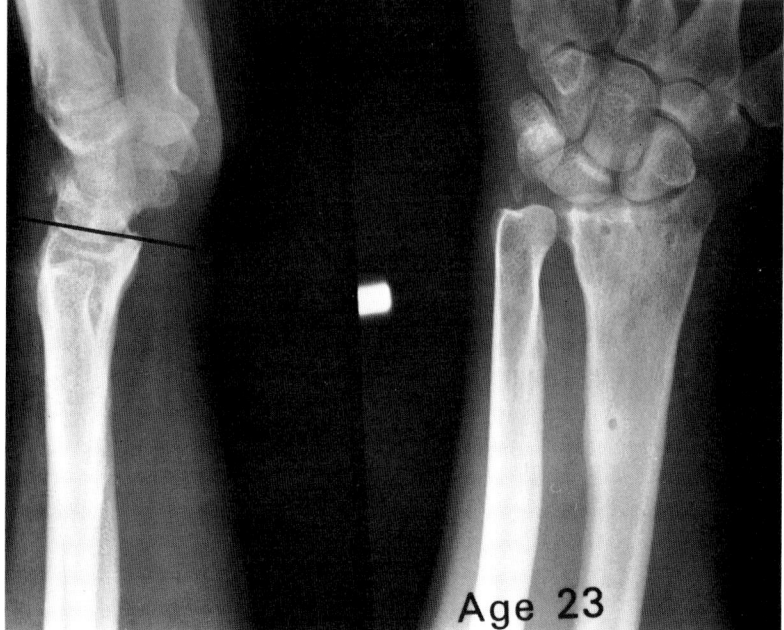

C

FIG. 14–89. A: Lateral view of a comminuted volar Barton's fracture with considerable subluxation. **B:** The fragments are in good position following plate and K wire fixation. **C:** Healed fracture following removal of the plate and screws. The distal radial angle is normal (*line*). There is slight ulnar minus variance with radiocarpal arthrosis.

extension and forearm pronation under compressive loading.

Treatment

Reduction by simple longitudinal traction as described earlier usually is readily achieved. Occasionally, impaction of the fracture fragments may prevent adequate closed reduction. The major difficulty with this injury, however, is maintenance of a perfect reduction. Cast treatment may be successful, particularly if the fracture is stable to a trial of gentle manipulation at the time of reduction. If so, the dorsal variety fracture should be immobilized in a long-arm cast in a position of forearm pronation and neutral position or slight wrist extension. Palmar flexion should be avoided, as this appears to increase the tendency of the carpus to translate dorsally with recurrence of the subluxation. The palmar Barton fracture should be immobilized in the opposite position, that is, in a position of forearm supination and neutral or slight palmar flexion of the wrist.

If an anatomic closed reduction is not achieved, or if the fracture conveys the impression of marked instability at the time of reduction, some means of internal fixation is advised. For the dorsal variety, Kirschner wires placed percutaneously or under direct vision will often suffice for this purpose. The more common palmar variety is probably best managed by an open procedure with application of a volar buttress-type plate (128) and additional screw or pin fixation as needed (Fig. 14-89). Occasionally, if the fracture is unstable but inappropriate for an open procedure, exoskeletal fixation as previously described may be indicated.

Complications

The same array of complications as outlined for the Colles' fracture may occur with this injury. The major late sequela of the Barton-type fracture, however, is residual radiocarpal subluxation and articular incongruity, leading to degenerative arthrosis of the wrist (Fig. 14-90). Evaluation of this injury is most easily accomplished with computed tomography (CT).

Chauffeur's Fracture (Radial Styloid Fracture)

The chauffeur's fracture refers to an intra-articular fracture of the distal radius chiefly involving the radial styloid. The fracture line typically originates at the junction of the scaphoid and lunate fossae on the radial articular surface and courses laterally in a transverse or oblique direction. It may also be known by the eponym *Hutchinson's fracture* (2,3). It is best appreciated radiographically on a PA projection (Fig. 14-91A). The lateral projection may reveal few if any abnormalities (Fig. 14-91B).

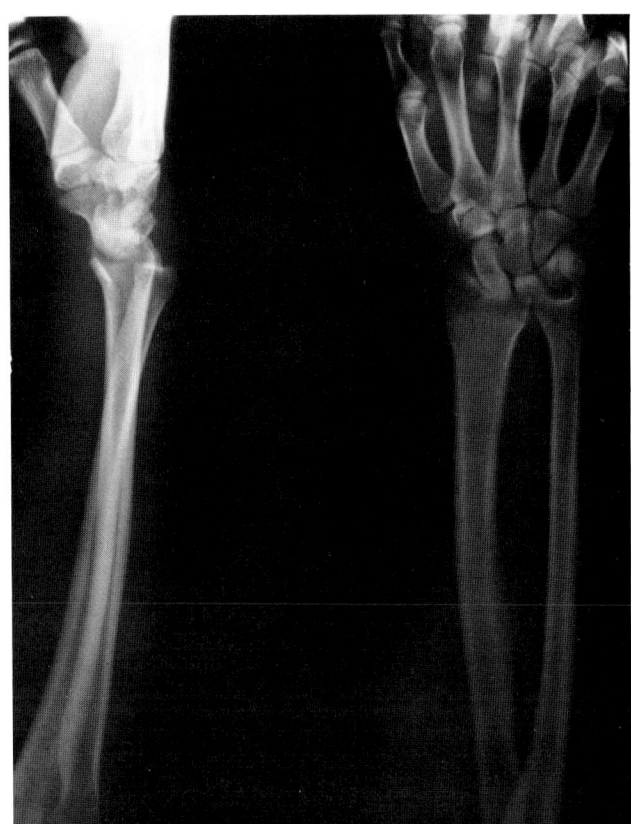

FIG. 14–90. Lateral (**A**) and PA (**B**) views of the forearm in a patient with an old Barton's fracture. Note the radiocarpal subluxation. There is also dorsal subluxation of the distal radioulnar joint.

Classification

This fracture may be simple or comminuted, displaced or undisplaced. By definition it is intra-articular. There should be no evidence of radiocarpal subluxation.

Mechanism of Injury

The likely mechanism of this fracture is direct axial compression transmitted through the scaphoid. Clinically, this injury was associated decades ago with the backfire of the starting crank of an automobile engine (127).

Treatment

If the fracture is nondisplaced or only slightly displaced (<1 mm articular depression), simple cast immobilization is sufficient. Because the brachioradialis tendon inserts on the radial styloid, an above-elbow cast with the elbow in 90° of flexion is advisable at least for the first 3 weeks. Usually 6 weeks is sufficient for complete bony union. If the fracture is moderately displaced,

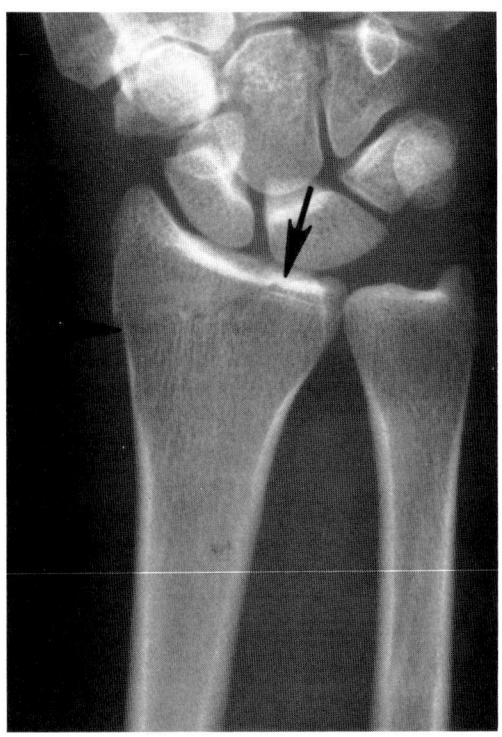

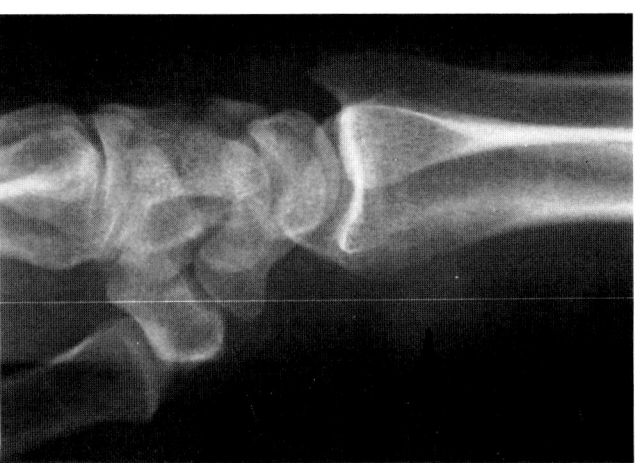

FIG. 14–91. A: PA view of the wrist demonstrating a typical chauffeur's fracture (*arrows*). **B:** Lateral view of the wrist with chauffeur's fracture. Obliteration of the pronator fat stripe (*arrow*) is the only indication of injury.

A

B

manipulative reduction is required. If the fracture is stable, fixation may be possible with cast immobilization following reduction. However, in general, if reduction is required, percutaneous fixation with multiple Kirschner wires or open fixation with either Kirschner wires or screws is advised.

Complications

Complications are similar to those discussed for other groups of distal radius fractures.

Galeazzi Fracture (Piedmont Fracture)

The Galeazzi fracture is included in this section, although it frequently falls outside of the topography of the wrist. This eponym refers to a fracture of the radius that usually, but not always, involves the diaphysis at the junction of the middle and distal thirds with an associated subluxation of the distal radioulnar joint (2,122,178). The latter feature may not always be apparent at the time of initial injury and may not become apparent until treatment is under way (Fig. 14-92). Variants of the Galeazzi fracture include fractures involving the distal metaphysis (Fig. 14-93) or the more proximal diaphysis of the radius (Fig. 14-94) and cases involving fracture of the distal ulna in association with the radius injury. This injury is particularly important to recognize and differentiate from a Colles'-type fracture, since its

treatment is quite different. Routine PA and lateral projections of the forearm are usually adequate to make the diagnosis. However, localized views of the wrist in the AP and true lateral positions may be necessary to evaluate the distal radioulnar joint (Fig. 14-92).

Classification

The fracture may be comminuted, but usually it is a simple oblique or transverse fracture of the distal radial diaphysis. It may be initially nondisplaced. Displacement characteristically involves the distal radial fragment shortening and angulating in a radial direction by the pull of the brachioradialis (2). Usually only the displaced variety will exhibit significant radioulnar subluxation radiographically.

Mechanism of Injury

A fall onto the outstretched hand with hyperpronation of the forearm is the usual cause of this injury. Occasionally, a direct blow on the dorsiradial aspect of the wrist may produce the fracture.

Treatment

Hughston has pointed out that closed treatment is unsatisfactory in 92% of cases (154). Therefore, in nearly all

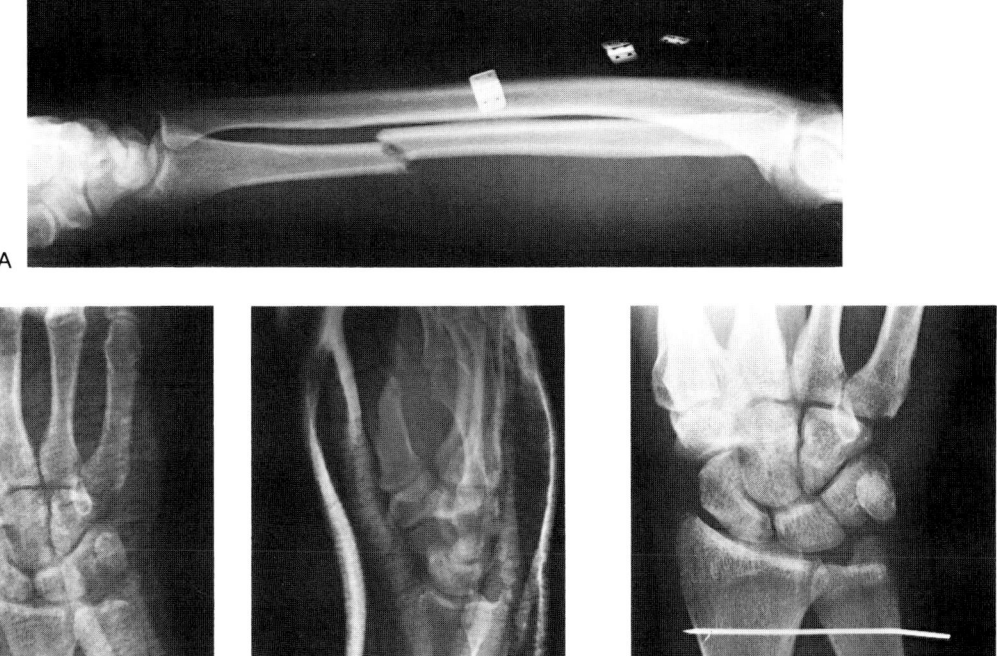

FIG. 14-92. Galeazzi fracture. **A:** Single view of the forearm demonstrates a fracture of the radial diaphysis. PA (**B**) and lateral (**C**) views following casting show incomplete reduction of the radius. The distal radioulnar subluxation is subtle but was recognized. **D:** The fracture was plated and the distal radioulnar joint internally fixed with a K wire.

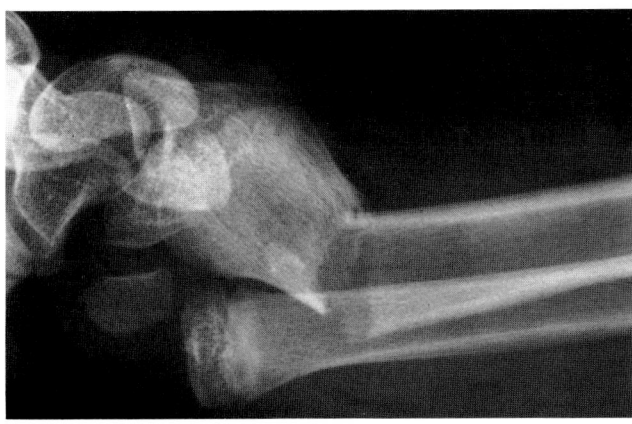

FIG. 14-93. Galeazzi variant. There is a fracture of the distal radius metaphysis with obvious dislocation of the distal radioulnar joint on the lateral view.

cases this fracture should be managed by reduction and internal stabilization. In the usual instance involving the shaft of the radius, open reduction and internal fixation of the radius with a compression plate is recommended. The distal radioulnar joint can then be reduced with closed technique using forearm supination and fixed percutaneously with a Kirschner wire (see Figs. 14-92 and 14-94). The forearm should be maintained in a position of supination for 6 weeks following the operation. Then it should be further protected for 3–6 weeks by a short-arm cast or removable splint. Some authors advocate open repair of the distal radioulnar joint in such cases. If the injury is a variant of the typical Galeazzi fracture and involves the distal radial metaphysis, a compression plate may prove unsatisfactory for fixation. In such instances, reduction followed by Kirschner-wire or exo-

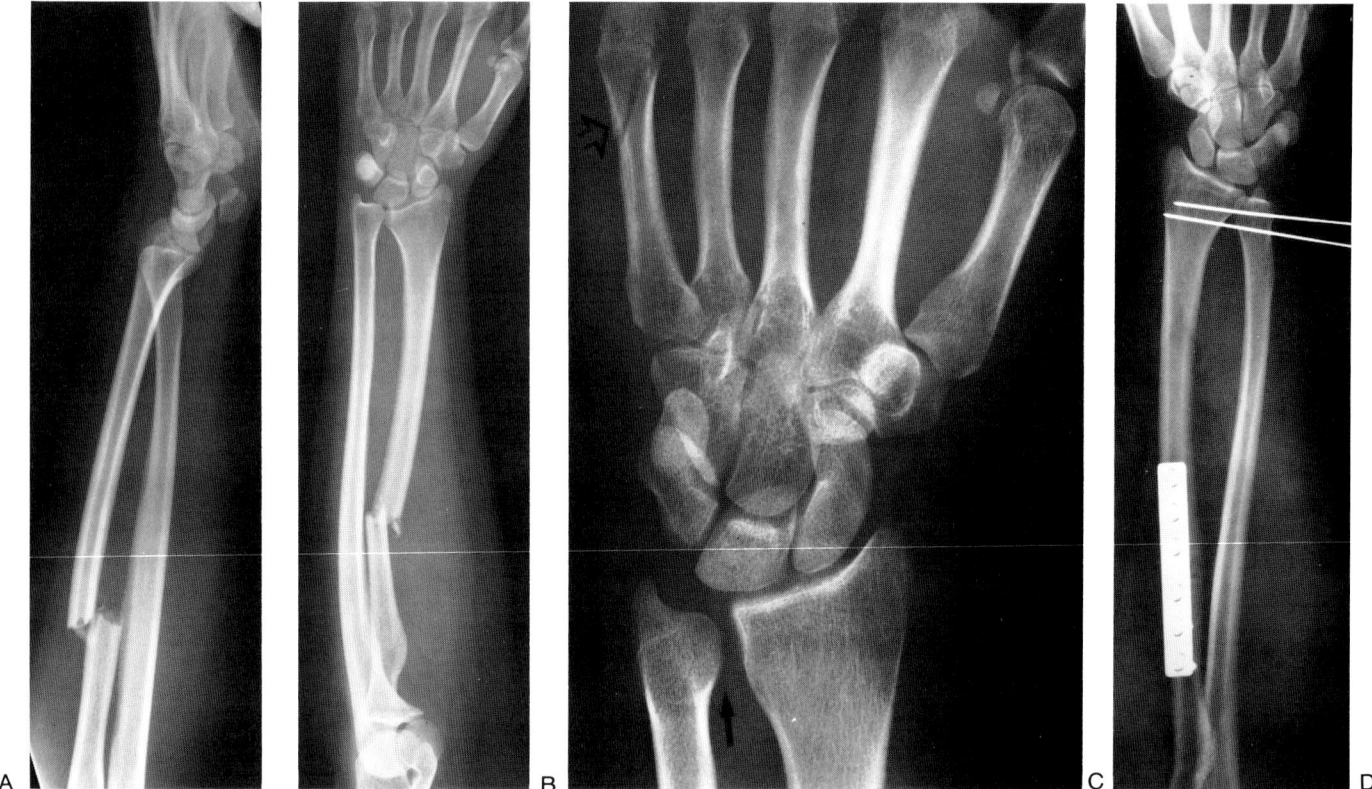

A   B   C   D

FIG. 14–94. Galeazzi variant. **A:** AP and lateral (**B**) views of the forearm demonstrate a proximal radial fracture. **C:** The AP view of the wrist makes the distal radioulnar subluxation (*black arrow*) more obvious (widened). There is also an oblique fracture of the fifth metacarpal (*open arrow*). **D:** The fracture is internally fixed with plate and screws and the distal radioulnar joint with K wires.

skeletal fixation may be best. Again, distal radioulnar joint reduction by forearm supination and percutaneous fixation should not be overlooked.

Complications

The most frequent complication of the Galeazzi fracture is malunion of the radius and residual subluxation of the distal radioulnar joint. This results most often from inadequate treatment, usually because of failure to recognize the differences between this fracture and either the Colles' or Smith variety. In contrast to the injuries mentioned above, delayed union or non-union is not unusual (154). If the fracture is seen late, chronic symptomatic subluxation of the distal radioulnar joint may require distal ulna excision (125).

In addition to the fracture groups mentioned above, variations of any of these involving an accompanying fracture of the distal ulna can be seen. Strictly speaking, these are *distal both-bone forearm* fractures. Most often these represent an injury similar to the Galeazzi fracture, with bony rather than ligamentous damage to the distal ulna. Similar treatment principles as discussed earlier apply in this group as well.

Dislocations about the Distal Radius

Dislocations of the distal radioulnar joint, or, rarely, the radiocarpal joint, can be seen in the absence of an accompanying fracture of the distal radius.

Distal Radioulnar Joint—Dorsal Dislocation

This is the most common type of dislocation-subluxation of the distal ulna (121,148,151). The usual cause is a hyperpronation injury to the wrist (97). Clinically, the patient maintains the forearm in a position of moderate pronation and resists supination. The distal ulna is usually dorsally prominent (179). Radiographic evaluation may reveal only subtle abnormalities. On a true lateral view of the wrist, the distal ulna should appear dorsally displaced. Minor degrees of forearm rotation may obscure this finding, however. Perhaps of greater significance is the PA projection, which suggests overlap, widening, or incongruity of the distal radioulnar joint (Fig. 14-93) (219). Images in the axial plane (CT or MRI) may be useful in diagnosing these injuries. If the dislocation is seen early, closed treatment by forearm supination and maintenance of this reduction through approximately 6 weeks of long-arm cast immobilization is usually satisfactory (2,97). Occasionally, closed reduction is not successful, particularly if treatment is delayed. In such cases, open reduction, temporary Kirschner-wire fixation, and repair or reconstruction of the damaged ligamentous structures may be indicated (156).

Distal Radioulnar Joint—Volar Dislocation

This injury results from a hypersupination stress to the forearm (13,225). Clinically, the patient presents with the forearm maintained in supination. The wrist appears narrowed in the lateral plane, and there may be a prominence or fullness over the palmar ulnar aspect of the wrist. Radiographic evaluation should suggest palmar displacement of the distal ulna on the lateral view and overlap of the distal radius and ulna in the frontal plane (Fig. 14-95). Reduction may be more difficult in this case than in the dorsal counterpart to this injury. It should be carried out by forearm supination with direct pressure in a dorsal direction over the displaced head of the ulna. Maintenance of reduction by long-arm cast immobilization with the forearm in a position of mild pronation should be continued for 6 weeks. If irreducible, open reduction and repair or reconstruction should be carried out.

Radiocarpal Dislocation

In the absence of significant bony injury to the distal radius or as a variant of a perilunate dislocation, radiocarpal dislocation is extremely rare (131). Displacement of the carpus in both the palmar and dorsal directions has been more commonly reported with perilunate dislocation (2,3).

Carpal Fractures

Fractures of the carpus frequently involve multiple bones or a single bone in association with significant ligamentous injury. The possibility of such a combination of injured structures must be carefully kept in mind when evaluating these fractures.

Scaphoid

The scaphoid is the most frequently fractured carpal bone (115,126,139,152,218). Scaphoid fractures account for 70% and 55% of all carpal injuries in the Mayo and Böhler series, respectively (2,3). Whether justified, the prognosis for these injuries has a sinister reputation. Union rates ranging from 50% to 95% have been reported (139). Furthermore, one must be vigilant to rule out or recognize a "transcaphoid-perilunate dislocation"

(to be discussed later) when evaluating the fractured scaphoid. Failure to recognize significant concomitant soft tissue injury may lead to serious errors in management. Although rare, associated injuries of the radial head have been reported. Attention to this more obvious area of symptoms can lead to overlooking scaphoid fractures (138).

If nondisplaced, fractures of the scaphoid may be difficult to detect on routine radiographs. The minimum requirements include PA, lateral, and scaphoid views. Air-gap magnification, particularly of the oblique projection, may enhance detail. Changes in the navicular fat stripe, as mentioned earlier in the section "Routine Radiographic Techniques," may be noted. If a high index of clinical suspicion persists despite negative initial films, repeat x-ray evaluation at approximately 2 weeks following the injury may be indicated. Usually, but not always, a fracture line may be obvious at this stage. If there should still be some doubt as to the presence of a fracture following the second radiographic study, further evaluation using Tc-99m methyl diphosphonate bone scans and trispiral tomography may be indicated. Generally in such cases we recommend the use of a bone scan as a screening study and proceed with trispiral tomography only if the bone scan shows focal abnormality in the scaphoid region. Lack of an area of increased uptake in the carpus effectively rules out a fracture (150,183,186).

If the fracture is displaced, there is usually little difficulty in diagnosing the scaphoid fracture on routine radiographic views. However, trispiral tomography, particularly on the lateral plane, may be extremely helpful in assessing the degree of displacement or angulation of the fracture, the adequacy of an attempt at reduction, or the presence of any associated carpal instability patterns (Fig. 14-96). In general, most displaced scaphoid fractures involving the waist (middle third) of the bone will tend to exhibit angulation of the distal fragment in a palmar direction, with resultant foreshortening of the carpal height, and dorsiflexion-instability pattern of the proximal scaphoid fragment and accompanying lunate (202–204,213,230).

Classification

The scaphoid fracture is most often classified by the location of the fracture line and its direction (2,3,115,194). Both of these factors have a bearing on the prognosis as well as on the approach to treatment. The fracture may be classified according to location as a proximal third, middle third, distal third, or tuberosity type (Fig. 14-97). The prognosis for union is worst and the risk of ischemic necrosis of the proximal bony fragment is highest in the proximal third type. Those fracture lines involving the distal third of the bone and tuberosity have the best prognosis and have the least risk of

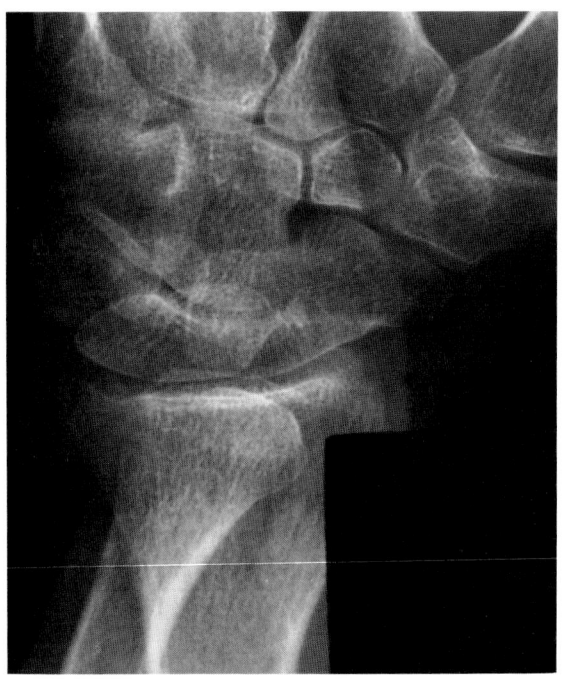

A

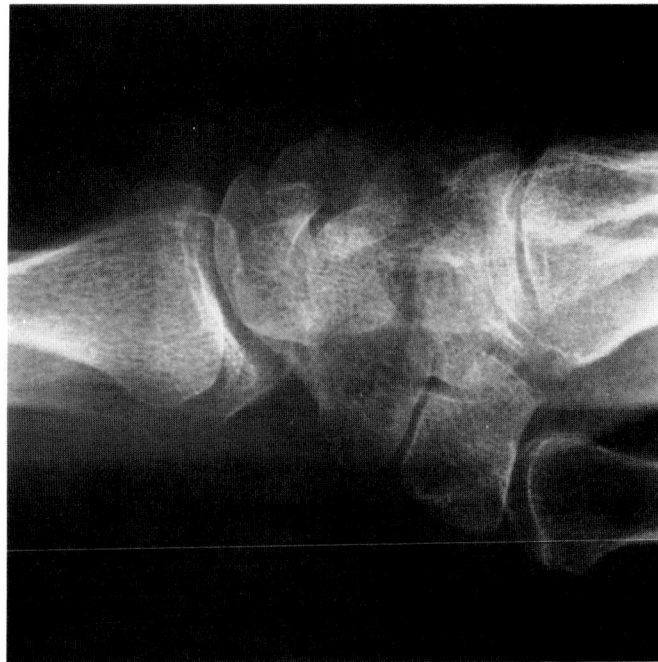

B

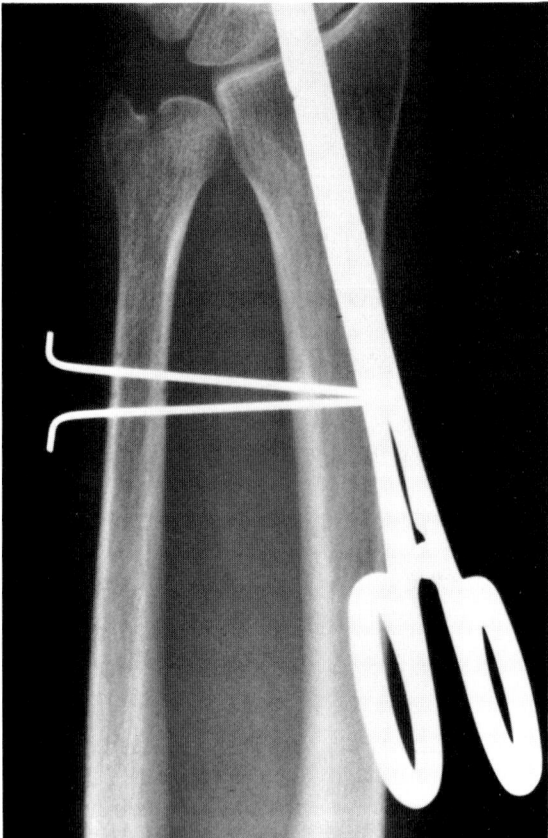

C

FIG. 14-95. Volar dislocation of the distal radioulnar joint. **A:** The oblique view shows marked overlap of the joint space. **B:** The ulna is in a volar position on the lateral view. Reduction was accomplished using K wire fixation (**C**). The towel clamp should have been adjusted prior to obtaining this operative film.

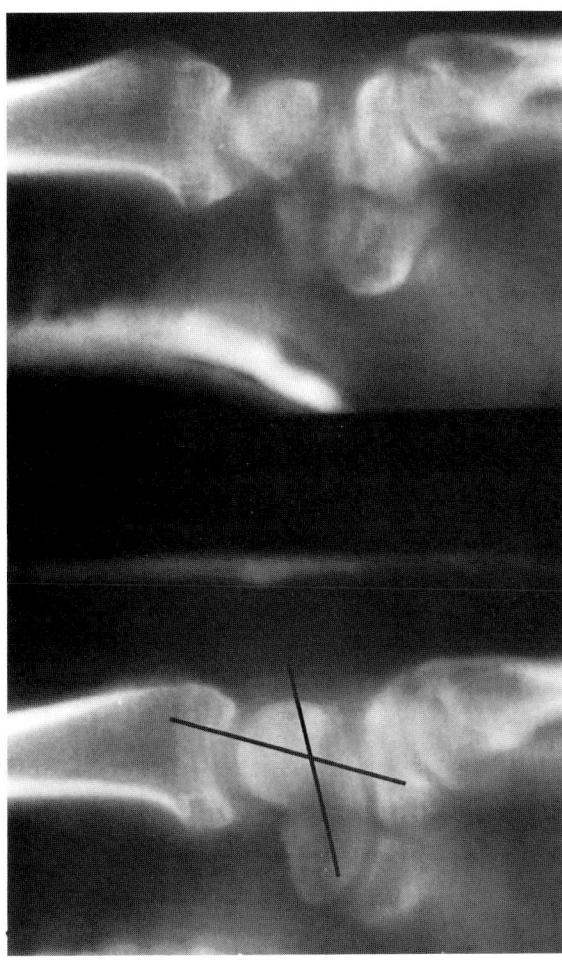

FIG. 14–96. Lateral trispiral tomograms demonstrate a scaphoid fracture with volar flexion ("humpback deformity") of the distal fragment.

osteonecrosis (Fig. 14-98). The middle third fractures involving the waist of the scaphoid are intermediate in terms of prognosis.

The direction of the fracture line has been classified by Russe into three types (Fig. 14-99) (194). Type I is basically perpendicular to the long axis of the wrist and oblique to the long axis of the scaphoid (Fig. 14-99A). Because it is perpendicular to the direction of the forces acting on it, most stresses acting on it are compressive with little shear. Thus, the situation is most favorable for

bony union. The Type II fracture line is perpendicular to the long axis of the scaphoid (Fig. 14-99B) and oblique to that of the wrist (Fig. 14-100). A small shear vector acts on fractures of this sort, but most of the forces favor compression of the fragments. Type III is least favorable, with the fracture line tending to parallel the long axis of the wrist (Fig. 14-99C). Stresses acting across the fracture tend to produce shearing vectors rather than compression. As a result, fracture displacement and non-union is highest with this type. Moreover, the Type III fracture is

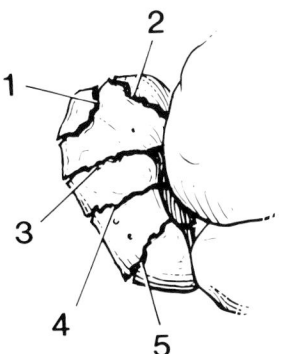

FIG. 14–97. Typical zones of fracture in the scaphoid. 1, capsular attachment or tubercle; 2, distal articular surface; 3, fracture of the distal third; 4, waist fracture; and 5, proximal pole fracture.

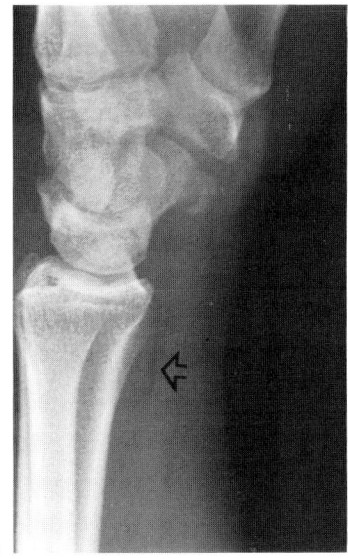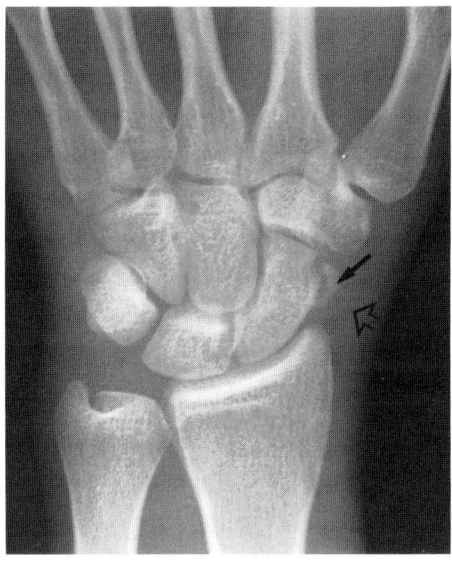

A

B

FIG. 14–98. Lateral (**A**) and PA (**B**) views of a scaphoid tubercle fracture (*black arrow*). Note the minimal displacement of the navicular fat stripe on the PA view (*open arrow*). The pronator fat stripe on the lateral view (*open arrow*) is not displaced.

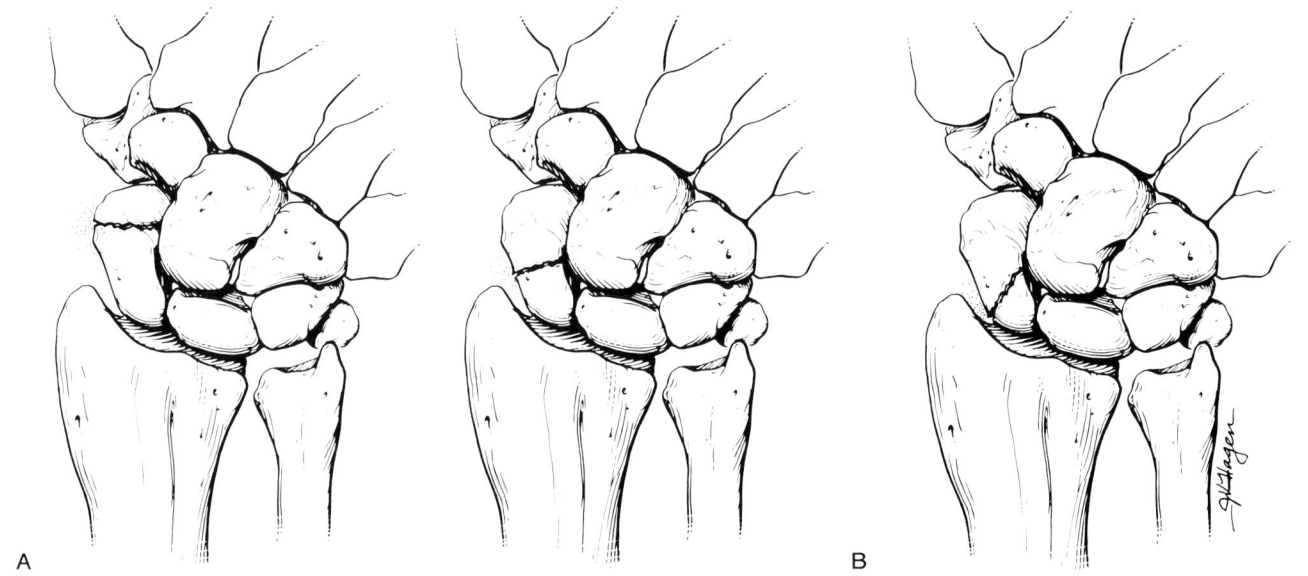

A

B

C

FIG. 14–99. Russe classification of scaphoid fractures. **A,** Type I; **B,** Type II; **C,** Type III.

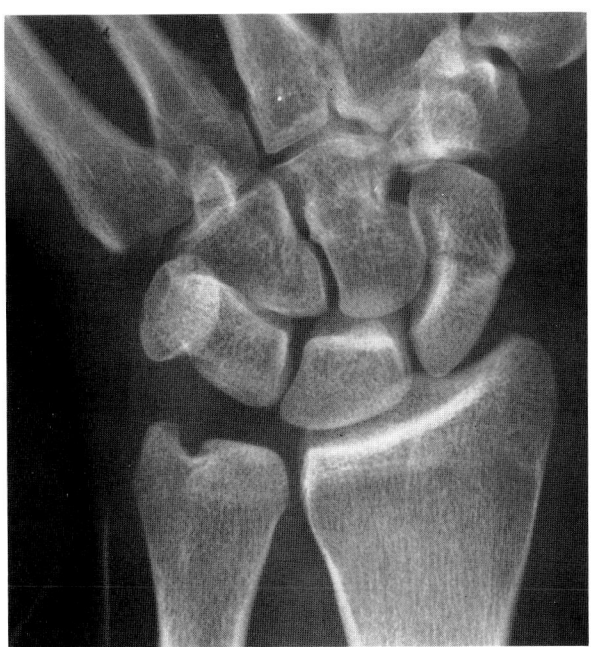

FIG. 14–100. PA view of Russe II scaphoid fracture. The fracture is perpendicular to the axis of the scaphoid and oblique to the long axis of the wrist.

most common with proximal third fractures. This further exacerbates the unfavorable prognosis.

In addition to location and direction of the fracture line, the presence of comminution or displacement should be noted in classifying such injuries. Both have a negative effect in terms of prognosis.

Mechanism of Injury

A fall onto the outstretched hand is the most common mechanism leading to a fracture of the scaphoid. Wrist hyperextension injuries with other causes (for example, vehicular accidents) may also be responsible. In the laboratory, fracture of the scaphoid is most consistently produced by wrist hyperextension in a position of radial deviation (220). Application of the deforming force more distally in the palm appears to produce a scaphoid fracture rather than a Colles'-type fracture.

Treatment

Treatment considerations will vary with the location of the fracture within the scaphoid bone, the degree of displacement, and the degree of associated soft tissue injury. The latter two factors are often related. In general, it is wise to consider all displaced fractures as inherently unstable, with a high percentage of these actually representing spontaneous, partially reduced transscaphoid-perilunate dislocations.

Except under unusual circumstances, all nondisplaced scaphoid fractures should be treated by cast immobilization (194,218). In the distal third fracture or tuberosity fracture, a short-arm cast that immobilizes the wrist in a neutral position and utilizes a thumb-spica extension to the base of the thumb nail to place the thumb in moderate palmar abduction is satisfactory. In general, with this fracture type, union will be complete in 4–8 weeks (139). Nondisplaced middle third and proximal third fractures present more of a challenge. Bony union requires more time, and avascularity of the proximal bone fragment must be considered. In the young individual with this fracture, an above-elbow cast with a similar thumb-spica extension is advised for the first 4–6 weeks. Thereafter, short-arm thumb-spica immobilization for 2–4 more months may be required. A small percentage of fractures will fail to unite even with this treatment. Such fractures may require further cast immobilization or bone grafting procedures to achieve union. In the older patient (i.e., over 50 years of age), an initial period of above-elbow cast immobilization is omitted because of concern for permanent limitation of the range of motion of the elbow.

The displaced fracture requires reduction. This is perhaps most easily achieved by longitudinal traction in finger traps followed by gentle manipulation. In all instances, once reduction is obtained, a clinical test for the stability of the fracture is central for guiding further management. If reduction is anatomic and post-reduction stability is achieved, then treatment as outlined earlier for the nondisplaced fracture is appropriate. Particular care in assessing post-reduction radiographs is important (Fig. 14-101). Restoration of the scaphoid outline on PA and oblique projections with maintenance of the normal carpal height is essential. In the lateral projection, palmar angulation of the distal fragment may be difficult to discern and is frequently overlooked. If this angulation remains, it may lead to healing in a "humpback" deformity (Fig. 14-96) and to secondary distortion of the intercarpal relationships (133). If routine lateral views leave room for doubt with regard to the adequacy of reduction in this case, trispiral tomographic evaluation may be indicated (Fig. 14-102).

If adequate reduction is possible but the reduction is unstable, a number of treatment options are possible. Above-elbow thumb-spica cast immobilization may be selected, but extreme vigilance is necessary for maintenance of reduction. This may require serial post-reduction radiographs. Alternatively, percutaneous Kirschner-wire fixation of the fracture or open reduction with screw or Kirschner-wire fixation may be appropriate (Fig. 14-103). Such unstable fractures may be frank or variants of forme fruste perilunate dislocations. As such, the extremely unstable variety may benefit from open repair of the injured ligaments (particularly the volar complex) in addition to fixation of the fracture.

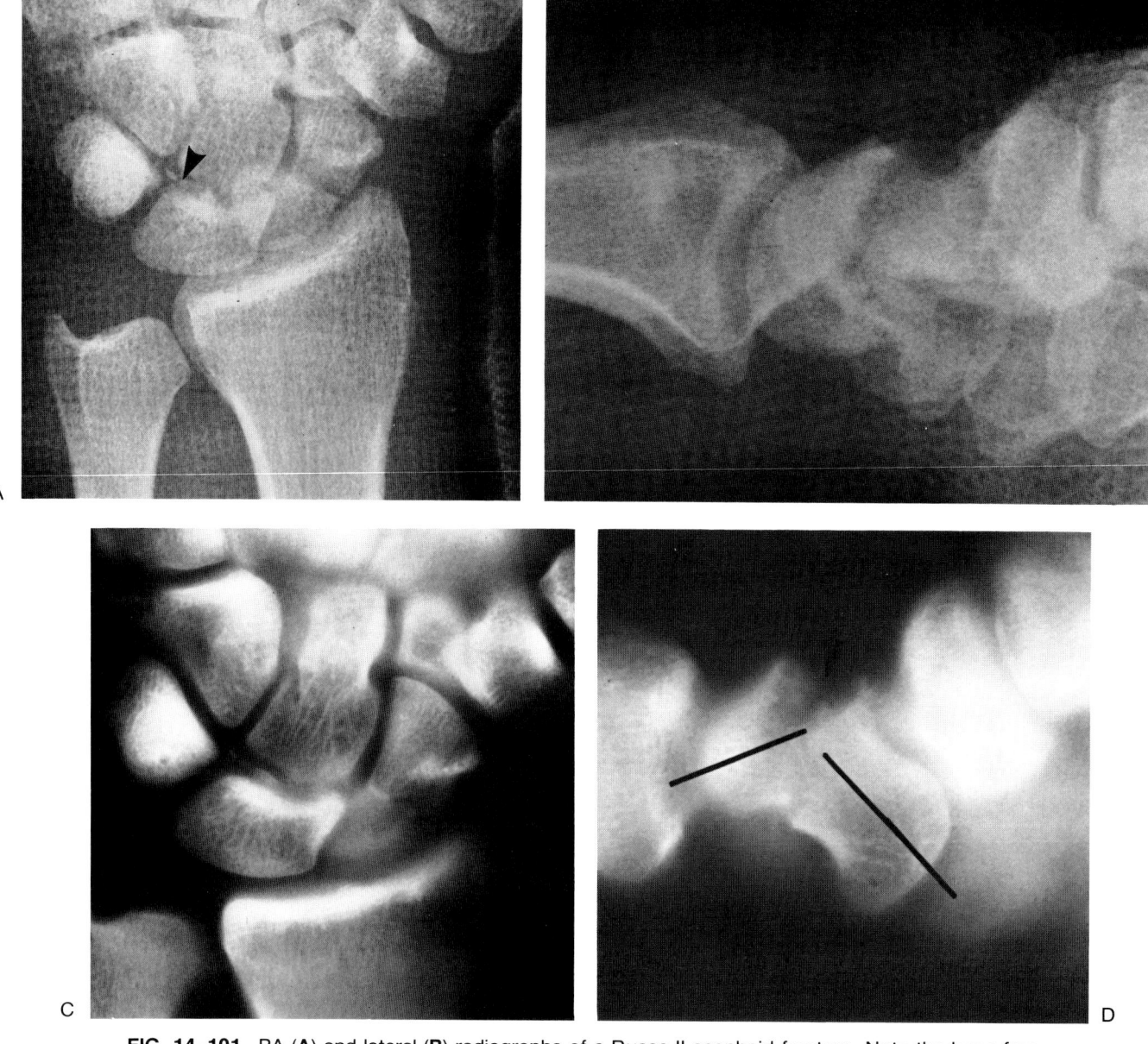

FIG. 14–101. PA (**A**) and lateral (**B**) radiographs of a Russe II scaphoid fracture. Note the bone fragments (*arrow*) distal to the lunate. AP tomogram (**C**) demonstrates osteochondral fragments from the proximal capitate. The proximal scaphoid fragment is out of plane with the distal fragment. Lateral tomogram (**D**) demonstrates dorsal separation with angular deformity.

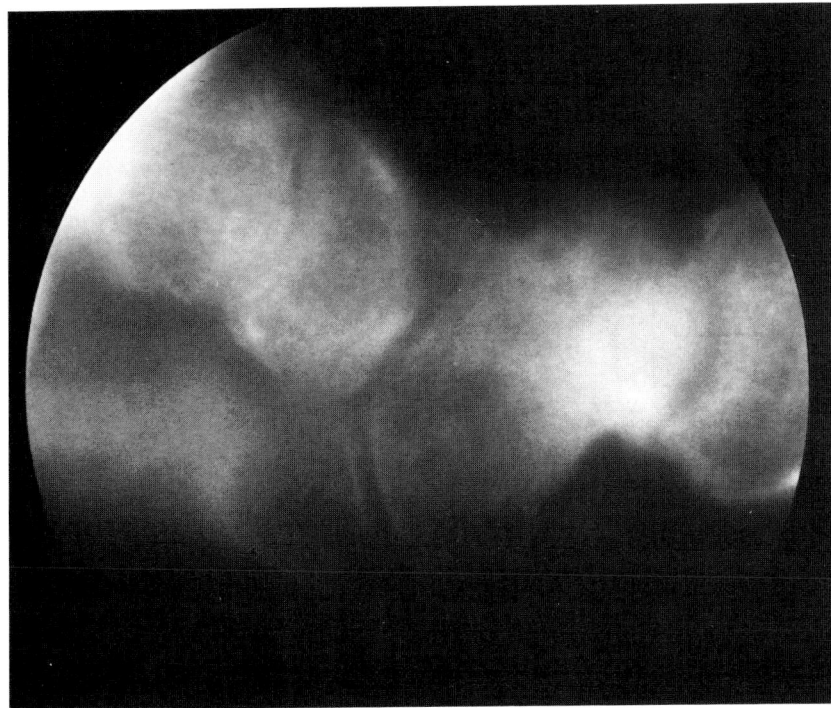

FIG. 14-102. Lateral trispiral tomogram following reduction of the scaphoid fracture. The fracture is healing. The proximal dense appearance is due to the thickening of the tomographic slice, which includes the radial styloid.

The unstable scaphoid fracture has a greater risk of non-union or delayed union (Fig. 14-104). If there appears to be little progress toward union after 3–4 months of such treatment, bone grafting or the application of electrical stimulation methods may be appropriate.

If adequate reduction is not possible by closed means, open reduction is indicated. Internal fixation as outlined earlier and possibly repair of associated disrupted ligaments should be carried out.

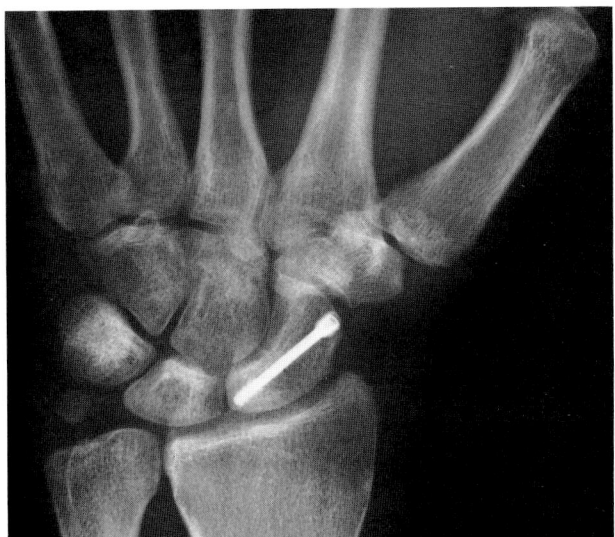

FIG. 14-103. Internal fixation of scaphoid fracture with a Herbert screw.

Complications

The scaphoid fracture is generally associated with a litany of complications (2,3,139,194,218). However, if recognized early, reduced adequately, and treated appropriately over a sufficient period, uneventful healing can be expected in over 90% of cases.

Delayed union is perhaps the most common complication and is defined generally as failure of union within 3 months of the initiation of cast immobilization. It must be recognized, however, that a significant percentage of scaphoid fractures require 6–12 months of cast or splint immobilization to achieve union (194,218).

Non-union probably occurs in fewer than 10% of cases but is more prevalent in fractures of the middle or proximal thirds of the bone (Fig. 14-105), in Russe Type III fractures (vertical direction), in comminuted fractures, and in fractures with unstable reductions. The most common preventable factors associated with non-union include delay of diagnosis and inadequate treatment. PA and lateral tomograms or flexion-extension lateral tomograms are usually adequate for diagnosis (202–204). However, MRI may be useful in this setting as well (102) (Fig. 14-106). Once non-union is established, its management usually takes the form of bone grafting or electrical stimulation modalities. The indications for one or the other of these approaches are not firmly established. If non-union persists despite either or both of these techniques, then further management, if indicated, may include radial styloidectomy, soft tissue arthroplasty of the

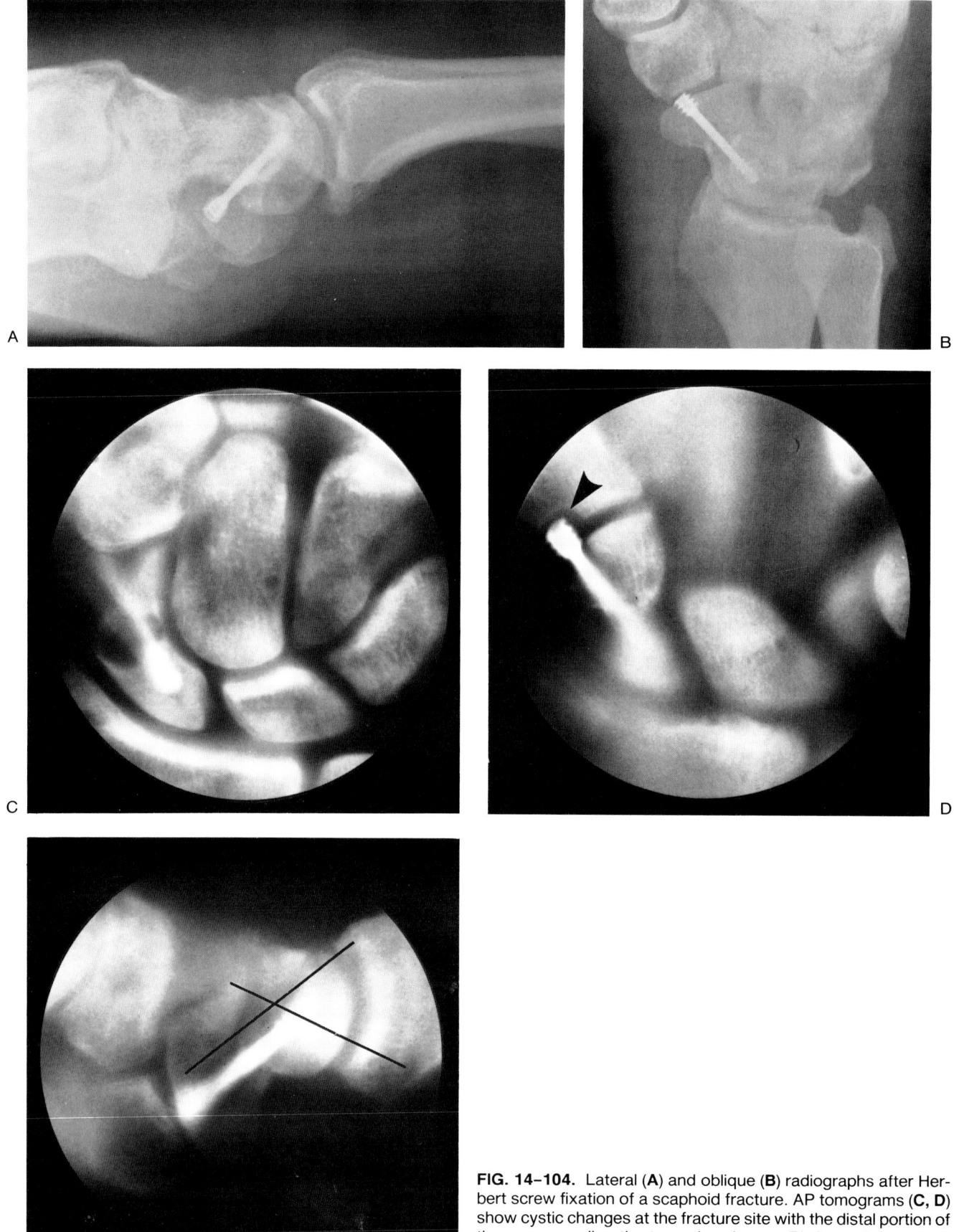

FIG. 14-104. Lateral (**A**) and oblique (**B**) radiographs after Herbert screw fixation of a scaphoid fracture. AP tomograms (**C, D**) show cystic changes at the fracture site with the distal portion of the screw eroding the trapezium (*arrow*, **D**). Lateral tomogram (**E**) shows ''hump back'' deformity due to dorsal separation of the fragments.

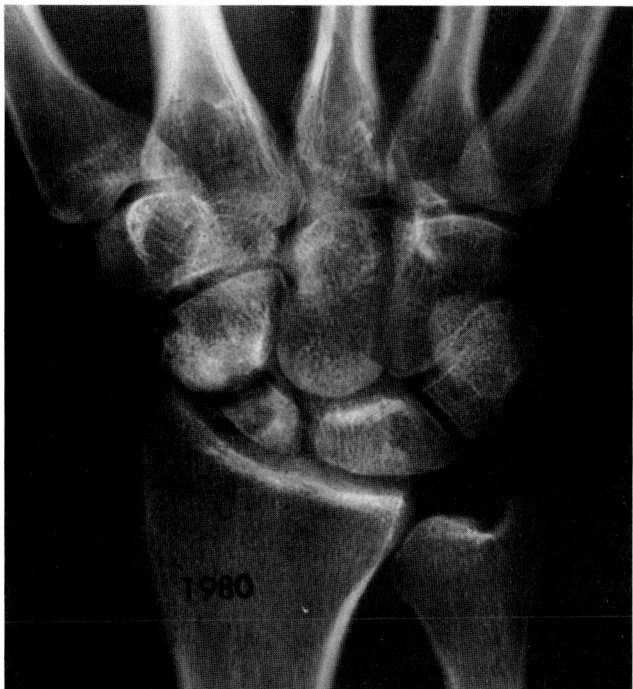

FIG. 14–105. PA view demonstrating an old ununited fracture of the proximal scaphoid.

pseudarthrosis site, scaphoid replacement arthroplasty, and limited wrist arthrodesis (2).

Malunion most frequently results from failure to recognize an inadequate reduction. Usually this takes the form of palmar angulation of the distal fragment, producing the so-called *humpback* deformity (Fig. 14-104). This situation may then lead to foreshortening of the carpal height, which in turn leads to an exaggerated scapholunate angle and a dorsal carpal instability pattern (133).

Avascular necrosis of the proximal scaphoid fragment is most prevalent with fractures involving the proximal third of the scaphoid (194). It may also be seen, but less frequently, in middle third fractures. It is distinctly unusual with fractures involving the distal third of the bone. Radiographically, this condition is characterized by increased radiopacity of the avascular portion (Fig. 14-107). MRI is useful in early assessment of healing and avascular necrosis (Fig. 14-108) (102,124). When such radiopacity is present, delayed union or non-union of the fracture is frequent. Revascularization occurs slowly over 1–2 years. Significant bony collapse of the avascular portion is unusual.

Radioscaphoid impingement or arthrosis may occur, particularly with malunited fractures or in those with a rather hypertrophic callus. It is most often between the tip of the radial styloid and the waist of the scaphoid (Fig. 14-109). If present, a limited radial styloidectomy or cheilectomy of the scaphoid may be indicated.

The other array of complications familiar to all wrist injuries, including limited wrist or digit range of motion, autonomic dysfunction syndrome (sympathetic dystrophy), and carpal tunnel syndrome, may also be seen.

Triquetrum

The triquetrum is the second most commonly injured carpal bone (108). Most often these are dorsal avulsion injuries presumably at the site of the ulnotriquetral liga-

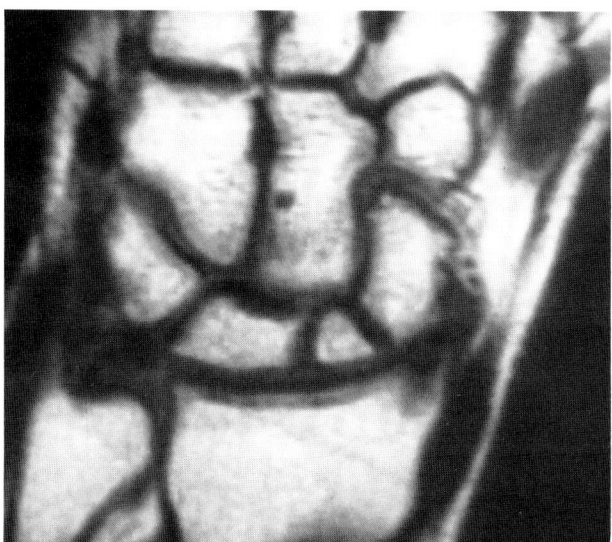

A

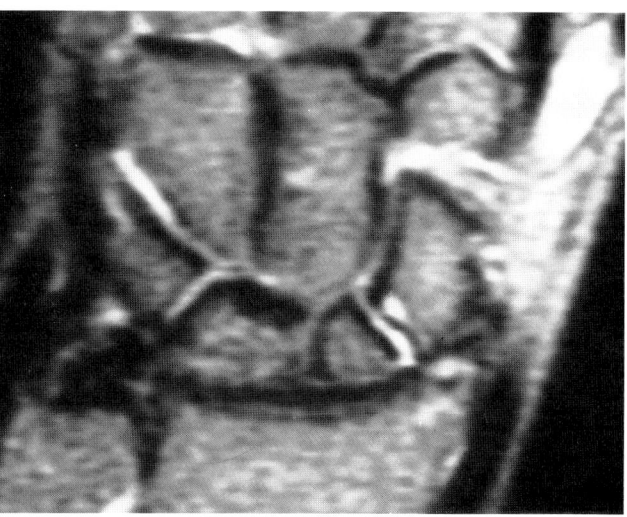

B

FIG. 14–106. Patient with previous scaphoid fracture referred to exclude avascular necrosis and non-union. Coronal SE 500/20 shows normal signal intensity in the proximal fragment excluding avascular necrosis. The fracture line is low intensity. ? fibrous or osseous tissue. SE 2000/60 image (**B**) shows high intensity in the fracture line due to fluid confirming the non-union (from 102, with permission).

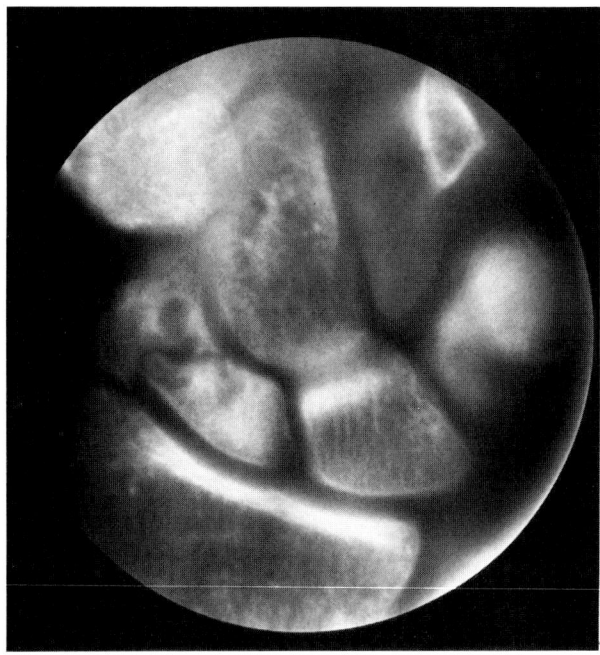

FIG. 14-107. PA trispiral tomogram with an ununited scaphoid fracture and avascular necrosis of the proximal fragment.

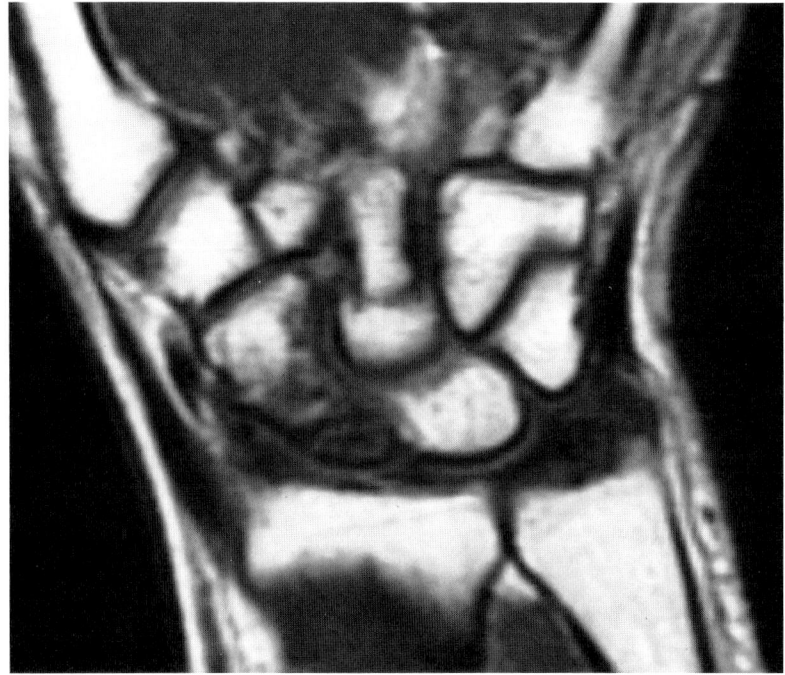

FIG. 14-108. SE 500/20 coronal image of a proximal scaphoid fracture demonstrating early avascular necrosis (AVN) of the proximal fragment.

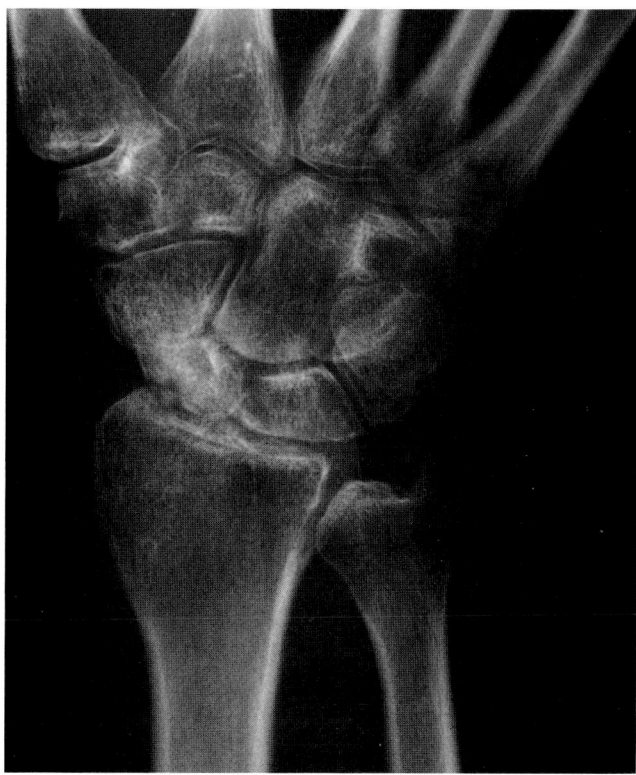

FIG. 14–109. Old fracture of the scaphoid with degenerative arthritis at junction of the radial styloid and scaphoid waist.

ment insertion. More rarely, fractures of the body of the triquetrum are seen (99). Usually these are nondisplaced, and often they are comminuted. The diagnosis is usually made by routine PA, lateral, and oblique wrist radiographs (Fig. 14-110). Trispiral tomograms may be useful, particularly to assess displacement of fractures involving the body. Treatment of the dorsal avulsion fracture is symptomatic. A short-arm cast immobilizing the wrist in slight extension for 4–6 weeks is usually adequate. Fractures of the body that are nondisplaced are best treated by a long-arm cast for 4–6 weeks followed by a short-arm cast for 2–6 additional weeks or until evidence of union is present. Significantly displaced fractures may be candidates for open reduction and internal fixation.

Lunate

Considerable confusion and disagreement exist regarding fractures of the lunate and their relation to Kienböck's disease (2,3,124,180). Some authors believe that the etiology of Kienböck's disease is a fracture of the lunate, whereas others believe that fracture and later fragmentation of the lunate is a consequence rather than a cause of Kienböck's disease. We believe that acute traumatic fracture of the lunate can occur and may or may not be followed by the typical radiographic findings of Kienböck's disease. We also believe that Kienböck's disease can be seen without a definite history of trauma and in the absence of radiographic evidence of lunate fracture. This condition will be discussed later in this chapter.

Fractures involving the body of the lunate may be extremely difficult to diagnose on routine radiographs. If a high index of clinical suspicion exists in spite of normal-appearing radiographs, further evaluation by trispiral tomography or bone scan may be warranted (140). The fracture line is usually disposed in the coronal plane (Fig. 14-111). The mechanism of injury of the lunate fracture is usually hyperextension. Direct axial compression has also been suggested. If the diagnosis is made in the absence of the typical radiographic changes suggesting Kienböck's disease, treatment is indicated. Nondisplaced fractures should be treated at least initially by long-arm cast immobilization. These fractures require careful vigilance to ensure that displacement does not occur from compressive loads within the cast. Because of the position of the lunate, compressive deforming forces as a result of finger motion are simply unavoidable. For this reason, some authors suggest treatment by external fixation-distraction across the wrist similar to that described for the unstable Colles' fracture (Fig. 14-81). Displaced fractures of the lunate are likely best managed by open reduction and internal fixation with Kirschner wires or miniature screws. The chief complication following fractures of the lunate is the development of Kienböck's sequelae, as discussed later in this chapter.

Pisiform

Fractures of the pisiform usually result from a blunt blow. This occurs when the base of the hypothenar eminence is struck in a direct fall or when the hand is used as an ill-advised hammer. The fracture may be comminuted or simple. Displacement is usually not marked because this bone is enveloped in the tendon of the flexor carpi ulnaris. Although routine radiographs may reveal a fracture line, the fracture is best visualized on a lateral projection with the wrist in a position of 30° supination (pisiform view) (Fig. 14-112). Closed symptomatic treatment in a short-arm cast is recommended (108). The major late complication is arthrosis of the pisotriquetral joint, which may require excision of the pisiform.

Hamate

Fractures of the hamate may involve the body (175), the dorsal aspect (140), the distal articular surface as a component of a carpometacarpal fracture-dislocation (150), or the hook (hamulus) (103,184,207). Fractures of the body are usually nondisplaced and can be diagnosed

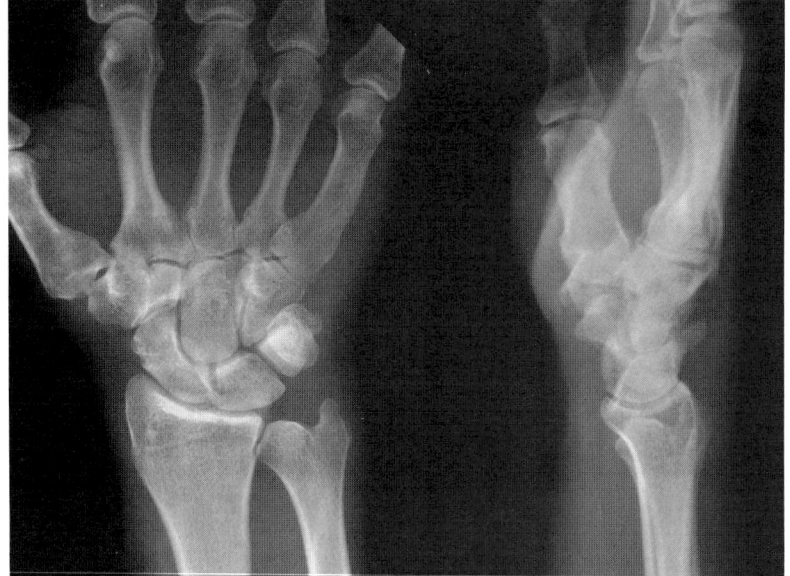

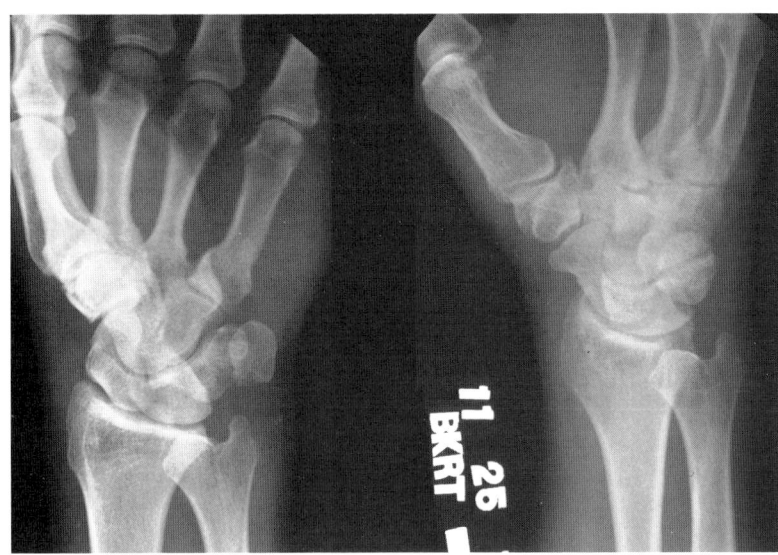

FIG. 14–110. Fractured triquetrum. PA (**A**), lateral (**B**) and both oblique views (**C, D**). The fracture is most clearly seen on the lateral view. There is associated soft tissue swelling.

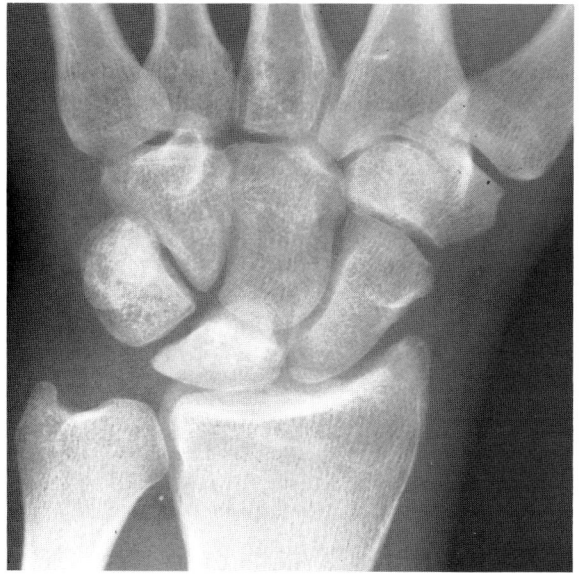

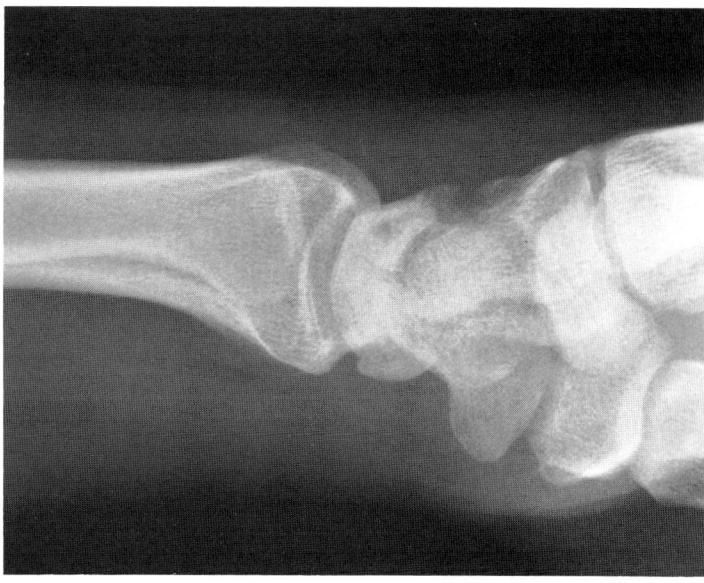

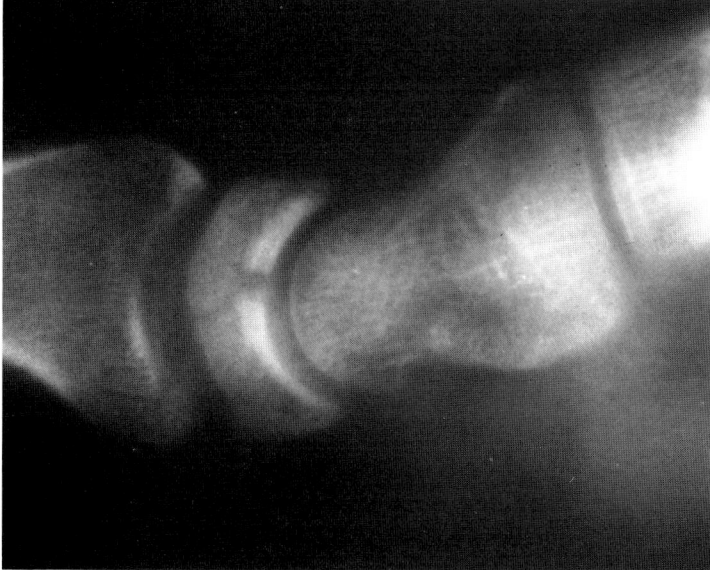

FIG. 14–111. AP (A) and lateral (B) views of the wrist show increased density of the lunate. The lateral tomogram (C) clearly demonstrates the fracture and flattening of the lunate due to associated Kienböck's disease.

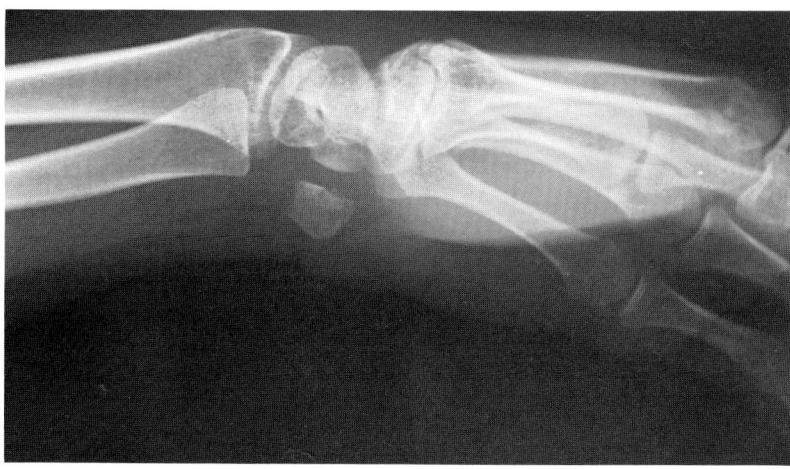

FIG. 14–112. Pisiform view of the wrist demonstrating a minimally displaced pisiform fracture.

using routine AP, lateral, and oblique radiographs. These are stable injuries and can generally be managed adequately by short-arm cast immobilization for 4–8 weeks. Complications are unusual. Fractures involving the distal articular surface as a component of a carpometacarpal dislocation are suggested by routine wrist radiographs. Accurate delineation of the fracture may require trispiral tomography (Fig. 14-113). These are unstable injuries and, hence, usually require internal fixation after closed or open reduction. The major late complication is degenerative arthrosis of the carpometacarpal articulation, particularly if the fracture heals with residual articular incongruity or joint subluxation.

Fracture of the hook (hamulus) is the most common injury to the hamate (108,110,111,184,205,207). This is generally believed to be an avulsion fracture, presumably caused by the pull of the transverse carpal ligament that inserts on the hook of the hamate. The majority of fractures occur at the base of the hook (207). It seems particularly prevalent in association with a dubbed golf swing and other racket sports (207,216). The diagnosis is difficult to make on routine radiographs. There are three useful radiographic signs that may be useful on the PA view. There may be absence of the hook, sclerosis in the region of the hook, or lack of the normal cortical ring (see normal appearance, Figs. 14-5 and 14-74A)(184). A carpal tunnel view may be helpful (Fig. 14-114A). Trispiral tomography is diagnostic in most instances; however, a localized bone scan may be useful in localizing the pathology prior to tomograms (Figs. 14-114B and C). Computed tomography may be useful in certain cases (207). Closed treatment by cast immobilization is unreliable for healing. Most authors recommend excision of the fractured fragment, although some suggest open reduction and internal fixation. Most complications of this injury result from failure to make the correct diagnosis. These include persistent pain, ulnar neuropathy, and attritional flexor tendon rupture (120).

Capitate

Capitate fractures may involve the body, the distal articular surface as a component of a carpometacarpal fracture-dislocation, or the proximal pole (2,3,94,108). Fractures involving the body occur most commonly through the middle third and are transverse (Fig. 14-115). They are usually the result of a hyperextension injury. A direct blow over the dorsum of the capitate may also be responsible. Comminution may be present. Routine PA and lateral radiographs are usually sufficient to arrive at a diagnosis. If the fracture is nondisplaced, short-arm cast immobilization for 6–8 weeks is usually adequate. If displaced, the fracture is likely to be unstable. In such cases, if reduction is adequate, vigilant cast immobilization may be successful. At least initially, a long-arm cast is advised in such cases. Alternatively, the unstable capitate fracture may be treated by internal fixation, usually with Kirschner wires. Complications include non-union, delayed union, and avascular necrosis of the proximal fragment. Fractures involving the distal articular surface are similar to those described for the same location in the hamate as part of the carpometacarpal dislocation. However, in contrast to the hamate, where carpometacarpal motion is desired following healing, the capitate-third metacarpal articulation should be stable with essentially no motion (9). Therefore, with extensive articular incongruity, treatment directed toward achieving an arthrodesis of the capitate-third metacarpal articulation may be justified.

Fractures of the proximal pole may be seen as isolated entities similar to middle third fractures as described earlier or as the so-called *naviculocapitate syndrome* (129,172,208). This injury, resulting from a hyperexten-

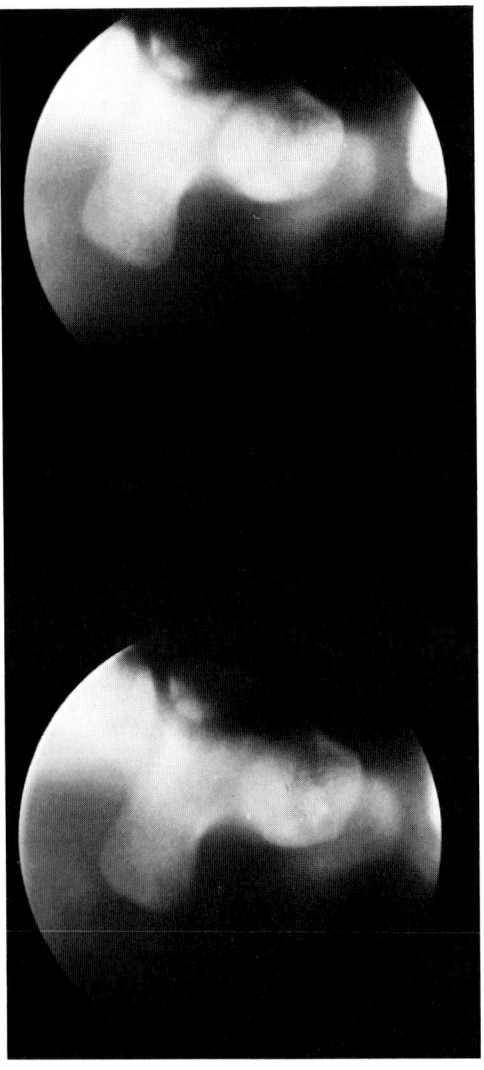

FIG. 14-113. Lateral trispiral tomogram of the wrist with a comminuted fracture of the doral aspect of the hamate.

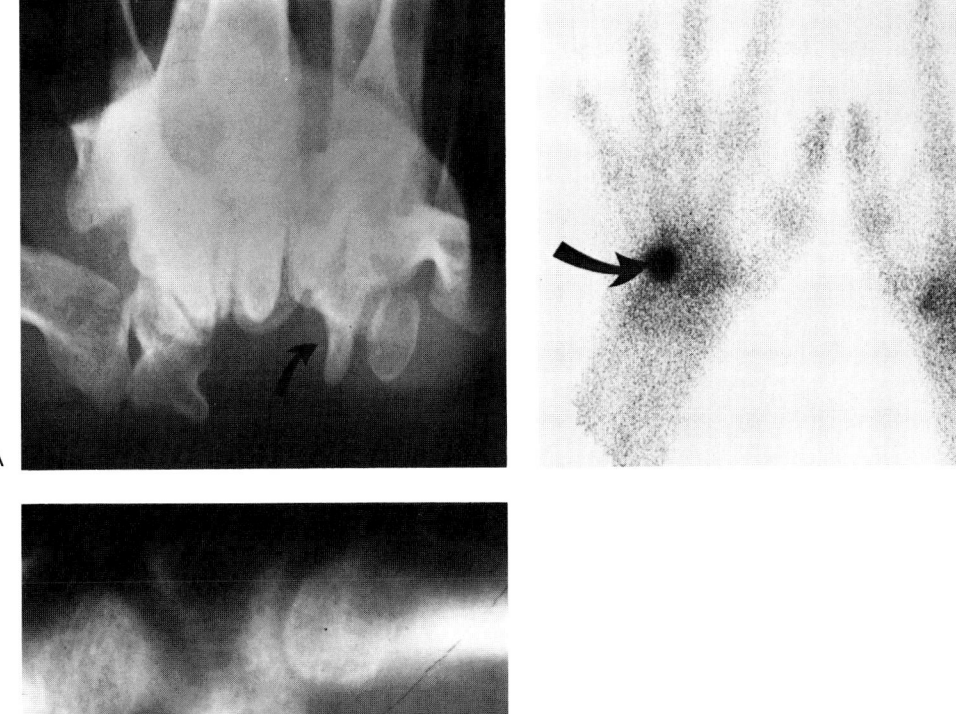

FIG. 14–114. Fracture of the hook of the hamate. **A:** The carpal tunnel view demonstrates the hook (*arrow*) clearly but a fracture is not definitely present. Follow-up isotope scan (**B**) with 99mTc demonstrates increased uptake in the region of the hamate hook (*arrow*). Trispiral tomograms (**C**) demonstrate the fracture (*arrows*) which has a Y configuration.

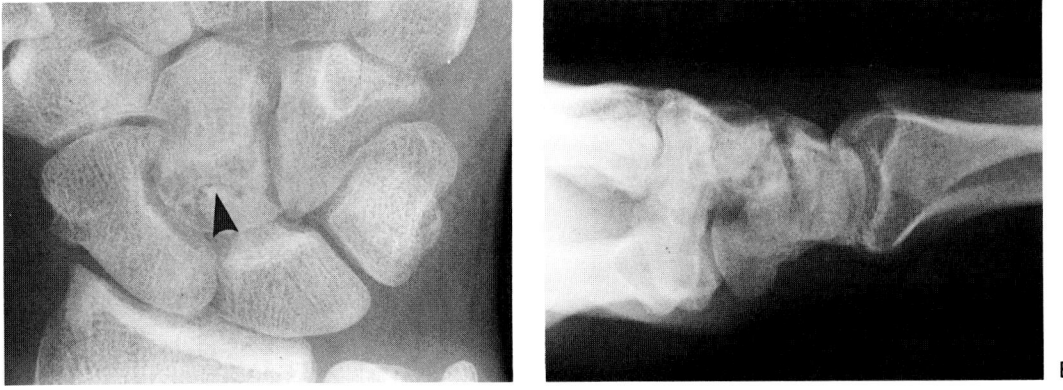

FIG. 14–115. Transverse fracture of the body of the capitate. The fracture is seen best on the PA view (*arrow*) (**A**) and difficult to detect on the lateral view (**B**).

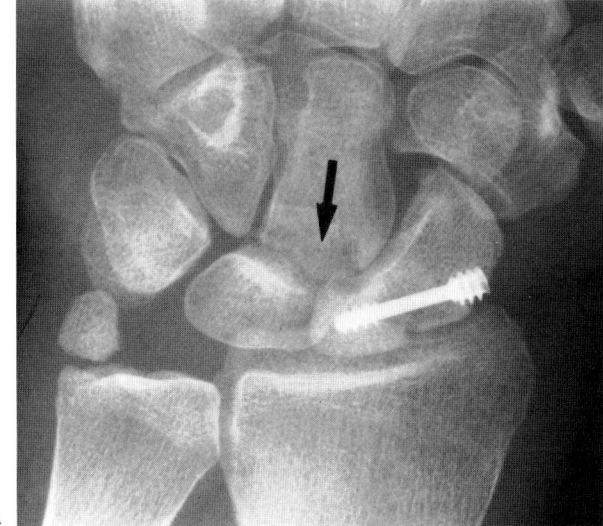
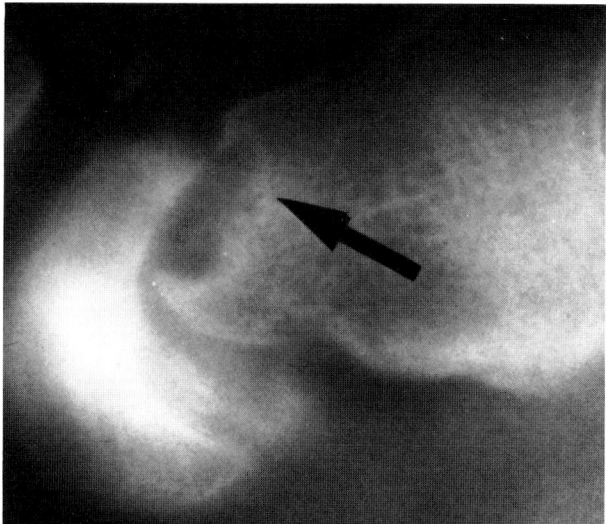

FIG. 14–116. **A:** PA view of the wrist following fixation of the scaphoid fracture. **B:** The capitate fracture (*arrow*) was clearly seen only with tomography.

sion force to the wrist, is probably a variant of a perilunate dislocation. With it, fracture of the scaphoid and the proximal pole of the capitate occurs. On spontaneous reduction, the latter rotates through 90° to 180°. Often this injury is overlooked, with the casual examiner directing attention to the scaphoid fracture only, and with details of the proximal capitate fragments being obscured on routine radiographs. Trispiral tomography or CT are diagnostic and should be carried out if there is any doubt regarding this syndrome (Fig. 14-116). Treatment requires open reduction and internal fixation of the capitate and scaphoid fractures. If the capitate fragment is extremely small, excision may be warranted. Avascular necrosis of the capitate fragment is not unusual. If seen late, excision of the fragment or capitolunoscaphoid arthrodesis may be indicated.

Trapezoid

Fractures of the trapezoid are uncommon and isolated dislocations are rare (2,3,108,153,158). They may be seen as a component of a carpometacarpal fracture-dislocation (150). In such instances, the comments directed to this same injury in the capitate apply. Detection on routine radiographs is difficult. Trispiral tomography or CT are usually indicated (141). It is not unusual to detect these subtle injuries when performing MR examinations (Fig. 14-117) to identify the cause of chronic wrist pain (102). The major goal of treatment is stability of the trapezoid-second metacarpal articulation. This may require arthrodesis.

Trapezium

Fractures of the trapezium involve the body, the margin, or the ridge (2,3,108,118,153). Those through the

body are usually vertical and may result from direct axial compression on the thumb, hyperextension of the first metacarpal, or a blow to the adducted thumb (Fig. 14-118). Comminution and displacement may be present. In addition to routine PA, lateral, and oblique radiographs, x-ray evaluation should include a true PA view of the first carpometacarpal joint and possibly trispiral tomograms. If the fracture is nondisplaced, short-arm thumb-spica cast immobilization with the thumb in moderate palmar abduction is usually adequate. If it is displaced, open reduction and internal fixation with the goal of anatomic articular reduction of both the scaphoid and the first metacarpal surfaces is recommended. The chief complication of this fracture is degenerative arthrosis of the basilar thumb joints.

Marginal fractures are not uncommon. Provided that

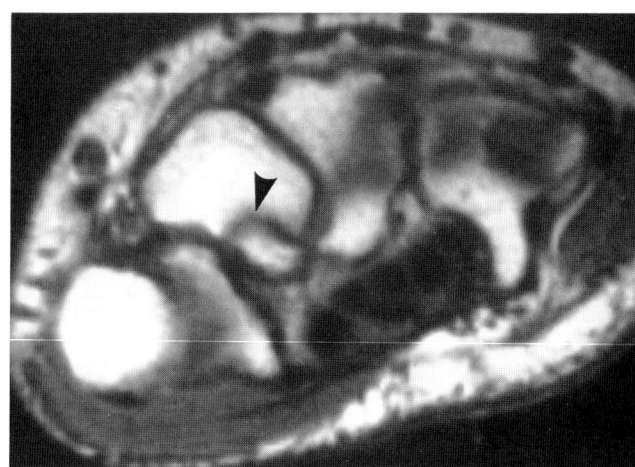

FIG. 14–117. Axial SE 500/20 image of the wrist in a patient with chronic post-traumatic pain. There is an undisplaced fracture (*arrow*) of the trapezoid.

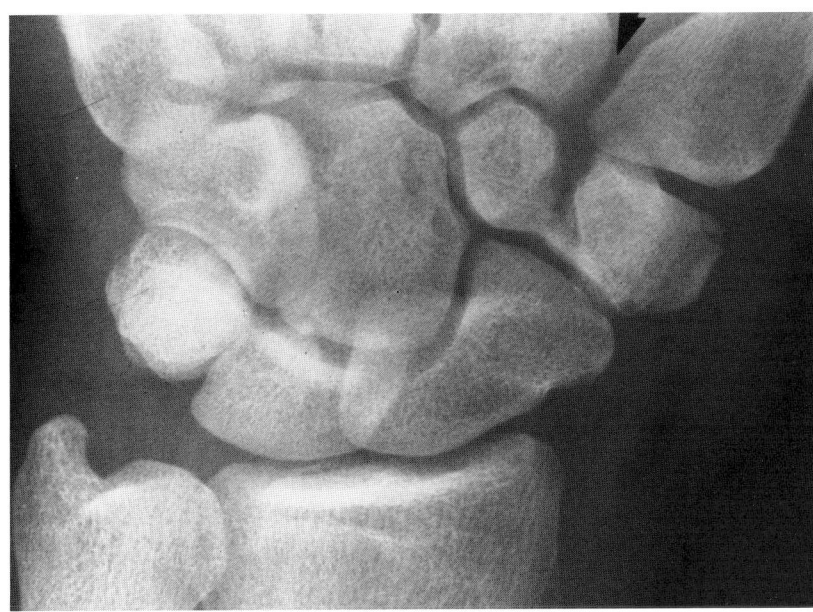

FIG. 14-118. Oblique view of the wrist. There is a fracture of the trapezium with associated swelling. Note the associated widening of the bases of the metacarpals (*arrow*) and joint of the trapezium and trapezoid.

they are not displaced, they are comparable in terms of treatment and prognosis to scaphoid tuberosity fractures (Fig. 14-119). If there is any displacement, careful radiographic scrutiny for evidence of subluxation of the joint should be carried out.

Fractures of the ridge of the trapezium are generally believed to be avulsion fractures at the site of the transverse carpal ligament insertion. These may be difficult to visualize on routine radiographic views but can usually be seen on carpal tunnel views or trispiral tomograms. In terms of prognosis and treatment, they may be similar to fractures of the hook of the hamate. If the fracture is displaced or seen late, excision of the fracture fragment may be indicated. Dislocations of the trapezium are rare and usually associated with other hand and wrist injuries (211).

Carpal Dislocations

Dislocations of the carpus are uncommon but most frequently are associated with a perilunate injury or a variant of this injury (134,146,158,170,178,195).

Dorsal Perilunate Dislocations and Variants

These injuries include a spectrum of findings varying with the degree of associated trauma and position of the force of impact on the wrist. Most are extreme hyperextension injuries resulting from a fall onto the dorsiflexed wrist (146,230).

Trans-scaphoid Perilunate Dislocation

This is the most common type of perilunate dislocation. It is also known as *de Quervain's fracture-*

dislocation. Typically, the lunate and proximal scaphoid fragment remain in articulation with the distal radius, while the remainder of the carpus and the distal scaphoid fracture are displaced in a dorsal direction (Fig. 14-120). Routine PA and lateral radiographs are usually adequate to suggest the injury. However, oblique views or tomograms may be necessary to clarify the diagnosis, particularly with regard to associated carpal fractures. Treatment requires reduction by closed or open means. Manipulative reduction is facilitated by strong longitudinal traction. The incidence of scaphoid malunion or

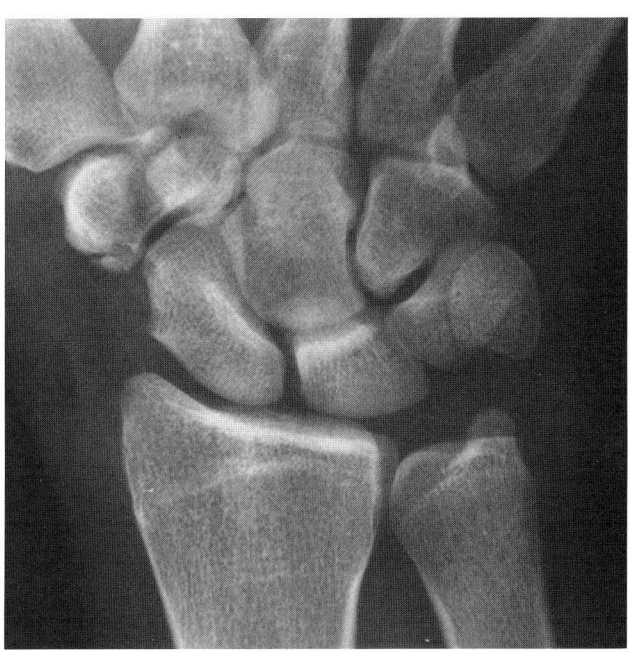

FIG. 14-119. PA view of the wrist with a ridge fracture of the trapezium. Note the air in the soft tissues indicating an open fracture.

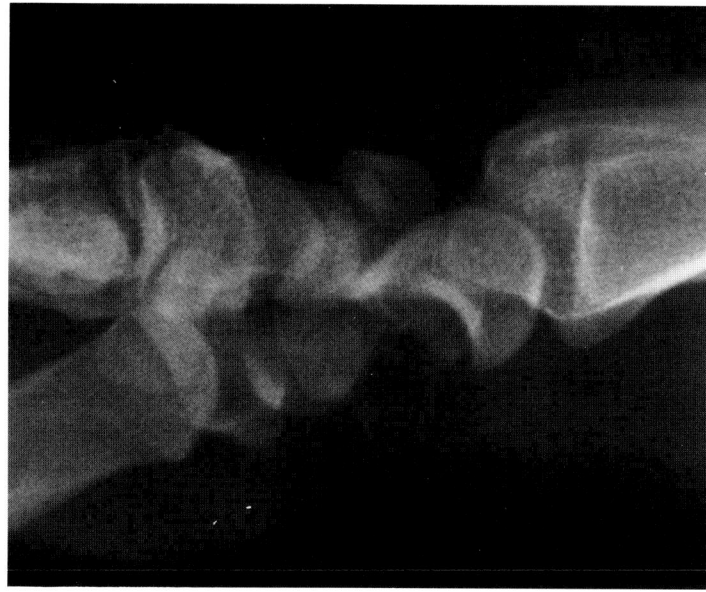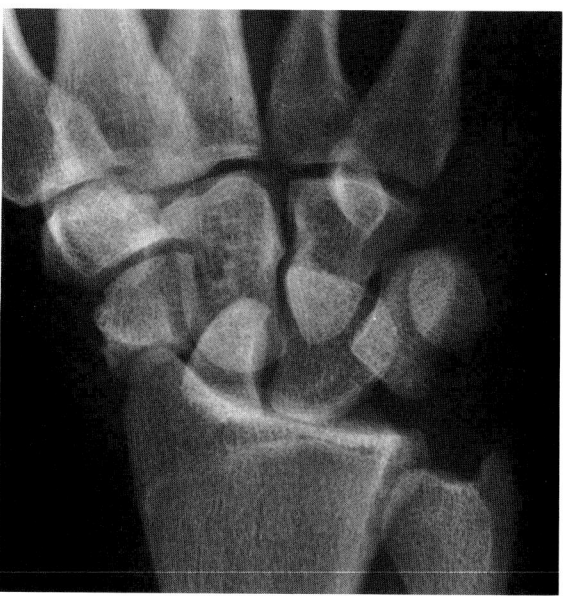

A   B

FIG. 14-120. Transcaphoid perilunate dislocation of the wrist. **A:** The lateral view demonstrates volar flexion of the lunate, which no longer articulates with the capitate. **B:** PA view more clearly shows the scaphoid fracture with rotation of the proximal fragment. The capitate appears to articulate with the distal radius due to its dorsal proximal position.

nonunion following this injury is appreciable. For this reason, unless a perfect and stable closed reduction is achieved, many authors advocate stable internal fixation with or without open repair of the disrupted or attenuated volar radiocarpal ligament complex (Fig. 14-121) (2,3).

In addition to scaphoid non-union or malunion, late complications and sequelae include carpal instability deformities, limited range of motion of the wrist, median neuropathy, late degenerative arthritis, and occasionally avascular bony necrosis.

Dorsal Perilunate Dislocation

This dislocation is essentially the same injury as the trans-scaphoid-perilunate dislocation but without the scaphoid fracture. The volar radiocarpal ligament complex is completely disrupted. The mechanism of injury and treatment principles are the same. The most significant late sequela is residual carpal instability of the DISI variety (see Figs. 14-9 and 14-10) (2,196).

Anterior (Volar) Lunate Dislocation

This injury is believed to represent a variant of the dorsal perilunate dislocation (191). Presumably it results from a spontaneous reduction of the dorsally displaced carpus, which essentially settles on the lunate, displacing it in a palmar direction (Fig. 14-122). Closed reduction of this injury may be more difficult and requires direct pressure over the displaced lunate in a dorsal direction in addition to longitudinal traction. The mechanism of injury and treatment principles are as outlined earlier.

Perilunate Dislocation with Multiple Fractures

These are simply variants of the trans-scaphoid-perilunate injury. These may include any element or combination of elements, encompassing transradial styloid, trans-scaphoid, transcapitate, transtriquetral, and transulnar-styloid-perilunate dislocation (224).

Volar Perilunate Dislocation and Variants

These injuries are extremely rare (2,3,96). Most commonly they are associated with violent trauma that produced hyperflexion of the wrist. They can involve any combination of associated fractures or may lead to a posterior (dorsal) lunate dislocation by a mechanism similar to that described earlier. Treatment should aim for perfect reduction. If the dislocation is unstable following reduction, internal fixation with Kirschner wires, with or without open repair of the disrupted ligaments, is recommended. Complications following these injuries are frequent and include carpal instability, limited range of motion, avascular bony necrosis, and degenerative arthritis.

Dislocations of the Carpus Other Than Perilunate

Although rare, dislocation of virtually every carpal bone has been described (156,176,186,211). These occur

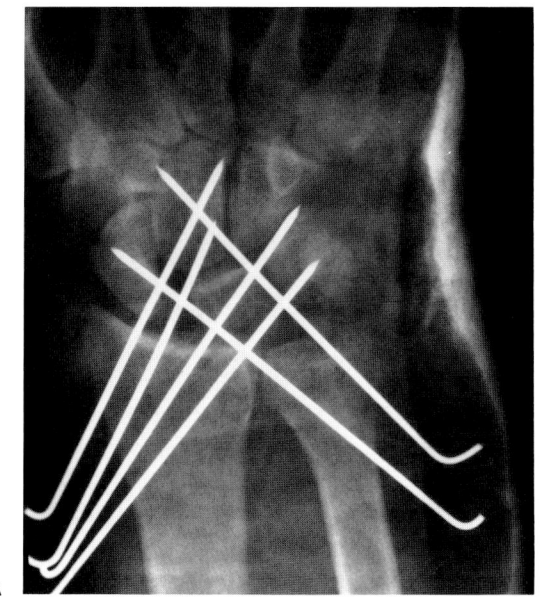 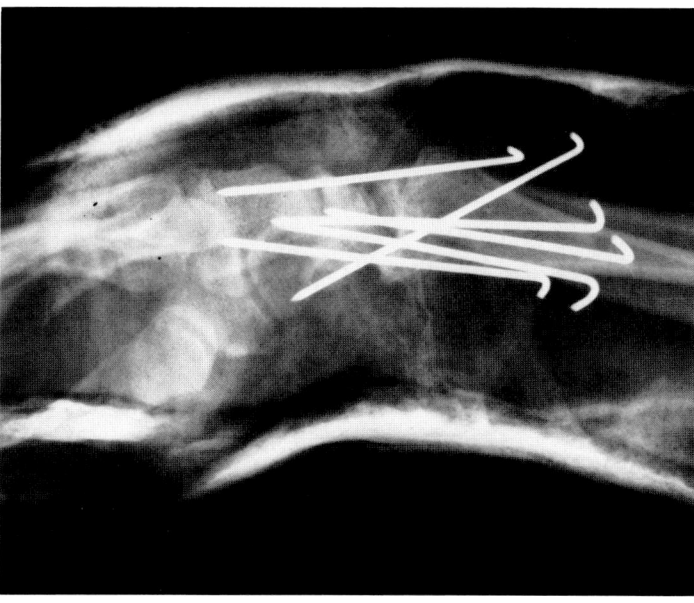

A   B

FIG. 14–121. PA (**A**) and lateral views (**B**) following reduction of a transcaphoid perilunate dislocation with K wires.

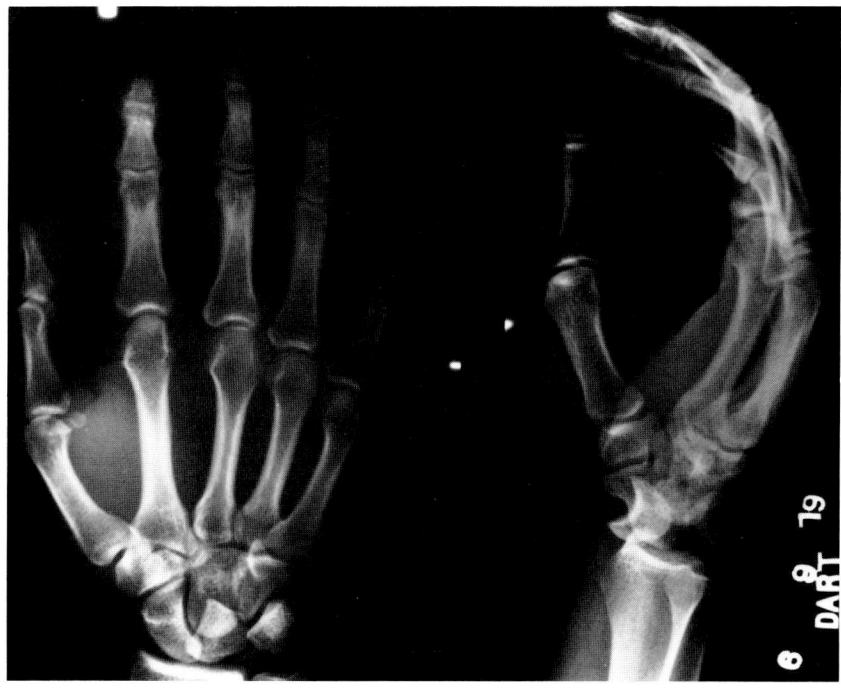

FIG. 14–122. PA (**A**) and lateral (**B**) views of an anterior lunate dislocation. The scaphoid and triquetrum are in near normal position in the PA view. The lunate has lost its normal relationship with the radius and the lunate appears triangular.

either as isolated entities or in combination with other carpal dislocations or fractures (Fig. 14-123). The most common nonperilunar carpal dislocations involve the trapezoid (144,163,207) and the trapezium (143,197, 199,211). Trapezoid dislocations occur most commonly in the dorsal direction, presumably from a hyperflexion stress to the second metacarpal. Palmar dislocations have also been described. Trapezial dislocations are most often associated with axial compression adduction injuries. Associated marginal fracture is common (211,227).

Diagnosis of subtle subluxation or dislocation may be difficult, especially when the typical scapholunate and lunate patterns described above are not present. Static instability (pattern present on neutral routine radiographs) and dynamic instability (patterns seen only with motion) may both exist. The latter are more easily appreciated with video fluoroscopic studies (Fig. 14-124) (100,106,204,213).

Carpometacarpal Dislocation

Carpometacarpal dislocation or subluxation is most often associated with an accompanying fracture of the distal carpal row or metacarpal base (Fig. 14-125). These injuries may be difficult to define accurately on routine radiographs. Multiple oblique views or trispiral tomograms are often helpful. As an isolated injury without fracture, carpometacarpal dislocations are rare (see Fig. 14-26) (2,133,163,177). Most commonly, they involve multiple rays or the border rays (153). The direction of displacement is usually dorsal, although volar dislocation has also been reported (181). These dislocations, particularly when involving the first or fifth metacarpal, may be grossly unstable (185). If the dislocations are re-

ducible but unstable, percutaneous fixation is recommended. If they are irreducible, open reduction with internal fixation and possibly soft tissue repair is advisable, particularly with the thumb ray.

Metacarpal Fractures

Fractures of the metacarpals, particularly the fourth and fifth, are common (3,7,193,204). In spite of this, errors of either over-/or undertreatment are not infrequent. Management considerations will depend upon a number of factors, which include the particular metacarpal involved, the type and location of the fracture line, the degree of displacement, the adequacy of rotatory alignment, and the presence of any associated soft tissue injury. In general, routine PA, lateral, and oblique radiographs are adequate for evaluation of these injuries. For both discussion and treatment purposes, metacarpal fractures should be considered in three subgroups: thumb, stable rays (second and third metacarpals), and mobile rays (fourth and fifth metacarpals). Within each of these groups, a similar fracture classification is applicable.

Thumb

The thumb metacarpal is highly mobile, with multiple degrees of freedom of motion at its basilar joint. Because of this freedom, considerable tolerance exists for fracture angulation and rotation. However, this same feature of high mobility of the basilar joint is offset by the requirement that the thumb transmit a high magnitude of compressive loads in pinch. This allows little tolerance for residual incongruity in the case of intra-articular fractures of the base.

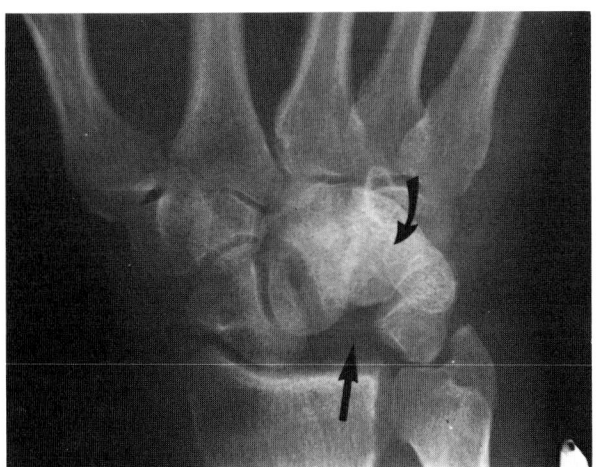
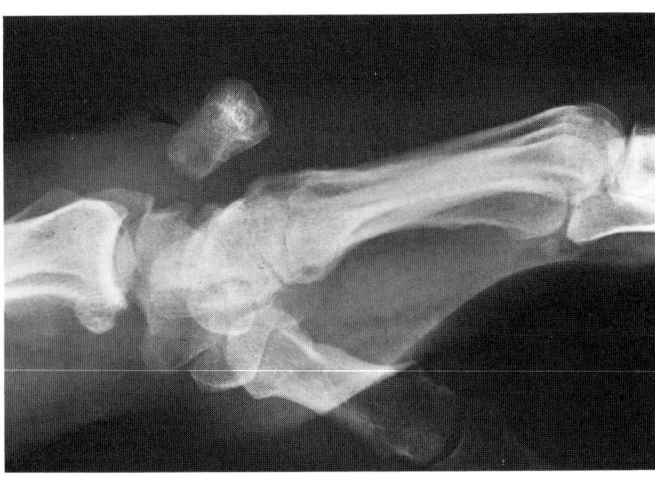

A   B

FIG. 14-123. Isolated dorsal lunate dislocation. The PA view shows absence of the lunate (*straight arrow*) with increased density (*curved arrow*) due to bone overlap. The lateral (**B**) view demonstrates the dorsally located lunate.

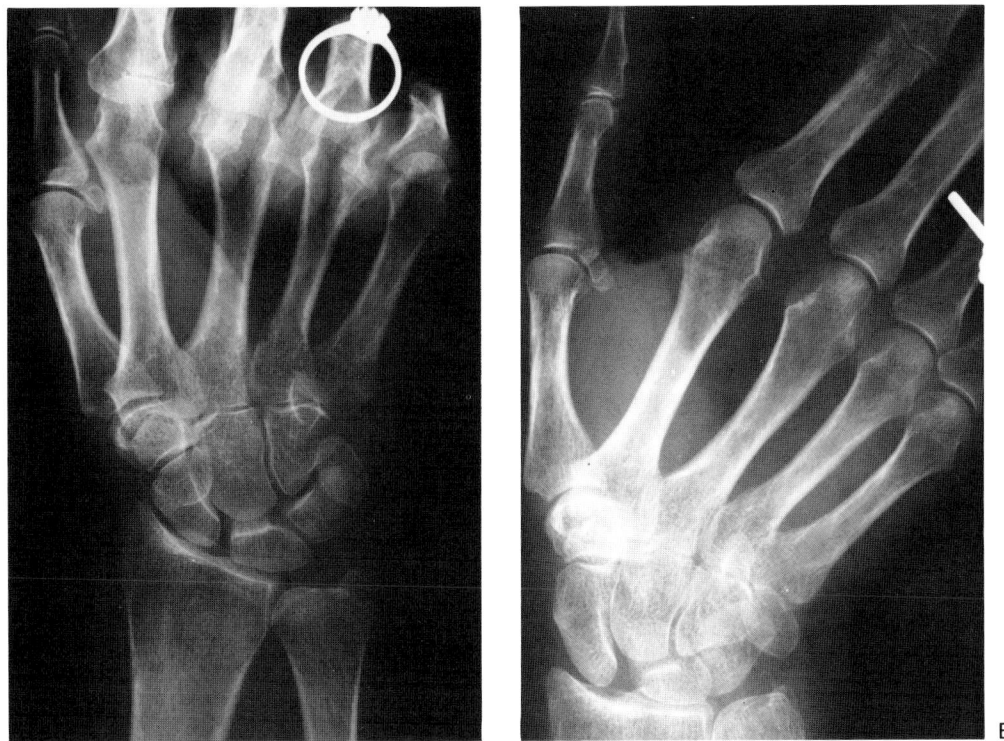

FIG. 14–124. PA clenched fist view (**A**) and ulnar deviation (**B**) monitored fluoroscopically clearly demonstrate scapholunate dissociation.

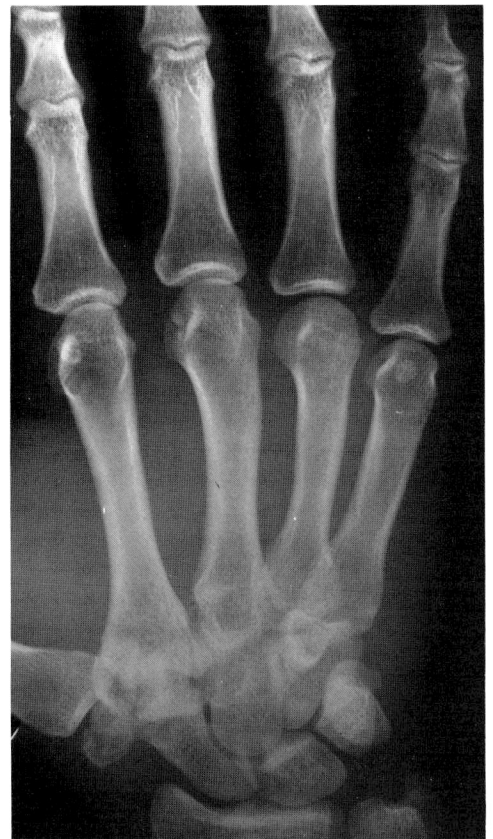

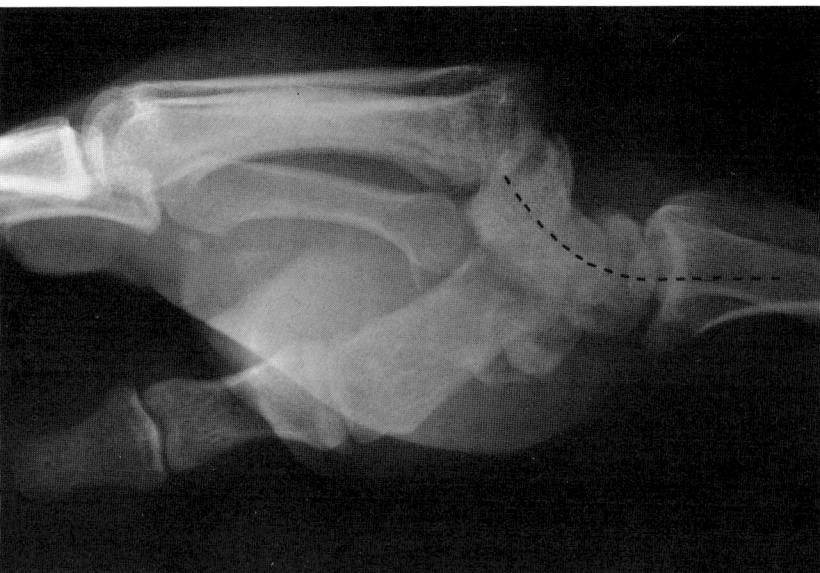

FIG. 14–125. Dorsal carpometacarpal (CMC) dislocation with an associated trapezial fracture. **A:** The PA view shows overlap of the CMC joints with comminution of the trapezium. The position of the metacarpals is better demonstrated on the lateral view (**B**).

Neck Fractures

These are uncommon. Displacement and instability are unusual. Symptomatic treatment by thumb-spica short-arm cast immobilization for 3–6 weeks is usually sufficient treatment.

Transverse Diaphyseal Fractures

These are also not common. Displacement may be present and require manipulative reduction. Angulation with the distal fragment flexed is usual. It should be corrected, although residual angulation of up to 20° may be acceptable. Rotatory alignment need not be anatomic provided there is not an excessive degree of clinical deformity. If the fracture is minimally displaced or stable following reduction, immobilization in a short-arm thumb-spica cast for 4–6 weeks is recommended. Unstable fractures may require percutaneous or open Kirschner-wire fixation. Continuous skeletal traction by a rubber band attached to a transverse Kirschner wire in the distal metacarpal fragment, which is anchored to an outrigger on a short-arm cast, may also be useful in certain cases. Irreducible fractures should be openly reduced and fixed with either Kirschner wires (147), tension-band wires, or plate and screws (101,119,167).

Spiral Diaphyseal Fractures

These are unstable more frequently than are transverse fractures. Internal fixation or skeletal traction is therefore often required. Otherwise these injuries do not differ from the transverse diaphyseal variety.

Extra-articular Proximal Metaphyseal Fractures

These fractures are relatively common (Fig. 14-126). They may be transverse or oblique and usually exhibit angulation in a dorsal direction. Displacement may be present. Angulation of up to 20° in the adult and 40° in the child is acceptable. Fractures of the transverse plane are usually readily reduced by longitudinal traction. Maintenance of reduction is usually possible through a well-molded thumb-spica cast that secures the thumb metacarpal in moderate palmar abduction and extension. Cast immobilization is continued for 4–6 weeks. The oblique fracture variety is more unstable and commonly exhibits a tendency toward proximal migration of the distal fragment. This injury is readily reduced by longitudinal traction, but it is often difficult to maintain at length by cast immobilization alone. Such fractures, therefore, not infrequently require percutaneous Kirschner-wire fixation or continuous skeletal traction, as described above.

Intra-articular Basilar Fractures

These are the most common fractures seen in the thumb metacarpal (3,7,193,204). They also are the most demanding in terms of treatment, with little leeway for anything but anatomic reduction of the articular surface. Two basic fracture types, each with an attached eponym, are seen in this group.

The first, or Bennett's fracture, is actually a fracture-subluxation of the first carpometacarpal joint. Characteristically, the fracture line is oblique and divides a smaller proximal fragment consisting of the volar (ulnar)

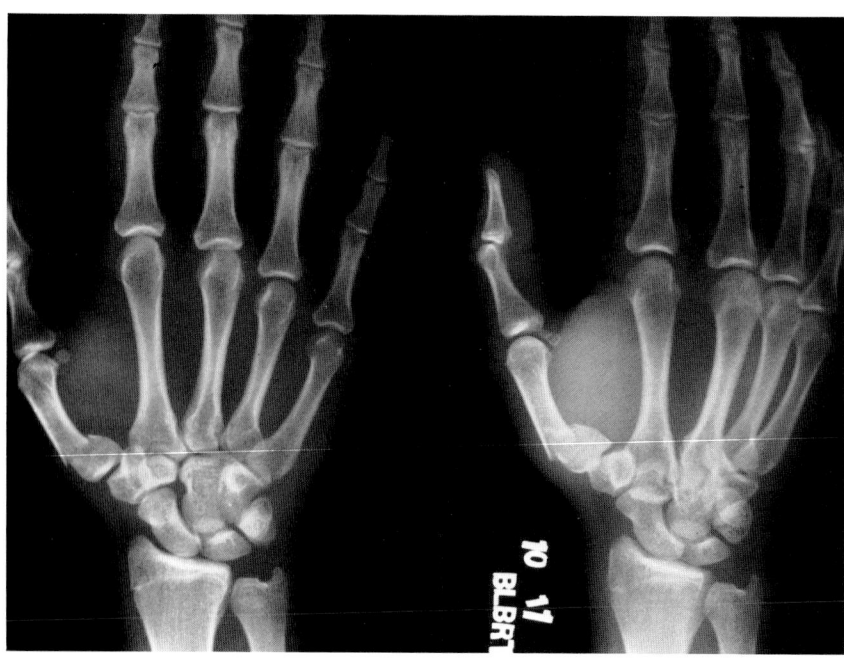

FIG. 14-126. PA (**A**) and oblique (**B**) views of the transverse slightly angulated fracture of the metaphysis of the first metacarpal.

lip of the first metacarpal base from the remainder of the metacarpal as the distal fragment (Fig. 14-127). The smaller proximal (volar or ulnar) fragment is anchored by the attached intermetacarpal and strong volar (ulnar) oblique ligament. It therefore remains undisplaced relative to the trapezium. But the larger distal fragment, consisting of essentially the entire first metacarpal, is characteristically unstable. It displaces proximally and falls into flexion. The proximal displacement is due primarily to the pull of the abductor pollicis longus and flexor pollicis longus tendons, while the fall into flexion is due to the action of the strong adductor pollicis muscle.

Reduction is usually possible by closed means and is accomplished by longitudinal traction on the thumb metacarpal accompanied by pronation. Maintenance of reduction by cast immobilization alone is very difficult and is unreliable. For this reason internal fixation with percutaneous-placed Kirschner wires is recommended (Fig. 14-128). The wires do not necessarily need to cross the fracture line or directly fix the smaller proximal (volar) fragment to the remainder of the metacarpal. Fixation of the base of the metacarpal to the trapezium is usually adequate. If anatomic reduction is not possible by closed means, open reduction and fixation by

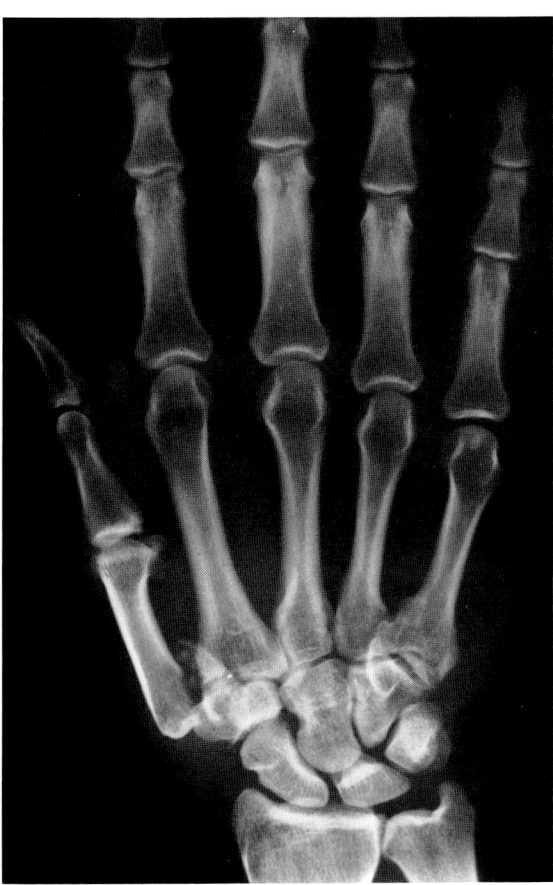

FIG. 14-127. Bennett's fracture seen on PA view of the hand.

Kirschner wires is indicated. Following reduction and internal fixation, a short-arm thumb-spica cast should be worn for 4–6 weeks.

The second type of intra-articular basilar fracture of the first metacarpal is the Rolando fracture. This is by definition a comminuted injury, usually with a *T* or *Y* condylar component (Fig. 14-129). The principles of management for the Rolando fracture are the same as in the Bennett type described earlier. The degree of comminution, however, may preclude reasonable internal fixation by either percutaneous or open means. In such cases, skeletal traction by a transverse Kirschner wire in the distal metacarpal may be indicated.

In all intra-articular fractures of the base of the first metacarpal, the major late complication is degenerative arthrosis of the first carpometacarpal joint. The risk of this complication is increased by residual articular incongruity or joint subluxation and is most frequent with highly comminuted injuries.

Stable Metacarpal Rays—Second and Third Metacarpals

The second and third metacarpals constitute the stable longitudinal axis of the hand. Because the position of these metacarpals is fixed with essentially no motion at the carpometacarpal joints, there is little compensatory potential to allow for fracture-rotation or angulation.

Neck Fractures

Neck fractures are relatively common and usually result from axial compression or from a blow over the dorsum of the affected metacarpal. Displacement may be present. Characteristically, the distal fragment falls into a position of palmar angulation as a result of the forces acting on the fracture from the intrinsic muscles and extrinsic flexor tendons (Fig. 14-130). Malrotation may be present. This is best assessed clinically rather than radiographically. Malrotation is characterized chiefly by overlap of the fingers on attempting to make a fist. In general, anatomic reduction of this fracture is required in the second and third metacarpals. Usually, this is readily achieved by longitudinal traction followed by a dorsally directed palmar pressure over the metacarpal head fragment and a palmarly directed dorsal pressure over the proximal fragment. If reasonably stable following reduction, the position can usually be maintained by application of a splint or cast. This secures the wrist in mild extension, the metacarpophalangeal joints in 60°–70° of flexion, and the proximal interphalangeal joints in 10°–15° of flexion. This position relaxes the deforming musculotendinous forces across the fracture site. If the position of reduction is moderately unstable, then percutaneous fixation with Kirschner wires may be indi-

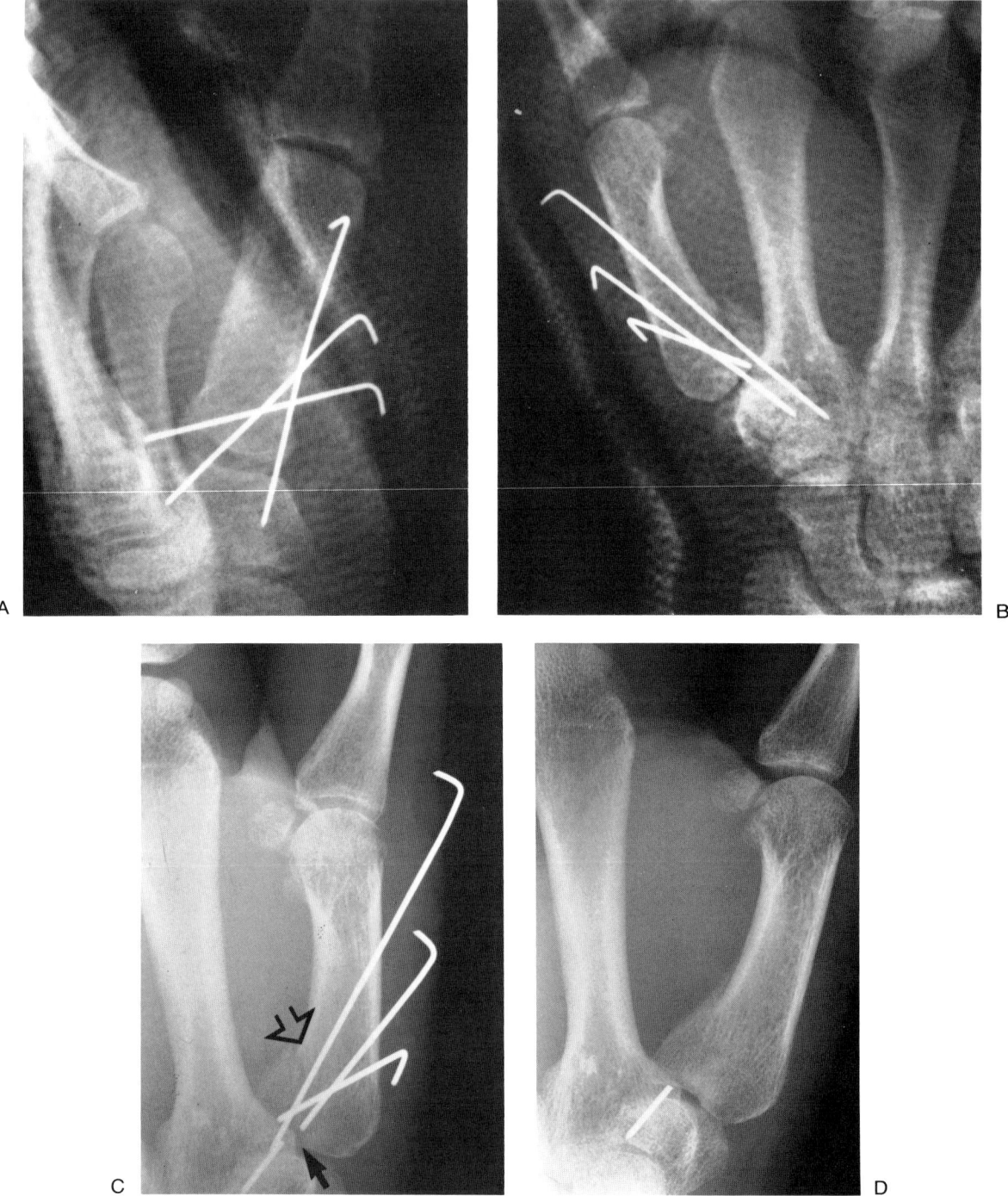

FIG. 14–128. Internal fixation of Bennett's fracture with K wires. PA (**A**) and lateral (**B**) views following reduction with 3 K wires and splints. Lateral view (**C**) 5 weeks following reduction shows good position of the fracture (*open arrow*) and articular surface. There is fracture of a K wire at the point (*black arrow*). **D:** Two months following reduction the fracture is healed.

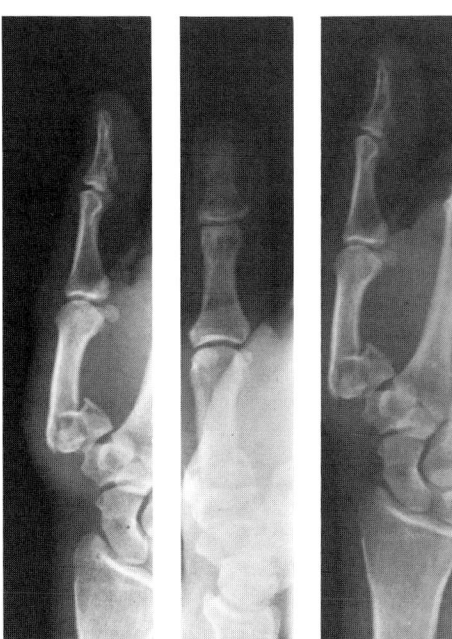

FIG. 14–129. Complex displaced intra-articular fracture (Rolondo type) of the first metacarpal base.

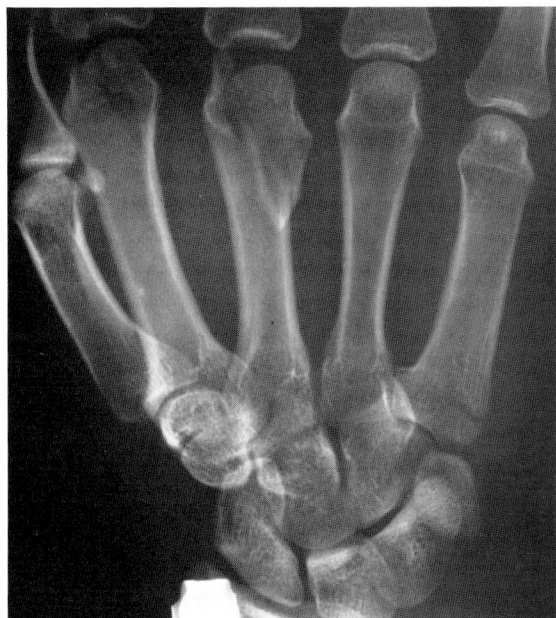

A

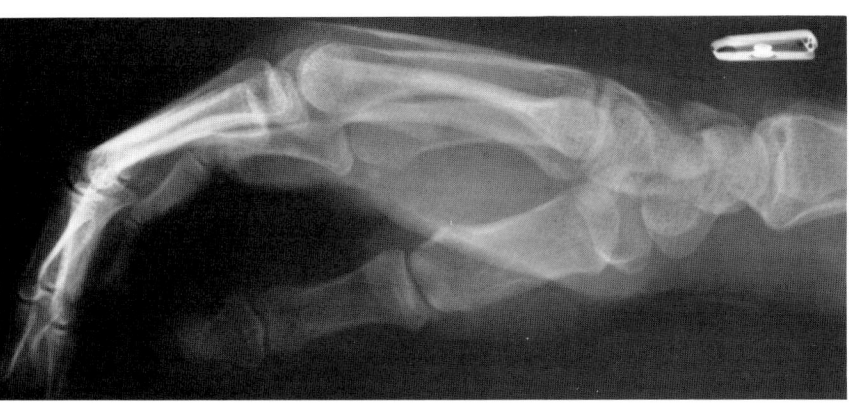

B

FIG. 14–130. PA (**A**), lateral (**B**), and oblique (**C, D**) views of the neck fractures of the second and third metacarpal necks extending into the articular surface. There is volar angulation of the second metacarpal, shortening of the third, and marked articular distortion. Note the subtle fracture of the base of the fifth metacarpal.

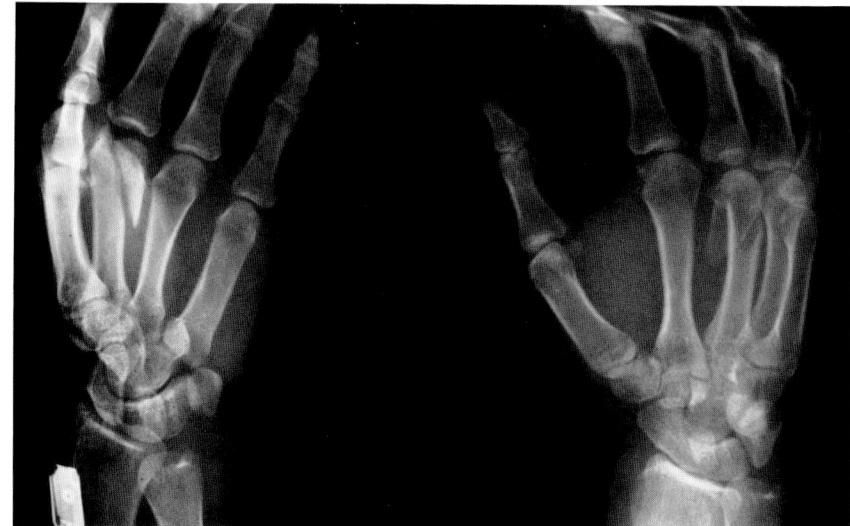

C   D   **FIG. 14–130.** (*Continued.*)

cated. Occasionally, open reduction and internal fixation may be necessary if adequate reduction is otherwise not possible or if there is significant accompanying soft tissue injury requiring local wound care or skin coverage. Following reduction, splint or cast immobilization is continued for 3–6 weeks.

Transverse Diaphyseal Fractures

These fractures are less common than fractures of the neck region. They present, however, the same array of problems regarding angulation or rotation. The treatment principles are essentially the same as those described in the preceding section.

Spiral Diaphyseal Fractures

These fractures are similar to transverse diaphyseal fractures but have a greater tendency toward shortening, instability, and malrotation.

Extra-articular Proximal Metaphyseal Fractures

Such fractures may be oblique or transverse and are usually stable. If there is not marked displacement and if rotation is satisfactory, symptomatic treatment by simple cast or splint protection for 3–4 weeks is satisfactory. The latter may permit metacarpophalangeal joint motion. Occasionally, open or closed reduction and internal fixation with multiple Kirschner wires may be necessary.

Intra-articular Basilar Fractures

These fractures are not common in the second and third metacarpals (Fig. 14-131). With such injuries, how-

ever, stability of the carpometacarpal joint is the goal of treatment. Therefore, if unstable and comminuted, internal fixation, possibly with an attempt at primary arthrodesis of the carpometacarpal joint, may be necessary.

Mobile Metacarpal Rays—Fourth and Fifth Metacarpals

Owing to the mobility of the carpometacarpal joints of the fourth and especially the fifth rays, a moderate degree of latitude for fracture-angulation is permissible in these metacarpals (3,7,204). For this reason anatomic reduction is less frequently necessary. However, malrotation or excessive displacement and shortening is not acceptable.

Neck Fractures

These are the most common metacarpal fractures and are particularly likely in the fifth ray. This injury is also known as the *boxer's fracture*, which implies that the common mechanism of injury is a direct axial compression force over the ulnar side of a clenched fist. Displacement usually is not excessive, but characteristically there is palmar angulation of the distal fragment (Fig. 14-132). The latter usually results from the deforming effects of the interosseous muscles and extrinsic digital flexors. Fracture-angulation in the lateral plane of up to 40° in the fifth metacarpal and up to 25° in the fourth is compatible with minimal functional limitation (3). Greater degrees of angulation may be accepted in the child with significant growth potential, provided that no malrotation is present. The lateral view is essential in determining the degree of angulation (Fig. 14-132C and D).

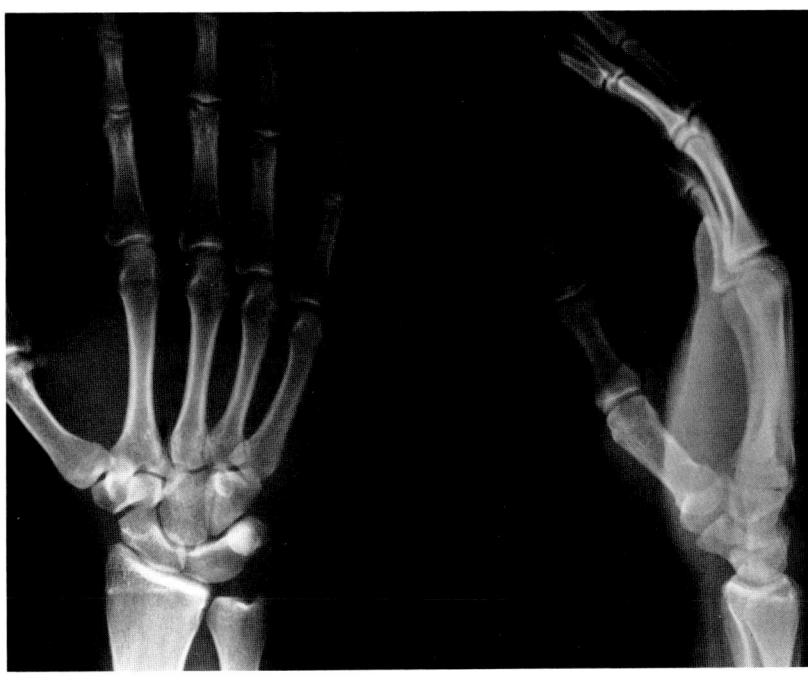

FIG. 14-131. PA (**A**) and lateral (**B**) views of an intra-articular fracture (*arrow*) of the base of the second metacarpal.

Reduction, when required, is generally not a problem. In the usual situation with fracture-angulation but otherwise no displacement, a dorsally directed pressure over the distal fragment with palmar counterpressure over the proximal fragment suffices. If complete displacement of the fracture is present, preliminary longitudinal traction may be necessary. Any malrotation must also be corrected with appropriate torsion on the distal bony fragment. Following reduction the ulnar two or three rays are immobilized in an ulnar gutter-type splint. This splint maintains the wrist in slight extension, the metacarpophalangeal joints in 60°–70° of flexion, and the interphalangeal joints in 10°–15° of flexion. Usually, splinting is continued for about 3 weeks, followed by an additional 2–3 weeks of removable splint protection. Cautious, active mobilization of the digits is permitted during this time. Grossly unstable fractures may require percutaneous internal fixation. This may be accomplished by the use of Kirschner wires passed transversely into the adjacent intact metacarpal or across the fracture site (Fig. 14-132D). This procedure is facilitated by the use of an image intensifier. If possible, the fixation hardware should avoid transfixing the metacarpophalangeal joint. Inability to achieve acceptable reduction by closed means, or extensive accompanying soft tissue injury, may be indications for open reduction and internal fixation with Kirschner wires or tension-band wires.

Transverse Diaphyseal Fractures

These fractures are less common but are associated with greater problems than injuries of the neck region (Fig. 14-133). Fracture union is less rapid, displacement and instability are more frequent, and angulation is less acceptable (3,7). The same principles of management as outlined for the neck fractures, however, are applicable to this injury.

Spiral Diaphyseal Injuries

These injuries are more prone to shortening, instability, and malrotation than transverse fractures of the mid-diaphysis (Figs. 14-134 and 14-135). It is not uncommon for multiple adjacent metacarpals to be affected. Internal fixation, either percutaneously or following open reduction, is frequently required.

Extra-articular Proximal Metaphyseal Fractures

These fractures are also not uncommon. They are usually impacted and stable and may be oblique or transverse. If there is no clinically apparent malrotation, reduction is rarely necessary. Because the interosseous muscles take their origin distal to the fracture, they do not represent a deforming force. Symptomatic treatment with a well-molded splint or short-arm cast that permits metacarpophalangeal joint range of motion is usually adequate.

Intra-articular Basilar Fractures

Such fractures are particularly prevalent in the fifth metacarpal (see Figs. 14-130 and 14-131). In many re-

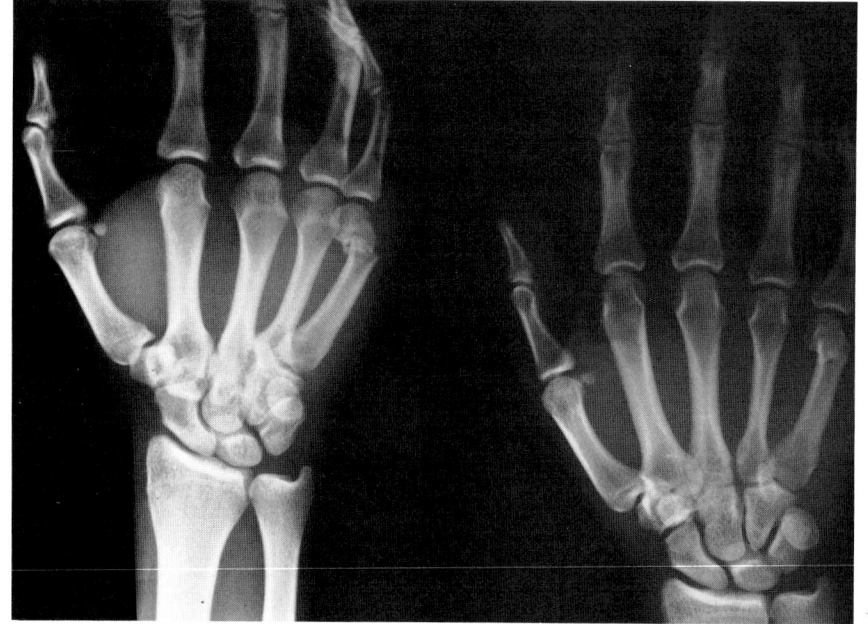

A

B

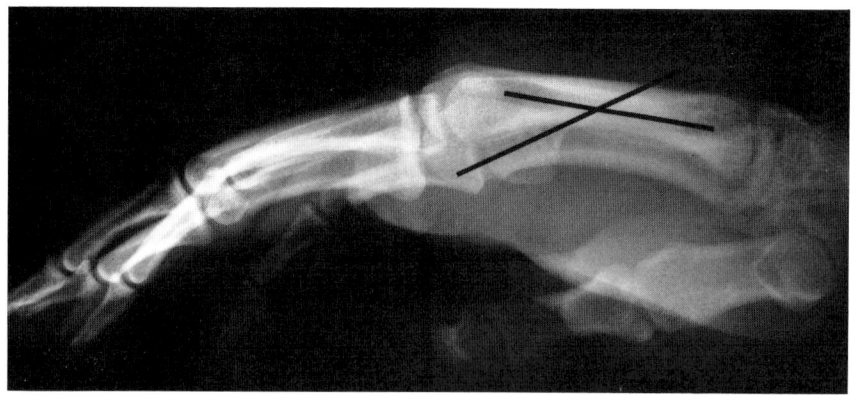

C

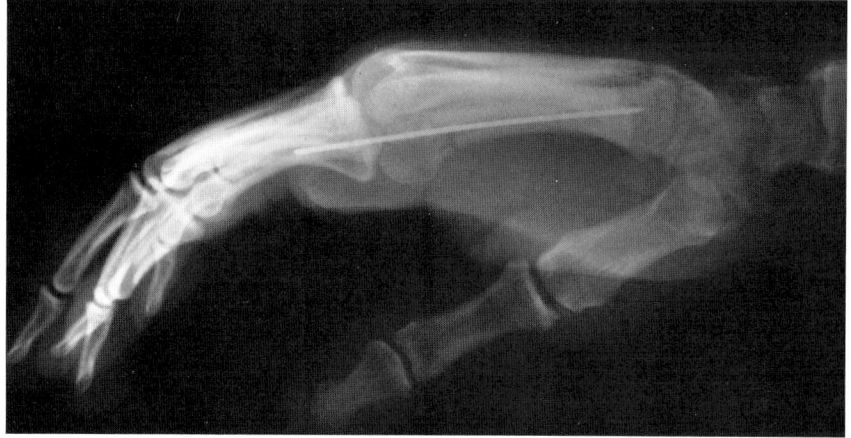

D

FIG. 14–132. Boxers fractures seen on the AP (**A**) and oblique (**B**) views. The degree of angulation is evaluated on the lateral view (**C**). Following reduction with K wire (**D**) there is no angulation.

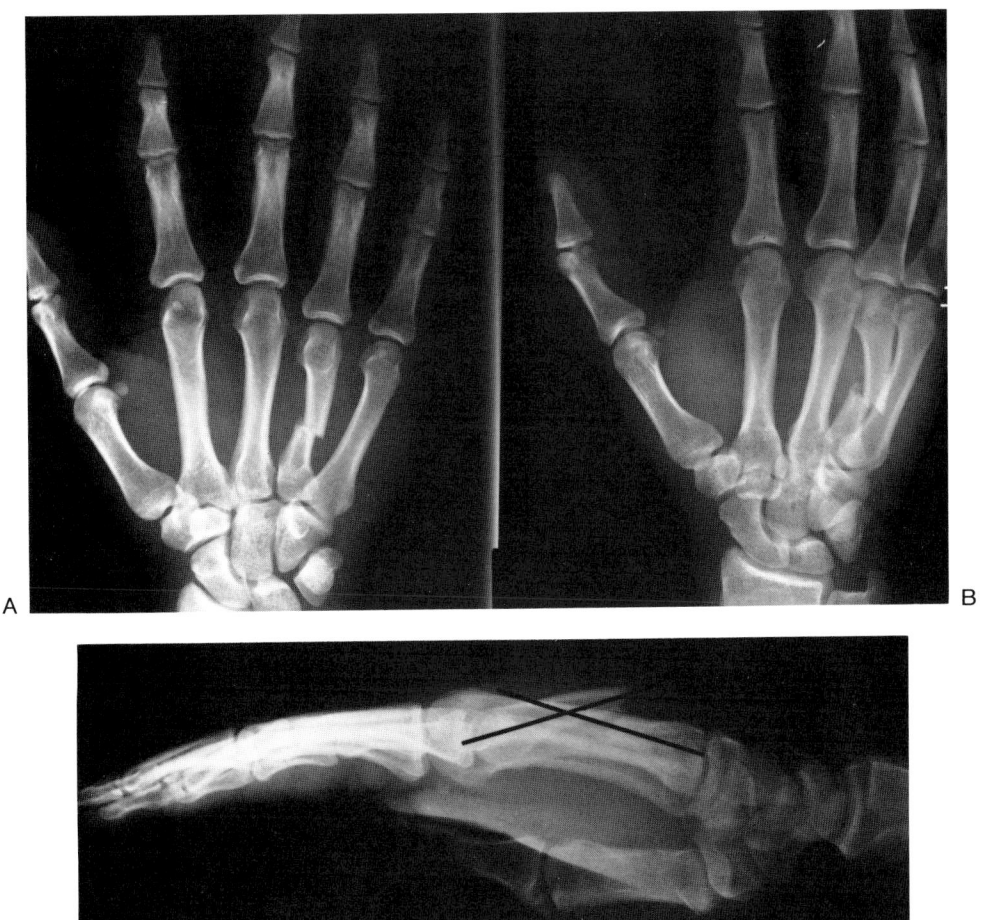

FIG. 14–133. AP (**A**), oblique (**B**), and lateral (**C**) views of a displaced fracture of the fourth metacarpal diaphysis with dorsal angulation.

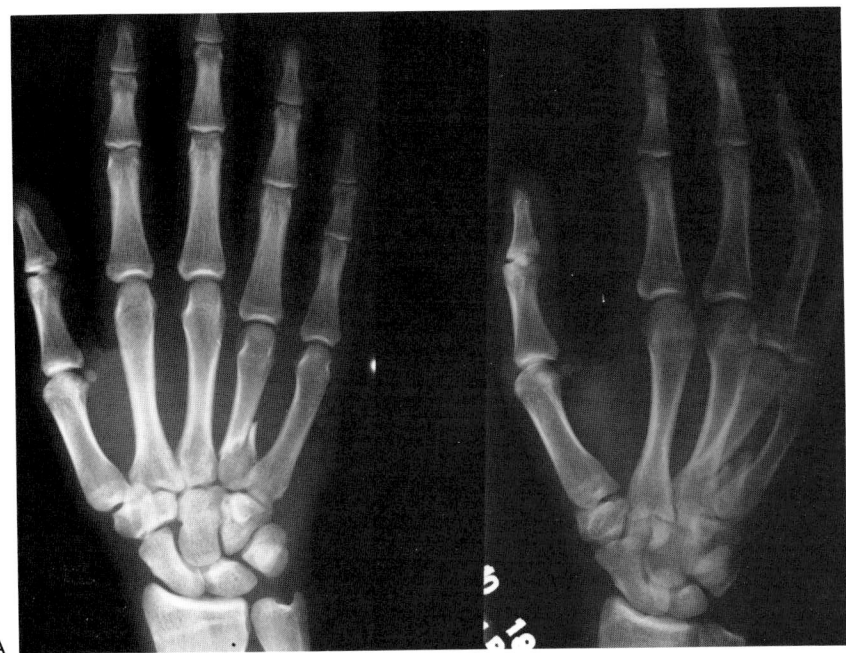

FIG. 14–134. PA (**A**) and oblique (**B**) views of the hand with an overriding, shortened fracture of the proximal fourth metacarpal.

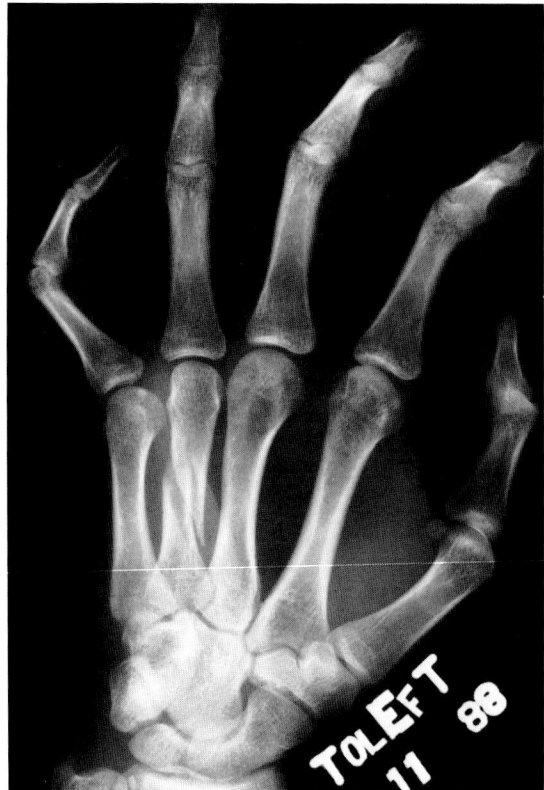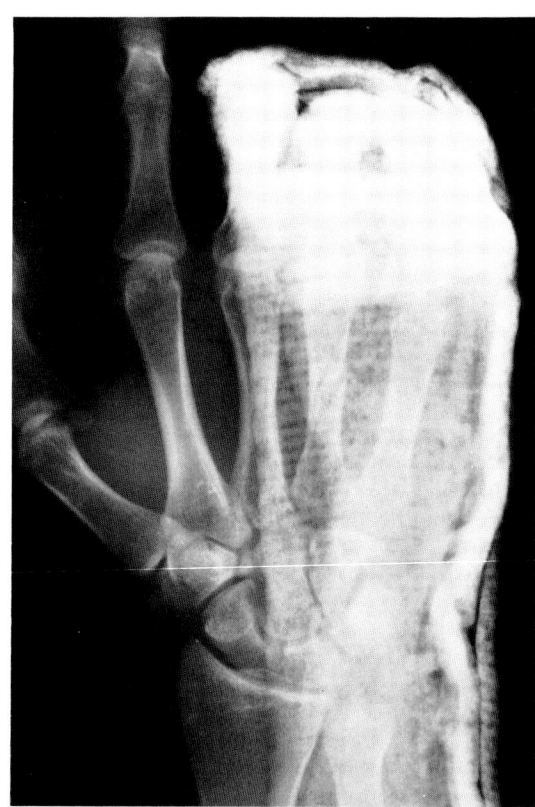

FIG. 14-135. Oblique view (A) of a spiral fracture of the fourth metacarpal with shortening and rotation. PA view (B) following reduction.

spects, this injury represents the fifth-ray counterpart of the Bennett fracture seen in the thumb (3,7). Instability, if present, usually results from the pull of the extensor carpi ulnaris tendon as it displaces the distal (metacarpal) fragment in a proximal direction. Treatment depends on the degree of articular incongruity and joint subluxation. In general, minor degrees of incongruity or subluxation are more tolerable in this case than with the same fracture type in the thumb metacarpal. However, greater amounts of articular incongruity and carpometacarpal joint subluxation are associated with greater risks of painful arthrosis. Therefore, an attempt at reduction is recommended for this injury when any obvious radiographic displacement is present. Except when impacted, this injury is frequently unstable. Therefore, percutaneous fixation with Kirschner wires should be used following reduction. In the nondisplaced or impacted fracture, immobilization for 3–4 weeks in an ulnar gutter-type splint, as previously described, or in a well-molded short-arm cast is usually satisfactory. In such cases, however, vigilant radiographic monitoring of the fracture for the first 2 weeks is advisable to be certain that displacement within the splint or cast does not occur.

Complications of Metacarpal Fractures

The chief complications of metacarpal fractures are limited range of motion, malunion, arthrosis, and non-

union. Limited joint range of motion is most commonly due to extension-contractures of the metacarpophalangeal joints and flexion-contractures of the proximal interphalangeal joints. These are often due to immobilization of the hand in an inappropriate position while awaiting fracture union. Occasionally, these contractures can result from pericapsular fibrosis consequent to post-traumatic autonomic dysfunction (sympathetic dystrophy, Sudeck's atrophy). Furthermore, limited range of motion may be due to peritendinous adhesions of the extensor tendons. These may result from either associated soft tissue injury or adherence of the tendons to the fracture site.

With proper management, malunion of the fracture is, for the most part, avoidable. Rotary malunion is the most frequent significant complication of this group. Arthrosis is mainly a complication of intra-articular fractures of the first or fifth metacarpal base. Non-union is unusual.

Metacarpophalangeal Joint Dislocations

Dislocations affecting the metacarpophalangeal joint are not frequent and usually are not accompanied by significant fracture. Occasionally, small chip fractures at the site of collateral ligament or volar plate insertion or small shear fractures of the metacarpal head may be seen in association with this injury. Radiographically the lateral view of the involved joint is most useful. Most often, the proximal phalanx is displaced dorsally relative to the metacarpal (3,98,160,168,193). Displacement in the opposite direction has rarely been reported (190,228).

Dorsal Metacarpophalangeal Joint Dislocation

Dorsal metacarpophalangeal joint dislocation usually results from a hyperextension injury (160,168). It is most common in the thumb, where it may or may not be associated with an injury to the collateral ligaments (Fig. 14-136) (3,107,117,200,209). The dislocation may be simple or complex, with the latter term indicating an irreducible injury. Usually the volar fibrocartilaginous plate of the metacarpophalangeal joint is disrupted at its proximal attachment on the metacarpal and travels with the proximal fragment. It may be an impediment to reduction.

Most dorsal dislocations of the thumb metacarpophalangeal joint are reducible by closed means. This is most safely accomplished by initially extending the proximal phalanx and then, while maintaining this position, translating the proximal phalanx in a palmar direction. Straight longitudinal traction on the digit may impale the volar plate within the joint, thus converting a simple dislocation to a complex one (3,168). It should therefore be avoided. On post-reduction x-rays, the joint space should be carefully evaluated. Incomplete reduction or widening of the joint space may indicate capsule or ligament interposition. Following satisfactory reduction, the joint is clinically tested for stability. The period of subsequent immobilization will depend on the degree of post-reduction volar and collateral ligament stability. If the joint is markedly unstable in extension, or if a complete collateral ligament disruption is suspected, immobilization for as long as 6 weeks in a thumb-spica cast may be advisable. Failure to achieve a satisfactory closed reduc-

tion is an indication for open reduction. The most frequent complication of this injury is limitation of metacarpophalangeal joint range of motion. The most disabling complication, however, is residual ulnar or radial collateral ligament instability (200) or residual joint subluxation.

Dorsal metacarpophalangeal joint dislocation of the finger is most common in the index digit (135,160,168). Unlike the thumb, a significant number of these injuries will not be amenable to closed reduction. The same reduction maneuver and the same precautions regarding longitudinal traction as outlined above are applicable to finger metacarpophalangeal joint dislocation. If closed reduction fails, it is likely that the metacarpal head is "buttonholed" by the volar plate, the natatory ligament, and the flexor tendons and lumbrical muscle of the affected digit (160). Open reduction of the complex dislocation is mandatory. Following reduction, the joint should be mobilized as early as the stability of the reduction permits. Preferably this should be within the first week. The most frequent late complication of dorsal metacarpophalangeal joint dislocation of the finger is limited range of motion. In contrast to the thumb, residual joint instability is infrequent and less of a functional impairment.

Volar Metacarpophalangeal Dislocation

Volar metacarpophalangeal dislocation is rare (Fig. 14-137). All reported cases have involved the fingers, and all have apparently been complex (228). The pathologic feature blocking reduction has been variously reported as either an entrapped volar plate (190) or a dorsal capsular flap (168,228). The mechanism of injury has been reported as either a hyperextension injury or a hyperflexion injury with a palmar translation force. Open reduction, identification of the pathologic features, and

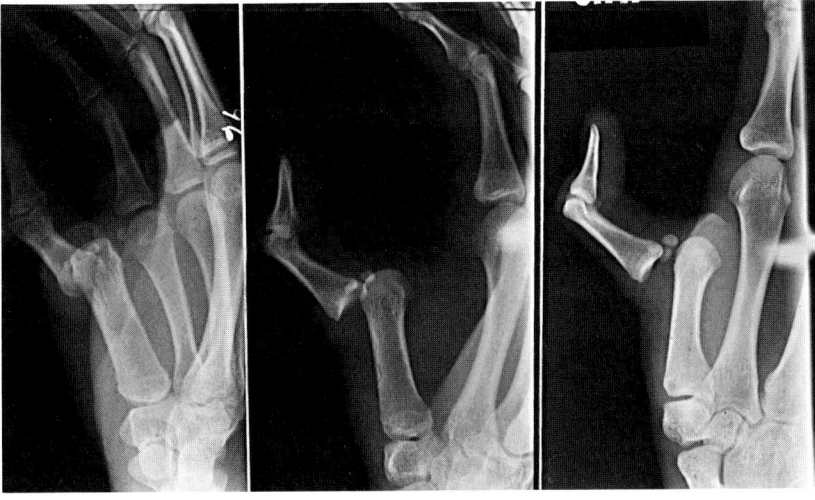

A,B,C

FIG. 14-136. Lateral, oblique, and AP views of a dorsal dislocation of the first MCP joint.

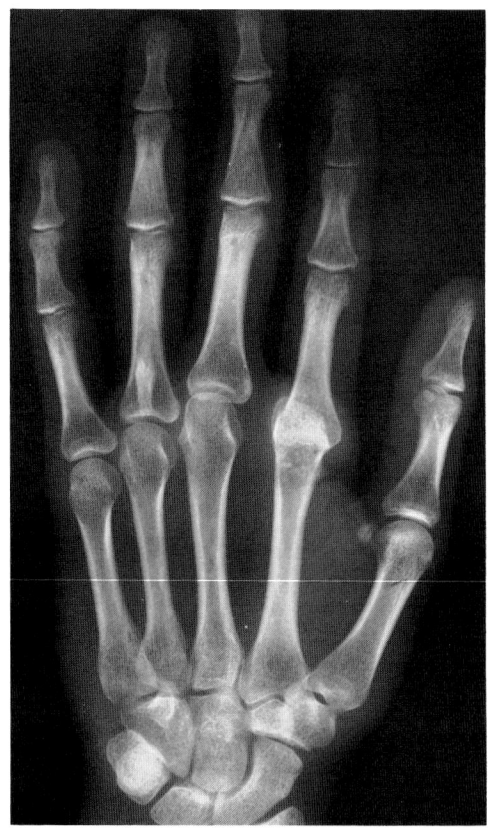

A

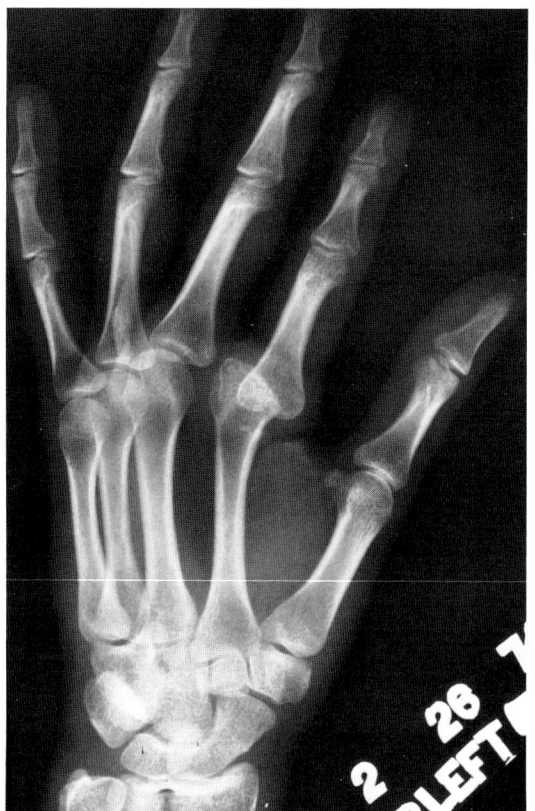

B

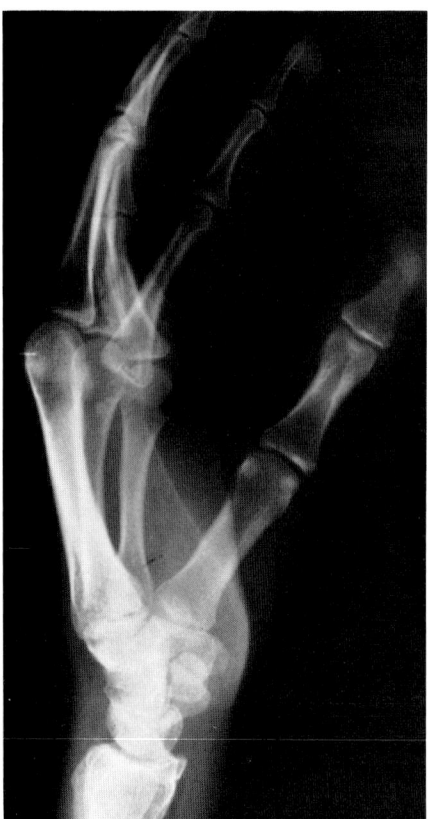

C

FIG. 14–137. Volar fracture dislocation of the second MCP joint seen in the PA (**A**) and oblique (**B**) views. The lateral view (**C**) is difficult to interpret due to the bony overlap. **D:** Reduction required an arthrodesis with K wire fixation.

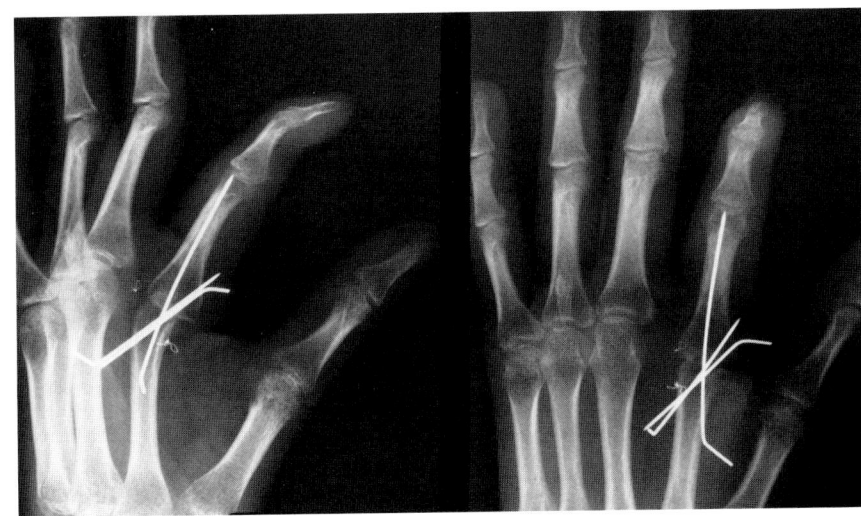

D

FIG. 14-137. (Continued.)

repair of disrupted structures is advisable. Often this injury is seen late and requires either arthroplasty or arthrodesis.

Phalangeal Fractures

As a group, fractures of the phalanges are the most common fractures involving the hand (3,7,109, 145,193,204,222). As in the case of the metacarpals, management will depend upon a number of considerations. These include the particular phalanx fractured, the type and location of the fracture line, the degree of displacement or rotation, and the presence of associated soft tissue injury. Routine PA and lateral radiographs are usually adequate to evaluate these injuries. If possible, the involved finger should be separated from the other fingers to prevent overlap (see Figs. 14-139C and 14-145). Localized views of the injured phalanx using dental x-ray film may provide greater clarity.

Proximal Phalanx

Fractures of the proximal phalanx are more common than those of the middle or distal phalanges (3). The adverse effects of malunion, shortening, and tendon adherence at the fracture site are more marked in the proximal phalanx than in the more distal fractures. The mechanism of injury in the proximal phalanx is widely varied and may include direct blows, sporting activities, falls, and vehicular injuries. Fractures of the proximal phalanx are best classified anatomically. Marked comminuted fractures may have features of more than one type.

Distal Fractures

Unicondylar and bicondylar fractures of the distal portion of the proximal phalanx may be nondisplaced

and appear innocuous (Fig. 14-138). However, they are frequently unstable as a result of traction on the fracture fragment from the attached collateral ligament. Furthermore, in the bicondylar type, compressive forces acting across the proximal interphalangeal joint can spread the two condyles apart. If nondisplaced, this fracture can often be adequately treated by splint protection. Com-

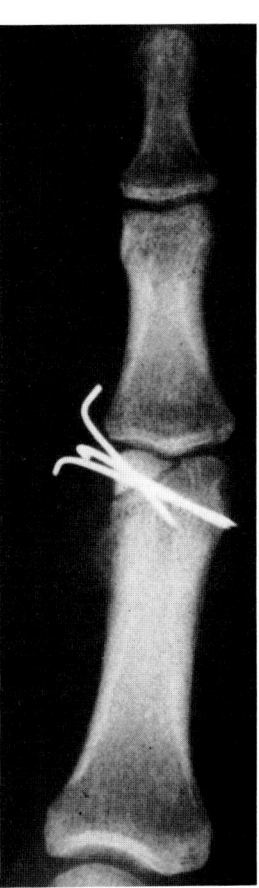

FIG. 14-138. PA view with K wire fixation of unichondylar fracture.

plete immobilization of the digit for the first 3 weeks, however, is necessary. This usually requires a short-arm cast with attached aluminum splint. When the injury involves the ulnar two rays, an ulnar gutter-type cast or splint is required. Careful radiographic monitoring of the fracture position during this time is advised. If the fracture is displaced, there is little allowance for deviation from the normal without adversely affecting joint function. In such cases open reduction and fixation with Kirschner wires (145) or wire loop (142,165) may be necessary (Fig. 14-138). Postoperative immobilization as outlined above should also be utilized. Protected motion of the digit may be initiated after 3 weeks. In most cases, part-time splinting and avoidance of vigorous activities should be continued until 6 weeks after the injury.

Supracondylar fractures are extra-articular. If markedly displaced, they may clinically mimic a joint dislocation. If nondisplaced, the fracture is usually stable. It may be managed as outlined above for the condylar injury. If the fracture is displaced, reduction may be difficult to obtain due to the small size of the distal fragment. However, if an anatomic reduction is accomplished, it is usually stable. If reduction is not possible by closed means, open reduction is indicated. In such cases or in cases of an unstable reduction, fixation by Kirschner wires (145) is indicated. Subsequent management is the same as outlined for the condylar fracture.

Diaphyseal Fractures

Transverse fractures of the diaphysis are quite common (Fig. 14-139). If the fractures are nondisplaced, they can almost always be managed by closed means. This usually requires a short-arm cast with an aluminum outrigger splint to maintain the wrist slightly extended, with the metacarpophalangeal joints flexed at 60°–70° and the interphalangeal joints flexed at 10°–15°. Angulation of the fracture, characteristically with the apex pointing in a palmar direction, is frequent (Fig. 14-140). This position results from the deforming forces of the intrinsic muscles, which act to flex the proximal fragment, and from the extrinsic extensor muscles, which act to extend the distal fragment. Angulation of more than

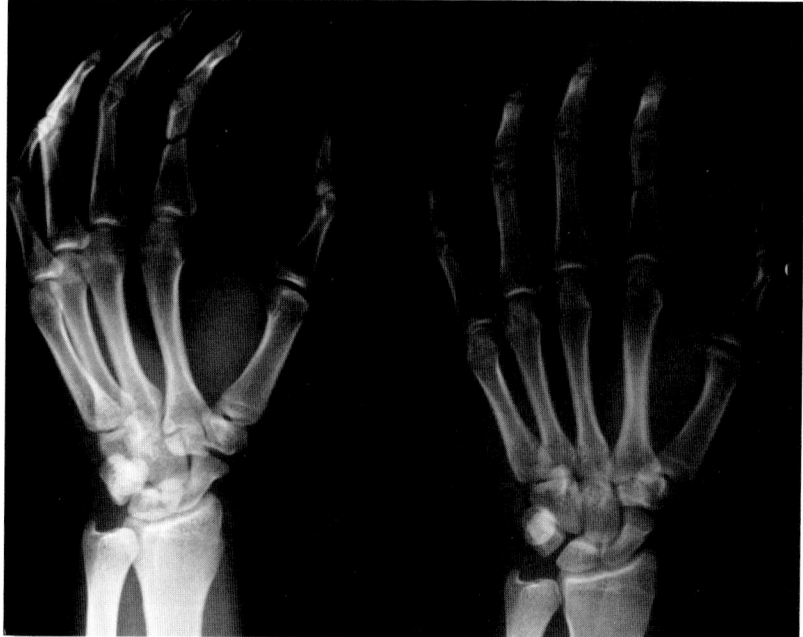

A   B

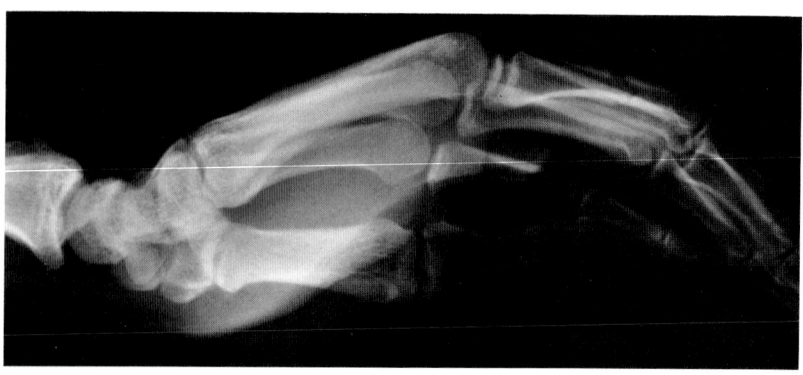

C

FIG. 14–139. Oblique (**A**) and PA (**B**) radiograph of an undisplaced fracture of the proximal phalanx of the index finger. The lateral view (**C**) shows no angulation at the fracture site.

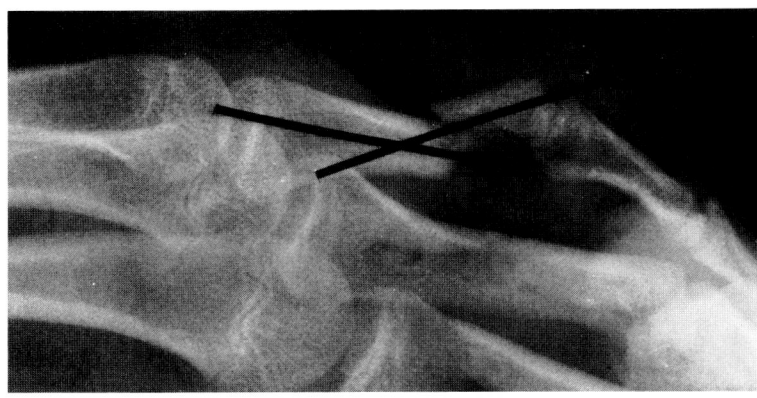

FIG. 14–140. Angulated fracture of the fifth proximal phalanx. The lateral view demonstrates volar angulation.

20° in the adult and 30° in the child should be corrected (3,7). If the fracture is otherwise not displaced, correction of the angulation and maintenance of reduction by an appropriate splint as outlined above are not difficult. If, however, the fracture is displaced as well as angulated, reduction may be difficult. It is most easily accomplished by applying longitudinal traction on the finger with the wrist extended, the metacarpophalangeal joints flexed, and the interphalangeal joints extended. Particular attention should be directed to proper rotary alignment of the digit. Once the fracture is reduced, closed treatment as outlined above usually suffices. If closed reduction cannot be obtained, or if it is markedly unstable following reduction, open reduction and internal fixation with Kirschner wires or a tension-band wire loop may be indicated (Fig. 14-141). Internal fixation may also be required in the unreliable patient or when significant associated soft tissue injury is present.

Spiral or oblique fractures of the diaphysis are more prone to shortening or malrotation than are the transverse variety. A very long spiral fracture may extend into the epiphyseal region and impair joint motion by producing a bony block (see Fig. 14-163). Although reduction of this fracture type is not usually difficult, maintenance of reduction may be a problem. If this is the case, internal fixation by percutaneous Kirschner wires is recommended (145). If open reduction is required, fixation by Kirschner wires, circlage wires, or small bone screws may be appropriate. The principles of management are otherwise similar to those described for the transverse diaphyseal fracture.

Proximal Fractures

Transverse fractures of the proximal metaphysis are common, particularly in the fifth digit in children. Dis-

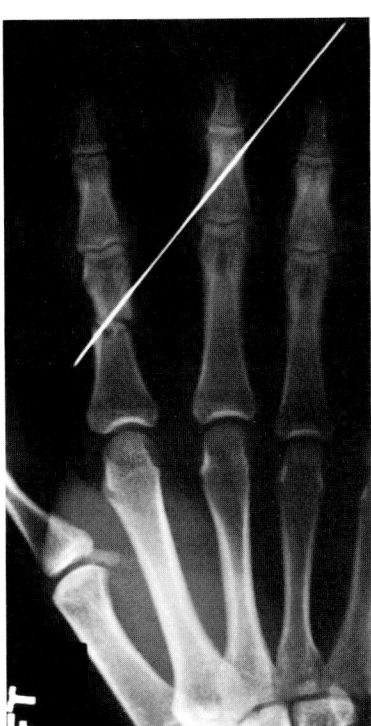
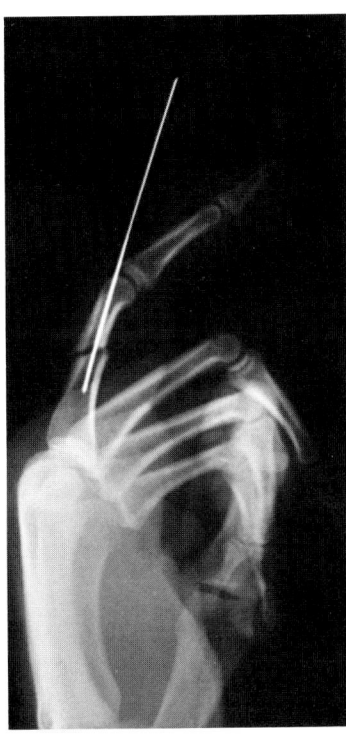

FIG. 14–141. Fracture of the proximal phalanx with K wire fixation. There is no angulation.

placement is usual, with angulation of the distal fragment dorsally and laterally and malrotation of the distal fragment in pronation. Closed reduction can usually be obtained. It is best carried out by maximally flexing the metacarpophalangeal joint to lock the small proximal fragment in position. The distal fragment may then be supinated and manipulated in a palmar and medial direction. Particular care should be taken to ensure proper rotatory reduction. Once reduced, this fracture is generally stable and should be immobilized for 3 weeks by a cast or splint in the position outlined in the preceding section. Continued part-time splint protection and limitation of activity are advisable until 6 weeks after the injury. Occasionally satisfactory closed reduction cannot be achieved. In such cases open reduction and internal fixation with Kirschner wires is recommended.

Proximal condylar fractures are more easily managed than their distal counterparts. They are usually insignificantly displaced and are often impacted and stable. If so, simple protection by taping the involved digit to its neighbor on the side of the injury may be adequate treatment. If the fragment is displaced (Fig. 14-142A), and particularly if it involves more than a third of the articular surface of the proximal phalanx, open reduction and internal fixation with Kirschner wires, a pullout suture, or a small bone screw may be necessary (Fig. 14-142B).

Proximal comminuted articular fractures are uncommon. This injury may or may not be stable. If the fracture is nondisplaced, motion of the involved metacarpophalangeal joint should be initiated as soon as the inherent stability of the fracture will permit. In such cases, the clinical outcome is usually favorable. If the fracture is displaced and it is feasible, an attempt to restore a congruous articular surface should be made. If the size of the major comminuted fragments is sufficient

to permit purchase by a Kirschner wire, open reduction may be advisable. Otherwise, longitudinal traction methods may be worthwhile, although some degree of residual arthrosis can be anticipated.

Middle Phalanx

For the most part, the spectrum of fracture types seen in the middle phalanx is similar to that described for the proximal phalanx with the exception of those occurring about the base. The same general treatment principles as outlined in the preceding section apply to the middle phalanx. Moreover, in some respects, management may be somewhat easier with middle phalangeal injuries. The more distal position of these fractures permits easier access for manipulative reduction and placement of percutaneous hardware. Furthermore, minor angulatory and rotatory deformity in the middle phalanx has less functional impact on the digit as a whole than a more proximally located deformity.

Volar Lip Proximal Base Fractures

In contrast to the proximal phalanx, the most common of the middle phalangeal fractures are those about the volar lip of the base. This fracture characteristically is associated with a direct axial "jamming" or hyperextension injury (3,7). It may be barely apparent radiographically (Fig. 14-143), or it may involve a sizeable portion of the proximal articular surface. If the latter is the case, when viewed laterally the fracture line characteristically courses obliquely in a dorsal and proximal direction. Treatment depends on the size of the bony fragment, the

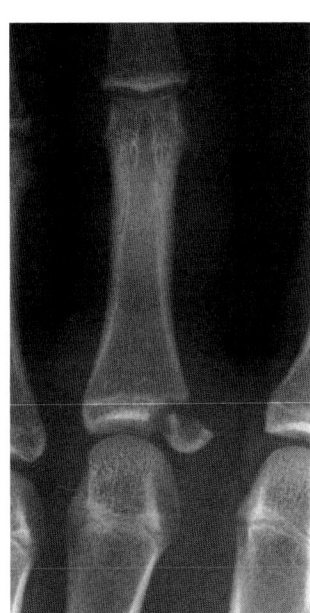

A

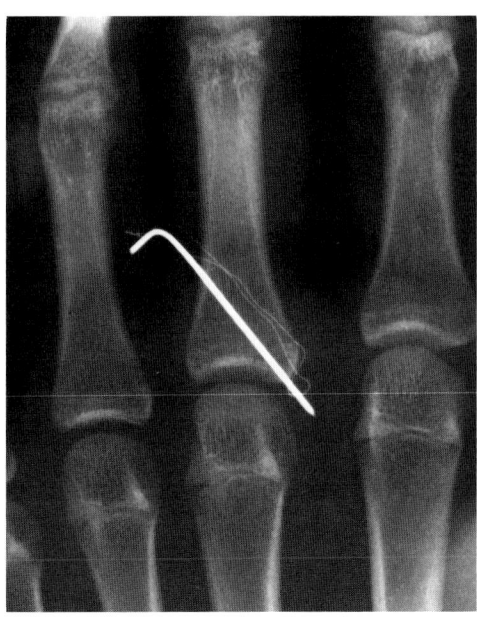

B

FIG. 14–142. PA view (A) demonstrates an intra-articular fracture of the base of the third proximal phalanx. B: Internal fixation with K wire shows the fragment in excellent position.

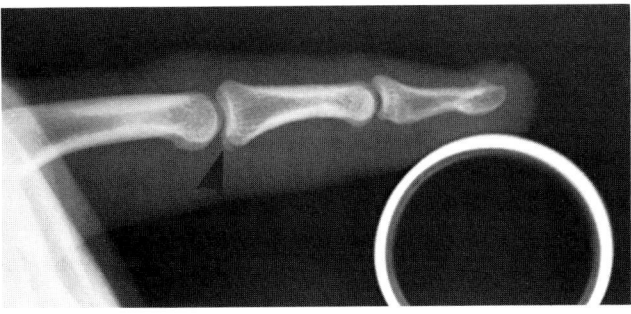

FIG. 14-143. Lateral view of the index finger demonstrating a small volar plate fracture of the middle phalanx (*arrow*).

degree of displacement, and the presence or absence of volar proximal interphalangeal joint instability.

The small chip fracture without dorsal subluxation or volar instability (Fig. 14-143) may be treated symptomatically with a monarticular finger splint to rest the proximal interphalangeal joint in 20°–30° of flexion. Range of motion exercise of the joint should be initiated early to prevent the development of flexion-contracture if there is no associated collateral ligament disruption. The recovery period with this injury may be surprisingly prolonged and depends upon the amount of associated traumatic joint synovitis.

The small chip fracture with either dorsal subluxation or significant volar instability of the proximal interphalangeal joint demands a considerably more vigilant management approach. In these cases, the avoidance of subluxation of the joint takes precedence over the radiographic appearance of the volar chip fracture (3,7,95,104,171). Indeed, the most significant pathologic lesion with this injury involves the volar fibrocartilaginous plate, which is not radiographically obvious (104). This injury must be maintained in the minimum degree of flexion to prevent dorsal proximal interphalangeal joint subluxation. If the joint is statically splinted in this flexed position, there is a substantial risk of residual joint contracture. Therefore, management by extension block splinting is recommended (3,7,171). This technique permits active proximal interphalangeal joint motion and full flexion but blocks extension just short of that that will allow dorsal joint subluxation. Over the 3–6-week period of treatment, the degree of extension block is progressively diminished commensurate with healing and re-establishment of volar stability.

Management of the large volar lip fracture (Fig. 14-144) will depend upon the same joint instability considerations as well as factors related to articular surface incongruity. In general, displaced or undisplaced fractures involving less than one-third of the articular surface may be managed in a manner similar to the small chip fracture. However, displaced fractures involving one-third or more of the articular surface should be reduced with restoration of the articular congruity by either closed or

open means (227). Following reduction, management by extension block splinting, as outlined above, is recommended. The nondisplaced volar lip fracture involving more than one-third of the articular surface is treated the same way.

The most significant complication of volar lip fractures of the middle phalanx is dorsal subluxation of the proximal interphalangeal joint (Fig. 14-144) (3,7). This subluxation may result from inadequate treatment, failure to recognize joint subluxation in the course of treatment, or incorrect treatment by immobilization of the joint in full extension. The consequence of a dorsally subluxed joint is painful limitation of proximal interphalangeal joint motion (95). An array of other complications may be seen with this fracture, the most common of which is limitation of joint motion as a result of capsular contracture. Late arthrosis as a result of a displaced articular fragment involving more than one-third of the joint surface or traumatic chondrolysis is not infrequent. Finally, recurrent locking of the proximal interphalangeal joint in hyperextension may result from mild volar instability in the absence of dorsal joint subluxation.

Dorsal Lip Proximal Base Fractures

This fracture of the middle phalanx is much less common than the volar lip variety. However, it also demands a cautious approach. Usually, this injury involves the insertion of the central extensor slip. If it is untreated or treated incorrectly, a boutonnière deformity of the proximal interphalangeal joint may result (7,193). This deformity is characterized by a flexion-contracture of the proximal interphalangeal joint and a hyperextension deformity of the distal interphalangeal joint due to an acquired imbalance of the extensor apparatus (Fig. 14-145). In addition to disruption of the extensor insertion into the middle phalanx, dorsal lip fractures may rarely be associated with volar subluxation of the proximal interphalangeal joint.

Appropriate management of the dorsal lip fracture will depend upon the size and degree of displacement of the fracture fragment, the integrity of the extensor mechanism, and the presence or absence of joint subluxation. The most frequent error of management is the failure to distinguish this injury from the volar lip variety and to apply a splint that maintains the joint in a flexed position. This will result in further compromise of the extensor apparatus and will encourage fracture-displacement as well as volar joint subluxation. A small fracture fragment with or without displacement and with a complete, active proximal interphalangeal joint extension can be managed by monarticular splinting of the proximal interphalangeal joint in complete extension for 3–4 weeks. A patient with a similar fracture who is unable to actively extend the proximal interphalangeal joint completely most likely has disruption of the extensor mechanism. If

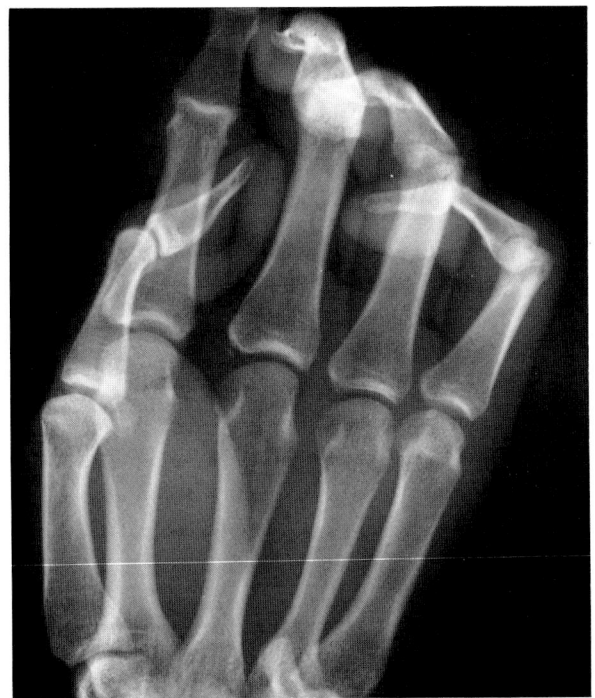

A

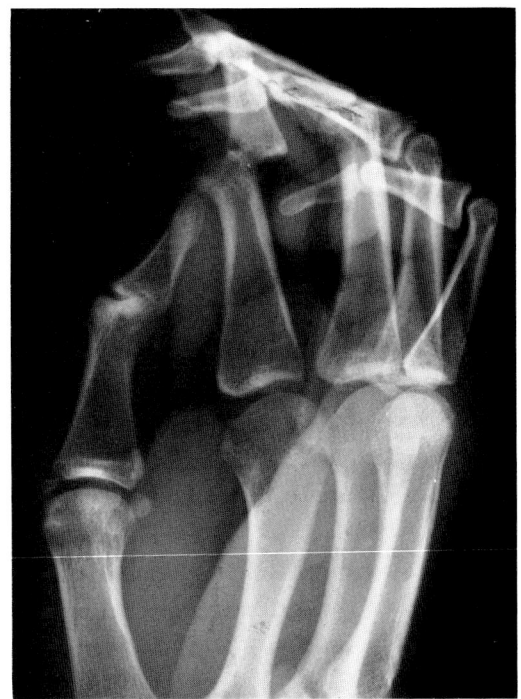

B

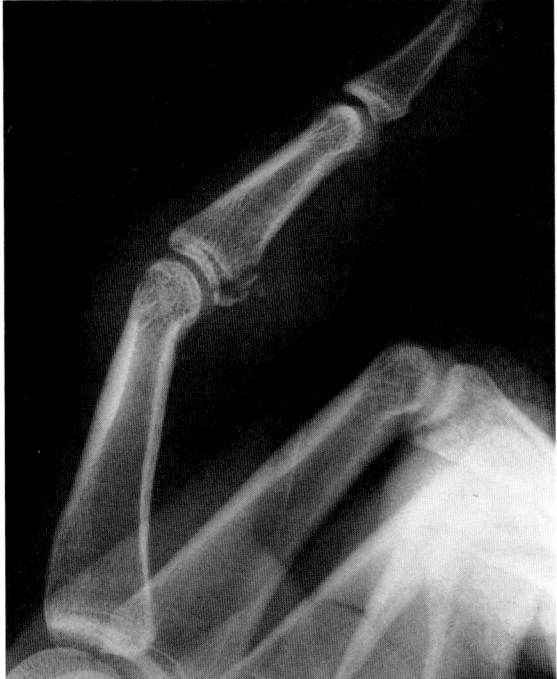

C

FIG. 14-144. AP (**A**) and oblique (**B**) views of the right hand reveal a dorsal dislocation of the second proximal interphalangeal (PIP) joint (*arrow*). There is also a chip fracture of the base of the third proximal phalanx and flexion deformity of the fifth PIP joint. Following reduction, the true lateral view (**C**) demonstrates the associated volar plate fracture.

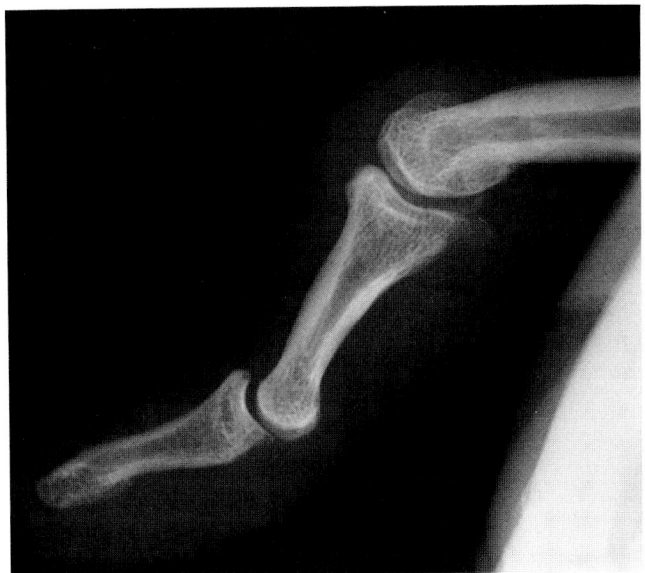

FIG. 14-145. Boutonière deformity.

maintenance of the joint in extension when it is passively straightened is possible, then management by splinting as described above is advised. In this case, however, splinting should be continued for at least 6–8 weeks. In the case of a large fracture fragment (over one-third of the articular surface), the fracture should be reduced closed, if possible, and splinted in extension until bony union is present. If closed reduction is not possible in patients unable to sustain the proximal interphalangeal joint in extension, or if volar proximal interphalangeal joint subluxation is present, then open reduction is recommended. Fixation of the dorsal lip fragment in such cases is usually possible with a pullout wire or with fine Kirschner wires. Complications of the dorsal lip fracture include joint contracture, boutonnière deformity, residual volar joint subluxation, and late joint arthrosis.

Comminuted Fractures of the Base

This injury may involve components of both dorsal and volar lip fractures as well as diffuse involvement of the proximal articular surface of the middle phalanx. Management considerations should be directed by restoration of a congruous articular surface without residual joint subluxation. Often this type of fracture may be so comminuted that little can be done to prevent late degenerative joint arthrosis. Treatment should be tailored to the patient and may include simple splinting, skeletal traction (95), or open reduction and internal fixation.

Distal Phalanx

Fractures of the distal phalanx are extremely common, but with few exceptions these require little in the way of treatment and are not associated with a high incidence of disabling sequelae.

Tuft Fractures

These fractures are the most frequent injury to the distal phalanx (Fig. 14-146). The true incidence of the fracture is unknown because it may not be accompanied by pain sufficient to warrant x-ray evaluation. Most often, the mechanism of injury is a blunt crush to the fingertip. Frequently these fractures are accompanied by a nail-bed laceration, a nail-root avulsion, or a subungual hematoma that may obscure the underlying bone injury. Displacement may be present, particularly if there is a significant nail-bed laceration. However, most cases are minimally displaced and comminuted. They are often well stabilized by the overlying nail plate and the strong fibrous septa that characterize the fingertip tuft. Treatment is symptomatic, usually utilizing a thimble-type splint, and should be directed to any accompanying nail-bed injury. The latter may exceptionally require a manual "compressive" reduction of the bony injury. Tenderness in the fingertip may persist for some time and bear little relationship to the progress of fracture union. Nonunion of the fracture may occur but is only rarely symptomatic. If it is, however, excision of the non-united fragment is usually curative.

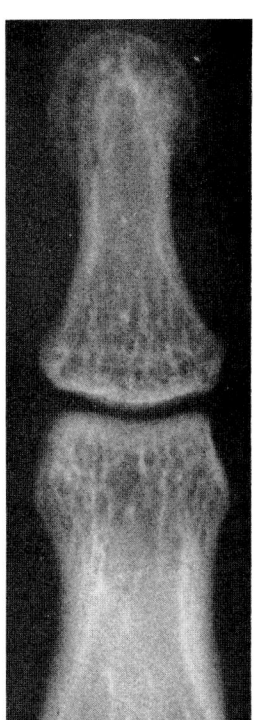
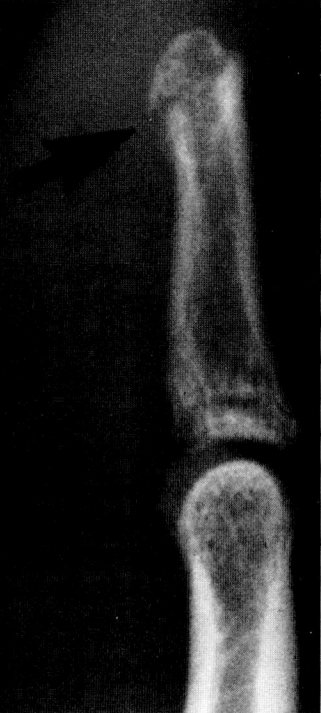

A B

FIG. 14-146. PA (A) and lateral (B) views of a minimally displaced tuft fracture of the distal phalanx.

Transverse Fractures

Transverse fractures of the distal phalanx are distinguished from tuft fractures by the absence of distal comminution. The mechanism of injury, however, is similar. These fractures are also often associated with nail-bed lacerations and nail-root avulsion. Reduction of the fracture usually facilitates management of the nail-bed injury. If the fracture is quite unstable, fixation with a fine smooth Kirschner wire may be helpful in the course of management of the nail-bed laceration. An awareness of this fracture is quite important, since it is usually an open injury with displacement of the nail root. The unwary may mistakenly interpret it as a mallet-finger deformity. In such cases, deep bony sepsis and a permanent nail deformity may result. Proper treatment requires thorough debridement, fracture reduction, relocation or excision of the nail root, and appropriate splinting.

Proximal Base Fractures

Like fractures of the middle phalanx, proximal base fractures of the distal phalanx are important. In contrast to the middle phalanx, however, the dorsal lip fracture of the distal phalanx is of the greatest clinical significance.

Dorsal Lip Fractures

Fractures of the dorsal lip of the distal phalanx constitute one of several members of the mallet-finger spectrum of injuries (Fig. 14-147). The terminal portion of the extensor apparatus of the finger is inserted into the dorsal lip region. Consequently, a displaced fracture will result in the inability to extend the distal phalanx completely. The mechanism of injury is most commonly a hyperflexion stress applied to the distal phalanx (3,7,193,222). Presumably in such a situation, avulsion of the dorsal lip of the distal phalanx results from the pull of the extensor tendon, or else rupture of the extensor tendon itself occurs. Treatment of this injury depends primarily upon the size of the dorsal lip fragment and the presence or absence of volar joint subluxation.

A small dorsal lip fragment constituting less than 30% of the articular surface of the distal phalanx can usually be managed with closed techniques. Acceptable reduction is generally possible by simple distal interphalangeal joint hyperextension. Some authors believe that radiographic reduction of the bony fragment is irrelevant to the clinical result. An initial period of 3–4 weeks of biarticular splinting, with the proximal interphalangeal joint in 20°–30° of flexion and the distal interphalangeal joint in maximum supple hyperextension, is our preference. This period is followed by monarticular splinting of the distal interphalangeal joint in complete extension or slight hyperextension for an additional 4–6 weeks. A further period of 3–4 weeks of monarticular night splinting is often helpful. The duration of splinting will vary but should be determined by the degree of tenderness at the fracture site, the integrity of distal interphalangeal joint extension, and the radiographic progress of fracture union.

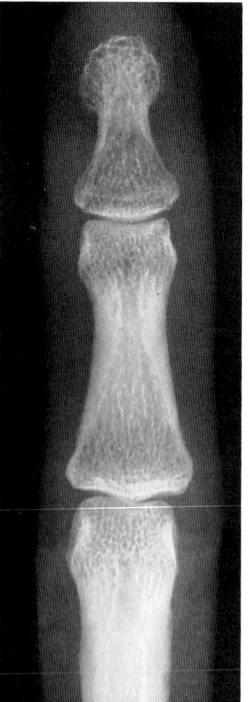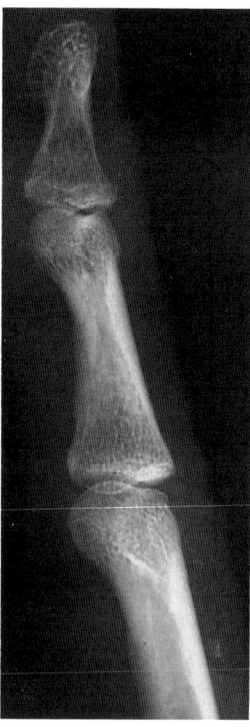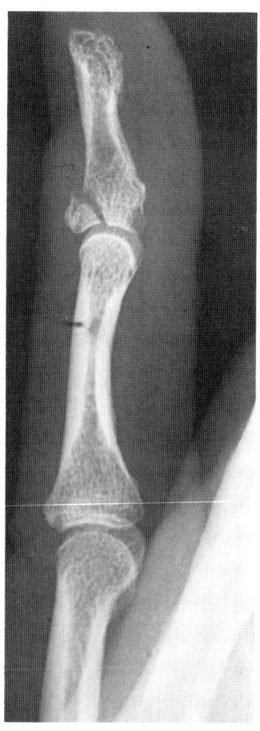

A B C

FIG. 14–147. PA (**A**), oblique (**B**), and lateral (**C**) views of the fourth finger. The dorsal plate fracture is clearly seen only on the lateral view.

Dorsal lip fractures involving 30% or more of the articular surface should be reduced with restoration of articular congruity. If a satisfactory reduction is possible by simple hyperextension of the distal phalanx, further closed management as outlined above is acceptable. Failure to achieve congruous articular reduction, however, may be an indication for open reduction and fixation of the fracture, either by a pullout wire or by a Kirschner wire. Rarely, volar subluxation of the distal phalanx may be associated with a large dorsal lip fracture. If this subluxation is present, the indications for open reduction and fixation are increased.

Volar Lip Fracture

Except in the thumb, volar lip fractures of the distal phalanx are unusual. They may or may not be associated with a large bony fragment and avulsion of the insertion of the flexor digitorum profundus tendon (Fig. 14-148) (164,189,223). If the latter occurs, dorsal subluxation of the distal interphalangeal joint may be present. Treatment usually depends on the presence or absence of associated flexor tendon injury. With an intact flexor tendon, simple monarticular symptomatic splinting of the distal interphalangeal joint in 20°–30° of flexion is usually sufficient. The length of splint protection will depend upon any associated collateral ligament injury and the degree of traumatic synovitis. Late complications are unusual. If there is associated flexor tendon injury, tenorrhaphy or open reduction of an attached bony fragment is indicated. Late complications may occur and are usually related to dysfunction of the flexor apparatus (164,189,223).

Comminuted Proximal Base Fractures

Comminuted fractures of the base of the distal phalanx may be seen. Treatment considerations are similar to those outlined for the same injury affecting the middle phalanx. However, in contrast to the middle phalanx, arthrodesis of the distal interphalangeal joint is often a viable and functionally satisfactory option in the highly comminuted fracture.

Complications of Phalangeal Fractures

General complications of phalangeal fractures are essentially the same as those involved in metacarpal fractures. These include limitation of range of motion, malunion, and non-union (3). Complications peculiar to specific fracture types have been discussed in the preceeding sections.

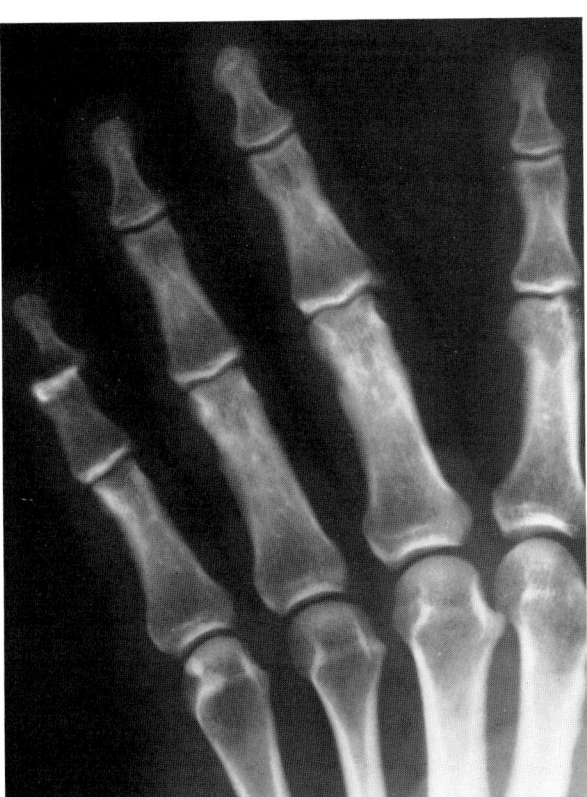
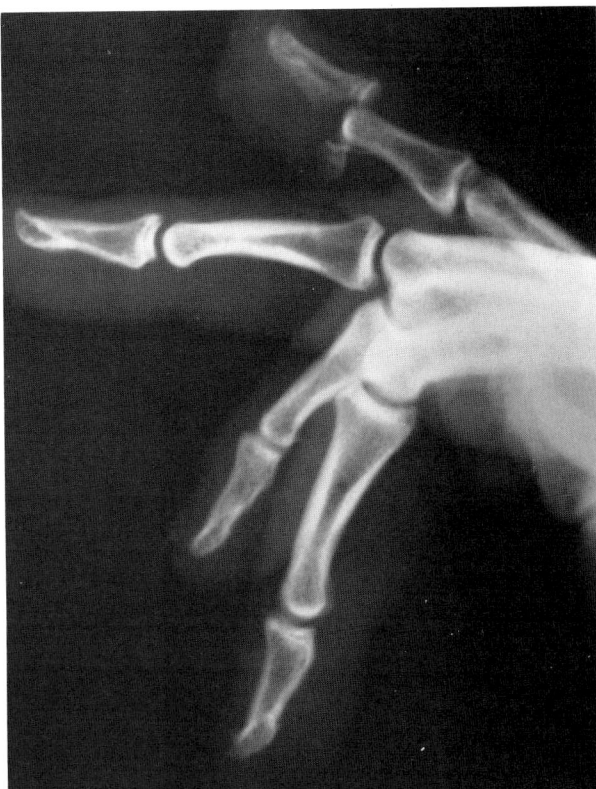

FIG. 14–148. PA (**A**) and lateral (**B**) views of a dorsal dislocation of the fifth distal interphalangeal joint with a volar plate fracture (50% of the articular surface).

Dislocations of the Interphalangeal Joints

Dislocations affecting the proximal interphalangeal joints are extremely common (3,7,171,193). Less frequently, this injury may occur in the distal interphalangeal joint. Often there may be accompanying bony injury, as in the dorsal or volar lip fractures of the middle phalanx discussed in the preceding sections. The dislocation almost always involves dorsal displacement of the middle on the proximal phalanx.

Dorsal Proximal Interphalangeal Dislocation

Dorsal proximal interphalangeal dislocation usually results from an axial compression or hyperextension injury to the fingertip (Fig. 14-149). In the absence of a displaced volar lip fracture, there is disruption of the volar cartilaginous plate (104) and varying degrees of collateral ligament injury. Occasionally, it is an open injury with a transverse palmar laceration. Reduction is usually possible by a maneuver identical to that described for dorsal dislocations of the metacarpophalangeal joints. Rarely the injury will be complex and require open reduction.

Following reduction, further management will be determined by the stability of the volar and collateral ligament structures. If the joint is stable in all planes, early mobilization is recommended, but the joint should be protected from repeat injury for at least 3 weeks. Collateral ligament instability may warrant splint immobilization of the proximal interphalangeal joint in 20°–30° of flexion for 2–3 weeks followed by an additional 2–3 weeks of "buddy taping" to the neighboring finger. Volar instability may warrant the treatment approach outlined earlier for volar lip fractures of the middle phalanx, which is associated with dorsal proximal interphalangeal joint subluxation.

The most common complication of this injury is a residual flexion-contracture due to periarticular fibrosis. The most significant complication, however, is unrecognized dorsal joint subluxation and secondary arthrosis (Fig. 14-150). Occasionally, recurrent volar instability may result with locking of the digit in hyperextension, as described for the middle phalanx volar lip fracture.

Volar Proximal Interphalangeal Joint Dislocation

Volar proximal interphalangeal joint dislocation is rare and almost always associated with a displaced dorsal lip fracture of the middle phalanx. It usually results from a hyperflexion injury to the digit. Treatment should be operative with repair of the disrupted bony and soft tissue structures.

Chronic Post-Traumatic Conditions

The vast majority of traumatic afflictions of the hand and wrist have been discussed in the preceding section. There are in addition to this, however, a number of conditions of radiologic significance that are chronic and post-traumatic in origin. These are diagnosed or become symptomatic after one or more minor traumatic events.

Madelung's Deformity

Madelung's deformity is characterized by an exaggerated ulnar and volar inclination of the articular surface of the distal radius (2). It is usually associated with a positive ulnar variance and a dorsal subluxation of the distal ulna (Fig. 14-151). This deformity results from a deficiency of longitudinal growth of the most ulnar aspect of the distal radius. Most cases are probably congenital as a variant of epiphyseal dysplasia. However, in some cases direct trauma to the physis of the distal radius with a resultant asymmetric arrest of growth has been postulated.

Regardless of etiology, the diagnosis of Madelung's deformity is often made on the basis of a wrist x-ray obtained because of the complaint of wrist pain. Frequently the pain will be of an insidious onset, but it may also follow relatively minor repetitive trauma. Occasionally the presenting clinical complaint will be related to deformity or limitation of wrist motion. Surgical correction of the established deformity is only occasionally indicated (2,3) and is limited to those cases with persistent wrist pain. This may involve excision of the subluxated distal ulna (150) or corrective osteotomy of the distal radius with or without distal ulna resection. If seen very early while the physis of the distal radius is still open, consideration can be given to radial dorsal epiphysiodesis or ulnar volar epiphysiolysis. Madelung's deformity may remain asymptomatic or only minimally symptomatic and be discovered as an incidental radiographic finding.

Tears and Disorders of the Triangular Fibrocartilage Complex

Tears of the triangular fibrocartilage complex may be diagnosed by wrist contrast arthrography or MRI (see MRI and Arthrography of the Wrist and Hand). These tears are characterized by communication of contrast material between the radiocarpal articulation and the distal radioulnar joint (see Figs. 14-58 and 14-61). The injury regularly occurs with certain more obvious conditions previously discussed (subluxation-dislocation of the distal radioulnar joint and most perilunate dislocations). However, triangular fibrocartilage complex tears

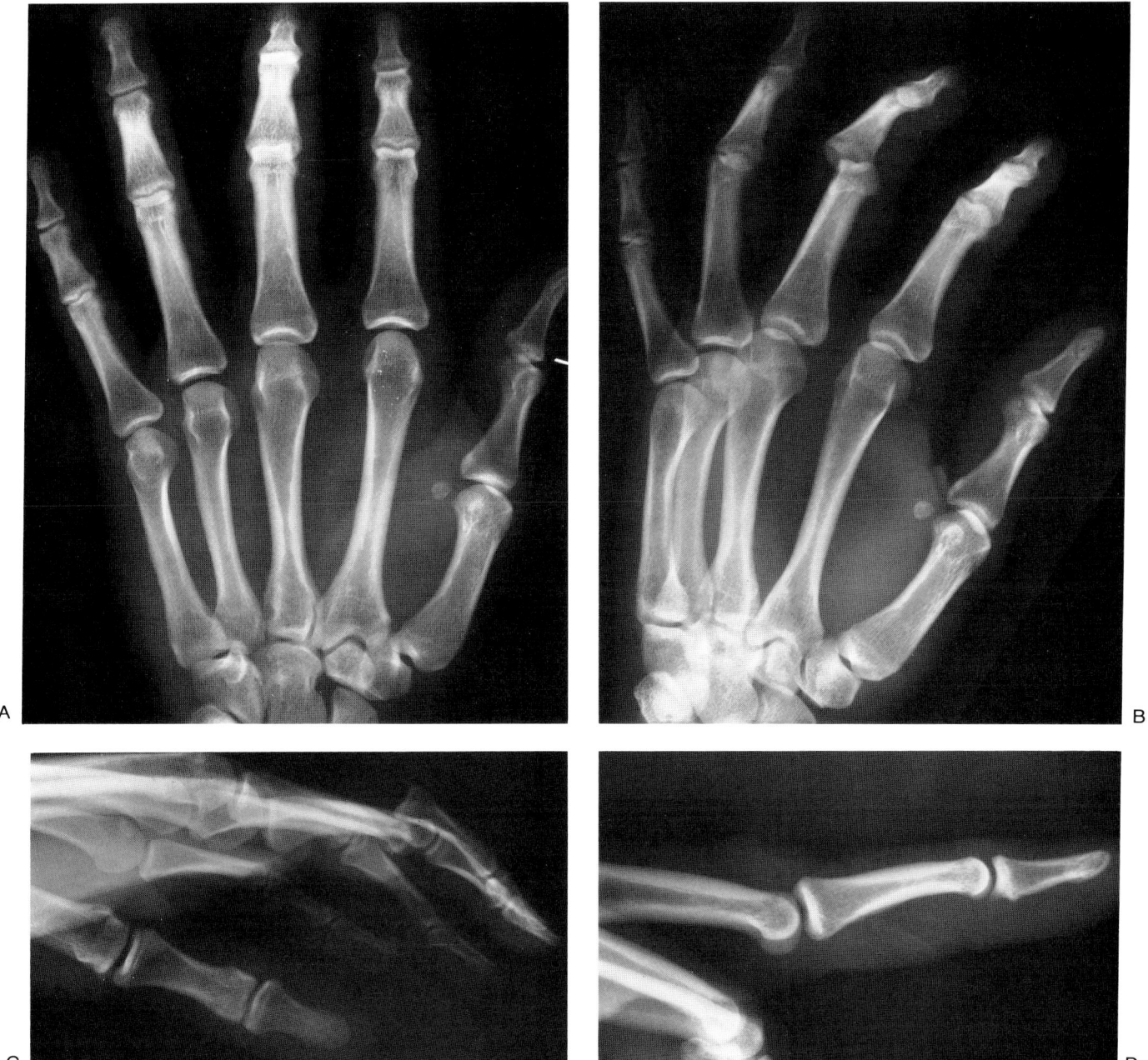

FIG. 14–149. PA (**A**), oblique (**B**), and lateral (**C**) views of the dorsal PIP joint dislocation of the third finger. The lateral view is most informative. **D:** Following reduction there are no fractures but the joint is hyperextended due to tearing of the volar capsule and plate.

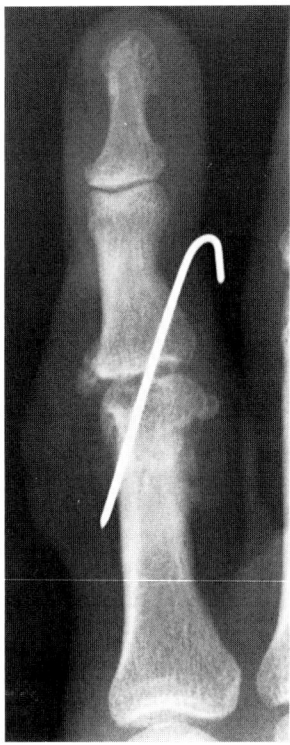

FIG. 14–150. PA view of the left small finger following repair of instability. Note the severe degenerative change from improper treatment of the previous dislocation.

are also common as an isolated entity (16,18). They may result from a single traumatic event or as an attritional tear from repetitive trauma. The true incidence of triangular fibrocartilage complex tears and the frequency of symptoms is unknown. The most common presenting complaint is pain over the ulnar aspect of the wrist with or without a "click," or crepitus. Treatment should be tailored to the patient and will range from symptomatic nonoperative management to surgical excision of the torn central fragment or repair of a peripheral rent (18).

Ulnolunate Abutment Syndrome

The ulnolunate abutment syndrome may present with normal radiographs. However, a positive ulnar variance (see Fig. 14-3) and perhaps reactive changes over the ulnar articulation of the lunate may be present. The latter is characterized by either bony sclerosis or intraosseous cyst formation and, if present, is best visualized by tri-spiral tomograms (Fig. 14-152). Typically with this condition, a bone scan may show increased scintillation activity about the ulnolunate region. In most cases a central perforation of the triangular fibrocartilage disk is present at the point of contact between the lunate and ulna (18). Presumably this perforation is the result of attritional changes and should not be mistaken as the primary pathology. The most common clinical presenta-

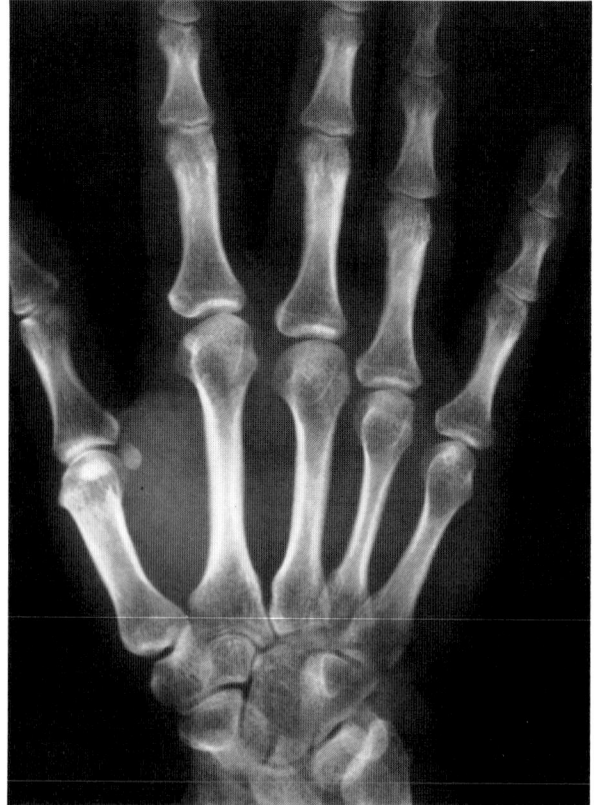

A

FIG. 14–151. Madelungs deformity: PA (**A**) and lateral (**B**) views demonstrate marked ulnar and volar angulation of the distal radial articular surface.

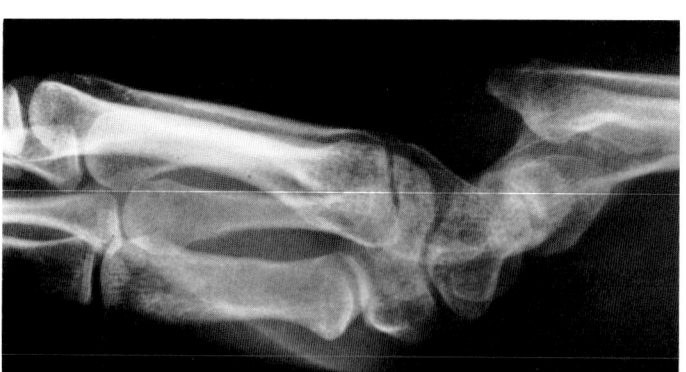

B

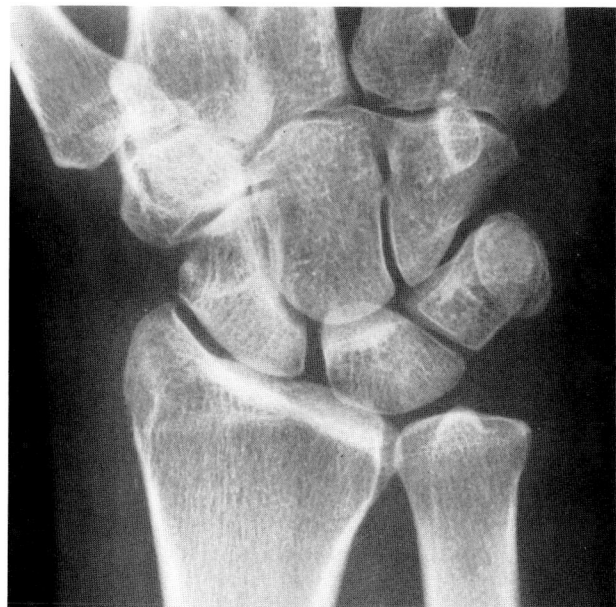
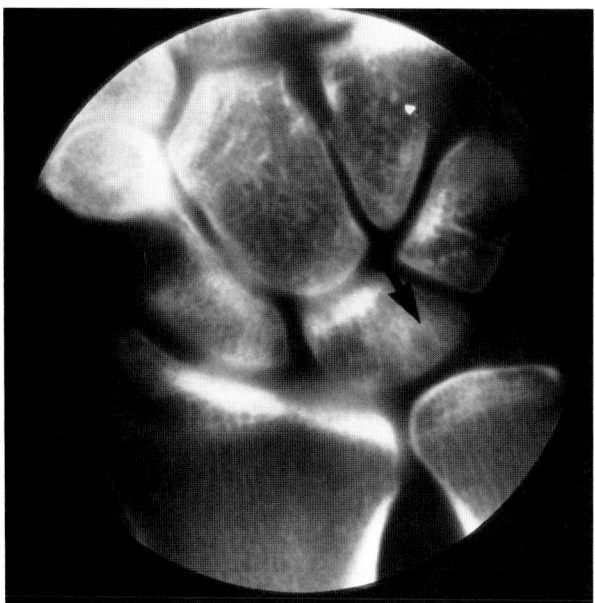

A B

FIG. 14-152. A: Normal PA view of the wrist. Tomogram (B) demonstrates sclerosis and cystic changes in the lunate due to ulnolunate abutment syndrome.

tion with the ulnolunate abutment syndrome is pain over the ulnar aspect of the wrist. Although symptoms may be heralded by a single traumatic event, more often they occur insidiously or with a history of minor repetitive trauma. In most cases, a trial period of nonoperative symptomatic treatment is warranted. However, if significant pain persists, surgical management by ulnar recession to a position of slight negative ulnar variance is warranted. In such cases, the triangular fibrocartilage perforation may be ignored.

Avascular Necrosis of the Lunate (Lunatomalacia, Kienböck's Disease) (237,238)

Kienböck's disease is not an uncommon cause of vague wrist pain, which may range from an annoying to a disabling degree. It may be associated with a single traumatic episode, and, if so, it is usually a result of a fall onto the outstretched wrist or a hyperextension injury. Conversely, the onset may be insidious or associated with repetitive minor trauma. In the early stages, routine radiographs may be normal. MRI is most sensitive and specific at this stage (see Fig. 14-59). Later progressive x-ray changes occur. These are characterized initially by increased radiodensity of the lunate relative to the remaining carpal bones (Fig. 14-153) (233). At this stage, MRI will show low signal intensity on both T1- and T2-weighted sequences. Later, fragmentation and flattening may be seen. These ultimately progress to reconstitution and secondary osteoarthritic changes (Fig. 14-154). In the later stages, routine radiographs are superior to MRI for purposes of classification. Lichtman has classified

these radiographic changes for treatment purposes into four stages, as outlined in Table 14-3 (241).

The course of the progression of these changes may be modified at any time, depending upon the speed of the revascularization process and the adequacy of bony reconstitution prior to marked collapse. Trispiral tomography is particularly useful for defining the radiographic changes (Fig. 14-154). Furthermore, in a few cases trispiral tomograms have revealed horizontal fracture lines following a traumatic episode prior to the development of the typical radiographic changes described above (232). This finding has led some to postulate an acute fracture with consequent injury to the intraosseous blood supply as the etiology of Kienböck's disease. An unusually high incidence of negative ulnar variance (5) has also been noted with this condition. This association has prompted others to postulate that the etiology of Kienböck's disease is a compression-stress concentration on the lunate by the distal radius without adequate ulnar support. Additionally, there are a number of cases without significant trauma, radiographic evidence of acute fracture, or negative ulnar variance. The etiology in these cases is unclear but appears in some way related to an intraosseous vascular insult. MRI is particularly useful for early diagnosis in this setting.

Clinically, most patients present with symptoms of wrist pain, but a relatively painless limitation of the wrist's range of motion or weakness of grip may also occur. With collapse of the lunate in later stages, symptoms of median neuropathy may predominate (232). Occasionally, the diagnosis is made as an incidental radiographic finding in a patient with an unrelated problem.

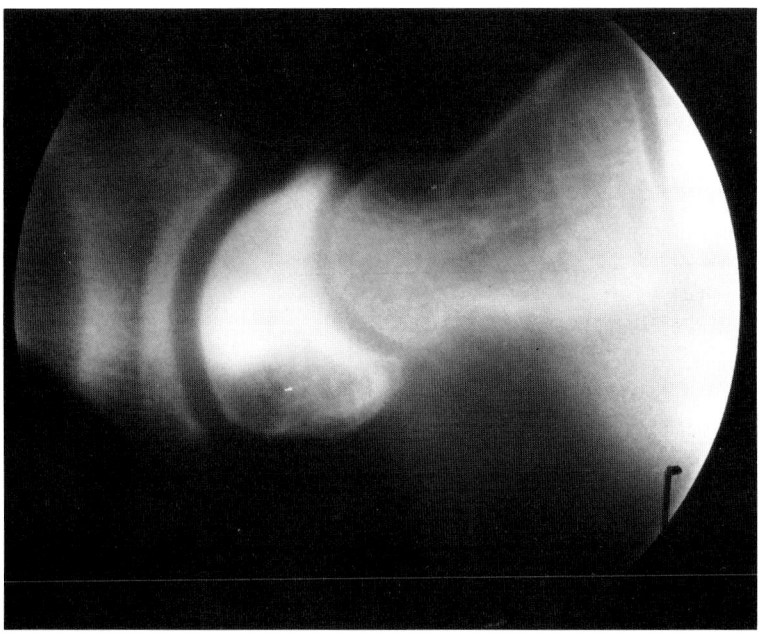

FIG. 14-153. Lateral trispiral tomogram with sclerosis of the lower lunate due to Kienböcks disease.

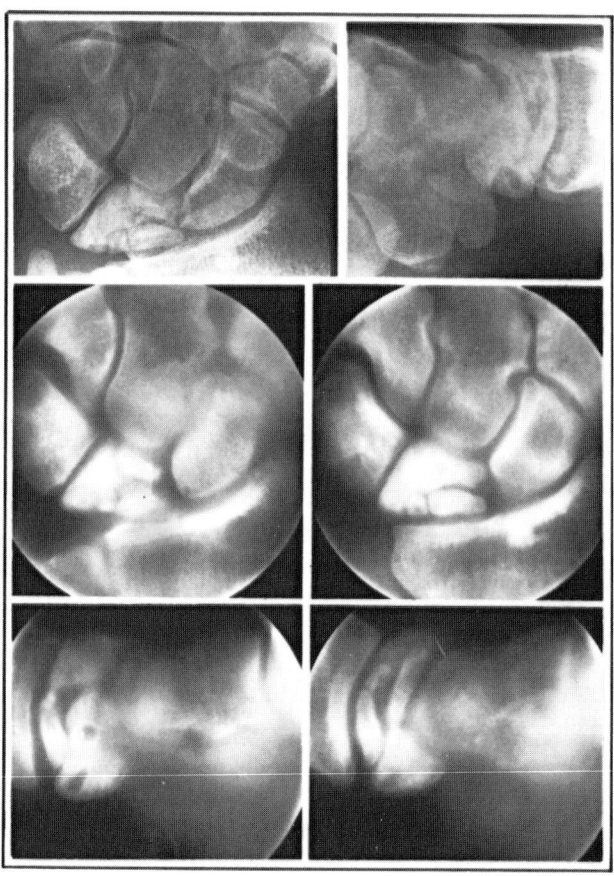

FIG. 14-154. AP and lateral trispiral tomogram with Stage III Kienböcks.

Treatment will vary with the stage of the disease and the severity of symptoms. Symptomatic nonoperative support is frequently adequate (see Fig. 14-59) (232,237). However, if symptoms persist and limit function, surgical management should be considered. If bony collapse is not extreme and secondary degenerative changes are not present, procedures to decrease compressive loads or to alleviate stress concentrations on the lunate appear to be efficacious. These procedures may involve ulnar lengthening (245,251), radial shortening (3,252), or scaphotrapezoidotrapezial arthrodesis (3). If limited perilunate degenerative joint changes are present, silastic or soft tissue lunate arthroplasty (232, 241,248) appears worthwhile. With more advanced de-

TABLE 14-3. *Lichtman classification of Kienböcks disease*[a]

Stage I	Normal radiographic architecture and bone density. May be linear or compression fracture.
Stage II	Increased sclerosis of lunate with normal size and shape.
Stage IIIA	Lunate collapse with proximal migration of the capitate and disruption of carpal architecture.
Stage IIIB	Stage IIIA with fixed rotation of the scaphoid.
Stage IV	As in Stage III with generalized degenerative changes.

[a] (241,252)

generative changes, total wrist arthroplasty, arthrodesis, or proximal row carpectomy (232,236) may be required.

Avascular Necrosis of the Scaphoid (Preiser's Disease)

Avascular necrosis of the proximal portion of the scaphoid following fracture is relatively frequent and has been discussed earlier in this chapter. However, in the absence of a fracture or dislocation, avascular necrosis of the scaphoid is rare (2,3). Radiographically, it is characterized by an increased radiopacity relative to the adjacent carpal bones (233). Low signal intensity is evident on T1-weighted MR images (Fig. 14-108). Later fragmentation, bony collapse, and secondary degenerative arthritis may occur. In all suspected cases, trispiral tomography using 1–2-mm cuts through the scaphoid should be carried out to rule out an unrecognized scaphoid fracture (see Fig. 14-107). Treatment principles are similar to those outlined for the lunate.

Scapholunate Dissociation

Scapholunate dissociation (Fig. 14-155, see also Fig. 14-124) is also not uncommon, but the diagnosis of this condition is frequently overlooked. For this reason it is often seen late, months or years after the original injury. Many authors regard scapholunate dissociation as the initial pathologic phase of the perilunate-dislocation spectrum of injuries (146,170). The mechanism of injury leading to scapholunate dissociation is usually one of wrist hyperextension resulting in at least a partial disruption of the volar radiocarpal ligament complex and scapholunate interosseous ligament.

Routine PA and lateral x-rays of the wrist may suggest the diagnosis but are often inadequate. For this reason, we recommend a series of seven x-ray projections to define or rule out the diagnosis of scapholunate dissociation. Video fluoroscopic evaluation is useful to assure proper positioning (234). This series (2,3,13,167,169) includes

"Palm-up" projections	1. full ulnar deviation of wrist
	2. neutral
	3. full radial deviation of wrist
	4. clenched-fist position
True lateral projections	5. full-wrist palmar flexion
	6. neutral
	7. full-wrist dorsal flexion

The diagnosis of scapholunate dissociation is made by any of a number of characteristic x-ray findings. The most important finding is a diastasis exceeding 2 mm between the scaphoid and the lunate on any of the PA projections (Fig. 14-156) (14). This finding has been given the eponym of *Terry Thomas sign* in recognition of the dental peculiarities of this British comedian (2). The first-compression view is perhaps the most important in this regard. Supportive findings on the PA view should include a "ring sign" of the scaphoid as a result of the x-ray shadow of the scaphoid tubercle when viewed vertically (Fig. 14-157) (59,134). The lunate may appear more triangular than quadrilateral. Furthermore, the opposing surfaces of the lunate and scaphoid may lose their parallel relationship and instead may appear to define a triangular space (Fig. 14-156). The carpal height is diminished. On the lateral projection of the wrist in neutral position, there is usually a dorsiflexion-instability pattern (see Fig. 14-10), and, in any of the lateral views, the scapholunate angle may approach 90°. The supportive x-ray findings are particularly helpful when the scapholunate diastasis on the PA view is equivocal or falls within normal ranges.

The treatment of scapholunate dissociation is almost always surgical, particularly in the young patient prior to development of secondary degenerative changes. A detailed discussion of the array of surgical management options available for this condition is beyond the scope of this chapter, however, most involve the principle of scapholunate reduction and stabilization by tendon repair, reconstruction, or intercarpal arthrodesis (Fig. 14-158) (244,249). If seen early and if a satisfactory closed

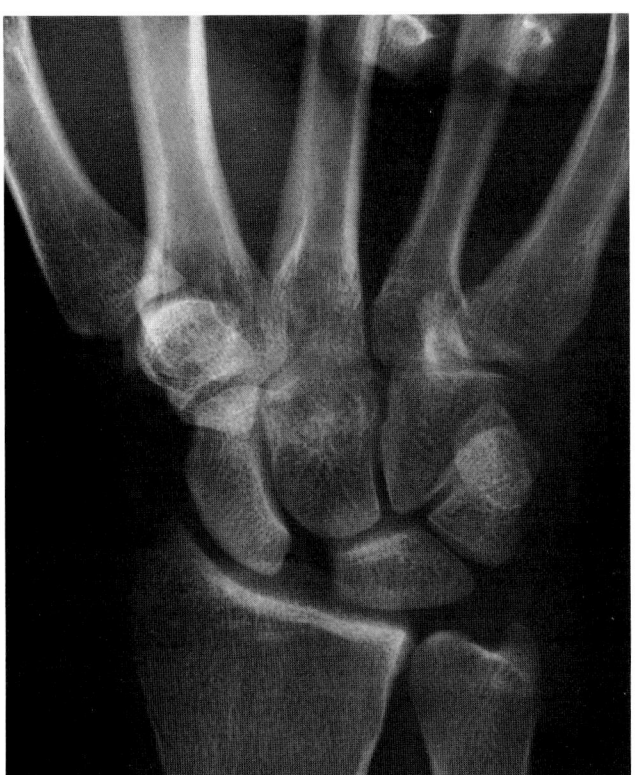

FIG. 14-155. PA view of the wrist with widening of the scapholunate space due to scapholunate dissociation.

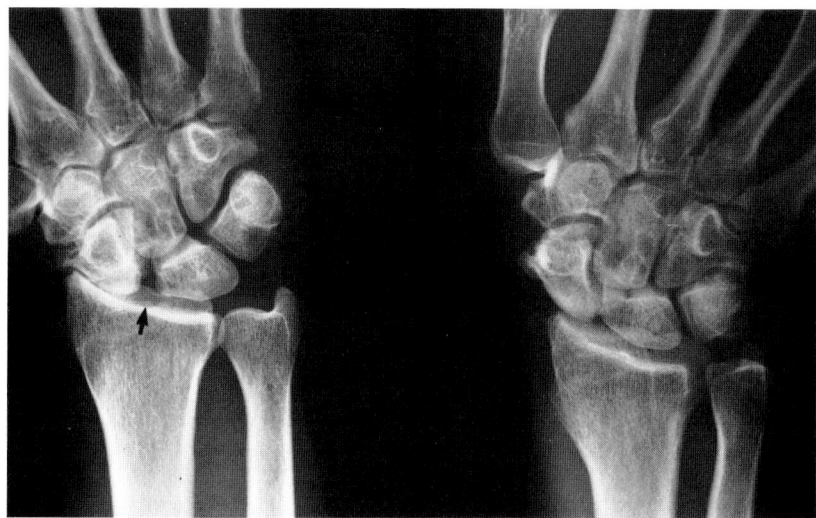

FIG. 14-156. Old wrist injury with scapholunate dissociation. There is a widening of the scapholunate space with radial deviation (**A**). The abnormality is less obvious with ulnar deviation of the wrist (**B**). Note the ring sign (*arrow*).

manipulative reduction can be achieved, percutaneous fixation with multiple Kirschner wires and prolonged cast immobilization may be appropriate. If the condition is seen late and particularly if it is accompanied by degenerative joint changes, treatment will depend upon the level of symptoms. If pain is relatively minimal and not disabling, symptomatic nonoperative management is satisfactory. Those with more marked symptoms may require limited or total wrist arthrodesis, wrist arthroplasty, or proximal row carpectomy.

Lunotriquetral Instability

Lunotriquetral instability is less clearly defined than scapholunate instability but may be more common than previously appreciated. The diagnosis is usually made on the basis of the seven-projection x-ray series previously described or by fluoroscopic examination of the wrist using cinematography or videotape. Unlike its scapholunate counterpart, a frank dissociation or diastasis between the lunate and triquetrum on the PA films is not often seen. However, on the lateral view, a volar flexion-instability pattern in neutral position and a marked diminution of the scapholunate angle to less than 30° on at least one view is highly suggestive of this condition (see Fig. 14-11) (2). Arthrographic demonstration of contrast-material communication between the proximal and midcarpal joints through the lunotriquetral interval helps support the diagnosis (see Fig. 14-61). The principles of management are similar to those outlined for scapholunate instability.

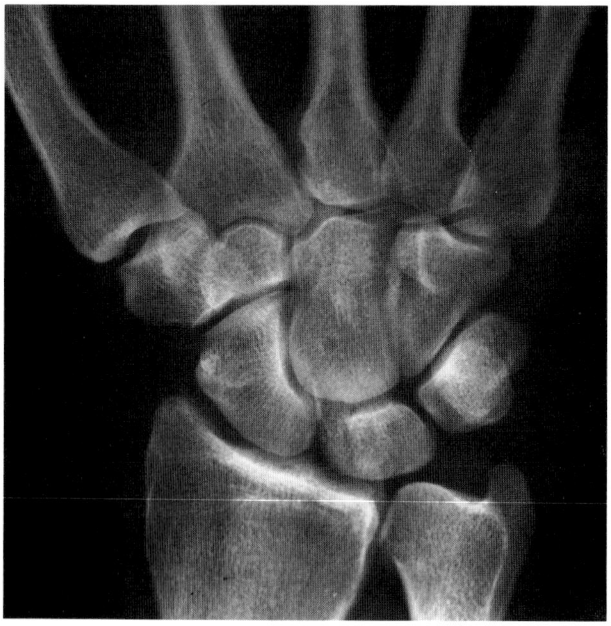

FIG. 14-157. PA view of the wrist showing a triangular scapholunate joint.

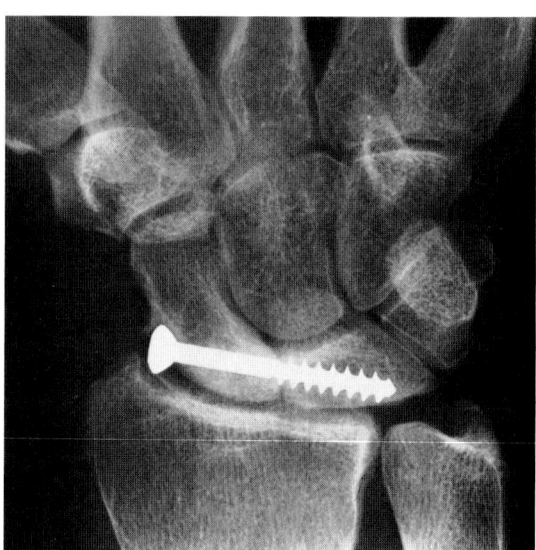

FIG. 14-158. PA view of the wrist following scapholunate arthrodesis with screw fixation.

Carpe Bosseau

Carpe bosseau is not a common deformity. It is clinically characterized by a firm mass or enlargement over the dorsum of the hand in the region of the second or third carpometacarpal joint (230,235). The mass may or may not be painful or locally tender and is frequently mistaken for a ganglion cyst. Most authors agree that the "apparent" mass is actually a hypertrophic lipping of the second or third carpometacarpal joint (Fig. 14-159). It is usually associated with an acquired post-traumatic laxity of the respective carpometacarpal joints (9). In some instances, this condition has been attributed to a nonunited chip fracture of the base of the second or third metacarpal, a congenital assessory ossicle (231,240), periostitis at the site of insertion of the radial wrist extensor tendons, or peritendinitis calcarea. If these latter etiologic factors occur, it is probably in the minority of cases. The carpe bosseau may be difficult to demonstrate on routine PA and lateral radiographs. Oblique projection views, however, are often helpful. Lateral trispiral tomograms, although providing excellent visualization of the second and third carpometacarpal regions, are usually not necessary. Treatment will vary with the individual. The condition may be asymptomatic and represent a diagnostic problem only. Those cases with relatively mild pain and tenderness or of recent onset may require only local steroid injection. This is particularly true if periositis or peritendinitis calcarea is thought to be an etiologic factor in the case. If pain is more marked and chronic, surgical treatment may be necessary. In such cases, excision of a non-united chip fracture or accessory

ossicle may be all that is required. However, in the more usual case in which the condition is due to carpometacarpal joint instability, arthrodesis of the involved carpometacarpal joint and dorsal cheilectomy of the hypertrophic marginal bone spur is the most reliable treatment (2,3,9).

Turret Exostoses of the Phalanges

A phalangeal turret exostosis is a dorsal bony prominence of the middle or proximal phalanx that occasionally may be confused with a neoplasm (3). It is post-traumatic in origin and is usually attributed to a blunt blow to the dorsum of the involved phalanx. It may result from ossification of a subperiosteal hematoma from any cause.

Boutonnière Deformity

The boutonnière deformity has been mentioned earlier in connection with fractures of the dorsal lip of the middle phalanx or volar dislocation of the proximal interphalangeal joint (Fig. 14-145). In most cases, this deformity is not associated with either fracture or dislocation and results instead from a soft tissue injury at the insertion of the extensor central slip over the proximal interphalangeal joint (104,193,204,243,246,247). The mechanism of injury may be (1) a hyperflexion stress to the proximal interphalangeal joint resulting in closed rupture of the extensor apparatus, (2) a gradual attenuation of the extensor apparatus from long-standing proxi-

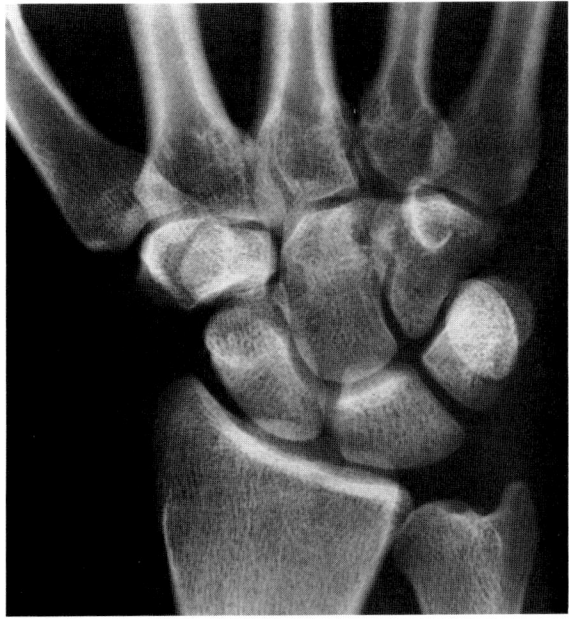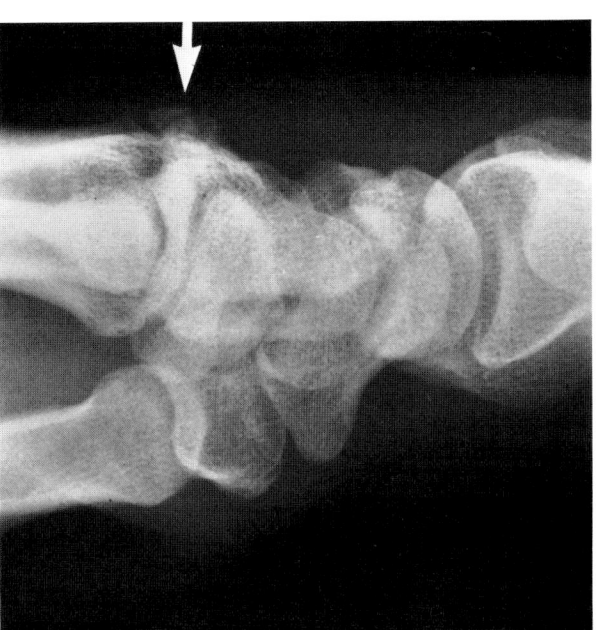

FIG. 14–159. AP (**A**) and lateral (**B**) view of the wrist demonstrating dorsal lipping of the second and third carpal metacarpal (CMC) joints (Carpe Bosseau).

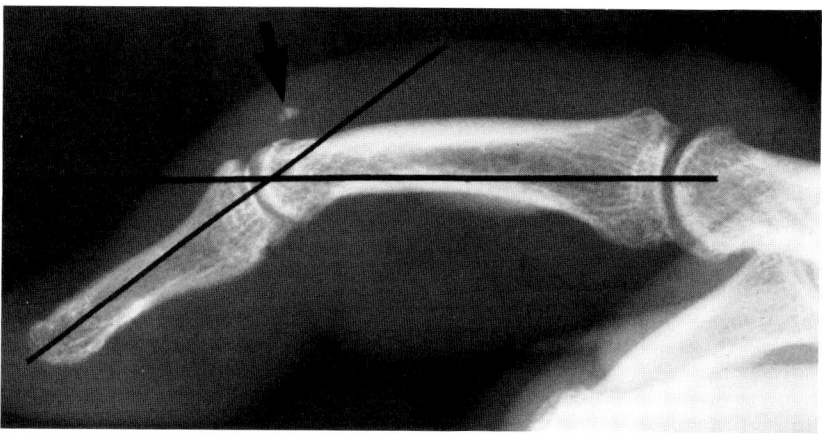

FIG. 14–160. Lateral view of the finger demonstrates a small dorsal chip with flexion of the distal interphalangeal (DIP) joint (mallet deformity).

mal interphalangeal joint synovitis, or (3) an open injury to the extensor apparatus over the proximal interphalangeal joint by penetrating trauma or a deep dorsal burn. The resultant deformity, when established, is characterized by a flexion-contracture of the proximal interphalangeal joint in association with a hyperextension-contracture of the distal interphalangeal joint. If the deformity is long standing, the secondary structural changes as a result of the joint contractures may be seen at either interphalangeal joint (239). The same principles of treatment outlined for nondisplaced small dorsal lip fractures of the middle phalanx apply to this injury in the acute or recent case. A discussion of treatment options for a chronic boutonnière deformity, however, is beyond the scope of this chapter.

Mallet Deformity (Baseball Finger)

Mallet finger deformity has been previously mentioned in connection with fractures of the dorsal lip of the distal phalanx (193,204,246). The same deformity is also frequently seen in the absence of fracture as a result of a rupture of the extensor tendon near its insertion into the distal phalanx. The mechanism of injury is usually a hyperflexion stress to the distal phalanx due to a blow to the tip of the finger. This injury is especially common in sports. The mallet deformity is characterized by a flexion posture of the distal phalanx (Fig. 14-160). There may be varying degrees of hyperextension of the proximal interphalangeal joint, particularly in individuals with volar laxity of this joint. The same treatment principles outlined for small dorsal lip fractures of the distal phalanx apply to this injury in the acute setting. A discussion of late reconstructive procedures for chronic deformities is beyond the scope of this chapter.

Avascular Necrosis of the Metacarpal Head

Rarely, avascular necrosis of the metacarpal head following trauma can be seen in the absence of fracture. It is

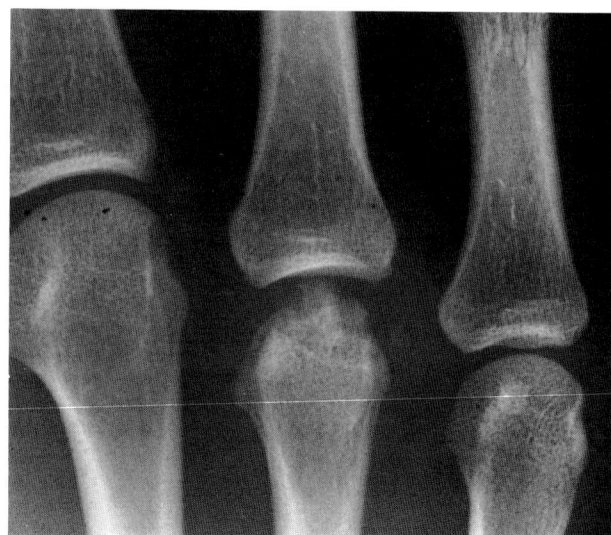 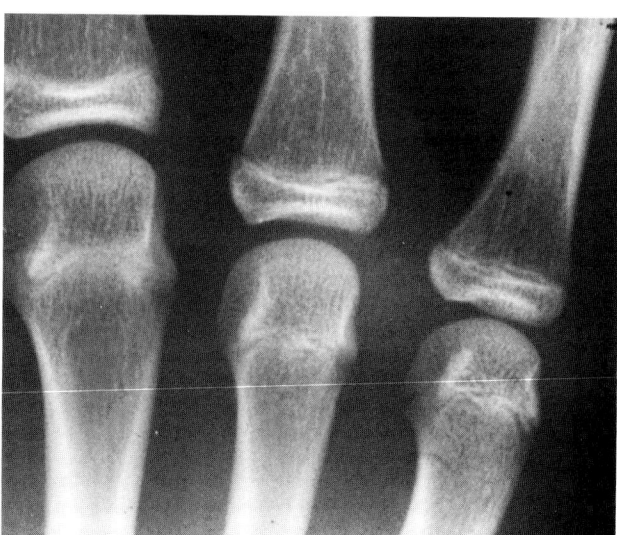

A   B

FIG. 14–161. A: PA view of the third to fourth metacarpal heads following a softball injury. There is no fracture. **B:** Eight months later there is avascular necrosis with collapse of the fourth metacarpal head.

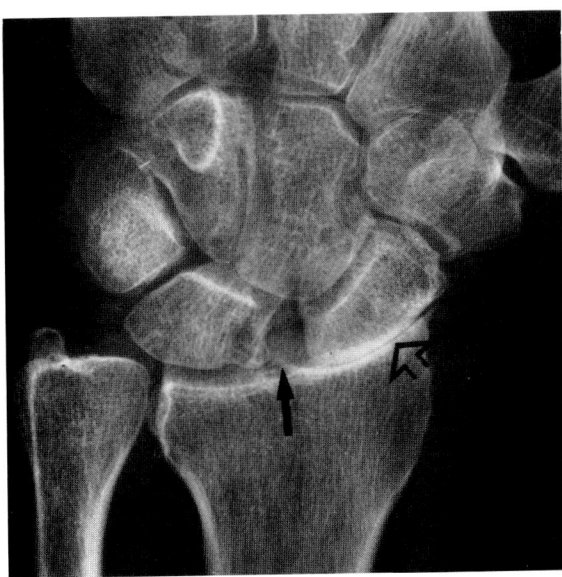

FIG. 14–162. PA view of the wrist with post-traumatic arthritis in the radiocarpal joint (*open arrow*) and an old scapholunate ligament tear with widening of the scapholunate joint (*black arrow*).

characterized radiographically by fragmentation and collapse of a portion of the metacarpal head (Fig. 14-161). Treatment will vary according to the digit involved, the age of the patient, and the extent of collapse and articular disruption.

Post-traumatic Degenerative Arthritis

Post-traumatic degenerative arthritis is common in the hand and wrist. It is particularly prevalent in the distal interphalangeal joints, the first carpometacarpal joint, the scaphotrapezial joints, and the radiocarpal articulation (Fig. 14-162). It may be seen, however, at any joint following an intra-articular fracture or unreduced subluxation. A detailed discussion of the arthritides is beyond the scope of this text and will therefore be omitted.

POST-TRAUMATIC RECONSTRUCTION

Most of the traumatic conditions of the hand or wrist discussed in this chapter require some form of early treatment. However, the treatment rendered may not always lead to a satisfactory outcome, and, in some instances, the injury may go unrecognized or be inappropriately managed. Therefore, secondary surgical reconstruction may be necessary. A detailed description of reconstructive techniques and their indications for specific post-traumatic conditions is beyond the scope of this text. In general, however, reconstruction for post-traumatic conditions in the hand or wrist may be cat-

egorized into the following four groups: osteotomy, soft tissue stabilization, arthrodesis, or arthroplasty. An awareness of the basic principles involved with each of these groups may be pertinent to radiographic interpretation.

Osteotomy

Osteotomy is usually required to correct malunion of fractures (Fig. 14-163). It may additionally be useful for correction of congenital abnormalities (symptomatic ulnar variance, Madelung's deformity), to alter bone alignment for joint motion or stress concentration (radial shortening in Kienböck's disease), to position bones in certain fixed postures for functional considerations, and at times to facilitate surgical exposure of an underlying structure. The term *osteotomy* simply implies the sectioning of a bone by any means. Following bone section, the position of the osteotomy is usually maintained by some means of internal fixation. In the small bones of the hand this is usually accomplished by smooth or threaded Kirschner wires. For longer bones, Steinmann pins of a similar configuration but of larger diameter than Kirschner wires may be used. Wire loops are applicable in certain situations and may be of the circlage type or the tension-band figure-of-8 type. The former usually is placed along the central axis of the bone, while the latter is placed eccentrically over the "tension" side of the bone (the side opposite to where compressive bending forces are expected). Occasionally small bone screws, miniplates (Fig. 14-164), or external fixators may be preferred. For larger bones (radius or ulna), Kirschner wires, Steinmann pins, or wire loops may also be used, but compression plates and screws are more common (Fig. 14-94). These may be of any length or configuration. The chief complication of radiographic significance for osteotomy is delayed union or non-union. Routine views are usually insufficient to evaluate union. Tomography provides improved detail. However, differentiation of non-union from fibrous union is difficult.

Arthrodesis

The term *arthrodesis* implies bony fusion of a joint. It may also be applicable to a psuedarthrosis site. In general, arthrodesis is most often required for stabilization of a painful joint of any cause. It may also be a useful procedure for stabilization of an unstable joint (Fig. 14-165), particularly in certain paralytic disorders. The means of fixation for arthrodesis are similar to the hardware devices described in the preceding section. Bone-graft material may also be utilized at the arthrodesis site. The chief complication of radiographic significance for arthrodesis is delayed union or non-union. The evaluation of either of these complications may be aided by tomography and occasionally by arthrography.

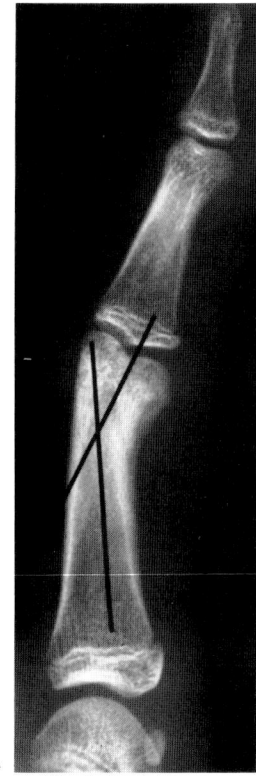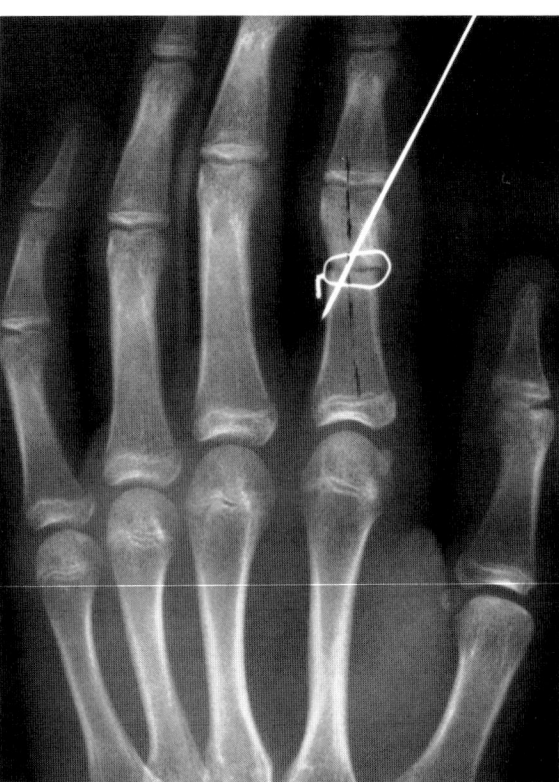

A B

FIG. 14–163. A: AP view of the left index finger with rotation and angular deformity due to an old fracture. **B:** The deformity was corrected with osteotomy using K wire and band fixation.

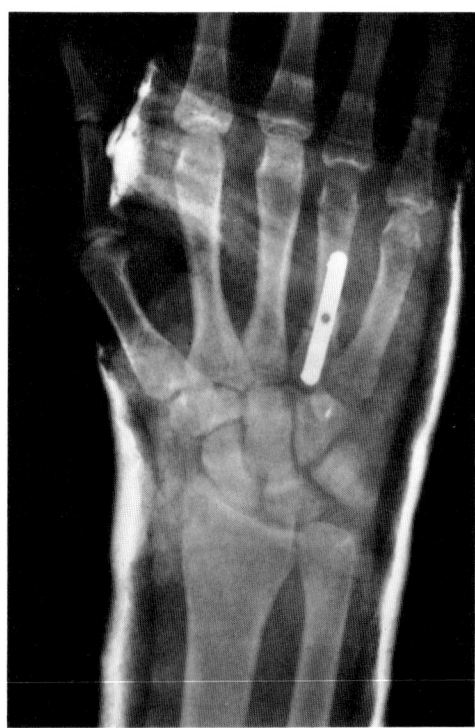

FIG. 14–164. Fracture of the proximal fourth metacarpal with mini plate and screw fixation.

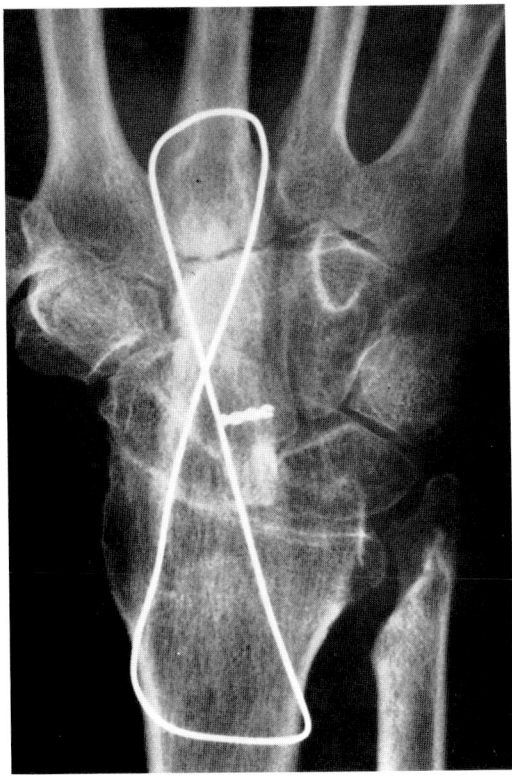

A

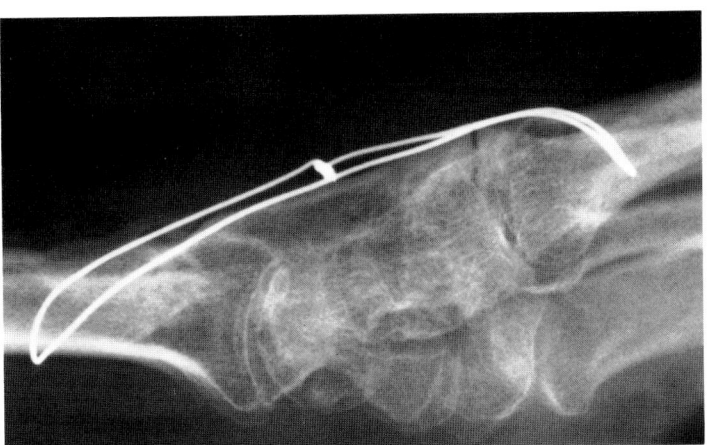

B

FIG. 14–165. PA (**A**) and lateral (**B**) views following arthrodesis of the wrist; bone graft dorsally with figure-of-8 wire.

Soft Tissue Stabilization

Soft tissue stabilization procedures are not infrequent. They are most often applied for reconstruction of symptomatic ligamentous disruptions (subluxation of the distal radioulnar joint [155], scapholunate dissociation [244,249], proximal interphalangeal-joint swan-neck deformity). The specific technique of soft tissue stabilization will vary widely. There are no particular radiographic features of such procedures.

Arthroplasty

Arthroplasty procedures utilized for salvage or reconstruction of the hand or wrist may be broadly categorized as resection or implant (prosthetic) arthroplasty. These are most frequently applicable for arthritic disorders, but they may also be required for reconstruction following post-traumatic articular incongruity or for correction of severe contractures. The more common resection arthroplasty procedures include excision of the distal ulna (Fig. 14-166) (125,255), proximal row carpectomy, excision of the trapezium (Fig. 14-167), or resection of metacarpal heads. Often some form of soft tissue interposition (e.g., a loop of tendon [254]) is used in conjunction with resection arthroplasty to prevent direct bone-to-bone contact or to minimize bony collapse into the resulting void.

A wide variety of implants are available for prosthetic arthroplasty. These fall into two broad categories: implants that act as spacers (248) and implants that act as true articulating surfaces or hinges (253). The spacer implants are more common and are more frequently used for metacarpophalangeal joint replacement (Fig. 14-168). The same type of implant is applicable for the purposes of proximal interphalangeal joint arthroplasty. Spacer implants are also available for total wrist replacement as well as lunate, scaphoid, trapezium, ulnar head, and first metacarpal base arthroplasty.

Articulating implants at this time appear to have a more limited application in the hand and wrist. In contrast to spacer implants, these generally require some means of stem-bone fixation. Usually this implies the use of methyl methacrylate cement or a porous surface-bone in-growth stem design. Articulating implant arthroplasty is most commonly utilized for metacarpophalangeal joint or total wrist replacement.

A variety of complications with radiographic significance may be noted with arthroplasty procedures. Excision arthroplasty may be associated with instability and subluxation of the pseudarthrosis. Prosthetic arthroplasty may be complicated by implant fracture, subluxation, or dislocation. Erosion of the implant through bone may be seen late, particularly when firm bone-stem fixation is used. Deep sepsis involving the prosthesis may be characterized by a lucent zone of bone rarefaction about the implant stem, soft tissue swelling, and at times

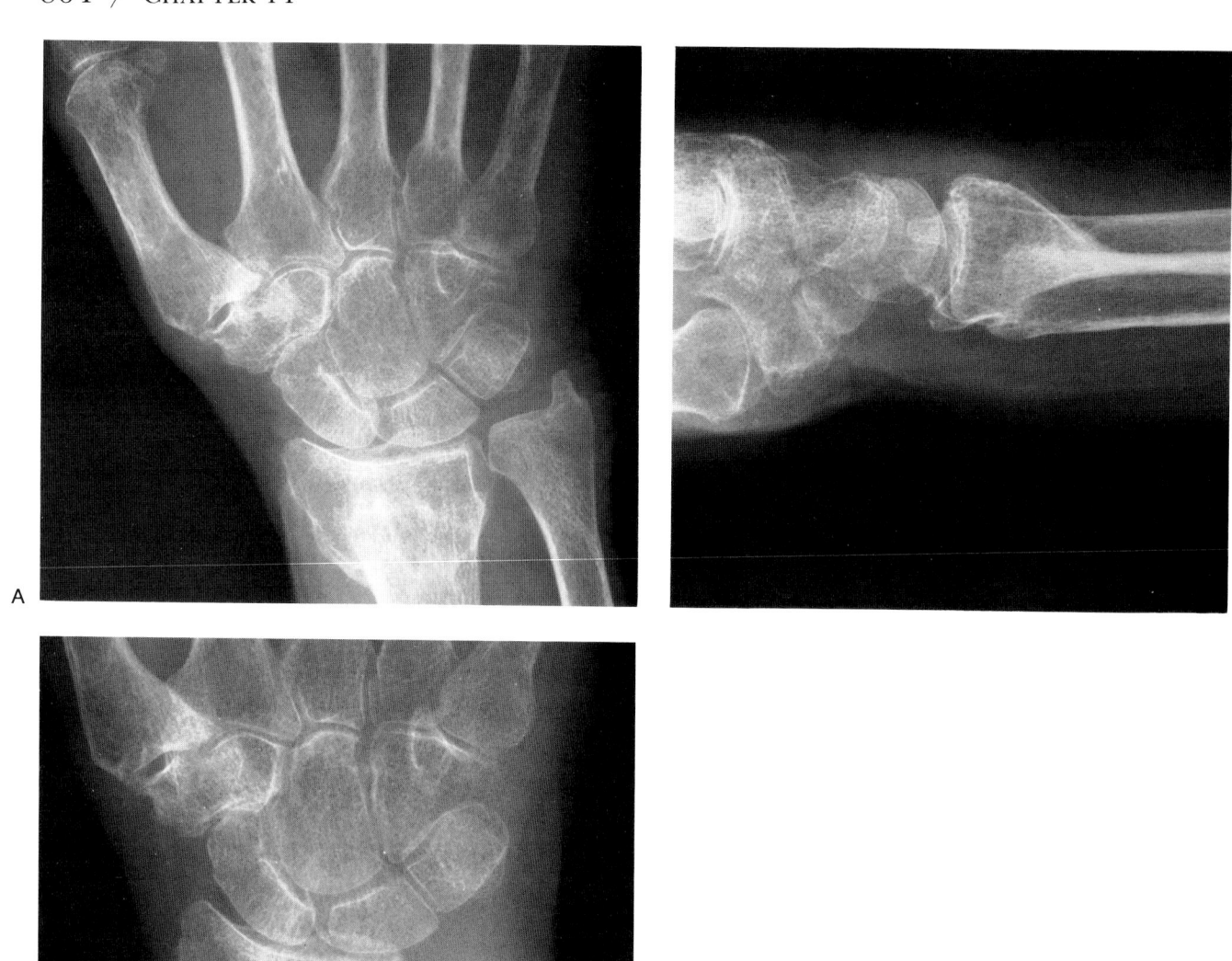

FIG. 14–166. PA (**A**) and lateral (**B**) views of an old distal radial fracture with shortening of the radius and positive ulnar variance. **C:** PA radiograph following resection of the distal ulna.

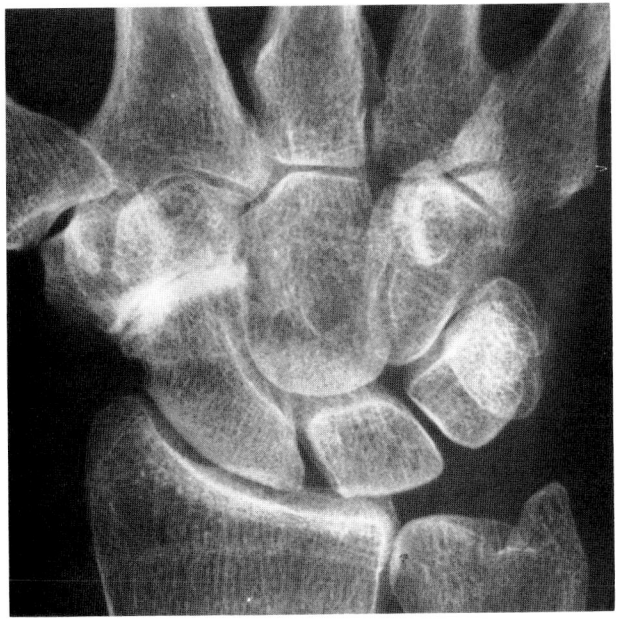

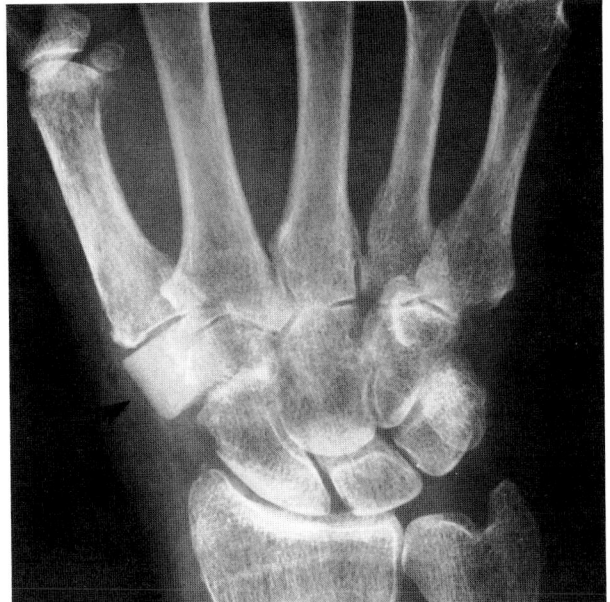

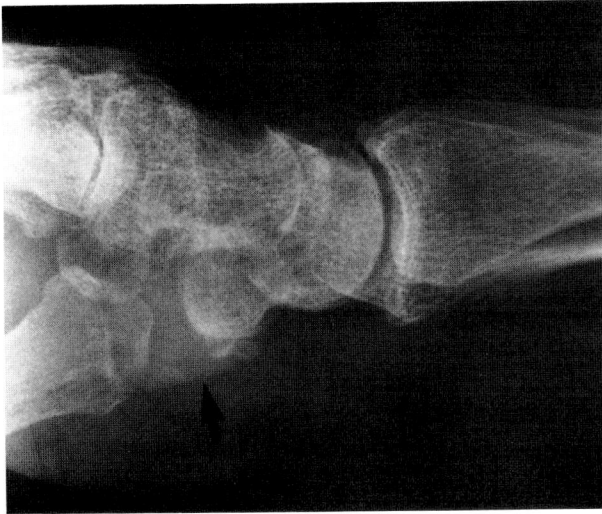

FIG. 14–167. A: PA view of the wrist with degenerative arthritis involving the scaphotrapezial articulation. PA (**B**) and lateral (**C**) views following prosthetic replacement (*arrow*).

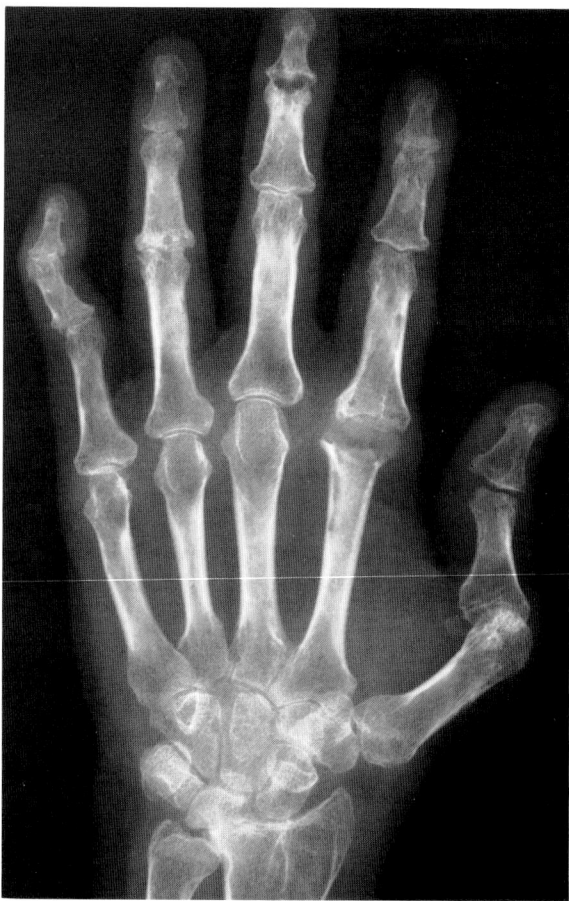

FIG. 14–168. PA view of the hand and wrist with metacarpophalangeal joint spacer (silicone) in place.

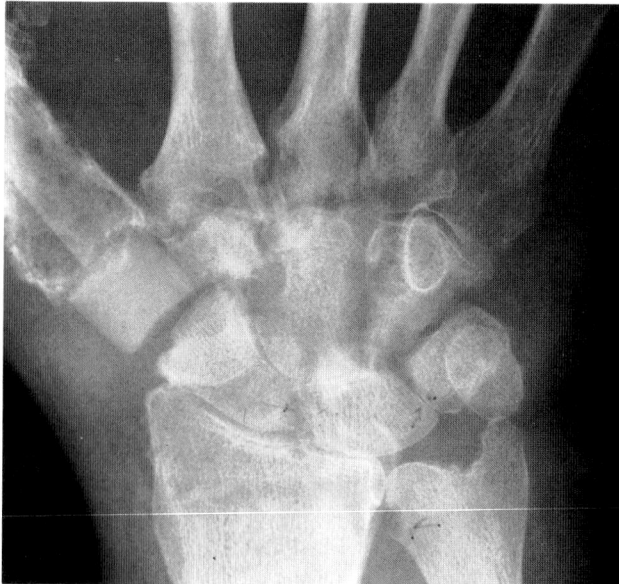

FIG. 14–169. Infected prosthesis: AP view of the hand demonstrates bone destruction and periosteal new bone around the implant due to infection. There are numerous erosions in the carpal bones due to infectious arthritis.

an exaggerated degree of periosteal ossification (Fig. 14-169).

SUMMARY

Trauma is the most common etiologic factor leading to disability in the hand and wrist. Judicious radiographic evaluation is required for accurate assessment in practically all but the most minor of such injuries. Frequently serial radiographic evaluation is essential for directing the course of treatment and for following the healing process. A meaningful radiographic evaluation requires a comprehensive knowledge of the normal radiographic anatomy, an overview of the spectrum of pathology, and an awareness of the usual mechanisms of injury, appropriate treatment options, and relevant array of possible complications.

REFERENCES

Anatomy

1. Bowers WH, Wolf JW, Nehil JL. The proximal interphalangeal joint volar plate. I. An anatomical and biomechanical study. *J Hand Surg* 1980;5:79–88.
2. Dobyns JH, Linscheid RL. Fractures and dislocations of the wrist. In: Rockwood CA Jr, Green DP, eds., 2nd ed., *Fractures in adults.* Philadelphia: J.B. Lippincott Co., 1984;411–509.
3. Dobyns JH, Linscheid RL, Beckenbaugh RD, et al. Fractures of the hand and wrist. In: Flynn JE, ed. *Hand surgery.* Baltimore: Williams & Wilkins Co., 1982.
4. Epner RA, Bowers WH, Guilford WB. Ulnar variance—the effect of wrist positioning and roentgen filming technique. *J Hand Surg* 1982;7:298–305.
5. Gelberman RH, Solomon PB, Jurist JM, Posch JL. Ulnar variance in Kienböck's disease. *J Bone Joint Surg* 1975;57:674–676.
6. Gilford WW, Bolton RH, Lambrinudi C. The mechanism of the wrist joint with special reference to fractures of the scaphoid. *Guy's Hosp Rep* 1943;92:52–59.
7. Green DP, Rowland SA. Fractures and dislocations in the hand. In: Rockwood CA Jr, Green DP, eds., 2nd ed., *Fractures in adults.* Philadelphia: J. B. Lippincott Co, 1984;313–409.
8. Hollinshead HW. *Anatomy for surgeons,* vol. 3. The Back and Limbs. New York: Harper and Rowe, 1982.
9. Joseph RB, Linscheid RL, Dobyns JH, Bryan RS. Chronic sprains of the carpometacarpal joints. *J Hand Surg* 1981;6:172–180.
10. Kaplan EB. *Functional and surgical anatomy of the hand,* 2nd ed. Philadelphia: J.B. Lippincott Co., 1965.
11. Kauer JMG. Functional anatomy of the wrist. *Clin Orthop* 1980;149:9–20.
12. Landsmeer JMF. The proximal interphalangeal joint. *Hand* 1975;7:30.
13. Lichtman DM, Schneider JR, Swafford AR, Mack GR. Ulnar midcarpal instability. Clinical and laboratory analysis. *J Hand Surg* 1981;6:515–523.
14. Linscheid RL, Dobyns JH, Beabout JW, Bryan RS. Traumatic instability of the wrist: Diagnosis, classification, and pathomechanics. *J Bone Joint Surg* 1972;54A:1612–1632.
15. Mayfield J, Johnson R, Kilcoyne R. The ligaments of the human wrist and their functional significance. *Anat Rec* 1976;185:417–428.
16. Mikic ZD. Age changes in the triangular fibrocartilage of the wrist joint. *J Anat* 1978;126:307–384.
17. O'Rahilly R. A survey of carpal and tarsal anomalies. *J Bone Joint Surg* 1953;35A:626–642.

18. Palmer AK, Werner FW. The triangular fibrocartilage complex of the wrist—anatomy and function. *J Hand Surg* 1981;6:153–162.
19. Seffafian S, Melamed JL, Goshgarian GM. Study of the wrist motion in flexion and extension. *Clin Orthop* 1977;126:153–159.
20. Taleisnik J. The ligaments of the wrist. *J Hand Surg* 1976;1:110–118.
21. Volz RG, Lieb M, Benjamin J. Biomechanics of the wrist. *Clin Orthop* 1980;149:112–117.
22. Youm Y, Flatt AE. Kinematics of the wrist. *Clin Orthop* 1980;149:21–32.
23. Youm Y, McMurthy RY, Flatt AE, Gillespie TE. Kinematics of the wrist. I. An experimental study of the radial-ulnar deviation and flexion-extension. *J Bone Joint Surg* 1978;60A:423–431.

Imaging Techniques

24. Abbitt PL, Riddervold HO. The carpal tunnel view: Helpful adjuvant for unrecognized fractures of the carpus. *Skel Radiol* 1987;16:45–47.
25. Ballinger PW. *Merrill's atlas of roentgenographic positions and standard radiologic procedures,* 5th ed. St. Louis: C.V. Mosby, 1982.
26. Belsole RJ, Quinn SF, Greene TL, Beatty ME, Rayhack JM. Digital subtraction arthrography of the wrist. *J Bone Joint Surg* 1990;72A:846–851.
27. Berger RA, Blair WF, El-Koury GY. Arthrotomography of the wrist. The palmar radiocarpal ligaments. *Clin Orthop* 1984;186:224–229.
28. Bernau A, Berquist TH. *Orthopedic positioning in diagnostic radiology.* Baltimore: Urban and Schwarzenberg, 1983.
29. Berquist TH. *MRI of the musculoskeletal system.* New York: Raven Press, 1990.
30. Berquist TH. The elbow and wrist. *Top Mag Res Imag* 1989; 1(3):15–27.
31. Blair WF, Berger RA, El-Khoury GY. Arthrotomography of the wrist: An experimental and preliminary clinical study. *J Hand Surg* 1985;10A:350–359.
32. Braunstein EM, Louis DS, Greene TL, Hankin FM. Fluoroscopic and arthrographic evaluation of carpal instability. *AJR* 1985;144:1259–1262.
33. Bowers WH, Hurst LC. Gamekeeper's thumb. Evaluation by arthrography and stress roentgenography. *J Bone Joint Surg* 1977;59A:519–524.
34. Brewerton DA. A tangential radiographic projection for demonstrating involvement of the metacarpal head in rheumatoid arthritis. *Br J Radiol* 1967;40:233–234.
35. Bridgman CF. Radiography of the carpal navicular bone. *Med Radiogr Photogr* 1949;25:104.
36. Burman M. Anteroposterior projection of the carpometacarpal joint of the thumb by the radial shift of the carpal tunnel view. *J Bone Joint Surg* 1958;40A:1156–1157.
37. Bush CH, Gillespie T, Dell PC. High-resolution CT of the wrist: Initial experience with scaphoid disorders and surgical fusions. *AJR* 1987;149:757–760.
38. Cone RO, Szabo R, Resnick D, Gelberman R, Taleisnick J, Gilula LA. Computed tomography of the normal radioulnar joints. *Invest Radiol* 1983;18:541–545.
39. Cone RO, Szabo R, Resnick D, Gelberman R, Taleisnick J, Gilula LA. Computed tomography of the normal soft tissues of the wrist. *Invest Radiol* 1983;18:546–551.
40. Crittenden JJ, Jones DM, Santarelli AG. Bilateral rotational dislocation of the carpal navicular. *Radiology* 1970;94:629–630.
41. Curtis DJ, Downey EF Jr. A simple first metacarpophalangeal stress test. *Radiology* 1983;148:855.
42. Downey EF, Curtis DJ. Patient induced stress test of the first metacarpophalangeal joint: A radiographic assessment of collateral ligament injuries. *Radiology* 1986;158:679–683.
43. Epner RA, Bowers WH, Guifford WB. Ulnar variance—The effect of wrist positioning and roentgen filming technique. *J Hand Surg* 1982;7:298–305.
44. Fisher MR, Rogers LF, Hendrix RW. A systematic approach to identifying fourth and fifth carpometacarpal joint dislocations. *AJR* 1983;140:319.
45. Fodor J III, Malett JC, Moulton J. Carpal tunnel ring artifact. *AJR* 1985;144:765–766.
46. Gandee RW, Harrison RB, Dee PM. Peritendinitis calcaria of the flexor carpi ulnaris. *AJR* 1979;133:1139.
47. Ganel A, Engel J, Oster Z, Farene I. Bone scanning in the assessment of fractures of the scaphoid. *J Hand Surg* 1979;4:540–543.
48. Gilula LA. Carpal injuries: Analytic approach and case exercises. *AJR* 1979;133:503–517.
49. Gilula LA. Mid carpal wrist arthrography. *AJR* 1986;146:645–646.
50. Gilula LA, Totty GW, Weeks PM. Wrist arthrography: The value of fluoroscopic spot filming. *Radiology* 1983;146:555–556.
51. Gilula LA, Weeks PM. Post-traumatic ligamentous instability of the wrist. *Radiology* 1978;129:641–651.
52. Gilula LA, Distouet JM, Weeks PM, Young LV, Wray RC. Roentgen diagnosis of the painful wrist. *Clin Orthop* 1984; 187:52–64.
53. Greyson ND, Tepperman PS. Three-phase bone studies in hemiplegia with reflex sympathetic dystrophy and the effect of disuse. *J Nucl Med* 1984;25:423–429.
54. Gruber L. Practical approaches to obtaining hand radiographs and special techniques in hand radiography. *Hand Clin* 1991; 7:1–20.
55. Gundry CR, Kursimoglu-Brahme S, Schwaighofer B, Kang HS, Sartoris DJ, Resnick D. Is MR better than arthrography for evaluating the ligaments of the wrist? In vitro study. *AJR* 1990;154:337–341.
56. Hardy DC, Totty WG, Reinus WR, Gilula LA. Posteroanterior wrist radiography: Importance of arm positioning. *J Hand Surg* 1987;12A:504–508.
57. Hart VL, Gaynor V. Roentgenographic study of the carpal canal. *J Bone Joint Surg* 1941;23:382–383.
58. Holder LE, Mackinnon SE. Reflex sympathetic dystrophy in the hands: Clinical and scintigraphic criteria. *Radiology* 1984;152: 517–522.
59. Howard FM, Fahey T, Wojcik E. Rotary subluxation of the navicular. *Clin Orthop* 1974;104:134–139.
60. Hudson TM, Caragal WJ, Kaye JJ. Isolated rotary subluxation of the carpal navicular. *AJR* 1976;126:601.
61. Kindynis P, Resnick D, Kang HS, Haller J, Sartoris DJ. Demonstration of the scapholunate space with radiography. *Radiology* 1990;175:278–280.
62. Lane CG. Detecting occult fracture of the metacarpal head: The Brewerton view. *J Hand Surg* 1977;2:131–133.
63. Lentino W, Lubetsky HW, Jacobson HG, Poppel MH. The carpal bridge view. *J Bone Joint Surg* 1957;39A:88–90.
64. Levinsohn EM, Palmer AK. Arthrography of the traumatized wrist. Correlation of radiography and the carpal instability series. *Radiology* 1983;146:647–651.
65. Levinsohn ME, Rosen DI, Palmer AK. Wrist arthrography: Value of the three-compartment injection method. *Radiology* 1991;179:231–239.
66. Levinsohn ME, Palmer AK, Coren AB, Zinberg E. Wrist arthrography: The value of the three compartment injection technique. *Skel Radiol* 1987;16:539–544.
67. Lewis OJ, Hamshire RJ, Buckneel TM. The anatomy of the wrist. *J Anat* 1970;106:539–552.
68. Magid D, Thompson JS, Fishman EK. Computed tomography of the hand and wrist. *Hand Clin* 1991;7:219–234.
69. Maloney MD, Sauser DD, Hanson EC, Wood VE, Theil AE. Adhesive capsulitis of the wrist. Arthrographic diagnosis. *Radiology* 1988;167:187–190.
70. Manaster BJ. Digital wrist arthrography: Precision in determining the site of radiocarpal-mid carpal communication. *AJR* 1986;147:563–566.
71. Manaster BJ. The clinical efficacy of the triple-injection wrist arthrography. *Radiology* 1991;178:267–270.
72. Mauer AH. Nuclear medicine in evaluation of the hand and wrist. *Hand Clin* 1991;7:183–200.
73. Mirro DE, Palmer NK, Levinsohn ME. Radiography and computerized tomography in the diagnosis of incongruity of the distal radioulnar joint. *J Bone Joint Surg* 1985;67A:247–252.

74. Mrose HE, Rosenthal DI. Arthrography of the hand and wrist. *Hand Clin* 1991;7:201–218.

75. Murry WT, Mueller PR, Rosenthal DI. Fracture of the hook of the hamate. *AJR* 1979;133:899.

76. Poznanski AK. Useful measurements in the evaluation of hand radiographs. *Hand Clin* 1991;7:21–36.

77. Protas JM, Jackson WR. Evaluating carpal instability with fluoroscopy. *AJR* 1980;135:137–140.

78. Quinn SF, Belsole RS, Green TL, Rayhack JM. Post-arthrography computed tomography of the wrist: Evaluation of the triangular fibrocartilage complex. *Skel Radiol* 1989;17:565–569.

79. Quinn SF, Murray W, Watkins T, Kloss J. CT for determining results of treatment of fractures of the wrist. *AJR* 1987;149:109–111.

80. Resnick D. Roentgenographic anatomy of the tendon sheaths of the hand and wrist: Tenography. *AJR* 1975;124:44.

81. Resnick D, Dalinka MK. Arthrography and tenography of the wrist. In: Dalinka MK, ed. *Arthrography.* New York: Springer-Verlag, 1980.

82. Rosenthal DI, Murray WT, Smith RJ. Finger arthrography. *Radiology* 1980;137:647.

83. Smith DK, Linscheid RL, Amadio PC, Berquist TH, Cooney WP. Scaphoid anatomy: Evaluation with complex motion tomography. *Radiology* 1989;173:177–180.

84. Stecher WR. Roentgenography of the carpal navicular bone. *AJR* 1937;37:704.

85. Tehranzadeh J, Davenport J, Pas MJ. Scaphoid fracture: Evaluation with flexion-extension tomography. *Radiology* 1990;176:167–170.

86. Terry DW, Ramin JE. The navicular fat stripe. A useful roentgen feature for evaluating wrist trauma. *AJR* 1975;124:25.

87. Tirman RM, Weber ER, Snyder LL, Koonce TW. Mid carpal wrist arthrography for detection of tears of the scapholunate and lunotriquetral ligaments. *AJR* 1985;144:107–108.

88. Wahlstrom O, Ekberg S, Hammerby S. Serial bone scanning of Colles fracture. *Arch Orthop Trauma Surg* 1983;102:11–17.

89. Wechsler RJ, Wehbe MA, Rifkin MD, Edeiken J, Branch HM. Computed tomography diagnosis of distal radioulnar subluxation. *Skel Radiol* 1987;16:1–5.

90. Weeks PM, Vanner MW, Stevens WG, Gayon D, Gilula LA. Three-dimensional imaging of the wrist. *J Hand Surg* 1985;10A:32–39.

91. White SJ, Lous DS, Braumstein EM, Hankin FM, Greene TL. Capitate-lunate instability. Recognition by manipulation under fluoroscopy. *AJR* 1984;143:361–364.

92. Yeager BA, Dalinka MK. Radiology of trauma to the wrist: Dislocations, fracture dislocations, and instability patterns. *Skel Radiol* 1985;13:120–130.

93. Zlatkin MB, Chis PC, Osterman AL, Schmoll MD, Dalinka MK, Kressel HY. Chronic wrist pain: Evaluation with high-resolution MR imaging. *Radiology* 1989;173:723–729.

Fractures and Dislocations

94. Adler JB, Shaftan GW. Fractures of the capitate. *J Bone Joint Surg* 1962;44A:1537–1547.

95. Agee JM. Unstable fracture-dislocations of the proximal interphalangeal joint of the fingers: A preliminary report of a new treatment technique. *J Hand Surg* 1978;3:386–389.

96. Aitkin AP, Nalebuff EA. Volar transnavicular perilunar dislocations of the carpus. *J Bone Joint Surg* 1960;42A:1051–1057.

97. Albert SM, Wohl MD, Rechtman AM. Treatment of the disrupted radio-ulnar joint. *J Bone Joint Surg* 1963;45A:1373–1381.

98. Baldwin LW, Miller DL, Lockhart LD, Evans EB. Metacarpophalangeal-joint dislocations of the fingers. *J Bone Joint Surg* 1967;49A:1587–1590.

99. Bartone NF, Grieco RV. Fractures of the triquetrum. *J Bone Joint Surg* 1956;38A:353–356.

100. Bellinghausen H, Gilula LA, Young LV, Weeks PM. Post-traumatic palmar carpal subluxation. *J Bone Joint Surg* 1983;65A:998–1006.

101. Belsole R. Physiologic fixation of displaced and unstable fractures of the hand. *Orthop Clin North Am* 1980;11:393–404.

102. Berquist TH. *MRI of the musculoskeletal system.* New York: Raven Press, 1990.

103. Bowen TL. Injuries of the hamate bone. *Hand* 1973;5:235–238.

104. Bowers WH. Management of small joint injuries in the hand. *Clin Orthop* 1983;14:798.

105. Bradway JK, Amadio PC, Cooney WP. Open reduction and internal fixation of displaced, comminuted intra-articular fractures of the distal end of the radius. *J Bone Joint Surg* 1989;71A:839–847.

106. Braunstein EM, Louis DS, Greene TL, Hankin FM. Fluoroscopic and arthrographic evaluation of carpal instability. *AJR* 1985;144:1259–1262.

107. Browne EZ, Dunn HK, Snyder CC. Ski pole thumb injury. *Plast Reconstr Surg* 1976;59:19–23.

108. Bryan RS, Dobyns JH. Fractures of the carpal bones other than lunate and navicular. *Clin Orthop* 1980;149:107–111.

109. Burton RJ. Fractures of the proximal phalanx of the finger. *Contemp Surg* 1977;11:32–37.

110. Cameron HU, Hastings DE, Fournasier VL. Fracture of the hook of the hamate. A case report. *J Bone Joint Surg* 1975;57A:276–277.

111. Carter PR, Eaton RG, Littler JW. Ununited fracture of the hook of the hamate. *J Bone Joint Surg* 1977;59A:583–588.

112. Conway WF, Destouet JM, Gilula LA, Bellinghausen HW, Weeks PM. The carpal boss: An overview of radiographic evaluation. *Radiology* 1985;156:29–31.

113. Cooney WP, Dobyns JH, Linscheid RL. Complications of Colles' fractures. *J Bone Joint Surg* 1980;62A:613–619.

114. Cooney WP, Beckenbaugh RD, Bryan RS, Dobyns JH. External minifixators: Clinical applications and techniques. In: Johnston M, ed. *Advances in external fixation.* Chicago: Year Book Medical Publishers, 1980.

115. Cooney WP, Dobyns JH, Linscheid RL. Fractures of the scaphoid: A rational approach to management. *Clin Orthop* 1980;149:90–97.

116. Cooney WP, Linscheid RL, Dobyns JH. External pin fixation for unstable Colles' fractures. *J Bone Joint Surg* 1979;61A:840–845.

117. Conrad RW, Goldner JL. A study of the pathological findings and treatment in soft-tissue injury of the thumb metacarpophalangeal joint. *J Bone Joint Surg* 1968;50A:439–451.

118. Cordrey LJ, Ferrer-Torells M. Management of fractures of the greater multangular. *J Bone Joint Surg* 1960;42A:1111–1118.

119. Crawford GP. Screw fixation for certain fractures of the phalanges and metacarpals. *J Bone Joint Surg* 1976;58A:487–492.

120. Crosby EB, Linscheid RL. Rupture of the flexor profundus tendon of the ring finger secondary to ancient fracture of the hook of the hamate: Review of the literature and report of two cases. *J Bone Joint Surg* 1974;56A:1076–1078.

121. Dameron TB. Traumatic dislocation of the distal radioulnar joint. *Clin Orthop* 1972;83:55–63.

122. Darrach W. Forward dislocation at the inferior radioulnar joint with fractures of the lower third of the radius. *Ann Surg* 1912;56:801.

123. Desser TS, McCarthy S, Trumble T. Scaphoid fractures and Kienböck's disease of the lunate: MR imaging with histopathologic correlation. *Mag Res Imag* 1990;8:357–361.

124. De Oliveira JC. Barton's fractures. *J Bone Joint Surg* 1973;55A:586–594.

125. Dingman PVC. Resection of the distal end of the ulna (Darrach operation). End-result study of 24 cases. *J Bone Joint Surg* 1952;34A:893–900.

126. Dunn AW. Fractures and dislocations of the carpus. *Surg Clin North Am* 1972;52:1513.

127. Edwards HC. Mechanism and treatment of backfire fracture. *J Bone Joint Surg* 1926;8:701–717.

128. Ellis J. Smith's and Barton's fracture—a method of treatment. *J Bone Joint Surg* 1965;47B:724–727.

129. Fenton RL. The naviculo-capitate fracture syndrome. *J Bone Joint Surg* 1956;38A:681–684.

130. Fernandez DL. Radial osteotomy and Bowers arthroplasty for malunited fractures of the distal end of the radius. *J Bone Joint Surg* 1988;70A:1538–1550.

131. Fernandez DL. Irreducible radiocarpal fracture-dislocation and radioulnar dissociation with entrapment of the ulnar nerve, artery, and flexor profundus II-V—case report. *J Hand Surg* 1981;6:456–461.

132. Fisher MR, Rogers LF, Hendrix RW, Gilula LA. Carpometacarpal dislocation. *CRC Crit Reviews Diag Imag* 1984;22:95–126.

133. Fisk GR. Carpal instability and the fractured scaphoid. *Ann Roy Coll Surg* 1970;45:63–77.

134. Fisk GR. An overview of injuries of the wrist. *Clin Orthop* 1980;149:137–144.

135. Flatt AE. Recurrent locking of an index finger. *J Bone Joint Surg* 1958;40A:1128–1130.

136. Frykman G. Fractures of the distal radius including sequelae—shoulder-hand-finger syndrome, disturbance in the distal radioulnar joint, and impairment of nerve function. *Acta Orthop Scand* (Suppl.) 1967;108:1–55.

137. Funk DA, Wood MB. Concurrent fractures of the ipsilateral scaphoid and radial head. *J Bone Joint Surg* 1988;70A:134–136.

138. Gelberman RH, Welock BS, Siegel DB. Fractures and non-unions of the carpal scaphoid. *J Bone Joint Surg* 1989;71A:1560–1565.

139. Gillespy T III, Stork JJ, Dele PC. Dorsal fracture of the hamate: Distinct radiographic appearance. *AJR* 1988;151:351–353.

140. Gilula LA, Destouet JM, Weeks PM, Young LV, Wray RC. Roentgen diagnosis of the painful wrist. *Clin Orthop* 1984;187:52–64.

141. Gilula LA, Hardy DC, Totty WG. Distal radioulnar joint arthrography. *AJR* 1988;150:864–866.

142. Gingrass RP, Fehring B, Matloub H. Intraosseous wiring of complex hand fractures. *Plast Reconstr Surg* 1980;66:383–394.

143. Goldberg I, Amit S, Bahar A, Seelenfreeval M. Complete dislocation of the trapezium. *J Hand Surg* 1981;6:193–195.

144. Goodman ML, Shankman GB. Update: Palmar dislocation of the trapezoid—a case report. *J Hand Surg* 1984;9:127–131.

145. Green DP, Anderson JR. Closed reduction and percutaneous fixation of fractured phalanges. *J Bone Joint Surg* 1973;55A:1651–1653.

146. Green DP, O'Brien ET. Classification and management of carpal dislocations. *Clin Orthop* 1980;149:55–72.

147. Grundberg AB. Intramedullary fixation for fractures of the hand. *J Hand Surg* 1981;6:568–573.

148. Hamlin C. Traumatic disruption of the distal radioulnar joint. *Am J Sports Med* 1977;5:93–96.

149. Hanks GA, Kolinak A, Bowman LS, Sebastianelli WJ. Stress fractures of the scaphoid. *J Bone Joint Surg* 1989;71A:938–941.

150. Hartwig RH, Louis DS. Multiple carpometacarpal dislocations: A review of four cases. *J Bone Joint Surg* 1979;61A:906–908.

151. Heiple KG, Freehafer AA, Van't Hof A. Isolated traumatic dislocation of the distal end of the ulna and distal radioulnar joint. *J Bone Joint Surg* 1962;44A:1387–1394.

152. Hill NA. Fractures and dislocations of the carpus. *Orthop Clin North Am* 1970;1:275–284.

153. Hsu JD, Curtis RM. Carpometacarpal dislocations of the ulnar side of the hand. *J Bone Joint Surg* 1970;52A:927–930.

154. Hughston JC. Fracture of the distal radial shaft—mistakes in management. *J Bone Joint Surg* 1957;39A:249–264.

155. Hui FC, Linscheid RL. Ulnotriquetral augmentation tenodesis: A reconstructive procedure for dorsal subluxation of the distal radioulnar joint. *J Hand Surg* 1982;7:230–236.

156. Immermann EW. Dislocation of the pisiform. *J Bone Joint Surg* 1948;30A:489–492.

157. Inque G, Inagaki Y. Isolated palmar dislocation of the trapezoid associated with attritional rupture of the flexor tendon. *J Bone Joint Surg* 1990;72A:446–448.

158. Johnson RP. The acutely injured wrist and its residuals. *Clin Orthop* 1980;149:33–44.

159. Jupiter JB. Fractures of the distal end of the radius. *J Bone Joint Surg* 1991;73A:461–469.

160. Kaplan EB. Dorsal dislocation of the metacarpophalangeal joint of the index finger. *J Bone Joint Surg* 1957;39A:1081–1086.

161. Knirk JL, Jupiter JB. Intra-articular fractures of the distal end of the radius in young adults. *J Bone Joint Surg* 1986;68A:647–659.

162. Lawlis JF, Gunther SF. Carpometacarpal dislocations. *J Bone Joint Surg* 1991;73A:52–58.

163. Leddy JP, Packer JW. Avulsion of the profundus tension insertion in athletes. *J Hand Surg* 1977;2:66–69.

164. Lewis HH. Dislocation of the lesser multangular: Report of a case. *J Bone Joint Surg* 1962;44:1412–1414.

165. Lister GD. Intraosseous wiring of the digital skeleton. *J Hand Surg* 1978;3:427–435.

166. Louis DS, Huebner JJ, Hankin FM. Rupture and displacement of the ulnar collateral ligament of the metacarpophalangeal joint of the thumb. *J Bone Joint Surg* 1986;68A:1320–1326.

167. Lucas GL. Internal fixation in the hand: A review of indications and methods. *Orthopedics* 1980;3:1083–1092.

168. MacLaughlin HL. Complex "locked" dislocations of the metacarpophalangeal joints. *J Trauma* 1965;5:683–688.

169. Maudsley RH, Chen SC. Screw fixation in the management of the fractured carpal scaphoid. *J Bone Joint Surg* 1972;54B:432–441.

170. Mayfield JK, Johnson RP, Kilcoyne RK. Carpal dislocations: Pathomechanics and progressive perilunar instability. *J Hand Surg* 1980;5:226–241.

171. McElfresh EC, Dobyns JH, O'Brien ET. Management of fracture-dislocation of the proximal interphalangeal joint by extension-block splinting. *J Bone Joint Surg* 1972;54A:1705–1711.

172. Meyers MH, Wells R, Harvey JP Jr. Naviculocapitate fracture syndrome. *J Bone Joint Surg* 1971;53A:1383–1390.

173. Mikic ZD. Galeazzi fracture-dislocations. *J Bone Joint Surg* 1975;57A:1071–1080.

174. Mikio T, Yamamuro T, Kotoura Y, Tsuji T, Shimizu K, Itakura H. Rupture of the extensor tendons of the fingers. *J Bone Joint Surg* 1986;68A:610–614.

175. Milch H. Fracture of the hamate bone. *J Bone Joint Surg* 1934;16:459–462.

176. Minami M, Hamazaki J, Ishii S. Isolated dislocation of the pisiform: A case report and review of the literature. *J Hand Surg* 1984;9:125–127.

177. Moore JR, Webb CA, Thompson RC. A complete dislocation of the thumb metacarpal. *J Hand Surg* 1978;3:547–549.

178. Morawa LG, Ross PM, Schock CC. Fracture and dislocations involving the navicular-lunate axis. *Clin Orthop* 1976;118:48–53.

179. Morrissy RT, Nalebuff EA. Dislocation of the distal radioulnar joint: Anatomy and clues to prompt diagnosis. *Clin Orthop* 1979;144:154–158.

180. Mouat TB, Wilkie J, Harding HE. Isolated fracture of the carpal semilunar and Kienböck's disease. *Br J Surg* 1932;19:577–592.

181. Nalebuff EA. Isolated anterior carpometacarpal dislocation of the fifth finger: Classification and case report. *J Trauma* 1968;8:1119–1123.

182. Nielsen PT, Hederboe J, Thommesen. Bone scintigraphy in the evaluation of fracture of the carpal scaphoid bone. *Acta Orthop Scand* 1983;54:303–306.

183. Normal A, Nelson J, Green S. Fracture of the hook of the hamate: Radiographic signs. *Radiology* 1985;154:49–53.

184. North ER, Eaton RG. Volar dislocation of the fifth metacarpal. *J Bone Joint Surg* 1980;62A:657–659.

185. Olsen N, Schousen P, Dirksen H, Christoffersen JK. Regional scintimetry in scaphoid fractures. *Acta Orthop Scand* 1983;54:380–382.

186. Parks JC, Stovell PB. Dislocation of the carpal scaphoid: A report of two cases. *J Trauma* 1973;13:384–388.

187. Peltier LF. Eponymic fractures: John Rhea Barton and Bartons fractures. *Surgery* 1953;34:960–970.

188. Peltier LF. Eponymic fractures: Robert William Smith and Smith's fractures. *Surgery* 1959;45:1035–1042.

189. Reef TC. Avulsion of the flexor digitorum profundus: An athletic injury. *Am J Sports Med* 1977;5:281–285.

190. Renshaw TS, Louis DS. Complex volar dislocation of the metacarpophalangeal joint: A case report. *J Trauma* 1971;12:1086–1088.

191. Rosado A. A possible relationship of radio-carpal dislocation and dislocation of the lunate bone. *J Bone Joint Surg* 1966;48B:504–506.

192. Rose-Innes AP. Anterior dislocation of the ulna at the inferior radioulnar joint. *J Bone Joint Surg* 1960;42B:515–521.

193. Ruby LK. Common hand injuries in the athlete. *Orthop Clin North Am* 1980;11:819–839.

194. Russe O. Fracture of the carpal navicular. *J Bone Joint Surg* 1960;42A:759–768.

195. Russell TB. Intercarpal dislocations and fracture-dislocations. A review of 59 cases. *J Bone Joint Surg* 1949;31B:524–531.

196. Sebald JR, Dobyns JH, Linscheid RL. The natural history of collapse deformities of the wrist. *Clin Orthop* 1974;104:140–148.

197. Seimon LP. Compound dislocation of the trapezium. *J Bone Joint Surg* 1972;54A:1297–1300.
198. Shall J, Cohn BT, Froimson AI. Acute compartment syndrome of the forearm in association with fracture of the distal end of the radius. *J Bone Joint Surg* 1986;68A:1451–1454.
199. Siegel MW, Hertzberg H. Complete dislocation of the greater multangulum (trapezium). *J Bone Joint Surg* 1969;51A:769–772.
200. Smith RJ. Post-traumatic instability of the metacarpophalangeal joint of the thumb. *J Bone Joint Surg* 1977;59A:14–21.
201. Smith DK, Gilula LA, Amadio PC. Dorsal lunate tilt (DISI configuration): Sign of scaphoid fracture displacement. *Radiology* 1990;176:497–499.
202. Smith DK, Linscheid RL, Amadio PC, Berquist TH, Cooney WP. Scaphoid anatomy: Evaluation with complex motion tomography. *Radiology* 1989;173:177–180.
203. Stahelin A, Pfeiffer K, Sennwald G, Segmuller G. Determining carpal collapse. *J Bone Joint Surg* 1989;71A:1400–1405.
204. Stark HH. Troublesome fractures and dislocations of the hand. *Inst Course Lect* 1970;19:130–149.
205. Stark HH, Jobe FW, Boyes JH, Ashworth CR. Fracture of the hook of the hamate in athletes. *J Bone Joint Surg* 1977;59A:575–582.
206. Stark HH, Chao E, Zemel NP, Rickard TA, Ashworth CR. Fracture of the hook of the hamate. *J Bone Joint Surg* 1989;71A:1202–1207.
207. Stein AH. Dorsal dislocation of the lesser multangular bone. *J Bone Joint Surg* 1971;53A:377–379.
208. Stein R, Siegel MW. Naviculo-capitate fracture syndrome. *J Bone Joint Surg* 1969;51A:391–395.
209. Stener B. Displacement of the ruptured ulnar collateral ligament of the metacarpophalangeal joint of the thumb. *J Bone Joint Surg* 1962;44B:869–879.
210. Stevanovic MV, Stark HH, Feller BC. Scaphotrapezoid dislocation. *J Bone Joint Surg* 1990;72A:449–452.
211. Swanson AB. Fractures involving the digits of the hand. *Orthop Clin North Am* 1970;1:261–274.
212. Talersnik J. Carpal instability. *J Bone Joint Surg* 1988;70A:1262–1268.
213. Tehranzadeh J, Davenport J, Pais MJ. Scaphoid fracture: Evaluation with flexion-extension tomography. *Radiology* 1990;176:167–170.
214. Thomas FB. Reduction of Smith's fractures. *J Bone Joint Surg* 1957;39B:463–470.
215. Thompson GH, Grant TT. Barton's fracture—reverse Barton's fracture: Confusing eponyms. *Clin Orthop* 1977;122:210–220.
216. Torisu T. Fracture of the hook of the hamate by a golf-swing. *Clin Orthop* 1972;83:91–94.
217. Vasilas A, Grieco RV, Bartone NF. Roentgen aspects of injuries to the pisiform bone and pisotriquetral injury. *J Bone Joint Surg* 1960;42A:1317–1328.
218. Verdan C, Narakas A. Fracture and pseudoarthrosis of the scaphoid. *Surg Clin North Am* 1968;48:1083–1095.
219. Vesley DG. The distal radioulnar joint. *Clin Orthop* 1967;51:75–91.
220. Weber ER, Chao EYS. An experimental approach to the mechanism of scaphoid waist fracture. *J Hand Surg* 1978;3:142–148.
221. Wehbe MA, Schneider LA. Mallet fractures. *J Bone Joint Surg* 1984;66A:658–669.
222. Weiss A, Weiland AJ, Moore R, Welges EFS. Radial shortening for Kienböck disease. *J Bone Joint Surg* 1991;73A:384–391.
223. Wenger DR. Avulsion of the profundus tendon insertion in football players. *Arch Surg* 1973;106:145–149.
224. Wesely MS, Barenfield PA. Trans-scaphoid, transcapitate, transtriquetral, perilunate fracture-dislocation of the wrist. *J Bone Joint Surg* 1972;54A:1073–1078.
225. Wesely MS, Barenfield PA, Bruno J. Volar dislocation of the distal radioulnar joint. *J Trauma* 1972;12:1083–1088.
226. White SJ, Louis DS, Braunstein EM, Hankin FM, Greene TL. Capitolunate instability. *AJR* 1984;143:361–364.
227. Wilson JN, Rowland SA. Fracture-dislocation of the proximal interphalangeal joint of the finger. Treatment by open reduction and internal fixation. *J Bone Joint Surg* 1966;48A:493–505.
228. Wood MB, Dobyns JH. Chronic, complex volar dislocation of the metacarpophalangeal joint. *J Hand Surg* 1981;6:73–76.
229. Yeager BA, Dalinka MK. Radiology of trauma of the wrist: Dislocations, fracture dislocations, and instability patterns. *Skel Radiol* 1985;13:120–130.

Chronic Post-traumatic Conditions

230. Artz TD, Posch JL. The carpometacarpal boss. *J Bone Joint Surg* 1973;55A:747–752.
231. Bassoe E, Bassoe HH. The styloid bone and carpe bosseau disease. *Am J Roentgenol* 1955;74:886–888.
232. Beckenbaugh RD, Shives TC, Dobyns JH, Linscheid RL. Kienböck's disease: The natural history of Kienböck's disease and consideration of lunate fractures. *Clin Orthop* 1980;149:98–106.
233. Bobechko WP, Harris WR. The radiographic density of avascular bone. *J Bone Joint Surg* 1960;42B:626–632.
234. Braunstein EM, Louis DS, Greene TL, Hankin FM. Fluoroscopic and arthrographic evaluation of carpal instability. *AJR* 1985;144:1259–1262.
235. Conway WF, Destouet JM, Gilula LA, Bellinghausen HW, Weeks PM. The carpal boss: An overview of radiographic evaluation. *Radiology* 1985;156:29–31.
236. Jorgensen EC. Proximal-row carpectomy. An end-result study of 22 cases. *J Bone Joint Surg* 1969;51A:1104–1111.
237. Kienböck R. Uber traumatische Malazie des Mondbeins und ihre Folgezustande: Entartungsformen and Kompressionsfrakturen. *Fortschr Geb Röntgen* 1910;16:77.
238. Kienböck R. Concerning traumatic malacia of the lunate and its consequences: Degeneration and compression fracture. *Clin Orthop* 1980;149:4–8.
239. Kleinert HE, Kasdan ML. Reconstruction of chronically subluxated proximal interphalangeal finger joint. *J Bone Joint Surg* 1964;47A:958–964.
240. Koostra G, Huffstadt AJC, Kauer JMG. The styloid bone. A clinical and embryological study. *Hand* 1974;6:185.
241. Lichtman DM, Mack GR, MacDonald RI. Kienböck's disease: The role of silicone replacement arthroplasty. *J Bone Joint Surg* 1977;59A:899–908.
242. Linscheid RL, Dobyns JH, Beckenbaugh RD, et al. Instability patterns of the wrist. *J Hand Surg* 1983;8:682–686.
243. Lovett WL, McCalla MA. Management and rehabilitation of extensor tendon injuries. *Orthop Clin North Am* 1983;14:811–826.
244. Palmer AK, Dobyns JH, Linscheid RL. Management of post-traumatic instability of the wrist secondary to ligament rupture. *J Hand Surg* 1978;3:507–532.
245. Persson M. Casual treatment of lunatomalacia, further experience of operative ulna lengthening. *Acta Chir Scand* 1950; 100:531–544.
246. Posner MA. Injuries to the hand and wrist in athletes. *Orthop Clin North Am* 1977;8:593–618.
247. Souter WA. The problem of boutonnière deformities. *Clin Orthop* 1974;104:116–133.
248. Swanson AB. Silicone rubber implants for the replacement of the carpal scaphoid and lunate bones. *Orthop Clin North Am* 1970;1:299–309.
249. Taleisnik J. Post-traumatic carpal instability. *Clin Orthop* 1980; 149:73–82.
250. Taleisnik J. Carpal instability. *J Bone Joint Surg* 1988;70A:1262–1268.
251. Tilberg B. Kienböck's disease treated with osteotomy to lengthen the ulna. *Acta Orthop Scand* 1968;39:359–368.
252. Weiss AC, Weiland AJ, Moore R, Wilgis EFS. Radial shortening for Kienböck disease. *J Bone Joint Surg* 1991;73A:384–391.

Post-traumatic Reconstruction

253. Beckenbaugh RD. New concepts in arthroplasty of the hand and wrist. *Arch Surg* 1977;112:1094–1098.
254. Froimson A. Tendon arthroplasty of the trapeziometacarpal joint. *Clin Orthop* 1970;70:191–199.
255. Lugnegard H. Resection of the head of the ulna in post-traumatic dysfunction of the distal radioulnar joint. *Scand J Plast Reconstr Surg* 1969;3:65–69.

Imaging of Orthopedic Trauma,
Second Edition, edited by T.H. Berquist,
Mayo Clinic © 1992. Published
by Raven Press, Ltd., New York.

CHAPTER 15

Imaging of Post-traumatic Infection

Thomas H. Berquist and Manuel L. Brown

Osteomyelitis, 871
  Imaging of Post-traumatic Osteomyelitis, 871
Soft Tissue Infection, 877

Surgical Reconstruction, 878
References, 879

Musculoskeletal infections may progress rapidly from their initial clinical presentation, or they may present with a slow, insidious course complicating previous trauma or the placement of an orthopedic device. Determining the extent of involvement is important in planning proper medical or surgical management.

OSTEOMYELITIS

It has been demonstrated that trauma causes generalized reduction in resistance to infection. Hematogenous osteomyelitis may develop more readily after growth plate fractures (43). However, most post-traumatic infections are related to fractures with extensive soft tissue injury or surgical techniques (11,18,29,32).

Lack of soft tissue covering causes the tibia to be particularly susceptible to open injury and infection. Therefore, it provides a useful model for discussion of post-traumatic infection. Gustilo and Anderson (20) demonstrated that the extent of soft tissue injury, vascular injury, and fracture stability were important factors. Infection may develop in up to 80% of these severe injuries (11).

Caudle and Stern (11) further classified open injuries (Type III) into three categories that impact prognosis. Type IIIA injuries have adequate soft tissue coverage despite extensive soft tissue laceration. Type IIIB lesions also have soft tissue laceration but periosteum is stripped exposing the underlying bone. Type IIIC lesions have

significant arterial injury that requires repair. The prognosis and number of surgical procedures required for final healing increases with more severe injuries (Type IIIC). Twenty-nine percent of Type IIIB lesions developed deep infection; 78% of Type IIIC lesions required early or late amputations (11).

Surgical reduction of fractures also increases the incidence of infection (29,32,34). This can occur with open reduction and internal fixation or use of external fixation devices and traction pins. The incidence of infections with external pin fixation is fairly low (~1%) when used with plaster compared to 8.2% with mechanical external fixation devices (18). Pin tract infections are usually related to soft tissue necrosis and pin motion (18,19,28). Detection of these infections is important because the impact on future treatment is significantly affected. For example, the presence of pin tract infection contraindicates further reduction with intramedullary nailing (28).

The offending organisms in post-traumatic osteomyelitis are similar to hematogenous osteomyelitis (29,32). However, anaerobic organisms may also be evident and prognosis is adversely affected. Hall et al. (22) noted treatment failures three times more frequently in post-traumatic anaerobic infections.

Imaging of Post-traumatic Osteomyelitis

Radiographic detection of infection following fracture or internal fixation can be difficult. The usually useful early signs of acute hematogenous osteomyelitis (soft tissue swelling or periosteal reaction) are usually not useful. Bone destruction is also difficult to evaluate in the presence of fracture line irregularity and bone remodeling

T. H. Berquist: Department of Diagnostic Radiology, Mayo Medical School, Mayo Clinic Jacksonville, Jacksonville, Florida 32224.
M. L. Brown: Department of Diagnostic Radiology, Mayo Medical School, Mayo Clinic, Rochester, Minnesota 55905.

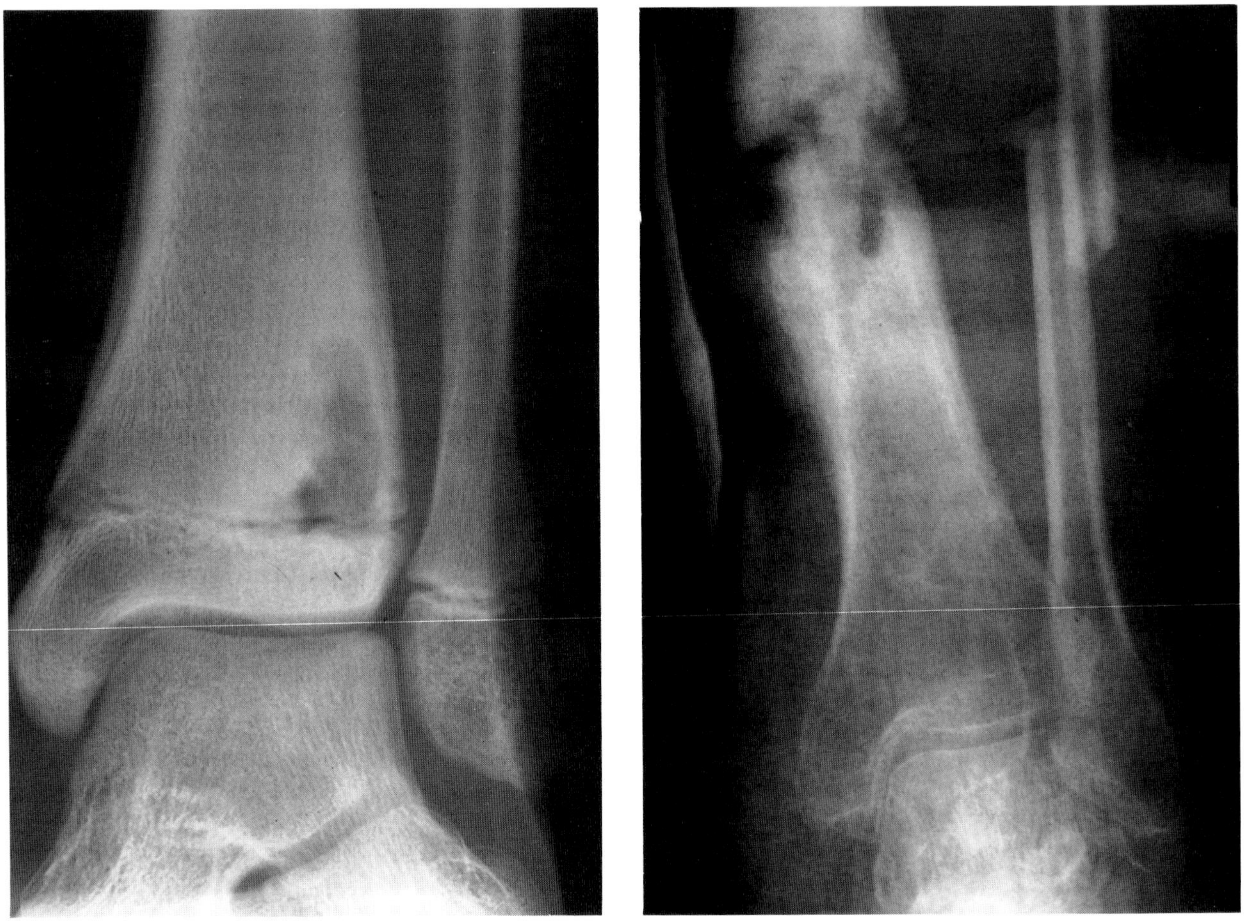

FIG. 15–1. A: AP radiograph of the ankle demonstrating the typical features of hematogenous osteo-myelitis. **B:** Fractures of the distal tibia and fibula with infection at the fracture site.

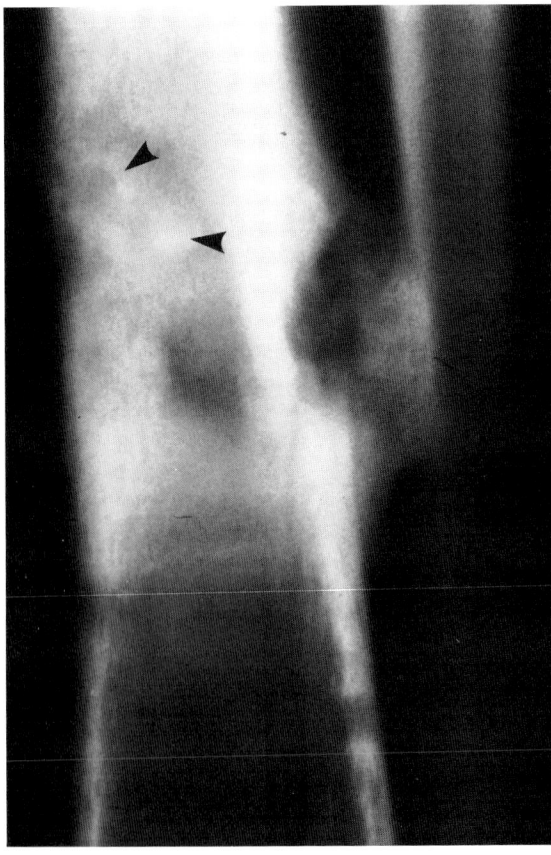

FIG. 15–2. Tomogram of an old tibial fracture with sequestra (*arrow*) in a lucent marrow defect due to active osteomyelitis.

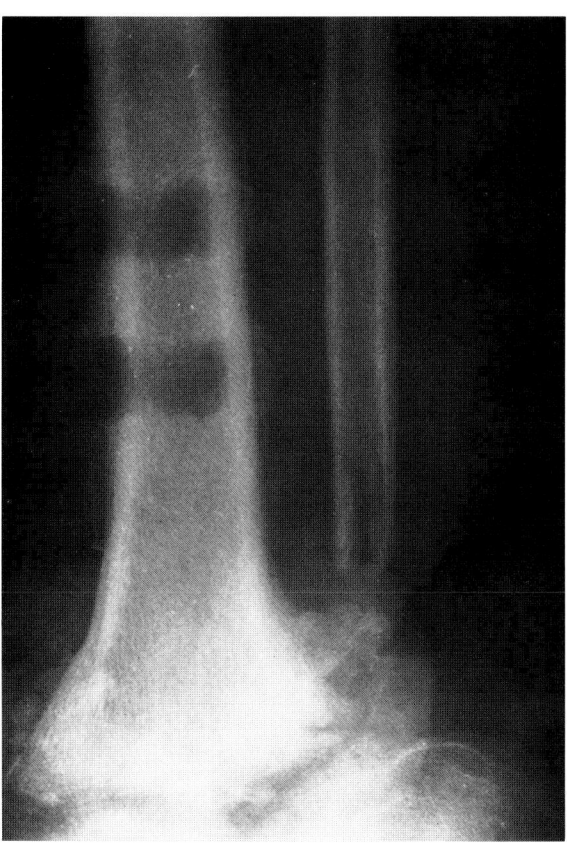

FIG. 15-3. Pin tract infections. Grossly expanded pin tracts with periosteal new bone in the distal tibia. Sequestra are not necessary for diagnosis when changes are this advanced.

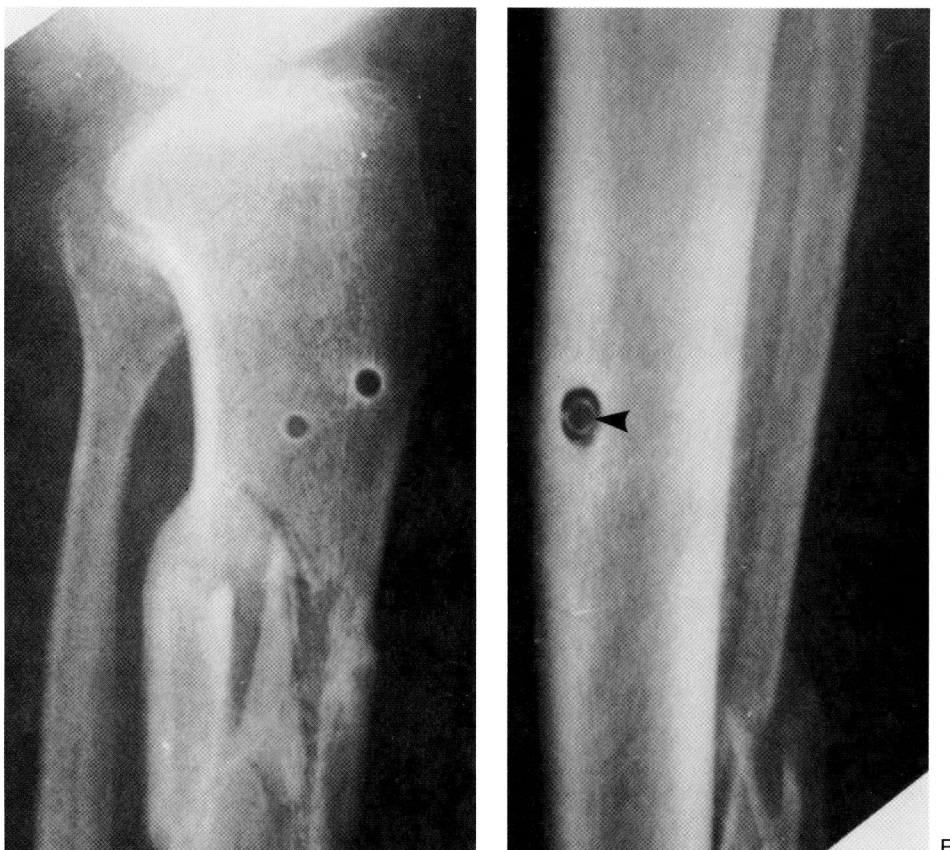

A

B

FIG. 15-4. Fluoroscopically positioned tibial radiographs for direct evaluation of old pin tracts. **A:** Normal pin tracts. **B:** Ring sequestra (*arrow*) (from 31, with permission).

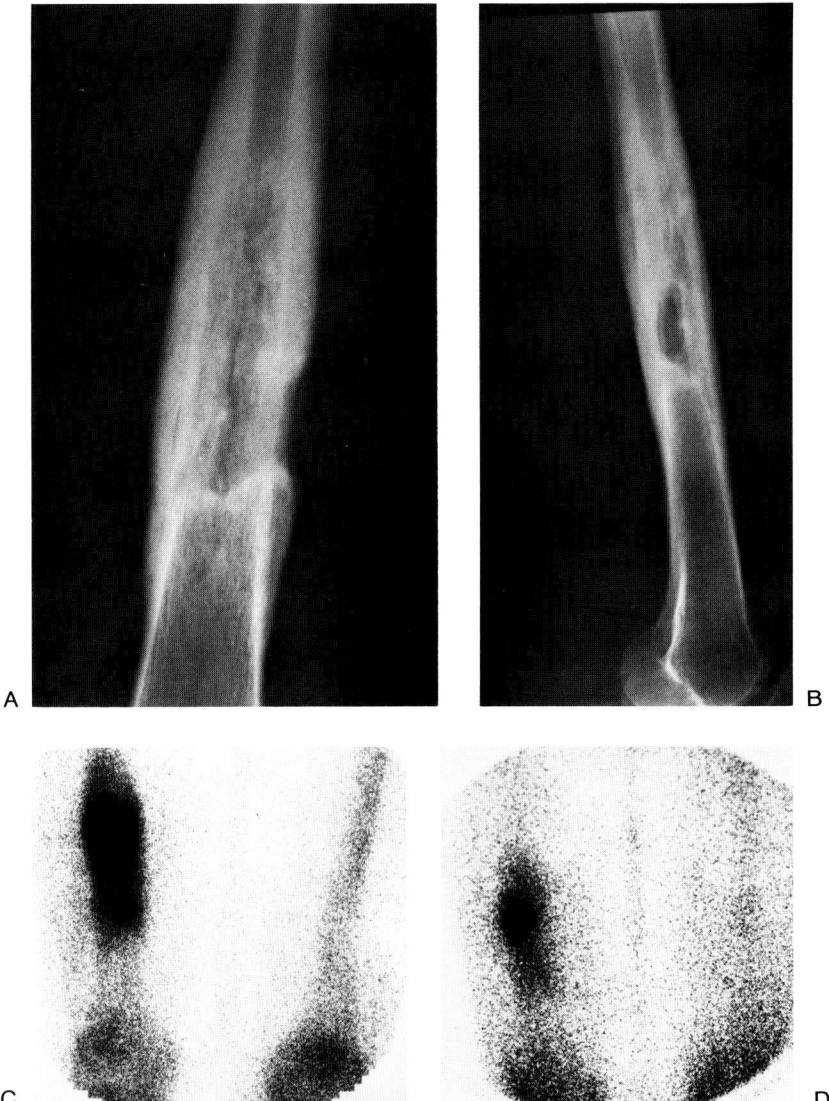

FIG. 15–5. AP (**A**) and lateral (**B**) radiographs of the femur demonstrating an old fracture deformity with previous curettage. Technetium-99m MDP (**C**) and gallium-67 (**D**) images show increased uptake in the region of the previous surgery. The uptake on the gallium image (**D**) is smaller and less intense than the technetium scan (**C**). Although this is less specific, infection was present.

(Fig. 15-1). Tumeh et al. (38) reported that the only specific radiographic feature of active infection was identification of sequestra. Sequestra are difficult to identify with routine radiography. Conventional or computed tomography (CT) are most useful in this setting (Fig. 15-2) (3,23,33,43).

Pin tract infections are a significant problem. Routine radiography and, on occasion, tomography are useful in defining the ring sequestrum associated with pin tract infection (19,31). Fluoroscopic positioning is useful with either technique to properly align the pin tract for optimal detection of the sequestra (Figs. 15-3 and 15-4) (31).

Radionuclide imaging is particularly useful in patients with suspected osteomyelitis. Conventional technetium-99m MDP images are sensitive and, when negative, ex-

clude the diagnosis of osteomyelitis (15,27). However, following fracture, increased tracer is expected and nonspecific (35).

Specificity has improved using gallium-67- or Indium-111-labeled white blood cells in conjunction with technetium-99m MDP studies. Tumeh et al. (37,38) described five patterns of uptake using combined gallium-67 and technetium-99m MDP scintigraphy. Pattern 1 patients demonstrate increased uptake with technitium scans and normal gallium-67 images. With the second pattern, there is diffuse uptake with both agents, and pattern 3 shows different geographic distribution but similar uptake intensity. Pattern 4 revealed similar uptake intensity and pattern. The most specific finding, pattern 5, was a gallium-67 study with more

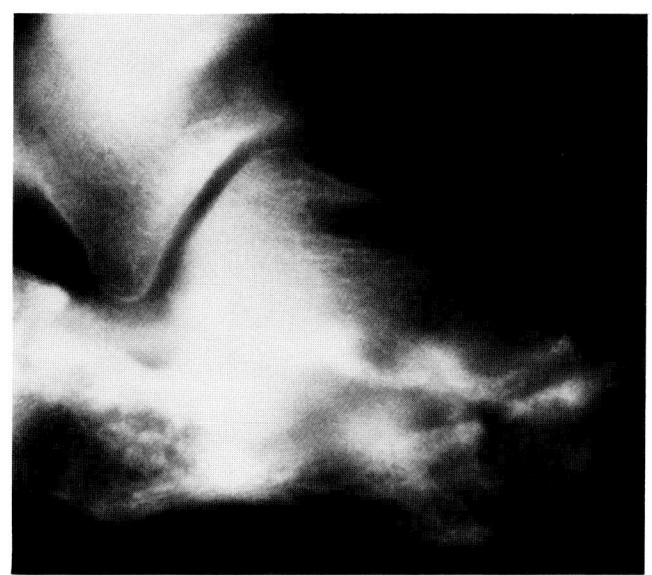
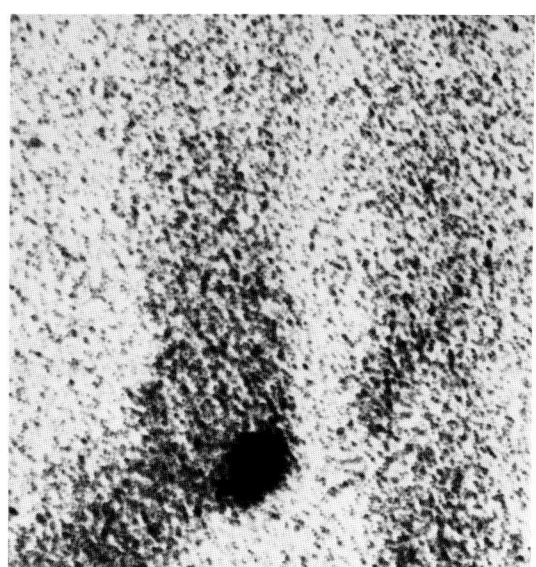

FIG. 15–6. A: Lateral tomogram of the calcaneus following fracture. **B:** Indium-111 white blood cell scan shows focal intense uptake due to osteomyelitis.

intensity compared to technetium-99m MDP (Fig. 15-5).

Indium-111 white blood cell studies are also useful in detecting subtle osteomyelitis (30,35). However, it is not unusual to note mild increased uptake following fracture in the absence of fracture (26). Combined studies are more useful (Fig. 15-6).

Magnetic resonance imaging (MRI) has also proved useful for evaluating infection. The examination of patients with infection (as with other musculoskeletal pathology) requires at least T1- (SE 500/20 or inversion recovery) and T2- (spin-echo with long TE [≥60] and TR [>2000]) weighted sequences (4,6,7,36). These sequences are needed to provide the necessary contrast between normal and abnormal tissue and to detect and characterize subtle abnormalities. T1-weighted spin-echo sequences (SE 500/20) can be performed quickly and provide high spatial resolution. Infection is demonstrated as an area of decreased signal intensity compared to the high signal intensity of normal marrow (Fig. 15-7). Changes in cortical bone, periosteum, and muscle are often less obvious. Inversion recovery sequences may detect more subtle changes but images are "noisier" and scans require more time (TR usually ≥2000). T2-weighted sequences (SE 2000/60) demonstrate infection as areas of high signal intensity. The second echo (2000/60) is ideal for distinguishing abnormal areas in cortical bone and soft tissues. Fat signal is reduced so areas of marrow inflammation show increased intensity compared to normal marrow (Fig. 15-7). In certain situations, more than two sequences may be required to improve tissue characterization. For example, short TI inversion recovery (STIR) sequences (Fig. 13-4) or chem-

ical shift imaging may provide valuable information about fat, water (cellular elements), or inflammatory changes in bone marrow (7).

The anatomic extent of osteomyelitis can be clearly demonstrated by MRI (4,6,7). The extent of disease, including detection of skip areas, is easily established using transaxial images in combination with either the sagittal or coronal images (Fig. 15-7). This information is particularly valuable in planning surgical debridement.

Compared to isotope scintigraphy, MRI was particularly useful in separating bone and soft tissue processes. Gallium-67- and Indium-111-labeled white blood cells are more specific for infection than technetium scans (5,21). Beltran et al. (5) compared technetium-99m MDP, gallium-67, and MRI in evaluating musculoskeletal infection. All techniques were equally effective in detecting osseous infection. However, MRI was more sensitive (100% compared to 69% for isotope scans) in identifying abscesses and distinguishing abscesses from cellulitis (Fig. 15-7).

The specificity of MRI in diagnosing osteomyelitis needs to be more clearly defined. Increased signal intensity in marrow, cortical bone, periosteum, and soft tissue is noted on T2-weighted, STIR, and gradient-echo (T2*) sequences. Decreased signal intensity is evident when T1-weighted sequences are used (5). Similar findings, however, have also been noted with neoplasms. A potentially useful image feature is the increased signal in medullary bone with a well-defined lucent margin (Fig. 15-8) (7). This observation has been noted with both infection and benign tumors (6,7). Infection must be present for several weeks to allow the reactive region in the medullary bone, which is responsible for this finding to occur.

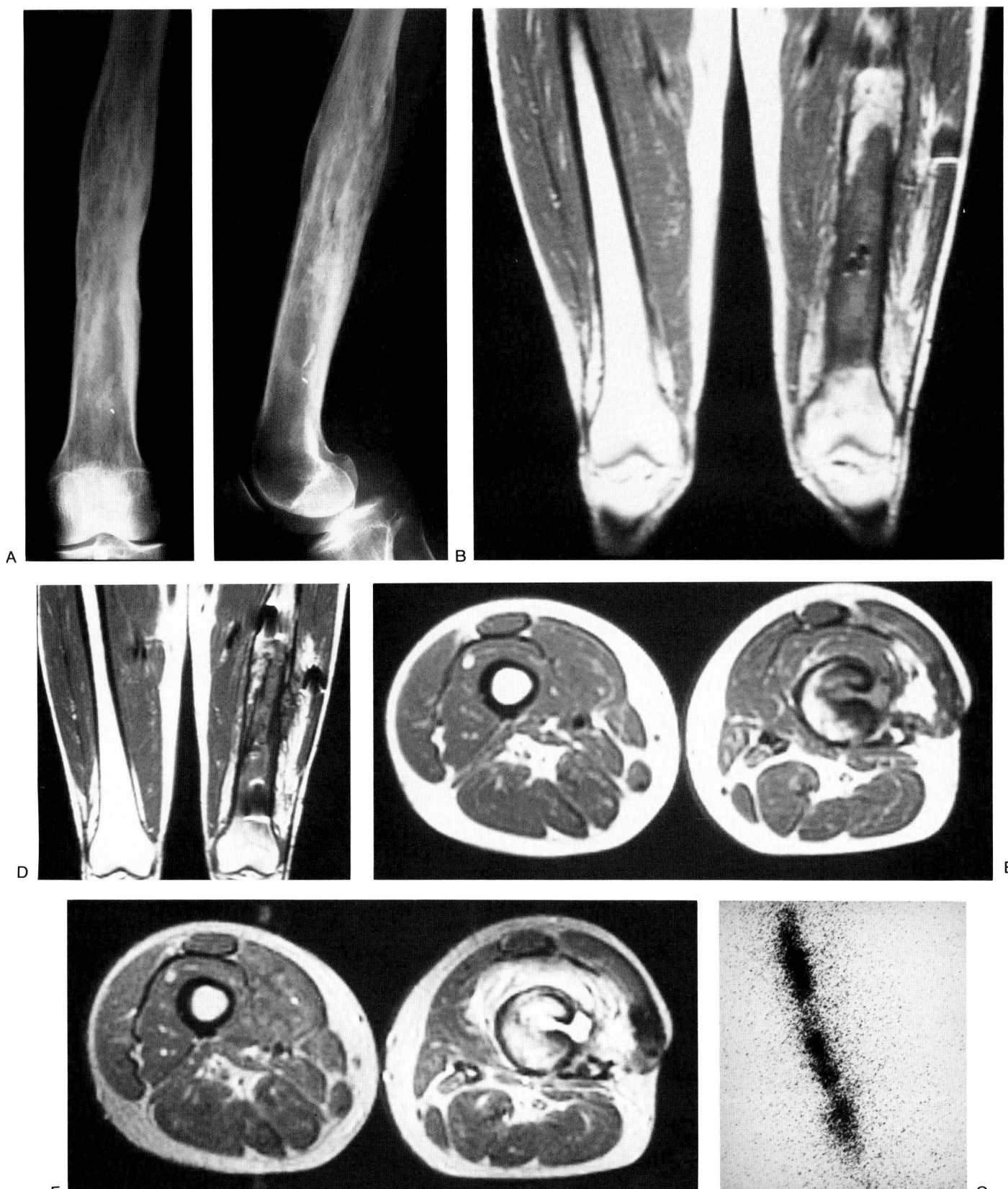

FIG. 15-7. AP (**A**) and lateral (**B**) radiographs demonstrate an old fracture deformity of the mid femur. Coronal SE 500/20 MR images (**C, D**) show a large area of decreased signal intensity in the distal femur. Note the metal artifact. Axial SE 2000/20 (**E**) and SE 2000/60 (**F**) images show soft tissue extension and abscess formation with soft tissue edema. Lateral indium-111 white blood cell (WBC) scan (**G**) shows diffuse uptake due to osteomyelitis, but the soft tissue changes are not detectable.

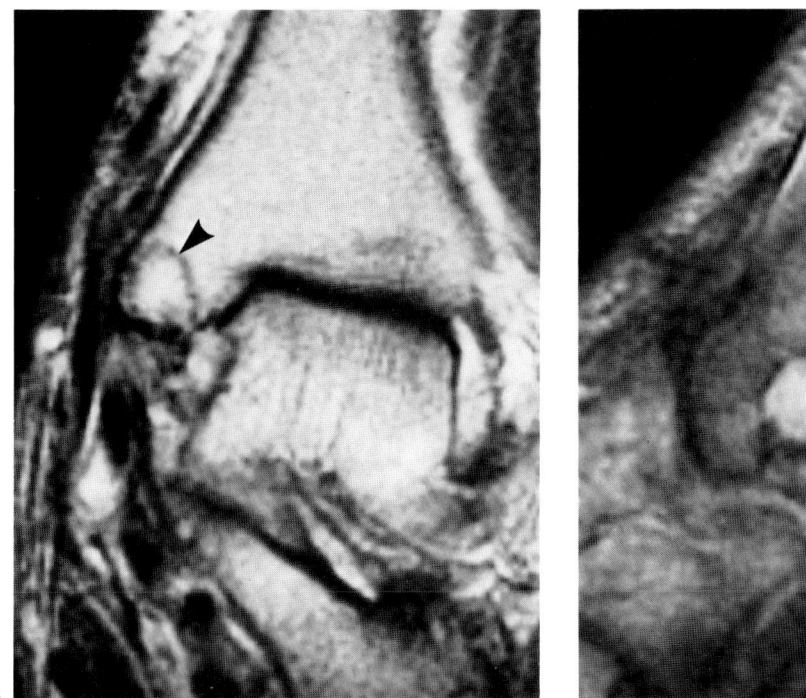
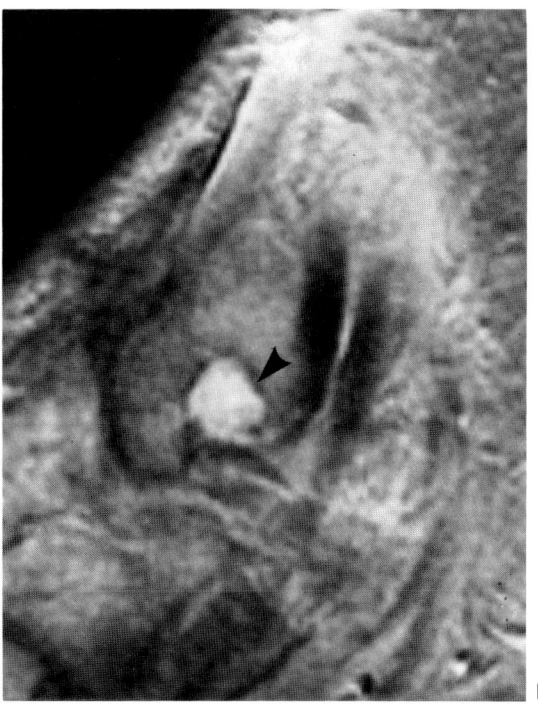

FIG. 15–8. Coronal (**A**) and sagittal (**B**) MR images demonstrate an area of increased signal intensity with a well-defined margin (*arrow*) due to osteomyelitis (from 7, with permission).

SOFT TISSUE INFECTION

The superior soft tissue contrast of MRI is ideally suited for identification of soft tissue inflammation and abscesses. Localization of the infected area, specifically the relationship to bone and neurovascular structures, is easily accomplished without injection of contrast medium (7,12). Both T1- and T2-weighted images are used to assist in defining the nature of the lesion and to define its extent. The signal intensity of abscess fluid may be inhomogeneous and high to intermediate signal intensity on T2-weighted STIR sequences (Fig. 15-9). Signal intensity varies slightly depending upon the protein content and necrotic debris in the abscess (7,9,13,41). Abscesses are typically similar to or of slightly lower inten-

sity than muscle on T1-weighted sequences (3,7,12). Gadolinium has been used to enhance the hyperemic margins or capsules of chronic abscesses. This technique may assist in improving the diagnostic specificity.

Reports suggest that MRI is more sensitive than CT for detection of abscesses (12). The choice of technique should be varied with the clinical setting. In patients with recent surgery or strong clinical indication of abscess formation, CT may be more useful. This is especially true if abdominal or pelvic abscesses are suspected and percutaneous drainage is considered. The examination and intervention can be accomplished at the same time. Patients who have subtle clinical findings and when extremity involvement is suspected are more appropriately evaluated with MRI.

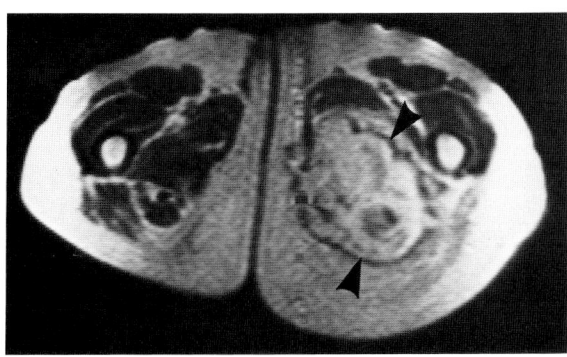

FIG. 15–9. Axial MR image demonstrating a large thigh abscess (*arrows*).

SURGICAL RECONSTRUCTION

A high percentage of patients with chronic osteomyelitis require surgical therapy for excision of necrotic or infected tissue. The use of free vascularized muscle, omental, and bone grafts is increasing in the treatment of patients with chronic osteomyelitis (2,16). Reconstructive procedures may be needed depending on the vascularity of adjacent tissue and the size and type of defect. There are several basic goals regardless of the tissue or technique used. These include (1) wound coverage, (2) obliteration of dead space (which may permit survival of existing organisms or provide a medium for recurrent infection), and (3) providing optimal vascular supply to the described area (2,16).

Preoperative assessment should include review of the necessary information and planning of the surgical approach; postoperative assessment should determine whether the surgical goals have been achieved. Preoperatively, MRI is an ideal way to assess the extent of bone and soft tissue involvement, as well as to detect skip areas. Preoperative images also serve as a valuable baseline to later determine whether the surgical goals are achieved.

MRI is well suited for evaluating defect coverage or dead space, residual infection, and hematomas or fluid collections that may serve as media for recurrent infection (Fig. 15-10). MRI is particularly useful in the evaluation of omental and muscle flaps (Fig. 15-10). Vascularized fibular grafts can be evaluated, but the small amount of marrow presents certain problems, since there is little fibular marrow to image in the axial plane.

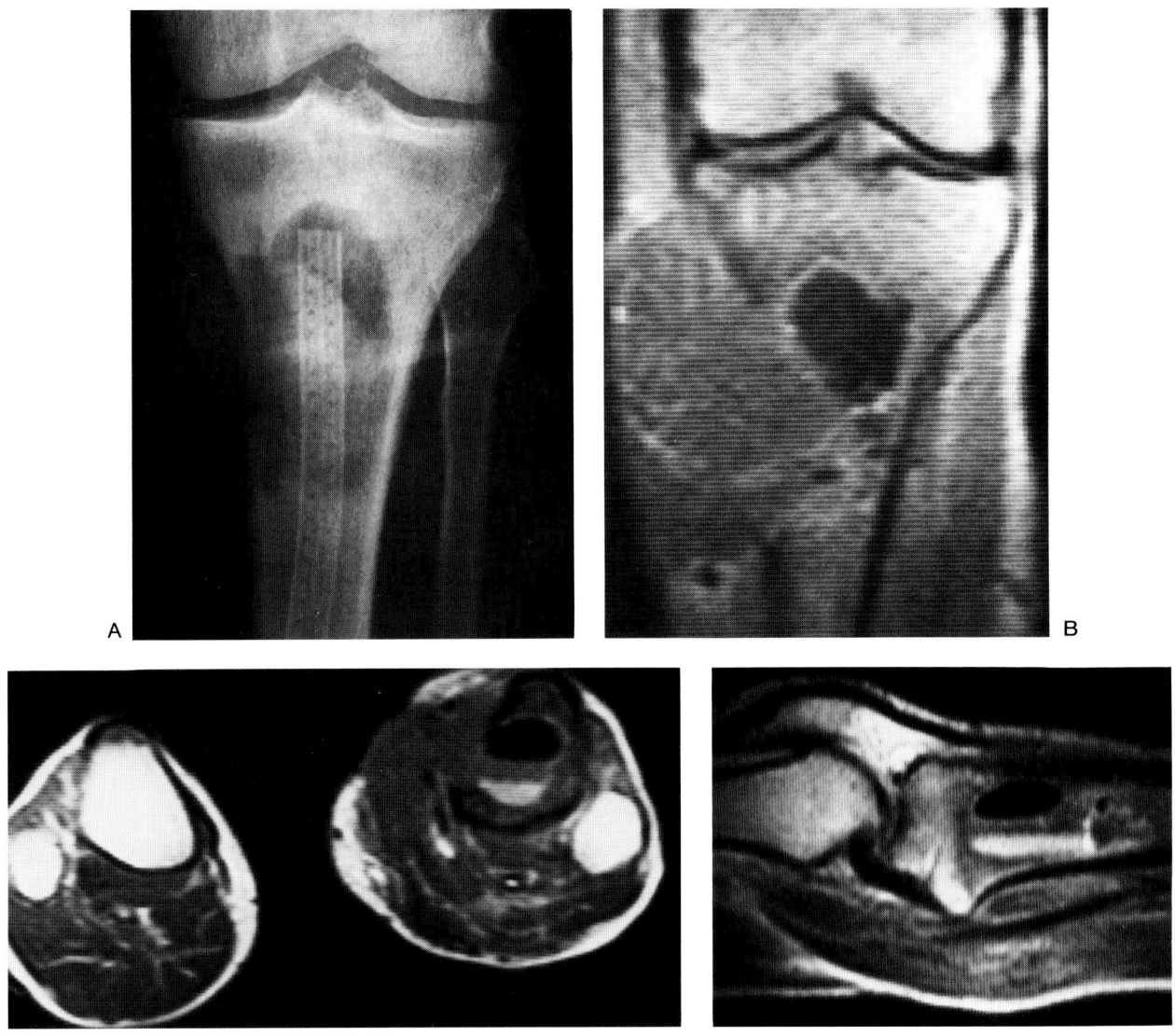

FIG. 15-10. Postoperative muscle flap for chronic osteomyelitis. **A:** AP radiograph following surgery. **B:** Coronal SE 500/20 images shows that the muscle flap does not completely fill the dead space. Axial (**C**) and sagittal (**D**) images demonstrate fluid-fluid levels in the dead space.

This can be improved by using coronal and sagittal views, which increase the marrow volume imaged and allow the position as well as the proximal and distal attachments of the grafts to be more easily evaluated.

Recently, Gd-DTPA has been used to confirm viability of vascularized grafts. Varnell et al. (39) demonstrated that viable grafts enhanced while those with early vascular occlusion did not enhance.

Further studies and follow-up of these patients will be needed to determine the effectiveness of MRI in evaluating viability and flow factors in the grafts. Spectroscopy may also play a role in graft evaluation, especially early ischemic changes.

REFERENCES

1. Al-Sheikh W, Sfakianakis GN, Mnaymneh W, et al. Subacute and chronic bone infections: Diagnosis using In-111, Ga-67, and Tc-99m MDP bone scintigraphy and radiography. *Radiology* 1985;155:501–506.
2. Arnold PG, Irons GB. Lower extremity muscle flaps. *Orthop Clin North Am* 1984;15:441–449.
3. Azouz EM. Computed tomography of bone and joint infections. *Can Assoc Radiol* 1981;32:102–106.
4. Beltran J, Nato AM, McGhee RB, Freedy RM, McCalla MS. Infections of the musculoskeletal system: High-field-strength MR imaging. *Radiology* 1987;169:449–454.
5. Beltran J, McGhee RB, Shaffer PO, et al. Experiment infections of the musculoskeletal system: Evaluation with MR imaging and Tc-99m MDP and Ga-67 scintigraphy. *Radiology* 1988;167:167–172.
6. Berquist TH, Brown ML, Fitzgerald RH, May GR. Magnetic resonance imaging: Application in musculoskeletal infection. *Mag Res Imag* 1985;3:219–230.
7. Berquist TH. *MRI of the musculoskeletal system,* 2nd ed. New York: Raven Press, 1990.
8. Bonakdarpour A, Gaines VD. The radiology of osteomyelitis. *Orthop Clin North Am* 1983;14:21–37.
9. Brown JJ, Van Sonnenberg E, Gerber KH, Strich G, Wittich GR, Slatsky RA. Magnetic resonance relaxation of percutaneously obtained normal and abnormal body fluids. *Radiology* 1985;154:727–731.
10. Brown ML, Komida CB, Berquist TH, Fitzgerald RH. An imaging approach to musculoskeletal infections. In: Berquist TH. *Imaging of orthopedic trauma and surgery.* Philadelphia: W.B. Saunders Co., 1986;731–753.
11. Caudle RJ, Stern PJ. Severe open fractures of the tibia. *J Bone Joint Surg* 1987;69A:801–806.
12. Chandnani VP, Beltran J, Morris CS, et al. Acute experimental osteomyelitis and abscesses: Detection with MR imaging versus CT. *Radiology* 1990;174:223–226.
13. Cohen JM, Weinreb JC, Moravilla KR. Fluid collections in the intraperitoneal and extraperitoneal spaces. Comparison of MR and CT. *Radiology* 1985;155:705–708.
14. Daoud A, Saighi-Bouaguina A. Treatment of sequestra, pseudarthrosis, and defects in the long bones of children who have chronic hematogenous osteomyelitis. *J Bone Joint Surg* 1989;71A:1448–1468.
15. Duszynske DO, Kuhn JF, Afshani E. Early radionuclide diagnosis of acute osteomyelitis. *Radiology* 1975;117:337–340.
16. Fitzgerald RH, Ruttle PE, Arnold PG, Kelly PJ, Irons GB. Local muscle flaps in the treatment of chronic osteomyelitis. *J Bone Joint Surg* 1985;67A:175–185.
17. Gohil VK, Dalinka MK, Edeiken J. The serpiginous tract: A sign of subacute osteomyelitis. *J Can Assoc Radiol* 1973;24:337–339.
18. Green SA. Complications of external skeletal fixation. *Clin Orthop* 1983;180:109–115.
19. Green SA, Ripley MJ. Chronic osteomyelitis in pin tracts. *J Bone Joint Surg* 1984;66A:1092–1098.
20. Gustilo RB, Anderson JT. Prevention of infection in treatment of one thousand and twenty-five open fractures of long bones. *J Bone Joint Surg* 1976;58A:453–458.
21. Gustilo RB, Mendoza RM, Williams DN. Problems in the management of Type III (severe) open fractures: A new classification of Type III open fractures. *J Trauma* 1984;24:742–746.
22. Hall BB, Fitzgerald RH, Rosenblatt JE. Anaerobic osteomyelitis. *J Bone Joint Surg* 1983;65A:30–35.
23. Helms CA, Jeffrey RB, Wing VW. Computed tomography and plain film appearance of bony sequestration: Significance and differential diagnosis. *Skel Radiol* 1987;16:117–120.
24. Kahn DS, Pritzka DP. The pathophysiology of bone infection. *Clin Orthop* 1973;96:12–19.
25. Kelly PJ. Osteomyelitis in the adult. *Orthop Clin North Am* 1975;6:983–987.
26. Kim EE, Pjura GA, Lowry PA, Goberty AH, Traina JF. Osteomyelitis complicating fractures: Pitfalls of 111-In leukocyte scintigraphy. *AJR* 1987;148:927–930.
27. Martin P. The appearance of bone scans following fractures including intermediate and long-term studies. *J Nucl Med* 1979;20:1227.
28. Mauer DJ, Merkow RL, Gustilo RB. Infection after intramedullary nailing of severe open tibial fractures initially treated with external fixation. *J Bone Joint Surg* 1989;71A:835–838.
29. May JW, Jupiter JB, Weiland AJ, Byrd HS. Clinical classification of post-traumatic tibial osteomyelitis. *J Bone Joint Surg* 1989;71A:1422–1428.
30. Merkel KD, Brown ML, Dewanjee MK, Fitzgerald RH. Comparison of Indium-labeled leukocyte imaging with sequential technetium-gallium scanning in diagnosis of low-grade musculoskeletal sepsis. *J Bone Joint Surg* 1985;67A:465–476.
31. Nguyen VD, London J, Cone O III. Ring sequestrum: Radiologic characteristics of skeletal fixation pin tract osteomyelitis. *Radiology* 1986;158:129–131.
32. Petty W, Spanier S, Shuster JJ, Silverthorne C. Influence of skeletal implants in incidence of infection. *J Bone Joint Surg* 1985;67A:1236–1244.
33. Quinn SF, Murry W, Clark RA, Cochran C. MR imaging of chronic osteomyelitis. *J Comp Assist Tomogr* 1988;12:113–117.
34. Resnick D, Niwayama G. *Diagnosis of bone and joint disorders,* vol. 3. Philadelphia: W.B. Saunders, 1988.
35. Seabold JE, Nepola JV, Conrad GR, et al. Detection of osteomyelitis at fracture non-union sites. Comparison of two scintigraphic methods. *AJR* 1989;152:1021–1027.
36. Tang JSH, Gold RH, Bassett LW, Seeger LL. Musculoskeletal infection in the extremities: Evaluation with MR imaging. *Radiology* 1988;166:205–209.
37. Tumeh SS, Aliabadi P, Weissman BN, McNeil BJ. Chronic osteomyelitis: Bone and gallium scan patterns associated with active disease. *Radiology* 1986;158:685–688.
38. Tumeh SS, Aliabadi P, Weissman BN, McNeil BJ. Disease activity in osteomyelitis. Role of radiography. *Radiology* 1987;165:781–784.
39. Varnell RM, Flint DW, Dalley RW, Maravilla KR, Cummings CW, Shuman WP. Myocutaneous flap failure: Early detection with Gd-DTPA-enhanced MR imaging. *Radiology* 1989;173:755–758.
40. Waldvogel FA, Medoff G, Schwartz MN. Osteomyelitis: A review of clinical features, therapeutic considerations, and unusual aspects. *N Engl J Med* 1970;282:198–206.
41. Wall SD, Fisher MR, Amparo EG, Hricak H, Higgins CB. Magnetic resonance imaging in the evaluation of abscesses. *AJR* 1985;144:1217–1221.
42. Whalen JL, Fitzgerald RH, Morrissy RT. A histological study of acute hematogenous osteomyelitis following physeal injury in rabbits. *J Bone Joint Surg* 1988;70A:1383–1392.
43. Wing VW, Jeffrey RB, Federle MP, Helms CA, Trafton P. Chronic osteomyelitis examined by CT. *Radiology* 1985;154:171–174.

*Imaging of Orthopedic Trauma,
Second Edition,* edited by T.H. Berquist,
Mayo Clinic © 1992. Published
by Raven Press, Ltd., New York.

CHAPTER 16

Stress Fractures

Thomas H. Berquist, Kay L. Cooper, and Douglas J. Pritchard

Radiographic Evaluation, 881
Distribution of Stress Fractures, 883
  Foot, 883
  Tibia, 886
  Fibula, 889
  Femoral Shaft, 889

Femoral Neck, 889
Pelvis, 890
Other Locations, 891
Summary, 893
References, 893

The term *stress fracture* has been applied to a variety of fractures that result from repetitive stress of a lesser magnitude than that required for an acute traumatic fracture. Daffner (13) states that a stress fracture results from muscular activity on bones rather than from direct trauma. Most stress fractures are fatigue fractures resulting from abnormal muscular tension on normal bone (13,18). These usually occur in the lower extremity in association with significant changes in physical activity. Fatigue fractures are commonly reported in military personnel (27,28,47). Insufficiency fractures occur when normal stress or muscle tension acts on bone with abnormal elastic resistance (9–13,16,18,54).

In the civilian population, the patient frequently gives a history of starting a new activity, such as track or jogging. Usually several weeks after starting the activity the patient notes local pain. Symptoms are usually relieved by rest. If the activity is continued, the pain generally increases (18). Table 16-1 lists the locations and related activity of common stress fractures.

Physical examination may reveal local tenderness or swelling over the fracture (4,18). Children may have slight temperature elevation (18). Clinically, most stress fractures arise distal to the knee. The importance of this finding lies mainly in the difficulty it presents for differentiating stress fractures from other entities. For example, stress fractures of the proximal tibia may result in

   T. H. Berquist: Department of Diagnostic Radiology, Mayo Medical School, Mayo Clinic Jacksonville, Jacksonville, Florida 32224.
   K. L. Cooper, D. J. Pritchard: Departments of Diagnostic Radiology and Orthopedic Surgery, Mayo Medical School, Mayo Clinic, Rochester, Minnesota 55905.

periosteal new bone formation, leading the physician to suspect a primary bone tumor. Similarly, if the metatarsal is involved, there may be exuberant periosteal reaction that suggests either osteomyelitis or tumor. In either case, the history of repetitive stress is helpful in suggesting the diagnosis. Table 16-2 lists clinical conditions that may simulate stress fractures (11,18,35).

RADIOGRAPHIC EVALUATION

There are multiple imaging techniques available for evaluating musculoskeletal conditions. Unfortunately, detection of stress fractures may be difficult in the early stages except with isotope studies (13,27). Recently, magnetic resonance imaging (MRI) has also demonstrated its sensitivity and specificity for early diagnosis of stress fractures (3). Early diagnosis is especially important with stress fractures of the femoral neck; displacement of these fractures can occur, resulting in a significant increase in morbidity (4).

Routine radiographs are almost always normal initially. Blickenstaff and Morris (4) described the phases of stress fractures. During the first 5–14 days osteoclastic resorption leads to local osteoporosis. This is followed by periosteal or endosteal callus. Swelling and increased vascularity accompany these changes. Continued activity results in fracture. The fracture defect may be primarily cortical or trabecular. Greaney and colleagues (27) reported isotope findings in 250 military personnel. Twenty-three percent of the fractures were considered cortical and 77% cancellous. Routine radiographs were positive in only 40% of cortical and 26% of trabecular

TABLE 16-1. *Common stress fractures*[a]

Location	Etiology	Reference
Foot		
Metatarsals	Marching	25,27,28,47
	Running	13,27
	Ballet	19,55
	Prior surgery	13,24
Calcaneus	Jumping	32
	Marching	
	Running	27,47,60
	Recent immobilization	57
Tarsals	Long distance runners	13,19,45
	Marching	13,19,45
Sesamoids	Standing, cycling, skiing	18,25
Tibia		
Proximal	Running	18,44
Mid	Ballet	6,14,19,20,21,43,55
Distal	Running	5,27,44,55,60
Fibula	Running	3,22,27,45
	Jumping (parachute)	28
Patella	Hurdling	13,19,21,27
Femur		
Shaft	Running (long distance)	13,29,37,44,48
Neck	Running (long distance)	4,13,17,44
	Ballet	19,60
Pelvis (Pubic arch)	Running	43,44
	Stooping	13,28
	Bowling	5
	Gymnastics	19
Spine		
Vertebral arch (lumbar)	Lifting	13,19
	Ballet	13
Spinous arch (C, T)	Clay shovelers	28
Ribs		
1st	Back packs	5,13,28
Lower	Golf, cough	13,50,60
Clavicle	Radial neck surgery, tic	13,28
Coracoid (scapula)	Trap shooting	53
Humerus	Baseball	5
Ulna	Baseball, pitchfork, wheelchair patients	13,28
Hook of hamate	Golf, tennis, baseball	5,13,56
Metacarpals	Weight lifting, gymnastics	44

[a] After (13) with permission.

stress fractures. Cortical fractures may present with endosteal or periosteal callus, with or without a lucent cortical defect (4,7). Tomography is often necessary to define a fracture line. Stress fractures in cancellous bone may appear as a hazy area of increased density or a sclerotic line due to trabecular compression (4).

Metabolic activity around stress fractures may allow isotope detection as early as 24 hours following the in-

TABLE 16-2. *Clinical conditions*

Simulating stress fractures
Neoplasm
Infection
Tendinitis
Ligament injury
Gout
Pseudogout
Vascular occlusive disease (claudication)

jury (27). The bone changes must progress to cause a 30–50% change in the bone density before radiographs will be positive. This usually takes 10–21 days.

Classification of stress fractures may be useful in certain cases. Wilson and Katz (60) categorized fractures according to their radiographic appearance. Type I fractures present with a lucent line with no associated periosteal reaction; Type II fractures reveal cancellous sclerosis and endosteal callus; Type III fractures have external callus; and Type IV fractures present with a mixture of Types I through III.

Devas (18) divided stress fractures into compression and distraction categories. Compression fractures are equivalent to torus fractures. These most commonly occur in children and elderly patients and are most often located in the femoral neck and tibia. Distraction fractures are similar to greenstick fractures and may be transverse, oblique, or longitudinal. The transverse frac-

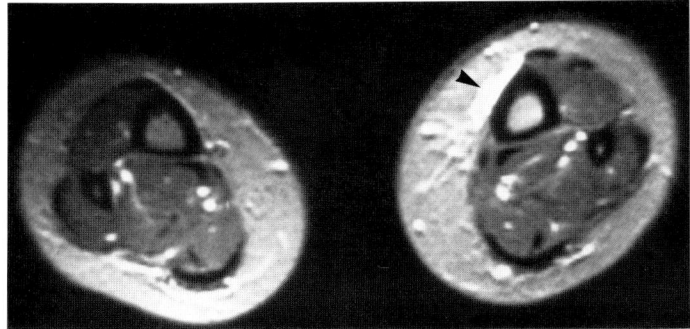

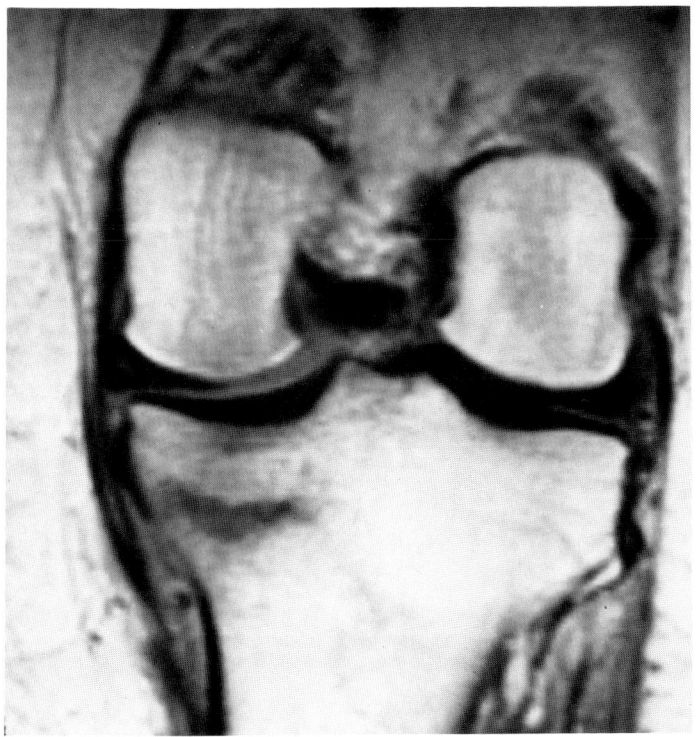

FIG. 16-1. Two patients (**A, B**) with tibial pain referred to rule out stress fracture. **A:** Axial SE 2000/60 image shows increased signal adjacent to the tibial cortex (*arrow*) due to periosteal and juxta periosteal inflammation. No fracture. **B:** Coronal MR image demonstrating an obvious upper tibial stress fracture.

tures are most significant in that complete fracture and displacement may occur.

Unfortunately, stress fractures differ in their appearance depending upon location. Therefore, early diagnosis and appearance are important mainly in determining which fractures are likely to displace (13,48).

Attempts at earlier radiographic diagnosis of stress fractures with the use of magnification techniques, xeroradiography, and tomography have been useful in certain cases (27,45,59). Computed tomography (CT) is useful for detection of longitudinal long bone stress fractures and insufficiency fractures in the pelvis (1,9–12,16). MRI is useful for early detection of stress fractures and differentiating stress fractures from other causes of bone pain. In the acute phase, reactive marrow changes lead to decreased signal on T1- and increased signal on T2-weighted sequences. Increased signal intensity is also evident using short T1 inversion recovery (STIR) and gradient-echo (T2*) sequences (3). The actual fracture line may also be evident, which provides the most specific diagnostic information. (Fig. 16-1).

Despite new imaging techniques, isotope studies using Tc-99m remain most useful in early detection of stress fractures (27). Greaney and colleagues (27) noted normal radiographs in 50% of their patients with stress fractures even during follow-up. Radiographic techniques, including CT and MRI, are still extremely important in determining the nature of isotope abnormalities. Differential diagnostic challenges may occur with osteogenic sarcoma, chronic osteomyelitis, and osteoid osteoma (13,21,35). Problems in diagnosis and treatment of stress fractures vary depending on the location and type of fracture.

DISTRIBUTION OF STRESS FRACTURES

Foot

Military recruits have provided a large, controlled population for the study of stress fractures. Wilson and Katz (60) studied 250 patients, and Greaney and colleagues

TABLE 16-3. *Distribution of stress fractures in three series (%)*

Location	Orava et al.[a] (142 patients)	Wilson & Katz[b] (250 patients)	Greaney et al.[c] (250 patients)
Foot			
Metatarsal	18.3	35.2	15
Calcaneus	—	28	23
Talus	—	—	7
Navicular	0.7	—	4
Tibia	53	24	39
Fibula	14.7	3.2	0
Femur	6.3	3.2	9
Pubic arch	1.4	0.4	—
Spine	0.7	1	—
Ribs	—	5.6	—
Ulna	0.7		3 (Patella, cuboid, and cuneiform)
Humerus	1.4		
Metacarpals	1.4		

[a] (44)
[b] (60)
[c] (27)

(27) examined 250 Marine recruits. Orava and colleagues (44) revealed stress fractures in 142 athletes and sportsmen. Although the statistics vary somewhat, most authors agree that stress fractures in the foot most commonly involve the metatarsals (51) (Table 16-3). "March" fractures are common in military recruits. Stress with marching is applied maximally to the second and third metatarsals (Fig. 16-2). Less commonly the fourth metatarsal is involved (18,51). Initial radiographs are usually normal. Follow-up films in 10–14 days often demonstrate a small lucent cortical defect or early periosteal change. Metatarsal stress fractures most commonly involve the mid- or distal shaft of the metatarsals (Fig. 16-3).

Metatarsal stress fractures are not uncommon in civilians (18,44). These are usually the result of a change in the patient's footwear, walking, or running habits. For example, a patient who is relatively sedentary may assume a job that requires increased standing or walking. Pain with weight bearing (24) may begin in the first few weeks after the change in activity. This pain is usually reproducible each time the activity is resumed. The pain is usually well localized. There is also an increased incidence of metatarsal stress fracture following bunionectomy (24).

Treatment of metatarsal stress fractures requires restriction of weight bearing. These fractures essentially never displace and are of little consequence once the diagnosis is established.

Wilson and Katz (60) noted calcaneal stress fractures nearly as frequently as metatarsal fractures. Calcaneal stress fractures were most common in the Greaney series (27). Associated stress fractures of the upper tibia medially were noted in 60% of military recruits (27). This has been partially attributed to running and marching in combat boots (25).

Calcaneal stress fractures occur less frequently in civilians, but again there seems to be an association between these fractures and footwear that increases heel stress. When asked to describe their pain, patients normally point to the medial and lateral sides of the heel rather than the plantar surface. Physical examination often reveals pain when the heel is squeezed.

Radiographically, a hazy or speckled appearance may be noted first. This usually progresses to a sclerotic band if stress continues (Fig. 16-4) (27,60). These findings may be more obvious using magnification technique. Trabecular stress fractures rarely produce periosteal

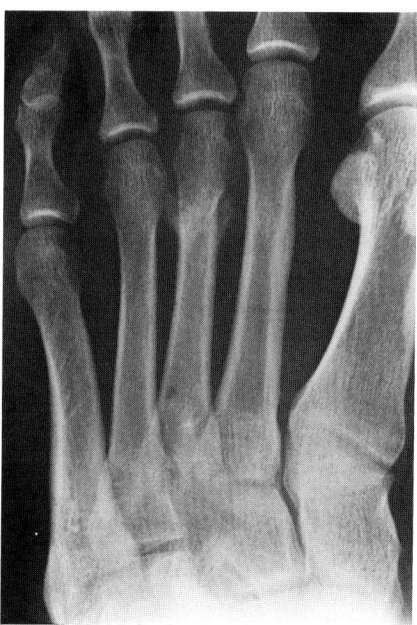

FIG. 16-2. AP radiograph of the foot demonstrating a typical healing stress fracture of the third metatarsal neck.

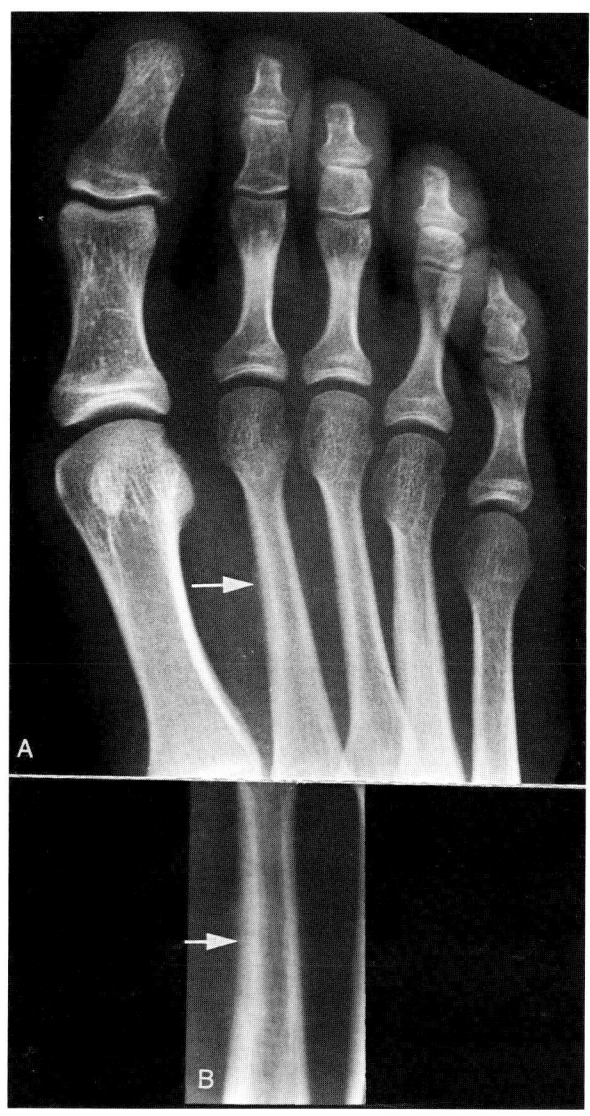

FIG. 16–3. AP radiograph of the foot (**A**) and localized view (**B**) demonstrating a subtle midshaft stress fracture (*arrow*) of the second metatarsal.

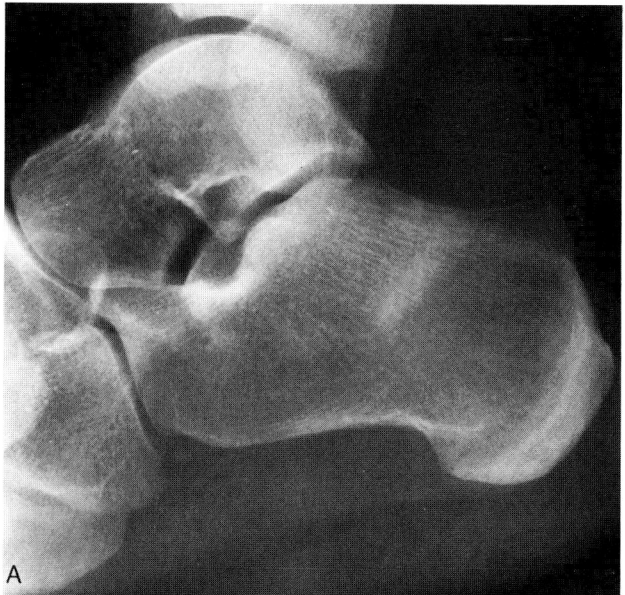
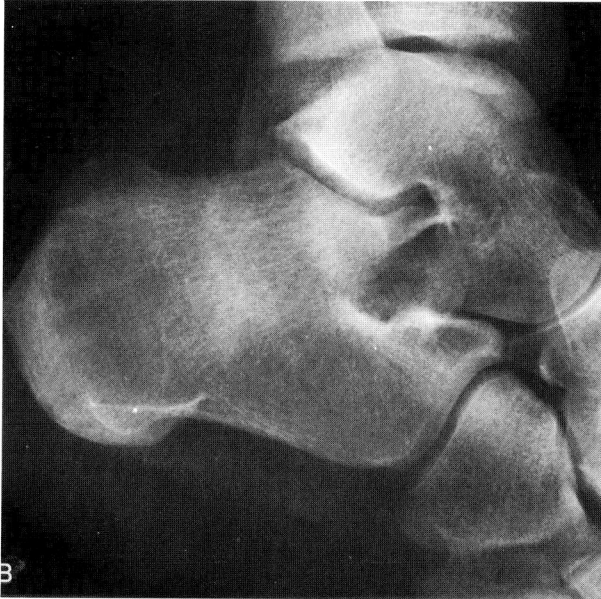

FIG. 16–4. Lateral (**A**) and oblique views (**B**) of the calcaneus demonstrate a band of sclerosis due to a stress fracture.

changes. Isotope scans will demonstrate a linear area of increased uptake. They may be positive within 24 hours and are almost invariably positive in 72 hours (27,40).

Treatment of calcaneal stress fractures is accomplished with a plastic heel cup and 4-inch foam rubber heel pad.

Stress fractures involve the tarsal navicular, talus, phalanges, and sesamoids less frequently (Tables 16-1 and 16-3) (44,45,59). Tarsonavicular stress fractures, common in runners, are particularly difficult to diagnose (26,45). Pavlov and colleagues (45) accomplished diagnosis of tarsonavicular fractures with isotope scans and tomography. Isotope studies (Tc-99m), especially with the plantar view, were useful in localizing the abnormality, while tomograms were useful in defining the fracture. Tomograms were performed in the dorsiplantar projection with slight dorsiflexion. This allows a more tangential examination of the navicular.

Most navicular fractures are sagittal and involve the mid- and medial third of the navicular (45,59). In a series reported by Torg and colleagues (59), treatment of navicular fractures was successful with non-weight bearing. However, simple restriction of activity led to non-union in 7 of 9 patients.

Tibia

Tibial stress fractures are common in both military and civilian populations (1,27,43,44,59,62). The inci-

dence of tibial stress fractures in the series reported by Greaney was 73% (27). Cortical involvement is much more common in the tibia. Tibial and calcaneal stress fractures have also been reported in patients with healing acute fractures (62).

Stress fractures may arise anywhere along the length of the tibia. Classically they occur on the posteromedial aspect of the proximal tibia at the junction of the metaphysis and diaphysis (Fig. 16-5). However, variations are not uncommon (Fig. 16-6). Ballet dancers often develop stress fractures in the midtibia (7,14,21,43). Following total knee replacement, fractures occur in the medial tibial plateau. These fractures are most often associated with malalignment and improper orientation of the component (Fig. 16-7) (49).

Almost any form of strenuous activity may precede stress fractures of the tibia; hence tennis, racquetball, and any form of running may be responsible. In the past, when the athlete first started training for a sport, leg pain was called "shin splints". It was recognized that this condition would not improve unless the activity was halted. Probably at least some of these cases were early stress fractures (see Fig. 16-1A). Isotope studies will be positive soon after symptoms begin if a stress fracture is present (27,40,46). Radiographs may remain negative for 2–3 weeks (27). The earliest findings may be subtle periosteal reaction. Tomograms often demonstrate the fracture line and assist in differentiating a stress fracture from a primary bone tumor. The latter condition may be

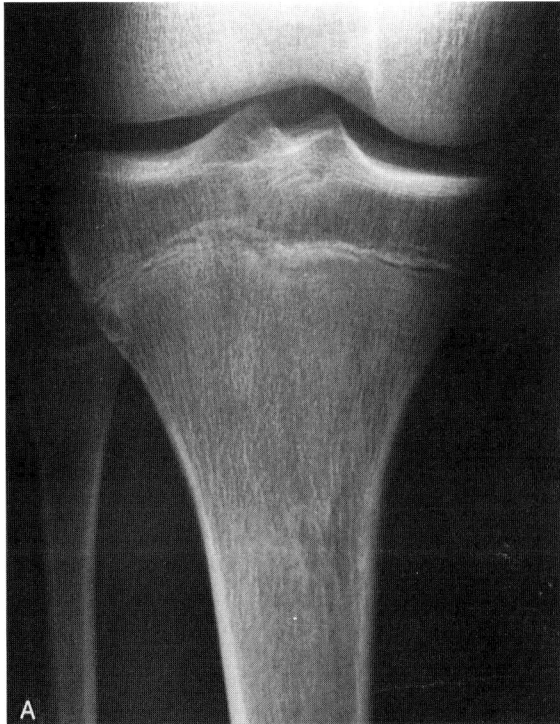
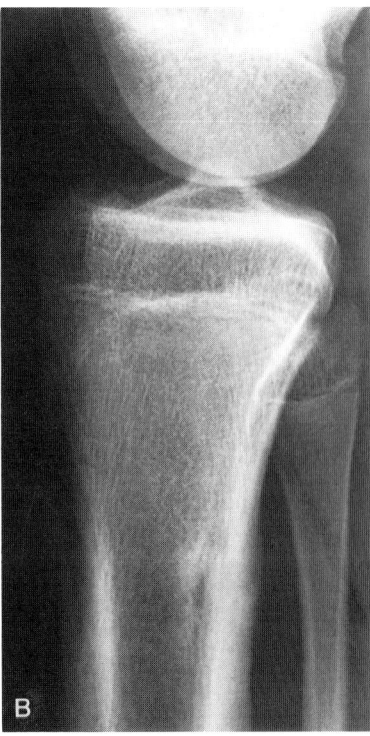

FIG. 16–5. AP **(A)** and lateral **(B)** views of the proximal tibia demonstrating atypical stress fracture at the posteromedial junction of the metaphysis and diaphysis. There is early periosteal reaction.

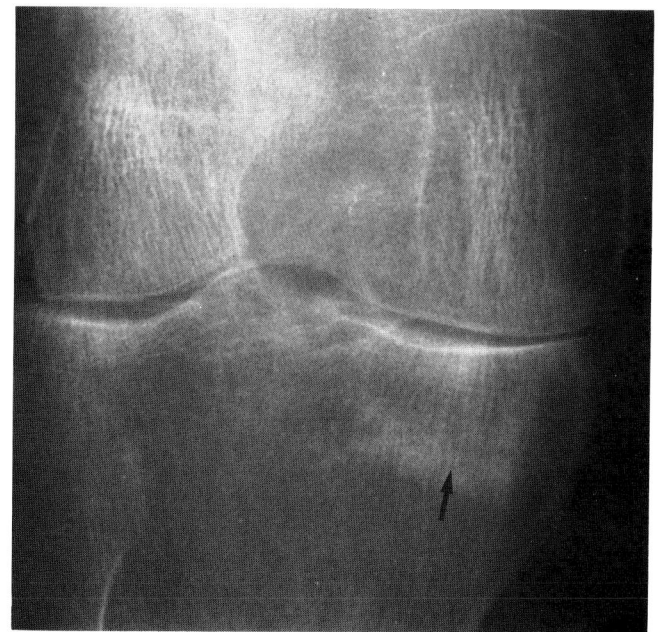

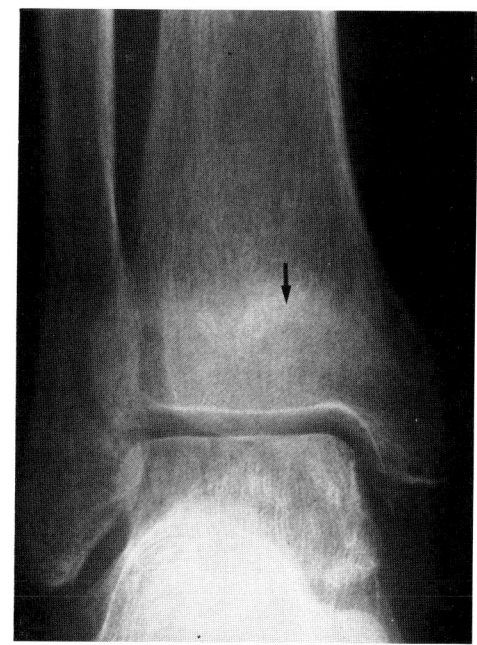

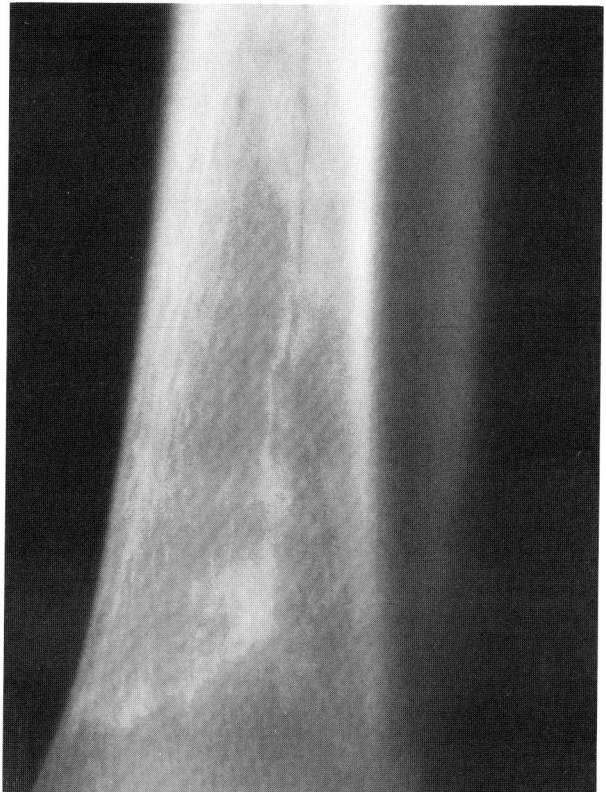

FIG. 16–6. A: AP view of the knee with trabecular condensation in the medial plateau due to a stress fracture. B: AP view of the ankle demonstrating a transverse metaphyseal stress fracture. C: Tomogram demonstrating a longitudinal stress fracture in the distal tibia.

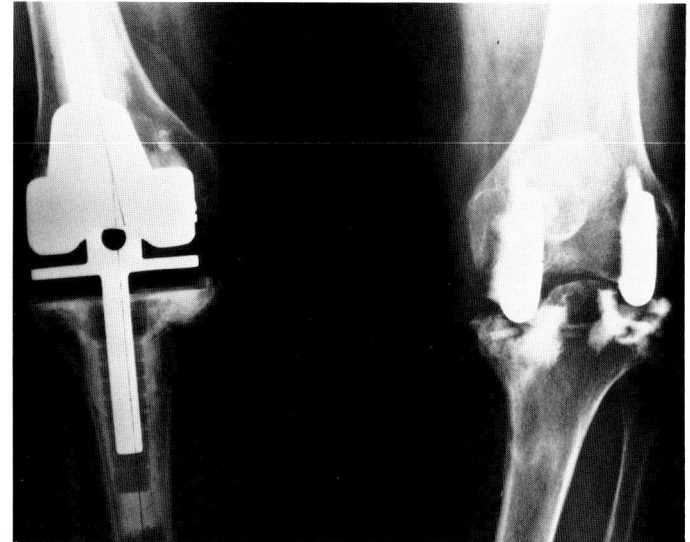
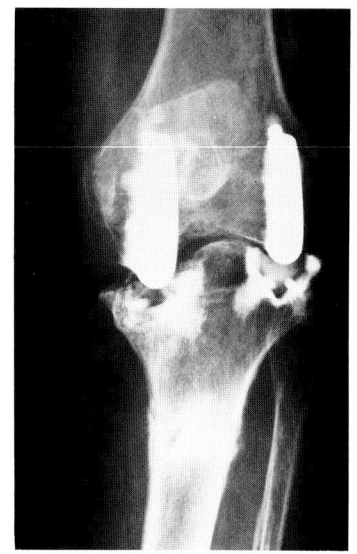
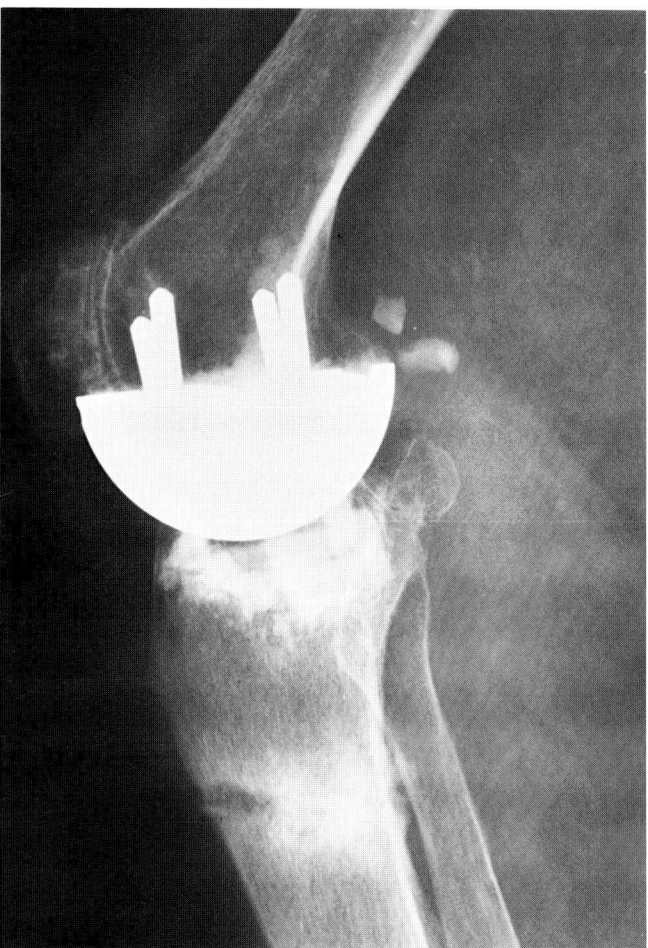

FIG. 16–7. Bilateral total knee arthroplasty. Pain left knee. Initial views (**A**) demonstrate sclerosis in the tibial plateau and periosteal changes in the medial tibia medially. There is also trabecular sclerosis. Six months later there is an obvious stress fracture in the upper tibia seen on the AP (**B**) and lateral (**C**) views.

difficult to differentiate from a stress fracture if there is no clear-cut history of change in physical activity (Fig. 16-8).

Usually the pain present with stress fractures is sufficient to cause patients to restrict their activities voluntarily. This may be the only treatment necessary. How-

ever, persistent pain with simple weight bearing may indicate the need for more aggressive therapy, such as crutches or even a long-leg cylinder cast. Radiographic changes may be helpful in making this decision concerning therapy. Hallel and colleagues (29) described tibial fractures as Grade I if periosteal reaction involved one

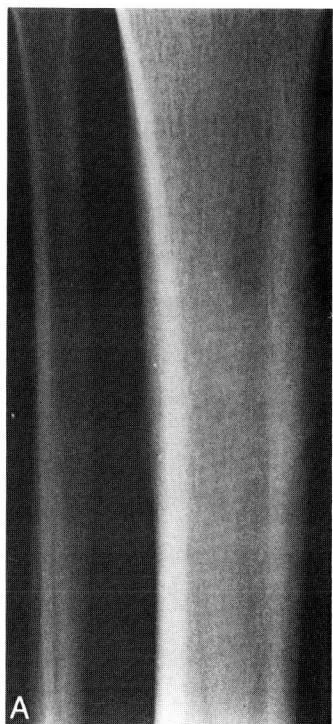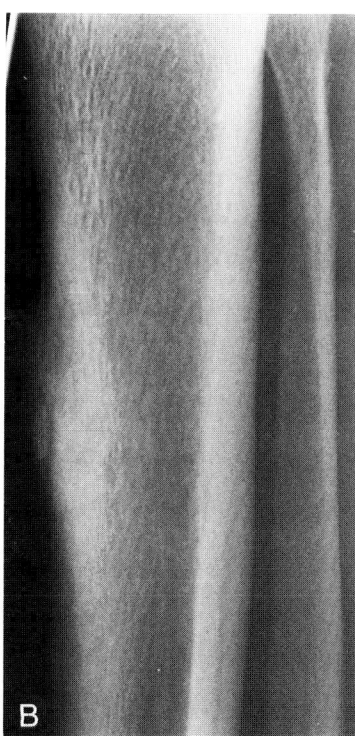

FIG. 16-8. AP (**A**) and lateral (**B**) views of the mid tibia. Osteosarcoma mimicking a stress fracture.

cortex, as Grade II if changes were circumferential, and as Grade III if the fracture was displaced. Tibial stress fractures rarely displace. However, Grade II fractures may require more aggressive therapy than the less extensive Grade I fracture.

Fibula

Stress fractures involve the fibula less frequently than the tibia. Orava (44) reported an incidence of 14.1% in 142 athletes with stress fractures. The fibula is a non-weight-bearing bone. Therefore, the fractures are due to muscle stress (18,60). This stress is most commonly applied with calf muscle contraction during running (18). Fibular fractures can usually be treated with reduction of the associated activity, since there are no weight-bearing stresses.

Femoral Shaft

Stress fractures of the femoral shaft are not common. Orava (44) reported an incidence of 2.8% in civilians. These fractures are more frequent in long-distance runners and occasionally in ballet dancers (8,36,37,55). Highly motivated, well-conditioned athletes tend to be at risk for this type of fracture (29,37). Luchini (37) reported femoral shaft fractures in long-distance runners who were totally asymptomatic prior to the fracture.

This was attributed to muscle fatigue that resulted in transfer of stress to the femoral shaft. Early recognition of this fracture is important, as displacement tends to occur (Fig. 16-9). Treatment of femoral shaft fractures may require open reduction and internal fixation if such displacement occurs.

Femoral Neck

Stress fractures of the femoral neck are more common than diaphyseal stress fractures (44). Detection may be difficult clinically (Fig. 16-10). The patient's pain will frequently be referred to the knee, and point tenderness may be difficult to elicit (18,48). Early diagnosis and treatment are essential, for progression of this type of fracture may lead to eventual displacement (4,18,29). Classification of femoral neck fractures is useful in determining which fractures tend to displace (4,18,42). Devas (19,20) classified fractures as transverse or compressive. Compression fractures occur at the base of the femoral neck medially (calcar). They often present with localized osteoporosis that progresses to periosteal callus formation. This type usually occurs in younger patients (42). Osteoid osteoma should be considered in this location as well. History and tomography are useful in differentiating these two conditions. Compression stress fractures usually do not displace and can be treated with non-weight bearing (42). Transverse fractures occur in older patients. Initially a defect in the superior cortex of the

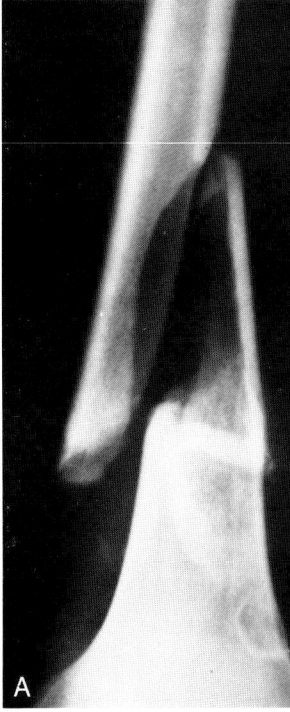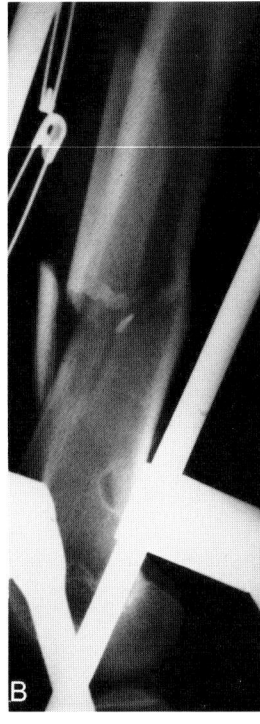

FIG. 16-9. AP (**A**) and lateral views (**B**) demonstrate a displaced comminuted stress fracture.

neck will be seen. This defect frequently progresses to a complete fracture and displacement. Devas noted displacement in 11 of 18 transverse fractures (Fig. 16-11) (11,12).

Blickenstaff and Morris (4) classified femoral neck fractures according to radiographic appearance. A Type I fracture demonstrated callus only. Type II fractures demonstrated a fine calcar fracture with or without extension across the femoral neck. Type III fractures were displaced. Blickenstaff and Morris noted that once a fracture line was visible, internal fixation was indicated. Patients with Type I fractures were treated conserva-

tively, requiring about 9.5 weeks of hospitalization. Displaced fractures healed without complication only 20% of the time. The average hospital stay in Type III fractures was 59 weeks. Complications included malunion, non-union, and vascular necrosis.

Pelvis

Stress fractures in the pelvis most frequently involve the pubic arch (5,13,18). They may be related to running, gymnastics, and bowling (Fig. 16-12) (4,8,11).

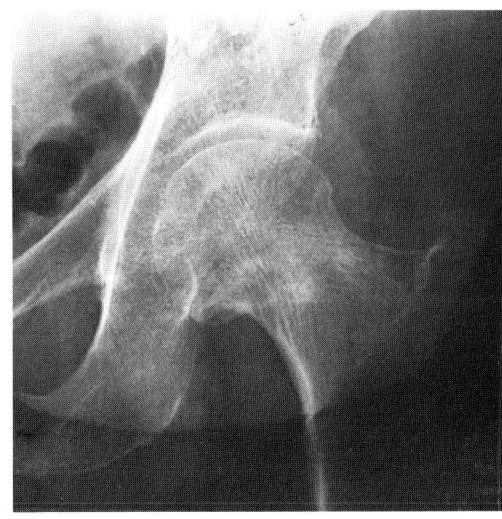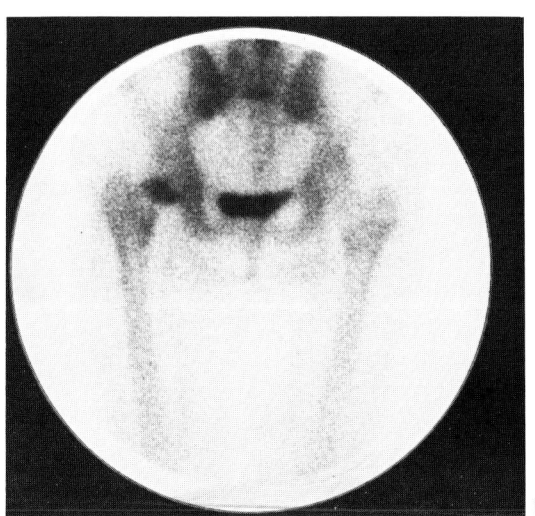

FIG. 16-10. A: AP view of the hip demonstrates sclerotic zones in the trabeculae of the neck. **B:** ^{99m}Tc scan clearly demonstrates the stress fracture.

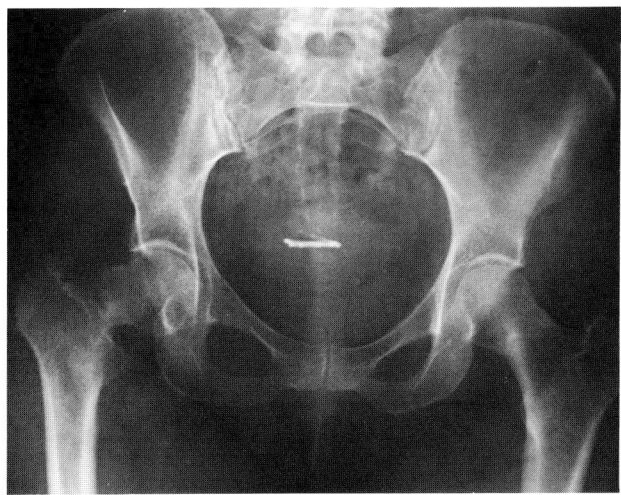

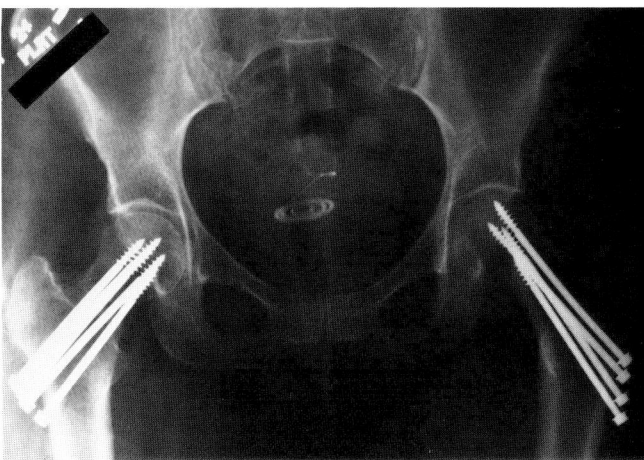

A

B

FIG. 16-11. **A:** AP view of the pelvis with bilateral femoral neck stress fractures. The fracture on the left is subtle. The fracture on the right is complete with varus displacement. **B:** Both fractures were treated with pin fixation.

Insufficiency fractures in this region are also common (38,41,54). These fractures are particularly common in elderly postmenopausal females, patients with rheumatoid arthritis, and in patients being treated with radiation or systemic steroids (9–12,16). Fractures are common along the pubic symphysis and more laterally in the pubic rami (9,11), in the sacrum, and supra-acetabular regions (10–12). Typically, radiographs (Fig. 16-13) demonstrate sclerotic zones or areas of condensation in the above areas. Multiple fractures are common. Radionuclide studies demonstrate the typical *H* pattern for sacral insufficiency fractures (11). Computed tomography is definitive, especially in patients with suspected pathologic fractures due to metastasis (10–12).

Pubic arch stress fractures tend to occur in older individuals. Patients frequently noticed pain in the groin or hip with weight bearing. Treatment consists of activity restriction or partial weight bearing with crutches.

Other Locations

Stress fractures in the spine and upper extremities are uncommon compared with the lower extremities (Table 16-1 and 16-3) (31,33,50,53,56). Stress fractures may occur in the spinous processes of clay shovelers and in the lumbar pars in patients who repeatedly lift heavy weights (13,18,27,54,60). Evaluation of the pars may be accomplished with isotope studies followed by localized (1–3-mm thick) tomograms. On occasion, CT scanning may be used to evaluate the posterior elements (Fig. 16-14). This technique is especially helpful in excluding other bone and soft tissue abnormalities. Magnetic resonance imaging may provide even better sensitivity in soft tissue abnormalities (3).

Upper-extremity stress fractures have been described in baseball players, golfers, and trap shooters (Table 16-1) (5,13). Stress fractures of the ribs due to chronic cough

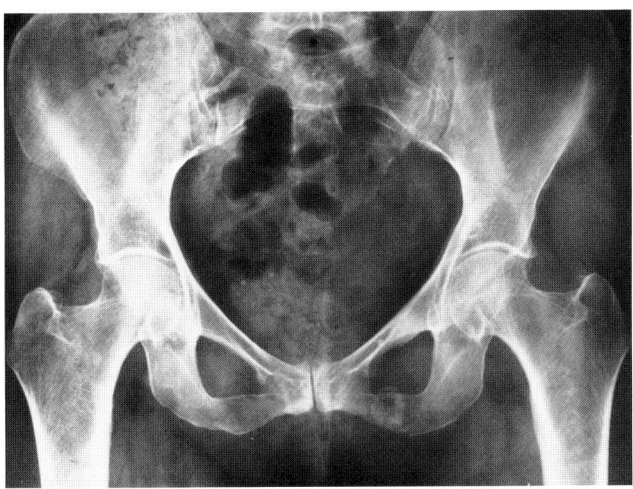

FIG. 16-12. AP view of the pelvis demonstrating healing stress fractures of both pubic rami on the left.

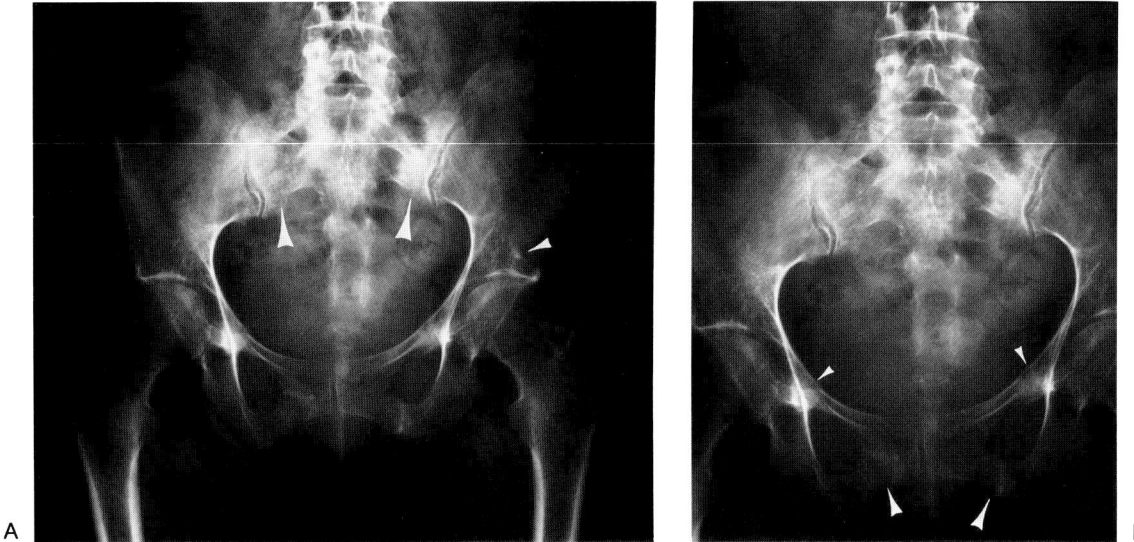

FIG. 16-13. AP view (**A**) and coned down views (**B**) of the pelvis demonstrating sacral, acetabular, and pubic insufficiency fractures (*arrows*).

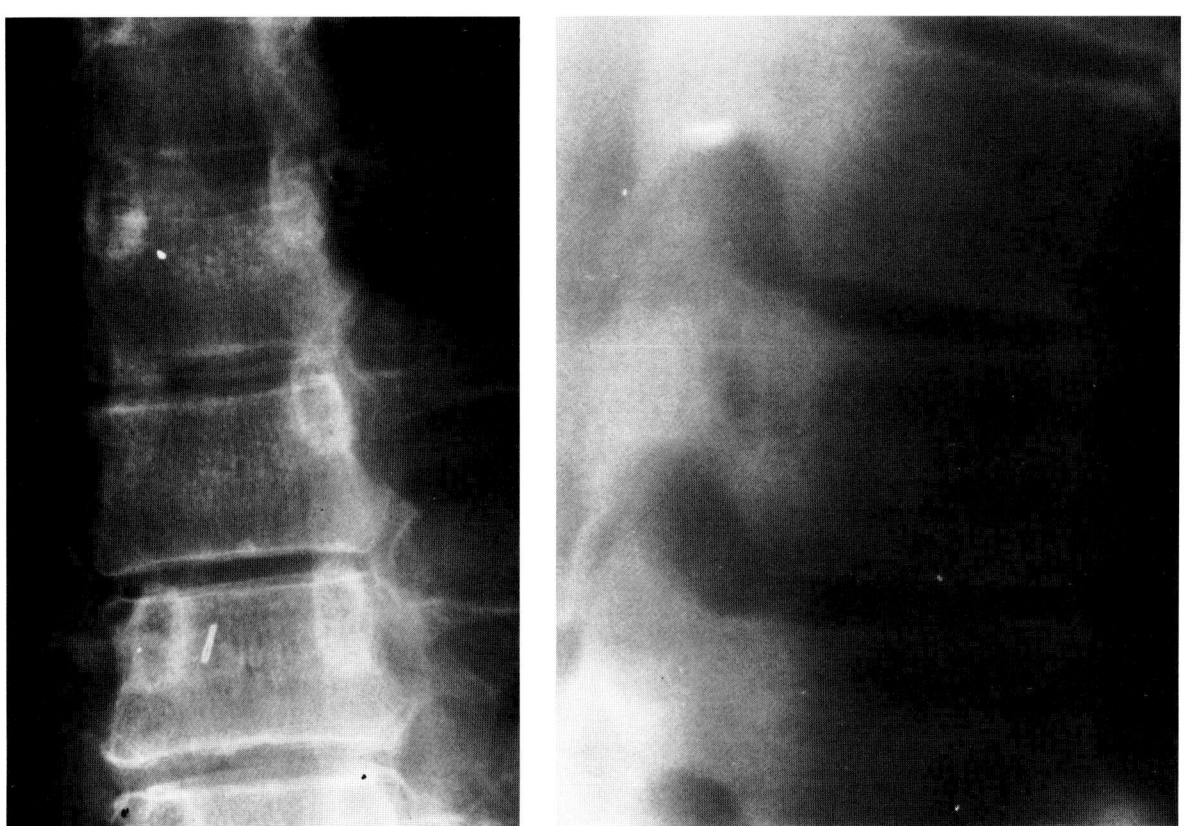

FIG. 16-14. Pedicle stress fracture in the thoracic spine following laminectomy. **A:** AP view of the spine demonstrating sclerosis of the pedicle. Lateral tomogram (**B**) and CT scan (**C**) demonstrate the changes to better advantage.

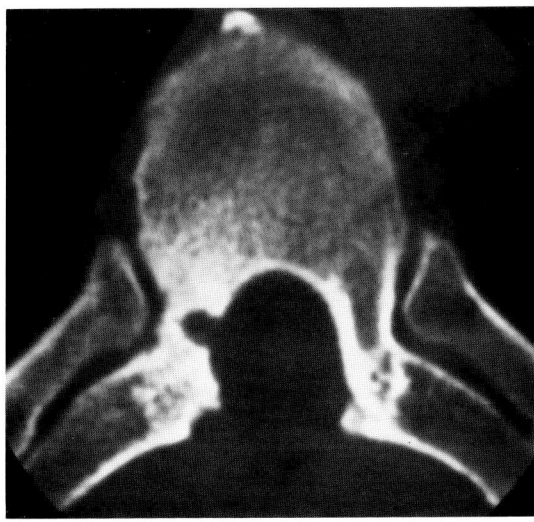

C

FIG. 16–14. (*Continued.*)

and to golfing have also been described. Fractures of the first ribs can develop after prolonged use of heavy back packs (5,13).

SUMMARY

The diagnosis of a stress fracture should be considered in patients presenting with pain after a change in activity, especially if the activity is strenuous and the pain is in the lower extremities. Since evidence of the stress fracture may not be apparent for weeks on routine radiographs, proper use of other imaging techniques will allow an earlier diagnosis (Fig. 16-15). Prompt diagnosis is especially important in the femur, where displacement may occur.

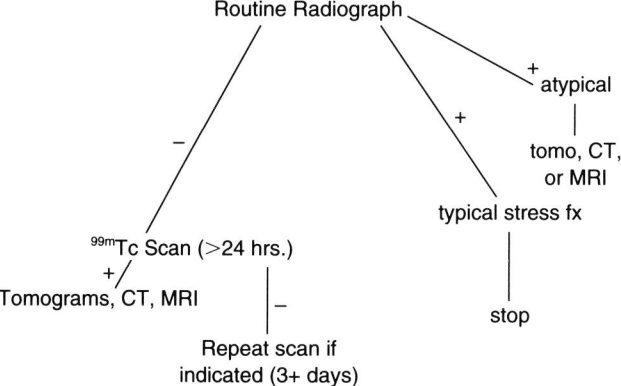

FIG. 16–15. Algorithm for imaging in patients with suspected stress fracture.

REFERENCES

1. Allen JG. Longitudinal stress fractures of the tibia: Diagnosis with CT. *Radiology* 1988;167:799–801.
2. Bargren JH, Tilson DH Jr, Bridgefort OE. Prevention of displaced fatigue fractures of the femur. *J Bone Joint Surg* 1971;53A:1115–1117.
3. Berquist TH. *MRI of the musculoskeletal system.* New York: Raven Press, 1990.
4. Blickenstaff LD, Morris JM. Fatigue fracture of the femoral neck. *J Bone Joint Surg* 1966;48A:61031–1047.
5. Bowerman JW. *Radiology and injury in sport.* New York: Appleton-Century-Crofts, 1977.
6. Burrows HJ. Fatigue fractures of the fibula. *J Bone Joint Surg* 1948;30B:266–279.
7. Burrows HJ. Fatigue infarction of the middle of the tibia in ballet dancers. *J Bone Joint Surg* 1956;38B:83–94.
8. Butler JE, Brown SL, McConnel BG. Subtrochanteric stress fractures in runners. *Am J Sports Med* 1982;10:228–232.
9. Casey D, Mirra J, Staple TW. Parasymphyseal insufficiency fractures of the os pubis. *AJR* 1984;142:581–586.
10. Cooper KL, Beabout JW, McLeod RA. Supraacetabular insufficiency fractures. *Radiology* 1985;157:15–17.
11. Cooper KL, Beabout JW, Swee RG. Insufficiency fractures of the sacrum. *Radiology* 1985;156:15–20.
12. Cooper KL. Insufficiency fractures of the sternum: A consequence of thoracic kyphosis. *Radiology* 1988;167:471–472.
13. Daffner RH. Stress fractures. *Skeletal Radiol* 1978;2:221–229.
14. Daffner RH. Anterior tibial striations. *AJR* 1984;143:651–653.
15. Darby RE. Stress fractures of the os calcis. *JAMA* 1967;200:1183–1184.
16. Desmet AA, Neff JR. Pubic and sacral insufficiency fractures: Clinical course and radiologic findings. *AJR* 1985;145:601–606.
17. Devas MB. Longitudinal stress fractures. *J Bone Joint Surg* 1960;42B:508–514.
18. Devas MB. *Stress fractures.* Edinburgh: Churchill Livingstone, 1975.
19. Devas MB. Stress fractures of the femoral neck. *J Bone Joint Surg* 1965;47B:728–738.
20. Devas MB. Stress fractures of the patella. *J Bone Joint Surg* 1960;42B:71–74.
21. Devas MB. Stress fractures in children. *J Bone Joint Surg* 1963;45B:528–541.
22. Devas MB, Sweetnan R. Stress fractures of the fibula. *J Bone Joint Surg* 1956;38B:818–829.

23. Farquharson-Roberts MA, Fulford PC. Stress fractures of the radius. *J Bone Joint Surg* 1980;62B:194–195.
24. Ford LT, Gilula LA. Stress fractures of the middle metatarsals following the Keller operation. *J Bone Joint Surg* 1977;59A:117–118.
25. Gilbert RS, Johnson HA. Stress fractures in military recruits—a review of twelve years' experience. *Milit Med* 1966;131:716–721.
26. Goergen TG, Venn-Watson EA, Rossman DJ, Resnick D, Gerler KH. Tarsal navicular stress fractures in runners. *AJR* 1981;136:201–203.
27. Greaney RB, Gerber FH, Laughlan RL. Distribution and natural history of stress fractures in US Marine recruits. *Radiology* 1983;146:339–346.
28. Grusd R. Pseudofractures and stress fractures. *Semin Roentgenol* 1978;13:81–82.
29. Hallel T, Amit S, Segal D. Fatigue fractures of the tibial and femoral shaft in soldiers. *Clin Orthop* 1976;118:35–43.
30. Hartley JB. "Stress" or "fatigue" fractures of bone. *Br J Radiol* 1943;16:255–262.
31. Kitchin ID. Fatigue fracture of the ulna. *J Bone Joint Surg* 1948;30B:622–623.
32. Kroening PM, Shelton ML. Stress fractures. *AJR* 1963;89:1281–1286.
33. Laferty JF, Winter WG, Ganilaro SA. Fatigue characteristics of posterior elements of vertebra. *J Bone Joint Surg* 1977;59A:154–158.
34. Lesniewski PJ, Testa NN. Stress fractures of the hip as a complication of total knee replacement. *J Bone Joint Surg* 1982;64A:304–306.
35. Levin DC, Blazena ME, Levina E. Fatigue fractures of the shaft of the femur: Simulation of malignant tumor. *Radiology* 1967;89:883–885.
36. Lombardo SJ, Benson DW. Stress fractures of the femur in runners. *Am J Sports Med* 1982;10:219–227.
37. Luchini MA, Sarokhan AJ, Micheli LJ. Acute displaced femoral-shaft fractures in long distance runners. *J Bone Joint Surg* 1983;65A:689–691.
38. Marmor L. Stress fracture of the pubic ramus simulating a loose total hip replacement. *Clin Orthop* 1976;121:103–104.
39. Martin LM, Bourne RB, and Rorabeck CH. Stress fractures associated with osteoarthritis of the knee. *J Bone Joint Surg* 1988;70A:77–1774.
40. Matin P. The appearance of bone scans following fractures, including immediate and long-term studies. *J Nucl Med* 1979;20:1227–1231.
41. McElwaine JP, Sheehan JA. Spontaneous fractures of the femoral neck after total replacement of the knee. *J Bone Joint Surg* 1982;64B:323–325.
42. Miller F, Wenger DR. Femoral neck stress fracture in a hyperactive child. *J Bone Joint Surg* 1979;61A:435–437.
43. Mussbaum AR, Treves ST, Micheli L. Bone stress lesions in ballet dancers: Scintigraphic assessment. *AJR* 1988;150:851–855.
44. Orava S, Puranen J, Ala-Ketola L. Stress fractures caused by physical exercise. *Acta Orthop Scand* 1978;49:19–27.
45. Pavlov H, Tord JS, Freiberger RH. Tarsal navicular stress fractures: Radiographic evaluation. *Radiology* 1983;148:641–645.
46. Prather JL, Nusynowitz ML, Snowdy HA, Hughes AD, McCortney WH, Bragg RJ. Scintigraphic findings in stress fractures. *J Bone Joint Surg* 1977;59A:869–874.
47. Protzman RR, Griffis CG. Stress fractures in men and women undergoing military training. *J Bone Joint Surg* 1977;59A:825.
48. Provost RA, Morris JM. Fatigue fracture of the femoral shaft. *J Bone Joint Surg* 1969;51A:487–498.
49. Rand JA, Coventry MB. Stress fractures after total knee arthroplasty. *J Bone Joint Surg* 1980;62A:226–233.
50. Rasad S. Golfer's fracture of the ribs. Report of 3 cases. *AJR* 1974;120:901–903.
51. Rogers LF, Campbell RE. Fractures and dislocations of the foot. *Semin Roentgenol* 1978;13:157–166.
52. Ross DJ, Dieppe PA, Watt I, Newman JH. Tibial stress fracture in pyrophosphate arthropathy. *J Bone Joint Surg* 1983;65B:474–477.
53. Sandrock AR. Another sports fatigue fracture. Stress fracture of the coracoid process of the scapula. *Radiology* 1975;117:274.
54. Schneider R, Kaye JJ. Insufficiency fractures of the long bones occurring in patients with rheumatoid arthritis. *Radiology* 1975;116:595–599.
55. Schneider HJ, King AY, Brownson JL, Miller EH. Stress injuries and development changes of lower extremities in ballet dancers. *Radiology* 1974;113:627–632.
56. Stark HH, Jobe FW, Boyes JH, Ashworth CR. Fracture of the hook of the hamate in athletes. *J Bone Joint Surg* 1977;59A:575–582.
57. Stein RE, Stelly FH. Stress fracture of the calcaneus in a child with cerebral palsy. *J Bone Joint Surg* 1977;59A:131–132.
58. Symeonides PP. High stress fractures of the fibula. *J Bone Joint Surg* 1980;62B:192–193.
59. Torg JS, Pavlov H, Cooley LH, et al. Stress fractures of the tarsal navicular. *J Bone Joint Surg* 1982;64A:700–712.
60. Wilson ES, Katz FN. Stress fractures. An analysis of 250 consecutive cases. *Radiology* 1969;92:481–486.
61. Young A, Kinsella P, Boland P. Stress fractures of the lower limb in patients with rheumatoid arthritis. *J Bone Joint Surg* 1981;63B:239–243.
62. Zlatkin MB, Bjorkengren A, Sartoris DJ, Resnick D. Stress fractures of the distal tibia and calcaneus subsequent to acute fractures of the tibia and fibula. *AJR* 1987;149:329–332.

Subject Index

A

Abdomen injury, pelvic fracture, 258–260
Abdominal aorta, 214
Abduction, 466
Abductor digiti minimi fascia, ultrasound, 14
Abductor digiti minimi muscle, 458–459
Abductor hallucis muscle, 458–459
Acetabular dome, cartilage damage, 249
Acetabular dome comminution, hip
    dislocation, 263
Acetabular dome fracture, 226
Acetabular fracture, 218, 227, 234, 251
    anterior, 226
    classification
        anterior and posterior column, 240
        femoral head position, 240
    complex, 243–244, 245
    computed tomography, 22
    elementary, 240–243, 244
    femur, 241
    lateral compression injury, 228, 230
Acetabular insufficiency fracture, 892
Acetabular labral tear, hip arthrography, 299,
    300, 301
Achilles insertion, calcaneal fracture, 549
Achilles tendon
    normal, 486, 502
    thickened, healed, 502
    ultrasound, 483
        normal, 86
Achilles tendon injury, 499–501, 502
Achilles tendon pain, chronic, 500
Achilles tendon tear, 89, 483, 486, 499–501,
    502
    calcaneal fracture, 553
    treatment, 501
Acromial spur, 610
Acromioclavicular arthrography, 625–626
Acromioclavicular dislocation, 643–644,
    645, 646
    classification, 644
    ossification, 646
    prognosis, 644
    separation, 645
Acromioclavicular joint, 584
    anatomy, 626
    ankle traction cuff, 594
    clavicle, 593
    disruption, 649
    injection, 626
    magnetic resonance imaging
        hypertrophy, 628
        supraspinatus compression, 628

radiography, 592, 593, 594
    stress views, 594
Acromioclavicular ligament, 644
Acromiohumeral distance, shoulder
    arthrography, 608
Acromion, 590, 643
    computed tomography, 606
    humeral head, 614
    osteophytic changes, 610
    shoulder arthrography, 608
Acromion fracture, 653
    undisplaced comminuted, 652
Adduction, 466
Adductor hallucis muscle, 459, 460
Adductor muscle injury, 329, 330
Adhesive capsulitis, shoulder arthrography,
    616–617, 618
    axillary recess, 617
    subscapularis recess, 617
Amipaque, myelography, 29
Anger-gamma camera, 17
Angiography, 26–28
    applications, 26
    equipment, 26–28
    indications, 28
    pelvic fracture, 27
    technique, 28
    treatment with, 26
Ankle, 453–571
    anterior tendon, 496
    arthritis, 495
    bone scanning, 483–484
        infection, 484
    computed tomography, 484–485
        positioning, 484–485
    deep muscles, 456
    fused posterior talar ossification center, 467
    imaging techniques, 468–492
    incomplete tear, 495–496
    injury, 492–505. See also Specific type
    lateral structures, 471
    lateral tendon, 496
    ligament injury, 492–496, 504
        sequelae, 496
    ligamentous structures, 461–462
    magnetic resonance imaging, 485, 486
        surface coils, 485
    muscle insertions, 454
    muscle origins, 454
    neurovascular anatomy, 456
    neurovascular structures, 491
    normal variants, 465
    osseous anatomy, 461–462

osteoarthritis, 524
osteomyelitis, 872
radiography, 468–469
    AP view, 468
    lateral view, 469
    mortise view, 470
    oblique views, 470, 471
    stress views, 470–475
Salter-Harris IV fracture, 42
soft tissue anatomy, 453–467
subtalar area, 471
supporting structures, 462, 463
talar shift, 495
tendon, 491
tendon injuries, 495–505
terminology, 465–466
tomography, 479–482
    motion artifact, 479–482
ultrasound, 482–483
varus stress view, 494
Ankle arthrography, 485–489
    ankle sprain, 495
    clinical applications, 487–489
    indications, 486
    normal anatomy, 487
    technique, 485–487
Ankle fracture, 505–557
    arthrodesis, 525
    cast immobilization, 517
    classification, 511–518
    clinical features, 509
    comminution of mid-fibula, 526
    complex, 526
    complications, 521–525, 526, 527
    compression plate, 519, 520
    high fibular fracture, 517
    instability, 521
    Lauge-Hansen classification, 512–518
    Lauge-Hansen Stage III pronation-lateral
        rotation injury, 519, 520
    Lauge-Hansen supination-adduction Stage
        I, 512, 513
    Lauge-Hansen supination-lateral rotation
        injuries, 512, 514
    malunion, 521
    marked syndesmosis involvement, 517
    neurovascular injury, 525, 526
    non-union, 521
    osteoarthritis, 521
    pronation-abduction injuries, 515, 516
    pronation-lateral rotation injuries, 515,
        516, 517, 519, 520
    radiography, 518–519

Ankle fracture, (contd.)
  reflex sympathetic dystrophy, 521
  ring concept, 509, 512
  supination-adduction injury, 512, 513
  supination-lateral rotation Stage II injury,
      514
    undisplaced, 517
  supination-lateral rotation Stage IV injury,
      515
  syndesmosis ossification, 525, 527
  syndesmosis screw, 519, 520
  treatment, 519–521
  Weber classification, 516–517
  Weber Type C2 fracture, 517
Ankle sprain, 488, 493–495
  ankle arthrography, 495
  differential diagnosis, 497
  talar dome fracture, 543
  tenography, 495
  treatment, 495–496
Ankylosing spondylitis, 199–201
  pseudarthrosis, 201
Annulus fibrosus, 100
Anterior arch, management, 163–164
Anterior body, 93, 94
Anterior column fracture, 243, 244
Anterior compression fracture
  T3, 171
  T4, 171
Anterior compression injury, 174
  pelvic fracture, 228, 230
Anterior cruciate ligament tear, 379
  criteria, 411
  hemarthrosis, 419
Anterior drawer sign, 381, 473
Anterior inferior chip fracture, vertebral
      body, 161
Anterior inferior iliac spine
  avulsion fracture, 232
  stress fracture, 304
Anterior interbody fusion, 187
Anterior ligament injury, 161
Anterior longitudinal ligament, 100, 101
Anterior lunate dislocation, 828, 829
Anterior process, compression fracture, 549
Anterior ring fracture, classification, 237
Anterior superior iliac spine, avulsion
      fracture, 232, 233
Anterior talofibular ligament tear, 488
Anterior tendon, 503
  injury, 505
  tenography, 492
Anterior ulnar collateral ligament, 675, 678
AO plate and screw
  fibula fracture, 443
  tibia fracture, 443
Apophyseal joint, 93, 101
Arachnoid, 103
Arm, 659–673
  anatomy, 659–663
  muscles, 659
  nerves, 662
  soft tissue injury, 673
  vessels, 662
Artery of Adamkiewicz, 101–103
Arthritis, 412
  ankle, 495

hip arthrography, 296–298
hip dislocation, 269
hip fracture-dislocation, 269
magnetic resonance imaging, 632
post-traumatic degenerative, 861
posterior pillar, 250
radial styloid, 821
scaphoid fracture, 821
scaphoid waist, 821
synovitis, 623
talar neck fracture, 533, 535
wrist arthrography, 794
Arthrodesis, 252
  ankle fracture, 525
  hand, 861, 863
  talar neck fracture, 536
  tibial plafond fracture, 521
  wrist, 861, 863
Arthrogram set, 31–32
Arthrographic suite, 32
Arthrography, 30–33
  articular cartilage, 620–623
  commonly studied joints, 31
  complications, 33
  contrast material, 33
  equipment, 31–32
  glenoid labrum, 620–623
  hip, 294–305
  pelvis, 294–305
  synovium, 620–623
Arthroplasty
  hand, 863–866
  wrist, 863–866
Arthrosis, scaphoid fracture, 819
Articular cartilage, 393, 396, 397, 614, 621
  arthrography, 620–623
  increased density, 623
  olecranon, 678
  osteoarthritis, 408
  thinning, 623
Articular condyle
  deforming rotation, 705
  lateral musculature, 705
  medial musculature, 705
Articular disorder, knee, 379–389
  arthrography, 389–417
  imaging, 389–424
Articular facet, regional differences, 96
Articular pillar fracture, 152, 154
Articulated endoprosthesis, femoral neck
      fracture, 278, 279
Artifact, magnetic resonance imaging, 23–24
Atlantoaxial dislocation, 133–136
  type I, 136
  type II, 136
  type III, 136
  type IV, 136
Atlantoaxial fusion, 164
Atlanto-occipital dislocation, 131
Atlanto-occipital region
  cervical spine fracture, 129–130
    management, 163
  cervical spine fracture-dislocation, 129–130
    management, 163
Atlas, 96, 97
  heterotopic ossification, 145
  impaction fracture, AP tomogram, 121

normal congenital cleft, 133
spinous process, 94, 95
Atlas fracture, 130–133
  AP odontoid view, 133
  avulsion fracture, 134
  incidence, 130
  Jefferson fracture, 128–129
  lateral view, 133
  management, 163–164
  neurologic complications, 133
  transverse ligament attachment avulsion,
      134
  types, 130
Atlas subluxation, 135
Atrophic non-union, humerus, 75
Avascular necrosis
  alcoholic, 278
  femoral head, 281
  femoral neck fracture, 278–281, 282–283
    stages, 279–280
  hip, 282
    staging, 279–280
  hip dislocation, 268
  hip fracture-dislocation, 268
  lunate, 789, 855–857
  metacarpal head, 860–861
  Moore prosthesis, 278
  patellar fracture, 367
  prosthesis, 278
  scaphoid, 857
  scaphoid fracture, 819, 820
  sclerosis, 280
  straight stem Moore prosthesis, 278
  subchondral lucency, 280
  talar neck fracture, 530–535
  talus, 523
Avascular non-union, 74, 75
Aviator's astragalus, 506
Avulsion fracture, 42, 43, 289
  anterior cruciate ligament, 382
  anterior inferior iliac spine, 232
  anterior superior iliac spine, 232, 233
  cuboid, 559
  hip, 232
  ilium, 232
  ischial tuberosity, 232
  ischium, 43
  pelvis, 232
  tibia, 376–377
Axillary recess, 623
Axis, 96, 98
  traumatic spondylolisthesis, 147
Axis fracture, 136–151
  body, 151
  incidence, 136
  location, 151
  management, 164–165

B
Bankhart lesion, computed tomography, 622
Barton's fracture type, 804–807
  classification, 804
  complications, 807
  mechanism of injury, 804–807
  treatment, 806, 807
Baseball finger, 860

Bateman-type bipolar endoprosthesis, femoral head fracture, 279
Bennett's fracture, 832–833
  internal fixation, 834
  K wire, 834
Biceps tendon, 613, 621, 634, 695
  absent, 619, 622
  incomplete, 700, 701
  inferior subluxation, 622
  irregularity, 619
  loose body, 619, 620
  medial subluxation, 619
  origin, 612
Biceps tendon arthrography, 617–620
  abnormalities, 619
Biceps tendon rupture, 700
Biceps tendon sheath, 614
Bicipital groove, 582, 619
  radiography, 597, 598, 599
Bifid spinous process, C4, 152, 154
Bimalleolar fracture, internal fixation, 519–521
Bioelectric potential, 55
Bipartite scaphoid, 755
Bladder rupture, pelvic fracture, 259
Blood flow, 49–50
  bone, 48–49
    regional differences, 49
    regulation, 49
Blood supply
  hip, 213–216
  pelvis, 213–216
Body part
  centimeter thickness, 3–6
  kilovoltage, 3–6
Bone
  blood flow, 48–49
    compression-plate fixation, 59
    intramedullary nail fixation, 62–63
    regional differences, 49
    regulation, 49
  electrical signal, 55–56
  material properties, 53
  morphological findings, 52
  nonisotropic nature, 53
  normal biomechanics, 52–53
  porosity, tibia fracture, 60
  vascular supply, 47–48
    anastomosis, 47–48
    cortical venous channels, 47
    emissary veins, 47
    metaphyseal arteries, 47
    nutrient artery, 47
    periosteal arteries, 47
    periosteal capillaries, 47
    vena comitans, 47
    venous drainage, 47
  vascularity
    bone scanning, 18
    skeletal scintigraphy, 18
  viscoelastic material, 53
Bone bruise, 40, 42
Bone graft, 74
  femoral shaft fracture, 326
  talar neck fracture, 536

Bone graft cervical fusion
  myelography, 31
  tomography, 31
Bone-inductive signal, 56–57
Bone plate, types, 57
Bone scanning, 16–19
  Anger-gamma camera, 17
  ankle, 483–484
    infection, 484
  applications, 17
  bone vascularity, 18
  collimator, 17
  femoral head, 19
  femur, 19
  hand, 779–782, 784
  infection, 19
  instrumentation, 17
  pelvis, 17
  radiopharmaceuticals, 16–17
  tibia, 18
  tomogram, 17
  trauma, 17–18
  vs. pelvic x-ray, 17
  wrist, 17, 779–782, 784
Bosworth's fracture, 506
Boutonière deformity, 849, 859–860
Bowing fracture, 40
  radius, 41
  ulna, 41
Boxer's fracture, 836, 838
Brachial artery, 663
  branches, 663
Bucket handle fracture, 238, 239
Bucket handle tear
  medial meniscus, 405
  meniscus, 401
Buckle fracture, sacrum, 236
Bursitis, 84
Bursography, 624–625
  rotator cuff tear, 625
  subacromial bursa, 624
Burst fracture
  classification, 181
  L3, 194
  L4, 191–192
  lumbar spine trauma, management, 188–190, 191–192
  mechanism of injury, 181
  multiple small fragments, 182
  subtle, 184
  thoracic spine trauma, management, 188–190, 191–192
  type A, 182
  vertebral body fracture, 156, 157

C

C1. See Atlas
C2. See Axis
C2 on C3, normal subluxation, 105
C3, 96, 99
C4, 96, 99
  bifid spinous process, 152, 154
  facet fracture, 155
C4-C5, disk space narrowing, 115
C5, 96, 99
  pedicle fracture, 152, 153

C5-C6 flexion compression injury, 122
C5-C6 interspace
  Lhermitte's sign, 165, 166
  ligamentous injury, 165, 166
C5 compression fracture, 123
C5 on C6, subluxation, 108
C6, 96, 99
  asymmetric fracture, 129
  compression, 129
  facet fracture, management, 168
  lamina fracture, 151, 152
  pillar fracture, 152, 154
C6 fracture, 158
C7, 96, 99
  compression fracture, 123
  spinous process, 94, 95
  spinous process fracture, 153
  swimmer's views, 108–109, 110
  T1, difference in size, 105
Calcaneal fracture, 463–464, 546, 546–557
  Achilles insertion, 549
  Achilles tendon tear, 553
  avulsion, 556
  calcaneocuboid joint, 552
  classification, 547, 549
  compression fracture, 550
  Essex-Loprestic classification, 547
  incidence, 549
  intra-articular, 556
    complex, 551, 554–555
  intra-articular tongue fracture, 550
  mechanism of injury, 547
  navicular compression, 551
  osteomyelitis, 875
  plate fixation, 554–555
  radiography, 547–552, 553
  Rowe classification, 546
  screw fixation, 554–555
  subtalar joint, 552
  sustentacular fragment, 554–555
  sustentaculum, 553
  sustentaculum involvement, 550
  treatment, 552–557
  vertical forces, 550
Calcaneal stress fracture, 884–886
Calcaneocuboid joint, calcaneal fracture, 552
Calcaneofibular ligament avulsion, flake fracture, 493
Calcaneofibular ligament tear, 489
Calcium, fracture healing, 51
Calf, 433–451
  compartment syndrome, 450, 451
  deep compartment, 455
  magnetic resonance imaging, 24
  nerves, 431–436
  neurovascular anatomy, 456–457
  soft tissue injury, 450–451
  vessels, 431–436
Calf fracture
  classification, 437–438
  management, 439–447
  mechanism of injury, 437–438
  radiography, 438–439
Calf muscle, 431
Cancellous screw, 58
Capitate, 751, 753
  lunate, 774

Capitate fracture, 785, 824–826
  scaphoid fracture, 826
Capitate injury, 824–826. *See also* Specific
    type
Capitellar avulsion fracture, 698
Capitellar fracture, 707–708, 709
  classification, 707–708
  impacted, 709
  K-wire, 708
  physical examination, 708
  radiography, 708, 709
  treatment, 708
  Type I, 707, 708
  Type II, 707
Capitellum, 683
Capitotriquetral ligament, 756
Capsulitis, hip arthrography, 298
Carpal bone, infectious arthritis, 866
Carpal dislocation, 827–830
Carpal fracture, 811–827
Carpal height, 753, 754
Carpal joint space, traction, 801
Carpal tunnel, 761, 778
Carpal ulnar distance, wrist, 752
Carpe bosseau, 859
Carpometacarpal dislocation, 830, 831
Carpometacarpal joint, 765
  1st, 775
  2nd, 775
  4th, 770, 775
  5th, 770, 775
Carpometacarpal joint dislocation, second to
    fifth, 764
Carpometacarpal ligament, 756–757
Carpus, 751
Carpus dislocation, 828–830
Cast brace technique, femoral shaft fracture,
    319
Cast immobilization, ankle fracture, 517
Casting, femoral shaft fracture, 319–320
Cervical spine
  clivus, 106
  flexion teardrop fracture dislocation,
    160–161, 163
  lamina, 106
  ligament, 100–101
  ligament anatomy, 101–103
  normal anatomic relationships, 106
  normal cervical lines, 107
  prevertebral fat stripe, 107
  retrotracheal soft tissues, 106
  subluxation, 45
Cervical spine fracture, 129–151
  atlanto-occipital region, 129–130
    management, 163
  management, 165–168
Cervical spine fracture-dislocation, 129–151
  atlanto-occipital region, 129–130
    management, 163
  management, 165–168
Cervical spine trauma, 123–169
  associated injuries, 161–163
  classification, 123–124
  hyperextension, 124, 127–128
    anterior inferior body fracture of C2, 151
    C2 pedicle fracture, 151

hangman's fracture, 127–128
  management, 168–169
hyperflexion, 124–127
  compressive, 126
  disruptive, 124–125
  flexion-rotation injuries, 124–126
  shearing, 126
  teardrop, 126
instability indicators, 127
management, 163–169
mechanism of injury, 123–129
radiography, 104–115, 123–124
  AP view, 109–111
  flexion/extension view, 113–115
  lateral, 104, 105–109, 110
  oblique views, 111, 112, 113
  odontoid view, 112
  pillar views, 112–113, 114
  thoracolumbar fracture, 162
  vertical-compression injury, 124, 128–129
Cervical vertebra, 94, 95, 96, 99. *See also*
    Specific type
Cervical vertebral body fracture
  incidence, 156
  location, 156
Chance fracture
  lumbar spine, 11
  tomography, 11
Chauffeur's fracture, 807–808
  classification, 807
  complications, 808
  mechanism of injury, 807
  pronator fat stripe, 808
  treatment, 807–808
Check-rein ligament, 757
Chest injury, pelvic fracture, 258–260
Chip fracture, vertebral body fracture, 156
Chondrocalcinosis, 792
  knee arthroscopy, 423, 424
Chondromalacia, 359–362, 413–414
  etiology, 360–361
  stages, 360
Chopart's fracture-dislocation, 506
Choport's joint, 557
Circlage wire, 366, 367
  femoral shaft fracture, 324
Clavicle
  acromioclavicular joint, 593
  computed tomography, 606
  erosions, 651
  muscle attachments, 580
  normal, 651
  osteology, 579, 580
  radiography, 592–595, 596
    AP views, 592–595
    oblique view, 595, 596
Clavicle fracture, 598, 646–650
  classification, 646–647
  middle third, 646
  non-union, 648, 650
  radiography, 647
  treatment, 648
  undisplaced, 645
Clavicle trauma, 598
Clay shoveler's fracture, 39
Coccyx fracture, 235

Collapse deformity, 753
  dorsal intercalated segment instability,
    753, 754
  volar intercalated segment instability, 753,
    754
Collateral ligament, 757
Colles' fracture, 796–802
  classification, 796–797
  complications, 802, 803
  external fixation, 801
  finger traction, 801
  Frykman classification, 796–797, 798, 799,
    800, 801
  mechanism of injury, 796
  metacarpal fracture, fifth, 802
  radial length, 802
  traction, 801
  treatment, 797–801
  ulnar tilt, 802
Colon, 215, 216
Common iliac artery, 214
Compartment syndrome, 84, 505
  calf, 450, 451
  thigh, 329–332
Complex rotary injury, lower lumbar spine,
    180
Compression fracture, 42, 43
  anterior process, 549
  calcaneus, 550
  cuboid, 559
  management, 186, 187
  T12, 194
  vertebral body fracture, 156, 157
Compression plate, ankle fracture, 519, 520
Compression-plate fixation, 57–58
  adverse effects, 60–62
  biomechanics, 59–60
  bone-blood flow, 59
  mechanism of action, 58–59
  morphologic findings, 59
  primary fracture healing, 59
  removal timing, 61
  vs. intermedullary nail fixation, 65–67
Compression screw
  medial head fracture, 722
  ulna fracture, 724
Computed tomography, 19–22
  acetabular fracture, 22
  acromion, 606
  ankle, 484–485
    positioning, 484–485
  Bankhart lesion, 622
  clavicle, 606
  coracoid, 606
  data collection method, 19–20
  equipment, 19–20
  foot, 484–485
    positioning, 484–485
  glenoid, 606
  hand, 778–779, 783
  Hill-Sachs lesion, 622
  hip, 226–227, 305
  hip arthroplasty, 25
  indications, 22
  knee, 401
  lumbar spine fracture, 21

medial clavicular lesion, 598, 606
odontoid fracture, type II, 120
partial volume effect, 20
pelvis, 226–227, 305
scanners, 19
scapula, 606
scapular fracture, 606
shoulder, 606–607
soft tissue injury, 305
spine, 119–121, 122
sternoclavicular lesion, 598, 606
stress fracture, 883
T4-T5 fracture subluxation, 122
techniques, 20–22
thoracic fracture, 122
vs. tomography, 120–121
wrist, 778–779, 783
x-ray beam, 20
x-ray dose, 20
Condylar fracture
    classification, 709–710
    comminuted Type II condyle fracture, 710
    comminuted Type II lateral fracture, 710
    complications, 711
    diagnosis, 710
    flexion limitation, 711
    mechanism of injury, 709
    posterior displacement, 711
    treatment, 710
    undisplaced lateral, 710
    varus angulation, 711
Condyle, anterior angulation, 676
Contrast material
    arthrography, 33
    Hypaque-M-60, 33
    Reno-M-60, 33
    Renografin-60, 33
Contusion, 83
Conus medullaris, 103
Coracoacromial arch, 590
Coracoclavicular ligament
    disruption, 645, 649
    rupture, 647
    screw fixation, 649
Coracoid, 590, 643
    computed tomography, 606
Coracoid fracture, 653
Coracoid stress fracture, 653
Cord syndrome, 170
Coronoid fracture, 723–725
    classification, 723–725
    radiography, 725
    treatment, 725
    types, 725
Cortical fracture, tibia, 42
Cortical screw, 58
Cotton's fracture, 506, 508
Cross-union
    forearm fracture, 745–747
    radius fracture, 745–747
    ulna fracture, 745–747
Cruciate ligament
    anterior, 338
        avulsion fracture, 382
        chronic laxity, 379
        fascicles, 338

injury, natural history, 379
        nerve supply, 339
        normal, 410
        tibial avulsion fracture, 382
        vascular supply, 339
    forces, 341–342
    knee, 338–340
    lateral rotation, 340
    normal, 393, 394, 395
    posterior, 338, 339
        normal, 409
        vascular supply, 339
    valgus stress, 339
    vascular supply, 339
Cruciate ligament injury, knee arthrography, 411
Crystalline synovitis, knee arthroscopy, 423, 424
Cuboid, 464
    avulsion fracture, 558, 559
    compression fracture, 559
    plantar dislocation, 559
Cuneiform, 464

D
Defect non-union, 74
Degenerative arthritis, scaphotrapezial articulation, 865
Degenerative cyst, ulna, 693
Degenerative joint disease, knee arthroscopy, 424
Degenerative meniscal lesion, 407–409
Degenerative subluxation, 161, 163
Deltoid ligament, rupture, 510
Depression fracture, 42
Diagnostic technique, 1–33
Diaphyseal fracture, 844–845
Digital subtraction angiography, 26–28
Discoid lateral meniscus
    biconcave type, 407
    multiple vertical tears, 405, 406
    slab type, 406, 407
Discoid meniscus, 405–407
    asymmetric anterior horn enlargement, 407
    types, 407
Disk, 100
    magnetic resonance imaging, 123
Disk herniation, myelography, 30
Disk space, 107, 108
Dislocation, description, 45
Disruptive hyperflexion injury, 124–125
Distal humerus fracture, 701–702
    classification, 701
    mechanism of injury, 701
    physical examination, 701–702
    treatment, 702
Distal interphalangeal joint, fifth, dorsal dislocation, 851
Distal phalanx
    comminuted proximal base fracture, 851
    dorsal lip fracture, 850–851
    proximal base fractures, 850
    transverse fractures, 850
    volar lip fracture, 851

Distal radial fracture, 796–810, 864
    distal radioulnar joint, 799
Distal radial metaphysis, 797
Distal radioulnar joint, 749, 755–756, 799, 809
    comminuted, 799
    dislocation, 809
    distal radial fracture, 799
    dorsal dislocation, 810–811
    volar dislocation, 811, 812
Distal radioulnar subluxation, 809, 810
Distal radius metaphysis fracture, 809
Distal second metatarsal, stress fracture, 511
Distal ulnar metaphysis, 797
Doppler ultrasound, 13, 15
Dorsal carpometacarpal dislocation, 831
Dorsal ganglion, 785
Dorsal interosseous muscle, 460
Dorsal lip fracture, 850–851
Dorsal lip proximal base fracture, 847–849
Dorsal lunate dislocation, isolated, 830
Dorsal perilunate dislocation, 827–828
Dorsal proximal interphalangeal joint dislocation, 852, 853, 854
Dorsal recess, 794
Dorsalis pedis artery, 526
Dorsiflexion, 465–466
Dupuytren's fracture, 506, 508
Dura, 103

E
Edema
    osteomyelitis, 876
    scaphoid fracture, 786
Elbow, 675–728
    anatomy, 675–680
    anterior fat pads, 686
        displacement, 698
    articulation, 675
    displaced extension supracondylar injury, 702
    imaging techniques, 680–696
    joint entrapment, 703
    ligament injury, 696–699, 700
    magnetic resonance imaging, 693–696
        coil selection, 694, 695
        image planes, 694–696
        patient positioning, 694, 695
        pulse sequences, 694–696
    muscle, 679
    neurovascular structures, 679–680
    normal valgus carrying angle, 699
    posterior dislocation, 696, 697
    posterior fat pads, 686
        displacement, 698
    radiography, 680–687
        AP view, 680, 681
        assessment, 685–687
        axial views, 682–685
        lateral view, 680–682, 683
        oblique views, 682, 683, 684
        radial head view, 682, 684
        stress views, 687
    soft tissue injury, 696–701

Elbow, (contd.)
  valgus stress, 703
  valgus stress view, 699
Elbow arthrography, 687–692
  abnormal, 690–693
  indications, 687
  normal, 689–690
  patient positioning, 689
  technique, 687–689
Elbow clicking, 691
Elbow fracture, 701–728. See also Specific
    type
Elbow pain, 691
Elbow trauma, 696–728
Electrical signal, bone, 55–56
Electrical stimulation, 74
  fracture non-union, 74, 75, 76, 77
Emphysema, 652
Ender nail
  femoral shaft fracture, 320, 323
  intertrochanteric fracture, 290–293
Endoprosthesis
  femoral head fracture, 279
  femoral neck fracture, 274–278
Endosteal callus
  fracture healing, 52
  intramedullary nail fixation, 63–64
Endosteum, fracture healing, 52
Endosteum periosteum, centrifugal flow of
    blood, 48
Enhanced through-transmission, 14
Epicondylar fracture, 702–704
  complications, 703–704
  mechanisms of injury, 702–703
Epicondyle articulation, 685
Equina compression, 191–192
Eversion, 466
Extensor carpi ulnaris tendon sheath, 783
Extensor digitorum longus muscle, 457–458
Extensor hallucis longus muscle, 457–458
Extensor muscle, ultrasound, 14
Extensor tendon, 786
External coil electrical stimulation device, 76
External fixation, 67–69
  Colles' fracture, 801
  complications, 69
  fibula fracture, 482
  indications, 67–69
  mechanical monitoring, 69
  tibia fracture, 482
External iliac artery, 214
Extra-articular proximal metaphyseal
    fracture, 832, 836, 837

F
Facet dislocation, 159–160
  bilateral, 159, 160
    management, 166, 167
  unilateral, 159–160
Facet fracture
  C4, 155
  C6, management, 168
  vertebral arch fracture, 155
Facet joint, 93, 101, 107, 108
  degenerative changes, 198
  flexion rotation injury, 179

fracture subluxation, lateral tomograms,
    121, 122
  widening, 115
Facet locking, 159–160
  bilateral, 159, 160
  unilateral, 159–160
Fat plane, 218
  gluteal, 213
  hip, 210, 213
  iliopsoas, 213
  obturator internus, 210
  pericapsular, 213
Fatigue fracture, 881
Femoral artery, 313
Femoral articular cartilage, normal, 412
Femoral condyle, normal articular cartilage,
    393, 395
Femoral head
  avascular necrosis, 281
  blood supply, 279
  bone scanning, 19
  hip dislocation, 261
    posterior impaction, 264
  skeletal scintigraphy, 19
  structural collapse, 281
Femoral head defect, 299
Femoral head fracture, 268
  Bateman-type bipolar endoprosthesis, 279
  endoprosthesis, 279
  non-union, 284
  Pipkin classification, 264, 265
    hip dislocation, 264
  subtrochanteric valgus osteotomy, 284
Femoral neck fracture, 226, 251, 267,
    269–284, 328
  articulated endoprosthesis, 278, 279
  avascular necrosis, 278–281, 282–283
    stages, 279–280
  classification, 269–270
  comminuted, 277
  complete displacement, 277
  complications, 278–284
  endoprosthesis, 274–278
  Garden Stage I, 270, 272
  Garden Stage II, 271, 274
  Garden Stage III, 271, 276
  greater trochanter, 272
  hip arthroplasty, 274
  impacted fracture, 273, 274
  lesser trochanter, 272
  location, 269
  Pauwel's classification, 270
  radiographic evaluation, 270–272
  stress fracture, 273, 274, 889–890, 891
  subcapital fracture, 273
  trabeculae, 272
  treatment, 272–278, 279
  undisplaced, 225
  unstable, 273–274
Femoral nerve, 313
Femoral shaft, 311, 312, 314
  blood supply, 311
  fracture description, 44
  muscle groups, 311, 313
  stress fracture, 889, 890
Femoral shaft fracture, 314–328
  angulation, 324

bilateral, 328
bone graft, 326
cast brace technique, 319
casting, 319–320
cerclage wire, 324
classification, 315–317
comminuted, 319, 321
  overriding, 316
comminuted midshaft, 328
complications, 326–328
displacement, 324
Ender nail, 320, 323
femoral neck fracture, 315
hip dislocation, 269
hip fracture-dislocation, 269
interlocking medullary nailing
  dynamic, 320, 322
  static, 320, 322
internal fixation, 320–326
  Küntscher intramedullary nail, 320, 321
ipsilateral hip injury, 327–328, 329
malunion, 327
mechanism of injury, 314–315
methyl methacrylate cement, 326
non-union, 327, 328
overriding, 321
plate fixation, 320–326
radiographic evaluation, 317–318
refracture, 326
rotation, 321
Rush pin, 320
spiral, 326
traction, 318–319, 321
treatment, 318–326
Type II, 315
vascular injury, 327
Winquist Type IV, 321
Femoral vein, 313
Femur fracture, 226, 246, 247, 311–332, 314
  acetabular fracture, 241
  anatomy, 311–314
  bone scanning, 19
  comminuted, 226
  comminuted fracture, 226
  comminuted overriding, 45
  comminuted overriding fracture, 45
  fracture non-union, 73
  fracture union, 72
  infection, 874
  ipsilateral fracture, 377–379
    classifications, 377, 379
    treatment, 377
  non-union, 76
  osteomyelitis, 876
  pathologic fracture, 43
  posterior acetabular fragment
    abduction, 241
    adduction, 241
  Richard's screw-plate, 292
  skeletal scintigraphy, 19
  soft tissue injury, 329–332
  supracondylar fracture, 367–370
    classification, 367–368
    comminuted, 369
    internal fixation, 369–370
    open reduction, 369–370
    treatment, 368–370

Fibula, 433–451
  musculoskeletal anatomy, 434, 435
  soft tissue injury, 450–451
  tomography, 10
Fibula fracture
  AO plate and screw, 443
  classification, 437–438
  comminuted, 439, 440, 441
  complications, 447–450
  distal, 440, 442
  external fixation, 482
  Fischer apparatus, 440, 443
  internal fixation, 482
  intramedullary nailing, 443, 444
  management, 439–447
  mechanism of injury, 437–438
  medullary rod, 445
  non-union, 447
  osteomyelitis, 872
  popliteal artery occlusion, 447, 449
  prognosis, 446–447
  radiography, 438–439
  stress fracture, 889
Fifth, metatarsal, metaphysis fracture, 566
Film labeling, radiography, 7
Filum terminale, 103
Finger
  index, 786
  middle, 766, 768
  third, 766
Finger traction, Colles' fracture, 801
Fischer apparatus
  fibula fracture, 440, 443
  tibia fracture, 440, 443
Fixation device
  classification, 70
  imaging, 69–71
Flake fracture, calcaneofibular ligament
      avulsion, 493
Flexion compression injury, 126, 158
Flexion-distraction injury, 175
  management, 186, 188, 189
Flexion-rotation injury, 124–126
  facet joint, 179
  laminar fracture, 179
  lower lumbar spine, 179
  lumbar spine trauma, 178, 179, 180
      management, 186–188
  thoracic spine trauma, 178, 179, 180
      management, 186–188
Flexion teardrop, 160–161
Flexion teardrop fracture, radiographic
      features, 161
Flexion teardrop fracture-dislocation
  cervical spine, 160–161, 163
  management, 169, 170
Flexor carpi radialis, 758
Flexor carpi ulnaris, 758
Flexor digiti minimi brevis muscle, 459, 460
Flexor digitorum brevis muscle, 458–459
Flexor digitorum longus muscle, 452–456
Flexor digitorum longus tendon, 459
  normal, 503
Flexor hallucis brevis muscle, 459, 460
Flexor hallucis longus muscle, 452–456
Flexor hallucis longus tendon, 459

Flexor muscle
  hand, 758, 759, 760
  wrist, 758, 759, 760
Flexor tendon, 786
Flexor tendon sheath, 793
Foot, 453–571
  accessory ossification centers, 465
  articular relationships, 475
  computed tomography, 484–485
      positioning, 484–485
  deep muscles, 456
  foreign bodies, 505
  imaging techniques, 468–492
  injury, 492–505
      ligament injuries, 492–496
  ligament injury, 504
  magnetic resonance imaging, 485, 486
      surface coils, 485
  muscle insertions, 454
  muscle origins, 454
  musculature, 458–461
  neurovascular supply, 460–461
  normal variants, 465
  radiography, 475–476
      AP view, 474, 475–476
      lateral view, 475
      oblique view, 475, 476
  soft tissue anatomy, 453–467
  stress fracture, 883–886
  tendon injuries, 495–505
  terminology, 465–466
Foot arthrography, 487–488
Foot fracture, 505–557
Foramen magnum, 103
Foramen transversarium, 96
Forearm, 731–747
  anatomy, 731–736
  anterior muscle attachments, 733
  arteries, 735
  muscle, 731, 732
  posterior muscle attachments, 734
  radiography, 734–736
  soft tissue injury, 646
Forearm fracture, 736–747
  classification, 736–737
  complications, 743–747
  cross-union, 745–747
  incidence, 738
  location, 738
  management, 737–743
  mechanism of injury, 736
Forefoot, AP view, 474
Fracture. See also Specific type
  angulation, 44, 45
      describing, 45
  cellular response, 51–52
  complete, 40
  displacement, 45
  endosteal blood supply, 50, 51
  illustration, 44
  incomplete, 40
  periosteal blood supply, 50, 51
  post-reduction views, 45–46
  radiography, 43–46
  types, 39–43. See also Specific type
  vascular dilatation function, 51

vascular proliferation, 49
vascular response, 49–51
Fracture-dislocation, radiography, 43–46
Fracture fixation, 57–71. See also Specific
      type
  imaging, 69–71
Fracture healing, 39–77
  biologic signs, 55
  biomechanical characteristics changes, 54
  biomechanical stages, 54, 55
  biomechanics, 53–57
  calcium, 51
  endosteal callus, 52
  endosteum, 52
  factors, 72
  Haversian canal, 52
  healing strength, 54
  inflammatory, 46–47
  mechanical forces, 54–55
  medullary vascular system, 50–51
  mesenchymal cell, 52
  osteogenic cell, 52
  oxidative metabolism, 51
  oxygen tension, 51
  periosteal callus, 52
  periosteum cambrum layer, 52
  phases, 46–47
  physiology, 49–52
  remodeling, 46–47
  reparative, 46–47
  Volkmann's canal, 52
Fracture non-union, 71–77
  classification, 73–74
  definition, 71
  diagnosis, 73–74
  electrical stimulation, 74, 75, 76, 77
  etiologic factors, 71–72
  femur, 73, 76
  humerus, 73
  pseudarthrosis, 71
  tibia, 73
  treatment, 74–77
Fracture union, 71–77
  definition, 71
  femur, 72
Fusion, 187
Fusion complications
  lumbar spine trauma, 190–194, 195
  thoracic spine trauma, 190–194, 195

G
Galeazzi fracture, 808–810
  classification, 808
  complications, 810
  mechanism of injury, 808
  radial shaft fracture, 742–743, 744
  treatment, 808–810
Gallium-67 citrate, 16
Ganglia, wrist arthrography, 794
Gastrocnemius muscle, 451–455
Gastrointestinal anatomy, 215, 216
Genitourinary injury, pelvic fracture,
      253–258, 259
  bladder injuries, 256–258, 259
  classification for urethral injuries, 256, 257
  urethra, 253, 257, 258

Genitourinary tract
  female, 215, 216
  male, 215, 216
Glenohumeral dislocation, 639–643
  anterior, 639–641
  complications, 642–643
  posterior, 641–642
  recurrence, 642
  superior and inferior, 642, 643
Glenohumeral joint, 582–584
  osteoarthritis, 589, 632
Glenoid, 590, 643
  computed tomography, 606
  humeral head, 639
Glenoid articular surface fracture, 606, 650, 651
Glenoid dysplasia, 634
Glenoid fracture, 640, 650–652
Glenoid labrum, 614, 621
  arthrography, 620–623
  normal, 632
  subscapularis recess, 613
Glenoid rim, 580, 600
  eburnation, 608, 610
Glenoid rim fracture, persistent anterior subluxation, 640
Glenoid tip, 580
Gluteal, fat plane, 213
Gosselin's fracture, 506, 509
Gracilis muscle, 340–341
Greater sigmoid notch, 677
Greater trochanter, 217
  femoral neck fracture, 272
Greater trochanter avulsion, 289
Greater tuberosity fracture, 640
  proximal humeral fracture, 636
  shoulder arthrography, 608
Greenstick fracture, 39, 40, 506
  ulna, 40, 41
Growth plate fracture, 40
  Salter-Harris type, 41
Guyon's canal, 761

H

Hamate, 751, 753
Hamate fracture, 821–824
Hamate hook, 770, 778
Hamate hook fracture, 824, 825
Hamate injury, 821–824
Hamstring muscle tear, 329
Hamstring tendon tear, 303, 305
Hamulus fracture, 824, 825
Hand, 749–866
  anatomy, 749–763
  arthrodesis, 861, 863
  arthroplasty, 863–866
  bone scan, 779–782, 784
  chronic post-traumatic conditions, 852
  computed tomography, 778–779, 783
  dorsal vascular anatomy, 762
  flexor muscle, 758, 759, 760
  imaging, 763–789
    anatomic region, 787
    imaging work-up, 787
    indication, 787
  infected prosthesis, 866

interosseous muscle, 759
joint capsule, 755–758
ligament, 755–758
magnetic resonance imaging, 782–789
  field of view, 782, 784
  image planes, 785–787
  positioning, 782
  pulse sequences, 785–787
  technique, 782–789
metacarpophalangeal joint spacer, 866
muscular anatomy, 758–761
neurovascular anatomy, 761–763
osteology, 749–755
osteotomy, 861, 862
post-traumatic reconstruction, 861–866
racket injury, 784
radiography, 763–764
  Brewerton view, 767, 770
  Burman view, 767, 771
  finger, 764–767
  lateral view, 764, 766, 771, 774, 775
  oblique view, 764, 765, 771–776
  PA views, 763–764, 765
  stress views, 767, 772
radionuclide imaging, 779–782, 784
soft tissue stabilization, 863
Sudeck's atrophy, 802
tendon, 760
tendon sheath, 760
tomography, 777–778, 782
volar vascular anatomy, 762
Hand arthrography
  abnormal, 795, 796
  normal anatomy, 794, 795
  technique, 794–795
Hangman's fracture, 145–147, 148
  associated findings, 132
  categories, 147, 148
  incidence, 132
  type I, 147, 148, 149
  type II, 147, 148, 149
  type III, 147, 148, 149
  upper thoracic spine, 150, 151
Harrington rod instrumentation, 187, 188
Haversian canal, fracture healing, 52
Head injury, pelvic fracture, 258–260
Heinig view, radiography, 598
Hemarthrosis, anterior cruciate ligament tear, 419
Hematoma, 83–84
  imaging, 86–87
  plantaris muscle tear, 89
  thigh, 89
  ultrasound, 86, 87
Hemorrhage, 83
  imaging, 86–87
  medial capsule, 419
  pelvic fracture, 227
  thigh, 87, 88
Herbert screw, scaphoid fracture, 817
  humpback deformity, 818
Hill-Sachs lesion
  computed tomography, 622
  radiography, 599, 600
Hind foot, 463–464
  architecture, 479

Hip
  anatomy, 207–216
  avascular necrosis, 282
    staging, 279–280
  avulsion fracture, 232
  computed tomography, 226–227, 305
  fat plane, 210, 213
  fragmentation of posterior cortex, 284
  ilium, 207–209
  imaging, 216–227
  innominate bone, 207–209
  ischium, 207–209
  ligament, 210–213
    anterior, 212
    articulations, 210–213
    motion, 210
    posterior, 212
    type, 210
  muscle insertions, 213
  neuroanatomy, 214, 216
  periarticular anatomy, 210, 213
  pubis, 207–209
  radiography, 216–227, 222–227
    AP view, 222
    Judet view, 223, 224
    lateral view, 224–225
    oblique view, 217, 225
  skeletal anatomy, 207–210
  soft tissue injury, 294
    arthrography, 294–305
  subcapital fracture, 44
  ultrasonography, 305
  vascular anatomy, 213–216
Hip arthrography
  acetabular labral tear, 299, 300, 301
  arthritis, 296–298
  capsulitis, 298
  contrast agent, 295, 296
  filming technique, 295, 296
  iliopsoas bursa, 299, 301
  indications, 294, 295, 296–305
  inflammatory joint disease, 296
  injection site, 295
  Legg-Calvé-Perthes disease, 298
  loose body, 298–299
  normal anatomy, 295, 296
  osteochondritis dissecans, 298
  osteonecrosis, 298
  post-traumatic joint disease, 296
  pubic symphysis, 303, 304–305
    injection technique, 303
  sacroiliac joint, 303, 304–305
    injection technique, 303
  snapping tendon syndrome, 299–303
  synovial chondromatosis, 298–299, 300
  synovial evaluation, 298
  technique, 295–296
Hip arthroplasty, 251
  computed tomography, 25
  femoral neck fracture, 274
  magnetic resonance imaging, 25
Hip dislocation, 260–269
  acetabular dome comminution, 263
  anterior, 264, 265, 266
    classification, 264
  arthritis, 269
  avascular necrosis, 268

central, 260–261
classification, 261–264
complications, 268–269
femoral head, 261
    posterior impaction, 264
femoral head fracture, Pipkin
    classification, 264
femoral shaft fracture, 269
incidence, 260
intra-articular fragment, 263
posterior, 260, 261–264
radiographic evaluation, 264–267, 268
sciatic nerve, 269
Thompson-Epstein Type I, 262
Thompson-Epstein Type II, 262
treatment, 267–268
Hip fracture-dislocation, 260–269
anterior, 264, 265, 266
arthritis, 269
avascular necrosis, 268
central, 260–261
classification, 261–264
complications, 268–269
femoral shaft fracture, 269
incidence, 260
posterior, 260, 261–264
radiographic evaluation, 264–267, 268
sciatic nerve, 269
treatment, 267–268
Hip pain, chronic, 299, 300
Hoffmann-Vidal apparatus, 246, 247
Humeral articulation, 677
Humeral fracture, 701–712
classification, 636
proximal. See Proximal humeral fracture
Humeral head, 590, 641, 643
acromion, 614
glenoid, 639
normal cartilage, 634
proximal humeral fracture, 636
scapular spine, 643
sclerosis, 623
Humeral head dislocation, 637
Humeral head fracture-dislocation, 638
Humeral head spur, 608, 610
Humeral shaft, 659
Humeral shaft fracture, 663–672
callus, 668
classification, 663–666
complications, 670
delayed treatment, 667–670, 671
initial management, 666–667, 668, 669,
    670
levels, 664
mechanism of injury, 663–666
mid-shaft, 668
muscle forces, 664
non-union, 666–670, 671
    callus, 671
    Hoffman apparatus, 671
    methyl-methacrylate, 672
    osteoporosis, 672
    plate fixation, 672
    Rush rod fixation, 672
    screw fixation, 672
overriding spiral midshaft, 668
plate fixation, 669

radiography, 666, 667
screw fixation, 669
Humeral subluxation, 634
Humeroacromial distance, shoulder
    arthrography, 608
Humeroacromial space, reduction, 602
Humeroulnar articulation, widening, 700
Humerus, 659–673, 675, 676
anatomy, 659–663
anterior, 660
atrophic non-union, 75
blood, 663
distal, 685
fracture non-union, 73
lateral projection, 676
muscle insertions, 659, 660, 661
osseous anatomy, 676
osteology, 582
physeal lines, 635
posterior, 659, 661
radius, 696
scapular spine, 643
soft tissue injury, 673
ulna, 696
Hypaque-M-60, contrast material, 33
Hyperemia, scaphoid fracture, 786
Hyperextension
cervical spine trauma, 124, 127–128
    anterior inferior body fracture of C2, 151
    C2 pedicle fracture, 151
    hangman's fracture, 127–128
    management, 168–169
    lamina fracture, 151, 152
lumbar spine trauma, 179–181, 184
thoracic spine trauma, 179–181, 184
Hyperflexion
cervical spine trauma, 124–127
    compressive, 126
    disruptive, 124–125
    flexion-rotation injuries, 124–126
    shearing, 126
    teardrop, 126
lumbar spine
    force axis, 171
    posterior complex distraction, 173
    thoracolumbar junction, 173–175
    wedge fractures, 171–173, 174, 175
thoracic spine
    force axis, 171
    posterior complex distraction, 173
    thoracolumbar junction, 173–175
    wedge fractures, 171–173, 174, 175
Hyperflexion fracture-dislocation, 160–161
Hyperflexion injury, 108
Hyperflexion teardrop injury, 126
Hypertrophic non-union, 73–74
tibia, 76, 77
Hypervascular non-union, 74
Hypothena muscle group, 760–761

I
Iliac spine, 217
Iliac tuberosity, 209
Iliopsoas, fat plane, 213
Iliopsoas bursa, hip arthrography, 299, 301
Iliopsoas tendon, snapping, 302

Ilium, avulsion fracture, 232
Ilium fracture, 218, 226
Impaction fracture
C1, AP tomogram, 121
femoral neck fracture, 273, 274
Impression defect, lateral femoral condyle,
    383
Indium-111-labeled autologous white blood
    cell, 16–17
Infection
bone scanning, 19
skeletal scintigraphy, 19
surgical reconstruction, 878–879
Infectious arthritis, carpal bone, 866
Inferior pubic ramus fracture, 234
transverse, 232
Inflammatory joint disease, hip
    arthrography, 296
Instability, ankle fracture, 521
Insufficiency fracture, 42–43, 881
Interlocking medullary nailing, femoral shaft
    fracture
dynamic, 320, 322
static, 320, 322
Intermuscular septa
lateral, 659, 661
medial, 659, 661
Internal fixation
Bennett's fracture, 834
bimalleolar fracture, 519–521
femoral shaft fracture, 320–326
    Küntscher intramedullary nail, 320, 321
fibula fracture, 482
radial head fracture, 717
tibia fracture, 482
trimalleolar fracture, 519–521
Internal iliac artery, 214
Interosseous fascia, ultrasound, 14
Interosseous membrane, 433, 732
Interosseous muscle
hand, 759
wrist, 759
Interpedicular distance
increased, 116
widening, 183
Interphalangeal joint, 755
ligamentous support, 757
Interphalangeal joint dislocation, 571, 852
dorsal proximal, 852, 853, 854
volar proximal, 852
Intertrochanteric fracture, 284–287
classifications, 285
comminuted, 293
complications, 287
Ender nailing, 290–293
instability, 286
methacrylate, 292, 293
myeloma, 292, 293
type I, 290
unstable, treatment, 290, 291
Interventional fluoroscopic suite, 32
Intra-articular basilar fracture, 832–833, 834,
    835, 836, 837–840
Intra-articular loose body, 414
Intra-articular tongue fracture, calcaneus, 550
Intramedullary nail fixation, 62–67
biomechanics, 64

Intramedullary nail fixation, (contd.)
  bone-blood flow, 62–63
  breaking, 64
  complications, 64–65
  endosteal callus, 63–64
  fibula fracture, 443, 444
  fluted nail, 64
  intramedullary reaming, 64
  loose-fitting, 62
  morphologic findings, 63–64
  periosteal callus, 63–64
  tibia fracture, 443, 444
  tight-fitting, 62
  types, 62
  vs. plate fixation, 65–67
Intraosseous ligament, 731
Intraperitoneal rupture, 259
Inversion, 466
Iophendylate, myelography, 29
Ipsilateral fracture
  femur, 377–379
    classifications, 377, 379
    treatment, 377
  tibia, 377–379
    classifications, 377, 379
    treatment, 377
Ischial fracture, 226
Ischial tuberosity, avulsion fracture, 232
Ischium, avulsion fracture, 43

J
Jefferson fracture, 132
  asymmetrical involvement, 134
  atlas, 128–129
  mechanism of injury, 133
Joint capsule, 393, 396, 397, 755–758
  hand, 755–758
  pigmented villonodular synovitis, 422
  wrist, 755–758
Joint space, osteoarthritis, 408
Jones fracture, 506, 509, 566, 568

K
K-wire
  Bennett's fracture, 834
  capitellar fracture, 708
  talar fracture, 531
  tibial plafond fracture, 523
  transcaphoid perilunate dislocation, 829
Kermath Versitome system, 2, 8–9
Kienböck's disease, 855–857
  Lichtman classification, 856
  lunate fracture, 821, 823
  lunate injury, 821, 823
Knee, 333–433. See also Meniscus; Patella
  anatomy, 333–341
  anterior ligamentous structures, 340
  articular abnormalities, 411–414
    degenerative changes, 411, 412, 413
  articular disorder, 379–389
    arthrography, 389–417
    imaging, 389–424
  biomechanics, 341–344
  combined rotatory instabilities, 386–387
  computed tomography, 401

cruciate ligament, 338–340
  distended, 395
  Fairbanks changes, 335
  forces, 341
    joint deformity, 342–343
  joint load, 343
  lateral ligamentous structures, 336–338
  ligament abnormality, 409–411, 412
    magnetic resonance imaging, 409–411
  ligament anatomy, 392
  ligamentous restraints, 341, 342
  ligaments, 335–340
  lipohemarthrosis, 347
  loose body, 414
  magnetic resonance imaging, 26, 399–401
    gadolinium, 399
    normal anatomic variants, 399–401
    pitfalls, 399–401
    positions, 399
    pulse sequences, 399
    three-dimensional acquisitions, 399
  medial aspect, 335
  medial ligamentous structures, 335–336
  meniscal anatomy, 392
  muscles, 340–341
  osseous anatomy, 333–334
  periarticular disorder
    arthrography, 389–417
    imaging, 389–424
  posterolateral aspect, 337
  radiography, 344–352
    AP view, 344, 345
    electronic pressure indicator, 351
    lateral view, 344–346, 347
    normal, 344
    notch view, 348, 350
    oblique view, 346–350
    patellar views, 349, 350
    Settegast technique, 349
    stress views, 350–352
    valgus stress view, 351
    varus view, 351
  rotatory instability, 384–386
    tests, 384–385
  Salter-Harris fracture, 352
  single-plane instability, 383–384
  snapping syndrome, 415–417
  soft tissue injury, 379–389
  straight instability, 383–384
  synovial abnormalities, 414, 415
  synovial disease, 400
  synovial plica, 414
  ultrasonography, 401
  vascular supply, 341
Knee arthrography
  approach, 389
  complications, 399
  contrast medium, 389
  cruciate ligament injury, 411
  errors in interpretation, 397
  film techniques, 389
  indications, 389
  injection techniques, 389–390
  lateral collateral ligament, 411
  meniscal abnormality, 401–402
  meniscal tear, 402–405
  needle placement, 389–390
  normal anatomy, 390–394, 395

overlying semimembranous bursa, 397, 398
  pitfalls, 397–399
  positioning errors, 397
  stress device, 390, 391
  technique, 389
Knee arthroplasty, bilateral total, 888
Knee arthroscopy, 417–424
  accuracy, 417
  chondrocalcinosis, 423, 424
  crystalline synovitis, 423, 424
  degenerative joint disease, 424
  equipment, 418
  evaluation, 418–424
  indications, 417
  loose body, 421
  meniscal lesion, 420–421
  meniscal tear, peripheral, 421
  meniscus injury, 420
  osteochondritis dissecans, 422, 423
  patellar disorder, 423–424
  plicae, 420
  routine preparation, 418
  synovial disorder, 423, 424
  synovial fold, 420
Knee flexion, 353–355
  patella, 358
Knee fracture, 363–379
  subtle intra-articular, 40
Knee ligamentous injury, 379–389
  diagnosis, 380–381
  natural history, 379–380
  sites, 380
  treatment, 387–389
  types, 380
Knee motion, restraints, 334
Knee pain, 352
Kyphosis, 187
Kyphotic deformity, 172, 195

L
L1
  AP view, 119
  compression, 118
  cortical collapse, 118
  posterior arch fracture, 178
  transverse fracture, 118
  transverse process, 94, 96
L1 on L2 slice fracture-dislocation, 189–190
L2
  AP view, 119
  oblique fracture, 184
  transverse process, 94, 96
L2 lamina, transverse fracture, 177
L2 pedicle, transverse fracture, 177
L3
  AP view, 119
  burst fracture, 194
  transverse process, 94, 96
L3 compression, 175
L4
  burst fracture, 191–192
  transverse process, 94, 96
L5
  pars defect, 197
    bilateral, 198
  transverse process, 94, 96

L5 facet, pedicle fracture, 185
L5 on S1 dislocation, spondylolysis, 196
Lamina, 93
Lamina fracture
  C6, 151, 152
  flexion rotation injury, 179
  hyperextension, 151, 152
Laminar space, normal, 109
Laminography, 7
Lateral capsule tear, 692
Lateral collateral ligament, knee
    arthrography, 411
Lateral compression injury
  acetabulum fracture, 228, 230
  ramus fracture, 228, 230
  sacrum fracture, 228, 230
Lateral epicondyle
  avulsion injury, 703
  posterior bony landmarks, 702
Lateral femoral condyle, 347
  chronic anterolateral rotatory instability,
    383
  impression defect, 383
  osteochondral fracture, 364
Lateral malleolus, transverse avulsion
    fracture, 512, 513
Lateral meniscus
  normal, 391, 392, 396
  posterior horn, 393, 394
    anatomy, 391–393
    complex tear, 405
Lateral supracondylar ridge, 659, 660, 661
Lateral tendon, tenography, 490–491
LeFort's fracture, 506, 510
Leg
  anterior compartment musculature,
    457–458
  anterolateral muscles, 431, 457–458
    neurovascular anatomy, 458
  compartments, 436–437
  neurovascular supply, 436
  posterior musculature, 453–457
Legg-Calvé-Perthes disease, hip
    arthrography, 298
Lennox-Hill brace, ligamentous instability,
    388
Lesser trochanter
  avulsion, 289
  femoral neck fracture, 272
  fracture, 225
Lesser tuberosity, proximal humeral fracture,
    636
Lhermitte's sign, 165, 166
Ligament, 755–758. See also Specific type
  cervical spine, 100–101
  hand, 755–758
  hip, 210–213
    anterior, 212
    articulations, 210–213
    motion, 210
    posterior, 212
    type, 210
  imaging, 87
  pelvis, 210–213
    anterior, 210, 211
    articulations, 210–213
    posterior, 210, 211
    type, 210

Ligament injury. See also Specific type
  ankle, 504
  elbow, 696–699, 700
  foot, 504
Ligament of Testut, 756
Ligament sprain, classification, 85
Ligamentous disruption, 188
Ligamentous instability, Lennox-Hill brace,
    388
Ligamentum flavum, 100, 101
Light color, phosphor material, 3
Linear tomography, 7, 8
Lipohemarthrosis, 40
  knee, 347
Lisfranc fracture-dislocation, 506, 510
  patterns, 561
Lisfranc injury
  complications, 568
  missed, 564
  partial incongruity laterally, 563
  radiography, 563–568
  treatment, 568
Loose body
  biceps tendon, 619, 620
  hip arthrography, 298–299
  knee arthroscopy, 421
  osteoarthritis, 421
  posterolateral compartment, 419
  suprapatellar pouch, 421
Lordotic curve, loss, 108
Lower cervical C3-C7 fracture, 151–161
Lower cervical spine fracture, 151–161
Lower cervical spine fracture-dislocation,
    157–161
Lower cervical spine subluxation, 157–161
  degenerative, 161, 163
Lower cervical spine trauma, management,
    165
Lower lumbar spine
  complex rotary injury, 180
  flexion rotation injury, 179
Lower thoracic fracture, 186
Lumbar spine, 169
  AP view, 116, 117, 118
  hyperflexion
    force axis, 171
      posterior complex distraction, 173
      thoracolumbar junction, 173–175
      wedge fractures, 171–173, 174, 175
  lateral view, 116, 117
  oblique views, 116–119
  radiography, 115–119
    vertebral bodies, 115
  scotty dog view, 119
  tomography, 11
Lumbar spine fracture
  Chance fracture, 11
  computed tomography, 21
  myelogram, 21
Lumbar spine trauma, 169–194
  bursting fracture, management, 188–190,
    191–192
  flexion-rotation injury, 178, 179, 180
    management, 186–188
  fusion complications, 190–194, 195
  hyperextension injury, 179–181, 184
  management, 185–194
  mechanism of injury, 170–185

shear injury, 181, 184
  management, 190–193
  vertical compression injury, 178–179,
    181, 182, 183
Lumbar vertebra, 94, 95, 96–99
Lumbrical muscle, 459, 758
Lunate, 751
  avascular necrosis, 789, 855–857
  capitate, 774
  dorsal portions, 779
  dorsal rotation, 780
  radius, 829
  triangular, 829
Lunate fracture, Kienböck's disease, 821, 823
Lunate injury, 821, 823
  Kienböck's disease, 821, 823
Lunatomalacia, 855–857
Lunotriquetral instability, 858

M
Madelung's deformity, 852, 854
Magnetic resonance imaging, 22–26
  acromioclavicular joint
    hypertrophy, 628
    supraspinatus compression, 628
  ankle, 485, 486
    surface coils, 485
  arthritis, 632
  artifact, 23–24
  calf, 24
  clinical applications, 25–26
  coil selection, 24
  disk, 123
  elbow, 693–696
    coil selection, 694, 695
    image planes, 694–696
    patient positioning, 694, 695
    pulse sequences, 694–696
  external fixation devices, 24
  foot, 485, 486
    surface coils, 485
  hand, 782–789
    field of view, 782, 784
    image planes, 785–787
    positioning, 782
    pulse sequences, 785–787
    technique, 782–789
  hip arthroplasty, 25
  imaging parameters, 25
  knee, 26, 399–401
    gadolinium, 399
    normal anatomic variants, 399–401
    pitfalls, 399–401
    positions, 399
    pulse sequences, 399
    three-dimensional acquisitions, 399
  meniscal tear, 26, 403, 405
  metallic implants, 23, 24
  osteomyelitis, 632
  patellar ligament, 411, 412
  patient positioning, 24
  patient selection, 23–24
  pelvis, 305
  pulse sequence, 25
  quadriceps tendon ligament, 411, 412
  rhabdomyolysis, 90

Magnetic resonance imaging, (contd.)
  shoulder, 626–633
    applications, 628–633
    capsular abnormalities, 630–632
    image planes, 626, 627
    impingement syndrome, 628–630
    inflammatory disorders, 632–633
    osseous disorders, 633, 634
    patient positions, 626
    rotator cuff tear, 628–630
    techniques, 626, 628
    trauma, 628–630
  shoulder capsule, 630–632
  shoulder dislocation, 631
  soft tissue injury, 305
  spinal cord, 123
  spine, 121–123
  stress fracture, 883
  techniques, 23
  thigh, post-traumatic hematoma, 25
  tibial stress fracture, 26
  wrist, 782–789
    field of view, 782, 784
    image planes, 785–787
    positioning, 782
    pulse sequences, 785–787
    technique, 782–789
Magnification radiography, 11–12. See also
      Radiography
  advantages, 12
  equipment, 11
  limitations, 12
  magnification principles, 11, 12
  wrist, 13
Maisonneuve's fracture, 506, 510
Malgaigne fracture, 238, 239
Malleolar fracture, 522
Malleolus, ossicle, 466
Mallet deformity, 860
Malunion
  ankle fracture, 521
  proximal humerus fracture, 636, 637, 638
  talar neck fracture, 535
March fracture, 506
Medial capsule
  disruption, 383
  hemorrhage, 419
Medial clavicular lesion, computed
      tomography, 598, 606
Medial collateral ligament tear, 351, 675, 678
  complete, 411
  partial, 411
Medial compartment pain, chronic, 412
Medial condyle, osteochondral defect, 348
Medial epicondyle, 675–679, 684, 685
  avulsion, 703
  ligamentous disruption, 698
  posterior bony landmarks, 702
Medial epicondyle fracture, 700
Medial femoral condyle, patellofemoral pain,
      413
Medial force inversion injury, 558
Medial gastrocnemius tear, 449, 450
Medial head fracture
  compression screw, 722
  ulna fracture, 722
Medial malleolar fracture, talar neck
      fracture, 534

Medial malleolus, loss of reduction, 523
Medial meniscus, 334–335
  bucket handle tear, 405
  complex peripheral tear, 402
  double contrast technique, 396
  mid portion, 398
  normal, 391, 392, 396
  posterior, partial peripheral tear, 398
  posterior horn
    flap tear, 419
    horizontal tear, 402
    radial tear, 405
Medial navicular fracture, 559
Medial tendon, 503
  tenography, 491–492
Medial tendon injury, 501–505
  treatment, 501–505
Median nerve, 663, 761
  compression, 787
Mediopatellar plicae, 414, 415
Medullary rod
  fibula fracture, 445
  tibia fracture, 445
Medullary vascular system, fracture healing,
      50–51
Meniscal abnormality, knee arthrography,
      401–402
Meniscal cyst, 409
Meniscal lesion, knee arthroscopy, 420–421
Meniscal recess, 397, 398
Meniscal tear, 403
  bucket handle tear, 401
  central (radial) tear, 402
  knee arthrography, 402–405
  knee arthroscopy, peripheral, 421
  magnetic resonance imaging, 26, 403, 405
  radial tear, 401
  subtle horizontal tear, 408
  tibial condyle fracture, 370
  undisplaced vertical, 401
  undisplaced vertical tear, 401
  vertical tear, 402
Meniscectomy, arthroscopic partial medial,
      420
Meniscus. See also Knee; Patella.
  anatomy, 334–335
  degenerative lesion, 407–409
  functions, 334
  medial. See Medial meniscus
  osteoarthritis, 408
Meniscus injury, knee arthroscopy, 420
Mesenchymal cell, fracture healing, 52
Metacarpal, 753–755
  2nd, 833
    extra-articular proximal metaphyseal
        fracture, 836
    intra-articular basilar fracture, 836
    neck fracture, 833–836
    spiral diaphyseal fracture, 836
    transverse diaphyseal fracture, 836
  3rd, 833
    extra-articular proximal metaphyseal
        fracture, 836
    intra-articular basilar fracture, 836
    neck fracture, 833–836
    spiral diaphyseal fracture, 836
    transverse diaphyseal fracture, 836
  3rd to 5th, overlap, 765

  4th, 836
    extra-articular proximal metaphyseal
        fracture, 837
    intra-articular basilar fracture, 836,
        837–840
    neck fractures, 836–837, 838
    spiral diaphyseal injury, 837, 839, 840
    transverse diaphyseal fracture, 837, 839
  5th, 810, 836
    extra-articular proximal metaphyseal
        fracture, 837
    intra-articular basilar fracture, 836,
        837–840
    neck fractures, 836–837, 838
    spiral diaphyseal injury, 837, 839, 840
    transverse diaphyseal fracture, 837, 839
Metacarpal base
  first, 778
    complex displaced intra-articular
        fracture, 835
  second, intra-articular fracture, 837
Metacarpal dislocation, fifth, 765
Metacarpal fracture, 830–840
  complications, 840
  fifth, Colles' fracture, 802
Metacarpal head, 755, 770
  avascular necrosis, 860–861
Metacarpophalangeal joint, 755, 766
  ligamentous support, 757
Metacarpophalangeal joint dislocation,
      840–843
  dorsal, 841, 842
  volar, 841–843
Metacarpophalangeal joint spacer
  hand, 866
  wrist, 866
Metacarpophalangeal ligament, 757
Metaphysis, 794
Metatarsal, 560
  1st, lateral displacement, 562
  2nd, lateral displacement, 562
  5th, fracture, 556
  proximal second, stress fracture, 43
Metatarsal base, 5th
  fracture, 565, 568
  normal epiphysis, 565
  normal physis, 565
  normal tuberosity, 565
Metatarsal fracture, 568–571
  proximal fifth, 566, 568
  radiography, 571
  second, 558
    healed, 564
  stress fracture, 884, 885
    treatment, 884
  treatment, 571
Metatarsal head, first, 481
Metatarsal neck, stress fracture, third, 884
Metatarsal phalangeal joint
  first, 481
  fourth, lateral dislocation, 568
Metatarsophalangeal joint dislocation, 571
Methacrylate, intertrochanteric fracture, 292,
      293
Methyl methacrylate cement, femoral shaft
      fracture, 326
Metrizamide, myelography, 29
Microfracture, 40

Midcarpal articulation, 749
Midcarpal joint
　dorsal dislocation, 774
　scapholunate tear, 793
Midfoot, 464–465, 560
　lateral injury, 559
Midfoot fracture
　classification, 557
　isolated tarsal fracture, 557
　mechanism of injury, 557
　radiography, 557–560
　treatment, 560
Midfoot fracture-dislocation
　classification, 557
　isolated tarsal fracture, 557
　mechanism of injury, 557
　radiography, 557–560
　treatment, 560
Monteggia fracture, 39
Monteggia lesion, 725–728
　classification, 725, 726
　complications, 728
　mechanism of injury, 726
　radial head dislocation, 742, 743
　radiography, 726, 727
　results, 728
　treatment, 726, 727
　ulnar shaft fracture, 743
Moore prosthesis, avascular necrosis, 278
Muscle
　imaging, 87
　ultrasound, normal, 86
Muscle flap, osteomyelitis, 878
Musculocutaneous nerve, 659
Myelography, 28–30
　Amipaque, 29
　bone graft cervical fusion, 31
　contrast agents, 29
　disk herniation, 30
　indications, 30, 31
　Iophendylate, 29
　lumbar spine fracture, 21
　Metrizamide, 29
　nerve root, 30
　normal myelographic anatomy, 29–30
　Pantopaque, 29
　spinal canal, 30
　spinal cord, 29–30
　technique, 29
　thoracic spine, 30
Myeloma, intertrochanteric fracture, 292, 293
Myositis ossificans, 84
　imaging, 87

N
Navicular, 464
Navicular compression, calcaneal fracture,
　551
Navicular fat stripe
　scaphoid tubercle fracture, 814
　wrist, 773
Naviculocapitate syndrome, 824–826
Nerve injury, 84
Nerve root, myelography, 30
Non-union fracture
　ankle fracture, 521
　clavicle fracture, 648, 650

humeral shaft fracture, 666–670, 671
　callus, 671
　Hoffman apparatus, 671
　methyl-methacrylate, 672
　osteoporosis, 672
　plate fixation, 672
　Rush rod fixation, 672
　screw fixation, 672
　olecranon osteotomy, 724
　proximal humerus fracture, 636, 637, 638
　scaphoid, cystic, 787
　scaphoid fracture, 817–819, 820
　supracondylar fracture, 724
　talar neck fracture, 535
　ulna fracture, 724
Nucleus pulposus, 100

O
Oblique fracture, L2, 184
Obturator fat stripe displacement, 236
Obturator foramen, 209
Obturator internus, fat plane, 210
Obturator ring fracture, double, 235
Occipital-atlantal relationship, normal, 131
Occipital condyle, horizontal fracture, 130
Occipitocervical dislocation, management,
　163
Odontoid
　chronic changes, 145
　normal variants, 139, 144
　sclerosis, 141
Odontoid fracture, 136–145
　Anderson and D'Alonzo's classification,
　　138–145
　associated lower cervical spine fractures,
　　145, 147
　chip fracture, 145
　combination fracture, 145, 146
　computed tomography, type II, 120
　management, 164
　retropharyngeal soft tissue swelling, 138
　skull fracture, 145, 146
　tomography, type II, 120
　type I, 138–140
　type II, 138–142
　　comminuted, 142
　　sclerotic margins, 141
　　ununited, 141
　type III, 138, 139, 142–144
　　anteriorly displaced, 143
　　undisplaced, 142
　　ununited, 144
　variations, 145, 146
Olecranon, 677, 685
　articular cartilage, 678
　posterior bony landmarks, 702
Olecranon fossa, 685, 699
　fixation devices, 707
Olecranon fracture, 718–721
　classification, 718, 719
　comminuted, 720
　displaced
　　complications, 723
　　intramedullary fixation, 721
　　results, 723
　　tension band wiring, 721
　　treatment, 721–723

mechanism, 718
　radiography, 718, 721
　treatment, 718–721
Olecranon osteotomy
　non-union, 724
　supracondylar fracture, 724
Operative fixation, indications, 69
Os odontoideum, 139–145
Os supranaviculare, 468
Os supratrochlear dorsale, 692
Ossicle
　malleolus, 466
　normal, 233
Osteoarthritis
　ankle, 524
　ankle fracture, 521
　articular cartilage, 408
　glenohumeral joint, 589, 632
　joint space, 408
　loose body, 421
　meniscus, 408
　patellar fracture, 366–367
　shoulder, 589, 632
Osteochondral compression fracture,
　comminuted, 537
Osteochondral defect, medial condyle, 348
Osteochondral fracture, 363, 632
　lateral femoral condyle, 364
　patella, 421
Osteochondritis dissecans, 413
　hip arthrography, 298
　knee arthroscopy, 422, 423
Osteogenic cell, fracture healing, 52
Osteogenic cell differentiation
　biologic factors, 53
　mechanical factors, 53
Osteoid osteoma, 605
Osteology
　clavicle, 579, 580
　hand, 749–755
　humerus, 582
　scapula, 579–582
　wrist, 749–755
Osteolysis, post-traumatic, 651
Osteomyelitis
　ankle, 872
　classification, 871
　edema, 876
　etiology, 871
　femur, 876
　fibia fracture, 872
　fracture calcaneus, 875
　imaging, post-traumatic, 871–877
　magnetic resonance imaging, 632
　muscle flap, 878
　pathogens, 871
　soft tissue edema, 876
　surgical reconstruction, 878–879
　tibial fracture, 872
Osteonecrosis, hip arthrography, 298
Osteoporosis, 246
　Sudeck's atrophy, 802
Osteotomy
　hand, 861, 862
　wrist, 861, 862
Overlapping pisiform, 751
Oxidative metabolism, fracture healing, 51
Oxygen tension, fracture healing, 51

P

Palmar articular surface, 794
Palmar recess, 794
Pantopaque, myelography, 29
Paraspinal soft tissue, 116, 117
Patella. *See also* Knee
    biomechanics, 353–355
    bipartate, 365
    double contrast arthrogram, 397
    fragmentation, 353, 354
    knee flexion, 358
    osteochondral fracture, 421
    shapes, 353, 354
    stabilizers, 353
    vascular supply, 353
Patella alta, 356
Patella infra, 356
Patellar dislocation, 362–363
    chronic recurrent lateral, 361
    factors predisposing, 362
    natural history, 362–363
    treatment, 363
Patellar disorder, 352–363
    knee arthroscopy, 423–424
Patellar displacement, lateral, assessment, 359
Patellar facet, patellofemoral pain, 413
Patellar fracture, 364–367
    avascular necrosis, 367
    comminuted, 365
    displaced transverse, 364
    modified tension band technique, 366, 367
    osteoarthritis, 366–367
    patellectomy, 367
    treatment, 365–336
    treatment results, 366–367
    types, 364
Patellar instability, 362–363
    factors predisposing, 362
Patellar ligament, magnetic resonance
        imaging, 411, 412
Patellar subluxation, 359, 362–363
    factors predisposing, 362
    natural history, 362–363
    recurrent, 362
        pathologic changes, 362
    treatment, 363
Patellar tracking disorder, 413–414
Patellectomy
    partial, 367
    patellar fracture, 367
    total, 367
Patellofemoral angle, lateral, 358
Patellofemoral arthralgia, 359
Patellofemoral contact annex, 353, 354
Patellofemoral index, 358
Patellofemoral joint
    anatomy, 353
    examination, 353–359
    radiography, 355–359
Patellofemoral pain
    etiology, 360–361
    medial femoral condyle, 413
    patellar facet, 413
    surgical treatment, 361–362
    treatment, 361
Patellofemoral pain syndrome, 359–362
Patellofemoral relationship, 356

Pathologic fracture, 42, 43
    femur, 43
Pedicle, 93, 95
Pedicle fracture, 147
    C5, 152, 153
    L5 facet, 185
    vertebral arch fracture, 152
Pedicle stress fracture, 893
Pelvic fracture, 226, 227–260
    abdomen injury, 258–260
    adjacent fractures, 253, 255
    angiography, 27
    anterior compression injury, 228, 230
    avulsion fracture, 232
    bladder rupture, 259
    chest injury, 258–260
    class I, 228–236
        treatment, 244–246
    class II, 236–238
        treatment, 246
    class III, 238–240
        treatment, 246–247, 248
    class IV, 240–244, 245
        treatment, 247–252
    classification, 228–231
    complex, 239, 244, 245, 248
        age distribution, 228
        etiology, 227
        mortality rate, 227
    complications, 252–260
        delayed, 260
    Connally-Hedberg classification, 228
    distant fractures, 253, 255
    genitourinary injury, 253–258, 259
        bladder injuries, 256–258, 259
        classification for urethral injuries, 256,
            257
        urethra, 253, 257, 258
    head injury, 258–260
    hemorrhage, 227
    Key and Conwell classification: Kane
            modification, 231
    neurologic complications, 253, 256
    pelvic hemorrhage, 252–253, 254
        angiographic embolization, 253
    radiography, 27
    sacral fracture, 256
    severe compound, 252
    severity, 227
    shear injury, 228–231
    stress fracture, 890–891, 892
    Tile-Pennal classification, 228
    treatment, 244–252
    unstable, 246, 247
    vertical shearing forces, 255
    Watson-Jones classification, 228
Pelvic hemorrhage, pelvic fracture, 252–253,
        254
    angiographic embolization, 253
Pelvis, 314
    anatomy, 207–216
    bone scanning, 17
    computed tomography, 226–227, 305
    ilium, 207–209
    imaging, 216–227
    innominate bone, 207–209
    ischium, 207–209

    ligament, 210–213
        anterior, 210, 211
        articulations, 210–213
        motion, 210
        posterior, 210, 211
        type, 210
    magnetic resonance imaging, 305
    neuroanatomy, 214, 216
    normal, 218
    periarticular anatomy, 210, 213
    pubis, 207–209
    radiography, 216–222
        AP angled views, 219, 220
        AP view, 216–219
        lateral view, 219–222
    skeletal anatomy, 207–210
    skeletal scintigraphy, 17
    soft tissue injury, 294
        arthrography, 294–305
    ultrasonography, 305
    vascular anatomy, 213–216
Periarticular anatomy
    hip, 210, 213
    pelvis, 210, 213
Periarticular disorder, knee
    arthrography, 389–417
    imaging, 389–424
Periarticular tendon snapping syndrome, 415
Pericapsular fat plane, 213
Perilunate dislocation, with multiple
        fracture, 828
Periosteal callus
    fracture healing, 52
    intramedullary nail fixation, 63–64
Periosteal vessel, 436
Periosteum cambrum layer, fracture healing,
        52
Peroneal artery, 436
    occlusion, 526
Peroneal nerve, 436
Peroneal tendon dislocation, 497
Peroneal tendon injury, 496–499
    treatment, 499
Peroneal tendon rupture, 497–499
Peroneal tendon sheath, 491
Peroneus tertius muscle, 457–458
Pes anserine bursitis, 415, 416
Pes anserinus muscle, 340–341
Phalangeal fracture, 568–571, 843–851, 851
    distal phalanx, 849, 849–851
    middle phalanx, 846–849
        dorsal lip proximal base fracture,
            847–849
        volar lip proximal base fracture, 846–849
    proximal phalanx, 843–846
        distal fractures, 843–844
        proximal fracture, 845–846
    radiography, 571
    stress fracture, 997
    third proximal, 567
    treatment, 571
Phalanx
    middle, 755
        dislocation, 45
    radiography
        axial calcaneal view, 478–479
        lateral calcaneal view, 479

lateral view, 476, 477
oblique view, 476, 477
sesamoid views, 479, 481
subtalar views, 479, 480
third to fifth, overlap, 765
turret exostosis, 859
Phosphor material
light color, 3
system speed, 3
Physeal fracture, 40
Pia mater, 103
Piedmont fracture, 808–810
classification, 808
complications, 810
mechanism of injury, 808
treatment, 808–810
Pigmented villonodular synovitis, joint
capsule, 422
Pillar fracture, 152–155
asymmetry, 153
C6, 152, 154
non-union, 250
radiographic signs, 154, 155
types, 153
Pilon fracture, 506
Pin tract infection, tibia, 873
ring sequestra, 873
Pisiform, 777, 778
Pisiform fracture, 821, 823
Pisiform injury, 821, 823
Pisiform-triquetral articulation, 775
Pisotriquetral joint, 792
Planography, 7
Plantar dislocation, cuboid, 559
Plantar fascitis, 505
Plantar flexion, 465
Plantar interosseous muscle, 460
Plantaris muscle, 451–455
Plantaris muscle tear, hematoma, 89
Plate fixation
calcaneal fracture, 554–555
femoral shaft fracture, 320–326
humeral shaft fracture, 669
Plicae, knee arthroscopy, 420
Pneumothorax, 647
Popliteal artery occlusion, fibula fracture,
447, 449
Popliteal cyst, ultrasound, 15, 16
Popliteus muscle, 452–456
Post-traumatic infection, imaging, 871–879
Post-traumatic joint disease, hip
arthrography, 296
Post-traumatic syrinx, spinal cord, 122
Posterior acetabular fragment, femur
abduction, 241
adduction, 241
Posterior arch, management, 163–164
Posterior arch fracture, 132, 181
Posterior column fracture, 241, 242
Posterior decompression, 187
Posterior ligament injury, 157–159, 160
Posterior longitudinal ligament, 100, 101
Posterior margin fracture
classification, 181
type II, 182
Posterior neural arch, 93, 94

Posterior pillar
arthritis, 250
non-union, 250
Posterior pillar fracture, non-union, 250
Posterior tibial artery, occlusion, 526
Posterior tibial avulsion fracture, 519
Posterior tibial tendon injury, 501
treatment, 501–505
Posterior tibial tendon, normal, 503
Posterior tibial tendon tear, 504
Posterolateral compartment, loose body, 419
Posteromedial rotatory instability, 384–386
Pott's fracture, 506, 511
Pre-styloid recess, 792
Preiser's disease, 857
Prevertebral fat stripe, 106, 107
Profunda brachii artery, 663
Pronation, 466
Pronator fat stripe
chauffeur's fracture, 808
radial fracture, 774
scaphoid tubercle fracture, 814
Prostate, 215, 216
Prosthesis, avascular necrosis, 278
Proximal humeral fracture, 635–639
classification, 636
complications, 636
four major anatomic fragments, 635
greater tuberosity, 636
humeral head, 636
incidence, 636
lesser tuberosity, 636
malunion, 636, 637, 638
non-union, 636, 637, 638
Rush rod, 637
Proximal phalanx, 755
Proximal radius fracture, 712–717, 810
classification, 712–716
complications, 717
mechanism of injury, 712
radiography, 712–716
results, 717
treatment, 712–717
Proximal tibiofibular joint, pain, 417
Pseudarthrosis, 195
ankylosing spondylitis, 201
fracture non-union, 71
Pubic bone, 209
Pubic insufficiency fracture, 892
Pubic ramus fracture, 219, 228–229, 234, 267
inferior, 232, 234
stress fracture, 246
superior, 232
transverse, 232
Pubic symphysis, 209, 217
hip arthrography, 303, 304–305
injection technique, 303
Pubic symphysis diastasis, 238, 248
Pulmonary contusion, 647

Q
Q-angle, measurement, 355
Quadratus plantae muscle, 459
Quadricep injury, 329, 330
Quadriceps muscle, 340

Quadriceps tendon ligament, magnetic
resonance imaging, 411, 412
Quadriceps tendon tear, 412

R
Radial collateral ligament, ultrasound, 14
Radial deviation, 781
Radial diaphysis, 809
Radial fragment, 740
Radial head, 684
anterior dislocation, 727
dislocation, Monteggia lesion, 742, 743
resection, 718
Radial head fracture, 40
comminuted, 716
impacted, 714
internal fixation, 717
posterolateral dislocation, 697
Type I, 713
Type II, 713, 715
Type III, 713
Type IV, 713
undisplaced, 713
Radial head fracture-dislocation, 716
Radial head fragment, displacement, 697
Radial length, Colles' fracture, 802
Radial nerve, 659
Radial shaft fracture, 40
Galeazzi fracture, 742–743, 744
minimally displaced, 739
Radial styloid fracture, 782, 807–808
arthritis, 821
chip fracture, 776
classification, 807
complications, 808
mechanism of injury, 807
scaphoid fracture, 817
soft tissue swelling, 776
treatment, 807–808
Radial tear, meniscus, 401
Radial tuberosity, 740
Radiation protection, radiography, 7
Radiocapitate ligament, 756
Radiocapitellar alignment, 683
Radiocapitellar articulation, 685
Radiocapitellar relationship, 686
Radiocarpal articulation, 749
Radiocarpal dislocation, 811
Radiocarpal joint, 792, 799, 861
radial fracture, 798
ulnar pain, 793
wrist pain, 793
Radiographic magnification unit, 11
Radiographic trauma unit, 2
Radiography, 107. See also Magnification
radiology
acromioclavicular joint, 592, 593, 594
ankle, 468–469
AP view, 468
lateral view, 469
mortise view, 470
oblique views, 470, 471
stress views, 470–475
ankle fracture, 518–519
bicipital groove, 597, 598, 599
calcaneal fracture, 547–552, 553

Radiography, (*contd.*)
  calf fracture, 438–439
  capitellar fracture, 708, 709
  cervical spine trauma, 104–115
    AP view, 109–111
    flexion/extension view, 113–115
    lateral, 104, 105–109, 110
    oblique views, 111, 112, 113
    odontoid view, 112
    pillar views, 112–113, 114
  clavicle, 592–595, 596
    AP views, 592–595
    oblique view, 595, 596
  clavicle fracture, 647
  coronoid fracture, 725
  elbow, 680–687
    AP view, 680, 681
    assessment, 685–687
    axial views, 682–685
    lateral view, 680–682, 683
    oblique views, 682, 683, 684
    radial head view, 682, 684
    stress views, 687
  equipment, 2–3
  exposure factors, 3–5
  exposure times, 7
  fibula fracture, 438–439
  film labeling, 7
  focal spot, 5, 7
  foot, 475–476
    AP view, 474, 475–476
    lateral view, 475
    oblique view, 475, 476
  forearm, 734–736
  fracture, 43–46
  fracture-dislocation, 43–46
  hand, 763–764
    Brewerton view, 767, 770
    Burman view, 767, 771
    finger, 764–767
    lateral view, 764, 766, 771, 774, 775
    oblique view, 764, 765, 771–776
    PA views, 763–764, 765
    stress views, 767, 772
  Heinig view, 598
  Hill-Sachs lesion, 599, 600
  hip, 216–227, 222–227
    AP view, 222
    judet view, 223, 224
    lateral view, 224–225
    oblique view, 217, 225
  humeral shaft fracture, 666, 667
  knee, 344–352
    AP view, 344, 345
    electronic pressure indicator, 351
    lateral view, 344–346, 347
    normal, 344
    notch view, 348, 350
    oblique view, 346–350
    patellar views, 349, 350
    Settegast technique, 349
    stress views, 350–352
    valgus stress view, 351
    varus view, 351
  Lisfranc injury, 563–568
  lumbar spine, 115–119
    vertebral bodies, 115

  metatarsal fracture, 571
  midfoot fracture, 557–560
  midfoot fracture-dislocation, 557–560
  Monteggia lesion, 726, 727
  olecranon fracture, 718, 721
  patellofemoral joint, 355–359
  pelvic fracture, 27
  pelvis, 216–222
    AP angled views, 219, 220
    AP view, 216–219
    lateral view, 219–222
  phalanageal fracture, 571
  phalanx
    axial calcaneal view, 478–479
    lateral calcaneal view, 479
    lateral view, 476, 477
    oblique view, 476, 477
    sesamoid views, 479, 481
    subtalar views, 479, 480
  post-reduction interpretation, 45–46
  proximal radius fracture, 712–716
  radiation protection, 7
  radius, 734–736
  rotator cuff tear, 607
    chronic, 609
  scapula, 590–592
    AP view, 590, 591
    lateral view, 590–592
  shoulder, 586–605
    acromial changes, 601, 603
    AP views, 587, 588
    apical oblique view, 601, 602
    axillary view, 590, 591
    impingement, 601, 602
    posterior oblique view, 587, 589
    scapular Y-view, 587, 590
    standard projections, 587, 588
    Stryker notch view, 599–601
    transthoracic lateral view, 587–590
    West Point view, 600
  sternoclavicular joint, 595–597, 598
  T and Y condylar fracture, 705–706
  tarso-metatarsal fracture-dislocation, 563–568
  thoracic spine, 115–119
    vertebral bodies, 115
  thumb, 767, 769
  tibia fracture, 438–439
  ulna, 734–736
  ulna fracture, 718, 721
  wrist
    carpal tunnel view, 776, 778
    dorsal tangential view, 776, 779
    PA view, 767–771, 774
    pisiform view, 776, 777
    scaphoid view, 776
Radiolunotriquetral ligament, 756
Radionuclide imaging
  hand, 779–782, 784
  spine, 123
  wrist, 779–782, 784
Radioscaphoid impingement, scaphoid fracture, 819
Radioscapholunate ligament, 756
Radioulnar articulation, 684
Radioulnar joint, 774, 791
  distal, evaluation criteria, 783

  ulnar pain, 793
  wrist pain, 793
Radioulnar joint fracture, 782
Radius, 731, 731–747
  anatomy, 731–736
  humerus, 696
  lunate, 829
  normal neck-shaft angles, 712
  proximal, 677
  radiography, 734–736
  soft tissue injury, 646
  ulna, 696
    enface, 750
    pronation, 734
    supination, 734
Radius fracture. *See also* Specific type
  bowing fracture, 41
  complications, 743–747
  cross-union, 745–747
  distal, 775
  distal fragment pronation, 741
  management, 737–743
  moderately displaced, 741
  pronator fat stripe, 774
    displaced, 775
  proximal. *See* Proximal radius fracture
  proximal shaft, 745
  radiocarpal joint, 798
  subtle, 775
  synostosis, 745
  torus fracture, 40, 41
  undisplaced, 739
Ramus fracture, lateral compression injury, 228, 230
Real-time scanner, 12–13
Rectum, 215, 216
Reflex sympathetic dystrophy, ankle fracture, 521
Reno-M-60, contrast material, 33
Renografin-60, contrast material, 33
Retrolisthesis, 198
Retropharyngeal soft tissue swelling, odontoid fracture, 138
Reverse Monteggia fracture, 742
Rhabdomyolysis, 84
  imaging, 87–90
  magnetic resonance imaging, 90
Rheumatoid arthritis, ultrasound, 15, 16
Richard's screw-plate, femur, 292
Ridge fracture, trapezium fracture, 827
Rotary fixation, Fielding-Hawkins classification, 135, 136
Rotation, external, 466
Rotator cuff
  calcification, 610
  muscles, 583
Rotator cuff tear, 610, 612
  bursography, 625
  radiography, 607
    chronic, 609
  shoulder arthrography, 608, 609, 614–616
Rush pin, femoral shaft fracture, 320
Rush rod
  proximal humerus fracture, 637
  trimalleolar fracture, 519, 521

S

Sacral insufficiency fracture, 892
Sacroiliac joint, hip arthrography, 303,
    304–305
  injection technique, 303
Sacrum, 94, 99–100, 210
  AP view, 119, 120
  lateral view, 119, 120
Sacrum fracture, 234, 236
  buckle fracture, 236
  lateral compression injury, 228, 230
  pelvic fracture, 256
  transverse fracture, 232
Sagittal fracture, vertebral body fracture, 157,
    158
Salter-Harris II fracture, tibia metaphysis, 42
Salter-Harris IV fracture, ankle, 42
Sartorius muscle, 340–341
Scaphoid, 751, 775, 780, 781
  avascular necrosis, 857
  dorsal portions, 779
  non-union, cystic, 787
Scaphoid tracture, 811–819, 820, 821
  arthritis, 821
  arthrosis, 819
  avascular necrosis, 819, 820
  capitate fracture, 826
  classification, 811–815
  complications, 817–819, 820, 821
  edema, 786
  Herbert screw, 817
  humpback deformity, 813, 818
  hyperemia, 786
  mechanism of injury, 815
  non-union, 817–819, 820
  osteochondral fragments, 816
  radial styloid, 817
  radioscaphoid impingement, 819
  Russe classification, 813, 814
  Russe II, 815, 816
  subtle, 786
  treatment, 815–817, 818
  volar flexion, 813
  zones, 813
Scaphoid tubercle fracture
  navicular fat stripe, 814
  pronator fat stripe, 814
Scaphoid waist, arthritis, 821
Scapholunate angle, 751, 753, 774
Scapholunate arthrodesis, screw fixation, 858
Scapholunate axis, normal, 752
Scapholunate dissociation, 791, 831, 857–858
Scapholunate joint
  scapholunate ligament tear, 861
  triangular, 858
Scapholunate ligament disruption, 792
Scapholunate ligament instability, chronic,
    792
Scapholunate ligament tear, 782
Scapholunate space
  triangular configuration, 792
  widened, 773
Scapholunate tear, midcarpal joint, 793
Scaphotrapezial, 775
Scaphotrapezial articulation, degenerative
    arthritis, 865

Scapula
  computed tomography, 606
  dorsal musculature, 581
  osteology, 579–582
  radiography, 590–592
    AP view, 590, 591
    lateral view, 590–592
  ventral musculature, 581
Scapula fracture, 650–653
  body, 651
  computed tomography, 606
  lower glenoid, 651
  neck, 651
Scapular spine
  humeral head, 643
  humerus, 643
Sciatic nerve, 213, 314
  hip dislocation, 269
  hip fracture-dislocation, 269
Sclerosis, ulnolunate abutment syndrome,
    855
Screen-film combination, 2–7
  body part, 3–6
  intensifying screen, 3
  manufacturing processes, 3
  patient size, 3–6
  relative speed index, 3
  selection, 2
Screw fixation
  calcaneal fracture, 554–555
  coracoclavicular ligament, 649
  humeral shaft fracture, 669
  scapholunate arthrodesis, 858
  talar fracture, 531
  talar neck fracture, 532
Seatbelt injury, 175, 177, 178
  vs. flexion-distraction injury, 175
Segond fracture, tibia, 376–377
Semimembranous bursa, enlarged, 398
Semimembranous muscle, sites of
    attachment, 340, 341
Semitendinosus muscle, 340–341
Sesamoid bone, 755
  stress fracture, 997
Sesamoid fracture, 481
Shear injury
  lumbar spine trauma, 181, 184
    management, 190–193
  pelvic fracture, 228–231
  thoracic spine trauma, 181, 184
    management, 190–193
Shepherd's fracture, 506, 511
Shoulder, 579–653
  anatomy, 579–586
  articular anatomy, 582–584
  Bankhart lesion, 620
  bicipital groove, 588
  biomechanics, 584–586
  computed tomography, 606–607
  dislocation, 620
    magnetic resonance imaging, 631
  displaced greater tuberosity fracture, 620
  greater tuberosity fracture, 634
  Hill-Sachs lesion, 604
  imaging techniques, 586–635
    compared, 630, 631

magnetic resonance imaging, 626–633
  applications, 628–633
  capsular abnormalities, 630–632
  image planes, 626, 627
  impingement syndrome, 628–630
  inflammatory disorders, 632–633
  osseous disorders, 633, 634
  patient positions, 626
  rotator cuff tear, 628–630
  techniques, 626, 628
  trauma, 628–630
neurovascular anatomy, 584, 585, 586
osteoarthritis, 589, 632
osteology, 579–582
radiography, 586–605
  acromial changes, 601, 603
  AP views, 587, 588
  apical oblique view, 601, 602
  axillary view, 590, 591
  impingement, 601, 602
  posterior oblique view, 587, 589
  scapular Y-view, 587, 590
  standard projections, 587, 588
  Stryker notch view, 599–601
  transthoracic lateral view, 587–590
  West Point view, 600
recurrent anterior dislocation, 604
superior dislocation, 643
tomography, 605
tuberosity, 588
ultrasonography, 605–606
Shoulder arthrography
  acromiohumeral distance, 608
  acromion, 608
  adhesive capsulitis, 616–617, 618
    axillary recess, 617
    subscapularis recess, 617
  complications, 624
  double-contrast examinations, 611, 612
  entry site, 611
  greater tuberosity, 608
  humeroacromial distance, 608
  indications, 607
  normal, 612–614
  pitfalls, 623–624
  radiographic technique, 611
  rotator cuff tear, 608, 609, 614–616
  single-contrast technique, 611, 612
  techniques, 611–612
Shoulder arthroscopy, 633–635
Shoulder bursa, 584
Shoulder capsule, magnetic resonance
    imaging, 630–632
Sigmoid notch, 749, 750
Sinus tarsi, 480
Skeletal scintigraphy, 16–19
  Anger-gamma camera, 17
  applications, 17
  bone vascularity, 18
  collimator, 17
  femoral head, 19
  femur, 19
  infection, 19
  instrumentation, 17
  pelvis, 17
  radiopharmaceuticals, 16–17
  tibia, 18

Skeletal scintigraphy, (contd.)
  tomogram, 17
  trauma, 17–18
  vs. pelvic x-ray, 17
  wrist, 17
Skull, retropharyngeal soft tissue, 107
Skull fracture, odontoid fracture, 145, 146
Smith fracture type, 802–804
  classification, 803, 804
  complications, 804
  juxta-articular, 803
  mechanism of injury, 803–804
  Thomas classification, 804
  treatment, 804
Snapping syndrome, knee, 415–417
Snapping tendon syndrome, hip
      arthrography, 299–303
Soft tissue edema, osteomyelitis, 876
Soft tissue infection, 877
Soft tissue injury, 83–90
  arm, 673
  calf, 450–451
  categories, 83–84
  classification, 84–85
  computed tomography, 305
  elbow, 696–701
  femur, 329–332
  fibula, 450–451
  healing, 85
    acute inflammatory phase, 85
    remodeling phase, 85
    reparative phase, 85
  hip, 294
    arthrography, 294–305
  humerus, 673
  imaging, 86–90
  knee, 379–389
  magnetic resonance imaging, 305
  overuse, 84, 85
  pelvis, 294
    arthrography, 294–305
  thigh, 329–332
  tibia, 450–451
  ultrasonography, 305
Soft tissue stabilization
  hand, 863
  wrist, 863
Soleus muscle, 451–455
  accessory, 455
  edema, 450, 451
Space of Poirier, 756
Spinal artery, 101
Spinal canal, myelography, 30
Spinal cord
  magnetic resonance imaging, 123
  myelography, 29–30
  normal, 186
  post-traumatic syrinx, 122
Spinal cord disruption, 169
Spinal nerve, 103
Spine, 93–201. See also Specific type
  anatomy, 93–103
  computed tomography, 119–121, 122
  imaging, complications following
      treatment, 194
  ligamentous anatomy, 100–101
  magnetic resonance imaging, 121–123

  neurovascular anatomy, 101–103
  osteology, 93–96
  radionuclide scanning, 123
  sprain, management, 165, 166
  stress fracture, 891
  three columns, 108, 109
  tomography, 119–121, 122
  trauma radiographic evaluation, 103–123
Spinous process, 107, 108
Spinous process fracture, 152, 153, 154
  C7, 153
Spiral diaphyseal fracture, 832, 836
Spiral diaphyseal injury, 837, 839, 840
Spondylolisthesis, 194–199
  etiology, 195
  grading system, 196, 197
  radiographic evaluation, 196–198
  treatment, 198–199
Spondylolysis, 194–199
  etiologic theories, 194–195
  L5 on S1 dislocation, 196
  radiographic evaluation, 196–198
  treatment, 198–199
Sprain, 84
  spine, management, 165, 166
Standing potential, 55
Steffee Plote, 194
Stellate fracture, 551
Sternoclavicular dislocation, 644–646
  anterior, 644–646
  classification, 646
  complications, 646
  posterior, 644–646
  treatment, 646
Sternoclavicular joint, 584
  normal, 648
  radiography, 595–597, 598
  subluxation, 648
Sternoclavicular lesion, computed
      tomography, 598, 606
Straddle fracture, 238, 239
Straight stem Moore prosthesis, avascular
      necrosis, 278
Strain, 84
Strain-generated potential, 55
Stratigraphy, 7
Stress fracture, 42, 43, 881–893
  anterior inferior iliac spine, 304
  classification, 882
  computed tomography, 883
  differential diagnosis, 882
  distal second metatarsal, 511
  distribution, 883–893
  etiology, 882
  femoral neck, 889–890, 891
  femoral neck fracture, 273, 274
  femoral shaft, 889, 890
  fibula, 889
  foot, 883–886
  location, 882
  magnetic resonance imaging, 883
  metatarsal neck, third, 884
  pelvis, 890–891, 892
  phalanx, 997
  physical examination, 881
  proximal second metatarsal, 43
  pubic ramus, 246

  radiography, 881–883
  related activity, 882
  sesamoid, 997
  spine, 891
  talus, 997
  tarsal navicular, 997
  tibia, 376–377
  tibial pain, 883
  treatment algorithm, 893
  upper-extremity, 891–893
Stress-generated potential, 55
Stryker notch view, 604
Styloid bone, 755
Subacromial bursa, bursography, 624
Subacromial spur, 602, 603
Subcapital fracture, 224
  hip, 44
Subcoracoid anterior dislocation, 639
Subluxation
  cervical spine, 45
  description, 45
  facet joint, lateral tomograms, 121, 122
Subscapularis, 613
Subscapularis bursa, 613
Subscapularis recess, 623
Subtalar dislocation, 544–546
  diagnosis, 544–546
  treatment, 546
Subtalar joint, 480
  calcaneal fracture, 552
  overlap, 475
  subluxation, 530
  talar fracture, 532
  talar neck fracture, 536
Subtalar joint arthrography, 487–488
Subtrochanteric fracture, 287–289, 314
  Boyd and Griffin classification, 287–289
  classifications, 287
  comminuted, 288
  complications, 289, 294
  Fielding classification, 287
  long side plate, 289
  Seinsheimer classification, 287, 289
  sliding screw, 289
  treatment, 293–294
  Zickel nail, 293
Subtrochanteric valgus osteotomy, femoral
      head fracture, 284
Sudeck's atrophy, 525
  hand, 802
  osteoporosis, 802
  wrist, 802
Sulcus angle, 358
Supination, 466
Supinator fat stripe, 686
Supracondylar bone, 675
Supracondylar fracture, 701–702
  classification, 701
  crossed K-wires, 702
  extension type, 701
  femur, 367–370
    classification, 367–368
    comminuted, 369
    internal fixation, 369–370
    open reduction, 369–370
    treatment, 368–370
  flexion-type, 701

mechanism of injury, 701
non-union, 724
olecranon osteotomy, 724
physical examination, 701–702
treatment, 702
Supracondylar process, 659, 662
Suprapatellar bursa, effusion, 346
Suprapatellar pouch, loose body, 421
Supraspinatous tendon, normal, 634
Supraspinatus outlet view, 603
Supratellar plicae, 414, 415
Sustentacular fragment, calcaneal fracture, 554–555
Sustentaculum, calcaneal fracture, 553
Syndesmosis ossification, ankle fracture, 525, 527
Syndesmosis screw, ankle fracture, 519, 520
Synostosis
    radius fracture, 745
    ulna fracture, 745
Synovial chondromatosis, hip arthrography, 298–299, 300
Synovial disease, knee, 400
Synovial disorder, knee arthroscopy, 423, 424
Synovial fold, knee arthroscopy, 420
Synovial plica, knee, 414
Synovitis, arthritis, 623
Synovium, arthrography, 620–623
System speed, phosphor material, 3

T
T and Y condylar fracture, 704–707
    classification, 704–705
    clinical evaluation, 705
    complications, 706–707
    mechanism of injury, 704
    radiography, 705–706
    treatment, 706
T1
    C7, difference in size, 105
    swimmer's views, 108–109, 110
T3
    anterior compression fracture, 171
    compression, 172
T4
    anterior compression fracture, 171
    compression, 172
    wedge fracture, 173
T4-T5 fracture subluxation
    computed tomography, 122
    tomography, 122
T5 on T6, anterior subluxation, 116
T6, paraplegia, 193
T6 on T7 dislocation, 193
T9, complete neurological deficit, 193
T12
    burst fracture, 116
    compression, 183
    compression fracture, 194
Talar body fracture, 537–538
    types, 537
Talar dislocation, 544–546
    diagnosis, 544–546
    talar dome, 545
    talectomy, 545
    treatment, 546

Talar dome, 470
    talar dislocation, 545
Talar dome fracture, 538–544
    ankle sprain, 543
    classification, 541
    complications, 542–544
    diagnosis, 541–543
    etiology, 538
    mechanism of injury
        lateral, 540, 541
        medial, 540
    medial, 544
    treatment, 542
Talar fracture
    comminuted, 507
    displaced, 531
    K-wire fixation, 531
    screw fixation, 531
    subtalar dislocation, 531
    subtalar joint, 532
    type, 529
Talar fracture-dislocation, 529
Talar head fracture, 537–538
Talar neck fracture, 527–537
    arthritis, 533, 535
    arthrodesis, 536
    avascular necrosis, 530–535
    bone graft, 536
    classification, 527
    comminuted, 530
    complications, 530–537
    Hawkins Type I, 529
    incidence, 529
    malunion, 535
    management, 527, 530, 531
    medial malleolar fracture, 534
    non-union, 535
    radiographic diagnosis, 527–530
    screw fixation, 532
    subtalar joint, 536
    tibiotalar joint, 536
    types, 527, 529
Talar neck fracture-dislocation
    incidence, 529
    type, 529
Talar process fracture, 537–538
Talar shift, ankle, 495
Talectomy, talar dislocation, 545
Talocalcaneal joint, posterior aspect, 480
Talonavicular joint, subluxation, 530
Talonavicular joint fracture-dislocation, 507 558
Talus, 463–464, 525–527
    avascular necrosis, 523
    blood supply, 528
    stress fracture, 997
Tarsal fracture, 557
Tarsal joint, overlap, 474
Tarsal joint arthrogram, 487–488
Tarsal navicular, stress fracture, 997
Tarsometatarsal fracture-dislocation, 560–568
    complications, 568
    radiography, 563–568
    treatment, 568

Tarsometatarsal joint
    bony anatomy, 561
    ligamentous anatomy, 561
Teardrop fracture, vertebral body fracture, 156, 157
Tendon
    hand, 760
    imaging, 87
    ultrasound, normal, 86
    wrist, 760
Tendon injury
    ankle, 495–505
    elbow, 700–701
    foot, 495–505
Tendon sheath
    hand, 760
    wrist, 760
Tenography, 490
    ankle sprain, 495
    anterior tendon, 492
    aspirations, 492
    diagnostic injection, 492
    indications, 492
    lateral tendon, 490–491
    medial tendon, 491–492
    normal anatomy, 490–492
    technique, 490–492
Tenosynovitis, 84
Thenar eminence, 759–760, 761, 795
Thigh, 311–332
    anatomy, 311–314
    compartment syndrome, 329–332
    fascial compartments, 311, 313
    hematoma, 89
    hemorrhage, 87, 88
    magnetic resonance imaging, post-traumatic hematoma, 25
    overuse syndrome, 331
    soft tissue injury, 329–332
Thigh abscess, 877
Thigh pain, chronic, 327
Thoracic aorta, tear, 193
Thoracic compression fracture, 173
Thoracic dislocation, 184
Thoracic fracture
    computed tomography, 122
    tomography, 122
Thoracic fusion, 195
Thoracic spine
    compression fracture, 43
    cross-table technique, 115, 116
    hyperflexion
        force axis, 171
        posterior complex distraction, 173
        thoracolumbar junction, 173–175
        wedge fractures, 171–173, 174, 175
    kyphotic curve, 169
    myelography, 30
    radiography, 115–119
    vertebral bodies, 115
Thoracic spine trauma, 169–194
    bursting fracture, management, 188–190, 191–192
    flexion-rotation injury, 178, 179, 180
        management, 186–188
    fusion complications, 190–194, 195
    hyperextension injury, 179–181, 184

Thoracic spine trauma, (contd.)
  management, 185–194
  mechanism of injury, 170–185
  shear injury, 181, 184
    management, 190–193
  vertical compression injury, 178–179, 181, 182, 183
Thoracic vertebra, 94, 95, 99
Thoracolumbar fracture, cervical spine trauma, 162
Thoracolumbar junction, columns, 171
Thumb, 769, 830
  extra-articular proximal metaphyseal fracture, 832
  intra-articular basilar fracture, 832–833, 834, 835
  neck fractures, 832
  radiography, 767, 769
  spiral diaphyseal fracture, 832
  transverse diaphyseal fracture, 832
Tibia, 433–451
  anatomy, 433–435
  blood-supply systems, 436
  bone scanning, 18
  fracture non-union, 73
  hypertrophic non-union, 76, 77
  musculoskeletal anatomy, 434, 435
  pin tract infection, ring sequestra, 873
  skeletal scintigraphy, 18
  soft tissue injury, 450–451
  tomography, 10
  traction pin, 319
Tibia fracture. See also Specific type
  AO plate and screw, 443
  avulsion fracture, 376–377
  bone porosity, 60
  classification, 437–438
  comminuted, 439, 440, 441
  complications, 447–450
  cortical fracture, 42
  distal, 440, 442
  external fixation, 482
  Fischer apparatus, 440, 443
  internal fixation, 482
  intramedullary nailing, 443, 444
  ipsilateral fracture, 377–379
    classifications, 377, 379
    treatment, 377
  management, 439–447
  mechanism of injury, 437–438
  medullary rod, 445
  minor, 437
  non-union, 447
  osteomyelitis, 872
  prognosis, 446–447
  radiography, 438–439
  Segond fracture, 376–377
Tibia metaphysis, Salter-Harris II fracture, 42
Tibial artery, posterior, 436
Tibial avulsion fracture, anterior cruciate ligament, 382
Tibial condyle fracture, 370–377
  associated injuries, 370
  classification, 370–372
  diagnosis, 370
  incidence, 372

lateral instability in extension, 373–374
  management, 372
  mechanism of injury, 372, 373
  meniscus tear, 370
  nonoperative treatment, 372–373
  operative treatment, 373–376
  permanent disability, 373
  treatment, 370
Tibial diaphysis, circulation, 48
Tibial marrow fracture, 42
Tibial nerve, 436
Tibial pain, stress fracture, 883
Tibial plafond fracture, 517–518, 522
  arthrodesis, 521
  K-wire reduction, 523
  Ovadia classification, 517–518
  treatment, 521
Tibial plateau fracture, classification, 370, 372
Tibial screws, trimalleolar fracture, 519, 521
Tibial stress fracture, 376–377, 886–889
  magnetic resonance imaging, 26
Tibialis anterior muscle, 457–458
Tibialis posterior muscle, 452–456
Tibiofibular articulation, 347
Tibiofibular syndesmosis, 433
Tibiofibular synovial joint, 433
Tibiotalar joint, 472
  talar neck fracture, 536
Tillaux fracture, 506, 511
Toe, overlap, 477
Tomography, 7–11. See also Computed tomography
  ankle, 479–482
    motion artifact, 479–482
  blurring, 7–8, 9
  bone graft cervical fusion, 31
  Chance fracture, 11
  commonly used motions, 7, 8
    orthopedic tomography, 8–9, 10, 11
  equipment, 7
  fibula, 10
  hand, 777–778, 782
  Kermath Versitome system, 2, 8–9
  linear, 7, 8
  lumbar spine, 11
  odontoid fracture, type II, 120
  orthopedic indications, 8
  section thickness, 7–8
  shoulder, 605
  spine, 119–121, 122
  T4-T5 fracture subluxation, 122
  thoracic fracture, 122
  tibia, 10
  vs. computed tomography, 120–121
  wrist, 777–778, 782
Torus fracture, 40, 236
  radius, 40, 41
  wrist, 40, 41
Trabecular compression, 714
Trabecular sclerosis, 888
Trachea, normal, 648
Traction
  carpal joint space, 801
  Colles' fracture, 801
  femoral shaft fracture, 318–319, 321

Traction pin, tibia, 319
Transcaphoid perilunate dislocation, 827–828, 829
  K wire, 829
Transcondylar fracture, 701–702
  classification, 701
  mechanism of injury, 701
  physical examination, 701–702
  treatment, 702
Transducer, 12
Transmission ultrasonography, 13
Transverse acetabular fracture, 241, 243
  undisplaced, 241–243
Transverse diaphyseal fracture, 832, 836, 837, 839
Transverse fracture
  inferior pubic ramus, 232
  L2 lamina, 177
  L2 pedicle, 177
  sacrum, 232
  superior pubic ramus, 232
Transverse ligament tear management, 164
Transverse process, 93
  overlapping, 156
Transverse process fracture, 155, 156, 181, 185
  multiple, 185
Trapezium, 778
Trapezium fracture, 782, 831
  ridge fracture, 827
  undisplaced, 826
Trapezium injury, 826–827
Trapezoid, 751, 753
Trapezoid fracture, 826
Trapezoid injury, 826
Traumatic spondylolisthesis
  axis, 147
  Effendi type I, 149
Triangular cartilage tear, 793
Triangular fibrocartilage complex, 755–756
Triangular fibrocartilage complex disorder, 852–854
Triangular fibrocartilage complex tear, 788, 852–854
Triangular fracture, vertebral body fracture, 156, 157
Triceps avulsion, 700
Trimalleolar fracture
  internal fixation, 519–521
  Rush rod, 519, 521
  tibial screws, 519, 521
Triquetrum, 751
  dorsal portions, 779
Triquetrum fracture, 822
  chip, 805
Triquetrum injury, 819–821, 822
Trochanteric fracture, 284–294. See also Specific type
  classification, 284–289
  complications, 294
  treatment, 289–294
Trochlea, 683, 685
  fragmentation, 532
Trochlear sulcus, 683
Tuft fracture, 849
Turret exostosis, phalanx, 859

U

Ulna, 677, 699, 731, 731–747, 750
  anatomy, 731–736
  bowing fracture, 41
  degenerative cyst, 693
  greenstick fracture, 40, 41
  humerus, 696
  radiography, 734–736
  radius, 696
    pronation, 734
    supination, 734
  radius enface, 750
  soft tissue injury, 646
Ulna fracture, 718–721, 799
  bridging callus, 746
  classification, 718, 719
  comminuted, 722, 727
  complications, 743–747
  compression screw, 724
  cross-union, 745–747
  displaced, 722
  distal fragment pronation, 741
  linear component, 722
  management, 737–743
  mechanism, 718
  medial head fracture, 722
  moderately displaced, 741
  non-union, 724
  proximal shaft, 745
  radiography, 718, 721
  segmental, 727
  synostosis, 745
  treatment, 718–721
  undisplaced, 739
Ulnar articulation, 677
Ulnar capsular tear, 795
Ulnar collateral ligament, ultrasound, 14
Ulnar collateral ligament tear, 795
Ulnar deviation, 781
Ulnar nerve, 663, 761
Ulnar pain, 796
  radiocarpal joint, 793
  radioulnar joint, 793
Ulnar shaft fracture, Monteggia lesion, 743
Ulnar styloid fracture, 782
Ulnar styloid tendon sheath, 796
Ulnar sulcus articulation, 685
Ulnar tilt, Colles' fracture, 802
Ulnar trochlear articulation, 685
Ulnar variance, 750, 864
  negative, 750
  neutral, 750
  positive, 750
Ulnocarpal articulation, 755–756
Ulnohumeral joint fracture-dislocation, 716
Ulnolunate abutment syndrome, 852–853
  cystic changes, 855
  sclerosis, 855
Ulnotriquetral ligament, 756
Ultrasound, 12–16
  abductor digiti minimi fascia, 14
  Achilles tendon, 483
    normal, 86
  ankle, 482–483
  enhanced through-transmission, 14
  extensor muscle, 14

fluid vs. solid tissue, 13–14, 15
  hematoma, 86, 87
  hip, 305
  interosseous fascia, 14
  knee, 401
  muscle, normal, 86
  musculoskeletal applications, 13–16
  orthopedic applications, 13–16
  pelvis, 305
  popliteal cyst, 15, 16
  popliteal fossa, 14–15
  radial collateral ligament, 14
  real-time scanner, 12–13
  rheumatoid arthritis, 15, 16
  shoulder, 605–606
  soft tissue injury, 305
  tendon, normal, 86
  transducer, 12
  ulnar collateral ligament, 14
Uncinate process fracture, vertebral body
    fracture, 156–157
Unichondylar fracture, 843
Upper thoracic spine, hangman's fracture,
    150, 151
Upper thoracic spine fracture, 176
Urethra, 215, 216
Urethra injury, 253, 257, 258
  classification, 257
  fistula, 258
Urethral rupture, 258

V

Valgus, 466
Valgus stress, cruciate ligament, 339
Valgus stress view, 472
Varus, 466
Varus stress view, 472
  ankle, 494
Vascular injury, femoral shaft fracture, 327
Vascular supply, bone, 47–48
  anastomosis, 47–48
  cortical venous channels, 47
  emissary veins, 47
  metaphyseal arteries, 47
  nutrient artery, 47
  periosteal arteries, 47
  periosteal capillaries, 47
  vena comitans, 47
  venous drainage, 47
Venous plexus, 103
Vertebra, 93, 94. *See also* Specific type
  arterial anatomy, 101–103, 104
  ossification centers, 94
  unfused ossification, 93, 94
  venous anatomy, 101–103, 104
Vertebral arch fracture, 151–155
  facet fracture, 155
  incidence, 151
  location, 151
  pedicle fracture, 152
Vertebral artery, 101
Vertebral body, 93, 95
Vertebral body compression, 177
Vertebral body fracture, 155–157
  anterior inferior chip fracture, 161

burst fracture, 156, 157
  chip fracture, 156
  compression fracture, 156, 157
  incidence, 155, 156
  location, 155, 156
  management, 169, 170
  radiographic presentation, 155–156
  sagittal fracture, 157, 158
  teardrop fracture, 156, 157
  triangular fracture, 156, 157
  uncinate process fracture, 156–157
  wedge fracture, 156, 157
Vertebral disk. *See* Disk
Vertebral foramen, 103
Vertical cleft fracture, 244, 245
Vertical compression injury
  cervical spine trauma, 124, 128–129
  lumbar spine trauma, 178–179, 181, 182,
    183
  thoracic spine trauma, 178–179, 181, 182,
    183
Vertical tear, meniscus, 402
Vesicorectal pouch, 215, 216
Volar lip fracture, 851
Volar lip proximal base fracture, 846–847,
    848
Volar lunate dislocation, 828, 829
Volar perilunate dislocation, 828
Volar plate, 757, 794
Volar plate fracture, 768, 851
Volar proximal interphalangeal joint
    dislocation, 852
Volar radial recess
Volkmann's canal, fracture healing, 52
Volkmann's ischemic contracture, 702

W

Wedge fracture
  differential diagnosis, 173
  radiographic fractures, 172
  T4, 173
  vertebral body fracture, 156, 157
West Point view, 604
Winquist Type I fracture, 314
Wrist, 749–866
  anatomy, 749–763
  arcs, 774
  arthrodesis, 861, 863
  arthroplasty, 863–866
  bone scan, 17, 779–782, 784
  carpal ulnar distance, 752
  chronic post-traumatic conditions, 852
  computed tomography, 778–779, 783
  dorsal compartments, 791
  dorsal ligaments, 757
  dorsal vascular anatomy, 762
  extensors, 759
  flexor muscle, 758, 759, 760
  imaging, 763–789
    anatomic region, 787
    imaging work-up, 787
    indication, 787
  intercompartmental communications, 791
  interosseous muscle, 759
  joint capsule, 755–758

Wrist, (contd.)
  magnetic resonance imaging, 782–789
    field of view, 782, 784
    image planes, 785–787
    positioning, 782
    pulse sequences, 785–787
    technique, 782–789
  magnification radiography, 13
  metacarpophalangeal joint spacer, 866
  motion studies, 777, 780, 781
  muscular anatomy, 758–761
  navicular fat stripe, 773
  neurovascular anatomy, 761–763
  normal lateral view, 752
  osteology, 749–755
  osteotomy, 861, 862
  palmar ligaments, 756

  post-traumatic arthritis, 861
  post-traumatic reconstruction, 861–866
  radiography
    carpal tunnel view, 776, 778
    dorsal tangential view, 776, 779
    PA view, 767–771, 774
    pisiform view, 776, 777
    scaphoid view, 776
  radionuclide imaging, 779–782, 784
  skeletal anatomy, 751
  skeletal scintigraphy, 17
  soft tissue stabilization, 863
  Sudeck's atrophy, 802
  tendon, 760
  tendon sheath, 760
  tomography, 777–778, 782

  torus fracture, 40, 41
  volar vascular anatomy, 762
Wrist arthrography, 789–794
  abnormal, 790–794
  arthritis, 794
  ganglia, 794
  normal anatomy, 790, 791, 792
  technique, 789–790, 791
  trauma, 790–794
Wrist fracture, 782
Wrist pain
  post-traumatic, 791
  radiocarpal joint, 793
  radioulnar joint, 793

Z
Zickel nail, subtrochanteric fracture, 293